Atlas of Amputations and Limb Deficiencies

Surgical, Prosthetic, and Rehabilitation Principles

FIFTH EDITION

Atlas of Amputations and Limb Deficiencies

Surgical, Prosthetic, and Rehabilitation Principles

FIFTH EDITION

EDITORS

Joseph Ivan Krajbich, MD, FRCS(C)
Staff Orthopaedic Surgeon
Shriners Children's
Associate Professor
Department of Orthopaedics and Rehabilitation
Oregon Health and Science University
Portland, Oregon

Michael S. Pinzur, MD, FAAOS
Professor of Orthopaedic Surgery and Rehabilitation
Department of Orthopaedic Surgery and Rehabilitation
Loyola University Health System
Maywood, Illinois

COL Benjamin Kyle Potter, MD, FAAOS, FACS
Norman M. Rich Professor and Chair
Uniformed Services University – Walter Reed Department of Surgery
Uniformed Services University of the Health Sciences F. Edward Hebert School of Medicine
Chief Orthopaedic Surgeon, Amputee Patient Care Program and Director, Musculoskeletal Oncology
Director, Department of Defense Limb Optimization and Osseointegration Program
Department of Orthopaedics
Walter Reed National Military Medical Center
Bethesda, Maryland

Phillip M. Stevens, MEd, CPO, FAAOP
Prosthetist/Orthotist
Hanger Clinic
Adjunct Assistant Professor
Division of Physical Medicine and Rehabilitation
University of Utah
Salt Lake City, Utah

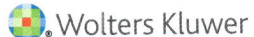

Wolters Kluwer

Philadelphia · Baltimore · New York · London
Buenos Aires · Hong Kong · Sydney · Tokyo

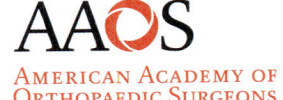

AMERICAN ACADEMY OF
ORTHOPAEDIC SURGEONS

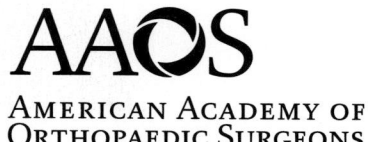

Board of Directors, 2023-2024

Kevin J. Bozic, MD, MBA, FAAOS
President

Paul Tornetta III, MD, PhD, FAAOS
First Vice President

Annunziato Amendola, MD, FAAOS
Second Vice President

Michael L. Parks, MD, FAAOS
Treasurer

Felix H. Savoie III, MD, FAAOS
Past President

Alfonso Mejia, MD, MPH, FAAOS
Chair, Board of Councilors

Joel L. Mayerson, MD, FAAOS
Chair-Elect, Board of Councilors

Michael J. Leddy III, MD, FAAOS
Secretary, Board of Councilors

Armando F. Vidal, MD, FAAOS
Chair, Board of Specialty Societies

Adolph J. Yates, Jr, MD, FAAOS
Chair-Elect, Board of Specialty Societies

Michael P. Bolognesi, MD, FAAOS
Secretary, Board of Specialty Societies

Lisa N. Masters
Lay Member

Evalina L. Burger, MD, FAAOS
Member at Large

Chad A. Krueger, MD, FAAOS
Member at Large

Toni M. McLaurin, MD, FAAOS
Member at Large

Monica M. Payares, MD, FAAOS
Member at Large

Thomas E. Arend, Jr, Esq, CAE
Chief Executive Officer (ex-officio)

Staff

American Academy of Orthopaedic Surgeons

Anna Salt Troise, MBA, *Chief Commercial Officer*

Hans Koelsch, PhD, *Director, Publishing*

Lisa Claxton Moore, *Senior Manager, Editorial*

Steven Kellert, *Senior Editor*

Wolters Kluwer Health

Brian Brown, *Director, Medical Practice*

Tulie McKay, *Senior Content Editor, Acquisitions*

Stacey Sebring, *Senior Development Editor*

Erin E. Hernandez and Sean Hanrahan, *Editorial Coordinators*

Erin Cantino, *Product Marketing Manager*

Catherine Ott, *Production Project Manager*

Stephen Druding, *Manager, Graphic Arts & Design*

Margie Orzech-Zeranko, *Senior Manufacturing Coordinator*

TNQ Technologies, *Prepress Vendor*

Atlas of Amputations and Limb Deficiencies: Surgical, Prosthetic, and Rehabilitation Principles, Fifth Edition

The material presented in the fifth edition of the **Atlas of Amputations and Limb Deficiencies: Surgical, Prosthetic, and Rehabilitation Principles** has been made available by the American Academy of Orthopaedic Surgeons (AAOS) for educational purposes only. This material is not intended to present the only, or necessarily best, methods or procedures for the medical situations discussed, but rather it is intended to represent an approach, view, statement, or opinion of the author(s) or producer(s), which may be helpful to others who face similar situations. Medical providers should use their own, independent medical judgment, in addition to open discussion with patients, when developing patient care recommendations and treatment plans. Medical care should always be based on a medical provider's expertise that is individually tailored to a patient's circumstances, preferences and rights.

Some drugs or medical devices demonstrated in AAOS courses or described in AAOS print or electronic publications have not been cleared by the US Food and Drug Administration (FDA) or have been cleared for specific uses only. The FDA has stated that it is the responsibility of the physician to determine the FDA clearance status of each drug or device he or she wishes to use in clinical practice and to use the products with appropriate patient consent and in compliance with applicable law.

Furthermore, any statements about commercial products are solely the opinion(s) of the author(s) and do not represent an AAOS endorsement or evaluation of these products. These statements may not be used in advertising or for any commercial purpose.

All rights reserved. No part of this publication may be reproduced, stored in a retrieval system, or transmitted, in any form, or by any means, electronic, mechanical, photocopying, recording, or otherwise, without prior written permission from the publisher.

ISBN: 978-1-975184-45-2

Library of Congress Control Number: Cataloging in Publication data available on request from publisher.

Printed in Mexico

Published 2024 by the
American Academy of Orthopaedic Surgeons
9400 West Higgins Road
Rosemont, Illinois 60018

Copyright 2024 by the American Academy of Orthopaedic Surgeons

Editors

Atlas of Amputations and Limb Deficiencies: Surgical, Prosthetic, and Rehabilitation Principles
Fifth Edition

Joseph Ivan Krajbich, MD, FRCS(C)
Staff Orthopaedic Surgeon
Shriners Children's
Associate Professor
Department of Orthopaedics and Rehabilitation
Oregon Health and Science University
Portland, Oregon

Michael S. Pinzur, MD, FAAOS
Professor of Orthopaedic Surgery and Rehabilitation
Department of Orthopaedic Surgery and Rehabilitation
Loyola University Health System
Maywood, Illinois

COL Benjamin Kyle Potter, MD, FAAOS, FACS
Norman M. Rich Professor and Chair
Uniformed Services University – Walter Reed Department of Surgery
Uniformed Services University of the Health Sciences F. Edward Hebert School of Medicine
Chief Orthopaedic Surgeon, Amputee Patient Care Program and Director, Musculoskeletal Oncology
Director, Department of Defense Limb Optimization and Osseointegration Program
Department of Orthopaedics
Walter Reed National Military Medical Center
Bethesda, Maryland

Phillip M. Stevens, MEd, CPO, FAAOP
Director, Clinical and Scientific Affairs
Hanger Inc.
Austin, Texas
Adjunct Assistant Professor
Division of Physical Medicine and Rehabilitation
University of Utah
Salt Lake City, Utah

Contributors

Rashmi Agarwal, MD
Assistant Professor
College of Medicine
Texas A&M University
Department of Orthopaedic Surgery
Baylor Scott and White Health
Temple, Texas

Sonya Agnew, MD
Associate Professor, Division of Plastic and Reconstructive Surgery
Program Director, Plastic Surgery
Department of Orthopaedic Surgery and Rehabilitation
Loyola University Medical Center
Section Chief, Division of Plastic Surgery
Hines VA Medical Center
Hines, Illinois

Michael Aiona, MD, FAAOS
Orthopedic Surgeon
Shriners Children's
Assistant Professor
Department of Orthopaedics and Rehabilitation
Oregon Health and Science University
Portland, Oregon

COL Joseph F. Alderete, MD
Director, Musculoskeletal Oncology
San Antonio Military Medical Center
San Antonio, Texas

Edward A. Athanasian, MD, FAAOS
Chief Emeritus, Hand and Upper Extremity Service
Hospital for Special Surgery
Professor of Clinical Orthopaedic Surgery
Weill Cornell Medical College
New York, New York

David J. Baty, CPO, LPO
Director, Fabrications Services
Hanger Inc.
Austin, Texas

Mark David Beachler, CP
Chief of Orthotic and Prosthetic Services
Walter Reed National Military Medical Center
Bethesda, Maryland

Christopher Bibbo, DO, DPM, FAAOS, FACS, FACFAS
Head of Foot and Ankle Surgery
International Center for Limb Lengthening
Assistant Director, Foot and Ankle Deformity Correction and Orthoplastics Fellowship
Rubin Institute for Advanced Orthopedics
Sinai Hospital of Baltimore
Baltimore, Maryland

John T. Brinkmann, MA, CPO/L, FAAOP(D)
Associate Professor
Department of Physical Medicine and Rehabilitation
Northwestern University
Chicago, Illinois

Helena Burger, MD, PhD
Full Professor
Department of Physical and Rehabilitation Medicine
Faculty of Medicine
University Rehabilitation Institute
Ljubljana, Slovenia

Josef A. Butkus, MS, OTR/L
Occupational Therapy Supervisor
Walter Reed National Military Medical Center
Bethesda, Maryland

Stephen Butler, MBBS(Hons), FRACS(Orth), FAOrthA, PFET(Hand Surgery)
Consultant Hand and Wrist Surgeon
Queensland Children's Hospital
Brisbane, Australia

Federico Canavese, MD, PhD
Professor, Department of Pediatric Orthopedic Surgery
Jeanne de Flandre Hospital
Faculty of Medicine Henri Warembourg
Lille University
Lille, France

Jill Cannoy, PT, DPT
Board Certified Pediatric Clinical Specialist
Physical Therapist
Orthotics and Prosthetics
Children's Healthcare of Atlanta
Atlanta, Georgia

Kevin Carroll, MS, CP, FAAOP(D)
Vice President of Prosthetics
Hanger Clinic
Austin, Texas

Michael K. Carroll, PhD, CPO, FAAOP(D)
Chief, Orthotic and Prosthetic Clinical Services
Orlando VA Healthcare System
Assistant Professor
Department of Medical Education, College of Medicine
University of Central Florida
Orlando, Florida

Paul S. Cederna, MD
Chief, Section of Plastic Surgery
Robert O'Neal Professor of Plastic Surgery
Professor of Biomedical Engineering
Section of Plastic Surgery
Department of Biomedical Engineering
University of Michigan
Ann Arbor, Michigan

W. Lee Childers, PhD, CP
Senior Scientist
Extremity Trauma and Amputation Center of Excellence (EACE)
Center for the Intrepid
Brooke Army Medical Center
San Antonio, Texas

Helen Cochrane, MSc, CPO(c)
Assistant Professor
Program Director
Master of Science in Prosthetics and Orthotics
Department of Rehabilitation Science and Technology
University of Pittsburgh
Pittsburgh, Pennsylvania

Contributors

Sheila A. Conway, MD, FAAOS, FAOA
Professor and Vice Chair of Education
Department of Orthopaedic Surgery
University of Miami
Miller School of Medicine
Miami, Florida

Colleen P. Coulter, PT, DPT, PhD, PCS
Adjunct Professor
Department of Rehabilitation Medicine
Emory University School of Medicine
Atlanta, Georgia

Robin C. Crandall, MD, FAAOS
Orthopedic Surgeon
Limb Deficiency Clinic
Shriners Children's Twin Cities
Woodbury, Minnesota

Mark T. Dahl, MD, FAAOS
Professor, Department of Orthopaedic Surgery
University of Minnesota
Minneapolis, Minnesota

Charles d'Amato, MD, FRCSC
Orthopaedic Surgeon
Shriners Children's
Portland, Oregon

Todd DeWees, MHA, CPO
Manager, Department of Orthotics and Prosthetics
Shriners Children's
Portland, Oregon

Michael P. Dillon, PhD, BPO(Hons)
Professor, Department of Physiotherapy, Podiatry, Prosthetics and Orthotics
La Trobe University
Melbourne, Victoria, Australia

Kim Doolan, BS
Consultant, Kim Doolan Consulting
Milford, New Hampshire

Israel Dudkiewicz, MD, MHA
Associate Professor
Division of Rehabilitation
Sheba Medical Center, Tel-Hashomer
Sackler School of Medicine
Tel Aviv University
Tel Aviv, Israel

Gregory A. Dumanian, MD
Chief of Plastic Surgery
Department of Surgery
Stuteville Professor of Surgery
Feinberg School of Medicine
Northwestern University
Evanston, Illinois

LTC Tobin Thomas Eckel, MD, FAAOS
Associate Professor
Department of Surgery
F. Edward Hebert School of Medicine
Uniformed Services University of the Health Sciences
Bethesda, Maryland

Jorge A. Fabregas, MD, FAAOS
Orthopaedic Surgeon
Department of Orthopaedic Surgery and Sports Medicine
Children's Healthcare of Atlanta
Atlanta, Georgia

Christopher Fantini, MSPT, CP, BOCO
National Program Manager
VA Orthotic, Prosthetic and Pedorthic Clinical Services
Rehabilitation and Prosthetic Services
United States Department of Veterans Affairs
Bronx, New York

Stefania Fatone, PhD, BPO(Hons)
Professor, Department of Rehabilitation Medicine
University of Washington
Seattle, Washington

James Robert Ficke, MD, FAAOS, FACS
Robert A. Robinson Professor and Chair
Department of Orthopaedic Surgery
Johns Hopkins Medicine
Baltimore, Maryland

Sandra Fletchall, OTR/L, CHT, MPA, FAOTA
Manager, Department of Burn Rehabilitation
Firefighters' Regional Burn Center
Memphis, Tennessee

Jonathan A. Forsberg, MD, PhD, FAAOS
Attending Orthopaedic Oncologist
Department of Surgery
Memorial Sloan-Kettering Cancer Center
New York, New York

Krister Freese, MD, FAAOS
Assistant Professor
Shriners Children's
Portland, Oregon

Robert S. Gailey, PhD, PT, FAPTA
Professor, Department of Physical Therapy
Director, Functional Outcomes Research and Evaluation Center
University of Miami Miller School of Medicine
Coral Gables, Florida

Donald A. Gajewski, MD, MBA, FAAOS
Musculoskeletal Oncologist
Department of Orthopedic Surgery
Mission Hospital
Asheville, North Carolina

Ignacio Gaunaurd, PT, PhD, MSPT
Associate Professor
Department of Physical Therapy
University of Miami Miller School of Medicine
Coral Gables, Florida
Research Health Scientist
Bruce W. Carter VA Medical Center
Miami, Florida

Andrew G. Georgiadis, MD, FAAOS
Associate Professor
Department of Orthopaedic Surgery
University of Minnesota
Minneapolis, Minnesota

Brian J. Giavedoni, MBA, CP, LP
Manager, Orthotics and Prosthetics
Children's Healthcare of Atlanta
Atlanta, Georgia

Frank A. Gottschalk, MD*
*Deceased

Carson Harte, HDip
Chief Executive Officer
Exceed Worldwide
London, England

Zach Harvey, CPO
Regional Upper Limb Prosthetic Specialist
Hanger Clinic
Englewood, Colorado

Brad D. Hendershot, PhD
Facility Research Director
Research and Surveillance Division
Department of Defense-Veterans Administration Extremity Trauma and Amputation Center of Excellence
Walter Reed National Military Medical Center
Associate Professor
Department of Physical Medicine and Rehabilitation
Uniformed Services University of the Health Sciences
Bethesda, Maryland

Contributors

Rebecca Hernandez, CPO, LPO
Prosthetist, Children's Healthcare of Atlanta
Atlanta, Georgia

Annie Hess, CP
National Upper Limb Prosthetic Specialist
Hanger Clinic
Clayton, North Carolina

James T. Highsmith, MD, MS
Dermatologist
Dermatology Surgery Institute
Lutz, Florida

M. Jason Highsmith, PhD, PT, DPT, CP, FAAOP
National Director
US Department of Veterans Affairs
Rehabilitation and Prosthetic Services
Orthotic, Prosthetic and Pedorthic Clinical Services
Washington, DC
Professor, University of South Florida
Morsani College of Medicine
School of Physical Therapy and Rehabilitation Sciences
Tampa, Florida
Physical Therapist
US Army Reserves (SP Corps)
32nd Medical Brigade
319th Minimal Care Detachment
Pinellas Park, Florida

Wendy Hill, BScOT
Research Occupational Therapist
Atlantic Clinic for Upper Limb Prosthetics
University of New Brunswick
Fredericton, New Brunswick, Canada

R. Scott Hosie, CPO
Director of Clinical Education
Fillauer Motion Control
Salt Lake City, Utah

Sabrina Jakobson Huston, CPO
Orthotist/Prosthetist
Pediatric Orthotics and Prosthetics
Shriners Children's
Portland, Oregon

Brad M. Isaacson, PhD, MBA, MSF, PMP
Chief of Research and Operations
Musculoskeletal Injury Rehabilitation Research for Operational Readiness (MIRROR)
Uniformed Services University of the Health Sciences
Associate Professor
Department of Physical Medicine and Rehabilitation
Uniformed Services University of the Health Sciences
Bethesda, Maryland

Craig Jackman, CPO, FAAOP
National Upper Limb Prosthetic Specialist
Hanger Clinic
Austin, Texas

Brian Kaluf, CP, FAAOP
Director of the Salt Lake City Research Hub
Ottobock Healthcare
Salt Lake City, Utah

Heather Kong, MD, FAAOS
Pediatric Orthopedic Surgeon
Shriners Children's
Portland, Oregon

Stephen J. Kovach III, MD, FACS
Herndon B. Lehr Endowed Associate Professor of Plastic Surgery
Associate Professor of Surgery, Division of Plastic Surgery
Associate Professor of Surgery, Department of Orthopaedic Surgery
Chief of Plastic Surgery
Penn Presbyterian Medical Center
Director, Microsurgery Fellowship
University of Pennsylvania Health System
Philadelphia, Pennsylvania

Joseph Ivan Krajbich, MD, FRCS(C)
Staff Orthopaedic Surgeon
Shriners Children's
Associate Professor
Department of Orthopaedics and Rehabilitation
Oregon Health and Science University
Portland, Oregon

Anat Kristal, PhD, MScPT
Assistant Professor
Department of Physical Therapy
University of Miami Miller School of Medicine
Coral Gables, Florida

Debra Latour, OTD, MEd, OTR/L
Doctoral Experiential Capstone Coordinator
Assistant Professor
College of Pharmacy and Health Sciences
Division of Occupational Therapy
Western New England University
Springfield, Massachusetts

Peter Jeffrey Laub, MD
Chief Integrated Plastic Surgery Resident
Division of Plastic Surgery
Department of Surgery
Loyola University Stritch School of Medicine
Maywood, Illinois

L. Scott Levin, MD, FAAOS, FACS
Professor of Surgery
Division of Plastic Surgery
Department of Orthopaedic Surgery
Hospital of the University of Pennsylvania
Philadelphia, Pennsylvania

Terry R. Light, MD, FAAOS, FACS, FAOrthA
Professor and Emeritus Chair
Department of Orthopaedic Surgery and Rehabilitation
Loyola University Stritch School of Medicine
Maywood, Illinois

Robert D. Lipschutz, CPO, BSME
Certified Prosthetist/Orthotist
Mary Free Bed Rehabilitation Hospital
Grand Rapids, Michigan
Assistant Professor
Department of Physical Medicine and Rehabilitation
Feinberg School of Medicine
Northwestern University
Chicago, Illinois

Blair A. Lock, MS, PE
Chief Executive Officer
Coapt, LLC
Chicago, Illinois

Contributors

Motasem A. Al Maaieh, MD
Associate Professor of Orthopaedic Surgery
Director of Spine Oncology
Spine Surgery
Musculoskeletal Oncology
Miller School of Medicine
University of Miami
Jackson Memorial Hospital
Miami, Florida

Ellen J. MacKenzie, MSc, PhD
Dean, Bloomberg Distinguished Professor
Johns Hopkins Bloomberg School of Public Health
Baltimore, Maryland

Matthew J. Major, PhD
Research Health Scientist
Jesse Brown VA Medical Center
Chicago, Illinois
Edward Hines, Jr. VA Hospital
Hines, Illinois
Associate Professor
Department of Physical Medicine and Rehabilitation
Feinberg School of Medicine
Department of Biomedical Engineering
McCormick School of Engineering
Northwestern University
Evanston, Illinois

Catherine B. McClellan, PhD
Pediatric Psychologist
Medical Staff
Shriners Children's
Portland, Oregon

Lakeya S. McGill, MA, PhD
Postdoctoral Fellow
Department of Physical Medicine and Rehabilitation
Johns Hopkins University School of Medicine
Baltimore, Maryland

Samir Mehta, MD, FAAOS
Associate Professor
Department of Orthopaedic Surgery
University of Pennsylvania
Philadelphia, Pennsylvania

Danielle H. Melton, MD
Associate Professor
Department of Physical Medicine and Rehabilitation
University of Colorado, School of Medicine
Anschutz Medical Campus
Aurora, Colorado

Matthew J. Mikosz, CP, LP
National Upper Limb Prosthetic Specialist
Hanger Clinic
Southington, Connecticut

Laura A. Miller, PhD, CP
Research Scientist and Prosthetist
Center for Bionic Medicine
Shirley Ryan AbilityLab
Associate Professor
Department of Physical Medicine and Rehabilitation
Feinberg School of Medicine
Northwestern University
Chicago, Illinois

LTC Matthew E. Miller, MD
Director, Graduate Medical Education
Assistant Professor
Department of Rehabilitation
Walter Reed National Military Medical Center
Bethesda, Maryland

Brian Monroe, CPO
National Upper Limb Prosthetic Specialist
Hanger Clinic
Austin, Texas

Amy M. Moore, MD
Professor and Chair
Department of Plastic and Reconstructive Surgery
The Ohio State University Wexner Medical Center
Columbus, Ohio

Sara J. Morgan, CPO, PhD
Clinical Scientist
Department of Research
Gillette Children's Specialty Healthcare
St. Paul, Minnesota
Affiliate Assistant Professor
Department of Rehabilitation Medicine
University of Minnesota
Minneapolis, Minnesota

Stewart G. Morrison, MBBS
Bob Dickens Paediatric Orthopaedic Research Fellow
Department of Paediatrics
The University of Melbourne
Melbourne, Australia

Munjed Al Muderis, MB ChB, FRACS, FAOrthA, DMedSc
Clinical Professor
School of Medicine
Clinical Discipline Head-Orthopaedics and Sports Medicine MQHealth
Macquarie University
Sydney, Australia

Mark David Muller, CPO, MS, FAAOP
Department Chair / Program Director
Department of Orthotics and Prosthetics
California State University Dominguez Hills
Carson, California

George Peter Nanos III, MD, FAAOS
Associate Professor
Department of Orthopaedic Surgery
Johns Hopkins University School of Medicine
Baltimore, Maryland

Harvey Naranjo, COTA/L
Assistant Professor
Department of Rehabilitation
Walter Reed National Military Medical Center
Uniformed Services University of the Health Sciences
Bethesda, Maryland

LeRoy H. Oddie, CP, MBA, CLCP
Clinical Specialist
Integrum, Inc.
San Francisco, California

Chinmay S. Paranjape, MD, MHSc
Orthopedic Surgeon
Rady Children's Hospital
University of California, San Diego
San Diego, California

Paul F. Pasquina, MD
Chair, Department of Rehabilitation
Uniformed Services University of the Health Sciences
Walter Reed National Military Medical Center
Bethesda, Maryland

Branden Petersen, BS, CP, LP
West Zone Upper Limb Prosthetics Clinical Leader
National Upper Limb Program
Hanger Clinic
Watertown, New York

Terrence M. Philbin, DO
Orthopedic Surgeon
Orthopedic Foot and Ankle Center
Worthington, Ohio

Michael S. Pinzur, MD, FAAOS
Professor of Orthopaedic Surgery and Rehabilitation
Department of Orthopaedic Surgery and Rehabilitation
Loyola University Health System
Maywood, Illinois

David J. Polga, MD, FAAOS
Orthopedic Surgeon
Orthopaedic Trauma and Adult Reconstruction Surgery
Department of Orthopaedic Surgery
Marshfield Clinic Health System
Marshfield, Wisconsin

COL Benjamin Kyle Potter, MD, FAAOS, FACS
Norman M. Rich Professor and Chair
Uniformed Services University – Walter Reed Department of Surgery
Uniformed Services University of the Health Sciences F. Edward Hebert School of Medicine
Chief Orthopaedic Surgeon, Amputee Patient Care Program and Director, Musculoskeletal Oncology
Director, Department of Defense Limb Optimization and Osseointegration Program
Department of Orthopaedics
Walter Reed National Military Medical Center
Bethesda, Maryland

Lisa Prasso, PT, DPT
Physical Therapist
Military Advanced Training Center
Walter Reed National Military Medical Center
Assistant Professor
Department of Physical Medicine and Rehabilitation
Uniformed Services University of the Health Sciences
Bethesda, Maryland

Mark E. Puhaindran, MBBS, MMED, MRCS, FAMS
Senior Consultant and Head
Department of Hand and Reconstructive Microsurgery
National University Hospital
Singapore

Kevin Quinn, MSPO, CPO
Certified Prosthetist and Orthotist
Rise Prosthetics and Orthotics
Denver, Colorado

Robert Radocy, MS
Physical Education and Recreation
Founder and Executive Vice President
Fillauer TRS Inc.
Boulder, Colorado

Ellen M. Raney, MD, FAAOS
Affiliate Professor Orthopaedics and Rehabilitation
Oregon Health and Science University
Shriners Children's
Portland, Oregon

LTC David E. Reece, DO
Director, Clinical Operations
Assistant Professor
Department of Rehabilitation
Walter Reed National Military Medical Center
Bethesda, Maryland

Linda Resnik, PT, PhD, FAPTA
Research Career Scientist
Providence VA Medical Center
Professor, Department of Health Services, Policy and Practice
School of Public Health, Brown University
Providence, Rhode Island

John Rheinstein, CP, FAAOP(D)
Clinic Manager
Lower and Upper Limb Prosthetic Specialist
Hanger Clinic
Austin, Texas

David B. Rotter, CPO
President, David Rotter Prosthetics, LTD
Joliet, Illinois

MAJ Ean Saberski, MD
Plastic Surgeon
Department of General Surgery
Walter Reed National Military Medical Center
Bethesda, Maryland

Michael Schmitz, MD, FAAOS
Chief, Orthopedic and Sports Medicine Center
Children's Healthcare of Atlanta
Atlanta, Georgia

Phoebe Scott-Wyard, DO, FAAP, FAAPMR
Assistant Clinical Professor
Department of Orthopedics, Division of Pediatric Rehabilitation
University of California, San Diego
San Diego, California

Scott B. Shawen, MD
Adjunct Associate Professor of Surgery
Department of Surgery and Rehabilitation
Wake Forest University School of Medicine
Winston-Salem, North Carolina

Ryan Sheridan, MS, CPO, FAAOP
National Upper Limb Prosthetic Specialist
Hanger Clinic
Austin, Texas

Jaimie T. Shores, MD, FACS
Associate Professor
Hand Surgery Fellowship Director
Director of Upper Extremity Transplantation
Plastic and Reconstructive Surgery and Orthopaedic Surgery
Johns Hopkins University School of Medicine
Baltimore, Maryland

Jason M. Souza, MD, FACS
Associate Professor
Department of Plastic and Reconstructive Surgery
Department of Orthopaedics
The Ohio State University
Columbus, Ohio

Gerald E. Stark, PhD, MSEM, CPO/L, FAAOP
Director of Clinical Affairs
Contributing Faculty Member
Ottobock Patient Care
University of Tennessee at Chattanooga
Chattanooga, Tennessee

Phillip M. Stevens, MEd, CPO, FAAOP
Director, Clinical and Scientific Affairs
Hanger Inc.
Austin, Texas
Adjunct Assistant Professor
Division of Physical Medicine and Rehabilitation
University of Utah
Salt Lake City, Utah

Siobhán Strike, PhD
Associate Professor
School of Life and Health Sciences
University of Roehampton
London, England

CDR Scott M. Tintle, MD, FAAOS
Chief Hand Surgery/Fellowship Director
Department of Orthopaedic Surgery
Walter Reed National Military Medical Center
Bethesda, Maryland

Ian P. Torode, MD, FRACS*
*Deceased

Jack E. Uellendahl, CPO
Clinical Education Consultant
Hanger Clinic
Austin, Texas

Contributors

Benjamin D. Umbel, DO
Fellow, Foot and Ankle Surgery
Department of Orthopedic Surgery
Duke University
Durham, North Carolina

Francois J. Van Der Watt, CPO, LPO
Clinician/Owner
Van Der Watt Prosthetics and Orthotics
Greenwood, Arkansas

Anna D. Vergun, MD, FAAOS
Associate Professor
Division Chief of Pediatric Orthopedics
Department of Orthopedic Surgery
University of North Carolina, Chapel Hill
Chapel Hill, North Carolina

Stephen T. Wegener, MA, PhD
Director, Division of Rehabilitation Psychology and Neuropsychology
Professor, Department of Physical Medicine and Rehabilitation
Johns Hopkins University School of Medicine
Baltimore, Maryland

Rebecca C. Whitesell, MD, MPH, FAAOS
Pediatric Orthopedic Surgeon
Department of Pediatric Orthopedics
Mary Bridge Children's Hospital
Tacoma, Washington

Shane R. Wurdeman, PhD, CP, FAAOP(D)
Director of Clinical Research
Clinical and Scientific Affairs
Hanger Clinic
Austin, Texas

Vivian J. Yip, OTD, MA, OTR/L
Occupational Therapist
Physical Medicine
University of California, Los Angeles
Los Angeles, California

Preface

The fifth edition of the *Atlas of Amputations and Limb Deficiencies: Surgical, Prosthetic, and Rehabilitation Principles* represents the continued commitment of the American Academy of Orthopaedic Surgeons to patients with congenital or acquired limb loss and the medical professionals who dedicate their lives to optimizing the functional independence of this patient population.

The recent conflicts have continued to bring amputees and the challenges that they face to the front pages of our newspapers and magazines. We have again leaned heavily on our military colleagues to bring together in one text the latest surgical, prosthetic, and rehabilitation methodologies, many of which were developed or refined over the past 2 decades. In addition to the need to meet simple, daily functional requirements, this very motivated and demanding group of patients has inspired the recognition of newly evolving techniques and tools to promote sports participation and advanced rehabilitation. There is a new and expanded focus on such rehabilitation, which is now viewed as a continuous, integrated process.

The sections on advanced nerve interventions, such as targeted muscle reinnervation and osseointegration, have been expanded because the science of these techniques has evolved and advanced since the publication of the fourth edition of this text. An expanded section on pediatrics focuses on current approaches and considerations for treating this special group of patients.

Although all of the chapters in this fifth edition have been revised, we hope, in particular, that the new and expanded chapters will enhance the book's usefulness to all members of the treatment team, including surgeons (whether general, vascular, pediatric, plastic, or orthopaedic); prosthetists; physiatrists; physical, occupational, and recreational therapists; biomedical engineers; rehabilitation nurses; social workers; and individuals with limb loss and their families. The goals of this comprehensive text are, ultimately, to enhance and advance the care of those living with congenital or acquired limb loss. The dedicated involvement of all members of the treatment team is essential to the success of this process.

The support of the Board of Directors of the American Academy of Orthopaedic Surgeons has made this volume possible and is gratefully acknowledged. The contributions of the authors and editors have been enhanced by the work and commitment of the Academy's publications staff. We trust that the reader will find this volume a valuable educational resource.

Joseph Ivan Krajbich, MD, FRCS(C)
Michael S. Pinzur, MD, FAAOS
COL Benjamin Kyle Potter, MD, FAAOS, FACS
Phillip M. Stevens, MEd, CPO, FAAOP

Contents

Section 1: General Principles

1. General Principles of Amputation Surgery 3
   Sonya Agnew, MD; Peter Jeffrey Laub, MD; Michael S. Pinzur, MD, FAAOS

2. General Principles of Postoperative Residual Limb Management 13
   Frank A. Gottschalk, MD; Michael S. Pinzur, MD, FAAOS

3. General Principles of Limb Salvage Versus Amputation in Adults 21
   Christopher Bibbo, DO, DPM, FAAOS, FACS, FACFAS; David J. Polga, MD, FAAOS; Samir Mehta, MD, FAAOS; Stephen J. Kovach III, MD, FACS

4. Prosthetic Gait: Biomechanical Analysis and Clinical Assessment 43
   John T. Brinkmann, MA, CPO/L, FAAOP(D); Siobhán Strike, PhD

5. Kinesiology of the Upper Limb 67
   Terry R. Light, MD, FAAOS, FACS, FAOrthA

6. Wartime Amputations 75
   Donald A. Gajewski, MD, MBA, FAAOS

7. Prosthetic Rehabilitation in Less-Resourced Settings 85
   Helen Cochrane, MSc, CPO(c); Carson Harte, HDip

8. General Rehabilitation Principles and Strategies for the Upper Limb Amputee 97
   Josef A. Butkus, MS, OTR/L; Danielle H. Melton, MD

9. General Rehabilitation Principles and Strategies for the Lower Limb Amputee 117
   Israel Dudkiewicz, MD, MHA; Lisa Prasso, PT, DPT

Section 2: Upper Limb

10. Upper Limb Body-Powered Components 129
    Annie Hess, CP

11. Harnessing and Controls for Upper Limb Body-Powered Prostheses 149
    David B. Rotter, CPO

12. Upper Limb Externally Powered Components 165
    LeRoy H. Oddie, CP, MBA, CLCP

13. Control Options for Upper Limb Externally Powered Components 183
    R. Scott Hosie, CPO; Blair A. Lock, MS, PE

14. Partial Hand Amputation: Surgical Management 191
    Edward A. Athanasian, MD, FAAOS; Mark E. Puhaindran, MBBS, MMED, MRCS, FAMS

15. Partial Hand Amputation: Prosthetic Management 201
    Jack E. Uellendahl, CPO; Matthew J. Mikosz, CP, LP

16. Wrist Disarticulation and Transradial Amputation: Surgical Management 211
    George Peter Nanos III, MD, FAAOS

17. Wrist Disarticulation and Transradial Amputation: Prosthetic Management 223
    Christopher Fantini, MSPT, CP, BOCO; Gerald E. Stark, PhD, MSEM, CPO/L, FAAOP

18. Elbow Disarticulation and Transhumeral Amputation: Surgical Management 239
    CDR Scott M. Tintle, MD, FAAOS

19. Elbow Disarticulation and Transhumeral Amputation: Prosthetic Management and Design 247
    Gerald E. Stark, PhD, MSEM, CPO/L, FAAOP; Christopher Fantini, MSPT, CP, BOCO

Contents

20 Amputations About the Shoulder: Surgical Considerations 261
COL Joseph F. Alderete, MD

21 Amputations About the Shoulder: Prosthetic Management 275
Branden Petersen, BS, CP, LP

22 Bilateral Upper Limb Prostheses 285
Jack E. Uellendahl, CPO

23 Targeted Muscle Reinnervation for Enhanced Prosthetic Control 301
Jason M. Souza, MD, FACS; Gregory A. Dumanian, MD

24 Advanced Nerve Management Techniques for Management and Prevention of Pain 311
Jason M. Souza, MD, FACS; Paul S. Cederna, MD; Amy M. Moore, MD

25 Targeted Muscle Reinnervation: Prosthetic Management 319
Craig Jackman, CPO, FAAOP; Brian Monroe, CPO; Ryan Sheridan, MS, CPO, FAAOP

26 Upper Limb Prosthetic Training and Occupational Therapy 329
Sandra Fletchall, OTR/L, CHT, MPA, FAOTA

27 Upper Limb Adaptive Prostheses for Vocation and Recreation 341
Robert Radocy, MS; Debra Latour, OTD, MEd, OTR/L

28 Functional Aesthetic Prostheses: Upper Limb 363
Matthew J. Mikosz, CP, LP; Kim Doolan, BS

29 Brachial Plexus Injuries 375
MAJ Ean Saberski, MD

30 Hand Transplantation 391
CDR Scott M. Tintle, MD, FAAOS; Jaimie T. Shores, MD, FACS, L. Scott Levin, MD, FAAOS, FACS

31 Outcome Measures in Upper Limb Prosthetics 401
Laura A. Miller, PhD, CP; Linda Resnik, PT, PhD, FAPTA

Section 3: Lower Limb

32 Prosthetic Foot and Ankle Mechanisms 417
Matthew J. Major, PhD; Phillip M. Stevens, MEd, CPO, FAAOP

33 Prosthetic Knee Mechanisms 431
Matthew J. Major, PhD; Phillip M. Stevens, MEd, CPO, FAAOP

34 Partial Foot Amputations and Disarticulations: Surgical Management 443
Terrence M. Philbin, DO; Benjamin D. Umbel, DO

35 Partial Foot Amputation: Prosthetic Management 453
Michael P. Dillon, PhD, BPO(Hons); Stefania Fatone, PhD, BPO(Hons)

36 Ankle Disarticulation and Variants: Surgical Management 463
LTC Tobin Thomas Eckel, MD, FAAOS; Scott B. Shawen, MD

37 Ankle Disarticulation and Variants: Prosthetic Management 469
Phillip M. Stevens, MEd, CPO, FAAOP; David J. Baty, CPO, LPO

38 Transtibial Amputation 477
James Robert Ficke, MD, FAAOS, FACS

39 Transtibial Amputation: Prosthetic Management 485
W. Lee Childers, PhD, CP; Shane R. Wurdeman, PhD, CP, FAAOP(D)

40 Knee Disarticulation: Surgical Management 499
Michael S. Pinzur, MD, FAAOS; COL Benjamin Kyle Potter, MD, FAAOS, FACS

41 Knee Disarticulation: Prosthetic Management 507
Phillip M. Stevens, MEd, CPO, FAAOP; David J. Baty, CPO, LPO

42 Transfemoral Amputation: Surgical Management 517
Frank A. Gottschalk, MD; COL Benjamin Kyle Potter, MD, FAAOS, FACS

43 Transfemoral Amputation: Prosthetic Management 529
Mark David Muller, CPO, MS, FAAOP

44 Hip Disarticulation and Transpelvic Amputation: Surgical Management 547
   Sheila A. Conway, MD, FAAOS, FAOA; Motasem A. Al Maaieh, MD

45 Hip Disarticulation: Prosthetic Management 557
   Phillip M. Stevens, MEd, CPO, FAAOP; David J. Baty, CPO, LPO

46 Bilateral Lower Limb Amputation: Prosthetic Management...................... 567
   *Michael K. Carroll, PhD, CPO, FAAOP(D); Kevin Carroll, MS, CP, FAAOP(D);
   John Rheinstein, CP, FAAOP(D)*

47 Osseointegration: Surgical Management...................................... 581
   Munjed Al Muderis, MB ChB, FRACS, FAOrthA, DMedSc; Jonathan A. Forsberg, MD, PhD, FAAOS

48 Prosthetic Management of Osseointegration................................. 595
   Phillip M. Stevens, MEd, CPO, FAAOP; Mark David Beachler, CP

49 Physical Therapy Management of Adult Lower Limb Amputees 605
   Robert S. Gailey, PhD, PT, FAPTA; Anat Kristal, PhD, MScPT; Ignacio Gaunaurd, PT, PhD, MSPT

50 Adaptive Lower Limb Prostheses for Sports and Recreation 631
   Francois J. Van Der Watt, CPO, LPO

51 Outcome Measures in Lower Limb Prosthetics 641
   Brian Kaluf, CP, FAAOP; Sara J. Morgan, CPO, PhD

Section 4: Management Issues

52 Skin Pathologies Associated With Amputation 653
   James T. Highsmith, MD, MS; M. Jason Highsmith, PhD, PT, DPT, CP, FAAOP

53 Chronic Pain After Amputation 673
   LTC Matthew E. Miller, MD; Paul F. Pasquina, MD; LTC David E. Reece, DO

54 Secondary Health Effects of Amputation.................................... 685
   Paul F. Pasquina, MD; Brad D. Hendershot, PhD; Brad M. Isaacson, PhD, MBA, MSF, PMP

55 Surgical Management of Residual Limb Complications 695
   COL Benjamin Kyle Potter, MD, FAAOS, FACS

56 Psychological Adaptation to Limb Amputation............................... 707
   Lakeya S. McGill, MA, PhD; Ellen J. MacKenzie, MSc, PhD; Stephen T. Wegener, MA, PhD

57 Vocational and Recreational Considerations After Amputation................ 721
   Helena Burger, MD, PhD; Harvey Naranjo, COTA/L

Section 5: Pediatrics

58 The Child With a Limb Deficiency: Classification and Etiology 735
   Chinmay S. Paranjape, MD, MHSc; Anna D. Vergun, MD, FAAOS

59 Congenital Limb Deficiencies: Embryology, Genetics, and Associated Syndromes ... 741
   Ellen M. Raney, MD, FAAOS

60 Development of Locomotor Systems.. 749
   Phoebe Scott-Wyard, DO, FAAP, FAAPMR

61 Scientific, Technologic, Surgical, and Prosthetic Advances in
   Pediatric Limb Deficiency... 753
   Michael Schmitz, MD, FAAOS; Rebecca Hernandez, CPO, LPO

62 Gait Analysis in the Child With a Limb Deficiency......................... 759
   Michael Aiona, MD, FAAOS

63 Psychological, Social, and Socioeconomic Aspects of Limb Deficiencies 769
   Catherine B. McClellan, PhD

64 Principles of Amputation in Children 779
   Chinmay S. Paranjape, MD, MHSc; Anna D. Vergun, MD, FAAOS

65 Role of Limb Lengthening in the Pediatric Amputee 789
   Mark T. Dahl, MD, FAAOS; Stewart G. Morrison, MBBS; Andrew G. Georgiadis, MD, FAAOS

Contents

66 Traumatic Amputations of the Lower Extremity in Children and Adolescents 799
Robin C. Crandall, MD, FAAOS

67 Congenital Longitudinal Deficiencies of the Upper Limb 819
Krister Freese, MD, FAAOS; Stephen Butler, MBBS(Hons), FRACS(Orth), FAOrthA, PFET(Hand Surgery)

68 Pediatric Hand Deficiencies 829
Krister Freese, MD, FAAOS; Rashmi Agarwal, MD

69 Upper Limb Prostheses for Children 843
Robert D. Lipschutz, CPO, BSME

70 Pediatric Physical Therapy 855
Colleen P. Coulter, PT, DPT, PhD, PCS; Jill Cannoy, PT, DPT

71 Occupational Therapy for Children With Upper Limb Deficiencies 867
Wendy Hill, BScOT; Vivian J. Yip, OTD, MA, OTR/L

72 General Principles of Limb Salvage Versus Amputations in Children 887
Federico Canavese, MD, PhD; Joseph Ivan Krajbich, MD, FRCS(C)

73 Prosthetic Considerations in the Pediatric Lower Limb Amputee 895
Brian J. Giavedoni, MBA, CP, LP

74 Hip Disarticulation and Hemipelvectomy in Children: Surgical and Prosthetic
Management 901
Joseph Ivan Krajbich, MD, FRCS(C); Todd DeWees, MHA, CPO

75 Transfemoral Amputations and Knee Disarticulation: Surgical Principles
and Prosthetic Management 913
Jorge A. Fabregas, MD, FAAOS; David B. Rotter, CPO

76 Congenital Deficiencies of the Femur 923
Joseph Ivan Krajbich, MD, FRCS(C); Ian P. Torode, MD, FRACS

77 Rotationplasty: Surgical Techniques and Prosthetic Considerations 937
Joseph Ivan Krajbich, MD, FRCS(C); Sabrina Jakobson Huston, CPO

78 Congenital Longitudinal Deficiencies of the Fibula 949
Michael Schmitz, MD, FAAOS; Rebecca Hernandez, CPO, LPO

79 Congenital Longitudinal Deficiency of the Tibia 959
Jorge A. Fabregas, MD, FAAOS; Rebecca C. Whitesell, MD, MPH, FAAOS

80 Syme, Boyd, and Transtibial Amputation in Children: Surgical and Prosthetic
Management 969
Heather Kong, MD, FAAOS; Rebecca Hernandez, CPO, LPO

81 Partial Foot Deficiencies in Children 979
Robin C. Crandall, MD, FAAOS

82 The Child With Multiple Limb Deficiencies 989
Chinmay S. Paranjape, MD, MHSc; Anna D. Vergun, MD, FAAOS

83 Lumbosacral Agenesis 997
Charles d'Amato, MD, FRCSC; Todd DeWees, MHA, CPO; Joseph Ivan Krajbich, MD, FRCS(C)

84 Terminal Bone Overgrowth 1007
Joseph Ivan Krajbich, MD, FRCS(C)

85 Athletics and Sports Programs for the Child With Limb Difference 1013
Kevin Quinn, MSPO, CPO; Zach Harvey, CPO

Index 1019

SECTION 1

General Principles

General Principles of Amputation Surgery

CHAPTER 1

Sonya Agnew, MD • Peter Jeffrey Laub, MD • Michael S. Pinzur, MD, FAAOS

ABSTRACT

Amputation should be viewed as the first step in the rehabilitation process for a patient with a limb that cannot be salvaged because of injury or disease. It is important for the treating surgeon to understand how an individual is affected by limb loss, the differing considerations in caring for those with upper versus lower limb amputations or amputations performed because of differing etiologies, and the nuances of treating children. Good surgical planning and familiarity with methods of managing possible complications will result in the best possible outcomes for patients.

Keywords: amputation; limb salvage versus amputation; principles of amputation

Introduction

During World War II, the perception of amputation changed from ablative failure surgery to the modern paradigm of amputation as the first step in rehabilitation. The effect that the destructive component of the injury or disease process has on the affected individual and the steps that can be taken to return them to, as close as possible, their preinjury or disease state need to be addressed using a modern evidence-based model for health care. It is important to discuss the components of limb loss that universally affect the amputee population and the unique characteristics of upper versus lower extremity amputation, amputation in the adult compared with the child, and some of the nuances associated with amputation for injury compared with infection or disease.

Effect of Amputation on Health-Related Quality of Life

The psychological effect of amputation on health-related quality of life has been best studied in trauma patients. The Lower Extremity Assessment Project was an observational study of more than 600 civilian patients who sustained mutilating lower extremity injuries, of whom more than 150 underwent amputation. Validated outcomes tools were used to achieve longitudinal observation of the effect of the injury on their quality of life. One of the most enlightening insights gained from this pivotal investigation was the appreciation that one of the most important factors for successful rehabilitation following traumatic amputation was family support structure.[1] Using insight gained from this observational study, the core investigators used similar tactics to evaluate amputees from Operation Enduring Freedom. The Military Extremity Trauma/Amputation Limb Salvage Study investigation provided further insight into these affected individuals, demonstrating that individuals with traumatic amputations had a high probability to exhibit severe symptoms of depression or posttraumatic stress disorder.[2]

This information provides modern evidence-based support that helps orthopaedic surgeons to objectively appreciate the obvious psychological effect that amputation has on the affected individual, both during the acute phase of injury and recovery, and the prolonged period of rehabilitation. The roles that depression and posttraumatic stress disorder play in each of the groups, whether it be the body image stresses affecting a child with a congenital amputation or a patient facing amputation for tumor, infection, or gangrene, can easily be extrapolated.[3]

The Upper Extremity as an Organ of Sensation and Prehension

The hand is a unique organ of prehension and sensation that helps differentiate humans from much of the rest of the animal kingdom. It is the special relationship between sensory input and functional prehension that makes amputation of the upper extremity far more disabling than amputation of the lower extremity. When planning reconstruction of the upper extremity following trauma, the orthopaedic surgeon must consider the negative effect that a prosthesis or orthosis has on the residual limb by both shielding the terminal

---

Dr. Pinzur or an immediate family member is a member of a speakers' bureau or has made paid presentations on behalf of Orthofix, Inc. and Stryker. Neither of the following authors nor any immediate family member has received anything of value from or has stock or stock options held in a commercial company or institution related directly or indirectly to the subject of this chapter: Dr. Agnew and Dr. Laub.

residual limb from its important role as a sensory probe with the world, and blocking the sight lines that are necessary to manipulate objects with a prosthetic terminal device.

Experience has demonstrated that a high percentage of patients reject even high-tech electronic-powered prostheses. They find that even the very sophisticated devices are perceived as being cumbersome and slow to respond to initiation of a task. Many patients will become proficient with a prosthesis and then use it only as a tool for performing necessary tasks. The fact that the prosthesis renders the upper extremity insensate shields the patient from proprioceptive feedback and demands continual visual monitoring to operate. Often, retention of a rudimentary post and palm that allows simple prehension is functionally superior to the most sophisticated prostheses.

The Lower Extremity as an Organ of Weight Bearing

The normal human foot is composed of more than 20 bones that allow the dual functions of a shock absorber at heel strike and a stable platform to allow propulsion at push-off. The ligaments that connect the bones of the foot are relaxed when the foot is loaded at heel strike. This unlocked position of the joints, combined with the unique durable cushioned plantar skin and subcutaneous fibrous connective tissue, allows the foot to dampen the effect of weight bearing. As the foot transitions from the unlocked load acceptance position of ankle dorsiflexion and foot supination at heel strike to the locked position of ankle plantar flexion and foot pronation at push-off, the foot is able to transition from an organ of dampening weight acceptance to a stable platform for propulsion at push-off.

Unlike the adaptable weight-bearing organ of the normal foot, an amputation residual limb is generally composed of one or two bones and a soft-tissue envelope that must interface with a prosthesis to mimic the organ functions of the normal foot. When surgically creating an amputation residual limb, surgeons need to be cognizant of these dual functions to create a terminal organ that will interface with a prosthesis to provide pressure-dissipating cushioning at loading and stability for push-off.

Metabolic Cost of Walking With an Amputation

The self-selected walking speed of a person is determined by multiple factors that allow them to optimize energy consumption during walking. People are most efficient when healthy and well rested, and least efficient when affected by illness or injury. Engineering professionals view the joints of the lower extremity as energy couples. Illness or injury to the limb makes the mechanical construct both less energy efficient and more prone to activity-related discomfort. Prosthetic joints are not as efficient as the original equipment. **Figure 1** depicts the metabolic/energy cost of walking with a prosthesis. The more proximal the level of amputation, the greater is the negative effect on function. Note that the transfemoral amputee uses very similar energy consumption during normal walking and maximum walking speed. Because these studies are performed in the laboratory, this is akin to having to run at all times.[4-7] It is further established that amputees tend to take a similar number of steps every day. This metabolic cost affects their daily lives, making amputees ration the number of steps they will take.[8]

Limb Salvage Versus Amputation

Several important questions should be addressed by the surgeon before making the decision to proceed with limb salvage versus amputation, regardless of the disease or injury indication. Experience in trauma has taught the surgeon that the best time to make that decision is at the time of injury. It becomes very difficult to convince a patient to remove a nonfunctional limb after a substantial effort has been made to take the path of functional limb salvage. Patients with poorly conceived reconstruction plans are often doomed to a life of poor function and chronic neurogenic regional pain.

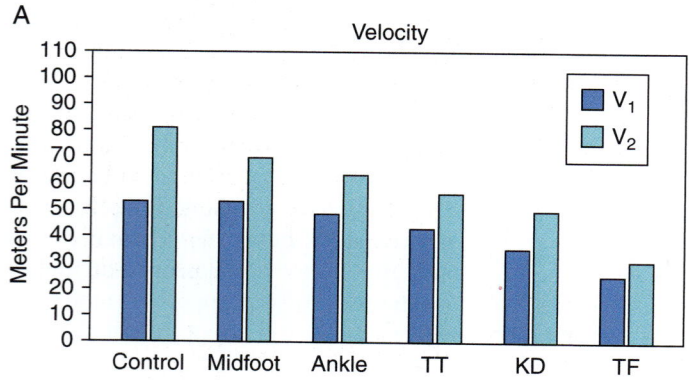
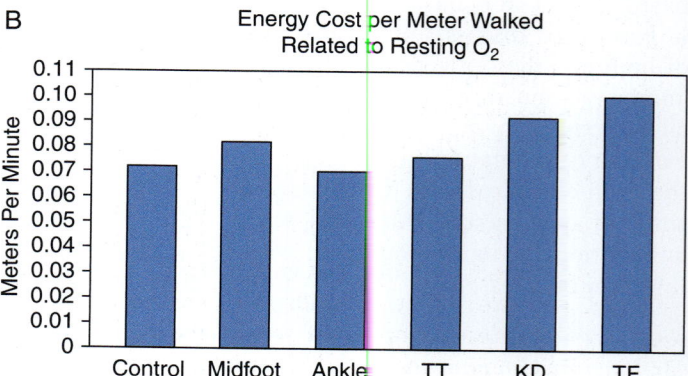

FIGURE 1 Bar graphs showing metabolic cost of walking with an amputation. **A,** Graph illustrates walking speed related to level of amputation. V_1 is a measure of self-selected walking speed, and V_2 is a measure of maximum walking speed. **B,** Graph showing oxygen consumption per meter walked as related to amputation level. Note that walking speed decreases and the energy cost of walking increases with more proximal amputation. KD = knee disarticulation, TF = transfemoral, TT = transtibial. (Reproduced with permission from Pinzur MS, Gold J, Schwartz D, Gross N: Energy demands for walking in dysvascular amputees as related to the level of amputation. *Orthopaedics* 1992;15[9]:1033-1037.)

The questions to be addressed in the trauma bay, the diabetic foot clinic, or the oncology clinic are:

- Will limb salvage outperform amputation and prosthetic limb fitting?
  The surgeon should have a realistic expectation of what the functional outcome will be with either limb salvage or amputation. It is unlikely that every patient will achieve the best result that the surgeon has ever achieved. Most surgeons will achieve a bell-shaped curve of clinical outcomes for a given set of clinical parameters, with most patients being in the middle of the curve. When initiating a treatment plan, the surgeon and the patient should have a realistic expectation whichever course is taken.
- What is the cost of limb salvage?
  Beyond the financial costs and the resources consumed during limb salvage treatment, the other costs to the patient must be considered. These include the lost wages from being out of work, the depletion of financial reserves, time lost from work, and the emotional costs associated with the multiple necessary surgeries.
- What are the risks?
  When establishing a risk assessment for limb salvage versus amputation, the surgeon should consider factors beyond a simple determination of surgical-associated morbidity. The risks of the multiple necessary surgeries and anesthesia, the potential for sepsis, the time necessary for rehabilitation, and the potential for narcotic addiction also should be considered. When each of these questions is addressed before the initiation of treatment, the decision often becomes more straightforward.

Amputation Level Selection

In the modern outcomes-oriented environment, it is clear that retention of limb length is closely correlated with optimal functional outcomes. When planning amputation surgery, the surgeon should strive to retain as many functional joints and residual limb length compatible with available tissue and prosthetic limb fitting. The most difficult decisions arise when the surgeon is required to choose between a longer residual limb length with a poor soft-tissue envelope and a more proximal amputation level with a more optimal residual limb. Results of the Lower Extremity Assessment Project study would suggest that the poor functional outcomes of the 17 knee disarticulations were due to suboptimal amputation residual limbs as opposed to poor ability to use a prosthesis. When the data were closely scrutinized, it was determined that most of the knee disarticulations performed in the Lower Extremity Assessment Project study were performed within the zone of injury and had poor soft-tissue envelopes. Those patients would likely have fared better with an optimally performed transfemoral amputation.[1]

The Terminal Organ of Weight Bearing

Bioengineering professionals view weight bearing as the transfer of load between the amputation residual limb and the prosthetic socket. The ground reaction force vector is applied to the amputation residual limb directly in disarticulations at the knee or ankle levels and thorough total surface bearing in the transosseous transfemoral or transtibial amputation levels. Orthopaedic surgeons use the terms direct load transfer, or end-bearing in disarticulations, and indirect load transfer, or total surface bearing in transosseous amputation levels (**Figure 2**).

End-bearing disarticulations behave much like normal weight transfer in a sound limb. Long bones are expanded at the level of the metaphysis to create a larger surface area for distribution of the weight-bearing load, and composed of low–elastic modulus cancellous bone to dissipate the impact of loading. A cushioned end pad acts to substitute for the dampening and cushioning function of the durable plantar tissue of the foot. Because the actual bony loading is similar to normal, prosthetic socket fit is not crucial. This is a valuable feature in patients with significant volume fluctuations, for example, renal failure, where the socket can be adjustable to compensate for volume changes[9,10] (**Figure 2, A** and **Figure 3**).

The bioengineering concept of indirect load transfer is better known in the prosthetic world as total surface bearing. This method of prosthetic socket construction is used in transosseous amputation levels where the surface area of the terminal bone is small and the bone is composed of higher stiffness cortical bone (**Figure 2, B**). The theoretic concept is to unload the small surface area of the stiff cortical bone of the terminal tibia in the transtibial amputation level and terminal femur in the transfemoral level. By flexing the knee 7° to 10° in the transtibial prosthesis and adducting the femur in the transfemoral prosthesis, pressure can be taken away from the distal end of the bone and distributed over the entire surface area of the residual limb.[11,12] To accomplish this task, prosthetic socket fit becomes crucial. If the patient loses as few as 5 lb, pain or ulceration overlying the prominent terminal cortical bone can develop. If the patient gains weight, they will not be able to fit the prosthetic socket.[9,10] The residual bone of transosseous amputees normally pistons during weight bearing. When the soft-tissue envelope of the residual tibia or femur is composed of mobile muscle and full-thickness normal skin, the bone will piston within the soft-tissue envelope. When the soft-tissue envelope is adherent to the bone, the pistoning occurs between the skin and the prosthetic socket, creating shear forces that lead to blisters and skin breakdown. This is best addressed surgically by creating an optimal soft-tissue envelope. When the skin of the amputation residual limb is adherent to the bone, the prosthetist will attempt to compensate by using some form of a silicone liner as an interface between adherent skin and the prosthetic socket (**Figure 4**).

The Soft-Tissue Envelope

The residual bone of an amputation residual limb serves as a platform for load transfer in lower extremity amputation and a lever arm to drive an upper

Section 1: General Principles

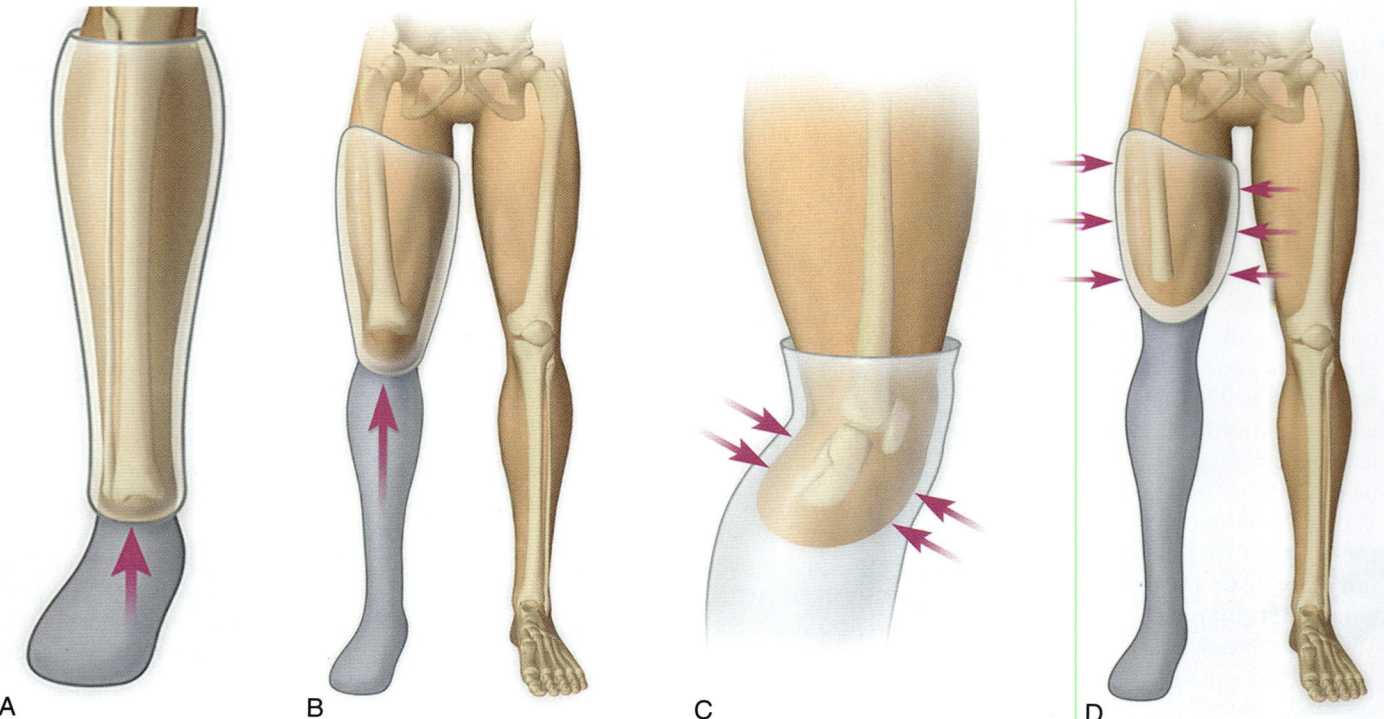

FIGURE 2 Illustrations depicting direct load transfer, that is, the end-bearing method of weight bearing, in disarticulation amputations at the Syme ankle disarticulation (**A**) and knee disarticulation (**B**) amputation levels. Illustrations depict the concept of indirect load transfer, or total surface bearing, which is the method of weight bearing at the transtibial (**C**) and transfemoral (**D**) amputation levels.

extremity prosthesis. The soft-tissue envelope serves as a cushion to dampen the effect of weight bearing and prevent tissue breakdown over bony prominences during prosthetic use. The optimal soft-tissue envelope is composed of mobile muscle and full-thickness skin (**Figure 4**).

The first step in creating a terminal organ of weight bearing is the removal of all nonviable tissue. This process should be completed without consideration of the reconstruction, as retaining marginal tissue leads to less favorable outcomes. Once all nonviable tissue is removed, all viable tissue should be retained to ensure retention of as much normal tissue for reconstruction as possible. When performing amputation for infection or trauma, the reconstruction is often performed at a second surgical stage to allow the zone of injury, in trauma, to recover, and to ensure infection-free margins when the surgery is being performed for infection or gangrene.

When staging amputation surgery for trauma or infection, the safest option is open wound management with either a vacuum-assisted wound closure device or moist gauze dressings. If there is redundant viable-appearing residual tissue, a reasonable alternative wound management option is provisional loose wound closure without tension. A planned staged return to surgery allows takedown of the provisional wound closure, secondary débridement, and formal creation of a durable cushioned soft-tissue envelope. The use of skin traction should be avoided, as the traction adds further insult to the zone of injury. Definitive wound closure in trauma is delayed until the zone of

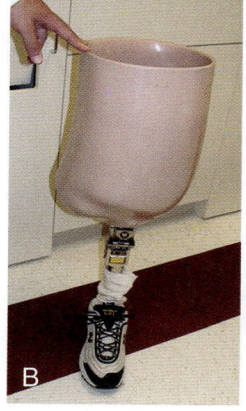 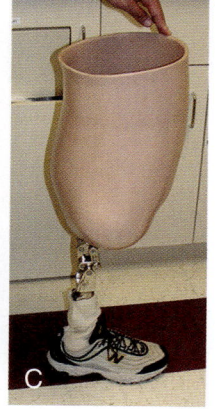

FIGURE 3 A, Clinical photograph from a patient with morbid obesity who has diabetes and renal failure and significant residual limb volume fluctuation that would have made transtibial prosthetic fitting very difficult. **B** and **C,** Photographs of the volume-adaptable knee disarticulation end-bearing prosthesis that allowed the patient to achieve functional ambulation.

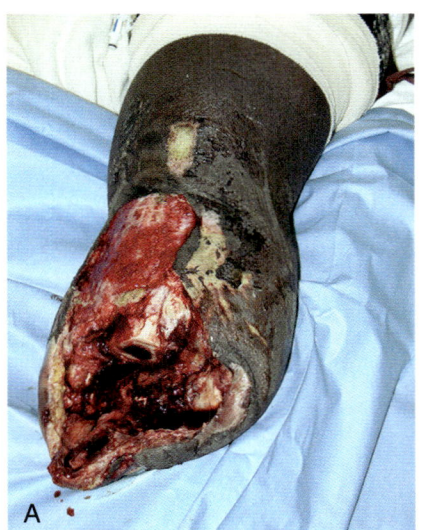
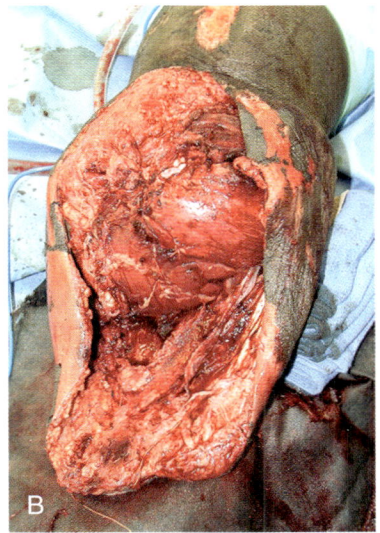
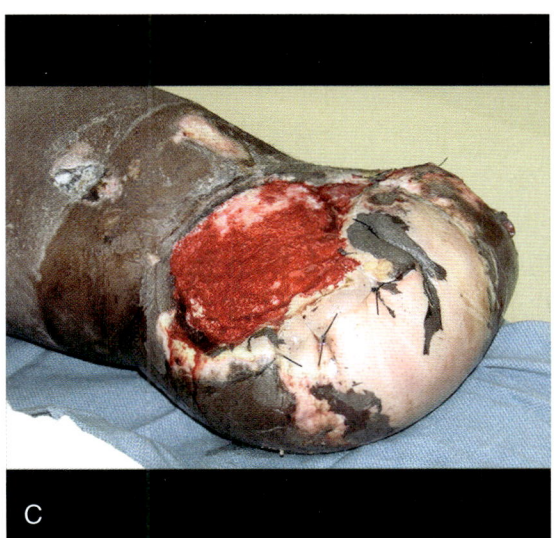
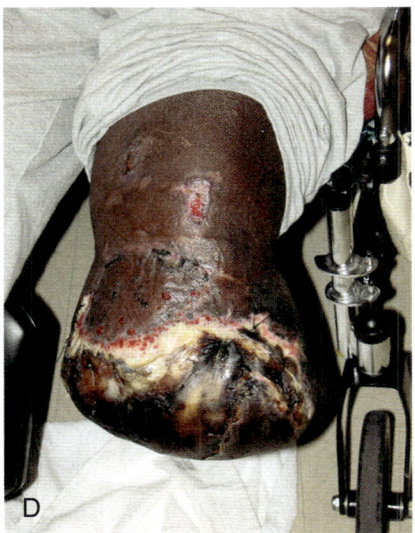
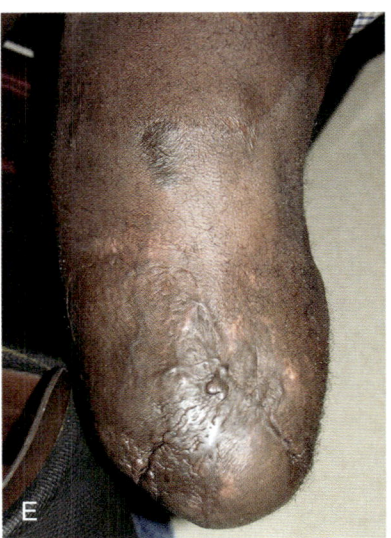

FIGURE 4 **A**, Clinical photograph from a young male who sustained a mutilating limb injury that was initially managed with an open transtibial amputation. **B**. Clinical photograph shows the initial attempt to create a cushioned gastrocnemius soft-tissue envelope for the residual tibia. The retained skin that had been degloved at the time of the original injury eventually died. **C**, Clinical photograph demonstrates the area of granulation tissue overlying the weight-bearing region of the anterior tibial shaft. Before the availability of silicone gel prosthetic socket liners, this region of the residual tibia would not have been able to tolerate the shear forces associated with weight bearing. **D**, Clinical photograph obtained following split-thickness skin grafting at the time of preparatory prosthetic limb fitting. **E**, Clinical photograph obtained 1 year following amputation. Note that the soft-tissue envelope has matured, allowing the patient to return to running sports, using a prosthesis.

injury recovers from the crush and traction insult of the injury.

When performing amputation for tumor, the first consideration is the creation of adequate tumor margins, whether they be transverse or compartment-based. Creation of the soft-tissue envelope and the residual limb is only determined after obtaining adequate tumor margins.

Socket Interface in Upper Extremity Amputation

Intimate prosthetic socket fit in the upper extremity is crucial for different considerations than in lower extremity amputation. Although the patient will not bear weight, intimate fit is necessary to drive the socket through space and establish leverage for performing tasks (**Figure 5**). Attempts should be made to maintain as much length as possible, based on the available muscle that will be used to create the soft-tissue envelope. Muscle groups should be attached to the residual bone at a relatively normal resting tension. This allows the retained muscles to create an electromyography signal that can be used to drive a myoelectric prosthetic motor.

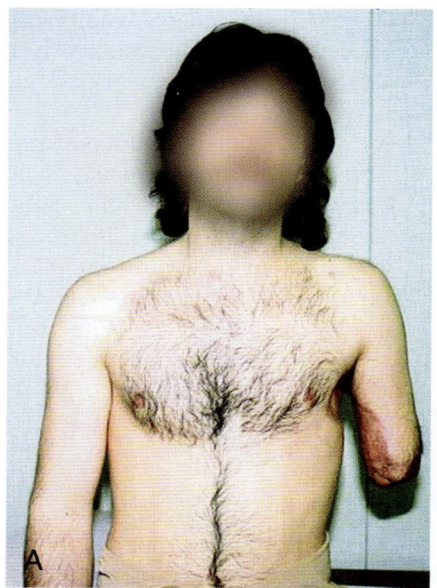 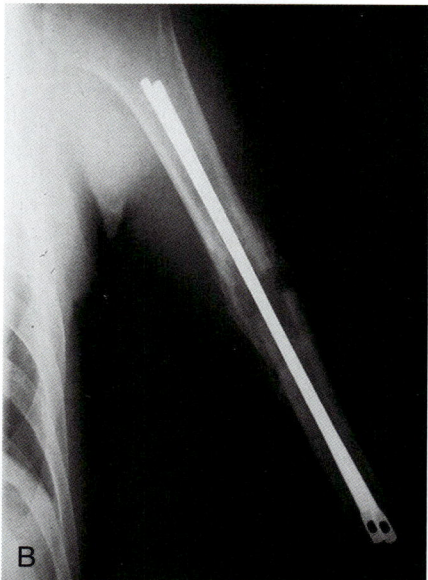 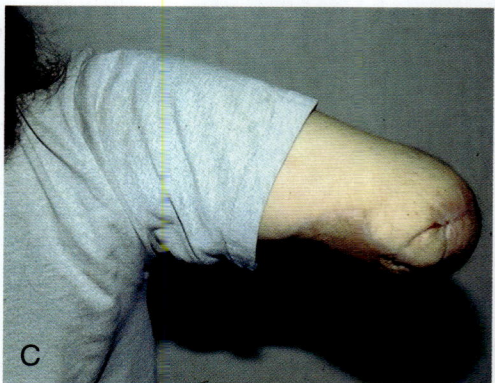

FIGURE 5 **A**, Clinical photograph shows a patient who sustained a crush injury that required transhumeral amputation. **B**, The radiograph demonstrates the fracture fixation that allowed retention of sufficient humeral length to allow functional prosthetic limb fitting. **C**, Clinical photograph demonstrates the limb length retention allowed sufficient surface area to achieve prosthetic socket suspension and leverage to drive the prosthesis through space.

Tissue Management

Experience, rather than evidence, has provided generally accepted principles in creating amputation residual limbs. The use of tourniquets has not been effectively studied in amputation surgery. Accepted practice is to avoid the use of tourniquets in limbs that have previously undergone vascular surgery or angioplasty. When a tourniquet is used, it should be deflated before wound closure to obtain control of bleeding. Arteries should be ligated with suture ligatures, that is, stick ties, to avoid late bleeding from a simple ligature that is extruded by the pulsations of the artery. Venous bleeding can be controlled by simple ligature, metal vascular clips, or electrocautery.

In creating a transosseous residual limb, soft-tissue stripping from bone should be limited to the amount required to create the soft-tissue envelope. Excessive periosteal stripping should be avoided to avoid late prominent periosteal bone formation. Bone necrosis from thermal burning with power saws can generally be avoided by cooling the bone with cool saline during the bony transection.

Once muscles within the zone of injury have recovered from trauma, they should be attached to bone at as close to normal tension as possible. In order, flexor and extensor muscle groups should be attached to the bone (radius and ulna for transradial amputation and humerus for transhumeral amputation) at normal resting muscle tension. Attaching the muscles to bone at normal resting tension creates a normal physiologic cushion, allows the muscles to drive the limb through space in a pattern that most closely mimics normal, and allows creation of an optimal electromyography signal to drive a myoelectric prosthesis.[6,7,13]

Crushing nerves with clamps should be avoided, even when there are plans to resect the crushed section of nerve. Crush is likely a major factor for the development of phantom limb or residual limb pain following amputation. The best practice is to gently grasp a nerve with a gauze sponge, apply gentle traction, and transect proximally with a fresh, sharp scalpel blade. Although a neuroma will develop in every transected nerve, a neuroma embedded in muscle is less likely to develop late sensitivity.

Native full-thickness skin is far more durable than any coverage obtained with grafting or healing by secondary intention. All viable skin should be retained for use in construction of the eventual functional amputation residual limb. When full-thickness skin is not available, options of healing by secondary intention must be considered, with or without the use of a vacuum-assisted wound closure device, skin grafting, or plastic surgery soft-tissue transfer.

Targeted Muscle Reinnervation

Surveys have shown that 80% to 91% of lower extremity amputees have functional or lifestyle-limiting pain.[14-17] Complex peripheral and central neural pathways contribute postamputation pain often classified as residual limb pain, phantom limb pain, and neuroma pain. Residual limb pain involves discomfort related to the soft-tissue envelope of an amputation residual limb and is generally attributed to suboptimal pressure point offloading and soft-tissue envelope. Phantom limb pain is incompletely understood but thought to stem from a complex interplay of aberrant peripheral and central nervous system. Centrally, the areas of somatosensory cortex responsible for the amputated limb exhibit activation when nearby adjacent parts are activated or stimulated.[18] Neuroma pain is estimated to account for 25% of all postamputation pain.[19,20] When a peripheral nerve lacks a distal target, axons sprout haphazardly within a disorganized topography of neural cells in a dense collagen matrix.[21] Hyperexcitability and spontaneous discharge from the neuroma manifest as localized allodynia and chronic reproducible pain.

Historically, numerous surgical and nonsurgical techniques have been described for the management of pain in amputees with variable success.[18] Despite a multitude of advances and techniques, there is no consensus on the optimal surgical management for postamputation pain.[22-24] Excision of painful neuromas, transposition into muscle or bone, and silicone capping yield inconsistent results and high reoperation rates for painful neuromas and phantom limb pain. These techniques share a passive approach to nerve management by aiming to bury the nerve in healthy tissue.[25] Targeted muscle reinnervation (TMR) is a paradigm shift toward active nerve management by capitalizing on the relentless regenerative potential of nerve to manage neuromas and, in the acute setting, prevent neuromas. Recent high-quality prospective studies evaluating TMR have shown favorable and consistent outcomes at managing and preventing neuroma and phantom limb pain.[26-29]

TMR was originally pioneered by the translational work of Dumanian and Kuiken for improved control of myoelectric upper extremity prostheses.[30-32] Their work initially focused on coapting motor nerve residual limbs from amputated muscles to remaining muscles to clarify and amplify electromyographic signals for improved myoelectric prosthesis control. Long-term follow-up of the patients treated with TMR revealed prevention of postamputation pain when performed at the same time as amputation and drastic reductions in pain for patients who underwent delayed TMR.[33] Currently, the main indication for TMR in lower extremity amputees is to prevent the development of neuroma and phantom limb pain at the time of amputation and to reduce chronic pain in established amputees.

Fundamentally, TMR restores continuity to sensory nerves that lack a distal target, aptly described by Dumanian et al as giving nerves "somewhere to go and something to do."[26] In TMR for lower extremity amputees, the transected ends of sensory serves are coapted to the terminal motor nerves of nearby muscles. Providing a target for the sensory nerves to innervate, sprout axons, and regenerate epineurium promotes organized proliferation of nerve. This process restores normal nerve architecture on a histologic level, thus preventing the formation of hyperexcitable and spontaneously discharging neuromas.[34]

Multiple studies demonstrated that TMR can provide durable and marked pain reduction in amputees. Compared with standard neuroma excision and burying in muscle, a recent randomized clinical trial of 28 patients with chronic postamputation pain demonstrated a 3.7-point reduction in pain on a 10-point scale for patients treated with TMR.[13] Prospective analysis has shown a 2.7/10 daily pain reduction for patients undergoing TMR for chronic pain in addition to statistically significant improvements in functional outcomes.[35] Other retrospective reviews have shown similar clinically and statistically significant success after TMR for amputation pain.[27,36]

Compared with patients who underwent general amputation, patients who undergo TMR concurrently with amputation experience less intense and less frequent neuroma symptoms, leading some centers to use TMR at the time of initial amputation.[37] A multi-institutional cohort study found that TMR at the time of index amputation was associated with a threefold high odds of decreased pain across multiple measurements.[37] Studies of TMR done at the same time of upper extremity amputation have documented similar results.[33,38]

Postamputation pain is most frequently experienced in trauma patients; therefore TMR may be most beneficial in this population.[19,39] Primary or secondary TMR in patients with oncologic and diabetic amputations has demonstrated improvement in pain as well.[26,28,29,33]

Caution should be taken in patients with uncontrolled medical issues such as osteomyelitis, residual limb pain from soft-tissue envelope ischemia, or chronic wounds. Pain from ischemic neuropathy and pain at rest are not addressed by TMR. Patients with diffuse, poorly localized pain are less likely to benefit from TMR.

Technique Principles

- Preoperative planning: TMR may be performed on an outpatient basis using loupe magnification, tourniquet, and regional blocks.[26,27,40] TMR can be performed concurrently with amputation (primary TMR) or on established amputees with chronic pain (secondary or delayed TMR).
- Sensory nerve identification: For patients with chronic neuromatous pain, careful preoperative examination reveals problem nerves with palpation eliciting pain in the sensory distribution of the nerve. For patients undergoing TMR at the time of initial transfemoral amputation or transtibial amputation, nerves known to generate painful neuromas are selected for TMR. In the transfemoral amputation, they are the common peroneal, tibial, saphenous, and posterior femoral cutaneous nerves. These are dissected and prepared for transfer to nearby motor points. Peroneal and posterior femoral nerves are targeted with the biceps femoris, whereas the saphenous nerve is transferred to the vastus medialis. Tibial components of the sciatic nerve are coapted to motor nerve endpoints in the semitendinosus or semimembranosus.[41,42] In the transtibial amputation, they are tibial deep and superficial peroneal, medial and lateral sural, and saphenous nerves. **Figure 6** illustrates typical nerve transfers in a transtibial amputation via one-incision or two-incision approaches.
- Motor point identification: A disposable biphasic nerve stimulator

Amputee with Chronic Pain

One-Incision Approach

Sensory Nerve	Motor Nerve Target
*Common peroneal →	Lateral gastrocnemius
*Lateral sural →	Lateral gastrocnemius
*Medial sural →	Soleus or medial gastrocnemius
*Tibial →	Soleus

Two-Incision Approach

Sensory Nerve	Motor Nerve Target
*Deep peroneal →	Tibialis anterior
*Superficial peroneal →	Extensor digitorum longus
*Lateral sural →	Lateral gastrocnemius
*Medial sural →	Soleus or medial gastrocnemius
*Tibial →	Soleus

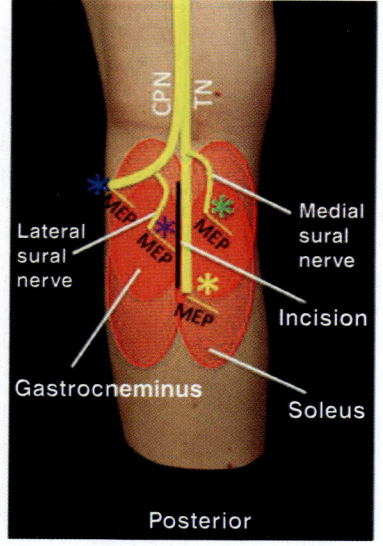
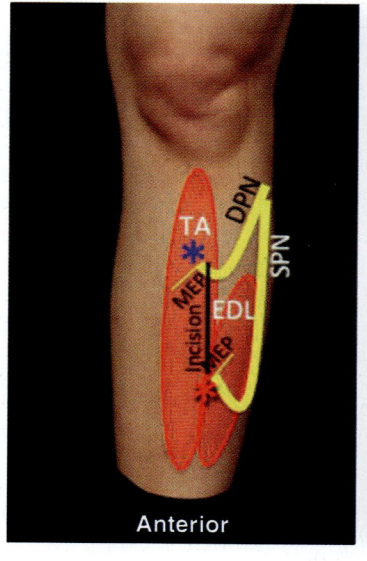
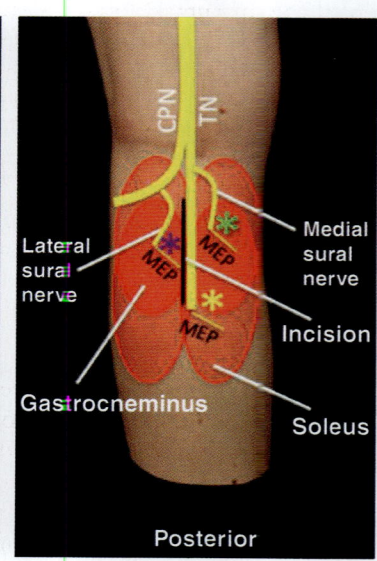

FIGURE 6 Schematic example of nerve transfers for targeted muscle reinnervation of transtibial amputation.

is used to identify motor nerve endpoints. Regional blocks do not preclude identification of motor targets as the nerve stimulator acts directly on the nerve-muscle unit. Muscle or parts of muscle will undergo tetanic contraction when stimulated nearby. Tourniquet deflation during this part of the surgery may be required for reliable motor point detection.[43] The motor nerve is dissected free and sharply transected near its insertion to the muscle. In transtibial amputations, preservation of the motor branches from the deep peroneal nerve to the lateral compartment is preferred to avoid atrophy and problems with prosthetic wear.
- Neurorrhaphy: Axons of the peripheral nerve residual limb are coapted with 6-0 and 8-0 nonabsorbable monofilament suture in a tension-free fashion. Size mismatch is expected and has no bearing on the outcome. Aberrant sprouting can be prevented using absorbable suture to pull a muscle envelope up around the coaptation.
- Postoperative care: Patients are instructed on edema control and to avoid prosthesis wear for 4 to 6 weeks to allow for appropriate soft-tissue healing.

Managing patient expectations is important when pursuing TMR for a patient. Patients who have lived with chronic pain for years should be counseled to expect pain reduction but not elimination. Instrumentation on painful nerves often results in transient worsening of pain in the early postoperative period, and the benefits typically take 3 to 6 months to fully realize.[26,28-40]

Amputation in Children

There are several considerations that make amputation in children different from amputation in adults. Epiphyseal growth centers in amputated limbs will generally achieve less limb length than in a contralateral normal limb. When planned appropriately, temporizing with provisional prostheses is often a valuable component of a well-conceived longitudinal treatment plan.

Bony overgrowth is a common complication of transosseous amputation in growing children. Surgery to resect painful bony overgrowth is a common necessity of the longitudinal management of this patient population. Various surgical techniques to limit bony overgrowth have not been universally successful in preventing this annoying complication.

Outcomes Following Amputation

The rehabilitative process should start before surgery in elective amputation, and as soon as possible following trauma. The amputation surgeon should use similar methods of preoperative planning as those used by fracture or joint replacement surgeons. Each step of the amputation process should be accomplished with a reasonable surgical plan. Early transfer training and ambulation with crutches or a walker should be accomplished before prosthetic limb fitting. Peer counseling has been extremely valuable in dealing with the inevitable posttraumatic stress disorder that follows amputation.[3,35,44,45]

SUMMARY

Surgeons have learned that amputation surgery should be considered as the first step in the rehabilitation of a patient where amputation is determined to offer a more favorable clinical outcome than limb salvage. The principles of amputation surgery should address the creation of a residual limb that is optimized for interfacing with the external environment.

References

1. Bosse MJ, MacKenzie EJ, Kellam JF, et al: An analysis of outcomes of reconstruction or amputation of leg-threatening injuries. *N Engl J Med* 2002;347(24):1924-1931.
2. Doukas WC, Hayda RA, Frisch M, et al: The Military Extremity Trauma Amputation/Limb Salvage (METALS) study. *J Bone Joint Surg Am* 2013;95(2):138-145.
3. Available at: http://www.amputee-coalition.org/inmotion/oct_07/intro_npn.html.
4. Pinzur MS, Gold J, Schwartz D, Gross N: Energy demands for walking in dysvascular amputees as related to the level of amputation. *Orthopaedics* 1992;15(9):1033-1037.
5. Fisher SV, Gullickson G: Energy cost of ambulation in health and disability: A literature review. *Arch Phys Med Rehabil* 1978;59(3):124-133.
6. Breaky J: Gait of unilateral below-knee amputees. *Orthot Prosthet* 1976;30:17-24.
7. Pinzur MS, Asselmeier M, Smith DG: Dynamic electromyography in active and limited walking below-knee amputees. *Orthopaedics* 1991;14(5):535-538.
8. Available at: http://www.amputee-coalition.org/inmotion/sep_oct_09/evidence_based_care.pdf.
9. Pinzur MS: Current concepts: Amputation surgery in peripheral vascular disease. *Instr Course Lect* 1997;46:501-509.
10. Pinzur MS, Smith DG, Guedes S, Pinto MA, Schon LC: Controversies in amputation surgery. *Instr Course Lect* 2003;52:445-454.
11. Tucker CJ, Wilken JM, Stinner PDJ, Kirk KL: A comparison of limb-socket kinematics of bone-bridging and non-bonebridging wartime transtibial amputations. *J Bone Joint Surg Am* 2012;94(10):924-930.
12. Schiff A, Havey R, Carandang G, et al: Quantification of shear stresses within a transtibial prosthetic socket. *Foot Ankle Int* 2014;35(8):779-782.
13. Gottschalk F, Kourosh S, Stills M: Does socket configuration influence the position of the femur in above-knee amputation? *J Prosthet Orthot* 1989;2:94-102.
14. Smith DG, Ehde DM, Legro MW, Reiber GE, del Aguila M, Boone DA: Phantom limb, residual limb, and back pain after lower extremity amputations. *Clin Orthop Relat Res* 1999;361:29-38.
15. van der Schans CP, Geertzen JHB, Schoppen T, Dijkstra PU: Phantom pain and health-related quality of life in lower limb amputees. *J Pain Symptom Manage* 2002;24(4):429-436.
16. Ephraim PL, Wegener ST, MacKenzie EJ, Dillingham TR, Pezzin LE: Phantom pain, residual limb pain, and back pain in amputees: Results of a national survey. *Arch Phys Med Rehabil* 2005;86(10):1910-1919.
17. Schley MT, Wilms P, Toepfner S, et al: Painful and nonpainful phantom and stump sensations in acute traumatic amputees. *J Trauma* 2008;65(4):858-864.
18. Flor H: Phantom-limb pain: Characteristics, causes, and treatment. *Lancet Neurol* 2002;1(3):182-189.
19. Ducic I, Mesbahi AN, Attinger CE, Graw K: The role of peripheral nerve surgery in the treatment of chronic pain associated with amputation stumps. *Plast Reconstr Surg* 2008;121(3):908-914.
20. Pierce RO, Kernek CB, Ambrose TA: The plight of the traumatic amputee. *Orthopedics* 1993;16(7):793-797.
21. Woo SL, Kung TA, Brown DL, Leonard JA, Kelly BM, Cederna PS: Regenerative peripheral nerve interfaces for the treatment of postamputation neuroma pain: A pilot study. *Plast Reconstr Surg Glob Open* 2016;4(12):e1038.
22. Poppler LH, Parikh RP, Bichanich MJ, et al: Surgical interventions for the treatment of painful neuroma: A comparative meta-analysis. *Pain* 2018;159(2):214-223.
23. Decrouy-Duruz V, Christen T, Raffoul W: Evaluation of surgical treatment for neuropathic pain from neuroma in patients with injured peripheral nerves. *J Neurosurg* 2018;128(4):1235-1240.
24. Bowen JB, Wee CE, Kalik J, Valerio IL: Targeted muscle reinnervation to improve pain, prosthetic tolerance, and bioprosthetic outcomes in the amputee. *Adv Wound Care (New Rochelle)* 2017;6(8):261-267.
25. Eberlin KR, Ducic I: Surgical algorithm for neuroma management: A changing treatment paradigm. *Plast Reconstr Surg Glob Open* 2018;6(10):e1952.
26. Dumanian GA, Potter BK, Mioton LM, et al: Targeted muscle reinnervation treats neuroma and phantom pain in major limb amputees: A randomized clinical trial. *Ann Surg* 2019;270(2):238-246.
27. Souza JM, Cheesborough JE, Ko JH, Cho MS, Kuiken TA, Dumanian GA: Targeted muscle reinnervation: A novel approach to postamputation neuroma pain. *Clin Orthop Relat Res* 2014;472(10):2984-2990.
28. Mioton LM, Dumanian GA, Shah N, et al: Targeted muscle reinnervation improves residual limb pain, phantom limb pain, and limb function: A prospective study of 33 major limb amputees. *Clin Orthop Relat Res* 2020;478(9):2161-2167.
29. Valerio IL, Dumanian GA, Jordan SW, et al: Preemptive treatment of phantom and residual limb pain with targeted muscle reinnervation at the time of major limb amputation. *J Am Coll Surg* 2019;228(3):217-226.
30. Kuiken TA: Targeted muscle reinnervation for real-time myoelectric control of multifunction artificial arms. *J Am Med Assoc* 2009;301(6):619-628.
31. Kuiken TA, Dumanian GA, Lipschutz RD, Miller LA, Stubblefield KA: The use of targeted muscle reinnervation

for improved myoelectric prosthesis control in a bilateral shoulder disarticulation amputee. *Prosthet Orthot Int* 2004;28(3):245-253.

32. Hijjawi JB, Kuiken TA, Lipschutz RD, Miller LA, Stubblefield KA, Dumanian GA: Improved myoelectric prosthesis control accomplished using multiple nerve transfers. *Plast Reconstr Surg* 2006;118(7):1573-1578.

33. Pet MA, Ko JH, Friedly JL, Mourad PD, Smith DG: Does targeted nerve implantation reduce neuroma pain in amputees? *Clin Orthop Relat Res* 2014;472(10):2991-3001.

34. Kim PS, Ko JH, O'Shaughnessy KK, Kuiken TA, Pohlmeyer EA, Dumanian GA: The effects of targeted muscle reinnervation on neuromas in a rabbit rectus abdominis flap model. *J Hand Surg Am* 2012;37(8):1609-1616.

35. Smith DG, Michael JW, Prusakowski PE, et al: Outcomes measures in lower limb prosthetics. *J Prosthet Orthot* 2006;18:6.

36. Michno DA, Woollard ACS, Kang NV: Clinical outcomes of delayed targeted muscle reinnervation for neuroma pain reduction in longstanding amputees. *J Plast Reconstr Aesthet Surg* 2019;72(9):1576-1606.

37. Alexander JH, Jordan SW, West JM, et al: Targeted muscle reinnervation in oncologic amputees: Early experience of a novel institutional protocol. *J Surg Oncol* 2019;120(3):348-358.

38. O'Brien AL, Jordan SW, West JM, Mioton LM, Dumanian GA, Valerio IL: Targeted muscle reinnervation at the time of upper-extremity amputation for the treatment of pain severity and symptoms. *J Hand Surg Am* 2021;46(1):72.e1-72.e10.

39. Hanley MA, Ehde DM, Jensen M, Czerniecki J, Smith DG, Robinson LR: Chronic pain associated with upper-limb loss. *Am J Phys Med Rehabil* 2009;88(9):742-751.

40. Lanier ST, Jordan SW, Ko JH, Dumanian GA: Targeted muscle reinnervation as a solution for nerve pain. *Plast Reconstr Surg* 2020;146(5):651e-663e.

41. Fracol ME, Janes LE, Ko JH, Dumanian GA: Targeted muscle reinnervation in the lower leg: An anatomical study. *Plast Reconstr Surg* 2018;142(4):541e-550e.

42. Agnew SP, Schultz AE, Dumanian GA, Kuiken TA: Targeted reinnervation in the transfemoral amputee: A preliminary study of surgical technique. *Plast Reconstr Surg* 2012;129(1):187-194.

43. Bowen JB, Ruter D, Wee C, West J, Valerio IL: Targeted muscle reinnervation technique in below-knee amputation. *Plast Reconstr Surg* 2019;143(1):309-312.

44. Available at: http://www.amputee-coalition.org/support-groups-peer-support/certified-peer-visitor-program/.

45. Smith DG, Berke GM: Post-operative management of the lower extremity amputee. *J Prosthet Orthot* 2004;16:3.

General Principles of Postoperative Residual Limb Management

CHAPTER 2

Frank A. Gottschalk, MD* • Michael S. Pinzur, MD, FAAOS

ABSTRACT

Various postoperative management protocols have been used over the years to care for postoperative wounds and residual limbs after amputation. The most successful protocols have been those using modern soft dressings, including negative-pressure incision and wound dressings. Compression dressings and various types of rigid dressings, including removable rigid dressings, are applied over the incision dressings and help reduce postoperative edema. Some of the newer postoperative dressings are impregnated with silver ions. The goal of each type of dressing is to improve wound healing and shorten the time to prosthesis fitting.

Keywords: compressive dressings; hydrofiber dressings; incision and wound dressings; negative-pressure dressings; protective dressings

Introduction

The management of immediate and early postoperative wounds and residual limb care is generally not well described in surgical texts. The goal of such care is to ensure uncomplicated healing in as short a time as possible. Because many lower limb amputations are a consequence of diabetes mellitus and vascular disease, wound healing problems are common and may subsequently result in a more proximal-level amputation. Traumatic amputations may have unrecognized tissue damage, and wound care is paramount to subsequent satisfactory healing. The minimization of wound healing issues begins at the time of surgery by removing dead, nonviable, and infected tissues and ensuring the adequate viability of remaining tissues. Soft tissue (muscle, fascia, and subcutaneous tissue) and skin closure without tension is key to reducing the potential for wound breakdown and failure to heal.

Over the past several years, scientific articles have been published that document the superiority of one method of wound care over another. Several studies have noted that some form of rigid or supportive dressing is better than soft dressing alone.[1-4] Various types of postoperative management are currently in use, with some incorporating modifications from older methods. Immediate postoperative management encompasses the application of initial wound or incision dressings and coverings and more sophisticated applications of compressive, elastic support, and/or rigid dressings. After the initial postoperative care, various additional coverings are used, all of which are intended to aid in protecting the residual limb and assisting amputee mobility. The use of various soft-tissue dressings to "shape the residual limb" has been invoked in the past; however, the shape of the residual limb is determined by the quality of the surgery and the length of the bone and soft-tissue flaps, not by the bandages and wrappings. The use of rigid dressings in the early postoperative period helps to reduce trauma to the residual limb and minimize tissue breakdown, which may help in reducing edema. The application of ice packs to the end of the residual limb may also contribute to edema reduction.

Incision and Wound Dressings

In general, postoperative wound dressing of the amputated limb may be divided into the following categories: soft dressings, negative-pressure wound dressings, hydrofiber dressings, compressive dressings, protective dressings, and rigid dressings.

Soft Dressings

Soft dressings traditionally have been used to cover the residual limb after surgery. Their role is to cover the suture line and wrap the limb to hold the incision dressings in place. Gauze wraps do not reduce edema, nor do they affect the shape of the residual limb. Residual limb shape is determined at the time of surgery and is affected by muscle, soft tissue, skin flaps, and, in certain areas, by the shape and length of the bones, such as the tibia and fibula or radius and ulna.

Soft dressings include cotton or polyester gauze pads and wrapping with cotton gauze rolls or conforming polyester rolls.[1] These dressings are used to hold wound and incision coverings in place, but they do not provide support for the residual limb. The dressings are

---

Dr. Pinzur or an immediate family member is a member of a speakers' bureau or has made paid presentations on behalf of Orthofix, Inc. and Stryker.

*Deceased.

permeable and help absorb drainage from the incision, but they do not provide a substantial degree of wound protection.[1,2] Soft dressings are ubiquitous in their use and inexpensive. Wrapping gauze rolls over the end of the residual limb frequently requires some expertise to ensure even distribution of pressure being applied to the surgically created residual limb. Major disadvantages of soft dressings are that they tend to loosen and require reapplication as frequently as every 3 to 4 hours. These dressings may provide padding when a compressive sleeve or rigid dressing is required.

Petroleum-impregnated gauze is frequently applied to the incision site at the conclusion of the surgical procedure, and it is then covered with regular gauze. Some form of wrap (often a gauze roll or elastic wrap) is then applied. Many surgeons use these dressings instead of rigid dressings because they prefer to view the incision site on a daily basis, although it has been shown that this is often unnecessary.[3]

In 1980, Kane and Pollak[4] reported no statistical difference in narcotic use among patients with amputations resulting from vascular causes who were treated with soft dressings or those who were fitted with an immediate postoperative prosthesis (IPOP); however, the analgesic protocols at that time were different from those in current use. They noted no statistical difference in wound necrosis and infection between the two methods. The authors noted that 56% of the patients fitted with the IPOP became prosthesis users compared with 22% of the patients treated with soft dressings; however, it is not known if there was a selection bias based on their perceived rehabilitation potential. They were not able to identify either beneficial or harmful effects of the IPOP on early healing or functional clinical outcomes after amputation.

Negative-Pressure Wound Dressings

Negative-pressure wound dressings (also known as vacuum-assisted closure dressings) are becoming more widely used and are commonly applied in orthopaedic surgery for open wounds

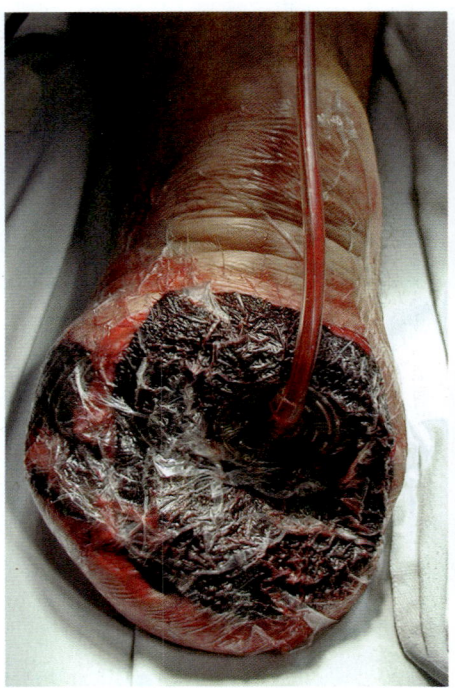

FIGURE 1 Photograph of a residual limb after an open transtibial amputation. A negative-pressure dressing covers the wound.

associated with fractures, after wound débridements, and before skin closure, as well as for contaminated and infected wounds when closure is contraindicated (**Figures 1** and **2**). These devices use open-pore foam to fill the wound cavity, an occlusive wound dressing, suction tubing, and a suction device. A wound-healing mechanism of action of negative-pressure wound dressings is the bringing together of the wound edges by the suction distributed through the foam sponge.[5,6] Another healing mechanism of action, which has been determined by finite element computer analysis, is the 5% to 20% strain that negative-pressure wound dressings produce across the healing tissues. This strain promotes cell division and proliferation, growth factor production, and angiogenesis.[6] Other reported benefits of negative-pressure wound dressings are removal of edema fluid and exudate from the extracellular space and removal of inflammatory mediators and cytokines, whose prolonged effect can hinder the ability of the microcirculation to support damaged tissue. Another positive factor in wound healing is reduction of wound

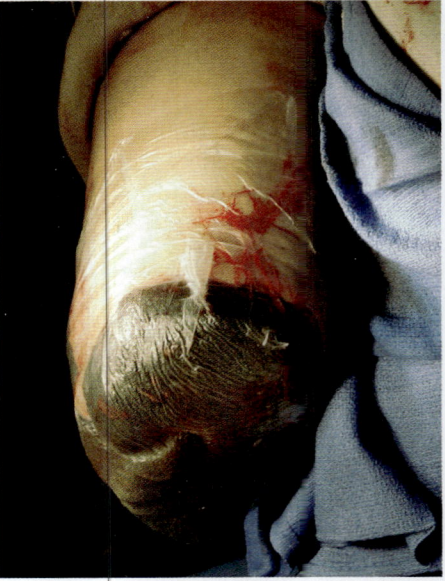

FIGURE 2 Photograph of a residual limb after an open transfemoral amputation. A negative-pressure wound dressing was applied at the end of the first-stage surgery.

desiccation and enhanced formation of granulation tissue. There is convincing evidence to support the hypothesis that the reduction of lateral tension and hematoma, coupled with an acceleration of the elimination of tissue edema, are the main beneficial mechanisms of action of negative-pressure wound therapy over the incision site.[7]

Over the past several years, there has been an increased frequency of managing residual limb wounds with negative-pressure dressings applied over the incision site at the conclusion of surgery (**Figures 3** and **4**). Applying these dressings to closed incisions reduces the relative risk of infection.[8] A randomized controlled trial demonstrated a decrease in postoperative seromas after the application of incisional negative-pressure wound dressings after total hip arthroplasty.[9] A study by Hansen et al[10] confirmed that negative-pressure dressings reduced or eliminated incisional drainage after hip arthroplasty, and no adverse effects were reported. Negative pressure set between 50 and 125 mm Hg helps to reduce edema and decrease incisional drainage.[6] Negative-pressure incisional dressings are kept in place for 3 days and may be reapplied or discarded. If no additional fluid collects

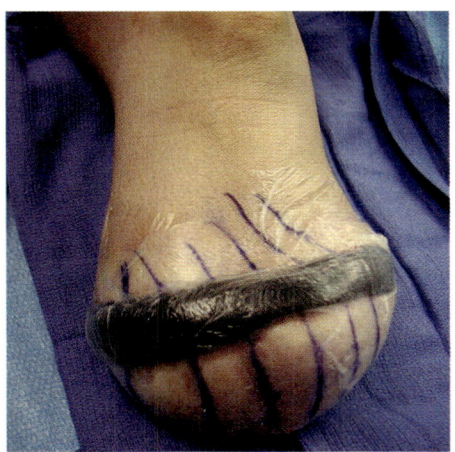

FIGURE 3 Photograph of a residual limb after a transtibial amputation. An incisional negative-pressure dressing was applied immediately postoperatively.

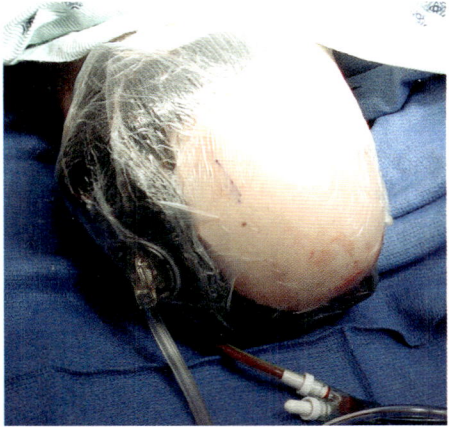

FIGURE 4 Photograph of a residual limb after a transfemoral amputation. An incisional negative-pressure wound dressing was applied at wound closure.

in the canister over a 12-hour period, it is recommended that the dressing be discontinued. However, it is likely that, because of the decreased wound-edge tension created by the negative-pressure dressing, there is often no measurable fluid accumulation in the collection reservoir. Recent studies have noted that the benefits of negative-pressure dressings may be associated with edema reduction, increased blood flow, and increased granulation tissue in the wound.[6,7] After 3 to 5 days of postoperative negative-pressure wound therapy, healing time may be reduced, and there is evidence of a reduced incidence of wound healing complications and a reduced frequency of infections.[7] Karlakki et al[7] reported the existence of good evidence for incisional negative-pressure wound therapy in orthopaedic surgery because of the frequency of patient comorbidities and the substantial incidence of infection. Brem et al[11] reported that incisional negative-pressure wound therapy may reduce the risk of delayed wound healing and infection after severe trauma and orthopaedic interventions. In some instances, a rigid dressing may be placed over the negative-pressure wound dressing on the residual limb for added protection.[12]

Negative-pressure wound dressings also can be used over open wounds before definitive skin closure in situations such as traumatic amputations and in the presence of infection when a two- or three-stage amputation is planned.[13] For open wounds, a new negative-pressure dressing is applied at the second-stage surgery. Two studies reported good results with the application of a custom, topical negative-pressure dressing for open amputations.[14,15]

Hydrofiber Dressings

Hydrofiber wound dressings consist of soft nonwoven sodium carboxymethylcellulose fibers integrated with ionic silver. This is a moisture-retention dressing, which forms a gel on contact with wound fluid and has the antimicrobial properties of ionic silver.[1,16]

After the use of a negative-pressure dressing, a hydrofiber with silver dressing may be applied over the incision (**Figure 5**). This dressing can remain in place for up to 7 days and may cover sutures. Because the dressing is impervious to water, patients may shower with the dressing in place. There has been renewed interest and research in using ionic silver (the oxidized active state of silver) as a prophylactic antimicrobial agent in wound dressings because of its broad-spectrum antibacterial range.[16] The gel promotes a moist wound-healing environment but absorbs any wound exudate and contains it away from the wound. Because of the antimicrobial effect of silver, this dressing has the potential to reduce postoperative infections.[1] Cutting et al[17] reported that the silver in the hydrofiber dressing provides a certain amount of resistance to infection. In a randomized study of acute surgical wounds in 100 patients, the performances of hydrofiber and alginate dressings were compared.[18] Ninety-two percent of patients randomized to the hydrofiber dressing were found to experience less pain (mild or none) compared with 80% of those who received alginate dressings. Similarly, 84% of patients who had hydrofiber dressings were pain free at 1 week postoperatively compared with 58% of those treated with alginate dressings. Although statistical significance was not shown, the authors concluded that hydrofiber dressings consistently performed better than the alginate dressings.

Compressive Dressings

Compressive dressings consist of elastic and conforming dressings. The original compressive dressing was an elastic bandage or sleeve. Newer materials have been developed to apply more uniform pressure over the residual limb. These dressings apply a measure of compression to the limb and help control postoperative edema.[19,20] The most basic compression dressing is the elastic wrap, which should be applied in a figure-of-8 configuration, with the most pressure applied distally to proximally (**Figure 6**). Applying uniform pressure is difficult with this method, so the wraps have to be reapplied every 4 to 6 hours. Volume reduction takes more time in the first 2 weeks after surgery with elastic compression dressings compared with rigid dressings and is not as effective.[21,22] Another form of elastic dressing is an elastic shrinker or sock, which has built-in elasticity and is rolled onto the limb[23] (**Figure 7**). The socks are available in various sizes and materials, are provided by a prosthetist, and may be kept in place throughout the day and night for as long as required. They are helpful at night to reduce edema when a prosthesis has been fitted and is doffed after daily use. In shorter residual limbs, a suspension belt may be required to hold the shrinker sock in place.

Section 1: General Principles

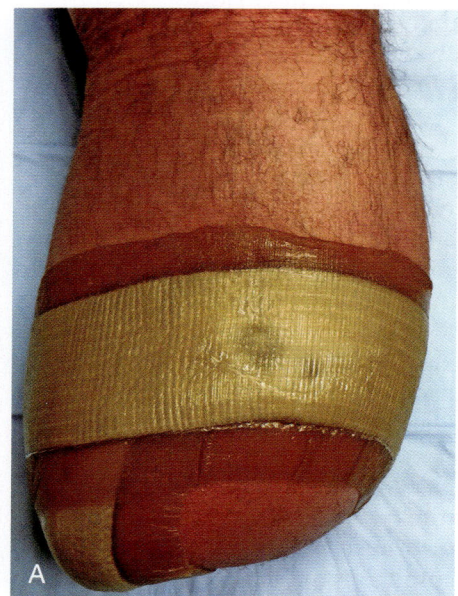
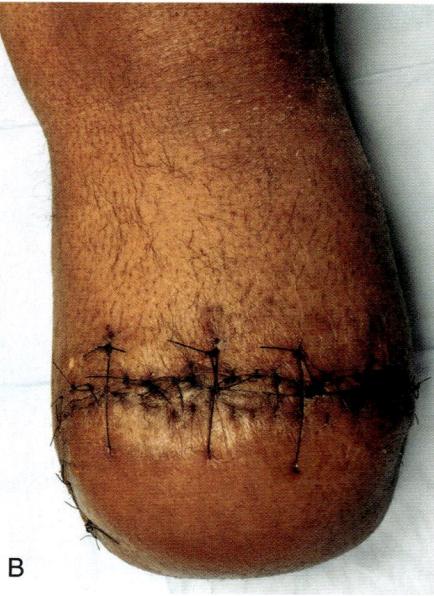

FIGURE 5 Photographs of a hydrofiber dressing in place over a transtibial amputation incision (**A**) and the incision site 10 days after surgery (**B**).

Compression devices to help reduce edema include polymer gel socks and thermoplastic and silicone liners[24,25] (**Figures 8** and **9**). These devices are rolled onto the limb and stay in place because of their compressive force and associated evenly distributed shear friction. They are more effective in edema reduction than elastic bandages. The liners also are used within the prosthetic socket and may provide suspension assistance in addition to padding.

A technique that is now rarely used after amputations is the Unna paste dressing, a mixture of zinc oxide, calamine, gelatin, and glycerin that is applied over successive layers of residual limb bandages that have been applied in a figure-of-8 configuration.[26,27] After 24 hours, a semirigid, inextensible dressing is formed that prevents edema. The dressing may be used for any level of amputation. This type of dressing was previously used primarily by physical therapists and physical medicine and rehabilitation physicians, but it has fallen out of favor because of newer materials and techniques.

Protective Dressings

Protective dressings include rigid and semirigid dressings and pneumatic postamputation mobility (PPAM) aids. These dressings are designed to protect the residual limb in the immediate postoperative period and are used only for a limited time until edema of the residual limb has decreased and provisional wound healing has occurred.

Rigid Dressings

Plaster or fiberglass rigid dressings are recommended for transtibial and more distal amputations in the lower limb and for transradial and more distal amputations in the upper limb. Rigid dressings are kept in place for 5 to 7 days by a suspension strap[28] (**Figure 10**). A rigid dressing is applied in the operating room by the surgeon or prosthetist, with appropriate padding over the bony prominences. The rigid dressing is removed after 5 to 7 days, and may be replaced if required. At the time of removal, the wound can be evaluated. In a review of the published literature, Smith et al[2] reported that several studies demonstrated that patients treated with plaster cast dressings had substantially quicker rehabilitation times and less edema compared with those treated with soft gauze dressings. The authors also noted that patients treated with prefabricated prostheses had substantially fewer postoperative complications and required fewer revisions to a higher level compared with those treated with soft gauze dressings. A retrospective study by Sumpio et al[28] noted that transtibial amputations managed with a rigid dressing as opposed to a soft dressing had significantly quicker healing times ($P = 0.02$) as measured by the time needed before prosthesis casting. Of 151 patients analyzed, 60 were treated with soft dressings and 91 with rigid dressings. Patients with a soft dressing had a statistically increased prevalence of

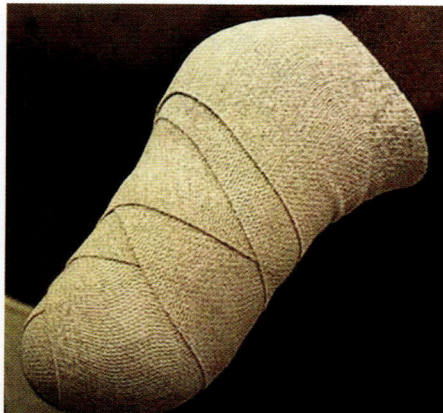

FIGURE 6 Photograph of a residual limb wrapped with a figure-of-8 elastic compressive bandage after a transtibial amputation.

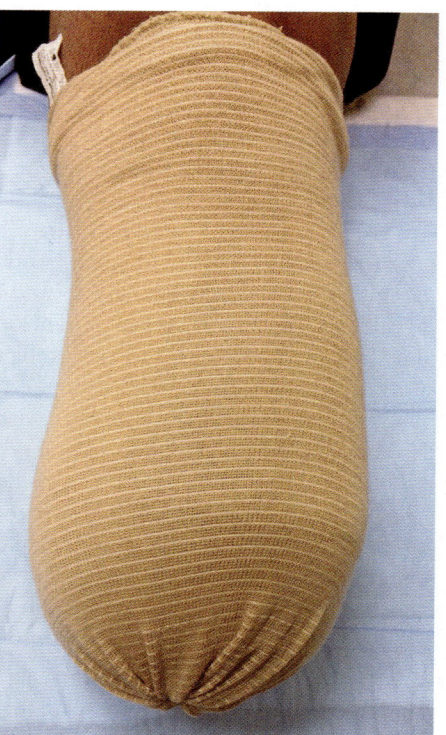

FIGURE 7 Photograph showing a tubular elastic sock rolled over a residual limb after a transtibial amputation.

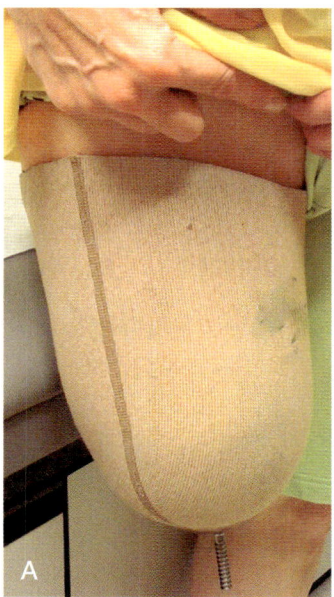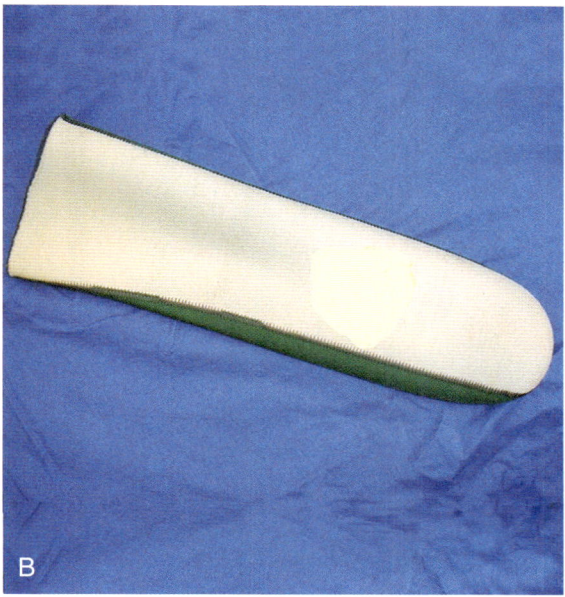

FIGURE 8 Photographs of a thermoplastic liner in place over a transfemoral amputation (**A**) and a tubular liner for a transtibial amputation (**B**).

diabetes mellitus, hypertension, and chronic renal failure compared with the rigid dressing group. The two groups did not show any significant differences with regard to complications caused by infection or cellulitis. Patients with rigid dressings healed in a median time of 76 days compared with 127 days for the group treated with soft dressings. Fifty percent of patients treated with a rigid dressing had an initial casting for a prosthesis within 43 days compared with 75 days for those receiving a soft dressing.

A 2005 study reported an improvement in the time to delivery of the prosthesis when a rigid dressing was used.[19] In comparison with the elastic bandaging method, the use of a rigid dressing resulted in a statistically significant shorter period from amputation to the delivery of the first regular prosthesis (110 days versus 50 days, respectively) and a decreased risk of knee flexion contracture. Other studies have confirmed that rigid dressings are preferable to soft dressings for treating patients with transtibial amputation and result in substantially shorter times from amputation to casting or fitting of a prosthesis.[20,29,30]

Vigier et al[31] noted that rigid dressings helped promote healing in open wounds of residual limbs associated with transtibial amputations for vascular disease, as well as leading to shorter hospital stays. In 2010, Johannesson et al[25] evaluated outcomes using rigid dressings and silicone compression liners in a standardized surgical and rehabilitation program for 217 individuals who had undergone transtibial amputation for peripheral vascular disease. The authors reported a reduction in morbidity in patients treated by a dedicated team using a protocol requiring a rigid dressing for 5 to 7 days postoperatively and subsequent incremental applications of a silicone liner to apply residual limb compression. Prosthetic fitting was achieved in 119 of the patients (55%), and 76 of those patients (64%) achieved good function. Of the 217 patients in the study, 51% had diabetes, more than 75% could walk before amputation, and approximately 50% were living in an elderly care nursing home. The reamputation rate (amputation to a higher level) during the first year was 8.2%.

The use of rigid dressings may be limited by application difficulties and gaining access to the incision. In a 2008 study, Johannesson et al[32] compared the use of a removable vacuum-formed rigid dressing and a conventional rigid plaster of Paris dressing in 27 patients treated with transtibial amputation. The authors found that a vacuum-formed removable rigid dressing appears to achieve results similar to those of a conventional rigid dressing regarding time to prosthetic fitting and a patient's function with a prosthesis.

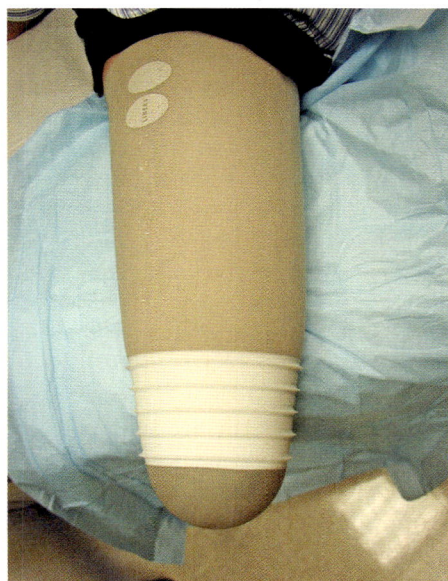

FIGURE 9 Photograph of a transfemoral silicone liner with rings for vacuum suspension.

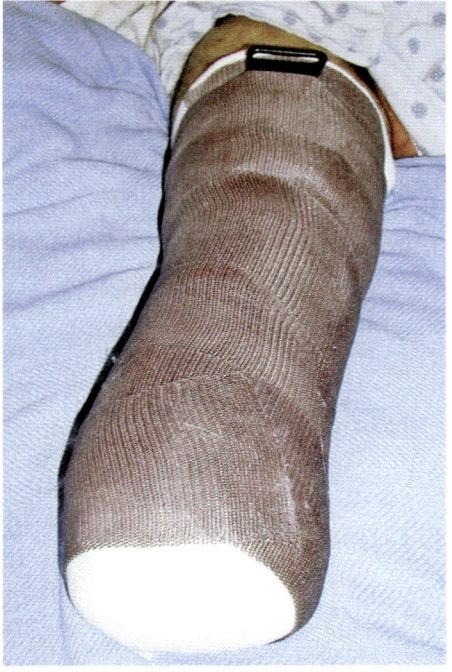

FIGURE 10 Photograph of a rigid dressing with an outer covering of fiberglass on a residual limb after a transtibial amputation. The device for the suspension strap is seen at the anterior brim.

Section 1: General Principles

Removable Rigid Dressings

Removable rigid dressings are most frequently used after transtibial amputations and are easy to apply and use (**Figure 11**). A removable rigid dressing is a transtibial cast that is suspended using an outer layer of stockinette and held by a supracondylar femoral cuff. This technique is an effective method for postoperative, preprosthetic, and prosthetic care of patients who have undergone transtibial amputation.[33] Removable rigid dressings allow additional shrinker socks to be applied as edema in the residual limb decreases.[34] The removable rigid dressing is used for 2 to 3 weeks in preparation for fitting with a preparatory prosthesis.

Commercially available rigid removable dressings can be applied over some version of a compression dressing (**Figure 12**). These devices allow the use of inexpensive readily available gauze and elastic compression under a protective shell that can prevent the development of a knee flexion contracture following transtibial amputation.[35]

A 2005 randomized controlled study of 50 patients with a dysvascular transtibial amputation reported that primary wound healing of the residual limb occurred approximately 2 weeks earlier in patients treated with a removable rigid dressing compared with those treated with a standard soft dressing.[36] Both dressing types were applied immediately postoperatively and were only removed for wound dressing changes. There were no significant differences in the two groups in time to prosthetic fitting, length of hospital stay, incidence of residual limb breakdown, and time needed for volume stabilization of the residual limb. The authors proposed that removable rigid dressings protect the new residual limb from trauma while permitting regular wound access, care, and assessment.

Although upper limb amputations are less frequent than those for the lower limb, removable rigid dressings have a place in the treatment of these patients. The principles of wound care are the same, and timely healing is a major goal.

Immediate Postoperative Prosthetic Limb Fitting

IPOP use has been recommended for mobilizing patients immediately after amputation surgery. A rigid dressing is applied after an incisional dressing has been placed. Adequate padding over bony prominences (such as the fibular head, tibial crest, and patella) is essential, and a pylon and foot are incorporated below the cast[30] (**Figure 13**). A prosthetist should ensure correct alignment of the IPOP, and patient mobilization should be supervised by a therapist. Initially, partial weight bearing is permitted for a few minutes at a time with a gradual increase as the patient is able to cooperate and regain strength. Cast changes are necessary when edema has decreased and there is a volume discrepancy between the residual limb and the cast. For patients to be considered for an IPOP fitting, certain requirements should be met, including preoperative ambulatory status, no evidence of active infection, good motivation, willingness to comply with the required postoperative protocol, and good healing potential.[40] Incision breakdown with the IPOP fitting technique has been noted, and its use has become less popular. One study reported that skin breakdown was higher in the IPOP group of patients than in the non-IPOP group, but the need for revision surgery was lower.[30]

A consensus conference in 2003 demonstrated limited benefits at 6 months with immediate prosthetic limb fitting. This has led to the current approach of early postoperative prosthetic limb fitting that initiates

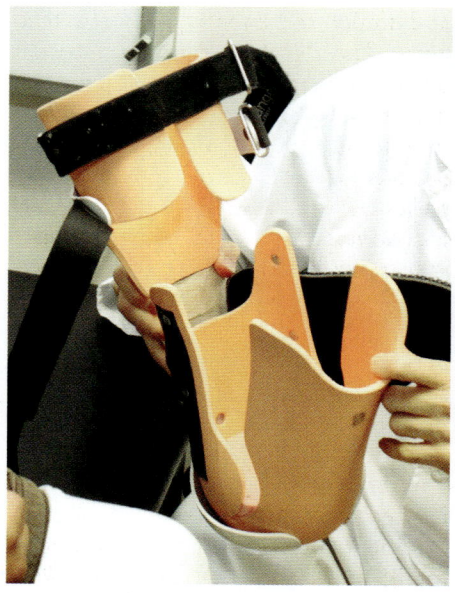

FIGURE 12 Photograph of a prefabricated rigid removable dressing. This dressing can be applied over soft dressings. (Courtesy of John Rheinstein, CP, FAAOP(D), Hanger Clinics, Austin, TX.)

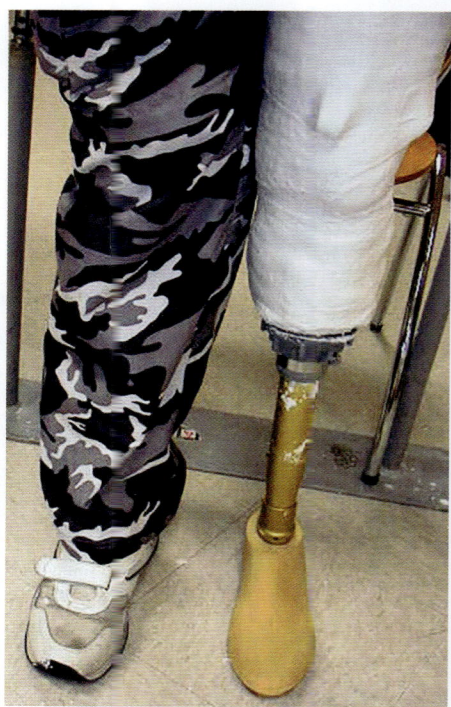

FIGURE 13 Photograph of an immediate postoperative prosthesis made using a plaster cast and prosthetic foot.

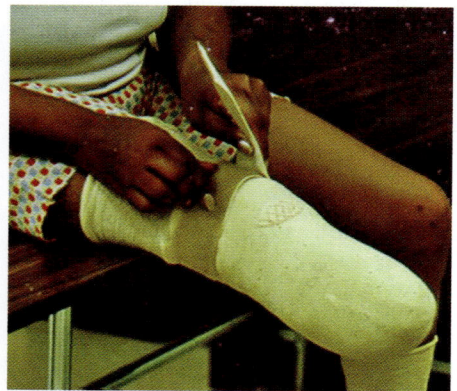

FIGURE 11 Photograph of an individual applying a supracondylar femoral suspension strap over an outer stockinette.

prosthetic limb fitting at 2 to 4 weeks following surgery when the surgical wound appeared to be secure.[2]

Postoperative Pneumatic Systems

The initial popularity and enthusiasm of pneumatic systems seen in the 1980s has substantially declined, and there have been no scientific articles published in the past 10 years regarding their routine use. Pneumatic sleeves are not used in the United States but are used sporadically in the United Kingdom, Europe, and Australia.

In the early 2000s, a pneumatic IPOP system was advocated for the mobilization of lower limb amputees. This prefabricated pneumatic system was applied in the operating room at the time of wound closure.[36] The average time to custom prosthetic limb fitting was 8.1 weeks (range, 4 to 16 weeks). Another study reported on a removable, adjustable, prefabricated IPOP with pneumatic air bladders inflated to 20 to 30 mm Hg.[37] In a study by Schon et al,[38] 19 patients fitted with an IPOP were compared with a retrospective matched control group of 23 patients with soft dressings. Eleven patients in the soft-dressing group required revision procedures, whereas no patients in the IPOP group required surgical revision. The pneumatic systems were used until the wound was healed; a custom prosthesis was then applied at an average of approximately 3 months after the amputation surgery. For a variety of reasons, 11 patients were able to use the temporary device for only 14 days or less; however, this was not considered a failure of the technique.

Although the PPAM aid is not used in the United States, the device is used in select Scottish, Scandinavian, and Australian settings.[39] The PPAM aid helps to reduce residual limb edema; allows reeducation of postural reactions, balance, and gait; and prepares the residual limb for a standard prosthetic socket. It can be placed over a soft dressing, an elastic wrapping, or a plaster cast. It is initially used for a very limited amount of time on a daily basis and under the supervision of a therapist. The PPAM aid is designed for partial weight bearing. With progress, use of the PPAM aid is increased over time to achieve longer weight-bearing periods in the early postoperative period. The PPAM aid is suitable for individuals with knee disarticulations and transtibial and long transfemoral amputations. A disadvantage of the PPAM aid is that it does not allow a patient with a transtibial amputation to flex or extend the knee during walking.[39] An alternative device was developed that allows for knee flexion; however, no functional differences between the two devices were noted.[39]

Pneumatic devices were purported to be superior to rigid cast IPOP because they are lighter in weight, allow for better compression control, and permit easy removal for incision inspection.[2] Despite these early claims, they are infrequently used and have been superseded by modern postoperative amputation dressings.

SUMMARY

Because soft dressings for amputation wounds do not provide adequate protection, the use of dressings that are more compressive and protective is generally recommended. With the advent of improved materials and techniques, rigid and removable rigid dressings are considered superior for the immediate postoperative care of patients with transtibial and transradial amputations. Negative-pressure wound therapy is valuable for the first few days after surgery and is followed by an appropriate alternative dressing. Modern dressings reduce edema, enhance wound healing, and facilitate early mobilization. This allows for accelerated, definitive prosthetic fitting and initiation of gait training. In individuals with an upper limb amputation, postoperative residual limb management is vital to early prosthetic fitting and subsequent daily use of a prosthesis. In the United States, current postoperative residual limb management after amputation involves the use of modern treatment techniques, removable rigid devices, systems for edema control and wound protection, and no or protected weight bearing until incision and wound healing are achieved.

References

1. Sood A, Granick MS, Tomaselli NL: Wound dressings and comparative effectiveness data. *Adv Wound Care (New Rochelle)* 2014;3(8):511-529.
2. Smith DG, McFarland LV, Sangeorzan BJ, Reiber GE, Czerniecki JM: Postoperative dressing and management strategies for transtibial amputations: A critical review. *J Rehabil Res Dev* 2003;40(3):213-224.
3. Barnes R, Souroullas P, Chetter IC: A survey of perioperative management of major lower limb amputations: Current UK practice. *Ann Vasc Surg* 2014;28(7):1737-1743.
4. Kane TJ III, Pollak EW: The rigid versus soft postoperative dressing controversy: A controlled study in vascular below-knee amputees. *Am Surg* 1980;46(4):244-247.
5. Putnis S, Khan WS, Wong JM: Negative pressure wound therapy: A review of its uses in orthopaedic trauma. *Open Orthop J* 2014;8:142-147.
6. Huang C, Leavitt T, Bayer LR, Orgill DP: Effect of negative pressure wound therapy on wound healing. *Curr Probl Surg* 2014;51(7):301-331.
7. Karlakki S, Brem M, Giannini S, Khanduja V, Stannard J, Martin R: Negative pressure wound therapy for management of the surgical incision in orthopaedic surgery: A review of evidence and mechanisms for an emerging indication. *Bone Joint Res* 2013;2(12):276-284.
8. Stannard JP, Gabriel A, Lehner B: Use of negative pressure wound therapy over clean, closed surgical incisions. *Int Wound J* 2012;9(suppl 1):32-39.
9. Stannard JP, Volgas DA, McGwin G III, et al: Incisional negative pressure wound therapy after high-risk lower extremity fractures. *J Orthop Trauma* 2012;26(1):37-42.
10. Hansen E, Durinka JB, Costanzo JA, Austin MS, Deirmengian GK: Negative pressure wound therapy is associated with resolution of incisional drainage in most wounds after hip arthroplasty. *Clin Orthop Relat Res* 2013;471(10):3230-3236.
11. Brem MH, Bail HJ, Biber R: Value of incisional negative pressure wound therapy in orthopaedic surgery. *Int Wound J* 2014;11(suppl 1):3-5.

12. Sumpio BJ, Cordova AD, Mahler D, Sumpio BE: Use of negative pressure wound therapy in healing below knee amputation in patients with chronic venous insufficiency and/or Charcot disease. *Angiol Open Access* 2013;1(2):1-3.

13. Stannard JP, Volgas DA, Stewart R, McGwin G Jr, Alonso JE: Negative pressure wound therapy after severe open fractures: A prospective randomized study. *J Orthop Trauma* 2009;23(8):552-557.

14. Guyver PM, Mountain AJ, Jeffery SL: Application of topical negative pressure for traumatic amputations. *Ann R Coll Surg Engl* 2013;95(3):226-227.

15. Penn-Barwell JG, Fries CA, Street L, Jeffery S: Use of topical negative pressure in British servicemen with combat wounds. *Eplasty* 2011;11:e35.

16. Barnea Y, Weiss J, Gur E: A review of the applications of the hydrofiber dressing with silver (Aquacel Ag) in wound care. *Ther Clin Risk Manag* 2010;6:21-27.

17. Cutting K, White R, Hoekstra H: Topical silver-impregnated dressings and the importance of the dressing technology. *Int Wound J* 2009;6(5):396-402.

18. Foster L, Moore P, Clark S: A comparison of hydrofibre and alginate dressings on open acute surgical wounds. *J Wound Care* 2000;9(9):442-445.

19. van Velzen AD, Nederhand MJ, Emmelot CH, Ijzerman MJ: Early treatment of trans-tibial amputees: Retrospective analysis of early fitting and elastic bandaging. *Prosthet Orthot Int* 2005;29(1):3-12.

20. Alsancak S, Köse SK, Altınkaynak H: Effect of elastic bandaging and prosthesis on the decrease in stump volume. *Acta Orthop Traumatol Turc* 2011;45(1):14-22.

21. Punziano A, Martelli S, Sotgiu V, et al: The effectiveness of the elastic bandage in reducing residual limb volume in patients with lower limb amputation: Literature review [Italian]. *Assist Inferm Ric* 2011;30(4):208-214.

22. Nawijn SE, van der Linde H, Emmelot CH, Hofstad CJ: Stump management after trans-tibial amputation: A systematic review. *Prosthet Orthot Int* 2005;29(1):13-26.

23. Manella KJ: Comparing the effectiveness of elastic bandages and shrinker socks for lower extremity amputees. *Phys Ther* 1981;61(3):334-337.

24. Graf M, Freijah N: Early transtibial oedema control using polymer gel socks. *Prosthet Orthot Int* 2003;27(3):221-226.

25. Johannesson A, Larsson GU, Ramstrand N, Lauge-Pedersen H, Wagner P, Atroshi I: Outcomes of a standardized surgical and rehabilitation program in transtibial amputation for peripheral vascular disease: A prospective cohort study. *Am J Phys Med Rehabil* 2010;89(4):293-303.

26. MacLean N, Fick GH: The effect of semirigid dressings on below-knee amputations. *Phys Ther* 1994;74(7):668-673.

27. Wong CK, Edelstein JE: Unna and elastic postoperative dressings: Comparison of their effects on function of adults with amputation and vascular disease. *Arch Phys Med Rehabil* 2000;81(9):1191-1198.

28. Sumpio B, Shine SR, Mahler D, Sumpio BE: A comparison of immediate postoperative rigid and soft dressings for below-knee amputations. *Ann Vasc Surg* 2013;27(6):774-780.

29. Churilov I, Churilov L, Murphy D: Do rigid dressings reduce the time from amputation to prosthetic fitting? A systematic review and meta-analysis. *Ann Vasc Surg* 2014;28(7):1801-1808.

30. Ali MM, Loretz L, Shea A, et al: A contemporary comparative analysis of immediate postoperative prosthesis placement following below-knee amputation. *Ann Vasc Surg* 2013;27(8):1146-1153.

31. Vigier S, Casillas JM, Dulieu V, Rouhier-Marcer I, D'Athis P, Didier JP: Healing of open stump wounds after vascular below-knee amputation: Plaster cast socket with silicone sleeve versus elastic compression. *Arch Phys Med Rehabil* 1999;80(10):1327-1330.

32. Johannesson A, Larsson GU, Öberg T, Atroshi I: Comparison of vacuum-formed removable rigid dressing with conventional rigid dressing after transtibial amputation: Similar outcome in a randomized controlled trial involving 27 patients. *Acta Orthop* 2008;79(3):361-369.

33. Taylor L, Cavenett S, Stepien JM, Crotty M: Removable rigid dressings: A retrospective case-note audit to determine the validity of post-amputation application. *Prosthet Orthot Int* 2008;32(2):223-230.

34. Wu Y, Keagy RD, Krick HJ, Stratigos JS, Betts HB: An innovative removable rigid dressing technique for below-the-knee amputation. *J Bone Joint Surg Am* 1979;61(5):724-729.

35. Reichman JP, Stevens PM, Rheinstein J, Kreulen CD: Removable rigid dressings for postoperative management of transtibial amputations: A review of Published Evidence. *PM R* 2018;10(5):516-523.

36. Deutsch A, English RD, Vermeer TC, Murray PS, Condous M: Removable rigid dressings versus soft dressings: A randomized, controlled study with dysvascular, trans-tibial amputees. *Prosthet Orthot Int* 2005;29(2):193-200.

37. Pinzur MS, Angelico J: A feasibility trial of a prefabricated immediate postoperative prosthetic limb system. *Foot Ankle Int* 2003;24(11):861-864.

38. Schon LC, Short KW, Soupiou O, Noll K, Rheinstein J: Benefits of early prosthetic management of transtibial amputees: A prospective clinical study of a prefabricated prosthesis. *Foot Ankle Int* 2002;23(6):509-514.

39. Scott H, Condie ME, Treweek SP, Sockalingam S: An evaluation of the Amputee Mobility Aid (AMA) early walking aid. *Prosthet Orthot Int* 2000;24(1):39-46.

General Principles of Limb Salvage Versus Amputation in Adults

CHAPTER 3

Christopher Bibbo, DO, DPM, FAAOS, FACS, FACFAS •
David J. Polga, MD, FAAOS • Samir Mehta, MD, FAAOS •
Stephen J. Kovach III, MD, FACS

ABSTRACT

The decision to attempt limb salvage of an injured or diseased limb requires good clinical judgment, knowledge of the pathologic process that put the limb in jeopardy, and an understanding of the social and psychological profile of the patient. Each patient must be treated as an individual, based on current medical and physiologic status. The functional potential of a salvaged limb must be evaluated. Retention of a painful limb that is not used by the patient is to be avoided. However, retention of a limb that may be used to assist even with wheelchair locomotion deserves an attempt at salvage. A nonpainful limb, even with minimal function, may be of significant psychological value to the patient. A few of the factors that require consideration are the patient's premorbid conditions, psychosocial factors, desires and expectation, social support network, and accessibility to reconstruction services. Knowledge of the general principles of limb salvage versus amputation will aid in providing optimal treatment for these patients.

Keywords: amputation; extremity; flaps; limb salvage; trauma

Introduction

A limb (primarily a lower limb) that is at risk for amputation and being considered for salvage may be simplistically categorized to primarily possess a vascular, infectious, tumorous, or trauma-related etiology. In reality, however, these categories often overlap, increasing the degree of difficulty to achieve limb salvage; unfortunately, difficulties in healing and recovery after an amputation can escalate concurrently.

The general principles of limb salvage versus amputation in adults mandate that the first consideration is always life over limb. Dire circumstances are most commonly encountered in patients with serious infections or multiple traumatic injuries. If limb salvage is contemplated, the surgical team must weigh whether the treatment required for salvage is worse than the condition or the disease state. For example, if salvage of a limb with extensive tibial osteomyelitis is being considered in a patient who is frail, elderly, and has diabetes, the possibility of organ failure, irreversible functional decline, and a stiff nonfunctional limb may indicate amputation as the prudent option. The adage "burn no bridges" is especially important for the at-risk limb. Any procedure must be executed with deference to subsequent surgical interventions: how step one will affect steps two, three, and so forth. An essential component to the overall treatment strategy is that backup management plans must be in place in the event of a change in the patient's condition.

The principles of limb salvage versus amputation in adults—whether in acute, chronic, or staged settings—mandate the assessment of several key issues that immediately and secondarily surround the patient's symptoms, including the patient's physiologic reserve and medical comorbidities; arterial, venous, and lymphatic patency (vascular status); neurologic and psychological/psychiatric statuses;

Dr. Mehta or an immediate family member is a member of a speakers' bureau or has made paid presentations on behalf of Bioventus, DePuy, a Johnson & Johnson Company, and Smith & Nephew; serves as a paid consultant to or is an employee of Smith & Nephew and Synthes; has received research or institutional support from Becton-Dickinson and Synthes; and serves as a board member, owner, officer, or committee member of the AO Foundation and the Orthopaedic Trauma Association. Dr. Kovach or an immediate family member is a member of a speakers' bureau or has made paid presentations on behalf of Becton Dickinson, Integra LifeSciences, and WL Gore. Neither of the following authors nor any immediate family member has received anything of value from or has stock or stock options held in a commercial company or institution related directly or indirectly to the subject of this chapter: Dr. Bibbo and Dr. Polga.

functional potential and quality of life; surgical site considerations and surgical procedures available from the surgical team or teams; and the availability of multidisciplinary resource teams during the immediate perioperative and rehabilitative phases of treatment. The key assessments in all patients are physiologic reserve, medical comorbidities, and vascular status.

Physiologic Reserve and Medical Comorbidities

A patient must have adequate physiologic reserve to withstand limb salvage. Moreover, all correctable organ system pathologies (eg, renal, endocrine, cardiac, and hepatic) must be addressed to maximize healing of both limb salvage and amputation procedures. The most commonly encountered conditions are acute metabolic and cardiac issues resulting from the circumstances of acute settings, as well as age-related conditions. A patient's nutritional health and immune competence also must be evaluated to improve healing and help prevent complications caused by infection[1,2] (Table 1). These parameters should be identified, with appropriate management strategies initiated immediately. However, because timing often is critical in limb salvage procedures and amputations, complete correction of immune and nutritional deficits often is not feasible; correction must simply be initiated and continued throughout the perioperative period and through hospital discharge.

Vascular Status

The principles of evaluating and managing peripheral vascular disease are particularly important because adequate vascularity is a critical factor when deciding on limb salvage or amputation. Adequate arterial inflow is mandatory for all patients undergoing limb salvage, whether in the setting of infection, trauma, the immediate coverage of defects after tumor resection (Figure 1), or complications from external beam radiation. Patients with peripheral vascular disease often are elderly, have diabetes, and/or are smokers and may have preexisting cardiac disease. Thus, these patients have important risk factors for perioperative complications. These risk factors must be evaluated (eg, cardiac stress testing), and the patient's health status should be maximized (eg, catheterization, control of hypertension, and diabetes). Venous outflow also may be diminished in these patients, so adequate planning must be undertaken if limb salvage is planned (eg, saphenous mapping for an arterial-venous loop to provide a vascular axis for a free flap). Peripheral vascular disease typically is progressive, and multiple peripheral vascular revisions may be required. The use of limb salvage in this setting may be guided by the surgeon's experience, direct input from the patient, and a global assessment of quality of life if multiple major revisions are required.

Considerations for Limb Salvage or Amputation

Peripheral Vascular Arterial Disease

Adequate arterial blood supply to the tissues is necessary for normal tissue metabolism and healing, and arterial inflow must be adequate before limb salvage or amputation can be considered. The less complex Fontaine classification and the more inclusive Rutherford classification of peripheral vascular arterial disease are useful screening tools that use patient symptoms and objective measures (arterial pressures) to allow stratification of patients with preexisting peripheral vascular arterial disease (Table 2).

Newer classification schemes for predicting outcomes have been presented and are being validated.[3] However, the most basic and often simplest methods to help determine successful healing after limb salvage or amputation are still the direct physical examination and an arterial evaluation. Arterial assessment includes both noninvasive and invasive evaluations. Physical examination of pulses along with a bedside Doppler examination are quick and easy initial examinations. Arteriography, computer-assisted arteriography, and magnetic resonance arteriography are evaluation tools to better assess and plan the technical execution of a surgical procedure and have their relative merits (Table 3). Transcutaneous oxygen measurements are supplemental and of greater use in the noninvasive evaluation of chronic wound healing potential. Such measurement provides information pertaining to a site-specific area but has limitations when edema is present and is highly operator dependent; its greatest utility is when amputation is selected and data on healing potential are desired at a certain level of amputation. All of these evaluations, however,

TABLE 1 Laboratory Evaluation of Immune and Nutritional Parameters to Help Predict Healing Response to Injury and Surgery

Laboratory Value	Commonly Accepted Normal Range or Threshold	Comments
Prealbumin	Severe risk: <10 mg/dL Moderate risk: 10-17 mg/dL	Overall protein-energy malnutrition; one of the most rapidly changing nutritional parameters to follow in the acute setting.
Albumin	3.5-5.5 g/dL	Overall protein-energy malnutrition; acute trends indicate improvements in nutrition.
Total protein	5.5-8.0 g/dL	Global protein-energy nutrition status of the patient.
Total lymphocyte count	Malnutrition: <1,500 cells/mm^3	Protein-energy malnutrition and immune status; low values are considered ominous for healing complications that may not be able to be treated acutely.
Total cholesterol	Severe risk: <50 mg/dL At risk: <150 mg/dL	Overall caloric malnutrition; very low values indicate severe malnutrition, which requires intensive nutritional supplementation; at risk for mortality.

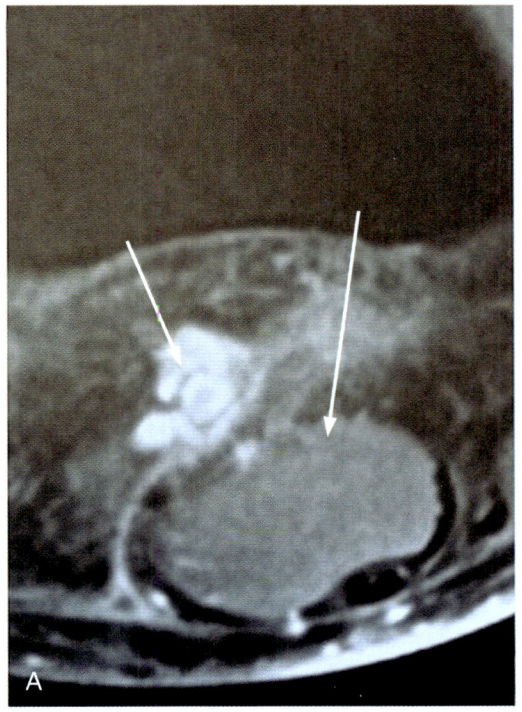 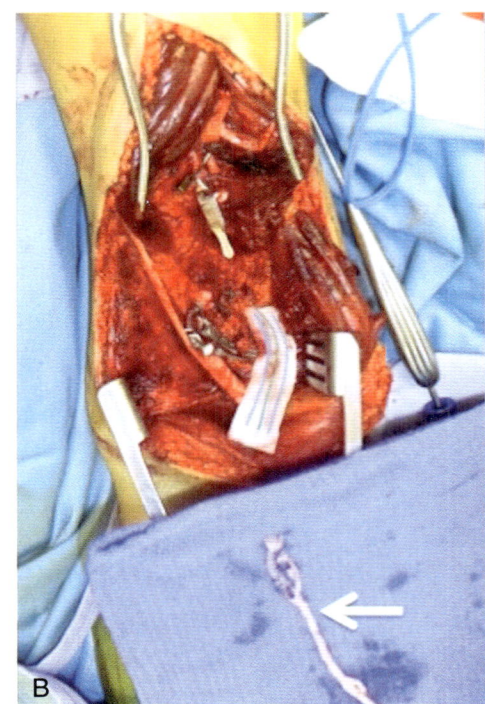 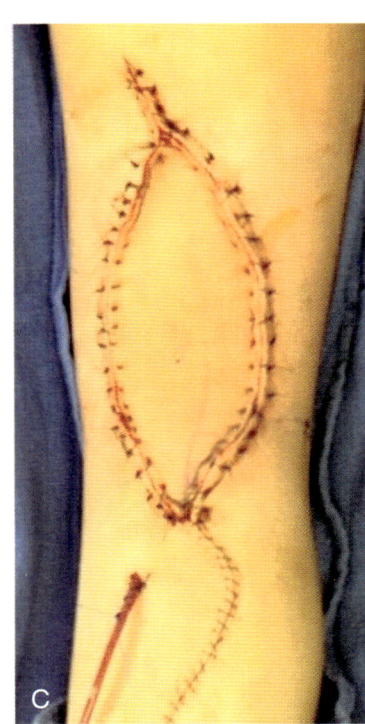

FIGURE 1 **A**, Magnetic resonance image of a popliteal fossa tumor (long arrow) involving the popliteal vessels (short arrow). **B**, Intraoperative photograph of the defect after tumor and vessel resection: clamps are on the arterial residuums, and a saphenous vein graft (arrow) will be used. **C**, Photograph of the final reconstruction for limb salvage that used reversed saphenous vein for arterial and venous reconstruction, sural nerve grafts for motor nerve reconstruction, and anterolateral thigh free flap for coverage of the soft-tissue defect. (Courtesy of Stephen J. Kovach III, MD, Philadelphia, PA.)

TABLE 2 Classifications of Peripheral Vascular Arterial Disease

Fontaine Classification		Rutherford Classification		
Stage	**Clinical Findings**	**Grade**	**Category**	**Clinical Findings**
I	Asymptomatic	0	0	Asymptomatic
IIa	Mild claudication	I	1	Mild claudication
IIb	Moderate to severe claudication		2	Moderate claudication
III	Ischemic rest pain		3	Severe claudication
IV	Ulcer/gangrene	II	4	Ischemic rest pain
		III	5	Minor tissue loss
			6	Major tissue loss

TABLE 3 Tools for Arterial Evaluation

	Doppler Examination	CTA	MRA	Arteriography
Indication	Evaluation of flow beyond pulse palpation.	Evaluation of arterial inflow when Doppler examination is limited or preoperative planning requires investigation of arterial lumen.	Same as CTA.	Same as CTA and when percutaneous interventions are being considered.
Utility	Easily performed by clinician at bedside with simple handheld Doppler device to determine phasicity of arterial flow and augmentation of flow by checking retrograde filling of the arterial tree. Advanced color flow and velocity gradients can identify occult intimal lesions.	Evaluation of major arterial network to determine patency of vessels for preoperative planning; especially useful in patients not suited for MRI. Easier to interpret than MRA.	Same as CTA; longer time for image acquisition and more difficult in extremity arterial evaluation.	Fine details and runoff (operator dependent). To enhance healing, stenting with or without mechanical ablation of lesions can be performed to maximize flow velocity across stenotic areas before limb salvage or amputation.

CTA = computer-assisted arteriography, MRA = magnetic resonance arteriography

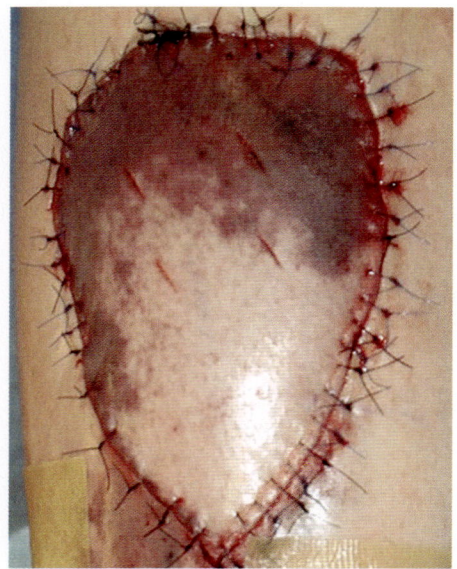

FIGURE 2 Postoperative photograph of partial flap necrosis secondary to poor venous outflow. (Courtesy of Christopher Bibbo, DO, FAAOS, FACS, Baltimore, MD. All rights reserved.)

must be tempered with experience and sound clinical judgment.

Venous outflow is important to control chronic tissue changes as well as the health of tissues in the immediate perioperative period of limb salvage (eg, free tissue transfers) (**Figure 2**). Surrogate methods to improve venous return and reduce edema, such as intermittent gradient compression devices, frequent medical wraps (eg, calamine/ gelatin paste dressings), and compression stockings, are vital to improving venous return and preventing chronic adverse tissue changes. In the immediate postoperative period of limb salvage (after free-tissue transfers to maintain an amputation level or salvage an entire limb), mild elevation, adequate pharmacologic anticoagulation, and dangling protocols assist in preventing venous occlusion, which, if severe, can result in microanastomotic arterial thrombosis.

Limb edema often is caused by multiple factors, including venous insufficiency, reperfusion overload, and cardiac, renal, and primary/secondary lymphatic insufficiency. The effects of chronic edema resulting from any of the primary causes can be compounded by a secondary etiology as well as poor nutrition (low serum albumin/protein level, resulting in low serum oncotic pressure). Regardless of the cause, edema is believed to result in a relative reduction of local tissue oxygen perfusion, thus potentiating poor healing. Edema may delay wound healing or result in tissue ulceration.[4] In most patients, temporary control of edema can be obtained during tissue healing; however, in certain patients (eg, those with Milroy disease, those treated with radiation, or patients who have undergone lymph node dissection), edema in the lower limb may impede successful limb salvage.

Patients who have undergone a mastectomy or axillary dissection may have chronic edema in the upper limbs. Primary lymphatic patency should be investigated in the setting of massive refractory edema that is uncontrolled by medical maximization and standard control methods, such as manual edema control programs, edema pumps, and garments. Preoperative investigations include dye-based and scintigraphic lymphangiograms. Although in its infancy, vascularized lymph node transfer may be helpful in controlling massive edema in patients with refractory edema that impedes healing after limb salvage or amputation.[5]

Nerve Injury and Psychological and Psychiatric Conditions

Acute nerve injury is most likely to occur in patients as the result of a traumatic injury or in those with musculoskeletal tumors as a result of the oncologic resection. Acute nerve injury is not a reliable predictor of success or failure of either limb salvage or amputation.[6] In general, nerve transections are amenable to direct grouped fascicular repair. The recovery of nerve injuries is expected at a rate of 1 mm/day. Nerve injuries that pose special problems in patients with trauma are segmental nerve loss (**Figure 3**) and severe brachial plexopathies with nerve

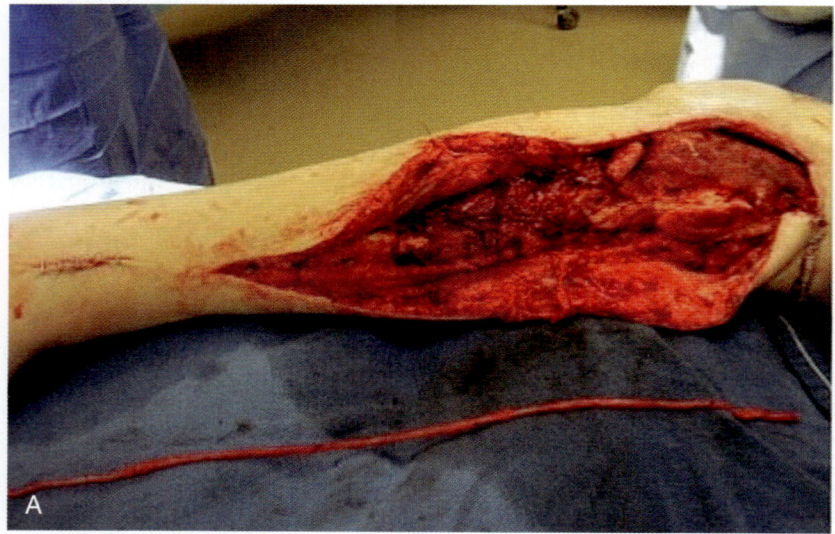
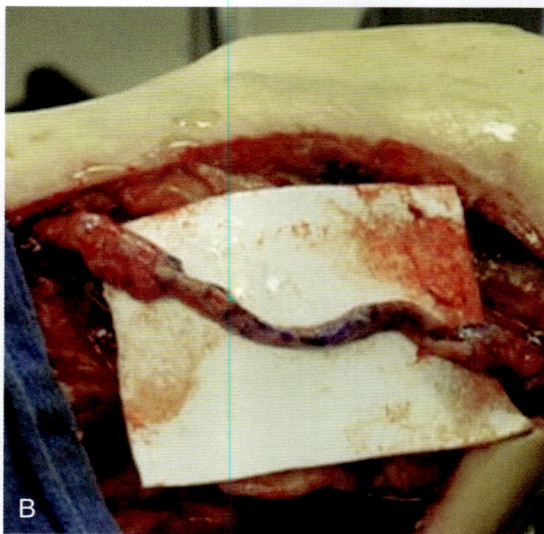

FIGURE 3 Intraoperative photographs of a full-length sural nerve graft (**A**), which was divided into three cables for grouped fascicular repair (**B**) in a patient with traumatic segmental loss of the common peroneal nerve after an open knee dislocation. (Courtesy of Christopher Bibbo, DO, FAAOS, FACS, Baltimore, MD. All rights reserved.)

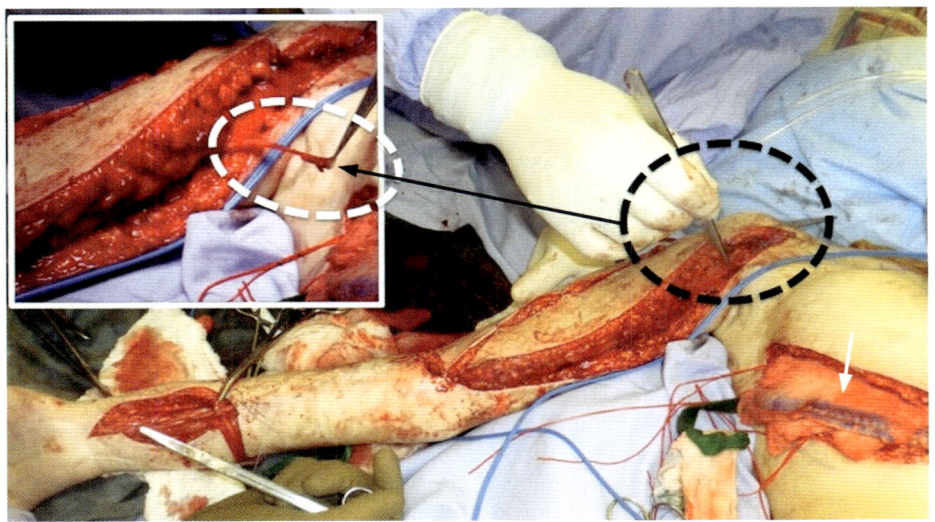

FIGURE 4 Intraoperative photograph of arm reconstruction with a functional gracilis free-tissue flap. Motor branch to gracilis muscle (inset, white dashed circle) is anastomosed to the proximal musculocutaneous nerve using subcostal nerve grafts (white arrow). Arterial and venous vessels are microanastomosed to branches of the brachial vessels. (Courtesy of L. Scott Levin, MD, FAAOS, FACS, Philadelphia, PA.)

root avulsion. Nerve transfer and grafting techniques are available that will produce good functional results in the upper limb.[6]

The loss of nerve segments in a mutilated lower limb is problematic. These cases require specialized techniques, including free vascularized nerve transfers, in situ nerve transfers, and muscle and tendon transfers or tenodesis. In a patient being treated with a limb salvage protocol in whom vascular, bony, and soft-tissue issues have been successfully managed or who has a limb with only an isolated nerve injury, strong consideration should be given to the continuation of limb salvage efforts. This is especially true if some motor function is anticipated. Pure sensory deficits in a lower limb in an otherwise supple limb are not necessarily indications for amputation. Appropriate bracing and skin protection measures may allow the limb to assist in functional ambulation. Salvage should be given even greater consideration in an upper limb because of the devastating nature of upper limb amputations, especially if a lower limb amputation is already present.

The treatment of a patient with a limb with isolated, long-segment nerve loss can be managed with grouped fascicular nerve grafting accompanied by a long recovery period; however, there is the potential for irreversible muscle wasting. In patients with nerve loss accompanied by composite tissue loss (nerve plus bone, muscle, and skin) or late loss of function, free functional muscle transfers have become a valuable tool for accomplishing limb salvage[7-16] (**Figure 4**). Newer techniques of nerve free flaps may be considered in both the lower and upper extremity (**Figure 5**).

Patients with chronic pain syndrome (type I or II) who experience trauma or massive infection require special consideration. In these patients, the limb may have substantial tissue changes and limited function before the traumatic injury or the onset of infection. In addition to the physical state of the limb, these patients frequently have substantial psychological disability that manifests as anxiety or depressive disorders, including posttraumatic stress disorder (axis I disorder), which may be compounded by their current traumatic injury (axis III disorder).[17] These patients should undergo a thorough neuropsychiatric evaluation as part of the global salvage versus amputation evaluation. The patient's psychological and psychiatric profile weighs heavily into the equation that determines functional recovery and overall quality of life. In up to 50% of patients with type I chronic pain syndrome, pain will worsen with amputation;[18] nevertheless, the patient may elect amputation after thorough counseling (**Figure 6**). Limb salvage procedures can also result in substantial additional physiologic stress for these patients, deterioration of their mental health status, and worsening of their pain syndrome. However, appropriate multidisciplinary counseling, careful planning, and realistic expectations

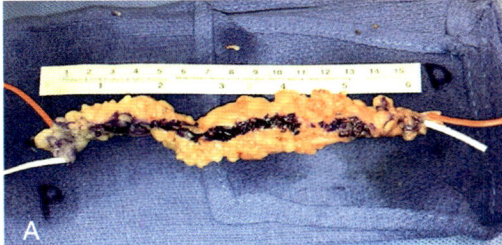

FIGURE 5 Images of nerve free flap. Intraoperative photograph of an arterialized (reverse flow) saphenous vein and nerve free flap for reconstruction of a long segment of both the dorsalis pedis artery and deep peroneal nerve after resection of aggressive tumor. **A**, Harvested free flap (P = proximal margin, D = distal margin). **B**, Free flap in situ (white arrow). (Courtesy of Christopher Bibbo, DO, FAAOS, FACS, Baltimore, MD. All rights reserved.)

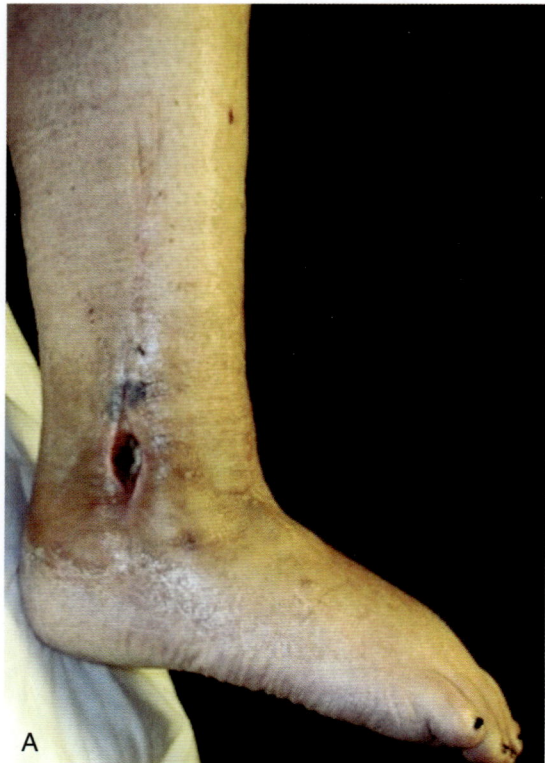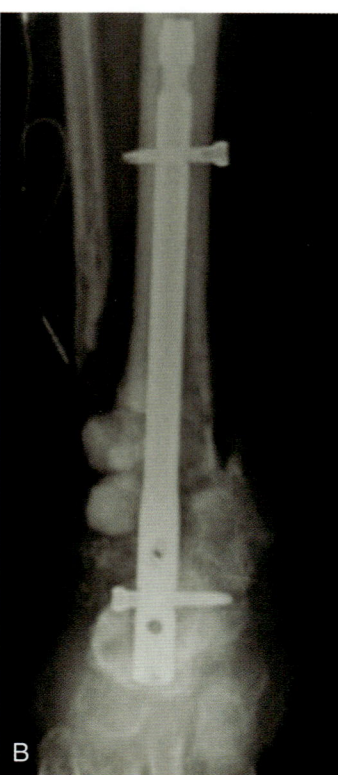

FIGURE 6 Clinical photograph (**A**) and AP radiograph (**B**) of the infected lower limb of a 38-year-old patient with type I chronic pain syndrome who smokes and had five surgeries for polymicrobial drug-resistant osteomyelitis (staged as Cierny-Mader type B-IV). The patient elected transtibial amputation. (Courtesy of Christopher Bibbo, DO, FAAOS, FACS, Baltimore, MD. All rights reserved.)

can achieve reasonable outcomes after limb salvage.

Unique considerations also apply to patients who sustain complete spinal cord injuries or severe closed head injuries. In patients with paraplegia, the level of injury, overall limb function, and the care setting are critical in determining whether to proceed with limb salvage or amputation. For example, if the patient has the potential to use a standing aid, or the limbs assist with sitting and balance, salvage should be considered. Limb salvage of an upper limb is warranted in patients with paraplegia because the upper limb often is the patient's last resource for independent function. Patients with paraplegia or quadriplegia with an at-risk limb require thorough evaluation. If the limb is a liability to the patient's near-term overall health or survival, amputation may be the best option (**Figure 7**). Patients with closed head injuries and an expected poor recovery must be evaluated and treated in the acute setting (life over limb), but the long-term sequelae of their brain injuries, including useful functional status, must be considered.

Patients with progressive neurologic conditions who have little chance of having a functional or useful limb require a preemptive psychological and psychiatric evaluation along with a global assessment of future quality of life, with or without the limb. The surgeon must remember that all patients value an intact body image, which directly affects mental health and global quality of life. Thus, the value of a psychological and psychiatric evaluation and an open dialogue with the surgical team, which concentrates on realistic goals, outcomes, and patient desires, are vitally important. In situations in which limb preservation or amputation is required to preserve life, the surgical team may have to make a decision without input from the patient.

Functional Potential and Quality of Life

The assessment of future limb function is made by the treating orthopaedic surgeon in conjunction with input from the physical medicine and rehabilitation teams. Typically, motor function and patient motivation are the key factors in achieving optimal function and quality of life. The patient's perception of their future quality of life may be strongly influenced by the surgical team leader's expertise and experience; therefore, it is important that the surgeon provide an unbiased assessment of the pros and cons of limb salvage and amputation.

Multidisciplinary Resources

Complex limb salvage or major amputation surgery requires a comprehensive, sophisticated set of surgical services, including trauma, oncologic, orthopaedic, plastic reconstructive, and vascular disciplines. Ancillary services, including physical medicine rehabilitation, prosthetics and orthotics, physical and occupational therapy, psychology, psychiatry, and discharge planning also should be available to aid the patient throughout their hospitalization and during the rehabilitation phases of recovery.

Infection in an Adult

The need to consider limb salvage in the setting of musculoskeletal infections is common. Severe necrotizing infections may occur in otherwise healthy patients, but patients who are immunocompromised are more likely to have an at-risk limb and systemic sepsis. In addition, these patients often have diabetes and poor glucose control. Other at-risk subgroups include patients with pharmacologic immune suppression, such as those who have had a solid organ transplant and are steroid dependent; those receiving tumor necrosis factor suppression and interleukin-6 suppression for conditions such as rheumatoid arthritis or Crohn disease; and patients with cancer. Infection control is essential because continued infection results in tissue death and local and regional arterial and venous

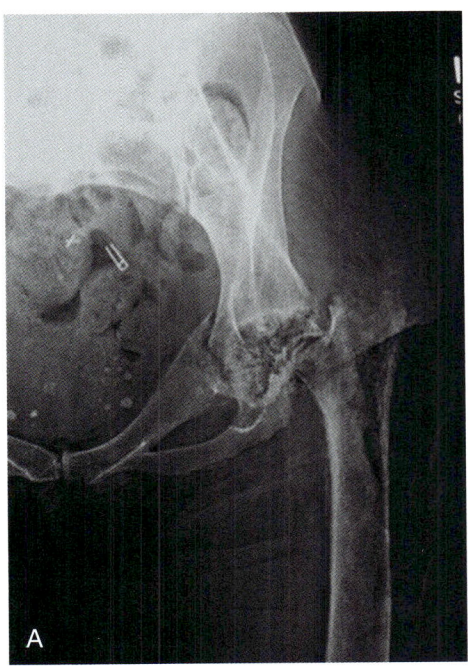
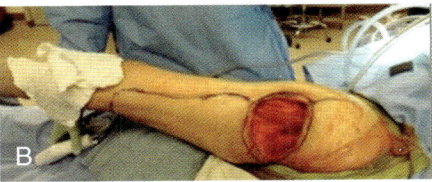
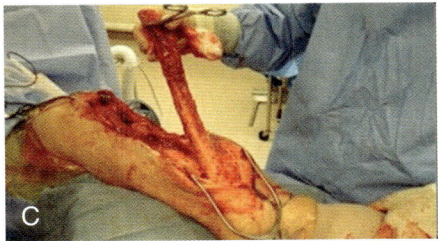
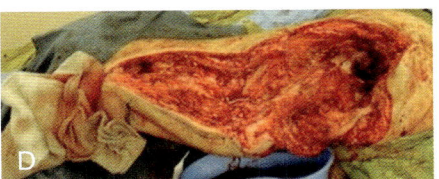
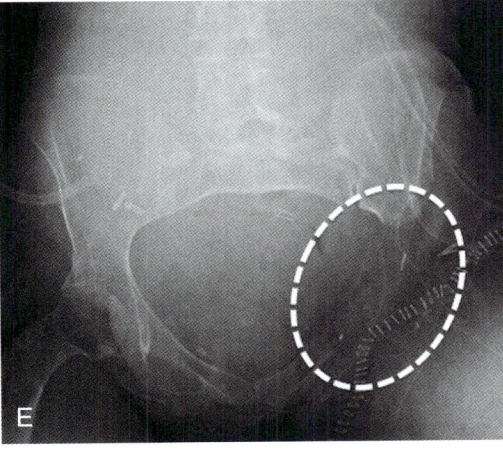
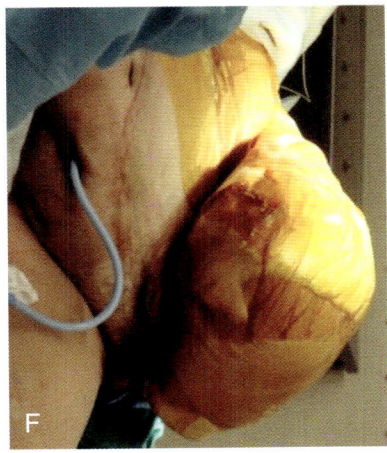
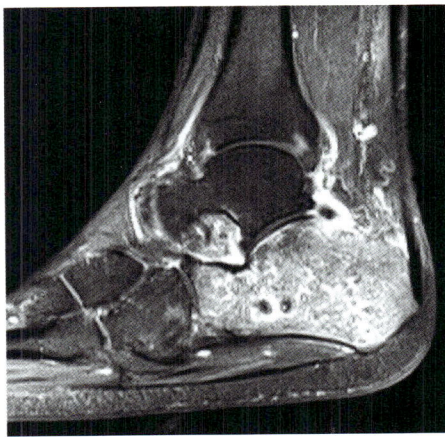

FIGURE 8 Magnetic resonance image of a massive calcaneal blastomycosis, with concomitant involvement of the spleen, liver, and skin, in an immunocompromised patient. A staged reconstruction of the calcaneus using multiple débridements, fluconazole/voriconazole antifungal beads, and massive autologous bone grafting resulted in salvage of the patient's foot. (Courtesy of Christopher Bibbo, DO, FAAOS, FACS, Baltimore, MD. All rights reserved.)

FIGURE 7 A, Pelvic radiograph from a patient with septic T5-level paraplegia with massive recurrent decubitus ulcers (after failure of previous rotation flaps), diffuse osteomyelitis, pathologic fracture of the hip and acetabulum, and fixed ankle and knee flexion deformity. Intraoperative photographs show the massive decubitus ulcer that extended to the hip joint and pathologic fracture (**B**), enucleation of the infected femur (**C**), and creation of the thigh fillet flap (**D**). **E**, Final AP radiograph of the internal hemipelvectomy resection and creation of the pelvic sling with biologic mesh (dashed circle). **F**, Final intraoperative photograph of the pelvic resection margins and inset thigh fillet flap. The flap is made slightly large to re-create the silhouette of a limb, as well as provide redundant tissue for possible future needs. (Courtesy of Christopher Bibbo, DO, FAAOS, FACS, Baltimore, MD. All rights reserved.)

thrombosis, which perpetuate the process of tissue necrosis.

Bacterial infections remain the most common type of infections, whether the primary source is the integument or muscle.[19] Direct extension of the infection into other tissues can be rapid, especially in necrotizing infections. The immediate goals of limb salvage are to halt further spread of the infection (thus limiting systemic toxicity and the amount of local tissue destruction) and preservation of the integrity of the major and secondary vessels of the limb.

Fungal infections are suspect for underlying immune suppression and may involve soft tissue and bone and disseminate to internal organs. Fungal infections in patients who are immunocompromised may be extremely difficult to eradicate and often have high morbidity and mortality rates, necessitating consideration of amputation. However, if the patient has adequate physiologic reserve to tolerate multiple wide débridements and long-term antifungal therapy and the potential for use of a functionally salvageable limb, then attempts at limb salvage are warranted (**Figures 8** and **9**).

When acute or chronic osteomyelitis is present, thorough débridement is needed. The patient's comorbidities and the extent of the osseous infection are critical factors when undertaking limb salvage for osteomyelitis. The Cierny-Mader classification for chronic adult osteomyelitis (**Table 4**) provides categoric descriptive items that should be considered; however, this tool cannot dictate treatment plans. The key assessments as outlined in this chapter also must be examined. Evaluation tools for osteomyelitis include plain radiographs and indium-111/technetium dual-window scans with spot CT and MRI.

The most reliable method for the diagnosis of osteomyelitis is the

Section 1: General Principles

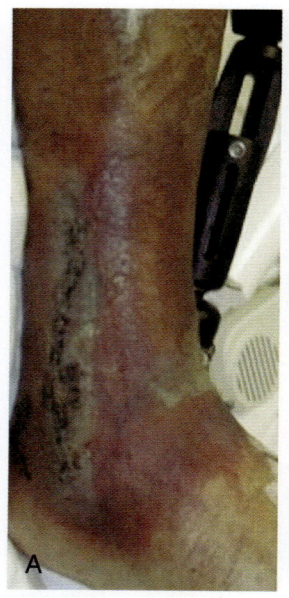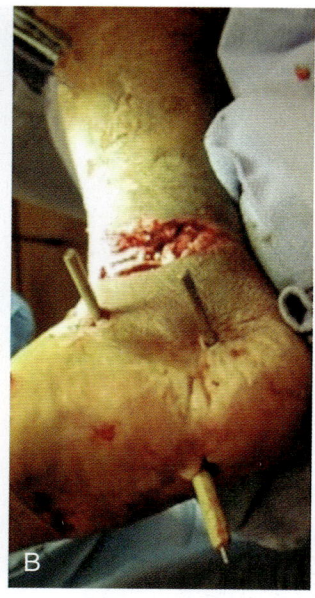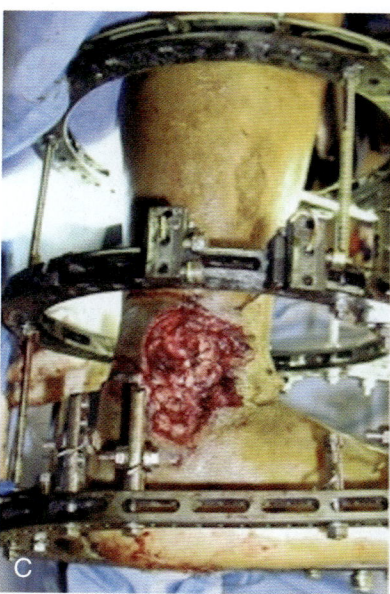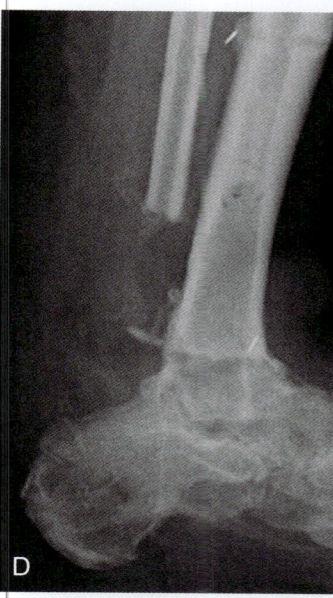

FIGURE 9 Images of an extensive mucormycosis infection developed in the lower limb of a patient with type 1 diabetes after an open ankle fracture. **A**, Preoperative photograph of the limb. Purpuric skin discoloration may be seen in mucormycosis infections along with dark discoloration of the deep soft tissues. Intraoperative photographs of the limb salvage procedure that included multiple débridements and an amphotericin rod and beads, parenteral liposomal amphotericin, wide resection of the involved skin and bone, followed by a peroneus brevis flap (**B**) and use of a fine-wire frame (**C**). **D**, Final radiograph showing successful limb salvage with tibiotalar fusion. (Courtesy of Christopher Bibbo, DO, FAAOS, FACS, Baltimore, MD. All rights reserved.)

analysis of deep bone cultures surgically obtained from a patient who has not been given antibiotics for 5 to 7 days before the specimen is obtained. Osteomyelitis is a biologically complex disease. Deep bone specimens must be obtained because surface areas will be heavily contaminated. Specimens should be sent for aerobe, anaerobe, acid-fast, and fungal cultures. Specimens with negative cultures should be held for bacterial 16S polymerase chain reaction testing and, if appropriate, 18S polymerase chain reaction testing for fungal infections. However, patients with the most complex cases of osteomyelitis may still warrant limb salvage, even if an unstable soft-tissue envelope is present (**Figure 10**).

Infection in the Upper Limb

Infections of the upper limb are less common, with hand infections comprising the bulk of upper limb infections. Nonetheless, upper limb amputations are very disabling, so every effort should be made to preserve an infected limb. In patients with diabetes, upper limb infections are extremely serious, especially when osteomyelitis is present. Multiple staged irrigations and débridements, stabilization, and restoration of bone and soft-tissue integrity are needed (**Figure 11**).

Infected joint prostheses with nonhealing wounds that expose the implant present a considerable challenge to successful limb salvage. However, diligent care and adherence to the principles of adequate débridements, culture-specific antibiotics, bony stabilization, and wound coverage may allow the limb to be salvaged; more challenging cases may require flap coverage (**Figures 12** and **13**) or late functional free-flap tissue transfers (**Figure 4**).

Because the upper limb has highly specialized functions, limb salvage is the preferred option if feasible (**Figure 14**), even in circumstances that may have prompted an amputation if it were in the lower extremity.[20] When salvage is not possible, amputation and prosthetic fitting should be considered. In the past, upper limb prostheses provided limited function; however, current techniques to augment function, such as targeted muscle reinnervation techniques, hold promise for

TABLE 4 Cierny-Mader Classification of Adult (Chronic) Osteomyelitis

Anatomic Location	Type A Host	Type B Host	Type C Host
I = Medullary II = Superficial III = Localized IV = Diffuse	Healthy patient; normal response to stress and trauma; normal response to infection	Comorbidities compromise both healing and the response to treatment	Comorbidities so severe that treatment is worse than disease; treatment is to observe and palliate or amputate

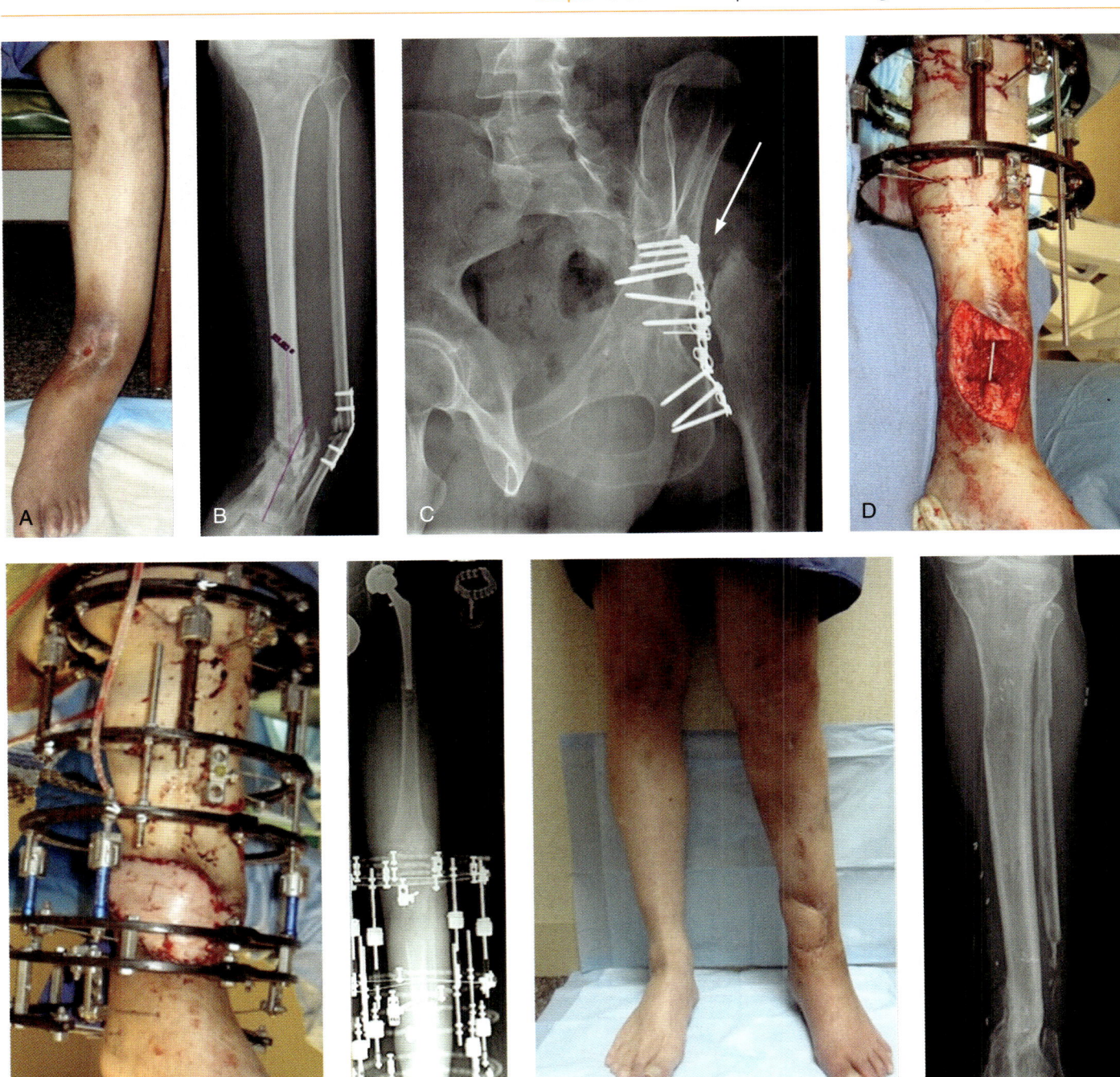

FIGURE 10 Images demonstrate limb salvage in a 35-year-old man who has alcohol use disorder and smokes and who has tibial osteomyelitis and an unstable soft-tissue envelope. **A**, Clinical photograph of the unstable soft-tissue envelope. **B**, AP radiograph shows diffuse grade IVB osteomyelitis. **C**, Oblique radiograph shows posttraumatic osteonecrosis of the femoral head and neck (arrow). **D**, Intraoperative photograph of the proximal tibial ring block for proximal tibial distraction osteogenesis. Soft-tissue and bone resection margins are seen at the distal third of the leg. **E**, Intraoperative photograph of the reverse sural flap coverage over the soft-tissue defect. **F**, Full-length radiograph of the limb with knee reconstruction in progress. A total hip arthroplasty was performed to regain hip function and limb length from the contribution of the pelvic girdle. **G**, Postoperative final clinical photograph after full healing of the bone and soft tissue. **H**, Final postoperative AP radiograph. The bifocal Ilizarov method of distal compression and proximal distraction osteogenesis restored bone length and alignment. (Courtesy of Christopher Bibbo, DO, FAAOS, FACS, Baltimore, MD. All rights reserved.)

Section 1: General Principles

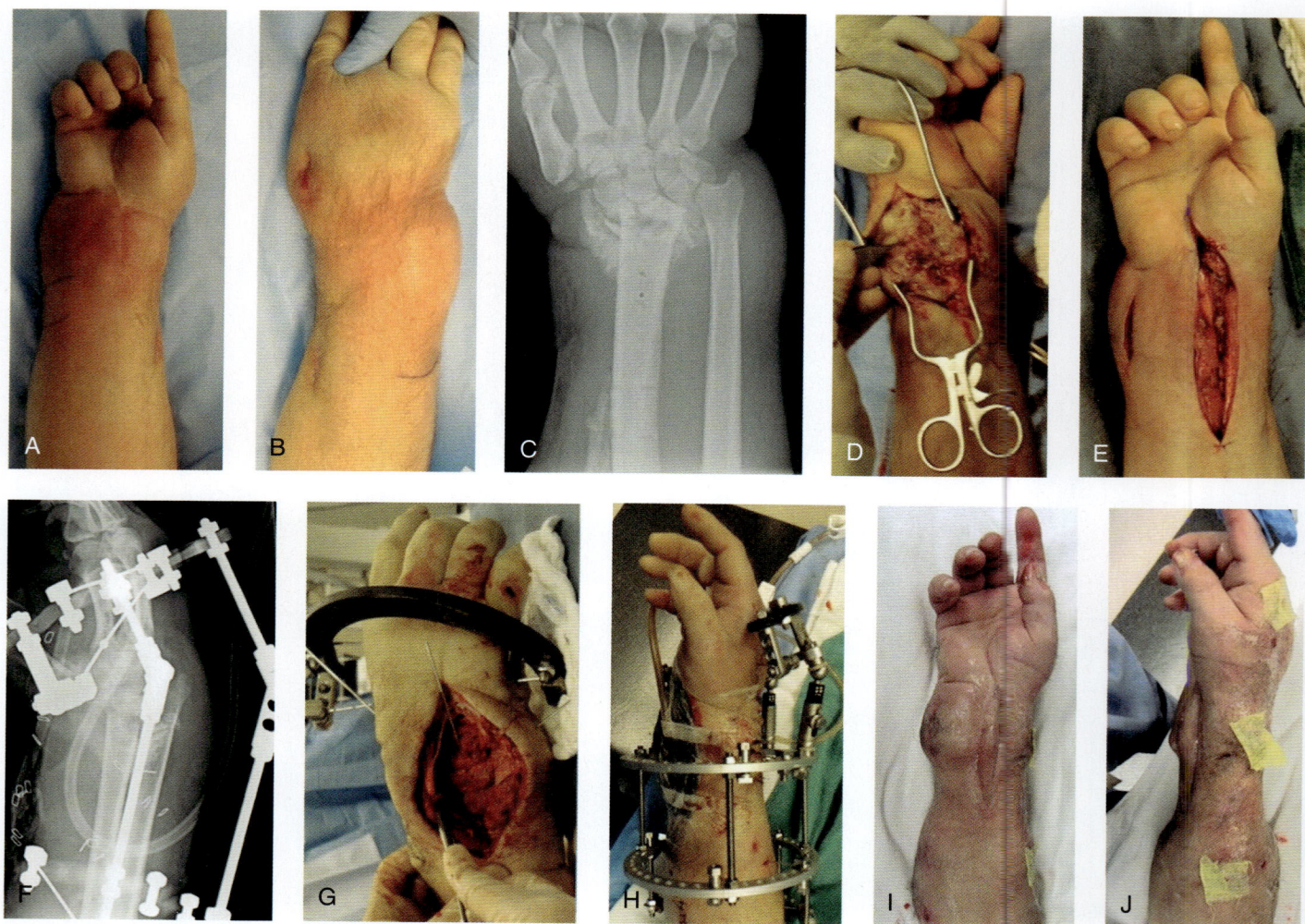

FIGURE 11 Images showing diffuse osteomyelitis and sepsis that developed in a 74-year-old right-hand-dominant patient with type 1 diabetes after three failed attempts at stabilization of a distal radius fracture. Clinical volar (**A**) and dorsal (**B**) photographs of the infected hand and distal forearm. **C**, AP radiograph of the wrist demonstrating diffuse osteomyelitis. **D** and **E**, Intraoperative photographs of wide débridements of soft tissue and bone. **F**, Radiograph shows Ilizarov stabilization. **G**, Intraoperative photograph of pan-wrist fusion after administration of parenteral antibiotics and obtaining negative bone cultures. **H**, Conversion to a hinged external ring fixator with distractive/compressive struts. Negative-pressure dressing is seen on the volar wrist surface. **I** and **J**, Final postoperative photographs show successful limb salvage after healing of the volar skin grafts. Osseous union allowed removal of the external fixator, which was followed by aggressive edema reduction and hand therapy. (Courtesy of Christopher Bibbo, DO, FAAOS, FACS, Baltimore, MD. All rights reserved.)

regaining motor group function that will facilitate the improved use of upper limb prostheses.[21]

Foot Infection in Patients With Diabetes

Diabetic foot infections in patients 65 years or older occur at a rate of 6%, with a concordant 11% mortality rate that increases to approximately 22% after a lower limb amputation.[22] Diabetic ulcers range in severity from an ulcer at the tip of a toe to massive ulcers with infection of an entire limb (Figure 15). Aggressive débridements, the use of negative-pressure dressings (including antibiotic/antiseptic instillation), hyperbaric oxygen therapy, and proper management of diabetes have been successful in salvaging the foot in most patients with diabetes who have foot infections. However, many patients with diabetes and foot infections are challenging to treat because of multiple preexisting medical comorbidities. These patients require metabolic control and optimization of cardiovascular health and peripheral vascular system functions to allow successful limb salvage. Medical management is needed to control blood glucose levels, and dialysis needs and electrolyte balance must be optimized. The patient should be carefully evaluated for cardiac disease; a low threshold for perfusion stress testing and catheterization is warranted. If the patient does not have adequate physiologic reserve and the reversal of coexisting medical comorbidities is not possible, then primary amputation should be considered. However, in the absence

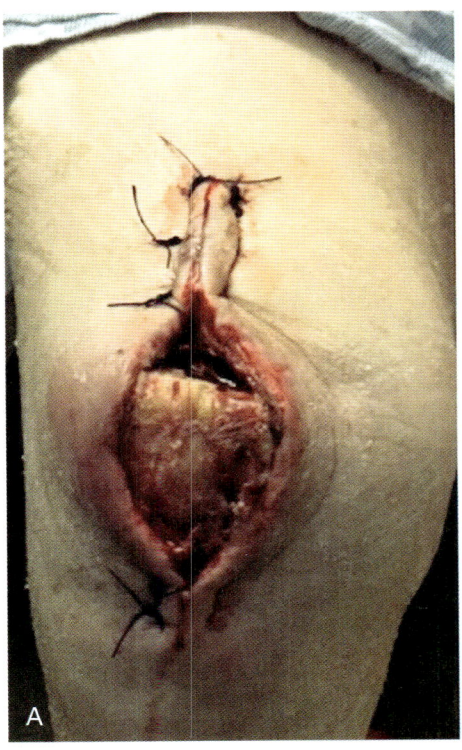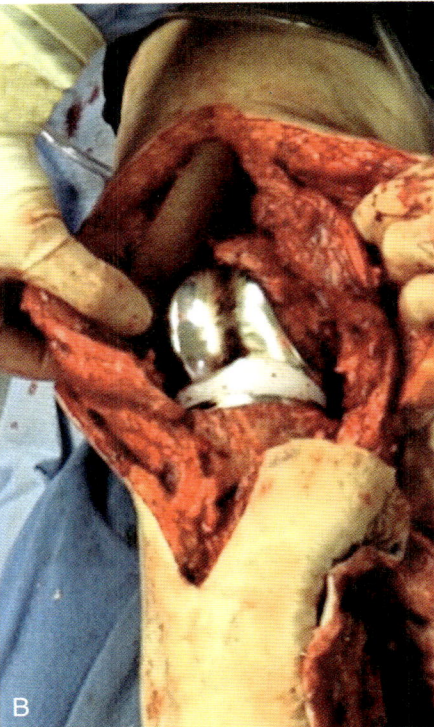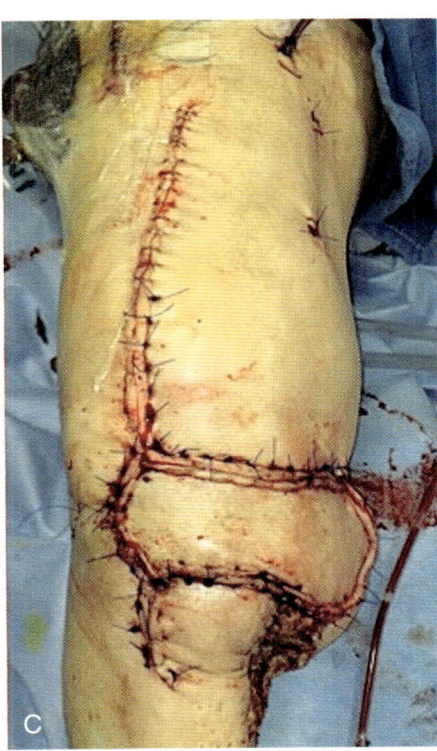

FIGURE 12 Intraoperative photographs of an acutely exposed and infected but well-fixed total knee arthroplasty with a soft-tissue defect (**A**), managed with extensive débridement and polyethylene insert exchange (**B**), and an extended medial gastrocnemius myocutaneous flap (**C**). (Courtesy of Christopher Bibbo, DO, FAAOS, FACS, Baltimore, MD. All rights reserved.)

of contraindications, limb salvage can achieve positive results, allowing a patient to have a useful limb for locomotion in the home or community.

If limb salvage is planned for an infected lower limb, it is necessary to ensure that the limb has adequate vascularity and will be useful to the patient (eg, helping to propel a wheelchair or allowing full ambulation). It is important that the salvage procedure does not create circumstances that will place the limb or the patient's life at future risk. For example, when multiple toes require amputation, resulting in a foot with one or two toes, the salvaged toes, foot, and limb are at greater risk of injury and infection. In this setting, isolated toe salvage may not be prudent, and a higher-level amputation (eg, transmetatarsal) may provide a more durable, stable limb.

Efforts for salvage or amputation to the transtibial level are encouraged.[23-26] However, even in patients with diabetes and peripheral vascular arterial disease, limb salvage by methods such as free tissue transfer can result in good long-term results after revascularization; thus, amputation is not the automatic choice in all patients with dysvascular disease or diabetes.[27] Recent advances in the use of offloading external fixation after flap reconstruction in limb salvage in patients with diabetes can maintain patient mobility while allowing reconstructions to heal.[28] Likewise, with the use of external fixator-based immediate postoperative prosthesis (X-Prosthesis; PostOp Innovations), patients who have had a major lower extremity amputation may be able to bear weight immediately (**Figure 16**).

Charcot Neuroarthropathy in Patients With Diabetes

Charcot neuroarthropathy is a debilitating disorder that affects up to 2.5% of patients with diabetes. First described in patients with tabes dorsalis, it is now recognized as a complex problem that involves neuropathy, an overall altered metabolic state that results in an imbalance of the neurohumoral regulatory mechanisms of the bones and joints of the foot and the ankle. On a cellular basis, an inciting event appears to trigger cell signaling pathways, resulting in an imbalance of osteoclastic and osteoblastic activity.[29] If the patient has substantial loss of bone mineral density, a neuropathic dislocation will develop and frank Charcot bone destruction may ensue,[30] causing loss of periarticular bony stability, joint destruction, and varying degrees of collapse of the foot and the ankle.

Protected weight bearing and strict control of diabetes will cause the process to enter a resolution phase, with the final outcome from the Charcot process resulting in a spectrum of resultant deformities. If altered weight bearing and poor control of diabetes remain untreated, skin breakdown, ulceration, and soft-tissue and bony infections may result. Limb salvage is an option in patients with Charcot neuroarthropathy, even when severe open wounds and bone loss are present (**Figure 17**). In the experience of the lead author of

Section 1: General Principles

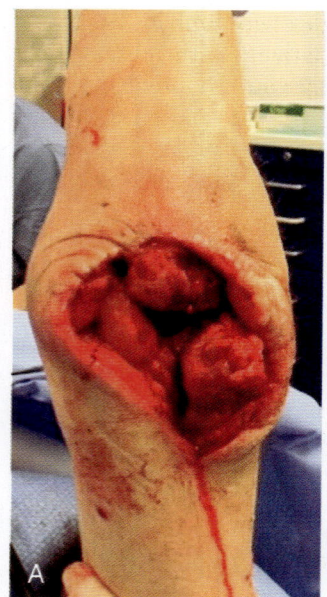
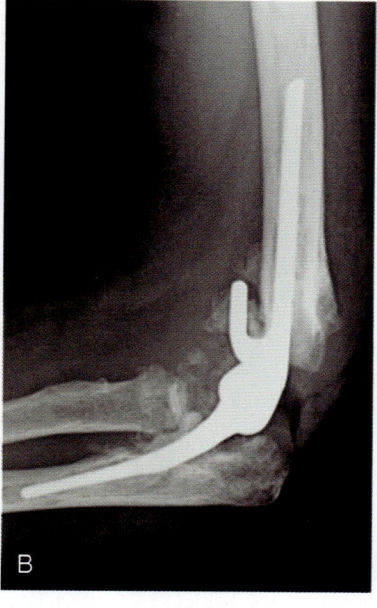
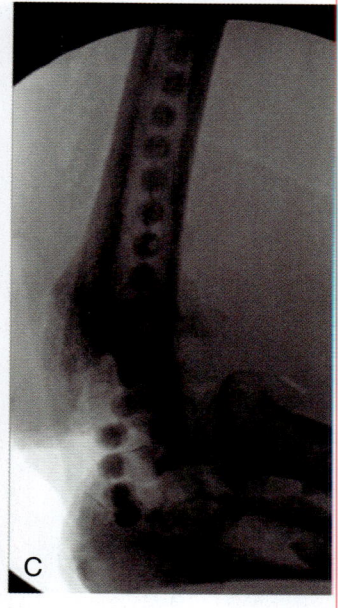
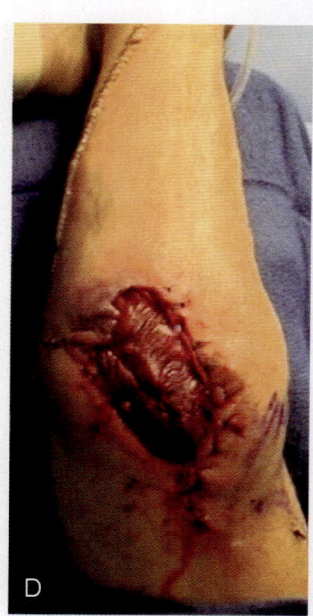
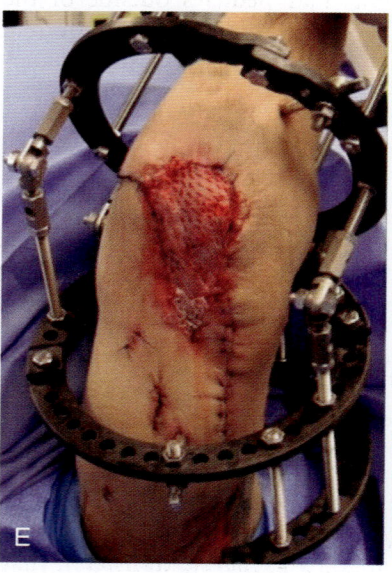
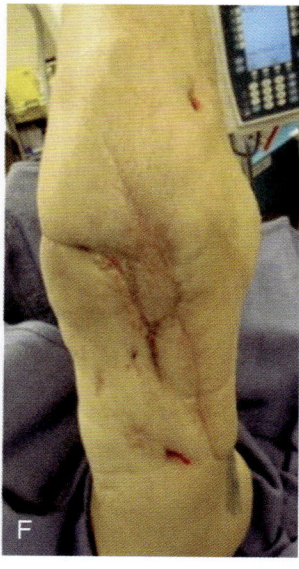

FIGURE 13 Images from an 84-year-old man with Parkinson disease who had a massive nonhealing infected elbow wound on his nondominant upper limb after total elbow arthroplasty. **A**, Clinical photograph of the chronically infected elbow wound that exposed the arthroplasty implant. **B**, Lateral radiograph shows the loose, infected elbow arthroplasty. **C**, Lateral fluoroscopic image after bony and soft-tissue débridements, removal of the infected implant, and insertion of antibiotic-impregnated polymethyl methacrylate beads. **D**, Intraoperative photograph. After control of the acute infection, a flexor carpi ulnaris muscle rotation flap was used to reduce the deep potential space and provide a base for resurfacing the soft-tissue defect of the elbow. **E**, Intraoperative photograph. A split-thickness skin graft was placed over the flexor carpi ulnaris muscle flap, and an Ilizarov ring fixator was applied to stabilize the elbow reconstruction. This method was important to counteract the patient's elbow tremor and relieve pressure on the soft-tissue reconstruction. **F**, Final photograph of the healed elbow reconstruction. (Courtesy of Christopher Bibbo, DO, FAAOS, FACS, Baltimore, MD. All rights reserved.)

this chapter (CB), the management of physiologic parameters (namely blood glucose control) is of utmost importance for acute and long-term success.

Physiologic Reserve and Comorbidities

In the setting of acute necrotizing or purulent infections, the first consideration is preservation of life over limb. It should be recognized that the use of antibiotics or antifungal medications with their attendant toxicities, multiple débridements with blood loss, and the possibility of multiple future reconstructive surgeries place great stress on a patient, especially an elderly patient with major medical comorbidities. However, in many of these patients, successful limb salvage can be obtained with proper medical and surgical management. Whether to proceed with limb salvage or amputation is highly dependent on the presence of a coexisting multidrug-resistant infection (eg, osteomyelitis), the degree of bone loss, and diabetes control. The potential for meaningful limb use must be considered; it must be remembered that in many instances, even the use of a limb to assist with wheelchair locomotion should be considered valuable. As in nearly all settings, when the treatment of a pathology becomes worse than the disease itself, then interceding with amputation must be entertained.

Musculoskeletal Tumors

Physiologic Reserve and Comorbidities

Patients with cancer who are faced with limb salvage or amputation are unique in that primarily pathologic lesions and the stage of the lesion determine the appropriate treatment option. Patients undergoing adjuvant or neoadjuvant chemotherapy or radiation may become acutely ill and malnourished, but this is a short-term

Chapter 3: General Principles of Limb Salvage Versus Amputation in Adults

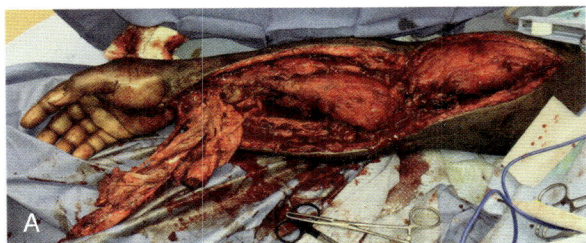

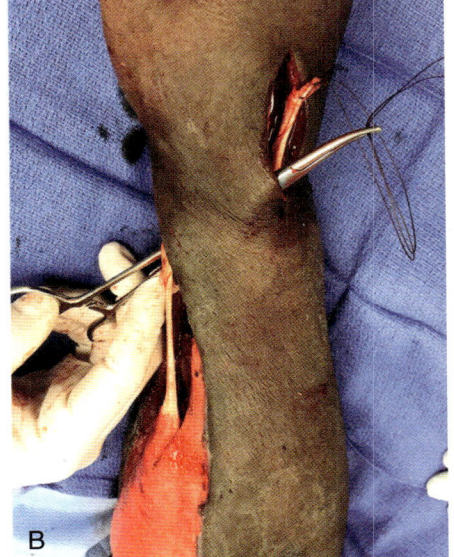

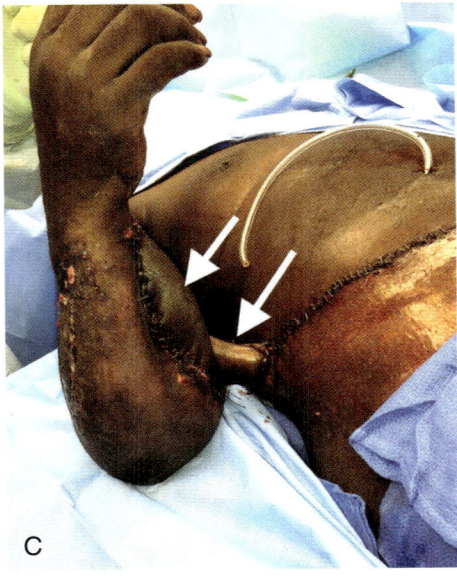

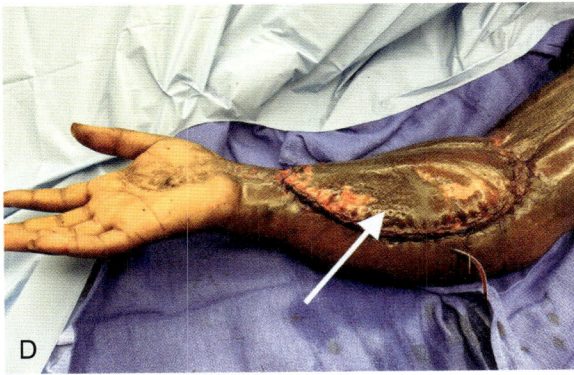

FIGURE 14 Photographs of upper extremity salvage in a patient with COVID-19 sepsis, hypercoagulability, capillary leak syndrome resulting in compartment syndrome. **A**, Necrotic medial nerve and volar forearm muscles. **B**, Tendon transfer. **C**, Abdominal tubed flap (white arrows) to cover volar forearm. **D**, Final flap inset (white arrow) after reconstruction after division of flap pedicle. (Courtesy of Christopher Bibbo, DO, FAAOS, FACS, Baltimore, MD. All rights reserved.)

with a single-stage limb salvage procedure. In patients with musculoskeletal oncology who are physiologically unable to meet the challenge of limb reconstruction, primary amputation below the pelvic girdle may be the best option.

Arterial, Venous, and Lymphatic Patency

The timing of external beam radiation therapy in relation to reconstructive limb salvage is important. A balance must be struck with early neoadjuvant external beam radiation versus adjuvant radiation because local or free-tissue flap reconstruction in radiated fields is difficult and prone to complications. Thus, larger flaps with vascular pedicles outside of the field of radiation may be required. Brachytherapy may allow for the concentrated application of radiation, limit the field of exposure, and be performed in the single-setting treatment of musculoskeletal sarcomas.

Neurologic Status

When major motor nerves are sacrificed during an oncologic resection, tendon transfer or extensive bracing often is required. If radiation therapy is not required, it is possible that free functional muscle transfers can be used to provide function.[7-16] However, if extensive postoperative radiation is likely to result in postradiation fibrosis of a functional muscle transfer, it may be best to consider other acute reconstructive techniques or delay a free functional muscle transfer.

Sensory nerve preservation is usually of less concern, but techniques using local flaps with sensory nerve splitting and transfer have been successful in providing soft-tissue coverage and protective sensation.[32]

Functional Potential and Quality of Life

The patient's quality of life is a critical determinant when considering limb salvage in a patient with cancer. Influential factors include the type of cancer, the oncologic stage and grade of the sarcoma, 5- and 10-year

complication and is correctable with dietary supplements. In contrast, patients with tumor recurrence may require multiple rounds of chemotherapy over a long treatment period. The use of anthracycline-based agents often results in irreversible cardiomyopathy; however, with the exception of those with Ewing sarcoma, most patients in need of limb salvage have not been treated with an anthracycline-based agent unless they were enrolled in an experimental protocol.[31] Peripheral neuropathy related to cisplatin-based chemotherapy is not an indication for amputation. The patient with musculoskeletal sarcoma usually is otherwise healthy (unless associated with a multiple neoplastic syndrome), and reconstructive efforts are usually immediate

Section 1: General Principles

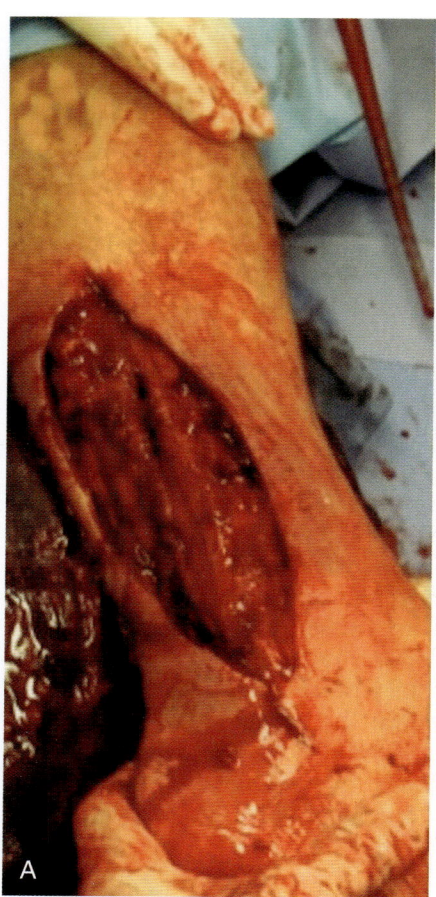 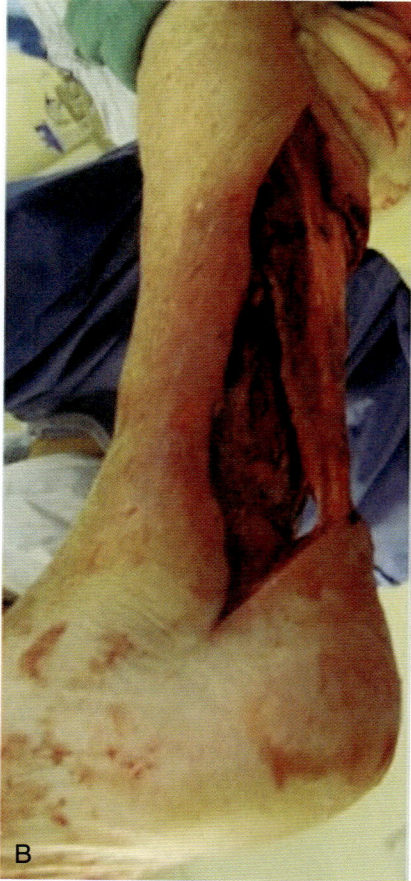 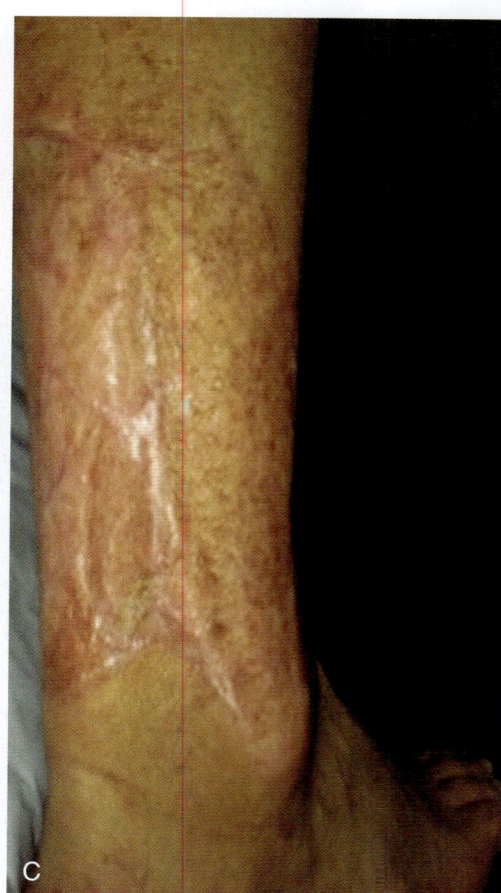

FIGURE 15 **A**, Intraoperative photograph of a necrotizing infection in a patient who has type 1 diabetes, vascular disease, and renal failure. **B**, Intraoperative photograph of the final wound after débridements and culture-specific antibiotics. **C**, Clinical photograph of successful limb salvage after protection in a fine-wire external fixator and the use of collagen-based ingrowth matrix, negative-pressure dressings, and skin grafting. (Courtesy of Christopher Bibbo, DO, FAAOS, FACS, Baltimore, MD. All rights reserved.)

survival rates for the involved cancer, and the patient's age and preoperative functional capacity. Although the surgical and medical care of patients with musculoskeletal tumors can be challenging, there is often time for more planning and more certainty in expected outcomes in this patient population. In addition, advances in the perioperative management of patients with tumors[33,34] as well as refinements in limb salvage implants have made limb salvage a goal among orthopaedic oncologists and reconstructive surgeons[35] (**Figure 18**). A multidisciplinary team approach that includes an orthopaedic oncologist, a reconstruction surgeon, a medical oncologist, a general medicine practitioner, a radiation oncologist, a physical therapist, and a prosthetist can best manage these complex cases.

Trauma

Physiologic Reserve and Medical Comorbidities

The decision to proceed with limb salvage or amputation in a patient who sustains a severe traumatic injury is clinically challenging. Clinicians typically determine the overall magnitude of injury to a limb based on the fracture pattern, degree of soft-tissue injury, level of contamination, and vascular status (**Figures 19** through **22**). Occasionally, decision making is simplified if the patient is in extremis and emergent amputation (often a complete amputation) contributes to saving the patient's life (**Figure 23**).

The decision to salvage or amputate a severely injured lower limb has long been a vexing problem. The Lower Extremity Assessment Project (LEAP) study evaluated the outcomes of lower limb salvage versus amputation in patients sustaining high-energy injuries.[36] Data from the study challenged previous paradigms in that outcomes for limb salvage or amputation may be more influenced by a patient's socioeconomic status, personal resources, and overall psychosocial health than by the degree of bodily injury alone.[36] Thus, limb injuries that often were determined to be either salvageable or requiring amputation are now evaluated on a spectrum that considers socioeconomic factors, outpatient resources, premorbid conditions, the magnitude of the injury, and potential therapeutic interventions. When a patient's life is not at risk, the decision between limb salvage and early amputation is based on multiple factors and is individualized to the patient. Although the American

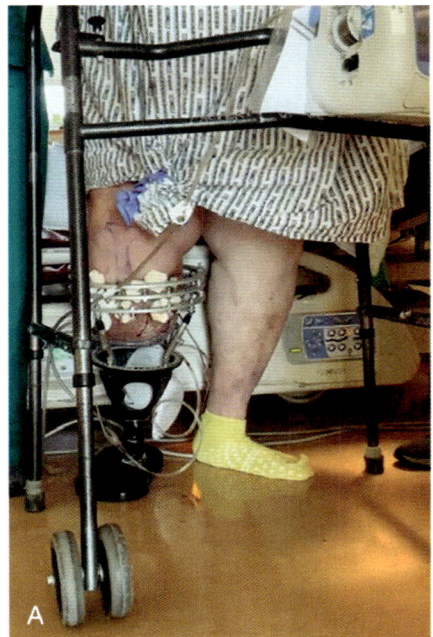 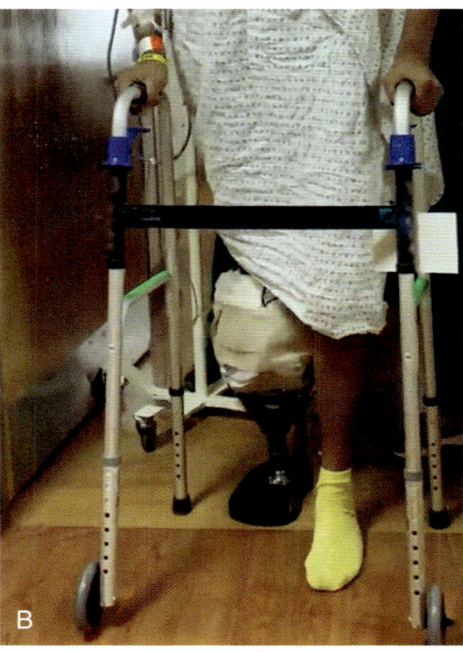

FIGURE 16 **A**, Photograph from a patient with morbid obesity and diabetes on postoperative day 1 after transtibial amputation and negative-pressure wound dressing therapy beginning weight-bearing ambulation training on an external fixator-based immediate postoperative prosthesis. **B**, Photograph from a patient with diabetes on postoperative day 2 of a transtibial amputation ambulating independently with an external fixator-based immediate postoperative prosthesis. (A, X-Prosthesis; PostOp Innovations, Fallston, MD. B, X-Prosthesis; Courtesy of Christopher Bibbo, DO, FAAOS, FACS, Baltimore, MD. All rights reserved.)

Academy of Orthopaedic Surgeons has published clinical practice guidelines to help clinicians guide treatment decisions,[37] it is not considered a rigid protocol and some choices remain controversial. Attempts to develop a scoring system to determine whether limb salvage versus early amputation would provide a better patient outcome have been unsuccessful.[38,39] Therefore, the clinician and patient must evaluate all variables to determine the best course of treatment for each individual case.

Arterial Injury

Early vascular assessment and a recognition of arterial disruption are critical for successful limb salvage. Prolonged ischemia times result in irreversible cell damage and death that may be so extensive that amputation is required. Arterial inflow may be caused by arterial transection, thrombosis, or physical interruption by a displaced fracture. Thus, it is essential that the injured limb be provisionally reduced to lower the risk of deformity

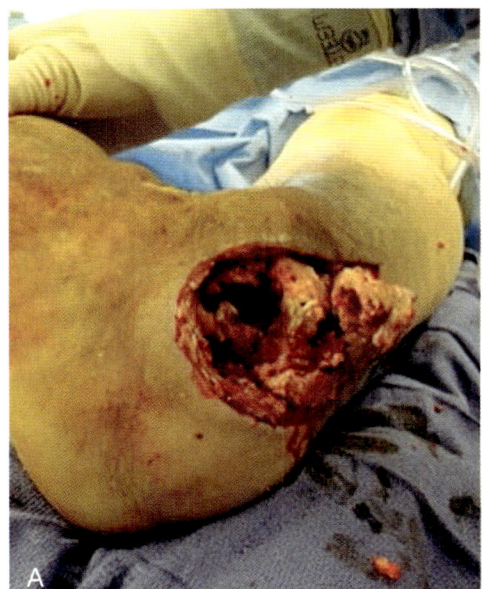 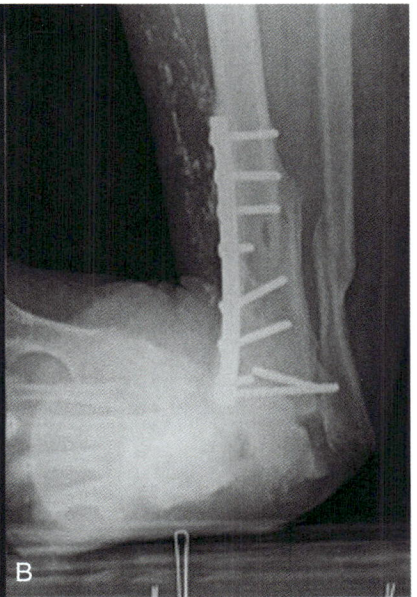 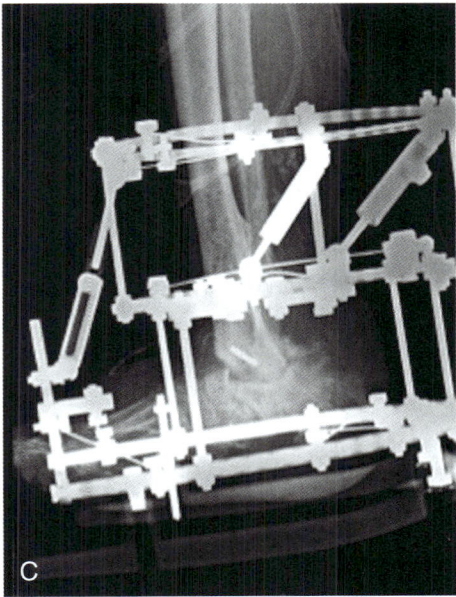

FIGURE 17 Images from a patient with ankle Charcot neuroarthropathy with a deep, infected soft-tissue wound and osteomyelitis that was successfully managed with débridements, antibiotics, tibiocalcaneal fusion, and fine-wire external fixation. **A**, Intraoperative photograph of the lateral left ankle demonstrates severe ankle varus instability and the extent of the wound. **B**, AP weight-bearing radiograph of the left ankle shows the severe varus instability. **C**, Lateral radiograph demonstrates configuration of the fine-wire ring external fixator that was applied immediately after extensive débridement. The external fixator allowed immediate partial weight-bearing mobilization. (Courtesy of Christopher Bibbo, DO, FAAOS, FACS, Baltimore, MD. All rights reserved.)

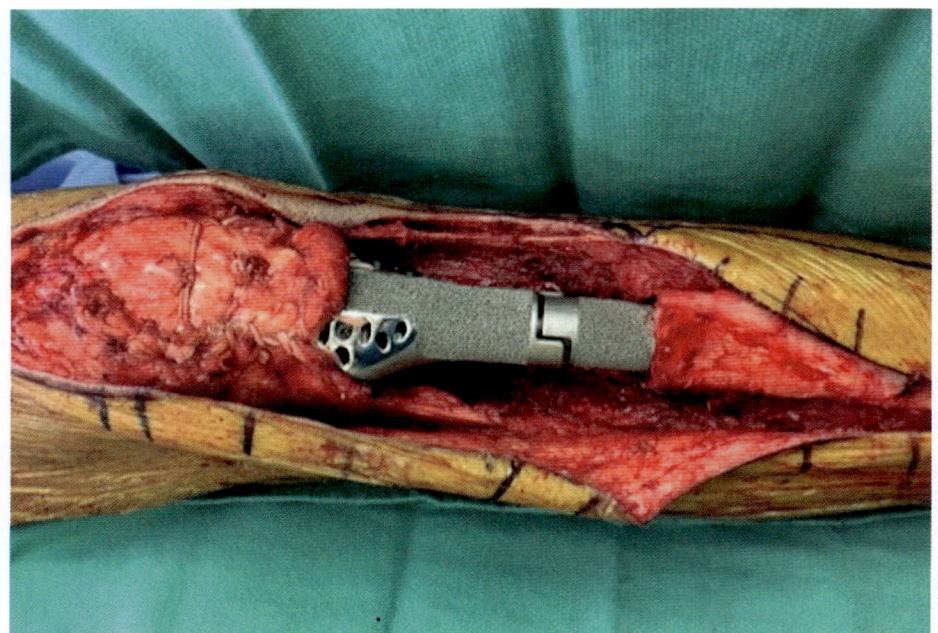

FIGURE 18 Intraoperative photograph of a proximal tibia modular prosthesis for limb salvage. Wounds were closed and covered with medial and lateral gastrocnemius flaps and skin graft. (Courtesy of David A. Ehrlich, MD, Philadelphia, PA.)

that may cause blood vessels to kink (**Figure 19**).

The primary assessment of the patient also should include checks for pulses, skin temperature, and capillary refill at and below the zone of injury. A Doppler probe is used to evaluate nonpalpable pulses, listen for bruits (audible sounds associated with waveform changes), and determine the ankle-brachial index. An ankle-brachial index less than 0.9 in an otherwise healthy young adult (no history of peripheral arterial vascular disease or diabetes) indicates a potential vascular injury and requires further analysis.[40] Such analysis may include a noninvasive color Doppler ultrasonography, computer-assisted arteriography, or arteriography. A doubling of the flow velocity across the area of injury indicates an occult intimal lesion. When concern for vascular injury exists, a vascular surgeon should be consulted.

The time from vascular injury to reperfusion of the tissues is a factor often considered when attempting limb salvage. It is generally thought that revascularization becomes a relative contraindication after 6 hours from the time of injury.[41,42] Limb ischemia is so critical in patients with trauma that ischemia times beyond 6 hours elevate the severity of injury on several injury scoring systems.[43-45] However, the role of collateral flow states in major axial arterial injuries can influence outcomes and should be considered on a case-by-case basis.

In the setting of unstable fractures and vascular injury, there is no universal agreement on the sequence of fracture stabilization versus vascular repair.[46,47] The logical approach is to perform the most expedient sequence of orthopaedic or vascular procedures to temporarily stabilize or reperfuse the limb, followed by more definitive procedures.

Neurologic Status

Peripheral nerve injury is common with limb trauma and becomes increasingly more likely with the increasing severity and volume of soft-tissue injuries. Often, a complete neurologic examination of the limb can be difficult in the acute setting (eg, the presence of a decreased Glasgow Coma Scale score, intubation, or massive soft-tissue injury with limb deformity), and a cursory baseline examination is all that is afforded. Surgical exploration and

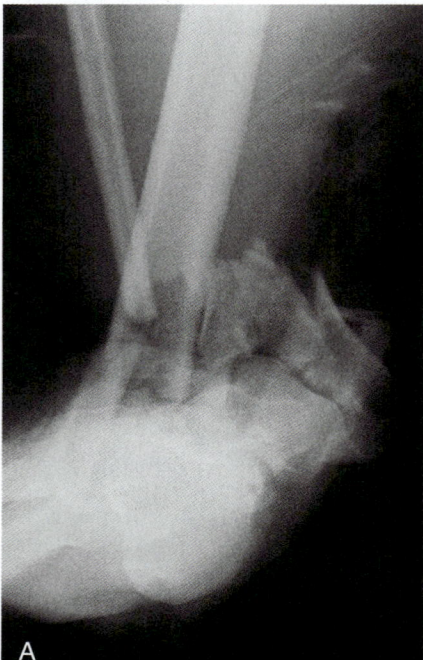
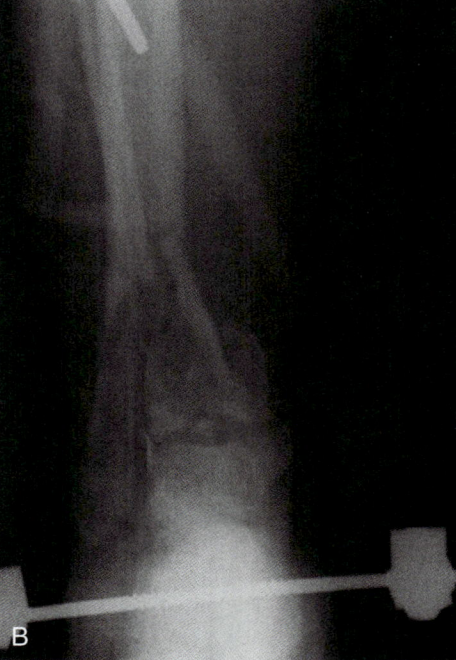

FIGURE 19 AP radiographs of a high-grade pilon fracture. **A**, Loss of pulses is seen. Immediate reduction and traveling traction provided return of pulses and provisional stabilization and restoration of leg length (**B**). (Courtesy of Christopher Bibbo, DO, FAAOS, FACS, Baltimore, MD. All rights reserved.)

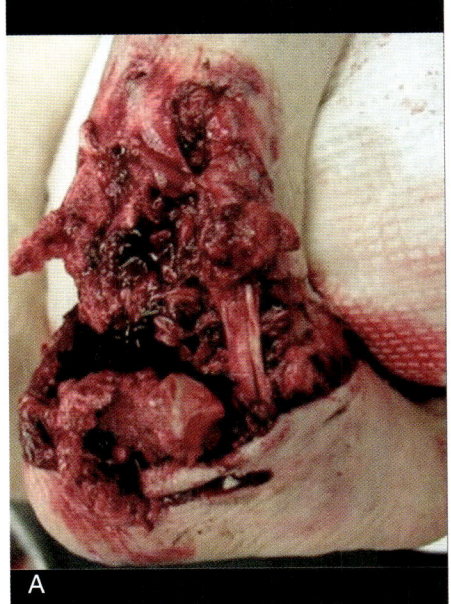 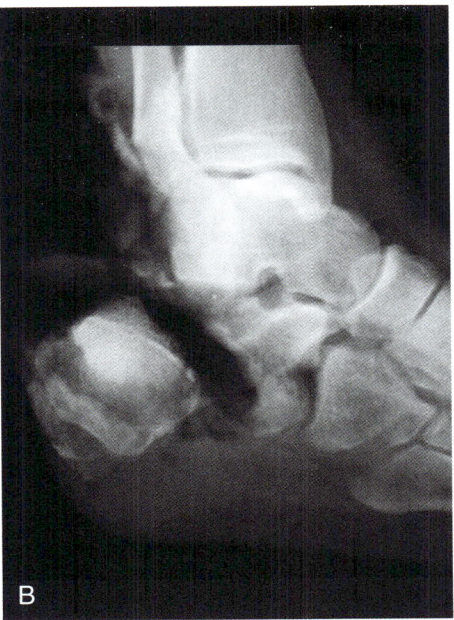

FIGURE 20 Intraoperative photograph (**A**) and lateral radiograph (**B**) of traumatic injury to the foot resulting in a high-grade Tscherne soft-tissue injury with open ankle and calcaneus fractures; note degloving of the skin distally. This patient had a history of one-vessel runoff (a single-vessel limb), and the wound was highly contaminated. Amputation was elected as final management in the subacute setting. (Courtesy of Christopher Bibbo, DO, FAAOS, FACS, Baltimore, MD. All rights reserved.)

inspection are critical, as well as follow-up secondary survey examinations.

Loss of plantar foot sensation was thought to be an important factor in deciding between limb salvage and amputation. However, Bosse et al[48] reported that, based on health-related quality-of-life activities and the percentage of individuals returning to work at 12 or 24 months after amputation, loss of plantar sensation alone should not be considered as a factor for deciding between limb salvage and amputation in patients with severe lower limb trauma. The authors concur that loss of sensation and in many cases loss of selected motor functions are not rigid criteria to proceed with lower extremity amputation.

Functional Potential and Quality of Life

Data from the LEAP Study Group have shown that previous predictive scoring systems (eg, the Mangled Extremity

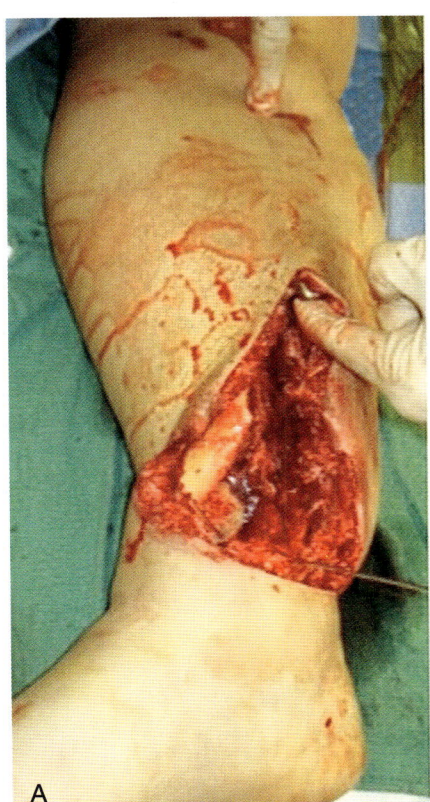 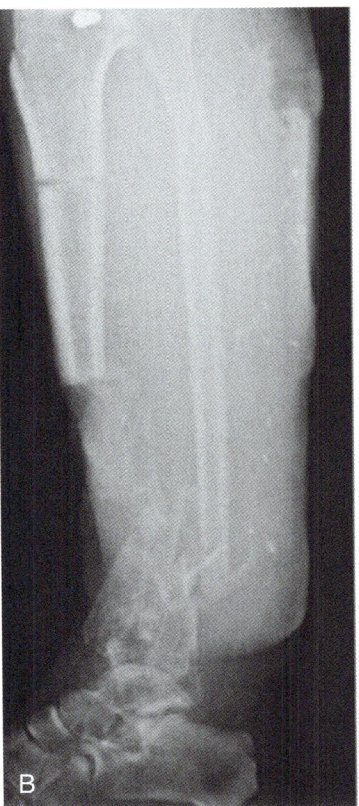 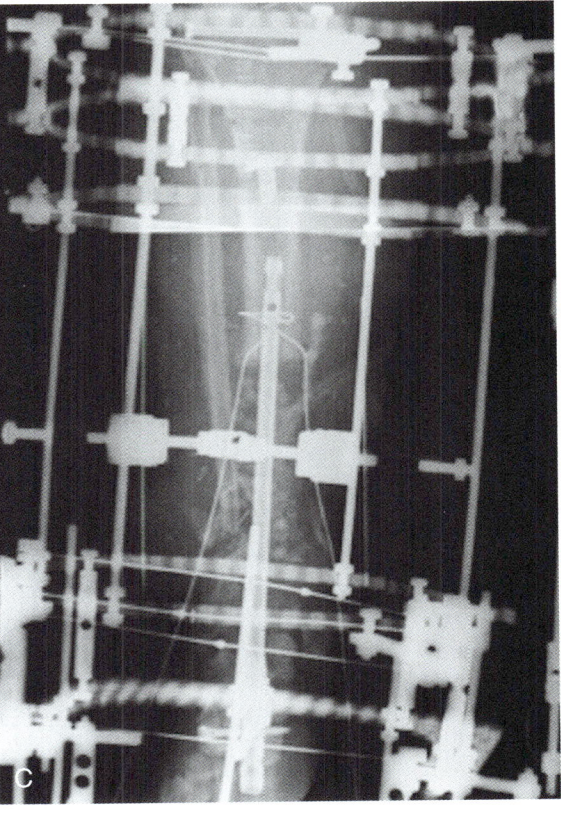

FIGURE 21 **A**, Intraoperative photograph of a severe degloving injury of the distal tibia. **B**, Lateral radiograph best demonstrates loss of the distal tibia. **C**, AP radiograph obtained after serial débridements of contaminated and subsequently infected bone; bone transport was performed over a temporary intramedullary nail using the Weber technique. (Courtesy of Christopher Bibbo, DO, FAAOS, FACS, Baltimore, MD. All rights reserved.)

Section 1: General Principles

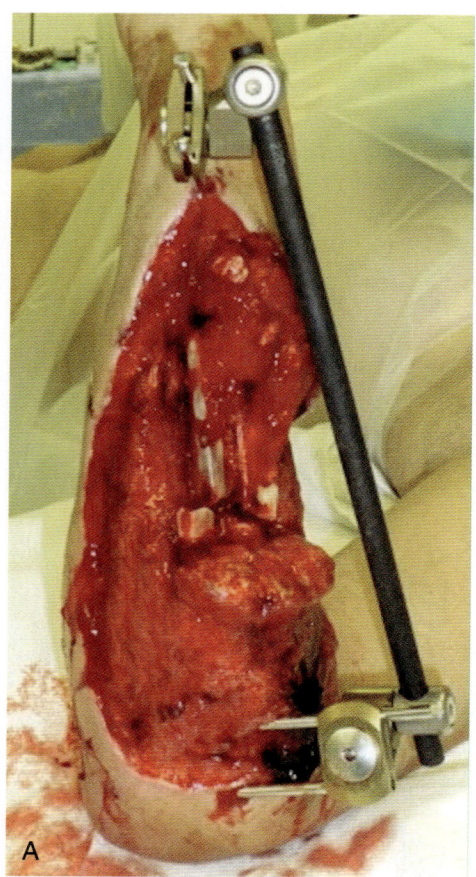 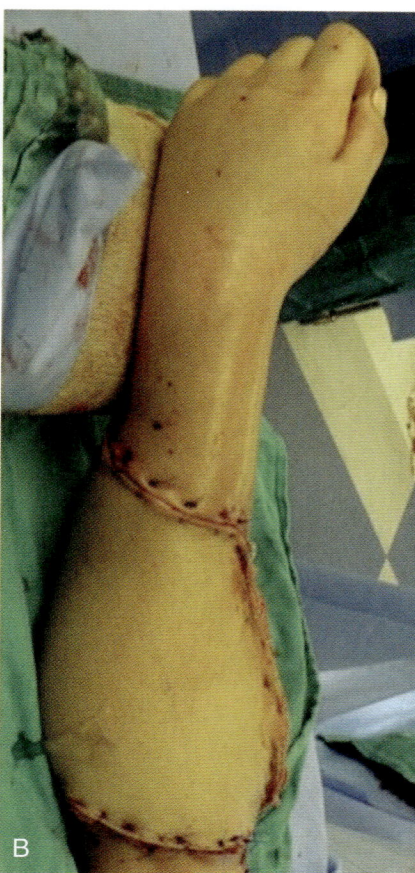

FIGURE 22 **A**, Intraoperative photograph of a mangled upper limb. **B**, Photograph of the limb after serial débridements, fixation of radial and ulnar fractures with locking plates, and soft-tissue coverage with an anterolateral thigh free flap. (Courtesy of Stephen J. Kovach III, MD, Philadelphia, PA.)

Severity Score) have little use, and limb salvage may have outcomes equivalent to amputation in properly selected patients.[49-53] The data indicate that outcomes are influenced by the following factors: rehospitalization for a major complication, less than a high school education, a household income below the federal poverty line, nonwhite race, no insurance or Medicaid coverage, a poor social support network, a low level of self-efficacy, smoking, and legal system involvement for injury compensation.[49-53]

Similar to the LEAP study, the Military Extremity Trauma Amputation/Limb Salvage (METALS) study sought out functional outcomes following high-energy lower extremity trauma sustained during active military duty.[54] The baseline characteristics of the study participants, as well as a high percentage of blast injuries being the mechanism of injury, differed from those of the civilian population included in the LEAP study. Despite these differences, it was hypothesized that outcomes between limb salvage and amputation would be similar. However, in this retrospective cohort study, those treated with amputation appeared to have better functional outcomes than those treated with limb salvage based on Short Musculoskeletal Function Assessment scores. The authors discussed several potential explanations for the outcome difference between groups but cautioned interpretation of the results due to the potential for selection bias based on study design. They did not believe the current data were sufficient enough to support amputation over limb salvage.

Availability of Multidisciplinary Resources

A resource-intensive process is required for the treatment of patients who sustain severe, limb-threatening, traumatic injuries—whether limb salvage or amputation is undertaken. A variety of medical practitioners are involved with the care of these patients, starting soon after the injury and throughout the course of treatment. Rehabilitation efforts for these patients have not been the subject of extensive research, and efforts have traditionally focused on return of physical function. Although rehabilitation is certainly an important area of emphasis, experience from the LEAP Study Group has indicated that mental health also should be given attention during a patient's recovery.[55]

The determinants of patient satisfaction identified in the LEAP study offer areas on which to focus rehabilitation efforts and resources. Five factors were identified and significantly associated with patient satisfaction 2 years after injury: faster walking speed, a higher physical function score on the Sickness Impact Profile, lower pain intensity, no depression, and return to work.[55] Beyond the acute hospital setting, a skilled set of therapists, qualified rehabilitation and long-term acute care facilities, and a system for long-term patient follow-up are mandatory. Rehabilitation efforts for these patients need to emphasize not only physical function but also mental health. Patients in the LEAP study with unmet physical therapy needs were less likely to exhibit improvement on physical functional tests when compared with those with adequate therapy.[56] A postulation as to improved outcomes in amputees in the METALS study centered on an early, focused rehabilitation program for this group.[54] The presence of depression and posttraumatic stress disorder in both patients with limb salvage and those with amputation had an effect on outcome. Early recognition and intervention for treatment of these psychosocial risk factors should be another area of emphasis in the care of these patients.

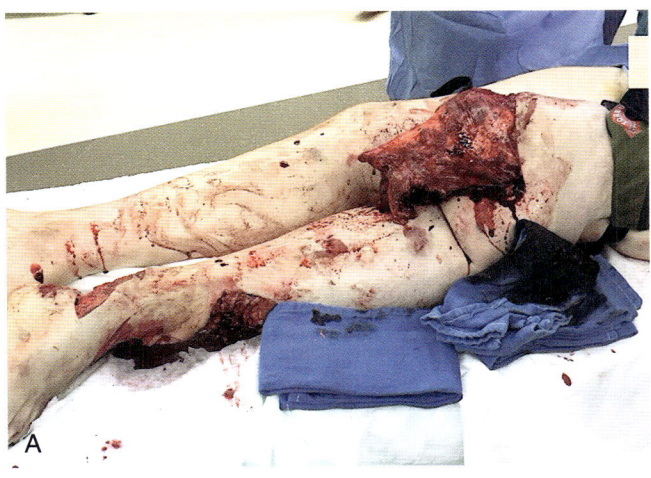
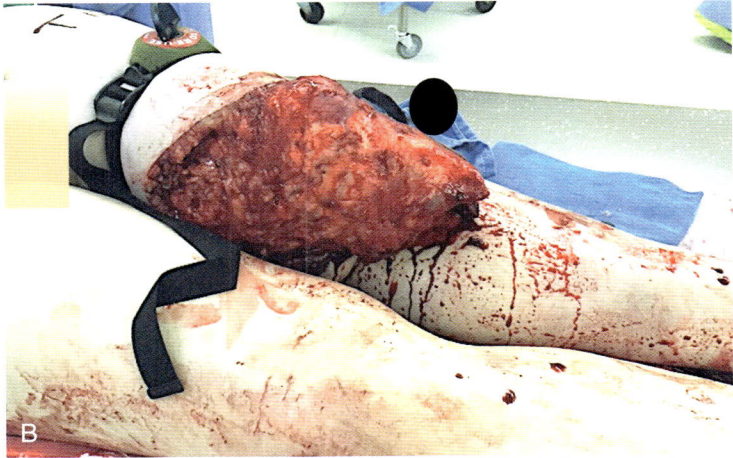
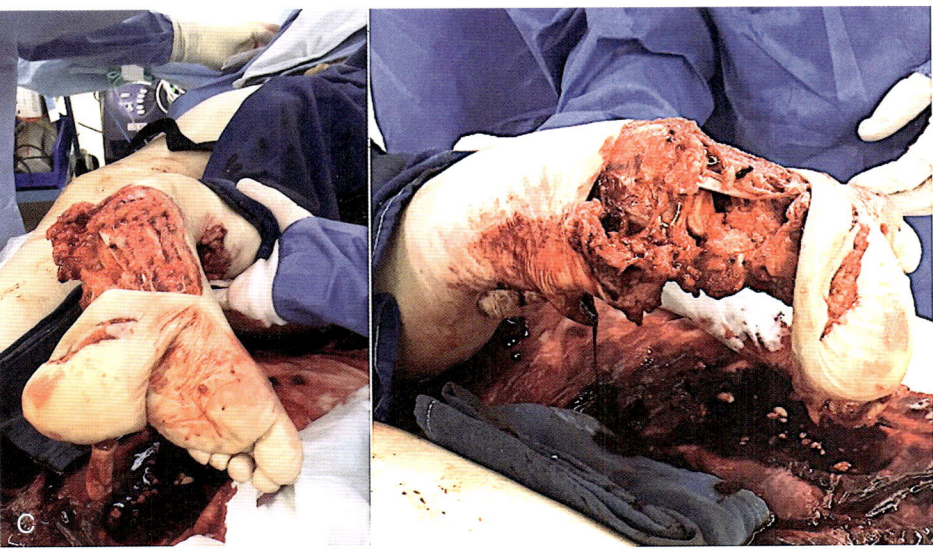
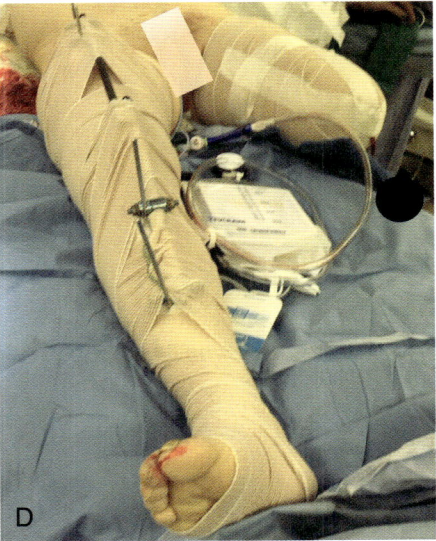

FIGURE 23 Images from a 61-year-old man with preexisting liver disease involved in a motorcycle crash. Injuries included a pneumothorax, liver laceration, and closed head injury. Musculoskeletal injuries included left hip dislocation/acetabular fracture (**A**), a closed right supracondylar femur fracture (**B**), and severe degloving from above the knee to the foot with associated segmental tibial shaft/pilon/calcaneal fractures with an associated injury to the superficial femoral artery (**C**). External fixation of the right limb and immediate transfemoral guillotine amputation was performed (**D**) and assisted with the overall resuscitation of the patient. (Courtesy of David J. Polga, MD, FAAOS, Marshfield, WI. All rights reserved.)

SUMMARY

Regardless of the injury or the underlying disease process, decision making for limb salvage versus amputation is complex. Other than a patient in extremis requiring an emergent, life-saving amputation, few clear guidelines exist. The patient's status, including psychosocial and premorbid functional status, along with the soft-tissue, bone, vascular, and neurologic status of the injured or diseased limb must be considered. In general, after appropriate counseling regarding the anticipated treatment course and outcomes, erring on the side of limb salvage is preferred for most patients, but the goals are individualized. Acceptable functional outcomes for complex limb salvage using advanced surgical techniques are feasible for most patients. Each patient must be evaluated individually in the decision making for limb salvage or amputation. Surgeon experience and judgment is still the most important factor in deciding whether to proceed with limb salvage or amputation. Recently described novel techniques to allow immediate ambulation after lower extremity amputation even during phases of active wound care (**Figure 16**) and recent significant advancements in prosthetic designs have allowed for amputees to experience enhanced functionality after amputation.

References

1. de Luis DA, Culebras JM, Aller R, Eiros-Bouza JM: Surgical infection and malnutrition. *Nutr Hosp* 2014;30(3):509-513.
2. Chow O, Barbul A: Immunonutrition: Role in wound healing and tissue regeneration. *Adv Wound Care (New Rochelle)* 2014;3(1):46-53.
3. Zhan LX, Branco BC, Armstrong DG, Mills JL Sr: The Society for Vascular Surgery lower extremity threatened limb classification system based on Wound, Ischemia, and Foot Infection (WIFI) correlates with risk of major amputation and time to wound healing. *J Vasc Surg* 2015;61(4):939-944.

4. Jockenhöfer F, Gollnick H, Herberger K, et al: Aetiology, comorbidities and cofactors of chronic leg ulcers: Retrospective evaluation of 1 000 patients from 10 specialised dermatological wound care centers in Germany. *Int Wound J* 2016;13(5):821-828.

5. Patel KM, Lin CY, Cheng MH: A prospective evaluation of lymphedema-specific quality-of-life outcomes following vascularized lymph node transfer. *Ann Surg Oncol* 2015;22(7):2424-2430.

6. Moore AM, Franco M, Tung TH: Motor and sensory nerve transfers in the forearm and hand. *Plast Reconstr Surg* 2014;134(4):721-730.

7. Estrella EP: Functional outcome of nerve transfers for upper-type brachial plexus injuries. *J Plast Reconstr Aesthet Surg* 2011;64(8):1007-1013.

8. Jang YJ, Park MC, Hong YS, et al: Successful lower extremity salvage with free flap after endovascular angioplasty in peripheral arterial occlusive disease. *J Plast Reconstr Aesthet Surg* 2014;67(8):1136-1143.

9. Giessler GA, Schmidt AB: The functional peroneus brevis as a third muscle component in the osteomyocutaneous fibula free-flap system. *J Plast Reconstr Aesthet Surg* 2013;66(5):e137-e140.

10. Wechselberger G, Pichler M, Pülzl P, Schoeller T: Free functional rectus femoris muscle transfer for restoration of extension of the foot after lower leg compartment syndrome. *Microsurgery* 2004;24(6):437-441.

11. Wechselberger G, Ninkovic M, Pülzl P, Schoeller T: Free functional rectus femoris muscle transfer for restoration of knee extension and defect coverage after trauma. *J Plast Reconstr Aesthet Surg* 2006;59(9):994-998.

12. Moschella F, D'Arpa S, Pirrello R, Cordova A: Posterior compartment of the lower leg reconstruction with free functional rectus femoris transfer after sarcoma resection. *J Plast Reconstr Aesthet Surg* 2010;63(3):e269-e272.

13. Muramatsu K, Ihara K, Miyoshi T, Yoshida K, Hashimoto T, Taguchi T: Transfer of latissimus dorsi muscle for the functional reconstruction of quadriceps femoris muscle following oncological resection of sarcoma in the thigh. *J Plast Reconstr Aesthet Surg* 2011;64(8):1068-1074.

14. Fansa H, Plogmeier K, Feistner H, Schneider WJ: Plasticity and function: The fate of a free, neurovascular muscle graft ten years post-reconstruction. *J Reconstr Microsurg* 1997;13(8):551-554.

15. Lin CH, Lin YT, Yeh JT, Chen CT: Free functioning muscle transfer for lower extremity posttraumatic composite structure and functional defect. *Plast Reconstr Surg* 2007;119(7):2118-2126.

16. Innocenti M, Abed YY, Beltrami G, Delcroix L, Balatri A, Capanna R: Quadriceps muscle reconstruction with free functioning latissimus dorsi muscle flap after oncological resection. *Microsurgery* 2009;29(3):189-198.

17. American Psychiatric Association: *Diagnostic and Statistical Manual of Mental Disorders*, ed 5. American Psychiatric Publishing, 2013.

18. Bodde MI, Dijkstra PU, Schrier E, van den Dungen JJ, den Dunnen WF, Geertzen JH: Informed decision-making regarding amputation for complex regional pain syndrome type I. *J Bone Joint Surg Am* 2014;96(11):930-934.

19. Bibbo C, Patel DV, Mackessy RP, Lin SS, Barricella RL: Pyomyositis of the leg with early neurologic compromise. *Pediatr Emerg Care* 2000;16(5):352-354.

20. Bibbo C: Reconstruction of COVID-19-related compartment syndrome with massive soft tissue necrosis. *Wounds* 2021;33:99-105.

21. Cheesborough JE, Smith LH, Kuiken TA, Dumanian GA: Targeted muscle reinnervation and advanced prosthetic arms. *Semin Plast Surg* 2015;29(1):62-72.

22. Margolis DJ, Malay DS, Hoffstad OJ, et al: *Incidence of diabetic foot ulcer and lower extremity amputation among Medicare beneficiaries, 2006 to 2008: Data points #2. Data Points Publication Series*. Agency for Healthcare Research and Quality, 2011. Available at: http://www.ncbi.nlm.nih.gov/books/NBK65149/. Accessed October 1, 2015.

23. Bibbo C, Nelson J, Fischer JP, et al. The versatility of the anterolateral thigh free flap in lower extremity limb salvage for trauma. *J Orthop Trauma* 2015;29(12):563-568.

24. Bibbo C, Ehrlich DA, Levin LS, Kovach SJ: Maintaining level of lower extremity amputation with tissue transfers. *J Surg Orthop Adv* 2016;25(3):137-148.

25. Bibbo C: Modification of the Syme amputation to prevent postoperative heel pad migration. *J Foot Ankle Surg* 2013;52(6):766-770.

26. Bibbo C, Newman AS, Lachman RD, Levin LS, Kovach SJ: A simplified approach to reconstruction of hemipelvectomy defects with lower extremity fillet free flap that minimizes flap ischemia time. *J Plast Reconstr Aesthet Surg* 2015;68(12):1750-1754.

27. Kallio M, Vikatmaa P, Kantonen I, Lepäntalo M, Venermo M, Tukiainen E: Strategies for free flap transfer and revascularisation with long-term outcome in the treatment of large diabetic foot lesions. *Eur J Vasc Endovasc Surg* 2015;50(2):223-230.

28. Bibbo C: A novel limb salvage technique of external fixation protection of lower extremity plastic reconstructions with immediate postoperative ambulation (Bibbo flap and frame technique). *Clin Pediatr Med Surg* 2021;38:55-71.

29. Jeffcoate WJ, Game F, Cavanagh PR: The role of proinflammatory cytokines in the cause of neuropathic osteoarthropathy (acute Charcot foot in diabetes. *Lancet* 2005;366(9502):2058-2061.

30. Herbst SA, Jones KB, Saltzman CL: Pattern of diabetic neuropathic arthropathy associated with the peripheral bone mineral density. *J Bone Joint Surg Br* 2004;86(3):378-383.

31. Benjamin RS, Wagner MJ, Livingston JA, Ravi V, Patel SR: Chemotherapy for bone sarcomas in adults: The MD Anderson experience. *Am Soc Clin Oncol Educ Book* 2015;35:e656-e660.

32. Bibbo C: Plantar heel reconstruction with a sensate plantar medial artery musculocutaneous pedicled island flap after wide excision of melanoma. *J Foot Ankle Surg* 2012;51(4):504-508.

33. Bibbo C, Patel DV, Benevenia J: Perioperative considerations in patients with metastatic bone disease. *Orthop Clin North Am* 2000;31(4):577-595, viii.

34. Benevenia J, Bibbo C, Patel DV, Grossman MG, Bahramipour PF, Pappas P: Inferior vena cava filters prevent fatal pulmonary emboli in orthopaedic cancer patients. *Clin Orthop Relat Res* 2004;426:88-92.

35. Kang S, Han I, Kim S, Lee YH, Kim MB, Kim HS: Outcomes after flap reconstruction for extremity soft tissue sarcoma: A case-control study using propensity score analysis. *Eur J Surg Oncol* 2014;40(9):1101-1108.

36. MacKenzie EJ, Bosse MJ: Factors influencing outcome following limb-threatening lower limb trauma: Lessons learned from the Lower Extremity Assessment Project (LEAP). *J Am Acad Orthop Surg* 2006 14(10 Spec No.):S205-S210.

37. AAOS Clinical Practice Guideline: *Limb Salvage or Early Amputation*,

2019. Available at: https://www.aaos.org/globalassets/quality-and-practice-resources/dod/limb-salvage-or-early-amputation-1-16-20.pdf. Accessed February 25, 2023.

38. Ly TV, Travison TG, Castillo RC, et al. Ability of lower-extremity injury severity scores to predict functional outcome after limb salvage. *J Bone Joint Surg Am* 2008;90(8):1738-1743.

39. Sheean AJ, Krueger CA, Napierala MA, et al. Evaluation of the mangled extremity severity score in combat-related type III open tibia fracture. *J Orthop Trauma* 2014;28(9):523-526.

40. Lynch K, Johansen K: Can Doppler pressure measurement replace "exclusion" arteriography in the diagnosis of occult extremity arterial trauma? *Ann Surg* 1991;214(6):737-741.

41. Lange RH, Bach AW, Hansen ST Jr, Johansen KH: Open tibial fractures with associated vascular injuries: Prognosis for limb salvage. *J Trauma* 1985;25(3):203-208.

42. Lange RH: Limb reconstruction versus amputation decision making in massive lower extremity trauma. *Clin Orthop Relat Res* 1989;243:92-99.

43. Russell WL, Sailors DM, Whittle TB, Fisher DF Jr, Burns RP: Limb salvage versus traumatic amputation: A decision based on a seven-part predictive index. *Ann Surg* 1991;213(5):473-480.

44. Johansen K, Daines M, Howey T, Helfet D, Hansen ST Jr: Objective criteria accurately predict amputation following lower extremity trauma. *J Trauma* 1990;30(5):568-572.

45. Howe HR Jr, Poole GV Jr, Hansen KJ, et al: Salvage of lower extremities following combined orthopedic and vascular trauma: A predictive salvage index. *Am Surg* 1987;53(4):205-208.

46. Fowler J, Macintyre N. Rehman S, Gaughan JP, Leslie S: The importance of surgical sequence in the treatment of lower extremity injuries with concomitant vascular injury: A meta-analysis. *Injury* 2009;40(1):72-76.

47. Halvorson JJ, Anz A, Langfitt M, et al: Vascular injury associated with extremity trauma: Initial diagnosis and management. *J Am Acad Orthop Surg* 2011;19(8):495-504.

48. Bosse MJ, McCarthy ML, Jones AL, et al: The insensate foot following severe lower extremity trauma: An indication for amputation? *J Bone Joint Surg Am* 2005;87(12):2601-2608.

49. Gregory RT, Gould RJ, Peclet M, et al. The mangled extremity syndrome (M.E.S.): A severity grading system for multisystem injury of the extremity. *J Trauma* 1985;25(12):1147-1150.

50. MacKenzie EJ, Bosse MJ, Kellam JF, et al: Early predictors of long-term work disability after major limb trauma. *J Trauma* 2006;61(3):688-694.

51. MacKenzie EJ, Bosse MJ, Pollak AN, et al: Long-term persistence of disability following severe lower-limb trauma: Results of a seven-year follow-up. *J Bone Joint Surg Am* 2005;87(8):1801-1809.

52. MacKenzie EJ, Bosse MJ, Kellam JF, et al: Characterization of patients with high-energy lower extremity trauma. *J Orthop Trauma* 2000;14(7):455-466.

53. Bosse MJ, MacKenzie EJ, Kellam JF, et al: An analysis of outcomes of reconstruction or amputation after leg-threatening injuries. *N Engl J Med* 2002;347(24):1924-1931.

54. Doukas WC, Hayda RA, Frisch HM, et al: The Military Extremity Trauma Amputation/Limb Salvage (METALS) study: Outcomes of amputation versus limb salvage following major lower-extremity trauma. *J Bone Joint Surg Am* 2013;95(2):138-145.

55. O'Toole RV, Castillo RC, Pollak AN, MacKenzie EJ, Bosse MJ, LEAP Study Group: Determinants of patient satisfaction after severe lower-extremity injuries. *J Bone Joint Surg Am* 2008;90(6):1206-1211.

56. Castillo RC, MacKenzie EJ, Archer KR, et al: Evidence of beneficial effect of physical therapy after lower-extremity trauma. *Arch Phys Med Rehabil* 2008;89(10):1873-1879.

Prosthetic Gait: Biomechanical Analysis and Clinical Assessment

John T. Brinkmann, MA, CPO/L, FAAOP(D) • Siobhán Strike, PhD

ABSTRACT

An understanding of gait is essential for maximizing the mobility and function of the user of lower limb prostheses. Instrumented and observational gait analysis is valuable for guiding clinical decisions and in assessing treatment outcomes. A detailed understanding of the kinematic (motion) and kinetic (force) patterns of the hip, knee, and ankle during walking in individuals without limb absence will aid the clinician in restoring a competent, efficient, and adaptable gait pattern in prosthesis users and improve functional performance in real-world locomotive tasks. Gait deviations in prosthesis users are complex and dynamic and influenced by the level of limb loss and the prosthetic components chosen by the clinician. Understanding how patient factors (eg, strength and range of motion) and prosthetic factors (eg, fit and alignment) influence gait is essential for effective prosthetic care.

Keywords: gait analysis; gait deviations; joint kinetics and kinematics; observational gait assessment; prosthetic alignment

Introduction

The overall goal of rehabilitation after lower limb amputation is to support a level of function commensurate with the individual's functional capabilities before amputation. Walking is a common activity of daily living and regaining walking ability is a high priority for most individuals following an amputation.[1,2] Successful walking involves transporting the body safely and efficiently from one place to another. To achieve this, each limb must support the body in turn and advance forward while transitioning weight bearing from one limb to the other. During prosthetic gait this is achieved by matching, as closely as possible, the patient's preamputation kinetic and kinematic gait parameters. However, practitioners should expect that structural asymmetries caused by amputation will result in kinetic and kinematic asymmetries even after successful rehabilitation.[3,4]

Prosthetic gait that deviates excessively from normal parameters can have detrimental physical and functional effects, including inappropriate distribution of forces on the residual limb, increased loading of the contralateral limb, and increased energy expenditure.[5-7] Long-term altered biomechanics can contribute to the development of orthopaedic problems, including osteoarthritis.[8,9] Gait deviations should be minimized as much as possible to mitigate these deleterious effects.

Gait deviations are observed and addressed by applying established clinical principles and professional judgment to arrive at the most appropriate gait pattern for each individual. Instrumented gait analysis (IGA) can be used to identify, quantify, and understand the effect of lower limb absence and can facilitate appropriate prescription and clinical decision-making for patients. This chapter explores the mechanics of walking, determined through IGA, to explain the changes that occur when using a prosthesis. The relationship between these biomechanical principles, important clinical phenomena determined through observational gait assessment, and prosthetic implications are discussed throughout the chapter.

Biomechanical Goals of Human Locomotion

To be able to progress stably and efficiently, the lower limbs act as a system of rotating elements coupled in series. Each segment stores and releases energy through passive absorption of strain energy or through active muscle activation. The linked segments, known as the kinematic chain, enhance the range of motion and overall load-bearing capacity of the body. This results in a multifaceted, complex system. Prosthetic replacement of an absent limb alters

---

John T. Brinkmann or an immediate family member serves as a board member, owner, officer, or committee member of the American Academy of Orthotists and the Prosthetists. Neither Dr. Strike nor any immediate family member has received anything of value from or has stock or stock options held in a commercial company or institution related directly or indirectly to the subject of this chapter.

This chapter is adapted from Queen RM, Orendurff M: Amputee gait: normal and abnormal and Brinkmann, JB, Stevens PM: Clinical considerations of observational gait analysis, in Krajbich JI, Pinzur MS, Potter BK, Stevens PM, eds: *Atlas of Amputations and Limb Deficiencies: Surgical, Prosthetic, and Rehabilitation Principles*, ed 4. American Academy of Orthopaedic Surgeons, 2016, pp 69-95.

this highly coordinated system and can alter an individual's ability to move effectively.

Progression

The ultimate goal of walking is to be able to move the body forward using the intact body segments and the prosthesis for support and to enable propulsion. The body's center of mass (CoM) follows a wave-like sinusoidal motion. The body descends forward from its maximum height during single support to the low point during double support, and then must be lifted forward and upward again to rise from double support to the subsequent single-limb support. An input of energy from both limbs through concentric muscle contractions is required to enable the step-to-step transition, with the trail leg pushing and the lead limb pulling the body onto the lead limb. Eccentric muscle contractions act to control the body as it falls sequentially from one limb to the other. By understanding the primary mechanisms by which the muscles and joints act to enable progression, the requirements of the prosthesis and how its alignment can influence progression can be understood. Adequate step length, achieved through foot clearance in swing, is required for effective progression. The length and frequency of each step determine walking speed, which is a key measure of rehabilitation and functional capability. The speed of walking reduces with higher levels of amputation and less responsive prostheses.

Stability

Progression can only be accomplished if the limbs can support the body in single support and can safely transfer load from one limb to the other. To be able to walk, the stance foot must be stable on the floor and the swinging limb must be able to clear obstacles. Stability is challenged during walking because the body is top heavy and the body segments are constantly moving, so dynamic stability is required for effective walking. The reduced proprioception and altered walking pattern of people with lower limb absence has been associated with poorer balance and responsiveness to perturbations[10] and increased fall risk.[11] This is heightened by inability to compensate and adapt to changing walking surfaces.[12] A prosthesis must be sufficiently stiff to enable stable contact with the floor and sufficiently compliant to enable progression. In an attempt to reduce the risk of falling, prosthesis users evoke a larger margin of stability compared with people with no disability.[13]

A more recent interpretation of stability also includes analyzing the variability of the repeating signal, which can indicate fluctuations between gait cycles.[14,15] Slight differences between gait cycles are normal as one stride rarely exactly matches the next stride because of the highly complex and coordinated link-segment human body. Some variability is desirable as it allows for adaptations to the environment. However, too much variability between stride cycles has been associated with inefficiency and falling.[11,16] Furthermore, if there is little variability between movement cycles (every stride is similar to the ones before and after) the walker is unable to adapt to different stimuli or to the changes in the environment, such as a nudge or changing surface, and may lose confidence when walking in the community. The effect of limb absence, prosthetic componentry, and alignment on gait variability is not well understood. Further research is required to determine the appropriate healthy thresholds of variability which is neither too great (leading to inefficiency and poor balance control) nor too low (leading to reduced ability to adapt to the environment).[14]

Efficiency

To be sustainable, walking must not be too tiring. In normal walking, the interplay between kinetic and potential energy through the gait cycle, coupled with synergistic muscle contractions across joints, along with making use of muscle stretch during an eccentric contraction before a concentric contraction (the stretch-shortening cycle), reduces the metabolic cost required to progress the body. The energy cost of walking increases with more proximal levels of limb absence as a consequence of the missing anatomy, and can be influenced by prosthetic technology. Habitual self-selected walking speed can be used as an indicator of efficiency as energy expenditure is normally lowest at this speed.

When walking with a prosthesis, impaired control, poor proprioception, muscle absence and weakness, and pain all may challenge the body's ability to achieve an efficient and symmetrical step-over-step walking pattern. The prosthesis should make use of all the force and energy resources both internal and external to the body, to enable progression which is energy efficient but not at the cost of maintaining a stable base of support. The level of amputation, mechanics and alignment of the prosthesis and the type and fit of the socket will affect walking ability and efficiency. For example, the gait deviations observed during transfemoral prosthetic gait are more common and more noticeable than those associated with transtibial prosthetic gait. The relatively bony nature of the transtibial limb generally facilitates control of the prosthesis, and the redundant soft tissues of the transfemoral limb often present a challenge in achieving consistent prosthetic control. In addition, the shortened anatomic lever arm of the more proximal residual limb, the increased lever arm of the prosthesis, and additional loss of muscular control of the residual limb further reduce a patient's ability to control their gait pattern while wearing a transfemoral prosthesis. This is evident throughout the gait cycle and across all planes, but in particular in the coronal plane instabilities common at the transfemoral level, and in the challenges in maintaining sagittal plane knee stability during standing and ambulation.

Phases of the Gait Cycle

Walking is a cyclic activity–the movement is repeated over and over and ideally should be symmetrical between the two limbs. The gait cycle is used to give a framework for analysis. It is now well accepted that the gait cycle starts and ends with initial contact of one foot with the floor. A **stride** is defined from initial contact of one foot to the next initial contact of that foot, whereas a **step** is initial contact of one foot to the initial contact of the other foot. Step is the term often used clinically to describe the portion of this cycle when the limb is in the swing phase. For more clarity, the swing and stance phases of a step should be described explicitly when referring to a step.

The gait cycle is broadly divided into two phases: stance and swing. The stance phase is defined by the foot being in contact with the ground and swing is defined by the foot moving through the air. The stance phase comprises approximately 60% of the gait cycle and the swing phase about 40%. Single support is defined as only one foot is in contact with the ground while the contralateral limb is in swing. There are two periods of double support, when both limbs are in stance, each comprising about 10% of the gait cycle. (Double support distinguishes walking from running, which has no double support and involves a period of flight when neither foot is in contact with the support surface.) The first double support phase is frequently known as the loading phase whereas the second double support phase is frequently called the propulsion phase (**Figure 1**).

Different subphasing systems are used and the two most common are Perry's five phases of stance and three of swing[17] and Kirtley's three phases of stance and two phases of swing[18] (**Figure 1**). Kirtley's phases are becoming more popular, make the dynamic walking theory (outlined in the next section) easier to conceptualize, and allow a sensible interpretation of the coordination of both limbs as they achieve their tasks simultaneously. Loading of the ipsilateral limb, which is in front of the CoM, causes it to decelerate. At the same time, the contralateral limb is in propulsion, accelerating the CoM. This interaction has been established as important to achieving progression.

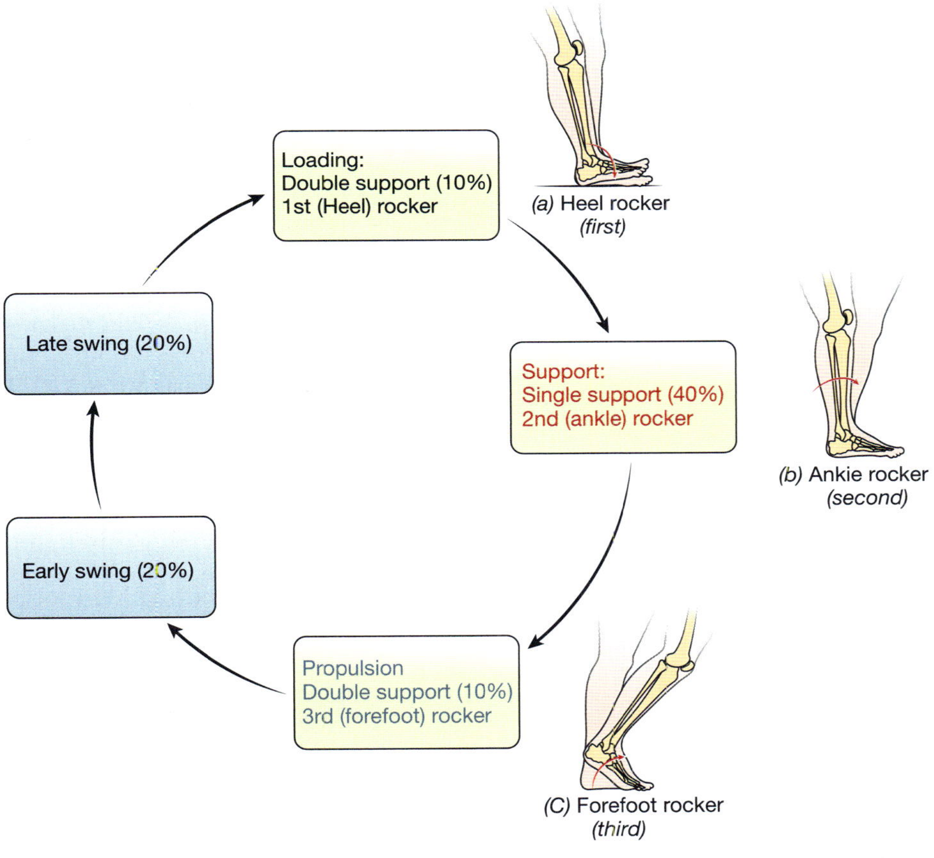

Theoretical Models of Gait

Different models have been used to analyze how individuals walk, and the simplest models consider the movement of the CoM. Horizontal and vertical velocity are not constant. During loading, the lead limb is in front of the CoM and acts to decelerate it and to ensure the forward motion of the trunk. The muscles of the lead limb must contract to accelerate the body forward and upward. This process costs energy. After World War II, one of the earliest quantitative gait analyses of normal and prosthetic gait described six determinants of gait[19] to explain these energy changes. This analysis detailed the individual and integrated requirements of joint rotations and suggested that the limbs act to minimize the vertical movement of the CoM. However, although this model is conceptually useful, it is not generally used because it is limited in application—the energy cost of walking is not fully explained using this model because the CoM oscillates more than the model predicts.

Cavagna et al[20] developed an alternative model, which considered the body as an inverted pendulum. The CoM moves in an arc-like trajectory while sitting on top of a rigid pendulum (the leg) during stance, using gravitational potential energy for forward progression. Although this is an informative model, the energy cost of walking is much greater than the model suggests. This indicates the limitations of considering the limbs as nonjointed rods and highlights the importance of flexion and extension at the joints to achieve efficient progression.

The dynamic walking model has recently gained widespread acceptance[21] (**Figure 2**). This model highlights the importance of the step-to-step transition

FIGURE 1 Illustration of the subphases of the gait cycle. Loading begins with ipsilateral initial contact and ends with contralateral foot off. It is the first period of double support. Support is defined by the period of single support. Propulsion is defined by the second period of double support and begins with contralateral initial contact and ends with ipsilateral foot-off. Swing begins at foot-off and ends with initial contact and is split into two phases, determined by knee flexion and knee extension. Perry outlined the importance of the rockers to successful walking and this is detailed in the text. (Drawings reprinted with permission from Abu-Faraj ZO, Harris GF, Smith PA, Hassani S: Human gait and clinical movement analysis, in Webster JG, ed: *Wiley Encyclopedia of Electrical and Electronics Engineering*, ed 2. John Wiley & Sons, 2015, pp 1-34.)

between each single support. The transition emphasizes the need to redirect the CoM velocity when moving from one leg to the next. This model makes a convincing argument that the push from the trailing limb in late stance balances the braking from the leading limb in early stance to allow a smooth transition from one limb to the next. This theory provides a useful framework to understand why the limbs act as they do and why particular compensatory mechanisms are adopted or pathologies result. For example, the theory explains why the energy cost of walking is higher for people using a prosthesis as the trailing prosthetic limb cannot push the leading, contralateral intact limb into its stance. The intact leading limb experiences higher forces and increased energy contributions to enable the step-to-step transition. Because the prosthesis does not effectively accelerate the body over the intact side, the intact side has to work harder and experiences greater forces to compensate.[22]

The acceleration of the center of mass is reflected in the ground reaction force (GRF) which has direction and magnitude, represented by a vector (GRV). The body's momentum is related to the impulse (force × time) generated under the feet. The vertical acceleration of the CoM can be interpreted through the vertical GRF (vGRF)[22,23] (**Figure 3**). The higher magnitude of the forces on the intact limb[24] (**Figure 3**, dotted lines) may be a reason for loading-related comorbidities such as joint pain and osteoarthritis at joints of that limb.[25] This illustrates the limited capacity of the prosthesis to replace the active contractions by the muscles to accelerate the body when walking, evidenced by the lower magnitude of vGRF (**Figure 3**, solid lines). A value of 10 N/kg equates to almost one body weight (BW). In walking, magnitudes of a little over 10 N/kg are typical, and these will increase with faster walking and reduce with slower walking. Magnitudes of approximately 15 to 25 N/kg are experienced during jogging and running, while values of over 30 N/kg may be experienced when landing from a jump.

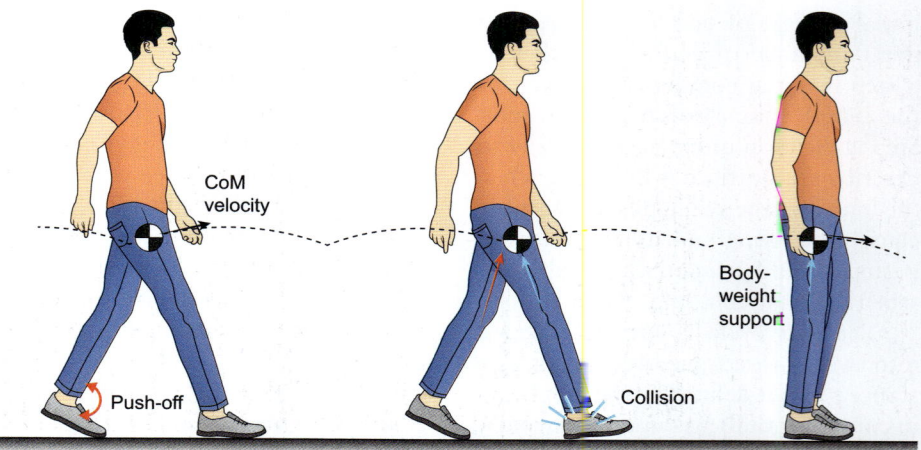

FIGURE 2 Illustration of the dynamic walking model. This model suggests that most of the energy to achieve progression is achieved through passive leg dynamics. The collision of the lead leg reorients the trajectory of the center of mass (CoM) from downward to upward. The collision causes energy to be lost and this is replaced through the positive work completed by the trailing leg, highlighting the requirements for the step-to-step transition. Push-off from the trailing limb (first person) enables rollover onto the leading limb (middle person) to enable single support with a high CoM (last person). (Reprinted from Kuo AD, Donelan JM: Dynamic principles of gait and their clinical implications. *Phys Ther* 2010;90[2]:157-174, by permission of Oxford University Press.)

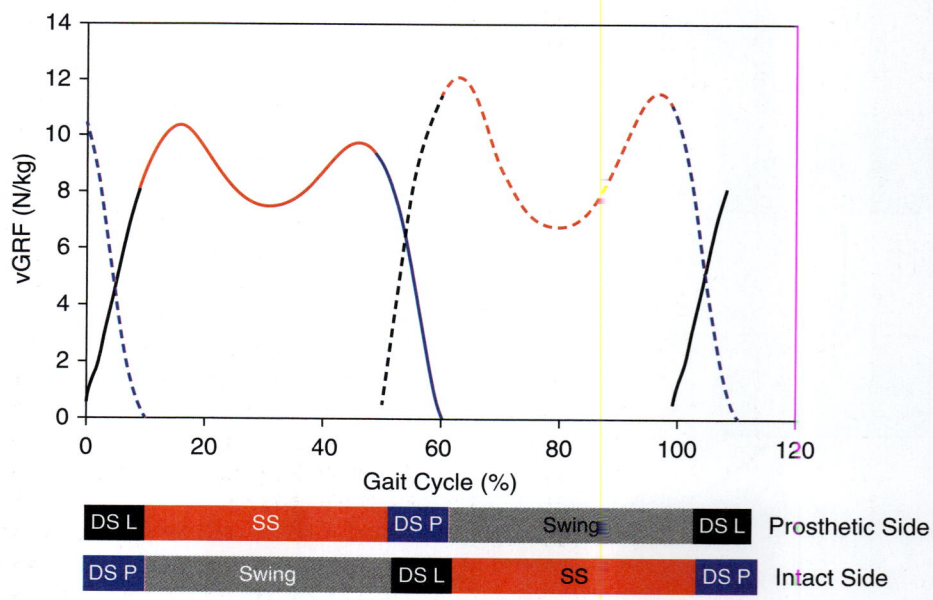

FIGURE 3 Graph illustrating vertical ground reaction force (vGRF) for the prosthetic (solid line) and intact (dotted) sides of one person with a transtibial amputation (TTA) walking at their self-selected habitual speed. When the limb is in stance the vGRF increases as the limb is loaded. The forces are lower on the prosthetic side compared to the intact side (see text for an explanation). The reduced peak on the prosthetic side during the propulsion (DS P) phase may be related to the increased peak on the intact side during the loading phase (DS L). The black portion of the signal relates to the loading double support phase (DS L), the red portion to single support (SS) and the blue portion to the propulsion double support phase (DS P). When the limb is in swing, no forces are recorded as the limb is not in contact with the ground.

Instrumented Gait Analysis

Walking is the most common activity of daily living and also one of the most researched human movements, allowing a relatively good understanding of how the anatomy and mechanics work to produce movement. Using quantitative IGA (objective measurement of specific variables) has enhanced understanding of how missing anatomic segments can be more effectively replaced. Gait analysis allows identification of the causes of altered joint actions and how different prosthetic designs affect them. More sophisticated prostheses,[24] better fitting sockets,[26] and greater attention to appropriate alignment[27] have resulted in improved walking patterns for prosthesis users.

Four main types of data can be recorded, often simultaneously, depending on the level of sophistication of the IGA system: temporospatial, kinematics, kinetics, and electromyography. Of these, temporospatial variables are the least complicated and expensive to collect and analyze but are not able to identify the cause of the deviation. Kinematic variables relate to those that can be seen—linear and angular (joint) displacement, velocity, and acceleration. These require a video and/or (electro)goniometer to record the motion. Careful placement of the equipment is required to acquire valid and reliable data. Kinetic data require the measurement of forces. Quantifying kinetic data requires expensive equipment and specialist training for interpretation. However, this allows a better understanding of the cause and effect of the deviation. Electromyography data quantify the timing and intensity of the muscle contraction and also require specialist training and equipment. Excellent resources on how to collect and interpret gait data are available.[17,18,28-30]

Practitioners in most clinical settings do not have access to three-dimensional IGA and must rely on unassisted observation as the primary method for identifying pathologic gait patterns. Several limitations are inherent in observational assessment. First, many factors that influence gait are not directly observable. For example, the pressure of the residual limb against the socket and the corresponding joint moments caused by those pressures can only be directly observed using equipment and methods not available in most clinical settings. Second, observational gait assessment also has been demonstrated to have limited validity and reliability for gait-related events in neuromuscular and musculoskeletal pathologies.[31,32] Studies focused specifically on individuals using lower limb prostheses have confirmed this limitation.[33] However, because resources and expertise are limited, observational gait assessment and clinical judgment remain the primary strategies for assessing prosthetic gait clinically. With a proper understanding of the mechanics of the gait cycle, the relationship between joint moments, and the influence of prosthetic alignment, many commonly observed deviations can be resolved effectively using these clinical strategies.

Analyzing the temporal (time) and spatial (distance) characteristics of the gait cycle allows the practitioner to determine the quality of the walking performance. Along with age,[34] strength,[35] rehabilitation,[36] engagement with physical activity,[37] prosthetic components,[38] time and experience using the prosthesis,[39] the environment, and performing secondary tasks all have been shown to affect the temporospatial variables.

Walking speed can easily be calculated by measuring the time it takes to complete a defined distance using simply a stopwatch and measuring tape. Different lengths of walk can be used, depending on ability. Typically, walking speed is determined over 10 m. For example, if a person takes 11 s to complete 10 m, their average walking speed is $10/11 = 0.91$ m.s^{-1}. Walking speed is determined by the stride length and the stride frequency. A **stride** includes two steps. Step length is defined by the distance the limb moves forward in front of the supporting limb (**Figure 4**). The right step is defined by initial contact of the left foot to initial contact of the right foot, that is, the foot advancing during swing defines the step.

Average stride length can be quantified by dividing the distance walked by the number of strides. If a person takes seven strides to cover 10 m, their average stride length is $10/7 = 1.43$ m. If the step length is symmetrical, then a step length is half the stride length.

Step length and time asymmetries are common in prosthetic gait and indicate that the remaining limbs and the prosthesis are not able to completely replace the function of the missing anatomy.[40,41] Some common causes of differences associated with the prosthesis are detailed in the next section.

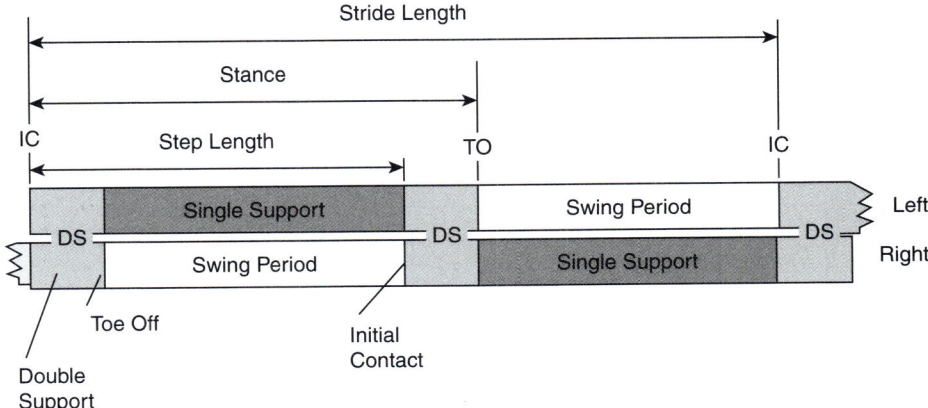

FIGURE 4 Illustration of the temporal and spatial characteristics of the gait cycle. The amount of time that an individual spends in each phase depends on walking speed and asymmetry between the limbs. When walking slowly, the time in stance increases and the time in swing decreases. People with a unilateral prosthesis usually spend less time in support and have a shorter intact limb step length.

Prosthetic Step Length Asymmetries

Disruptions in the stance and swing ratio are common in prosthetic gait. Step length asymmetries are best observed in the sagittal plane. They can be observed as shortened steps on either side, corresponding with shortened stance periods on the contralateral side. Uneven arm swing, which is often observed during prosthetic gait, may be related to unequal step lengths caused by pain during ambulation or other factors. Clinically, the root causes for the asymmetrical step must be correctly identified in each case, and may not be completely correctable.

A short step on the nonprosthetic side is more common because the prosthetic foot and ankle cannot actively plantarflex, which limits heel rise and push-off. More mobile feet and ankles and those with dynamic energy return can mitigate this and allow a more symmetrical gait when aligned properly and of the correct stiffness. The shortened contralateral step also often results from the patient's reluctance to maintain full body weight on the prosthesis. During propulsion phase on the prosthetic side the contralateral step is shortened by placing the foot on the ground earlier. This is particularly common early in the gait training process, and the patient should be trained to take smaller, more symmetrical steps. Less frequently, a shortened prosthetic step length may be observed. This is often the result of a flexion contracture of the contralateral knee that prevents full extension in terminal swing.

Step length asymmetries are commonly observed during transfemoral prosthetic gait. Sagittal knee stability is of paramount concern as patients transition into the support phase on their prosthetic side and begin to load their prostheses. A large prosthetic step increases the knee flexion moment on the prosthetic side during loading and can decrease knee stability. By taking a shorter prosthetic step patients can reduce the knee flexion moment and achieve greater knee control and stability. Patients may even exhibit a step-to-step gait pattern on the prosthetic side, never advancing the prosthetic foot further forward than the contralateral foot. This increases the knee extension moment on the prosthetic side, increasing stability during the support phase. Because of stability concerns, prosthesis users are often reluctant to shift their weight fully onto their prostheses and allow their body weight to transfer from the heel to the toe of the prosthetic foot throughout the stance phase. In this case, a shortened stance phase on the prosthetic side and a shortened nonprosthetic step allow the patient to offload the prosthesis earlier as they transition to the contralateral (nonprosthetic) limb.

Hip flexion contractures, which are very common at the transfemoral level, prevent the hip on the affected side from attaining sufficient extension to allow a full-length sound side step. Unfortunately, it is very common for this lack of range of motion to not be properly accommodated for in the socket alignment (insufficient initial socket flexion), and this improper alignment is a common source of step length asymmetries observed clinically. Gait training, hip range of motion, and proper alignment all are crucial to maintaining step length asymmetry at the transfemoral level.

At the transtibial level, where knee stability is often less of a concern, patient confidence in the support provided by their sound limb during the stance phase results in them taking a longer step with their prosthetic limb and a relatively shorter step with the nonprosthetic limb. This deviation is especially common in newer amputees and can become habitual if not identified and corrected early in gait training. Improvements may be seen with time, training, and improved confidence in the prosthesis. However, poor habits developed during initial gait training can be very difficult to correct later. During gait training, more emphasis should be placed on step asymmetry achieved by a relatively shorter step on both sides, and developing the habit of loading the prosthetic foot in mid and terminal stance, rather than on a large initial step on the prosthetic side. Instructing the patient to take their first step with the nonprosthetic limb can help them develop confidence in the support provided by the prosthesis during terminal stance.

Kinematics and Kinetics of Gait

In the 1980s to 1990s three seminal research teams codified the gait cycle, highlighting the variables that are commonly used to complete a clinical gait analysis (joint angles, moments, and powers) and their interpretation.[17,28,42] Kinematic variables typically describe the joint angles (**Figure 5, A** through **C**) through the gait cycle, whereas kinetic variables relate to the joint moments (**Figure 5, D** through **F**) and powers (**Figure 5, G** through **I**). IGA systems which involve motion capture and force plates allow quantification of the kinematics and kinetics of gait. These variables are interpreted in the context of the requirements of each subphase of the gait cycle (**Figure 1**) and the mechanisms that are required to meet these demands.

Internal joint moments indicate the net force of the muscles that act to cause rotation at the joint. These muscle moments resist the inertial forces/moments produced by the external GRV. If the joint velocity and moment are in the same direction, a concentric contraction is occurring at the joint. Positive power indicates this type of contraction. When muscles contract concentrically (shortening) they act as accelerators and energy generators. If the joint velocity and moment are in opposite directions, an eccentric contraction is occurring. When muscles contract eccentrically (lengthening) they act as decelerators and energy absorbers. A negative power indicates an eccentric contraction. For example, in single support, the ankle is dorsiflexing while the plantarflexors are contracting. As the joint velocity and moment are in opposite directions, a negative power burst indicates this eccentric contraction by the plantarflexors to control the progress of the leg over the foot during the second ankle rocker, known as A1S. However, in late single support and double support propulsion, the ankle is plantarflexing with an internal plantarflexor moment. The velocity and moment are in the same direction and a positive power burst indicates this concentric contraction to lift the limb into swing and shift the weight onto the contralateral limb, known as A2S.

The specific power bursts in the sagittal plane (**Figure 5, G** through **I**: A1S, A2S, K1–4S, H1–3S) and in the frontal plane (H1–2F) were detailed by Winter[28] and Gage[42] and are referred to in the following sections. Their research highlighted the key variables associated with effective walking gait, though the relative contribution of these variables is still controversial, particularly with respect to the relative importance of the ankle push-off power in the propulsion phase. Sagittal plane angles, moments, and powers are often the focus of walking research because the movement is greatest in this plane, to enable forward progression.

The effect of reduced motion and function of the prosthetic ankle can be seen in the reduced angles, moments, and powers at the knee and hip.[43] The ankle, knee, and hip joint angles indicate reduced range of motion on the prosthetic side throughout the gait cycle (**Figure 5, A** through **C**). Joint moments indicate reduced moments on the prosthetic side, particularly at the ankle (**Figure 5, D**) and knee (**Figure 5, E**) which has been associated with reduced strength because of long-term disuse.[35] Joint powers indicate reduced powers on the prosthetic side, particularly at the ankle (**Figure 5, G**), indicating the inability of the prosthesis to actively alter the joint orientation, which limits the user's ability to walk at different speeds.[44]

The Loading Phase

During double support loading, the limb must be able to accept weight and transition from the trailing leg (**Table 1**). The limb usually contacts the ground with the heel, with the ankle slightly dorsiflexed (**Figure 5, A**: 0° to 10°), the knee slightly flexed (**Figure 5, B**: 5° to 15°), and the hip flexed (**Figure 5, C**: 30° to 40°). The GRV is behind the ankle and knee and in front of the hip, tending to cause the ankle to plantarflex and the knee and hip to flex. As the foot rolls to foot flat, the ankle slightly plantarflexes, which is controlled by the dorsiflexors contracting eccentrically (creating an internal dorsiflexion moment) to control the lowering of the foot to the floor (**Figure 5, D**). Plantar flexion of the foot during this phase has been described by Perry[17] as the first rocker.

Knee flexion is controlled by eccentric contraction of the extensors (creating an internal knee extension moment) (**Figure 5, B, E,** and **H**). This serves as a power-absorbing mechanism (K1S) that facilitates the smooth foot-to-foot transition (**Figure 5, H**). The hip extends as a result of a concentric contraction by the hip extensors (H1S), actively pulling the body up toward single support (**Figure 5, G** and **I**).

In the frontal plane, the motion primarily occurs at the hip joint. Here, as the GRV passes medial to the joint, the hip abductors contract to maintain a stable pelvis and minimize pelvic drop (H1F).

If the push-off from the contralateral limb is not effective, the joints on the limb in the loading phase must compensate to enable the transition to the limb and to enable the body to rise up into single support. This is most obvious at the hip, with increases in H1S and to a lesser extent H1F.

Prosthetic Gait During Loading Phase

Prosthetic feet have differing properties and thus will influence the loading phase differently. The soft cushion heel of the solid ankle, cushion heel foot, or a foot with a single (sagittal plane) axis mimics the eccentric action of the dorsiflexors during loading, and allows for some shock absorption. A prosthetic foot with a soft heel also reduces the knee flexion moment during loading. A dynamic heel component compresses and stores energy, and this can aid in transition load onto the keel of the foot. All of these design features can result in a more natural first rocker. However, a softer heel shortens the prosthesis during loading, and can result in excessive vertical lowering of the CoM and an asymmetrical gait pattern. Excessive heel softness also can be problematic by increasing the knee extension moment during midstance and compromising the transition to terminal stance.

A firm heel of the prosthetic foot or shoe increases the knee flexion moment during loading. This often results in a shortened prosthetic step to avoid the GRV passing too far posterior to the knee, causing instability, and also limits the knee flexion required to achieve foot flat during the first rocker. For those users who do not shorten the step, a large push-off contralaterally by the intact limb is required to enable the step-to-step transition.

Prosthetic Foot Rotation

Axial rotation of the prosthesis on the residual limb is generally evident by the position and movement of the foot during loading. Rotational control of the transfemoral prosthesis in early stance is affected by the fleshy nature of the residual limb and the comparative lack of underlying bony anatomy, as well as the strength of the remaining musculature. Rotation can be caused by a socket that is either too loose (allowing motion between the socket and residual limb) or too tight (in response to muscle contractions). External rotation of the foot during the loading phase may occur if the heel of the foot or the shoe is too stiff. Ischial containment transfemoral sockets include aggressive proximal contours that may be uncomfortable, causing the patient to don the prosthesis in a rotated position to improve comfort. Accordingly, appropriate transverse plane alignment proximally at the level of the socket should be established, with subsequent positioning of the knee and foot in relation to the properly positioned socket. Chronic rotational problems, or a prosthesis position that alternates between internal and external rotation, may be indicative of poor hip control, and may require strengthening and gait retraining to resolve. Episodic, inconsistent rotation of the prosthesis may be caused by movement of the socket on a soft, fleshy residual limb.

Aberrant Stance Flexion

Limited and controlled knee flexion of 10° to 15° is desirable during the

Section 1: General Principles

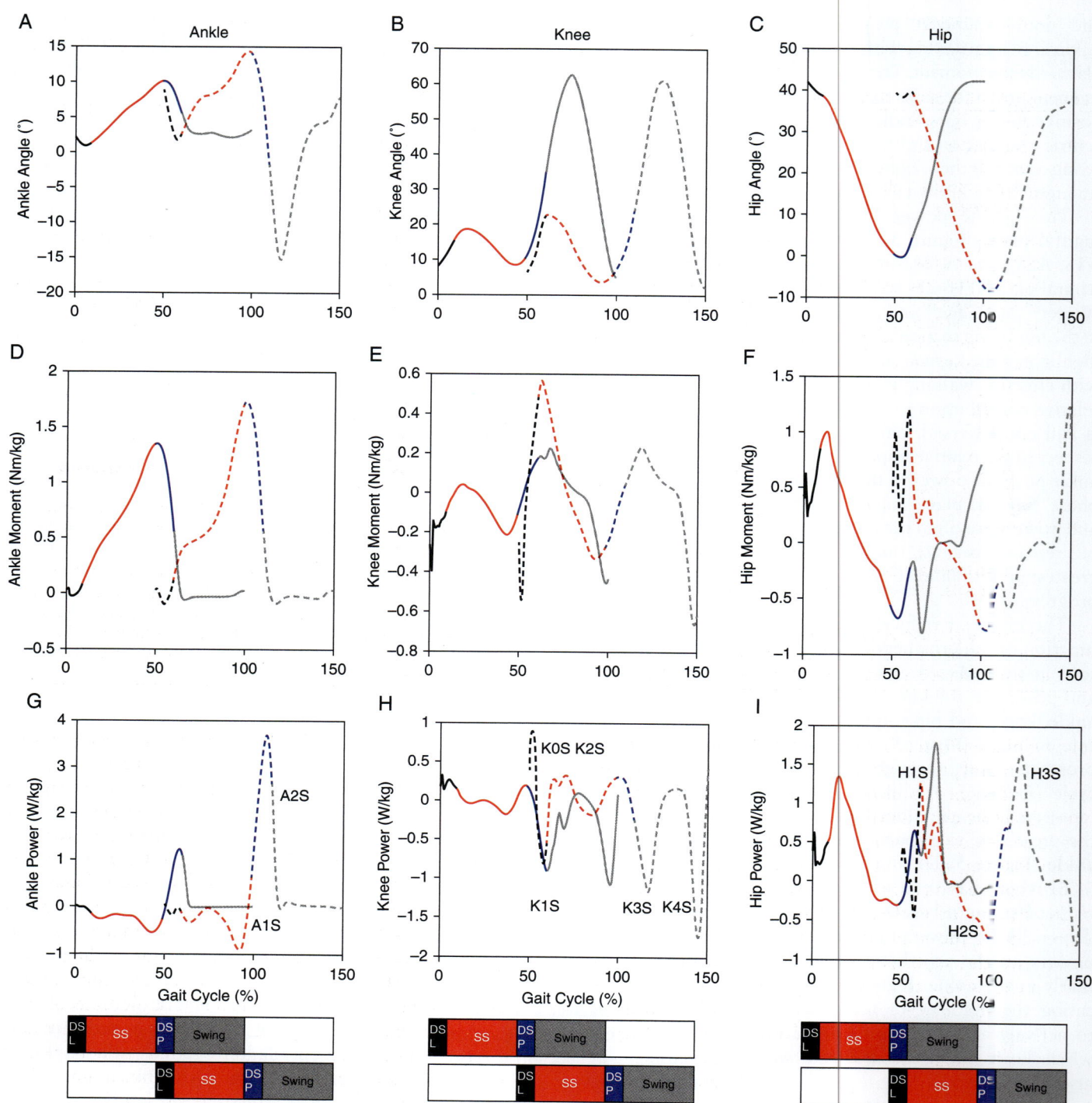

FIGURE 5 Graphs illustrating the mean ankle, knee, and hip joint angles (**A** through **C**), moments (**D** through **F**), and powers (**G** through **I**) for the prosthetic (solid) and intact (dashed) limbs for patients with a transtibial amputation wearing a dynamic prosthesis ($n = 23$). Loading (DS L) is colored black, single support (SS) is red, and propulsion (DS P) blue. Swing is colored gray. The data are presented to indicate the joint actions in time—when the prosthetic limb is in loading (solid black), the intact limb is in propulsion (dashed blue). Positive values indicate dorsiflexion and knee and hip flexion (**A** through **C**); ankle internal plantarflexor, knee and hip internal extensor moments (**D** through **F**); concentric contractions at the joints (**G** through **I**). Key power bursts are indicated according to the convention for the intact side.

TABLE 1 Loading and Propulsion Phases: Task Requirement and Key Mechanisms, Deviations, and Adaptations to Achieve the Requirement

Loading (0%-10% of the Gait Cycle)	Propulsion (50%-60% of the Gait Cycle)
Overall phase requirement: • Safe contact with floor • Absorb shock • Accept load onto the limb • Active load bearing Joint mechanics: The external ground reaction force vector (GRV) causes an external plantarflexor, knee and hip flexor moment which is counteracted by an internal dorsiflexor moment which controls the plantar flexion and lowers the foot to the floor; knee and hip extensor moment which stop the limb from collapsing. The H1S power burst extends the hip and helps to raise the body over the stance limb. 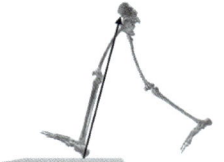 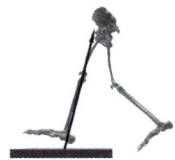 Intact side (left) loading shows the position of the GRV relative to the joints. The muscles about the joints contract to stop the limb from collapsing. Prosthetic side (right) shows how the reduced step length influences the magnitude and direction of the GRV. A longer step may increase the external moment at the knee and compromise joint stability.	Overall phase requirement: • Facilitate initial contact of the other limb • Initiate advancement into swing • Weight shift Joint mechanics: Powerful concentric plantarflexor contraction (A2S) helps to propel the limb into swing. Eccentric knee extensor contraction controls knee flexion (K3S). Hip concentric flexor contraction (H3) helps to propel the limb into swing. 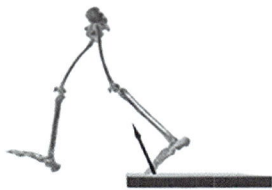 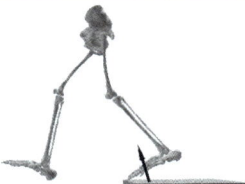 Intact side (left) shows the relatively large GRV. The ankle muscles produce A2S, propel the body into the next stance phase and accelerate the limb into swing. Prosthetic side (right) shows the reduced push-off power from the prosthetic side which may not accelerate the body sufficiently to counteract the deceleration caused by the leading limb's foot contact and this is costly in both mechanical and metabolic terms. Foot stiffness influences heel rise and may also cause drop-off—the knee suddenly and prematurely flexes.

loading phase (**Figure 5**). Achieving this in transfemoral prosthetic gait requires a knee unit designed to allow this motion. Several factors can contribute to excessive knee flexion moments and motion during loading, including excessive dorsiflexion of the foot, excessive transtibial socket flexion, an excessively posterior placement of the foot underneath the socket (which lengthens the heel lever), and an excessively stiff prosthetic heel. A similar effect is seen when an individual changes the shoe of the prosthesis to one with a higher heel, which places the socket in a more flexed position and inclines the shank. Patients wearing a transtibial prosthesis with limited ability to eccentrically contract their knee extensors during the loading phase, either because of quadriceps weakness or because of the resultant discomfort created in the socket, can also exhibit excessive knee flexion during this phase. Individuals with shorter residual limb lengths have a shorter lever available to control the prosthesis and are more prone to anterior distal tibial pressures in the socket, both of which can exacerbate this problem.

Although less frequently observed, reduced or absent knee flexion during the loading phase can be problematic, and in extreme cases hyperextension may be observed. Excessive extension of the socket, an excessively anterior foot placement beneath the socket (which lengthens the toe lever), excessive plantar flexion, or an excessively stiff prosthetic keel all are prosthetic factors that can contribute to this deviation. Alternatively, the patient may voluntarily or involuntarily limit knee flexion early in stance as a way of compensating for weak quadriceps. Reducing the knee flexion moment by forcibly maintaining an extended knee position helps to prevent inadvertent buckling of the knee.

Different prosthetic knees have different properties that will influence the loading phase. A passive knee must be fully extended at initial contact to ensure stability. This is frequently achieved through a shortened prosthetic step length. The knee remains extended during stance, necessitating the user to raise the CoM higher and quicker, which results in an inefficient step-to-step transition. This requires increased contribution from the contralateral (nonprosthetic) limb while it is in the propulsion phase. Some knee mechanisms include a stance flexion feature, which allows limited and controlled flexion during the loading phase. A stance flexion feature minimizes the need for the user to raise the center of mass as high or quickly. A microprocessor-controlled knee permits a more refined stance flexion that enables a more effective step-to-step transition.[45,46]

The Support Phase

During single support, the limb must be able to support the body without losing balance or collapsing (**Table 2**). Safe swing of the contralateral limb also must be enabled. The GRV passes from behind to in front of the ankle and knee and from in front of the hip to behind it. As the body moves forward over the stable foot, ankle dorsiflexion

Section 1: General Principles

TABLE 2 Support and Swing Phases: Task Requirement and Key Mechanisms, Deviations, and Adaptations to Achieve the Requirement

Support (0%-10% of the Gait Cycle)	Swing (50%-60% of the Gait Cycle)
Overall phase requirement: • Maintain a stable base of support, balance and avoid limb collapse • Facilitate swing of the contralateral limb • Enable forward progression	**Overall phase requirement:** • Advance the limb forward to enable progression • Avoid trips and stumbles • Safely prepare the limb for stance
Joint mechanics: The external ground reaction force vector (GFV) passes from behind to in front of the knee and hip which prevents their collapse and minimizes energy expenditure. The trunk passes in front of the ankle, and the plantarflexors contract eccentrically (A1S) to control the dorsiflexion of the second rocker.	**Joint mechanics:** The ankle dorsiflexes to bring the foot into neutral to avoid its tripping while the knee flexes to shorten the limb. Toward the end of the phase a large eccentric contraction by the knee flexors (K4S) slows the shank to prepare for touchdown.
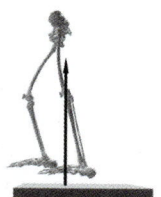 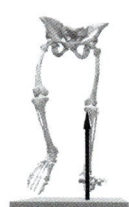	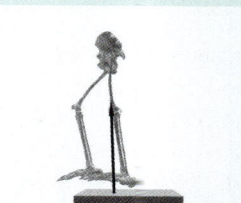
On the prosthetic side sagittal plane (left), the stiffness of the prosthesis and its alignment will influence the location of the GRV as it passes along the foot. Knee instability can be caused by too much dorsiflexion or a knee joint that is positioned too far anteriorly. On the prosthetic side frontal plane (right), the GRV passes medial to the hip. Lateral trunk lean toward the prosthetic side prevents the pelvis and trunk from dropping and assists swing side clearance. Fitting the socket to bear load down the lateral shaft of the femur and strengthening the muscles can reduce this deviation.	Pistoning of the residual limb out of the socket at the beginning of the phase may be because of poor socket fit or residual limb shape changes. This can cause discomfort, skin damage, and compromise toe clearance. Typical deviations to ensure toe clearance include circumduction, vaulting, hip hiking, and trunk lean. The amount of knee flexion will affect the toe clearance and the duration of the swing phase.

(**Figure 5**) is controlled by an eccentric contraction of the plantarflexors (A1S, **Figure 5, G**). This is frequently known as the second rocker.[17] After a small concentric contraction by the knee extensors to extend the knee (K2S), the muscles about the knee do not contract because the GRV passes in front of the knee, keeping the joint stable (**Figure 5, E**). The hip continues to extend as the body passes over the foot (**Figure 5, C**) and this is controlled by the hip flexors eccentrically contracting (H2S, **Figure 5, I**). In the frontal plane, the GRV passes medial to the limb and an eccentric contraction by the hip abductors controls the pelvic drop, an important factor to enable the contralateral limb to swing through.

Prosthetic Gait During Support Phase

Prosthetic sockets must appropriately support the residual limb and load-tolerant areas during loading and support phases of gait to prevent excessive distal movement within the socket. Excessive distal motion during loading can be caused by inappropriate socket contours or overall looseness, and can contribute to discomfort, skin breakdown, and gait deviations. Movement of the residual limb too far distally into the socket may be observed if the residual limb has lost volume (and no longer matches the socket volume) and the socket does not support the residual limb appropriately as it is loaded. Residual limb volume typically reduces significantly for the first 18 to 24 months following amputation, but daily volume fluctuations occur even long after amputation. In common socket designs, daily residual limb volume fluctuations can be accommodated by the addition of socks. Consistent volume reduction may require modifications to the socket size, which is often achieved by the addition of padding. Extreme daily volume fluctuations may require a design that allows the patient to make significant changes to socket size. A new, properly fitted socket may be required in cases of extreme volume reduction.

Some prosthetic feet and ankles dorsiflex during the support phase, mimicking the second rocker. Depending on the shape of an energy storing and return foot, different magnitudes of energy can be stored in the spring of the prosthesis during this phase as the shank moves in front of the ankle (A1S). The stiffness of the prosthetic foot will influence this movement, and thus the effectiveness of the second rocker and the energy stored and available for use in the next phase (**Figure 5, G**).

Knee Instability

Patients with a transfemoral amputation must activate the hip extensors to maintain voluntary control of the knee flexion moment during the loading and support phases. If voluntary control is insufficient or unavailable (because of weakness or improper training), knee stability is dependent only on the inherent stability of the knee design and the alignment of the components. Knee instability can be caused by excessive foot dorsiflexion, a prosthetic heel that is too stiff, or a knee joint positioned too far anteriorly in relation to the socket. Proper selection of the knee control mechanism and alignment is essential for all patients, and particularly those with weak hip extensors or shorter limb lengths who have less voluntary control of the knee unit.

Lateral Trunk Bending

Excessive lateral trunk bending toward the prosthetic side is commonly observed during transfemoral prosthetic gait. In able-bodied ambulation the hip abductors of the stance limb stabilize the pelvis, preventing it from dropping toward the swing side. This assists in clearance of the swing limb and reduced energy expenditure by limiting lateral trunk bending. This mechanism is compromised when amputation severs the distal attachment of the adductor musculature and when the femur is allowed to move laterally within the socket. The abducted position of the hip joint relaxes the abductor musculature, resulting in even less force available to stabilize the pelvis. The reduced adduction musculature (and often weakness), abduction of the hip, and the shortened lever arm of the femur all result in less effective stabilization of the hip joint in adduction. Patients frequently compensate by actively bending their trunk laterally toward the prosthetic side during stance. This action elevates the contralateral pelvis, facilitating swing phase clearance. It also positions the CoM closer to the prosthetic foot, reducing the force pulling the pelvis on the contralateral side toward the floor. This lateral lean also reduces the pressure that the distal lateral end of the femur exerts on the socket.

Assuming a well-fitting socket in which the lateral shaft of the femur is loaded rather than the distal end, with proper training many transfemoral prosthesis users can learn to shift their weight at their hips rather than at their trunk to restore a more balanced gait. However, for individuals with shorter residual limbs or weak hip abductors, some degree of lateral trunk bending may be inevitable.

Excessive lateral trunk bending will occasionally be seen in patients using a transtibial prosthesis during single-limb stance on the prosthetic limb. This typically occurs when a patient is not fully loading their prosthesis, either because of socket discomfort or inadequate training or experience. It may also be a compensation for weak ipsilateral hip abductors, as in the case of transfemoral prosthesis users. If the underlying causes of this deviation are not addressed early in prosthetic gait training for both transtibial and transfemoral prosthesis users, a fixed gait pattern may be established.

Coronal Plane Knee Instability

A modest varus moment at the knee during midstance is generally desirable in transtibial gait, as this mimics normal gait and loads pressure-tolerant areas of the residual limb. Slight inset of the foot beneath the socket is an effective way to create the desired varus moment. Deviations from this pattern may be caused by improper prosthetic alignment or socket fit. General looseness or an excessive medial/lateral dimension of the socket allows the residual limb to move within the socket, and can result in an excessive varus moment. An excessive varus moment may be caused by an excessively inset position of the prosthetic foot beneath the socket. Similarly, an excessive valgus moment may be caused by a prosthetic foot that has been insufficiently inset. (Except in rare cases, prosthetic feet should not be outset, or positioned laterally to the midpoint of the socket, as this can create a valgus moment.) Excessive socket abduction can cause an excessive varus moment, and excessive socket adduction can cause an insufficient varus moment. Changes in step width also can affect the frontal plane moments. For example, as novice walkers gain more confidence and progressively narrow the step width, they begin to experience increasing varus moments. In contrast, a cautious walker who widens the step width when not using an assistive device (such as a walker) may experience a valgus moment at the knee.

The extreme sensitivity of the perineal region increases the challenges of achieving an optimal fit and coronal plane stabilization within a transfemoral socket. No specific socket design, including ischial containment, ensures adequate control of the femur and effective coronal plane stabilization, and subischial designs can provide appropriate coronal plane control. Each socket must be carefully designed to provide optimal control for each patient.

The Propulsion Phase

During this phase, the limb must be able to push the body onto the contralateral limb (which is in loading) and lift into swing. The heel rises as the ankle concentrically plantarflexes (A2S, **Figure 5, G**) and weight shifts forward onto the contralateral limb. This active push-off is well established to be important for forward progression[23,47,48] and is known as the third rocker.[49] Although there remains some controversy as to the relative importance of this action, there is no dispute that is a required element of effective gait.

During propulsion, knee flexion is controlled by eccentric contraction by the knee extensors (K3S, **Figure 5, H**). This flexion is coordinated with the ankle plantar flexion and heel rise (**Figure 5, A**) to control the limb length and to smoothen the movement of the CoM during the step-to-step transition. The knee extensors provide knee stability and enable the push from the ankle while the knee is flexing. Soon after the ankle has actively plantarflexed to push the body over onto the contralateral limb, the hip begins to flex to pull the limb into swing. The active flexion as a result of the hip flexors concentrically contracting (H3S, **Figure 5, I**) is important for initiating swing and completing the transition into single support contralaterally. When using a prosthesis, the reduced ankle push-off power at A2S is compensated for by an increased hip flexor power at H3S, and contralaterally H1S is increased to enable the step-to-step transition (**Figure 5, G and I**).

Prosthetic Gait During Propulsion Phase

Most commercially available prosthetic feet do not provide active concentric plantar flexion contraction at A2S, so push-off on the prosthetic side is reduced (**Figure 5, G**). Because plantar-flexion past neutral is not possible, the third rocker cannot be mimicked. The lift-off of the prosthetic side limb into swing is generally achieved through increased hip flexion and a higher H3S power burst (**Figure 5, C and I**). When using a dynamic (energy storing and return) prosthetic foot, some of the energy that has been stored earlier in stance is returned to accelerate the limb into swing, but this is not equivalent in magnitude to that generated by intact plantarflexors. This remains a critical problem because the push-off power from the prosthetic side does not accelerate the body sufficiently to counteract the deceleration caused by the leading limb's contact with the ground. The resulting loss of momentum in the step-to-step transition is costly in both mechanical and metabolic terms. Early research on powered ankles has shown some benefit from these prostheses to improve gait,[50] but their cost, weight, and limited battery life limit their commercialization currently. When using a passive prosthetic knee mechanism, some knee flexion, controlled by the hip extensors, may be evident and can be improved by training. The timing of knee flexion in terminal stance can be affected by the design and adjustment of the knee mechanism, but is ultimately controlled by the user. A microprocessor-controlled knee can better mimic and control the knee flexion and enable a more realistic and efficient propulsion phase.[45,46,51]

In transtibial gait, premature heel rise can be caused by two opposite malalignments. In the first case, an excessive toe lever increases the extension moment at the knee, and may cause difficulty in forward progression over the foot in mid to late stance on the prosthetic side. To overcome the excessive extension moment, the patient may forcibly roll over the toe of the prosthetic foot, causing the heel to leave the ground earlier in the gait cycle than it normally would. This deviation often corresponds to a patient report of excessive knee extension or hyperextension, and can cause increased exertion during ambulation. Alternatively, the patient may not overcome an excessive knee extension force, which causes the heel to remain on the ground longer in stance.

In the second case, an insufficient toe lever can cause early heel rise as a result of the knee flexion that occurs in terminal stance when the toe lever is insufficient to adequately support the body. "Drop off" in terminal stance (during the propulsion phase) may be observed, as the knee flexes and the heel leaves the ground early in response to inadequate keel stiffness. This deviation often corresponds with a patient report of excessive knee flexion, and can result in abrupt loading of the contralateral limb. This abrupt loading may lead to the premature development of osteoarthritis of the knee and hip.[22,52] Published evidence has consistently supported the position that the stiffer, dynamic resistances associated with energy storage and release in prosthetic feet reduce the drop-off experienced at the end of single-limb support on the prosthesis, with an associated reduction on the loading rate of the sound side limb.[22,53] However, research also indicates that patients prefer a more flexible (compliant) foot with less resistance to rollover during terminal stance, rather than a stiffer foot that may provide more energy storage and return.[54,55] The practitioner must balance the goals of biomechanical optimization and patient preference when selecting components and aligning the prosthesis.

The Swing Phase

During this phase, the limb must advance forward to complete the step, which requires toe clearance in mid swing. At toe-off the ankle returns to a neutral position and remains in neutral throughout swing. From mid swing, the knee extends from its flexed position to near full extension at the end of the phase to prepare for the next ground contact (**Figure 5, B**). The hip flexes through swing from its position of extension at foot-off to flexion at initial contact (**Figure 5, C**) and this is largely completed without any active muscle contractions (**Figure 5, I**). Toward the end of swing, a large eccentric contraction by the knee flexors (K4S, **Figure 5, H**) slows the shank to prepare it for touch down. This slowing reduces the energy lost as the foot contacts the ground. If there is a risk of tripping when the foot is close to the floor, compensation may be induced to shorten the limb and ensure a safe swing.

Prosthetic Gait During Swing Phase

The weight of the prosthesis will affect the swing phase, and a heavy prosthesis, which is more difficult to lift into swing, will swing faster than a lighter prosthesis. For individuals with a bilateral limb absence, the inability to compensate between limbs results in shorter steps, greater trunk involvement, and high energy cost. The trade-off between mobility and stability is more difficult to achieve in these cases.

Excessive Pistoning

Pistoning is the term commonly used to describe vertical movement of the residual limb in relation to the socket, and can be observed during early and mid swing when the residual limb pulls out of the socket. A modest amount of pistoning is to be expected with some suspension methods, including both cuff strap and anatomically contoured socket suspension systems. In other systems, visible pistoning is atypical and warrants further investigation. For example, excessive pistoning when incorporating suction suspension or locking liners may indicate a mechanical flaw or failure of a suspension component. A moderate amount of pistoning may be tolerated by the patient, and patients may prefer a particular suspension method that is less effective at minimizing pistoning but has other beneficial features, such as ease of donning.[26,56,57] Pistoning must be addressed when it causes problematic residual limb pressures, compromises toe clearance, or results in other excessive compensations (excessive vaulting, hip hiking, or trunk lean).

Toe Clearance Strategies

If a patient is concerned about toe clearance they may adopt circumduction, vaulting, hip hiking, or trunk lean strategies. These deviations are common at the transfemoral level because there is less voluntary control of the timing and magnitude of knee flexion to ensure adequate toe clearance. Circumduction involves excessive abduction as the hip flexes during swing phase, which effectively shortens the prosthesis to facilitate toe clearance. Vaulting involves contralateral ankle plantar flexion as the patient rises on the toe of the contralateral foot to lengthen the contralateral limb, raising the pelvis as the prosthesis is in swing. Hip hiking or lateral trunk lean to the contralateral side may be used to elevate the pelvis on the prosthetic side to improve toe clearance. These strategies are seen among both transtibial and transfemoral prosthesis users, and may initially be a result of inexperience and a lack of confidence. For more experienced users, they may persist as an individual walking preference. Deviations intended to ensure toe clearance should be identified and addressed early in the rehabilitation process because they often can become an established compensation strategy that is difficult to improve once they become habitual.

Any actual or functional increase in length of the prosthesis should be considered and addressed when these deviations are observed. Causes of functional lengthening include a prosthetic foot aligned in too much plantar flexion, inadequate suspension (excessive pistoning), insufficient knee flexion, excessive knee extension assist, and excessive prosthetic knee alignment stability. A patient who lacks confidence in the stability of the prosthetic knee, whether because of inexperience or unstable alignment, may adopt one of these toe clearance strategies because they allow the knee to be held in extension during swing to prepare for stable loading. The swing resistance settings of a prosthetic knee mechanism directly affect the magnitude and timing of knee flexion and therefore toe clearance. Knee function should be adjusted to ensure adequate and appropriately timed toe clearance.

Excessive Heel Rise

The swing phase heel rise (which is directly related to the magnitude of swing phase knee flexion) observed in the transfemoral prosthetic gait should match that observed in the contralateral limb. Heel rise increases at faster gait speeds because of the stronger forces acting on the prosthesis. If swing resistance adjustability is available, it can be adjusted until the heel rise of the prosthesis matches that of the sound limb. In mechanical, constant-friction knee designs, heel rise can be modestly adjusted by increasing or decreasing the friction of the knee joint. However, this friction setting remains the same for both swing flexion and extension, and these knee mechanisms will only adapt to very small changes in velocity while the patient is walking. Once the appropriate level of swing resistance has been established, increased walking speeds result in increased heel rise and other gait disruptions. For this reason, these knee designs should only be prescribed for individuals who walk at only one speed. Variable cadence is only functionally possible if the knee mechanism includes hydraulic or pneumatic fluid control of knee flexion resistance. The inherent characteristics of fluid flow make fluid knee cylinders a well-established means of regulating the resistance to knee flexion (and consequently the amount of heel rise) during swing phase. In these designs, resistance to flexion increases in response to the increased walking speeds.

Excessive Terminal Impact

Terminal impact is the physical phenomenon of the knee mechanism reaching full extension in terminal swing. Frequently, patients prefer to experience a distinct terminal impact as it provides confirmation that the knee has reached full extension, ensuring knee stability as body weight is transferred to the prosthesis. This impact, though unsightly and inconsistent with the behavior of the contralateral knee, provides users with a sense of certainty that the prosthesis is in a stable position beneath them. The amount of terminal impact preferred will vary from patient to patient depending on walking experience and confidence in the prosthesis. Just as resistance mechanisms exist to modulate the amount of knee flexion observed in early swing, similar mechanical and fluid mechanisms exist to adjust the rate and magnitude of knee extension in late swing. An extension assist is used to facilitate knee extension, but may also create an excessive terminal impact. Inadequate swing phase resistance or excessive extension assist can cause excessive terminal impact. A knee extension assist mechanism also resists knee flexion. Precise resistance and assistance adjustments are often required to balance control of knee flexion in early swing with knee extension in late swing. Mechanical, constant-friction knee mechanisms represent a significant disadvantage in achieving the appropriate balance of resistances, because the flexion and extension resistance cannot be adjusted independently. Many fluid-controlled knees allow separate adjustment of swing flexion and extension resistance, allowing increased refinement of knee function to achieve a more appropriate gait pattern.

Whips

The prosthetic knee and foot should track along the line of progression as the prosthesis moves through the swing phase. Deviations in the transverse plane from this ideal are described as whips, and are often the product of poor alignment of the knee axis or the whole prosthesis. A prosthetic knee axis that is aligned in excessive internal rotation creates a lateral whip in which the rising heel deviates laterally during early and mid-swing extension. In contrast, a knee axis aligned in excessive external rotation creates a medial whip in which the rising heel deviates medially. A prosthesis donned in excessive internal or external rotation also can create a visible whip by malaligning the knee joint axis. This situation can occur because of inexperience donning the prosthesis or as an intentional effort by the user to increase the comfort of the prosthesis by changing the orientation of the socket brim. As with foot rotation during stance phase, swing phase whips can be the product of a poorly fitting socket. Rotational instabilities are a common problem for transfemoral prosthesis users because of the fleshy nature of the residual limbs and the lack of supporting bony structures within the socket. Clinically, whips are usually consistent motions, and episodic and inconsistent rotation indicates problems with socket fit.

Prosthetic Dynamic Alignment

Prosthetic components are assembled in a particular spatial relationship to each other, which is commonly referred to as the alignment of the prosthesis. Dynamic alignment involves observation of the ambulating patient and optimization of the spatial relationship of the components. Dynamic alignment involves integrating the practitioner's observational assessment and user feedback to detect and reduce common patterns of pathologic gait (deviations) that indicate the need to change the spatial orientation of the components in established ways. Research has demonstrated that, although prosthesis users are able to accurately sense and report changes in prosthetic function resulting from changes in alignment, these reports are less accurate for angular alignment changes of less than 6° and translational alignment changes of less than 20 mm.[58,59]

Although different goals for prosthetic alignment have been suggested, no single optimal alignment has been objectively measured or described.[60] Rather, studies have demonstrated that a range of alignments are acceptable to both patients and prosthetists.[60-62] Although the reduction of asymmetries is a legitimate goal, not all parameters of gait reach the same level of symmetry when a prosthesis is optimally aligned for a particular patient.[63] In addition, a direct relationship between kinetic and kinematic changes should not be assumed.[4] There is evidence that patients consider overall function more important than the presence or degree of gait deviation, so prosthetists must use clinical judgment in determining which deviations should be minimized to ensure optimal long-term health and function.[64]

After confirming the appropriateness of the overall fit and function of the prosthesis, the prosthetist refines the alignment during multiple walking trials. For maximum safety, initial ambulation should occur with the patient supported by parallel bars. Ambulation should then proceed within the clinical environment, using the appropriate assistive devices when needed. Although initial walking trials are usually performed on level terrain, they can also include negotiation of common environmental barriers and terrains, provided that the patient's safety and comfort are ensured. Practitioners must be aware of patient fatigue and residual limb sensitivity during dynamic alignment since these factors impact gait. Alignment is often modified during follow-up visits to ensure that it is appropriate for the patient's current function.

Observational Gait Analysis Tools

Several strategies can be employed to improve gait assessment and dynamic alignment. Advances in hardware and software have made high-definition video recording technology readily accessible to most clinicians. Use of high-quality video (with adequate lighting and correct camera placement) has been shown to improve the reliability of observational gait assessment.[65] A software program with analysis tools has been shown to increase interrater reliability when assessing patients with neuromuscular disorders, and a similar benefit may exist when assessing the gait of prosthesis users.[66] Unassisted observational gait assessment and assessment enhanced by the use of a software program have been shown to allow reliable determination of initial contact and foot-off during prosthetic gait, indicating that both techniques are useful for assessing temporal and spatial parameters.[67] The use of checklists and gait scores has been shown to improve observational gait assessment. The Prosthetic Observational Gait Score (a modification of the Edinburgh Gait Score) was developed to aid prosthetists during observational gait assessment. As with most gait scores, the intraobserver reliability of the Prosthetic Observational Gait Score is greater than the interobserver reliability.[68] Components that record socket reaction moments can assist practitioners in making alignment decisions, and good agreement has been found between alignment using an instrumented component and traditional methods.[69] Because of the similarity with alignments achieved using conventional methods, the instrumented component may be most appropriate for challenging cases or when alignment is performed by less experienced prosthetists.

Factors Affecting Gait Patterns

Patient Factors

Many patients receive a prosthesis after a period of prolonged debilitation, functional status commonly changes over time, and comorbidities affect various aspects of health and function. For these reasons it is especially important for the rehabilitation team to assess how strength, range of motion, and other health factors may contribute to a poor gait pattern. Refinements to alignment and other aspects of prosthetic design are necessary to support each patient's current function as these factors change over time. Many factors related to gait are

TABLE 3 Alignment Adjustments to Affect Toe and Heel Levers

	To Increase	To Decrease
Toe lever	Plantarflex foot	Dorsiflex foot
	Lengthen foot	Shorten foot
	Stiffen keel	Soften keel
	Soften heel	Firmer heel
	Extend socket	Flex socket
	Move foot anterior	Move foot posterior
Heel lever	Dorsiflex foot	Plantarflex foot
	Firmer heel	Soften heel
	Flex socket	Extend socket
	Move foot posterior	Move foot anterior
	Raise heel of shoe	Lower heel of shoe

best addressed through rehabilitation and training rather than adjustments to the prosthesis and are best assessed and addressed in collaboration with a physical therapist.

Prosthetic Factors

Each component of a prosthesis can contribute directly or indirectly to the gait pattern of the patient. The prosthetist is responsible for ensuring that the fit of the prosthetic socket and the associated suspension mechanism are optimal and support the function of the patient. Alignment changes should not be used to address socket fit problems, and advanced components do not obviate the need for proper alignment. In addition, the functional characteristics of the foot, ankle, and knee components can substantially affect the patient's gait pattern and must be selected appropriately. Factors as seemingly benign as the height and density of a shoe's heel can affect the orientation of the foot in the sagittal plane, alter the location of GRFs, and affect proximal joint moments. All relevant factors should be carefully considered during the evaluation, fitting, and alignment process.

During ambulation, GRFs act on the prosthetic foot creating rotational moments between the prosthesis and the residual limb. Different orientations of prosthetic components in relation to each other change the magnitude and direction of these rotational forces, causing different joint and socket reaction moments.[70] Such alignment variations can cause observable kinematic changes, gait deviations, and gait improvements.[71,72] Because these moments affect prosthetic gait in predictable ways, certain gait deviations are commonly observed as a consequence of specific malalignments.[73] Identification of these deviations can guide the prosthetist in adjusting the alignment to reduce inappropriate moments and optimize the gait pattern. Gross malalignments in each plane should be reduced when they are observed. Because sagittal plane malalignments can substantially affect coronal plane moments, it is advisable to finalize the sagittal plane alignment first, followed by the coronal plane alignment.[74]

The spatial orientation of components in a prosthesis is commonly described according to angular and linear relationships. Angular relationships in the sagittal plane involve socket flexion, foot dorsiflexion, socket extension, and foot plantar flexion. In the coronal plane, the angular relationship involves socket abduction, foot eversion, socket adduction, and foot inversion. Linear relationships include anterior and posterior translation of the components in the sagittal plane and medial and lateral translation in the coronal plane. Transverse plane orientation involves internal or external rotation from the line of progression.

As they relate to the prosthetic foot, the design and alignment of prosthetic components impact heel and toe levers and therefore the direction and magnitude of the moments (**Table 3**).

The gait deviation charts (**Tables 4 and 5**) identify appropriate goals, as well as common deviations and their causes during each phase of gait.

Section 1: General Principles

TABLE 4 Transtibial Gait Deviation Chart

Phase	Goals	Deviation	Prosthetic Factors	Patient Factors
Initial contact and loading response	Knee in 5°-10° flexion; equal step length	No knee flexion	Insufficient heel lever: heel too soft, heel of shoe too long, foot too anterior	Weak knee extensors - patient maintains knee in extension for stability
			Insufficient socket flexion or excessive plantar flexion	
			Anterior/distal residual limb pain	
		Excessive knee flexion (>10°)	Suspension maintains knee in excessive flexion (suprapatellar bar or tight cuff strap)	Knee or hip flexion contracture
				Hip or knee extensor weakness
			Excessive heel lever: Heel too firm, heel of shoe too high, foot too posterior	
			Socket too flexed or foot too dorsiflexed	
			Flexion contracture not accommodated	
		Unequal step length	Faulty suspension (limits knee ROM)	Habit
	Smooth knee flexion of 20°	Abrupt or uncontrolled knee flexion	Excessive heel lever: heel of foot or shoe too firm, heel of shoe too high, foot too posterior	Weak knee extensors
	Appropriate heel compression (3/8" for SACH)		Shoe does not allow sufficient SACH heel compression	
			Excessive dorsiflexion or socket flexion	
	Minimal pistoning	Insufficient knee flexion	Insufficient heel lever: heel too soft, heel of shoe too low, foot too anterior	Excessive use of knee extensors (habit)
		Knee remains extended and patient rides the heel through to midstance	Insufficient socket flexion or excessive plantarflexion	
		Excessive motion of residual limb in socket	Loose socket or inadequate support contours	Insufficient sock ply
Midstance	Vertical pylon; 1/2" of lateral thrust of socket and pylon	Excessive genu varum moment, excessive lateral thrust, laterally leaning pylon	Foot too inset	
	2-4" width of base of support		Socket ML too large	
			Excessive socket abduction; insufficient socket adduction	
			Excessive relative outset of foot	
	Limited lateral trunk lean	Insufficient varus moment	Excessive socket adduction; insufficient socket abduction	
		Medially leaning pylon	Insufficient foot inset or actual outset of the foot	
		Narrow base of support	Foot too inset	Wide stance to increase base of support and stability
		Wide base of support	Foot too outset	Wide stance to increase stability
		Lateral trunk bending toward the prosthetic side	Prosthesis too short	
			Residual limb pain	
			Prosthesis too long	
			Foot too outset	

Atlas of Amputations and Limb Deficiencies, Fifth Edition

Phase	Normal observation	Deviation	Possible causes
Terminal stance	Smooth heel-off. After heel-off, knee begins to flex to prepare for toe-off	Drop-off—abrupt knee flexion	Insufficient toe lever: keel too soft, foot too posterior; Excessive socket flexion, excessive dorsiflexion
		Hill climbing	Excessive toe lever: keel too stiff, foot too anterior; Insufficient socket flexion or excessive plantar flexion; Foot too long
		Excessive knee extension moment, delayed knee flexion	Knee flexion contracture not accommodated; Weak quadriceps or hip extensors
		Early or delayed heel-off	Early—insufficient toe lever; delayed—excessive toe lever
Pre-swing	Smooth transfer of body weight to the sound side; Adequate socket suspension into swing	Socket drops away from the residual limb	Inadequate suspension; Insufficient sock ply
Swing phase	Smooth acceleration in the heel of the foot; Adequate toe clearance	Medial/lateral whip	Improper alignment of cuff suspension tabs; Socket donned in rotation; Mal-alignment of femur or hip in transverse plane
		Excessive pistoning	Inadequate suspension
		Inadequate toe clearance at midswing	Prosthesis too long; Inadequate suspension; Limited knee flexion; Muscle weakness or lack of gait training

ML = medial-lateral, ROM = range of motion, SACH = solid ankle, cushion heel

Section 1: General Principles

TABLE 5 Transfemoral Gait-Deviation Chart

Phase	Goals	Deviation	Prosthetic Factors	Patient Factors
Initial contact and loading response	Knee stability; Equal step length; Smooth, controlled plantar flexion; Foot remains in the line of progression	Knee instability	Excessive heel lever: heel of shoe or foot too firm, heel of shoe too high, foot too posterior	Weak hip extensors
			Foot too dorsiflexed	
			Knee alignment instability (knee center on or anterior to TA line)	
			Insufficient socket flexion (hip flexion contracture not accommodated)	
		Short step (swing extension) on prosthetic side	Knee instability	Habit to reduce knee flexion moment
		Short stance duration on prosthetic side (uneven timing)	Excessive initial socket flexion	Patient chooses to limit weight bearing on the prosthesis
			Painful socket results in quick weight transfer to sound side	Insecurity: muscle weakness, lack of balance
			Insufficient friction or extension assist can cause excessive heel rise and prolonged swing	
		Long prosthetic step; longer swing (step forward) on prosthetic side	Alignment stability may be a factor, if the knee buckles too easily	
			Insufficient socket flexion (contracture not accommodated)	
		Foot slap (rapid toe descent)	Insufficient plantarflexion resistance, heel too soft	Patient forcibly contacting the walking surface to assure knee stability
		External rotation of foot during LR	Heel too firm	Patient applied excessive knee extension force and pressure on heel to ensure knee stability
			Socket rotation: poor suspension, loose socket; too tight on gluteus, tight medial/posterior wall angle (quad)	Week hip musculature
			Anterior/medial brim pressure	
			Poor suspension resulting in socket rotation	
		External rotation of foot throughout swing/stance	Excessive external rotation alignment of foot	

Phase	Normal	Deviation	Cause
Midstance	Vertical pylon in coronal plane Normal width base of support (2-4") Limited lateral trunk lean	Abducted gait (prosthesis held away from the midline)	Proximal medial brim pressure/pain — Weak or contracted abductors
			Ramus pressure: high medial wall, inaccurate contour, adductor roll — Short residual limb
			— Patient insecurity (lack of balance)
		Pain at distal lateral femur	Hip abduction contracture
		Lateral wall does not provide adequate femoral support	Common in bilateral cases to increase stability
		Prosthesis too long	Flexion contracture causing anterior tilt of pelvis and ramus pressure
		Excessive socket abduction alignment	
		Pelvic band too far from the ilium	
		Locked knee	
		Excessive lateral trunk lean (compensated Trendelenburg; excessive bending laterally from the midline, generally to the prosthetic side)	Prosthesis too short — More commonly associated with weakness than alignment
			Excessive foot outset — Weak or contracted abductors
			Insufficient socket adduction; excessive socket abduction — Short residual limb
			Wide ML socket dimension — Habit (to improve balance)
			Lateral wall does not provide adequate femoral support — Weak hip extensors or abdominals; lean engages lumbar erector spinae
			ML instability
			Pain at lateral distal femur
			Painful medial wall/brim: ramus pressure, adductor roll
		Toe in/toe out	Improper transverse plane foot alignment
		Knee instability	Failure to limit dorsiflexion can lead to inadequate knee control.
		Excessive medial lean or thrust	Foot too lateral
			Excessive socket adduction
			Socket ML too large
		Excessive lateral lean or thrust	Foot too medial
			Excssive socket abduction
			Socket ML too large

(Continued)

Section 1: General Principles

TABLE 5 Transfemoral Gait Deviation Chart (Continued)

Phase	Goals	Deviation	Prosthetic Factors	Patient Factors
Terminal stance	Center of gravity follows a smooth arc without noticeable rise and fall of the head. Normal stance duration on sound side without excessive lumbar lordosis	Pelvic rise (hill climbing; extension moment in terminal stance delaying knee flexion)	Excessive toe lever: keel too firm, foot too anterior, foot too plantarflexed; Heel too soft	
		Drop-off (excessive pelvic drop with forward progression)	Insufficient toe lever: keel to soft, foot too posterior, foot too dorsiflexed	
		Excessive lumbar lordosis and trunk extension	Insufficient socket flexion (hip flexion contracture not accommodated); Improperly shaped ischial seat—painful ischial bearing; Insufficient anterior/posterior support from socket; Improperly shaped ischial seat cause forward rotation of pelvis to avoid pressure on ischium	Hip flexion contracture (lordosis allows longer swing phase on contrx side); Short residual limb; Weak hip extensors or abdominals (lordosis is used to compensate for weak musculature)
		Rotation on toe	Hip flexion contracture not accommodated	Limited hip flexion ROM; pelvis rotates to allow longer swing phase on contrx side
		Excessive forward trunk flexion (throughout stance)	Gait aids too short; Unstable knee joint	Habit (for stability); Hip flexion contracture
Pre-swing	Smooth hip and knee flexion	Inadequate or delayed knee flexion	Excessive knee flexion resistance or extension assist; Prosthesis aligned with too much stability; Excessive toe lever: keel too stiff, foot too posterior or socket too anterior	
Initial and midswing	Socket remains secure on the residual limb. Heel rise equal to contralateral limb. Hip, knee, and foot swing through line of progression. Center of gravity smoothly reaches the summit on its path over the prosthetic foot	Socket drops away from residual limb	Inadequate suspension	
		Medial whip	Knee axis in excessive external rotation; Socket donned with too much external rotation; Socket contours do not accommodate contracting muscles; Loose socket; Silesian belt worn too tight	Weak musculature; Soft tissue rotating around femur
		Lateral whip	Knee axis in excessive internal rotation; Socket donned with too much internal rotation; Socket contours do not accommodate contracting muscles; Loose socket	
		Excessive heel rise (excessive knee flexion early in swing phase)	Insufficient knee flexion resistance or extension assist	Forceful hip flexion to ensure knee extension in terminal stance
		Insufficient heel rise	Excessive knee flexion resistance or extension assist	Fear or insecurity—patient limits knee flexion

Phase	Observation	Prosthetic causes	Amputee causes
	Circumduction	Prosthesis is too long; Excessive knee alignment stability; Excessive knee flexion resistance or extension assist; Inadequate suspension (excessive pistoning); Locked knee; Socket too loose (excessive pistoning); Socket too tight or foot too plantarflexed (prosthesis is functionally too long); Pressure on medial brim	Fear (keeps knee extended during swing to ensure stability at IC/LR); Inadequate hip flexion; Abduction contracture
	Vaulting (rising on the toe of the contralateral foot permitting the amputee to swing the prosthesis through to clear the toe with little knee flexion)	Prosthesis is too long; Excessive knee alignment stability; Excessive knee flexion resistance or extension assist; Inadequate suspension (excessive pistoning); Locked knee; Socket too loose (pistoning); Socket too tight or foot too plantarflexed (prosthesis is functionally too long)	Fear—keeps knee extended during swing to ensure stability at IC/LR; Habit—to ensure toe clearance
	Uneven arm swing (arm on prosthetic side held close to body)	Socket discomfort	Fear, poor balance, habit
Terminal swing	Excessive terminal impact	Insufficient knee friction; Excessive extension assist; Worn/absent extension bumper	Patient strongly and deliberately extends hip for proprioceptive feedback at full extension
	Smooth and quiet deceleration to reach full extension		

IC/LR = initial contact/loading response, LR = loading response, ML = medial-lateral, ROM = range of motion, TA = trochanter to ankle

Summary

Understanding normal gait and the common features of gait when walking with a prosthesis is an important foundation for clinical assessment and prosthetic treatment. Efficient and stable progression is enabled through the complex coordination of the joints of both limbs. A thorough understanding of normal gait, including the aim of locomotion and the joint mechanics informs the clinicians' understanding of the common aberrant patterns exhibited by individuals walking with a prosthesis. When determining the effect of a prosthesis on gait, it is important to examine the effect across both lower limbs as the effect of the prosthesis is not isolated to a single joint or just to the prosthetic side. Assessment and optimization of the gait of patients using lower limb prostheses is a qualitative clinical task, requiring close collaboration between the patient, prosthetist, and other members of the rehabilitation team. Interpreting the common gait deviations within this framework is a necessary part of effective clinical management, enhancing clinical decision-making, clinical care, and the development of prosthetic components. Adopting a methodical approach to dynamic alignment, using a structured assessment tool, and incorporating video assessment can aid prosthetists in achieving an acceptable alignment that minimizes gait deviations and supports the activity level of the patient.

References

1. Wurdeman SR, Stevens PM, Campbell JH: Mobility Analysis of AmpuTees (MAAT I): Quality of life and satisfaction are strongly related to mobility for patients with a lower limb prosthesis. *Prosthet Orthot Int* 2018;42(5):498-503.
2. Davie-Smith F, Coulter E, Kennon B, Wyke S, Paul L: Factors influencing quality of life following lower limb amputation for peripheral arterial occlusive disease: A systematic review of the literature. *Prosthet Orthot Int* 2017;41(6):537-547.
3. Winter DA, Sienko SE: Biomechanics of below-knee amputee gait. *J Biomech* 1988;21(5):361-367.
4. Childers WL, Kogler GF: Symmetrical kinematics does not imply symmetrical kinetics in people with transtibial amputation using cycling model. *J Rehabil Res Dev* 2014;51(8):1243-1254.
5. Pinzur MS, Cox W, Kaiser J, Morris T, Patwardhan A, Vrbos L: The effect of prosthetic alignment on relative limb loading in persons with trans-tibial amputation: A preliminary report. *J Rehabil Res Dev* 1995;32(4):373-377.
6. Schmalz T, Blumentritt S, Jarasch R: Energy expenditure and biomechanical characteristics of lower limb amputee gait: The influence of prosthetic alignment and different prosthetic components. *Gait Posture* 2002;16(3):255-263.
7. Jia X, Suo S, Meng F, Wang R: Effects of alignment on interface pressure for transtibial amputee during walking. *Disabil Rehabil Assist Technol* 2008;3(6):339-343.
8. Gailey R, Allen K, Castles J, Kucharik J, Roeder M: Review of secondary physical conditions associated with lower-limb amputation and long-term prosthesis use. *J Rehabil Res Dev* 2008;45(1):15-29.
9. Lloyd CH, Stanhope SJ, Davis IS, Royer TD: Strength asymmetry and osteoarthritis risk factors in unilateral trans-tibial amputee gait. *Gait Posture* 2010;32(3):296-300.
10. Vanicek N, Strike S, McNaughton L, Polman R: Postural responses to dynamic perturbations in amputee fallers versus nonfallers: A comparative study with able-bodied subjects. *Arch Phys Med Rehabil* 2009;90(6):1018-1025.
11. Lamoth CJC, Ainsworth E, Polomski W, Houdijk H: Variability and stability analysis of walking of transfemoral amputees. *Med Eng Phys* 2010;32(9):1009-1014.
12. Hak L, Van Dieën JH, Van Der Wurff P, et al: Walking in an unstable environment: Strategies used by transtibial amputees to prevent falling during gait. *Arch Phys Med Rehabil* 2013;94(11):2186-2193.
13. Guaitolini M, De Marchis C, Rinaldi M, et al: Kinematic gait analysis in amputees for functional evaluation of dynamic stability. *Gait Posture* 2017;52:2.
14. Parker K, Hanada E, Adderson J: Gait variability and regularity of people with transtibial amputations. *Gait Posture* 2013;37(2):269-273.
15. Hordacre BG, Barr C, Patritti BL, Crotty M: Assessing gait variability in transtibial amputee fallers based on spatial-temporal gait parameters normalized for walking speed. *Arch Phys Med Rehabil* 2015;96(6):1162-1165.
16. Dingwell JB, Cusumano JP: Nonlinear time series analysis of normal and pathological human walking. *Chaos* 2000;10:848-863.
17. Perry J: Normal and pathological gait, in American Academy of Orthopaedic Surgeons, ed: *Atlas of Orthotics*, ed 2. CV Mosby, 1985, pp 76-111.
18. Kirtley C: *Clinical Gait Analysis: Theory and Practice*. Churchill Livingstone, 2006.
19. Saunders JB, Inman VT, Eberhart HD: The major determinants in normal and pathological gait. *J Bone Joint Surg Am* 1953;35-A(3):543-558.
20. Cavagna GA, Thys H, Zamboni A: The sources of external work in level walking and running. *J Physiol* 1976;262(3):639-657.
21. Kuo AD: The six determinants of gait and the inverted pendulum analogy: A dynamic walking perspective. *Hum Mov Sci* 2007;26(4):617-656.
22. Morgenroth DC, Segal AD, Zelik KE, et al: The effect of prosthetic foot push-off on mechanical loading associated with knee osteoarthritis in lower extremity amputees. *Gait Posture* 2011;34(4):502-507.
23. Adamczyk PG, Kuo AD: Mechanisms of gait asymmetry due to push-off deficiency in unilateral amputees. *IEEE Trans Neural Syst Rehabil Eng* 2015;23(5):776-785.
24. Grabowski AM, D'Andrea S: Effects of a powered ankle-foot prosthesis on kinetic loading of the unaffected leg during level-ground walking. *J Neuroeng Rehabil* 2013;10:49.
25. Morgenroth DC, Medverd JR, Seyedali M, Czerniecki JM: The relationship between knee joint loading rate during walking and degenerative changes on magnetic resonance imaging. *Clin Biomech* 2014;29(6):664-670.
26. Gholizaleh H, Abu Osman NA, Eshraghi A, Ali S: The effects of suction and pin/lock suspension systems on transtibial amputees' gait performance. *PLoS One* 2014;9(5):e94520.
27. Zhang T, Bai X, Liu F, Fan Y: Effect of prosthetic alignment on gait and biomechanical loading in individuals with transfemoral amputation: A preliminary study. *Gait Posture* 2019;71:219-226.
28. Winter DA: *Biomechanics and Motor Control of Human Gait*. University of Waterloo Press, 1987.
29. Baker R: Gait analysis methods in rehabilitation. *J Neuroeng Rehabil* 2006;3:4

30. Baker R: Gait analysis, in Wnek G, Bowlin G, eds: *Encyclopedia of Biomaterials and Biomedical Engineering,* ed 2. CRC Press, 2015.
31. Toro B, Nester C, Farren P: A review of observational gait assessment in clinical practice. *Physiother Theory Pract* 2003;19(3):137-149.
32. Rathinam C, Bateman A, Peirson J, Skinner J: Observational gait assessment tools in paediatrics – a systematic review. *Gait Posture* 2014;40(2):279-285.
33. Saleh M, Murdoch G: In defence of gait analysis. Observation and measurement in gait assessment. *J Bone Joint Surg Br* 1985;67(2):237-241.
34. Ko SU, Hausdorff JM, Ferrucci L: Age-associated differences in the gait pattern changes of older adults during fast-speed and fatigue conditions: Results from the Baltimore longitudinal study of ageing. *Age Ageing* 2010;39(6):688-694.
35. Sibley AR, Strike S, Moudy SC, Tillin NA: The effects of long-term muscle disuse on neuromuscular function in unilateral transtibial amputees. *Exp Physiol* 2020;105(3):408-418.
36. Wong CK, Ehrlich JE, Ersing JC, Maroldi NJ, Stevenson CE, Varca MJ: Exercise programs to improve gait performance in people with lower limb amputation: A systematic review. *Prosthet Orthot Int* 2016;40(1):8-17.
37. Lin S-J, Winston KD, Mitchell J, Girlinghouse J, Crochet K: Physical activity, functional capacity, and step variability during walking in people with lower-limb amputation. *Gait Posture* 2014;40(1):140-144.
38. Gitter A, Czerniecki JM, DeGroot DM: Biomechanical analysis of the influence of prosthetic feet on below-knee amputee walking. *Am J Phys Med Rehabil* 1991;70(3):142-148.
39. Barnett CT, Polman RCJ, Vanicek N: Longitudinal changes in transtibial amputee gait characteristics when negotiating a change in surface height during continuous gait. *Clin Biomech* 2014;29(7):787-793.
40. Fridman A, Ona I, Isakov E: The influence of prosthetic foot alignment on trans-tibial amputee gait. *Prosthet Orthot Int* 2003;27(1):17-22.
41. Isakov E, Burger H, Krajnik J, Gregoric M, Marincek C: Influence of speed on gait parameters and on symmetry in trans-tibial amputees. *Prosthet Orthot Int* 1996;20(3):153-158.
42. Gage JR: *Gait Analysis and Cerebral Palsy.* Blackwell Scientific Publications, 1991.
43. Strike SC: Gait and ergonomics: Normal and pathological, in Kumar S, ed: *Ergonomics for Rehabilitation Professionals.* CRC Press, 2009, pp 137-171.
44. Silverman AK, Fey NP, Portillo A, Walden JG, Bosker G, Neptune RR: Compensatory mechanisms in below-knee amputee gait in response to increasing steady-state walking speeds. *Gait Posture* 2008;28(4):602-609.
45. Howard CL, Wallace C, Perry B, Stokic DS: The utility of the single-subject method for comparison of temporal-spatial gait changes between a microprocessor and non-microprocessor prosthetic knees. *Prosthet Orthot Int* 2020;44(3):133-144.
46. Stevens PM, Wurdeman SR: Prosthetic knee selection for individuals with unilateral transfemoral amputation: A clinical practice guideline. *J Prosthet Orthot* 2019;31(1):2-8.
47. Lehmann JF: Push-off and propulsion of the body in normal and abnormal gait. Correction by ankle-foot orthoses. *Clin Orthop* 1993;288:97-108.
48. Meinders M, Gitter A, Czerniecki JM, Mienders Gitter A, Czerniecki JMM: The role of ankle plantar flexor muscle work during walking. *Scand J Rehabil Med* 1998;30(1):39-46.
49. Perry J: *Gait Analysis: Normal and Pathological Function.* SLACK Inc., 1992.
50. D'Andrea S, Wilhelm N, Silverman AK, Grabowski AM: Does use of a powered ankle-foot prosthesis restore whole-body angular momentum during walking at different speeds? *Clin Orthop Relat Res* 2014;472(10):3044-3054.
51. Ramstrand N, Nilsson KA: A comparison of foot placement strategies of transtibial amputees and able-bodied subjects during stair ambulation. *Prosthet Orthot Int* 2009;33(4):348-355.
52. Morgenroth DC, Gellhorn AC, Suri P: Osteoarthritis in the disabled population: A mechanical perspective. *Pharm Manag PM R* 2012;4(5 suppl):S20-S27.
53. Hafner BJ, Sanders JE, Czerniecki J, Fergason J: Energy storage and return prostheses: Does patient perception correlate with biomechanical analysis? *Clin Biomech* 2002;17(5):325-344.
54. Raschke SU, Orendurff MS, Mattie JL, et al: Biomechanical characteristics, patient preference and activity level with different prosthetic feet: A randomized double blind trial with laboratory and community testing. *J Biomech* 2015;48(1):146-152.
55. Shepherd MK, Rouse EJ: Comparing preference of ankle–foot stiffness in below-knee amputees and prosthetists. *Sci Rep* 2020;10(1):16067.
56. Gholizadeh H, Abu Osman NA, Eshraghi A, Ali S, Razak NA: Transtibial prosthesis suspension systems: Systematic review of literature. *Clin Biomech* 2014;29(1):87-97.
57. Gholizadeh H, Osman NAA, Eshraghi A, et al: Transtibial prosthetic suspension: Less pistoning versus easy donning and doffing. *J Rehabil Res Dev* 2012;49(9):1321-1330.
58. Hobson DA: *Powered Aid for Aligning the Lower-limb Modular Prosthesis.* Bulletin of the Prosthetics Research, Fall 1972.
59. Boone DA, Kobayashi T, Chou TG, et al: Perception of socket alignment perturbations in amputees with transtibial prostheses. *J Rehabil Res Dev* 2012;49(6):843-853.
60. Geil MD: Variability among practitioners in dynamic observational alignment of a transfemoral prosthesis. *J Prosthet Orthot* 2002;14(4):159-164.
61. Zahedi MS, Spence WD, Solomonidis SE, Paul JP: Alignment of lower-limb prostheses. *J Rehabil Res Dev* 1986;23(2):2-19.
62. Sin SW, Chow DHK, Cheng JCY: Significance of non-level walking on transtibial prosthesis fitting with particular reference to the effects of anterior-posterior alignment. *J Rehabil Res Dev* 2001;38(1):1-6.
63. Chow DH, Holmes AD, Lee CK, Sin SW: The effect of prosthesis alignment on the symmetry of gait in subjects with unilateral transtibial amputation. *Prosthet Orthot Int* 2006;30(2):114-128.
64. Kark L, Simmons A: Patient satisfaction following lower-limb amputation: The role of gait deviation. *Prosthet Orthot Int* 2011;35(2):225-233.
65. Fatone S, Stine R: Capturing quality clinical videos for two-dimensional motion analysis. *J Prosthet Orthot* 2015;27(1):27-32.
66. Borel S, Schneider P, Newman CJ: Video analysis software increases the interrater reliability of video gait assessments in children with cerebral palsy. *Gait Posture* 2011;33(4):727-729.
67. Peterson MV, Ewins D, Shaheen A, Catalfamo Formento PA: Evaluation of methods based on conventional videography for detection of gait events. *IFMBE Proceedings.* Springer, 2015.

68. Hillman SJ, Donald SC, Herman J, et al: Repeatability of a new observational gait score for unilateral lower limb amputees. *Gait Posture* 2010;32:39-45.
69. Chen CWJ, Heim W, Fairley K, et al: Evaluation of an instrument-assisted dynamic prosthetic alignment technique for individuals with transtibial amputation. *Prosthet Orthot Int* 2016;40(4):475-483.
70. Kobayashi T, Orendurff MS, Zhang M, Boone DA: Effect of alignment changes on sagittal and coronal socket reaction moment interactions in transtibial prostheses. *J Biomech* 2013;46(7):1343-1350.
71. Boone DA, Kobayashi T, Chou TG, et al: Influence of malalignment on socket reaction moments during gait in amputees with transtibial prostheses. *Gait Posture* 2013;37(4):620-626.
72. Yang L, Solomonidis SE, Spence WD, Paul JP: The influence of limb alignment on the gait of above-knee amputees. *J Biomech* 1991;24(11):981-997.
73. Neumann E: State-of-the-science review of transtibial prosthesis alignment perturbation. *J Prosthet Orthot* 2009;21(4):175-193.
74. Kobayashi T, Orendurff MS, Zhang M, Boone DA: Effect of transtibial prosthesis alignment changes on out-of-plane socket reaction moments during walking in amputees. *J Biomech* 2012;45(15):2603-2609.

Kinesiology of the Upper Limb

CHAPTER 5

Terry R. Light, MD, FAAOS, FACS, FAOrthA

ABSTRACT

Since the human upper limbs are unnecessary for ambulation, they are free to explore and interact with the environment to gather sensory information, prehension, object manipulation, pushing, and carrying. The mobility of the shoulder, elbow, and wrist orient the hand in space and allow the hand to access body surfaces and orifices for self-care, hygiene, and nutrition. Prehensile and nonprehensile activities require limb stability, mobility, and power.

Keywords: grip; kinesiology; pinch; prehension

Introduction

From an evolutionary perspective, when primates stood on their hind limbs the upper limbs were freed from weight bearing. The upper limbs of upright primates are thus able to function as both organs of prehension and as sensory probes of their environment. Many seemingly simple hand functions are only possible through the integration of the entire body, the upper limb, and the hand.

Kinesiology considers motion as it occurs under living conditions, analyzing mechanical forces on the body in motion. Motion is studied as activities are performed against extrinsic forces, such as gravity, or against the resistance of objects that are grasped, pushed, or hurled by the upper limb. Steindler[1] emphasized that in many situations, muscles are primarily used to achieve "stabilization and equilibrium rather than free motion." Steindler also identified that the muscle contraction necessary to stabilize the skeleton is often not apparent as visible joint motion, yet these unseen muscle forces play an essential role in maintaining musculoskeletal equilibrium. This chapter focuses on the major pattern of upper limb activity and details the mechanical and nonmechanical factors essential to humans in efficient task performance. Sensory function, muscle strength, and skeletal stability are essential to effective integrated function.

Trunk Stability

Prehensile activity depends upon the stability of the trunk. Trunk or core stability creates the potential to create multiple integrated spheres of influence (**Figure 1**). Proximal limb stability, essential for secure hand placement, demands more than shoulder control. Spinal stability with attendant trunk control is essential to free the upper limb to perform effective prehensile activity. If the arms are being used to hold crutches or a walker, the hands cannot be spared for other activity. The paralyzed patient who uses a wheelchair may be unable to fully use his hands in the presence of trunk instability. Many wheelchair-bound patients are relatively well balanced in a static sitting position but become unstable by the simple forward shift of their center of gravity as they reach forward. This may occur when the combined mass of the upper limb and the object being held is shifted anterior to their sitting center of gravity. The arm must be retracted, and the object surrendered, or individuals risk tumbling out of the wheelchair. Many individuals will hook one arm over the back or the side of the chair for stability, sacrificing the opportunity for bimanual function. If hip or spinal extensor muscles are ineffective, the wheelchair-confined patient must be stabilized by a reclining backrest, retaining strap, or other spinal support so that both upper limbs can he free to reach away from the body.

Limb Mobility

Effective functioning of the upper limb requires flexibility and mobility as well as stability. The hand should be able to reach the mouth, hair, and perineum as well as the front of the body. Kapandji[2] delineated seven degrees of freedom of the upper limb as it positions the hand in space. The shoulder possesses three degrees of freedom, the elbow one, and the wrist and forearm have three, rotation, flexion/extension, and radioulnar deviation.

Shoulder

Because the shoulder is the most proximal joint, it plays the primary role in limb orientation. The shoulder's substantial mobility is enhanced by the

---

Dr. Light or an immediate family member serves as a board member, owner, officer, or committee member of the American Society for Surgery of the Hand.

This chapter is adapted from Pinzur MS: Kinesiology of the upper limb, in Krajbich JI, Pinzur MS, Potter BK, Stevens PM, eds: *Atlas of Amputations and Limb Deficiencies: Surgical, Prosthetic, and Rehabilitation Principles*, ed 4. American Academy of Orthopaedic Surgeons, 2016, pp 97-113.

Section 1: General Principles

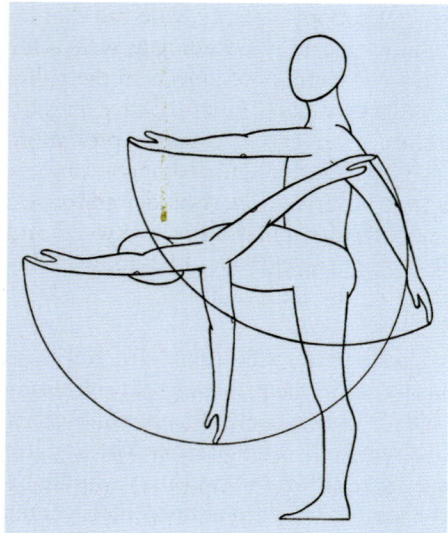

FIGURE 1 Schematic demonstration that the field of motion of the upper limb is defined by the length of the limb. A combination of hip and knee joint flexion is needed for the hand to reach the lower limb below the upper thigh.

The shoulder girdle musculoskeletal complex provides attachment and suspension of the upper limb from the axial skeleton. The glenohumeral, acromioclavicular, and sternoclavicular joints, as well as the scapulothoracic interface govern shoulder mobility. The sternoclavicular joint is the sole point of direct contact of the upper limb appendicular skeleton with the axial skeleton. Motion through the sternoclavicular and acromioclavicular joints allows scapulothoracic motion either alone or combined with glenohumeral movement.

Scapular motion may be described in terms of the change in position of the scapula relative to the thorax.[3] Scapular elevation and depression are readily appreciated. Upward scapular rotation is motion in which the inferior angle of the scapula moves anterolaterally, tilting the glenoid articular surface upward. Downward scapular rotation is the opposite motion, in which the inferior angle moves medially, tilting the articular surface of the glenoid downward. Scapular protraction refers to laterally and forward motion of the scapula around the thorax. Scapular retraction implies scapular movement medially and posteriorly about the thorax.

The normal glenohumeral joint flexes 180° and extends 60° (**Figure 2**). During the first 30° of shoulder abduction, the scapula is stabilized against the thorax so that all abduction takes place at the glenohumeral joint.[4] Through the arc from 30° to 180°, every 2° of glenohumeral motion is associated with 1° of scapulothoracic motion.[5] Thus, in full 180° of abduction, 130° of motion occurs at the glenohumeral joint while 50° of motion takes place at the scapulothoracic interface (**Figure 3**).

Elbow

The elbow has a single primary arc of motion: flexion and extension. Constraint of the elbow arc is governed by the osseous contour of the olecranon and the trochlea and stabilizing ligaments. Recurrent dislocation of this constrained joint is infrequent. Because the elbow has a single arc of motion, it has been likened to a caliper functioning to regulate the distance between the hand and the trunk. The flexibility

modest constraint in the articulation of the spherical humeral head with the shallow glenoid fossa. Flexion and extension occur around the transverse or coronal axis, abduction and adduction about the sagittal axis, and internal and external rotation about the vertical axis. Since the shoulder is loosely constrained by its bony configuration, it is particularly vulnerable to dislocation when soft-tissue constraints have been disrupted and to subluxation when musculo-tendinous coapting forces have been altered by paralysis or weakness (eg, a cerebrovascular accident).

The most frequently used arc of shoulder motion is in front of the body, a domain that allows visual input to optimize effective hand function. A greater arc of motion is employed for other bodily activities. Shoulder abduction is necessary for the hand to access the scalp for combing one's hair. Shoulder abduction is not necessary for feeding or washing. Internal shoulder rotation is usually employed for posterior perineal hygiene. Combined shoulder extension and adduction can also be used to access the posterior perineum if an individual is unable to internally rotate the shoulder.

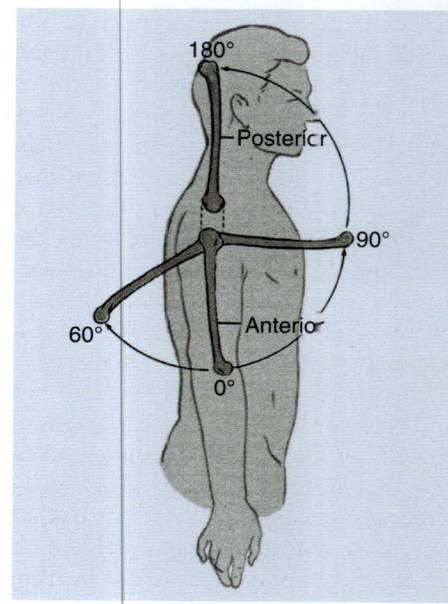

FIGURE 2 Schematic drawing showing 180° of flexion and 60° of extension at the glenohumeral joint.

of the elbow to alter the length of the limb is critical to fundamental self-care activities including feeding and perineal care.

The biceps muscle has been termed the primary feeding muscle since it both flexes the elbow and supinates the forearm to bring the hand to the mouth. Biceps muscle strength should

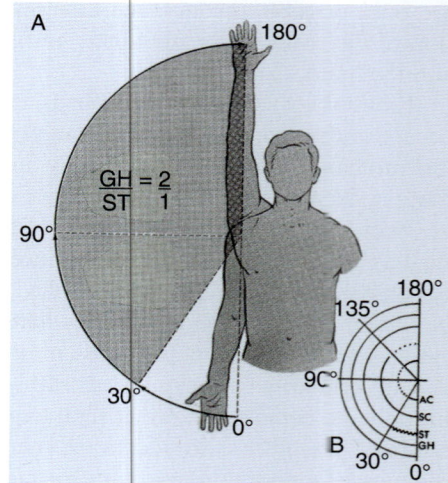

FIGURE 3 Schematic drawing showing motion in the shoulder. Elevation of the shoulder from 0° to 180°. From 0° to 30°, the motion is mostly glenohumeral. From 30° to 180° one third of the motion is scapulothoracic and two thirds of the motion is glenohumeral.

be sufficient to lift the weight of the hand, forearm, and any object in the grasp of the hand against the force of gravity.[5] Although gravity may allow elbow extension in the absence of an active triceps muscle, it is essential that passive elbow extension be preserved if the limb is to be capable of reaching the perineum. Active elbow extension is necessary for reaching or placing the hand overhead as well for locomotion using a walker or propelling a wheelchair.

When triceps function is absent but full passive elbow motion is preserved, the elbow may be temporarily locked in a stable hyperextended position by shifting the weight of the trunk to that side. This strategy creates a stable limb by shifting the axis of weight bearing from the shoulder to the hand slightly posterior to the hyperextended elbow.[6] The locked elbow position is particularly useful for transfer activity in paralyzed individuals. The limb is stable to axial load as long as the elbow remains extended.

Forearm

The forearm and wrist are defined by three degrees of freedom that govern the orientation of the hand: forearm rotation, wrist flexion–extension, and wrist radial and ulnar deviation. The proximal and distal radioulnar articulations allow forearm pronation and supination. Though the interosseous space between analogous points on the radius and ulna is generally maintained throughout rotation, the space is maximal in neutral rotation and slightly narrowed in pronation (**Figure 4**).[7]

Because the olecranon of the ulna is stabilized against the humerus proximally, forearm rotation appears to occur as the radius (with the attached carpus and hand) rotates around the ulna. More precisely observed, the elbow is a loose hinge allowing rotation or rocking. When the forearm moves from pronation to supination, the distal ulna shifts radially and the ulna flexes (**Figure 5**). Pronation is the ideal position for body weight support activity, whereas supination is important in feeding as well as for balanced support of objects in the palm. Shoulder abduction is effective in substituting for absent forearm pronation. The usual strategy for compensating for a lack of supination, shoulder adduction and carpal supination is awkward and less effective since shoulder adduction is hindered by the trunk.

Wrist

Both dorsiflexion and palmar flexion as well as radial and ulnar deviation occur through the radiocarpal and intercarpal joints (**Figure 6**).[8] A limited degree of rotation is possible at the wrist, principally at the radiocarpal articulation. Because wrist dorsiflexion passively tightens the finger flexors by the tenodesis effect, dorsiflexion is an essential posture for strong grip activities. The ability of the wrist to passively palmar flex to release digital grip is important in hands possessing limited active motor units. In ulnar deviation the thumb becomes aligned with the long axis of the radius, a particularly effective posture for holding tools.

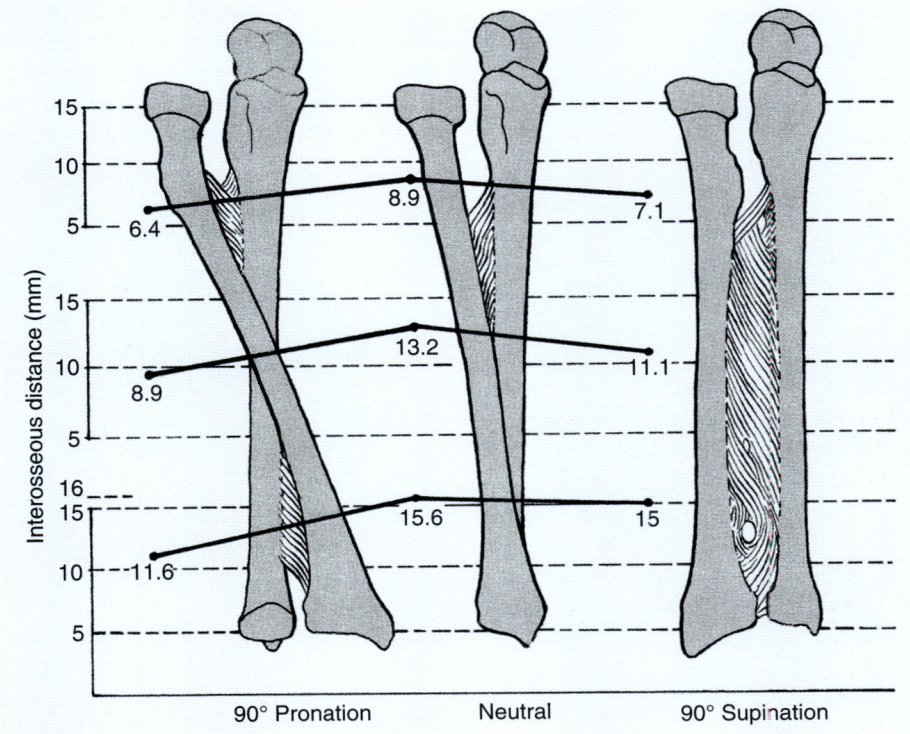

FIGURE 4 Schematic drawing showing radioulnar distance in pronation, supination, and neutral rotation. The distance between analogous points on the radius and ulna is least in pronation and maximal in neutral rotation. (Data from Christensen JB, Adams JP, Cho KO, et al. A study of the interosseous distance between the radius and ulna during rotation of the forearm. *Anat Rec*. 1968;160:261-271.)

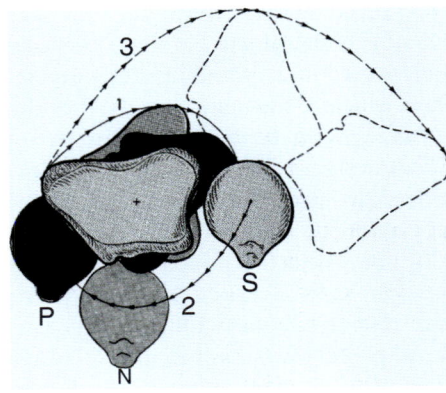

FIGURE 5 Schematic drawing of rotation of distal radio-ulnar joint from pronation (P) through neutral (N) to supination (S) is demonstrated by Arc 2. The axis of rotation of the distal radioulnar joint is in the distal volar-ulnar corner of the distal ulna. As the forearm moves from pronation to supination the distal ulna shifts radial-ward while the elbow extends a few degrees. Arc 1 demonstrates the arc needed if the ulna rotated about the radius while Arc 3 demonstrates the displacement if the ulna was fixed with the radius rotating about the distal ulna.

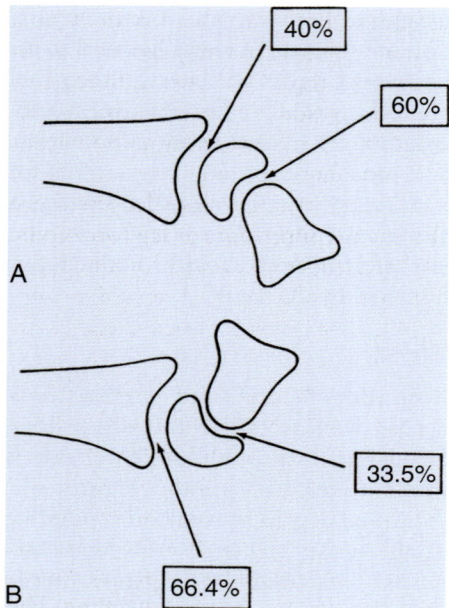

FIGURE 6 Schematic drawing demonstrating the contributions to wrist flexion and extension of both the radiocarpal and midcarpal joints. **A**, Sixty percent of flexion is midcarpal and 40% is radiocarpal. **B**, A total of 33.5% of extension occurs at the midcarpal joint, while 66.4% occurs at the radiocarpal joint. (Reproduced with permission from Sarrafian SK, Melamed JL, Goshgarian GM: Study of wrist motion in flexion and extension. *Clin Orthop Relat Res* 1977;126:153-159.)

A tenodesis effect is present whenever an innervated or denervated musculotendinous unit traverses more than one joint. When the tension on a muscle is increased by the altered posture of one joint, there will be a reciprocal effect on the tension across adjacent joints. For example, when the wrist is extended the flexor tendons are stretched around the palmar aspect of the wrist. The tension on the finger flexor tendon is increased, and the fingers are passively pulled into a posture of increased flexion at the metacarpophalangeal and interphalangeal joints.

It has been observed that many hand activities result in motion in a plane that begins in dorsiflexion and radial deviation and moves into palmar flexion and ulnar deviation. This arc of motion has been termed "dart-throwing" motion. Combined dorsiflexion and radial deviation is driven by the extensor carpi radialis brevis and longus, while flexion and ulnar deviation are primarily driven by the flexor carpi ulnaris.

Characteristic wrist motion has been studied in test subjects as they performed 52 standardized tasks.[9] The normal functional range of the wrist was determined to be from 5° of palmar flexion to 30° of dorsiflexion and from 10° of radial deviation to 15° of ulnar deviation. Culinary skills required only 24° of flexion–extension and 17° of radioulnar deviation, with an average centroid of 12° dorsiflexion and 5° ulnar deviation. Eleven other activities of daily living required an average arc of 35° of flexion–extension and 20° of radioulnar deviation, with average centroids of 10° dorsiflexion and 1° ulnar deviation.

The extent of reach of each finger is dictated by the motion at the metacarpophalangeal and interphalangeal joints and the length of the metacarpal and phalanges. Together they subtend an arc that is best described as an equiangular spiral (**Figure 7**).

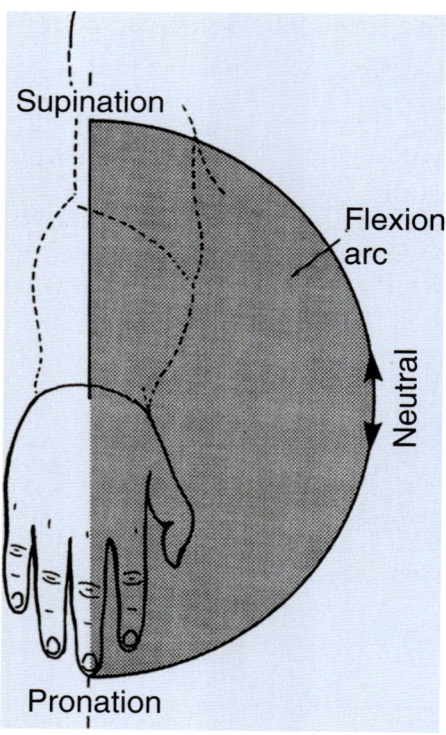

FIGURE 7 Schematic drawing of the field of motion of the wrist and fingers. The action envelope of the fingers, E_4, traces an equiangular spiral. The field of the finger is within E_3 with the wrist extended projecting forward with the wrist maximally flexed.

Hand

Within the hand, the metacarpophalangeal joints of the fingers as well as the carpometacarpal joint of the thumb are the least constrained joints. The metacarpophalangeal joints of the fingers allow flexion, extension, radial and ulnar deviation, while the saddle-shaped basilar joint of the thumb allows flexion, extension, radial abduction, palmar abduction, adduction, and rotation. This arrangement is analogous to the arm since the most proximal joint, the shoulder joint, is the least constrained and thus allows the distal segment to subtend a maximal arc. The interphalangeal joints of the thumb and fingers are restricted to flexion and extension, whereas the metacarpophalangeal joint of the thumb can flex and extend and, to a limited degree, rotate.

Thumb

Several terms are applied to precisely describe the motions of the thumb (**Figure 8**). Flexion and extension occur at both the metacarpophalangeal and interphalangeal joints. Thumb adduction is motion of the thumb metacarpal at the carpometacarpophalangeal joint toward the center of the palm as defined by the middle finger

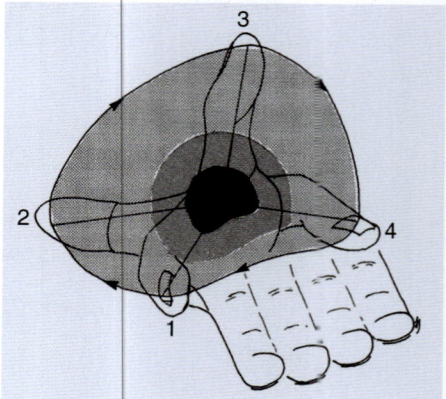

FIGURE 8 Schematic drawing demonstrating the field of motion of the thumb. The basic motions are 1 to 2, extension and radial abduction in the palmar plane; 2 to 3, abduction in the plane perpendicular to the palm with pronation; 3 to 4 flexion, adduction, and further pronation to oppose the thumb pulp to that of the ring or small finger; 4 to 1, extension with supination; 1 to 4, flexion, adduction, and pronation.

metacarpal powered by the adductor pollicis muscle. Radial abduction occurs at the carpometacarpal joint. The movement of the thumb metacarpal away from the palm of the hand is in the plane defined by the palm. Palmar abduction is carpometacarpal motion of the thumb away from the palm in a plane perpendicular to the palm. Retroposition is motion of the thumb from palmar abduction toward a balanced resting posture.

Thumb rotation occurs at both the carpometacarpal and metacarpophalangeal joints. Thumb supination occurs when the thumb metacarpal and proximal phalanx rotates toward a position in which the nail of the extended thumb lies in the same plane as the nail of the extended fingers. Thumb pronation is rotation in which the thumb metacarpal and proximal phalanx rotates away from the plane of the other metacarpals. *Opposition* (**Figure 9**) is a complex composite motion that occurs through both the carpometacarpal and metacarpophalangeal joints. Thumb carpometacarpal pronation, carpometacarpal palmar abduction, metacarpophalangeal joint flexion, and metacarpophalangeal joint pronation are integrated to allow the palmar pulp surface of the thumb to directly face the pulp of each of the fingers. The abductor pollicis brevis is the most powerful intrinsic muscle in the hand contributing to opposition.

Impediments to Function and Motion

Systemic disease can limit the sphere of upper limb activity. The respiratory cripple often rests on the elbows on a table when seated so that the shoulder girdle muscles are available to assist in respiration. Pulmonary dysfunction has an adverse effect on hand function, since in the wheelchair-bound respiratory cripple the hands are limited to functioning within a markedly constrained area dictated by a table or forearm rests that support the forearm. Objects can be manipulated only if they are directly in front of the individual.[5]

Soft-tissue constraints are particularly important for the most mobile joint of the upper limb, the shoulder. Although gravity tends to compress or co-apt joints of the lower limb, the sheer weight of the hand and arm affected may distract the shoulder with compromised musculotendinous balance.

The Hand as a Sensory Probe

The hand acts as a probe able to detect pressure, texture, temperature, moisture, vibration, and pain in its environment. Sensation is critical to hand function. Individuals routinely bypass skin areas of compromised sensation, preferring to use functional patterns that incorporate skin regions with best sensation. For example, a patient with median sensory loss may ignore a well-controlled thumb, choosing instead to use side-to-side pinch between the sensate ulnar side of the ring and the sensate little finger.

The ability to perceive deep pressure allows an appropriate grasp force to be adjusted and maintained on an object. Compromised pressure sensibility will often result in objects being unexpectedly dropped even though flexor muscles are uncompromised. Regulation of the strength of pinch and grip is dictated primarily by sensory nerve endings within the pulp of the digit rather than by muscle spindle fiber tension.[10] In lower motor neuron lesions (eg, a nerve laceration) sensory loss is accompanied by a loss of sweating. The absence of sweat reduces friction at the fingertips and further increases the difficulty of securing objects between denervated digits. By contrast, in upper motor neuron lesions (eg, spinal cord injury) sweating is preserved.

Normal sensory awareness implies a synthesis of visual and tactile information. This normal overlap allows the typist to feel the keys of the computer keyboard while watching the results on screen. Such integration of multiple sensory cues provides optimum hand function. When one form of sensory input is impaired, overlapping input may partially compensate for the impairment. Individuals with loss of tactile awareness may be able to partially compensate for their loss by directly viewing their hand. Conversely, blind persons can focus on the sensory cues of Braille letters to compensate for the absence of sight. An unexpected explosion may instantly deprive the youngster playing with fireworks, the laboratory technician working with chemicals, or the soldier in combat of both sight and tactile feedback from their hands. These unfortunate individuals are deprived of robust sensory awareness, since their ability to compensate for visual loss through tactile clues is severely compromised.

Objects may be grasped bimanually if the distal portions of the residual upper limbs can be brought together. Techniques of prosthetic management

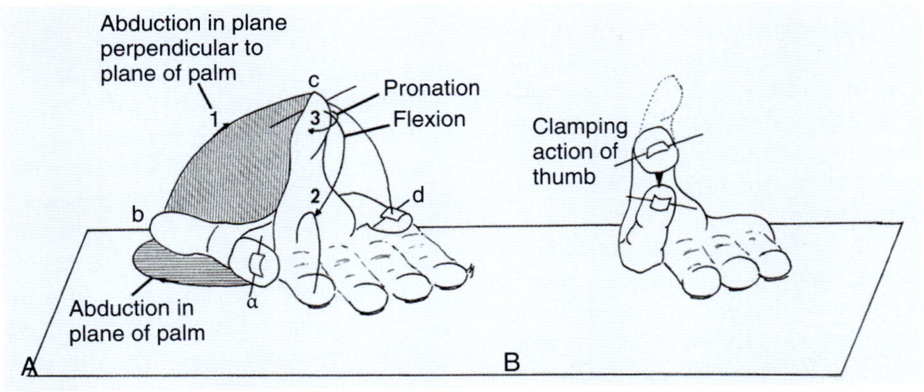

FIGURE 9 Schematic drawings of thumb opposition. **A**, Initially the first web space is widened by thumb extension (a to b). The thumb is then abducted through the curve (b to c) bringing the thumb perpendicular to the plane of the hand (1). Flexion (2) and pronation (3) through the carpometacarpal and metacarpophalangeal joints rotates the distal phalanx pulp to broadly face the pulp of one or more of the fingers (c to d). **B**, In full opposition, the nails of the thumb and fingers are nearly parallel.

must be reconsidered in the blind patient. Prosthetic devices that cover the skin of the residual limb of a blind individual may further hamper function by rendering the terminal portion of the residual limb insensate. The Krukenberg reconstruction[11] is an operative procedure that has been suggested for blind individuals that have lost both hands. The procedure divides the forearm bones apart. The musculature is separated into radial and ulnar components and the two bones are surfaced with sensate skin, providing an opportunity for these patients to regain single-limb prehension as the radius and ulna separate and converge under active motor control.

Gloves can be a mixed blessing. Although they may be covered by a surface with greater friction that shields against high-frequency vibrations,[12] gloves substantially alter the quality of sensory input by eliminating direct skin contact and thus lead to the inadvertent use of abnormally high grip pressures.[13]

Nonprehensile and Prehensile Activity

Classifications of upper limb activities often focus upon prehensile activity in which objects are grasped or pinched between the fingers and the palm and thumb. Important nonprehensile activities should not be overlooked since the fingers and hand can transmit substantial force by tapping, pushing, or punching. Force is focused when individual digits tap, scratch, or strike keyboard keys. The upper limb also functions in a limited number of activities that do not require participation of the hand itself. The fingers may be used for a pushing or blocking maneuver, whereas the forearm can provide support for an object secured against the chest.

The entire upper limb may function as a nonprehensile unit while maintaining its structural integrity under axial loading. Nonprehensile activities may involve the hand as a passive force transmitter. Protraction, the process by which objects are pushed away from the body, requires stability across the shoulder and elbow. Active elbow extension is coupled with forward flexion of the shoulder to provide the impetus for motion. The magnitude of force transmitted in this fashion is variable. Only a minimum amount of force may be required to push open a swinging door. In such an activity the momentum of the entire trunk acts through the stabilized upper limb, with augmentation provided by the triceps as it extends the elbow as the door swings open. A greater force transmitted across the flattened palm is required to support body weight, by both the exercising athlete doing push ups and the paraplegic performing transfers. In the latter situation the individual must exert considerable force through the upper limb to move his or her body weight against the force of gravity. The boxer's punch is an example of passive force transmission through the clenched fist;[10] the force originates at the shoulder and elbow and passes across the stabilized wrist to the hand to the body of his opponent.

Prehension is the process by which the hand grasps and releases an object.[10] Cerebral control is required to approach an object, to initiate grasp, and to incorporate sensory feedback to modulate the force of grip and to precisely release the grip.[3] Effective prehension demands that the object is held securely over time. Although the length of time that the object is grasped may be as short as the moment the ball rests in the juggler's palm between tosses, the time must be sufficient for friction to develop between the object and the skin for the momentary interruption of motion and the maintenance of control. By contrast, a handball impacting against the palm of a moving hand is redirected in a nonprehensile manner.

Napier[14] further categorized prehensile activity as either power or precision activities and has delineated the characteristics of these two modes of hand functioning. Although some activities are clearly a mixture of both, and few activities fall into neither category, this distinction is useful in analyzing requirements for the restitution of upper limb functional capabilities.

Power Grip

In power grip an object is secured in a three-sided clamp, between the palmar surface of partially flexed fingers, the palm, and the palmar surface of the thumb. The adducted thumb provides counter pressure and buttresses the object.[10]

In precision grip an object is pinched between the distal phalangeal palmar aspects of the opposing thumb and fingers.

Power grip often requires maintaining the stability of an object while movement occurs at the shoulder, elbow, or wrist. An example of this would be the use of a hammer to drive a nail. The hammer is forced securely against the palm by the flexed fingers and is further stabilized by the adducted thumb. It is the movement of the shoulder, elbow, forearm, and wrist that guides it to firmly strike the nail.

By contrast, precision grip often involves the manipulation of an object held in the hand. An example would be the surgeon's manipulation of a micro needle holder. Optimum function occurs when the surgeon is relaxed and comfortably seated with the forearm supported. In this posture proximal support is maximized and fine alterations of intrinsic and extrinsic muscle firing are combined for ideal performance. In precision activities the fingers are generally positioned in flexion. Small objects are held between the thumb and the index and middle fingers. The degree of abduction at the metacarpophalangeal joint of the index and middle fingers depends on the size of the object being held. As the size of the object increases, more ulnar digits are added to buttress and stabilize the grasp. Very small objects, such as marbles, may be held between the thumb and the index finger. Precision activities usually involve pulp-to-pulp grip, with the palmar surfaces of the finger and thumb facing each other. This posture supplies the brain with maximum sensory input from the pulp surfaces, which are high in sensory end organs.

Precision prehensile activities may be subclassified as either palmar, tip, or lateral pinch. Palmar pinch occurs when the pulp of the thumb is opposed to the pulps of the index and middle fingers. Tip pinch involves opposition of the tip of the thumb to the tips of the index and middle fingers. The contact area is much greater in pulp than in tip pinch. Lateral pinch, also referred to as key pinch, involves the pressure of the thumb pulp against the lateral aspect of a finger, usually the index finger.

Because palmar pinch is the most used pattern of prehension, it was initially suggested that surgical reconstruction after spinal cord injury should attempt to reproduce this pattern. Experience has demonstrated, however, that the restitution of lateral pinch is a more useful and realistic goal for the severely impaired individual.[15]

Tools used in precision activities are designed for a radial-based grip, whereas those used in power activities are designed for an ulnar-based grip.[9]

Not all activities fall into the power grip or precision grip category. An exception is the use of chopsticks. This requires an intermediate grip[16] that incorporates digital positioning midway between the typical power and precision postures. Another would be the thumbless grip, in which an object such as a cigarette is held between adducted fingers. The hook grip is a form of prehensile activity in which the fingers, but not the thumb, are curled around an object. Hook grip requires a balance between the extrinsic flexors and extensors. Prolonged power is often necessary since the hook grip is often used for carrying objects such as a suitcase. Hook grip is also used for pulling actions as when opening a refrigerator door.

Muscle Strength

Muscles may function either to stabilize a body part without movement of a joint, isometric contraction, or to move the joint by isotonic contraction, in which the muscle belly shortens. Several upper limb muscle groups function in concert to statically position the forearm allowing other muscles to contract so that the hand can perform the desired prehensile activity. Many hand and forearm muscles function primarily to pre-position the digital skeleton in a posture that will enable other muscle groups to contract and effect a desired motion. Pre-positioning activities require less absolute strength than do muscles that forcefully secure objects within the grasp of the hand.

The force a muscle exerts is proportional to the resting cross-sectional area of muscle fibers, with the force approximating 3.65 kg/cm^2 of muscle. A relative scale of the work capacity of extrinsic muscles has thus been calculated.[17] The flexor carpi ulnaris (19.6 N/m) and the brachioradialis (18.7 N/m) are the strongest forearm muscles, whereas the palmaris longus, extensor pollicis longus, and abductor pollicis longus are the weakest (1.0 N/m). The flexor carpi radialis (7.8 N/m), each of the three wrist extensors, extensor carpi radialis longus, extensor carpi radialis brevis, and extensor carpi ulnaris (8.8 to 10.8 N/m), and the pronator teres (11.8 N/m) all have an intermediate potential. The flexors digitorum profundi as a group have a work capacity of 44.1 N/m. They interpose combine to yield a substantial potential force (26.5 N/m) that is further amplified by combined lumbrical input (4.9 N/m).

When one is contemplating either tendon transfer or orthotic substitution of missing musculotendinous units, it is important to define the strength requirements of the missing function. By separating muscle activities into stabilizing, pre-positioning, and active impacting subgroups, one is better able to choose an appropriate motor or orthotic substitution.

For example, although opposition of the thumb is vital to effective precision activity, relatively little motor power is necessary to reposition the thumb in space. Since it requires but minimal power, this essential function can be satisfactorily restored using a variety of tendon transfers of weak motors or simple orthotic devices. Conversely, to draw the thumb toward the middle metacarpal, an essential component of a strong power grip, employs the adductor pollicis, an extremely powerful muscle. Unfortunately, there are no effective active orthotic substitutions for this muscle. At best, in the absence of an active adductor pollicis muscle function, tendon transfer substitution can increase lateral pinch power to only 50% of normal.[18]

Muscles with intermediate-level strength can function well in some activities but will fail in other roles. For example, although a relatively weak muscle transferred to the triceps may function effectively in pre-positioning the hand in front of the body or in helping to comb one's hair, it will be insufficient to allow a tetraplegic individual to actively elevate the body when attempting to transfer their body from bed to chair.

Pathologic Hand Deformity

The analysis of established hand deformities demonstrates several important concepts. Each musculotendinous unit will influence the posture of each joint that it traverses, and the magnitude of that effect will be influenced by the position of the musculotendinous unit relative to the center of axis of rotation of the given joint. The digital flexors illustrate this effect. The deep and superficial flexors of the fingers (flexors digitorum profundus and superficialis) have a secondary influence on wrist motion and contribute to wrist flexion. This tendency must be counteracted by active wrist extension if wrist position is to be maintained in a stable posture and finger flexor tendon excursion is used with optimum strength. Though wrist and finger flexors are innervated by the median and ulnar nerves, the loss of radial innervated wrist extensors substantially diminishes grip strength.

When a flexion contracture of a soft-tissue structure (eg, musculotendinous unit) traverses two joints, a seesaw-like phenomenon will occur. As one joint is extended, increased tension will be placed on the abnormally taut volar musculotendinous unit and the second joint will be passively pulled into flexion. Conversely, when the second joint is extended, the first joint will then be flexed. It will be impossible to extend both joints fully at the same time. This phenomenon is often seen in forearms affected by cerebral palsy, stroke, or Volkmann contracture.

Optimum volitional joint position control requires at least two musculotendinous units acting in a reciprocal direction through each plane of intended joint motion. Balance must be preserved at each articulation. Collateral ligaments and joint configuration may constrain the planes of motion to a single arc, such as occurs at the elbow and the interphalangeal joints. When these constraints are weakened, as in rheumatoid arthritis, joints are particularly vulnerable to deformation, subluxation, or dislocation. When a single musculotendinous unit traverses two or more joints, a deformity of one joint may lead to reciprocal deformity of adjacent joints.

An example of this pathophysiologic interaction is the evolution of joint deformity of the rheumatoid thumb.[19] In the most common deformity (Nalebuff Type I) synovitis begins at the metacarpophalangeal joint. The extensor apparatus becomes stretched locally while at the same time loss of joint support (collateral integrity) allows volar subluxation of the proximal phalanx. The loss of extensor integrity creates a motor imbalance that results in a posture of chronic metacarpophalangeal flexion. This tends to tighten the extensor pollicis longus and relax the flexor pollicis longus, with the ultimate evolution of a position of interphalangeal joint hyperextension.

Implications for Upper Limb Prosthetic Prescription

Effective prostheses should improve function sufficiently to justify covering sensate normal skin. The importance of preserving remaining sensation cannot be overestimated. A prosthesis that obscures or prevents exposure of sensate skin may be discarded. Prehensile patterns must be based on remaining sensate skin rather than on predetermined patterns of normal functioning.

An upper limb prosthesis should not obscure visual cues. Since full pronation blocks vision, the prosthetic terminal device should probably be positioned in a neutral position to facilitate visual control.

The weight of an upper extremity prosthesis is also an important consideration, particularly in a paralyzed or weakened limb.

SUMMARY

The full potential of the upper limb is best realized when the upper limb functions in concert with the entire body. The trunk provides proximal limb stability while the shoulder maximizes limb mobility. The elbow regulates the distance of the hand from the trunk while the orientation of the hand is controlled at the forearm and wrist level. Optimum function of the hand depends on cerebral integration of sensory input, both tactile and visual. Treatment should aim at harnessing the potential of the impaired limb without compromising remaining sensibility or motor power.

References

1. Steindler A: *Kinesiology of the Human Body.* Charles C Thomas Publisher, 1955.
2. Kapandji I: Architecture and functions of the hand, in Tubiana R, ed: *The Hand.* W.B. Saunders Co., 1981.
3. Hollingshead W: *Anatomy for Surgeons,* in *The Back and Limbs,* ed 3. Harper & Row, Publishers, 1982, vol 3.
4. Bunch W, Keagy R: Basics of upper limb orthotics, in Bunch WH, Keagy RD, eds: *Principles of Orthotic Treatment.* The C.V. Mosby Co, 1976:Chap 5.
5. Inman V, Sanders M, Abbot C: Observations on the function of the shoulder joint. *J Bone Joint Surg* 1944;26:1.
6. Perry J: Normal upper extremity kinesiology. *Phys Therapy* 1978;58:265.
7. Christensen JB, Adams JP, Cho KO, et al: A study of the interosseous distance between the radius and ulna during rotation of the forearm. *Anat Rec* 1968;160:261-271.
8. Sarrafian SK, Melamed JL, Goshgarian GM: Study of wrist motion in flexion and extension. *Clin Orthop Relat Res* 1977;126:153-159.
9. Palmer AK, Werner FW, Murphy D, Glisson R: Normal wrist motion; A biomechanical study. *J Hand Surg* 1985;10(1):39-46.
10. Flatt A: Kinesiology of the hand, in Reynolds FC, ed: *American Academy of Orthopaedic Surgeons: Instructional Course Lectures.* The C. V. Mosby Co, 1961, vol 18.
11. Swanson A: The Krukenberg procedure in the juvenile amputee. *J Bone Joint Surg* 1964;46A:1540.
12. U.S. Department of Health and Human Services: *Vibration Syndrome.* NIOSH Current Intelligence Bulletin No. 38, 1983.
13. Tichauer ER, Gage H: Ergonomic principles basic to hand tool design. *Am Indus Hygiene Assoc J* 1977;38:622.
14. Napier JR: The prehensile movements of the human hand. *J Bone Joint Surg* 1956;388:902.
15. Moberg E: *The Upper Limb in Tetraplegia.* Georg Thieme Verlag, 1978, p 11.
16. Kamakura N, Matsuo M, Ishii H, Mitsuboshi F, Miura Y: Patterns of static prehension in normal hands. *Am J Occup Ther* 1980;34(7):437.
17. Von Lanz T, Wachsmuth W: *Praktische Anatomie.* Springer Verlag, 1959. Cited in Boyes J. *Bunnell's Surgery of the Hand,* ed 4. J.B. Lippincott, 1964.
18. Smith R: Extensor carpi radialis brevis tendon transfer for thumb adduction. *J Hand Surg* 1983;8(1):4.
19. Nalebuff E: Diagnosis, classification, and management of rheumatoid thumb deformities. *Bull Hosp Joint Dis* 1967;29:119.

Wartime Amputations

Donald A. Gajewski, MD, MBA, FAAOS

CHAPTER 6

ABSTRACT

Amputations are among the most severe limb injuries seen in military combat. Caring for personnel with such severe traumatic injuries is a two-stage procedure involving initial care at a forward medical facility to remove the damaged limb to prevent infection and save the patient's life, and later definitive care provided after the patient is transported to another medical facility. Advances in care over decades of wars and conflicts have led to the increased survival of personnel with limb amputations. Specialized care centers staffed by surgeons, nurses, prosthetists, and therapists have been established by the US military to provide a team approach to caring for combat personnel with amputations, with the goal of returning each injured patient to the best possible health and function.

Keywords: combat amputations; Korea; Operation Enduring Freedom; Operation Iraqi Freedom; US amputee care program; Vietnam; World War II

Introduction

Compared with the typical battle casualty, amputations represent a small but important group of combat casualties that require longer hospital stays, more surgical care, and prosthetic fitting. The wars of the 20th and 21st centuries have found surgeons relearning the principles of care for individuals with amputations in a combat setting. The techniques and special postoperative care for these patients are not routinely taught in surgical training programs in the United States. Such personnel often are the most severely injured patients seen on the battlefield and require priority care at forward surgical echelons.

Conflict can occur without warning, and military surgeons could be treating battle casualties with little or no preparation. It is the goal of any military surgeon to be prepared to treat any battle casualty that arises, which means minimizing morbidity and mortality, even with a large number of patients. Preparedness therefore involves the ability to not only treat battlefield casualties but also instruct others on the care of such patients.

Personnel with amputations have historically been a substantial clinical problem for military surgeons because of (1) the severity of injury, (2) high morbidity, and (3) long hospital stays. Very few surgeons have extensive experience caring for individuals with amputations in civilian practice, thus making the study of this type of injury paramount for military surgeons to provide the best care for their patients. During every conflict in the 20th and 21st centuries, there has been a steep learning curve concerning the care of individuals with amputations.

The latest surgical techniques from civilian practice often are inappropriately applied to personnel who must be transported from a combat zone. The goals of initial care must take into account the deleterious effects of evacuation; thus, any initial surgery should prepare the soldier (or civilian) for the trauma of transportation. In the case of personnel with amputations, wound closure often is attempted to provide a residual limb so that a prosthesis may be fitted as soon as possible. As documented in World War I, World War II, and the Vietnam War, early wound closure in battlefield hospitals was shown to dramatically increase complication rates.

During the recent past, the Army Medical Department has assumed responsibility for other missions (eg, refugee care). The care of refugees and patients who are not US or allied soldiers, and therefore are not evacuated, has changed the traditional role of military surgeons. For such patients, both initial and definitive care currently occurs in the combat theater. Patient factors also are variable, including being of any age or sex and having a variety of nutritional and health problems. Prosthetic fitting of the amputated limb also is highly variable and depends on the resources of the international community, involved nongovernmental organizations, and the healthcare resources of the patient's nation.

Neither Dr. Gajewski nor any immediate family member has received anything of value from or has stock or stock options held in a commercial company or institution related directly or indirectly to the subject of this chapter.

This chapter is adapted from Gajewski DA, Dougherty PJ: Wartime amputations, in Krajbich JI, Pinzur MS, Potter BK, Stevens PM, eds: *Atlas of Amputations and Limb Deficiencies: Surgical, Prosthetic, and Rehabilitation Principles*, ed 4. American Academy of Orthopaedic Surgeons, 2016, pp 115-124.

Evolution of US Military Care

Mechanisms of Injury

During the American Civil War, gunshot wounds were the main cause of injury leading to amputation (75%), with the remainder of the injuries caused by artillery projectiles (fragments or grapeshot).[1,2] By World War I, artillery shell fragments were the most common cause of injury leading to amputation. Artillery and shell fragments were the major cause of injury during World War II, but Hampton[3] noted that the prevalence of land mines contributed to the number of patients with limb loss in Italy.

Indications for Surgery

Early in the American Civil War, amputations were recommended under the following conditions: crush injury, nerve or blood vessel injury, gunshot fracture with extensive comminution, a major open joint injury accompanied by a fracture, or extensive soft-tissue injury.[4,5] Surgery was recommended as soon as possible within the primary period of the first day, before the development of sepsis.

By 1863, as surgical techniques evolved and surgeons became more experienced, indications for amputation became more refined. Gunshot fractures of the femur were not always necessarily an indication for amputation. In 1863, Moses[6] reported a 12.9% incidence of amputation associated with long-bone fractures for the battles near Chattanooga, Tennessee. Hodgen[7] and Lidell[8] reported good results in treating gunshot fractures of the lower limbs with Hodgen splints. Hodgen himself, who treated survivors of the long evacuation from the battlefield to a large hospital in St. Louis, Missouri, thought that amputation should be performed only for those patients who had injuries to joints, blood vessels, or nerves. Swinburne[9] advocated amputation surgery for a partial or complete traumatic amputation, extensive soft-tissue injury associated with nerve or blood vessel injury and denuded bone, the loss of a major blood vessel, or compound fractures of the knee or ankle joint. Most gunshot fractures were managed nonsurgically during the Civil War, and a variety of splints were developed to treat patients with these fractures.[7,8]

During World War I, the indications for surgery also changed. Speed,[10] who was with the Base Hospital (Chicago Unit) in France in 1918, reported on 121 amputations. The indications for surgery were severe fractures, gas gangrene, sepsis, secondary hemorrhage, and trench foot. The most common level was transfemoral amputation (58.6%). Speed[10] recommended an open circular amputation with longitudinal skin slits up the side of the residual limb.

Evacuation Hospital No. 8 reported 151 amputations in 4,714 battle injuries (3.2%) from September 13 to November 13, 1918. Of these, 62% were for gas gangrene, 33.7% for trauma, and 10.5% for sepsis. Again, transfemoral amputations were the most prevalent (39%).[11]

By World War II, the indications for surgery were primarily for the direct effects of trauma, with a partial or complete traumatic amputation being the most common reason for amputation; completion of the amputation was the initial procedure performed. Major vascular repair had not yet been developed, and up to 20% of limb losses were caused by vascular injuries. Infection had declined as a major indication for surgery, possibly because of the widespread use of antibiotics.[3,12,13]

Surgical Techniques

Various amputation techniques were reported during the Civil War. The Army Medical Museum recorded 253,142 casualties in the Civil War; 20,559 patients (8.1%) had major limb amputations (those proximal to the wrist or the ankle). In this series, transfemoral amputation was the most common amputation level. The open circular (or flapless) technique was most commonly used. For transtibial amputations, flaps were used in 1,720 patients (58.8%), and the open circular technique was used in 1,206 patients (41.2%). The total overall mortality of these patients was 35.7%.[14]

During World War I, various techniques were attempted for amputation surgery. The United States officially declared war in 1917, but the Red Cross had been providing medical units to France since the beginning of the war in 1914. In 1918, a hospital center was established in Savenay, France, with Evacuation Hospital No. 8 as its core unit. An amputation service was established at that hospital to care for people with amputations who would be returning to the United States. The goals of this service were to provide skin traction, wound care, and physical therapy. A program of early ambulation with fitting of a temporary prosthesis, with a design based on the experience of Belgian physicians, also was instituted at Savenay, and approximately 20% of the returning personnel with amputations were initially fitted there.[11,15] Of the 550 individuals with amputations examined at Savenay, 58% were treated using the open circular technique, 30% using the flap technique with delayed primary closure, and 11% using primary or delayed primary closure alone.[11] Of the residual limbs that were closed, 25% needed to be reopened because of infection.

After patients were stabilized, they were evacuated to the United States. In the continental United States, five hospitals were designated as amputation centers to consolidate the resources of surgeons, prosthetists, physical therapists, and nurses. The team approach, which is currently used, had its origin at these specialty centers during World War I.[16]

Kirk,[17] who became the US Army Surgeon General during World War II, wrote about his experiences in caring for personnel with amputations at two hospitals, where he treated approximately 1,700 patients. He advocated the open circular technique for war casualties for two reasons: (1) its simplicity and (2) preservation of the maximum residual limb length, both of which allowed wide drainage to manage infection and enabled earlier transport of the patient. Surgical procedures were staged, and definitive surgical closure was performed when the patient was stable and in a stable environment. Kirk[17] noted that at least 95% of the patients who arrived from overseas with open residual limbs needed additional care before prosthetic fitting. Most residual limbs were edematous and had unhealed areas. Other problems included bony protrusion and infection (most often from *Streptococcus*, *Staphylococcus*, *Proteus*, and Klebs–Löffler bacillus species).[17]

Early in World War II, military surgeons relearned the lessons from previous conflicts. Patients who did not have skin traction after open circular amputations experienced bony protrusion and needed reamputation, with the resultant loss of residual limb length. Amputations in which the skin had been closed were seldom successful because of infection. After the attack on Pearl Harbor, Hawaii, amputated limbs managed with delayed primary or primary closure became infected and required amputation at a higher level (LT Peterson, MD, unpublished data, 1946).

Early in World War I, because of his experience, Kirk was instrumental in developing policies to care for personnel with amputations. In 1942, the lack of success with early wound closure led Kirk[18] (before becoming Surgeon General) to reemphasize the open circular amputation technique. The technique at this time was characterized by amputating at the lowest level of viable soft tissue, allowing the skin to retract, and successively cutting layers of muscle and bone more proximally to produce a concave residual limb. The open residual limb permitted wide drainage to prevent infection. Postoperatively, the patient was to be maintained in continuous skin traction to prevent the retraction of soft tissues. A repair or plastic closure of the residual limb was then performed for patients with an adherent scar. In a later article, Kirk and McKeever[12] emphasized that the open circular technique was a two-stage procedure that required a second surgery for wound closure.

Prosthetic Devices

There was no standardized prosthetic fitting or rehabilitation for Civil War soldiers with amputations. Minor[19] recommended that the artificial limb should have the following characteristics: the same size and shape as the limb being replaced; constructed of light, strong, and durable materials; and "well fitting to the residual limb." Minor[19] thought that the Anglesey and Bly legs (patented in 1805 and 1858, respectively) were most appropriate because both had an ankle joint. Palmer legs (created by Benjamin Palmer in 1846), which had a solid ankle, also were popular. It is not known how many soldiers used prostheses because many people with lower limb amputations walked with ambulatory aids, such as crutches, rather than wearing a prosthesis. During the Civil War, Otis and Huntington[14] reported that 40 to 60 patients with knee disarticulations were fitted for a prosthesis.

During World War I, several improvements were made in the care and prosthetic fitting of soldiers with limb loss. First, a program of early fitting with a plaster temporary prosthesis was tried in France.[15] Wilson,[15] who was in charge of the amputee service at Savenay where a limited program of early walking was instituted for people with lower limb amputations, believed that if the wound was clean, a patient could begin ambulating after 2 to 3 weeks. At this time, the patient was fitted with a temporary prosthesis consisting of a socket and a frame. The frame could be prefabricated and needed a minimum of fitting, and the socket was generally made from plaster of Paris and molded to relieve wound pressure. Wilson[15] believed that early ambulation promoted wound healing, caused residual limb shrinkage, improved morale, and decreased the time to permanent prostheses. For upper limb amputations, body-powered grasping hooks were developed and used.[17,20,21]

Before World War II, no national research program, either military or civilian, existed to investigate the quality of artificial limbs. Initially, the military believed that such a program was the responsibility of the Veterans Administration, which had long-term responsibility for personnel with amputations. However, the Veterans Administration procured nearly all its prostheses from commercial manufacturers and therefore lacked its own experienced prosthetists and engineers.

At the request of the US Surgeon General in February 1945, the National Research Council established a Committee on Artificial Limbs. Paul E. Klopsteg of Northwestern University in Evanston, Illinois, chaired the committee. The goals of the committee were to assist the Army, the Navy, and the government in procuring the best prostheses to meet the demands of World War II personnel.[22,23] In addition, the committee sponsored studies on the mechanical behavior of both normal and artificial limbs; studied existing prostheses; and directed research toward improving, simplifying, and standardizing artificial limbs as much as possible. This included investigating potential new materials to manufacture limbs, studying the art of limb fitting, and training the patient in its use. These studies and research resulted in improvements in upper limb prostheses, including improvements in the use of plastics; the testing of many different joints; and the use of rubber, fabric, and bonding methods that were recommended by the National Bureau of Standards.[22-24]

At the University of California, basic research was conducted on gait and the use of muscles to power an upper limb prosthesis; the latter was known as a cineplastic operation. Lower limb studies focused on identifying the elements of normal gait, principles that are still in current use. This research, started during World War II, was ongoing for several years and led to substantial improvements in prostheses.[22-26]

The Vietnam Experience

The experiences of World War II and the Korean War were not routinely taught to surgeons before they were deployed to Vietnam. Consequently, the treatment of personnel with amputations in forward hospitals was not standardized and occasionally compromised patient care, especially in the earlier stages of the Vietnam War. As casualties increased, amputation centers in the continental United States slowly began to handle the specialized care required by these patients.

The incidence of amputations at surgical hospitals in Vietnam ranged from 4.5% to 5.6%. Most patients had either partial or complete traumatic amputations that were caused by their injuries, necessitating only completion of the residual limb. Trauma was the primary indication for amputation in more than 90% of the patients in Vietnam, followed by vascular complications (6%) and infection (3%).[27-31]

Late amputations were performed in cases of infection, from either an open fracture or a failed vascular repair. Schmitt and Armstrong[29] reported that 186 of 485 amputations (38%) performed at Clark Air Force Base in the Philippines were late amputations. The precise number of late amputations performed because of osteomyelitis is not known.

The Wound Data and Munitions Effectiveness Team recorded 98 significant amputations in their series (RF Bellamy, MD, personal communication). Of these, 35 patients died before reaching medical care, and one patient died of wounds after reaching medical care, a mortality rate similar to that caused by land mine injuries in the Bougainville Campaign during World War II.

Valley Forge Army General Hospital Experience

Amputations caused by land mines and booby traps occurred in 62% of the patients examined at Valley Forge Army General Hospital (Alcide M. LaNoue, MD, Ft. Leavenworth, KS, unpublished data, 1971). Land mines in Vietnam were unconventional devices made from other ordnance or improvised from local materials. Transtibial (40%) and transfemoral (27% to 31%) amputations were the most common. According to data of the Wound Data and Munitions Effectiveness Team, patients who had lost more than one limb comprised 16% of the battlefield casualty admissions at Valley Forge Army General Hospital and 19% of the patients who were received alive at a medical treatment facility. It is unknown if this increase was the result of improved medical care, which preserved the most severely injured, or if there was a change in the type of weapons used against American troops.

Although the recommended technique at this time was an open circular amputation with postoperative skin traction, as in previous wars, this technique was not always used. In his series of 410 patients received at Valley Forge Army General Hospital between 1969 and 1970, LaNoue reported that 41% of the transtibial amputations had skin closure before evacuation, and this group incurred a 56% failure rate because of gross infection. He also found that the time from injury to the prosthetic fitting increased from 9 to 11 months when closure was performed before evacuation (Alcide M. LaNoue, MD, Ft. Leavenworth, KS, unpublished data, 1971).

LaNoue also reported an 88% failure rate for Syme ankle disarticulations performed in the combat theater, necessitating conversion to amputation at the transtibial level. This failure occurred because the heel pad was partially devascularized by removal of the hindfoot. Rather, LaNoue recommended that the hindfoot be left intact and that simple wound débridement be performed for forefoot injuries, leaving the choice of definitive amputation to the receiving physician. The devascularized heel flap did poorly when a patient was transferred from Vietnam to the United States.

LaNoue concluded that initial amputations in the combat theater should follow three principles: (1) maximum length should be preserved, and definitive procedures should be ignored until a stable environment can be provided; (2) if a definitive procedure was necessary, the environment must be stabilized and the evacuation deferred; and (3) skin traction must be maintained on all residual limbs wherever possible.

A substantial number of US Army personnel from Vietnam received treatment at Letterman, Fitzsimons, Walter Reed, Brooke, and Valley Forge Army General Hospitals.[32] Only Valley Forge Army General Hospital, however, established an amputation service that combined the skills of a physical therapist, a surgeon, and a prosthetist on one team. A staff psychiatrist was added to the team in January 1971.[33] The goals of treatment in these hospitals were to provide residual limb healing, ambulation training (for lower limb amputations) or training in activities of daily living (for upper limb amputations), an initial prosthesis, and a medical board that would allow for medical retirement.

By 1969, the number of people with amputations had become large enough to justify a separate service at Valley Forge Army General Hospital. Patients evacuated from Vietnam were placed with other amputees, evaluated, and started on a program of residual limb healing and physical therapy. Later, patients were fitted with a temporary prosthesis to walk or perform activities of daily living. Because the numbers were substantial, these individuals were widely studied. The treatment of individuals with amputations generally followed a series of successive stages, as follows: (1) wound healing, (2) preprosthetic training, (3) the fitting of provisional prostheses, and (4) the fitting of permanent prostheses. Patients generally progressed from one stage to the next in sequential order. Each member of the treatment team was responsible for a specific stage. During wound healing, the surgeon provided most of the care. During preprosthetic training, primarily therapists worked with the patient. The prosthetist gradually became involved during the provisional and permanent prosthetic stages.[34]

An innovative early ambulation program was initiated at Valley Forge Army General Hospital to shorten the stages of rehabilitation, based on the program used by Wilson[15] during World War I. Patients ambulated earlier, even on open residual limbs, which allowed them to become upright sooner in an effort to attain an earlier proprioceptive sense. Moreover, weight bearing on lower limb amputations reduced swelling. The hard socket allowed for compression of the residual limb and decreased edema, which was thought to allow earlier prosthetic fitting. The psychological benefits associated with being upright sooner and earlier independence were well documented. The team approach of the amputation service at Valley Forge Army General Hospital was not always possible for the general orthopaedic service. The entire team followed a patient's progress from admission to discharge, providing comprehensive care to the patient and, ultimately, better patient functionality.

Long-Term Follow-Up

A review of the records of 484 personnel with battlefield amputations who were treated at Valley Forge Army General Hospital was performed to document the level of amputation, indication for initial surgery, and mechanism of injury.[34-36] The most common level of limb loss seen was a unilateral transtibial amputation, a trend that started in World War II, but there was a higher proportion of those with multiple limb loss (15.9%) than other studies, probably because Valley Forge Army General Hospital was a referral hospital where the more severely wounded patients were concentrated.

Sixty-four percent of the patients with a transtibial amputation were injured by land mines or booby traps. Small arms fire, exploding munitions, and rocket-propelled grenades accounted for the other amputations. Trauma was the indication for amputation in 89.5% of the patients, followed by vascular injury (8.4%) and infection (1.9%).[34]

To determine the lifetime effects of wartime limb loss (approximately 28 years after injury), patients from Valley Forge Army General Hospital were surveyed regarding their prosthetic history and family life, including marriage and children; the number of additional surgeries since the initial amputation; psychiatric history, including membership in Alcoholics Anonymous and marriage counseling; other injuries; and work history.[34-36]

Transtibial Amputations

Of the 123 patients with transtibial amputation eligible for the follow-up study, 72 (59%) were available for follow-up and divided into two groups.[34] One group had isolated transtibial amputations, and the second group had at least one other major injury (polytrauma), defined in this study as a major lower limb long-bone fracture; burns over more than 20% of the body surface area; and/or substantial head, face, chest, or abdominal wounds. Most of the patients (44) were in the second group. A comparison of employment, marriage, and family factors showed no significant difference between the two groups. However, the reported incidence of psychological care differed significantly ($P < 0.001$) between the two groups, with only 21% of the first group seeking help compared with 50% of the second group.[34]

All respondents were currently wearing prostheses, with the first group averaging 15.9 hours per day and the second group, 15.7 hours. Most respondents reported that they had changed prostheses, specifically 78.5% of the first group and 72% of the second group. The most commonly reported changes were in the foot ($n = 22$), suspension ($n = 20$), liner ($n = 18$), and socket ($n = 8$). The average number of prostheses used since the first permanent prostheses were fitted was 7.89 (range, 3 to 30) in the first group and 8.84 (range, 4 to 30) in the second group. Patients reported an average of 1.94 surgical procedures since their initial amputation (range, 0 to 13), with 1.36 in the first group and 2.32 in the second group.[34]

The use of an osteoplastic technique (Ertl technique) for transtibial limb loss has been advocated for young, active patients. An Ertl osteoplasty produces an end-bearing residual limb by creating a bony synostosis between the tibia and the fibula at the distal end of the residual limb. The technique was originally described as creating a periosteal sleeve bridge or tube between the most distal end of the tibia and fibula, then filling this tube with bone graft to create a bone bridge at the distal bone of the residual limb. Proponents of this technique think that it produces a better end-bearing residual limb, with better prosthetic wear. Subsequent modifications to this technique include using a fibular strut and orthopaedic hardware for fixation of the bone. One important aspect of the technique, which is often ignored, is that it provides good soft-tissue coverage of the residual limb, including myodesis and/or myoplasty.

Deffer et al[37] reported that the Ertl procedure resulted in a more stable and durable residual limb. Comparison with other transtibial amputations was not documented however, and the definitive benefits of this level of amputation compared with the conventional transtibial amputation remain unclear. The Ertl procedure was performed in 42 patients (63%), 19 in the first group and 23 in the second group.[34] One patient reported undergoing bone block removal because of pain. The Medical Outcomes Study 36-Item Short Form (SF-36) scores for the first group were not significantly different ($P < 0.01$) from the controls. Patients in the second group were significantly different in all areas ($P < 0.01$). Currently, results are inconclusive regarding whether this technique should be used in every young patient undergoing transtibial amputation.[34,38,39]

Transfemoral Amputations

A review of records by Dougherty[36] showed that 59% of the patients with transfemoral amputations were injured by land mines and booby traps. Indications for surgery were trauma in 61.8% of the patients, failed vascular repair in 29.2%, and infection in 8.7%. The average time to Valley Forge Army General Hospital was 4.4 weeks and to pylon fitting was 4 weeks, with permanent prosthetic fitting at an average of 7 months. At follow-up, an average of 28 years after injury, 51% of those alive and eligible for the study agreed to answer the questionnaire. Of those, 93% are or were married, 91.3% are or have been employed, and 85% have children.

The average number of surgical procedures on the residual limb since the initial amputation was 2.4.[36] Six patients (13%) did not at that time wear a prosthesis; the others wore a prosthesis an average of 13.5 hours per day and hade owned an average of 13.8 prostheses since their initial fitting. Of those who wore a prosthesis, half had changed their prescription since the initial fitting. Twenty-four patients (52%) reported seeking psychological care, including Alcoholics Anonymous and marriage counseling. The SF-36 scores were significantly lower than those of a control group ($P < 0.05$) in all categories except mental health.

Bilateral Transfemoral Amputations

Thirty patients (6.2%) in the follow-up study were identified as having bilateral transfemoral amputations.[35] Of these patients, 26 were injured by land mines or booby traps. Other mechanisms of injury included artillery or mortar fire (three patients) and machine gun fire (one patient). The indications for surgery were trauma in 53 (88%) of 60 residual limbs and infection in the remaining seven limbs. The medical records indicated that postoperative skin traction was used in fewer than 50% of the patients. Three patients also sustained an upper limb amputation, with one at the wrist, one above the elbow, and one below the elbow. Documentation of shock and resuscitation attempts was incomplete, but the records of 14 patients indicated that an average of 23.7 units of blood had been transfused.

Patients arrived at Valley Forge Army General Hospital an average of 4.5 weeks after injury. The records of 23 patients showed that they were fitted with pylons or stubbie feet an average of 8.3 weeks after injury (range, 3 to 20 weeks). The records of 17 patients showed that they were fitted with permanent prostheses an average of 6.5 months after injury (range, 3 to 12 months).

Three patients died after leaving Valley Forge Army General Hospital, and 23 of the remaining 27 (85.2%) agreed to answer the questionnaire and complete the SF-36 form. Sixteen of the 23 (69.5%) were employed outside the home even though they had adequate compensation from the Veterans Administration to maintain a modest lifestyle. Twenty-one (91.3%) were or had been married, and 20 (87%) had children. Five patients (21.7%) reported the use of mental health services.[35]

Five patients (21.7%) reported that they still wore a prosthesis for an average of 7.7 hours per day. Ten others (43.4%) reported using their prostheses an average of 12.8 years after leaving Valley Forge Army General Hospital. Five patients reported using prostheses primarily for "going out."

The SF-36 scores of those with bilateral transfemoral amputations did not differ significantly from those of a control group except in the area of physical function. It is not clear why the SF-36 scores for this group were higher than those of the other groups. One explanation might be the small number of patients. Another explanation might be the lower proportion of patients in the other groups who were eligible to participate in the study. Finally, an error in the methodology is a possibility.

Operations Iraqi Freedom and Enduring Freedom

The wars in Iraq and Afghanistan saw the lowest fatality rate from combat wounds of any conflict in American history.[40] Although much of this can be attributed to improvements in protective equipment, the development of an in-theater trauma system has undoubtedly contributed to improved outcomes for service members injured on the battlefield.[41] In addition, all deploying surgical teams prepared themselves for combat casualty care at the Army, Navy, or Air Force Trauma Training Centers, which are associated with renowned civilian level 1 trauma hospitals. Tactical combat casualty care and emergency war surgery courses also were available to deploying surgeons. Operations Iraqi Freedom and Enduring Freedom also saw the development of far-forward surgical resuscitation teams that provided surgical and critical care to the most severely wounded service members as close to the point of injury as possible. In addition, these operations saw the implementation of the Critical Care Aeromedical Transport Team, which has the capability of evacuating stabilized, critically ill patients while providing en route care and continued resuscitation.[42] These advances have unarguably led to the increased survival of personnel with amputations who may have succumbed to their injuries in previous conflicts.[43]

In these recent military operations, the most common mechanism of injury for major limb amputations was a blast injury, mostly in the form of improvised explosive devices. Of all the military casualties in Operations Iraqi Freedom and Enduring Freedom, 70.5% of individuals sustained a major limb injury, with amputation comprising 7.4% of all major limb injuries.[44] Transtibial amputations were the most common, accounting for 41.8% of all amputations, followed by transfemoral amputations at 35.5%. Thirty percent of military personnel sustained multiple amputations, and 14% of all amputations involved the upper limbs. Ten percent of all military personnel underwent amputation more than 90 days after the date of injury (late amputation), either because of patient wishes or complications with attempted limb salvage.[45] It should be noted by the care team that these late amputation patients have a higher prevalence of wound complications when compared with patients who elect early amputations. Melcer et al showed that late amputations had a significantly higher osteomyelitis rate (53%) than early amputations. Additionally, patients undergoing late amputations had significantly more psychologic diagnoses than patients undergoing either early amputation or limb salvage.[46] In 2001, the US Army, under the guidance of the Army Surgeon General, consolidated the care of personnel with amputations in specialized centers located at Walter Reed Army Medical Center in Washington, DC, and Brooke Army Medical Center in San Antonio, Texas. The US Navy established a third center at the Balboa Naval Hospital in San Diego, California, with the intent of providing care to personnel who were from the West Coast. At each center, a multidisciplinary team from more than a dozen specialties was brought together to address not only the physical needs of the wounded service member but also the psychological, social, vocational, and spiritual needs of soldiers, sailors, airmen, and Marines.[47] Because of this specialized care, soldiers from these recent conflicts have seen the highest rate for return to duty (16.5%) in recent history.[48] Special Forces soldiers were significantly more likely to return to duty (58%), despite having amputation levels and Injury Severity Scores similar to those of all other military personnel sustaining amputation. Interestingly, none of these high-level operators were found to have post-traumatic stress disorder as a disabling condition, suggesting a difference in motivation, resources, and/or opportunities for an operator to return to duty.[49]

Current Concepts

In-Theater Care

The initial goal of the combat surgeon in treating a traumatic battlefield amputation is to prevent infection and save the patient's life while preserving as much residual length as possible. The indications for immediate amputation in the combat theater are near-complete or partial amputation, irreparable vascular injury or failed vascular repair with an ischemic limb, life-threatening sepsis because of local infection, or a patient in extremis with severe soft-tissue and bone injury to the limb.[50] If a patient has a catastrophic limb injury but has a viable limb and is physiologically stable, amputation should not be performed in the combat theater solely because of predicted limb dysfunction. In this case, serial débridement of the wounds to prevent infection and stabilize the limb should take place until the patient arrives in the continental United States. At that time, the patient can participate in the decision for amputation, which psychologically may help the patient accept their limb loss.

The most common mechanism of injury for a traumatic amputation is a blast injury, and the high energy of this mechanism should be respected. The zone of injury is much more proximal and broader than appreciated at first glance. Thorough débridement should be performed, which includes extending wounds with longitudinal incisions to check for debris that may have traveled proximally through tissue planes. The treating physician should have knowledge of standard amputation incisions to facilitate future definitive closure. An improperly placed incision for initial débridement may change the definitive closure when the patient returns to the continental United States for continued care. Guillotine amputations should not be performed; rather, open, length-preserving amputations, preserving all healthy tissue, should be performed to leave the maximum number of treatment options for the surgeon providing definitive care. Any distal tissue can be considered a "flap of opportunity" and can aid in the definitive closure, saving not only length but also potentially a joint level.[50]

Amputation length should not be determined by proximal ipsilateral fractures. All proximal fractures should be stabilized before patient transport for potential salvage of optimum residual limb length.[51] Antibiotic beads should be considered in heavily contaminated, deep wounds. Invasive mold infection should be suspected in patients who sustain high transfemoral amputations while on foot patrol and have received large volumes of blood transfusion during resuscitation.[52] These wounds should be packed open with a topical adjunct, such as Dakin solution (dilute sodium hypochlorite solution).

Evacuation Care

Although the transport times between echelons of care are predictably short, the accepting surgeon should always consider a repeat débridement after the patient's arrival at the treatment facility. The zone of injury, which may initially have been limited, can rapidly declare itself during transfer of the patient from one treatment facility to another and between serial procedures. The application of a negative-pressure wound dressing should be at the discretion of the surgeon and should be avoided in complex, massive wounds in which the seal would be difficult to maintain (**Figure 1**). Otherwise, this dressing has been shown to be not only feasible in an intercontinental air evacuation system but also preferred by both flight crews and patients.[53]

Definitive Care

After arrival at the definitive treatment facility, serial débridement is continued until the wound is ready for definitive closure. All means should be used to preserve limb length, keeping in mind, however, that a stable soft-tissue envelope is the most important factor in a patient's ability to wear and ambulate in a prosthesis. Skin traction may not work if there is a tenuous soft-tissue envelope that precludes the use of benzoin for traction. A negative-pressure wound dressing is a good substitute for skin traction when used in conjunction with elastic bands (vessel loops) that are applied under tension in a zig-zag pattern (Roman sandal pattern) along the skin edge. As the negative-pressure dressing assists with fluid evacuation and edema control, the vessel loops provide skin traction, gradually bringing the wound edges closer. Free tissue transfers and skin grafting also should be considered to preserve length in a combat amputation, but may have the disadvantage of sensation loss, thus resulting in pressure sores in areas of prosthesis contact. Advances in prosthetic liner and socket technology have decreased the complications commonly seen in these insensate tissues.[54]

Rehabilitation

The concept of multidisciplinary amputation care learned at Valley Forge Army General Hospital during the Vietnam War was mirrored during the conflicts in the Global War on Terror. Three facilities, the Military Advanced Training Center at Walter Reed Army Medical Center (now known as Walter Reed National Military Medical Center), the Center for the Intrepid at Brooke Army Medical Center, and the Comprehensive Combat and Complex Casualty Care Center at Naval Medical Center San Diego all focused on a holistic, family-centered care program. The goal was to return the service member to the highest quality of life regardless of injuries. Using specialized care centers also allowed for a strong peer visitation and mentorship program, providing accessible, constant peer support and camaraderie.[55]

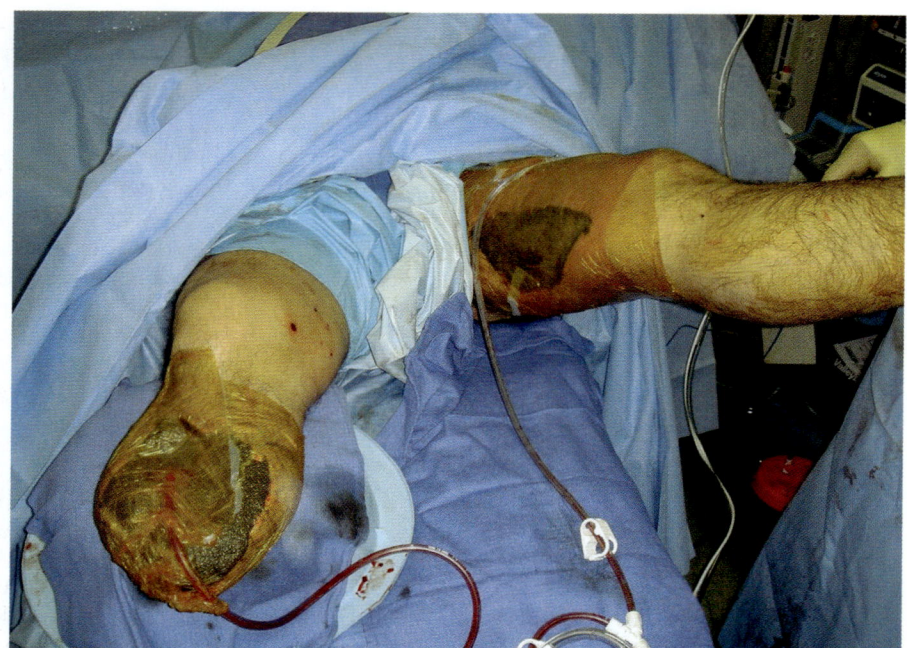

FIGURE 1 Clinical photograph showing the use of negative-pressure wound therapy to separate a wound from the environment. This patient was subsequently treated with a tissue-sparing amputation after injury by a mortar explosion. (Reproduced from Covey DC, Richardson MW, Powell ET, Mazurek MT, Morgan SJ: Advances in the care of battlefield orthopaedic injuries. *Instr Course Lect* 2010;59:427-435.)

Revision Surgery

Both elective and nonelective complication rates are high in combat amputations. Tintle et al[56] showed that there was a 53% revision surgery rate in patients sustaining a major lower limb amputation. Postoperative wound infection was the most common at 27%, followed by symptomatic heterotopic ossification (24%), neuromas (11%), scar revision (8%), and myodesis failure (6%). Revision surgery can be psychologically challenging to a patient who has made great strides in rehabilitation only to have this progress stopped or delayed by additional surgery and recovery time. Therefore, it is important to counsel patients on this high revision surgery rate during the initial hospitalization and further inform them that, other than surgery for infections, they are commonly the ones requesting the revision surgery.

SUMMARY

Amputations are among the most severe limb injuries seen in war. Care for personnel with amputations has been an important clinical concern for the military in every major conflict in the 20th and 21st centuries. Because few surgeons or medical teams have substantial clinical experience in caring for such patients, lapses or inconsistencies occur. In addition, the techniques and requirements for patients evacuated from overseas hospitals differ from those required by patients treated in civilian hospitals.

War surgery for amputations is a two-stage procedure. Initial care to remove the limb, prevent infection, and save the patient's life is provided at a forward hospital. Length-preserving amputations should be performed, avoiding guillotine amputations and skin traction. After stabilization, the patient continues along the evacuation chain, undergoing additional débridements at every echelon of care. The patient should be treated with a negative-pressure wound dressing when possible.

As demonstrated in previous conflicts, there is a clear need for amputation centers that specialize in the care of personnel evacuated from a combat theater. The main advantages of this consolidation of efforts include maintaining the clinical skills of the nursing staff, prosthetists, therapists, and surgeons to facilitate complete healing of the residual limb; fitting with a provisional prosthesis; rehabilitation; and fitting with a satisfactory permanent prosthesis. Specialized care centers have been established by the US military to provide a team approach to caring for combat personnel with amputations, with the goal of returning these individuals to maximal health and function.

References

1. Fisher GJ: Report of fifty-seven cases of amputations, in the hospitals near Sharpsburg, MD, after the Battle of Antietam, September 17, 1862. *Am J Med Sci* 1863;45(89):44-51.
2. Letterman J: *Medical Recollections of the Army of the Potomac*. Appleton and Company, 1866.
3. Hampton J: Amputations, in Cleveland M, ed: *Orthopaedic Surgery in the Mediterranean Theater of Operations*. US Government Printing Office, 1957, pp 245-270.
4. Gross SD: *A Manual of Military Surgery*. JB Lippincott, 1861, pp 74-89. (Reprinted by Norman Publishing, 1988.)
5. Hamilton FH: *A Practice Treatise on Military Surgery*. Bailliere Brothers, 1861, pp 165-189. (Reprinted by Norman Publishing, 1989.)
6. Moses I: Surgical notes of cases of gunshot injuries occurring near Chattanooga, TN. *Am J Med Sci* 1863;48:344-366.
7. Hodgen JT: On the treatment of gunshot fractures of the femur and tibia. *Am Med Times* 1863;8:169-170.
8. Lidell JA: Correspondence. *Am Med Times* 1863;8:102-103.
9. Swinburne J: Amputations. *Am Med Times* 1863;6:149-150.
10. Speed K: Base hospital amputations in war. *J Am Med Assoc* 1918;71(4):271-274.
11. Weed FW, ed: Surgery. Vol XI. US Government Printing Office, 1927, pp 687-712.
12. Kirk NT, McKeever FM: The guillotine amputation. *J Am Med Assoc* 1944;124(15):1027-1030.
13. Cleveland M: Amputations, in *Surgery in World War II: Orthopedic Surgery in the European Theater of Operations*. US Government Printing Office, 1956, pp 155-167.
14. Otis GA, Huntington DC: *The Medical and Surgical History of the War*

of the Rebellion: Part II. Vol 2. US Government Printing Office, 1883, pp 1-614, 870-871.

15. Wilson PD: Early weight-bearing in the treatment of amputations of the lower limbs. *J Bone Joint Surg Am* 1922;4:224-247.

16. Callender GR, Coupal JF, Section JF: *Surgery*. Vol XII. US Government Printing Office, 1929, pp 407-461.

17. Kirk NT: *Amputations*. WB Conkey, 1924.

18. Kirk NT: Amputations in war. *J Am Med Assoc* 1942;120(1):13-16.

19. Minor JM: *Report on Artificial Limbs*. New York Academy of Medicine, 1861, pp 1163-1180.

20. Office of the Surgeon General: Instruments and appliances: Temporary artificial limbs. *Mil Surg* 1918;42:490-498.

21. Office of the Surgeon General: The relation between the amputation and the fitting of the artificial limb. *Mil Surg* 1918;42:154-168.

22. Klopsteg PE: The functions and activities of the committee on artificial limbs of the National Research Council: A preliminary report. *J Bone Joint Surg Am* 1947;29(2):538-540.

23. Conn H, Magnuson PS, Wilson PD: Report of civilian consultants committee on army amputation services. *Mil Surg* 1946;98:52-57.

24. Brodbeck JA: Experiment with the suction socket for transfemoral amputees. *Bull US Army Med Dep* 1947;7(4):408-411.

25. Kissane MM: A light-weight end-bearing thigh bucket. *Bull US Army Med Dep* 1947;7(4):406-407.

26. Thomas A: Anatomical and physiological considerations in the alignment and fitting of amputation prostheses for the lower extremity. *J Bone Joint Surg Am* 1944;26:645-659.

27. Byerly WG, Pendse PD: War surgery in a forward surgical hospital in Vietnam: A continuing report. *Mil Med* 1971;136(3):221-226.

28. Jones EL, Peters AF, Gasior RM: Early management of battle casualties in Vietnam: An analysis of 1,011 consecutive cases treated at a mobile army surgical hospital. *Arch Surg* 1968;97(1):1-15.

29. Schmitt HJ Jr, Armstrong RG: Wounds causing loss of limb. *Surg Gynecol Obstet* 1970;130(4):682-684.

30. Seligson D, Bailey R: Traumatic amputations: A Vietnam experience. *Clin Orthop Relat Res* 1976;114:304-306.

31. Wilber MC, Willett LV Jr, Buono F: Combat amputees. *Clin Orthop Relat Res* 1970;68:10-13.

32. Mayfield GW: Vietnam war amputees, in Burkhalter WE, ed: *Surgery in Vietnam: Orthopedic Surgery*. US Government Printing Office, 1994, pp 131-153.

33. Frank JL: The amputee war casualty in a military hospital: Observations on psychological management. *Int J Psychiatry Med* 1973;4(1):1-16.

34. Dougherty PJ: Transtibial amputees from the Vietnam War: Twenty-eight-year follow-up. *J Bone Joint Surg Am* 2001;83(3):383-389.

35. Dougherty PJ: Long-term follow-up study of bilateral above-the-knee amputees from the Vietnam War. *J Bone Joint Surg Am* 1999;81(10):1384-1390.

36. Dougherty PJ: Long-term follow-up of unilateral transfemoral amputees from the Vietnam war. *J Trauma* 2003;54(4):718-723.

37. Deffer PA, Moll JH, LaNoue AM: The Ertl osteoplastic transtibial amputation (Proceedings). *J Bone Joint Surg Am* 1971;53:1028.

38. Tintle SM, Keeling JJ, Forsberg JA, Shawen SB, Andersen RC, Potter BK: Operative complications of combat-related transtibial amputations: A comparison of the modified Burgess and modified Ertl tibiofibular synostosis techniques. *J Bone Joint Surg Am* 2011;93(11):1016-1021.

39. Keeling JJ, Shawen SB, Forsberg JA, et al: Comparison of functional outcomes following bridge synostosis with non-bone-bridging transtibial combat-related amputations. *J Bone Joint Surg Am* 2013;95(10):888-893.

40. Gawande A: Casualties of war: Military care for the wounded from Iraq and Afghanistan. *N Engl J Med* 2004;351(24):2471-2475.

41. Eastridge BJ, Jenkins D, Flaherty S, Schiller H, Holcomb JB: Trauma system development in a theater of war: Experiences from Operation Iraqi Freedom and Operation Enduring Freedom. *J Trauma* 2006;61(6):1366-1372.

42. Mason PE, Eadie JS, Holder AD: Prospective observational study of United States (US) air force critical care air transport team operations in Iraq. *J Emerg Med* 2011;41(1):8-13.

43. Bellamy RF: A note on American combat mortality in Iraq. *Mil Med* 2007;172(10):i, 1023.

44. Stansbury LG, Lalliss SJ, Branstetter JG, Bagg MR, Holcomb JB: Amputations in U.S. military personnel in the current conflicts in Afghanistan and Iraq. *J Orthop Trauma* 2008;22(1):43-46.

45. Krueger CA, Wenke JC, Ficke JR: Ten years at war: Comprehensive analysis of amputation trends. *J Trauma Acute Care Surg* 2012;73(6 suppl 5):S438-S444.

46. Melcer T, Walker J, Bhatnager V, Richard E, Sechriest V, Galarneau M: A comparison of fout-year halth outcomes following compat amputation and limb salvage. *PLoS One* 2017;12(1):e0170569.

47. Gajewski D, Granville R: The United States armed forces amputee patient care program. *J Am Acad Orthop Surg* 2006;14(10 Spec No.):S183-S187.

48. Stinner DJ, Burns TC, Kirk KL, Ficke JR: Return to duty rate of amputee soldiers in the current conflicts in Afghanistan and Iraq. *J Trauma* 2010;68(6):1476-1479.

49. Belisle JG, Wenke JC, Krueger CA: Return-to-duty rates among US military combat-related amputees in the global war on terror: Job description matters. *J Trauma Acute Care Surg* 2013;75(2):279-286.

50. US Government Printing Office: *Emergency War Surgery: Fourth United States Revision*. US Government Printing Office, 2013.

51. Gordon WT, O'Brien FP, Strauss JE, Andersen RC, Potter BK: Outcomes associated with the internal fixation of long-bone fractures proximal to traumatic amputations. *J Bone Joint Surg Am* 2010;92(13):2312-2318.

52. Warkentien T, Rodriguez C, Lloyd B, et al: Ivasive mold infections following combat-related injuries. *Clin Infect Dis* 2012;55(11):1441-1449.

53. Fang R, Dorlac WC, Flaherty SF, et al: Feasibility of negative pressure wound therapy during intercontinental aeromedical evacuation of combat casualties. *J Trauma* 2010;69(suppl 1):S140-S145.

54. Crowe CS, Impastato KA, Donaghy AC, Earl C, Friedly JL, Keys KA: Prosthetic and orthotic options for lower extremity amputation and reconstruction. *Plast Aesthet Res* 2019;6:4.

55. Potter BK, Scoville CR: Amputation is not isolated: An overview of the US Army Amputee Patient Care Program and associated amputee injuries. *J Am Acad Orthop Surg* 2006;14(10 Spec No.):S188-S190.

56. Tintle SM, Shawen SB, Forsberg JA, et al: Reoperation after combat-related major lower extremity amputations. *J Orthop Trauma* 2014;28(4):232-237.

Prosthetic Rehabilitation in Less-Resourced Settings

Chapter 7

Helen Cochrane, MSc, CPO(c) • Carson Harte, HDip

ABSTRACT

A less-resourced setting has been defined as a geographic area with limited financial, human, and infrastructure resources. These conditions are common in low-income and middle-income countries and can represent a substantial barrier to the delivery of appropriate prosthetic services. Access to services, policies, funding, human resources, and prosthetic technologies may differ in less-resourced settings compared with conditions in some high-income countries. It is helpful to be aware of common commercially available prosthetic systems used in these challenging environments along with current technologic advances.

Keywords: assistive technology; barriers to prosthetic services; education prosthetics orthotics; less-resourced settings/low-income countries; prosthetics

Introduction

A less-resourced setting (LRS) has been defined as a geographic area with limited financial, human, and infrastructure resources. These conditions are common in low-income and middle-income countries but can also exist in some high-income countries.[1] Assistive technologies, such as prosthetic devices to help individuals with disabilities attain mobility, achieve equal opportunities, enjoy human rights, and live with dignity, are limited in these settings.[2-10]

The World Report on Disability from the World Health Organization (WHO) and the World Bank indicates that more than one billion individuals around the world live with disabilities.[3] Conservative population-based estimates suggest that 0.5% of any population may benefit from prosthetic or orthotic services;[3,5,9,11] in Africa, Asia, and Latin America; this includes an estimated 30 million individuals.[11] In many LRSs, the prevalence of disabilities is reported as higher than in well-resourced settings[10,12] and is expected to increase.[3,5] Irrespective of the setting, individuals with disabilities are known to have poorer health outcomes, lower educational attainment, reduced social and economic participation, and higher overall rates of poverty than those without disabilities.[3] Individuals from typical at-risk groups such as women, the elderly, those with limited education, and the unemployed also are considered to be at increased risk of disabilities.[3] These trends suggest a cycle of exclusion and a profound effect on those with disabilities living in an LRS.[10]

Access to appropriate, affordable, sustainable prosthetic services is important in mitigating this effect and presents challenges in LRSs. Appropriate services require collaboration among a spectrum of key stakeholders, including governments, funding agents, educators, industry, private enterprise, service providers, and the users of prosthetic services. Additional requirements include addressing the shortfall of adequately trained professional workforce and access to appropriate technology.[13]

Access to Prosthetic Services

The service and delivery of prosthetic devices in LRSs is provided by a range of stakeholders, which varies from country to country. The individual responsibilities between stakeholders within each country are unique and depend on the resources and capacities of the contributors. Services from referral through follow-up are often in short supply. They are commonly centralized in large cities and are usually located at a substantial distance from many potential users.[2]

Three major institutional donors, Deutsche Gesellschaft für Internationale Zusammenarbeit GIZ (formerly GTZ), the United States Agency for International Development (USAID), and The Nippon Foundation, have provided substantial ongoing support to improve access to assistive technology and monitor and evaluate the effect of investment in prosthetic orthotic services. Their input has generated activity in education, technology transfer, and services.

An impact assessment in East Africa by USAID indicated that its grants had a positive effect on the establishment of

---

Helen Cochrane or an immediate family member serves as a board member, owner, officer, or committee member of International Society of Prosthetics and Orthotics and Orthotics Prosthetics Canada. Carson Harte or an immediate family member serves as a paid consultant to or is an employee of Exceed Social Enterprise; and serves as a board member, owner, officer, or committee member of International Society for Prosthetics Orthotics.

services, the appropriateness of service delivery, and on the lives of individuals with disabilities.[14]

In South East Asia, the effect of The Nippon Foundation's long-term investment in establishing professional prosthetic orthotic education and services in six countries was found to have transformed the lives of users and their families, enabling greater independence, participation, and inclusion. The investment is a starting point for prosthetics and orthotics services and should improve its reach through development of better referral and increased awareness. Despite these investments, there persists a broad lack of understanding of the benefits and needs of assistive technologies; a failure of infrastructure to procure, produce, and maintain devices; and the absence of a properly trained workforce.[6]

In addition to major institutional donors, one of the most significant contributors to services, education, and technology in LRSs is the International Committee of the Red Cross (ICRC) through its Physical Rehabilitation Programme in low-income, conflict, or postconflict settings.

In 2020 alone the organization delivered 174,711 assistive devices; of those, 12.5% were prostheses representing the fitting of 21,874 services users.[15]

Policy and Funding

Many countries have an existing legislative framework related to disability and/or rehabilitation. As of 2018, 175 United Nations Member States have ratified the Convention on the Rights of Persons with Disabilities.[16] However, systematic barriers exist in the implementation of laws, including a lack of strategic planning, health infrastructure, health information systems, and communication strategies. These barriers are further compounded by a lack of agencies responsible for administering, coordinating, and monitoring complex referral systems, as well as inadequate consultation with individuals with disabilities.[3]

The provision of assistive technology for mobility has often been a low priority for governments. In a global survey of 114 countries on the equalization of opportunities for individuals with disabilities, 50% had not passed relevant legislation, 48% had no policies related to providing assistive technology, and 36% had not allocated fiscal resources to develop and supply assistive devices.[2]

The United Nations Convention on the Rights of Persons with Disabilities has been an important step toward providing an accountability framework for governments. Articles 4, 20, and 26 of the Convention specifically require member states to ensure access to assistive technology that is provided by trained professionals.[4]

In recent years, advocating for and advancing access to appropriate, affordable services for all users of assistive technology including prostheses has risen in priority for the global community. In January 2018 the Seventy-First World Health Assembly adopted the resolution that sets a global mandate to improve access to assistive technology. This resolution obliges member states to include assistive technology in universal health coverage as an integral part of achieving the Sustainable Development Goals, reducing the burden of noncommunicable diseases, contributing to the WHO's comprehensive mental health plan and in tackling the other major contributors to global burden of disease.[17]

The resolution has cemented the following actions:

- the Global Cooperation on Assistive Technology[18] (GATE)
- the WHO Priority Assistive Products list including prostheses[19]
- ATscale's[20] Product Narrative on Prostheses[21] and a prosthetic components market analysis[22]

To further support these aims, the WHO has developed tools to assess system-level capacity to deliver assistive technology; measure the need, demand, and barriers; and to measure the effect of assistive technology on individuals.[23]

In 2006, key stakeholders from 35 organizations and agencies agreed to a common approach to improve access to good-quality services for individuals with disabilities. *The Prosthetic Orthotic Programme Guide,*[5] which was endorsed by the International Society for Prosthetics and Orthotics (ISPO), provides support to international and local aid organizations involved in supporting the establishment and development of prosthetic and orthotic services in low-income settings. The guide recommends considering the following principles (among others): Ensure that the project has been proposed by or is supported by government; support the establishment of services that provide both prosthetic and orthotic devices; build local capacity in both technical and managerial aspects within the program; promote the ideal that services should be open for all; work closely with carefully selected local partners and owners of the service; build services on existing systems with respect to such considerations as staff compensation and the procurement of materials; carefully consider the selection of technology and components (ie, consider technology already in use in the country, realistic expectations for cost, availability, clinical capacity, and technical capacity); and promote continuous evidence-based research.[5]

These guiding principles are considered key to developing services that are cost effective and sustainable. These principles are echoed in a 2011 joint position paper published by WHO and USAID on the provision of mobility devices in LRSs and the WHO Standards for Prosthetic and Orthotic Services,[13] which encourage a comprehensive approach to service delivery.[2]

The 2017 Standards for Prosthetics and Orthotics Services with accompanying implementation guidelines aim to assist member states in setting up, improving, or transforming the delivery of services.[13,24] Building on previous work the Standards urges member states to include prosthetic/orthotic services in universal healthcare as an important step in achieving the Sustainable Development Goals.[13]

Funding limitations persist as a challenge frequently encountered in LRSs,[2] where individuals with disabilities reportedly pay for more than 50% of the cost of assistive technologies.[25] Because disability is bidirectionally linked to poverty,[3] the challenge of funding prosthetic services should not be underestimated. Studies indicate that individuals with disabilities have higher costs of living, higher health care expenditures,[3,26] fewer assets, and worse living conditions.[3] In low-income countries with a per capita income as low as $664 USD,[27] it would be reasonable to suggest that the cost of prosthetic devices may be unaffordable for most individuals with disabilities.

In 2014, WHO issued a concept note on its GATE initiative to increase access to assistive technology. This concept note stated that the assistive technology industry is essentially a monopoly; the cost of products is overly high and does not take advantage of economies of scale; and global issues exist regarding limited funding for development and production, weak or nonexistent procurement systems, the absence of safety measures, and inadequate servicing and user training in LRSs.[6]

In the USAID impact assessment of East Africa, researchers reported that in Tanzania, Kenya, and Uganda (the three target countries), constraints related to cost, supply chain, and limited availability of consumables had a substantial effect on services.[14] These countries reported heavy reliance on international, nongovernmental, and/or charitable organizations to fund services, which, anecdotally, is also considered to be true in other LRSs.

It is important that funding agents understand the complexities of providing prosthetic and orthotic services. Appropriate, sustainable services are considered a long-term endeavor and may require input or support over many decades to achieve acceptable results. Short-term assistance for users of prosthetic and orthotic services may generate few or no lasting results. In short-term endeavors, after a device wears out, beneficiaries may consider themselves to be in a worse situation than before having the device. ISPO recommended that the long-term objectives be prioritized over the narrower goal of supporting a large number of individuals as quickly as possible.[5]

Human Resources

Training a professional workforce is important for the delivery of appropriate services.[2-4,11,14,28] The lack of professionally trained personnel is a barrier to providing appropriate services. Similarly, continuing education for existing personnel is insufficient.[2] In the 2005 United Nations survey on equalization opportunities for individuals with disabilities, 37 countries reported that no action had been taken to train personnel in rehabilitation, and 56% reported that the medical knowledge of health care clinicians related to disability had not been updated.[2]

The current and projected shortfall of an appropriately trained workforce is reported to be a significant risk to access to appropriate prosthetic services. The 2017 WHO Service Standards stated that "Without an increase in the number of personnel, access to prosthetics and orthotics services would remain inadequate, uncertain or even at crisis point.[13]" According to the WHO's implementation guide, an estimated 5 to 10 prosthetic orthotic clinicians per million population are needed as a minimum, with high-income countries usually having a ratio of 15 to 20 per million population. In addition, it was recommended that each clinician be supported by two nonclinicians.[13]

Because of the long recognized need for appropriate training in LRSs, WHO and ISPO have worked together on international standards and guidelines for training personnel. The first joint guidelines were developed in 1991 and have since been supplemented and strengthened by detailed standards on education and training written by ISPO.

To date 36 programs and 2 pathways in 27 countries, in both less-resourced and well-resourced settings, are recognized by ISPO as meeting the standard for training in prosthetic and orthotic occupations.[29] These accredited programs/pathways represent 51 different education programs at various levels of training.

The standards consider differences in educational settings and the need for services. The standards also provide a reference for appropriate training levels for professionals to ensure that safe, appropriate care is provided, irrespective of the resources in a given setting. Training is stratified into three categories[30] (**Table 1**): The two clinical categories include Prosthetist Orthotist as the training level aimed at clinical leadership and advancing services; Associate Prosthetist Orthotist as the training level aimed at general clinical service delivery; and Prosthetic Orthotic Technician as the nonclinical training level aimed at technical fabrication of devices without providing clinical interventions.[30]

The importance of standards in education is exemplified by investigations in settings where standards have not been implemented. When individuals without formal training provide prosthetic services in LRSs, poor outcomes have been reported. A 2010 study in the Philippines found that of

TABLE 1 International Society for Prosthetics and Orthotics (ISPO) Occupation Classifications

ISPO Occupation Classification	Short Description
Prosthetist/Orthotist	The training level aimed at the full breadth of clinical service, leadership, advancing models, and/or methods of service delivery.
Associate Prosthetist/Orthotist	The training level aimed at general clinical service delivery.
Prosthetic/Orthotic Technician	The training level aimed at technical design and fabrication of devices without providing clinical intervention.

Reproduced with permission from International Society for Prosthetics and Orthotics. ISPO Education Standard for prosthetic/orthotic occupations. 2018. https://www.ispoint.org/wp-content/uploads/2022/02/ispo_standards_nov2018_sprea.pdf. Accessed February 9, 2019.

1,494 patients with an amputation who had been screened, 122 (8.2%) had a prosthesis, and these individuals attended the screening because their prosthesis needed to be adjusted or replaced because of poor quality or fit.[31] Field tests in two countries where service providers had received 3 weeks of training (but were not formally trained to international standards) identified that the recipients of such services were less intensive users with fewer jobs and that the craftsmanship of the provided devices was generally considered to be poor.[32] These findings support the need for formally trained professionals to provide prosthetic services to ensure that resources and outcomes are optimized.

Prosthetic Technologies in LRSs

A variety of prosthetic technologies exists and are widely used in well-resourced settings for many clinical and user-initiated goals. Research and development of new or improved prosthetic designs over the past 3 decades have focused largely on these relatively affluent and resource-rich settings.[25] With the expiration of patents on certain prosthetic or orthotic devices, a new trend has begun in which products using technologies developed for well-resourced settings are being manufactured and distributed in low-income and middle-income countries, with the potential to decrease cost and increase availability. However, in many LRSs, these designs remain cost prohibitive and are often impractical for application in local environments and user activities[6,28] (**Figure 1**).

A recent Prosthetic Components Landscape Analysis Report by ATscale identified 95 prosthetic suppliers. The investigators shortlisted 34 suppliers to survey about their engagement in low-income and middle-income countries. Suppliers indicate that high-income countries remain the majority of their business. Wide variance in the cost of components was reported to exist with transtibial prosthetic kits ranging from $77 USD to $450 USD and transfemoral kits ranging from $188 USD to $540 USD. Many of the suppliers were considered to be generic manufacturers, providing lower cost clones of older technology. Eighty percent of those responding to the survey indicated they were certified by the International Standards Organization (ISO). However, only 35% of suppliers reported using a third-party laboratory to test components, and responses from participants suggest that many organizations were not certified under the standards related to structural testing but under administrative certification. The report calls for standardized testing, quality assurance measures, and in-country regulatory frameworks ensuring quality while allowing generic manufacturers to contribute to the supply chain.[22]

Access to materials and equipment is limited in LRSs. Research and development is needed to identify technologies, materials, methods, and equipment that are cost effective and do not adversely affect the quality of services.[5]

Concerns have been raised about the ethical standard of research conducted in LRSs. Lack of mandatory ethical review common in many LRSs should not be seen as an opportunity to circumvent ethical practice in research. To guide researchers in planning appropriate studies, ISPO and the Exceed Research Network have jointly prepared a position paper that outlines expected steps that researchers should take to comply with the principles of respect for the person, beneficence, and justice.[33]

Frequently, the cost of importation is high and the demand for devices may be low because of poor awareness or limited purchasing capacity.[2] For most LRSs, prosthetic services are delivered on a small scale, often using novel, indigenous designs (**Figure 2**) and donated or recycled materials and parts.

In many countries, prostheses are classified as single-use devices and are considered appropriate for a single user only. Reusing a device without approval by the licensed manufacturer of the device is prohibited by law because it potentially reduces performance or effectiveness and presents risks to the user and treating staff, including mechanical failure and cross

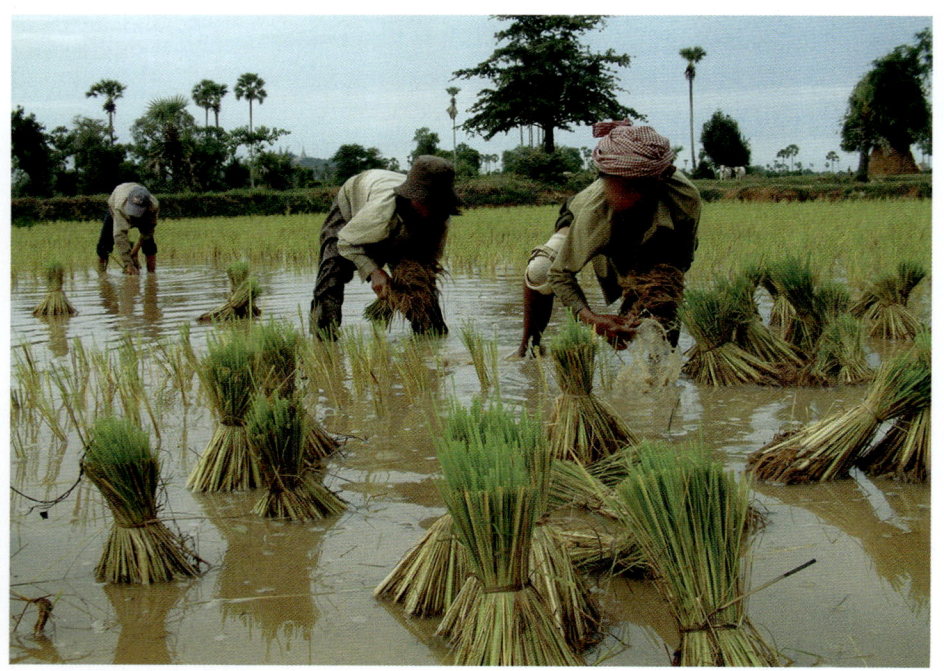

FIGURE 1 Uneven terrain, high humidity, mud, and wet conditions (in various combinations) are common in less-resourced settings. Photograph shows the user of a transtibial prosthesis harvesting rice in a wet and muddy Cambodian field. (Courtesy of Robert Joiner, Wellington, New Zealand.)

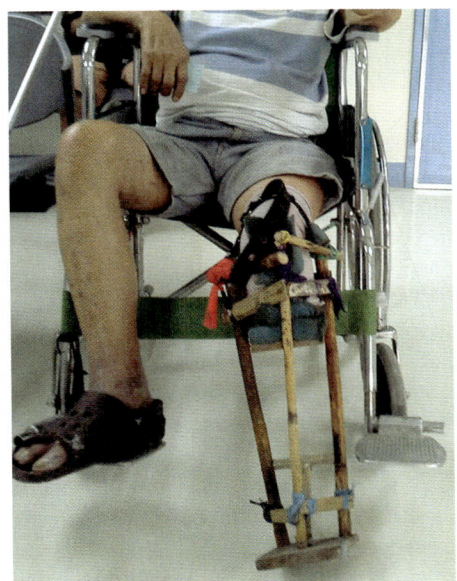

FIGURE 2 Photograph shows a homemade transtibial prosthesis. (Courtesy of Christine Joy Lao Dee, RTRP, RN, CPO, Manila, Philippines.)

contamination.[34] Despite such restrictions implemented in well-resourced settings, secondhand components (and even complete devices) are sometimes reused in LRSs. These items are recycled to extend the useful life of the technology or to provide limbs for individuals who otherwise would have no access to prostheses. This model of service may seem appealing, but it can be problematic for individuals receiving prosthetic devices and for the long-term sustainability of services. Parts are often not interchangeable and the ability to repair or refurbish parts can be almost nonexistent. Individuals who provide such services often have little or no training and may lack the capabilities to safely and appropriately assess, assemble, fit, and/or align devices. The technology often cannot be repaired or replaced in the future, leaving the user with no prosthesis or a relatively basic or unsafe device. Collectively, this approach to service delivery can potentially do more harm than good.[5]

The report of the Seventy-First World Health Assembly affirmed that adequate regulation is lacking, and deficiencies of context-appropriate designs and use of parts that cannot be repaired or replaced locally contribute to high rates of abandonment. In addition, those from poorer sectors of society are forced to rely on high volumes of low-quality products that are inappropriate for the user and their setting, delivered through donations and charitable models.[16]

Ikeda et al[9] reviewed research and outcome measures in resource-limited environments and reported that lack of durability is a persistent problem. In addition, although a few specific benchmarks exist for lower limb prosthetic interventions, no upper limb benchmarks could be identified.

As a result of concerns of the international community, the ISO, with support from ISPO, developed ISO 10328 (prosthetics standard for structural testing) to ensure safety and assist in the development of prosthetic devices.[35] This minimum standard is considered an important safety benchmark that all prosthetic components delivered in LRSs should be in compliance with.[13]

In the 1996 Consensus Conference on Appropriate Prosthetics Technology for Developing Countries,[36] the use of international and national manufacturing standards was considered to be essential and important in settings without ready access to services. Some technologies designed for use in LRSs, such as the ICRC systems, the Limbs International Knee (**Figure 3**), and the Alimco limb systems, have met this standard. Encouragingly, a few additional systems and components are in the testing phase.

Jensen and Heim[37] reported the ISPO protocol and assessment system for clinical and technical interventions as one of the most common outcome measures used for lower limb prosthetic devices in LRSs. It describes quality standards that are attainable, and encourages providers to achieve those standards.[9]

Feet

Prosthetic feet have long been reported as the prosthetic part most likely to fail in LRSs.[36] Durability has been cited as the most important factor for the

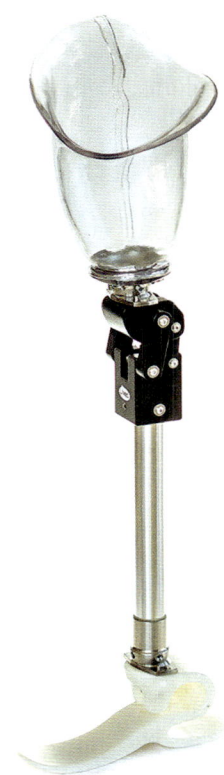

FIGURE 3 Photograph of a Limbs International transfemoral prosthesis with a Niagara foot. (Courtesy of Roger V. Gonzalez, PhD, PE, El Paso, TX.)

prescription and/or selection of prosthetic feet, especially in barefoot or open shoe walking conditions. Conditions related to climate that are common in many LRSs such as heat, moisture, and exposure to ultraviolet light negatively affect the durability of prosthetic feet. Several prosthetic feet designed for use in LRSs have been tested in industry-standard static-proof tests and cyclical loading tests with acceptable results. However, LRS field tests have demonstrated that these functional working environments can result in a lower level of durability than that identified by laboratory tests alone.[9,32,35]

In 2013, a review by Ikeda et al[9] reported that polyurethane prosthetic feet were not recommended for tropical environments. Vulcanized rubber prosthetic feet offered improved durability and therefore were preferred for tropical environments. Prosthetic feet designed for use in LRSs such as the Niagara foot (**Figure 4**) met the

Section 1: General Principles

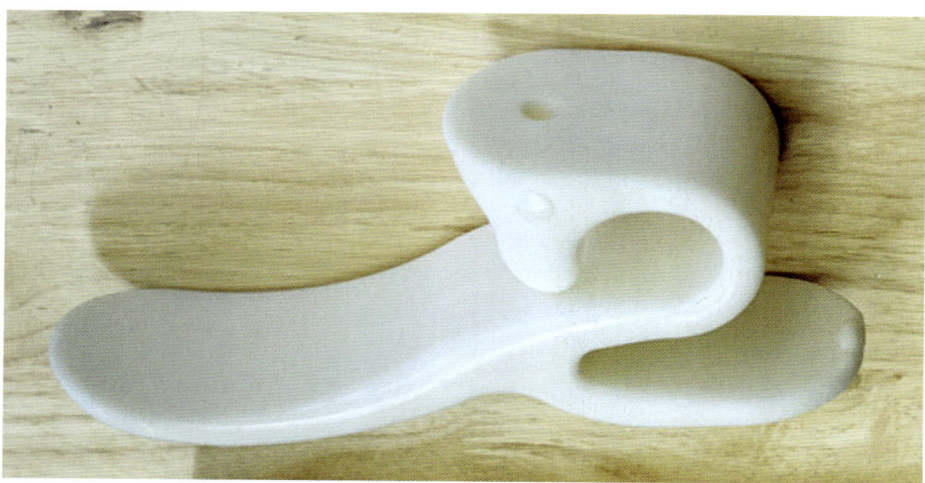

FIGURE 4 Photograph of the Niagara foot prosthesis. (Courtesy of Roger V. Gonzalez, PhD, PE, El Paso, TX.)

outlined needs associated with cost, simplicity, and durability, although field tests suggested that the durability of the cover may need improvement.[9]

Knees

Some low-cost prosthetic knees that take advantage of existing design principles have been tested for use in LRSs and are showing potential for improving function and stability at a low cost (**Figure 5**); however, independent tests are still needed to verify results.[9]

Prosthetic Systems

Considering the scope of the potential market for prosthetic componentry in LRSs, only a few specifically designed prosthetic systems exist. Two of the main designs used in such settings are the ICRC Polypropylene Technology and the Jaipur System.

International Committee of the Red Cross

In 1979, to provide services in conflict areas and LRSs, the ICRC launched its Physical Rehabilitation Programme. The aim of the program was to deliver good-quality, sustainable services that promoted the use of technology appropriate to the specific contexts in which the organization operates. The goal was to deliver devices that were durable, comfortable, and easy for patients to use and maintain; easy to learn and repair; standardized, but compatible with the climate in different regions of the world; low cost, but modern and consistent with internationally accepted standards; and easily available regarding the supply chain.

Following early efforts to use locally available raw materials for component manufacture, the ICRC began using polypropylene sockets in 1988. In 1991, the first prosthetic knee joint was produced in Cambodia, followed by work in Colombia to develop a range of injection-molded polypropylene prosthetic kits to standardize the organization's various projects.[38]

Both lower limb and upper limb systems are available. Simple, comprehensive manuals are available describing fabrication and bench alignment of the systems. Most levels of amputation can be addressed with the simple range of modular kits (**Figures 6** and **7**). Parts are standardized, interchangeable, durable, of midrange cost, and can be ordered internationally. The modular design facilitates an efficient supply chain and is easy to fabricate, adjust, maintain, and repair.

In the ICRC system, each socket is created from an individual cast and positive plaster model. For transfemoral sockets, a quadrilateral design is encouraged because the wrap-draped polypropylene socket generally does not allow for the frame socket design to be used effectively with the ischial and ischial/ramal containment sockets.

Transfemoral sockets are suspended using either a standard or modified Silesian belt. A valve for suction suspension may be used where appropriate, but prescribing suction suspension in tropical climates should be considered carefully. Although some individuals can successfully use suction suspension in a tropical climate, heat and humidity can diminish the skin-socket interface required to maintain suspension. Muddy, wet, irregular terrain associated with many rural areas and some urban areas can result in distraction forces that are higher than usually expected, especially during the tropical rainy season. In such instances, it can be difficult to maintain suspension through suction alone.

The lower limb systems use solid ankle cushion heel–style feet. The transtibial kits (**Figure 8**) include attachment/alignment couplings and a pylon. The transfemoral kit (**Figure 9**) adds a manually locking, single-axis knee joint (**Figure 10**). Also, a single-axis hip joint is available for more proximal amputation levels. Ankle disarticulation and knee disarticulation can be addressed with the system using a modified foot or knee joint with a low-profile attachment coupling.

In the lower limb system, a wide range of alignment adjustments are possible through the attachment/alignment couplings. This includes convex/concave disks for tilt/shift, as well as sliding surfaces for shifting and rotation (**Figure 11**). The various sections are locked in place during alignment using bolts and secured with plastic welding after the alignment process is complete. Allowing for alignment changes from standard bench alignment throughout the dynamic alignment process and even after the prosthesis is fitted represents an important functional advantage in achieving optimized and energy-efficient gait.

The upper limb system offers body-powered split-hook terminal devices (**Figure 12**) and passive hands in a range of sizes. The transradial prosthesis can be used with a self-suspending

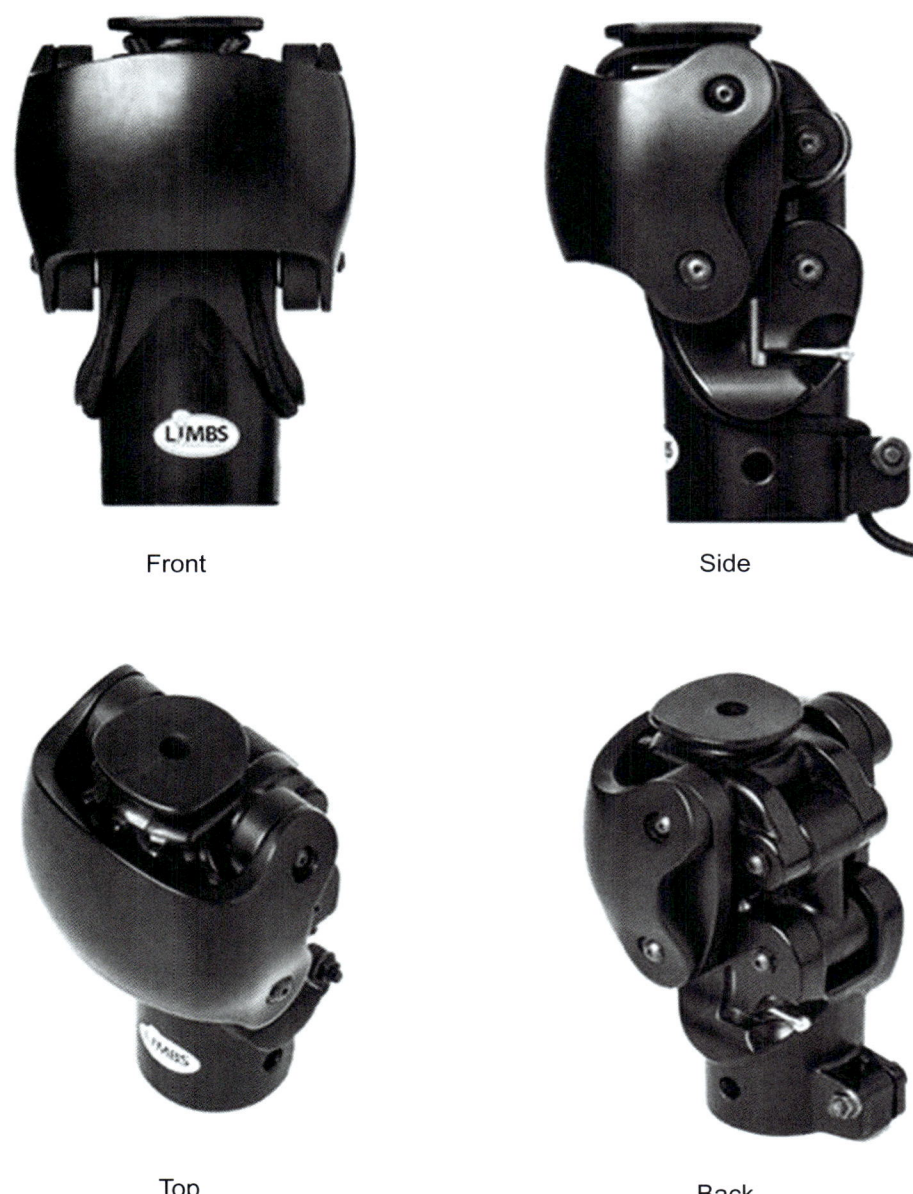

FIGURE 5 Photographs of the Limbs International Knee, formerly known as the LeTourneau Engineering Global Solutions Knee. (Courtesy of Roger V. Gonzalez, PhD, PE, El Paso, TX.)

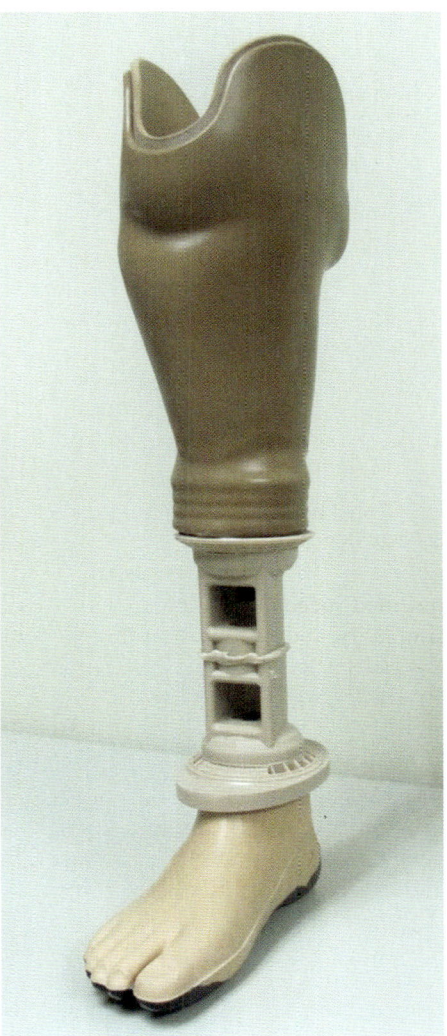

FIGURE 6 Photograph of an International Committee of the Red Cross transtibial prosthesis ready for bench alignment. (Courtesy of Helen Cochrane CPO(c), MSc, Manila, Philippines.)

socket or with harness suspension, double-wall construction for fabrication of the forearm, a control harness as appropriate, and a bicycle brake cable acting as a control cable to connect the harness to the terminal device. The transhumeral system uses a manual locking elbow (**Figure 13**) and standard socket designs, harnessing, and control systems.

Although the ICRC scaled back its involvement in the production of prosthetic (and orthotic) components, the system continues to be manufactured and sold to nongovernmental organizations via private vendors. The cost for this system is generally less than for other commercially available prosthetic parts. Sockets are typically drape-formed from polypropylene sheets, which limits the range of raw materials that must be stored. The need for chemical storage and the regulation of ambient temperature frequently associated with composite/lamination materials, which can be a challenge in LRSs, is also reduced. These simple, standardized manufacturing methods can improve the consistency of outcomes, resulting in lighter and more durable prostheses than can be achieved and maintained by locally made devices fabricated in LRSs.

Another benefit is that the interchangeable parts can be used across many amputation levels, further limiting the range of materials that must be kept in inventory. This simplifies the supply chain, and for organizations that import parts, this system offers a simple, cost-effective way to manage high-volume individual needs. Studies

Section 1: General Principles

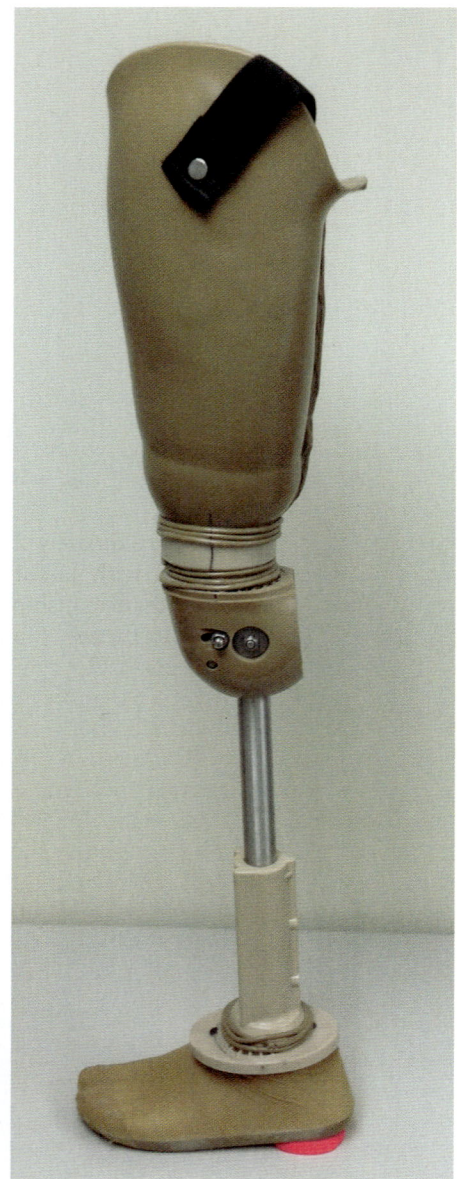

FIGURE 7 Photograph of a transfemoral prosthesis using an International Committee of the Red Cross single-axis manual locking knee, a solid ankle cushion heel foot, and Silesian suspension. (Courtesy of Helen Cochrane, CPO(c), MSc, Manila, Philippines.)

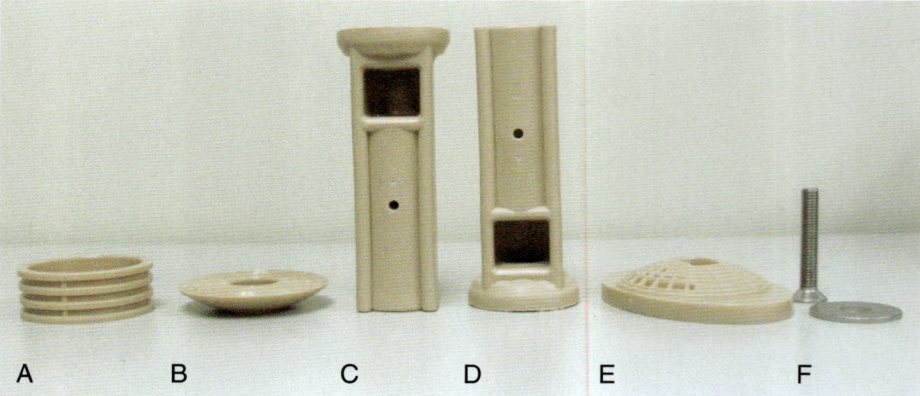

FIGURE 8 Photograph of an International Committee of the Red Cross transtibial prosthesis kit, which includes a socket attachment cup (**A**), an alignment disk with a flat superior surface and convex inferior surface (**B**), a two-part pylon with a concave alignment coupling (**C** and **D**), a foot attachment coupling with a convex superior surface for alignment and a flat inferior surface for solid ankle cushion heel foot attachment (**E**), and a foot bolt (**F**). (Courtesy of Helen Cochrane, CPO(c), MSc, Manila, Philippines.)

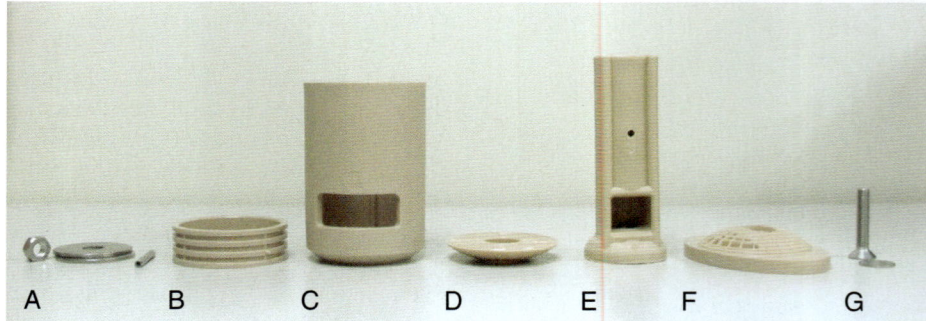

FIGURE 9 Photograph of an International Committee of the Red Cross transfemoral prosthesis kit, which includes a socket attachment plate (**A**), an attachment coupling for a long transfemoral amputation (**B**), an attachment cup for a short transfemoral amputation (**C**), an alignment disk with a flat superior surface and a convex inferior surface (**D**), a distal pylon attachment with a concave alignment coupling (**E**), a foot attachment coupling with a convex superior surface for alignment and a flat inferior surface for solid ankle cushion heel foot attachment (**F**), and a foot bolt (**G**). (Courtesy of Helen Cochrane, CPO(c), MSc, Manila, Philippines.)

of prosthetic systems in LRSs indicate that the ICRC system is appropriate for both transtibial and transfemoral applications.[9]

Jaipur Foot

The Jaipur foot is part of a prosthetic limb system linked with several prosthetic/orthotic centers in India. It has

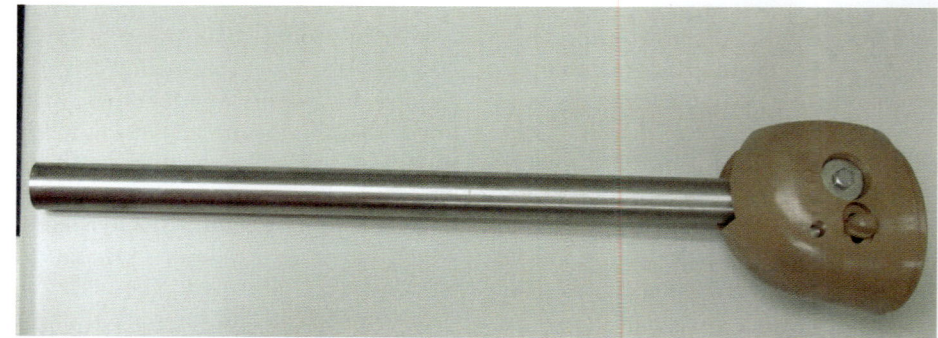

FIGURE 10 Photograph of a manual locking knee. (Courtesy of Helen Cochrane, CPO(c), MSc, Manila, Philippines.)

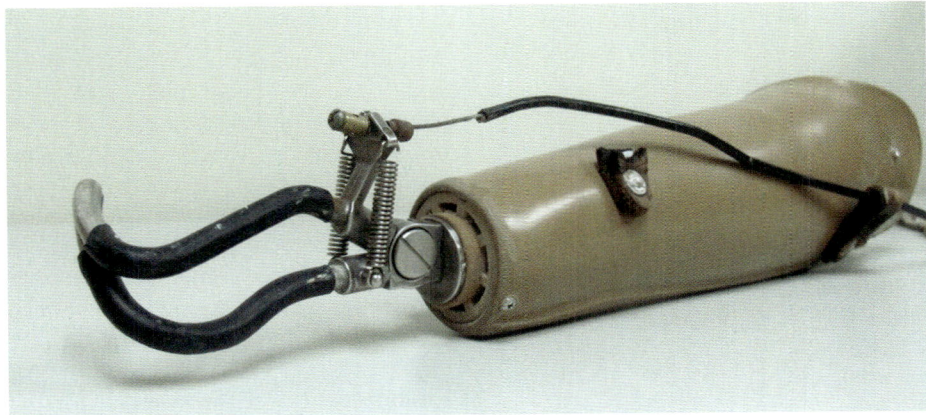

FIGURE 12 Photograph of an International Committee of the Red Cross transradial prosthesis with a split hook terminal device. (Courtesy of Helen Cochrane, CPO(c), MSc, Manila, Philippines.)

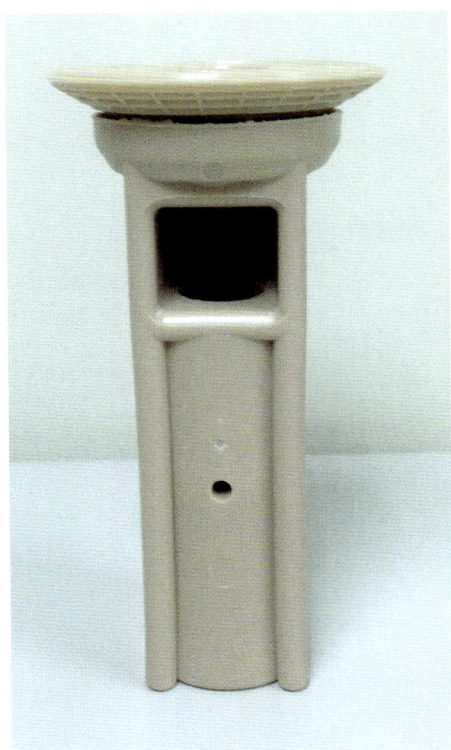

FIGURE 11 Photograph of an International Committee of the Red Cross transtibial concave pylon and alignment disk with a convex surface for tilting and a sliding surface for shifting. (Courtesy of Helen Cochrane, CPO(c), MSc, Manila, Philippines.)

also been used within short-term international fitting camps in other countries.

The Jaipur foot (**Figure 14**) was first developed in 1968 to meet the sociocultural needs of individuals with disabilities in India. The foot was designed to allow the user to squat; sit cross-legged; walk on uneven terrain; work in wet, muddy fields; and walk without shoes. The foot does not have a central keel and aims to allow a wide range of motion through the foot-ankle assembly. This vulcanized rubber foot is reported to be waterproof. Its design is culturally appropriate, low cost, and widely used in India.[39] It has higher rates of deformation in independent static loading tests and higher rates of delamination when compared with other feet during cyclical load tests.[32] However, the technical quality of the Jaipur foot can be considered acceptable and is better than that observed and reported by ISPO for some solid ankle cushion heel foot designs aimed at low-income countries.[39]

The Jaipur transtibial prosthetic system uses high-density polyethylene pipes for both the socket and shank and is an exoskeletal design (**Figure 15**). The system is designed for quick fitting (usually within 1 day) but offers limited dynamic alignment and maintenance. The Jaipur transfemoral prosthesis is also fabricated from high-density polyethylene pipes and offers a single-axis knee with or without a lock.[39]

In a study in three countries that examined 172 individuals with transtibial amputation approximately 2 years after being provided with Jaipur transtibial prostheses, craftsmanship and fit were poor in 56% of cases.[40] In another study that examined 72 transfemoral prosthesis users in the same three countries approximately 2.5 years after being provided with Jaipur transfemoral prostheses, craftsmanship and fit were assessed as being poor in 86% of cases.[41] Fabrication and fitting in the three projects were performed by individuals who had limited background training in prosthetics. The outcome was considered unsatisfactory both

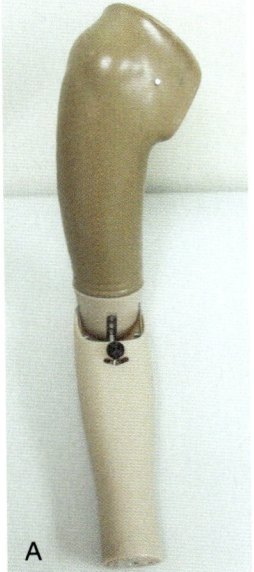
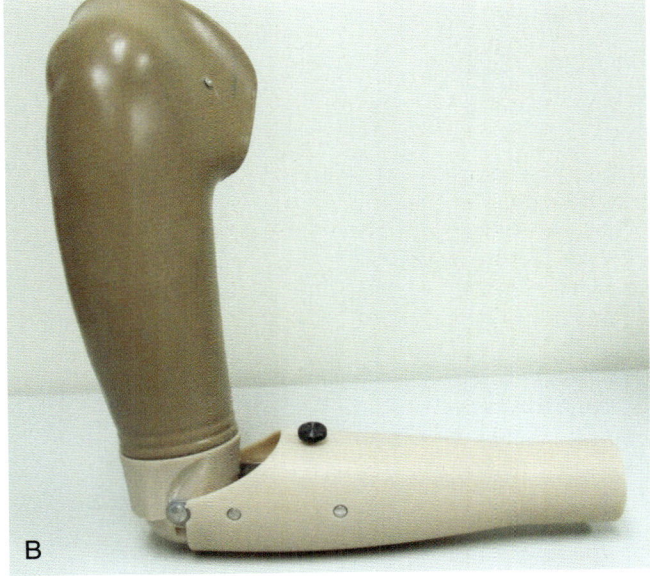

FIGURE 13 Photographs show anterior (**A**) and lateral (**B**) views of an International Committee of the Red Cross transhumeral prosthesis with a manual locking elbow. (Courtesy of Helen Cochrane, CPO(c), MSc, Manila, Philippines.)

Section 1: General Principles

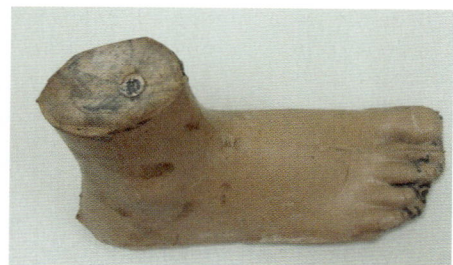

FIGURE 14 Photograph of a Jaipur prosthetic foot. (Courtesy of Helen Cochrane, CPO(c), MSc, Manila, Philippines.)

technically and clinically. This was considered a reflection of the inadequacies of the prosthetic construction and the inadequate training of those involved in fitting and fabrication of the devices.[40,41]

The Jaipur foot program has been working to improve its components, as shown by involvement with a polycentric knee, which improves stability in stance and improves gait when compared with single-axis designs.[39]

SUMMARY

A LRS is usually a low-income or middle-income geographic area that is at a stage of economic and/or social development in which resources are insufficient to meet the needs of a population. There are many strategies that can be used to help meet the needs of individuals who could benefit from prosthetic services in an LRS. When resources are scarce, optimizing the efficiency of services is vital. Training a professional workforce is essential for the delivery of appropriate services; WHO and ISPO have developed international standards and guidelines for such training. Because the range of appropriate, available technology and access to materials and equipment are limited in an LRS, further research and development are needed to identify technologies, materials, methods, and equipment that are cost effective and do not adversely affect the quality of services provided to individuals with prosthetic and orthotic needs. In recent years global policy has seen considerable action to promote access to quality services which now needs to be followed by investment in the implementation of policy.

References

1. *Executive Summary: Guidelines on the Provision of Manual Wheelchairs in Less Resourced Settings.* NCBI Bookshelf, 2008. http://www.ncbi.nlm.nih.gov/books/NBK143785/#fm.s8. Accessed March 10, 2015.
2. World Health Organization, United States Agency for International Development: *Joint Position Paper on the Provision of Mobility Devices in Less Resourced Settings.* World Health Organization, 2011.
3. World Health Organization, The World Bank: *World Report on Disability.* World Health Organization, 2011.
4. United Nations: Convention on the rights of persons with disabilities. http://www.un.org/disabilities/convention/conventionfull.shtml. Accessed March 15, 2015.
5. Prosthetic and orthotics programme guide: Implementing P&O services in low-income settings. https://www.motivation.org.au/wp-content/uploads/2016/02/po-programme-guide-final-version.pdf. Accessed March 10, 2015.
6. World Health Organization: Concept note: Opening the GATE for assistive health technology shifting the paradigm. http://www.ispoint.org/sites/default/files/gate_concept_note_1.pdf. Accessed March 10, 2015.
7. Borg J, Lindström A, Larsson S: Assistive technology in developing countries: A review from the perspective of the convention on the rights of persons with disabilities. *Prosthet Orthot Int* 2011;35(1):20-29.
8. Wyss D, Lindsay S, Cleghorn WL, Andrysek J: Priorities in lower limb prosthetic service delivery based on an international survey of prosthetists in low- and high-income countries. *Prosthet Orthot Int* 2015;39(2):102-111.
9. Ikeda AJ, Grabowski AM, Lindsley A, Sadeghi-Demneh E, Reisinger KD: A scoping literature review of the provision of orthoses and prostheses in resource-limited environments 2000-2010: Part two. Research and outcomes. *Prosthet Orthot Int* 2014;38(5):343-362.

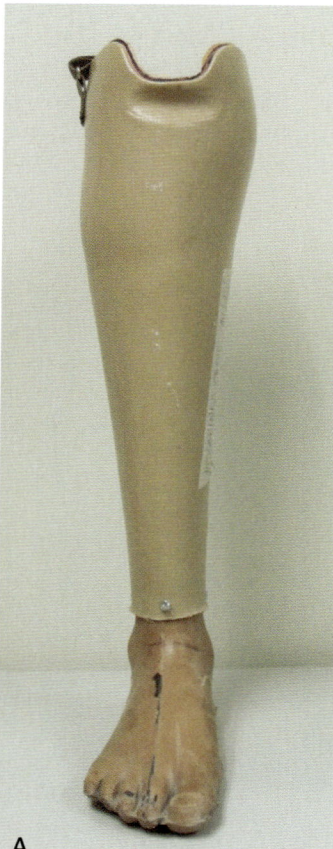
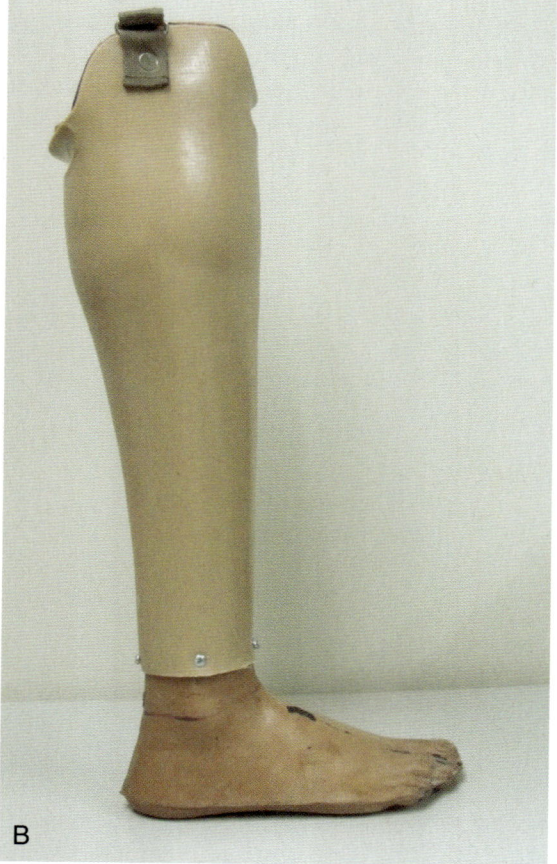

FIGURE 15 Photographs show anterior (**A**) and lateral (**B**) views of a Jaipur transtibial foot prosthesis. (Courtesy of Helen Cochrane, CPO(c), MSc, Manila, Philippines.)

10. Durocher J, Lord J, Defranco A: Disability and global development. *Disabil Health J* 2012;5(3):132-135.
11. World Health Organization, International Society for Prosthetics and Orthotics: Guidelines for Training Personnel in Developing Countries for Prosthetic and Orthotics Services. World Health Organization, 2005.
12. World Health Organization: *The Global Burden of Disease: 2004 Update*. World Health Organization, 2008.
13. World Health Organization: Standards for Prosthetic and Orthotics Services Provision Part 1 2017. https://apps.who.int/iris/bitstream/handle/10665/259209/9789241512480-part1-eng.pdf. Accessed March 8, 2023.
14. Sexton S, Shangali H, Munissi B: Prosthetic & orthotic impact assessment: East Africa Tanzania, Kenya and Uganda. The Impact of Training Personnel to the Minimum Standards ISPO Category I & II: Tanzania Training Centre for Orthopaedic Technologists. http://www.ispoint.org/sites/default/files/sections/partnership/ispo_impact_assessment_tatcoteast_africa_with_appendices.pdf. Accessed March 10, 2015.
15. International Committee of the Red Cross: Physical Rehabilitation Programme 2020: Annual Report. October 2021. Accessed September 15, 2021. https://www.icrc.org/en/publication/4528-physical-rehabilitation-programme-2020-annual-report
16. World Health Organization: *Improving Access to Assistive Technology—Seventy-First World Health Assembly* 2018, p 6. Accessed September 11, 2021. https://apps.who.int/gb/ebwha/pdf_files/WHA71/A71_21-en.pdf.
17. World Health Organization: *Improving access to assistive technology— Seventy-first World Health Assembly WHA71.8* 2018. Accessed September 15, 2021. https://apps.who.int/gb/ebwha/pdf_files/WHA71/A71_R8-en.pdf.
18. World Health Organization: Global Cooperation on Assistive Technology (GATE). https://www.who.int/news-room/feature-stories/detail/global-cooperation-on-assistive-technology-(gate). Accessed September 20, 2021.
19. World Health Organization: Priority Assistive Products List. http://www.who.int/phi/implementation/assistive_technology/low_res_english.pdf. Accessed June 1, 2016.
20. ATscale: The global partnership for assistive technology: A background. https://atscalepartnership.org/the-global-need-for-assistive-technology. Accessed January 12, 2023.
21. ATscale: Product narrative: Prostheses 2020. https://at2030.org/static/at2030_core/outputs/Prostheses_Product_Narrative_a11y_20200827.pdf. Accessed March 8, 2023.
22. ATscale: Increasing Access to Affordable Quality Prosthetic Components in LMIC Markets—A Market Landscape Analysis Report 2021. Available at: https://atscalepartnership.org/global-public-goods-1#prosthetics-device-landscape. Accessed February 27, 2023.
23. World Health Organization: Advancing data collection on assistive technology. https://www.who.int/tools/ata-toolkit. Accessed September 20, 2021.
24. World Health Organization: Standards for prosthetics and orthotics Part 2. Implementation manual 2017. http://apps.who.int/iris/bitstream/10665/259209/2/9789241512480-part2-eng.pdf?ua=1. Accessed September 06, 2021.
25. Pearlman J, Cooper RA, Krizack M, et al: Lower-limb prostheses and wheelchairs in low-income countries. *IEEE Eng Med Biol Mag* 2008;27(2):12-22.
26. Mitra S, Findley PA, Sambamoorthi U: Health care expenditures of living with a disability: Total expenditures, out-of-pocket expenses, and burden, 1996 to 2004. *Arch Phys Med Rehabil* 2009;90(9):1532-1540.
27. World Bank Group: Data: Low income. http://data.worldbank.org/income-level/LIC. Accessed March 10, 2015.
28. Harkins CS, McGarry A, Buis A: Provision of prosthetic and orthotic services in low-income countries: A review of the literature. *Prosthet Orthot Int* 2013;37(5):353-361.
29. International Society for Prosthetics and Orthotics: Education: Programmes. http://www.ispoint.org/programmes. Accessed March 10, 2015.
30. International Society for Prosthetics and Orthotics: ISPO Education Standard for Prosthetic/orthotic Occupations 2018. https://cdn.ymaws.com/www.ispoint.org/resource/resmgr/3_learn/ispo_standards_nov2018_sprea.pdf. Accessed September 06, 2021.
31. Bundoc JR: The challenge of "walking free" from disability. *Acta Med Philipp* 2010;44(2):13-16.
32. Jensen JS, Sexton S: Appropriate prosthetic and orthotics technologies in low income countries (2000-2010) 2010. http://www.ispoint.org/sites/default/files/archives/appropriate_prosthetic_orthotic_technologies_in_low_income_countries_2000-2010.pdf. Accessed March 10, 2015.
33. International Society for Prosthetics and Orthotics, Exceed Research Network: Ethical considerations and approaches for conducting clinical research studies related to prosthetics, orthotics and wheelchair technology in the low-and middle-income countries. 2021. https://cdn.ymaws.com/www.ispoint.org/resource/resmgr/docs/ethical_considerations_to_po.pdf. Accessed September 06, 2021.
34. Medicines and Healthcare Products Regulatory Agency: Single-use medical devices: Implications and consequences of reuse 2013. https://www.gov.uk/government/uploads/system/uploads/attachment_data/file/403442/Single-use_medical_devices_implications_and_consequences_of_reuse.pdf. Accessed March 10, 2015.
35. ISO: ISO 10328:2006. Prosthetics: Structural testing of lower-limb prostheses. Requirements and test methods. https://www.iso.org/obp/ui/#iso:std:iso:10328:ed-1:v1:en. Accessed March 10, 2015.
36. Day HJ: A review of the consensus conference on appropriate prosthetic technology in developing countries. *Prosthet Orthot Int* 1996;20(1):15-23.
37. Jensen JS, Heim S: Evaluation of polypropylene prostheses designed by the International Committee of the Red Cross for trans-tibial amputees. *Prosthet Orthot Int* 2000;24(1):47-54.
38. International Committee of the Red Cross: Manufacturing guidelines: Trans tibial prosthesis. Physical Rehabilitation Programme. https://www.icrc.org/eng/assets/files/other/eng-transtibial.pdf. Accessed March 10, 2015.
39. Jaipur Foot. http://jaipurfoot.org. Accessed March 15, 2015.
40. Jensen JS, Craig JG, Mtalo LB, Zelaya CM: Clinical field follow-up of high density polyethylene (HDPE)-Jaipur prosthetic technology for trans-tibial amputees. *Prosthet Orthot Int* 2004;28(3):230-244.
41. Jensen JS, Craig JG, Mtalo LB, Zelaya CM: Clinical field follow-up of high density polyethylene (HDPE)-Jaipur prosthetic technology for trans-femoral amputees. *Prosthet Orthot Int* 2004;28(2):152-166.

General Rehabilitation Principles and Strategies for the Upper Limb Amputee

CHAPTER 8

Josef A. Butkus, MS, OTR/L • Danielle H. Melton, MD

ABSTRACT

Rehabilitation for the population that has experienced upper extremity limb loss is vital to ensure the success of the individual. There is a variety of care that is considered standard but rehabilitation, clinician experience, and reimbursement are not uniform. Having experienced medical staff is essential to ensure successful rehabilitation, but care can vary given the relatively narrow patient population. Research is lacking in the field of limb loss, as is an overarching protocol that delivers the best outcomes for all patients. In many fields there just is not complete evidence-based research available and often the best resource is knowledgeable professionals or individuals who have seen the results firsthand. The factors involved in prosthetic acceptance are important for clinicians and individuals who have experienced limb loss to understand to eliminate barriers. Similar to navigating any complex health issue, there are many perspectives and options, but those in need do not always know what to expect. Success after limb deficiency is ultimately determined by the individual regardless of intervention or device. Individuals who take a proactive approach and advocate for their needs will likely achieve more satisfying outcomes. There are possible physical consequences for the patient who has experienced limb loss if poor habits develop with compensations after limb loss. The quality of the patient experience with medical care after limb loss may affect outcomes. It is important to highlight some of the best interventions, support, and training available for patients with upper limb deficiencies. A review of rehabilitation principles will serve to educate and assist clinicians and patients to maximize independence and navigate a successful return to an active lifestyle after upper extremity limb loss.

Keywords: limb loss rehabilitation; myoelectric or body-powered prosthetic limb; prosthesis; prosthetic training; upper extremity amputee

Introduction

Upper extremity limb loss is a devastating injury that interferes with the way a person interacts with almost everything in their environment. Imagine waking up and leaving for work with the use of only one arm. Almost every task involved in bathing, grooming, dressing, meal preparation, child care, carrying items, and driving is seamlessly integrated as a bimanual task, the individual performances of which have to change drastically. Rehabilitation is the best way to assist patients with limb deficiency in this transformational period. Prosthetic limbs offer an opportunity for return of some function, which in turn allows individuals to return to participation in meaningful activities. Rehabilitation is vital to ensuring the successful return of the individual to their environment with or without a prosthetic limb. A prosthesis needs to fit well, the control strategy and suspension need to be comfortable, prosthesis fitting needs to happen in a timely manner, the individual needs to have a good fit between function and the user task requirements, and the individual needs to understand how best to incorporate their new limb into tasks. There are many moving parts in the previous description, and this is why rehabilitation is so important to successful reintegration of the individual in all the activities they need to perform daily.

Role of Rehabilitation

The role of rehabilitation serves to guide individuals through a complex recovery and return them to an active engaged life. Many adjustments are required of the individual while dealing with pain, emotional challenges, and an incredibly stressful time. Some individuals are more resilient to dealing with the complexities of recovery, but the role of the clinicians is to accept them wherever they are mentally and compassionately support them through this transition. Individuals will need to determine what a prosthesis can offer them and be encouraged to identify what needs are the most important to them. Clinicians are there to educate, train, support, and encourage individuals with limb deficiency as they redefine how to interact with the environment.

Neither of the following authors nor any immediate family member has received anything of value from or has stock or stock options held in a commercial company or institution related directly or indirectly to the subject of this chapter: Josef A. Butkus and Dr. Melton.

Success With and Without a Prosthesis

Prosthetic limbs have their advantages and disadvantages, but nothing replaces the ability of a native hand. Individuals with limb deficiency should always be given the opportunity for a prosthesis and training to return to full bimanual performance. Robotic technology is advancing at an incredible rate, but nothing comes close to offering the range of motion, strength, sensation, and dexterity of the human hand. Occasionally, prosthesis users find that covering sensate skin with a prosthesis socket interferes with the function of a sensate residual limb. Sensation is very important to inform the individual about how much control they have over an object. Partial hand prostheses are uniquely challenging because they often cover sensate distal skin to gain more prosthetic device function, which is insensate. The same prosthesis does not work for everyone, all the time, in all situations. No one intentionally goes to sleep wearing their device. Everyone has a sliding scale of comfort with when and why they like to wear a prosthesis and when they do not. This also applies to specific terminal devices; a person would not want to wear a swimming terminal device to dinner with friends or take an electric arm kayaking. There are many needs to be met after losing an arm. Many factors go into determining what and when an individual with a limb deficiency may desire to incorporate a prosthesis. If someone learns to be comfortable performing tasks one-handed, then why would they put on an uncomfortable device that may not work perfectly all the time? Individuals need to see the value and purpose of wearing a device. If someone chooses not to wear an artificial limb, clinicians need to be supportive of that choice as well and facilitate independence as best as possible. A prosthesis may be too painful or limiting, but the clinician's role is to eliminate these barriers and help the individual find a system that may increase their function. Whether the individual chooses to wear a prosthesis or not is subjective if the clinicians have done their jobs. Factors involved in prosthetic acceptance and rejection will be discussed in greater detail in this section. There appears to be a limited window of time to learn how an artificial limb can add value to a patient's day and tasks.[1] Individuals can have a variety of motivators such as additional pinch to help them with tasks, a cosmetically identical device that goes unnoticed, a device with the most strength or versatility, or something that looks cool. Remarkably, it has been noted that individuals at the time of their amputation may be concerned about not being accepted by a potential partner because of their limb difference. This is another reason why people need to grieve, talk, voice concerns, identify negative self-talk, enhance coping skills, and accept their changes to move forward as Belon and Vigoda[2] summarized emotional adaptation for amputees in a 2014 review. The work of Elizabeth Kubler-Ross is apt for identifying stages of grieving and moving toward acceptance after amputation.[2,3] There are many factors involved in the adaptation of the person as they transition to life without an intact extremity, and clinicians need to be familiar with the complexities to best serve their clients.

Why a Prosthesis?

Clinicians assist an individual with limb deficiency to return to function after limb loss through education, support, training, and exposure to the appropriate tools at the right time. People with limb difference have a variety of options for a primary prosthesis, but the individual must see the value in its use. Whether it helps them function, is cosmetically appealing, does not draw undue attention, makes them feel whole again, helps them accomplish a meaningful task; all of these reasons help support a need of the individual. Clinicians should encourage the patient with developing this priority of needs of a prosthesis to ensure the device matches those needs. Ideally, clinicians would like to encourage the individual to explore the possibility of using a device to add a functional grasp to return bilateral upper extremity interactions. The clinician's goal for the patient is to achieve a certain level of dexterity, comfort, knowledge, and ability to make an informed choice. It is not always easy for an individual, who has recently undergone trauma, to be open-minded and assertive about all the factors involved in selecting, training, and wearing an artificial limb. Under the time-constrained cost-containment medical model, given the amount of one-on-one clinician time patients receive, how do clinicians distill the most important aspects of a medical issue and motivate them to take on these challenges? One of the biggest selling points for use of a prosthesis is the additional function. How does one hold their wallet to take out something without a prosthetic grasp? How does one carry a coffee and unlock a door with keys? Or hold vegetables in place while cutting them? Or tie shoes? Or carry a bag and put sunglasses on? The list goes on. Assisting an individual to achieve a level of competency with a prosthesis to make an informed decision is the best for which clinicians can strive. That is easier said than done as many moving parts, emotions, clinicians, reimbursements, appointments, and training need to come together in a relatively short amount of time. The individual with a limb deficiency and their family need to advocate for a high quality of care and the results they desire. Clinicians can encourage, educate, train, remove barriers, and assist the patient in their recovery, but ultimately the individual determines what course is the best fit for them.

Effects of Amputation

Repetitive stress disorders (RSDs) and musculoskeletal conditions (MSCs) of the intact limb are additional reasons for prosthesis use. In a retrospective cohort study of combat-related amputations by Cancio et al[4] in 2021, it was found that 1 year following amputation overuse upper limb conditions, neck and upper back conditions, lower limb conditions, and low back pain were more likely to develop in service members with upper limb amputations than in those who sustained minor combat-related injuries. Repetitive stress disorders such as carpal tunnel syndrome, cubital tunnel syndrome, radial tunnel syndrome, tendinopathies, and medial and lateral epicondylitis are some of the possibilities. Other overuse challenges may involve arthritis, ligamentous damage, rotator cuff tears, and muscle and tendon trauma. Another study identified that MSCs were 65% higher than in those without amputation.[5] If these individuals do not use a prosthesis, they are potentially at increased risk for MSCs and they may have very limited function while recovering from injury or surgery to the intact limb.[6] Good evidence identifies the link between limb loss and RSD or MSC, but there is not good evidence for the use of a prosthesis decreasing the burden on the intact upper extremity. There is a tendency for individuals with limb deficiency to use their teeth to assist with opening or stabilizing items. This is not advised because of the increased wear or damage to the teeth. Individuals with limb deficiency need to be educated in prevention of these secondary traumas through ergonomics education, workplace ergonomic assessment, activity modification, stretching, strengthening, and joint protection techniques. Yoga and Pilates-type exercises can be an excellent tool to promote proper alignment, symmetry, range of motion, strength, and endurance after limb loss. The use of a single upper extremity has been shown to increase the risk of repetitive stress disorders and/or musculoskeletal disorders; individuals need to be educated in prevention of these disorders, as well as the potential benefits of prosthesis use.

Learning to Use a Prosthesis

Individuals with limb deficiencies have varying levels of interest to train and rehabilitate in the use of a new prosthesis. Unfortunately for the individual with a limb deficiency, learning to use a prosthesis is a little more complicated than switching out a part. The clinician roles are clear as the physician prescribes the intervention, the prosthetist crafts a limb replacement device, and a therapist trains them in the application of the device. A prosthesis is essentially a tool, and some tools require more practice than others. A golf club is made to hit a golf ball, but the execution of the user is the main variable determining success. To become a skilled user of a golf club takes many hours of practice and education to do one thing: strike a ball. Learning how to use a prosthesis to assist with many tasks is more complicated, and the individual may have to adapt the task or tool to find success. Clinicians work hard to lead patients with limb deficiency to a level of competence with accuracy, knowledge of the device, dexterity, problem solving, and task adaptation, and the rest is up to the patient. Therapy is crucial to educate and inform quality use of the device by the user. Working with individuals going through major life stressors requires compassion, flexibility, and resilience of the clinician. When and where the individual wants to use the device is a personal choice. Engaged participation in therapies can be encouraged by matching the patient's personality and interests, assisting in solving problems, providing a safe atmosphere for patients to share their feelings, facilitating humor (the best coping technique), and finding mutual interests in common. To get the most engagement out of an individual, physicians themselves need to be engaged, enjoying their time, learning, sharing, and appreciating the individuals and work involved. Motivational interviewing skills are also a wonderful method to help meet a person where they are mentally, and gently develop aspects of what they are communicating into positive opportunities for growth with prosthesis use. Rehabilitation is vital for the patient to start thinking about when and how to use the prosthesis and ideally habituate its use in a number of daily tasks.

Prosthesis Preferences

Individuals with limb deficiency have a number of different interests when using a prosthesis. Some individuals prefer something that appears as close to lifelike appearance as possible but is passive and only used as a stabilizer without prehension. Other individuals prefer body-powered terminal devices and harnessing systems with the use of a Hosmer hook to allow fine pinch and to not occlude sight. Still other individuals prefer the power and harnessless myoelectric devices. More technologically advanced multiarticulating terminal devices that bridge design gaps are coming to the field every year, but there is not necessarily evidence that advanced devices have improved acceptance rates.[7] Myoelectric devices are also available with custom-painted silicone covers to appear real while offering the benefits of prehension. Activity-specific devices offer a more task-oriented approach to device selection. Individuals may choose one of these devices to use as their primary prosthesis to assist them with a specific need such as wheelchair transfers or wheelchair propulsion. For more information see details about activity-specific devices discussed later in the chapter. Typically, activity-specific devices are used for a particular sport or activity and then switched out for a more versatile prehension device once the sport or task is finished. For example, if someone uses a terminal device to assist with an afternoon of biking, it will help them bike, but would not be helpful if they stop to shop or eat because it does not have prehension. There are advantages and disadvantages to all prosthetic systems, which the patient should be educated on and consider their needs before receiving a prescription.

Prosthesis Acceptance

There are many factors involved in successful prosthesis acceptance. A study conducted with bomb blast survivors with upper extremity limb loss demonstrated that revision surgery to improve the residual limb improved prosthesis compliance from 19% before amputation to 87% after amputation.[8] This demonstrates that limb quality plays a crucial role in prosthesis acceptance. Education of individuals in the quality of their residual limb and changes that may happen over time could ensure more prosthesis acceptance. Malone et al refer to a golden period of prosthesis acceptance if a patient is fitted within 1 month of amputation.[1] This study goes on to state that the initial type of prosthesis did not matter for long-term acceptance, but the time frame was more important.[1] In another survey study, factors associated with prosthesis acceptance included having fewer than two complicating health factors and being employed.[9] The average speed of delivery of the prosthetic devices in this study was from 6.5 to 15.4 months after amputation. Fewer than two complicating factors, completion of high school education, employment during the time of amputation and review, rapid return to work, acceptance of the amputation by the time of review, and the perception that the prosthesis was expensive were factors associated with successful rehabilitation.[9] Biddiss and Chau[10] identified perceived need of prosthetic limb and satisfaction with the prosthetic technology as the most important aspects to acceptance. Factors that increase the likelihood of rejection include pain/discomfort, female sex, partial hand amputation, transhumeral amputation, non–full-time workers, and those with low satisfaction with health care and prosthetic options. Work seems to play a role as full-time employed individuals recorded 20% rejection versus part-time employed individuals at 35% rejection. The occupational roles with the most rejection, at greater than 40%, included students and homemakers.[10] There are many factors that can decrease the likelihood of prosthetic acceptance and practitioners can assist the patient in overcoming these. There is an opportunity to help individuals with limb deficiency benefit from prostheses over the life span but this depends on informed quality care. Biddiss and Chau described the importance of establishing need, enabling resources, involving the patient in the prescription process, and fostering peer support.[10] Another study from Austria identified that advanced prosthetics have not corresponded to increased acceptance.[7] Most of the participants in the study were myoelectric users and most complained about the poor comfort and weight of the devices.[7] Østlie et al identified primary prosthesis rejection and secondary or delayed prosthesis rejection as being highest in elderly, female patients whose amputations were more proximal.[11] The questionnaire based in Norway found less primary rejection (4.5%) than secondary rejection (13.4%) among the 224 participants. The rationale for rejection followed a similar theme of perceived need as well as dissatisfaction with comfort, function, and control.[11] The aforementioned items indicated the need for quality patient-centered care with experienced clinicians and maximization of comfort and function. Further research is needed to determine the causes of prosthetic rejections with current devices and health care delivery processes.

Meeting Clients' Needs

Individuals are confronted with challenges to many parts of their lives after amputation, and clinicians are there to support them in this transition. Faced with a loss of function, individuals must determine the best option to support their return to successful performance of tasks. Although a prosthesis may not be beneficial for everyone, it has a remarkable ability to assist function. There have been advances in upper extremity prosthetics devices, but this does not correlate to increased rates of acceptance.[7] Timeliness of prosthesis fitting, perceived need of a prosthesis, comfort, residual limb quality, and full-time employment all play a role in acceptance.[1,8-10] The key to success is finding a fit between the individual and a device that meets their needs to interact in their environment.

Postamputation Pain

Postamputation pain (PAP) encompasses the various types of pain that an amputee can experience. Under that umbrella term, phantom limb syndrome (PLS) is a unique phenomenon associated with limb loss.

Phantom Limb Syndrome

The concept of phantom sensations and pain dates back centuries, described a "ghost" pain from an amputated limb no longer present. The term phantom limb pain was coined to label the symptoms that patients experience after an amputation. Phantom limb syndrome (PLS) is a broader term used when referring to any sensation (pain or otherwise) localized distal to the amputated limb. People with limb loss experiencing PLS may describe feeling the hand or fingers present (sensation) or they may report pain (PLP) described as electrical, shooting, stabbing, burning, throbbing, cramping, numbness, or pins and needles (**Figure 1**). In severe cases, amputees with PLP report feeling as if their hand is being crushed and twisted, causing excruciating pain, which prevents them from sleeping or carrying out activities of daily living (ADLs).

PLS is thought to be neuropathic in nature, with the mechanism occurring along the sensory nervous system in three specific areas: supraspinal, spinal, and peripheral. Supraspinal involves pathways in the somatosensory cortex, which has been shown to reorganize the area in the brain mapped to the amputated limb as a result of the sensory input (the deafferentiated limb), termed neuroplasticity. In the spinal cord, the dorsal horn is reorganized after the peripheral nerve injury. The severed peripheral nerve results in axonal nerve damage initiating inflammation, subsequent regenerative sprouting of the nerve endings, and ultimately increased ectopic afferent input. The perceived experience is pain distal to the residual limb from this disrupted reorganized sensory feedback loop resulting in PLP.

Residual Limb Pain

Pain localized in the residual limb may be attributed to several causes, which include problems with the bone, soft tissue, or incision. Acutely, pain in the limb could be intrinsic pain from surgical manipulation of the soft tissue or may be due to an underlying infection, which may be accompanied by localized fever, tenderness, redness, or purulent drainage

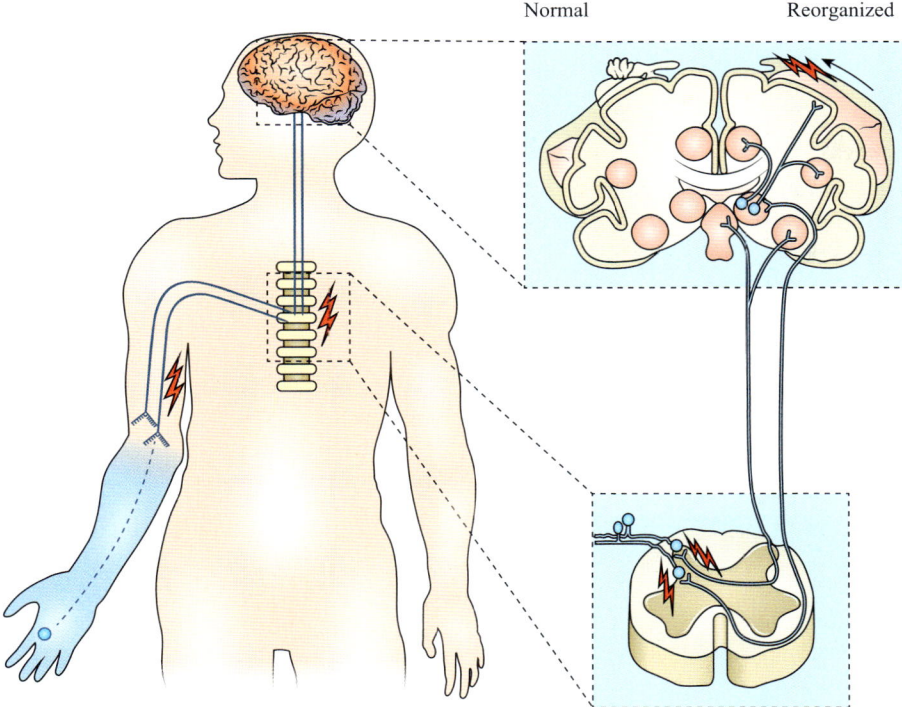

FIGURE 1 Schematic illustration depicting phantom limb pain. (Reprinted with permission from Flor H, Nikolajsen L, Staehelin Jensen T: Phantom limb pain: A case of maladaptive CNS plasticity? *Nat Rev Neurosci* 2006;7:873-881. Copyright © Nature Publishing Group.)

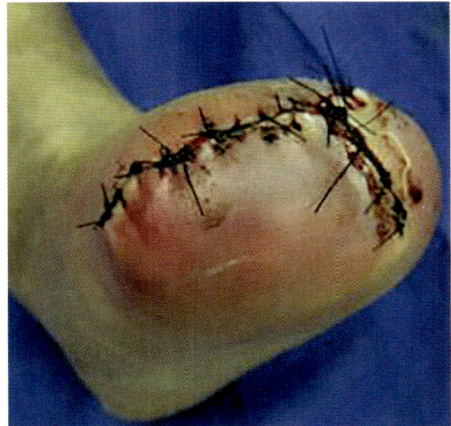

FIGURE 2 Clinical photograph showing residual limb healing.

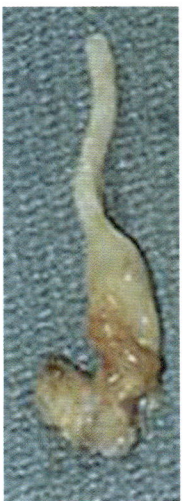

FIGURE 3 Photograph showing an excised neuroma: regenerated nerve bundle.

(**Figure 2**). In the subacute phase, muscle spasms result from surgical procedures performed to cover the distal end of the limb such as a myodesis, where the muscle is sewn into the bone to provide appropriate shape and structure in an ideal level of amputation.

Once the incision is healed, another common cause of intrinsic residual limb pain is the development of neuroma, which occurs when the peripheral nerves cut during the amputation tend to regenerate, forming a bundle of nerve endings (**Figure 3**). These neuromas produce neuropathic-type pain when the mass is palpated causing a sharp, electrical sensation radiating proximally along the nerve.

Residual limb pain may also result from causes external to the limb such as pressure from a dressing or a shrinker being too tight or from a prosthesis exerting uneven pressure in an anatomic area that is sensitive, such as the bony protuberance (humeral condyles) in the elbow.

Biomechanics of Abnormal Positioning

Pain can also arise from wearing or not wearing a prosthesis. Conventional body-powered prostheses have a cable harness system that relies on suspension around the shoulder/axilla region (**Figure 4**). Fitting and alignment are key to ensuring proper functioning and prevention of abnormal positioning, which might result in pain during use. Alternatively, many upper limb amputees choose not to wear a prosthesis or unfortunately do not have the resources to obtain a prosthesis. Regardless, studies have shown that not using a prosthesis places an upper limb amputee at risk for the development of overuse syndrome in the contralateral limb or in a joint proximal to the amputation. Additionally, in the case of traumatic traction injuries causing an amputation, for example, an arm pulled into a machine, damage to the brachial plexus could result in pain in the residual limb separate and apart from the amputation causing pain. Musculoskeletal pain in the cervical and thoracic spine can be from the biomechanics as a complication of an upper limb amputation, such as an overactive shoulder girdle musculature without the gravitational weight of an arm.

Other complications that can cause pain include abnormalities related to the bone, soft tissue, and skin interface. Examples include bone spurs or heterotopic ossification (**Figure 5**), joint contractures, and bony prominences post upper limb amputation. Skin complications include infections (bacterial, fungal), allergic reactions, and adherent skin grafting.

Pain Assessment

Evaluating pain in an amputee is critical to diagnosing and treating the various types and complications associated with upper limb loss. Aside from the standard visual analog pain scale,

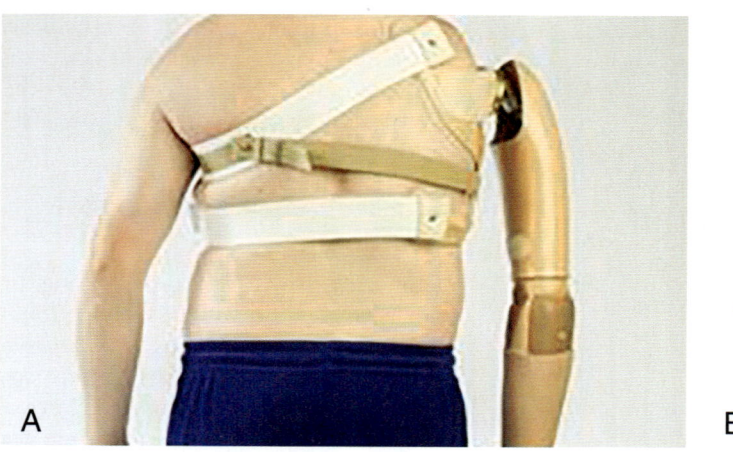
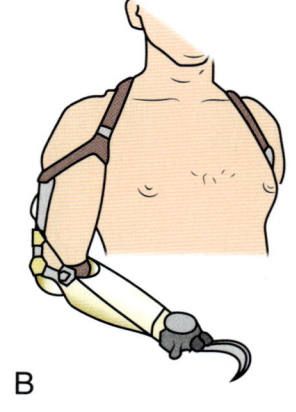
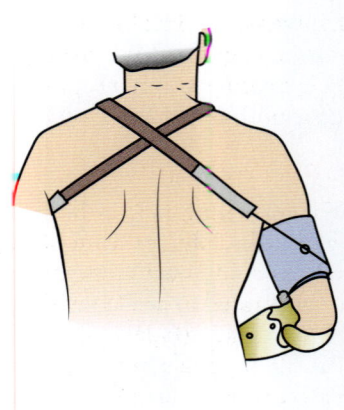

FIGURE 4 **A**, Photograph and (**B**) illustrations show prosthesis harnessing.

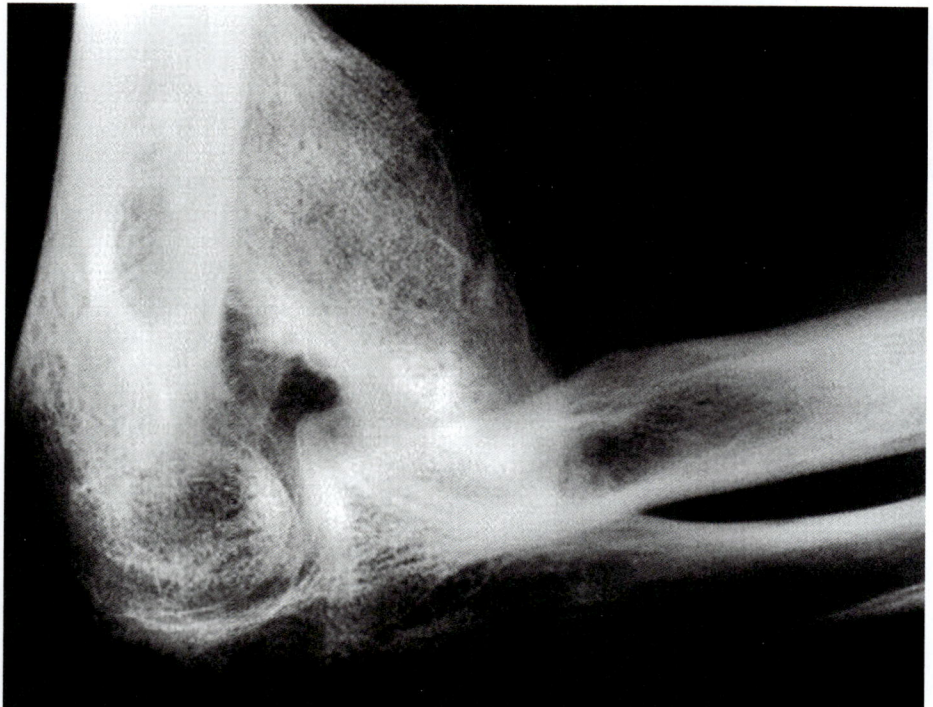

FIGURE 5 Radiograph showing heterotopic ossification.

asking specific questions about descriptors and locations of their pain assists with differentiating the various types of pain outlined previously that amputees can experience.

Screening for psychological issues such as depression, anxiety, sleep disorder, chronic pain, or any substance use history, both family and personal, is an important part of the initial assessment. Coping with limb loss often triggers or exacerbates preexisting psychological disorders and certainly affects one's ability to adjust to this life-changing diagnosis. Loss of an arm initially can be debilitating in basic daily functioning and independence. Adjusting to an upper limb amputation requires processing the five stages of grief (denial, anger, bargaining, depression, and acceptance), which can take years to achieve a healthy mental health outlook. Depending on the nature of the injury, posttraumatic stress disorder can contribute to the ability to cope with PAP and affect treatment options.

The initial workup for the management of PAP and the psychological issues of limb loss should include basic laboratory values that include a metabolic panel, complete blood count, and urine drug screening. Use of a pain contract, which requires the patient to obtain all medications related to pain, sleep, anxiety, or depression from one physician, should be a key part of the process. Frequent, often monthly, follow-up and monitoring with the physician monitoring program can identify any areas of concern and create a transparent dialogue between health care clinicians who treat amputees and their unique needs. Providing a pain and medication journal helps educate and focus the amputee with PAP to understand their treatment options.

Treatment for PAP is multifactorial, including pharmacologic options, desensitization techniques, modalities (heat/ice, mirror therapy, alpha stimulator, transcutaneous electrical nerve stimulator), invasive interventions (acupuncture, nerve blocks, botulinum toxin, radiofrequency ablation, spinal cord stimulators, and pain pumps), and surgical techniques (neuroma resection, targeted muscle reinnervation regenerative peripheral nerve interface).

Approaching PAP pharmacologically is a complex issue. The opioid crisis is at the forefront and must be acknowledged. Since 1999 when pain was classified as a vital sign, opioids or opioid derivatives have caused devastating statistics in loss of life and economic impact, including increased costs of healthcare, lost productivity, addiction treatment, and criminal justice involvement. Health care clinicians must recognize these risks and adjust their treatment options, particularly for those with upper limb loss.

Professional Roles

When treating upper limb amputees, an interdisciplinary team of health care professionals works together to provide an integrated approach with the patient at the center (**Figure 6**). Starting with identifying goals and expectations, the team can provide information to make informed decisions in their overall treatment plan including the necessary training for the best possible outcome. This becomes a lifelong education process in which the primary team consists of the physician (surgeon and/or physiatrist), occupational therapist (specializing in limb loss), and certified prosthetist (with expertise in upper limb prosthetic devices). There are other peripheral team members who might become key players depending on the individual treatment plan. Other individual disciplines could include a mental health specialist (psychiatrist, psychologist, counselor) or a resource expert (social worker, case manager, peer visitor).

A clinic dedicated to the upper limb amputee can provide a unique setting for individuals with upper limb amputations with a focused approach by the physician. The initial evaluation should include a discussion about the patient's goals, resources available, a preliminary education on prosthetic and assistive device technologies, as well as address the medical issues that often arise in the acute and subacute phases of managing limb loss. The assessment should include identifying comorbidities that may affect treatment options and any complications that will affect the overall function. And, as discussed, pain unique to upper limb amputees along with the psychological effect on upper limb amputees needs to be considered (**Figure 7**).

A physical examination must focus on the residual limb and the range of motion of the proximal joint of the limb and strength of the residual limb as well as overall strength and function of nonamputated limbs (**Table 1**). Any neurologic issue that affects the limb, including sensory feedback (sensation and proprioception) and cognitive status that might affect the ability to operate a prosthesis, is an important part of the evaluation. Complications affecting the soft tissue (bone spurs or heterotopic ossification) or skin interface (grafts or incisions) must be taken into consideration and documented in the medical record, which is used to justify the medical necessity of assistive and prosthetic devices.

Involving certified peer visitors early in the process can have a profound effect in the recovery of an upper limb amputee (**Figure 8**). Matching levels and backgrounds between the peer visitor and the patient is desirable if possible.

Caring for the upper limb amputee requires lifelong management and

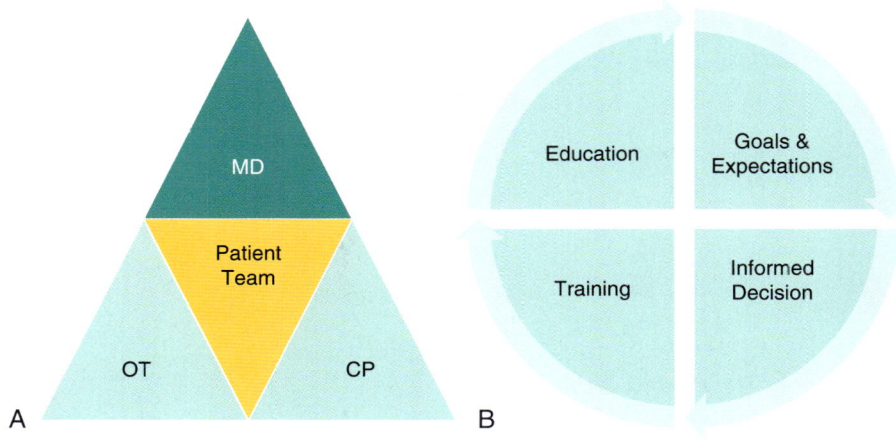

FIGURE 6 Schematic illustration showing the interdisciplinary team (**A**) and process (**B**). CP = certified prosthetist, MD = medical doctor, OT = occupational therapist.

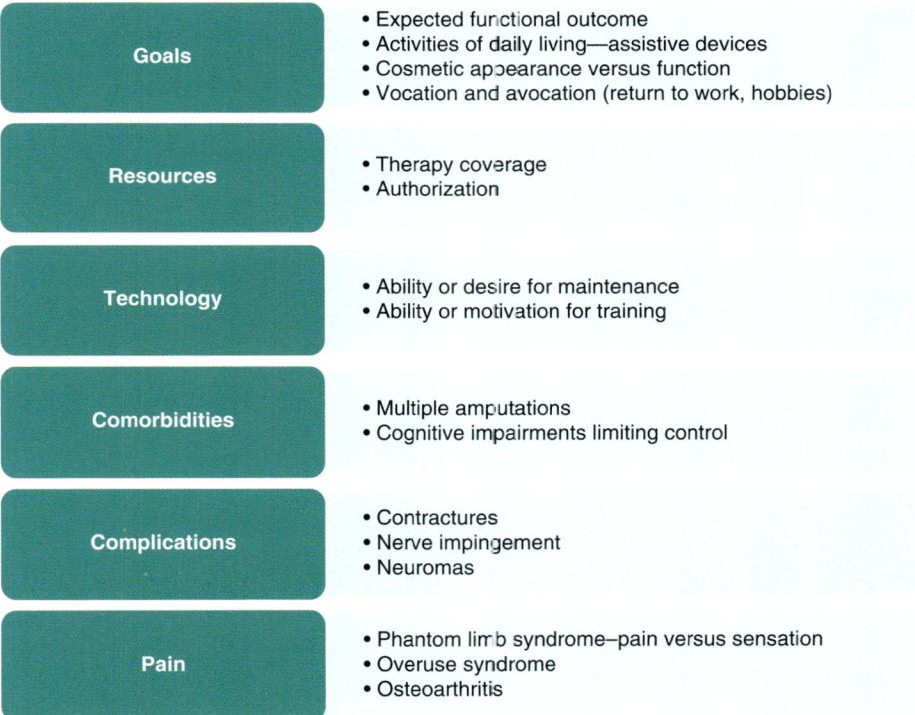

FIGURE 7 Illustration outlining the evaluation of the patient with limb loss.

Section 1: General Principles

TABLE 1 Key Components of the Physical Examination
- Residual limb evaluation - Range of motion - Neurologic (sensation, proprioception) - Cognitive evaluation - Strength (residual limb and nonamputated limbs) - Skin issues (grafts or incision) - Soft tissue (heterotopic ossification or bone spurs)

continuity of care to address the ongoing medical needs (**Figure 9**).

In an ideal situation, the team approach incorporates the occupational therapist and certified prosthetist to assist with the educational process. Using integrated communication to the team including functional assessments presumably provides the patient with information in choosing prosthetic devices to restore function meeting their goals and expectations (**Table 2**).

Prosthetic Limb Rehabilitation

Rehabilitation after limb loss is essential to returning to a full and active life (**Figure 10**). Smurr et al[12] proposed an excellent protocol of care for upper extremity limb loss and identified five stages through work with US service members returning from injuries sustained in Iraq and Afghanistan. This seminal work identified the standard of care for rehabilitation with the upper extremity limb loss population, and is an excellent resource for guiding rehabilitation. The following overview will examine these standards of care through a different lens, with a discussion of the progression through standard of care as initial care, intermediate rehabilitation, and integration of the prosthesis.

Initial Care
Healing
The initial care phase progresses from amputation surgery to training on basic prosthesis controls. Skin closure and wound healing are the first steps in having a viable residual limb to rehabilitate. Pain, wound care, edema management, and limb shaping are hallmarks of this initial care that all clinicians should be tracking. Wrapping

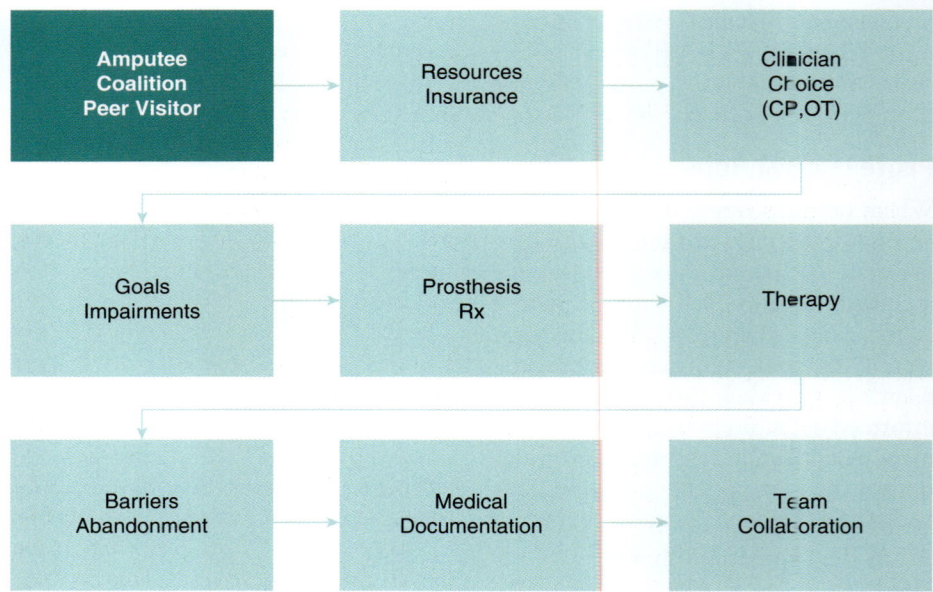

FIGURE 8 Chart outlining upper limb amputation prosthetic treatment evaluation. CP = certified prosthetist; OT = occupational therapist; Rx = prescription.

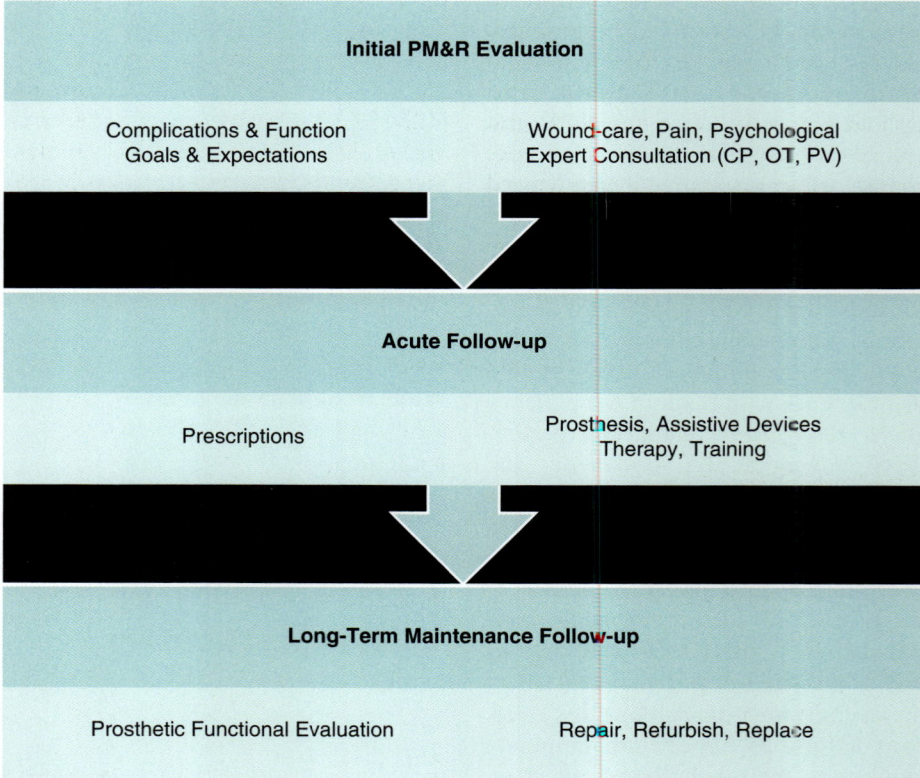

FIGURE 9 Schematic illustration showing the initial physical medicine and rehabilitation evaluation. CP = certified prosthetist; OT = occupational therapist; PM&R = physical medicine and rehabilitation; PV = peer visitor.

or tubular compressive garments help to move edema up and out of the residual limb to promote healing, shape the residual limb, and decrease pressure and pain at the healing site.

Elevation, closely monitored ice application, and lymphedema techniques can promote movement and reabsorption of edema fluid. Once edema has started to reduce, active movement for

TABLE 2 Patient Education
- Types of prostheses
- Impairments (activities of daily living)
- Expectations
- Goals (function/appearance)
- Process
- Resources (insurance)
- Timeline

available joints should commence to tolerance. It is a requirement to be aware of any tissue healing issues and prevent any suture dehiscence or interfere with any intravenous treatment or nerve block. As the individual begins to heal and reduce in volume, progress to more inclusion of the residual limb can be made.

Incorporation of Residual Limb With Daily Tasks

Incorporation of the residual limb in tasks as early as possible is important. Incorporation allows the patient to view the limb as an assist, instead of an area of the body to be left alone and ignored because of pain. Sometimes looking at the residual limb can remind the patient of trauma and bring on overwhelming emotions. If the individual lost both arms, then they absolutely must get their residual limbs involved to take an active role in their self-care. If the individual has lost their dominant extremity, then change of dominance retraining must begin at this point. Individuals should be encouraged to use the residual limb for stabilizing a plate while eating, picking up pillows, supporting a cell phone or tablet, and stabilizing items for drinking. Adding a universal cuff (**Figure 11**) will allow a stable pocket for tool use and fine motor interactions that are essential for individuals with bilateral limb deficiency. Custom adaptations may be necessary for individual bathing and toileting needs (**Figures 12** through **14**).

Adaptations for drinking tube devices, pain-controlled analgesia buttons, and cell phone or tablet holders can improve independence and allow patients to gain a sense of control. Large open loops made of low-temperature thermoplastic or splinting material can assist with tasks such as urinal manipulation. Clinicians should ensure the individual has a way to touch their face and scalp if there is bilateral involvement. Clinicians may want to incorporate splinting to form a cone type or Velcro strapped interface to assist with self-care.

Adaptive equipment should be introduced to assist in function at this point. Items including Dycem or nonslip materials to stabilize plates or containers for opening; suction brush to allow scrubbing of the intact hand or arm; long-handled sponge or rocker knife to allow for stabilizing an item during cutting;

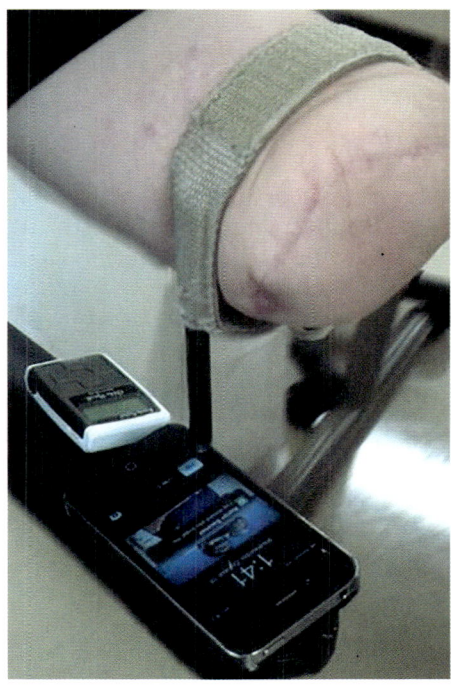

FIGURE 11 Photograph showing the universal cuff with capacitive touch stylus.

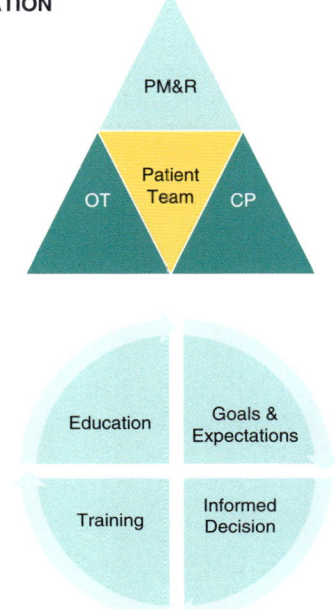

FIGURE 10 Schematic illustration showing prosthesis and rehabilitation. CP = certified prosthetist, OT = occupational therapist, PM&R = physical medicine and rehabilitation physician, PV = peer visitor.

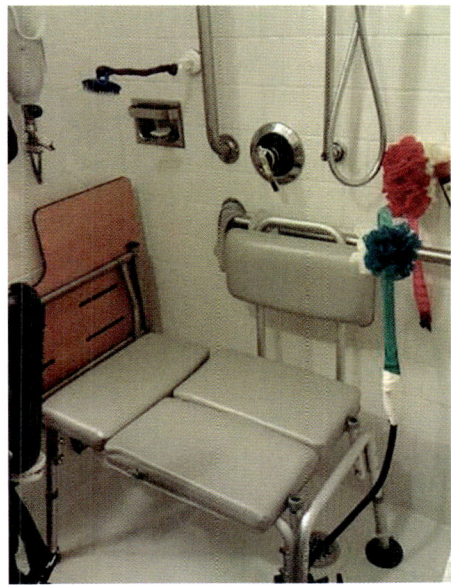

FIGURE 12 Photograph showing the adapted shower setup with a gooseneck scrubber. (Courtesy of Josef Butkus, MS OTR/L.)

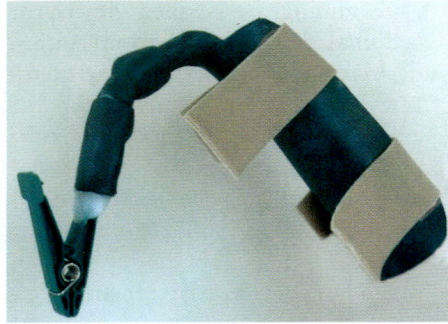

FIGURE 13 Photograph showing a toileting device.

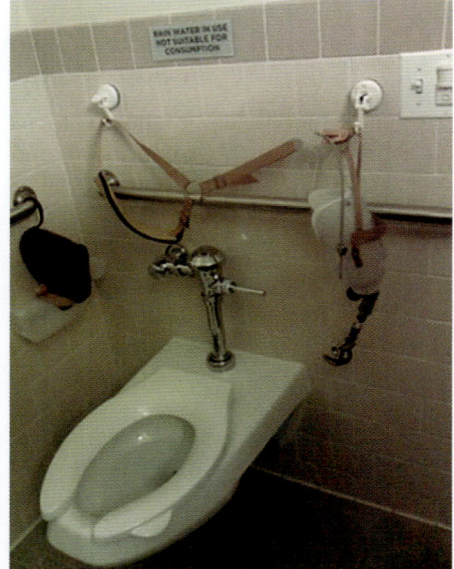

FIGURE 14 Photograph showing a toileting arm and adapted urinal. (Courtesy of Josef Butkus, MS OTR/L.)

use of a hydration pack; adapted clothing with Velcro in the seams; and use of a fanny pack or shoulder bag to access or store important items are especially useful. Incorporation of a residual limb helps add function and serves to normalize the limb again.

Exercise and Desensitization

Exercise and desensitization tasks should follow when tolerated. Range of motion is important to reestablish to prevent formation of scar tissue, which limits joint movement. Proximal musculature, given joint and nerve integrity, can be exercised with general exercises such as elbow flexion/extension, scapular protraction/retraction, arm circles, and neck movements. The shoulder should be exercised and stretched in all available motions including flexion/extension, abduction/adduction, horizontal abduction/horizontal adduction, and especially the easily forgotten internal/external rotation. External rotator muscles, which are already at a strength disadvantage, will be under heavy stress once a prosthesis is fitted. These active motions are a type of desensitization, but should also include sweeping, rubbing, and tapping the residual limb as well. A general guide to desensitize is to tell the patient to give a gentle pressure and increase if tolerable to allow their body to process and normalize the sensation. As time progresses they should be able to tolerate greater pressure or sharpness. If a patient is squeezing their limb very hard, they are likely giving it too much sensation and the goal is to visualize gentle massaging of a sore muscle. If the residual limb is unbandaged, the patient can use desensitization sticks with a variety of textures on different sticks in order to get all sensory receptors in the skin to recognize normal touch again. Combining exercise with function is an excellent way to address many aspects in on exercise. Combining desensitization and holding objects with bilateral upper extremities is a great way to exercise and desensitize. Individuals can accomplish this by squeezing a ball between intact and residual upper extremity limbs to perform exercises. Exercises such as shoulder flexion and performing trunk rotation or diagonal motions while holding a ball will promote bilateral integration and symmetry. Learning how and where a residual limb can support an object is very useful. Range of motion, desensitization, and endurance help to build a strong foundation for prosthesis training.

Education

Many items are addressed in this initial phase, and not to be overlooked is the opportunity to educate the individual about prostheses. Topics of discussion can include:

- How prosthetics realistically assist function
- How to protect and decrease stress on an intact limb
- The importance of humor in recovery
- The importance of peer support and success stories
- Casting and prosthesis fitting process
- Prosthesis suspension types
- How to best exercise, stretch, and strengthen
- Educate about the muscles involved in the operation of devices
- How myoelectric prostheses operate
- How myoelectrics can identify a switch (quick/slow, co-contraction, double/triple impulse)
- Pattern recognition systems such as CoApt and Motion Plus from Otto Bock
- Clarify that although there are more devices and control systems available, using microvolts traveling in muscles to act as switches is not a perfect system. Errors happen and precise control is not guaranteed
- Review safety and situations that would be dangerous, such as holding on to heavy machinery without a way to automatically release
- Types of terminal devices for body-powered or myoelectric prostheses
- Advantages and disadvantages of different terminal devices
- Scar massage
- Adaptive equipment

Education can help frame what to expect for the patient. It is always important for the patient to generate questions to help tailor information to their personal interests and concerns. Education is an invaluable part of assisting individuals with limb deficiencies build their knowledge as they prepare to regain function.

Preparation for a Prosthesis

Before receiving a prosthesis it is a good time to tune up the skills needed to perform well with the device. Scar massage is important to start once the skin is closed to ensure good mobility of the scar and prevention of a bulky scar. Silicone liners also improve the scar through light pressure and maintaining moisture. The physician should ensure that the residual limb is desensitized and available joints have been strengthened to tolerate the weight of the device. To exercise the residual limb the occupational therapist can manually resist motion, and resistance bands, cuff weights, or a cable machine attached to a D-ring on an ankle cuff strap also can be used. For body-powered arms it is very important to strengthen scapular protraction/retraction, shoulder flexion, shoulder abduction, and external rotation motions against resistance. For myoelectric arms there should be good control and endurance of myoelectric sites and demonstration of the applicable switch between different motions. The myoelectric arm will be heavier at the distal end, so strengthening is important for lifting the device. Shoulder strength and endurance are important to lift as well as operate a body-powered prosthesis. Myoelectric muscle sites need to have good endurance to tolerate hour-long sessions of therapy in the coming weeks. The Otto Bock as well as I-limb from Ossur make good myoelectric training devices, software, and offer training for staff and individuals on their respective websites. Good preparation for a prosthetic device sets an individual with a limb deficiency on the path for a smooth transition into using a prosthesis.

Initial Prosthesis Training

Initial device fitting is an important time and barriers need to be removed to gain success from the start. It is important to have the patient know just what to expect with the device. The patient will likely try on a check socket after the initial casting to ensure that it is a good fit without too much pressure on the residual limb. Once the patient has been fitted with an artificial arm, the physician needs to make sure all the components are working accurately. If there is pain, movement, or lack of control, it is important to return to the prosthetist as soon as possible to make the necessary corrections. If poor myoelectric control or material issues persist, the individual may start to lack confidence in the device. Tasks to perform after initial fitting include:

- Passing objects from the intact hand to the prosthesis in a variety of positions
- Operation of all joints
- Education on how to make minor adjustments to the artificial arm
- Skin checks and wearing schedule
- Begin working on experimenting with how to incorporate the terminal device with tasks such as tying a lacing board, beading a string, opening containers, holding a bag in which to place an item, opening/closing a bread bag, opening and placing objects in a Ziploc bag
- Practice holding objects while interacting with the other hand
- Working on light touch to prevent squeezing an object too hard
- Rote grasp and release at different distances and elevations
- Examine the differences in control of grasp in these different locations

Challenges in the Initial Phase
Body Powered
- Opening the body-powered terminal device with full flexion of the elbow. This is caused by increased friction on the pull cord and sheathing with more angles of flexion
- Opening device behind back or behind shoulder because of limited ability to get force on the pull cord, also known as excursion
- Finding additional motions to increase excursion of the pull cord

Myoelectric
- Accuracy testing: 12 motions are performed with the clinician noting these were correct, the wrong motion performed/stalls with number of attempts, or individual was unable to perform. The individual (1) opens the device three-fourths of the full finger extension, (2) supinates 180°, (3) closes hand to one-fourth extension, and (4) pronates 180°. This is repeated three times and the occupational therapist should cue the patient to the next motion, so the patient is not guessing. The clinician can make a list of 1 to 12, mark when there is an error or delay, and obtain a percentage of accuracy by dividing errors from the 12 motions. It becomes very clear what movements the individual is having difficulty with
- Closing on or releasing an object without looking
- Moving as slowly as possible
- Determining the smallest object the terminal device can pick up with a multiarticulating hand (nonhook-type terminal device) and what position relative to the table the hand must rest

Assessment
- Box and blocks
- Patient-specific functional status
- Disabilities of the Arm, Shoulder and Hand (DASH) or QuickDASH
- Orthotics Prosthetics User Survey (OPUS) Upper Extremity Functional Status
- Myoelectric accuracy testing (intermediate challenges discussed next).

The initial training should focus on getting comfortable, education, and operating the device efficiently in bilateral tasks.

Intermediate Phase

The intermediate phase is characterized by establishing fluidity. Ideas that should be incorporated are prepositioning, establishing a normal quality of motion with assistance of mirrors, dexterity, increased wearing schedule, and more automatic performance with the terminal device. Individuals using prostheses at this point are coached through discussion of how and why they use the device to build the awareness of prosthetic performance. The occupational therapist should introduce the idea of the patient analyzing the problems inherent in the task, rather than focusing purely on the function of the device itself. It is always good at this point to remind the individual that there is no completely right answer or only one way to perform a task. There are many options, and the goal is to try performing tasks a variety of ways and see what fits for that individual. For example, in the case of tying shoelaces, how many pinches are optimal? Where and when does it help the individual to pinch with the prosthesis? What parts of the task are essential to pinch? What aspects of the task are more cumbersome to involve the terminal device? Is there an optimal position to perform the task? How fast can they perform it? Other tasks that can be used to review these practices include making simple meal kits of foods such as soup or cookies, measuring and pouring ingredients for a recipe, cutting fruit or vegetables, making a skewer of marshmallows or fruit, folding clothes or towels, or putting clothes on hangers. Dexterity is particularly important in establishing perceived need for the patient. If the prosthesis is known to help with a certain part of a task quickly, then it helps overall efficiency of the task. Getting items in and out of the prosthesis to the other hand quickly is one of the primary skills for all task performance. The art of prosthetic training comes in the knowledge of how to adapt the task rather than what the prosthesis alone can do to establish fluid performance.

Therapeutic Relationship

Building a good relationship between the clinician and individual is essential to allow this open dialogue about how they perform these tasks of personal choice. The way someone performs a task is personal and rarely talked about. For example, if someone is critiqued about how they use utensils while eating, will that person be receptive to that information? Likely not. These are established patterns of physical performance that are automatic and can be considered a part of an individual's personality. The point is that critiques of any kind can be unsettling, invoke a personal history of unwelcome criticism, and be perceived as competitive or insensitive. Clinicians need to be attuned to the individual's openness with discussing these aspects of performance. Clinicians can grade or change the amount of observation or perceived attention to the task they give to the individual's performance. With sensitive individuals it might be necessary to set them up and walk away to allow them to go through their own process of practice and discovery. Humor is an excellent way to help a patient relax and experiment with their new device. The individual can be asked if they are open to feedback or discussing the performance. Individuals need to feel they are doing well and improving to engage and dig deeper to improve performance. The clinician needs to be attuned to the individual's body language, level of comfort or frustration, processing speed, and how best to offer information to support them while learning new skills. Clinicians and individuals with limb deficiency need to have a supporting relationship to get the most benefit from training.

Activity Analysis

The most eloquent use of a prosthesis involves comprehensive knowledge of task performance, and understanding when and how to incorporate this terminal for what gain. Ideally this problem solving will happen in real time with limited delay, but to do that, the patient needs to be very familiar with the performance of a wide variety of tasks. What if an item is wet and slippery? What if an item may crush with the activation of a grip? Occupational therapists in their education learn to analyze task performance and identify all performance components and skills that are required to complete a task.[13] This is also done to examine if a person with limited abilities will be successful and how the occupational therapist may be able to adapt or grade the task to help them be successful. This training assists the occupational therapist in breaking down all the components involved and how to grade or change the task to improve the individual's opportunities for success. This insight gives occupational therapists advanced knowledge and anticipatory skills to determine if the individual will succeed with a particular task given the skills and challenges of a task. For example, if an item is too small to manipulate easily, the occupational therapist may make the handle larger or find a way to keep this part stable. If items are too small to see, the clinician can provide a magnifying glass. If an item moves too easily upon manipulation, placing it on a nonslip surface or use of a device to stabilize it may assist them. A successful occupational therapist can regularly find the challenge that is just right for their patient.[14] This indicates that the task is not too hard, or too difficult, but just right to motivate them to focus on building their skills while having a sense of accomplishment.

Coaching Prosthesis Task Performance

The intermediate phase involves a number of training aspects coming together to maximize knowledge of the devices, tasks, and efficiency to be applied across many situations. The individual with a limb deficiency should be aware of the advantages and disadvantages of all of their terminal devices and start showing a preference for the device used daily. The individual should be encouraged to keep an open mind about what terminal device may help the most with individual tasks, but inevitably they will choose a primary terminal device and system. Individuals in therapy should focus on running through a variety of tasks with the prosthesis to see how it can be incorporated into the situation, adapting the task and discuss the performance. The Unilateral Upper Extremity Amputation: Activities of Daily Living Assessment provides an excellent sample of activities to perform with patients[15] (**Figure 15**). Coaching and discussions about the limitations of the device or challenges of the task should be the focus of these sessions. If poor control is more the issue, then therapy should be remediated to look at biofeedback with myosite activation, isolation, and practice. The prosthetist has more options to help with obtaining more distinct signals and the clinicians should collaborate often. If pain is the issue, more breaks or a better fitting socket may be needed. If strength and endurance are the limitation, then more time should be spent doing resistive exercise or

Name:	Age:	Occupation:	Date(s) of Test:
Therapist:	Sex:	Type of terminal device:	

RATING GUIDE KEY:

0 Impossible	1 Accomplished with much strain, or many awkward motions	2 Somewhat labored, or few awkward motions	3 Smooth, minimal amount of delays and awkward motions

ACTIVITIES OF DAILY LIVING	0	1	2	3	ACTIVITIES OF DAILY LIVING	0	1	2	3
PERSONAL NEEDS:					**GENERAL PROCEDURES:**				
Don/doff pull-over shirt					Turn key in lock				
Dress button-down shirt: cuffs and front					Operate door knob				
Manage zippers and snaps					Place chain on chain lock				
Don/doff pants					Plug cord into wan outlet				
Don/doff belt					Set time on watch				
Lace and tie shoes					**HOUSEKEEPING PROCEDURES:**				
Don/doff pantyhose					Perform laundry				
Tie a tie					Fold clothes				
Don/doff brazier					Set up ironing board				
Don/doff glove					Iron clothes				
Cut and file finger nails					Hand wash dishes				
Polish finger nails					Dry dishes with a towel				
Screw/unscrew cap of toothpaste tube					Load and unload dishwasher				
Squeeze toothpaste					Use broom and dustpan				
Open top of pill bottle					Operate vacuum cleaner				
Set hair					Use wet and dry mop				
Take bill from wallet					Make bed				
Open pack of cigarettes					Change garbage bag				
Light a match					Open/close jar				
Don/doff prosthesis					Open lid of can				
Perform residual limb care					Cut vegetables				
EATING PROCEDURES:					Peel vegetables				
Carry a tray					Manipulate hot pots				
Cut meat					Thread a needle				
Butter bread					Sew a button				
Open Milk Carton					**USE OF TOOLS:**				
DESK PROCEDURES:					Saw				
Use phone and take notes					Hammer				
Use pay phone					Screw drivers				
Sharpen pencil					Tape measure				
Use scissors					Wrenches				
User ruler					Power tools: drill, sander				
Remove and replace ink pen cap					Plane				
Fold and seal letter					Shovel				
Use paper clip					Rake				
Use stapler					Wheel barrel				
Wrap package					**CAR PROCEDURES:**				
Use computer: typing, access Internet					Open and close doors, trunk and hood				
Demonstrate handwriting					Perform steps required to operate vehicle				
COMMENTS:					**COMMENTS:**				

FIGURE 15 An example of a rating guide: the Unilateral Upper Extremity Amputation: Activities of Daily Living Assessment. (Reprinted with permission from Smurr LM, Gulick K, Yancosek K, et al: Managing the upper extremity amputee: A protocol for success. *J Hand Ther* 2008;21(2):160-176. Adapted with permission from Springer-Verlag: Atkins DJ: Adult upper-limb prosthetic training, in Atkins DJ, Meier RH, eds: *Comprehensive Management of the Upper-Limb Amputee*. Springer, 1989, p 49.)

talking with the prosthetist to find ways to decrease stress on the residual limb. As a patient starts to be more dexterous and perform more fluidly patterns of use will emerge. These techniques will be applied from one task to another and identifying and discussing them will assist in efficient task performance. Prosthesis users benefit from knowing as many ways to use the device as possible. They can then apply these strategies in real time as they come across new and novel tasks.

Intermediate Phase Challenges

- Performing tasks without sight
- Involve multitasking to increase the cognitive load with such tasks as making a multi-course meal or performing an assembly task while telling a story
- Unilateral performance: Ideally individuals will not need to perform tasks unilaterally but it makes them think about how they can use the device on its own and build the skill
- Jenga blocks challenge to identify how to pinch without putting any leverage on the block; having the tines meet flat on the block rather than twisting the block
- Playing Connect 4 without use of the intact upper extremity
- Eating a snack and drinking unilaterally
- Throwing or catching cornhole bean bags are good to practice problem solving
- Grasping objects in motion, to improve anticipation and coordination, ie, rolling/catching a ball on a table, or sliding/catching a block across the table
- Stacking blocks
- Polyvinyl chloride pipe structures.
- Complex construction tasks such as K'nex, Lego, or erector sets
- Small engine repair
- Sewing or needlepoint
- Shopping and wallet management
- Home-level tasks: Opening packages, hanging pictures, grocery shopping, vacuuming/sweeping, laundry, dishes, cleaning windows, lawn care, filing/organizing, wrapping presents, and cleaning

Body-Powered Topics

- Changing pull cable length when and if needed
- Locking pull cord strapping in place with stitches or safety pins to prevent slipping
- Adjusting or fixing certain parts (strapping, padding)
- Light touch and use of gravity to allow light pinch to rotate pegs
- Improvising fixes to device

Assessment

- Continue assessments from initial prosthetic training
- Nine-hole peg test (only with a hook-type terminal device)
- Jebsen-Taylor Hand Function Test
- University of New Brunswick Test of Prosthetics Function
- Assessment of capacity for myoelectric control

Integration Phase

Integration is the phase where training and task analysis come together for the individual and their long-term incorporation of the prosthesis. The wearing schedule for the device is typically throughout the working day or all day. Therapy should focus on personal goals for specific activities, elimination of barriers, fine-tuning problem solving, and adaptation of tasks as needed. The individual works to incorporate the device into all tasks, whether ADLs, instrumental ADLs, work, leisure, fitness, or sports activities.

Meaningful Activities

Meaningful activities are particularly important in this stage. Being completely absorbed in a task, or "in flow," is naturally self-healing and does not allow people to think about things other than the task in the moment.[16] Examples of flow activities can be, but are not limited to, reading, playing sports, exercise, yoga, videogaming, playing musical instruments, singing, cooking, sewing, gardening, and working on construction projects.[16] Independence with ADLs is essential to recover an individual's self-dignity and autonomy, but ADLs are not what someone does for fun. Sometimes it is a challenge to coax out what might be important to an individual with an upper limb deficiency through questions, for example: If you had a day off work without home responsibilities, what would you do? Did you have any hobbies or other interests before you settled into your current occupation or before starting a family? If you could vacation anywhere and do anything what would you do? If you won the lottery what would you do with your time? Everyone gets caught up in the maintenance of career, social, and family life, and a quality work-life balance is often forgotten. Recovering from an injury naturally provides an opportunity to look at how an individual spends limited time and offers a chance to consider whether that time should be spent doing other things. Often individuals who have experienced trauma report that the injury made them automatically start prioritizing their lives differently than before the accident. It is important to encourage individuals to give themselves space to allow more happiness in their life, especially as they may be dealing with pain, disturbed sleep, physical changes, relationship changes, and emotional struggles. Taking time to step away from habitual tasks and elucidating what is most important to them can benefit the individual over the long term. Now that the individual has additional challenges, how are they going to alter the equation so that they can still find happiness and emotional balance? This process provides the patient an opportunity to look at incorporating the prosthesis into some positive life changes.

The Move to Independent Training

As the integration stage progresses, prosthesis work will largely occur outside of the clinic as the individual works to find the best way to incorporate the device. The prosthesis user continues to benefit from checking in with clinicians and peers to problem solve occasionally, but benefits most from trial, error, and adaptation on their own. This stage is akin to weaning from outpatient therapy for an orthopaedic injury. At this point the prosthesis user has a good level of comfort with their performance and works on their home exercises and activities to improve their skills.

Challenges at the Integration Phase

- Incorporating a device into favorite work, recreational, or leisure activity
- Ergonomic assessment of specific tasks to be performed
- Multitasking with the use of a prosthesis that adds more of a cognitive load, such as cooking a three-course meal and timing those aspects. Or, performing construction tasks while listening closely to a podcast and being quizzed by someone on the information
- Community tasks: getting gas, shopping, landscaping/gardening, painting, climbing ladders, changing light bulbs, setting up a television/computer, and participation in church or community tasks
- Long-term projects
- Selection of activity-specific arms or terminal devices
- Return to sports or fitness activities
- Finding new hobbies or sports to perform with the prosthesis
- Taking a weekend trip, and pack for independence with prostheses and adaptive equipment
- Planning a vacation and trying to anticipate all needs and adaptations

Assessment

There are a number of good evaluations available but no single measure captures all aspects of prosthetic limb performance and satisfaction. All the items discussed in the next section are validated for use with the upper extremity limb loss population, but many upper extremity evaluations are not. Also of note is that although assessments may be validated, they are likely not normed for the level of amputation or any demographic concerning amputation. More research in this area is required to establish what is an average performance of a test for a body-powered transradial user with Box and Blocks Test for example. Clinicians are left to compare the individual's performance themselves and rely on their knowledge of the performance to determine if there is potential to improve. The 33-item DASH questionnaire or the abbreviated 11-item QuickDASH measure the participant's perceived ability to complete tasks.[17] Basic dexterity tests such as the Box and Blocks test give good feedback to how quickly a user is performing.[18] The OPUS consists of five modules that allow patient-reported experience with prosthesis use.[19] These are publicly available and modules of particular significance are the OPUS upper extremity functional status and OPUS satisfaction.[19] Dexterity is a particularly valuable metric to the use of a prosthesis as it implies efficient performance. The Southampton Hand Assessment Procedure is another type of dexterity test to measure many types of prehension.[20] Other assessments such as the Patient Specific Functional Scale have the patient identify important tasks and rate their perceived satisfaction with those tasks.[21] The Jebsen-Taylor Hand Function Test combines dexterity with function by performing a few tasks such as turning over notecards, scooping and placing dry beans with a spoon, and picking up small, large, and heavy objects.[22] The University of New Brunswick Test of Prosthetics Function allows the opportunity for occupational therapists to rate skill and spontaneity through the performance of 10 bilateral tasks.[23] The Assessment of Capacity of Myoelectric Control requires a 12-hour training course and examines grasp, hold, release, and readjustment with a few set bimanual tasks.[24] The Assessment of Capacity of Myoelectric Control is graded for myoelectric terminal devices from videotape to examine aspects of control, fluidity, and the unique role of vision involved in task performance.[24] There are more evaluations available, but these measures have been found to be particularly useful to inform therapies. Formal evaluation tools add to the evidence base and may be drawn upon in the future for comparative analysis. In a field with very limited evidence-based practice, it is important for clinicians to do their part to build the evidence to benefit future generations with limb deficiency.

Adaptations

Adaptations involving self-care, kitchen tasks, work tasks, and leisure tasks are outlined in **Table 3**.

In the past, prosthetic devices were prescribed using a linear approach of starting with a conventional body-powered prosthesis (**Figure 16**). In an effort to address the high abandonment rate of upper limb prosthesis, there has been a paradigm shift in how prosthetic devices are prescribed using a goal-oriented approach instead (**Figure 17**). The phase Limb Restoration and Optimization has become commonly used in the management and care of amputations. Restoring a person with limb loss to their prior level of function and optimizing their abilities to achieve their greatest potential should be the goal of the health care team. This ideal functional outcome likely requires access to a comprehensive team approach involving surgeons, rehabilitation specialists (PM&R physicians), therapists, and prosthetists. The ideal timeline for an upper limb amputation may resemble the depiction in **Table 4**. From the acute care throughout an amputee's life, managing amputations is a life-long process and requires continuity of care.

Depending on the individual and if any complications occur, a person with upper limb amputation(s) needs to have continued access to specialists throughout their life. They may benefit from a surgical evaluation that could involve evaluation for certain surgical techniques that have the potential to optimize an amputated limb with the most appropriate technology, which often requires specialized rehabilitation with therapists who have experience and expertise in training amputees for prosthetic use.

TABLE 3 Adaptations for Prosthesis Wear

Self-Care
- Nonslip material
- Rocker knives/fork combinations
- Cutting off the nasal cannula from oxygen tubing to provide a long-distance straw
- Use of a pump to dispense containers contents
- Automatic dispensers
- Wall-mounted power toothbrush that rotates
- Wall-mounted or table-mounted hair dryer
- Adapted switches
- Wall-mounted arm/back/chest scrubbers
- Wall-mounted comb/brush
- Head scrubber to assist with applying shampoo to the head
- Bidets
- Universal cuff or cuffs fitted for residual limbs
- Prosthetic arms for the shower
- Use of a long-handled sponge for bathing, a long-handled sponge to apply sunscreen/lotion to the affected side
- Elastic or alternative shoelaces
- Touch capacitive stylus or prosthetic fingers
- Button hooks

Kitchen Tasks
- Adapted cutting boards with nails or walls to hold items to be cut in place
- Razor-type mail openers for opening bags
- Cutting board vices
- Push-to-operate choppers
- Electric jar openers
- One-handed can openers
- Rocker knives
- Mounted clips for chip bags
- Cutting board mounted toggle clamps
- Funnels
- Pot handle holders to keep the pot in place on the stove
- Rubber mat or suction cups for sink for washing dishes
- Battery-powered dish scrubber
- Guillotine paper cutter
- Mounted table top platform spring-loaded scissors to open bags

Custom Adaptations
- Compressive foam, splinting material, or three-dimensional printing to provide a matching handle for better control
- Custom platform charger, rubber or silicone attachments to the terminal device to keep accessories in place
- Coband or rubber to increase friction of terminal device pinch
- Surgical tubing on metal tines to prevent scratching and increase friction

Community Level
- Shoulder bag, fanny pack, or shoulder sling pack for wallet and other essentials (the affected pocket side is not accessible to a prosthesis)
- Local adaptive sports organizations
- Amputee Coalition of America

Work Tasks
- Assistive Technologist (Rehabilitation Engineering and Assistive Technology Society of North America)
- One-handed keyboard, one-handed typing programs
- Change of dominance writing training
- Ergonomic assessment to decrease unilateral stress
- Proper desk chair with forearm support to eliminate pressure on carpals
- Voice to text
- Neutral forearm mouse
- Foot mouse
- Dictation software

TABLE 3 Adaptations for Prosthesis Wear (Continued)

Leisure
Adapted gaming (Microsoft Xbox controller, extremely customizable)
Customized performance of leisure tasks
Local interest-based clubs such as photography groups that may have knowledge and be willing to assist in adapting equipment
Online blog groups or MeetUp groups
Seeking out the seasoned professionals in a specific task
Fitness
Hauling hooks
Cuff weights
Velcro cuff with D-rings for cable machines
Custom strapping that goes over the shoulder or chest for suspending weight from residual limb
Athletic trainers who specialize in working with individuals who have experienced limb loss
Note balance changes with running and biking
Sports
Sports-specific terminal devices
Adaptive gyms, trainers, and clubs
Adaptive sports organizations

Historical Linear Approach

Body Powered Conventional → Externally Powered Myoelectric → Activity Specific Sports, Avocational → Passive Cosmetic

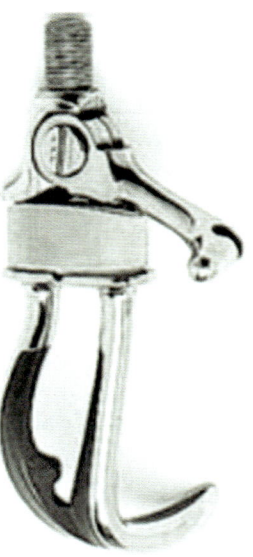
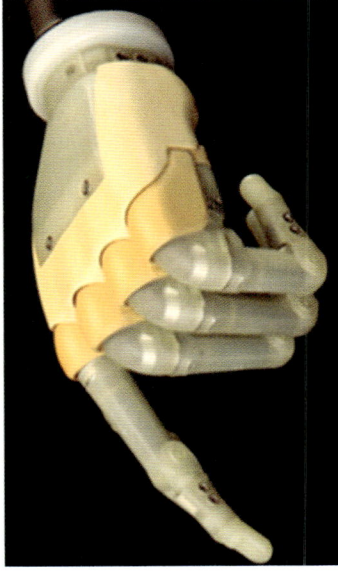
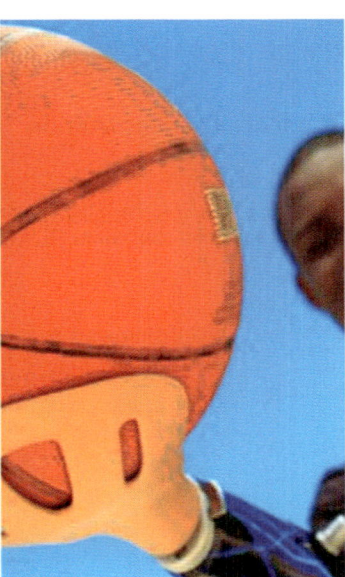
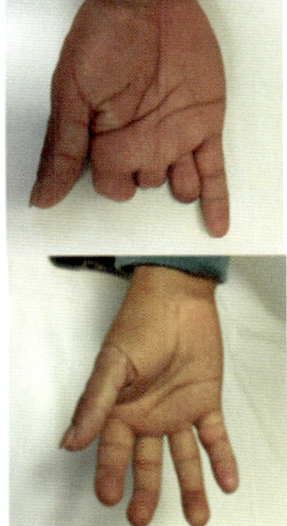

FIGURE 16 Images depicting the historical linear approach.

Section 1: General Principles

TABLE 4 Timeline: Acute Care to Lifelong Support

Amputation	Surgery	Early Rehabilitation	Pre-prosthetic Training	Rehabilitation Team Evaluation	Prosthetic Fitting	Training Therapy	Follow-up Adjustments
Range	Day 0	1-7 d	0-8 wk	0-8 wk	0-10 wk	0-24 wk	1-2 yr
Ideal	Preoperative consultation	POD1	POD1	2 wk PO	5 wk PO	8 wk PO	Life-long
Team members	Surgeon PMR	PMR OT CP	PMR OT CP	PMR OT CP	PMR OT CP	PMR OT CP	PMR OT CP

CP = certified prosthetist, OT = occupational therapist, PMR = physical medicine and rehabilitation (amputee rehabilitation physician), POD = postoperative day

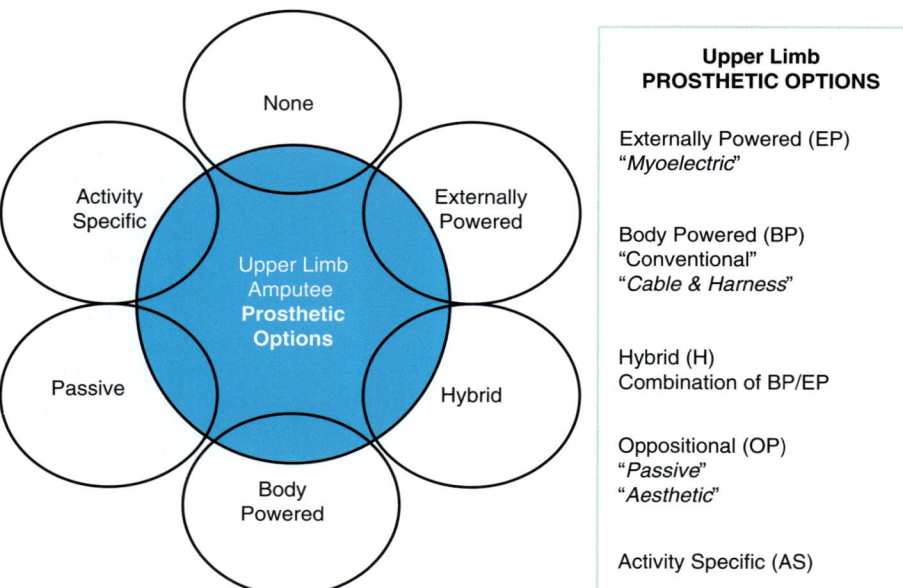

FIGURE 17 Diagram showing prosthetic options.

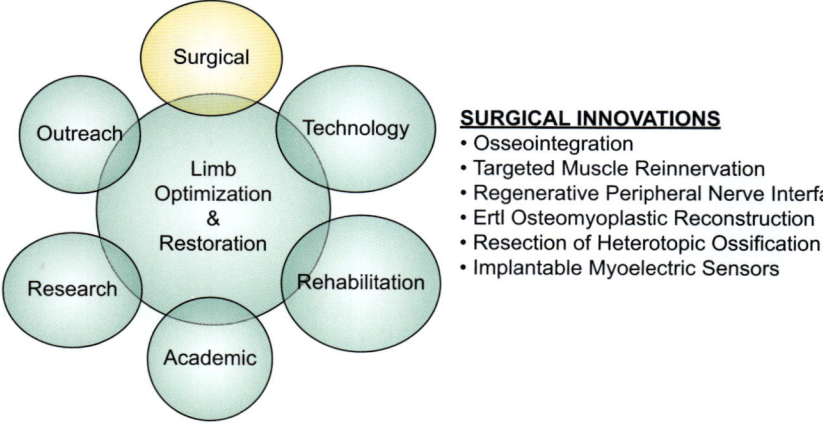

FIGURE 18 Diagram showing surgical innovations.

In actuality, the ideal care has many barriers and limitations including lack of resources and access to specialists. Often the academic settings have centers recognized for expertise in the care of limb loss and limb deficiency, and specifically related to this topic a specialization in the treatment of upper limb amputations. Limitations and barriers may be overcome with outreach programs, including virtual tools such as telehealth with specialized health care teams that extend access to care, especially for those challenged by logistical barriers. Another significant limitation for many people with limb loss includes suboptimal resources, particularly when it comes to access to technology. Reducing abandonment of prosthetic devices and following the guidelines outlined in this chapter will improve access to care and ensure resources are used to create the best possible outcome for people with upper limb amputations. Figure 18 is an illustration depicting an ideal limb restoration and optimization program.

SUMMARY

Recovering and returning to full function after an upper extremity amputation is a daunting process. The clinician's knowledge and experience are the foundation to good outcomes for individuals with limb deficiency. Education, training, support, and encouragement are needed for the individual with limb deficiency to achieve success. Many variables affect prosthetic acceptance and the clinician is able to best inform the individual in all options and new technologies that may be available. Matching the individual's needs with informed options best facilitates a return to a full and active lifestyle.

References

1. Malone JM, Fleming LL, Roberson J, et al: Immediate, early, and late postsurgical management of upper-limb amputation. *J Rehabil Res Dev* 1984;21(1):33-41.
2. Belon HP, Vigoda DF: Emotional adaptation to limb loss. *Phys Med Rehabil Clin N Am* 2014;25(1):53-74.
3. Kübler-Ross E: *On Death and Dying*. Macmillan, 1969.
4. Cancio JM, Eskridge S, Shannon K, Orr A, Mazzone B, Farrokhi S: Development of overuse musculoskeletal conditions after combat-related upper limb amputation: A retrospective cohort study. *J Hand Ther* 2021; May 16 [Epub ahead of print].
5. Postema SG, Bongers RM, Brouwers MA, et al: Musculoskeletal complaints in transverse upper limb reduction deficiency and amputation in the netherlands: Prevalence, predictors, and effect on health. *Arch Phys Med Rehabil* 2016;97:1137-1145.
6. Resnik L, Meucci MR, Lieberman-Klinger S, et al: Advanced upper limb prosthetic devices: Implications for upper limb prosthetic rehabilitation. *Arch Phys Med Rehabil* 2012;93:710-717.
7. Salminger S, Stino H, Pichler LH, et al: Current rates of prosthetic usage in upper-limb amputees - have innovations had an impact on device acceptance? *Disabil Rehabil* 2020;30:1-12.
8. Tintle SM, Baechler MF, Nanos GP, Forsberg JA, Potter BK: Reoperations following combat-related upper-extremity amputations. *J Bone Joint Surg Am* 2012;94(16):e1191-e1196.
9. Roeschlein RA, Domholdt E: Factors related to successful upper extremity prosthetic use. *Prosthet Orthot Int* 1989;13(1):14-18.
10. Biddiss E, Chau T: Upper-limb prosthetics: Critical factors in device abandonment. *Am J Phys Med Rehabil* 2007;86(12):977-987.
11. Østlie K, Lesjø IM, Franklin RJ, Garfelt B, Skjeldal OH, Magnus P: Prosthesis rejection in acquired major upper-limb amputees: a population-based survey. *Disabil Rehabil Assist Technol* 2012;7(4):294-303.
12. Smurr LM, Gulick K, Yancosek K, Ganz O: Managing the upper extremity amputee: A protocol for success. *J Hand Ther* 2008;21(2):160-175.
13. American Occupational Therapy Association: Occupational therapy practice framework: Domain and process (3rd ed.). *Am J Occup Ther* 2014;68(suppl 1):S1-S48.
14. Ayres J: *Sensory Integration and the Child: Understanding Hidden Sensory Challenges*, ed 25. Western Psychological Services, 2005.
15. Atkins DJ, Meier RH: *Comprehensive Management of the Upper-Limb Amputee*. 1989, Springer-Verlag, p 48.
16. Csikszentmihalyi M: *Flow: The Psychology of Optimal Experience*. Harper and Row, 1990.
17. Hudak PL, Amadio PC, Bombardier C: Development of an upper extremity outcome measure: The DASH. *Am J Ind Med* 1996;29:602-608.
18. Mathiowetz V, Volland G, Kashman N, Weber K: Adult norms for the box and block test of manual dexterity. *Am J Occup Ther* 1985;39(6):386-391.
19. Heinemann AW, Bode RK, O'Reilly C: Development and measurement properties of the Orthotics and Prosthetics Users' Survey (OPUS): A comprehensive set of clinical outcome instruments. *Prosthet Orthot Int* 2003;27:191-206.
20. Light CM, Chappell PH, Kyberd PJ: Establishing a standardized clinical assessment tool of pathologic and prosthetic hand function: Normative data, reliability, and validity. *Arch Phys Med Rehabil* 2002;83(6):776-783.
21. Horn KK, Jennings S, Richardson G, Van Vliet D, Hefford C, Abbott JH: The patient-specific functional scale: Psychometrics, clinimetrics, and application as a clinical outcome measure. *J Orthop Sports Phys Ther* 2012;42(1):30-42.
22. Jebsen RH, Taylor N, Trieschmann RB, Trotter MJ, Howard LA: An objective and standardized test of hand function. *Arch Phys Med Rehabil* 1969;50(6):311-319.
23. Sanderson ER, Scott RN, eds: *UNB Test of Prosthetic Function: A Test for Unilateral Amputees [test manual]*. Bio-Engineering Institute; University New Brunswick, 1985.
24. Hermansson LM, Fisher AG, Bernspång B, Eliasson AC: Assessment of capacity for myoelectric control: A new Rasch-built measure of prosthetic hand control. *J Rehabil Med* 2005;37(3):166-171.

General Rehabilitation Principles and Strategies for the Lower Limb Amputee

CHAPTER 9

Israel Dudkiewicz, MD, MHA • Lisa Prasso, PT, DPT

ABSTRACT

Lower limb amputation affects an average of 150,000 people per year in the United States and causes severe disability that may devastate a person's quality of life. The rehabilitation programs should be encoded to the International Classification of Functioning, Disability and Health. These rehabilitation programs should be started as soon as possible and have a multidisciplinary approach and include everything from pain management to assist with phantom pain prevention, psychological support to help process the loss of a limb, contraction prevention for ideal socket fit, range of motion to complete functional activities, muscle strengthening to promote proper gait mechanics, and activities of daily living. Initially these tasks should be completed at a wheelchair or crutch level and then, when cleared for weight bearing, be completed with the prosthesis donned. A major barrier that affects participation is accessibility. Rectifying this takes time and should be addressed in the early stages of rehabilitation. All disciplines and modalities should be taken into consideration to assist in the recovery from lower limb amputation including but not limited to traditional physical therapy, occupational therapy, hydrotherapy, behavioral therapy, and advanced technology such as virtual reality, gait laboratory assessments, or even dog-assisted therapy to facilitate the chances of success.

Keywords: International Classification of Functioning, Disability and Health (ICF); lower limb amputation; rehabilitation

Introduction

Lower limb amputation (LLA) can cause severe functional disability and negatively affect a person's quality of life. Most LLAs are induced by the combination of peripheral vascular disease and diabetes mellitus with an annual incidence in the United States of 120 new cases per 100,000 people: 20 of them are minor amputations (occurring distal to the ankle) and 100 are major amputations (ankle disarticulation or proximal).[1,2] Between 1990 to 2017, in Europe, there were between 16.7 and 27.9 new amputations per 100,000 people and in Australia between 31.4 and 41.9 per 100,000 people.[3] LLAs are mainly performed on an emergency basis, either to save a limb or to save a life when possible prehabilitation treatment should be initiated to improve function, independence, and quality of life.

It is important to outline the rehabilitation process according to the International Classification of Functioning, Disability and Health (ICF) principles. This will assist clinicians in understanding the main target of the rehabilitation plan of care to help patients achieve functional independence.

The ICF describes the parameters that affect human health (**Table 1**). It includes the body structure and function, activity, and participation according to the health condition (disorder or disease) and contextual factors (environmental and personal)[4] (**Figure 1**).

The rehabilitation program should incorporate all ICF principles to achieve full participation and return the patient to prior level of function with a prosthesis. Timing of the rehabilitation process is important for success and should focus on body function and structure (residual limb, etc) first, then proceed to activity and participation. Personal and accessibility issues can be deterrents that slow progress and prevent full recovery and therefore should be treated as soon as possible to manage, solve, and remove barriers.

The main ICF-related targets in LLAs are outlined in **Table 2**.

Health Conditions Associated With Amputation

The most common cause of LLA is diabetes mellitus, accounting for more than 80% of the cases.[5] These patients are at risk for further deterioration, with a 23% to 34.5% incidence of ipsilateral re-amputation and an 11.9% incidence of contralateral limb amputation within 1 year,[6,7] 17.8% after 2 years, 27.2% after 3 years, and 44.3% after 4 years[6] and with an overall mortality

---

Neither of the following authors nor any immediate family member has received anything of value from or has stock or stock options held in a commercial company or institution related directly or indirectly to the subject of this chapter: Dr. Dudkiewicz and Dr. Prasso.

Section 1: General Principles

TABLE 1 International Classification of Functioning, Disability and Health Parameters That Affect Human Health

Parameter	Definition
Body function	Physiologic functions of body systems (including psychological functions)
Body structure	Anatomic parts of the body such as organs, limbs, and their components
Impairments	Problems in body function or structure such as a significant deviation or loss
Activity	The execution of a task or action by an individual
Participation	Involvement in a life situation
Activity limitations	Difficulties an individual may have in executing activities
Participation restrictions	Problems an individual may experience in involvement in life situations
Environmental factors	The physical, social, and attitudinal environment in which people live and conduct their lives

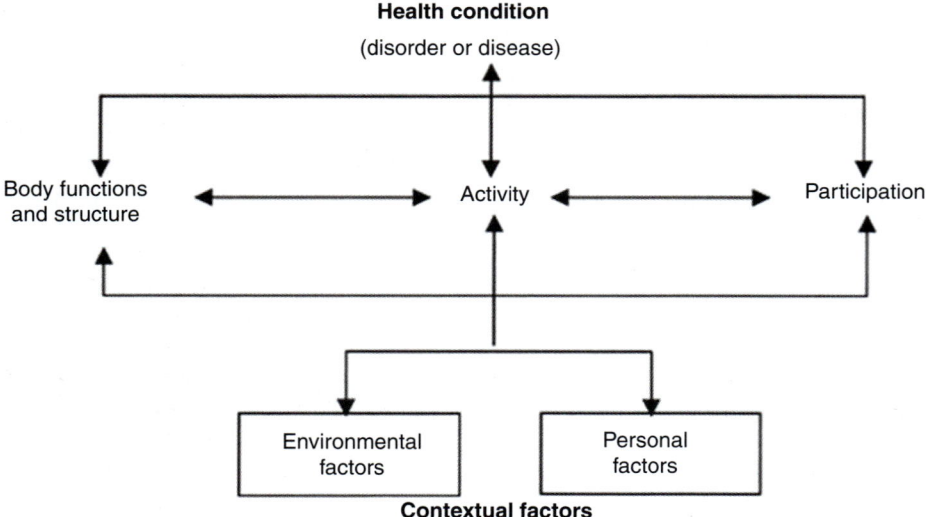

FIGURE 1 Algorithm of the International Classification of Functioning, Disability and Health model of disability.

TABLE 2 International Classification of Functioning, Disability and Health-Related Targets in Lower Limb Amputation

Parameter	Target
Health condition	General medical treatment and secondary prevention
Body structure	Pain management and residual limb treatment
Body function	Range of motion, contraction prevention, muscle strength, and balance
Activity	Practicing activities of daily living, wheelchair, and prosthesis fitting and training
Participation	Access home, work, education, and leisure
Contextual factors	
Personal	Profession, education, psychological, social, and family status
Environmental	Accessibility (stairs, elevators, ramps), transportation, house, and neighborhood

rate of 47.9%, 61.3%, 70.6%, and 62.2% at 1-, 2-, 3-, and 5-year follow-up, respectively.[8] These extreme numbers of diabetes-associated LLAs with high risk of deterioration make the need for secondary prevention (glucose balance, complication treatment, and engagement of diabetic foot program) a major part of the rehabilitation program.

Another issue that should be considered is the high prevalence of cardiovascular disease, especially myocardial ischemia and heart failure, in patients with diabetes mellitus. The presence of severe heart disease or heart failure may limit prosthetic rehabilitation because of the high energy expenditure rate. As an example, individuals who have undergone transfemoral amputation expend 30% to 60% more energy than nonamputees when completing activities of daily living and ambulation.[9]

Therefore, a clinical and, if needed, a laboratory assessment of heart function should be done prior to prosthetic rehabilitation to address possible cardiovascular barriers to care. In addition, kidney function should be screened because it can affect fluid accumulation, which influences the volume and shape of the residual limb.

Body Structure/The Residual Limb

The surgical site should be monitored and the patient educated about red flags that might indicate infection. Compression wrapping (using a figure-of-8 technique) or shrinkers should be used for volume management and limb shaping to optimize initial prosthetic fit and prepare the patient for functional success.

Pain can be a major barrier in the rehabilitation process and should be addressed with a multidisciplinary approach. Management of preoperative and postoperative pain increases success with prosthetic use and can reduce the possibility of the development of phantom limb pain (PLP), which is a predictor of poor functional outcomes.[10] PLP is one of the most common problems that affects quality of life; it decreases prosthetic use and can occur in 60% to 80% of patients.[11]

There are many theories about the etiology of PLP, including peripheral (ectopic impulses, structural changes of nerves, and alterations in neurotransmitter function), spinal (increased response of spinal cord neurons due to continued peripheral input, interference of the normal spinal inhibitory mechanisms, abnormal firing of neurons, and structural changes), and central (cortical remapping or reorganization and the neuromatrix theory) causes.[11,12]

Risk factors proposed for the development of PLP include severity of preamputation pain and postoperative pain due to infection or tissue ischemia,[13,14] improper prosthetic fit,[14] older patient age,[15] depression, and coping style characterized by excessive negative thoughts and emotions in relation to pain.[16,17] The connection between preoperative and postoperative pain can be seen in patients with diabetes and those with paraplegia who have reduced peripheral nociceptive inputs and hence less PLP.[18]

Patients with LLA-related pain are difficult to treat because many of them have a history of analgesic drug use, including opioids, and there is no single origin for the pain that can be induced.[19] The pain can be preoperative and postoperative ischemic pain, with intensity prior to amputation being a significant predictor of the development of chronic limb pain.[20,21] If residual limb pain does not improve in the first 2 weeks following surgery, complications such as infection, tissue necrosis, wound dehiscence, osteomyelitis, or neuroma formation should be suspected.[20,22-24] Therefore, such patients will benefit from the involvement of an acute pain service team and use of a multimodal analgesic regimen to optimize their pain management before and immediately after the amputation.[19] This is also useful in patients with PLP, as onset can occur 1 to 7 days postoperatively or later in the rehabilitation process.[10,20,22,23,25]

Body Functions

Limitations in joint range of motion complicate prosthetic usage. It is crucial to provide patient education on contracture prevention in early rehabilitation stages. Postoperative positioning is known to cause knee and hip flexion contractures. A patient with a transfemoral amputation should be guided to lie in a prone position if possible so that the hip is extended, in contrast to a patient with a transtibial amputation who should lie in a supine position or sit with an extended knee. Although it is much more comfortable, a pillow should not be placed under the knee because of the danger of the development of a knee flexion contracture (**Figure 2**). For patients who are not fully aware of their position or cannot cooperate, such as unconscious patients or those in intensive care units, a brace or cast should be considered.

If optimal residual limb length is preserved, the hip and knee range of motion will dictate walking quality, gait, and the type of prosthesis that can be used. The ideal hip range of motion that will maximize prosthetic usage and increase the likelihood of normal gait is between 0° to 10° extension and approximately 30° of flexion. The ideal knee range of motion for normal walking is between full extension and approximately 60° of flexion (90° to 100° for climbing stairs).[26] Flexion contracture more than 10° might be problematic for normal gait and may affect walking quality and prosthetic type and usage. Therefore, physiotherapy should be started as soon as possible in order to achieve a normal range of motion.

Muscle strength is also an important factor for walking, so isometric and isotonic muscle strengthening should be started as soon as possible, when the pain is under control. Hydrotherapy is another efficient tool for practicing even before prosthesis fitting.

The moment prosthesis fitting is done, balance training using a wobble board or similar tools should be started. Followed by gait training at different speeds and on various surfaces (regular, uneven, grass, sand, etc) and dual tasking activities/drills.

Physical Activity

There will be times a patient will not use their prosthesis for ambulation due to the higher energy demands (50% or higher in comparison with nonamputees).[9] There will be times when patients will be unable to use their prosthesis. Some reasons include changes in medical status, surgical revisions, prosthetic fit, or deterioration of function. Therefore, a proper wheelchair should be prescribed for every amputee, especially for those with transfemoral amputation or proximal amputation. To achieve maximum stability, the wheel axis should be relatively posterior because of the movement of the center of gravity toward the back due to the missing limb mass.

Although LLA usually does not affect cognition and upper limb function, difficulty with standing or stable walking, changing position from sitting to standing and vice versa, and lacking a free hand to carry something such as a cup of coffee when using crutches or a wheelchair can greatly affect the ability to perform activities of daily living (ADLs). Therefore, learning and practicing ADLs should be started as soon as possible, first from a wheelchair, progressing to crutches or canes, and later walking with the prosthesis.

The prosthesis type, fitting, and training quality are predictors of

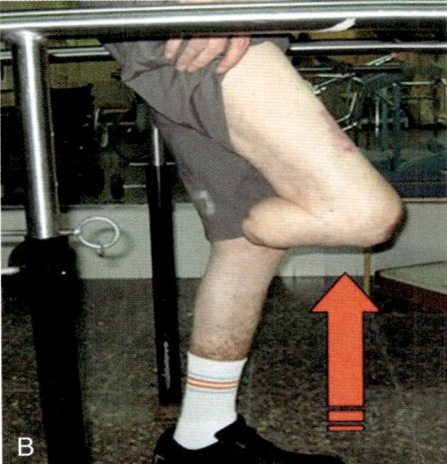

FIGURE 2 Photographs showing the development of contraction. **A**, Prolonged wheelchair sitting without maintenance of knee extension. **B**, Consequently in standing: Hip and knee flexion contractures can be seen. (Reprinted with permission from Orthopedic Rehabilitation Department, Rehabilitation Division, the Integrated Rehabilitation Hospital, Sheba Medical Center, Tel-Hashomer, Israel.)

Section 1: General Principles

TABLE 3 Medicare Functional Classification Levels

K-0	Does not have the ability or potential to ambulate or transfer safely with or without assistance
K-1	Has the ability or potential to use a prosthesis for transfers or ambulation in level surfaces at a fixed cadence
K-2	Has the ability or potential for ambulation with the ability to transverse low-level environmental barriers such as curbs, stairs, or uneven surfaces
K-3	Has the ability or potential for ambulation with variable cadence
K-4	Has the ability or potential for prosthetic ambulation that exceeds basic ambulation skills, exhibiting high impact, stress, or energy levels

rehabilitation success and return to ambulation. There are many prosthesis types that can range from simple setups such as a single-axis safety knee and solid ankle cushion heel foot, to highly sophisticated microprocessor and powered knees and ankles. Prosthetic prescription is done mainly in accordance with the five-level functional classification system (Medicare Functional Classification Levels) that was developed by the US Health Care Financing Administration and was adopted by Medicare[27] (**Table 3**).

The Amputee Mobility Predictor (AMPPRO and AMPnoPRO) was designed to measure an amputee's functional capabilities and to predict their ability to ambulate with a prosthesis in accordance with the Medicare Functional Classification Levels criteria. It can therefore be tested before prosthetic fitting to predict functional mobility with a prosthesis and justify componentry recommendations by the prosthetist. This outcome metric was proven to be a reliable and valid tool for the assessment of functional ambulation in lower limb amputees.[28]

Another outcome predictor is a multidisciplinary team specialized in LLA rehabilitation. Amputees who underwent specialized rehabilitation had motor Functional Independence Measure gains that were on average 8.0 points higher than those for amputees who underwent consultative rehabilitation.[29]

Participation

There are many factors that may restrict participation, such as type of career (physical or sedentary), prior physical and medical conditions, and motivation. However, the main barrier to full participation is accessibility. It involves all life activities and eras: home, workplace, educational facility (university or school), and social activities such as cinema, clubs, and sports and the transition between them. The amputee should have the ability to leave home independently, and to arrive and stay at the workplace, university, or other destination.

Participation in ADLs should be encouraged early because a patient's home might not be compliant with Americans with Disabilities Act regulations. Full home accessibility most likely means that the doors and corridors should be widened, stairs replaced by ramps or elevators, and toilets and bathrooms and any other room also should be modified to guarantee free and safe movement. Unfortunately, sometimes if the home cannot be adapted (technically or legally as in a rented house), the living place should be modified to an accessible one.

Not every occupation can accommodate an amputee, depending on the nature of work or the profession itself. For example, high-level physical performance or occupations that require climbing ladders might be problematic; therefore, another profession should be found if possible. Even when work is sedentary, there still might be barriers to resume work if adjustments are not made to the workplace to make it accessible for amputees (wheelchair, etc). Changes are not always possible or welcome and even if possible, time is needed to implement such changes. The same problem can exist in educational facilities and leisure institutions (theaters, clubs, cinema, etc.).

Work

Returning to work after an amputation is an issue of importance in the rehabilitation process. It can alter the patient's level of functioning; it can yield great benefits for the everyday routine, but it can also be accompanied by anxiety and fear, especially if the injury or the amputation was work related. Amputation affects the patient's mobility and therefore can be limiting in carrying out specific movements that might be required for work.[30] Even when these movements are achieved, they can be more energy consuming compared with a person without an amputation doing similar tasks. Transtibial amputation primarily limits ankle movement and proprioception of the prosthesis. This may limit patient participation in certain activities requiring climbing, kneeling, or squatting. Transfemoral amputation can also limit walking and standing and requires more energy to perform these movements. As for hip disarticulation, this generally will require more assistance with standing and will be even more energy consuming. It is important to note that not all amputees use prostheses, which will play a role in return to vocational activities. Pain, sensation limitations, and psychological difficulties can also affect the person's concentration and therefore their abilities. Schoppen et al[31] have stated the return-to-work ratio after amputation was approximately 79%, whereas Hebert and Burger[30] concluded that the return-to-work ratio varies between 43% and 100% in two-thirds of amputees studied. However, the percentage of amputees returning to the same job position is somewhat smaller.[32] The differences in return-to-work rates can be explained by the population tested, the method used, and the amputation etiology. Schoppen et al[31] have shown that amputees who changed their occupation after amputation were more likely to reintegrate into a job than amputees who stayed in the same job position. As for the time for reintegration to work, the results show variation between 9 months for transtibial amputation to 2.3 years in some studies, but 1 year can be somewhat of a consensus for estimated return to work, mainly because of issues with the residual limb and wound healing.[30] There is no conclusive evidence that amputation height affects the patient's ability to return to work.[30] Traumatic and work-related amputation, phantom, and residual limb pain all were found to be negative predicting factors for returning to work.[30] Age (45 years was found to be of significance), educational level, and sex (better for males) were found to affect the possibility of reintegration after amputation.[30] Emphasis on occupation during the rehabilitation program, work-related compensation, workplace accommodations, and adjustments all were found to increase the rate of return to work.[30]

Sports Participation

Sport and rehabilitation are strongly linked. Amputation affects the person's ability and mechanism for practicing different sports. Matthews et al[33] reviewed the literature regarding predicting factors for return to sport after amputation. It was found that it is difficult to determine age as a predicting factor because of the confounding effect of the general medical condition that is accompanied by older age. The use of a prosthesis was found to require as much as half of the maximum oxygen uptake for amputees and therefore physical status and exercise tolerance were found to be predictors for prosthesis use. Patients with better preamputation physical endurance have shown greater chances of returning to sport after amputation. Ability to stand on a single leg prior to the rehabilitation process was also attributed to better success in prosthetic use. It is worth noting that the aforementioned predictors might be a derivative of better general medical condition and physical strength instead of contributing factors. As for adverse predicting factors for walking ability, delayed residual limb wound healing, delayed commencement of rehabilitation process, and contractures in the residual limb were linked to reduced mobility and poor walking ability. As for the amputation characteristics, unilateral compared with bilateral amputation and level of amputation were found to affect the amputee's ability to return to sport after the rehabilitation process, with variations depending on the amputation itself. Also, among cognitive factors associated with the ability to use a prosthesis, memory was the only factor found to be statistically significant. In addition, sex was not found to be statistically significant, although males were more likely to take part in sports after amputation. Some studies, according to Matthews et al,[33] advise a cardiopulmonary and musculoskeletal checkup for amputees willing to participate in sports.

In a systematic review, Bragaru et al[34] estimated that 11% to 61% of amputees take part in sports after amputation. The type of sport participated in was influenced by prosthetic limb fitting, sex, and energy requirements. The most popular sports were fishing, swimming, golfing, walking, and cycling.

In addition, they reported that physical training as a part of the rehabilitation program yielded a shorter rehabilitation time for amputees. Patients who take part in sports after amputation were found to have better reported quality of life and higher self-esteem. As for adverse effects, sport injury rates for individuals after amputation were the same compared with those of the general population, although amputees have reported more muscle pain because of sports participation; as for prosthetic specifications, literature data suggest that prosthesis characteristics influence athletic performance.[34]

Driving

One of the key factors to achieve a successful rehabilitation is independent mobility. Driving is a way to create independence after amputation and therefore should be included as part of the rehabilitation process. Boulias et al[35] collected data from 123 patients with LLA who visited an outpatient amputation clinic. More than 80% of the patients had returned to driving. The average time to return to driving was 3.9 months after amputation. Of the driving patients, 81.8% have reported that they drive for several days every week. Men were significantly more likely to return to driving than women. Some of the factors that were found to reduce the likelihood of returning to driving were female sex, age, vascular disease, driving a few days a week or less, and right or bilateral amputation. The threshold for age that was found to predict the rate of return to driving was 55 years. Of the driving population, approximately 16% required automobile adjustments and most of those who had a manual transmission switched to automatic transmission. When asked about the factors preventing return to driving, it was found that preference not to drive or preference to use public transportation, fear or lack of confidence, other medical reasons, order from the physician, and family member concerns were the main reasons preventing patients from driving. Although reasons for difficulties with driving after amputation vary, the physical factor that affects the ability to operate the foot pedal can be of great importance. The loss of the leg and/or foot can make driving hazardous even if the foot itself remains intact and only strength, accuracy, or proprioception is lost. Engkasan et al[36] performed a survey of 90 patients after amputation and found a lower rate for return to driving of 45.6%, with a median time of 6 months for return to driving. The difference in both study results can be explained by the fact that the Engkasan et al survey included motorcycle drivers and that there was a lower percentage of individuals driving prior to amputation (51.1%). Another factor that might have contributed to the difference in the number of patients returning to driving stemmed from the population tested: Engkasan et al tested patients in Malaysia, whereas Boulias et al's population was Canadian. Also, the reasons for cessation of driving varied in their prevalence: prohibition by family member or physician was most prevalent but medical condition and fear or lack of confidence followed.

Other important personal contextual factors that should be considered are psychological, social, and family status. The duration of prosthetic training was affected by patient educational level ($P = 0.004$) and marital status ($P = 0.024$).[37]

Psychological/Mental Status

Amputation is an event accompanied by a lot of different emotions. Stress, anxiety, grief, and anger can be some of the feelings related to such a traumatic event. Therefore, it can be presumed that amputation greatly affects the amputee's life psychologically. In a study of sequelae of 23 patients who underwent LLA, Cavanagh et al[38] found a higher prevalence of psychiatric disorders such as posttraumatic stress disorder, general anxiety disorder, and major depression. It is worth noting that the rate of posttraumatic stress disorder was lower compared with earlier studies, such as the study by Martz and Cook,[39] which can be explained by the population for this study being patients who have undergone planned amputation because of their disease and therefore might be more prepared for the loss of the limb. This can be supported by the fact that when asked to rate their emotional preparedness on a scale of 1 to 10 the average result was 5.6. When the emotional reaction was examined, most of the patients experienced sadness, shock, and disappointment but also acceptance and trust in their caretaker. Pedras et al[40] showed that stress and anxiety symptoms were most prevalent 1 month after the amputation and decreased during a 10-month period, during which the most critical time was the first 6 months. Ali et al[41] reported that males were more likely to experience low self-esteem than females, which affected the psychological adjustments in a series of 100 case reports. van der Merwe et al[42] examined whether a late amputation following a failed limb salvage attempt would have a different result both psychologically and physically. Following interviews and questionnaires that examined results for 12 amputees, it was found that compared with early amputation, late amputation had no psychological effect.

In a study by Srivastava et al,[43] it was found that psychological intervention after amputation reduced anxiety and depression scores and was efficient, and its use was suggested in the rehabilitation process of lower leg amputees. In addition, in a comparison of intensive versus routine psychological treatment for patients with type 2 diabetes mellitus undergoing amputation, Amalraj and Viswanathan[44] found that intensive psychological treatment was more beneficial and had a better effect on the patients' quality of life as reported in questionnaires.

Miscellaneous Rehabilitation Methods

Virtual Reality

Virtual reality treatment for amputees, specifically for phantom sensations and related pain, is promising because there are no reported adverse effects, high accessibility, and high compliance because of the gaming nature of the treatment experience. In a proof-of-concept study, Murray et al[45] showed that immersive virtual reality treatment sessions for amputees with PLP led to decreased pain in at least one treatment session for all the patients tested ($n = 5$). In addition, virtual reality treatment appeared to show a sustained effect. Mercier and Sirigu[46] were able to show a beneficial effect in 8 male patients with PLP who underwent 8 weeks of virtual reality treatment sessions. These patients had an average 38% reduction of reported pain. Most of the patients tested reported pain reduction greater than 30% and this effect was found to be maintained 1 month postintervention. Virtual reality treatment has also been shown to have some efficacy over traditional distraction treatment. In a study conducted on 14 patients (7 lower limb amputees and 7 upper limb amputees), Cole et al[47] reported that relief of PLP was greater using virtual reality than distraction, therefore implying the beneficial effect of virtual reality in reducing PLP. Regarding the safety and efficacy of virtual reality treatment, in a study done by Rutledge et al[48] on 14 veterans who had undergone upper or lower amputation at least 6 months previously, it was found that a virtual reality treatment reduced the reported phantom sensation in almost all of the patients tested (13 of 14 patients) to less than 30% (4 of 14 patients); PLP was reportedly reduced by 50%, from 8 patients pretreatment to 4 patients posttreatment. Subjective measurements such as satisfaction and helpfulness were all reported to be high. No adverse effects were reported during the study and 4 of 14 patients showed continuing engagement and completed multiple virtual reality sessions with reported stable improvements.

A possible use of virtual reality for the rehabilitation of LLA was suggested by Phelan et al.[49] The virtual reality environment can be used for acceptance of fitting of the prosthesis, training for prosthesis use, and creating a safe and playful environment for the patient. Therefore, the use of virtual reality can be beneficial for prosthesis training to create a better rehabilitation process. In their study, Phelan et al used virtual reality to overcome difficulties of myoelectric signal recognition placed on a residual limb, which according to their data was shown to be beneficial. In addition, the experience of using virtual reality was perceived as engaging and further use and practice with the prostheses was encouraged. Patients using virtual reality reported the realism of the experience and the motivation for practicing translated to better results, which correlates with imaging findings. It was noted that the prosthetic arm was perceived as part of the body using the immersion virtual reality experience and no painful events were reported (**Figure 3**).

When reviewing the evidence presented here of the possible benefits of the use of virtual reality as a treatment for PLP and as a novel and valid option for rehabilitation in amputee populations, it is clear that the use of new technologies holds great promise for the rehabilitation of LLA. Nevertheless, validity trials and comparative studies are needed to build treatment protocols and for understanding the target population and for better understanding of virtual reality limitations.

Dog Services

Although less common in hospitals, dog services can be used as part of the rehabilitation program for amputees to practice balance, walk on uneven surfaces or changing ground conditions, and improve aerobic abilities (**Figure 4**). The main advantages of using dogs in a rehabilitation program are decrease

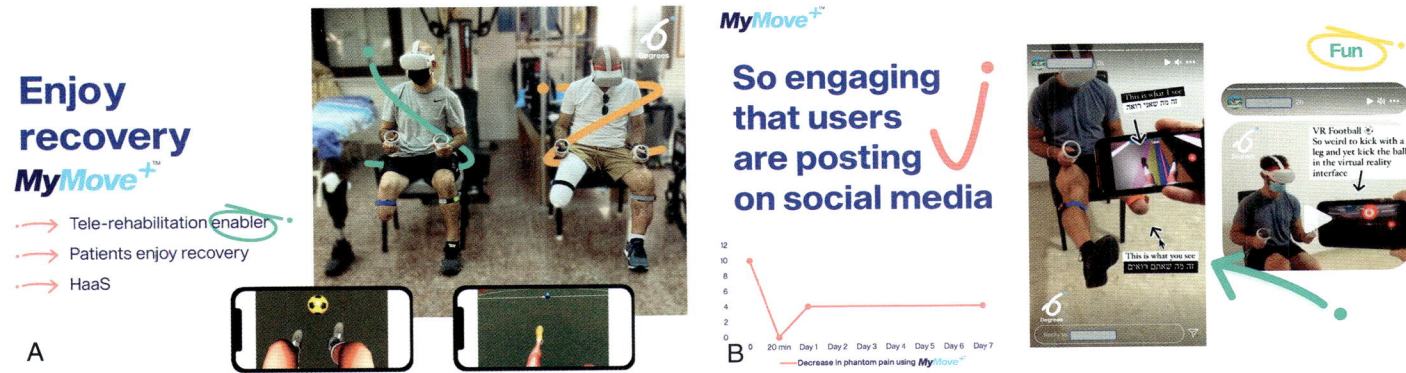

FIGURE 3 Photographs showing artificial intelligence-powered dedicated wearable device for remote rehabilitation and physiotherapy. **A**, Users playing virtual soccer. MyMove+ translating limb motion to full sensory experience. **B**, Using gamification to enhance fun and adherence in rehabilitation. (Reprinted with permission from 6Degrees LTD.)

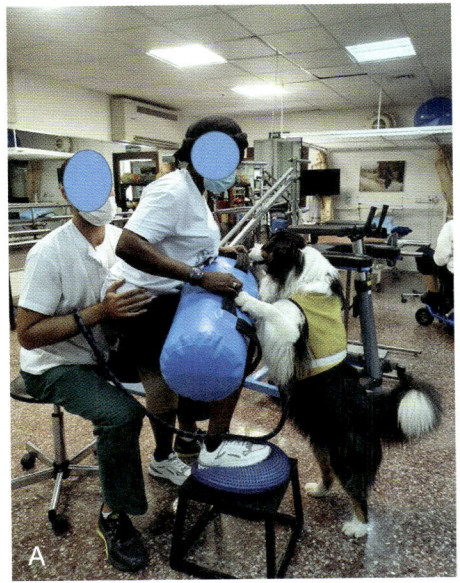 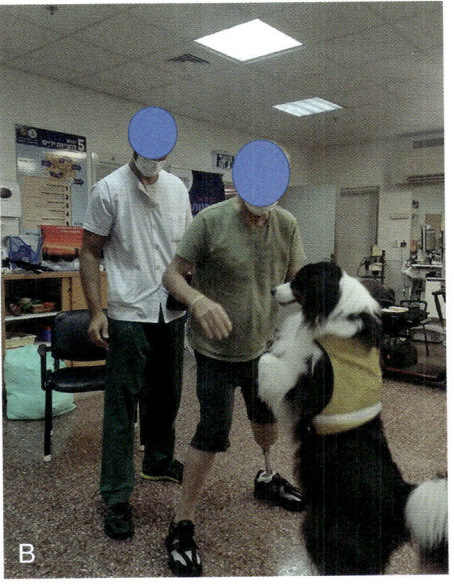

FIGURE 4 Photographs showing the use of service dogs. **A**, Practice to improve weight bearing on the prosthesis with the goal to improve stability and protective reactions in standing and walking. **B**, Practice weight transfer to the prosthesis in the coronal plane combined with external perturbation induced by the dog to improve stability in standing and walking. (Reprinted with permission from Orthopedic Rehabilitation Department, Rehabilitation Division, the integrated Rehabilitation Hospital, Sheba Medical Center, Tel-Hashomer, Israel.)

in anxiety and stress, decrease in pain, improved motivation and compliance, and increase in the training periods.[50,51]

Minor Amputations

Minor amputations may not require use of a prosthesis or other adaptive footwear for ambulation. Long periods of non–weight bearing or partial weight bearing (especially if a special shoe, cast, or walking boot is prescribed) decrease mobility, cause mood changes (depression), and negatively affect the quality of life. Because the chances for major reamputation are high (34.5% of minor amputations[7] and 30% of transmetatarsal amputation[52]), one of the main goals after minor amputation is to prevent further deterioration that may lead to major amputation.

SUMMARY

LLA is a growing problem that causes severe disability and affects every aspect of life. If not treated properly by a trained multidisciplinary rehabilitation team according to ICF principles, the chances of a patient returning to their previous lifestyle and being independent are very low. As for body function and structures, pain management, residual limb and wound care, secondary prevention, and psychological support should be started as soon as possible. These should be followed by physiotherapy, occupational therapy, and practicing ADLs. A mobility assessment such as the Amputee Mobility Predictor should be done early, and the patient fitted with a prosthesis and trained in its use when possible.

Although return to previous lifestyle activities is the last stage of the rehabilitation, it should be implemented as soon as possible because achieving environmental accessibility, even when there are no objections or financial issues, takes time and resources.

Because life is dynamic, aging, physiologic abilities, and performance decrease over time even when there are no complications or onset of new acute problems and in addition to the development of novel technologies. Therefore, continuous long-term follow-up programs should be advised and routinely performed.

References

1. Barnes JA, Eid MA, Creager MA, Goodney PP: Epidemiology and risk of amputation in patients with diabetes mellitus and peripheral artery disease. *Arterioscler Thromb Vasc Biol* 2020;40(8):1808-1817.
2. Kalbaugh CA, Strassle PD, Paul NJ, McGinigle KL, Kibbe MR, Marston WA: Trends in surgical indications for major lower limb amputation in the USA from 2000 to 2016. *Eur J Vasc Endovasc Surg* 2020;60(1):88-96.
3. Hughes WG, Goodall R, Salciccioli JD, Marshall DC, Davies AH, Shalhoub J: Editor's choice–trends in lower extremity amputation incidence in European Union 15+ countries 1990–2017. *Eur J Vasc Endovasc Surg* 2020;60(4):602-612.
4. World Health Organization: *Towards a Common Language for Functioning, Disability, and Health: ICF. The International Classification of Functioning, Disability and Health*. WHO, 2002.
5. Varma PS, Stineman MG, Dillingham TR, Erdman MJ: Physical Medicine and Rehabilitation Clinics of North America epidemiology of limb loss. *Phys Med Rehabil Clin N Am* 2014;25(1):1.
6. Ebskov B, Josephson P: Incidence of reamputation and death after gangrene of the lower extremity. *Prosthet Orthot Int* 1980;4(2):77-80.
7. Dillingham TR, Pezzin LE, Shore AD: Reamputation, mortality, and health care costs among persons with dysvascular lower-limb amputations. *Arch Phys Med Rehabil* 2005;86(3):480-486.
8. Stern JR, Wong CK, Yerovinkina M, et al: A meta-analysis of long-term mortality and associated risk factors following lower extremity amputation. *Ann Vasc Surg* 2017;42:322-327.
9. Genin JJ, Bastien GJ, Franck B, Detrembleur C, Willems PA: Effect of speed on the energy cost of walking in unilateral traumatic lower limb amputees. *Eur J Appl Physiol* 2008;103(6):655-663.
10. Anwar F: Phantom limb pain: Review of literature. *Khyber Med Univ J* 2013;5(4):207-212.
11. Chapman S: Pain management in patients following limb amputation. *Nurs Stand* 2011;25(19):35.
12. Siddle L: The challenge and management of phantom limb pain after amputation. *Br J Nurs* 2004;13(11):664-667.
13. Nikolajsen L, Jensen TS: Phantom limb pain. *Br J Anaesth* 2001;87(1):107-116.
14. Ahuja V, Thapa D, Ghai B: Strategies for prevention of lower limb post-amputation pain: A clinical narrative review. *J Anaesthesiol Clin Pharmacol* 2018;34(4):439.
15. Schug S: Acute neuropathic pain: Amputations, in *Acute Neuropathic Pain: Amputations*. Elsevier, 2008, pp 189-190.
16. Richardson C, Glenn S, Horgan M, Nurmikko T: A prospective study of factors associated with the presence of phantom limb pain six months after major lower limb amputation in patients with peripheral vascular disease. *J Pain* 2007;8(10):793-801.
17. Vase L, Nikolajsen L, Christensen B, et al: Cognitive-emotional sensitization contributes to wind-up-like pain in phantom limb pain patients. *Pain* 2011;152(1):157-162.
18. Flor H: Phantom-limb pain: Characteristics, causes, and treatment. *Lancet Neurol* 2002;1(3):182-189.
19. De Jong R, Shysh AJ: Development of a multimodal analgesia protocol for perioperative acute pain management for lower limb amputation. *Pain Res Manag* 2018;2018:5237040.
20. Nikolajsen L: Postamputation pain: Studies on mechanisms. *Dan Med J* 2012;59(10):B4527.
21. Hanley MA, Jensen MP, Smith DG, Ehde DM, Edwards WT, Robinson LR: Preamputation pain and acute pain predict chronic pain after lower extremity amputation. *J Pain* 2007;8(2):102-109.
22. Hsu E, Cohen SP: Postamputation pain: Epidemiology, mechanisms, and treatment. *J Pain Res* 2013;6:121-136.
23. Subedi B, Grossberg GT: Phantom limb pain: Mechanisms and treatment approaches. *Pain Res Treat* 2011;2011:864605.
24. Jackson MA, Simpson KH: Pain after amputation. *Contin Educ Anaesth Crit Care Pain* 2004;4(1):20-23.
25. Weeks SR, Anderson-Barnes VC, Tsao JW: Phantom limb pain: Theories and therapies. *Neurologist* 2010;16(5):277-286.
26. Rowe PJ, Myles CM, Walker C, Nutton R: Knee joint kinematics in gait and other functional activities measured using flexible electrogoniometry: How much knee motion is sufficient for normal daily life? *Gait Posture* 2000;12(2):143-155.
27. *HCFA Common Procedure Coding System HCPCS 2001*. US Government Printing Office, 2001, chap 5.3.
28. Gailey RS, Roach KE, Applegate EB, et al: The amputee mobility predictor: An instrument to assess determinants of the lower-limb amputee's ability to ambulate. *Arch Phys Med Rehabil* 2002;83(5):613-627.
29. Stineman MG, Kwong PL, Xie D, et al: Prognostic differences for functional recovery after major lower limb amputation: Effects of the timing and type of inpatient rehabilitation services in the Veterans Health Administration. *PM&R* 2010;2(4):232-243.
30. Hebert JS, Burger H: Return to work following major limb loss, in *Handbook of Return to Work*. Springer, 2016, pp 505-517.
31. Schoppen T, Boonstra A, Groothoff JW, van Sonderen E, Göeken LN, Eisma WH: Factors related to successful job reintegration of people with a lower limb amputation. *Arch Phys Med Rehabil* 2001;82(10):1425-1431.
32. Fisher K, Hanspal RS, Marks L: Return to work after lower limb amputation. *Int J Rehabil Res* 2003;26(1):51-56.
33. Matthews D, Sukeik M, Haddad F: Return to sport following amputation. *J Sports Med Phys Fitness* 2014;54(4):481-486.
34. Bragaru M, Dekker R, Geertzen JH, Dijkstra PU: Amputees and sports. *Sports Med* 2011;41(9):721-740.
35. Boulias C, Meikle B, Pauley T, Devlin M: Return to driving after lower-extremity amputation. *Arch Phys Med Rehabil* 2006;87(9):1183-1188.
36. Engkasan JP, Ehsan FM, Chung TY: Ability to return to driving after major lower limb amputation. *J Rehabil Med* 2012;44(1):19-23.
37. Chen MC, Lee SS, Hsieh YL, Wu SJ, Lai CS, Lin SD: Influencing factors of outcome after lower-limb amputation: A five-year review in a plastic surgical department. *Ann Plast Surg* 2008;61(3):314-318.

38. Cavanagh SR, Shin LM, Karamouz N, Rauch SL: Psychiatric and emotional sequelae of surgical amputation. *Psychosomatics* 2006;47(6):459-464.

39. Martz E, Cook DW: Physical impairments as risk factors for the development of posttraumatic stress disorder. *Rehabil Couns Bull* 2001;44(4):217-221.

40. Pedras S, Preto I, Carvalho R, Graça Pereira M: Traumatic stress symptoms following a lower limb amputation in diabetic patients: A longitudinal study. *Psychol Health* 2019;34(5):535-549.

41. Ali S, Waqar M, Anwar M, Zahid M, Sattar A, Arif M: Self-esteem as a predictor of psychological adjustment to limb loss: A case study of acquired limb amputation. *J Gandhara Med Dent Sci* 2021;8(3):53-59.

42. van der Merwe L, Birkholtz F, Tetsworth K, Hohmann E: Functional and psychological outcomes of delayed lower limb amputation following failed lower limb reconstruction. *Injury* 2016;47(8):1756-1760.

43. Srivastava K, Saldanha D, Chaudhury S, et al: A study of psychological correlates after amputation. *Med J Armed Forces India* 2010;66(4):367-373.

44. Amalraj MJ, Viswanathan V: A study on positive impact of intensive psychological counseling on psychological well-being of type 2 diabetic patients undergoing amputation. *Int J Psychol Couns* 2017;9(2):10-16.

45. Murray CD, Pettifer S, Howard T, et al: The treatment of phantom limb pain using immersive virtual reality: Three case studies. *Disabil Rehabil* 2007;29(18):1465-1469.

46. Mercier C, Sirigu A: Training with virtual visual feedback to alleviate phantom limb pain. *Neurorehabil Neural Repair* 2009;23(6):587-594.

47. Cole J, Crowle S, Austwick G, Henderson Slater D: Exploratory findings with virtual reality for phantom limb pain; from stump motion to agency and analgesia. *Disabil Rehabil* 2009;31(10):846-854.

48. Rutledge T, Velez D, Depp C, et al: A virtual reality intervention for the treatment of phantom limb pain: Development and feasibility results. *Pain Med* 2019;20(10):2051-2059.

49. Phelan I, Arden M, Matsangidou M, Carrion-Plaza A, Lindley S: Designing a virtual reality myoelectric prosthesis training system for amputees, in *Extended Abstracts of the 2021 CHI Conference on Human Factors in Computing Systems*, 2021, pp 1-7.

50. Colombo G, Buono MD, Smania K, Raviola R, De Leo D: Pet therapy and institutionalized elderly: A study on 144 cognitively unimpaired subjects. *Arch Gerontol Geriatr* 2006;42(2):207-216.

51. Bert F, Gualano MR, Camussi E, Pieve G, Voglino G, Siliquini R: Animal assisted intervention: A systematic review of benefits and risks. *Eur J Integr Med* 2016;8(5):695-706.

52. Thorud JC, Jupiter DC, Lorenzana J, Nguyen TT, Shibuya N: Reoperation and reamputation after transmetatarsal amputation: A systematic review and meta-analysis. *J Foot Ankle Surg* 2016;55(5):1007-1012.

SECTION 2

Upper Limb

Upper Limb Body-Powered Components

Annie Hess, CP

CHAPTER 10

ABSTRACT

Body-powered prostheses remain the most commonly prescribed category of upper limb prosthesis. A range of terminal devices, including both hooks and hands, is commercially available, along with a number of different wrist, elbow, and shoulder joints. A comprehensive understanding of the various features, benefits, and limitations of these component options will allow the rehabilitation team to match their detailed prosthetic recommendations to the needs and preferences of the individual user.

Keywords: body-powered components; cable-driven; conventional prosthesis; upper-limb prosthetic components

Introduction

Body-powered prostheses are the most commonly prescribed upper limb prostheses for individuals with amputations and limb differences. They have been used for centuries and remain popular among clinicians and users. In contrast to externally powered prostheses, which draw power from an external, nonanatomic source such as a battery to drive the motors of prosthetic components, body-powered prostheses use gross body movements to operate the prosthetic components. These motions increase the distance between two points on the body, and this linear increase is referred to as excursion. The excursion is captured with a harness and transmitted through a cable system to cause movement of the hand, hook, wrist, or elbow. For this reason, body-powered prostheses are sometimes referred to as cable-driven prostheses. Different components require various amounts of excursion to open, close, or otherwise operate.

Body-powered designs have remained popular over the years because they offer many advantages over other systems. They are low cost, lightweight, and reliable. Many users prefer their mechanical simplicity and predictable response. Because the user can feel the cable tension and force during operation, body-powered systems offer a level of proprioception not generally available with externally powered prostheses. These benefits, combined with the fine prehension offered by hooks, result in an extremely functional device for everyday tasks. Body-powered systems also are suitable for heavy-duty activities and for use in dirty, wet, and corrosive environments.

However, body-powered prostheses also have many disadvantages. Some methods of operating cable-controlled systems require substantial force and effort. Some harnessing approaches used to anchor the control cable can compress the axilla on the contralateral side, which can be uncomfortable and may lead to nerve compression over time. Individuals with a proximal limb absence usually find it difficult to generate the excursion and power necessary to operate a body-powered hand and elbow. Similarly, shorter limbs have reduced lever arms and smaller areas over which forces can be distributed, potentially resulting in difficulty generating the necessary operating power or creating discomfort from the extreme forces on the limb.

Despite these challenges, and even in the presence of advancing externally powered technologies, body-powered designs maintain an important place in the prescription of upper limb prostheses. A recent survey of clinicians reported that those with the most experience in upper limb prosthetics were less likely to think that body-powered prostheses were outdated.[1]

Terminal Devices

The terminal device is the most distal component of an upper limb prosthesis and is designed to replace the functions of the human hand. Terminal devices are available in many shapes, sizes, and designs, each with its own benefits, drawbacks, and specific uses. Passive terminal devices are static, whereas active terminal devices have some type of grasping capability.

Passive Prostheses

The terms passive and cosmetic are often used interchangeably, but they do not have the same meaning. The term passive is a functional description that indicates the terminal device or prosthesis does not have an actively controlled grasping capability. Cosmetic is a visual and aesthetic description indicating the terminal device or prosthesis is visually

---

Neither Annie Hess nor any immediate family member has received anything of value from or has stock or stock options held in a commercial company or institution related directly or indirectly to the subject of this chapter.

appealing or lifelike. A passive prosthesis may or may not be cosmetically appealing depending on its design and purpose. A prosthesis also may contain passive and active elements (eg, a body-powered terminal device with a passive elbow or shoulder).

Passive terminal devices include hands, mitts, and devices designed specifically for sports, recreation, or vocation. Specially shaped devices that facilitate targeted activities, such as swimming, playing baseball, or holding a nail, are included in this category because they do not have an active, cable-controlled grasp. Passive terminal devices are lightweight and typically do not require a harness; however, a harness may be needed in high-level amputations for suspension and stability.

Passive hands are available in various sizes, shapes, and configurations (**Figures 1** through **3**). Many passive hands have bendable or spring-loaded fingers that provide a static grasp when positioned appropriately by the contralateral hand. In some cases, the prosthetist can adjust the force required to open the hand to meet the needs of the patient. The natural appearance, lightweight design, and minimal (or no) harness are appealing to many patients. Most passive hands position the thumb and fingers in opposition, but other designs are available (**Figure 3**).

Despite lacking an active grasp, passive hands and other cosmetic prostheses can perform many important functions. Patients may use them to support and stabilize objects and to restore some bimanual activities. Utensils, tools, and grooming instruments can be wedged between the fingers and used effectively. The functional extension of the residual limb to anatomic length allows the patient to use the prosthesis to push, pull, carry, hold, and balance objects more easily. One study reported that, for nonmanipulative actions, passive prostheses were used functionally during everyday tasks as frequently as those with an active grasp.

Active Prehensor Devices

The two primary characteristics to consider when choosing a terminal device with active prehension are the mode of operation and the shape of the device. Body-powered systems have a voluntary-opening (VO) or voluntary-closing (VC) mode of operation or control strategy. These designations refer to the resting state of the terminal device and whether it opens or closes when the user pulls on the control cable.

VO terminal devices are closed at rest, and pulling on the control cable opens the device. Grip strength is a product of the force generated by the rubber bands or springs holding the terminal device closed and remains constant unless the device is held open and modulated by the user. In contrast, VC

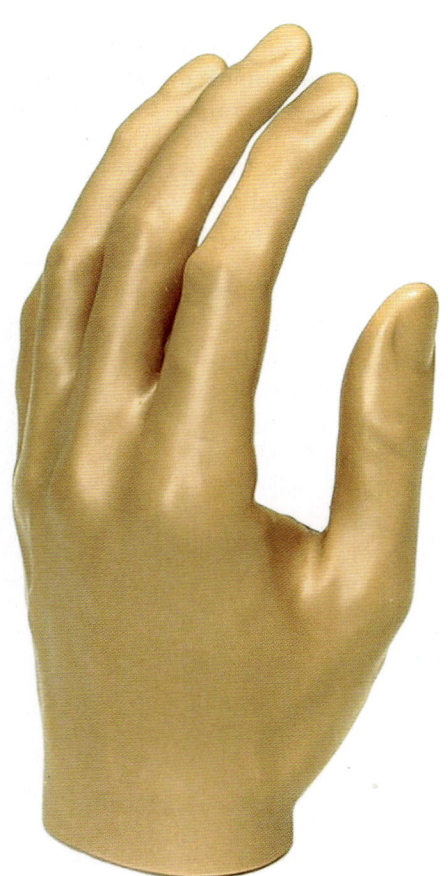

FIGURE 1 Photograph of an adult Standard Passive Hand. (Courtesy of Fillauer, Chattanooga, TN.)

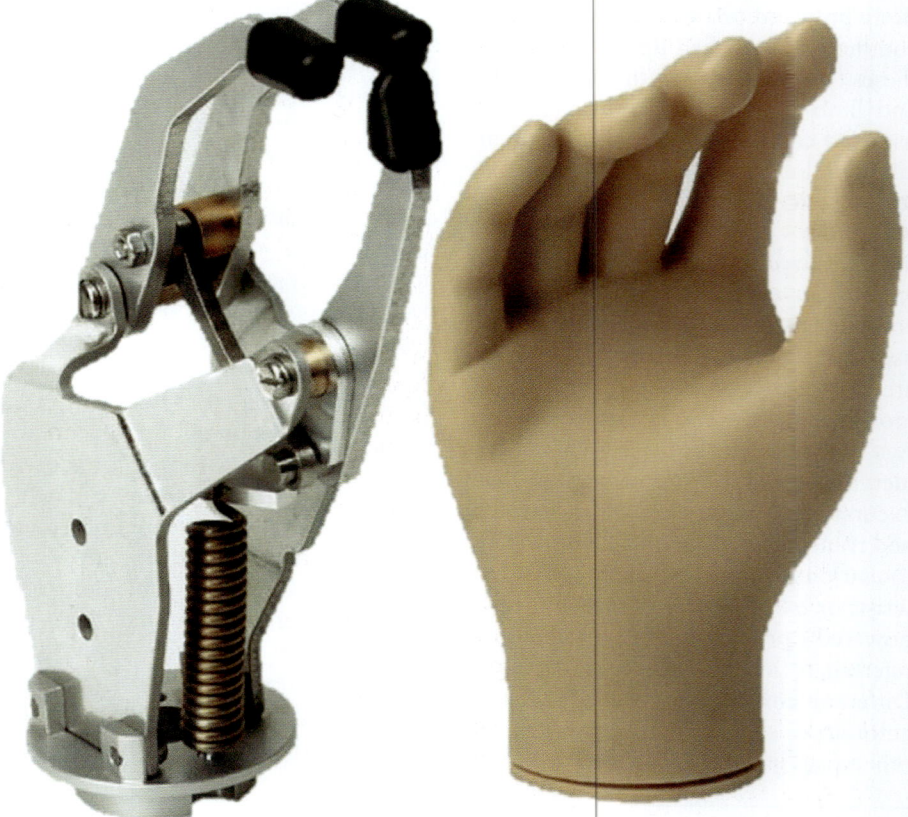

FIGURE 2 Photograph of a passive Spring Hand with a 3-Jaw-chuck internal frame that can be opened with the contralateral hand. When released, spring tension will close the fingers. (Reproduced with permission from Steeper, Leeds, UK.)

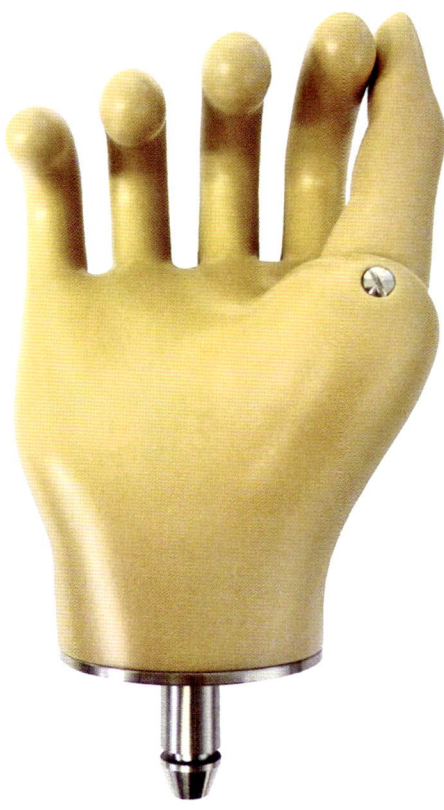

FIGURE 3 Photograph of the Steeplon Hand with static, curved fingers and the passive thumb in radial abduction to allow lateral or key grip. This hand is also available with hinged wooden fingers. (Reproduced with permission from Steeper, Leeds, UK.)

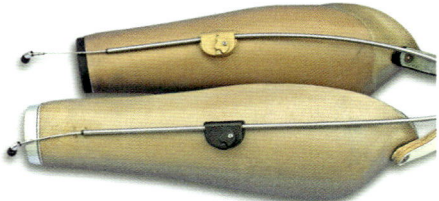

FIGURE 4 Photograph of the Sure-Lok voluntary closing locking mechanism. (Courtesy of Fillauer TRS Inc., Boulder, CO.)

terminal devices are naturally open at rest and are pulled closed by the control cable. Grip strength is determined by the amount of tension the user exerts on the control cable, which allows continuously variable grip strength.

Both strategies have advantages and disadvantages. The grip strength of VO terminal devices must be configured to provide the strongest grasp that the user needs and can repeatedly generate through the harness and control cable. This factor has important implications because every time users open the terminal device they must overcome the full grip strength of the device irrespective of the strength needed for a given task. In addition, when handling delicate objects, users must maintain appropriate tension on the cable to prevent crushing the object within its grasp. These related requirements can lead to fatigue, muscle strain, and compression of the contralateral axilla.

Higher pinch forces can be achieved in VC systems, because they are not limited by rubber bands or springs. The pinch force can be light or strong because it is determined by the user rather than the mechanical design. In addition, the graded prehension in proportion to applied effort may offer greater proprioception than other control mechanisms. Manipulation of delicate items often requires less overall work because the user needs only to maintain sufficient tension to hold an object and can relax the tension without fear of crushing it.

If the VC terminal device does not contain an associated locking mechanism, the user must apply continuous cable tension to maintain grasp. Although this process is normal physiologically, some patients find this requirement objectionable and prefer other terminal devices. This drawback can be addressed with a system such as the Sure-Lok Voluntary Closing Locking Mechanism (TRS). A small switch on the forearm of the unit clamps down on the cable and holds the terminal device in the desired prehensile position (**Figure 4**).

Although overall power requirements for VC systems may be lower, excursion requirements are greater because, whereas VO systems can be opened only part way with minimal excursion and still be useful for many activities, VC systems require full excursion to closely approximate the opposing grip surfaces in a similar manner. Therefore, care should be taken when prescribing VC systems for patients with more proximal amputations who desire active elbow control. The harness design also must conserve as much excursion as possible. Acceptance for VC terminal devices has been greatest in children and individuals with unilateral transradial amputation, particularly those with long residual limbs.

Members of the rehabilitation team should understand that the choice between a VO and a VC terminal device is not merely a selection of device characteristics. Rather, it will affect the entire mode of operation of the prosthesis across all of the user's activities.

VO Hooks

The original split-hook design was created in 1912 by David W. Dorrance, an upper limb amputee, to provide active prehension as opposed to the then-traditional, passive C-shaped pirate hook. The split-hook design has two fingers or tines that meet side by side and hold objects between them.

VO hooks vary in construction materials, size, configuration, coating options, and tension mechanisms. An extensive variety of VO hook is available (**Figure 5**). Although VO hooks were originally made of stainless steel, aluminum hooks have become increasingly common because of their reduced weight and are sufficient for most users. For individuals who require a more durable material than aluminum but find steel too heavy, titanium constructs are available. As material technology and manufacturing improve, hooks are becoming available in composite materials that are lightweight and resistant to corrosion (**Figure 6**).

Hooks are available in a range of infant to adult sizes. The most common shape is the canted design, which allows users to roll objects into their grasp with good visibility, but this design is less suited to picking up very small objects such as pins (**Figure 5, A**). An alternative style has a symmetric, rounded interior with lyre-shaped fingers, which are better suited for grasping cylindric objects and picking up small items; however, it can partially obstruct the user's ability to see what they are manipulating from some angles (**Figure 5, B**). Because most amputees find the canted approach satisfactory, the lyre shape tends to be more commonly prescribed for individuals with bilateral upper limb amputations for use on the nondominant side

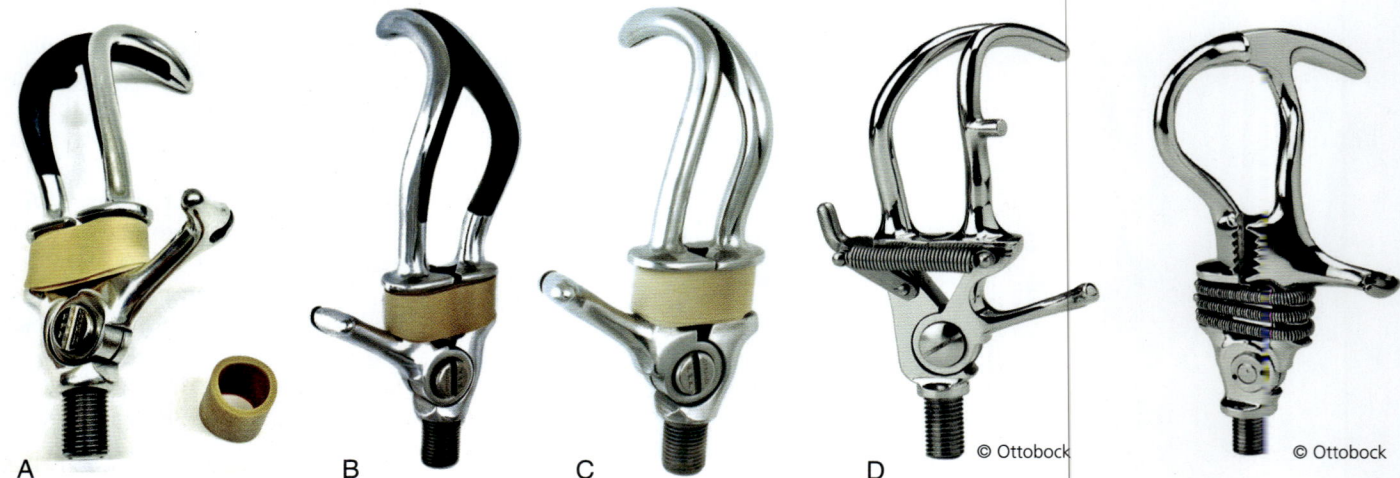

FIGURE 5 Photographs show voluntary-opening hooks. **A**, An example of the most commonly prescribed design of a split hook is the aluminum Model 5XA Hook (Fillauer) with canted and nitrile-lined fingers. **B**, The Model 555 Hook with lyre-shaped, nitrile-lined fingers. **C**, The Model 5 Hook, a stainless steel hook with canted fingers and no lining. **D**, The Cable-Activated Hook (left) and All-Purpose Hook (right) show two types of spring tension closures. (Panels B and C, Courtesy of Fillauer, Austin, TX, and Panel D, Courtesy of Ottobock.)

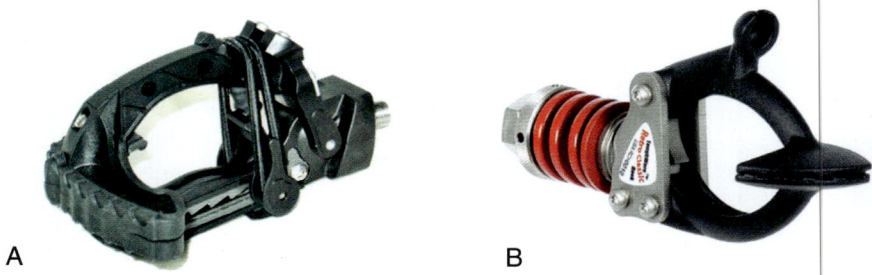

FIGURE 6 Photographs of hooks made of composite materials. **A**, The Vari-Pinch Prehensor with composite construction and a variable tension knob. **B**, The Retro Classic Hook with corrosion-resistant finish and spring closure. (Courtesy of ToughWare Prosthetics, Westminster, CO.)

to provide an alternative prehension pattern optimized for cylindric objects. The combination of one canted hook and one lyre-shaped hook offers the individual with bilateral upper limb loss the ability to grasp objects with different shapes.

A variation on the canted design is the farmer's hook, characterized by a wider opening than other hooks to facilitate holding shovel handles and similar objects (**Figure 7, A**). This type of heavy-duty, stainless steel hook is commonly prescribed as a terminal device for adult men who perform manual labor. The specialized fingers have several subtle contours that facilitate holding, grasping, and carrying objects such as buckets, chisels, knives, and carpentry tools. This design is also available with a back-lock feature, which allows the hook to be opened only by a cable pull; the fingers cannot be pried apart. This feature prevents the hook from opening inadvertently when grasping or lifting a heavy load and ensures that the hook remains closed without additional effort from the user (**Figure 7, B**).

Variation also exists in the gripping surfaces of VO hooks. The most common is a replaceable nitrile coating that lines the inner surface of the hook to increase the tackiness and compressibility of the gripping area (**Figure 5, A**). Pediatric hooks can be coated with a polyvinyl chloride plastic or covered with removable rubber sheaths to protect the user and the environment from incidental abrasions that occur from rubbing against the hook (**Figure 8**). In some instances, users prefer uncoated hooks because the gripping surface is less prone to degradation over time (**Figure 5, C**).

The most common means of creating hook tension is with rubber bands (**Figure 5, A through C**), although some hooks use springs (**Figure 5, D and Figure 6, B**). It is generally accepted that one rubber band creates approximately 1.5 lb of grip force. The application of additional or replacement rubber bands is somewhat difficult and is facilitated by a specialty tool; many patients defer this procedure to their treating prosthetist. Tremendous variability exists in the amount of hook tension preferred by an individual user. The desire for increased grip strength must be balanced by the realization that, in VO designs, a patient must overcome the hook's maximum

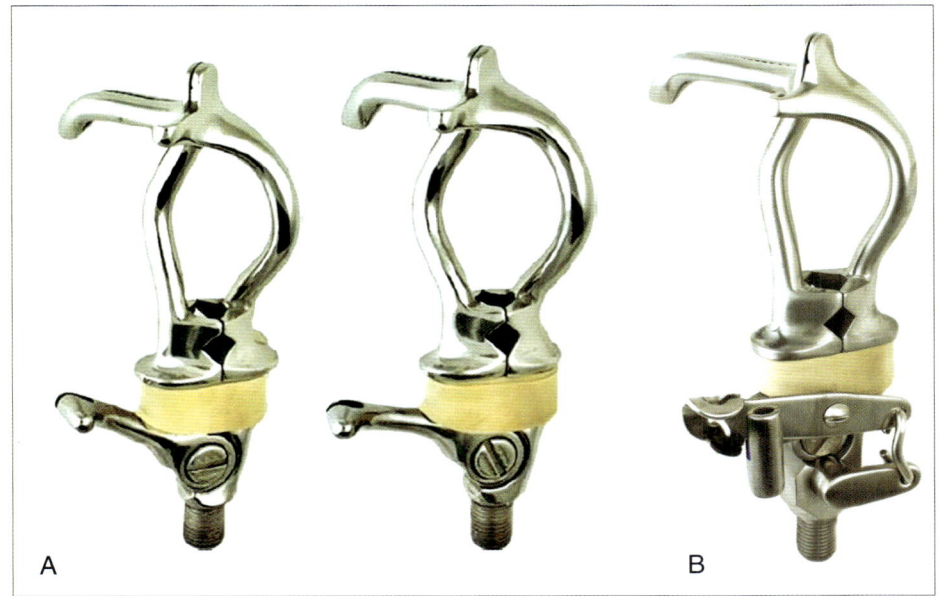

FIGURE 7 Photographs of farmer's hook terminal devices. **A**, The Model 7 Work Hook (left) and the Model 7LO Work Hook (right). **B**, The Model 6 Work Hook with backlock feature. (Courtesy of Fillauer, Chattanooga, TN.)

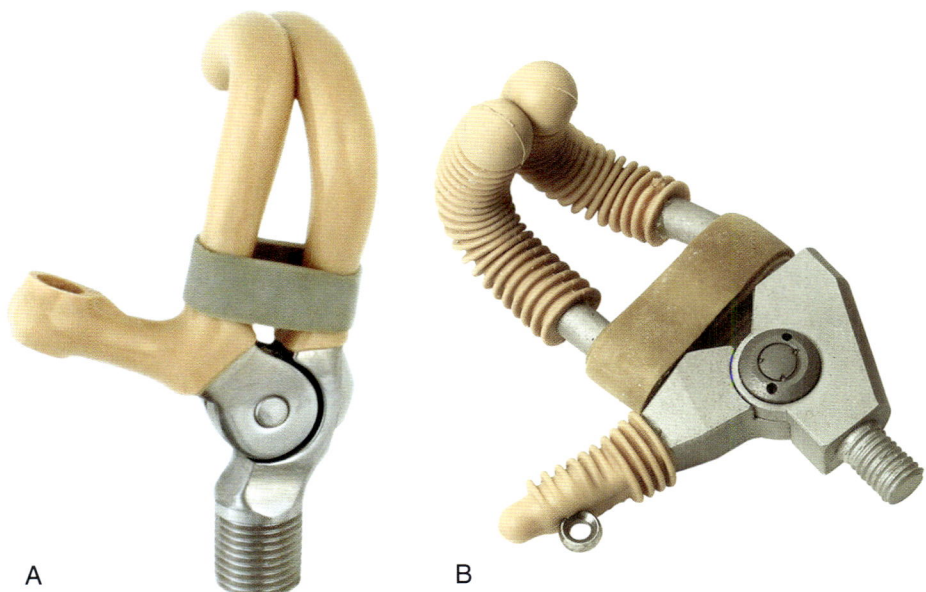

FIGURE 8 Photographs showing pediatric vinyl-coated hooks. **A**, The Model 12P Hook (Fillauer), a pediatric size hook coated with a polyvinyl chloride plastic coating. This hook is also available in smaller (Model 10P) and larger (Model 99P) sizes. **B**, A pediatric hook with removable rubber sleeves and a tie connection. (Panel B reproduced with permission from Steeper, Leeds, UK.)

grip strength every time the hook is opened, regardless of the grip strength required for the task.

Alternatively, several variations of adjustable-tension VO hooks are commercially available. Two-load hooks allow the user to choose between two prehensile strengths by positioning a switch at the base of the hook (**Figure 9**). In a related strategy, the Retro Classic Hook (ToughWare Prosthetics) and the Vari-Pinch Prehensor (V2P; ToughWare Prosthetics; **Figure 6**) allow the user to choose among several prehensile strengths with knobs or sliders on the underside of the device. In addition to this mechanical adjustment, the Vari-Pinch Prehensor allows the user to exchange elastic bands to further modulate the available grip strength. As in two-load hook designs, these features allow users to maintain a low cable tension when a reduced pinch force is sufficient, with the ability to raise this force when necessary.

Most hooks have a cable attachment for a ball terminal, but some have a ring for tying a nylon cord or a Spectra Cable (Allied-Signal) (**Figures 5, A and 8, B**).

Section 2: Upper Limb

VC Hooks

The Grip 3 Prehensor and Adept series (TRS) of terminal devices are unique prehensors available for adults and children in aluminum, steel, and titanium versions with or without a urethane coating. They feature multiple cylindric gripping surfaces within the fingers for gross grasping. Fine prehension is provided by the fingertips (**Figure 10**). Patient acceptance has been highest among children and sports-minded adults whose primary concern is function.

The Army Prosthetic Research Laboratory (APRL) Hook (Fillauer) is a split hook with lyre-shaped, replaceable aluminum fingers (**Figure 11**). An internal locking mechanism automatically engages when closed around an object and cable tension is removed. To unlock the grasp and open the hook, the user must apply a pull force greater than was used to close it. The inherent problem with this design is that a user holding a delicate object or another person's hand must close the hook slightly further to release the grasp. If the user already had a firm grip, it is possible to damage a delicate object or hurt the other person. The user can choose between two possible opening ranges of 0 to 1.375 inches (3.49 cm) or 0 to 3 inches (7.62 cm) by flipping a small switch on the base of the unit. A smaller range permits faster grasp and release and requires less excursion to fully close. Unfortunately, the mechanical complexity of this device makes it costly to manufacture and prone to breakdown.

The Equilux hook (Toughware) can switch between VO and VC operation. Rotating a lever at the base of the device changes the line of cable pull, allowing the user to choose what strategy to use for each task (**Figure 12**).

Hands

Although several body-powered hands are available, few are used as active terminal devices. These hands have many drawbacks, including frictional loss of force, glove restriction of motion, limited pinch force, and contours that block visual inspection. These factors substantially limit their usefulness for tasks requiring grasp and release.

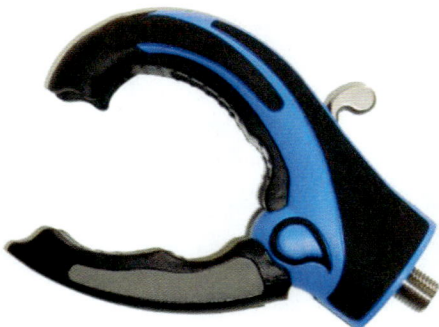

FIGURE 10 Photograph of the voluntary-closing Grip 5 Prehensor. (Courtesy of Fillauer TRS Inc., Boulder, CO.)

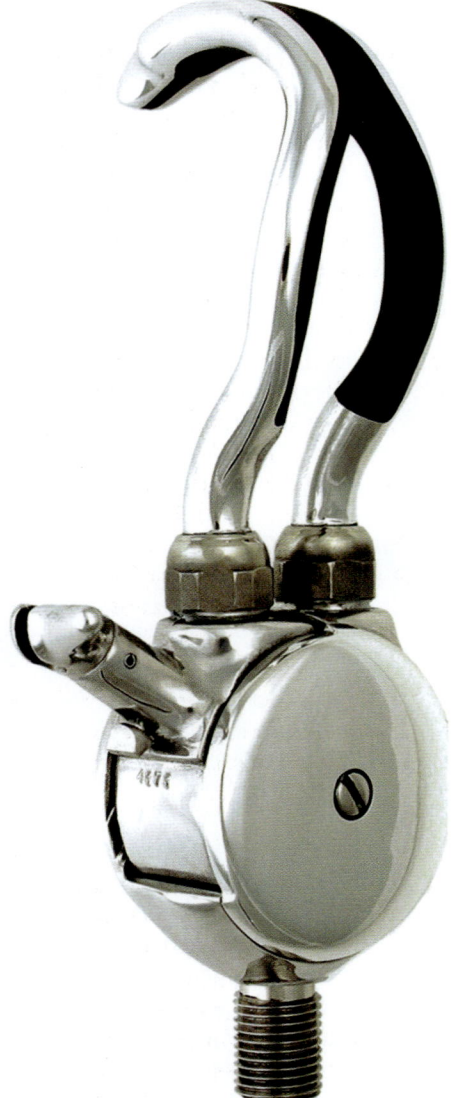

FIGURE 9 Photograph of the Sierra 2-Load Voluntary Opening Hook. (Courtesy of Fillauer, Chattanooga, TN.)

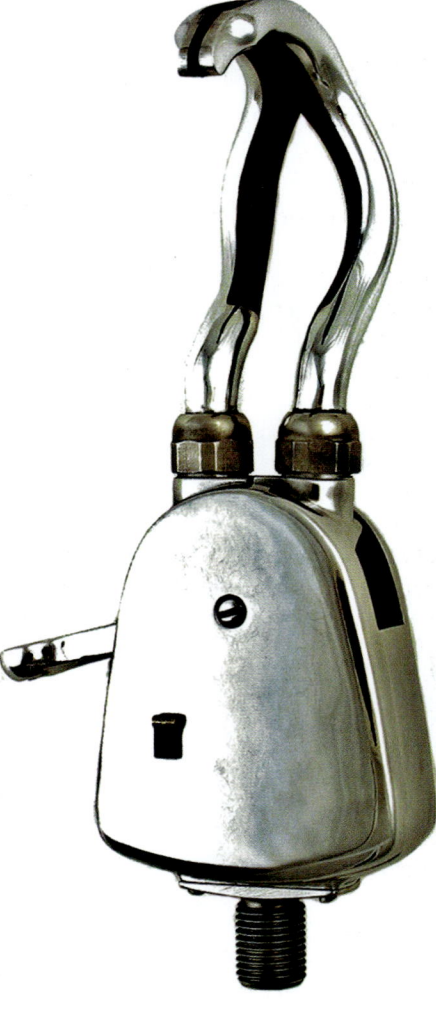

FIGURE 11 Photograph of the Army Prosthetic Research Laboratory (APRL) Voluntary Closing Hook. (Courtesy of Fillauer, Chattanooga, TN.)

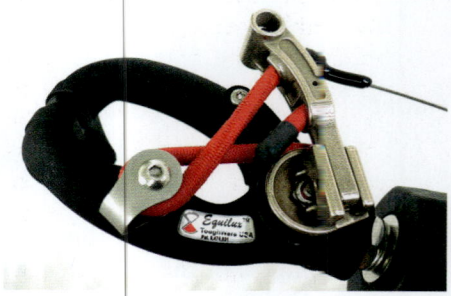

FIGURE 12 Photograph of the Equilux VO/VC Terminal Device with mechanism allowing users to switch between voluntary opening and voluntary closing control. Currently set for voluntary opening. Pivoting the thumb of the terminal device converts the unit to a voluntary closing configuration. (Courtesy of ToughWare Prosthetics, Westminster, CO.)

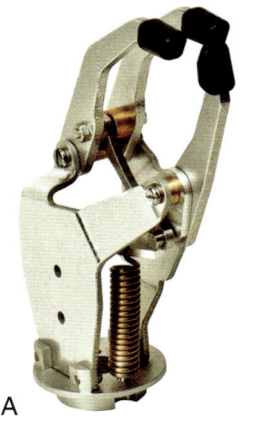 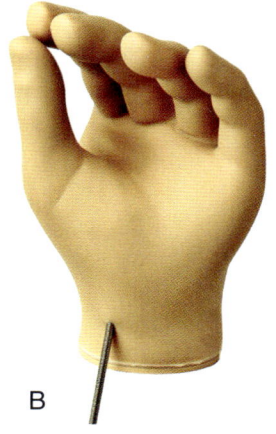 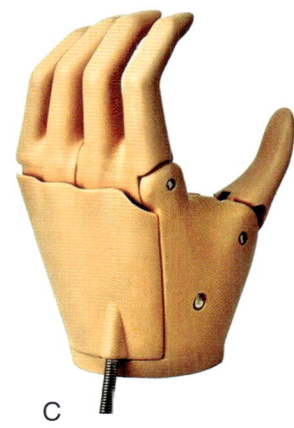

FIGURE 13 Photographs of cable-operated hands. **A**, An example of a three-jaw chuck internal hand mechanism. **B**, A three-jaw chuck body-powered hand with palmar cable exit. **C**, A pediatric cable-operated hand with five moving fingers and dorsal cable exit. (Reproduced with permission from Steeper, Leeds, UK.)

Many individuals with recent loss of an upper limb desire an interchangeable hand for social occasions in addition to a utility hook for general use; this request is the most common indication for prescribing a body-powered hand. Hooks require a longer cable length than hands because of their different attachment points, so a user intending to interchange the two must be provided with a hook-to-hand adapter cable that extends the control cable for hook use.

Body-powered hands are rarely appropriate for those with bilateral upper limb loss because of their functional limitations. Externally powered hands offer far greater pinch force and improved grasp-release function and are preferable when maximum prosthetic hand function is required.

Most cable-operated hands have the thumb and the first two fingers moving in a three-jaw chuck prehension pattern (**Figure 13**, A). Often, the metal structure of the three fingers is covered by a plastic hand shell (**Figure 13**, B). These first three fingers open and close the hand shell, and the fourth and fifth fingers move passively with the others. Some designs have a solid outer layer with three to five moving digits when the hand opens and closes (**Figure 13**, C).

Body-powered hands are heavier, less versatile for handling objects, and block the user from seeing the object during manipulation. They cannot fit into pockets or grasp buttons and zippers. The three-jaw chuck grip pattern positions the thumb to line up between the first two fingers, but is not directly opposed to either one. This makes it much more difficult to pick up small objects because the thumb and first finger do not meet to form a stable pinch surface.

Body-powered hands are less efficient than hooks because of frictional energy losses in the hand mechanism, so an equivalent amount of input force results in a lower output pinch force. As a result, both VO and VC hands require more power to operate than VO or VC hooks. A few studies have compared activation forces and efficiency and found that hooks outperform hands in most instances.[3,4] Most VO hooks obtain a pinch force of more than 20 N, with the ability to generate a greater force with the addition of rubber bands. None of the hands achieved a grip force greater than 18 N, and most forces were less than 15 N. The gloves used to cover the hands further increase the effort required for operation.[3] VC hands were also found to be inefficient, because the substantial frictional losses during hand operation require increased activation force and work by the user.[4]

Hands are sized by the circumference of the palm. Smaller hands have a smaller maximum opening width, and fewer objects can be grasped. The control cables can exit on the palmar (**Figure 13**, B) or dorsal (**Figure 13**, C) aspect of the hand. Some hands allow the cable to be rerouted through the threaded stud and interior of the socket, resulting in a more cosmetic prosthesis; however, this method of routing eliminates the ability to interchange the hand with a hook.

VO Hands

Several manufacturers offer VO hands with standard internal aluminum or nylon frames covered by a soft plastic shell. In some models, the pinch force is adjustable. Some are also available with automatic back-locking mechanisms that lock the fingers in the closed position to prevent inadvertent opening. Alternatively, hands may be constructed with a hard, solid exterior. Thumbs that move away from the other fingers, either during opening or by virtue of a wider, stationary position, allow for a greater opening width (**Figures 14** and **15**).

VC Hands

VC hands theoretically offer the same advantage of graded prehension as hooks, but the frictional losses in the mechanism are much greater. As a result, the user must exert more effort to close the hand and much of the control is lost. As with all cable-driven hands, the thick fingers block visual feedback at the fingertips, and the cosmetic glove further impedes motion. To compensate for the increased force

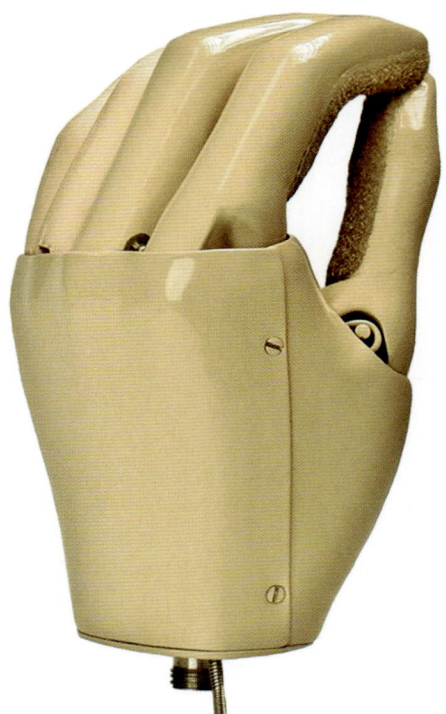

FIGURE 14 Photograph of the Sierra Voluntary Opening Hand with a rigid exterior. The first and second fingers move in a three-jaw chuck pattern with an automatic back lock and a two-position stationary thumb. (Courtesy of Fillauer, Chattanooga, TN.)

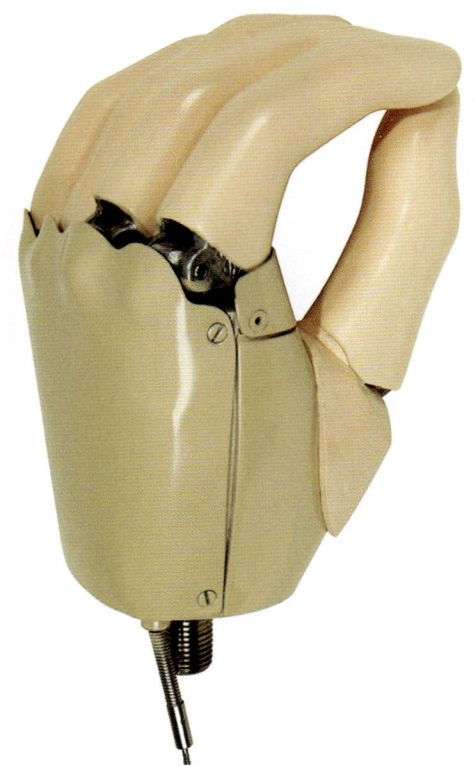

FIGURE 15 Photograph of the Dorrance Mechanical Hand, with a thumb that moves away from the other two fingers when opening to create a wider opening width. (Courtesy of Fillauer, Chattanooga, TN.)

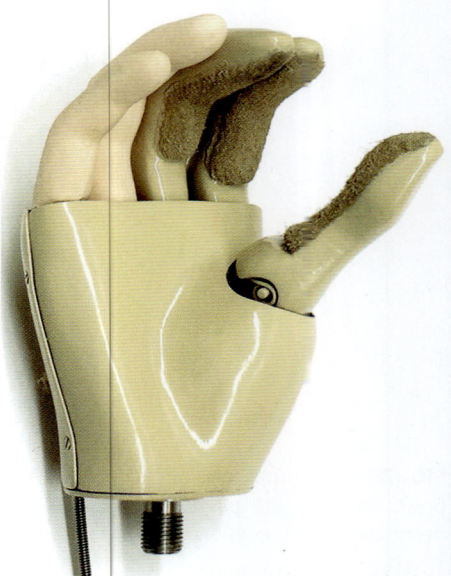

FIGURE 16 Photograph of the Army Prosthetic Research Laboratory (APRL) Voluntary Closing Hand (Fillauer) with the fingers closed and the thumb in the open position.

required for closing, some VC hands have a locking mechanism to maintain grasp after closure. After the user releases tension, a second cable-pull releases the lock and the hand opens. Several manufacturers offer VC hands with the familiar three-jaw chuck grip pattern.

The APRL hand, like the hook, features the same back-locking mechanism that automatically engages to prevent opening when cable tension is released. It also shares the same disadvantage of requiring increased grip force before the fingers will release. Like the Sierra Voluntary Opening Hand (Fillauer; **Figure 14**), it has a two-position thumb for opposition to the first two fingers or to create a wider opening width (**Figure 16**). Pushing the thumb inward toward the palm from its open position secures the thumb in the closed position. Slightly pushing it in again will release the lock, and the thumb will spring into the open position. The thumb of the APRL hand can be detached and used as a two-position opposition post in partial hand prostheses.

Cosmetic Gloves

A cosmetic glove protects the hand mechanism from contamination and provides the external appearance of the prosthesis. It is applied over the shell of a passive or mechanical hand and must be replaced at regular intervals when it deteriorates from wear. Prefabricated or custom-made gloves are available and vary in material, thickness, appearance, and detail.

Prefabricated gloves are the least costly and most commonly prescribed covering. The glove is chosen based on hand size, and the approximate skin tone is matched to the patient from color swatches available from each manufacturer. Gloves are available in generic male, female, adolescent, and child contours across a range of skin tones (**Figure 17**). Male and female gloves of the same size differ in nail, hair, and vein appearance.

Prefabricated, off-the-shelf gloves have improved in quality in recent years. Many are now made of silicone instead of easily stained polyvinyl chloride and are available with more sophisticated color depth and realistic skin texture. Some product lines have a wider selection of skin tones, with optional artistic painting of hair and fingernail details that add more customization and realism. Some manufacturers offer gloves in longer lengths that extend to the elbow. When used with an internal cable hand, these gloves can offer improved cosmesis, but they restrict full pronation and supination unless cut and separated at the wrist.

Gloves from different manufacturers may not be compatible with hands made by other manufacturers, even when the hand size is technically the same. Differences in finger shape, orientation, and length result in extra material in the palm, web space, or fingertips. This allows movement of the glove over the hand shell and creates wrinkling in the palm or sponginess at the fingertips, which can further impede hand function.

Custom-made gloves offer the most natural appearance. They are handmade from a sculptured reverse copy of the

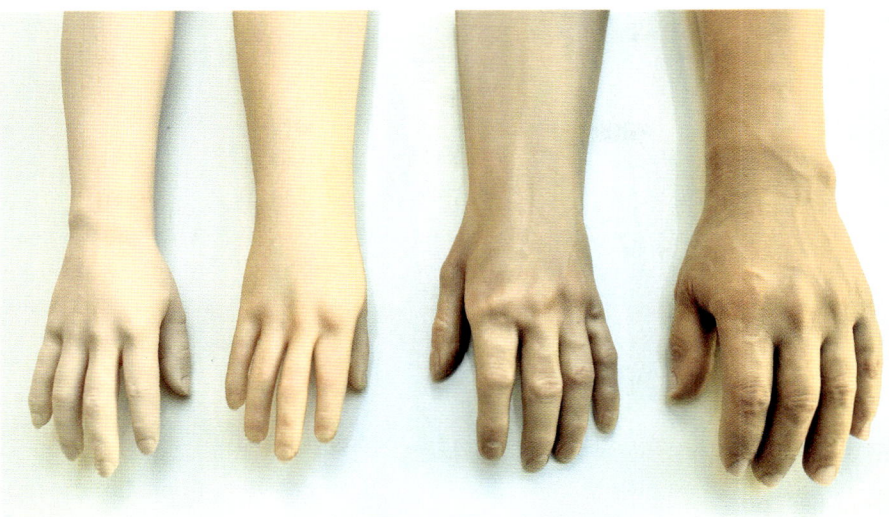

FIGURE 17 Photograph showing prefabricated gloves. From left: Female Silicone Glove (Fillauer) Female MCV Glove (Fillauer); Male MCV Glove (Fillauer); Male Silicone Glove (Regal). (Courtesy of Fillauer, Chattanooga, TN and Regal Prosthesis Ltd., Hong Kong.)

remaining hand. Skin tones and color may be matched in person or by using a calibrated photograph of the noninvolved side. Hairs and other details are applied individually or painted on.

Wrists

The purpose of the wrist unit is to attach the terminal device to the prosthesis and allow appropriate positioning for activities. Wrist units primarily facilitate pronation and supination, but some permit flexion, extension, or other movements.

To position the terminal device in the most functional orientation for a given task, the patient must have a full range of wrist rotation. The degree of voluntary pronation and supination the amputee can produce depends on the preserved anatomy and length of the residual limb and how well its movements are transmitted through the prosthesis to the terminal device. When an amputation occurs through the proximal half of the forearm, little or no voluntary pronation or supination can be captured by the socket. In the case of longer limbs, an ill-fitting socket that allows the limb to rotate inside it will not effectively translate anatomic motion into useable motion of the prosthesis. Self-suspending, supracondylar socket designs can also restrict rotation because the epicondyles lock the socket in a certain orientation. Amputees usually compensate for any loss of wrist rotation by adjusting their body position, often through shoulder movement.

Terminal devices are connected to the wrist unit by one of two mechanisms. The most common is a threaded stud that extends from the base of the terminal device and screws into the prosthetic wrist. European manufacturers sometimes use a baseplate mechanism with a plunger that inserts into the wrist unit and is held in place by a variety of mechanisms. Some terminal devices and wrist units are available with either option, but the two mechanisms are not compatible with each other.

Some wrist types are available in round and oval shapes. Oval shapes provide a smoother transition to the socket for long transradial amputation levels (**Figure 18**). If used with a prosthetic hand with an oval base, there will be a smooth, even contour to the prosthesis when it is in neutral rotation. When the hand is rotated into pronation or supination, however, a noticeable prominence will be seen at the wrist because the geometries are no longer congruent. Many hands have a round base to align with the more common round wrists; these hands have irregular contours when used with oval wrists.

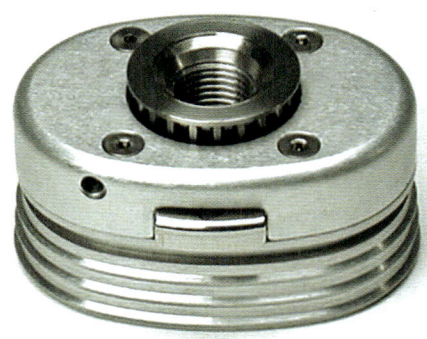

FIGURE 18 Photograph of an oval quick-disconnect wrist unit. (Courtesy of Fillauer, Chattanooga, TN.)

Friction Wrists

The simplest wrist units use friction to hold the terminal device in place. The user manually positions the terminal device wherever it is preferable along the 360° rotational axis. A set screw or spacer washers are adjusted so that sufficient friction is applied to prevent rotation of the terminal device under encountered loads, but manual rotation of the device is still possible with the uninvolved hand. Bilateral amputees may pre-position such friction wrists by striking one terminal device against the other or by gripping a stable object such as a table edge and rotating the device into the desired position. Friction wrist units are available in aluminum or stainless steel in a full range of infant, child, and adult sizes. Variable friction wrist units are durable and economical but, by nature of their simple design, do not provide a consistent resistance to rotation. Friction is generated by a rubber washer that compresses and applies increasing resistance to rotation as the terminal device is screwed in. Progressively less resistance is applied as the terminal device is unscrewed from the wrist unit and as the mechanism wears out (**Figure 19**).

Constant-Friction Wrists

Constant-friction wrist units generally are preferred because they provide constant friction throughout their range of rotation (**Figure 20**). Most units of this type use a recessed, nylon-threaded opening that is machined to accept the threaded posts of standard terminal devices. Turning a small set screw in the body of the wrist causes the nylon thread to be tightened evenly against the stud of the terminal device, thus creating constant friction. When the threads wear out, the insert can be replaced to restore function. Designs that use a mechanical wedge to apply pressure to the terminal device stud tend to resist wear and thermal breakdown better than nylon inserts (**Figure 21**). Constant-friction wrist units are available in several styles, round and oval configurations, and in a range of sizes. Although low-profile friction wrists are available for longer residual limbs, the standard length of the threaded stud on the terminal device may need to be shortened to facilitate their use.

In a unique approach, one type of constant-friction wrist allows the user to manually adjust the degree of friction by simply rotating the exterior housing to regulate the pressure on the friction mechanism around the end of the terminal device (**Figure 22**).

Because friction wrist units do not lock, they may present difficulties for users who engage in work or avocational activities that exert high rotational loads on the terminal device. Friction joints of all kinds can be difficult to keep in proper adjustment and tend to permit unwanted rotation when subjected to very high torsional loading.

Quick-Disconnect Wrists

Quick-disconnect wrists are named for their ability to facilitate rapid exchange of different terminal devices. However, even if this function is not necessary, they are often used because they can freely rotate for positioning and lockdown in the desired degree of supination or pronation. More locking positions allow a more precise positioning of the terminal device.

The most common design consists of an adapter that is screwed onto the base of each terminal device and inserted into the prosthetic wrist until it engages against an initial stop. This first, unlocked position permits free rotation and positioning but prevents the terminal device from falling out of the wrist unit. An additional axial force into the wrist activates a geared mechanism that securely locks the terminal device in the desired orientation. Pressing a lever releases the adapter to the unlocked position that allows free rotation. A heavier pressure ejects the adapter and terminal device from the wrist (**Figure 23**).

An alternative ring-type quick-change wrist uses a similar adapter, but the locking mechanism is operated by rotating the outer housing (**Figure 24**). Turning the ring in one direction unlocks and releases the terminal device from the wrist. Rotating it the other direction locks the terminal device in place. This mechanism is slightly less durable than the button type, and it is very difficult for bilateral users to operate.

Other quick-disconnect designs use a baseplate and plunger rather than a screw-on adapter. These wrists use a different locking mechanism in which a combination of ball bearings and a snap blade fit into holes or detents in the baseplate of the terminal device (**Figure 25**).

Friction disconnect wrists combine a user-adjustable, constant-friction

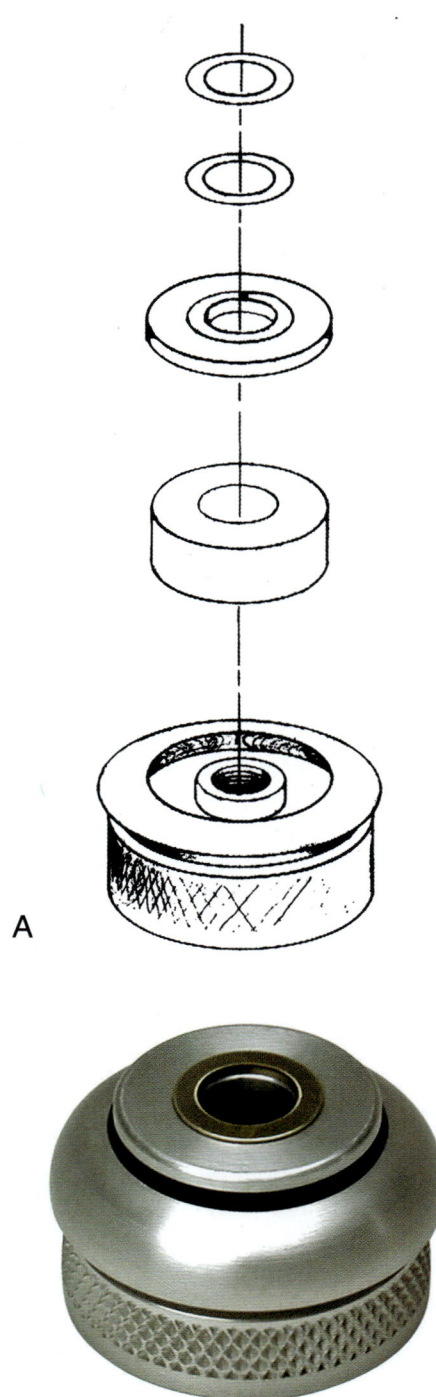

FIGURE 19 **A**, Illustration of the Economy Wrist, which has a variable friction mechanism that uses compression on inner rubber washers to provide friction and resistance to rotation. **B**, Photograph of the Economy Wrist. This device also is available with metal extensions to facilitate use in trial prostheses or for socket lamination for extra strength. (Courtesy of Fillauer, Chattanooga, TN.)

Chapter 10: Upper Limb Body-Powered Components

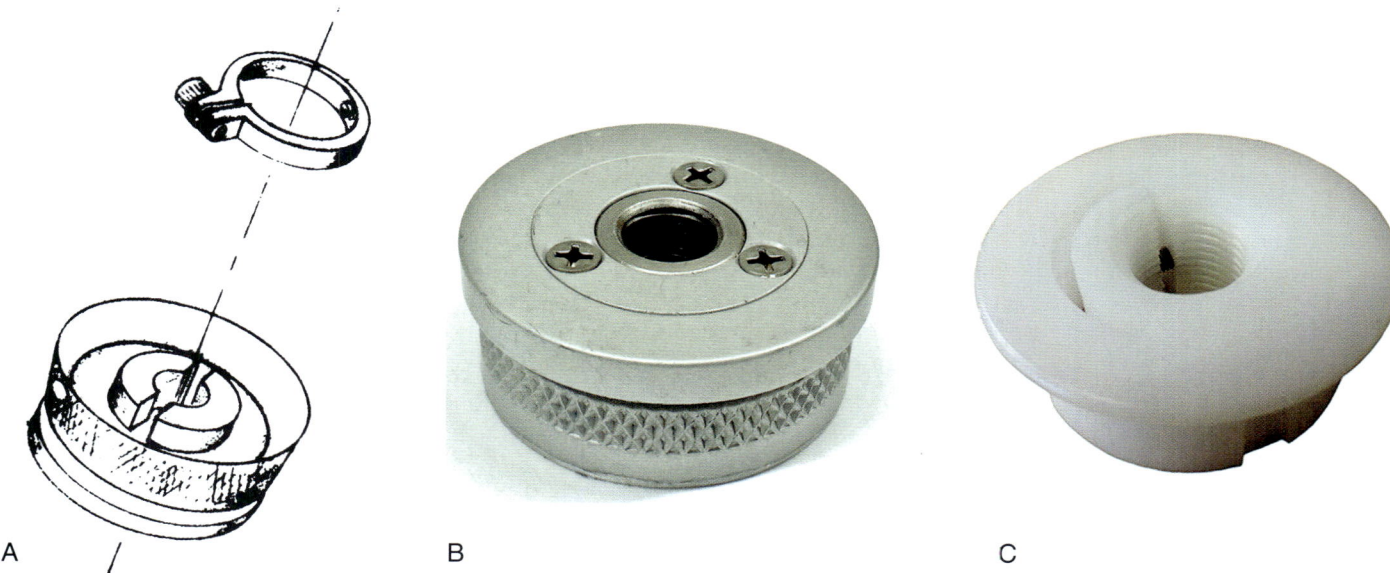

FIGURE 20 **A**, Illustration of a Hosmer constant-friction wrist mechanism. A clamp assembly tightens evenly around the mechanism that receives the threaded stud of the terminal device, providing constant friction that can be adjusted with a set screw. **B**, Photograph of a round WE Friction Wrist (Fillauer), which also is available in an oval shape. **C**, Photograph of a Delrin Wrist. (Panel C reproduced with permission from Steeper, Leeds, UK.)

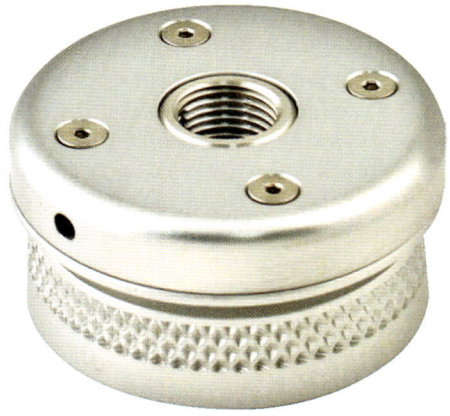

FIGURE 21 Photograph of the WedgeGrip Wrist. This constant-friction wrist uses a metal wedge that is resistant to breakdown. (Courtesy of Fillauer, Chattanooga, TN.)

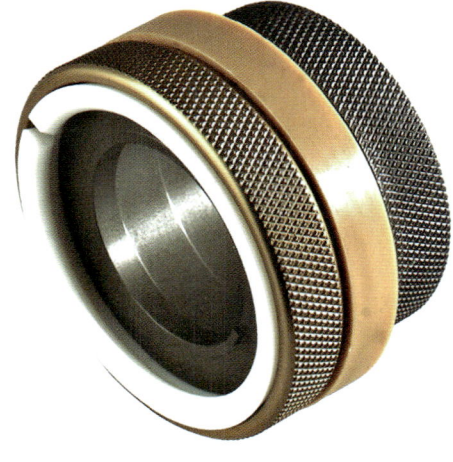

FIGURE 22 Photograph of a constant-friction wrist unit. (Reproduced with permission from Steeper, Leeds, UK.)

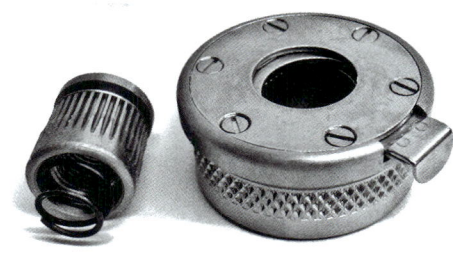

FIGURE 23 Photographs showing the FM Quick Change Wrist (right) with an adapter (left) (Fillauer).

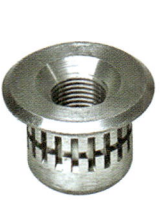 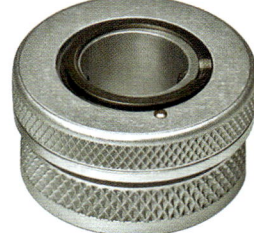

FIGURE 24 Photographs of a ring-type quick-change wrist (right) with an adapter (left). (Courtesy of Fillauer, Chattanooga, TN.)

Flexion Units

Wrist flexion is particularly useful for activities at the midline, such as toileting, eating, shaving, and dressing. For many users, such activities are usually performed more easily with the unaffected hand than with a prosthesis. The prosthetic forearm can also be biased radially (preflexed) and toward the midline (canted) to reduce or eliminate the need for a wrist with full flexion capability. For these reasons, flexion wrists were not traditionally prescribed for the unilateral amputee unless a restricted range of motion is present in the more proximal joints or on the contralateral side. However, some studies suggest that wrist flexion can improve performance, speed, and ease of use of the prosthesis for those without additional pathologies.[5-7]

mechanism with the free-rotation quick-disconnect feature (**Figure 26**). These units benefit users who like adjustable friction but need easy interchange of terminal devices.

Rotational Wrists

Rotational wrists facilitate hands-free positioning of the terminal device (**Figure 27**). Pressing a lever releases a lock and causes spring-loaded pronation. If the lever is held down, the wrist remains in free rotation, and a cable pull will supinate the terminal device to the desired position. Releasing the lever locks the wrist in 1 of 18 locking positions.

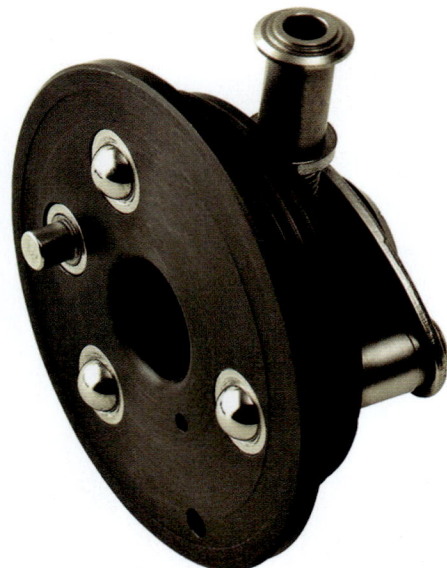

FIGURE 25 Photograph of a heavy-duty wrist unit (referred to as the Zed Rotary) that uses a baseplate and plunger-design quick-disconnect mechanism. (Reproduced with permission from Steeper, Leeds, UK.)

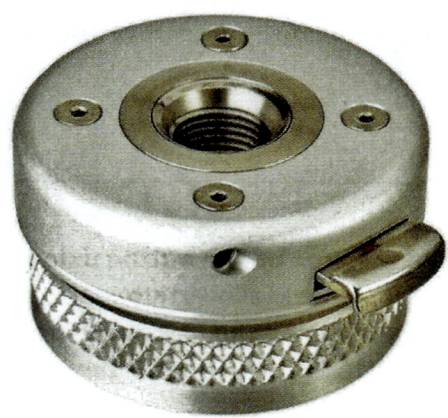

FIGURE 26 Photograph of the Friction Disconnect Wrist. (Courtesy of Fillauer, Chattanooga, TN.)

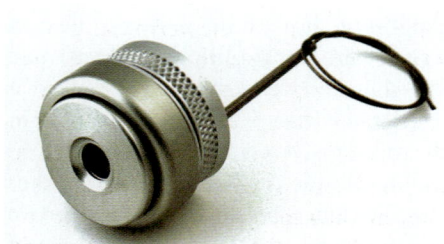

FIGURE 27 Photograph of the Rotational Wrist. (Courtesy of Fillauer, Chattanooga, TN.)

Restoring wrist flexion is essential for individuals with a bilateral upper limb amputation who perform all daily functions with prostheses. Because the mechanism adds weight at the distal end of the prosthesis, it is sometimes prescribed only for the dominant side. Flexion units are fully functional only with hooks, because the wide edges at the base of the hand base will hit most flexion wrist units and impede movement when flexion is attempted.

The Flexion Friction Wrist (Fillauer) contains a constant-friction mechanism for rotation inside a button-activated flexion hinge that permits

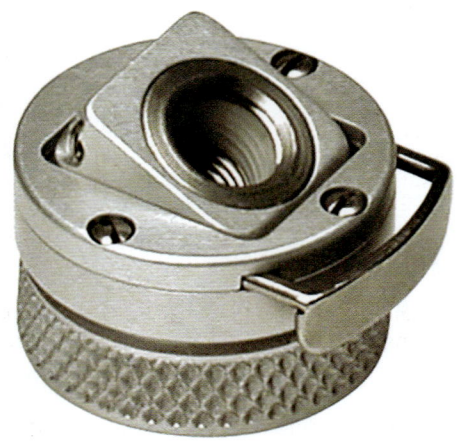

FIGURE 28 Photograph of the FW Flexion Friction Wrist. (Courtesy of Fillauer, Chattanooga, TN.)

manual pre-positioning of the hook in neutral, 30°, or 50° of palmar flexion (**Figure 28**). The Sierra Wrist Flexion Unit (Fillauer) is a dome-shaped device with similar locking flexion positions (**Figure 29**). Rotation with this unit occurs only if it is installed distally to another wrist unit, such as a friction or quick-disconnect unit. The entire unit rotates where it mounts to the second wrist, allowing the terminal device to be flexed in any direction around the 360° axis and to cover a wider work envelope than the first alternative. This can be advantageous for the bilateral amputee struggling to perform midline activities; however, the added weight and length from having two wrist units limit its applications. The MovoWrist Flex (Ottobock) combines locking rotation with locking wrist flexion and extension in a much lower-profile construct (**Figure 30**).

Most ball-and-socket joints offer infinite positioning in any direction, but are held in place only by friction. They do not lock, which poses a problem for a user engaging in more than just light duties. They are used most often in endoskeletal systems. An exception is found in the Robo-Wrist (Medical Bionics), an innovative locking ball-and-socket joint with a quick disconnect capability (**Figure 31**). The unique locking mechanism enables hundreds

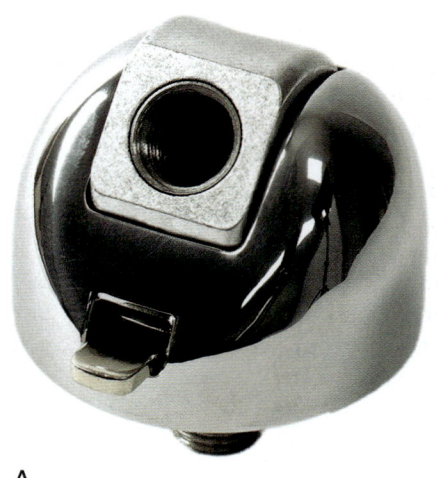
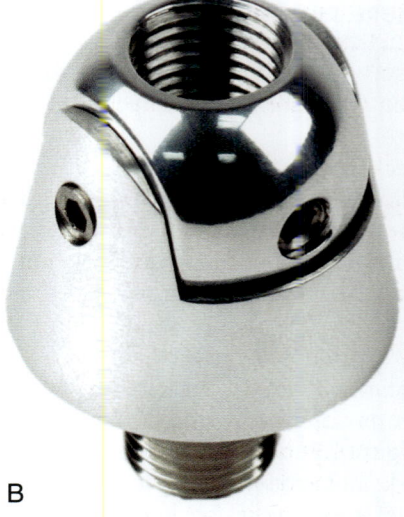

FIGURE 29 Photographs of the Sierra Wrist Flex Unit. **A,** The unit attaches to another wrist with a threaded stud. **B,** A pediatric version of the Sierra Wrist Flex Unit. (Courtesy of Fillauer, Chattanooga, TN.)

Chapter 10: Upper Limb Body-Powered Components

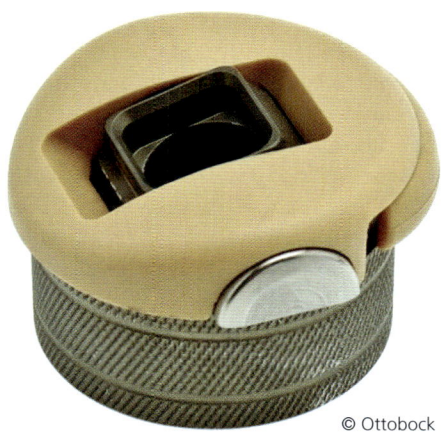

FIGURE 30 Photograph of the MovoWrist Flex. (Courtesy of Ottobock.)

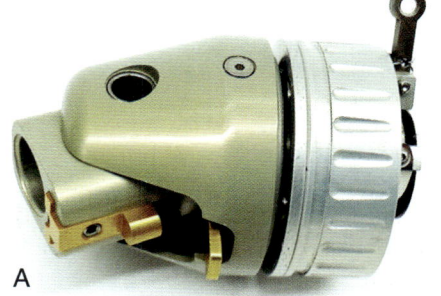 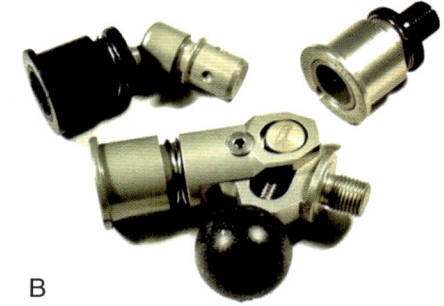

FIGURE 32 Photographs of devices in the N-Abler wrist series. **A**, The N-Abler V unit is a five-function wrist. **B**, The N-Abler II and accessories available for use alone or as distal attachments to the N-Abler V or another wrist unit. (Courtesy of Texas Assistive Devices, Brazoria, TX.)

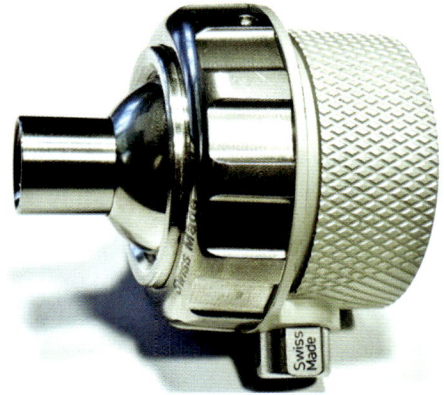

FIGURE 31 Photograph of the Robo-Wrist. This ball-and-socket wrist has quick-disconnect and locking capabilities. (Courtesy of Medical Bionics, Alberta, Canada.)

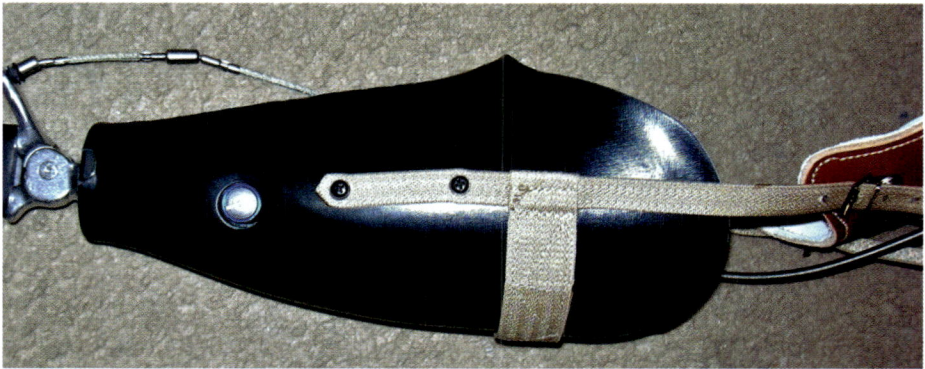

FIGURE 33 Photograph of hinges made of flexible polyethylene terephthalate on a transradial prosthesis. (Courtesy of Jim Skardoutos, C-Fab.)

of positions in varying degrees of rotation, flexion, and extension, along with radial and ulnar deviation up to 43° from the center in any direction.

Multifunction Wrists

The N-Abler V wrist unit (Texas Assistive Devices) combines the largest number of wrist functions. The unit is a five-function wrist combining spring-loaded pronation; cable-controlled supination; lever-activated flexion in 0°, 30°, or 50°; rotational locking; and a quick-disconnect mechanism. The spring-loaded rotation mechanism allows hands-free wrist positioning that is especially helpful for bilateral patients. Depressing a lever on the socket unlocks the wrist allowing it to pronate under the tension of an internal spring. To supinate, the user holds the lever down and pulls on the cable to overcome the spring tension and bring the hook back around. When the lever is released, the wrist rotation automatically locks again (**Figure 32**, A). The N-Abler II (Texas Assistive Devices) uses a ring-type quick-disconnect mechanism for locking rotation and a knob for precise, incremental adjustment of flexion and extension (**Figure 32**, B).

Midwest ProCad makes two-way and four-way locking wrist units that combine a locking QD wrist with additional flexion wrist units to provide numerous positioning options. The unit is fairly long and requires sufficient space and weight tolerance to accommodate.

Ultimately, the purpose of the wrist unit is to allow the user to position the terminal device in an orientation that maximizes assistance to the other hand when performing bimanual activities. Differences in a patient's anatomy, limb length, range of motion, comorbidities, and activities will influence wrist unit recommendations; such individual factors should be of primary consideration in prosthetic prescription.

Hinges for Transradial Prostheses

Flexible Hinges

Amputation through the distal third of the forearm usually preserves a limited amount of physiologic supination and pronation. Flexible hinges permit active use of this residual forearm rotation, thereby reducing the need for manual pre-positioning of the terminal device (**Figure 33**). Although flexible hinges of metal cable or leather are commercially available, custom-made flexible hinges made of polyethylene terephthalate webbing are most commonly used. They are attached proximally to the triceps pad and distally to the prosthetic forearm. Hinges of the proper length keep the socket secured onto the limb

Section 2: Upper Limb

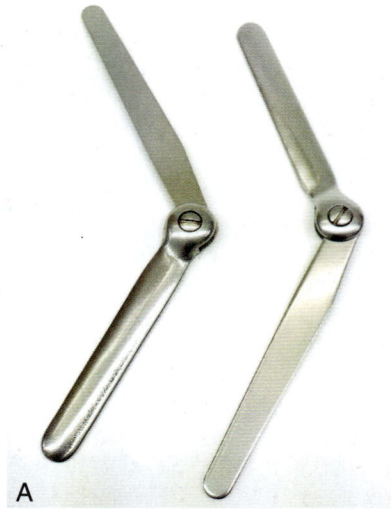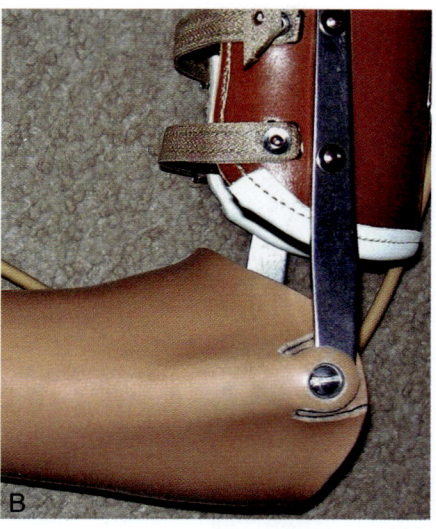

FIGURE 34 Photographs of single-axis hinges. **A**, A single-axis hinge provides axial and rotational stability between the prosthetic socket and the residual forearm. **B**, A transradial prosthesis with a single-axis hinge. (Courtesy of Jim Skardoutos, C-Fab.)

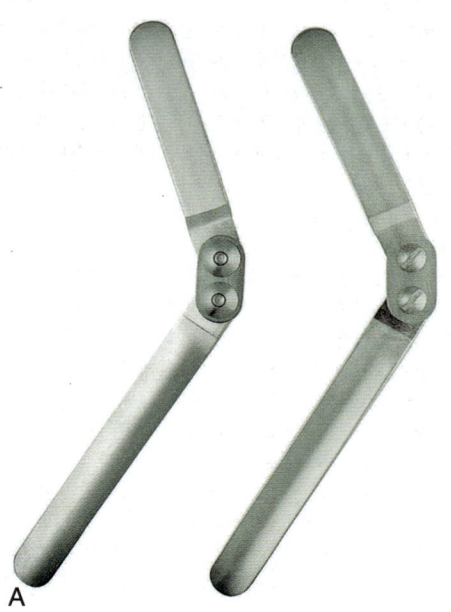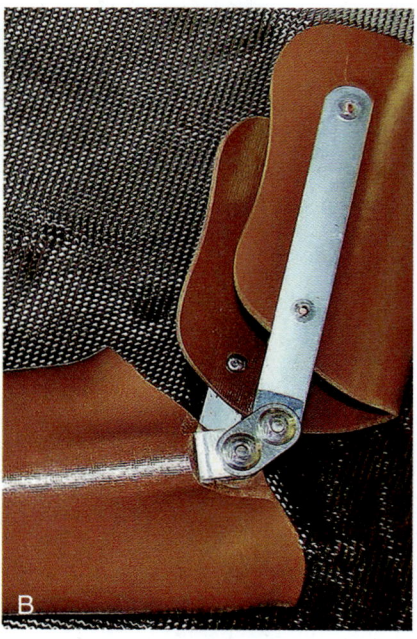

FIGURE 35 Photographs of Hosmer polycentric hinges (**A**), and the hinges installed on a transradial prosthesis (**B**). (Courtesy of Jim Skardoutos, C-Fab.)

when the elbow is flexed and prevent distal migration. Flexible hinges should permit at least 50% of the anatomic residual pronation and supination.

Rigid Hinges

An advantage of rigid hinges is their ability to stabilize the elbow and prevent rotation of the prosthesis during heavy loading. Because the forearm segment cannot rotate, the patient cannot use voluntary pronation and supination and must manually preposition the terminal device with a wrist mechanism. However, amputations at or above the level of the midforearm effectively eliminate the possibility of transmitting active supination or pronation to the terminal device, and the addition of rigid hinges would not substantially detract from the available range of motion. Rigid hinges add width at the elbow, and this added bulk often is visible in the lamination or through clothing.

Single-Axis Hinges

Single-axis hinges are designed to provide axial and rotational stability between the prosthetic socket and the residual forearm during active prosthetic use (**Figure 34**). Correctly aligned single-axis hinges should not restrict the normal flexion–extension range of motion of the anatomic elbow joint. The joints should be set in a modest amount of preflexion to load the stops of the joint when carrying heavy objects. This setting helps unweight the shorter residual limb and prevents hyperextension.

Polycentric Hinges

Short transradial limbs require that the anterior proximal trim line of the prosthetic socket be positioned close to the elbow joint for stability. The high anterior socket wall can restrict full elbow flexion resulting from the bunching of soft tissues in the antecubital region. Polycentric hinges reduce the tendency for bunching of the soft tissues by providing more room in the cubital area as the elbow is flexed, thereby increasing the potential range of motion at this joint (**Figure 35**).

Step-Up Hinges

Shorter amputation levels, immediately distal to the elbow joint, require a prosthetic socket with extremely high trim lines to provide adequate stability. Consequently, flexion of the anatomic elbow in the prosthesis is often restricted to 90° or less. If full range of elbow flexion is essential, step-up hinges may be used to overcome this limitation.

Step-up hinges require separation of the prosthetic forearm and socket, creating a split-socket prosthesis (**Figure 36**). Step-up hinges amplify the excursion of anatomic elbow joint motion by a ratio of approximately 2 to 1, such that 60° of anatomic elbow flexion causes the prosthetic forearm (and the terminal device) to move through a range of approximately 120°. However, this mechanism requires the user to exert twice as much force to flex the forearm. There are two types of step-up hinges: sliding action and geared joints. The sliding action step-up hinges have a variable amount of flexion amplification depending on

Chapter 10: Upper Limb Body-Powered Components

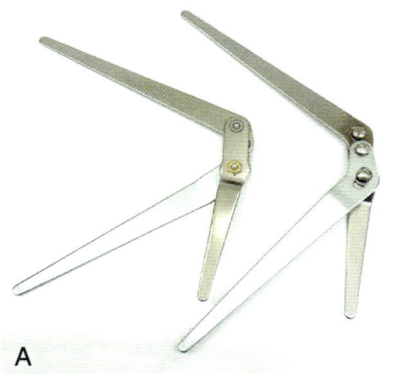
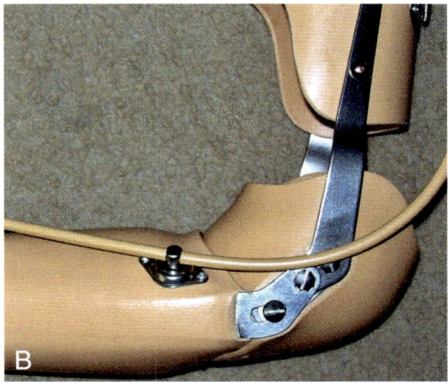

FIGURE 36 Photographs of sliding-action step-up hinges (**A**) and the hinges installed on a split-socket transradial prosthesis (**B**). (Courtesy of Jim Skardoutos, C-Fab.)

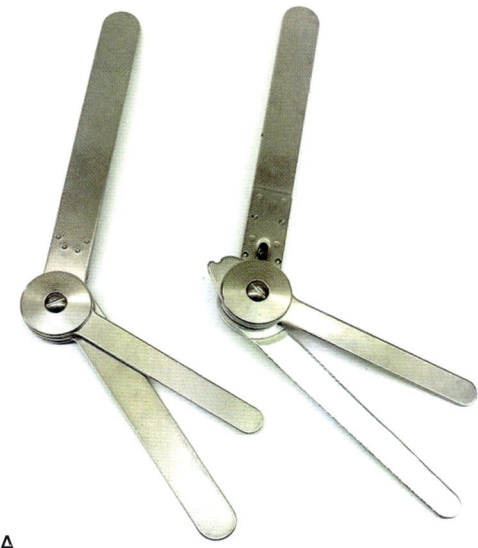
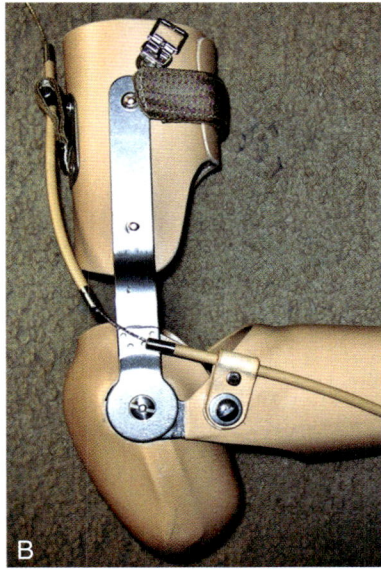

FIGURE 37 Photographs of locking hinges that are activated by the residual limb (**A**) and the hinges installed on a split-socket transradial prosthesis (**B**). (Courtesy of Jim Skardoutos, C-Fab.)

the position of the joint. At midrange, where most use occurs, the amplification is the greatest. Sliding action hinges require a split-housing cable system. Geared step-up hinges may use a standard Bowden cable system.

Residual Limb-Activated Locking Hinges

Amputees with the shortest transradial amputation levels often cannot operate a conventional transradial prosthesis because of inadequate strength, range of motion, or load bearing on the surface of the residual limb. Residual limb-activated locking hinges (**Figure 37**) address this issue by using movement of the residual limb to operate the locking hinges.

The prosthesis is cabled and controlled as a transhumeral prosthesis, and a split-socket design allows the short residual limb to control the hinge lock. When unlocked, glenohumeral flexion causes forearm flexion through a split-housing, dual-control cable system. The user locks the forearm in place by flexing the residual limb and split socket. Extension releases the lock and allows free swing of the elbow or positioning by the cable system with shoulder flexion.

Units for Elbow Disarticulation and Transhumeral Prostheses

Absence of the anatomic elbow joint requires a mechanical substitute that permits control of flexion and extension through a range of at least 135°. In addition, the unit must permit the user to lock and unlock the elbow at various points throughout the 135° arc. Body-powered elbows require up to 5 cm of cable excursion to position the elbow through its full arc of flexion range.

Outside-Locking Hinges

Outside-locking hinges are necessary for elbow disarticulation and long transhumeral limbs that do not have sufficient space for a traditional elbow unit (**Figure 38**). They are named for their position on the outside of the humeral condyles. The lock is usually installed on the medial side and can be controlled manually or by cable activation through shoulder movement. Outside-locking hinges are available from several manufacturers in standard, heavy-duty, and low-profile models and in a range of sizes.

Elbow Units

Whether an elbow unit can be used depends on the available distance or clearance between the end of the residual limb and the place where the anatomic elbow center should be located. Elbow joints vary in their proximal clearance height, but most are approximately 1.5 to 2.0 inches (3.8 to 5.0 cm). The practitioner also must allow for the thickness of any socket materials or suspension mechanisms and for access to the hardware for the friction adjustment of humeral rotation. Therefore, the guideline traditionally has been that transhumeral amputations approximately 5 cm proximal to the elbow joint permit the use of inside-locking elbow units.

Friction Elbows

Friction elbows are lightweight and simple to operate but require passive positioning of the forearm (**Figure 39**). For this reason, they can be appropriate for low-impact users, pediatric applications, cosmetic restorations, and in instances when brachial plexus injury or other factors preclude active elbow function.

The ENER-JOINT (TRS; **Figure 40**) is a passive, locking polyurethane joint

Section 2: Upper Limb

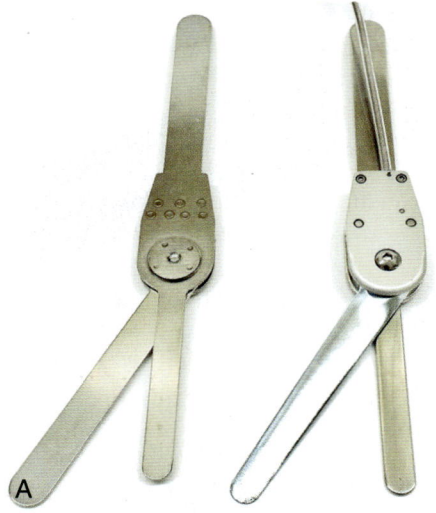

FIGURE 38 Photographs of outside-locking hinges. **A**, The Heavy-Duty Outside Locking Hinge (Fillauer) for use on a prosthetic device after a long transhumeral amputation or an elbow disarticulation. **B**, The standard Hosmer Outside Locking Hinge is shown installed on a transhumeral prosthesis. (Courtesy of Jim Skardoutos, C-Fab.)

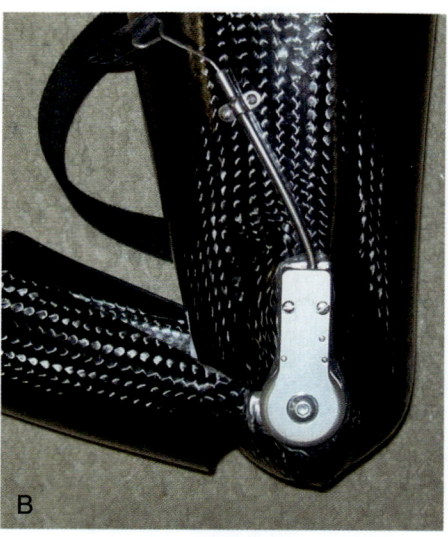

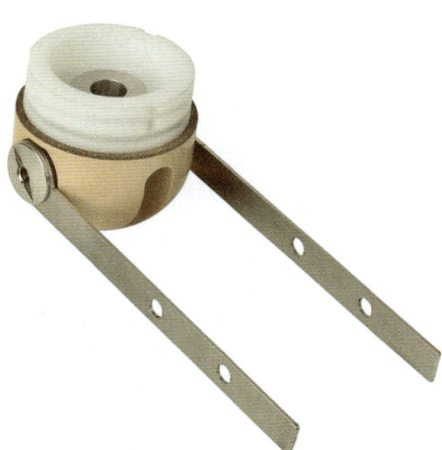

FIGURE 39 Photograph of the Pediatric Friction Elbow joint. (Reproduced with permission from Steeper, Leeds, UK.)

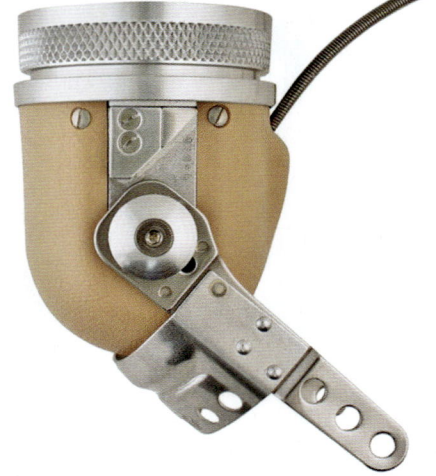

FIGURE 41 Photograph of the E-400 Elbow, an inside locking elbow unit. (Courtesy of Fillauer, Chattanooga, TN.)

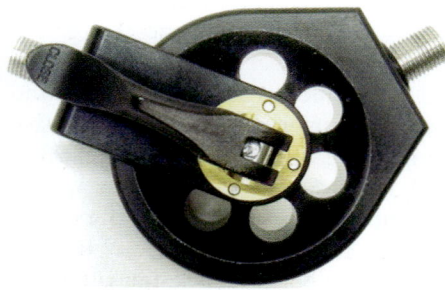

FIGURE 40 Photograph of the ENER-JOINT. This elbow joint is designed to absorb shock during high-impact activities. (Courtesy of Fillauer TRS Inc., Boulder, CO.)

that is designed to absorb shock during high-impact activities and dampen transmission of forces through the prosthesis to permit a more stable grip during certain activities, such as mountain biking and operating a chainsaw or jackhammer.

Inside-Locking Elbows

Inside-locking elbow units contain the joint and locking mechanism inside an outer shell and are installed distally to the residual limb. The elbow locking mechanism is usually triggered by a cable or string that exits through the anterior surface of the unit. The cable is traditionally connected to an elastic strap that runs over the top of the shoulder, and a small amount of excursion generated by shoulder movement locks and unlocks the joint. These elbows vary in the number of locking positions and range of flexion. As with all types of manual joints, more locking positions permit more precise positioning of the terminal device. In addition, all inside-locking units incorporate a proximal friction-held turntable that permits manual prepositioning of the prosthetic forearm to substitute for the loss of active external and internal humeral rotation.

The E-series elbows by Hosmer are available in three sizes and a heavy-duty version. They can be ordered in locking or friction versions (**Figure 41**). The Automatic Elbow (RSL Steeper) is similar but also has the unique ability to lock in humeral rotation in 30° increments (**Figure 42, A**). Some users prefer the simplicity of a passive locking elbow that can be passively positioned in the desired flexion angle and locked into position through a mechanism positioned on the forearm (**Figure 42, B**). Some manufacturers offer elbow units with additional features and integrated, prefabricated forearm shells that can simplify fabrication and reduce system weight.

Elbow Flexion Assists and Counterbalances

Elbows can incorporate flexion assists and counterbalances to reduce the force necessary for elbow flexion. Some units are added to the elbow as an additional component, whereas others incorporate the mechanism into an elbow–forearm combination.

Flexion assists work as a simple spring assist. Users can adjust the amount of flexion assist by manually increasing the tension upon the spring. As the spring unwinds, it exerts less force, resulting in the most lifting force at full extension and less as the forearm is flexed (**Figure 43**).

A counterbalance mechanism is a spring-loaded cam mechanism that can be adjusted to completely compensate for the weight of the forearm, wrist,

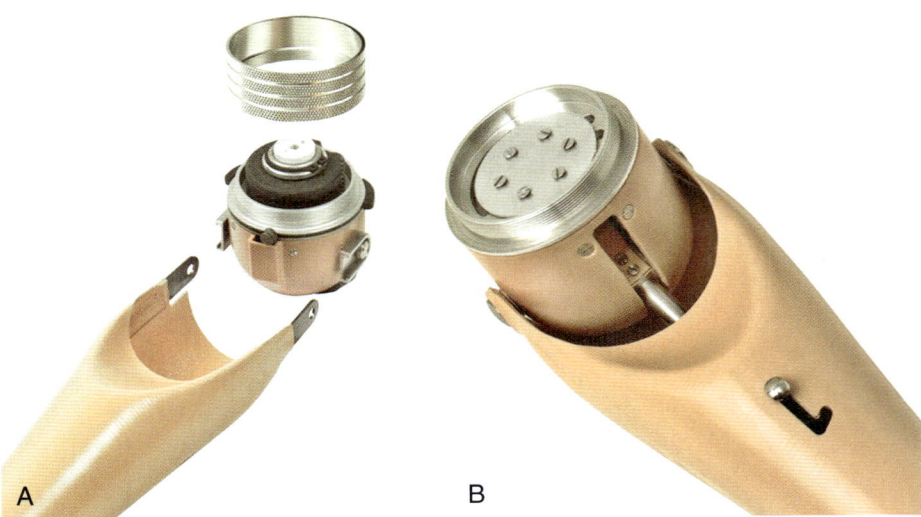

FIGURE 42 Photographs of prosthetic elbows. **A**, The Automatic Elbow unit, optional forearm shell, and lamination ring. **B**, The Manual Elbow in an adult size. This elbow locks with a knob on the forearm. (Reproduced with permission from Steeper, Leeds, UK.)

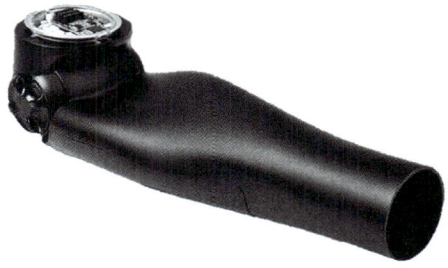

FIGURE 45 Photograph of Espire Hybrid Elbow with Counterbalance and electric lock. (Reproduced with permission from Steeper, Leeds, UK.)

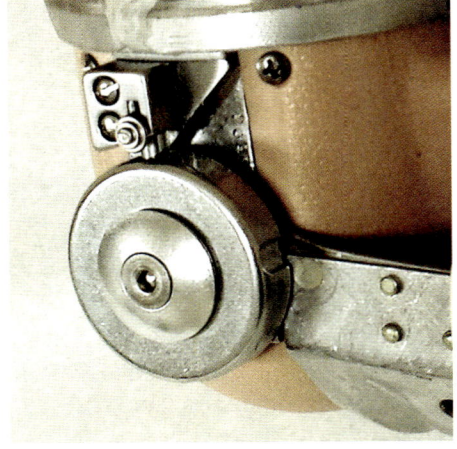

FIGURE 43 Photograph shows the Hosmer flexion assistance mechanism installed on the medial side of a left transhumeral prosthesis.

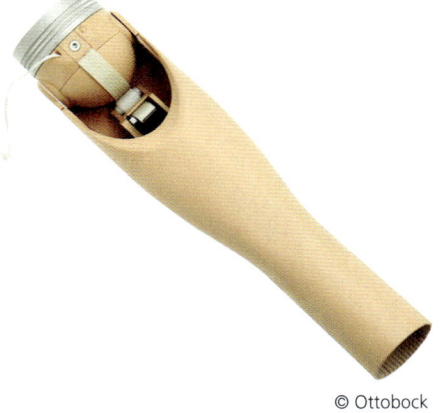

FIGURE 44 Photograph of the ErgoArm Plus. This device has an Automatic Forearm Balance for assistance in lifting, and a low clearance for longer residual limbs. Available in Body Powered and Hybrid Versions. (Courtesy of Ottobock.)

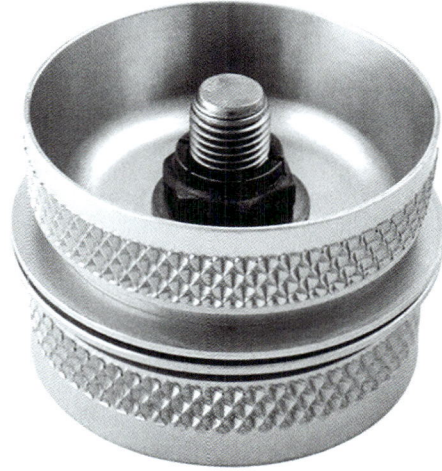

FIGURE 46 Photograph of a shoulder bulkhead. (Courtesy of Fillauer, Chattanooga, TN.)

and terminal device assembly during elbow flexion. It is designed to offset the effects of gravity by applying a lifting force in proportion to the flexion angle, increasing as the elbow reaches 90° and decreasing to full flexion or extension. The result is that the user perceives the same weight throughout the range of flexion. This feature can supplement the lifting power provided through a standard body-powered cable or it can be adjusted to facilitate ballistic flexion of the unit through gross body movements (**Figure 44**).

Reducing the force necessary for elbow flexion can permit subtle harnessing adjustments that require less excursion. In addition, the reduced strain on the limb may reduce shear forces between the socket and the skin.[8] Although optional, elbow flexion assistance components are prescribed routinely, particularly for use with heavier terminal devices.

Hybrid elbows are body-powered elbows that have been configured for use with externally powered components. Although elbow motion is still controlled with a cable, internal electronics and integrated wiring allow transmission of signals to the wrist and the terminal device. They incorporate a standard manual lock and/or an electric lock that uses an electromyographic signal or switch to lock the elbow in flexion (**Figures 44** and **45**).

Shoulders

Currently, all available shoulder joints rely on passive and strategic prepositioning to facilitate the optimal use of other prosthetic components. Most use occurs with the humeral segment vertical and the elbow near 90°. Users of a unilateral prosthesis may find minimal shoulder movement acceptable and appreciate the reduced weight and bulk from simplifying this joint.

Shoulder joints are generally classified according to the degree of motion allowed. The simplest design is termed a bulkhead, which consists of a circular unit integrated vertically to provide flexion and extension in the sagittal plane (**Figure 46**). Single-axis shoulder

Section 2: Upper Limb

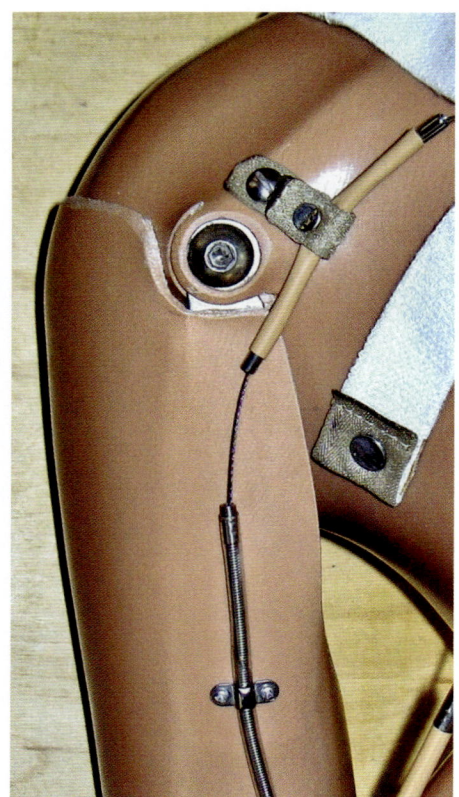

FIGURE 47 Photograph of a shoulder abduction hinge installed on a shoulder disarticulation prosthesis. (Courtesy of Jim Skardoutos, C-Fab.)

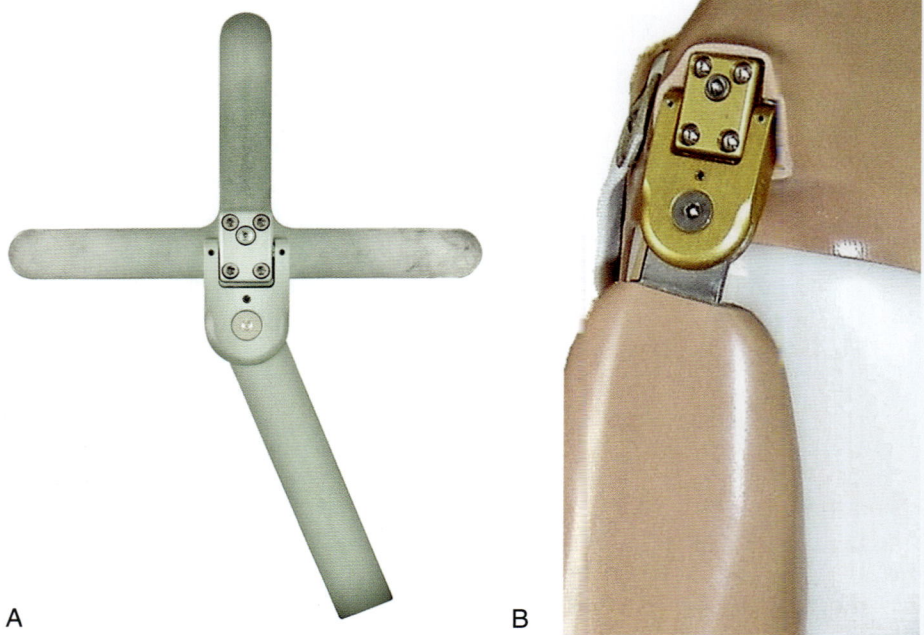

FIGURE 48 Photographs of a double-axis flexion-abduction hinge (**A**) and the hinge shown installed on a shoulder disarticulation prosthesis (**B**). (Panel A courtesy of Fillauer, Chattanooga, TN. Panel B courtesy of Jim Skardoutos, C-Fab.)

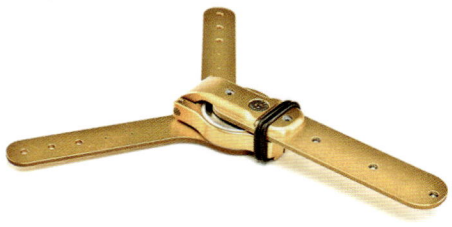

FIGURE 49 Photograph of the MovoShoulder Swing joint. (Courtesy of Ottobock.)

joints provide only abduction (**Figure 47**), and double-axis units provide abduction and flexion. Double-axis joints usually consist of a single-axis abduction hinge on top of a rotating plate that provides the flexion and extension (**Figure 48**). One double-axis shoulder joint unlocks in flexion/extension when abducted and locks when adducted. The user swings the arm to the side to unlock the joint, then swings it forward in flexion and adducts it to lock it in place (**Figure 49**).

The Universal Shoulder Joint (Fillauer) allows flexion in the sagittal plane, abduction in the coronal plane, and rotation about the humeral axis (**Figure 50**). It consists of a single-axis hinge with a threaded stud and friction wrist unit on both ends. One wrist unit is laminated into the shoulder socket facing outward, and the other attaches to the distal end of the shoulder unit to form the top of the humeral section. The hinge provides abduction in the coronal plane. The top wrist unit allows flexion and extension, and the bottom wrist unit permits humeral rotation.

The Axis Shoulder Joint (College Park) can stabilize a shoulder in 24 different flexion positions (**Figure 51**). This feature benefits individuals who wish to use the terminal device for upper quadrant activities such as reaching items on a high shelf. To position the joint in glenohumeral flexion, users will often unlock the shoulder joint and bend forward at the waist, allowing gravity to position the shoulder joint in relative flexion. A lock can be operated manually or by using an electrically powered switch. When the patient straightens at the waist, the prosthesis is positioned in relative shoulder flexion. A second, adjustable hinge with friction control provides abduction and adduction stabilization.

Other Socket Components

The nudge control unit is a paddle-shaped lever that can be pushed by the chin or a phocomelic digit or against environmental objects to provide a small amount of cable excursion (**Figure 52**). It is usually prescribed when other body motions are not available. Although originally designed to provide elbow locking and unlocking, it also can be adapted to operate other components, including flexion and rotation wrist units. The power and excursion required to operate the locking mechanism of a shoulder joint may necessitate the modification of a nudge switch with a lever extension.

The ELF Strap (TRS; **Figure 53**) is a rubberized extension designed to replace one of the functions of the triceps cuff in self-suspending, body-powered, transradial prostheses. It attaches to the posterior of the socket to provide an anchor point and stable routing for the control cable.

One unique, partially prefabricated design replaces the typical rigid forearm in favor of composite rods. The design significantly reduces weight, allows for easier adjustments, and absorbs torque and vibration (**Figure 54**).

Chapter 10: Upper Limb Body-Powered Components

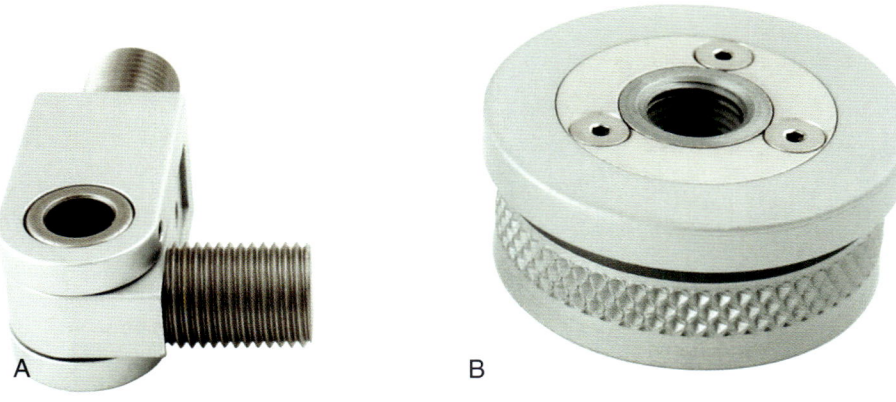

FIGURE 50 **A**, Photograph of the Universal Shoulder Joint. The abduction hinge joint is used between two wrist units, such as friction wrists (**B**), which are screwed onto both threaded studs of the hinge to provide humeral rotation and glenohumeral flexion and extension. (Courtesy of Fillauer, Chattanooga, TN.)

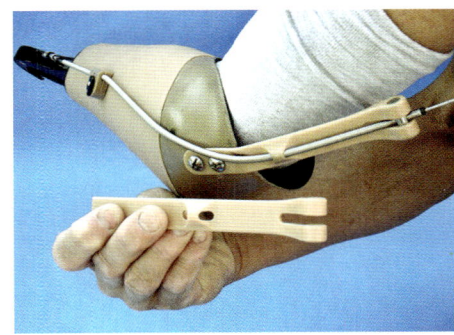

FIGURE 53 Photograph of an ELF Strap on a self-suspending transradial socket. (Courtesy of Fillauer TRS Inc., Boulder, CO.)

The International Transradial Adjustable Limb (ToughWare Prosthetics) is an off-the-shelf socket and suspension system for body-powered, VO transradial prostheses (**Figure 55**).

Endoskeletal Systems

Endoskeletal upper limb prosthetic systems are composed of tubular humeral and forearm elements, and the components allow for encasement in cosmetic foam covers (**Figure 56**). After final shaping and covering with a skin-colored stockinette or nylon, the completed prosthesis affords a high degree of cosmetic acceptability. In addition to improved cosmesis and softness, modular prostheses are lighter in weight than conventional artificial limbs. Three different endoskeletal upper limb prosthetic systems are currently available from Ottobock, RSL Steeper, and Fillauer.

Endoskeletal systems vary in exact components, connectors, mechanisms of movement, and durability, but they are usually passive and allow positioning with friction joints. Most allow rotation of different segments, and many use ball-and-socket joints. Any terminal devices with the standard thread can be used, although a cosmetic passive hand is usually chosen. Elbows may be passive or cable controlled, with or without locking capability. Shoulders are available in single-axis, double-axis, or ball-and-socket configurations.

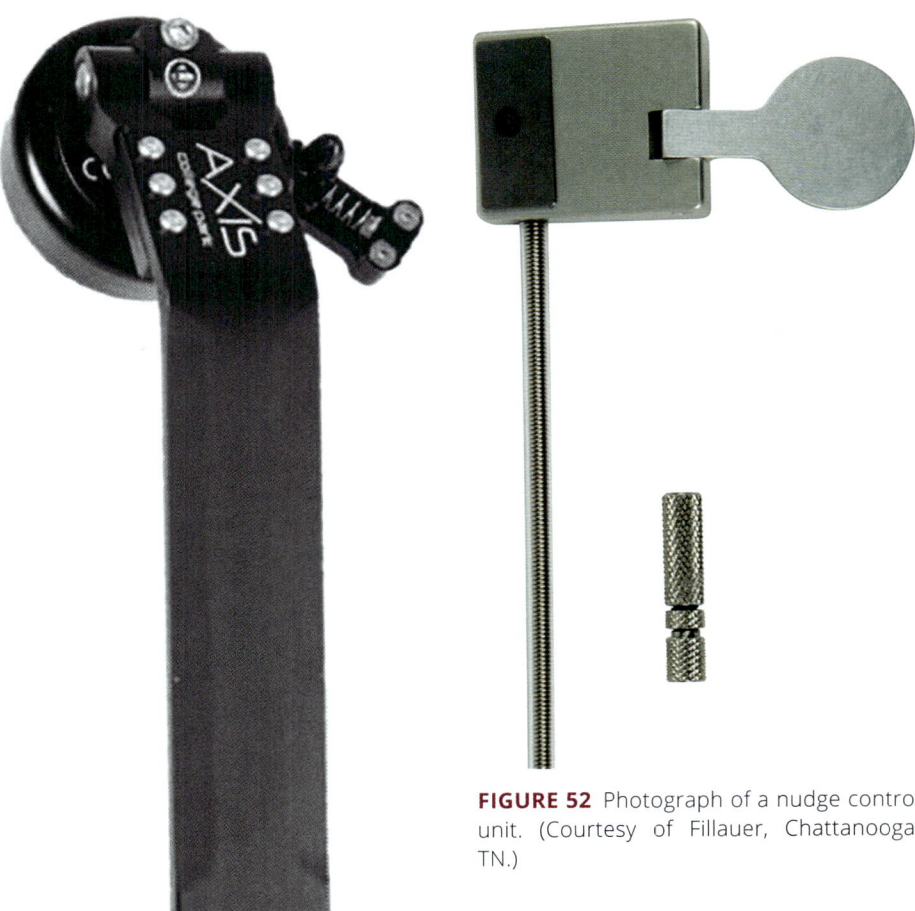

FIGURE 51 Photograph of Axis Locking Shoulder Joint. (Courtesy of College Park, Warren, MI.)

FIGURE 52 Photograph of a nudge control unit. (Courtesy of Fillauer, Chattanooga, TN.)

© 2024 American Academy of Orthopaedic Surgeons — Atlas of Amputations and Limb Deficiencies, Fifth Edition

Section 2: Upper Limb

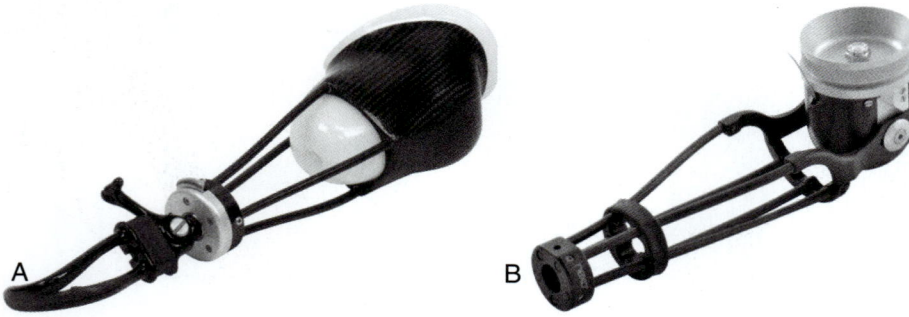

FIGURE 54 Photograph of the Nexo Series (**A**) Transradial (**B**) Transhumeral. (Courtesy of Fillauer, Chattanooga, TN.)

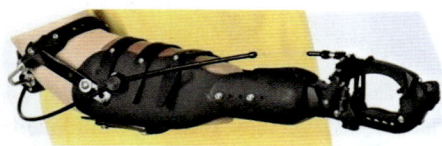

FIGURE 55 Photograph of the International Transradial Adjustable Limb. This device is an off-the-shelf socket and suspension system for body-powered, transradial prostheses. (Courtesy of ToughWare Prosthetics, Westminster, CO.)

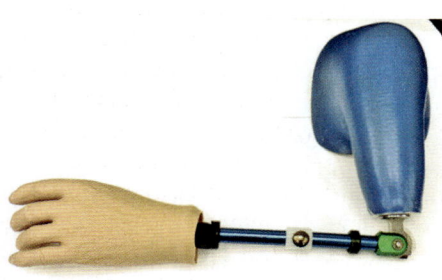

FIGURE 56 Photograph of an endoskeletal transhumeral prosthesis system. (Reproduced with permission from Steeper, Leeds, UK.)

SUMMARY

The main goal in providing a patient with a prosthesis is to enable the person to use the device as much as is needed to accomplish activities that are most important to that individual. Prosthetic use and acceptance is considerably increased when the user has an integral role in the selection process and is allowed to provide feedback during the fitting process. Acceptance or rejection may result from discomfort, a lack of desired function, appearance, or any number of reasons that the clinician may not anticipate. Therefore, it is important to include the user in any discussion about, and selection of, component choices. No body-powered or externally powered device can fully replace the human hand. Each of the components discussed in this chapter has its best applications, misuses, pros, and cons. Together, the clinician and patient must engage in a thorough discussion about these factors and must prioritize the patient's desired functions and ultimate goals.

References

1. Stark G: Upper limb prosthetic competency and characteristics among self-assessed novices-intermediates and experts-specialists. *J Assoc Pediatr Orthot Prosthet Clin* 2014;20(1):11-13.
2. Fraser CM: An evaluation of the use made of cosmetic and functional prostheses by unilateral upper limb amputees. *Prosthet Orthot Int* 1998;22(3):216-223.
3. Smit C, Bongers RM, Van der Sluis CK, Plettenburg DH: Efficiency of voluntary opening hand and hook prosthetic devices: 24 years of development? *J Rehabil Res Dev* 2012;49(4):523-534.
4. Smit G, Plettenburg DH: Efficiency of voluntary closing hand and hook prostheses. *Prosthet Orthot Int* 2010;34(4):411-427.
5. Kestner S: Defining the relationship between prosthetic wrist function and its use in performing work tasks and activities of daily living. *J Prosthet Orthot* 2006;18(3):80-86.
6. Kyberd PJ: The influence of passive wrist joints on the functionality of prosthetic hands. *Prosthet Orthot Int* 2012;36(1):33-38.
7. Bertels T, Schmalz T, Ludwigs E: Objectifying the functional advantages of prosthetic wrist function. *J Prosthet Orthot* 2009;21(2):74-78.
8. Miguelez J, Conyers D, Lang M, Gulick K: Upper extremity prosthetics, in Pasquina P, Cooper R, eds: *Care of the Combat Amputee*. Border Institute of Walter Reed Army Medical Center and Office of the Surgeon General, 2009, pp 607-640.

Harnessing and Controls for Upper Limb Body-Powered Prostheses

CHAPTER 11

David B. Rotter, CPO

ABSTRACT

Body-powered prosthetic devices are an effective method of controlling upper limb prostheses. Body-powered prostheses use body movements, which are captured with control straps and cables, to generate volitional movement. For those with bilateral involvement, body power is generally the preferred method of control because of the improved proprioception and reliability offered.

Keywords: figure-of-8 harness; force and excursion; prosthesis; transradial prosthesis

Introduction

Body-powered prostheses for the upper limb are controlled by harnessing, capturing movements from the patient's intact body segments. These movements, or control motions, become transferrable forces that actuate body-powered components, including prosthetic elbows and terminal devices. This is most often accomplished by a transmission of movement through a series of harness straps and cables that are circumferentially anchored at a fixed point on the body and create a reaction at targeted body-powered components.[1]

Despite exciting developments in externally powered prosthetic options, body-powered prosthetic devices continue to be relevant as a viable and effective means of controlling upper limb prostheses. For many patients with bilateral involvement, body power is the preferred method of control because of the improved proprioception and reliability offered.[2,3]

Body-powered prostheses have stood the test of time for a variety of reasons. They involve relatively lightweight, durable components that create consistent, dependable reactions every time they are used. Because there is no need for an external power source, the dependency on a source of electricity for recharging is eliminated. An important and often overlooked advantage is the sensory feedback provided to users of body-powered devices. The users can feel how much tension they are exerting through the socket and harness and can feel how much movement is taking place at the terminal device. This one-to-one relationship of movement to sensory feedback allows the user to know where the prosthesis is in space.[4]

From the earliest concepts to current practice, novel approaches of capturing body movements to control upper limb prostheses have been developed, refined, and subsequently taught to future generations of prosthetists. This chapter reviews basic harnessing and body power theory, discusses body-powered options at each major level of upper limb amputation, and describes the available movements used to actuate body-powered components. Alternative harnessing strategies designed to address more specific needs along with their clinical relevance are also discussed.

Finger Prostheses

The past decade has seen the development of many body-powered choices for patients with a partial hand amputation, with commercially available options for those missing single or multiple fingers. Five body-powered systems, the PIP Driver, MCP Driver, and Thumb Driver (Naked Prosthetics), the Partial M-Finger (Liberating Technologies), and the X-Finger (Didrick Medical), use forward flexion of the remnant finger to drive flexion of distal prosthetic segments. The durability and grip strength offered by these systems vary with the different mechanical systems (**Figures 1** through **3**).

PIP Driver

The PIP Driver is intended for finger amputations distal to the proximal interphalangeal joint, where sufficient length and flexion mobility of the residual middle phalanx remains. A proximal frame surrounds the proximal phalanx with a second frame surrounding the middle phalanx. Flexion and extension between these two frames are captured by a linkage joint that transmits flexion force and movement to a prosthetic distal interphalangeal joint, moving a prosthetic distal phalanx.

MCP Driver

The MCP Driver is intended for finger amputations approximating the PIP

David B. Rotter or an immediate family member serves as a board member, owner, officer, or committee member of the Association of Children's Prosthetic and Orthotic Clinics.

joint. Flexion of the metacarpophalangeal (MCP) joints is transmitted to distal prosthetic interphalangeal joints through a metal linkage system (**Figure 1**). Current manufacturing constraints are such that the optimal amputation length for such systems is just proximal to the PIP joint as this provides an optimal functional lever arm for the body segment driving the system, while leaving enough length distal to the amputation to fit the necessary length of the prostheses. Given its robust stainless steel construction, the MCP Driver is currently the most heavy-duty prosthetic solution at this amputation level.

Thumb Driver

Similar in some respects to the MCP Driver, the Thumb Driver is intended for amputations just distal to the MCP joint of the thumb. Driven primarily by movement at the carpometacarpal joint, and secondarily at the MCP joint of thumb, the Thumb Driver provides active flexion of a prosthetic interphalangeal (IP) joint and dynamic opposition against the remaining digits of the hand.

X-Fingers

The X-Finger system is intended for finger amputations distal to the metacarpophalangeal joint. It is anchored at the wrist joint with a linkage mechanism spanning the dorsum of the hand. As with the MCP Driver, flexion of the remnant fingers drives polycentric linkage mechanisms to flex the prosthetic fingertip. Variants for amputations both proximal and distal to the DIP joint are commercially available (**Figure 2**). The design of the X-finger is not as robust as that of the MCP Driver and it appears better suited to lighter duty applications.

Partial M-Fingers

The Partial M-Finger is also intended for finger amputation distal to the MCP. Similar in some respects to the MCP Driver, the M-Finger uses a cable system rather than a rigid linkage system, that is mounted on the dorsal surface of the hand. The mounting acts as the anchor, and metacarpophalangeal flexion creates cable tension that causes the partial finger element to flex volarly (**Figure 3**). Internal springs extend the interphalangeal joint in the absence of cable tension.

Partial Hand Prostheses

M-Fingers

M-Fingers use the movement of wrist flexion as the prime mover. As the user flexes the wrist, cables, which are anchored on a frame mounted proximal to the dorsal aspect of the forearm, are pulled. The frame acts as the anchor, and the action of wrist flexion acts to close the fingers about an object. The available force and excursion are both limited, making this type of prosthesis better suited for lighter duty applications (**Figure 4**).

Minnesota Split-Hand Prosthesis

The Minnesota split-hand device is an example of a prosthesis that uses wrist flexion and extension to activate a hinged, split hand. The hand is split at its base, making the thumb a stationary component, while the top section of the hand is activated with wrist flexion. Force and excursion are moderate to good with this type of device. It is appropriate for use in an individual with a congenital limb deficiency at the transcarpal level or a traumatic partial hand amputation (**Figures 5** and **6**).

Traditional Harnessing

Another option is the use of traditional body-powered terminal devices and a figure-of-8 harness for a partial hand amputee (**Figure 7**). This option can support carrying heavier loads as the durable construction of the terminal device can transmit considerable force through the broad surface area of the

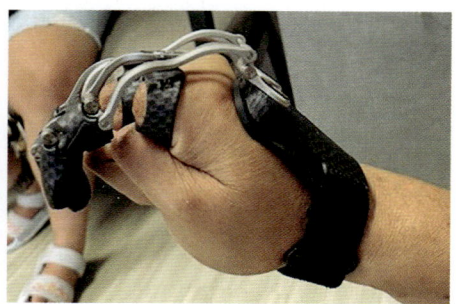

FIGURE 1 Photograph of an MCP Driver where flexion of the metacarpophalangeal joints is transmitted to distal prosthetic interphalangeal joints through a metal linkage system (Courtesy of Phillip M. Stevens, MEd, CPO, Salt Lake City, UT.)

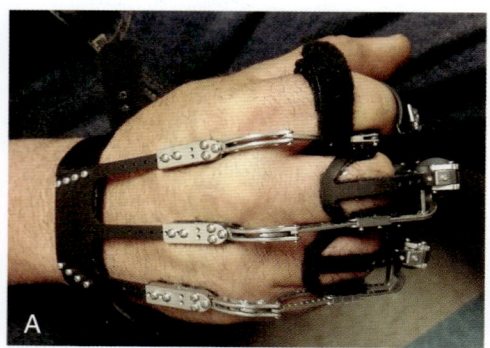 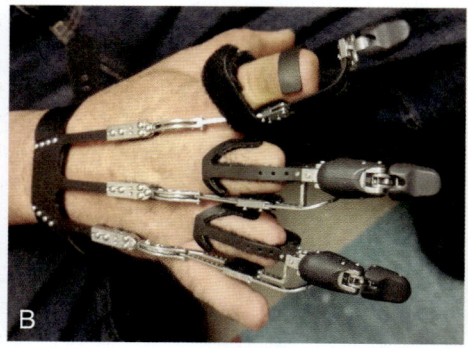 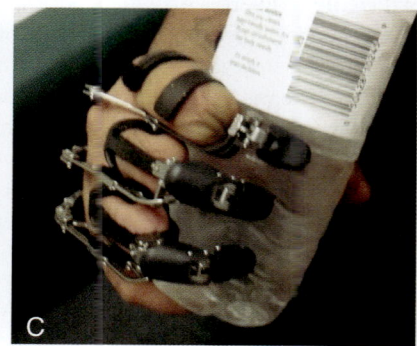

FIGURE 2 **A** through **C** illustrate how flexion at the metacarpophalangeal joint of the residual digits produces flexion at the interphalangeal joints of the prosthesis. (Courtesy of Phillip M. Stevens, MEd, CPO, Salt Lake City, UT.)

Chapter 11: Harnessing and Controls for Upper Limb Body-Powered Prostheses

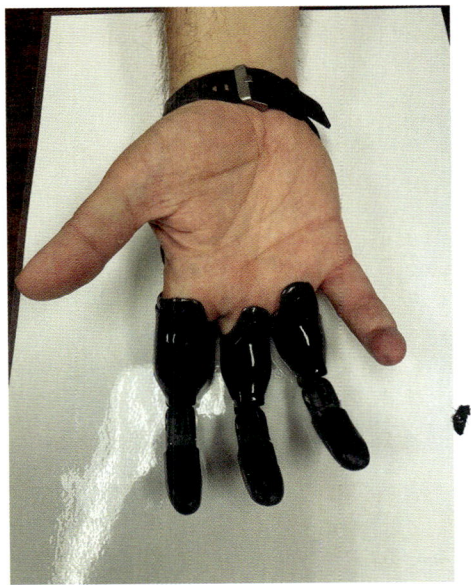
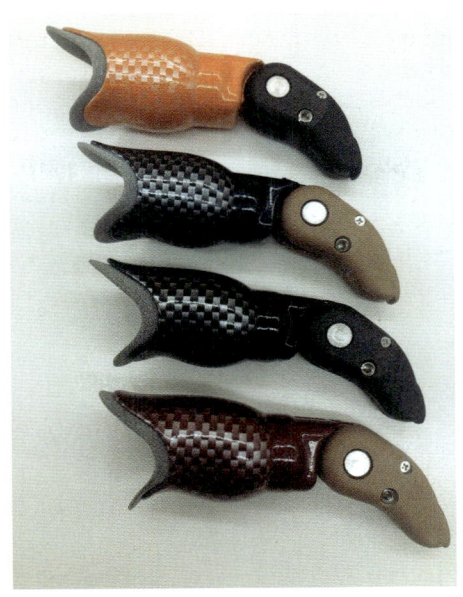
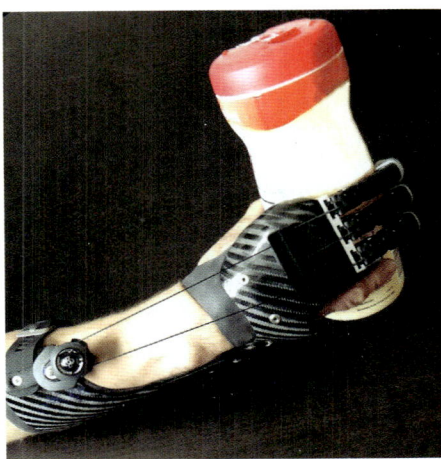

FIGURE 3 Photographs of the Partial M-Finger. In a device anchored at the wrist of the affected limb, metacarpophalangeal flexion creates the cable excursion needed to create interphalangeal flexion in the prosthesis. (Courtesy of Partial Hand Solutions, Southington, CT.)

FIGURE 4 Photograph of Partial Hand M-Fingers. Wrist flexion causes the cable to become taught, closing the fingers. (Courtesy of Partial Hand Solutions, Southington, CT.)

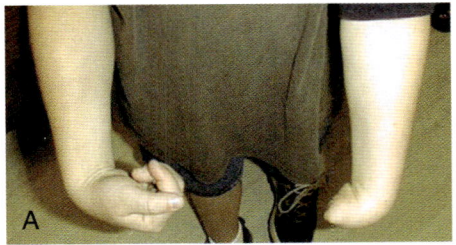
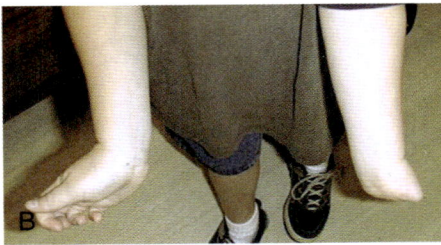
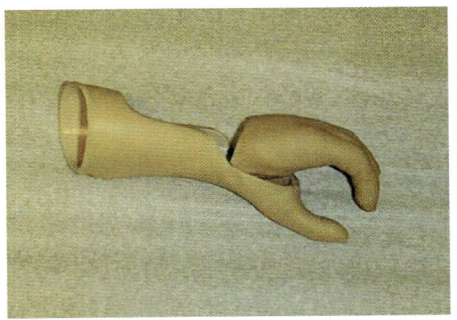

FIGURE 5 Photographs from a patient with a left partial hand amputation demonstrating residual wrist flexion (**A**) and extension (**B**) that can be used to actuate a body-powered, split-hand prosthesis. (Courtesy of David B. Rotter, CPO, David Rotter Prosthetics, LTD, Joliet, IL.)

FIGURE 6 Photograph of the Minnesota split-hand prosthesis. (Courtesy of David B. Rotter, CPO, David Rotter Prosthetics, LTD, Joliet, IL.)

harness. At this distal amputation level, the harness also allows the anatomic motions of wrist flexion and extension with full pronation and supination, which allows the user many options to position and then activate the prosthesis in space.

Transradial Applications

History

Artifacts and drawings have documented historical attempts at producing functional upper limb prosthetic devices. As early as the 16th century and continuing through the US Civil War, hook-like shapes were often fashioned as useful prosthetic implements for stabilizing, pulling, and carrying objects[5] (**Figures 8** and **9**). Patent filings in the 19th century document the use of body-powered control through a harness, such as William Selpho's 1857 patent for a body-powered prosthetic arm[6,7] (**Figure 10**).

The primary body-powered system still currently in use can be attributed to Dorrance's 1912 patent[8] of the split hook. The original hook design (**Figure 11**) was refined into multiple models and shapes and is currently sold by the Fillauer Corporation.[9] Both the Selpho and Dorrance designs demonstrate the use of a harness to both suspend and activate a cable that is pulled to open a terminal device.

Building on these original concepts, methods to efficiently transmit force through a harnessing system have been developed and refined. To better understand these concepts, it is useful to review force transmission and goals of efficiently harnessing a body-powered system.

Basic Concepts of Force Transmission

The goal when setting up body-powered prostheses is to create a transmission of force in the most efficient manner possible. To achieve this,

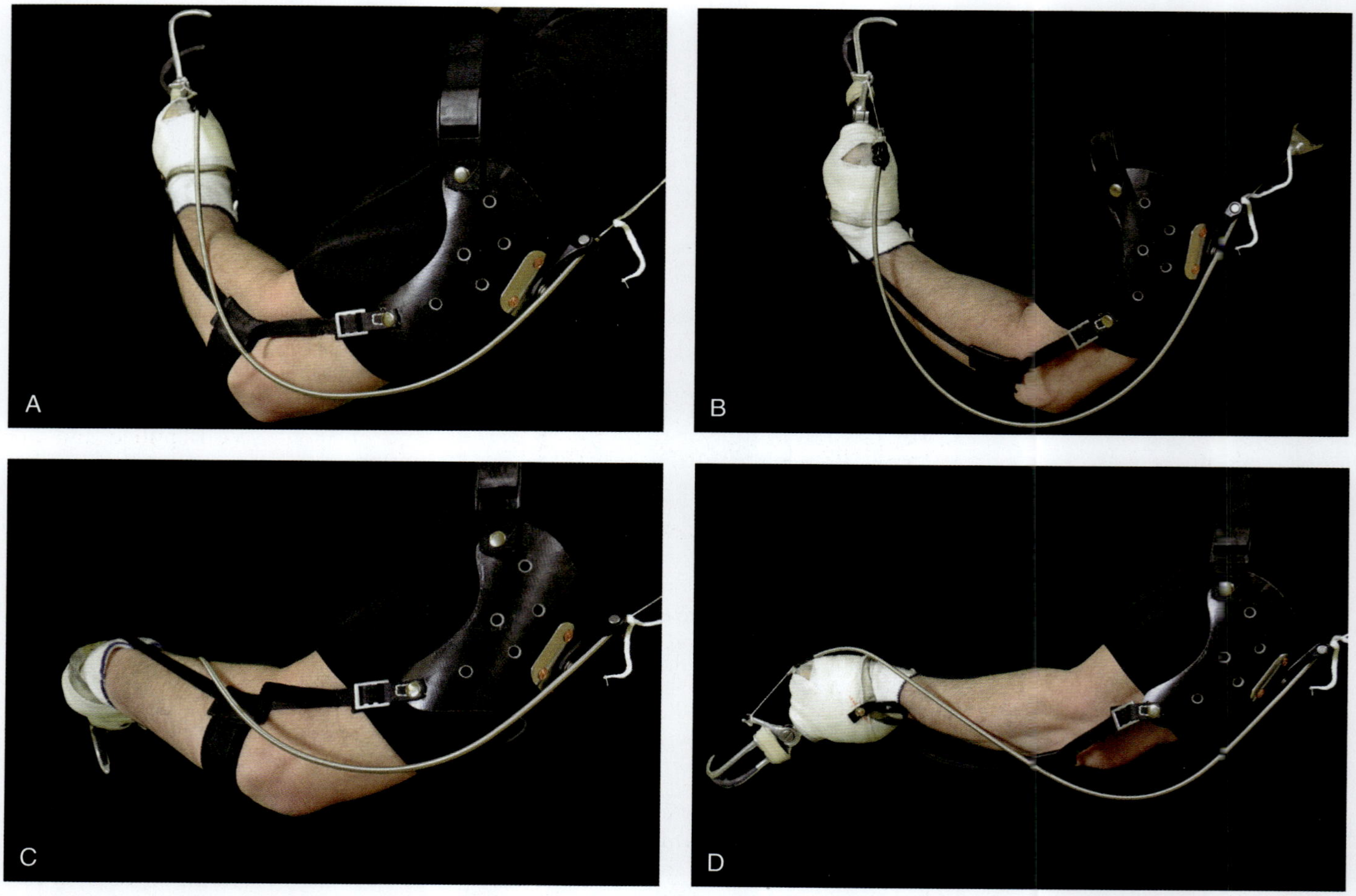

Section 2: Upper Limb

FIGURE 7 Photographs of traditional figure-of-8 harnessing of a partial hand prosthesis, which allows multiple degrees of freedom **A**, Full opening of the hook in the neutral position. Positioning the hook with wrist flexion (**B**), full pronation (**C**), and radial deviation and wrist extension (**D**). (Courtesy of David B. Rotter, CPO, David Rotter Prosthetics, LTD, Joliet, IL.)

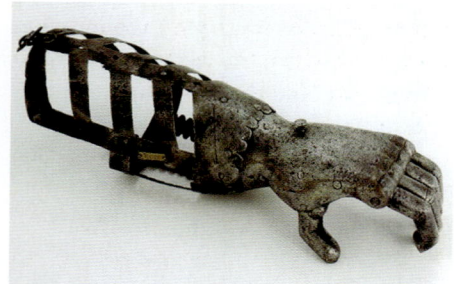

FIGURE 8 Photograph of Götz's artificial arm, 16th century, Weimar, Germany. (Courtesy of Peter Finer.)

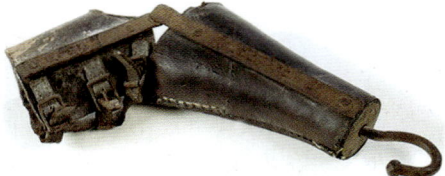

FIGURE 9 Photograph of a transradial prosthesis from the American Civil War era. (Courtesy of Hindman Auctions, Cincinnati, OH.)

the following criteria must exist. (1) The prosthesis must be securely suspended or anchored to the individual's body. (2) There must be a harness and cabling system designed to transmit body movements to efficiently activate a terminal device. (3) There must be an available power source in the form of movement generated by an intact body segment that can activate a body-powered component. (4) The body movement must be able to travel a sufficient distance to complete the action with adequate force to achieve the desired outcome.

Figure-of-8 Harness System

The figure-of-8 harness system has several key component parts (Figure 12).

Axilla Loop

The foundation of the figure-of-8 harness is the axilla loop, which is also known as the anchor because this portion of the harness acts to both suspend the prosthesis and provide a stable anchor for the user to generate power to activate the terminal device. The axilla loop is located through the contralateral deltopectoral groove.

Suspensior

The portion of the harness that is responsible for immediate vertical suspension is called the anterior suspensor

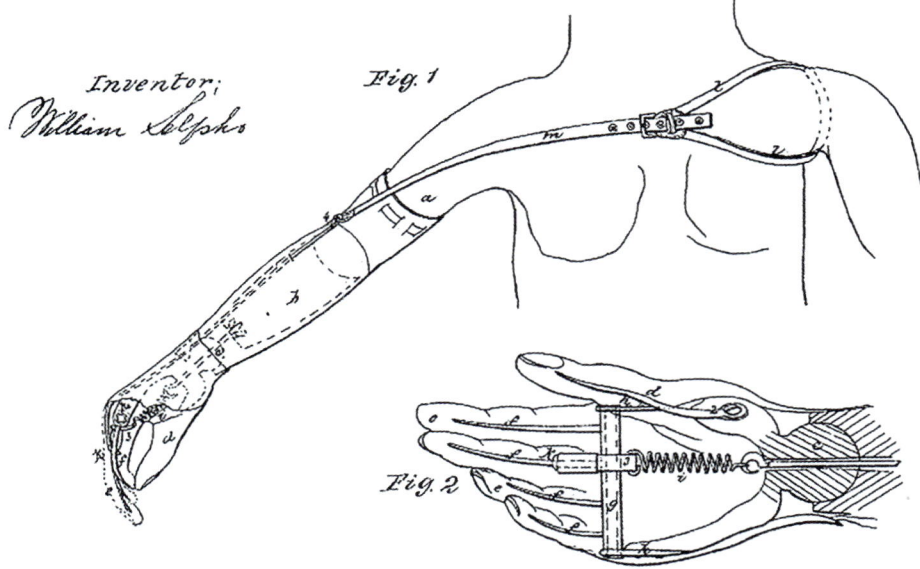

FIGURE 10 Patent drawing for a cable-controlled prosthesis filed in 1857. (Reproduced from Selpho W, inventor: Construction of artificial hands. US Patent 18021. August 18, 1855.)

strap. It starts at the anchor, which is located at the contralateral shoulder, and ascends superiorly and laterally until it reaches the ipsilateral deltopectoral groove. The strap descends and is attached to the inverted Y strap, which connects the harness to the proximal aspect of the triceps cuff.

Control Strap
The control strap travels from the proximal axilla loop across the inferior aspect of the ipsilateral scapula. This portion of the harness connects to the cabling system that ultimately activates the terminal device. The orientation of the strap is an approximate 45° angle that travels over the distal portion of the ipsilateral scapula. This strap is referred to as the control attachment strap.

Harness Center Point
There are two common methods for creating the center point of the harness—a static sewn point and a stainless steel ring juncture (**Figure 13**). The ring style is designed to offer more range and flexibility of movement. The optimum location of the center juncture point is at the midline and distal to the C7 vertebra.

Juncture Between the Harness and the Cable System
Attached to the end of the control attachment strap is the proximal end of a cable. The cable travels through a metal housing that acts to create a smooth and continuous fulcrum. To ensure the housing maintains its shape, it is anchored at two reaction points in the system. The reaction points consist of a proximal cross bar attached to the triceps cuff and a distal baseplate and retainer on the forearm of the prosthesis (**Figure 14**). This continuous cable approach is termed a Bowden housing cable system.

A key feature of the Bowden cable system is that it has a fixed length of cable housing. This ensures that the captured force and excursion at the harness are efficiently transferred to the terminal device. The two reaction points ensure that the housing maintains the same curvature as the prosthesis is being activated, functioning as a smooth and continuous fulcrum for the cable as it travels through it. With an appropriate amount of curvature, there is an optimal distribution of the friction caused by the cable traveling through the housing.[10]

Power Generation
The body movements available to activate a body-powered component are dependent on the level of amputation. As a general rule, the more distal the amputation, the more options remain available for body activation. At the transradial level, the two key movements in body-powered activation are glenohumeral flexion of the ipsilateral shoulder and biscapular abduction. In the former, as the upper arm translates forward with the harness anchored to the contralateral shoulder, the cable is pulled and the terminal device opens. Relaxing this movement allows the rubber bands on the voluntary-opening terminal device to close. This movement generates excellent force and is a key prime mover in body-powered activation (**Figure 15**).

With biscapular abduction, the user moves both scapulae in opposing directions. This widens the back and thereby creates tension on the cable that opens the terminal device. This movement is very useful when operating close to the body and when the user desires to open the terminal device while keeping it in a stationary position (**Figure 16**).

The movements of glenohumeral flexion and biscapular abduction can be used discreetly or simultaneously in combination. The activation movement chosen depends largely on the location in space at which the user would like to activate the terminal device.

The Relationship Between Force and Excursion
The power the body must generate to activate a terminal device is referred to as the activation force needed for activation. The distance the intact segment of the body must travel is known as the activation excursion needed for activation. These concepts are illustrated in the two previously described examples of body activation. Glenohumeral flexion produces both substantial force and excursion. The ipsilateral shoulder muscles generate excellent force and can travel a substantial distance.

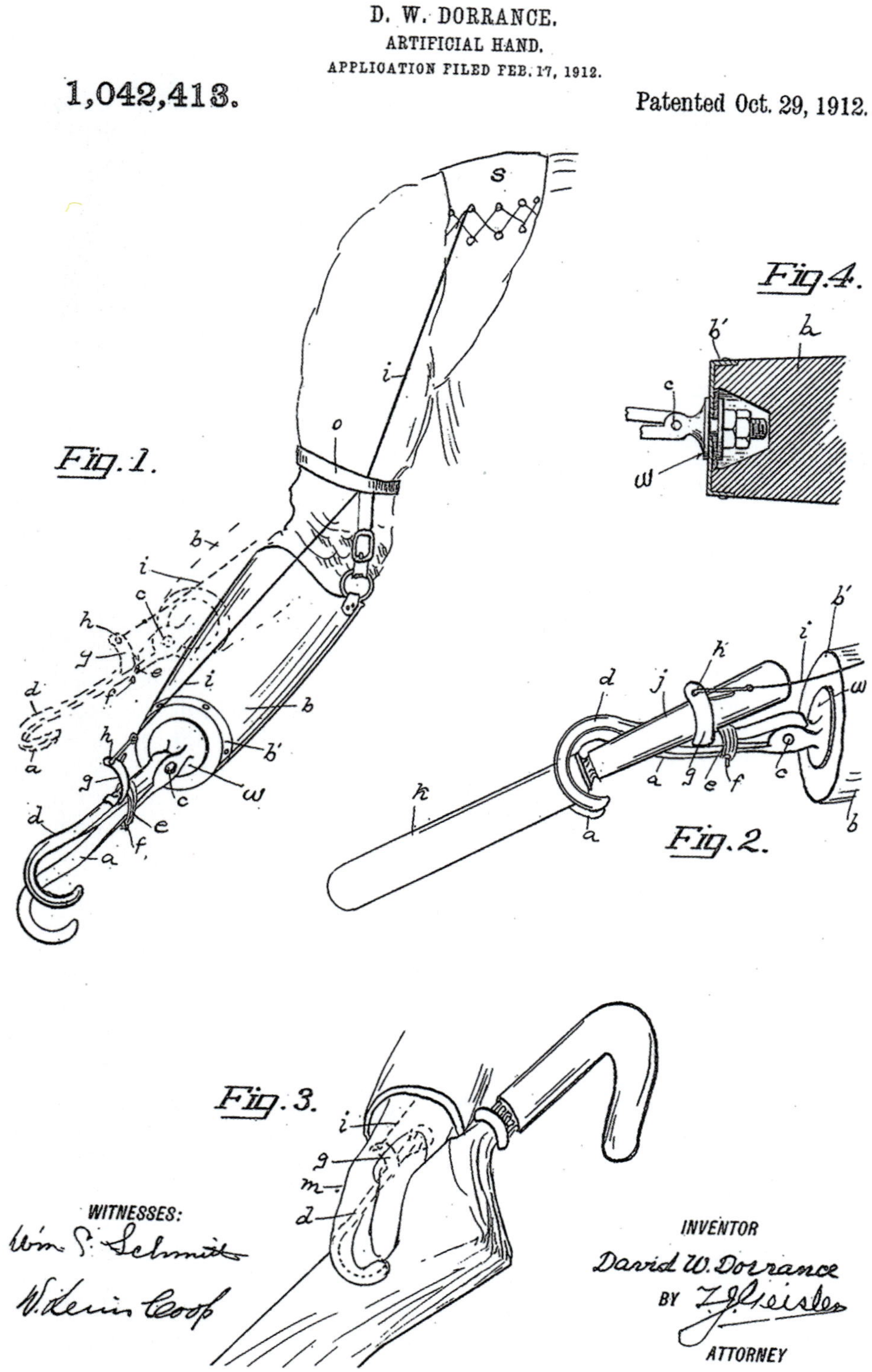

Section 2: Upper Limb

FIGURE 11 US patent drawing from David W. Dorrance's 1912 patent of the split hook. (Reproduced from Dorrence DW, inventor: Split hook. US Patent 1042413.1912.)

In contrast, biscapular abduction generates good force but more limited excursion because the two scapulae can travel only for a short distance when generating the movement.[11]

The force-to-excursion quotient is less of an issue with more distal amputation levels because of the multiple sources of power and excursion available. However, this can become a constraint at more proximal levels of amputation when sources of power and excursion are more limited.

Complete Transradial System Activation

Figures 17 through 20 demonstrate the elements involved in the activation of a complete transradial prosthetic system in an individual with a bilateral transradial amputation. Action starts from a figure-of-8 harness that anchors the system (**Figure 17**). Beginning at a state of rest (**Figure 18**), ipsilateral glenohumeral flexion produces the force and excursion to open the hook (**Figure 19**). Alternatively, biscapular abduction can be used to activate the terminal device when positioned closer to the body (**Figure 20**).

In a resting position and in a fully activated position, the cable housing maintains a gentle curvature. An efficient system maintains this curvature throughout all motions. If the cable housing is too tight, unnecessary friction is created; this causes discomfort for the user and reduces efficiency. If the housing has too much curvature, more force is needed to activate the system and efficiency is lost. Regardless of the level of amputation or the complexity of the prosthetic system, these basic rules of cabling apply. To further promote efficiency, modern cabling systems can be set up using a Teflon (DuPont) lining inside the housing and efficient, tightly woven steel or spectra cable. These combinations act to minimize unwanted friction and improve the overall efficiency of the system.

Alternative Harnessing Options

Shoulder Saddle Harness

The purpose of a shoulder saddle harness configuration is to distribute pressure in locations other than the contralateral deltopectoral groove and the axilla. This design was constructed for individuals who do heavy lifting with their prostheses. Prolonged heavy loading can make wearing a traditional figure-of-8 harness very uncomfortable because there is constant stress pulling into the contralateral axilla. The shoulder saddle design shifts the weight to the ipsilateral shoulder and the contralateral chest wall. When constructing this type of harness, the goal is to

Chapter 11: Harnessing and Controls for Upper Limb Body-Powered Prostheses

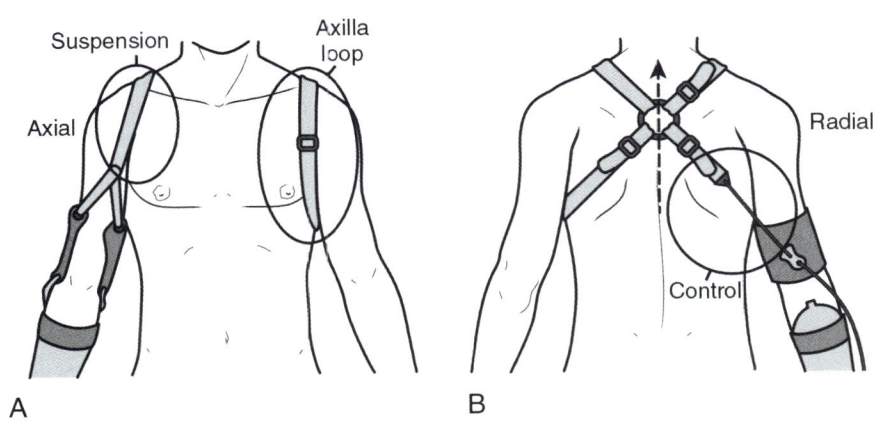

FIGURE 12 Component parts of a standard figure-of-8 harness. **A**, Anterior view. **B**, Posterior view.

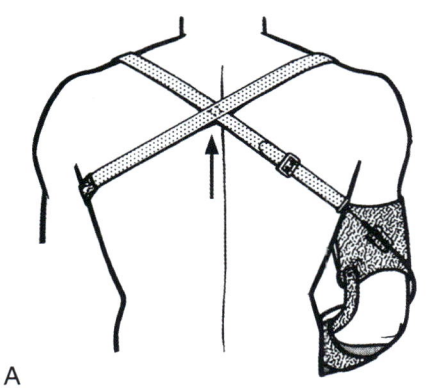 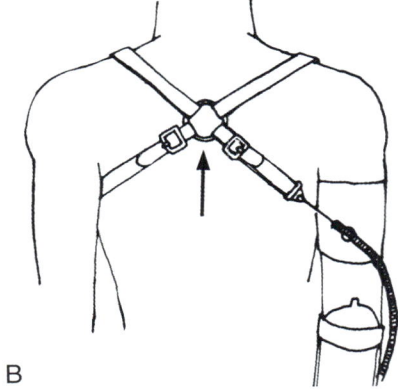

FIGURE 13 Illustrations showing two variations for creating the harness center point. The cross point can be sewn together (**A**) or connected by a ring (**B**). (Panel A reproduced with permission from Pursley RJ: Harness patterns for upper-extremity prostheses, in *American Academy of Orthopaedic Surgeons Orthopaedic Appliances Atlas. Artificial Limbs*. Ann Arbor, MI, JW Edwards, 1960, vol 2, pp 105-128. Panel B reproduced with permission from *Below and Above Elbow Harness and Control System*. Northwestern University Prosthetic-Orthotic Center, 1966.)

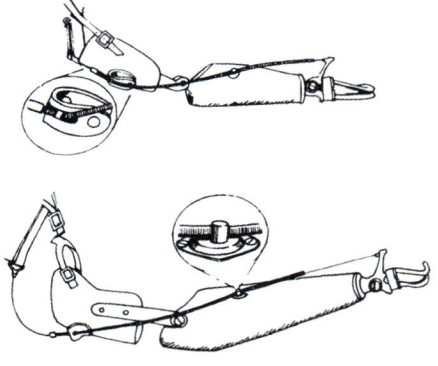

FIGURE 14 Illustration of the cross bar and attachment tab emanating from the triceps cuff (top illustration) and baseplate and retainer on the forearm of the prosthesis (bottom illustration). (Reproduced with permission from *Below and Above Elbow Harness and Control System*. Northwestern University Prosthetic-Orthotic Center, 1966.)

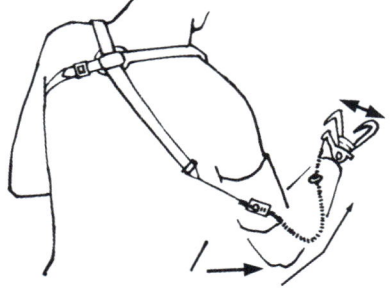

FIGURE 15 Illustration demonstrating that glenohumeral flexion is a primary control motion for body-powered prostheses. (Reproduced with permission from *Below and Above Elbow Harness and Control System*. Northwestern University Prosthetic-Orthotic Center, 1966.)

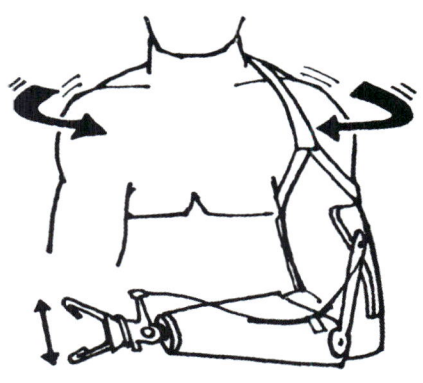

FIGURE 16 Illustration demonstrating bilateral scapular abduction, which represents an additional control motion for body-powered prostheses. (Adapted with permission from *Below and Above Elbow Harness and Control System*. Northwestern University Prosthetic-Orthotic Center, 1966.)

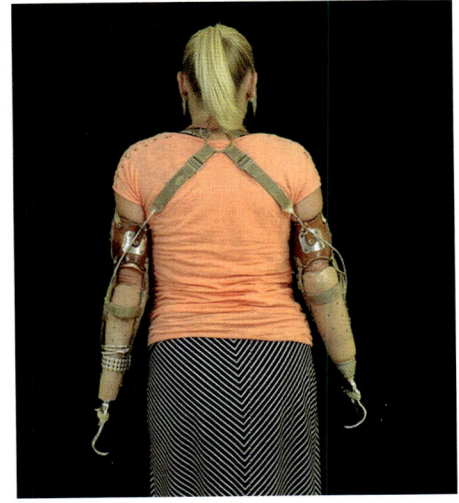

FIGURE 17 Posterior photographic view of an individual with bilateral transradial prostheses. (Courtesy of David B. Rotter, CPO, David Rotter Prosthetics, LTD, Joliet, IL.)

ensure that there is adequate surface area on the saddle and chest strap to distribute the pressure where it can be comfortably tolerated (**Figure 21**).

Chest Strap: Michigan Roller Variant

A variation on the shoulder saddle design is the Michigan roller harness, which uses cable and housing instead of static straps to attach to the triceps cuff. The purpose of this harness design is to allow a greater degree of unrestricted movement about the ipsilateral shoulder (**Figure 22**).

Section 2: Upper Limb

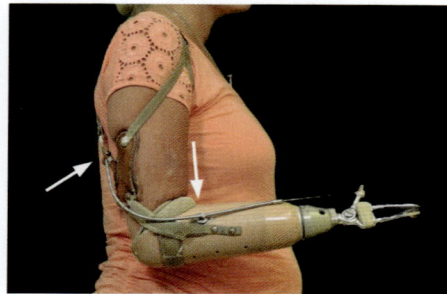

FIGURE 18 Photograph of a patient with a transradial prosthesis in the resting state. Ipsilateral glenohumeral flexion produces the force and excursion needed to open the hook. The arrows point to the two reaction points, one on the triceps cuff and one on the socket. (Courtesy of David B. Rotter, CPO, David Rotter Prosthetics, LTD, Joliet, IL.)

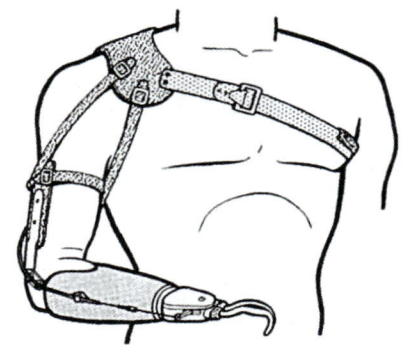 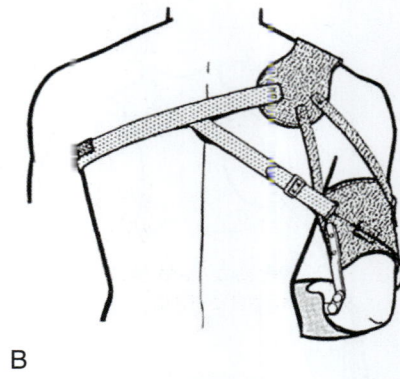

FIGURE 21 Illustrations showing the anterior (**A**) and posterior (**B**) views of a shoulder harness for a transradial prosthesis.

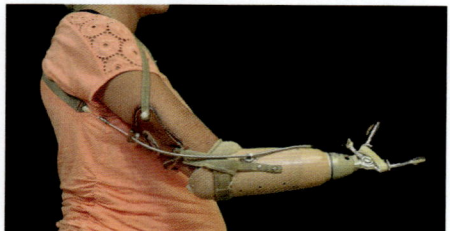

FIGURE 19 Photograph of a prosthesis in which the terminal device has been opened as a result of glenohumeral flexion. (Courtesy of David B. Rotter, CPO, David Rotter Prosthetics, LTD, Joliet, IL.)

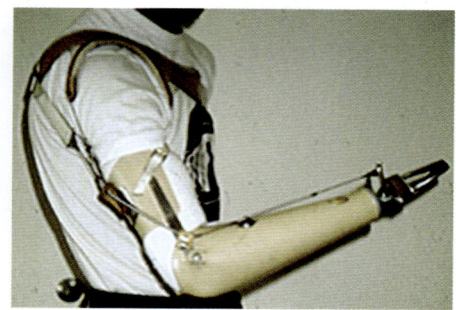

FIGURE 22 Photograph of a patient wearing a transradial Michigan roller harness. (Courtesy of Jack E. Uellendahl, CPO, Hanger Clinic, Phoenix, AZ.)

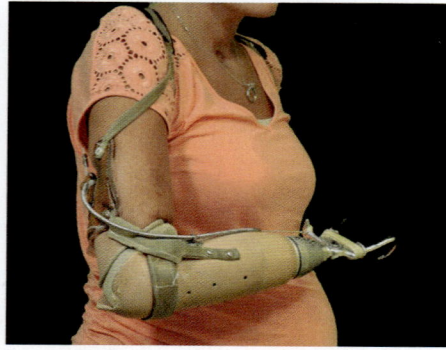

FIGURE 20 Photograph demonstrating activation of a terminal device using biscapular abduction, which allows the hook to stay close to the body. (Courtesy of David B. Rotter, CPO, David Rotter Prosthetics, LTD, Joliet, IL.)

Chest Strap: Distal Strap Variant

A harness design with a distal strap is intended to position the center of pressure on the contralateral chest wall, well distal to the axilla. This heavy-duty harness distributes most of the weight over the saddle portion of the harness. The additional straps ensure the counterforce point on the contralateral chest wall stays distal to the axilla (**Figure 23**).

Figure-of-9 Harness

A figure-of-9 harness is used when the socket is designed to be self-suspending. Self-suspension can be accomplished through a variety of socket designs, including an anatomic supracondylar suspension or pin suspension using a roll-on liner. Because the harness is not needed to suspend the socket, the anterior suspensor strap is eliminated, giving the harness the look of the number nine (**Figure 24**).

When using a figure-of-9 harness, the primary body-powered activation movements remain glenohumeral flexion and biscapular abduction. Based on his personal experience using voluntary-closing devices, prosthetic designer Bob Radocy identified alternative methods of terminal device activation, including elbow flexion (**Figure 25**). To take advantage of these alternative movements, the reaction point is placed on the posterolateral aspect of the socket, close to the juncture where elbow flexion and extension take place. This allows a fine pinch movement that can be used to regulate the pressure exerted on an object with a voluntary-closing terminal device.

Another use of the figure-of-9 concept is the Ipsilateral Scapular Cutaneous Anchor System, developed by Debra Latour, a registered occupational therapist. Latour, who herself has a congenital transradial limb deficiency and has been a lifelong prosthesis user, devised the Anchor to relieve the need for a harness loop around the contralateral axilla while still maintaining body-powered activation. Using medical-grade adhesive, a plastic tab is adhered to the ipsilateral aspect of the user's back, medial to the scapula. A tab on the plastic connects to the harness that activates the prosthesis (**Figure 26**). Pilot data have found this cutaneous anchor system to perform equally to the more traditional figure-of-9 harness in terms of force perception and control when using a voluntary closing terminal device, suggesting its use as a viable harness alternative.[12]

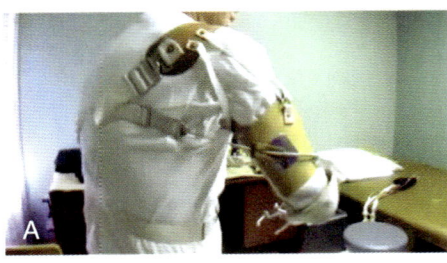
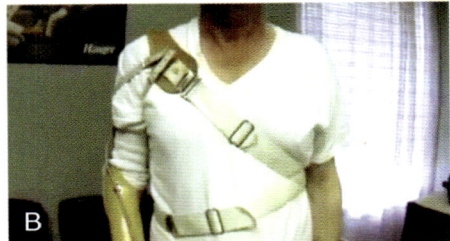

FIGURE 23 Posterolateral (**A**) and anterior (**B**) photographic views of a variation on the shoulder saddle harness that uses a distal circumferential strap to position the chest strap well distal of the contralateral axilla. (Courtesy of Jack E. Uellendahl, CPO, Hanger Clinic, Phoenix, AZ.)

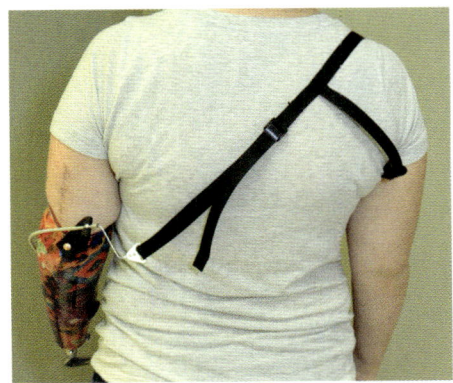

FIGURE 24 Posterior photographic view of a patient wearing a figure-of-9 harness used with a self-suspending transradial prosthesis. (Courtesy of Jack E. Uellendahl, CPO, Hanger Clinic, Phoenix, AZ.)

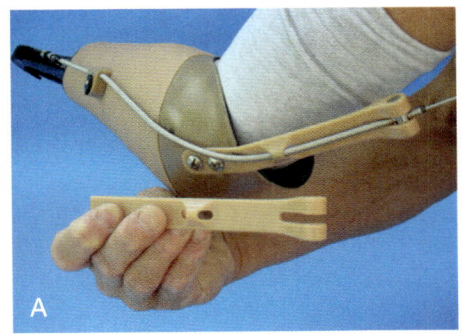
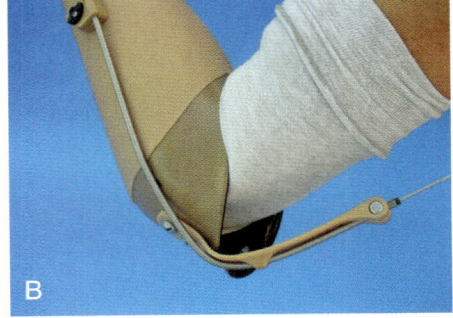

FIGURE 25 **A** and **B**, Photographs of a figure-of-9 socket and harnessing variation that allows the use of elbow flexion as a prosthetic control motion. (Courtesy of Bob Radocy, MS, Fillauer TRS, Boulder, CO.)

Transhumeral Applications

Mechanism of Control

A harness designed for the patient with a transhumeral amputation must control both elbow and terminal device function. Unlike the transradial user who has the remaining degrees of freedom of both the anatomic shoulder and elbow, the transhumeral prosthesis user has only anatomic shoulder function remaining.

Traditionally, an individual with a transhumeral prosthesis is required to operate the device in sequence. The user must first position the forearm in a desired location using the function of the prosthetic elbow. Once the forearm is positioned, the user can then activate the terminal device. The following three discrete actions must take place to accomplish the full sequence: (1) the user must position the elbow in space, (2) the user must lock the elbow, and (3) the user can then activate the terminal device.

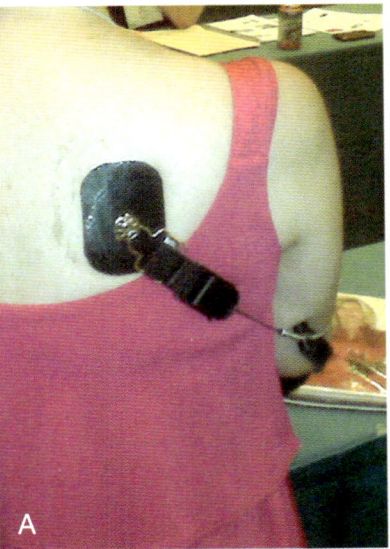
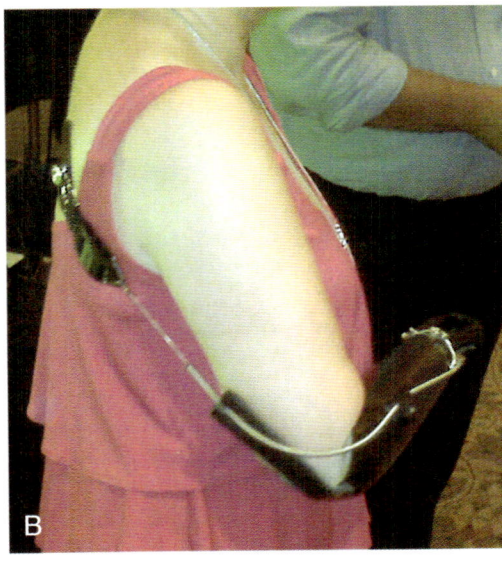

FIGURE 26 Posterior (**A**) and lateral (**B**) photographic views of an individual wearing the Ipsilateral Scapular Cutaneous Anchor System (the Anchor), a body-powered cabling technique that eliminates the need for a harness by the temporary adherence of an anchor point near the ipsilateral scapula. (Courtesy of David B. Rotter, CPO, David Rotter Prosthetics, LTD, Joliet, IL.)

Sequence of Actions

The primary control motions for the user of a transhumeral prosthesis are glenohumeral flexion and biscapular abduction. These movements are used to perform both elbow flexion and terminal device activation, which can be accomplished using a single cable that is responsible for the two actions. This is achieved by splitting the cable housing system to create a fairlead cable system (**Figure 27, A**). The cable housing is split just above and below the prosthetic elbow joint. As glenohumeral flexion is applied, the distance between the two split housings becomes smaller, causing the prosthetic elbow to flex (**Figure 27, B**).

When the elbow is prepositioned, the second action (elbow locking) must take place. In traditional positive locking elbow joints, an elbow lock cable works in a reciprocal fashion when pulled. Cycling between locking and unlocking allows the same body motion to achieve both functions. Body-powered motions commonly used to activate elbow locking include scapular depression, glenohumeral extension, and glenohumeral abduction.

The anterior suspensor of the transhumeral harness is designed to both assist in the suspension of the prosthesis and act as the reaction point for the elbow lock. This is accomplished by attaching the elbow lock cable to the anterior suspensor strap and fashioning the strap from a combination of rigid and elastic strapping materials (**Figure 28**). When the user applies the motions of glenohumeral abduction, glenohumeral extension, and scapular depression, the elbow lock cable anchored in the elbow unit becomes elongated, causing it to cycle. Relaxing that motion allows the elastic component of the anterior suspensor to rebound and return the cable to the original position. Using this sequence of motions, the user can alternate the elbow from unlocked to locked and repeat as needed (**Figure 29**).

After the elbow is locked, the same cable that flexed the elbow into position is used to activate the terminal device. The user must use additional glenohumeral flexion and biscapular abduction to activate the terminal device (**Figure 30**). Compared with transradial applications, nearly double the amount of excursion is required to complete the sequence of actions. Residual limb length strongly affects the ability to successfully complete these sequences. Longer residual limbs generally allow the user enough force and excursion to successfully complete

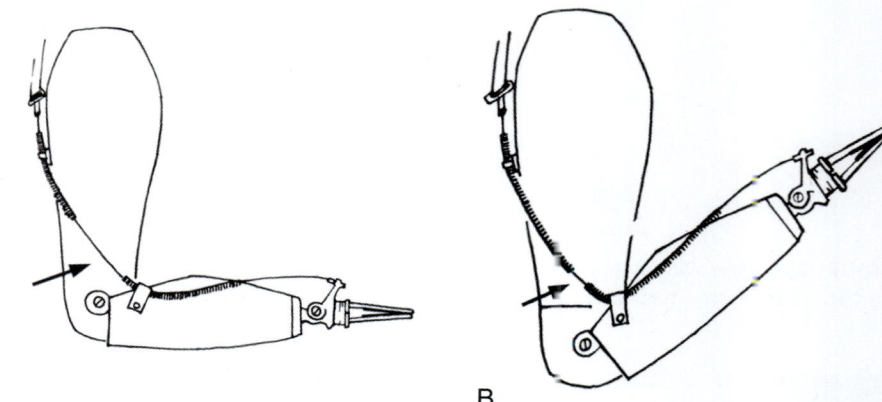

FIGURE 27 Illustrations of a split-housing cable used in a transhumeral application. **A**, Cable (arrow) in elongated position (elbow extended). **B**, Cable (arrow) in shortened position (elbow flexed). (Reproduced with permission from *Below and Above Elbow Harness and Control System*. Northwestern University Prosthetic-Orthotic Center, 1966.)

the sequence at the end range of flexion. Patients with shorter transhumeral residual limbs are less likely to complete the end range action because of insufficient available excursion. A well-fitting, intimate socket is especially important for these patients to ensure that the limited excursion available is captured.

The force-to-excursion quotient in transhumeral harnessing can be influenced by how the cable system is attached. The elbow flexion attachment tab on the forearm portion of the transhumeral prosthesis affects this ratio. There is an inverse relationship of force to excursion, depending on how close or how far the elbow axis is to the elbow flexion attachment tab (**Figure 31**). As the tab is mounted more distally and anteriorly to the elbow joint, less force is required to flex the elbow, but greater excursion is needed. Mounting the tab closer to the joint reduces the required excursion, but it increases the amount of force needed to flex the elbow. An average placement and good starting point of the elbow flexion attachment tab is a distance of 30 mm (1.25 inches) distal and 20 mm (0.79 inches) anterior to the elbow joint center.

Shorter residual limb lengths have both reduced available excursion and surface area on the residual limb to absorb the application of actuation forces. In such instances, excursion can be reduced by placing the elbow flexion attachment tab closer to the

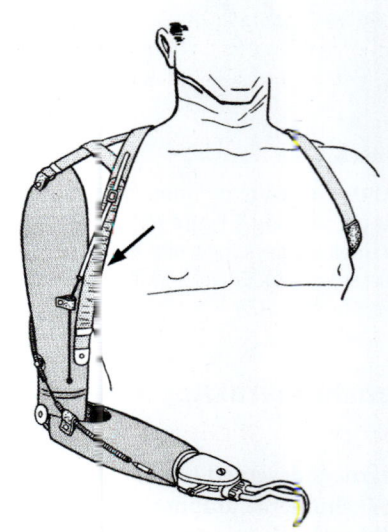

FIGURE 28 Illustration of an anterior suspensor strap (arrow) fabricated from rigid and elastic materials, allowing the elbow lock to cycle. (Reproduced with permission from Pursley RJ: Harness patterns for upper-extremity prostheses, in *American Academy of Orthopaedic Surgeons Orthopaedic Appliances Atlas. Artifical Limbs*. Ann Arbor, MI, JW Edwards, 1950, vol 2, pp 105-128.)

elbow axis of rotation if an elbow flexion assist or Automatic Forearm Balance (Ottobock) is used to offset the increases in the required elbow flexion forces.

Rotational Considerations

The amount of force and excursion captured by the prosthesis is influenced by the intimacy of the socket and harness

Chapter 11: Harnessing and Controls for Upper Limb Body-Powered Prostheses

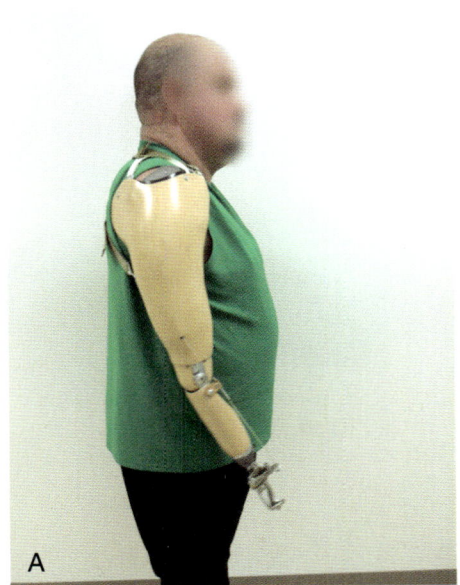 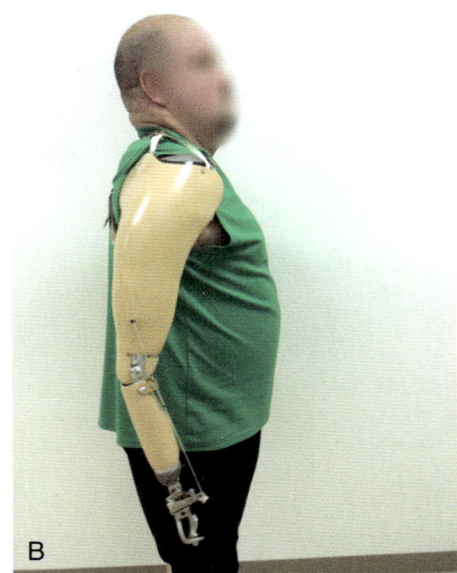 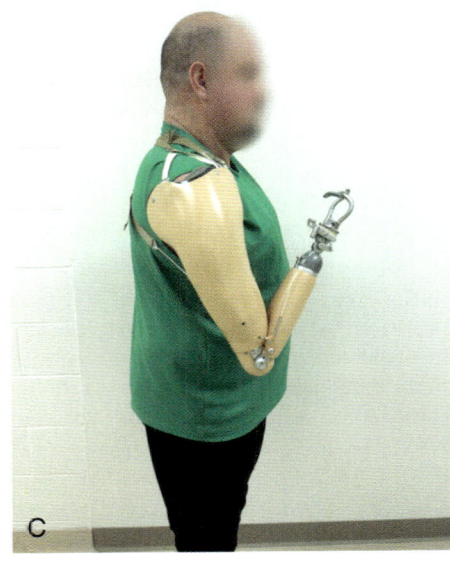

FIGURE 29 Photographs of a patient obtaining the desired elbow flexion angle through control cable excursion (**A**), unlocking the elbow through glenohumeral extension and abduction (**B**), and positioning the elbow in the desired flexion angle (**C**). (Courtesy of David B. Rotter, CPO, David Rotter Prosthetics, LTD, Joliet, IL.)

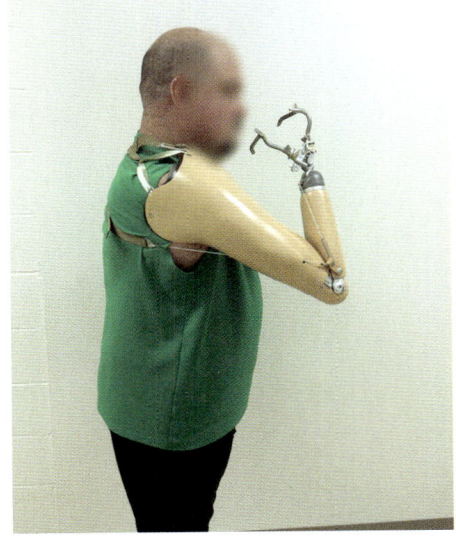

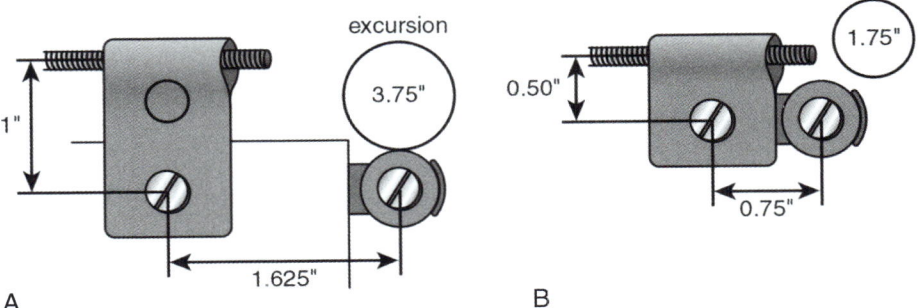

FIGURE 30 Photograph of a patient who, having obtained an advanced amount of elbow flexion angle through control cable excursion, must generate additional control cable excursion to open the hook. (Courtesy of David B. Rotter, CPO, David Rotter Prosthetics, LTD, Joliet, IL.)

FIGURE 31 Illustrations demonstrating the effect of the elbow tab placement relative to the elbow joint and the resultant force and excursion requirements. **A**, As the tab is mounted further from the elbow joint, less force is required but greater cable excursion is needed. **B**, As the tab is mounted closer to the elbow joint, the system requires greater force but less cable excursion.

fit. The anterior suspensor strap and additional lateral suspensor straps function to ensure this intimacy of fit in transhumeral applications while helping to control the rotation of the socket on the user's residual limb (**Figure 32**). When activating the control attachment strap, the socket will want to externally rotate. This can be controlled with a socket that contours proximally around the stable structure of the shoulder girdle. As pressure is applied through the cable system, the posterior aspect of the scapula resists a tendency for the socket to externally rotate. A well-fitting harness ensures that the socket is snugly held to the user's anatomy, making certain the socket is best positioned to resist unwanted external rotation. A loosely fitting harness can detract from the desired control. A well-fitting socket and harness work together maintaining the prosthesis in the user's desired orientation.

Capturing Maximum Power and Excursion

Two common approaches are used to lower the line of pull of the control attachment strap. The purpose of these strategies is to span a greater surface area of the back and capture more power and excursion. Traditionally, a double ring modification can be used to lower the line of pull of the control attachment strap to take advantage of a more optimal position of the strap on the user's back (**Figure 33, A**). More recently, the Biomechanically Aligned Harness Anchor (TRS) has been developed to lower the line of pull for the control

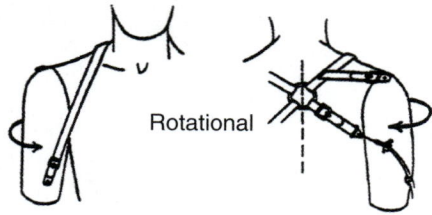

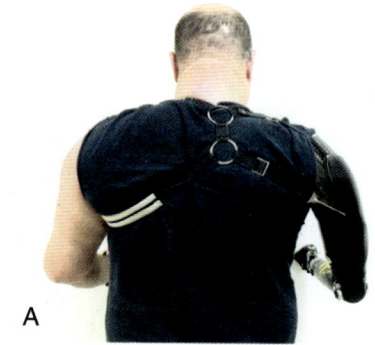

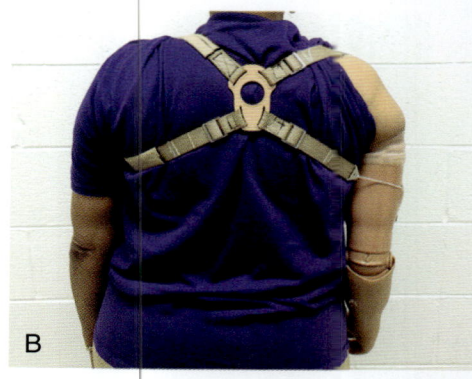

FIGURE 32 Illustration of the anterior suspensor strap (left) and an additional lateral suspensor strap (right). These straps provide an intimate fit and help control the tendency of the prosthetic socket to externally rotate (arrows). (Reproduced with permission from *Below and Above Elbow Harness and Control System*. Northwestern University Prosthetic-Orthotic Center, 1966.)

FIGURE 33 Photographs of patients wearing two different approaches to lower the line of pull of the control attachment strap. **A**, A double harness ring. **B**, The Biomechanically Aligned Harness Anchor. (Courtesy of David B. Rotter, CPO, David Rotter Prosthetics, LTD, Joliet, IL.)

attachment strap to take advantage of a better line of force transmission[13] (**Figure 33, B**). This anchor has the added benefit of encouraging lower placement of the superior center point, which can be helpful for patients whose anatomic shape encourages the standard steel ring to encroach proximally on the C7 vertebra and cause discomfort.

In a more elaborate approach, a figure-of-8 harness can be modified with a horizontal strap that crosses the back. The inferior cross-back strap is designed to harness more surface area of the back for the control attachment strap. This has the effects of stabilizing the anchor for the control attachment strap and lowering the line of pull to take advantage of the broad aspect of the back to generate power.

Transhumeral prosthesis users who are unable to obtain adequate excursion to achieve full terminal device activation in full elbow flexion may benefit from the addition of an inferior cross-back strap modification to the harness. Taking advantage of a better line of pull can maximize both power and excursion output. The inferior cross-back strap limits unwanted migration of the control attachment strap and keeps it firmly anchored in the broad powerful area of the user's back. The modification may allow individuals with shorter residual limbs to fully open the terminal device at full elbow flexion (**Figure 34**).

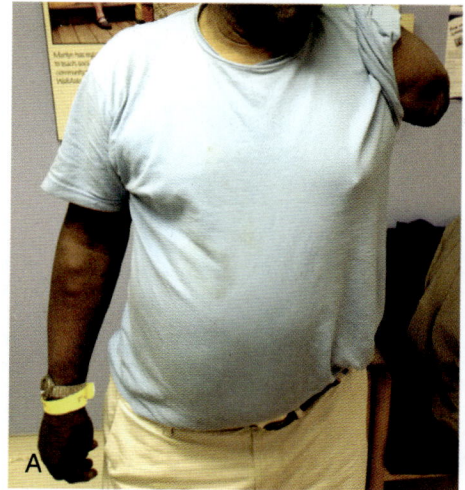

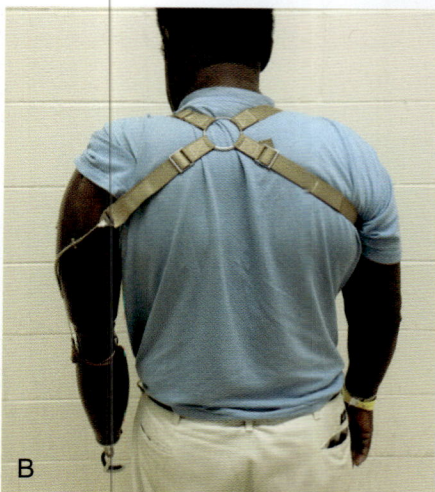

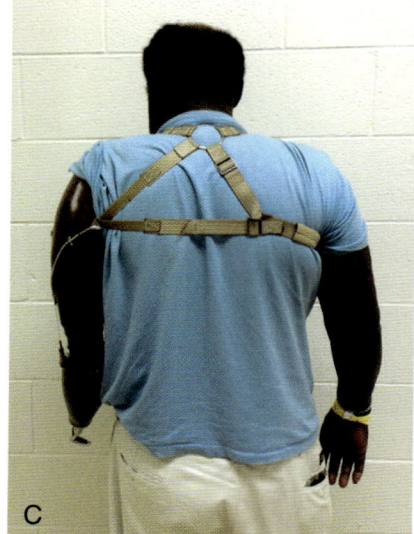

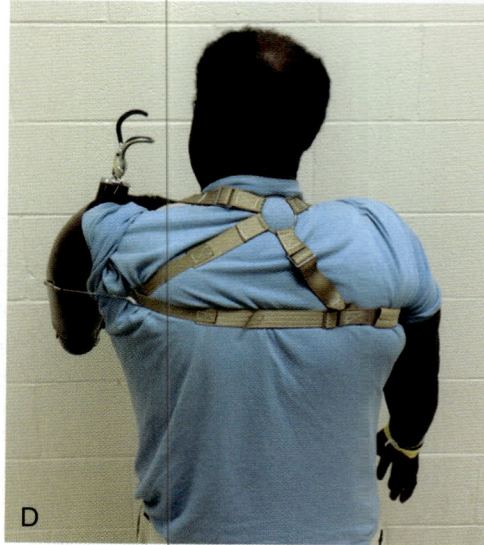

FIGURE 34 Photographs of a patient with a short transhumeral amputation (**A**) who was initially fitted with a figure-of-8 harness (**B**). The addition of a cross-back strap (**C**) ensured a better, more consistent line of pull and allowed full opening of the terminal device at full elbow extension (**D**). (Courtesy of David B. Rotter, CPO, David Rotter Prosthetics, LTD, Joliet, IL.)

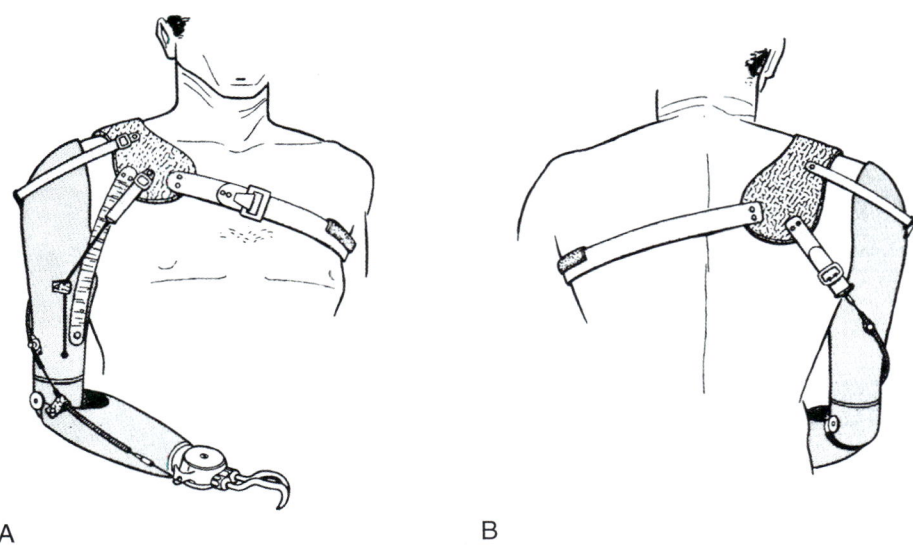
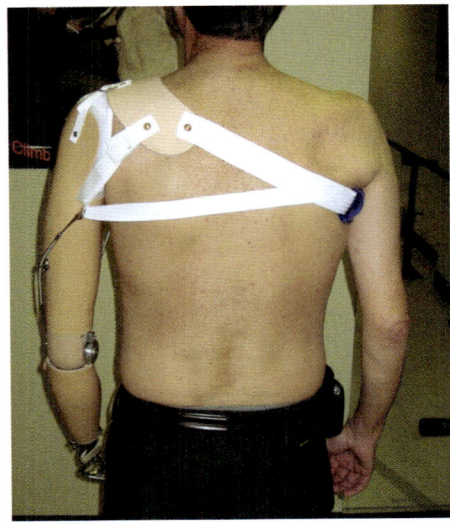

FIGURE 35 Illustrations of anterior (**A**) and posterior (**B**) views of a transhumeral application of a shoulder saddle harness. (Reproduced with permission from Pursley RJ: Harness patterns for upper-extremity prostheses, in *American Academy of Orthopaedic Surgeons Orthopaedic Appliances Atlas. Artificial Limbs*. Ann Arbor, MI, JW Edwards, 1960, vol 2, pp 105-128.)

FIGURE 36 Photograph demonstrating the use of the Z-strap modification to mimic the beneficial effects of a cross-back strap in a transhumeral, shoulder saddle harness design. (Courtesy of Jack E. Uellendahl, CPO, Hanger Clinic, Phoenix, AZ.)

Shoulder Saddle

Similar to its use in a transradial application, the shoulder saddle in transhumeral harnessing is used to achieve the goal of dispersing the pressure of suspension from the contralateral deltopectoral groove to the ipsilateral shoulder and contralateral chest wall. This application is appropriate for patients who use their prostheses for heavy lifting. Although this configuration has good load-bearing properties, it is less efficient for transmitting force and excursion. The placement of the anchor points does not allow the user to engage as effectively in force transmission as has been described previously. Glenohumeral flexion, ipsilateral scapular abduction, and the addition of chest expansion are used. Because the cross-back strap sits in a more inferior position than in previously described examples, the user can expand the rib cage to help engage the anchor strap to complement ipsiscapular abduction and glenohumeral flexion (**Figure 35**).

In an alternative application, the transhumeral shoulder saddle can increase excursion and power by including a Z-strap modification. Similar to the cross-back strap, the Z-strap modification takes advantage of the broad aspect of the user's back, allowing the user to generate more power and excursion (**Figure 36**).

Shoulder Saddle: Michigan Roller Variant

The Michigan roller harness is also used in transhumeral applications. Cable housing runs across the shoulder saddle and houses the cable that suspends the prosthesis. Similar to a transradial application, the purpose of this harness is to create unimpeded smooth movement as the user engages in forward flexion and return extension.

Alternative Transhumeral Harnessing Strategies

Alternative harnessing variations and strategies have been used to achieve the goals of capturing effective force and excursion while maintaining comfort for the user who cannot tolerate pressure in the contralateral axilla. Similar to transradial applications, these techniques lower the anchor point of the harness below the contralateral axilla using a distal circumferential strap.

Y Split

By using a Y split in the harness, the anterior branch travels superiorly to act as the suspensor, whereas the inferior branch travels laterally and connects anteriorly to form the anterior cross-chest strap. The cross-chest strap travels inferior to the user's xiphoid. This approach is appreciated by female users who desire a cosmetic harnessing option that does not have a strap crossing proximal to the breasts that can be seen when wearing low-cut clothing. The control attachment strap is anchored at the fork of the Y split (**Figure 37**). In a variation, the Y split on the user's back captures suspension and control because the inferior Y split acts as the control attachment strap.

Triple Control Harness

The Triple Control Harness (Ottobock) isolates three movements to perform three different functions. The anterior suspensor is responsible for elbow locking and unlocking, the center strap is responsible for terminal device opening and closing, and the inferior strap is responsible for elbow activation. By isolating the discreet movements of glenohumeral flexion for elbow activation and biscapular abduction for terminal device activation, both functions can be used simultaneously.

Bilateral Transhumeral Applications

Similar to harnessing at the transradial level, an axilla loop component is not needed for a bilateral harness. Rather,

Section 2: Upper Limb

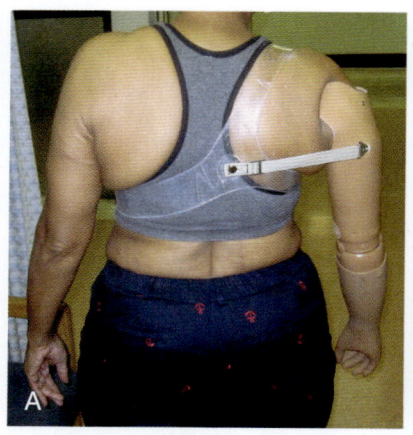
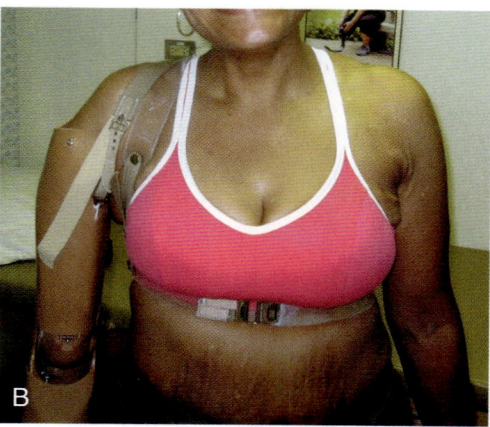

FIGURE 37 Posterior (**A**) and anterior (**B**) photographic views of an alternative harness strategy used to position the contralateral chest strap well distal to the contralateral axilla. This approach is appreciated by females because the strap runs distal to, rather than across, breast tissue. (Courtesy of David B. Rotter, CPO, David Rotter Prosthetics, LTD, Joliet, IL.)

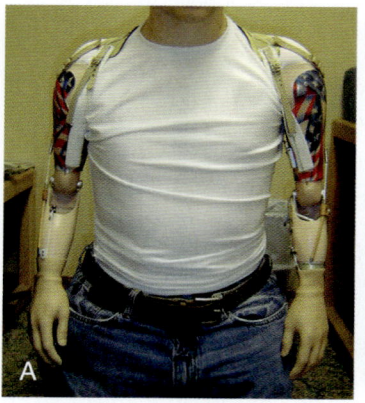
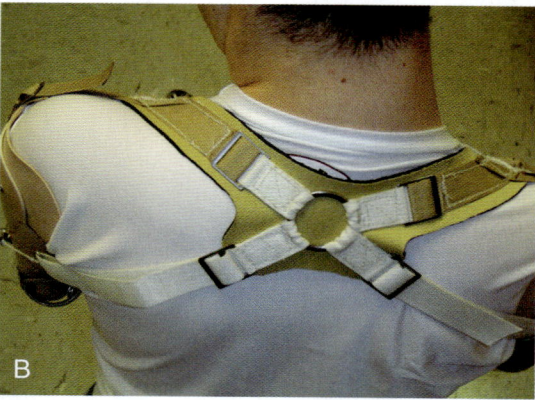

FIGURE 38 Anterior (**A**) and posterior (**B**) photographs of a patient demonstrate bilateral body-powered transhumeral harnessing. (Courtesy of David B. Rotter, CPO, David Rotter Prosthetics, LTD, Joliet, IL.)

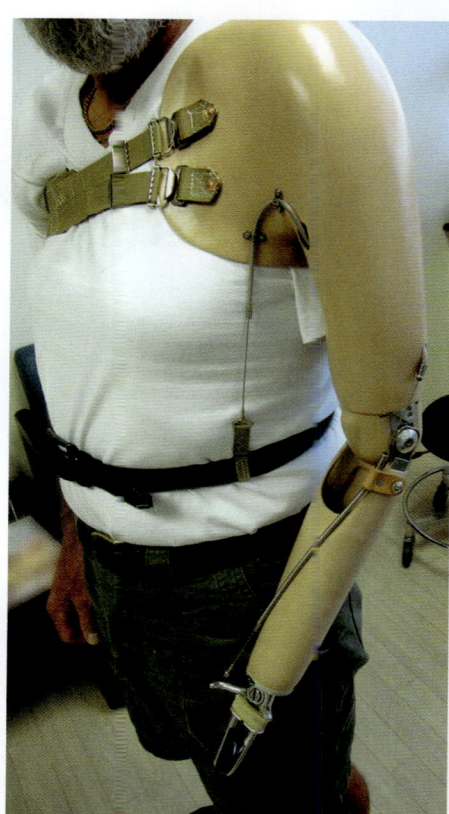

FIGURE 39 Photograph of a patient using a distal waist strap as an anchor point for the elbow lock cable, routed through a retainer positioned at axillary height. This approach allows scapular elevation as a control motion for elbow locking and unlocking for a shoulder disarticulation prosthesis. (Courtesy of David B. Rotter, CPO, David Rotter Prosthetics, LTD, Joliet, IL.)

the two prostheses anchor each other (**Figure 38**).

Shoulder Disarticulation Applications

Harnessing for a body-powered prosthesis at the shoulder disarticulation level is challenging because the sources available for generation of force and excursion are limited. With the absence of the humerus, the powerful and effective movement of glenohumeral flexion is no longer present. The movements available for elbow and terminal device activation are limited to biscapular abduction and chest expansion.

The elbow lock function must also be approached with a different strategy because glenohumeral abduction and glenohumeral extension are not possible. With appropriate prosthetic design, scapular elevation can be used to activate elbow locking. This movement is possible only if there is sufficient anchoring of the elbow lock strap. To accomplish this, a strap is fashioned that travels across the user's midsection, between the inferior ribs and superior to the iliac crest. The elbow lock cable runs proximally through cable housing mounted to the anterior socket wall at axillary height and then reflects distally where it connects, through a control strap, to the waist strap (**Figure 39**). Alternately, the elbow lock control strap can be clamped to the users belt or pants using a suspender style clip.

The Use of Pulleys

Pulleys have been used in a variety of applications to create a mechanical advantage for a given action, and the same concepts of leverage can be applied in body-powered harnessing. When excursion amplification is needed, the control cable runs through a pulley that is connected to the harness. This configuration doubles the required amount of force at the control cable to create the same overall movement but reduces the excursion required. This pulley configuration is used when there is sufficient force present but a limited amount of excursion is available (**Figure 40**).

For example, when using biscapular abduction as a control motion with a shoulder disarticulation prosthesis, the motion generates good power but has limited excursion. Using a pulley, the configuration allows the user to generate approximately double the amount of cable travel per the amount of

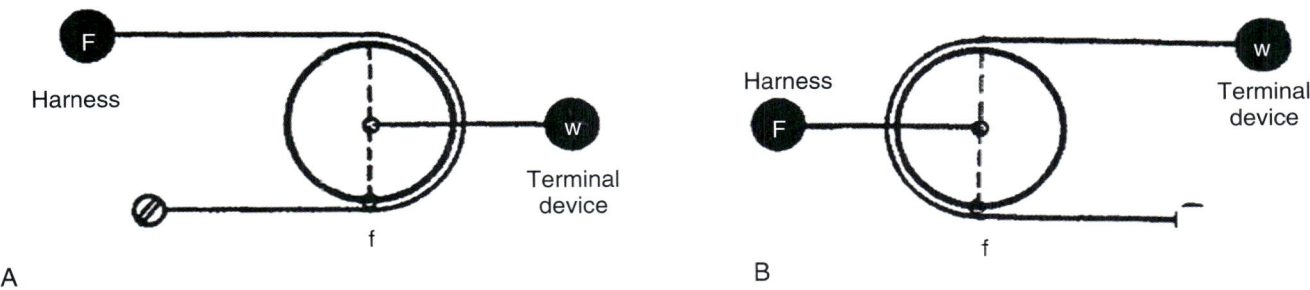

FIGURE 40 Illustrations of the use of pulleys to create force and excursion amplifiers in body-powered harnessing. **A**, A force amplifier is used when ample excursion is available. **B**, An excursion amplifier is used when ample force is available. (Reproduced with permission from *Below and Above Elbow Harness and Control System*. Northwestern University Prosthetic-Orthotic Center, 1966.)

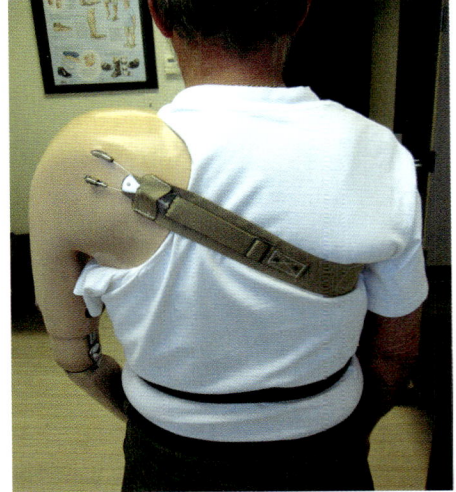

FIGURE 41 Photograph showing an excursion amplifier in the harnessing of a body-powered shoulder disarticulation prosthesis. (Courtesy of David B. Rotter, CPC, David Rotter Prosthetics, LTD, Joliet, IL.)

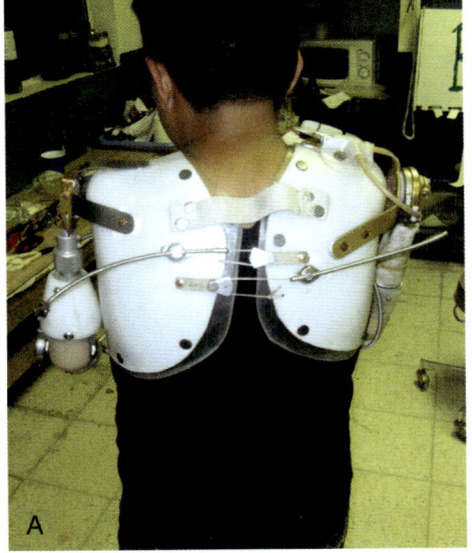

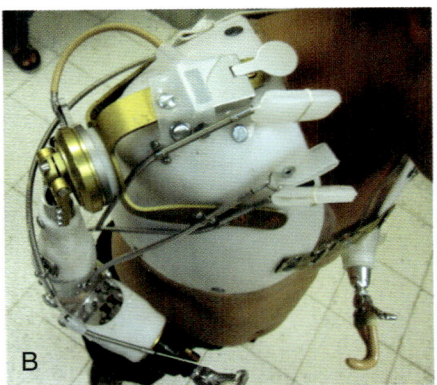

FIGURE 43 **A**, Photograph of a patient wearing a bilateral body-powered shoulder disarticulation prostheses. The bilateral excursion amplifiers control elbow flexion and terminal device prehension. **B**, Photograph showing a nudge switch and series of mouth pull switches that are used to control the shoulder lock, five-function wrist lock, elbow lock, and elbow turntable lock. (Courtesy of David B. Rotter, CPO, David Rotter Prosthetics, LTD, Joliet, IL.)

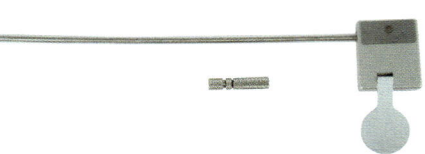

FIGURE 42 Photograph of a nudge switch that is used when a control motion cannot be provided through a harness. (Courtesy of Fillauer, Chattanooga, TN.)

biscapular abduction and chest expansion exerted (**Figure 41**).

In the opposite, less common application of force amplification, the control cable runs through a pulley that is connected to the terminal device. This configuration doubles the required amount of excursion of the control cable to create the same overall movement but reduces the force required. This configuration is used when ample excursion is available and the chosen action requires substantial force.

Nudge Control

If sufficient excursion or force is unavailable using harnessing options, a nudge control device allows the individual to use the chin to push down on a lever to create an action (**Figure 42**).

Harnessing a Bilateral Shoulder Disarticulation

It should be noted that, when possible, it is preferable to use a combination of body-powered and externally powered components when fitting a patient with bilateral shoulder disarticulation. There are, however, some instances in which some individuals with bilateral shoulder disarticulation do not have access or resources to be fit with externally powered components. In such cases, the prosthetists should creatively use the body-powered resources that are available. An example of such a device is shown in **Figure 43, A**. Two excursion amplifiers are mounted opposing each other on the posterior aspect of the sockets. This split-socket design maximizes the individual's ability to use maximum biscapular

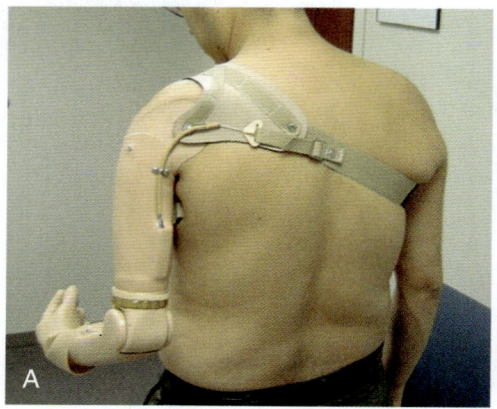
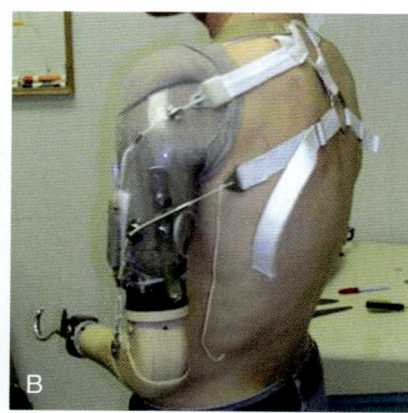

FIGURE 44 Photographs showing the application of body-powered control motions to control electric components. **A**, A linear potentiometer is used to control the position of an electric elbow using glenohumeral extension and biscapular abduction. **B**, In this hybrid setup with a triple control harness, the anterior suspensor strap controls a manual elbow lock, the middle strap controls an electric switch regulating the position of an electric hook, and the distal strap provides body-powered control of the elbow position. (Panel A courtesy of David B. Rotter, CPO, David Rotter Prosthetics, LTD, Joliet, IL. Panel B courtesy of Ryan Spill, CP/LP, Cincinnati, OH.)

abduction and chest expansion. This control motion enables movement of the elbows and terminal devices. It should be noted that the elbow must be locked on one side or this configuration will cause both elbows to flex simultaneously. The practical application of such devices uses one side as the prime mover of the system, with the other side primarily used in positional assistance. Many switches and nudge controls are necessary to activate the many elements of these types of body-powered devices (**Figure 43, B**).

Harnessing and Externally Powered Switches

The same motions available to an individual for activating a body-powered prosthesis can be used to activate switch controls responsible for activating electric components. For example, biscapular abduction and glenohumeral flexion are frequently used to pull a linear potentiometer rather than using a body-powered cable to operate an electric elbow (**Figure 44, A**). The advantage of this control strategy is that it gives the user positional feedback as he or she initiates the movement to pull the switch. It also requires substantially less force to initiate the movement. The same principles can be applied in more elaborate harnessing schemes (**Figure 44, B**).

SUMMARY

Body-powered devices continue to be effective tools for patients with upper limb amputations. As further advances are made in externally powered control, it is critical that continued developments of body-powered components and strategies are not overlooked or abandoned. There will always be a need for body-powered devices in the developing world, and these devices continue to prove their merit in the industrialized world.

References

1. Pursley RJ: Harness patterns for upper-extremity prostheses. *Artif Limbs* 1955;2(3):26-60.
2. Carey SL, Lura DJ, Highsmith MJ: Differences in myoelectric and body-powered upper limb prostheses: Systematic literature review. *J Rehabil Res Dev* 2015;52(3):247-262.
3. Hashim NA, Abd Razak NA, Abu Osman NA, Gholizadeh H: Improvement on upper limb body-powered prostheses (1921-2016): A systematic review. *Proc Inst Mech Eng H* 2018;232(1):3-11.
4. Simpson DC: The choice of control system for the multi-movement prosthesis: Extended physiological proprioception (EPP), in Herberts P, Kadefors R, Magnusson R, Peterson I, eds. *The Control of Upper Extremity Prostheses and Orthoses*. Thomas, 1974, pp 146-150.
5. Garber M: The perfect 3,000-year-old toe: A brief history of prosthetic limbs. *Atlantic* 2013. http://www.theatlantic.com/technology/archive/2013/11/theperfect3-000-year-old-toe-a briefhistory-of-prosthetic-limbs 281653/. Accessed September 14, 2015.
6. Kuniholm J: Prosthetic history: The body-powered arm and William Selpho. http://openprosthetics.ning.com/profiles/blogs/prosthetic-history-the. Accessed September 1, 2015.
7. William S, inventor. US patent US18021 A August 18, 1857. http://www.google.com/patents/US18021. Accessed September 15, 2015.
8. Dorrance DW, inventor. Artificial hand. US patent US1042413 A October 29, 1912. http://www.google.com/patents/US1042413. Accessed September 14, 2015.
9. Hosmer products: Hooks. https://fillauer.com/products/hosmer-5x-hook/. Accessed February 2, 2023.
10. Johnson K, Musicus M, Davis AJ: Upper extremity prosthetic sockets, suspension systems, and component option to fulfill prescription criteria in Spires MC, Kelly BM, Davis AJ, eds: *Prosthetic Restoration and Rehabilitation of the Upper and Lower Extremity*. Demos Medical Publishing, 2014, pp 179-194.
11. *Below and Above Elbow Harness and Control System*. Northwestern University Prosthetic-Orthotic Center, 1966.
12. Hichert M, Plettenburg DH: Ipsilateral scapular cutaneous anchor system: An alternative for the harness in body-powered upper-limb prostheses. *Prosthet Orthot Int* 2018;42(1):101-106.
13. BAHA: Better performance for BP prosthesis wearers. http://www.oandp.com/articles/NEWS_2006-11-27_02.asp. Accessed September 15, 2015.

Upper Limb Externally Powered Components

LeRoy H. Oddie, CP, MBA, CLCP

CHAPTER 12

ABSTRACT

Externally powered prosthetic components are a viable solution for individuals with upper limb amputation or paralysis. Because there are many possible component combinations, selection of an optimal combination can be challenging. Factors to consider in the selection of powered upper limb components include availability, weight, cost, cosmesis, power requirements, noise, durability, repairability, and compatibility, along with the patient's limb length, gadget tolerance, hand dominance, and the anticipated environments where the prosthesis will be used. Upper limb–powered prehensors, wrists, elbows, and shoulders can be characterized by the mechanical joint type, degree(s) of freedom, joint impedance, and power requirements. By comparing these characteristics with the lost anatomic function and unique requirements of the user, an appropriate combination of externally powered and/or body-powered prosthetic and orthotic components may be prescribed.

Keywords: externally powered prostheses; hybrid prostheses; myoelectric prostheses; myoelectric orthosis; powered orthosis

Introduction

There have been steady advancements in the field of externally powered upper limb orthotic and prosthetic components. In large part, the field of orthotics and prosthetics has benefited from technological developments of other industries in areas of electronics, software, communication standards, batteries, actuators, manufacturing methods, material science, and mobile communication devices. Consequently, current externally powered upper limb orthoses and prostheses offer increased hand dexterity, longer battery life, more intuitive control, increased function, and new methods of user interaction.[1]

Although the focus here is primarily on prosthetic components, nonmodular powered upper limb orthoses are commercially available for individuals with upper limb paralysis. Consequently, the terminology focuses on prosthetic components and amputees, yet is also applicable to individuals with upper limb paralysis. Discussion of powered upper limb orthoses is included at the end of the chapter.

The intact upper limb effortlessly performs both fine and gross motor tasks and even subtly contributes to communication.[2,3] It should be remembered that the intact upper limb is marvelously capable of a minimum of 28 simultaneous degrees of freedom (DOF),[4] with sightless proprioception (including position, heat, moisture, and pressure), with substantial strength for gross motor tasks and delicate dexterity for fine motor tasks, all with seemingly unlimited energy and unconscious control in a visually appealing, lightweight, waterproof package with self-healing properties.

In contrast, the upper limb prosthesis is primarily restricted to a supportive role, is often underactuated, and is generally limited to performing gross motor functions. All upper limb prosthetic components are engineering exercises in compromise, with limitations in power, size, aesthetics, strength, cost, and durability. As prosthetic functionality is increased, the cost, weight, and complexity of the components are also increased.[5] In addition, media reports often highlight outcomes of new prosthetic technologies, with no inclusion of important limitations; therefore, older prosthetic technology, which may not only be appropriate but may represent the best solution, is often ignored.[6] Thus, the expectations of individuals with upper limb amputations and their families may be greater than a prosthetist is capable of providing. The clinical team and the prosthetist must carefully inculcate realistic functional and aesthetic expectations as early in the rehabilitation process as possible.

Because upper limb prosthetic components are modular and highly compatible, a large number of component combinations are possible. In addition, these components are often complex in design and function, requiring

Neither LeRoy H. Oddie nor any immediate family member has received anything of value from or has stock or stock options held in a commercial company or institution related directly or indirectly to the subject of this chapter.

This chapter is adapted from Beachler MD, Oddie LR: Upper limb externally powered components, in Krajbich JI, Pinzur MS, Potter BK, Stevens PM, eds: *Atlas of Amputations and Limb Deficiencies: Surgical, Prosthetic, and Rehabilitation Principles*, ed 4. American Academy of Orthopaedic Surgeons, 2016, pp 175-191.

prosthetists to remain abreast of technological developments and consult with prosthetic manufacturers and other prosthetists who specialize in upper limb components. Prosthetists who are inexperienced in treating patients with complex upper limb amputations should consider referral to a prosthetist who specializes in upper limb care. Many manufacturers of upper limb prostheses employ prosthetists and/or occupational therapists with upper limb expertise who can serve as valuable resources.

Factors to Consider in Component Selection

Selecting the ideal combination of components is arguably the most difficult aspect in the provision of prostheses for upper limb amputees. Factors to consider in the selection of powered upper limb components include availability, weight, cost, cosmesis, noise, durability, repairability, and component compatibility, as well as patient-related factors such as limb length, gadget tolerance, and the environments where the prosthesis will be used.

Availability

Because the market for powered upper limb components is small, there are substantial product gaps such as the lack of powered wrists with multiple DOF. With knowledge of both what is and what is not commercially available, prosthetists and occupational therapists specializing in the care of individuals with upper limb amputation can serve as excellent resources for recommending appropriate prosthetic components.

Weight

Weight is an important factor in selecting an upper limb prosthesis. Multiple surveys have indicated that excessive weight is a cause for prosthesis abandonment.[7,8] Powered upper limb components inherently have more mass than other upper limb components because the sources of actuation (motors) and power (batteries) are usually contained within the prosthesis. However, this increased weight often results in increased function, which may be a priority for some users. Because weight tolerance is dependent on the strength of the individual amputee, weight is more likely to affect smaller individuals. Decreases in component mass are seldom proportional to decreases in component size.

Importantly, not all component weight is equal. Static weight (component weight measured on a scale)[9] does not equate to functional weight (the weight of the device perceived by the amputee during use). The more proximal the placement of the weight, the less the user perceives it. Depending on the length of the residual limb and component selection, the prosthetist can strategically decrease functional weight. For example, in a patient with a short transhumeral amputation, the prosthetist may place the battery proximal to the prosthetic elbow or on the posterior side of the socket, rather than within the forearm where the additional weight would decrease elbow capacity and increase perceived weight with humeral flexion. The overall functional and static weight must be considered when selecting a suspension method as heavier components may eliminate the preferred methods from consideration. Generally, less weight is preferable as less weight is often perceived as increased comfort.

Cost

The costs of powered prosthetic components are substantially greater than body-powered alternatives. Often, the end user does not pay for the prosthesis because the prosthetist is reimbursed by a third-party payer such as Medicare, private insurance, or workers' compensation. However, third-party payers may provide only one prosthesis during the lifetime of an amputee or may not cover the cost of powered prosthetic components because such technologies are considered experimental or investigational.[10] In addition, the amputee's medical coverage may change and the future costs of replacements and/or repairs must be considered. Because cost is not always reflective of function, more expensive components should not be selected unless they are a superior solution for the user's needs. Similarly, costs should not be a limiting factor unless available financial resources are exceeded. A long-term perspective should be used when considering costs because higher initial costs may provide justification for reduced future costs.[11] Knowledge of local and state laws and insurance regulations and the amputee's financial situation should be understood before a prosthesis is prescribed as some component costs may exceed available funding.[1,5,12]

Cosmesis

The importance of cosmesis (lifelike appearance) is highly personal and often culturally influenced.[13] Some amputees desire prostheses with a lifelike appearance, preferring detailed custom silicone prostheses, even to the point of sacrificing essential function.[13] Other amputees recognize that achieving a lifelike appearance with a prosthesis is challenging and thus prefer prosthetic designs which are far from lifelike. Other amputees adopt an intermediate position in which lifelike appearance is appreciated, but a prosthesis that does not draw the attention of a casual observer is also acceptable.[14]

Cosmesis can be further differentiated into static and dynamic cosmesis. Static cosmesis, which is the appearance of the prosthesis when not in motion, may be convincing to the casual observer. However, dynamic cosmesis considers the visual normalcy of both movement and appearance.[15] Dynamic cosmesis is not limited to the appearance of prosthetic components, but also considers how naturally the residual anatomic movement appears, such as the lack or minimization of compensatory movements.[16,17] Dynamic cosmesis often supersedes static cosmesis in importance because unnatural movement will alert the casual observer that the prosthesis is not a natural limb. Dynamic cosmesis may also refer to the motion of a powered prosthetic component, such as direct synchronous supination movement of a wrist rotator in contrast to the smooth motion of the anatomic forearm.[18]

Noise

For some individuals, noise can be just as important as cosmesis. Noise can draw undesirable attention to the prosthesis, diminishing realism.[19] For such individuals, demonstration of powered components before prescription can identify if actuator noise levels are tolerable.

Durability

The importance of durability varies by individual needs. Individuals with upper limb amputations who work in occupations involving manual labor require durable prosthetic components. Unlike the anatomic arm, all prosthetic components lack self-healing properties and have a limited useful life that necessitates eventual replacement. In general, powered upper limb components are less durable than body-powered components. In some instances, it may be challenging to pay for or to obtain reimbursement by third-party payers for the repair and replacement of powered components. The amputee should be encouraged to take personal responsibility in caring for their prosthesis to reduce both the cost and inconvenience of repairs.

Repairability, Warranty, and Service

In some instances, powered upper limb prosthetic components may require repair by the manufacturer. In such cases, consideration must be given to how the amputee will perform essential *activities of daily living* (ADLs) and *instrumental activities of daily living* (iADLs) while repairs are made. Solutions may include loaner components from the manufacturer for the duration of the repair, or the provision of a secondary spare prosthesis.

Component Compatibility

Because upper limb prostheses are assembled from various components, the patient's outcome will only be as successful as the compatibility of such components. Because there is only a limited number of manufacturers making upper limb prosthetic components,[20] the available selection of components is limited, and compatibility between components from different manufacturers cannot be assumed. Some manufacturers only ensure compatibility between their own prosthetic components, whereas other manufacturers develop products with the specific purpose of overcoming the incompatibility problem. If there is incompatibility between components, third parties may offer solutions, but the effect on warranty periods should be considered.

Component compatibility can manifest itself in several forms. The most obvious is mechanical compatibility. The quick-disconnect–type wrists made by several manufacturers allow interchangeability with most externally powered terminal devices, although a formal industry standard has not been established. Although most upper limb components have mechanical compatibility, they may not be electrically compatible. Components may operate at different voltages or the connecting cables may not be compatible. Some manufacturers offer adapter cables to enable electrical compatibility. Given the complexity of upper limb components and potential compatibility issues, a prosthetist with upper limb expertise is valuable in understanding appropriate component combinations, whether mechanical or electrical.

Limb Length

The length of the residual limb can have a substantial effect on the selection of appropriate components and, subsequently, available functions. In general, the restored prosthetic limb segments should be matched as closely as possible in function and cosmesis to the contralateral limb in those with unilateral upper limb loss.[21] In patients with bilateral upper limb amputation, anthropomorphic ratios serve as a guide, and left/right limb segment symmetry should be restored if possible.[21] In elective amputations or revision surgical procedures, the clinical team should consider the length of potential components when planning the amputation length.

For transradial amputations, there is a trade-off between a longer limb that preserves wrist supination and pronation and a shorter limb that allows space for wrist components with flexion features or powered pronation and supination. For transhumeral procedures, a length 12 cm (4.72 inches) shorter than an elbow disarticulation is ideal to permit selection of any elbow components. Although powered elbows can accommodate amputations as long as 5 cm (1.97 inches) short of elbow disarticulation, longer lengths are less desirable because the humeral segment may be longer than ideal.[22] Elbow disarticulations and transhumeral amputations that are less than 5 cm shorter than elbow disarticulations will require a body-powered elbow or outside hinges.

Gadget Tolerance

An amputee may have a physical or cognitive limitation (referred to as *gadget tolerance*) that prevents the use of a prosthesis, or possibly a particular prosthetic component. Each amputee's ability to adjust emotionally to wearing and using a prosthesis is unique and dependent on their personality and psychological stage of loss.[23] As prosthetic components become more complex, a higher gadget tolerance is needed. Modern upper limb–powered prosthetic components have many features, which makes them highly adjustable; however, such components may require interaction with mobile phones, computers, or other devices to access all of the possible features. For example, a prosthetic hand may offer several dozen possible grip patterns, but may require the user to interact with an external device such as a mobile phone to access a certain grip pattern. In addition, all powered prosthetic components currently require battery power, often requiring daily or intraday charging with frequent use. Some amputees may not have the cognitive or physical ability to access the desired features and/or may not be willing or responsible enough to charge batteries daily. For such amputees, simpler externally powered and/or body-powered components may be more appropriate.

Environmental Factors

Powered components have environmental limitations preventing their use in certain situations. Batteries and electronic components can be damaged or compromised by temperature extremes and water exposure. Although some components may be water resistant, most components are not waterproof, and wet environments should be avoided. Sand, dirt, or particle exposure also may compromise function or increase wear rates.[24] If an amputee frequently encounters such adverse environments, the manufacturer's specifications for the selected component should be consulted to ensure component warranties will not be voided with normal use.

Ancillary Equipment

Unlike body-powered prostheses, which require only the power of the amputee, externally powered prostheses require additional equipment for setup, maintenance, and use. Prosthetists and occupational therapists need testing equipment to determine if viable EMG signals are detectable, to refine EMG sensor placement within a prosthetic socket, and to provide muscle training. A computer, tablet, or mobile phone with appropriate software may be necessary for programming the features of microprocessor components. Demonstration tools are available for actuating prehensor devices to demonstrate component function to the amputee before component prescription (**Figure 1**). Amputees may also need a smartphone or other mobile device to actuate additional programmable modes. Although the patient's access to software typically does not incur additional costs, hardware costs should be considered when providing powered components.

Preparatory Fitting

Because of many factors involved in component selection and the possibility of prosthesis abandonment, a preparatory fitting can be a highly effective tool to ensure the amputee is capable of using the selected components and that their functions are suited to their needs.

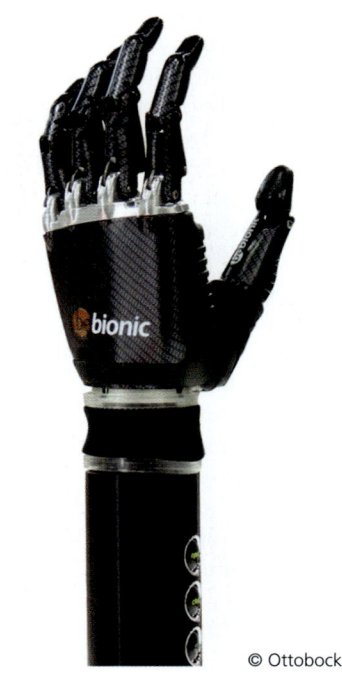

FIGURE 1 Photograph of a demonstration tool and anthropomorphic multiple-degrees-of-freedom bebionic hand. Prosthesis manufacturers can provide clinicians with prosthetic components so that function can be demonstrated to a patient before component prescription. (Courtesy of Ottobock.)

A diagnostic socket (test or check socket) not only ensures appropriate socket fit, but also allows component alignment, lengths, and electrode placement to be adjusted.[25] After powered components have been prescribed, component manufacturers should be consulted to determine if demonstration components or no-obligation trial periods are available to permit flexibility in selecting the final components.

Hybrid Configurations

Upper limb prostheses can be classified into the three broad categories of oppositional cosmetic restoration, body-powered, or externally powered; however, hybrid designs, with body-powered, passive, and/or externally powered components, are commonly prescribed for patients. Hybrid prostheses combine the advantages of both body-powered and externally powered designs, particularly for individuals with high-level and/or bilateral upper limb amputations.[26] Hybrid prostheses may reduce weight, provide simultaneous control of multiple DOF, reduce costs, increase grasping force and lifting capacities, and/or permit finer motor control.[26] However, hybrid prostheses also may compromise working envelopes and increase harnessing requirements.

In higher level upper limb amputations, the critical deciding factor in hybrid prosthesis design is often the choice of whether to power the elbow or the prehensor. Although both configurations are feasible, powering the prehensor seems to be the most advantageous choice.[27] As the number of possible hybrid configurations is vast, an in-depth discussion is beyond the scope of this chapter. However, some hybrid upper limb components are discussed as appropriate.

Characteristics of Externally Powered Components

Joint Types

Joints are essential for functional movement. To understand how prosthetic components mimic the anatomic upper limb, it is helpful to describe the function of the anatomic joints from the perspective of simple mechanical joints (**Figure 2**). Anatomic upper limb joints may be revolute with one DOF, universal with two DOF, or spherical with three DOF.[28] In addition, various joints can be combined in series or in parallel to increase the available DOF.[29]

Joint Impedance (Compliance)

In the anatomic limb, joint impedance (resistance to external force) varies depending on the task. Although variable impedance is feasible for powered prosthetic components, it is very inefficient. Consider the elbow holding a book while reading. The impedance of the arm equals the force of the gravity acting on the book and forearm. In a mechanical system with continuously variable impedance, continual energy would be required to maintain elbow joint position. To conserve energy resources, prosthetic components typically adopt a dual-state impedance control with low impedance (free motion) to move the joint to a desired position

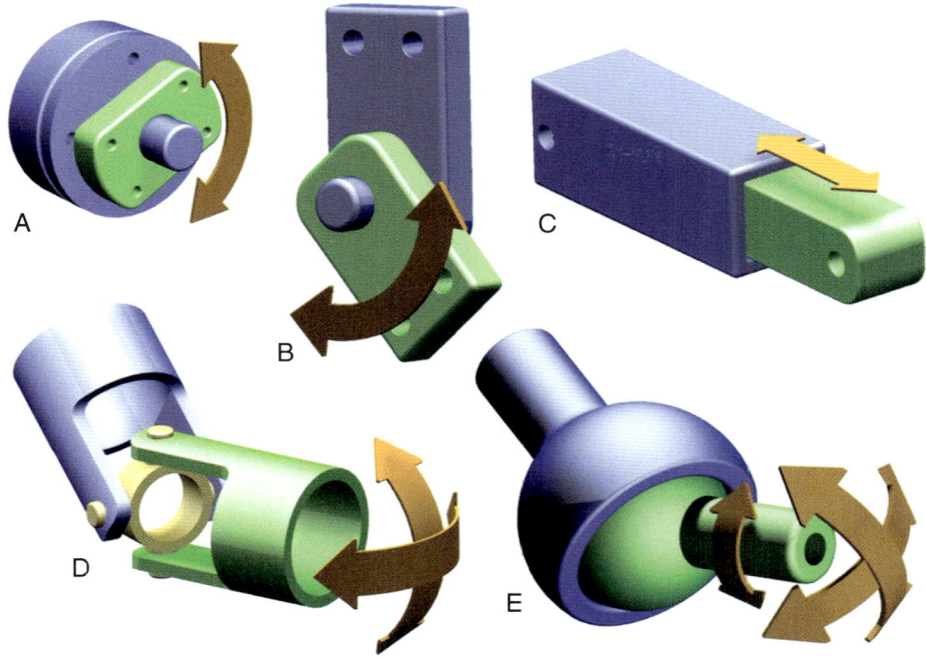

FIGURE 2 Illustrations of various types of mechanical joints. Revolute joints have one degree of freedom and can be arranged as rotator (**A**) or flexor (**B**) joints. **C**, A prismatic joint has one degree of freedom and is capable of linear motion. **D**, A universal joint has two degrees of freedom. **E**, A spherical joint has three degrees of freedom. (© 2015 IEEE. Reprinted, with permission, from Bajaj N, Spiers A, Dollar A: *State of the art in prosthetic wrists: commercial and research devices.* Presented at IEEE International Conference on Rehabilitation Robotics (ICARR), 2015. https://www.eng.yale.edu/grablab/pubs/Bajaj_ICORR2015.pdf. Accessed September 12, 2021.)

and high impedance to lock a joint into position.[30] Other prosthetic components, such as the multiaxial wrist, have a spring-loaded impedance, returning the joint to a neutral position after an external force is removed. To prevent actuator damage, some components have clutch mechanisms to allow low impedance (break-away) after a predetermined force is exceeded.

Movement Quality

Movement quality can refer to the extent to which the movement of powered actuators replicates lifelike motion. Many upper limb component actuators have crude singular velocity movements, which fall substantially short of the natural rapid accelerations and decelerations of normal human movement. In addition, it is common for amputees to overshoot the desired joint position, which increases task time and cognitive load and may lead to user frustration. As technology advances, the quality of movement of prosthetic components may receive more attention, improving functional outcomes and behavioral appearance.

External Power Source

Although unusual power sources, including compressed gas, rocket fuel, methanol, spinal fluid, and implantable glucose fuel cells, have been considered, all current available powered components rely on battery power.[31,32] A user may tolerate daily battery charging but may find intraday battery replacement inconvenient, particularly if the second battery must be carried in-person. Typical daily battery use expectancy should be considered in component prescription as the charging frequency may influence prosthesis acceptance.

Battery performance is dependent on several variables. Battery technology determines the relative power density, with lithium-ion batteries being the current standard. High power density is preferred because longer performance can be achieved with a similar weight. From a user's perspective, it is desirable to have a battery last an entire day before requiring recharging. The capacity of various batteries can be evaluated by comparing the milliamp-hour (mA h) rating, with a higher number representing increased time performance.[26]

Polymer batteries are packaged in a soft pouch, which decreases weight and rigidity. These batteries are advantageous for prosthetic applications because multiple thin flexible cells may be strategically located, such as proximally placed cells that are contoured to the socket to decrease perceived functional weight (**Figure 3**). Polymer batteries are not the same as lithium-polymer liquid electrolyte batteries, although both lithium-ion and lithium-polymer chemistries are available in flexible polymer packaging.[33]

Powered prosthetic systems may operate at differing voltages. For prostheses with multiple powered components, the voltage of one component may vary from another to maximize actuator performance. For example, the elbow requires much higher torque than the thumb or fingers because of the substantially longer forearm lever. To accommodate such complexity, dual-voltage batteries are available, or (less preferably) two batteries may be used.

User convenience is affected by battery type and placement. Some batteries are internal and must be recharged using a charging port before the prosthesis is useable. Other batteries are external (removable) to permit a charged replacement battery to be used while the depleted battery is being recharged. Batteries should be placed as proximally as possible to diminish perceived functional weight and maximize actuator capacity. Proprietary batteries may offer increased performance, but come at the expense of limited local availability. Battery charging times may become a factor if the amputee is not willing to carry a second battery when the capacity is insufficient for a full day of use.

Prehensors

The compactness of the hand and its many functions make it difficult to replicate in a powered prosthetic prehensor. To adequately replicate the core grasps of the human hand, a prosthetic hand-like prehensor requires atleast three or four DOF: two for the thumb, one for the index finger, and one for the remaining three digits.[6] Limited space availability restricts the size and number of motors available for use. Thus, prosthetic hands are often underactuated, attempting to provide similar function with fewer DOF and/or actuators.[34]

Electrically powered prehensors were developed more than a half a century ago and remain commercially available in several forms. Anthropomorphic prehensors take the general form of an anatomic human hand (**Figures 4** and **5**), whereas nonanthropomorphic prehensors may be formed in the shape of a hook or gripper (**Figures 6** through **8**). Initially, prehensors only provided one DOF, with two or three digits in opposition.[35] Recent developments in powered prehensor devices have focused on more anatomically influenced functional designs with the thumb and fingers having multiple DOF (**Figure 9**).

Similar to other powered components, most prehensor control strategies have proportional and digital control variants and are programmable to the user's needs, whether using a single-site or dual-site control scheme. Regardless of type, all prehensors are limited to basic grasp functions, without independent control of digits. For example, although complex hands may offer several dozen grasps and/or gestures, hand function does not allow for complex behaviors such as independent digit control when typing or playing an instrument.

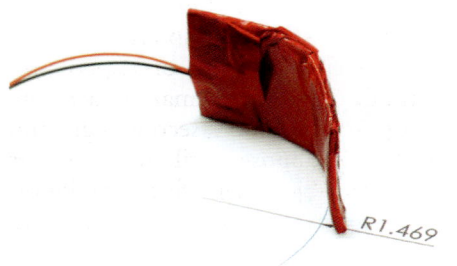

FIGURE 3 Photograph of the FlexCell Mini, a flexible lithium-ion polymer battery for use in upper limb prostheses. (Reproduced with permission from Infinite Biomedical Technologies.)

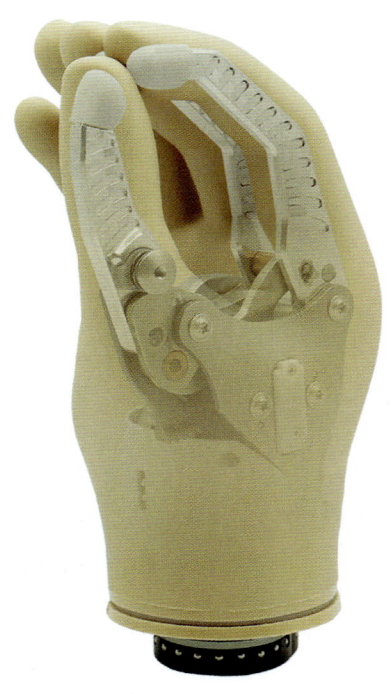

FIGURE 4 Depiction of the Myo Kinisi, an anthropomorphic single-degree-of-freedom prehensor. (Reproduced with permission from Steeper, Leeds, UK.)

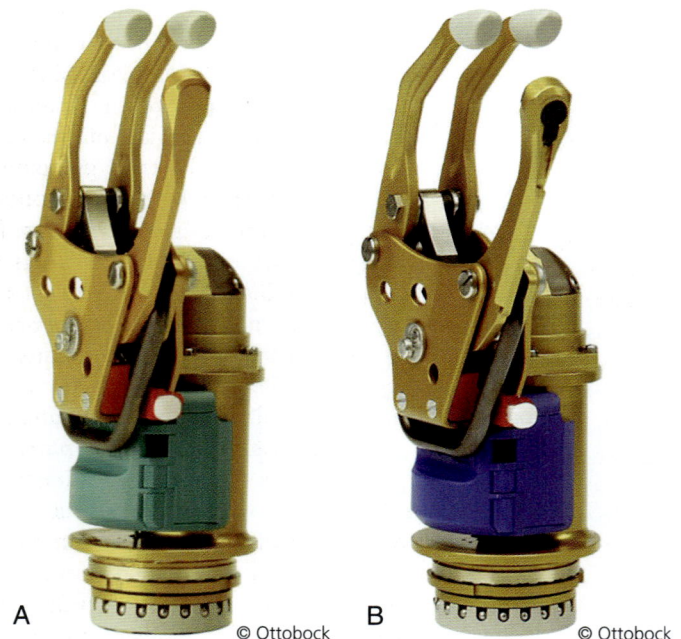

FIGURE 5 Photographs of the MyoHand VariPlus Speed (**A**) and the SensorHand Speed (**B**) without hand shells, examples of anthropomorphic single-degree-of-freedom prehensors. (Courtesy of Ottobock.)

articulation located at the MCP joints and the carpometacarpal (CMC) joint, respectively (**Figures 4** and **5**). Simple hands are typically constructed of an inner actuator mechanism, an outer hand-shaped form, and a cosmetic glove as a cover. Simple hands generally have one or two motors to oppose the thumb against the first and second digits. The third and fourth digits are passive and follow the motion of the first and second digits.

As the digits and thumb of simple hands are oriented in fixed palmar opposition, they are limited to a single palmar prehension grasp (also referred to as three-jaw chuck or tripod prehension). To form palmar prehension, the tips of the thumb, second digit, and third digit oppose until they close or secure an object. This fixed configuration allows for powerful, consistent, and durable thumb and digit operation when grasping. Objects may be grasped using the palmar distal aspect of the digits for a more precise-type grasp or by using a combination of the palmar aspect of the digits and palm to create a power or cylindrical grasp.[36]

The functionality of simple hands has been increased with the addition of intelligent grasp functions. Sensors located in the thumb tip or actuator transmission can limit grasp force or detect an object slipping and rapidly respond with increased grasping force. Examples of prosthetic hands with intelligent grasping are the SensorHand Speed (Ottobock) and the Motion Control ProPlus Hand with Force Limiting Auto Grasp (Fillauer). Intelligent grasping substantially increases user function, prevents dropping objects, and permits grasping of delicate objects. These types of hands should be considered when prescribing simple hands as amputees have substantial proprioception deficits.

Although simple hands may not be appropriate for all amputees because of their limited grasp capability, they remain an appropriate option for many individuals. Simple hands are appropriate for both dominant and nondominant hand loss as the prosthesis primarily provides a supportive role with basic grasp functions. Simple

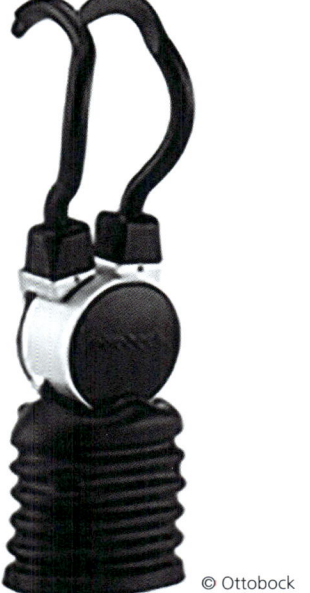

FIGURE 6 Photograph of the AxonHook, an example of a nonanthropomorphic prehensor with revolute, angular opening and closing mechanisms. (Courtesy of Ottobock.)

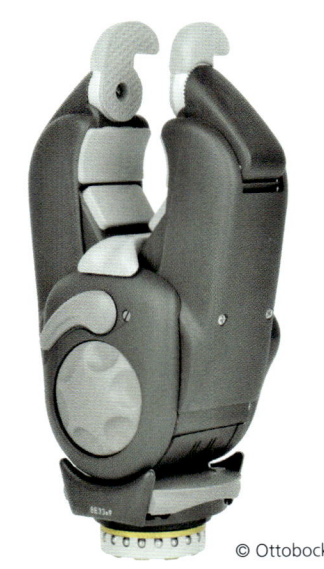

FIGURE 8 Photograph of the System Electric Greifer DMC Plus, a nonanthropomorphic prehensor. (Courtesy of Ottobock.)

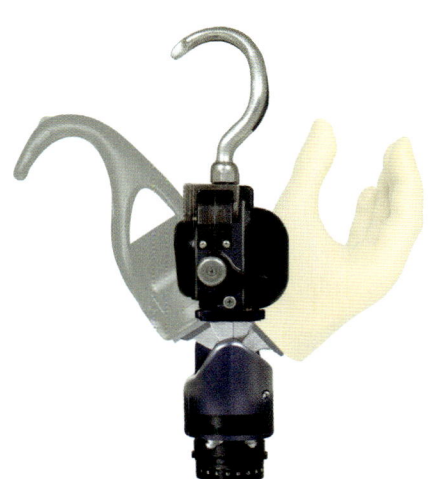

FIGURE 7 Depiction of the Motion Control Powered Flexion Wrist, a powered flexion/extension wrist, depicted with compatible powered prehensors. (Reproduced with permission from Fillauer, LLC.)

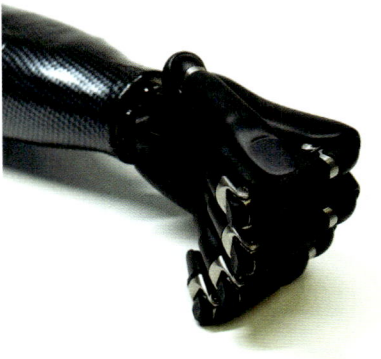

FIGURE 9 Photograph of the VINCENTevolution4, www.vincentsystems.de, a powered prehensor with thumb and fingers with multiple degrees of freedom. (Copyright Vincent Systems GmbH.)

Single Degree of Freedom: Anthropomorphic Prehensors

Anthropomorphic prehensors with one DOF (simple hands) were the first commercially available electrically powered hands. Current designs more closely mimic the shape of the human hand and have revolute joints with one DOF, with simple opening and closing prehension. The mechanical digits and thumb interphalangeal joints are rigid, with

Anthropomorphic prehensors are available in various sizes to improve cosmesis and minimize unnecessary weight. In individuals with a unilateral amputation, the width of the contralateral metacarpophalangeal (MCP) joints is typically measured to determine the appropriate hand size.

hands provide unsurpassed durability because of their simplicity and, when funding is limited, simple hands offer a more economical choice. The function of simple hands may be increased with the addition of passive radial/ulnar deviation and/or wrist flexion/extension units.

Single Degree of Freedom: Nonanthropomorphic Prehensors

Nonanthropomorphic powered prehensors (utility prehensors) were influenced by the desire to overcome functional deficits associated with simple hands. Utility prehensors, often referred to as electric hooks or grippers, are similar to simple hands as they simply open and close. Utility prehensors have one or two motors and a single-DOF rigid orientation of revolute joints for oppositional grasping. These prehensors sacrifice cosmesis for robust design, higher prehensor pinch force, and increased visual feedback for finer motor skills and heavy-duty work.[35]

Utility prehensors provide basic tip, lateral, and cylindrical grasping. The opening and closing configuration of these prehensor devices varies, with the System Electric Greifer DMC Plus (Ottobock) having a parallel opening and closing mechanism with a relatively large opening (**Figure 8**), whereas the AxonHook (**Figure 6**) and the Motion Control Electric Terminal Device (**Figure 7**) have revolute, angular opening and closing mechanisms. Both the System Electric Greifer DMC Plus and the Motion Control Electric Terminal Device feature a safety release lever to disengage the fingers from the gear train and passively release the grip of the device. The Motion Control Electric Terminal Device is also available with Force Limiting Auto Grasp. Utility prehensors may have additional functions, including passive radial/ulnar deviation and/or wrist flexion/extension.

Multiple Degrees of Freedom: (Multiarticulate) Anthropomorphic Prehensors

Recent developments in myoelectric anthropomorphic multiarticulating prehensors (complex hands) have resulted in a new generation of more anatomically influenced designs with increased function. Complex hands have more than one DOF, with multiarticulating thumbs and digits. Complex hands substantially increase the number of functional grasping patterns available to the user, with some having more than 30 unique grasps and/or gestures.

Unlike the singular palmar prehension of simple hands, complex hands add lateral prehension, permitting the thumb to be oriented in multiple planes. Research on uninjured hands reported that palmar prehension was the most widely used static grasp, whereas lateral prehension was the most dominant dynamic grasp.[26] From the lateral and palmar thumb positions, many more power and precision grasps may be accessed. Additional thumb and digit configurations are possible beyond grasps and are classified as gestures. Examples of unique gestures include index finger pointing for typing, the shaka (hang loose) sign, the OK sign, or the thumbs-up sign. Many complex hands allow the creation of custom gestures and grasps for each user.

Although accessing many grasps and gestures can increase the functional outcomes of the user, ease of access may become a limiting factor.[36] The gadget tolerance of the user should be carefully considered when prescribing complex hands because the user's tolerance may need to be fairly high, depending on the number of grasps and gestures available and how many will be used. Equally important is how easily and rapidly the grasps and gestures can be accessed.

There are multiple ways to access the various grasps and gestures of complex hands. Coordinated triggers, including hold-open and co-contraction input signals, allow the user to switch grasps. In the VINCENTevolution4 hand (Vincent Systems), a single trigger allows sequential access to all of its grasps and gestures (**Figure 9**). The bebionic hand (Ottobock) allows access to grasps and gestures with an external switch mounted on the back of the hand and/or an input trigger (**Figure 1**). The grasps and gestures of the i-Limb Quantum (**Figure 10**) can be accessed with multiple input triggers, mobile devices, Grip Chip proximity chips (Össur), or with a designated input trigger followed by coordinated prosthesis movements (i-mo intelligent motion gesture control; Össur).

In addition to grip chips, the Morph2 system (Infinite Biomedical Technologies) can be placed inside the socket proximal to the prosthetic wrist, providing proximity chip/tag compatibility for many complex hands (**Figure 11**). Desired grasps or gestures can be easily and quickly accessed when the prosthesis is positioned within the sensitivity of a strategically placed proximity chip/tag (eg, accessing an index finger pointing gesture when near a keyboard for typing). The user is also able to access additional grasps by manually stalling the desired finger(s) during actuation or manually moving the thumb, as is done with the bebionic hand.

Although complex hands have much more functional capacity than simple hands, their designs may limit their application. With five to six motors, compared with the single motor of

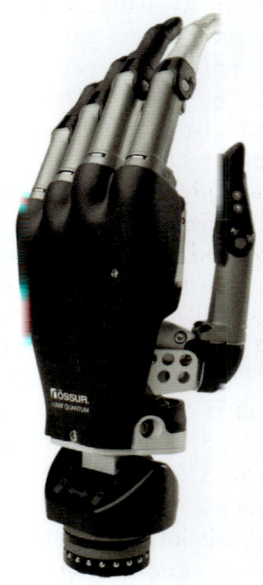

FIGURE 1 Photograph of the i-limb Quantum hand with a flexion/extension wrist. This complex hand has fingers and thumbs with multiple degrees of freedom. (Reproduced with permission from Össur.)

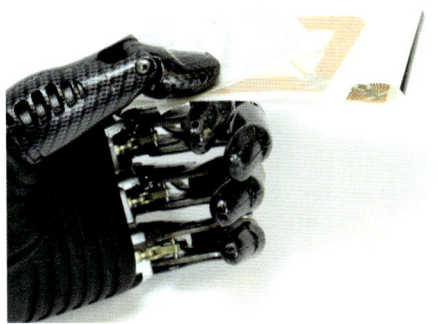

FIGURE 11 Photograph of the Morph2 system, a radiofrequency identification proximity tag system that allows easy access to desired grasps and gestures. It can be used with various multiarticulating hands. (Reproduced with permission from Infinite Biomedical Technologies.)

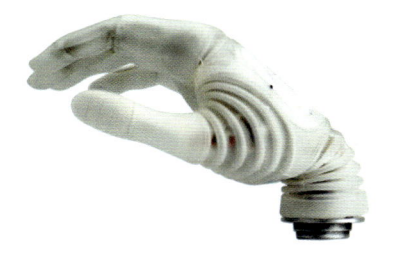

© Ottobock

FIGURE 12 Photograph of the Michelangelo Hand with wrist flexion and extension. This complex hand has fingers with one degree of freedom and a thumb with two degrees of freedom. (Courtesy of Ottobock.)

simple hands, opposition forces may be decreased and there may be an increase in electric current draw, increasing intraday battery depletion. However, larger capacity batteries, up to 2,000 mA h and 7.4 V, are available to increase usage time if space and weight tolerance permit. With many more points of articulation, plastic instead of metal frames, and/or a decrease in thickness, complex hands are not as durable as simple hands. While a few heavy duty multi-articulate hands have recently become commercially available, manufacturers generally recommend complex hands be limited to light-duty or medium-duty activities. These factors should be considered when prescribing such anthropomorphic prehensors.

An in-depth description of each complex hand design, characteristics, and features is beyond the scope of this chapter, particularly as there are many sizes and variations available. However, four commercially available complex hands will be briefly described: the Michelangelo Hand (**Figure 12**), the bebionic hand (**Figure 1**), the i-Limb Ultra hand (**Figure 10**), and the VINCENTevolution4 hand (Vincent Systems; **Figure 9**).

The Michelangelo Hand is unique from other complex hands because of its simpler finger mechanisms. Although this hand has fingers with one DOF, the thumb increases function beyond that of simple hands as it has two DOF, representing the anatomic thumb CMC joint. Each finger consists of one single rigid lever, with one revolute joint providing articulation similar to the MCP joint of the human hand.[37,38] All five fingers are actuated simultaneously by two electric motors driving a cam mechanism. Unlike the fingers, the thumb may accomplish multiarticulate motion, with two revolute joints arranged in series to mimic the anatomic thumb CMC joint. A small electric motor pre-positions the thumb in either palmar or lateral prehension before performing a task.[36] Although the Michelangelo Hand is not compatible with other quick-disconnect prehensors, the AxonHook is available as an interchangeable utility prehensor, and the optional AxonRotation wrist rotator (Ottobock) provides powered pronation/supination.

Unlike the Michelangelo Hand, the i-Limb Ultra, the bebionic, and the VINCENTevolution4 hands have fingers and thumbs with multiple DOF. Unlike the three DOF of anatomic fingers, the fingers of these complex hands are individually actuated with two revolute single-DOF joints (small hand sizes may have only one DOF).[36] Generally, digits two through five articulate similarly to the anatomical MCP joint and distally at a single interphalangeal joint, representing both proximal interphalangeal and distal interphalangeal anatomic joints.[37] The fingers of multiarticulating digit hands curl when flexed, allowing them to conform around the object being grasped. These hands, excluding some smaller versions, typically have five to six motors, with one motor to independently actuate each finger.

The thumbs of multiarticulating digit hands differ from the fingers in that each has one revolute joint for circumduction to mimic the CMC joint and one revolute joint for flexion/extension to mimic the anatomical MCP joint. The bebionic hand has an additional single-DOF revolute joint to mimic the interphalangeal flexion/extension articulation of the human thumb. The thumbs of multiarticulating digit hands have the ability for circumduction into opposed palmar or nonopposed lateral positions, increasing the number of functional hand grasping options.[38] Thumb circumduction pre-positioning may be accomplished with an actuator or manually by the user, depending on the type of prosthetic hand.

The fingers of some multiarticulating digit hands are not coplanar; instead, they are arranged in an arc to adduct during flexion, providing better grasp of spherical objects or thin objects, such as a credit card between the fingers. Conversely, the overall width across the fingers increases as the fingers abduct during extension. To protect multiarticulating fingers and drive mechanisms, each hand is available with a cosmetic glove and has built-in compliance to permit joint articulation when an unexpected force is applied.[37]

Many of the complex hands also have an option to increase user function with the addition of wrist function, such as manual radial/ulnar deviation and/or wrist flexion/extension (**Figures 10 and 12**).

3D Printed Prosthetic Hands

As digital scanners, 3D printers, and CADCAM systems have become more accessible, alternative technological approaches are becoming available, namely 3D printed upper limb prostheses. Although the focus of this chapter is on individual powered prosthetic components assembled together modularly, integrated upper limb powered prostheses are now available. Examples include the Hero Arm (Open Bionics, **Figure 13**) and the TrueLimb (Unlimited Tomorrow, **Figure 14**).

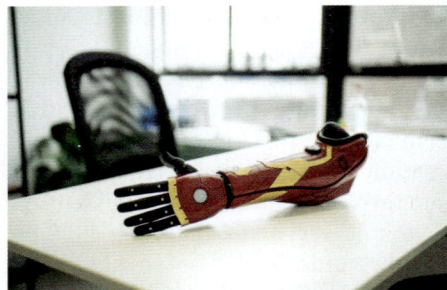

FIGURE 13 Photograph of the Hero Arm, a 3D printed powered prosthesis. (Reproduced with permission from Open Bionics.)

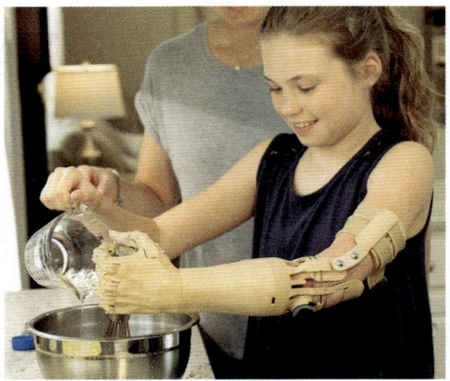

FIGURE 14 Photograph of the True Limb, a 3D printed powered prosthesis. (Reproduced with permission from Unlimited Tomorrow.)

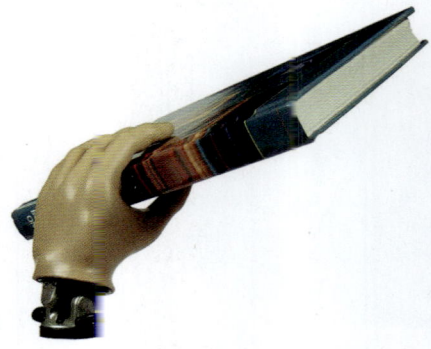

FIGURE 15 Photograph of the anthropomorphic one-degree-of-freedom Motion Control ProHand with Multi-Flex Wrist. This spring-loaded wrist provides flexion and extension and radial ulnar deviation. (Reproduced with permission from Fillauer, LLC.)

These prostheses are functionally similar to traditional components and thus an in-depth review is beyond the scope of this chapter. However, as they are 3D printed, integrating the socket into a monolithic or modular design, 3D printed prostheses may offer several advantages, such as the ability to create more aesthetically pleasing designs and unique shapes/structures (eg, ventilated socket), which would be prohibitively costly with traditional fabrication methods. At the time of this publication, independent research validating the safety, efficacy, and long-term durability of 3D printed upper limb prostheses is lacking. However, 3D printed upper limb prostheses are likely to become more prevalent in the O&P market as clinicians continue to adopt new technology.

Wrist Components

The recent technological advances in upper limb–powered prostheses have primarily focused on the anthropomorphic prehensors, increasing the number of DOF and grasp patterns. However, it is also important to consider the functional role of the anatomic wrist and forearm. Although the human hand is the most functional part of the upper limb, its dexterity is highly dependent on wrist function, particularly for tasks requiring manipulation. For example, many hand grasp patterns would either be useless or require exaggerated compensatory movement from the proximal joints and torso if it were not for the exceptional positioning capabilities of the wrist.[29,39,40] Although research and development of prosthetic wrist components have demonstrated increased function, commercially available options offer limited functionality.[28] In a survey, transradial amputees ranked improved wrist function as third of the four highest desired functions, whereas transhumeral amputees ranked it as second of the four highest desired functions.[41]

Prosthetic wrists not only mimic anatomic wrist motion, but also provide functional requirements unique to individuals with upper limb amputations. Prosthetic wrists reduce compensatory movements that may occur in the elbow, shoulder, and/or torso.[29,39,40] The reduction of compensatory movements is highly desirable because it may increase user comfort and reduce the risk of secondary complications, including overuse injuries.[42,43] In addition, prosthetic wrists may increase socket comfort because of decreased reaction forces exerted on the residual limb.[5]

Characteristics of Prosthetic Wrists

Just as anatomic wrist function occurs in both the hand and forearm, prosthetic wrist function may occur in several components, including the forearm, wrist, and/or prehensor. For example, an amputee may have wrist function with two DOF, with supination/pronation in the wrist component and flexion/extension in the prehensor (**Figure 15**). For this chapter, prosthetic wrist motion includes all wrist motion regardless of where it mechanically occurs, as function supersedes component location in restoring user needs.

Prosthetic wrists may offer one, two, or all three DOF in various axial configurations. In their simplest form, externally powered wrists provide at least one wrist DOF with a rotation-based quick-disconnect mechanism. Additional DOF may increase function through improvement of hand placement and object manipulation, but such increased function will likely come at the expense of increased weight, length, complexity, and cost. Longer transradial residual limbs may have space constraints that further limit the possible DOF.

For powered upper limb components, most prehensors connect using a quick-disconnect wrist, an unofficial industry standard connection common to all externally powered prehensors (excluding the Michelangelo Hand and the AxonHook). The quick-disconnect wrist enables easy exchange of prehensor devices; it is composed of a female housing in the prosthetic forearm that secures to a male ball retention mechanism in the prehensor. The quick-disconnect wrist provides power and communication for the prehensor using a male coaxial plug in the wrist and a mating female connector in the terminal device. The quick-disconnect wrist releases by rotating the prehensor clockwise or counterclockwise approximately 330° until it releases.

A prehensor may be inserted into the quick-disconnect wrist in any rotational orientation, requiring 330° rotation from the initial position for release. Although prosthetic hands are not frequently interchanged with other hands, they are frequently interchanged with nonanthropomorphic prehensors, such as converting from a hand for social situations to a utilitarian prehensor for occupational tasks and/or hobbies. The externally powered quick-disconnect wrist is not the same as a body-powered quick-disconnect wrist. The former has a larger diameter and requires a unique coupler to connect body-powered terminal devices to an externally powered wrist base.

The range of motion (ROM) of prosthetic wrists may vary by amputation level and is accomplished by various mechanical forms. Prosthetic wrists typically have less ROM in both flexion/extension and radial/ulnar deviation than that observed in anatomic wrists; however, all prosthetic quick-disconnect wrists exceed anatomic function in supination/pronation as they rotate a minimum of 300°. The three DOF of the anatomic wrist may be mimicked mechanically using several joint mechanisms in various configurations.

Prosthetic wrist motion may be passive or active, with the latter requiring external power. The joint impedance varies by joint motion. Passive wrist motion may have minimal impedance (free, unlocked), moderate impedance (friction), high impedance (locked), or minimal impedance with a centering force (spring-loaded). The supination and pronation of the quick-disconnect wrist has moderate impedance, with indexed positions every 15°. As the quick-disconnect wrist does not have a locking feature, powered prehensors have limited supination/pronation stability, even with active wrists.

Control strategies for passive wrists impose a relatively low cognitive burden as the positioning of the prosthetic wrist may be rapidly achieved and is typically maintained for the duration of a task. In addition, some passive wrists adapt to applied forces, moving from a neutral spring-loaded position when force is applied and then returning to the neutral position when the force is removed; this strategy further reduces cognitive burden. Passive wrists typically provide dual-state impedance with free and locked indexed positions that allow the prehensors to be prepositioned as desired, then secured during tasks.[43] For such wrists, the unilateral amputee may position the prehensor using the intact hand, by nudging the prehensor against an object, or by securing the prehensor to the object and using compensatory motion to achieve the desired position. For passive supination/pronation of a quick-disconnect wrist, the unilateral amputee often positions the wrist with the intact hand as this is the most rapid method.

To use an active wrist, there are frequently insufficient control sites to offer simultaneous control, although such control is possible in a hybrid design or with advanced surgical techniques such as targeted muscle reinnervation. Subsequently, control strategies for active wrists may impose a higher cognitive burden as the amputee must mode shift active control sequentially from the prehensor to the wrist and vice versa.[44]

Powered wrist function is currently limited to single-DOF supination/pronation (**Figure 16**). Although powered wrist rotators may provide continuous motion exceeding 360°, limiting the supination/pronation end points using software may increase user function by preventing overshooting the ROM typically used for accomplishing ADLs. The AxonRotation wrist rotator returns to a natural hand position after not being used for a set amount of time. Although wrist rotators can provide substantial actuation torque, rotational stability is limited to the friction of the quick-disconnect wrist mechanism. In preparing for elective amputations, the length of a powered wrist rotator should be considered if its use is anticipated as such components are substantially longer than other wrist components.

Discussion

It is easy to overlook the importance of wrist function in positioning the prehensor for optimal function. Restoration of wrist function is not only essential for bilateral amputees,[21] but also provides benefits for unilateral amputees. Examples of common ADLs/iADLs that may benefit from the increased functionality of a wrist with multiple DOF include threading a belt, tucking in a shirt, eating, operating a zipper, removing a wallet from a back pocket, hammering a nail into a wall, opening a door, holding a cup, driving a car, tying shoelaces, holding a clipboard, and carrying objects in the hand.[29,39,45] For amputations at or proximal to the short transradial level, full wrist function is desirable and should be provided if the user tolerates the additional weight. For longer transradial amputations, the user's residual supination/pronation may be sufficient, eliminating the burdens associated with the space requirements, power, cost, and weight that accompany restoration of full ROM.

When the provided wrist function is limited to passive supination/pronation of the quick-disconnect wrist, it should be placed in an optimal orientation to minimize unnecessary compensatory motions of the shoulder and elbow. Such optimal orientation may not be perpendicular to the elbow axis. Although research on anatomic wrist function during ADLs/iADLs suggests an orientation in ulnar deviation and extension as the most important alignment considerations,[41,45] the optimal wrist orientation for ADLs/iADLs has yet to be identified as none of the tested wrist orientations systematically decreased compensatory motions.[17]

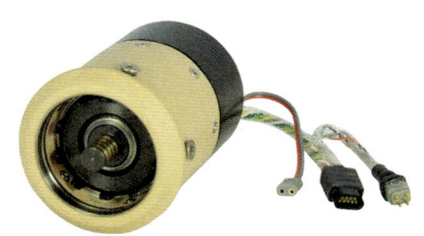

FIGURE 16 Photograph of the MC ProWrist Rotator, which allows supination and pronation. (Reproduced with permission from Fillauer, LLC.)

As prosthetic wrists currently do not mimic the three DOF provided by the anatomic wrist, the question of which DOF to restore is important. Although priorities are not clearly defined, research indicates that wrist flexion/extension substantially improves prosthesis usefulness in more activities and with a more natural motion.[5] However, consideration may be given to sacrificing hand function to increase wrist function as research indicates that complex prosthetic hands cannot be fully functional with a simple wrist rotator. Instead, a simple hand combined with an advanced wrist may provide similar function at a substantially reduced cost.[19]

Certain movements, such as those required for ADLs/iADLs, would not be possible without prosthetic wrist function, such as using wrist flexion to tuck a shirt into pants.[5,40] Even the restoration of two DOF may prove insufficient as wrist flexion/extension are not sufficient to enable all essential activities.[40] However, the combination of flexion/extension and supination/pronation enables amputees to perform many tasks commonly taken for granted.

Elbow Components

The elbow is the simplest of the anatomic arm joints to mimic mechanically, requiring only single-DOF forearm flexion/extension. However, the elbow has substantially higher force requirements than the wrist and hand because of the proportionally longer forearm lever. Elbow function presents design challenges for powered prosthetic elbows as speed and torque are often competing mechanical design goals, particularly when weight is a priority.

Functionally, the elbow effectively increases or decreases arm length, positioning the hand closer or farther from the body.[46] The elbow is essential for many ADLs/iADLs, permitting the hand to perform tasks close to the body, including bathing, toileting, brushing teeth, and holding a mobile phone. The elbow also extends arm length to permit tasks away from the body, including steering a car, typing, and shaking hands. The elbow also bridges the gap between distant objects and the body, which is essential for tasks such as eating and opening doors.

The anatomic elbow has dynamic control, providing slow movement throughout its ROM, maintaining a flexed position, or supporting partial body weight while increasing or decreasing arm length.[46] The elbow is equally adept at rapidly changing its position, actively or passively (with gravity).

Although it may be easy to increase prosthetic elbow actuator torque, it is difficult to simultaneously keep the elbow lightweight and/or retain fast actuation. To statically maintain a flexed position, prosthetic elbows must continuously draw electric current or increase both complexity and weight with clutch mechanisms. Thus, although the anatomic elbow is functionally simple, mechanical replication requires design compromises.

In addition, although the anatomic elbow has only one DOF, the prosthetic elbow adds an additional DOF, providing humeral internal/external rotation proximal to the elbow joint. The soft tissue of the transhumeral residual limb, coupled with the cylindric shape of the residual humerus, precludes an effective coupling to permit transfer of residual humeral rotation to the prosthesis. Many transhumeral socket designs inhibit anatomic humeral rotation to enhance socket comfort and increase socket stability.

Characteristics of Prosthetic Elbows

As the elbow is essential for ADLs/iADLs, all prosthetic elbows seek to mimic anatomic elbow function. Prosthetic elbows are one-DOF revolute joints, with ROM from 0° (full extension) up to 150° (maximum flexion). Actuation is provided by body power or electric motors (**Figures 17** and **18**); the latter being capable of higher torque, but increasing the overall weight of the prosthesis. Most electric motors are housed in the proximal elbow segment to reduce functional weight and increase lift capacity, although some may be located in the forearm.

Prosthetic elbows suitable for use with externally powered prostheses

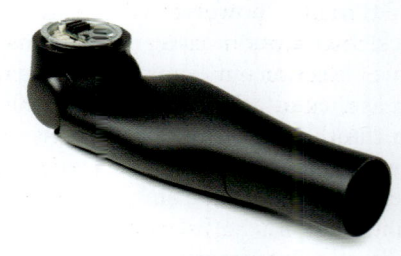

FIGURE 17 Image of the Steeper Espire Elbow providing one revolute degree of freedom. (Reproduced with permission of Steeper.)

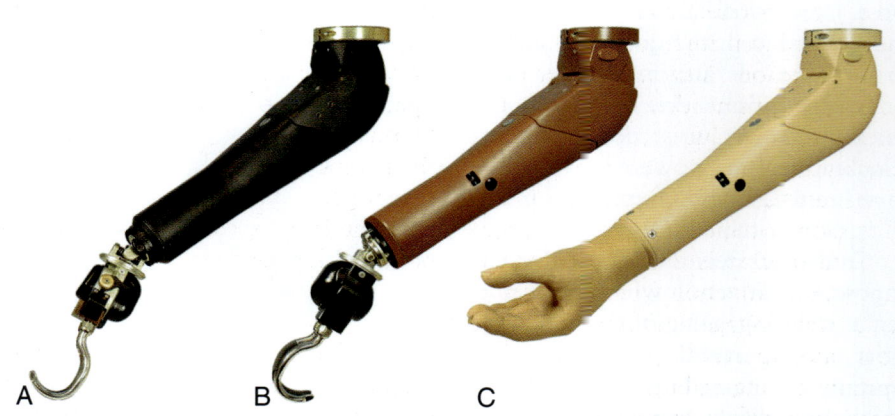

FIGURE 18 Photographs of prosthetic elbow components. **A**, The Utah Hybrid Arm. **B**, The Utah Arm 3. **C**, The Utah Arm 3+. (Reproduced with permission from Fillauer, LLC.)

may be divided into two general categories, body-powered and externally powered elbows. Body-powered elbows that are compatible with externally powered components may be referred to as hybrid elbows. Such hybrid elbows are similar to traditional body-powered elbows as they harness glenohumeral flexion and/or biscapular abduction for elbow flexion. They differ as they require cable routing for powered batteries, inputs, and/or prehensors.

Hybrid elbows may be further distinguished by the type of elbow lock they provide, body-powered (with a harness) or electrical (with switches or myoelectric inputs). Hybrid elbows are advantageous when weight, cost, strength, ROM, and/or limb lengths are concerns. However, as body-powered elbow flexion requires 11.5 cm (4.53 inches) or more of cable excursion, hybrid elbows have a limited working envelope.[21]

Externally powered elbows actuate elbow motion using a combination of electric motors, transmissions, clutches, and flexion-assist mechanisms. Although an in-depth discussion of elbow drivetrain characteristics is beyond the scope of this chapter, several features will be discussed. Typically, brushless electric motors are used because of their increased power density and durability. To optimize motor power, externally powered elbows may use a higher voltage than found in prehensors, necessitating battery accommodation. A flexion-assist mechanism may be present (also available in hybrid elbows) to provide a counterbalance to the gravitational force on the forearm and prehensor. Although a flexion-assist mechanism adds to the overall weight, the live lift (active lift force) capacity is increased and shear forces on the residual limb are decreased.[21]

Although elbow function during powered motion is commonly considered, passive function when the limb is not actively engaged in prehensile tasks is also an important consideration. For example, during ambulation, prosthetic elbows may offer a free-swinging mode to permit natural arm swing and reduce the extent to which the weight of the elbow disrupts the motion of the user's gait. However, direct drive designs likely draw electric current when in free-swinging mode.

As some control strategies only permit operation of one DOF at a time, the user often positions the elbow to a desired position before switching to prehensor control. When not under control, a mechanism must stabilize the elbow position. Although flexion-assist devices aid in stabilization, they lack sufficient force to lock the elbow. Functional elbow stabilization may come from a locking mechanism or from an anti-backdrive motor. The latter may decrease battery capacity, even though no elbow motion occurs. Elbow stability when locked determines the static lift capacity or the maximum weight the user may lift while the elbow is in a locked position (without overriding protective clutch mechanisms).

All commercially available prosthetic elbows provide passive humeral rotation using a one-DOF revolute joint that is perpendicular to the elbow axis. The humeral rotational joint is positioned proximal to the elbow joint, providing internal/external rotation. Joint impedance is typically moderate (user-adjustable friction). Whether joint friction will be adjusted internally or externally should be considered in the prosthesis design, as the former may require an aperture for access. Although it would be mechanically possible to include forearm supination/pronation along with humeral rotation in a prosthetic elbow joint, this option is not offered in any of the commercially available products. Experimental, powered humeral rotational components have been developed; however, because active control of this movement is a lower priority than other functional deficits, these components are not likely to become commercially available until control bandwidth is increased.[47]

Discussion

Powered elbows may be appropriate for many amputees. The most important advantage is the elimination of control harnessing for elbow joint actuation, with a subsequent increase in wearing comfort and expansion of the working envelope. Users with short residual limbs, limited strength, and/or limited ROM may benefit from powered elbows, particularly because of the increased lifting capacity. However, some users may find the increased weight, limited battery capacity, and/or lack of simultaneous elbow and prehensor control too burdensome.

Functional differences, including maximum flexion angle, live lift capacity, weight, flexion speed, and compatibility with the desired prehensors, may be considered when distinguishing between prosthetic elbows. The maximum flexion angle determines how close the user can bring the prehensor to their face, such as when eating, without the need for compensatory motion. Live lift capacity determines the maximum weight of objects that can be actively picked up by the elbow; this characteristic is of particular importance for bilateral prosthesis users. The weight of the prosthesis may also be a determining characteristic.

Although powered elbow control strategies are similar to those of prehensors with proportional and digital sequential control variants, hybrid elbows offer an advantage worthy of mention for transhumeral amputees. By using a body-powered harness to control elbow flexion in parallel with the myoelectric signals of the biceps and triceps for prehension, simultaneous two-DOF elbow control and prehensor control may be achieved. However, although simultaneous control is gained, many advantages of myoelectric prostheses (such as an expanded working envelope and increased live lift capacity) are lost with increased harnessing requirements. Although it is also possible to have a hybrid combination of a body-powered prehensor with an externally powered elbow, such configuration is less common.

Shoulder Components

Shoulder disarticulation and other higher level amputations are uncommon.[48] There are few commercially available prosthetic shoulder component options, none of which provides actively powered humeral flexion/extension or abduction/adduction. Although actively controlled shoulder components have been developed, the commercially available shoulder components only have passive actuation and are similar to those used with body-powered prostheses.[49,50] A shoulder component with an electric lock actuator is available, enhancing function for those with high-level amputations and providing essential function for bilateral amputees if mechanical release levers are not a viable option.

Prosthetic shoulder components offer two DOF, with flexion/extension and adduction/abduction. Anatomic humeral rotation is not provided as prosthetic elbows provide this DOF. The shoulder component may be functionally described as a revolute low-impedance (free-swinging) joint with 36 high-impedance (locking) positions (at every 10°) for the flexion/extension axis. In adduction/abduction, the joint has a second revolute axis with user-adjustable impedance (friction) positioned perpendicular to and functioning in parallel with the flexion/extension axis. An optional abduction ratchet is available to permit incremental abduction positioning and may be disengaged when friction adjustment is preferred. The shoulder component may be adapted for use with endoskeletal or exoskeletal systems and has a central aperture for proximal electrode and/or battery cabling.

Although joint activation for both axes is passive, the user may activate an electric lock actuator to change the flexion/extension axis from locked to free swinging. To passively position the flexion/extension axis, the user activates the electric lock actuator using an appropriate input (such as a switch or myosite) and activates trunk flexion to facilitate gravity-assisted humeral flexion to achieve the desired shoulder flexion/extension. After the desired position is attained, the user again activates the electric lock actuator to secure the joint in the next extension increment. During ambulation, the flexion/extension axis may remain unlocked for natural, passive arm swinging motion.

Powered Upper Limb Orthoses

Traditionally, powered upper extremity components have been limited to prostheses. However, powered upper limb orthoses are now commercially available, so an overview is warranted.[51] Although exoskeletal robotic control technologies are available, this discussion is limited to orthoses with voluntary control, similar to powered upper limb prostheses.

Powered upper limb orthoses are functionally similar to powered upper extremity prostheses as both are intended to restore function (ADLs/iADLs) to the upper extremity. However, there are several unique differences in the application of the orthotic and prosthetic devices because of considerations such as scarcity, interfacing, and the pathomechanics involved in dysfunction.

The most perfunctory difference in these populations is the presence or absence of intact musculoskeletal anatomy to interface with the device; the arm and hand remain intact in individuals with upper limb paralysis, whereas a void exists in cases of amputation. This limits the possible placement of powered components in an orthosis, requiring greater compromise in mechanisms working around the user's intact anatomy. Building an orthosis around the limb as opposed to building a prosthetic limb where mechanisms can be placed within the prosthetic limb, adds bulk to the user. However, there is a more complicated relationship between added componentry and potential bulk with a present but dysfunctional limb.

In the instance of the one currently available myoelectric elbow-wrist-hand-finger orthosis (**Figure 19**), motor housings are mounted externally to both the grasp and elbow elements, each of which contributes two powered DOF to the system. One more DOF is facilitated with friction (ulnar/radial deviation), while two are achieved with a multipositional lock (forearm supination/pronation and wrist flexion/extension). Minimizing these components also minimizes interference during use. By design, a prosthetic hand needs no consideration of anatomic alignment of the fingers to produce a functional grasp: that work is done out of the box. With an orthosis, the value and ability of a simple grasp are directly influenced by the maximal aperture of the grasp, which is user-dependent based on their finger length. Opportunities exist to lengthen the fingers and thumb post externally, but those too come with a compromise of increased bulk, reduced tactile feedback, and an absence of accommodation. The

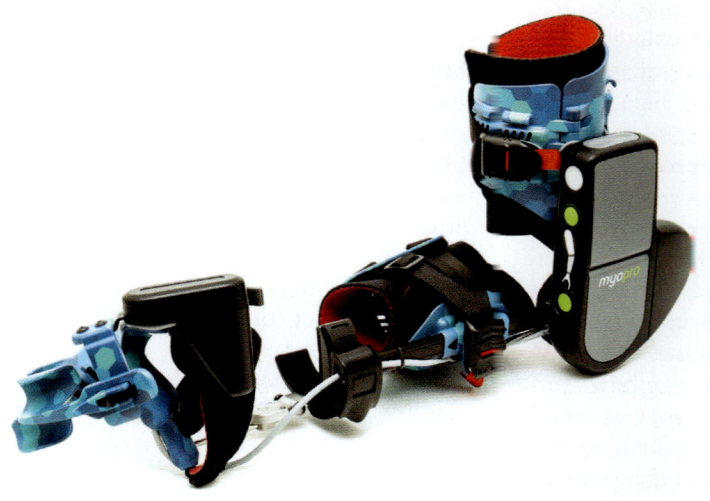

FIGURE 19 Photograph of the MyoPro 2+ Motion G, a powered upper limb orthosis with a powered elbow and hand and passive multiarticulating wrist. (Reproduced with permission from Myomo, Inc.)

lack of DOF is not a significant determinant of function, as conventional, mechanical, two-DOF prosthetic hooks are still archetypical for high-activity, heavy-duty ADL applications.

Another consideration is the power requirements of a system that has to produce unknown amounts of force to create functional motion. A prosthetic system satisfies the forces required for a relatively narrow range of potential component weights. The combined weight of an existing forearm and hand approximates 2% to 2.5% of total body weight.[52] If the user is a stout 250 lb man with a flaccid upper extremity, the device would be required to lift the 6.3 lb of his anatomy below the elbow. Co-contraction or unmitigated peripheral stretch reflex arcs can cause the user to produce force antagonistic to the intended motion actively. These considerations contribute to variable consistency in ROM capabilities, especially at the elbow. Conversely, provided the user is not dysfunctional from a progressive disease, it is expected that whatever muscles are being used to facilitate motion inside the myoelectric elbow-wrist-hand-finger orthosis may become stronger through normal physiologic mechanisms. Any strength and control restored to the muscles that normally produce motion will offload the motor's work requirement.

For example, if a client with a 6.3 lb arm is capable of producing enough work to neutralize the weight of their arm but not lift it, that is a force that the motor does not have to lift. A user capable of producing some flexion at their elbow will have the full strength of the myoelectric elbow-wrist-hand-finger orthosis motor supplementing their motion.

In addition, the electromyographic (EMG) signals in amputees are often normal in magnitude, although some traumatic amputations have strength deficits, which can exclude their myoelectric candidacy, whereas there is a broad spectrum of EMG signal levels in individuals with upper limb paresis/paralysis. For example, the existing upper limb may be flaccid or hypertonic, and there may be muscle strength imbalances or coactivation. Because of this variety in clinical presentation, the sensitivity (gain) of the EMG sensors found in myoelectric orthoses can be adjusted through proprietary software, magnifying the existing signal by a magnitude of 100,000× if needed. This software can be accessed on an ongoing basis by both the user and their clinician to ensure optimum response.

Another consideration is the modularity of powered prosthetic systems compared with powered orthotic systems. Powered upper limb prosthetic components are often modular/interchangeable (open system), and prosthetic systems balance component specialization by making segments modular. In contrast, the currently available powered upper limb orthosis is one contiguous system and is only available completely fabricated (closed system). Modularity is not a feature of powered orthoses. Thus, clinicians are limited to selecting a complete orthosis and cannot interchange powered components or control systems from other manufacturers. This limits the ability to use alternative myosites and control inputs (eg, nudge control, pull switches, etc), although alternative myosites can still be explored for users with insufficient EMG signal strength, and the orthosis can be customized to meet user-specific needs. Because powered orthoses as a concept are still in their infancy, it is expected that more options will become available over time.

Candidate considerations are similar in both populations. Clinicians must carefully consider functional restoration potential (ADLs/IADLs), weight, cost, cosmesis, noise, durability, repairability, component compatibility, and patient-related factors such as gadget tolerance and the environments in which the orthosis will be used. Similarly, patient management between these two groups is comparable. Each system will need adjustment to both the physical attributes of the device and the programming as the user increases their wear-time of the device, attempts new functional tasks, and encounters normal wear and tear.

Clinicians must be considerate of comorbidities that are either absent in or differently affect amputees. For example, some diagnoses resulting in paralyzed upper limbs present with insensate or dysvascular limbs. The prosthetic element that interacts with the environments is inorganic and durable, whereas in an orthosis, the hand is the terminal device. The application of powered forces may incur user injury: either excessive because of lack of sensory feedback or mechanical degradation that the impaired vascular system cannot sustain. Additionally, such diagnoses may present with excessive tone and/or spasticity. Thus, careful consideration must be given to the forces of the orthosis interface, which will be more localized than those experienced through a prosthetic socket.

The application of powered components to upper limb orthoses is long overdue as a possible means to restore ADLs/iADLs in individuals with upper limb paralysis. In many ways, the application of powered orthoses is similar to, although a bit more complicated than, prosthetic management with similar devices. In addition to the functional gains while using an upper limb orthosis, it is also worth noting the therapeutic impact of myoelectric upper limb orthoses. For users with neurologic impairments, unable to independently move or use their arm(s), a powered orthosis can provide a means to facilitate repeatable, active movement, enhance neurorehabilitation, and increase independence with a variety of gross motor and bilateral tasks. Current independent research supports these outcomes and speaks to the overall increase in quality of life for users of these orthoses. Clinicians are encouraged to complete a thorough assessment to determine candidacy for a myoelectric orthosis, bearing in mind the differences in application with prosthetic users.

SUMMARY

Powered prosthetic components have advanced substantially over the past decade, particularly with the recent commercial availability of multiarticulating digit hands. It is hoped that the advanced powered wrist and shoulder components that have been developed for research will soon become commercially available. Despite the advancements, much work is still needed to restore individuals with upper limb amputations to biologic normal states.

As more complex components become available, it will become increasingly difficult for clinicians to remain abreast of individual component features. Understanding the important functional characteristics of upper limb orthotic and prosthetic components may help clinicians to combine such components synergistically to achieve an optimal prosthetic solution for their patients.

Acknowledgment

The author thanks the authors of previous editions of the *Atlas of Amputations and Limb Deficiencies: Surgical, Prosthetic, and Rehabilitation Principles* for laying a foundation for this chapter.

References

1. Trachtenberg MS, Singhal G, Kaliki R, Smith RJ, Thakor NV: Radio frequency identification: An innovative solution to guide dexterous prosthetic hands. *Annu Int Conf IEEE Eng Med Biol Soc* 2011;2011:3511-3514.
2. Krauss RM, Chen Y, Chawla P: Nonverbal behavior and nonverbal communication: What do conversational hand gestures tell us? *Adv Exp Soc Psychol* 1996;28:389-450.
3. Hostetter AB: When do gestures communicate? A meta-analysis. *Psychol Bull* 2011;137(2):297-315.
4. Martin J: Focus on upper extremity: Future of upper-limb design. Clinical perspectives of the DARPA RP09 Program. *The Academy Today* 2008;4(3). http://www.oandp.org/AcademyTODAY/2008Jun/3.asp. Accessed October 23, 2015.
5. Sears HH, Iverson E, Archer S, Jacobs T: Wrist innovations to improve function of electric terminal devices. Proceedings of the MEC'08 Conference, UNB, 2008. http://dukespace.lib.duke.edu/dspace/handle/10161/2814. Accessed October 23, 2015.
6. Weir RF, Childress DS: Research trends for the twenty-first century, in Meier RH, Atkins DJ, eds: *Functional Restoration of Adults and Children with Upper Extremity Amputation.* Demos Medical Publishing, 2004, pp 353-361.
7. Biddiss E, Chau T: Upper-limb prosthetics: Critical factors in device abandonment. *Am J Phys Med Rehabil* 2007;86(12):977-987.
8. Gaine WJ, Smart C, Bransby-Zachary M: Upper limb traumatic amputees: Review of prosthetic use. *J Hand Surg Br* 1997;22(1):73-76.
9. Jones ME, Steel JR, Bashford GM, Davidson IR: Static versus dynamic prosthetic weight bearing in elderly trans-tibial amputees. *Prosthet Orthot Int* 1997;21(2):100-106.
10. Myoelectric upper limb prostheses: Policy. Aetna website. http://www.aetna.com/cpb/medical/data/300_399/0399.html. Accessed October 23, 2015.
11. Meier RH, Esquenzai A: Prosthetic prescription, in Meier RH, Atkins DJ, eds: *Functional Restoration of Adults and Children With Upper Extremity Amputation.* Demos Medical Publishing, 2004, pp 159-164.
12. Godfrey S: Workers with prostheses. *J Hand Ther* 1990;3(2):101-110.
13. Ritchie S, Wiggins S, Sanford A: Perceptions of cosmesis and function in adults with upper limb prostheses: A systematic literature review. *Prosthet Orthot Int* 2011;35(4):332-341.
14. Weir RF, Grahn ED, Duff SJ: A new externally powered, myoelectrically controlled prosthesis for persons with partial-hand amputations at the metacarpals. *J Prosthet Orthot* 2001;13(2):26-31.
15. Lippay AL: External power and the amputee: An engineer's view. *Inter-Clin Info Bull* 1968;7(5):7-12.
16. Abd Razak NA, Abu Osman NA, Kamyab M, Wan Abas WA, Gholizadeh H: Satisfaction and problems experienced with wrist movements: Comparison between a common body-powered prosthesis and a new biomechatronics prosthesis. *Am J Phys Med Rehabil* 2014;93(5):437-444.
17. Landry JS, Biden EN: Optimal fixed wrist alignment for below-elbow, powered, prosthetic hands. MEC 99: Proceedings of the 1999 MyoElectric Controls/Powered Prosthetics Symposium Fredericton, New Brunswick, Canada, August, 1999. http://dukespace.lib.duke.edu/dspace/handle/10161/4921. Accessed October 23, 2015.
18. Abd Razak NA, Abu Osman NA, Gholizadeh H, Ali S: Development and performance of a new prosthesis system using ultrasonic sensor for wrist movements: A preliminary study. *Biomed Eng Online* 2014;13:49.
19. Kyberd PJ, Lemaire ED, Scheme E, et al: Two-degree-of-freedom powered prosthetic wrist. *J Rehabil Res Dev* 2011;48(6):609-617.
20. Caldwell RR, Lovely DF: Commercial hardware for the implementation of myoelectric control, in Muzumdar A, ed: *Powered Upper Limb Prostheses: Control, Implementation and Clinical Application.* Springer, 2004, pp 55-71.
21. Migaez J, Conyers D, MacJulian L, Culick K: Upper extremity prosthetics, in Lenhart MK, ed: *Textbooks of Military Medicine: Care of the Combat Amputee.* Office of the Surgeon General, Department of the Army, United States of America and US Army Medical Department Center and School, 2009, pp 607-640.
22. Sears HH: External-power for the transhumeral amputee, in Meier RH, Atkins DJ, eds: *Functional Restoration of Adults and Children With Upper Extremity Amputation.* Demos Medical Publishing, 2004, pp 199-206.
23. Westie KS: Psychological aspects of spinal cord injury. *Clin Prosthet Orthot* 1987;11(4):225-229.
24. Atkins DJ: Functional skills training with body-powered and externally powered prostheses, in Meier RH, Atkins DJ, eds: *Functional Restoration of Adults and Children With Upper Extremity Amputation.* Demos Medical Publishing, 2004, pp 139-158.
25. Hubbard S, Heim W, Naumann S, Glasford S, Montgomery G, Ramdial S: Powered upper limb prosthetic practice in paediatrics, in Muzumdar A, ed: *Powered Upper Limb Prostheses: Control, Implementation, and Clinical Application.* Springer, 2004, pp 85-115.
26. Weir RF, Sensinger JW: Design of artificial arms and hands for prosthetic applications, in Kutz M, ed: *Standard Handbook of Biomedical Engineering and Design.* McGraw-Hill, 2003, pp 32.1-32.61.
27. Bagesteiro LB, Sainburg RL: Handedness: Dominant arm advantages in control of limb dynamics. *J Neurophysiol* 2002;88(5) 2408-2421.
28. Bajaj N, Spiers A, Dollar A: State of the art in prosthetic wrists: Commercial and research devices. Presented at IEEE International Conference on Rehabilitation Robotics (ICARR), 2015. http://www.eng.yale.edu/grablab/pubs/Bajaj_ICORR2015.pdf. Accessed October 23, 2015.

29. Zinck A, Kyberd P, Hill W, et al: *A study of the use of compensation motions when using prosthetic wrists.* Proceedings of the MEC'08 Conference, UNB, 2008. http://hdl.handle.net/10161/2827. Accessed October 23, 2015.

30. Burger H, Marincek C: Upper limb prosthetic use in Slovenia. *Prosthet Orthot Int* 1994;18(1):25-33.

31. Sensinger J, Pasquina PF, Kuiken T: The future of artificial limbs, in Lenhart MK, ed: *Textbooks of Military Medicine: Care of the Combat Amputee.* Office of the Surgeon General, Department of the Army, United States of America and US Army Medical Department Center and School, 2009, pp 721-730.

32. Adams BD, Grosland NM, Murphy DM, McCullough M: Impact of impaired wrist motion on hand and upper-extremity performance. *J Hand Surg Am* 2003;28(6):898-903.

33. Brodd RJ, Kazuo T: Lithium-ion cell production processes, in van Schalkwijk W, Scrosati B, eds: *Advances in Lithium-ion Batteries.* Kluwer Academic Publishers, 2002, pp 267-288.

34. Kyberd PJ, Clawson A, Jones B: The use of underactuation in prosthetic grasping. Mechanical Sciences open access. http://pf-mh.uvt.rnu.tn/132/1/The_use_of_underactuation_in_prosthetic_grasping.pdf. Accessed October 23, 2015.

35. Heckathorne CW: Components for electric-powered systems, in Smith DG, Michael JW, Bowker JH, eds: *Atlas of Amputations and Limb Deficiencies: Surgical, Prosthetic, and Rehabilitation Principles,* ed 3. American Academy of Orthopaedic Surgeons, 2004, pp 145-171.

36. Pröbsting ED, Kannenberg A, Conyers DW, et al: Ease of activities of daily living with conventional and Multigrip Myoelectric Hands. *J Prosthet Orthot* 2015;27(2):46-52.

37. Belter JT, Segil JL, Dollar AM, Weir RF: Mechanical design and performance specifications of anthropomorphic prosthetic hands: A review. *J Rehabil Res Dev* 2013;50(5):599-618.

38. Waryck B: *Comparison of two myoelectric multi-articulating prosthetic hands.* Proceedings of the MEC'11 Conference, UNB, 2011. http://hdl.handle.net/10161/4740. Accessed October 23, 2015.

39. Carey SL, Highsmith J, Maitland ME, Dubey RV: Compensatory movements of transradial prosthesis users during common tasks. *Clin Biomech* 2008;23(9):1128-1135.

40. Bertels T, Schmalz T, Ludwigs E: Objectifying the functional advantages of prosthetic wrist flexion. *J Prosthet Orthot* 2009;21(2):74-78.

41. Atkins DJ, Heard SC, Donovan WH: Epidemiologic overview of individuals with upper-limb loss and their reported research priorities. *J Prosthet Orthot* 1996;8(1):2-11.

42. Datta D, Selvarajah K, Davey N: Functional outcome of patients with proximal upper limb deficiency: Acquired and congenital. *Clin Rehabil* 2004;18(2):172-177.

43. Jones LE, Davidson JH: Save that arm: A study of problems in the remaining arm of unilateral upper limb amputees. *Prosthet Orthot Int* 1999;23(1):55-58.

44. Williams TW: Control of powered upper extremity prostheses, in Meier RH, Atkins DJ, eds: *Functional Restoration of Adults and Children With Upper Extremity Amputation.* Demos Medical Publishing, 2004, pp 207-224.

45. Alley RD, Sears HH: Powered upper limb prosthetics in adults, in Muzumdar A, ed: *Powered Upper Limb Prostheses: Control, Implementation, and Clinical Application.* Springer, 2004, pp 117-145.

46. Connolly BH, Montgomery P: *Therapeutic Exercise in Developmental Disabilities.* SLACK Inc., 2005, p 369.

47. Electronic prosthetic innovations. *O&P Business News* 1999;8(23).

48. Dillingham TR, Pezzin LE, MacKenzie EJ: Limb amputation and limb deficiency: Epidemiology and recent trends in the United States. *South Med J* 2002;95(8):875-883.

49. Troncossi M, Gruppioni E, Chiossi M, Cutti AG, Davalli A, Parenti-Castelli V: A novel electromechanical shoulder articulation for upper-limb prostheses: From the design to the first clinical application. *J Prosthet Orthot* 2009;21(2):79-90.

50. Lipschutz RD, Kuiken TA, Miller LA, Dumanian GA, Stubblefield KA: Shoulder disarticulation externally powered prosthetic fitting following targeted muscle reinnervation for improved myoelectric control. *J Prosthet Orthot* 2006;18(2):28-34.

51. Heather T, Peters SJ, Page AP: Giving them a hand: Wearing a myoelectric elbow-wrist-hand orthosis reduces upper extremity impairment in chronic stroke. *Arch Phys Med Rehabil* 2017;98(9):1821-1827.

52. Plagenhoef S, Evans FG, Abdelnour T: Anatomical data for analyzing human motion. *Res Q Exerc Sport* 1983;54(2):169-178.

Control Options for Upper Limb Externally Powered Components

CHAPTER 13

R. Scott Hosie, CPO • Blair A. Lock, MS, PE

ABSTRACT

The task of an upper limb prosthesis is to move a terminal device into a position to grasp or hold an object, and then move that object into a different position. Various input devices can be used to control these motions. Electromyographic (EMG) signals have become the most common method of controlling externally powered prostheses. Conventional myoelectric systems have been used for decades and now myoelectric pattern recognition software is becoming more commonplace. In situations where there are no EMG signals, linear potentiometers, touch pads, or even simple on/off switches may be employed. With higher level amputations, up to three powered degrees of freedom may be incorporated into a prosthesis. These multiple degrees of freedom systems may used EMG-base triggers, mechanical switches or pattern recognition to switch control from one joint to another. With the growing popularity of multiarticulating hands, there is a need to switch between grip patterns. This may be accomplished by EMG triggers, buttons, switches and/or pattern recognition.

Keywords: alternative proportional control, degree of freedom, myoelectric control, pattern recognition

Introduction

The human hand is designed to hold and manipulate objects. The arm moves the hand into a position to grasp an object and then position it elsewhere in space. These actions may be as simple as moving a spoon from a bowl of soup to the mouth, grasping a child's hands to swing them in the air, or something as complex as a surgeon manipulating a scalpel. The arm coordinates multiple joints at the same time to quickly position the hand in a specific orientation. This is accomplished by complex joints, muscles, and the nervous system working seamlessly together. Indeed, a large portion of the brain is dedicated to the movement of the hand and arm.[1]

Building a prosthetic replacement for such a complex, coordinated system is a challenge. For example, removing wrist functionality results in a significant reduction in terminal device orientation. The prosthesis user must now compensate through gross body movements to achieve otherwise standard body motions. Accessing the face for instance, requires far greater shoulder and elbow movement when wrist function is not available.[2]

Learning to manage a prosthetic device using a body motion not normally associated with a natural movement requires intensive learning and skill development. In the case of a body-powered transradial prosthesis, using shoulder flexion to open a split hook device is not intuitive. Much the same as learning to eat with a nondominant hand, it is going to take practice. Intuitive control is important when learning to incorporate a prosthesis into daily function.

Because of this nonintuitive control, slow positioning, limited work envelope, and a loss of degrees of freedom, a prosthetic wearer will often compensate with other, more direct movements. These compensatory motions may require a greater range of motion and/or increased forces that the body does not normally encounter. The result is overuse and repetitive use injuries over the wearer's lifetime.[3]

The goal for controlling the externally powered prosthesis is to minimize compensatory body motions and maximize intuitive learning.

Conventional Myoelectric Control

Electromyographic (EMG) signals are a superimposed collection of minute, electrical impulses given off by the polarization/depolarization of muscle fibers during contraction.[4] These EMG signals can be measured at the surface of the skin, amplified, then used to

---

R. Scott Hosie or an immediate family member serves as a paid consultant to or is an employee of Fillauer Motion Control. Blair A. Lock or an immediate family member serves as a paid consultant to or is an employee of Coapt LLC and has stock or stock options held in Coapt LLC.

This chapter is adapted from Kyberd P, Bush G, Hussaini A. Control options for upper limb externally powered components. In: Krajbich JI, Pinzur MS, Potter BK, Stevens PM, eds. *Atlas of Amputations and Limb Deficiencies: Surgical, Prosthetic, and Rehabilitation Principles*. 4th ed. American Academy of Orthopaedic Surgeons, 2016, pp 193-201.

control a prosthetic device. This has become the most common method of control for externally powered prostheses since the 1970s.

Muscle signals (contractions) can be measured and their amplitude equated to the strength and speed of a prosthetic device's motion. A weaker signal can be coded to move the device slowly, while a stronger muscle contraction will cause the device to move more quickly. When a wearer wants to grasp an object, they can target it with a strong signal (muscle contraction) to get the device into place, then reduce the muscle contraction to gently grasp the object. The ability to control the prosthesis in this way is called proportional control. Proportional control is extremely advantageous for users of externally powered upper limb prostheses.[5]

Electrodes

To detect muscle signals, conductive metal electrodes are placed in contact with the skin. EMG signals at the skin surface fall in the microvolt to millivolt range, and with such small signals the contact between the skin and electrode must be very intimate. Most commercially available devices employ bipolar measurement between two electrode contacts (and sometimes a third for grounding reference) (**Figure 1**). These electrodes are connected to a processor/amplifier (**Figure 2**). The processor examines the signal and filters out what may likely be interference. This interference may be caused by a variety of influences in the environment. Fluorescent lights, microwave ovens, and cell phones are three of a plethora of common items encountered in daily life that can cause interference. Failure to filter this could easily cause the unintentional motion of a device, crushing a can, or dropping a delicate object. The amplifier increases the signal from microvolts to volts that can be more easily processed by the main controller of the prosthetic device.

Most modern commercially available electrode amplifiers provide a clean, filtered signal. Many also have an accessible gain potentiometer to allow adjustment of the amplification.

Controller

The signal is sent from the electrode amplifier to the device controller. This microprocessor provides adjustment of signal amplification, threshold adjustment, control schemes, and use of alternative input devices. With multiple degree of freedom systems, input switching from one device to another is accomplished by the controller.

Amplification

The strength of the EMG signals can vary greatly. The controller can be adjusted to further amplify a weak signal or balance the signal between two antagonistic muscles. The amplification (gain) can then be adjusted so the wearer feels the same muscle contraction is necessary to move the device in either direction, eg, to open/close a prosthetic hand. This adjustment is important. If the gain adjustment is set too high (excessive amplification) the wearer will not be able to control the hand, and it will immediately close and crush an object. Once the gain is lowered there will be improved proportional control.

Threshold

In addition to intentional muscle movement, there are also resting and/or artifact signals. Resting signals are the constant, low level of contraction our muscles are constantly maintaining. Artifact signals are contractions that inadvertently happen, for example, when moving the next proximal joint. These signals can be ignored by adjusting the threshold level in the controller. Typically, the threshold level is kept low since increasing that level decreases proportionality.

Digital User Interface

With prosthesis controllers, a digital user interface provides access to make adjustments. Each prosthetic manufacturer designs their own user interface to communicate with their devices. The platform may be a laptop computer, an iOS, or Android handheld device.

Direct Control Strategies

As myoelectric control strategies become increasingly nuanced and creative, it's important to distinguish these emerging strategies from the comparatively simpler direct control strategies. In such strategies, electrodes are assigned to and positioned over a targeted muscle belly such that there is a direct relationship between the activation of a given muscle and a targeted movement of the prosthesis. The most common direct control strategies are dual- and single-site control.

Dual-Site Control

There are many advantages with myoelectric control, one being the coordinated nature of using muscle contractions to control a closely

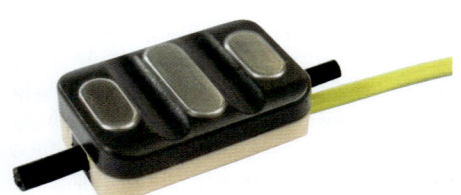

FIGURE 1 Photograph showing an electrode/amplifier. (Courtesy of Össur, Ossur Americas, Orange County, CA.)

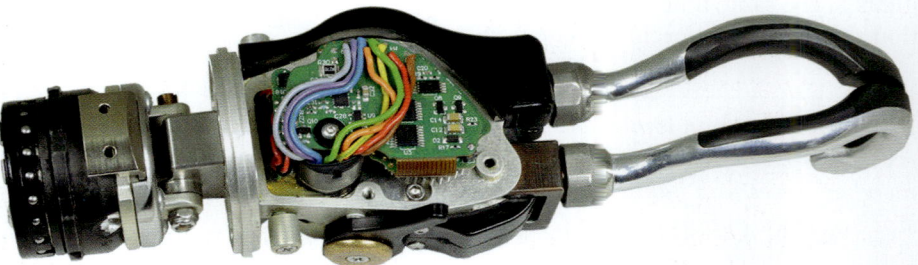

FIGURE 2 Photograph showing an integrated controller in the Fillauer Motion Control ETD. (Courtesy of Fillauer Motion Control, Salt Lake City, UT.)

associated movement in the prosthesis. In dual-site control it is common to assign control movements to antagonistic muscles, matching control signals to native biologic movements to the extent possible. For example, in the case of a transradial level amputation, remnant wrist extensors can control opening a prehensile device, while remnant wrist flexors close the device, much the same as with an intact limb. At the more proximal amputation level, dual-site control of multiple joint systems may be required through inputs that will be described shortly. For example, at the transhumeral amputation level remnant elbow extensors are commonly assigned control of both elbow extension and opening of a prehensile device, while remnant elbow flexors are commonly assigned control of both elbow flexion and the closing of the prehensile device. Through sophisticated systems, these two sites can also provide wrist pronation and supination. Control systems strive to allow the user to control three degrees of freedom as intuitively as possible.

Single-Site Control

In some cases, only one useable muscle site can be found. This may be because of a degloving injury, severe burns, or neurological trauma. The challenge is creating a system where the wearer can control two directions of motion, for example, a hand open/close or elbow flexion/extension with only one signal. For situations like this, several software algorithms have been developed to assign an action to a single muscle contraction.

Alternating Control

With alternating control, a single-site system receives the signal, and the device moves in one direction (eg, open). The wearer relaxes and the next signal causes the device to move in the opposite direction (eg, close). While not as intuitive as dual-channel control, speed is still proportional. The relax time is adjustable, allowing the wearer to still target the object and adjust the grasp force accordingly.

Voluntary Opening/Closing

With voluntary opening control, the hand will open with a signal, and closes with relaxation. With voluntary closing it is the opposite, as a signal will close the hand proportionally and relaxation will open the hand to full open.

The advantage of this system is that control can be very intuitive. The disadvantage is that it is difficult to create voluntary opening control and not crush objects when the device closes to full pinch force. With voluntary closing, the hand is always unnaturally open when relaxed. Manufacturers have designed systems to address these issues.

Manufacturer-Specific Single-Site Control

Each manufacturer has developed unique ways to operate a myoelectric device with only one muscle signal. It is recommended to investigate each to determine the best approach for specific situations. Two specific examples are the Otto Bock Hi/Lo and Motion Control Single Site.

Otto Bock Double Channel Control Mode

With this algorithm the user generates a quick strong muscle to open the terminal device and a slow, mild muscle to close. This is not a proportional signal and to grasp the object tighter, the user continues to give a signal until the object is grasped to the desired force.

Motion Control FLAG

FLAG is an optional feature on Motion Control terminal devices. In single-site control, the device is placed in alternating control. A long, open signal is generated, and this activates the FLAG feature. The next signal closes the device to about 2 lb (1 kg) of pinch force. A quick signal above and back below the threshold increases the pinch force by about two more pounds. The wearer can pulse up to 10 times to grasp an object tightly. A signal of greater than 1.6 seconds opens the device.

Alternative Proportional Control Inputs

There are situations when a patient may not have any EMG signal. This could be because of nerve damage such as a brachial plexus injury, complete degloving injury, or they may live in a very hot, humid environment where perspiration causes issues with EMG signals. Another indication for alternative inputs is a higher level amputation with multiple powered degrees of freedom. An alternative input can also be used to control a powered elbow, with EMG to control a terminal device.

Linear Potentiometer

For decades, persons with upper limb amputation/difference have used biscapular abduction and/or humeral flexion to operate body-powered devices. In reaching for an object these motions, while not entirely intuitive, are easy to learn. A linear potentiometer translates a linear pull into an electrical signal so that same body motion can be harnessed (**Figure 3**). Typically, only about 1 cm of excursion is required with negligible force necessary to pull the linear potentiometer. Linear potentiometers are not only position sensitive (eg, a position halfway in its excursion range translates to an elbow halfway in its range of motion) but also proportional. A fast pull will move an elbow quickly,

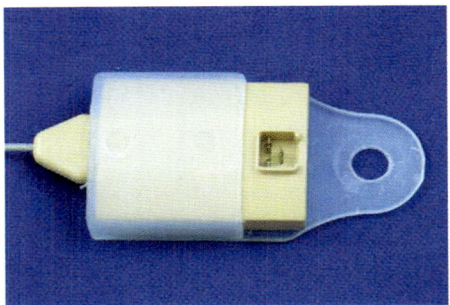

FIGURE 3 Photograph of a linear potentiometer, which is attached to one part of the socket by a fixture (right side) and across a joint via a cable (left side). (Reprinted from Kyberd P, Bush G, Hussaini A. Control options for upper limb externally powered components. In: Krajbich JI, Pinzur MS, Potter BK, Stevens PS, eds. *AAOS Atlas of Amputations and Limb Deficiencies*. 4th ed. American Academy of Orthopaedic Surgeons, 2018.)

a slower pull, more slowly. This may be an excellent option for a wearer moving from a body-powered device to an externally powered device as the motion is the same as they have previously learned.

A linear potentiometer can be incorporated into almost any type of harness. Shoulder saddle/chest strap harnesses are desirable in transhumeral limb loss cases as they support the weight of the prosthesis comfortably, however the drawback is lack of excursion. Requiring only a small amount of excursion, a linear potentiometer is useful in this application. When a wearer uses a linear potentiometer, the body motions are imperceptible and very natural.[6]

Force-Sensing Resistors

Force-sensing resistors (FSRs) are thin disks with conductors on each surface running at 90° to each other (**Figure 4**). Between these conductors is a resistive medium. As pressure (force) is placed on the disk, the two conductive surfaces come closer together, decreasing resistance. This resistance can be measured and translated to the motion of a device. Again, using an elbow as an example, pushing halfway down would translate to the elbow holding in a position halfway in its range of motion. Like the linear potentiometer, it is also proportional and pushing quickly translates into a fast motion, pushing slower causes a more controlled motion.

Since they are thin, FSRs may simply be mounted on the inside of a socket. The wearer can then use the residual limb inside the socket to press on the FSR. They are also manufactured in a protective case which improves proportionally of the FSR.

Since EMG control can sometimes be difficult with shoulder disarticulation cases, FSRs can be mounted anterior and posterior to the acromion process. Pushing on the anterior FSR would flex the elbow, the posterior FSR to extend it. They can also sense triggers such as a co-contraction for switching from one degree of freedom to another.

Control Strategies for Multiple Degrees of Freedom Systems

Powered elbows, powered wrist rotation, powered flexion wrists, and a multitude of powered terminal devices are all now available. The challenge becomes controlling each degree of freedom. Operating multiple degrees of freedom simultaneously, while desirable, requires multiple inputs and/or algorithmic complexity. Most wearers have dual-site control and controllers have a system of sequentially moving through each degree of freedom.

Simultaneous Control

The human hand/arm uses simultaneous control to quickly target and grasp an object. To provide this control in a prosthesis, each degree of freedom requires its own control input.

EMG Control

It is very difficult, if not impossible, for a wearer to generate multiple distinct muscle signals for simultaneous control of several powered joints. One alternate intervention is Targeted Muscle Reinnervation enabling additional myoelectric control sites. Described fully in a separate chapter, the severed nerves of the brachial plexus are identified and reinnervated in targeted muscle bellies in the remnant limb. These nerves corresponded to certain motions in the limb before amputation, allowing more native control of those prosthetic motions. The result is an increase in the number of distinct EMG sites that correspond to the natural function of the arm increasing intuitive prosthetic control.[7] Myoelectric pattern recognition is a candidate solution for simultaneous EMG control of prosthesis in the near future.

EMG/Alternative Input

Simultaneous control can also be obtained by mixing EMG inputs with alternate inputs. A common application is a powered elbow controlled with a linear potentiometer and the prehension device controlled with EMG. Using scapular abduction much the same as with a body-powered device, the wearer can flex the elbow while using EMG to operate the hand.

Sequential Control

For wearers of dual-site myoelectric control systems, control of multiple degrees of freedom requires switching control from one degree of freedom to the next. This could mean cycling through three degrees of freedom using the same switch, toggling between two degrees of freedom, or using different switches to go directly to a degree of freedom.[8]

EMG Switching

Several algorithms have been developed for switching between degrees of freedom. Co-contraction is a quick contraction of both muscles at the same time. Co-contraction is a muscle signal not commonly generated by wearers. Only by a deliberate, co-contraction signal does switching occur. New wearers experience crosstalk between two muscles that may cause inadvertent switching. This inadvertent switching can be rectified by adjustment of the digital user interface.

With Otto Bock 4-Channel control and Motion Control Fast Access switching, a quick contraction of one muscle immediately switches to a different

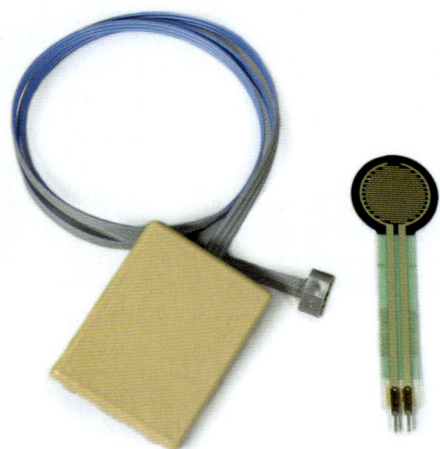

FIGURE 4 Photograph showing a force sensing resistor housed in a Touch Pad case. (Courtesy of Fillauer Motion Control, Salt Lake City, UT.)

degree of freedom, while with a slower impulse, control remains in the default degree of freedom. As an example, in a transradial system, initially the terminal device is active. With a quick contraction, the wrist will rotate. With a slower contraction, the terminal device is active. This is a very functional switching method as it results in instantaneous wrist rotation for quick prepositioning of the terminal device. The ease of difficulty of switching can be adjusted in the manufacturer's digital user interface balancing ease of switching and eliminating inadvertent switching.

Mechanical Switches

EMG switching algorithms are not intuitive and sometimes difficult to learn. There is also a limitation in the number of triggers available. External switches can also be employed. A bump switch can be mounted on the medial surface of the humeral section of a transhumeral prosthesis, and the wearer simply bumps the prosthesis against the chest wall to switch control to a different degree of freedom (**Figures 5** and **6**). They can also be mounted anteriorly on a shoulder disarticulation socket and bumped with the chin. Each time the switch is activated it can toggle between two degrees of freedom or sequentially progress between three degrees of freedom. Other options are cable pull switches and harness-mounted switches such as the Ottobock 9×14 (**Figure 7**).

For instance, an EMG switch might be used to unlock and elbow while a mechanical switch is used for hand/wrist switching. Finally, a switch may be employed to directly control a degree of freedom. The Ottobock rocker switch 9×25 may be mounted on the anterior portion of a shoulder disarticulation prosthesis (**Figure 8**). Using the chin on one side of the switch will pronate the wrist, the opposite side will supinate the wrist.

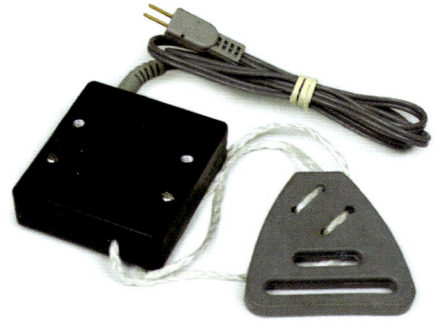

FIGURE 6 Photograph showing an elbow lock/unlock switch for a Utah Arm. (Courtesy of Fillauer Motion Control, Salt Lake City, UT.)

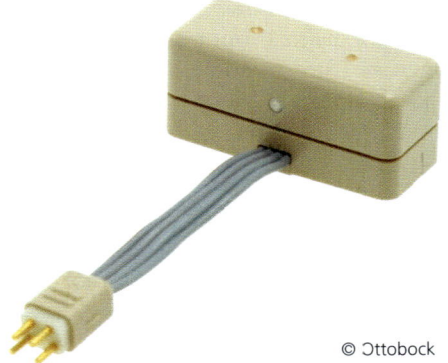

FIGURE 8 Photograph showing an Ottobock rocker 9×25 switch. (Courtesy of Ottobock.)

Pattern Recognition Myoelectric Control

An advanced alternative to dual- or single-site direct myoelectric control is myoelectric pattern recognition. Pattern recognition is a machine learning approach where computational algorithms running on the prosthesis' controller work to predict the user's motion and speed intent from a network of EMG signals. The electrode amplifiers required to do this are slightly different than the conventional ones as they pass the full fidelity of the EMG signal along to the processor, not simply the level/strength of the EMG signal. Additionally, pattern recognition typically requires more electrode amplifiers, commonly six to eight per prosthesis. The electrodes' location on the skin surface is not required to be as specific to muscle groups as with conventional myoelectric control.[9]

A functional advantage of pattern recognition is true, intuitive control of a prosthesis. That is, a user can employ their own natural perceptions of hand grasping patterns, wrist actions, etc. to be coordinated one-to-one with the matching prosthetic actuation. Thus, there is no requirement of sequential selection or mode switching common in conventional myoelectric control.

Another advantage of pattern recognition is that users can configure their own prosthesis control as needed by way of "teaching" or "calibrating" the system. During a calibration sequence, they let the algorithms record their desired EMG contraction pattern (as detected by the network of electrodes) for each specific prosthesis motion. Thereinafter, the algorithm monitors the network of EMG signals for patterns that match any of the recorded ones and correspondingly command the prosthesis to move.

With the increasing popularity of multifunction terminal devices and prosthetic arms with more than one powered component, pattern recognition is a clinically viable option that provides a solution to this complex control need.

Control of Multiarticulating Hands

Prehensile devices with multiarticulating fingers have gained popularity over the last several years. An adaptive grip

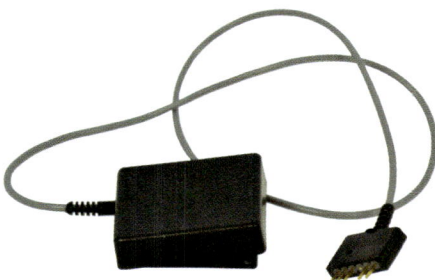

FIGURE 5 Photograph showing a high-profile wrist Bump Switch for hand/wrist switching. (Courtesy of Fillauer Motion Control, Salt Lake City, UT.)

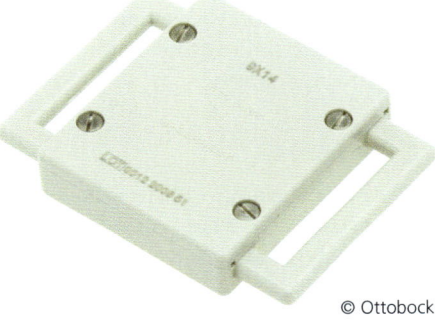

FIGURE 7 Photograph showing an Ottobock harness pull switch. (Courtesy of Ottobock.)

allows for a confident grasp without the high pinch force necessary in single degree of freedom hands. Additionally, the hand can be placed in specific pre-programmed grip patterns such as a power grasp or a lateral (key) grip. Most hands have multiple grasp patterns that can be programmed for a given user. However, access to these grasps is limited by the input constraints described throughout the chapter, allowing most users much more limited access to a smaller menu of preferred grasp patterns. Open/close can be accomplished with any of the inputs we have discussed. Control takes on added complexity in switching grip patterns. Manufacturers have come up with a variety of unique methods to switch grip patterns.

Grip Changes Through Myoelectric Triggers

A variety of EMG impulses can be trained and used with multiarticulating hands to change to a different grip pattern. These unique impulses are described as "triggers." A variety of novel triggers have been developed for use with multiarticulating hands set up with single- or dual-site myoelectric control. Intentional co-contraction, described earlier, is one example of a trigger. Other examples include a hold-open signal where the user fully opens their terminal device and sends an open signal of a second or more. With another trigger, double open, the user generates two successive open signals in a short period of time, which triggers a grip change. Using an EMG trigger allows the wearer to change grips without involving the contralateral limb. All multiarticulating hands have EMG triggers available to change grip patterns.

Grip Changes Through Pattern Recognition

Since pattern recognition myoelectric control allows a user to use natural, intuitive contraction patterns corresponding to prosthesis motions, users of this set up configure their two to four preferred grip patterns for control of the hand. When the hand is fully opened, the user makes their preferred EMG contraction (pattern) and the hand will close into that corresponding grip proportional to the overall signal level.

Grip Changes Through Physical Triggers

Thumb Position

Functionally, the position of the thumb commonly dictates the position of the fingers. In lateral grip, often the fingers are closed in a fist so the thumb can pinch on the index finger. When the thumb is in opposition, the fingers often close in power grasp, pincher, or a tripod grip. With some multiarticulating hands, the thumb position sets one or two grips which are toggled with an EMG trigger. When the thumb position is moved different grips are available.

Button Panel

With several hands, one or more buttons are conveniently placed on the dorsal surface of the hand. Pressing the button(s) can either toggle between two grips or sequentially move through more. The button may also double as an on/off switch.

Gesture Control

Inertial measurement units are electronic devices that sense movement. These are commonplace in cell phones and many other devices. When placed in a hand, they can sense movement from side to side, forward and backwards. A movement in one direction can then change the grip. Typically, there is a sequence such as hold the hand parallel with the floor, the patient gives a full open signal, then move the hand. This prevents common movement throughout the day from causing unintentional grip pattern changes.

SUMMARY

Initially, externally powered upper limb prostheses were entirely switch operated, with the user manually pulling or hitting a control pad or button. Since the advent of two-site myoelectric control, opening and closing a hand has become more intuitive. Pattern recognition systems now extend natural control to multiple degrees of freedom and multiple grip patterns in multiarticulating hands.[7]

Looking toward the future, targeted muscle innervation along with implanted electrodes shows promise.[8,10] With these systems, multiple inputs processed by pattern recognition will continue to expand control systems for externally powered upper limb systems. The increased acceptance of osseointegration and elimination of the limb/socket interface along with improved translation of body motions to the prosthesis will also improve function.[11] Finally, direct-to-nerve sensory feedback is showing great promise and is being designed to provide individuals with a sense of touch.[12]

These exciting future developments will eventually combine to provide improved function and quality of life for those with upper limb amputation and difference.

References

1. Dubuc B: *The motor cortex. The Brain from Top to Bottom.* McGill. https://thebrain.mcgill.ca/flash/d/d_06/d_06_cr/d_06_cr_mou/d_06_cr_mou.html. Accessed July 28, 2021.
2. Iversen E, Christenson J, Jacobs G, Hosie S: *Externally powered wrist flexion device. Myoelectric Controls Symposium.* University of New Brunswick, 2020.
3. Kyberd P, Bush G, Hussaini A: Control options for upper limb externally powered components, in *Atlas of Amputations and Limb Deficiencies*, ed 4. American Academy of Orthopaedic Surgeons, 2016, chap 14.
4. Raez MBI, Hussain MS, Mohd-Yasin F: Techniques of EMG signal analysis: Detection, processing classification and applications. *Biol Proced Online* 2006;8:11-35.
5. Sears HH, Shaperman J: Proportional myoelectric hand control: an evaluation. *Am J Phys Med Rehabil* 1991;70(1):20-28.
6. Lake C, Dodson R: Progressive upper limb prosthetics. *Phys Med Rehabil Clin N Am* 2006;17(1):49-72.
7. Kuiken TA, Li G, Lock BA, et al: Targeted muscle reinnervation for real-Time myoelectric control of multifunction artificial arms. *J Am Med Assoc* 2009;301:619-628.

8. Kyberd PJ, Holland OE, Chappell PH, et al: MARCUS: A two degree of freedom hand prosthesis with hierarchical grip control. *IEEE Trans Rehabil Eng* 1995;3(1):70-76.

9. Purushothaman G: Myoelectric control of prosthetic hands: State-of-the-art review. *Med Devices (Auckl)* 2016;9:247-255.

10. Pasquina P, Evangelista M, Carvalho A, et al: First-in-man demonstration of fully implanted myoelectric sensors for control of an advanced electromechanical arm by transradial amputees. *J Neurosci Methods* 2015;244:85-93.

11. Drew A, Taylor C, Tashjian R, Chalmers P, Henninger H, Bachus K: Initial stability of a percutaneous osseointegrated endoprosthesis with proximal interlocking screws for transhumeral amputees. *Clin Biomech* 2020;72:108-114.

12. Tyler D: Restoring the human touch: Prosthetics imbued with haptics give their wearers fine motor control and a sense of connection. *IEEE Xplore* 2016;53(5):28-33.

Partial Hand Amputation: Surgical Management

Edward A. Athanasian, MD, FAAOS
Mark E. Puhaindran, MBBS, MMED, MRCS, FAMS

ABSTRACT

Partial amputation of a finger, ray amputation, multiple ray amputation, and complete hand amputation may be required to treat patients after traumatic injury, infection, or in the setting of malignant bone and soft-tissue tumors. It is helpful to be familiar with the indications for amputation, surgical techniques, outcomes, potential pitfalls, and complications.

Keywords: double ray amputation; partial hand amputation; ray amputation; single ray amputation

Introduction

Amputations of fingers or portions of the hand may be required in the treatment of traumatic injury, infection, and tumor. Each patient has a unique clinical scenario, and treatment should be individualized to that patient and the injury or condition. A well-performed amputation may maximize patient function and appearance. This in turn may have a major effect on the patient's self-perception, socialization, and work capacity. In this chapter, we review the surgical techniques for different types of partial hand amputations, and look at recent developments that may help improve outcomes.

Single Ray Amputation

General Considerations

Single ray amputation is most commonly done for the treatment of infection, traumatic injuries, and, less frequently, malignant bone and soft-tissue tumors. Deficits produced by trauma can be limited to the affected digit or can extend more proximally into the metacarpus or the hand. Similarly, the surgical deficits that remain as a result of the oncologic requirements of resection or even infection control are sometimes unique and must be taken into consideration in surgical planning for definitive amputation and reconstruction. The status of the soft tissues and the need for coverage also must be considered. Fillet flaps and "spare parts" from distal amputated parts or adjacent digits can be extremely helpful in achieving wound closure or coverage.[1]

Index and small finger ray amputations are done by transecting the base of the metacarpal distal to the extensor carpi radialis and extensor carpi ulnaris, respectively. The middle ray is most commonly transected at the base of the metacarpal, with or without index ray transposition.[2] The ring finger ray is most commonly disarticulated at the carpometacarpal articulation, with the anticipation that the small finger ray base will migrate to the midline over time. Intermetacarpal ligament repair or reconstruction is critical to reduce the gap between digits as well as rebalance the adjacent digits following central ray amputation, and will improve cosmesis. The authors of this chapter prefer a middle ray amputation without transposition. Intermetacarpal ligament repair or reconstruction also avoids the risk of contamination of adjacent rays when the procedure is done because of malignancy.[3]

Outcome Considerations

When possible, it is imperative that the functional and cosmetic deficits produced by ray amputation be carefully reviewed with the patient before the surgical procedure. Emotional and psychological considerations should be addressed and expectations defined. Pictures demonstrating the anticipated result and appearance are helpful. Speaking to, or meeting with, an individual who had a ray amputation can be extremely beneficial. In some instances, psychological counseling is appropriate.

Neuroma at the transection site of the digital nerves is expected after all procedures. Most commonly, these neuromas are not particularly uncomfortable, with the exception of the index ray where painful neuromas occur in approximately 70% of patients. There is no widely accepted treatment method to reduce the risk of a painful digital neuroma after a ray amputation, and techniques to address painful neuromas are discussed later.

Grip strength is diminished by approximately 30% after ray amputation, although there can be great

---

Dr. Puhaindran or an immediate family member serves as a board member, owner, officer, or committee member of the Singapore Society for Hand Surgery. Neither Dr. Athanasian nor any immediate family member has received anything of value from or has stock or stock options held in a commercial company or institution related directly or indirectly to the subject of this chapter.

variation.[2,3] The routine reduction of grip strength should be discussed in advance with patients to provide realistic expectations. Patients commonly adapt well to this deficit.

The appearance of the hand after a well-done elective ray amputation can be excellent. Patients should be reassured preoperatively that the deficit of a single ray is not routinely noticed in human interactions, unless fingers are counted.

Preferred Techniques of This Chapter's Authors

Index Ray Amputation

In an index ray amputation, the dorsal incision is made and the flaps are elevated. The incision may be longitudinal (preferred) or a long V-flap. The extensor tendons are then transected, and interosseous muscles are mobilized extraperiosteally. Bone transection is performed distal to the insertion of the flexor carpi radialis.

For the volar incision, additional skin is taken radially when possible to facilitate closure. The V-incision is incorporated with a volar Bruner incision, which may need to be trimmed at final closure. Digital vessels are identified proximally, cauterized, and then transected. Digital nerves are identified, anesthetized with a local anesthetic, and transected. Flexor tendons are then transected, and the intermetacarpal ligament between the index ray and the middle finger ray is transected. The ray is rotated, and the remaining intrinsic musculature is transected. Skin is closed using nylon suture with attention to the distal radial flap first, followed by dorsal and palmar closures (**Figure 1**).

Middle Finger Ray Amputation

A middle finger ray amputation is similar to an index ray amputation. The proximal metacarpal is transected at the base of the diaphysis distal to the carpometacarpal ligaments. After removal of the ray, the intermetacarpal ligament is repaired using nonabsorbable suture or reconstructed using the A-1 pulley of the index and middle rays (**Figure 2**).

Ring Finger Ray Amputation

Ring finger ray amputation is similar to a middle finger ray amputation with the exception of routine disarticulation of the base of the ring finger metacarpal from the carpometacarpal joint. Care must be taken to avoid injury to the deep palmar arch and deep motor branch of the ulnar nerve, which are palmar to the base of the ring finger metacarpal and thus easily injured. Intermetacarpal ligament repair or reconstruction is important to adjust the balance of the small finger and for cosmesis. Over time, the base of the small finger metacarpal migrates radially to help reduce the defect produced by ring finger ray amputation (**Figure 3**).

Small Finger Amputation

Small finger ray amputation is entirely analogous to index ray amputation with similar incisions and skin flaps. Care must be taken to plan the ulnar-sided skin flap to facilitate closure. The bone is transected distal to the insertion of the extensor carpi ulnaris (**Figure 4**).

Alternative Surgical Techniques

Transposition of the index ray to the base of the middle ray is a well-accepted reconstruction technique after middle ray amputation. This broadens the first web space slightly and can reduce the tendency for index ray pronation after intermetacarpal ligament repair or reconstruction when transposition is not done. This procedure requires osteotomy of the index metacarpal base and open reduction and internal fixation of the index metacarpal diaphysis to the middle finger metacarpal base. Additional surgical time and risks of malrotation, nonunion, hardware removal, and theoretic expansion of the field of contamination (in the setting of malignant tumor resection) must be taken into consideration if transposition is being considered.

Rehabilitation

Bulky, soft compressive bandages are applied at the time of surgery. The digit range of motion is encouraged to the extent allowed by the level of pain, particularly metacarpophalangeal joint flexion and proximal interphalangeal joint extension. Supervised digit range of motion should be initiated between the first and second postoperative weeks. Sutures remain in place for 2 to 3 weeks. Recovery of range of motion should be the early emphasis of therapy. At week 6, strengthening is initiated. Palmar wound desensitization may be required in the first 3 months, after which incision-site sensitivity typically decreases. Full activity is allowed at 3 months, with continued improvement in strength and function expected for more than 1 year after surgery. Routine discussion of psychological well-being is incorporated into early postoperative physician visits.

Managing Complications

The management of complications should be considered at the time of surgery. Besides painful neuromas, other complications following single ray amputation include digit mal-alignment. To avoid this, digit alignment in extension and flexion must be critically assessed after intermetacarpal ligament repair and, particularly, reconstruction. It is possible to pronate radial-sided digits and supinate ulnar-sided digits during this repair. If done, this will affect the appearance, and could impair function.

Nonunion or malrotation after digit transposition will require additional intervention in the form of bone grafting or surgical correction of rotation.

Double Ray Amputation

General Considerations

Double ray amputation may be required for patients with major hand trauma, those with large tumors involving single rays that encroach on the adjacent ray, or in patients in whom a tumor is located in the space between individual rays. In some radiosensitive lesions, preoperative radiation can be considered in an attempt to reduce the size of the tumor. If adequate size reduction is achieved, it may be possible to convert a planned double ray amputation into a single ray amputation.

Chapter 14: Partial Hand Amputation: Surgical Management

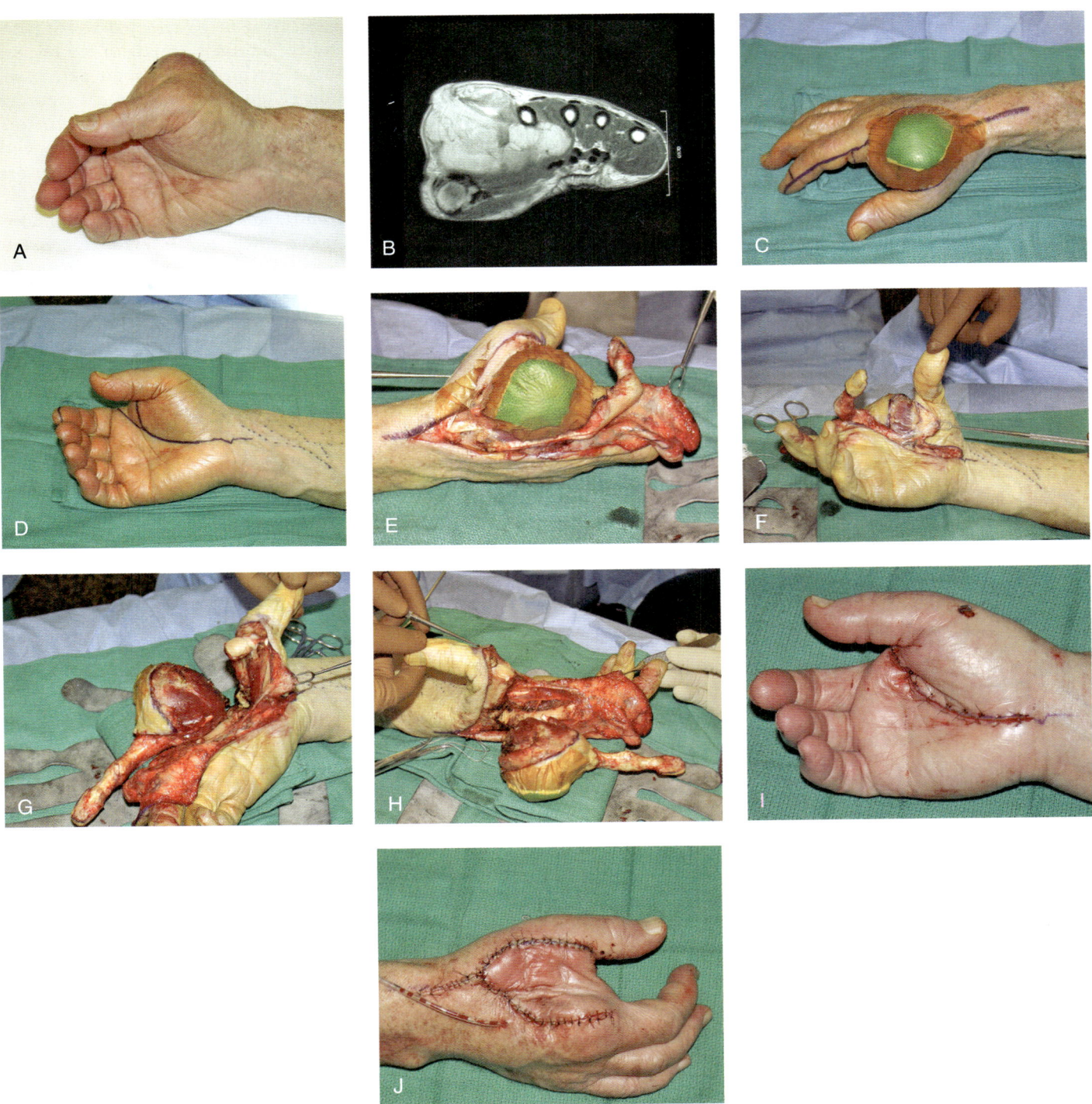

FIGURE 1 **A**, Clinical photograph of a liposarcoma involving the first web space. **B**, Axial MRI showing the lesion extending from the thumb metacarpal radially to the middle finger metacarpal ulnarly. The palmar barrier is the adductor pollicis. The dorsal disease fungating through the skin. **C** through **J**, Surgical photographs. **C**, The dorsal incision incorporates skin resection at the area of the fungating lesion, with a plan for an index fillet flap. **D**, The volar incision incorporates a fillet flap incision. The volar wrist veins are marked for a possible donor graft. **E**, A fillet flap is raised, and the radial dissection includes thumb metacarpal periosteum. **F**, Palmar dissection is done palmar to the adductor pollicis to allow adequate resection margin. The thumb is rotated radially to facilitate exposure. **G** and **H**, Dorsal views of the rotated thumb, fillet flap, and resection specimen. **I**, Volar appearance of the hand after closure, medial collateral ligament repair, and pinning. **J**, Dorsal appearance of the hand, with closure facilitated with a fillet flap.

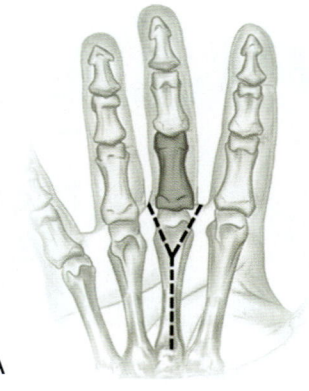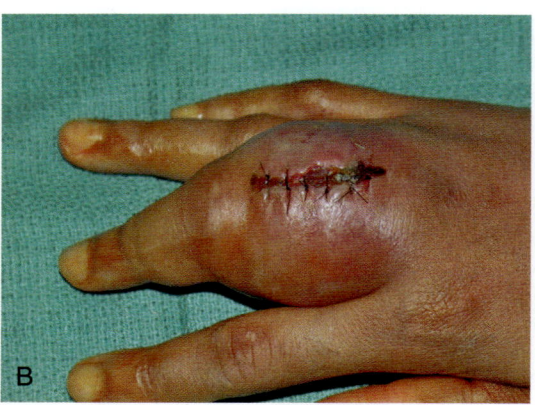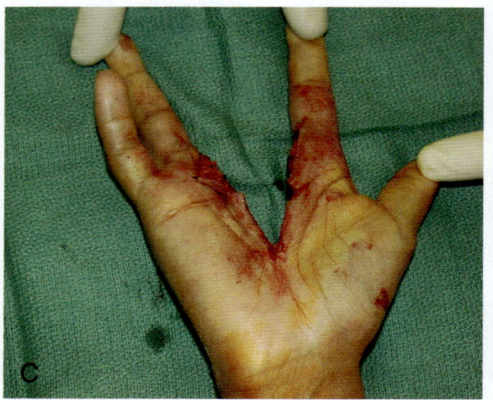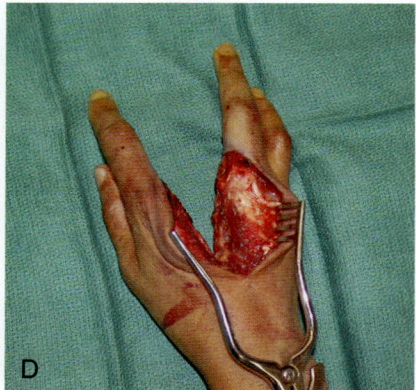

FIGURE 2 **A**, Illustration of a middle finger ray amputation. **B**, Clinical photograph of a large proximal phalanx tumor that required ray amputation. Surgical photographs of the volar incision (**C**) and the dorsal incision (**D**).

The preoperative physical examination should include the Allen test to confirm patency of the arterial arch and adequate perfusion of the digit. It is imperative to determine the patency of the superficial arch before double ray amputation when resection of the superficial vascular arch is being considered. Microsurgical capability is needed for vascular repair or grafting if indicated.

Outcome Considerations

Double ray amputation causes a much greater deficit in appearance compared with single ray amputation. This deficit is more commonly noted in routine interpersonal interactions and has a greater effect on a patient's perception of his or her appearance.[4,5]

Function after double ray amputation is also more severely affected than after single ray amputation. In one series of double ray amputation done to treat sarcomas, grip strength was reduced by approximately 75%.[4] Resection of the deep motor branch of the ulnar nerve, if required, also impairs thumb function and manual dexterity.

Preferred Techniques of This Chapter's Authors

When performing double ray amputation, incision placement is usually dictated by the location and extent of the tumor or the traumatic injury. Routine consideration of the use of a fillet flap from the uninjured or uncontaminated digit tissue should be incorporated into the surgical plan to facilitate coverage, if needed. If there is adequate tissue, ulnar- or palmar-based flaps may be used for ulnar double ray amputation. A large radial index flap will facilitate closure in radial-sided double ray amputation of the index and middle fingers (**Figures 5** and **6**).

Dorsal dissection is usually done first after completion of the dissection of any fillet flap. Extensor tendons are transected. Interosseous muscles that can be spared are dissected from the metacarpal to be resected at both the radial and ulnar aspects of the respective metacarpals. Metacarpal transection of both rays is done distal to the insertion of radial-sided wrist flexors and extensors at the index ray and ulnar-sided wrist flexors and extensors at the small finger ray.

Palmar dissection is determined by the extent of the lesion or trauma. The superficial palmar arch should be spared when possible. If this arch must be resected, the surgeon should be prepared to perform microsurgical repair or reconstruction of the arch if there is inadequate blood flow to the remaining digits. Transections of the flexor tendons and intrinsic muscles are needed to complete the amputation. Closure is performed using local flaps, a fillet flap, or (occasionally) distant coverage such as a radial forearm flap or a free flap.

Rehabilitation

Rehabilitation after double ray amputation of the hand is nearly identical to that for single ray amputation. The cosmetic deficit produced by double ray amputation is substantial. A passive prosthesis may be considered to improve appearance if this is important to the patient.

Managing Complications

Complications after double ray amputation are similar to those after single ray amputation. Double ray amputation for malignant bone and soft-tissue tumors is typically done for very large lesions. The extent of the resection may require extensive reconstruction, including tendon and bone reconstruction or repair. When perioperative radiation is used, for example in the treatment of soft-tissue sarcomas of the hand, then more complications are expected.[6] Problems with limited tendon excursion are more common after double ray amputation than single ray amputation, and subsequent tenolysis may be required.

Transmetacarpal Amputation

Elective transmetacarpal amputation is rarely performed. Even large distal tumors can be resected with either

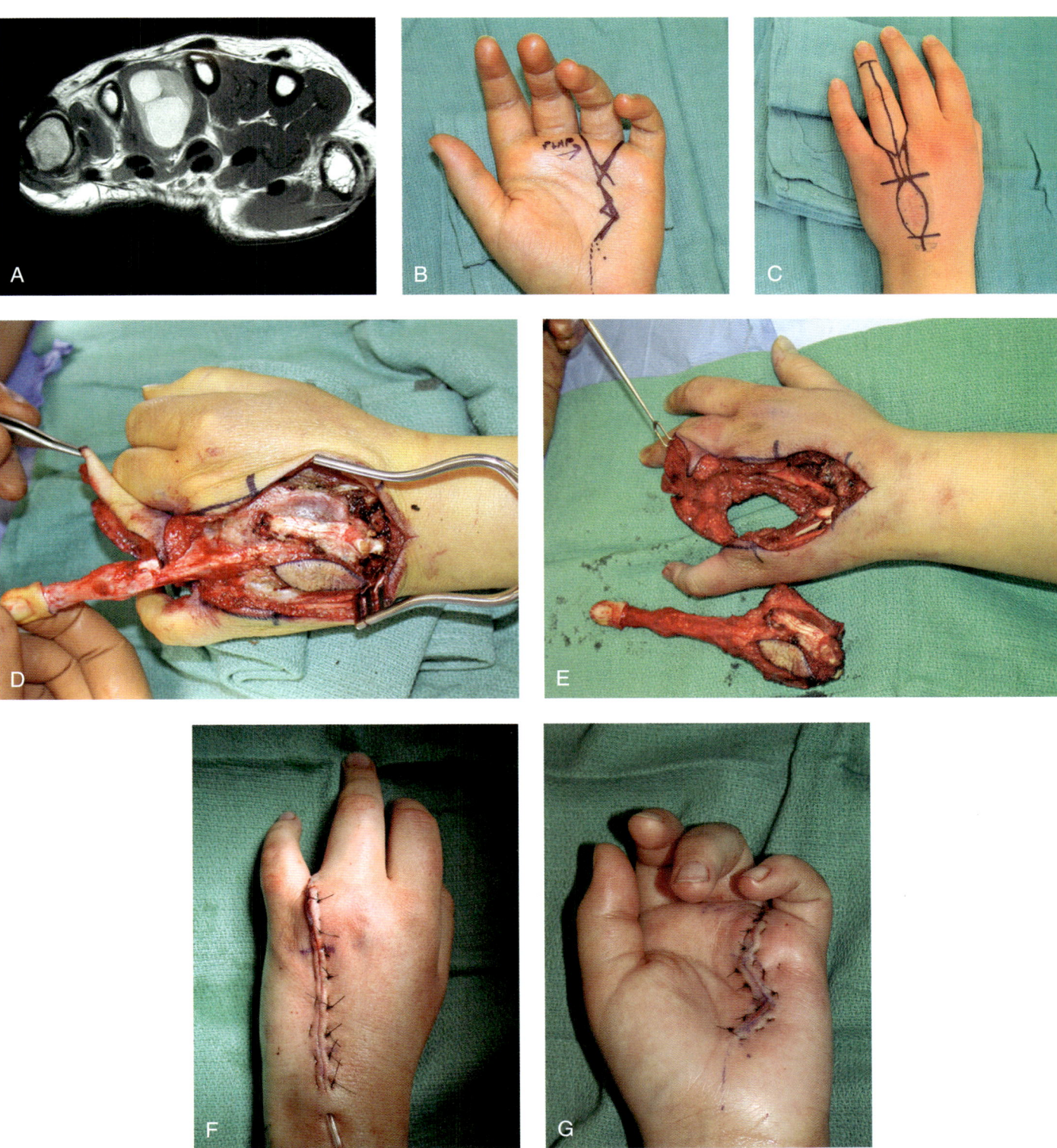

FIGURE 3 **A**, Axial MRI of a synovial sarcoma treated with a ring finger ray amputation and a middle finger metacarpal resection. **B** through **G**, Surgical photographs of the ring finger amputation. The plans for the volar incision with a fillet flap (**B**) and dorsal incision with a fillet flap (**C**) are marked on the hand. **D**, Dorsal dissection. **E**, The defect after the ray amputation with a fillet flap. The specimen has been disarticulated. Dorsal (**F**) and palmar (**G**) views of the hand after intermetacarpal ligament repair and wound closure.

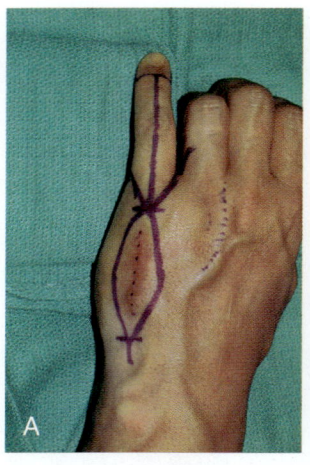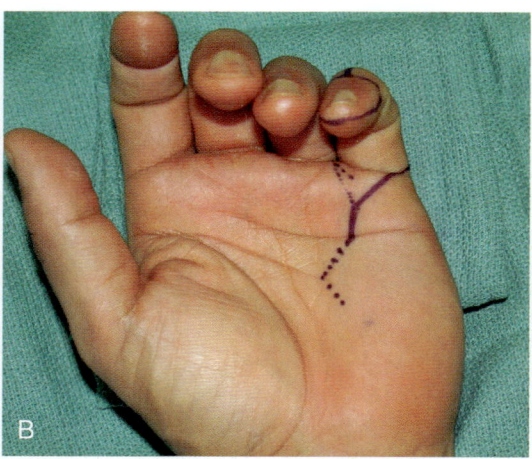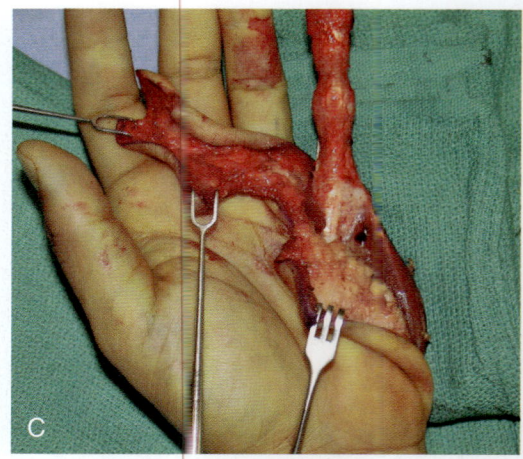
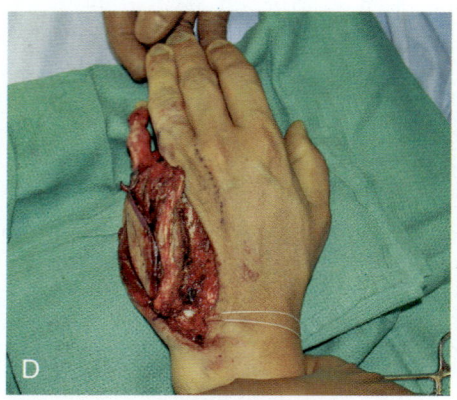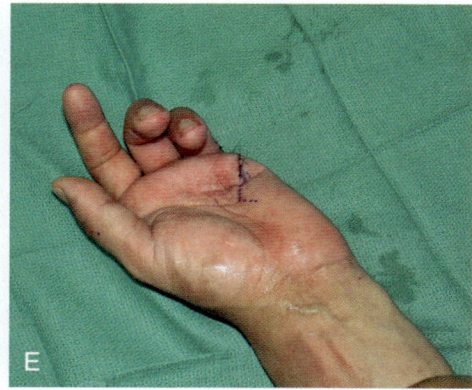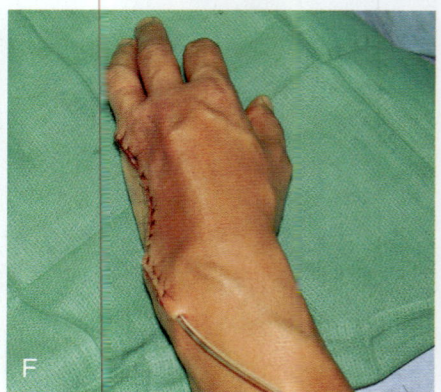

FIGURE 4 Surgical photographs of a fifth ray amputation with a harvest fillet flap. The planned dorsal incision (**A**) and palmar incision (**B**) are marked on the hand. **C**, The fillet flap is raised. **D**, The fifth ray is resected. Palmar (**E**) and dorsal (**F**) views of the hand after closure.

double ray or triple ray amputation. Preoperative radiation or chemotherapy can be used to decrease the tumor size to allow hand-sparing options at the time of definitive surgical treatment. If all four digit rays are contaminated by tumor, it is likely that there will be extension of the tumor into the carpal tunnel. In this setting, a more proximal level amputation is indicated.

Transmetacarpal amputation may be appropriate to treat some traumatic injuries. Every effort should be made to replant the amputated part, unless contraindicated. In severe crush injuries, it may not be possible to replant all digits. In this setting, the focus should be on the salvage of "spare parts" from the amputated digits and soft-tissue coverage, with a view to restore tip and side pinch, if needed with a staged toe-to-hand transfer.

Thumb Amputation
General Considerations
The thumb accounts for approximately 50% of hand function. A minimum requirement of thumb function is a stable post against which objects can be held. Function is improved if sensation is present or motion is possible.

Traumatic amputation of the thumb is considered a strong indication for replantation if possible. The success of thumb replantation may be limited in the setting of avulsion-type injuries.

Given the devastating effects of proximal level amputation of the thumb, there is an increased emphasis on thumb-sparing procedures when a sensate terminal thumb can be reconstructed.[7,8] If the entire thumb must be amputated at the metacarpophalangeal joint, proximal reconstruction options include toe-to-thumb transfer, index pollicization, and use of a passive prosthesis.

Interphalangeal Thumb Disarticulation
Interphalangeal thumb disarticulation is commonly done in the setting of melanoma, squamous cell carcinoma, and, less frequently, trauma. Two coverage options are generally considered. Volar-based flaps and fish-mouth incisions both yield excellent results.

Interphalangeal joint disarticulation is very well tolerated. Although the thumb is shortened, this rarely affects general functions such as gripping large objects, and there is only a small decrease in dexterity. Patients compensate well for any change in sensation, and will rely more heavily on the combination of visual and tactile sensations when handling small objects.

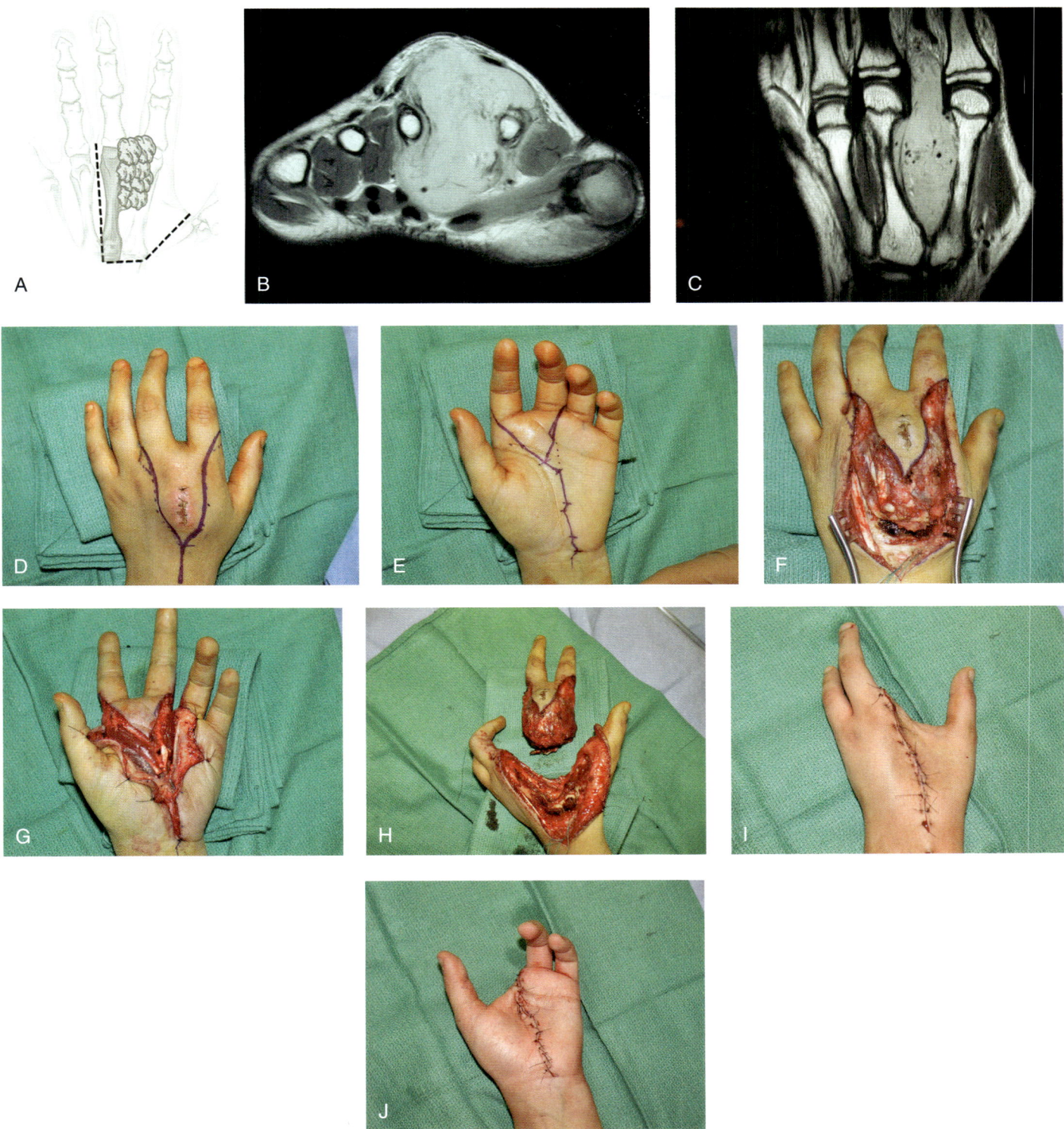

FIGURE 5 **A**, Illustration showing a planned index and middle ray resection for a malignant neoplasm. Axial (**B**) and coronal (**C**) MRIs demonstrating the extent of the malignant neoplasm. **D** through **J**, Photographs of the double ray amputation. The planned dorsal incision (**D**) and volar incision (**E**) are drawn on the hand. The hand after dorsal (**F**) and palmar (**G**) dissection. The resected specimen is removed (**H**). Dorsal (**I**) and palmar (**J**) views of the hand after closure.

Section 2: Upper Limb

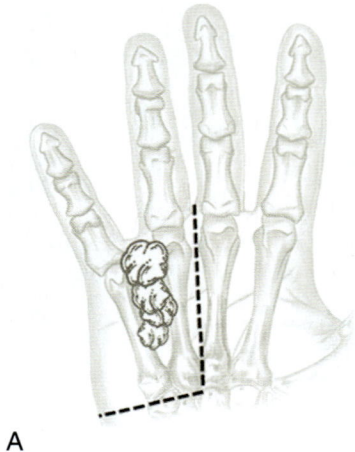
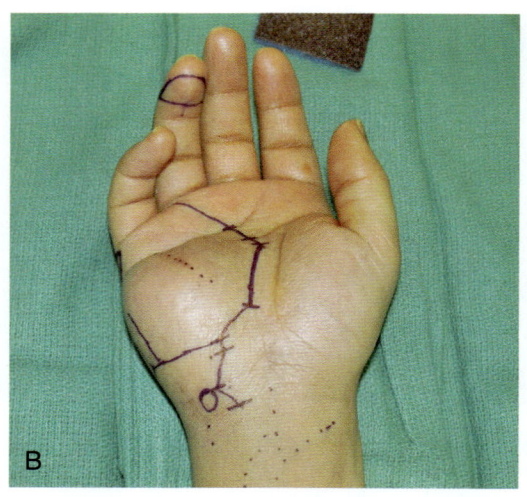
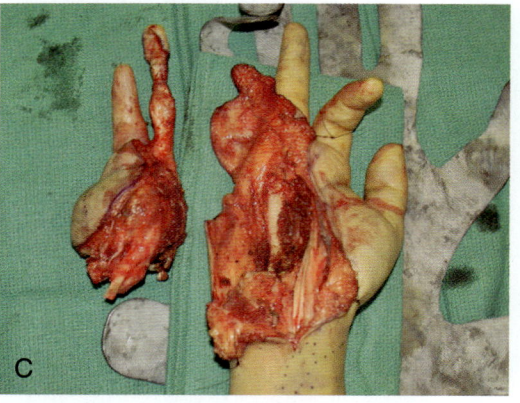
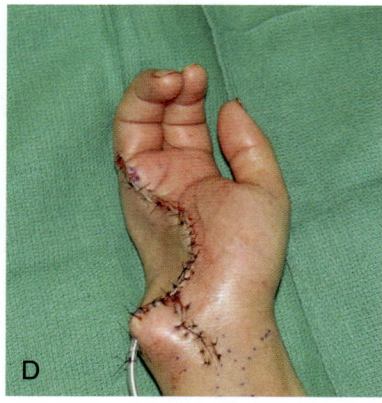

FIGURE 6 **A**, Illustration showing a planned ring and small finger ulnar double ray amputation for a soft-tissue tumor. **B** through **D**, Surgical photographs of the amputation. **B**, The volar incision with a fillet flap is marked on the hand. **C**, The ulnar double ray is resected with a ring fillet flap. The resection incorporated the flexor tendons to ring finger. **D**, Appearance of the hand after tendon reconstruction and direct closure using dorsal skin.

Preferred Techniques of This Chapter's Authors

In the experience of this chapter's authors, thumb lengthening has not been necessary after interphalangeal amputation.

Interphalangeal amputation coverage is often dictated by the extent of trauma or tumor. The use of a large volar flap is preferred when possible (**Figure 7**). If there is excessive palmar skin loss or contamination, fishmouth–type incisions are used.

A transverse incision is marked dorsally, often in line with the distal extensor crease. A palmar flap is marked with longitudinal extensions from the dorsal transverse incision, which will allow inclusion of the digital arteries and nerves in the volar flap. The dorsal incision is made first. Large dorsal veins are cauterized. The extensor mechanism is transected. The collateral ligaments are transected proximally from the proximal phalanx. The volar flap is elevated superficial to the flexor tendon sheath. The flexor tendon is transected at the level of the interphalangeal joint. The volar plate is transected, and the amputation is completed. Closure is performed using 5-0 nylon suture, with great care to approximate the volar flap without excessive tension, which may compromise blood flow.

Alternative Surgical Techniques

Aesthetic appearance is superior with a fish-mouth closure; however, sensation and padding are superior with a volar flap. More proximal level amputation through the distal portion of the proximal phalanx may be required for tumors extending into the interphalangeal joint or for more proximal level trauma.

Postoperative Care and Rehabilitation

A soft, bulky, lightly compressive thumb spica bandage is applied after surgery. Sutures are removed after 2 weeks. Physical therapy begins with range-of-motion and wound desensitization exercises. Activities are restricted for approximately 6 weeks and are then resumed as tolerated. Therapy can be very helpful in improving manual dexterity and the development of compensatory and adaptive techniques to facilitate function.

Managing Complications

Wound desensitization exercises supervised by a therapist are effective in reducing wound sensitivity, which tends to gradually lessen over time. Neuroma-related symptoms and phantom pain are possible but are uncommon after thumb interphalangeal disarticulation.

Metacarpophalangeal Disarticulation

When there is no other alternative, amputation at the metacarpophalangeal joint may be required.

Outcome Considerations

Metacarpophalangeal disarticulation of the thumb will result in a major functional deficit. Despite this deficit, some patients will choose to have no reconstructive procedures and will adapt and compensate as best as possible. If a toe-to-thumb reconstruction is being considered, it is best to stage the reconstruction after amputation done for malignant bone or soft-tissue tumors so that negative resection margins can be confirmed by definitive pathological analysis. Toe-to-thumb transfer in the setting of a positive margin will have a disease-dependent risk of local recurrence and might necessitate amputation of the transferred part.[9] If toe-to-thumb transfer is anticipated, it is wise to plan the soft-tissue flaps in advance so that additional uninjured, uncontaminated tissue can be spared at the time of disarticulation. This will facilitate subsequent closure at the time of reconstruction.

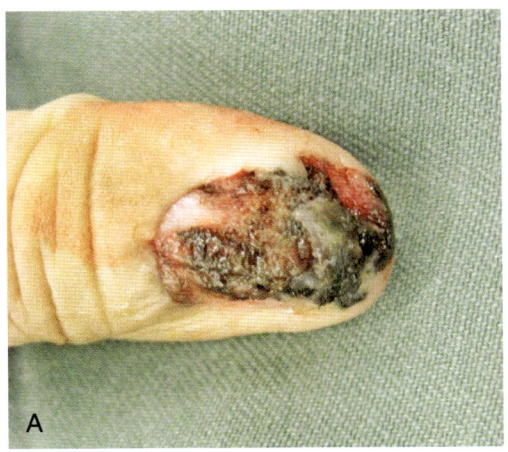
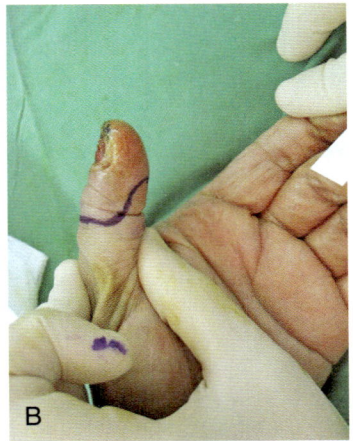
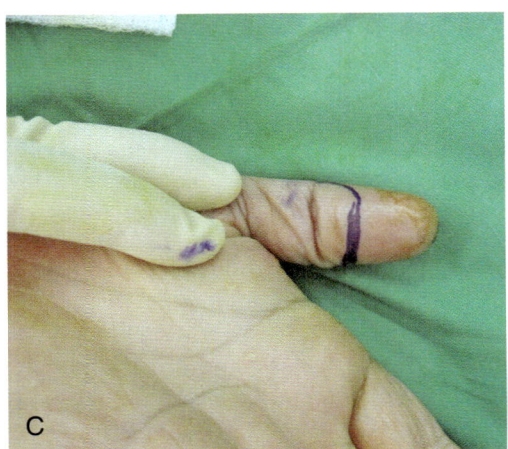
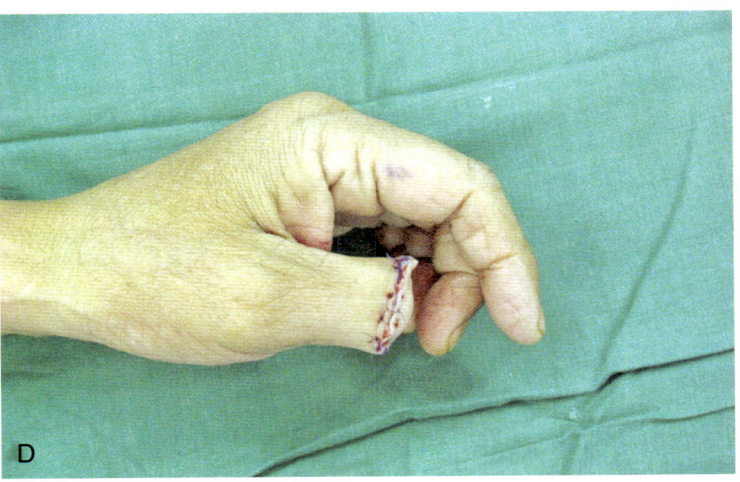
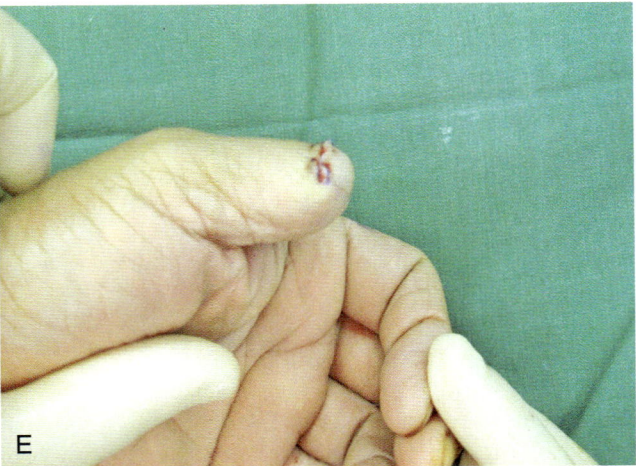

FIGURE 7 Photographs of a thumb interphalangeal disarticulation with volar flap closure. **A**, Subungual melanoma of the thumb is shown. Lateral (**B**) and palmar (**C**) views of the planned amputation and volar flap drawn on the thumb. Dorsal (**D**) and lateral (**E**) views of the thumb after the interphalangeal disarticulation and closure.

Index pollicization in children for congenital deformity often has an excellent final appearance. A pollicized index finger in an adult retains the appearance of a rotated index finger and does not have the same aesthetic result as seen in a child. Toe-to-thumb transfer is often preferred.

Preferred Techniques of This Chapter's Authors

Incisions are planned with the reconstructive procedure in mind. Fishmouth flaps are used, with longer flaps, when possible, if a toe-to-thumb transfer is anticipated.

The dorsal incision is made distal to the joint. Large veins are cauterized. Extensor tendons and sensory nerves are transected. The dorsal capsule is incised, and the collateral ligaments are transected. If a toe-to-thumb transfer is anticipated, larger remnants are left to allow ligament reconstruction and retain metacarpophalangeal joint stability after reconstruction. The volar flap incision is made. Digital nerves are identified, anesthetized, and transected. Digital arteries are cauterized and transected. The flexor pollicis longus and the volar plate are transected, and the amputation is completed. The wound is closed with 5-0 nylon suture.

Alternative Surgical Techniques

When a toe-to-thumb transfer is anticipated, nerves and vessels are tagged to facilitate identification at reconstruction. Vessels are ligated with hemoclips, and nerves and vessels are transected more distally.

Osseointegrated implants for the thumb have been described.[10] After amputation, a titanium peg is implanted into the distal metacarpal. After skin maturation, a passive prosthesis can be readily attached to the thumb metacarpal.

Postoperative Care and Rehabilitation

After surgery the hand is bandaged and the digits are kept free. Digit range of motion is encouraged. Sutures are removed after 2 weeks. Therapy can be beneficial for first web space stretching to avoid adduction contractures. A passive rigid prosthesis may be considered.

Neuroma Management in Partial Hand Amputations

Painful neuromas cause significant morbidity for patients following partial hand amputations. While many techniques have been described for surgical management, no single method has been shown to be superior.[11] Targeted muscle reinnervation and regenerative peripheral nerve interfaces) have shown good outcomes in patients with proximal amputations.[12,13] While the benefits are still being fully evaluated in patients with partial hand amputations, promising early results have been shown in some centers,[14,15] and we have also had positive early experience with some patients. By giving the transected nerve a target for regeneration mimicking a nerve repair, these procedures reduce the disorganized nerve sprouting that would otherwise occur, reducing the risk of the formation of painful neuromas. These techniques should be considered at the time of amputation, or as secondary procedures in patients with painful neuromas.

Improving Prosthetic Use in Partial Hand Amputations

The Starfish procedure, which involves intrinsic muscle transfers, was described to allow the generation of EMG signals for individual digital control on myoelectric prostheses. While this still involves a high level of prosthetic expertise not available in many centers worldwide, it can help to improve the functional outcomes, and reduce prosthesis abandonment, in patients with partial hand amputations.[16]

Outcomes of Partial Hand Amputations

Grip and pinch strength for patients with partial hand amputations vary greatly, depending on the digits affected, and the extent of amputation. While musculoskeletal complaints affecting the other limb, neck, and back appear to be no greater in patients with digit or partial hand amputations when compared with normal controls,[17] the presence of residuum sensations and limited range of motion of the wrist in these patients does predict their presence. Patients with partial hand amputations appear to have more pain interference with work, and were screened for higher levels of posttraumatic stress disorder when compared with patients with more proximal upper limb amputations.[18] The studies do highlight challenges faced by patients that may not be routinely addressed by treating surgeons, as well as emphasizing the need for aggressive pain management and avoidance of painful neuromas.

SUMMARY

Partial hand amputations may be performed to treat patients after traumatic injury, infection, or malignant bone and soft-tissue tumors. When possible, the functional and cosmetic deficits of the planned procedure should be discussed with the patient before surgery. Surgical considerations will depend on the etiology, the extent of the surgery (such as single ray, double ray, or thumb amputation), the status of soft tissues, and the general health of the patient. To obtain optimal outcomes, the surgeon should be familiar with established and alternative surgical techniques.

References

1. Talbot SG, Mehrara BJ, Disa JJ, et al: Soft-tissue coverage of the hand following sarcoma resection. *Plast Reconstr Surg* 2008;121(2):534-543.
2. Steichen JB, Idler RS: Results of central ray resection without bony transposition. *J Hand Surg Am* 1986;11(4):466-474.
3. Puhaindran ME, Healey JH, Athanasian EA: Single ray amputation for tumors of the hand. *Clin Orthop Relat Res* 2010;468(5):1390-1395.
4. Puhaindran ME, Athanasian EA: Double ray amputation for tumors of the hand. *Clin Orthop Relat Res* 2010;468(11):2976-2979.
5. Puhaindran ME, Steensma MR, Athanasian EA: Partial hand preservation for large soft tissue sarcomas of the hand. *J Hand Surg Am* 2010;35(2):291-295.
6. Rohde RS, Puhaindran ME, Morris CD, et al: Complications of radiation therapy to the hand after soft tissue sarcoma surgery. *J Hand Surg Am* 2010;35(11):1858-1863.
7. Puhaindran ME, Rothrock CP, Athanasian EA: Surgical management for malignant tumors of the thumb. *Hand (N Y)* 2011;6(4):373-377.
8. Goldner RD, Howson MP, Nunley JA, Fitch RD, Belding NR, Urbaniak JR: One hundred eleven thumb amputations: Replantation vs revision. *Microsurgery* 1990;11(3):243-250.
9. Buncke HJ, ed: *Microsurgery: Transplantation, Replantation. An Atlas Text*, ed 4. Lea & Febiger, 1991.
10. Lundborg G, Brånemark PI, Rosén B: Osseointegrated thumb prostheses: A concept for fixation of digit prosthetic devices. *J Hand Surg Am* 1996;21(2):216-221.
11. Poppler LH, Parikh RP, Bichanich MJ, et al: Surgical interventions for the treatment of painful neuroma: A comparative meta–Analysis. *Pain* 2018;159(2):214-223.
12. Dumanian GA, Potter BK, Mioton LM, et al: Targeted muscle reinnervation treats neuroma and phantom pain in major limb amputees: A randomized clinical trial. *Ann Surg* 2019;270(2):238-246.
13. Woo SL, Kung TA, Brown DL, Leonard JA, Kelly BM, Cederna PS: Regenerative peripheral nerve interfaces for the treatment of postamputation neuroma pain: A pilot study. *Plast Reconstr Surg Glob Open* 2016;4(12):e1038.
14. Daugherty THF, Bueno RA Jr, Neumeister MW: Novel use of targeted muscle reinnervation in the hand for treatment of recurrent symptomatic neuromas following digit amputations. *Plast Reconstr Surg Glob Open* 2019;7(8):e2376.
15. Hooper RC, Cederna PS, Brown DL, et al: Regenerative peripheral nerve interfaces for the management of symptomatic hand and digital neuromas. *Plast Reconstr Surg Glob Open* 2020;8(6):e2792.
16. Gaston RG, Bracey JW, Tait MA, Loeffler BJ: A novel muscle transfer for independent digital control of a myoelectric prosthesis: The starfish procedure. *J Hand Surg Am* 2019;44(2):163.e1-163.e5.
17. Bouma SE, Postema SG, Bongers RM, Dijkstra PU, van der Sluis CK: Musculoskeletal complaints in individuals with finger or partial hand amputations in the Netherlands: A cross-sectional study. *Disabil Rehabil* 2018;40(10):1146-1153.
18. Kearns NT, Jackson WT, Elliott TR, Ryan T Armstrong TW: Differences in level of upper limb loss on functional impairment, psychological well-being, and substance use. *Rehabil Psychol* 2018;63(1):141-147.

Partial Hand Amputation: Prosthetic Management

CHAPTER 15

Jack E. Uellendahl, CPO • Matthew J. Mikosz, CP, LP

ABSTRACT

Partial hand amputation is reported to be the most common upper limb amputation level in the United States. The hand has 29 joints, and approximately 25% of the motor cortex controls the 34 muscles that move the hand. Because these joints allow the hand to assume many postures and produce various grasping patterns, replacement with a prosthesis is challenging. Sensory feedback provides information about objects being grasped; loss or compromise of this feedback results in further disability. Trauma is the most common cause of partial hand amputation and often damages the remaining parts of the hand. Limited joint range of motion, malalignment of the remaining fingers, hypersensitivity or insensitivity, scarring, and a lack of strength in the remaining portions of the hand can be complicating factors. Prosthetic options for managing partial hand amputations have increased substantially in recent years.

Keywords: amputation; body-powered prosthesis; hand amputation; partial finger; partial hand; powered fingers; upper limb

Introduction

Partial hand amputation is the most common upper limb amputation level in the United States. In a review of hospital discharge records between 1988 and 1996, Dillingham et al[1] found that a mean of 18,496 individuals annually were reported to undergo upper limb amputations or have congenital limb deficiencies; 92% of these were below the wrist. Partial hand amputations have many possible presentations based on the large number of possible hand configurations that result from traumatic injury (**Figure 1**).

The hand is a marvelous tool. It has 29 joints, and approximately 25% of the motor cortex controls the 34 muscles of the hand. These joints allow the hand to assume many postures and produce a variety of grasping patterns. Therefore, prosthetic replacement is challenging. Sensory feedback provides information about objects being grasped; loss or compromise of this feedback results in further disability. Trauma is the most common cause of partial hand amputation and often damages the parts of the hand that remain. Limited joint range of motion, malalignment of the remaining fingers, hypersensitivity or insensitivity, scarring, and a lack of strength in the remaining portions of the hand may be complicating factors.[2]

Prosthetic options for managing partial hand amputations have increased substantially in recent years. The current prosthetic options and indications for their use are reviewed.

Clinical Considerations: Prosthetic Options

Prosthetic options can be divided into five categories: aesthetic, oppositional, activity-specific, body-powered, and externally powered. Not all options are available for all levels of partial hand absence. However, when evaluating a partial hand amputation, all options relevant to the amputation level should be reviewed. When deciding on the type of prosthesis to be used, considerations should include age, sex, occupation, degree of physical activity, gadget tolerance, type of amputation, functional goals, and unilateral versus bilateral involvement.[2]

Because the thumb is the most important finger, representing 40% of hand function, its presence and condition should be carefully evaluated.[3] Optimal management of the thumb should account for sensibility, stability, opposition, and length.[4] With partial thumb amputation, it is sometimes advantageous to restore length with a customized silicone finger prosthesis. However, this type of prosthesis will cover sensate skin and can impede function in instances in which comorbid missing fingers have been treated with a prosthetic replacement, which also provides no sensation (**Figure 2**). In this case, a short, sensate thumb may be more functional than a normal-length prosthetic thumb without normal sensation.

Additional options include surgical solutions. A partially amputated

---

Jack E. Uellendahl or an immediate family member serves as a paid consultant to or is an employee of Hanger Clinic and has stock or stock options held in Hanger Clinic. Neither Matthew J. Mikosz nor any immediate family member has received anything of value from or has stock or stock options held in a commercial company or institution related directly or indirectly to the subject of this chapter.

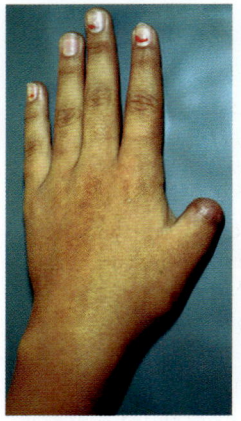 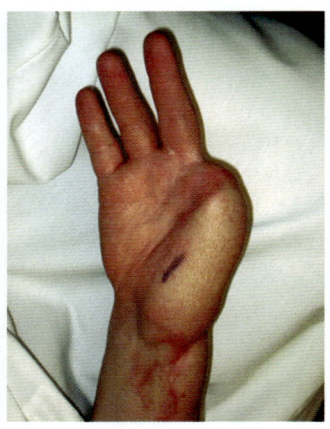 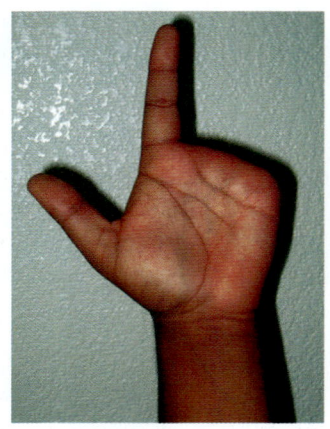
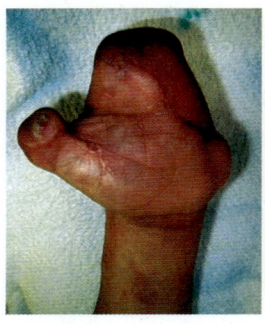 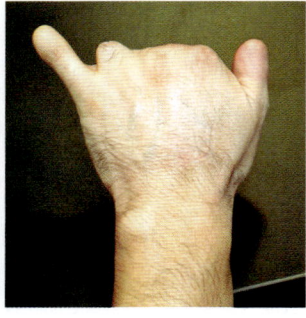 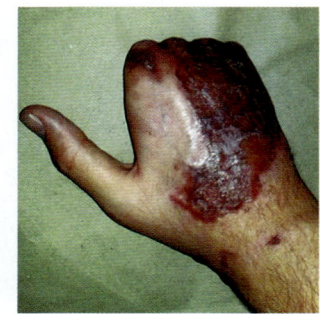

FIGURE 1 Photographs showing a variety of partial hand amputations.

thumb may be treated surgically with lengthening, web space deepening, toe transfer, pollicization, or osteointegration[5,6] (**Figure 3**). Such cases highlight the importance of early interaction among the patient, prosthetist, surgeon, and therapist in developing a treatment plan that optimizes a patient's outcome.

Component Considerations

Aesthetic Restoration

High-definition custom silicone prostheses are the best option to reproduce the natural appearance of the hand.[7] These prostheses are appropriate for all levels of partial hand amputation from fingertip to complete hand prostheses. The prosthesis is carefully matched in size, shape, surface detail, and color to the sound hand, which allows differences between the normal and prosthetic hand to go unnoticed by the casual observer (**Figure 4**). Silicone prostheses provide an extremely important psychological benefit in restoring body image.[7] The prostheses have a long history of use and are generally well accepted by patients.[7,8] They do not provide finger movement and are often referred to as passive prostheses. However, a study by Fraser[9] showed that, despite the lack of movement, these prostheses are used functionally when performing daily tasks. Passive silicone prostheses can provide opposition when some fingers remain and broaden the surface available for gripping stability. In addition, silicone prostheses protect sensitive or painful areas of the hand, with attendant improvements to manual function. Although silicone has good stain resistance, the material can be damaged if used for manual labor. Many individuals with partial hand amputations benefit from the use of an aesthetic prosthesis in addition to another type of prosthesis.

Opposition Prostheses

The primary goal of an opposition prosthesis is to provide opposition for intact fingers or the palm of the hand. These prostheses can be made of many materials but are usually strong, robust, and well suited for manual tasks (**Figures 4** through **6**). Most opposition prostheses are static, but some have joints that can be prepositioned on a task-specific basis, such as the CAPP Multi-Position Post (Hosmer), APRL thumb (Hosmer), and Vincent Finger Joint (Vincent Systems GmbH).

Activity-Specific Prostheses

In some cases, a prosthesis is needed to accomplish a specific function. The prosthesis may be constructed to hold and support a specific tool, with or without the contribution of any remaining digits (**Figure 7**). Alternatively, a

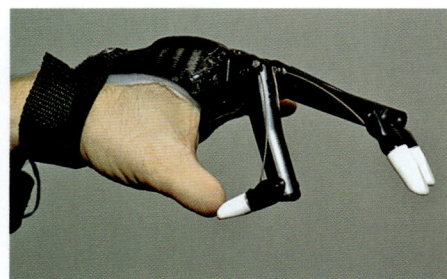

FIGURE 2 Photograph of a thumb that was left uncovered to preserve sensation while opposing three powered fingers. The little finger was also partially amputated and left uncovered.

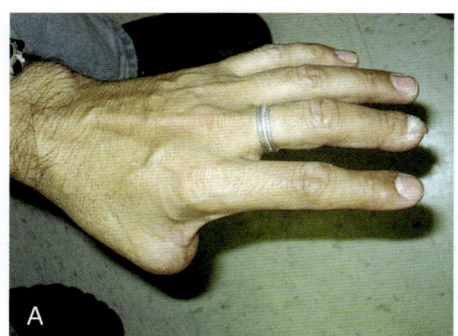 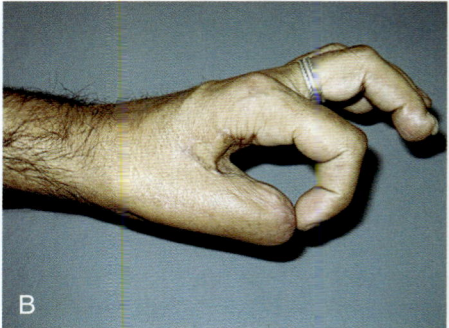

FIGURE 3 Preoperative (**A**) and postoperative (**B**) photographs of a thumb amputation that underwent bone lengthening and web space deepening to provide sufficient length for functional grasp.

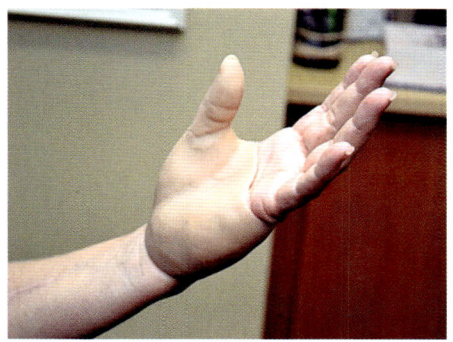

FIGURE 4 Photograph of a hybrid silicone and composite thumb prosthesis that provides good appearance and stability for functional opposition to the remaining fingers.

quick-disconnect mechanism can be fixed onto the palm of the remnant hand that allows attachment to a variety of commercially available tools and implements. At the partial finger amputation level, simple fingertip caps can extend the functional length of the residual finger to enable enhanced function (**Figure 8**). Collectively, these prostheses may allow participation in hobbies and sports and can be critical to performing job duties.

Body-Powered Prostheses

Body power refers to the use of force and excursion produced by more proximal joints to control a prosthesis. Because of the link between the controlled component and the proximal physiologic joints, body-powered control has the inherent advantage of providing proprioceptive feedback to the user regarding force, position, and speed of movement.[10] However, a possible disadvantage is that the required movements of the proximal joint segments may appear unnatural.[2] Body-powered prosthetic options are now available for nearly all levels of partial hand absences. Control is accomplished either through rigid linkages or through cables connecting the prosthetic joint(s) to a proximal intact joint. Examples of linkage-driven fingers are the Naked Prosthetic Finger (Naked Prosthetics; **Figure 9**) and the X-Finger (Didrick Medical; **Figure 10**).

Alternatively, the M-Fingers and Partial M-Fingers (Partial Hand Solutions) are cable driven. Partial M-Fingers use metacarpophalangeal (MCP) joint flexion to drive proximal interphalangeal joint flexion, whereas the distal interphalangeal joint is fixed (**Figures 11** through **13**). M-Fingers are designed for complete finger absence at or proximal to the MCP joints. Flexion at the MCP and proximal interphalangeal joints is actuated by wrist flexion; internal spring mechanisms return the joints to their extended positions with wrist extension[11] (**Figure 14**). Another body-powered option is a handihook-type device (**Figure 15**) in which a conventional hook terminal device, either voluntary opening or voluntary closing, is attached to a prosthetic socket in the palm of the partial hand prosthesis. The handihook is generally activated using a cable attached to a shoulder harness.[2,12]

Externally Powered Prostheses

Fitting externally powered devices to individuals with partial hand amputations is challenging. Because a portion of the physiologic hand remains, the space for any prosthetic mechanism is limited. Early efforts to develop externally powered options for partial hands were not made commercially available.[4,13-16] To fit the widest variety of partial hand configurations with externally powered options, the drive mechanism is best contained within the prosthetic finger itself. This allows for the successful fitting of amputations at or more proximal to the MCP level. The first powered fingers became commercially available in 2007 with the introduction of the i-limb hand (Össur). The fingers from the i-limb hand that were removed from the full hand and separately configured were referred to as ProDigits. The fingers were later redesigned for specific application to partial hand prostheses and renamed i-limb digits (Össur)[17] (**Figure 16**). Another system, the Powered Finger (Vincent Systems), became available in 2010[18] (**Figure 17**). Powered finger prostheses have demonstrated clinical efficacy for a wide variety of partial hand amputations and have become a mainstay in the prosthetic armamentarium.[2,19,20]

Powered finger prostheses are advantageous compared with body-powered devices because they require no force or excursion from the user; these devices are usually controlled using myoelectric signals or force-sensitive resistors. This can be an especially important consideration when the residual hand is sensitive to pressure. Prehension is maintained without continuous input control because the drive mechanism is not back drivable. Grip force is also generally greater with powered fingers than with the currently available wrist-driven options.

Although externally powered fingers do not provide feedback through the control system regarding finger

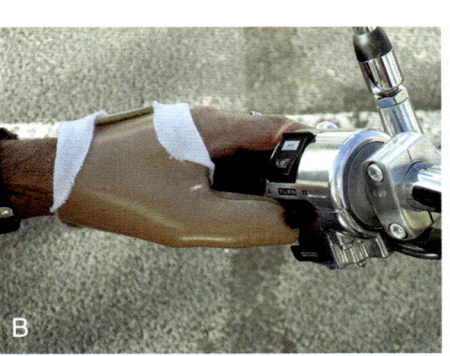

FIGURE 5 Photographs of a thumb amputated at the metacarpophalangeal joint (**A**) that was fitted with a rigid thumb opposition post (**B**).

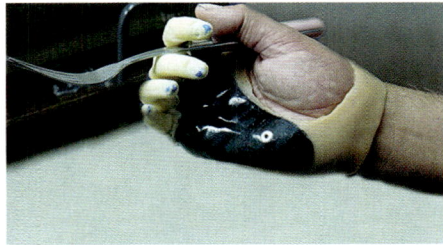

FIGURE 6 Photograph shows an opposition prosthesis during test fitting with the static fingers positioned for optimal function.

Section 2: Upper Limb

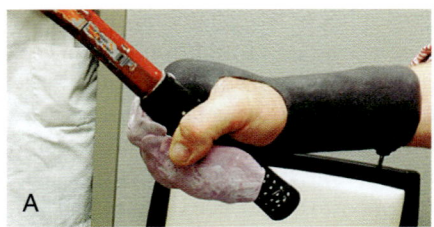 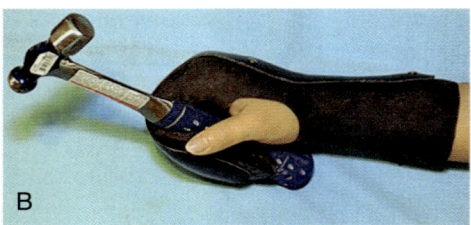

FIGURE 7 **A**, Photograph of an activity-specific static prosthesis during test fitting with a hammer for a farrier. **B**, Photograph of the completed hybrid prosthesis composed of silicone and prepreg carbon fiber, with a zipper for easy donning and doffing.

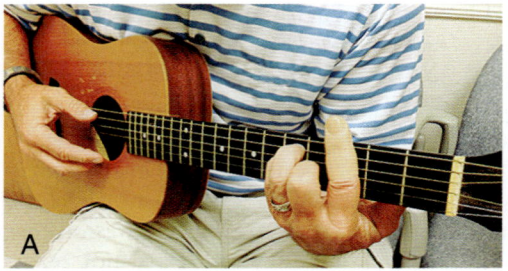 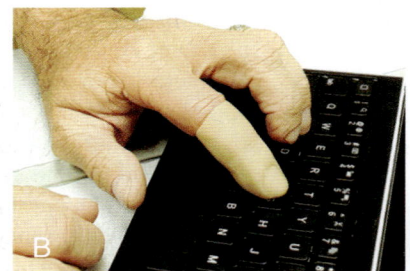

FIGURE 8 Photographs of an index finger prosthesis used for guitar playing (**A**) and typing (**B**).

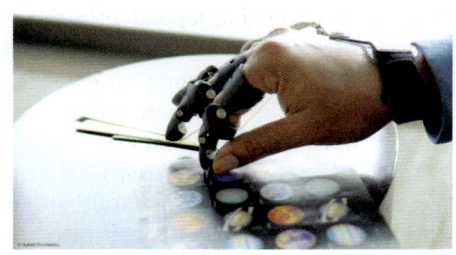

FIGURE 9 Photograph of a mechanical finger with distal interphalangeal joint flexion of the prosthesis driven by intact proximal interphalangeal flexion. (Courtesy of Naked Prosthetics, Olympia, WA.)

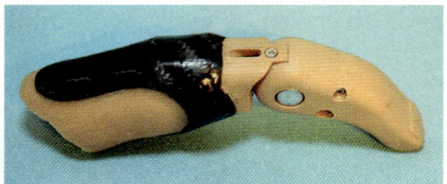

FIGURE 11 Photograph of a partial finger prosthesis with a silicone suction socket and prepreg carbon fiber, providing rigid stabilization and connection to a Partial M-Finger prosthesis (Partial Hand Solutions). (Courtesy of Elaine N. Uellendahl, CPE, Phoenix, AZ.)

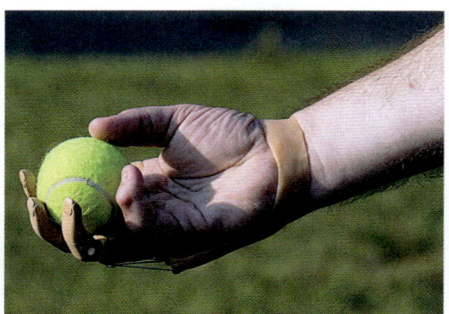

FIGURE 12 Photograph of a three-finger Partial M-Finger prosthesis (Partial Hand Solutions) showing the cables anchored to a silicone mounting system. Metacarpophalangeal joint flexion drives interphalangeal joint flexion, and internal springs return the fingers to extension. (Courtesy of the Hanger Clinic, Austin, TX.)

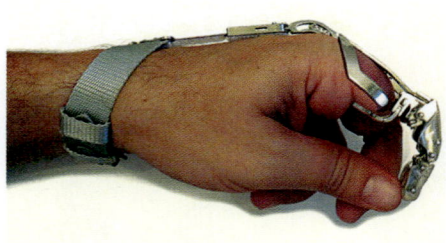

FIGURE 10 Photograph of a mechanical finger with distal interphalangeal joint and proximal interphalangeal joint flexion of the prosthesis, which are driven by intact metacarpophalangeal joint flexion. (Courtesy of Didrick Medical, Naples, FL.)

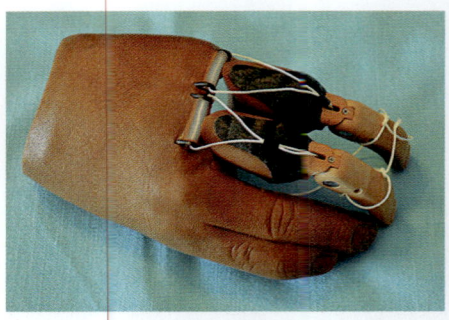

FIGURE 13 Photograph of a combination Partial M-Finger prosthesis (Partial Hand Solutions) that provides dynamic grasp for the index and middle fingers against the intact thumb, with the ring and little fingers replaced with static silicone fingers to provide a broader, more stable platform for grasp.

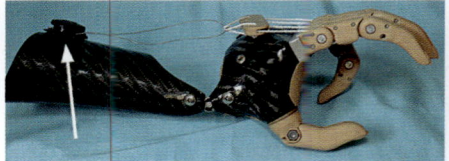

FIGURE 14 Photograph of a wrist-driven M-Finger prosthesis (Partial Hand Solutions). Wrist flexion drives all four fingers with a cable system in opposition to a passively positioned friction thumb. The cable tension can be adjusted using a quick-adjust knob (arrow).

force, position, and velocity the Vincent Powered Finger system offers feedback regarding finger force by means of vibration. The complete powered finger system includes the fingers, finger-mounting hardware, a microprocessor control unit, power supply, and control input(s). Because of the inherent space limitations at distal amputation levels, some of these components are housed on the forearm within a forearm cuff or a custom silicone socket (**Figures 18** and **19**). The motor for these powered fingers is housed in the proximal segment of the finger and drives the MCP joint, which is then used to drive a single interphalangeal joint via mechanical linkage.

Externally powered thumbs are manufactured by Össur and Vincent Systems. These thumbs do not articulate at the interphalangeal joint but are powered in flexion and extension at the MCP joint and can be passively rotated from a position opposed to the fingers or unopposed for lateral prehension (**Figure 20**). The control systems

Chapter 15: Partial Hand Amputation: Prosthetic Management

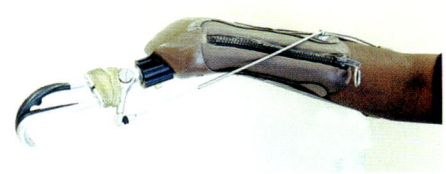

FIGURE 15 Photograph of the lower arm of an individual with carpometacarpal disarticulation who uses a body-powered handihook. The hook opening is actuated using a conventional shoulder harness. The hook is attached to a quick-disconnect adapter, allowing exchange of various tools in place of the cable-actuated hook. The prosthesis has a silicone socket with a zipper in a composite frame.

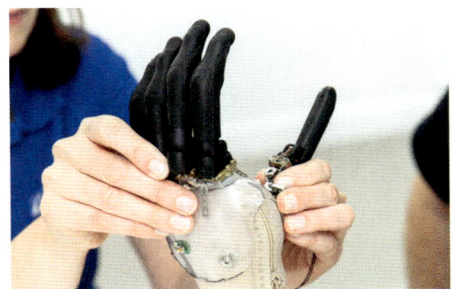

FIGURE 16 Photograph of an i-limb digit (Össur) with a motor in the proximal finger segment that drives the metacarpophalangeal (MCP) joint. MCP joint flexion is linked to proximal interphalangeal joint flexion with a string, and a spring provides extension at the proximal interphalangeal joint. The distal interphalangeal joint is fixed. Various fingertip lengths are available for finger sizing. (Courtesy of Össur.)

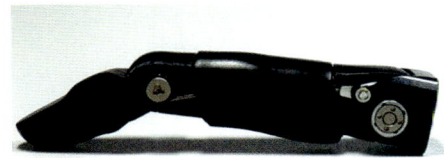

FIGURE 17 Photograph of the Powered Finger (Vincent Systems), which has a motor in the proximal finger segment that drives the metacarpophalangeal (MCP) joint. MCP flexion is linked to proximal interphalangeal joint flexion with a flexible metal strut that drives the proximal interphalangeal joint in flexion and extension. The distal interphalangeal joint is fixed. Various fingertip lengths are available for finger sizing.

are adjusted via wireless connections to a computer or a handheld device, where system parameters can easily be adjusted and real-time monitoring of patient control inputs can be viewed.

Control

Myoelectrodes and force-sensitive resistors are the most common types of control input used for powered fingers. Other types of control input devices include transducers and switches. Most users prefer dual-site proportional control, but single-site methods have been used successfully when only one control input is available. In the primary gripping pattern, all fingers are driven until motion is stopped either by contact with an object or when the mechanical stop is encountered. This provides a conformable grip (**Figure 21**). Because each finger is driven independently, it is possible to fix the position of some fingers and drive others. Selecting a grip mode in which the fingers are flexed and the thumb is active in the unopposed

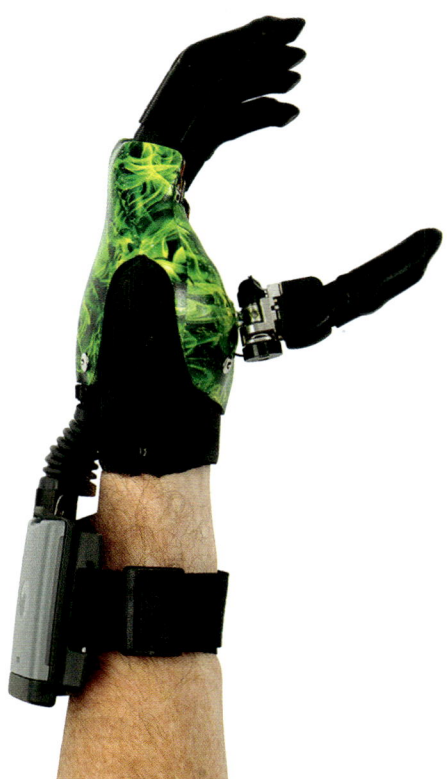

FIGURE 18 Photograph of a complete i-limb digits prosthesis (Össur), which uses a forearm cuff to house the battery cells, controller, and power switch. (Courtesy of Össur.)

position is useful for lateral prehension. A wide variety of additional grip patterns are possible, including a pointed index finger, which is valuable for keyboard use, and a trigger finger for the operation of spray bottles. Other grip patterns can be selected, generally by using a special control command such as co-contraction, a hold-open signal, or a rapid impulse signal from one of the available input sources.

Myoelectric control sites can be located either in the hand or in the forearm. Using the intrinsic muscles of the hand is often preferable because it allows finger control to be independent of wrist motion. Intrinsic muscles that have been used successfully include the thenar, hypothenar, and dorsal interossei muscles. When intrinsic hand muscles are not feasible as control sites, forearm muscles have been used with good results. With practice, most users achieve sufficient control of the fingers and wrist independently.

If a mobile feature of the remaining hand can be moved independently, control by force-sensitive resistors should be considered. If all fingers are missing and the thumb is amputated at the MCP joint, the mobile thumb metacarpal can be used to flex and extend the fingers by using the metacarpal to press against one force-sensitive resistor in the flexion direction and another force-sensitive resistor in the extension direction. In some instances, control has been achieved by mixing control inputs using one electrode and one force-sensitive resistor.

Using a separate control command to select each specific grip pattern is

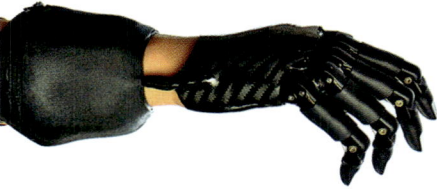

FIGURE 19 Photograph of a complete Powered Finger prosthesis (Vincent Systems) shows the batteries, controller, and charge port module housed in a custom silicone forearm cuff. These components are accessed through a zipper closure.

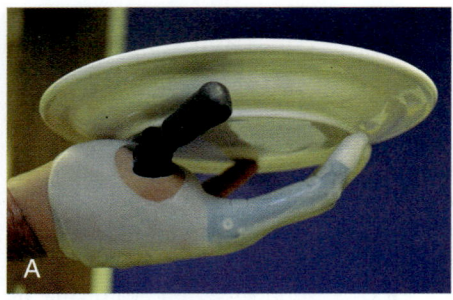
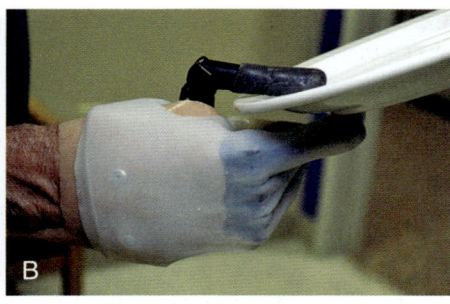

FIGURE 20 Photographs of an externally powered thumb prosthesis. **A**, Rotating the thumb to the unopposed position helps assume a flat hand to provide a stable, broad surface for holding plates, trays, or similar objects. **B**, Lateral prehension is achieved with the thumb in the unopposed position.

not ideal. Developing control strategies such as pattern recognition and implantable myoelectric sensors may eventually provide more intuitive control.[21-25]

Prosthesis Design

The prosthetic socket provides a stable connection to the residual limb, securely suspends the prosthesis, protects sensitive areas of the residual limb, and serves as a mount for the prosthetic components[2] (**Figure 22**). Materials used include rigid, laminated material; semirigid plastic; flexible thermoplastic; silicone, urethane, and expanded foam padding. For many partial hand prostheses, it is important to provide a soft flexible elastic interface so that bony prominences are protected, motion is not impeded by rigid edges, and the material can stretch to allow easy donning and doffing when bulbous limbs are involved. For these reasons, the preferred interface material of this chapter's authors is silicone that is structurally supported with composite plastic. With high-consistency silicone rubber, it is possible to design and fabricate silicone interfaces in which the material thickness, stiffness, and elasticity can be selectively controlled.[26,27] It also is possible to incorporate electrode mounts, screw attachments, zippers, and other hardware into the silicone interface. Custom silicone sockets have been reported to provide better comfort as well as the ability to protect fragile skin from breakdown compared with other materials.[28] The socket should not restrict limb motion at the wrist, thumb, or other remaining joints (**Figure 23**).

One of the most important features of the hand is sensation. The maximum amount of sensate skin should be exposed whenever possible.[5,16] In contrast, when the limb is hypersensitive, covering the skin can provide protection. These issues must be carefully evaluated and managed when planning the design of the prosthesis.

Partial Hand Limb Loss and 3D Printing

Three-dimensional (3D) printing technology has been around for many years, with the invention of stereolithography by Charles Hull in 1984.[30] More recently, the use of 3D printing has created a buzz in the field of prosthetics and orthotics. Many individuals with access to computers and low-cost printers have developed creative hand, partial hand, and finger designs. This has created new opportunities for clinicians with an interest in computer-aided design (CAD) to use their clinical and engineering knowledge to innovate and develop new designs for individuals with limb loss. **Figure 24** shows an example of a design created from a 3D scan of the patient's limb. There are many benefits to creating a design direct from a scan which include: using existing fingers to reference for alignment, creating precise socket wall thickness, and merging CAD files with organic shapes. The design shown in **Figure 25** uses a Partial M-Finger from Partial Hand Solutions, LLC, which was merged with the socket design. Alignment of the finger was precisely matched to the remaining fingers so optimal alignment can be achieved during the design process. Typically,

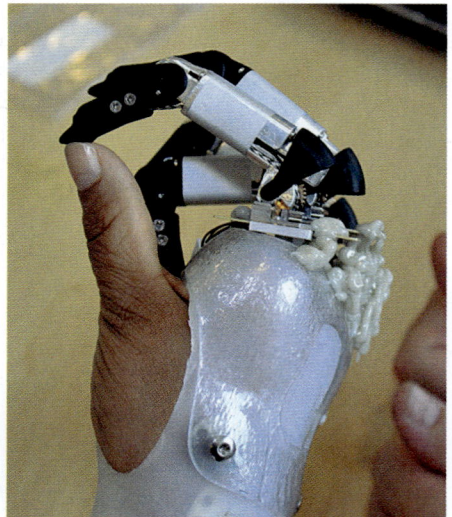

FIGURE 22 Photograph of a test fitting, with careful attention paid to finger alignment. Mounting frames are available that either group the fingers in a prearranged alignment to each other or allow the fingers to be individually positioned.

FIGURE 21 Photograph demonstrates individually powered fingers conformed around an irregularly shaped object, providing a secure grasp.

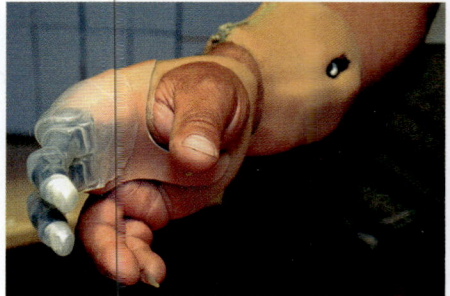

FIGURE 25 Photograph of a prosthesis designed to allow full motion of the intact thumb, ring, and little fingers as well as full wrist motion.

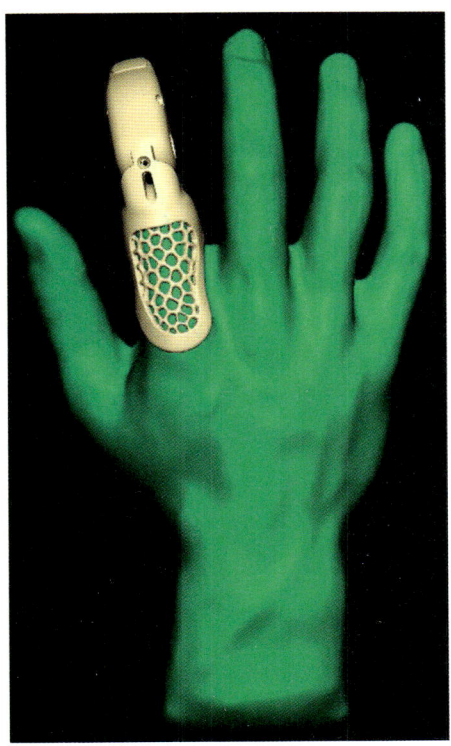

FIGURE 24 Rendering of an example of a design created from a 3D scan of the patient's limb.

this design would have a silicone interface and a rigid carbon fiber frame to support the finger base. Using the CAD design process, both the inner socket and outer frame can be designed together and printed with different materials. Designing the two together creates a precise fit when installing the inner socket to the outer frame. Now, with the ability to print medical-grade silicone, it is possible to design and print the entire device and very closely mimic the traditional process of fabricating a high-consistency rubber inner socket and carbon fiber frame. Custom cutouts or patterns can also be applied to the design to give the device a unique look and change the stiffness and flexibility of the frame if desired.

This process has been used with many of the currently available partial hand options and has been shown to be effective in all cases. Optimizing finger alignment in CAD allows the designer to precisely match the angle, rotation, and distance between fingers, and can easily adjust as needed. **Figure 25** shows a four-finger Titan Flex system aligned with this process. This process would consist of designing the inner socket and then the outer frame and trim each to the desired trimlines. The Titan flex mounts would then be installed and aligned to the appropriate location. Once all fingers are positioned, the fingers would be removed leaving the mounts in place. To connect the inner and outer frames together, mushroom-like extensions on the silicone can be designed with corresponding holes in the frame to allow the two to connect. Once all the design work is complete, each part can be sent to the corresponding printer for socket fabrication. Optimal print material for this design would be 35 shore silicone for the interface and nylon 12 for the frame. This process should not be considered unless the materials being used are properly tested for strength and durability before patient use.

The 3D process is also very useful when different components are being considered. This process allows the designer to prebuild the device to get a better assessment of what the finished device would look like and troubleshoot any potential design issues before fabrication. **Figure 26** shows a design using

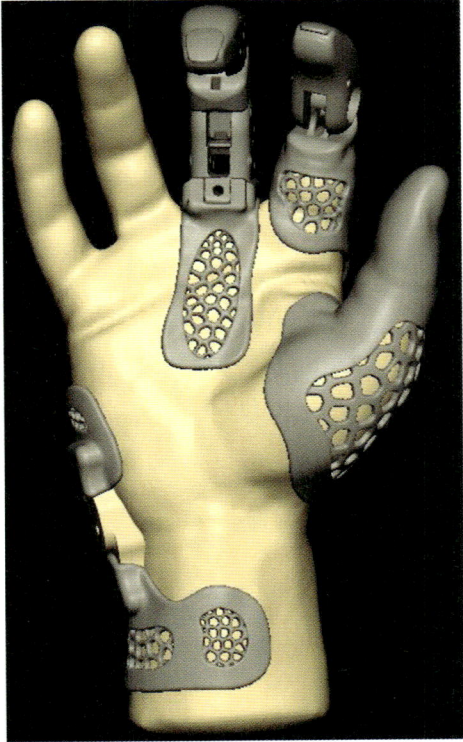

FIGURE 25 Rendering of a four-finger Titan Flex system aligned with this process.

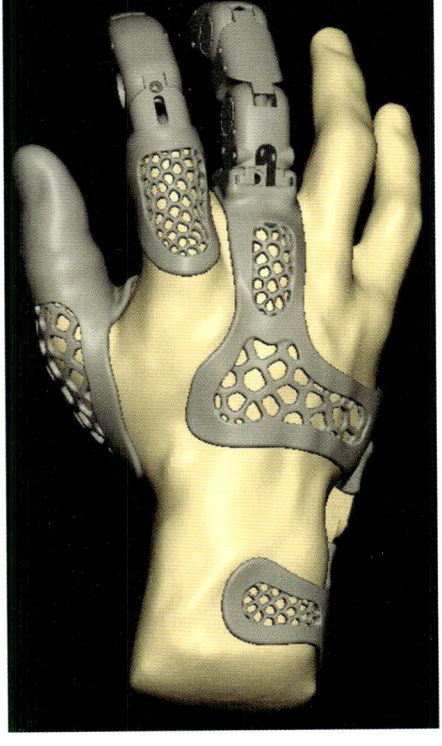

FIGURE 26 Rendering of a design using three different types of socket designs for various levels of amputation along with the appropriate component.

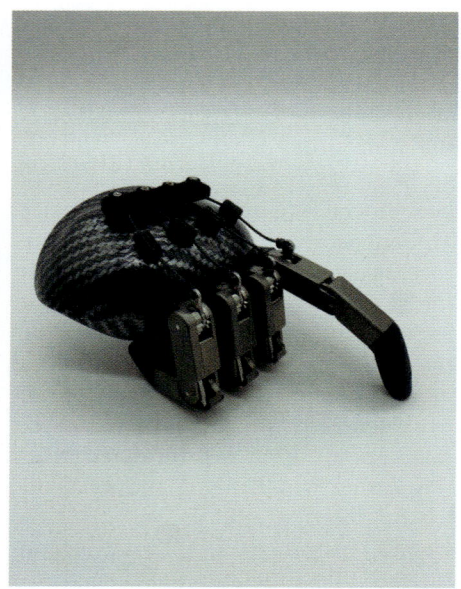 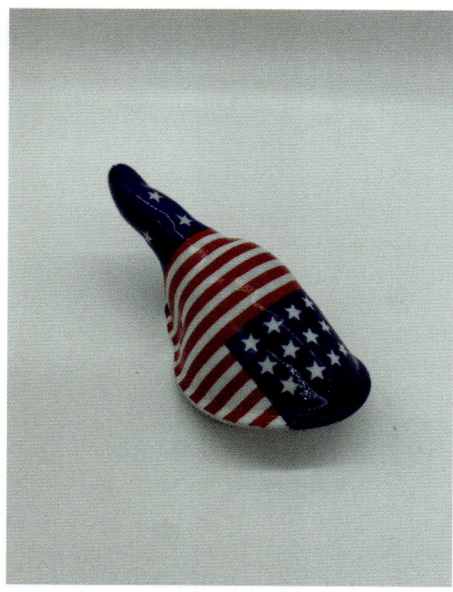 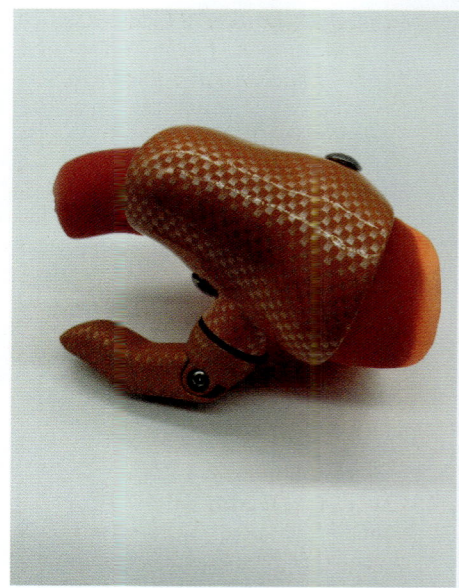

FIGURE 27 Photographs showing some examples of 3D printed devices with hydrographic coatings applied.

three different types of components. This system highlights a custom-designed thumb interphalangeal joint, a Partial M-Finger, and an M-Finger. This is also a very useful tool to show the patient or referral source so they can better assess the options presented to them. It is important to note that any device that is 3D printed should be thoroughly tested and evaluated for any patient use. There are many types of printers on the market today and a variety of potential issues can arise if caution is not taken to ensure all necessary precautions are considered before fitting any of these 3D printed designs.

There are also many finishing options to consider when using 3D printed devices. The application of hydrographic patterns can really personalize the device and add further customization to the prosthesis. **Figure 27** shows some examples of 3D printed devices with hydrographics coating applied.

In conclusion, 3D printing has been shown to be an effective option for orthotic and prosthetic professionals. It allows clinicians to develop creative designs and offer users alternatives to traditional methods. As 3D printing technology continues to evolve and new materials become available, more opportunities will arise to improve and develop new innovations.

SUMMARY

Currently, more prosthetic options exist for individuals with partial hand amputation than ever before; however, fitting the prosthesis is still challenging. The amputation is best managed by a team of knowledgeable professionals who can provide surgical, prosthetic, training, and counseling support. Appearance, function, and comfort should be carefully considered by both the patient and the team to determine the most appropriate prosthesis. Often, not all goals can be achieved with one prosthesis, and multiple devices are required. Surgical options may eliminate the need for a prosthesis in some patients; however, when a prosthesis is indicated, surgery should complement and optimize the successful use of the prosthesis. In all cases, a qualified therapist should educate the user regarding optimal function with and without a prosthesis to prevent potential overuse of the sound limb.[29]

References

1. Dillingham TR, Pezzin LE, MacKenzie EJ: Limb amputation and limb deficiency: Epidemiology and recent trends in the United States. *South Med J* 2002;95:875-883.
2. Uellendahl JE, Uellendahl EN: Experience fitting partial hand prostheses with externally powered fingers, in Parenti-Castelli V, Troncossi M, eds: *Grasping the Future: Advances in Powered Upper Limb Prosthetics*. Bentham Science, 2012, pp 15-27.
3. Engleberg A: *Guides to the Evaluation of Permanent Impairment*, ed 3. American Medical Association, 1988, pp 20-21.
4. Weir R: *An Externally-Powered Myoelectrically Controlled Synergetic Prosthetic Hand for the Partial-Hand Amputee* [thesis]. Northwestern University, 1989.
5. Ouellette EA, McAuliffe JA, Carneiro R: Partial hand amputations, in Bowker JH, Michael JW, eds: *Atlas of Limb Prosthetics: Surgical, Prosthetic, and Rehabilitation Principles*, ed 2. Mosby Year Book, 1992, pp 199-216.
6. Lundborg G, Brånemark P-I, Rosén B: Osseointegrated thumb prostheses: A concept for fixation of digit prosthetic devices. *J Hand Surg Am* 1996;21(2):216-221.
7. Pillet J, Mackin EJ: Aesthetic restoration, in Bowker JH, Michael JW, eds: *Atlas of Limb Prosthetics: Surgical, Prosthetic, and Rehabilitation Principles*, ed 2. Mosby Year Book, 1992, pp 227-235.
8. Pereira BP, Kour AK, Leow EL, Pho RW: Benefit and use of digital prostheses. *J Hand Surg Am* 1996;21(2):222-228.
9. Fraser CM: An evaluation of the use made of cosmetic and functional prostheses by unilateral upper limb amputees. *Prosthet Orthot Int* 1998;22(3):216-223.
10. Childress DS, Weir RF: Control of limb prostheses, in Smith DG,

Michael JW, Bowker JH, eds: *Atlas of Amputations and Limb Deficiencies: Surgical, Prosthetic, and Rehabilitation Principles*, ed 3. American Academy of Orthopaedic Surgeons, 2004, pp 173-195.

11. Mikosz MJ: Cable driven multiarticulating fingers providing compliant grasp for partial hand amputee, in *Proceedings of the 2008 MyoElectric Controls/Powered Prosthetics Symposium*. University of New Brunswick. Available at: http://hdl.handle.net/10161/2799. Accessed February 6, 2015.

12. Brown RD: An alternative approach to fitting partial hand amputees. *Orthot Prosthet* 1984;38(1):64-67.

13. Gow DJ, Douglas W, Geggie C, Monteith E, Stewart D: The development of the Edinburgh modular arm system. *Proc Inst Mech Eng H* 2001;215(3):291-298.

14. Putzi R: Myoelectric partial-hand prosthesis. *J Prosthet Orthot* 1992;4(2):103-108.

15. Biden E, Bush G, Olive M, Young W: Recent advances in the development of partial hand prostheses, in *Proceedings of the 1997 MyoElectric Control/Powered Prosthetics Symposium*. Available at: http://hdl.handle.net/10161/4896. Accessed February 9, 2015.

16. Lake C: Experience with electric prostheses for partial hand presentation: An eight year retrospective. *J Prosthet Orthot* 2009;21(2):125-130.

17. Gill H: *Experiences with ProDigits*, in *Proceedings of the 13th World Congress of the International Society for Prosthetics and Orthotics*. ISPO, 2010, p 730.

18. Schulz S: Introducing a new multiarticulating myoelectric hand system, in *Proceedings of the 13th World Congress of the International Society for Prosthetics and Orthotics*. ISPO, 2010, pp 598-599.

19. Atkins DJ: Congenital partial hand absence: What is the impact of fitting with an electric multi-articulating digit prosthesis. *ACPOC News* 2012;18(4):18-24.

20. Phillips SL, Harris MS, Koss L, Latlief G: Experience and outcomes with powered partial hand prostheses: A case series of subjects with multiple limb amputations. *J Prosthet Orthot* 2012;24(2):93-97.

21. Sensinger JW, Lock BA, Kuiken TA: Adaptive pattern recognition to ensure clinical viability over time, in *Proceeding of the 2008 MyoElectric Controls/Powered Prosthetics Symposium*. University of New Brunswick. Available at: http://hdl.handle.net/10161/2816. Accessed February 9, 2015.

22. Ahmad SA, Chappell PH: Surface EMG classification using moving approximate entropy and fuzzy logic for prosthesis control, in *Proceedings of the 2008 MyoElectric Controls/Powered Prosthetics Symposium*. University of New Brunswick. Available at: http://hdl.handle.net/10161/2760. Accessed February 9, 2015.

23. Hargrove L, Scheme E, Engelhart K, Hudgins B: A virtual environment assessment of a novel pattern recognition based myoelectric control scheme, in Proceedings of the 2008 MyoElectric Controls/Powered Prosthetics Symposium. University of New Brunswick. Available at: http://hdl.handle.net/10161/2784 Accessed February 9, 2015.

24. Farrell TR, Weir RF: A comparison of the effects of electrode implantation and targeting on pattern classification accuracy for prosthesis control. *IEEE Trans Biomed Eng* 2008;55(9):2198-2211.

25. Schorsch JF, Maas H, Troyk PR, DeMichele GA, Kerns DA, Weir RF: Multifunctional prosthesis control using implanted myoelectric sensors (IMES), in *Proceedings of the 2008 MyoElectric Controls/Powered Prosthetics Symposium*. University of New Brunswick. Available at: http://hdl.handle.net/10161/2811. Accessed February 9, 2015.

26. Schafer M: Prothetische Versorgungskonzepte nach partiellen amputationen im handbereich [German]. *Orthopadie Technik* 2009;60:584-595.

27. Uellendahl J, Mandacina S, Ramdial S: Custom silicone sockets for myoelectric prostheses. *J Prosthet Orthot* 2006;18(2):35-40.

28. Dodson RJ, Jowid B: The clinical application of an upper limb custom silicone interface: Observations of a case study. *J Prosthet Orthot* 2009;21(2):120-124.

29. Gambrell CR: Overuse syndrome and the unilateral upper limb amputee: Consequences and prevention. *J Prosthet Orthot* 2008;20(3):126-132.

30. Goldberg D: *History of 3D printing: It's Older Than You Are (This is, If You're Under 30)*. Available at: https://www.business2community.com/brandviews/autodesk/history-3d-printing-older-youre-30-01005930. Manufacturing Accessed April 13 2018.

Wrist Disarticulation and Transradial Amputation: Surgical Management

CHAPTER 16

George Peter Nanos III, MD, FAAOS

ABSTRACT

Amputation of an upper limb is a catastrophic event that frequently results from high-energy trauma in an otherwise young and healthy patient cohort. Transradial amputation and wrist disarticulation are the most frequently performed amputations in the upper limbs, report the highest prosthetic acceptance rates, and represent the amputation levels with the greatest functional potential. Preserved shoulder and elbow joints, a long lever arm, and forearm rotation allow the individual with an amputation below the level of the elbow to easily position the terminal prosthesis in space. There are, however, special considerations unique to amputations at these levels. It is helpful to be aware of surgical techniques to optimize residual limb length, prevent complications, and maximize the potential for future prosthetic use to achieve the best functional results for patients.

Keywords: amputation; transradial amputation; wrist disarticulation

Introduction

Amputation of an upper limb is a catastrophic event that frequently results from high-energy trauma in a young, otherwise healthy patient cohort.[1-3] Of the 1.6 million individuals in the United States living with limb loss in 2005, 34% (541,000) had upper limb loss; 92% of hospital discharges attributable to upper limb loss resulted from traumatic mechanisms of injury, 41,000 of which were proximal to the finger.[4,5] More than 2,200 major limb amputations have been performed as a result of injuries that occurred in US military conflicts over the past decade, including Operation Iraqi Freedom and Operation Enduring Freedom, and nearly 18% were upper limb amputations. Of the major upper limb amputations performed in military personnel to date for these conflicts, 50% were transradial and 10% were wrist disarticulations (John C. Shero, MHA, FACHE, Director, Extremity Trauma and Amputation Center of Excellence, unpublished data, September 2021). Amputations below the level of the elbow are the most frequently performed amputations in the upper limb; the transradial amputation is the most common level in both civilian and war-related traumatic injuries.[6]

The surgical principles of upper and lower limb amputations are quite similar, but key differences in morphology and function require special attention when considering upper limb amputation. The primary goal in lower limb amputation is to provide a well-padded, durable residual limb that facilitates weight bearing, maximizes ambulatory function, and minimizes energy consumption required for ambulation; the goals in upper limb amputation are to maximize precise function and provide a good cosmetic result. To ensure appropriate preoperative planning and optimal patient outcomes, the surgeon should be aware of prosthetic capabilities, prosthesis acceptance rates, and the functional outcomes associated with transradial amputations and wrist disarticulations.[7]

General Treatment Principles

An integrated team approach is vital to maximize amputee care. In addition to orthopaedic surgeons, specialists in trauma surgery, physical medicine, anesthesiology, pain management, rehabilitation, occupational therapy, physical therapy, mental health care, social work, nursing, and prosthetics should be involved in the care of patients with an upper limb amputation. Patient- and family-centered participation in the decision-making process enhances a patient's acceptance of the amputation and satisfaction with its outcome.[8,9] A multidisciplinary care approach is especially essential for patients with multiple limb amputations, which frequently occur after high-energy combat injuries. The patient often has numerous comorbid conditions and requires complex and comprehensive treatment.[10] Good functional outcomes and prosthetic acceptance rates can be expected with a well-coordinated rehabilitation protocol and timely prosthetic fitting.[11]

A good understanding of anatomy, adherence to sound orthopaedic surgical principles, and a systematic approach to the evaluation and treatment of the amputee are essential to achieve the best results.[12] In general,

Neither Dr. Nanos nor any immediate family member has received anything of value from or has stock or stock options held in a commercial company or institution related directly or indirectly to the subject of this chapter.

guillotine amputations should be avoided unless they are clinically indicated, which is uncommon. In traumatic amputations, all devitalized tissue should be meticulously débrided, taking special care to identify and protect all important neurovascular structures to maximize the final functional result.[13,14] Negative-pressure dressings are effective for staged surgical treatment because they limit the frequency of bedside dressing changes, improve pain control, and provide surgeons with greater flexibility when considering soft-tissue reconstruction options for more complex cases.[15,16] The timing of final amputation coverage or closure depends largely on surgeon experience, but a wound bed devoid of necrotic tissue and infection and a tension-free closure are critical to success.[17]

In general, preserving maximal limb length is preferred in upper limb amputations, but this goal must be balanced with consideration for wound-healing capacity and residual limb coverage, patient preference, rehabilitation potential, and local prosthetic expertise and availability. With increasing limb length and preservation of joints, enhanced positioning of the terminal residual limb and/or prosthetic device in space is achieved, allowing for the best functional results and improved outcomes. When considering amputation below the level of the elbow, the scope of the injury often determines the amputation level. The requirements and capabilities of prostheses for each amputation level must be understood and considered. Consultation with a prosthetist is recommended early in the decision-making process.

Concomitant fractures should be considered for surgical stabilization when functional limb length or joint preservation can be achieved, although higher complication rates can be expected. However, preservation of the established limb length at the time of fracture fixation is generally achieved.[18] Additional soft-tissue coverage options, including skin grafts and flaps, should be strongly considered when residual tissue flaps provide inadequate coverage for a distal amputation below the elbow and shortening the residual limb will diminish prosthetic fitting options and functional outcomes. This is perhaps most important in attempts to preserve the elbow joint but also when optimizing residual limb length for a transradial amputation. Using microvascular free tissue transfer in appropriately selected patients to maximize limb length and provide durable soft-tissue coverage has proved successful in upper limb amputations.[19-21] In the upper limb, indications for free tissue transfer include shoulder joint preservation by selecting a transhumeral amputation level, elbow joint preservation, and preservation of bone more than 7 cm below the shoulder or elbow. Relative indications include wrist joint preservation and skeletal preservation between 5 and 7 cm below the shoulder or elbow.[7,22] Although upper limb amputations that require skin grafts or flaps take longer to heal, the functional benefits of joint and/or limb-length preservation usually outweigh delays in rehabilitation and prosthetic fitting.

Careful attention to nerves and muscles is critically important in upper limb amputation because symptomatic neuromas are common.[23] Before final closure of an upper limb amputation, all involved sensory and motor nerves should be identified. All motor branches to muscle flaps within the surgical field also should be preserved to prevent muscle denervation that results in loss of muscle mass for limb padding and possible loss of sites for myoelectric signals. Nerves should undergo gentle traction neurectomy to locate neuromas away from the distal amputation myodesis or skin closure. Although more aggressive traction neurectomy was previously recommended for large peripheral nerves with motor function, preservation of additional nerve length while preventing more distal exposure of neuromas can ensure the possibility of future reconstructive surgery.

Stabilizing the musculotendinous units of the residual limb under physiologic tension at the time of amputation closure serves two main purposes. First, it facilitates robust coverage over the distal bone end, providing comfortable padding for the prosthetic socket while preventing painful bursa formation from mobile muscle units. Second, optimal contractility characteristics of the muscle are preserved, improving muscle signal quality and maximizing myoelectric control of a prosthesis, while also maximizing terminal residual limb control for a body-powered prosthesis. Myodesis, the process of attaching musculotendinous units directly to bone, is the surgical technique that provides the most stable construct over the distal bone end. Myodesis is typically performed by suturing the muscle and/or tendon to the bone end, usually through drill tunnels with braided nonabsorbable suture, or less commonly, to periosteum. Myoplasty, which attaches agonist muscles to antagonist muscles over the bone end to create physiologic tension, and myofascial closure, which sutures muscle and fascia together, are less stable constructs. These procedures may be indicated when myodesis cannot be achieved, for secondary muscles after primary myodesis, or to contour the remaining muscle bellies before closure. Although no data support the superiority of myodesis over myoplasty, myodesis is recommended in upper limb amputations to provide the most stable limb and best isolate muscle signals and myoelectric prosthetic control.

Wrist Disarticulation

The advantages of wrist disarticulation include preservation of forearm rotation when the distal radioulnar joint (DRUJ) is preserved, elimination of painful radioulnar convergence compared with transradial amputation, improved weight bearing directly through the terminal residual limb, enhanced functional length, and better prosthetic suspension. Historically, the main disadvantage of wrist disarticulation has been limited available prosthetic options because of the short working length and limited space available for the terminal device.[24] In 1972, before the introduction of modern wrist prostheses, a survey of US surgeons indicated a preference for distal transradial amputation over wrist disarticulation.[25] Even with recent advances in prosthetic design and materials, which have greatly improved function for an individual treated with wrist disarticulation, a preference remains in many amputation centers for revision to transradial amputation because of patient dissatisfaction with outcomes after wrist disarticulation.[7] Consultation with an upper limb prosthetist is highly recommended when a decision must be made between preservation of a wrist disarticulation or revision to a transradial amputation.

A successful wrist disarticulation requires a healthy, intact DRUJ.[1] Preservation of the triangular fibrocartilage complex and radioulnar ligaments facilitates stable pronation and supination, with an expected total arc of approximately 100° to 120°.[5,26,27] The thick palmar skin of the hand should be used for distal coverage, but often, skin flaps for final wound closure will be dictated by the injury.[1] The radial styloid should be saved for prosthetic suspension; it can be contoured to prevent prominence and skin irritation or breakdown at the prosthetic interface. The ulnar styloid is often excised to prevent soft-tissue prominence distally. It is crucial to perform myodesis of the flexor and extensor tendons to maintain tension in those muscles to provide necessary myoelectric prosthetic function. Important nerves to identify include not only the median and ulnar nerves, but also the superficial radial nerve, the palmar cutaneous branch of the median nerve, the dorsal ulnar cutaneous nerve, and possibly the terminal medial and lateral antebrachial cutaneous nerves. These nerves should be divided proximal to the level of amputation closure using gentle traction neurectomy and buried under muscle to prevent the development of painful neuromas. One exception is preservation of cutaneous nerves to a skin flap required for distal amputation coverage.[7] Additional nerve techniques, such as cauterization, suture ligation, and anesthetic injection, have been described but are not performed by the author of this chapter because of a lack of proven efficacy and theoretical concerns about exacerbating neuropathic pain.

Wrist Disarticulation: Surgical Technique

Surgery for wrist disarticulation is typically performed with the patient supine and under regional anesthesia. An indwelling peripheral nerve catheter placed intraoperatively can help control postoperative pain and aid in initial recovery. Initial dissection and amputation is performed using a tourniquet to allow accurate identification of all structures in a bloodless field. Under traumatic conditions, all available viable skin flaps are preserved and considered for final closure. If amputation is performed under elective conditions, skin flaps can be designed to allow the use of durable palmar skin over the distal residual limb. The radial and ulnar arteries are dissected free and double ligated. Large veins are typically ligated; small veins can be cauterized. Peripheral nerves are identified and dissected, including the median nerve, ulnar nerve, all branches of the dorsal sensory radial and ulnar nerves, and any terminal branches of the lateral and medial antebrachial cutaneous nerves. All cutaneous nerves to skin flaps intended for final closure should be preserved. Gentle traction neurectomy of all nerves is preferred to place them just proximal to the myodesis and the distal residual limb surface. This technique should minimize the likelihood of development of painful neuromas and preserve maximum nerve length for future limb reconstruction procedures. All crossing tendons are divided, followed by sharp amputation at the level of the radial and ulnar carpal joints, with great care taken to preserve the triangular fibrocartilage complex and the dorsal and palmar radioulnar ligaments to maintain DRUJ function. The radial styloid prominence should be assessed for minor bone contouring. The ulnar styloid is typically excised if prominent, but care should be taken to preserve the foveal attachment of the triangular fibrocartilage complex. The tourniquet is released, and strict hemostasis should be obtained before final amputation closure.

All hand and wrist flexor and extensor tendons are attached to the distal radius using braided, nonabsorbable suture through drilled tunnels, as is done in the myodesis technique. Myoplasty can then be performed for additional muscles to contour the residual limb, provide additional padding, and ensure maximum muscle working length (**Figure 1**). Skin flaps are closed in a tension-free manner in layers, with resorbable and nonresorbable monofilament sutures. Drains and/or incisional vacuum-assisted closure dressings can be placed according to surgeon preference and the clinical situation. The author of this chapter commonly uses incisional negative-pressure wound therapy for complex closure in combat-related amputations. Although the efficacy of incisional negative-pressure wound therapy has not yet been illustrated, it is thought to enhance wound healing and reduce postoperative wound dehiscence, seroma, and hematoma in higher risk patients.[28-30] Although dermal substitutes, skin grafts, and pedicle and free tissue flaps can be considered in cases in which primary skin closure cannot be obtained, in the practice of the author of this chapter, this typically indicates consideration of a more proximal transradial amputation level with similar functional outcomes.

Bulky gauze dressings are applied, followed by a compression dressing to minimize edema. Splints are typically not used, and certainly not above the elbow unless clinically indicated to prevent joint contracture. Postoperative elevation is recommended to reduce swelling and optimize the limb for prosthetic rehabilitation. The use of specialized elevation foam pillows helps improve patient compliance and minimizes pain.

Transradial Amputation

Transradial amputation is the most common major upper limb amputation and has the highest prosthetic acceptance rates of amputations performed in the upper limb.[6] Preserved shoulder and elbow joints, a long lever arm, and forearm rotation allow the individual with a distal transradial amputation to easily position the terminal prosthesis in space. Transradial amputation

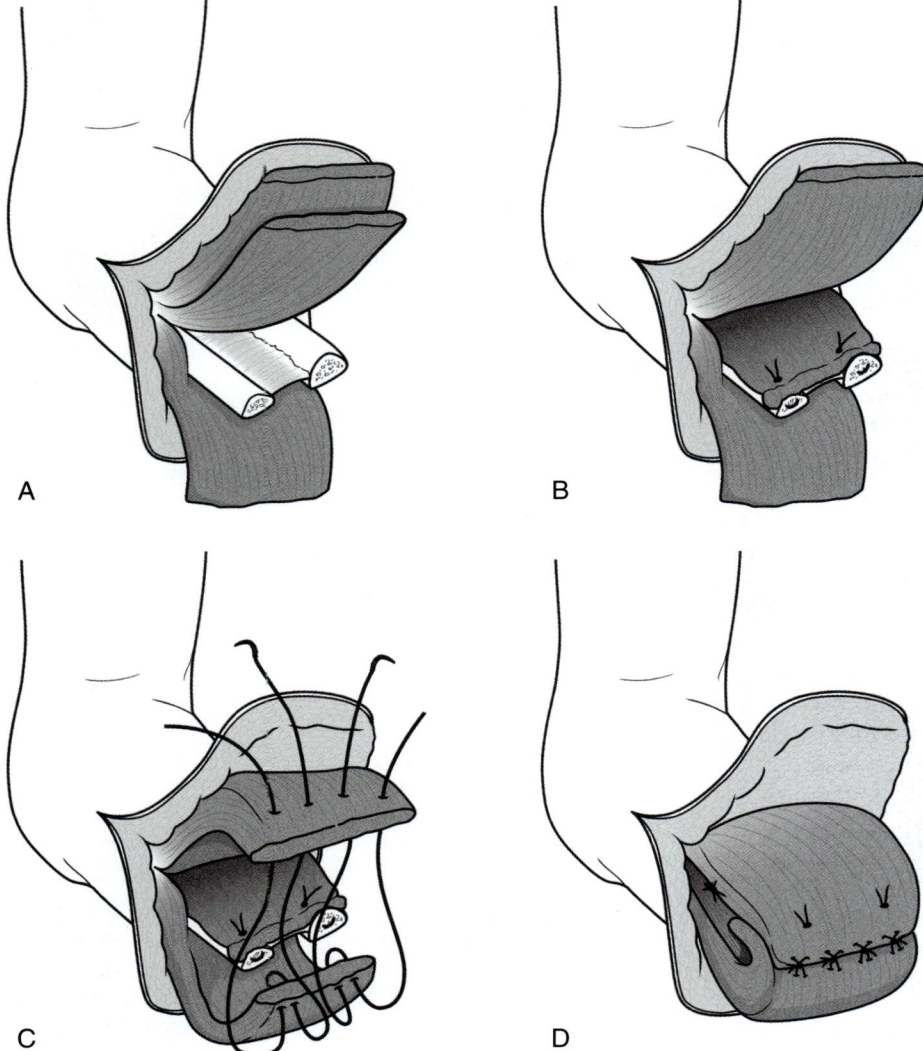

FIGURE 1 Illustrations of the myodesis technique for flexor and extensor musculotendinous units to bone with nonabsorbable suture through drill tunnels. **A** and **B**, Primary flexor and extensor muscles are sutured to bone. **C** and **D**, Myoplasty of additional muscles to the myodesis or antagonist muscle helps to contour the amputation for final closure, provides additional padding to the residual limb, and establishes remaining muscles at a physiologic working length for enhanced functional control of the prosthesis.

is cosmetically appealing because of the ability to fit body-powered or myoelectric prostheses with quick-disconnecting components, while maintaining equal limb lengths.

When practical, at least two-thirds of the forearm should be maintained. Removal of at least 6 to 8 cm of bone is recommended to provide a robust soft-tissue envelope and permit use of a wide variety of prosthetic options.[7] Soft-tissue interposition between the radius and ulna decreases the potential for painful convergence and instability. This is generally accomplished with the pronator quadratus for more distal amputation levels and can be performed more proximally with one interposed extensor and/or flexor tendon. Nerves are managed in the same manner as with wrist disarticulation; ensuring preservation of motor branches to muscles for myodesis maximizes myoelectric prosthesis function.

At least 5 cm of residual ulnar length is required to allow prosthetic fitting and elbow motion.[7] However, useful pronation and supination are not generally preserved when the planned amputation level is in the proximal third of the forearm and may affect use of a body-powered prosthesis.[1,8] At this proximal level, transfer of the distal biceps tendon to the proximal ulna should be considered.[26] The prosthetic and mechanical advantages of the transradial level, coupled with superior prosthetic acceptance rates, should prompt the surgeon to consider all reconstruction options, including free tissue transfer, to preserve an amputation at this level.

Transradial Amputation: Surgical Technique

Many of the surgical principles of transradial amputation (**Figure 2**) are similar to those of wrist disarticulation (**Figure 3**). The procedure is the same up to the step of applying gentle traction neurectomy of all of the nerves to place them just proximal to the myodesis and distal residual limb surface to minimize painful neuromas while preserving maximum nerve length. All crossing tendons and muscles are divided. To maximize length, bone cuts are performed with a cooled sagittal saw to preserve approximately two-thirds of forearm length, which is usually at least 6 to 8 cm from the radiocarpal joint. The tourniquet is released, and strict hemostasis should be obtained before final amputation closure. In cases of transradial amputation, the author of this chapter often uses thrombin spray and Gelfoam to help achieve hemostatic control in the event of a greater amount of cut muscle and exposed bone surfaces.

As with wrist disarticulation, after hemostasis is obtained, all hand and wrist flexor and extensor tendons and muscles are attached to the distal radius and ulna through drill tunnels using nonabsorbable, braided suture. Additional myoplasty can be performed to improve padding, allow adequate contouring of the residual limb, and to fix remaining musculotendinous units at physiologic working lengths. It is important to maintain the interosseous membrane to the extent possible and superimpose tissue between the

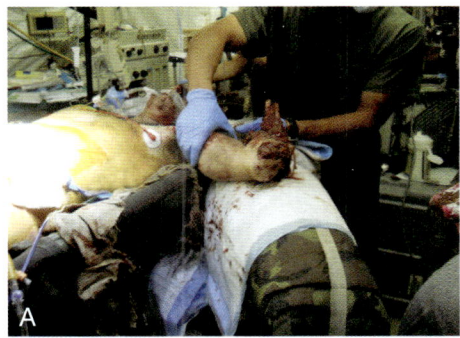 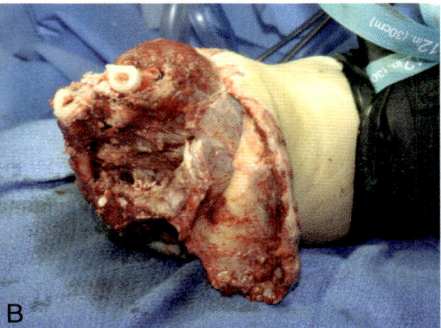 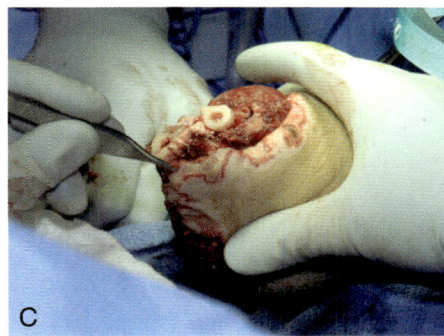
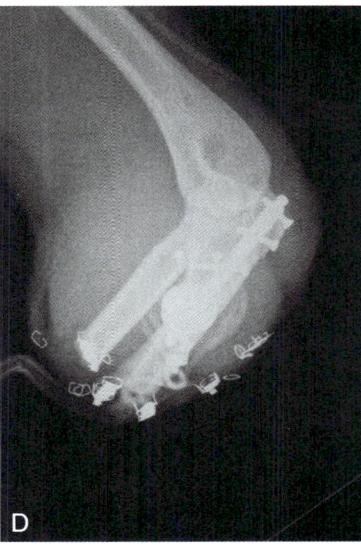 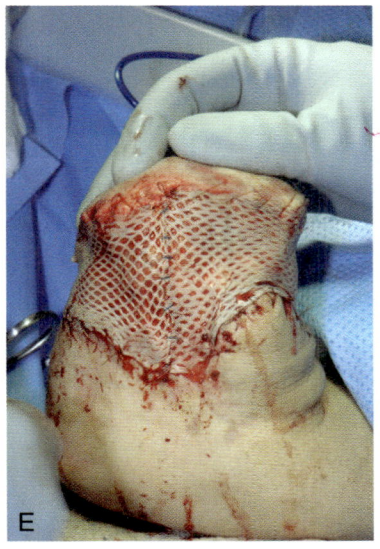

FIGURE 2 Images of a short, traumatic transradial amputation in a patient with multiple limb amputation secondary to injury from an improvised explosive device. The patient had a concomitant ulnar fracture and poor soft-tissue coverage. **A**, Photograph demonstrating initial amputation before débridement. Photographs obtained following serial débridement show that the amputation meets length requirements (**B**) but has inadequate soft-tissue coverage (**C**). **D**, Lateral radiograph showing ulnar fracture stabilized with internal fixation. **E**, Photograph showing soft-tissue coverage provided by a free vascularized anterolateral thigh flap and a biologic dermal substitute, followed by split-thickness skin grafting.

radius and ulna to prevent painful radioulnar convergence. When available, the pronator quadratus can be mobilized as necessary on its neurovascular pedicle, resulting in a functional muscle for interposition. If the pronator quadratus is not available, an extensor and/or flexor tendon is interposed proximally and attached using myodesis.[31] Skin flaps are closed in a tension-free manner in layers with resorbable and nonresorbable monofilament sutures. Drains and/or incisional vacuum-assisted closure dressings can be placed depending on the surgeon's preference and the clinical situation.

Dermal substitutes, skin grafts, and pedicle and free tissue flaps should be considered in cases in which primary skin closure cannot be obtained and maximum length preservation is preferred. Although dermal substitutes can increase cost, they provide a more durable skin graft and can positively affect prosthetic comfort and functioning.[32,33] Tissue flaps should be considered for elbow joint preservation when at least 5 cm of stable residual ulna remain.

Bulky gauze dressings are applied, followed by moderate compression dressing to minimize edema. Splints are typically not used to prevent iatrogenic joint contracture, especially above the elbow, unless clinically indicated. Postoperative elevation is recommended to reduce swelling and optimize the limb for prosthetic rehabilitation, and specialized foam pillows can help improve patient compliance and minimize pain. Early elbow joint range of motion is begun immediately postoperatively.

Additional Options for Neuroma Control

Chronic pain is a frequent complication of traumatic upper limb amputation, with a prevalence ranging from 7% to 49%. Pain may be more prevalent in patients with transradial amputations.[23] Although numerous sources of pain have been identified after amputation, the treatment of patients with neuroma deserves special attention when considering transradial amputation and wrist disarticulation.

Section 2: Upper Limb

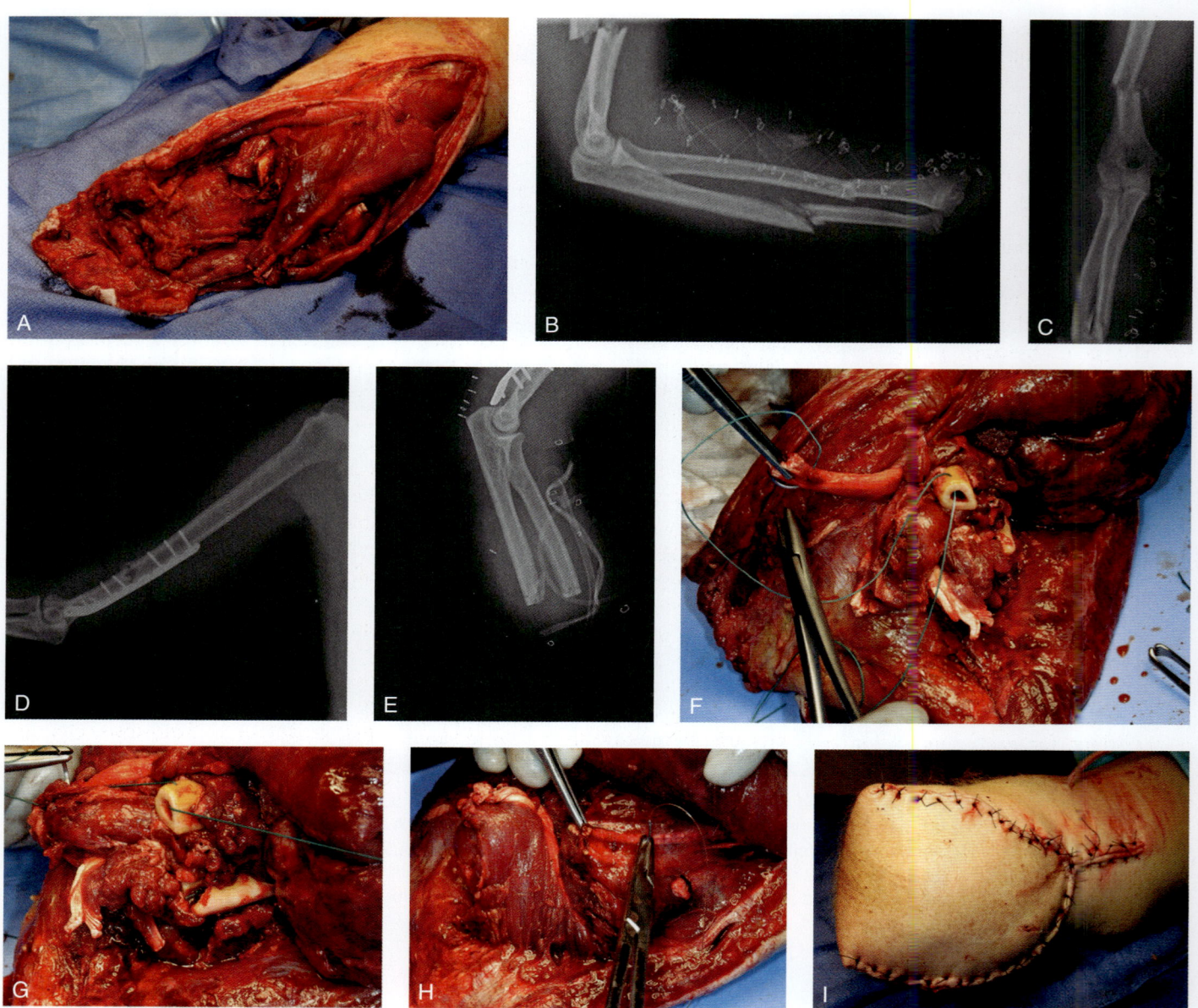

FIGURE 3 Images of the limb of a patient with a wrist-level disarticulation, concomitant radius and ulna shaft fractures, loss of distal musculotendinous units, and inadequate soft-tissue coverage. After discussion between the patient and the prosthetist, the patient elected a transradial amputation to allow robust myodesis, adequate distal padding, and primary skin closure. **A**, Photograph of wrist disarticulation after initial débridement demonstrates inadequate musculotendinous length and soft-tissue coverage. Lateral (**B**) and AP (**C**) radiographs of humeral shaft fracture and distal both-bone forearm fracture. Lateral (**D**) and AP (**E**) radiographs of fixation of a humerus fracture and amputation at the level of forearm fractures. **F**, Photograph showing myodesis of extensor and flexor tendons to bone through drill tunnels after revision of amputation to the level of the fractures. **G** and **H**, Photographs showing myodesis and myoplasty to provide adequate padding over the distal bone ends. **I**, Photograph showing primary skin closure that maintains adequate functional length of the residual limb.

Neuromas are an identifiable cause of chronic pain, which may diminish functional use of prostheses and delay return to daily activities and work. Numerous methods to manage painful neuromas have been described, including nerve repair and resection and nerve transposition with muscle implantation.[34-36] Although nerve repair can produce the best results, this treatment is not possible in an amputee. Simple neuroma excision appears to have the worst outcomes in amputees.[36] More recently, targeted muscle reinnervation (TMR) and regenerative peripheral nerve interfaces (RPNIs) have become established surgical techniques to treat patients with residual limb pain and phantom limb pain because of neuroma formation and can be performed at the time of a traumatic or elective amputation.[37-40] Although a complete discussion of TMR and RPNI is not within the scope of this chapter, given the wide prevalence of these techniques currently in amputation management, a discussion of the technique with an emphasis on muscle targets will be subsequently outlined for the transradial level.

Transradial TMR and RPNI Surgical Guide

Techniques for transradial TMR are described for both myoelectric functional benefit and neuroma control.[41,42] The principal goal of transradial TMR for myoelectric function is to establish thumb opposition and pinch, and to further improve intuitive intrinsic control of the prosthetic hand. RPNI can also be considered as a stand-alone procedure, or as an adjunct to TMR in the transradial amputation when the primary goal of the surgery is for neuroma control and a large number of sensory nerve donors are found, exhausting muscle motor targets.

A midline longitudinal incision is typically used when only performing TMR, but large volar and dorsal fish-mouth type flaps are used when TMR is performed for acute amputation or when distal amputation revision is indicated, which has been common. The median nerve, the ulnar nerve and its dorsal sensory branches, the sensory branches of the radial nerve, and the terminal branches of the lateral and medial antebrachial cutaneous nerves are identified. The median nerve and ulnar nerve are transected sharply as distal as possible to provide length for a tension-free reinnervation transfer. If transfer of the superficial branch of the radial nerve is also planned, this nerve is also transected sharply as distal as possible.

In a longer residual limb, muscle targets for the median nerve are the flexor digitorum superficialis or flexor digitorum profundus; in more proximal amputations, the pronator teres and the flexor carpi radialis can also be used. The ulnar nerve can easily be transferred to motor branches of the flexor carpi ulnaris, or alternatively, may be brought underneath the flexor digitorum superficialis to transfer to a motor branch to the flexor pollicis longus. This transfer has proven anatomically reliable in the experience of the author of this chapter, and further provides ulnar nerve animation of a muscle that is both relatively superficial and distal within the terminal residuum. If included, the superficial branch of the radial nerve can be transferred to the flexor digitorum profundus, flexor digitorum superficialis, the extensor carpi radialis longus, or the brachioradialis muscle. Alternatively, the superficial branch of the radial nerve or any large sensory nerve can be sutured to a section of denervated muscle to construct an RPNI to avoid risking unnecessary additional functional muscle denervation, or when additional nerve targets are not available.

Complications

Complications after amputation surgery distal to the elbow are frequent, especially with higher energy injury patterns such as those that occur in combat situations. Infection, wound dehiscence, skin breakdown, heterotopic ossification, joint contracture, painful neuromas, and myodesis failure have been reported with varied frequencies after both wrist disarticulation and transradial amputation.[23] It is common to have two or more complications that require surgical intervention.

In transradial amputations and wrist disarticulations, heterotopic ossification can cause painful bony prominences, bursa formation, a reduction of forearm rotation, or synostosis and complete arrest of forearm rotation, which reduces functional prosthetic use. Early resection of functionally limiting or painful heterotopic ossification and synostosis have effectively restored forearm rotation, improved function, and reduced pain.[23,43,44] The author of this chapter routinely excises heterotopic bone that limits forearm motion within 4 months of injury if the soft-tissue envelope is stable and the bone is mature on radiographic imaging. CT and three-dimensional modeling are important preoperative planning tools and can be used intraoperatively to guide surgical dissection in complex cases. Resecting heterotopic ossification is challenging. Emphasis must be placed on adequate exposure, identifying all neurovascular structures to prevent critical loss of functional muscle groups, and meticulous hemostasis. Single-dose postoperative radiation therapy or prophylactic NSAIDs have been used effectively to achieve a low risk of recurrence.[45]

Painful radioulnar convergence is a known complication of transradial amputation that results from loss of the DRUJ. The presentation is similar to that of a patient who has undergone distal ulna resection with radioulnar convergence. Symptoms include distal forearm pain with weight bearing and forearm rotation along with pain with squeezing of the forearm that compresses the radius to the ulna. Weight-bearing radiographs also can elucidate the problem. Interposition of an available muscle between the distal radius and ulna, as previously discussed, can help decrease or eliminate painful radioulnar convergence. Other techniques, such as allograft interposition, can be attempted if local soft tissue is inadequate, but this technique is not described in the literature for transradial amputation. Synostosis creation or revision to a more proximal level of amputation for short residual limbs can be considered (**Figure 4**).

Outcomes

The loss of one or both upper limbs is a devastating event. Currently, lost prehensile function and sensation are not adequately replaced using modern prosthetic technology. Although prosthetic acceptance rates are frequently discussed as an outcome measure, existing high-quality evidence is limited and outdated.

Prosthesis rejection rates for upper limb amputation are frequently reported to be 21% to 38%; larger studies typically report a rejection rate higher than 30%.[6,46-48] When excluding cosmetic prostheses, the rates are probably higher.[6,46-48] High rejection rates have been loosely associated with poor training, delayed prosthetic fitting, and more proximal amputations.[6] A 1995 survey of upper limb amputations reported limited usefulness, increased weight, and residual limb/socket discomfort as primary reasons

Section 2: Upper Limb

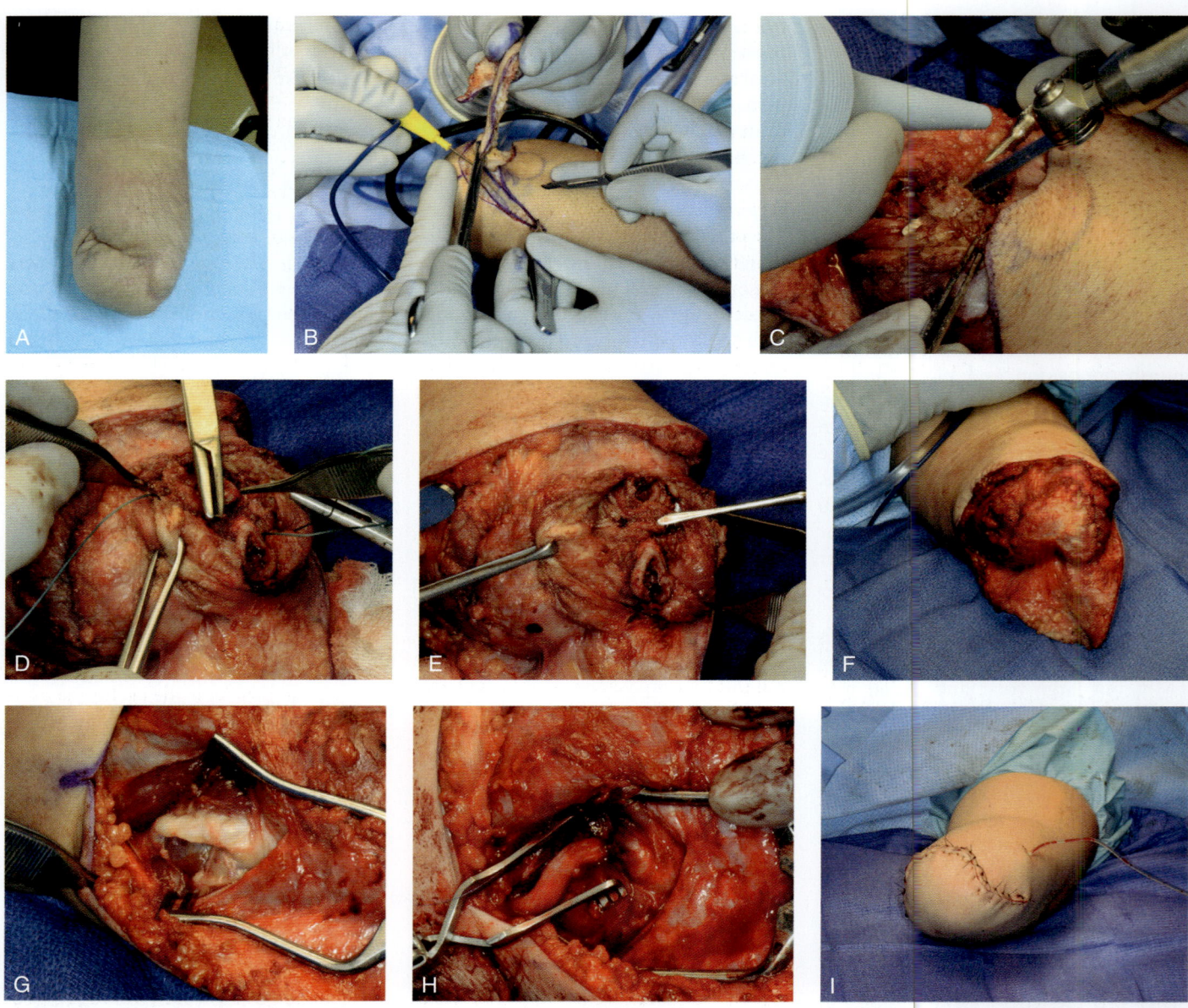

FIGURE 4 Photographs demonstrating surgical revision of a transradial amputation with a redundant soft-tissue envelope, failure of the myodesis, painful radioulnar convergence, heterotopic bone spurs, and a painful ulnar neuroma, resulting in decreased prosthetic use and function. **A**, Preoperative view of the limb. **B**, Excess skin is excised. **C**, Painful bone spurs at the distal radius and ulna are resected. The bone ends are contoured to eliminate sharp edges. **D**, Myodesis is performed through bone tunnels with nonresorbable heavy braided suture. **E**, Available muscle is sutured to bone between the radius and ulna to prevent painful radioulnar convergence. **F**, Additional myoplasty is performed to provide adequate distal padding and restore physiologic working length to the musculotendinous units to maximize myoelectric function. **G**, A painful ulnar neuroma is identified and resected. **H**, Targeted muscle reinnervation is performed from the ulnar nerve to the flexor carpi ulnaris muscle to treat a painful neuroma. **I**, Postoperative view of the limb.

for prosthesis rejection.[6] Factors associated with increased prosthetic acceptance include loss of the dominant limb, absence of pain in the residual limb, and early prosthetic fitting within 30 days of amputation.[6,11,49] Despite the incredible advancements of the past decade in upper limb prosthetics, rates of prosthetic acceptance have not improved substantively.[50]

Acceptance rates for prosthesis use are directly correlated with the level of amputation, with use increasing progressively at more distal levels of amputation, which correlates with higher functional scores.[6,11,46,51-53] The transradial amputation level has the highest reported prosthesis usage rates, ranging from 80% to 94%.[6,11,46,53] Transhumeral amputation acceptance rates range from 43% to 83%.[6,11] Shoulder disarticulation is associated with the lowest reported prosthesis acceptance rates. Increased prosthetic weight and complexity, decreased prosthetic functionality, and difficulty with suspension explain decreasing prosthetic acceptance rates with higher levels of amputation. Many patients are willing to function with only one upper limb rather than use a burdensome prosthetic device. Overall, these data further stress the importance of exhausting all surgical reconstruction options to preserve amputation levels distal to the elbow.

Most individuals who have undergone upper limb amputation are able to return to work, although one-half to two-thirds change their occupation to accommodate the limb loss.[6,11,26] Patients with transradial amputations have the highest rates of return to work.[6] In the military cohort, few upper limb amputees have been found fit for full duty irrespective of their amputation level, and even fewer return to active duty status. During recent conflicts, the overall return-to-duty rate has ranged from 8.3% to 16.5%.[7,54,55]

Current Innovations and Future Directions

Phenomenal innovations have occurred in surgical management and prosthetic advancement over the past decade. Many technologies have direct application to transradial amputation and wrist disarticulation. The surgical techniques of TMR and RPNI, in addition to well-established pain benefits, are now well studied surgical techniques to enhance myoelectric prosthetic function. Although hand allotransplantation indications are evolving, the transradial amputation level is the most common site of transplantation in the upper limb, with demonstrated improvements in function and quality of life in properly selected patients.[56-58] To improve outcomes for patients with transradial amputation or wrist disarticulation, technologies currently being studied include cortical- and peripheral-nerve–based prosthetic control, muscle signal recruitment, radiofrequency-controlled prostheses, advanced pattern recognition algorithms, improved suspension systems such as osseointegration, surgical agonist–antagonist myoneural interfaces to enhance proprioception and the search for functional haptic feedback sensory mechanisms.[59-61] In specific reference to osseointegration and agonist–antagonist myoneural interfaces, it should be noted that these technologies have yet to gain wide use at the transradial or wrist disarticulation level at the time of this writing and would refer the reader to descriptions of more proximal amputation levels within this publication. With the rapid advancement of emerging technologies to enhance upper limb prosthetic acceptance and function, it is important that the surgical team and treating institution develop a coordinated plan of education throughout the continuum of care. If institutional resources are inadequate, consideration should be given to transferring the patient to a center that specializes in amputation reconstruction and hand allotransplantation.[9]

SUMMARY

Transradial amputation and wrist disarticulation are the most frequently performed amputations in the upper limb, have the highest prosthetic acceptance rates, and represent the amputation levels with the greatest functional potential. Strict attention to skeletal preservation and soft-tissue stabilization will maximize the residual limb for future prosthetic use and/or novel reconstruction options. A multidisciplinary approach to patient care will maximize the clinical result, and a coordinated education program will ensure that the patient is well informed as new technologies and novel surgical procedures become available. Consideration should be given to transferring a patient to a higher level of care if local resources are not capable of providing the comprehensive reconstructive care necessary to maximize the patient's functional outcome.

References

1. Owens P, Ouellette EA: Wrist disarticulation and transradial amputation: Surgical management, in Smith DG, Michael JW, Bowker JH, eds: *Atlas of Amputations and Limb Deficiencies: Surgical, Prosthetic, and Rehabilitation Principles*, ed 3. American Academy of Orthopaedic Surgeons, 2004, pp 219-222.

2. Atroshi I, Rosberg HE: Epidemiology of amputations and severe injuries of the hand. *Hand Clin* 2001;17(3):343-350, vii.

3. Freeland AE, Psonak R: Traumatic below-elbow amputations. *Orthopedics* 2007;30(2):120-126.

4. Ziegler-Graham K, MacKenzie EJ, Ephraim PL, Travison TG, Brookmeyer R: Estimating the prevalence of limb loss in the United States: 2005 to 2050. *Arch Phys Med Rehabil* 2008;89(3):422-429.

5. Marchessault JA, McKay PL, Hammert WC: Management of upper limb amputations. *J Hand Surg Am* 2011;36(10):1718-1726.

6. Wright TW, Hagen AD, Wood MB: Prosthetic usage in major upper extremity amputations. *J Hand Surg Am* 1995;20(4):619-622.

7. Tintle SM, Baechler MF, Nanos GP III, Forsberg JA, Potter BK: Traumatic and trauma-related amputations: Part II. Upper extremity and future directions. *J Bone Joint Surg Am* 2010;92(18):2934-2945.

8. Pasquina PF, Bryant PR, Huang ME, Roberts TL, Nelson VS, Flood KM: Advances in amputee care. *Arch Phys Med Rehabil* 2006;87(3 suppl 1):S34-S43.

9. Veterans Affairs/Department of Defense Clinical practice guideline for the management of upper extremity amputation rehabilitation. Version 1.0-2014. http://www.guideline.gov/content.aspx?id=48529. Accessed January 1, 2015.

10. Harvey ZT, Loomis GA, Mitsch S, et al: Advanced rehabilitation techniques for the multi-limb amputee. *J Surg Orthop Adv* 2012;21(1):50-57.

11. Pinzur MS, Angelats J, Light TR, Izuierdo R, Pluth T: Functional outcome following traumatic upper limb amputation and prosthetic limb fitting. *J Hand Surg Am* 1994;19(5):836-839.

12. Nanos GP, Dromsky D, McKay PL: Arm and shoulder injuries, in Bone LB, Manczak C, eds: *Front Line and Extremity Orthopaedic Surgery: A Practical Guide*. Springer-Verlag, 2014, pp 133-141.

13. Attinger CE, Janis JE, Steinberg J, Schwartz J, Al-Attar A, Couch K: Clinical approach to wounds: Débridement and wound bed preparation including the use of dressings and wound-healing adjuvants. *Plast Reconstr Surg* 2006;117(7 suppl):72S-109S.

14. Bowyer G: Débridement of extremity war wounds. *J Am Acad Orthop Surg* 2006;14(10 spec no.):S52-S56.

15. Argenta LC, Morykwas MJ: Vacuum-assisted closure: A new method for wound control and treatment clinical experience. *Ann Plast Surg* 1997;38(6):563-576.

16. Couch KS, Stojadinovic A: Negative-pressure wound therapy in the military: Lessons learned. *Plast Reconstr Surg* 2011;127(suppl 1):117S-130S.
17. McKay PL, Nanos G: Initial evaluation and management of complex traumatic wounds, in Moran SL, Cooney WP III, eds: *Masters Techniques in Orthopaedic Surgery: Soft Tissue Surgery*. Lippincott Williams and Wilkins, 2009, pp 11-35.
18. Gordon WT, O'Brien FP, Strauss JE, Andersen RC, Potter BK: Outcomes associated with the internal fixation of long-bone fractures proximal to traumatic amputations. *J Bone Joint Surg Am* 2010;92(13):2312-2318.
19. Rohrich RJ, Ehrlichman RJ, May JW Jr: Sensate palm of hand free flap for forearm length preservation in non-replantable forearm amputation: Long-term follow-up. *Ann Plast Surg* 1991;26(5):469-473.
20. Wood MR, Hunter GA, Millstein SG: The value of stump split skin grafting following amputation for trauma in adult upper and lower limb amputees. *Prosthet Orthot Int* 1987;11(2):71-74.
21. Baccarani A, Follmar KE, De Santis G, et al: Free vascularized tissue transfer to preserve upper extremity amputation levels. *Plast Reconstr Surg* 2007;120(4):971-981.
22. Anderson RC, Nanos GP, Pinzur MS, Potter BK: Amputations in trauma, in Browner BD, Jupiter JB, Krettek C, Anderson PA, eds: *Skeletal Trauma: Basic Science, Management, and Reconstruction*, ed 5. Elsevier Saunders, 2014.
23. Tintle SM, Baechler MF, Nanos GP, Forsberg JA, Potter BK: Reoperations following combat-related upper-extremity amputations. *J Bone Joint Surg Am* 2012;94(16):e1191-e1196.
24. Lake C, Dodson R: Progressive upper limb prosthetics. *Phys Med Rehabil Clin N Am* 2006;17(1):49-72.
25. Tooms RE: Amputation surgery in the upper extremity. *Orthop Clin North Am* 1972;3(2):383-395.
26. Shawen SB, Doukas WC, Shrout JA, et al: *Combat Care of the Amputee*. Office of the Surgeon General, TMM Publications, 2009.
27. Taylor CL: The biomechanics of control in upper-extremity prostheses. *Artif Limbs* 1955;2(3):4-25.
28. Stannard JP, Atkins BZ, O'Malley D, et al: Use of negative pressure therapy on closed surgical incisions: A case series. *Ostomy Wound Manage* 2009;55(8):58-66.
29. Webster J, Scuffham P, Stankiewicz M, Chaboyer WP: Negative pressure wound therapy for skin grafts and surgical wounds healing by primary intention. *Cochrane Database Syst Rev* 2014;10:CD009261.
30. Zayan NE, West JM, Schulz SA, Jordan SW, Valerio IL: Incisional negative pressure wound therapy: And effective tool for major limb amputation and amputation revision site closure. *Adv Wound Care (New Rochelle)* 2019;8(8):368-373.
31. Bartoletta JJ, Israel JS, Rhee PC: Transradial amputation with pedicled quadratus interposition and advanced neuroma-prevention techniques. *J Hand Surg Am* 2021;46(12):1129.e1-1129.e8.
32. Helgeson MD, Potter BK, Evans KN, Shawen SB: Bioartificial dermal substitute: A preliminary report on its use for the management of complex combat-related soft tissue wounds. *J Orthop Trauma* 2007;21(6):394-399.
33. Foong DP, Evriviades D, Jeffery SL: Integra permits early durable coverage of improvised explosive device (IED) amputation stumps. *J Plast Reconstr Aesthet Surg* 2013;66(12):1717-1724.
34. Dellon AL, Mackinnon SE: Treatment of the painful neuroma by neuroma resection and muscle implantation. *Plast Reconstr Surg* 1986;77(3):427-438.
35. Mackinnon SE: Evaluation and treatment of the painful neuroma. *Tech Hand Up Extrem Surg* 1997;1(3):195-212.
36. Guse DM, Moran SL: Outcomes of the surgical treatment of peripheral neuromas of the hand and forearm: A 25-year comparative outcome study. *Ann Plast Surg* 2013;71(6):654-658.
37. Souza JM, Cheesborough JE, Ko JH, Cho MS, Kuiken TA, Dumanian GA: Targeted muscle reinnervation: A novel approach to postamputation neuroma pain. *Clin Orthop Relat Res* 2014;472(10):2984-2990.
38. Pet MA, Ko JH, Friedly JL, Mourad PD, Smith DG: Does targeted nerve implantation reduce neuroma pain in amputees? *Clin Orthop Relat Res* 2014;472(10):2991-3001.
39. Cheesborough JE, Souza JM, Dumanian GA, Bueno RA Jr: Targeted muscle reinnervation in the initial management of traumatic upper extremity amputation injury. *Hand (N Y)* 2014;9(2):253-257.
40. Valerio I, Schulz S, West J, Westenberg R, Eberlin K: Targeted muscle reinnervation combined with a vascularized pedicled regenerative peripheral nerve interface. *Plast Reconstr Surg Glob Open* 2020;8(3):e2689.
41. Morgan EN, Potter BK, Souza JM, Tintle SM, Nanos GP III: Targeted muscle reinnervation for transradial amputation: Description of operative technique. *Tech Hand Up Extrem Surg* 2016;20(4):166-171.
42. Pierrie SN, Gaston RG, Loeffler BJ: Targeted muscle reinnervation for prosthesis optimization and neuroma management in the setting of transradial amputation. *J Hand Surg Am* 2019;44:525.e1-525.e8.
43. Beingessner DM, Patterson SD, King GJ: Early excision of heterotopic bone in the forearm. *J Hand Surg Am* 2000;25(3):483-488.
44. Potter BK, Burns TC, Lacap AP, Granville RR, Gajewski DA: Heterotopic ossification following traumatic and combat-related amputations: Prevalence, risk factors, and preliminary results of excision. *J Bone Joint Surg Am* 2007;89(3):476-486.
45. Nauth A, Giles E, Potter BK, et al: Heterotopic ossification in orthopaedic trauma. *J Orthop Trauma* 2012;26(12):684-688.
46. Stürup J, Thyregod HC, Jensen JS, et al: Traumatic amputation of the upper limb: The use of body-powered prostheses and employment consequences. *Prosthet Orthot Int* 1988;12(1):50-52.
47. Raichle KA, Hanley MA, Molton I, et al: Prosthesis use in persons with lower- and upper-limb amputation. *J Rehabil Res Dev* 2008;45(7):961-972.
48. Bhaskaranand K, Bhat AK, Acharya KN: Prosthetic rehabilitation in traumatic upper limb amputees (an Indian perspective). *Arch Orthop Trauma Surg* 2003;123(7):363-366.
49. Malone JM, Fleming LL, Roberson J, et al: Immediate, early, and late postsurgical management of upper-limb amputation. *J Rehabil Res Dev* 1984;21(1):33-41.
50. Salminger S, Stino H, Pichler L, et al: Current rates of prosthetic usage in upper-limb amputees- have innovations had an impact on device acceptance? *Disabil Rehabil* 2022;44(14):3708-3713.
51. Heger H, Millstein S, Hunter GA: Electrically powered prostheses for the adult with an upper limb amputation. *J Bone Joint Surg Br* 1985;67(2):278-281.
52. Northmore-Ball MD, Heger H, Hunter GA: The below-elbow myo-electric prosthesis: A comparison of the Otto Bock myo-electric prosthesis with the

hook and functional hand. *J Bone Joint Surg Br* 1980;62(3):363-367.

53. Millstein SG, Heger H, Hunter GA: Prosthetic use in adult upper limb amputees: A comparison of the body powered and electrically powered prostheses. *Prosthet Orthot Int* 1986;10(1):27-34.

54. Stinner DJ, Burns TC, Kirk KL, Ficke JR: Return to duty rate of amputee soldiers in the current conflicts in Afghanistan and Iraq. *J Trauma* 2010;68(6):1476-1479.

55. Tennent DJ, Wenke JC, Rivera JC, Krueger CA: Characterisation and outcomes of upper extremity amputations. *Injury* 2014;45(6):965-969.

56. Foroohar A, Elliott RM, Fei L, et al: Quadrimembral amputation: Indications and contraindications for vascularized composite allotransplantation. *Transplant Proc* 2011;43(9):3521-3528.

57. Shores JT, Brandacher G, Lee WP: Hand and upper extremity transplantation: An update of outcomes in the worldwide experience. *Plast Reconstr Surg* 2015;135(2):351e-360e.

58. Petruzzo P, Dubernard JM: World experience after more than a decade of clinical hand transplantation: Update on the French program. *Hand Clin* 2011;27(4):411-416, vii.

59. Zlotolow DA, Kozin SH: Advances in upper extremity prosthetics. *Hand Clin* 2012;28(4):587-593.

60. Clites TR, Herr HM, Srinivasan SS, Zorzos AN, Carty MJ: The Ewing amputation: The first human implementation of the agonist-antagonist myoneural interface. *Plast Reconstr Surg Glob Open* 2018;6(11):e1997.

61. Cary MJ, Herr HM: The agonist-antagonist myoneural interface. *Hand Clin* 2021;37(3):435-445.

Wrist Disarticulation and Transradial Amputation: Prosthetic Management

CHAPTER 17

Christopher Fantini, MSPT, CP, BOCO • Gerald E. Stark, PhD, MSEM, CPO/L, FAAOP

ABSTRACT

The overall relative number of persons with upper extremity amputation is small, at an estimated 3% of the total amputation cohort in the United States. This poses a challenge for many clinicians to develop the experience and knowledge base to manage this cohort most effectively. However, given that transradial amputations are the most common major upper limb amputation performed and when combined with that of wrist disarticulation surgery, these amputations made up an estimated 60% of all major upper limb amputations among U.S. military personnel since the turn of the century, it is more likely a clinician will encounter these upper extremity major amputation levels than others. Individuals with amputation at the transradial level tend to use prostheses at a higher rate than those at other upper extremity levels. A clinical knowledge of limb length considerations, postoperative management, prosthetic interface design principles, suspension strategies, and control options are required to develop the most beneficial care plan for the patient.

| **Keywords:** prosthetic management; transradial; wrist disarticulation

Introduction

There were an estimated 2.2 million individuals living with limb loss in the United States in 2020.[1] The number of individuals with major upper limb loss, defined as through or proximal to the wrist joint, represent approximately 3% of the total amputee cohort in the United States, resulting in an estimated 66,000 individuals in 2020.[1] Common causes for upper limb loss include trauma, vascular infection, congenital absence, and malignant tumors (cancer). The most frequently performed major upper limb amputation occurs at the transradial (TR) level as a result of trauma.[1-3] TR and wrist disarticulation (WD) amputations made up an estimated 60% of all major upper limb amputations from injuries sustained by U.S. military personnel since the turn of the century.[2] Loss involving the upper extremity causes significant physical and psychosocial challenges that must be addressed to minimize any negative impact on a person's quality of life and participation in society. Interventions involving prosthetic devices are an important available tool to help address these needs.

Individuals who undergo amputations at the transradial level have more functional potential than those with more proximal amputations, and similarly show a much higher acceptance rate with using a prosthesis than those with upper extremity amputations at other levels.[4,5] Published data from the U.S. Department of Veterans Affairs shows TR and WD level prostheses represented approximately 74% of all active (ie, cable driven and externally powered) upper limb prostheses that were procured for veterans within the 7-year period from 2009 to 2016.[6]

Amputation Level Considerations

Trauma, as the primary cause of upper extremity amputation, results in rare opportunity for the patient, doctor, surgeon, and prosthetist to collaborate on surgical considerations upon initial amputation. Surgeons and doctors who deal with upper limb amputees should maintain a regular, open line of communication with a prosthetist experienced in fitting this cohort, so that general concepts and advancements in prosthetic fitting procedures can be shared.

Advantages of wrist disarticulation (**Figure 1**, A) amputation include: the preservation of the entire forearm for maximal mechanical leverage and load bearing; retention of up to 120°

Dr. Stark or an immediate family member serves as a paid consultant to or is an employee of Ottobock. Neither Christopher Fantini nor any immediate family member has received anything of value from or has stock or stock options held in a commercial company or institution related directly or indirectly to the subject of this chapter.

This chapter is adapted from Brenner JK: Wrist disarticulation and transradial amputation: prosthetic management, in Krajbich JI, Pinzur MS, Potter BK, Stevens PM, eds: *Atlas of Amputations and Limb Deficiencies: Surgical, Prosthetic, and Rehabilitation Principles*, ed 4. American Academy of Orthopaedic Surgeons, 2016, pp 233-241.

of active range of motion (ROM) with pronation/supination; eliminating the risk of impingement between the distal ulna and radius; and available use of the distal styloids as an anatomical suspension of a prosthetic device.

Although the preservation of full anatomic forearm length with WD is often considered advantageous for the patient for the reasons listed above, there are disadvantages which may contraindicate this level of amputation for consideration. WD amputations result in both limited choice of functional prosthetic options and aesthetic challenges with maintaining body symmetry. Insufficient space remains between the end of the limb and the prosthetic terminal device (TD) to both maintain proportional symmetry and allow use of a quick-disconnect wrist, which allows interchangeability of various TDs. In cases of unilateral amputations, this routinely results in a length discrepancy between the prosthesis and the sound limb. The result may create functional challenges with positioning the TD in space for activities at the body's midline and/or be aesthetically unacceptable to the patient. In bilateral WD cases, although prostheses may be made symmetrical in length even with use of quick-disconnect wrists, there are similar concerns as the devices would be disproportionately long as compared with the patient's body size. The additional length makes it more difficult to perform functional activities at the body's midline (eg, fastening a belt, buttoning a shirt, bringing food to the mouth, etc), requiring more compensatory trunk and shoulder movements. Further, the additional length may also result in the need for the amputee to purchase new clothing with longer sleeves to maintain desired appearances in public, adding wardrobe expense and inconvenience. If it is not expected that the patient will experience the advantages of WD resulting in retention of most of their natural pronation/supination ROM or adequate soft-tissue coverage and durability to support suspension over the distal styloids, then amputation at the TR level will likely better serve their needs.[7-10]

The TR amputation level (**Figure 1, B**), in contrast to WD, presents advantages including the potential for fitting various prosthetic designs, use of quick-disconnecting components, and is more likely to be aesthetically appealing, permitting the prosthesis to be made symmetrical in length to the sound side limb. TR amputations should aim to retain at least two-thirds of the forearm to provide optimal balance between forearm leverage, ROM in pronation/supination, and offer access to a wide variety of postoperative prosthetic options, including potential use of a quick-disconnect wrist unit to change TDs from hooks to hands and/or an electric wrist rotator to replace lost pronation/supination.[2,11] At least 5 cm of residual ulna is required to allow for prosthetic fitting and elbow motion.[2] A more distal transradial amputation results in a robust lever arm, allows for anatomical pronation/supination and preserved shoulder and elbow function, which allows the patient to more easily use the prosthesis to position the TD in space, for performing activities of daily living (ADLs).

Whenever possible, within the preoperative phase of care, the patient should be made aware of the advantages and disadvantages of undergoing a wrist disarticulation procedure versus a transradial amputation, so an informed team decision, centering on the patient as the lead influence, may be made. This will maximize the patient's functional recovery and quality of life after surgery.

Postoperative Prosthetic Management

Postoperative interventions include those common for other amputation levels: wound care, controlling extremity volume with compression wrapping or shrinkers, desensitization training, and scar management. Edema control, pain management, and residual limb shaping can be achieved through an immediate postoperative wound dressing and figure-of-8 compressive wrap. The patient may progress to early application of a shrinker or compression sleeve over the surgical dressing for continuous wear, as wound drainage resolves. Once postoperative sutures are removed the patient may be issued an appropriately sized shrinker or elastomer liner to attenuate limb volume and/or pain.

Desensitization techniques such as massage, limb tapping, vibration, and the use of desensitization media/textures may be used to address areas of residuum hypersensitivity. As tolerated, gradual load-bearing on the residuum should be initiated to help reduce residual and phantom limb pain and prepare the limb for use of a prosthesis.[10] It is beneficial for the patient to use the residual limb in active mobilization and stretching to reduce pain, maintain strength and ROM at the elbow and

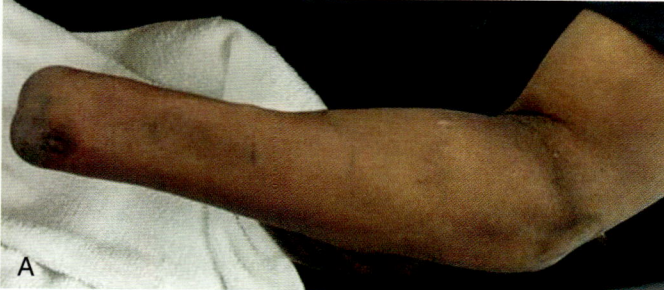 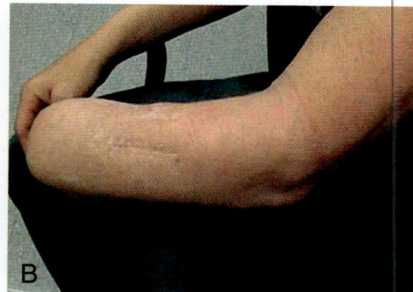 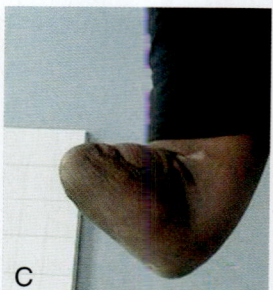

FIGURE 1 Examples of resulting residual limb lengths below the elbow. **A**, Wrist disarticulation. **B**, Mid-length transradial limb. **C**, Short transradial limb.

shoulder joints, and improve the potential for prosthetic function and use.

Early postoperative involvement of a trained peer visitor or peer support group can provide important psychosocial benefit to the patient.[10] Peer support provides an opportunity for patients to relate to one another and/or to disclose relevant emotions and experiences. Peers with experience relating to upper limb amputation can help the patient, as well as their caregiver(s), set realistic expectations, and provide insight to challenges yet to be faced. Connecting a patient with upper limb loss to a peer visitor, support group, or educational program may be accomplished through face-to-face programs or through telecommunication technology, which provides increased peer visitation access to individuals living in rural areas, who are otherwise often underserved with such opportunities.[10]

Early prosthetic fittings have been correlated with a higher level of successful outcomes with respect to device acceptance and use, suggesting prosthetic fittings should begin as early as within 30 days, or at least within 6 months, after amputation.[12-16] The importance of early training of patients using prostheses can not be overstated. The patient's exposure to quality training with the prosthetic device is another important factor that may be associated with successful outcomes of device acceptance and use.[10,13,17-20]

As the patient and clinical team develop short-term and long-term goals, education on the various prosthetic options for consideration should be provided to the patient as well as their family and/or caregiver(s), before the initiation of a prosthetic prescription. Prosthetic options can be divided into six categories: no prosthesis, aesthetic/semiprehensile, externally powered, body powered/cable-driven, hybrid, and special purpose. Traditionally, these items have been presented in a linear fashion, in literature and within prosthetics education curriculums, implying a hierarchical progression as to the prosthetic options considered for prescription. However, an alternate paradigm better illustrates the nonhierarchical patient-centered approach of considering all prosthetic

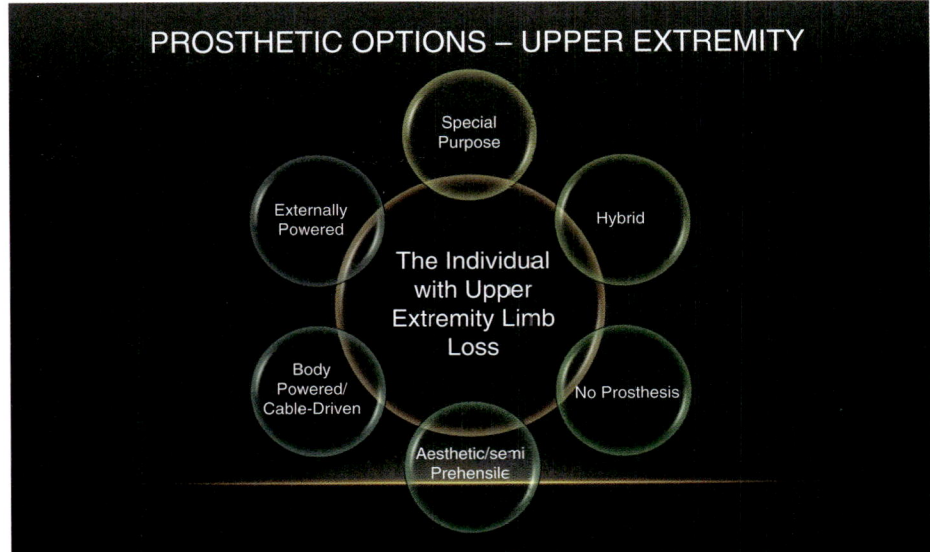

FIGURE 2 Diagram showing the nonhierarchical view of considering prosthetic options, better illustrating the patient-centered approach to decision-making than that of the hierarchical, linear model. (Adapted from Stevens PM, Highsmith MJ: Myoelectric and body power, design options for upper-limb prostheses: introduction to the state of the science conference proceedings. *J Prosthet Orthot* 2017;29(4S):P1-P3.)

options (**Figure 2**), at any point in the patient's stage of care.[21] Preprosthetic training should be initiated as necessary, corresponding to the type of prosthetic option selected to best match the needs of the patient.

Externally powered prosthetic designs, because of the creation of less shear and end-bearing forces on the residual limb, can be used earlier after amputation than body-powered designs. In some instances the process to identify electrode sites and initiate the training necessary for the operation of a myoelectric prosthesis may begin even before surgical wound closure is achieved. However, special consideration and attention is needed before fitting a myoelectric device on a residual limb that has not matured in volume. Myoelectric designs require an intimate fit with the limb to maintain sufficient electrode contact with the skin. The anticipated changes in volume of the residuum as it continues to heal in the immediate weeks and months after surgery will require multiple interface replacements to maintain proper functioning of the device, increasing the burden and potential frustration of the patient and/or their caregivers resulting from more frequent servicing and clinic visits.

There are sound therapeutic rationales to consider a body-powered prosthesis for a new TR or WD amputee. These include: desensitizing the limb through applied pressure between the residuum and interface during active use; controlling edema as the residual limb is shaped for a more definitive interface design; improvement of proximal joint ROM through active control of the TD; and accommodation of shape/volume changes in the residual limb as the healing process progresses, using the addition of socks, minimizing the frequency of interface replacements. In addition, the body-powered design offers proprioceptive feedback through the applied forces within the socket as tension is applied through the harness.

In the case where a passive prehensile prosthesis is the desired design, then the process of using a preparatory prosthesis is not necessary, since the active function of the device for dynamic use will be minimal.

Prosthetic Interface Considerations

The design of a transradial prosthetic interface is influenced by several factors including residual limb length and the selected prosthetic control strategy. Universal design goals for the prosthetic interface strive to comfortably spread load forces during active and static lift, maximize ROM, stabilize the prosthesis against rotary forces, and facilitate suspension on the residual limb. Patients with unilateral or bilateral amputations at this level should be able to independently don and doff their prosthesis(es) with relative ease.

Additionally, with self-suspending interface designs, the epicondyles, olecranon, and distal biceps tendon should be free of impingement or excessive pressure. The patient should be able to maintain prosthetic suspension passively without inadvertently losing suspension by flexing or extending the arm.

WD and long TR residual limbs permit a more distal interface trimline relative to the cubital fold, allowing for full ROM with elbow flexion. The interface should be made to intimately fit with the shape and contours of the distal forearm, specifically in the area of the distal interosseous space between the radius and ulna, which aids in more efficient translation of forearm rotation to the prosthetic TD. This produces an interface shape sometimes referred to as a "screwdriver fit," which stabilizes the interface to the residual limb as the amputee performs tasks requiring rotary forces, such as turning a doorknob, allowing the wearer to use up to 50% of their available ROM for pronation and supination of the prosthetic TD. The fundamentals of fitting the WD interface involve adequate loading along the ulnar shaft, proper medial/lateral dimension to transfer natural pronation and supination to the TD, and anatomical suspension over the radial and ulnar styloids. Some designs may remove parts of the interface that are not necessary. A common issue with upper and lower interface designs involves heat retention within a fully enclosed interface, which can lead to excessive perspiration and discomfort (**Figure 3**). Opening the interface by removing areas that are not crucial to the fundamental design aspects assists to minimize heat retention and moisture build up within the interface (**Figure 4**). In addition, fenestration of

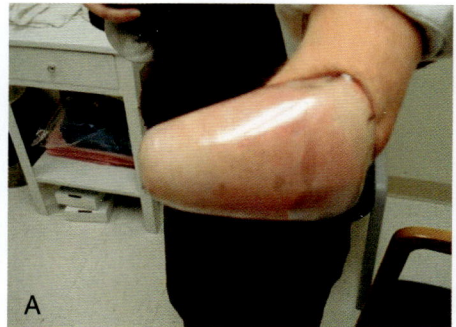 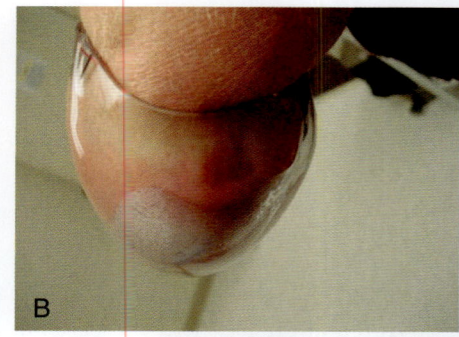

FIGURE 3 Clinical photographs of a diagnostic self-suspended hybrid interface design. **A**. Sagittal view showing an anterior trimline distal to the cubital fold for improved range of motion (no cubital bulging), relief over the anterior distal end and olecranon, as well as blanching of the skin over the supracondylar area. **B**. Posterior view showing blanching of the skin at the triceps bar as well as evidence of moisture fogging the diagnostic socket.

the interface also provides the advantage of accommodating increases in limb volume, as the uncovered soft tissue has space to expand without restriction. Yet another advantage is the resulting opportunity to use the advantages of direct forearm sensation with the external environment.

Short transradial limbs are more vulnerable to medial/lateral instability of the prosthesis on the limb. Muscle strength and ROM are also adversely affected with shorter limbs. Elbow stability, active range of motion (AROM), and weakness because of loss of leverage are all significant concerns to be addressed in the prosthetic design. Shorter TR amputations require a more proximal trimline of the interface up to the cubital fold and, depending on the suspension strategy, encompassing the epicondyles and olecranon, to maintain stability of the prosthesis with the limb (**Figure 5**). As a result, ROM at the elbow is often limited. Prostheses designed for short TR limbs may use rigid hinges, mounted on the outside of the interface. This improves stability between the residuum and interface, while maximizing the available surface area to distribute load forces. At this amputation level, the absence of natural

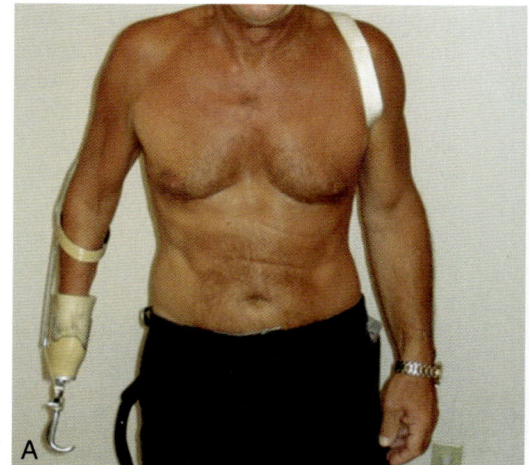 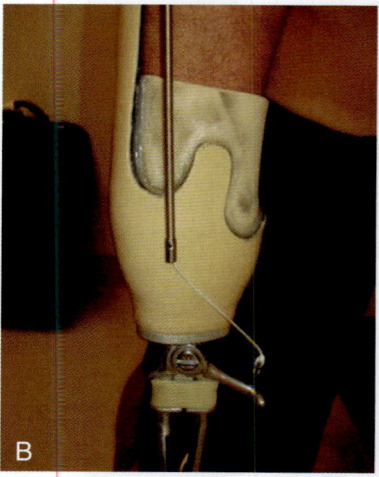

FIGURE 4 Clinical photographs of a modified self-suspended, body-powered wrist disarticulation interface with a figure-of-9 harness. **A**, The anterior, medial and lateral frame along the mid forearm is removed to reduce perspiration and improve sensory access to the environment through the sensate limb. **B**, Contours over the radial and ulnar styloids provide suspension via push-in donning. The interface frame provides load support on the ulnar shaft and provides a "screwdriver shape" over the distal forearm to enable use of natural wrist rotation to rotate the terminal device. The proximal trimline encircles the proximal forearm to provide stability.

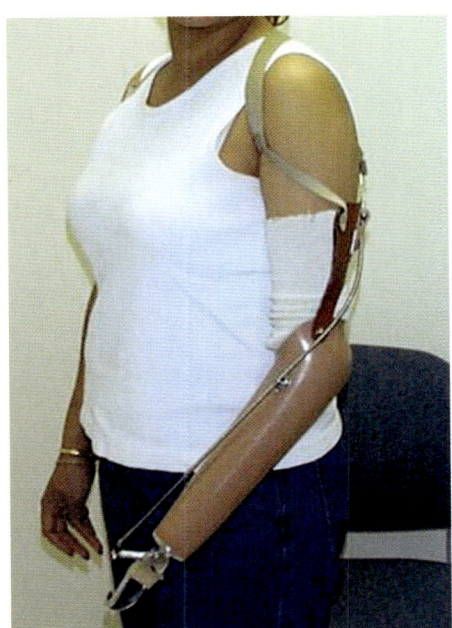

FIGURE 5 Clinical photograph of a body-powered transradial interface for a short residual limb, showing high trimlines enveloping the olecranon and epicondyles.

forearm rotation eliminates concern of the rigid hinges restricting any functional pronation/supination. There are four basic types of rigid hinges for transradial level prostheses: single-axis hinges, polycentric hinges, step-up hinges, and limb-activated locking hinges. Each has unique features that make them favorable under various circumstances which have been covered in various texts.[22]

Because of the short lever of the residual limb, efforts should be taken to keep the center of mass of the prosthesis as proximal to the elbow axis as possible, to minimize the muscle effort required to lift the prosthesis during active use. This is achieved via selection of a lightweight wrist and TD and/or shortening the overall length of the prostheses as compared with the anatomical limb length before amputation. In addition to providing better leverage, shortening the prostheses also facilitates the ability of the user to perform activities at midline where much of the ADLs occur. Shortened prostheses are especially beneficial to those with bilateral transradial amputations, as they optimize their ability to perform midline ADLs, thereby improving independence.

During lifting activities, with TR and WD prostheses, there is a force couple created which results in focused pressures on the distal radial and proximal ulnar aspects of the limb. When the WD or long TR prosthesis is intended for heavy-duty use, requiring lifting of larger loads, the ulnar trimline of the interface may extend up to, and even include, the olecranon to maximize the distribution of the load. Shorter TR level interfaces will often extend up to the triceps tendon. The anterior distal radius should be relieved so the vertical load, as elbow flexion occurs, is distributed to more proximal areas of the forearm.

Interface Suspension Options

Suspension is as equally an important and interrelated feature of the prosthetic interface as comfort. Resistance to distraction forces applied to the WD or TR prosthesis is accomplished through the employed suspension system, either that of a harness or a self-suspending interface design. Similar to interfaces for the lower extremity, upper limb interfaces are contoured to relieve pressure-sensitive areas and load pressure-tolerant areas of the limb. Inadequate suspension results in excessive forces in pressure-sensitive areas as the interface migrates on the limb causing potential discomfort to the patient. In addition, lack of appropriate suspension will have a negative impact on efficient voluntary control of the prosthesis, regardless of the control strategy used. Either of these effects, or in combination, may lead to patient frustration, demoralization of functional potential, and ultimately rejection of the device. However, a properly suspended prosthesis for the WD or TR amputee results in the potential for full functional independence and acceptance with use of prostheses.

Harness-Suspended Designs

Harness suspension uses an array of straps to attach the prosthesis to the wearer by distributing distraction forces over the shoulders and back. Harness-suspended WD or TR interfaces are well suited for prostheses that are intended for more rugged or heavy-duty use, where the wearer may carry heavier loads using the residual limb or expose the device to harsh environments (water/moisture, dirt, chemicals, vibration, etc) which may otherwise compromise suspension of the prosthesis or lead to frequent maintenance.

The two basic harness suspension designs used with WD and TR interfaces are the figure-of-8 design (**Figure 6**) and the shoulder saddle with chest

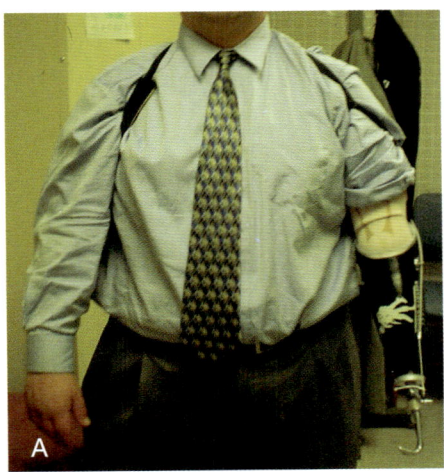 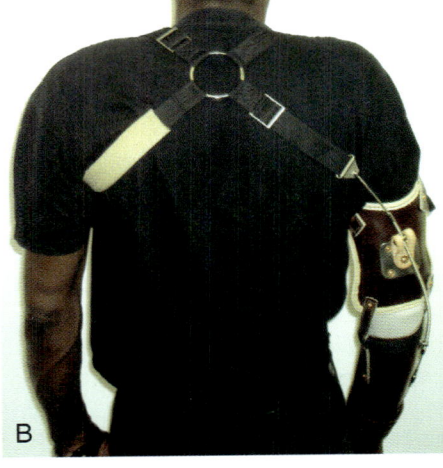

FIGURE 6 Photographs of a transradial figure-of-8 harness with flexible hinges. **A**, Anterior view. The anterior suspension strap, via the inverted Y connection to the triceps pad, carries the vertical load force applied to the prosthesis over the shoulder, to the posterior cross point of the harness. **B**, Posterior view, with a Northwestern ring cross point. The anterior suspensor strap runs over the ipsilateral shoulder to attach to the cross point. The contralateral axilla loop anchors the harness to suspend the prosthesis as forces are applied through the anterior suspension strap.

Section 2: Upper Limb

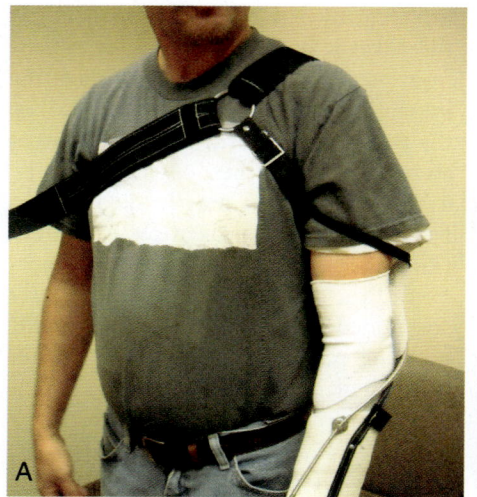
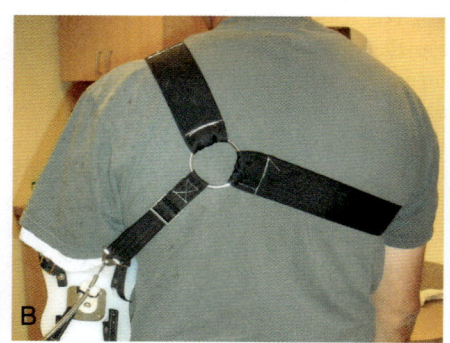
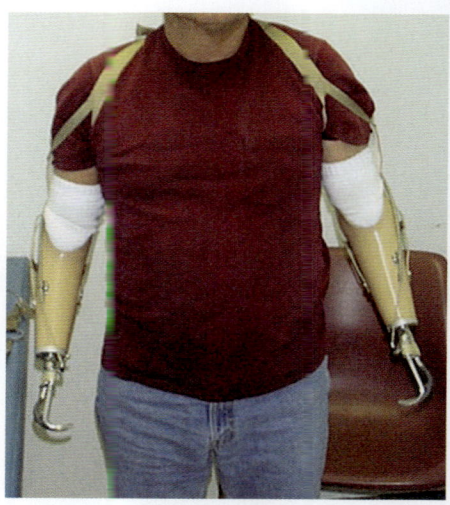

FIGURE 7 Photograph of a chest strap and shoulder saddle harness with flexible hinges. **A**, Anterior view. The anterior suspensor strap via the inverted Y connection to the triceps cup transfers the vertical load of the prosthesis to the ipsilateral shoulder saddle and contralateral chest wall. **B**, Posterior view with a Northwestern ring providing the anchor point for the control strap and cable. (Photo courtesy of Phil Stevens, MEd, CPO, FAAOP.)

FIGURE 8 Clinical photograph of bilateral transradial interfaces suspended with a figure-of-8 harness for mid-length residual limbs–anterior view. The anterior trimlines are lower to allow increased ROM with elbow flexion. The forearm lengths of the prostheses were made shorter than the anatomical limbs to facilitate better leverage and more readily reach the body's midline.

strap (**Figure 7**). The figure-of-8 harness design is the most commonly used for WD and TR cable-driven prostheses and is suitable for most daily activities, however the chest strap and shoulder saddle design may be a better option for those who frequently carry heavier loads using the prosthesis as well as for individuals who are uncomfortable with the contralateral axillary pressure exerted by a figure-of-8 harness. The chest strap and shoulder saddle may not be desirable for many female patients because of discomfort of the chest strap as well as its visibility under clothing with low neck lines.[7]

Harness suspension designs for WD and TR prostheses use elbow hinges which are designed to be either flexible or rigid. The hinges proximally attach to either a triceps pad, a half cuff, or a full cuff around the humerus and distally to the prosthetic forearm. Suspension is achieved via an anterior suspension strap or shoulder saddle which sits over the ipsilateral shoulder, and transmits forces from the interface through the proximal portion of the triceps pad or cuff to the cross point of the harness, where it attaches to the contralateral axilla strap, which either wraps around the contralateral shoulder (in the figure-of-8 design) or wraps around the torso to become the anterior chest strap (in the shoulder saddle/chest strap design). The contralateral axilla strap acts to anchor the harness for both suspension and cable-driven control of the TD. The axilla strap is often padded or augmented with flexible material to improve comfort. Figure-of-8 designs for bilateral WD and/or TR cases do not feature an axilla strap, as each anterior suspension strap (**Figure 8**) connects to the cross point and provides the anchoring counter force required to suspend the contralateral prosthesis (**Figure 9**).

Flexible hinges are preferred for WD, long TR, and bilateral TR amputees as they permit maximal transmission of the residual forearm rotation to the terminal device, minimizing the requirement for manual prepositioning by the amputee. These hinges are also preferred in pediatric cases so as not to limit developmental potential by restricting movement. Flexible hinges are made of webbing material, leather, or wire, while rigid hinges are of a metal pivot design. Rigid hinges are used for short residual limbs as well as prostheses intended for heavier workload use. They protect the very short residuum from excessive torque and prevent rotation of the interface on the residual limb; however they do not allow any anatomical pronation/supination.

Self-Suspended Designs

Self-suspended interface designs eliminate the need for harnessing to suspend the prosthesis. There are multiple strategies available for self-suspending designs. The most common and best

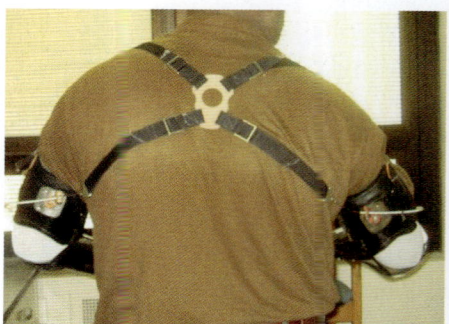

FIGURE 9 Clinical photograph of a bilateral transradial figure-of-8 harness showing the cable control straps with excessive slack, increasing the excursion necessary to fully open the TD. Tightening the cable control straps to move the cable hangars more proximal to the lateral-inferior border of the scapula reduces the cable excursion required to operate the TDs more efficiently.

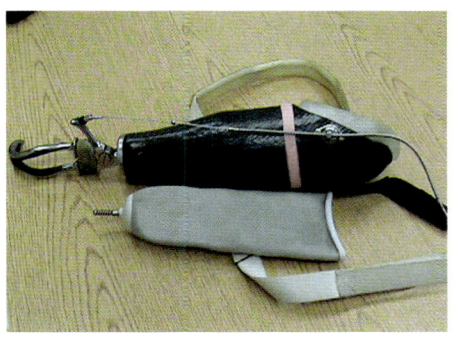

FIGURE 10 Photograph of a self-suspended body-powered design featuring a roll-on locking liner and a figure-of-9 harness for operation of the terminal device.

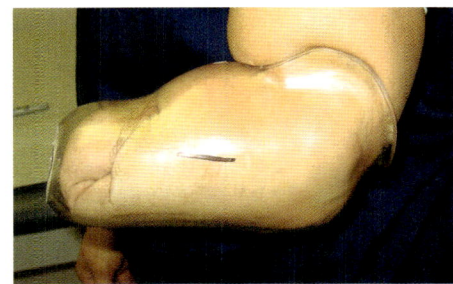

FIGURE 11 Photograph of a diagnostic Muenster interface, for a short transradial amputation. This socket is characterized by the use of anterior–posterior counterforce suspension with proximal trim lines extending into the cubital fold anteriorly and well above the olecranon posteriorly. A pull-sock and distal escape channel are required to pull the limb tissues through the narrowed opening and into the socket where they can then expand and fill the larger inner socket cavity. (Courtesy of Jack E. Uellendahl, CPO, Cave Creek, AZ.)

documented are anatomically suspended to the residual limb using contours designed over skeletal anatomy (ie, distal styloids of the radius and ulna for WDs; the epicondyles of the humerus for TR amputation levels). Many prosthetists, particularly those with little experience managing patients with upper limb amputation, may be tempted to first opt for strategies which promise to achieve suspension more easily, such as the use of gel liners (**Figure 10**), than with the modifications necessary for direct anatomical suspension. However, because of unique limb shapes, added thickness, rotation, accommodation of the distal attachment, and greater difficulty with electrode contact for myoelectric designs, many return to the direct loading of anatomical self-suspension techniques.

Anatomical self-suspension designs do present challenges for the prosthetist. The objective of securing the prosthesis is often counteracted by the need for comfort and maximized range of motion and it must be remembered that since the interface extends above the epicondyles it effectively blocks all pronation or supination which is compensated by using glenohumeral joint motion or wrist rotation components. The modification process involved in achieving anatomically self-suspended interfaces remains fairly involved, requiring attention to two key fundamental relationships common to all iterations of these designs: (1) the necessary balance of compression between the triceps bar and cubital/anterior trimline and (2) the height of the interface trimline and the resultant ROM available. Frequently, trimlines are lowered for improved comfort and/or ROM, only to lose suspension stability. However, the advantages of direct contact for loading and myo-electric control, minimized interface thickness, elimination of the harness, and relative ease of donning make it an attractive option.

Self-suspended interfaces use either a push-in or pull-in strategy of donning. Generally, longer TR or WD residual limbs favor a push-in method of donning the interface. When necessary, an evaporative lubricant, such as hand sanitizer, may be used to facilitate push-in donning. Designs for shorter TR limbs favor a pull-in donning method where the individual pulls their limb into the interface, using a pull sheath or stocking, to assure maximum contact between the interface and limb and encapsulate any excessive tissue. The shorter the limb, the more important it is to get as much residual limb tissue as possible, particularly distal to the cubital fold, into the interface and ensure the anterior counterforce to the triceps bar is applied to the limb as intended, maximizing comfort, stability, and control of the prosthesis. Modifications can be made, particularly for the case of the short transradial bilateral amputee, to create a looser fitting interface to allow a push-in method to don the interface, as this is easier for the bilateral amputee to independently manage than using a pull sheath or stocking. Though this comes at the cost of some stability between the prosthesis and limb, it may be outweighed by the increased independence with donning the prostheses for the bilateral patient with short TR residual limbs.

Muenster Design

The original anatomical TR self-suspension method was developed by Dr. Oscar Hepp and Dr. G.G. Kuhn in the mid-1950s for use with cosmetic passive arms at the University of Muenster, Germany, which was later introduced to the United States in 1958.[23] New York University published a fabrication manual for the Muenster method in 1965 in which it attempted to quantify the technique into a teachable method.[23] Originally used for body-powered cable systems, with a figure-of-9 harness for TD control, the NYU-Muenster design is well suited to short to very short unilateral transradial amputees (ranging from 1½ to 5½ inches).[23] The interface first introduced epicondylar suspension and encapsulation of the olecranon (**Figure 11**). To fit the shorter limb lengths, the NYU design uses relatively high anterior and posterior walls combined with a tight AP counterforce through the cubital fold with relief for the biceps tendon. This design limits the range of motion to 70° or from 35° to 105° and requires pull-in donning.[23] This limited range of motion was deemed acceptable at the time for short to very short unilateral amputees since the prosthesis was used at the extreme limits and then only as an assistive device. To accommodate this loss of motion the elbow is typically set in 35° of preflexion.[23]

The impression technique is fairly involved with the limb held at 90° of elbow flexion, the olecranon is cupped in the ball of the hand, the second, third, and fourth fingers applying triceps bar pressure, and the fifth finger and thumb curling in to make contact but not pressure with the epicondyles.

The opposite hand used the second and third fingers to load the cubital fold and create a biceps tendon relief. While this method produces relatively acceptable results for shorter limb lengths, the loss of range of motion continues to be problematic for individuals with longer limb lengths, who expected more functionality especially when combined with myoelectric systems.

Northwestern Design

The Northwestern interface design, originally described by Billock in 1974, features a more intimate medial-lateral fit over the anterior epicondyles as well as a drastically lower anterior trimline, approximately 45% of the overall length[24] (**Figure 12**). This design allows potential for full elbow ROM for longer limb lengths. Another difference is that the impression of the limb is taken with the limb at 45° of elbow flexion to capture the anatomic contours superior to the humeral epicondyles which are frequently distorted when the limb is held at 90° with the Muenster design (**Figure 13**, A through F).

Modification to the medial-lateral dimension is done anterior and posterior to the epicondyles, while allowing a slight channel to facilitate easy push-in, rather than pull-in, type donning. No modifications are made to distort the mold which would "disrupt the general contours of the amputation limb and displace the outlined areas of the olecranon process and humeral condyles."[24] The modifications are intended to rotate about the epicondyle to maintain suspension at 90°, full flexion, and full extension. The posterior triceps bar modifications, approximately ½ inch proximal to the olecranon, are not as high as for the Muenster, and so the extension range of motion is not inhibited while providing counter-pressure anteriorly. The radius of the modification is still abrupt enough to create tension over the olecranon to also provide counter-pressure to the anterior trim line. This feature is often obviated by excessive relief or flaring. Similar modifications have been described and reintroduced by more recent self-suspension methods to provide this necessary suspensory function. Overall, the Northwestern design greatly simplifies the impression technique and modification required, making easy push-in donning possible, which is especially beneficial to those with dexterity issues or bilateral patients. Many prosthetists use slight modifications to this procedure, primarily greater premolding of the epicondyles and anterior trimline pressure for fleshy patients, but invariably risk deforming the anatomy as expressed by Billock.

Otto Bock Muenster

The Otto Bock Muenster interface design, originally developed in the late 1970s, combines the suspension security of the Muenster interface with the increased range of motion of the Northwestern design. The design, in effect, modifies the Muenster by applying the Northwestern principles of an anterior M-L pressure over the anterior epicondyles, and ranges the casting impression from full flexion to full extension. The impression employs a proximal splint pattern that cups well over the epicondyles, but drops over the cubital fold and posterior trimline to allow a much greater range of motion than the Muenster (**Figure 14**, A). A rope splint, narrowed at the cubital fold, is pulled tightly over the apex of the olecranon (**Figure 14**, B). This creates an extremely secure fit and results in relief for the cubital tissue by pushing into the cubital fold, but requires pull-in type donning. Anteriorly a biceps tendon cubital tissue relief was borrowed from the Muenster, but this was molded as the patient flexed and extended the impression throughout their range of motion. This highly successful design continues to be used today with slight modifications to the impression procedure. These modified designs accentuate the anatomic contours even more to achieve, what is hoped to be, better suspension, rotation control, and range of motion, and optimized myoelectric function. Some have been presented in the literature. The Compression Release Stabilized (CRS) interface (**Figure 15**) and Anatomic Contoured Control Interface (ACCI) described by Alley, and the Transradial Anatomic Contour Interface (TRAC) described by Miguelez, accentuate the anterior pressure, cubital loading, biceps tendon relieve, and triceps bar counterforce found in the original Otto Bock Muenster.[2-27]

Although the preceding interfaces have distinct characteristics, many prosthetists employ hybrid approaches of these various principles depending on the patient's limb length, presentation, and functional goals. The longer limb lengths, 55% or more, can benefit from the dropped anterior trimline and

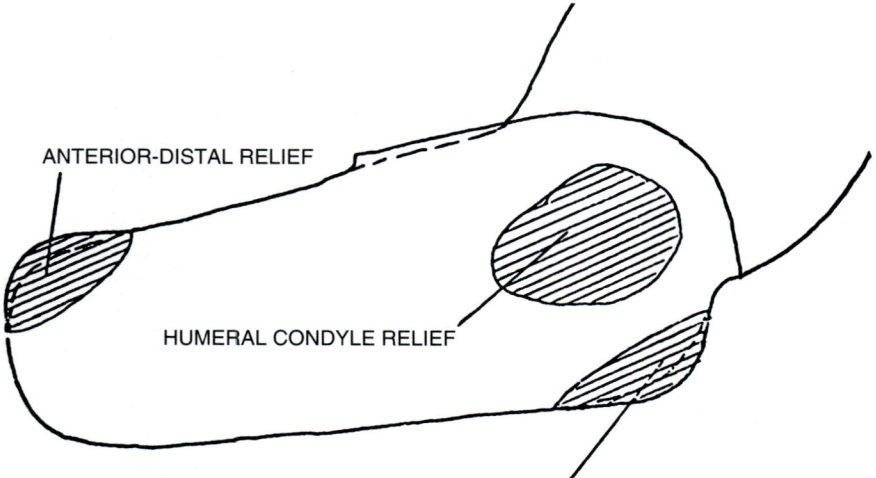

FIGURE 12 Picture from John Billock's original description of the Northwestern design showing the relief that is more posteriorly directed on the condyles and olecranon. (Reproduced from Billock J: The Northwestern University supracondylar suspension technique for below elbow amputations. *Orthot Prosthet* 1972; 26[4]:16-23.)

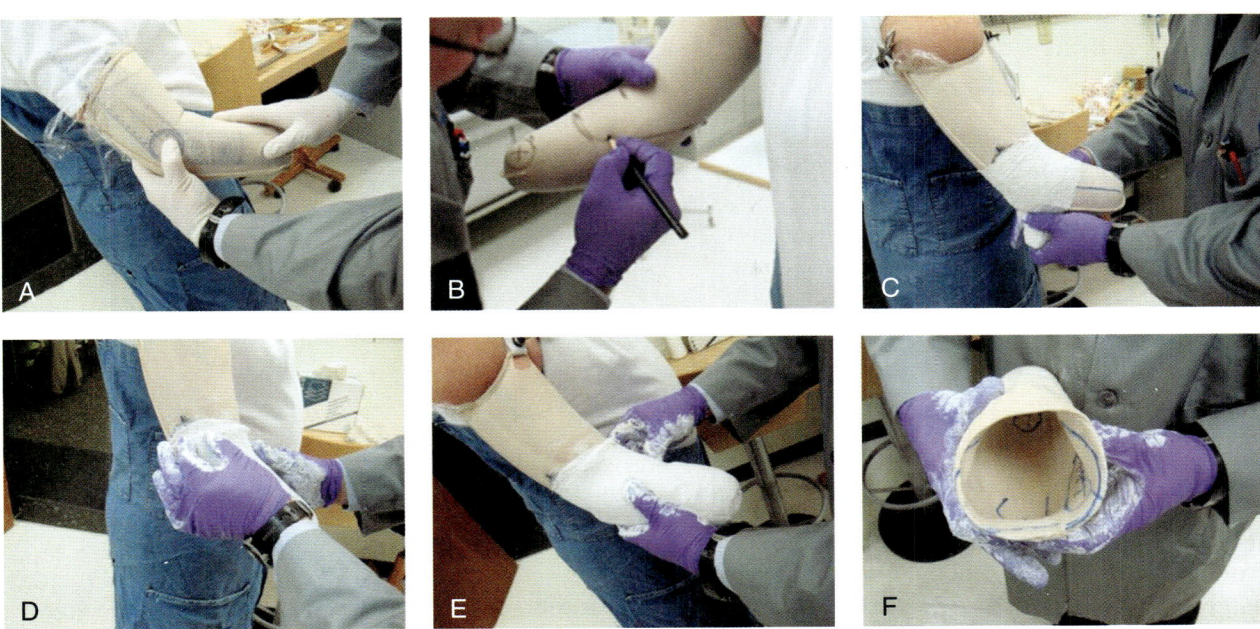

FIGURE 13 Photographs showing techniques for taking a transradial casting impression for the Northwestern interface design: Impression casting for the Northwestern interface design. **A**, During casting, the patient is instructed to hold the limb at 45°. **B**, Trimlines are marked: anterior trimline is drawn up to half the forearm length to the distal end, depending desired level of cubital loading; posterior trimline is 18 mm proximal to the olecranon; and medial lateral trimlines are 25 mm proximal to the epicondyle borders. **C**, Limb is completely wrapped with two to three layers of 3 inches elastic plaster. Patient maintains the limb at 45°. **D**, Once the elastic plaster is set, one to three layers of 4 inches rigid plaster is added and trimlines and contours are defined around the olecranon, epicondyles to simulate interface loading. **E**, The clinician defines the anterior using the thumb tips to define the load areas and trimline. Pressure is also applied over the longitudinal axis of the arm to define the "screwdriver" shape (not shown). **F**, The cast is carefully removed. The triceps bar will deform when removed and will need to be pushed back into position. The final shape should be triangular with loading contours at the olecranon and epicondyles.

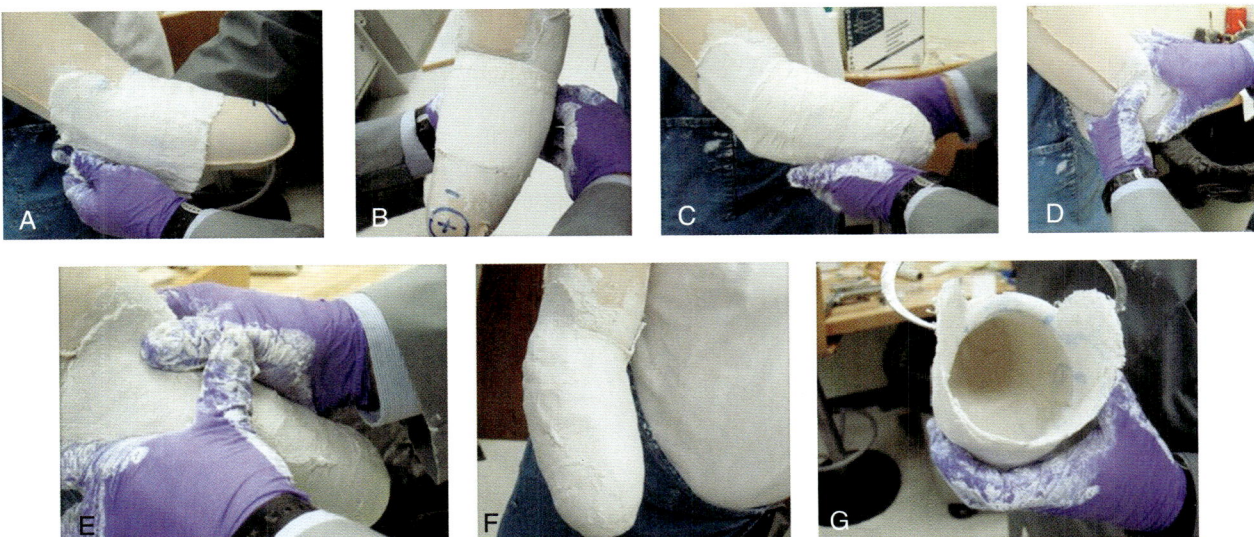

FIGURE 14 Photographs showing techniques for taking a transradial casting impression for the Otto Bock-Muenster interface design: **A**, The proximal splint pattern that encapsulates the epicondyles, while dropping over the cubital fold and posterior trimline. **B**, A cubital reinforcement rope splint is placed immediately below the cubital trimline mark. **C**, Elastic bandage is wrapped around the cubital fold mark. **D**, The anterior trimline is firmly held down against the radius while the other hand is used to tightly mold around the epicondyles and olecranon as the limb is held at greater than 90° of flexion. **E**, As the plaster sets, the cast is further flexed to resistance and extended to resistance as the proximal brim is held firmly in place. This dynamic casting process creates the added ROM lacking in the Muenster design. **F**, Before removal of the cast, the cast impression is inspected for proper shape and rigidity. The cast should be rigid before removal. **G**, The impression is examined for an appropriately formed triangular proximal shape.

Section 2: Upper Limb

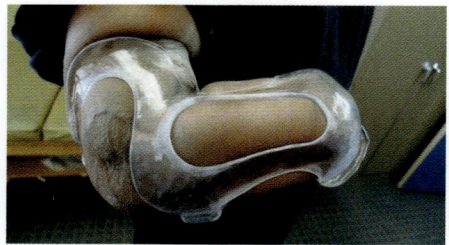

FIGURE 15 Clinical photograph of a diagnostic socket for a Compression Release Stabilized design featuring alternating areas of compression and soft-tissue release from the interface. The recurring principles espousing the relationship between the triceps bar and anterior cubital counterpressure are used to maintain suspension. Similar to the Muenster design, this particular fit requires a pull-in donning technique to ensure soft tissue fills the fenestration anteriorly to prevent cubital bunching from limiting ROM.

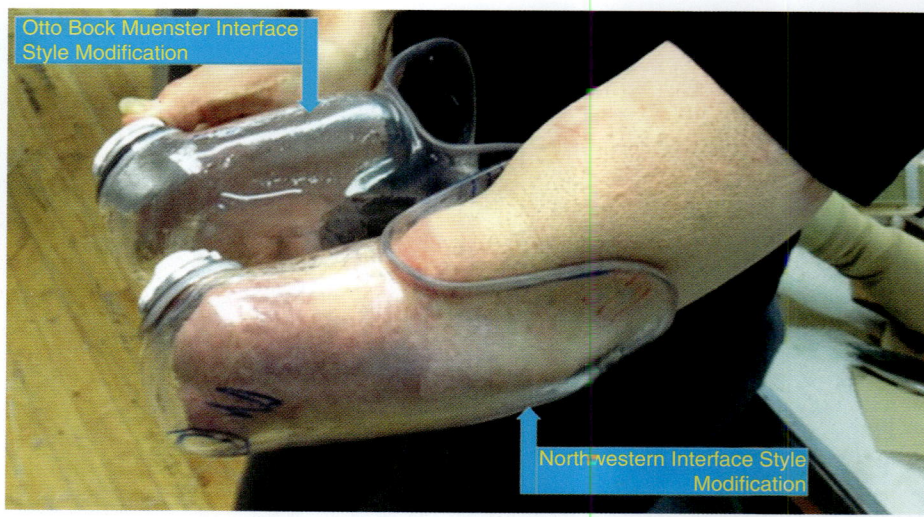

FIGURE 16 Clinical photograph of diagnostic interfaces comparing the trimlines and contours of Muenster and Northwestern designs. The patient is wearing the Northwestern diagnostic interface. Blanching of the soft tissue reveals the loading along the along the trimline.

increased range of motion of the NU design. Shorter limb lengths, 50% to 30%, benefit from the greater A-P cubital loading and suspension characteristics of the Otto Bock Muenster without sacrificing too much motion. Very short limbs, 30% or less, may require a more classic Muenster-type interface with higher anterior and posterior trimlines, sacrificing ROM to insure greater suspension security. The delineation between the different limb lengths is not a definitive one, but rather indicates the degree to which the different features are added or lessened.

Interface Evaluation

Regardless of the interface design chosen (**Figure 16**), the prosthetic goals remain the same. The prosthesis should be secure and comfortable, throughout the range of motion. The range of motion should be maximized, but not at the expense of secure suspension. Relief should be provided for comfortable loading axially, at 90°, and full extension. The patient should be able to easily don and doff the prosthesis independently without excessive impingement on the epicondyles or olecranon. The patient should be able to maintain suspension passively without inadvertently losing suspension by flexing or extending the arm.

In full extension the proximal ulna area has the tendency to pull away from the interface wall. A certain amount of gapping is acceptable since a well-loaded triceps bar, especially with a firm triceps tendon, causes this gapping naturally. Too much gapping may be a result of a posterior trimline that is too high or an anterior opening at the cubital fold that is too wide. Also, relief should be directed more proximally at the posterior epicondyle with some loading at the trimline to provide comfortable loading at full extension (**Figure 17**, A).

In full flexion, the distal radial area and proximal ulnar area are loaded respectively (**Figure 17**, B). If the triceps bar is placed incorrectly or it is too narrow the olecranon may pop out of its modification and the interface will migrate distally. This may also happen if there is excessive cubital fold pressure because the trimline is too high or the cubital tissue has not been accommodated. Typically a heavier pressure in the cubital fold will protrude proximally to the trimline and effectively block flexion. With different self-suspending methods the anterior trimline can be lowered or the cubital bulge can be accommodated by pulling it into the interface. Because of this pull-in donning is often chosen in varying degree for more proximal amputations where cubital bunching can be an issue. The biceps tendon does move anteriorly and should be accommodated in the anterior trimline.

At 90° the anterior epicondylar modification combined with the

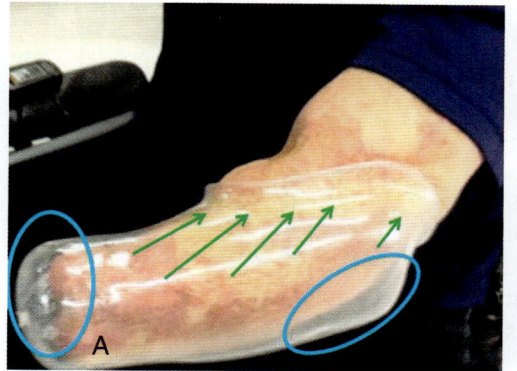 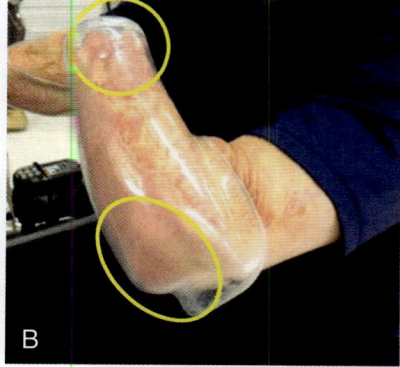

FIGURE 17 Clinical photographs of the evaluation of a diagnostic Northwestern interface design with reliefs and counterforce identified. **A**, At full elbow extension: blue circles indicate areas of appropriate relief/gapping to allow ranging into elbow flexion, green arrows highlight areas of the anterior counterforces to the pressure from the triceps bar. **B**, At full elbow flexion: the yellow circles indicate areas where the olecranon and distal limb fill the void seen in **A**.

anterior trimline loading provides the suspension. Obviously it is important to locate the epicondylar modifications accurately for comfort and relief. During elbow flexion the load areas must rotate concentrically about the epicondyle and not impinge during flexion or extension. Often patients indicate that the olecranon is impinged at 90° because of the counter-rotation that occurs when the hand is loaded or on a table top. For this reason a relief hole may be cut for the olecranon, first described as the "Three-Quarter Socket Type" by William Sauter.[28] Other designs have taken the Sauter modification concept further by opening up the interface to leave more of the residuum uncovered, including the medial and lateral epicondyles (**Figure 18**), to alleviate not only impingement, but, as previously mentioned, the discomfort and skin irritation that may result from perspiration in an enclosed interface environment.

Alternate Interface Designs

Advancements in materials (**Figure 19**), including bio-elastomers, have made prosthetic use much more comfortable, but result in different suspension characteristics. Given that the original Northwestern and Muenster sockets were designed for relatively stiff laminated interfaces, adjustments at the trimlines may be needed to account for a greater amount of tension and elastic bending associated with more elastic interfaces. Because of the flexibility of the newer bio-elastomers, more aggressive contours are possible and may explain the modifications presented in the CRS, ACCI, and TRAC designs.

Several novel socket designs have emerged with the growing use of high-consistency rolled (HCR) silicone. Short transradial residual limbs have historically necessitated management with high proximal trimlines that limit elbow motion as described earlier. A socket alternative at this limb length is a custom silicone socket with an integrated humeral suspension sleeve (**Figure 20**). The silicone sleeve is reflected distally over the rigid outer socket to facilitate donning. Once the limb is well-seated within the silicone socket the sleeve is rolled proximally

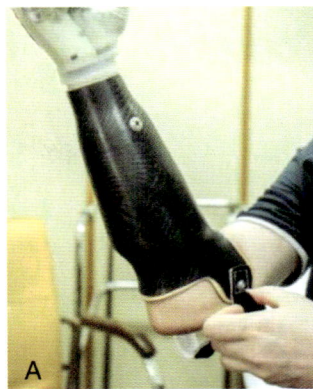 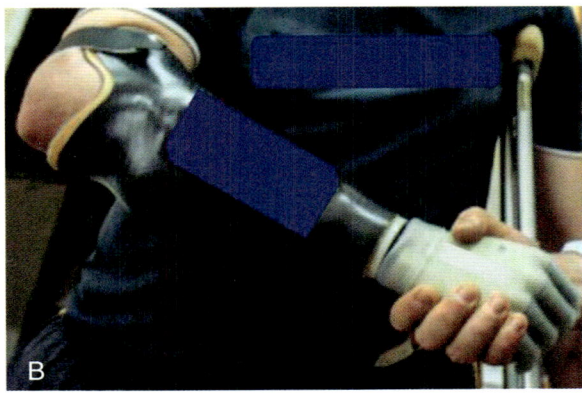

FIGURE 18 Photographs (**A**) and (**B**) illustrate a definitive self-suspended myoelectric prosthesis interface using an open design exposing the olecranon and epicondyles with a padded dacron strap acting as the triceps bar. This alternate design enables the patient to more easily push into the interface while allowing adjustability to increase or decrease tension over the olecranon. Some suspension security is sacrificed as it is reliant on the integrity of the strap, but the ease of donning and added comfort over the olecranon may outweigh the cost for some patients.

onto the upper arm where it establishes a proximal seal. A distal one-way air valve is often integrated into the distal aspect of the socket to permit the evacuation of any residual air.

Because this design suspends the prosthesis using suction, there is no need to secure an aggressive purchase over the bony contours of the elbow. Rather, the rigid trimlines need only

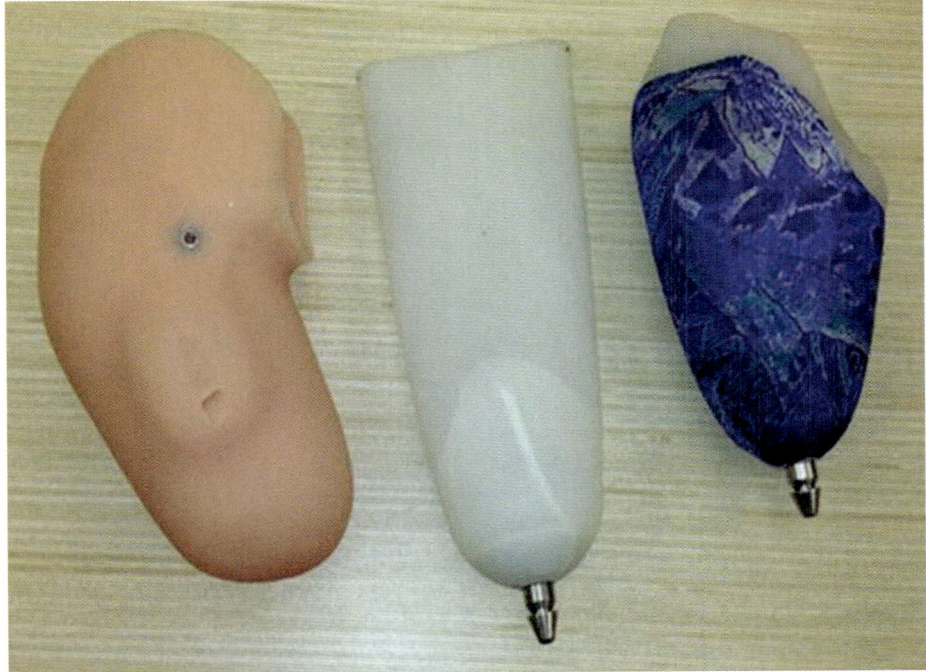

FIGURE 19 Photograph of sample elastomer liners. Liners may be used for added comfort as well as a mode of suspension. From left to right: a custom silicone interface for use with a myoelectric prosthesis. The patient uses evaporative lubricant to push-in to the interface, which is attached to the prosthetic frame via threaded screws embedded into the liner; a cylindrical locking liner which is rolled on to the residual limb is then pushed into a prosthetic frame to engage with a locking mechanism housed inside, achieving suspension; similarly, a liner which has been trimmed to minimize ROM limitations as the lower trimlines of the elastomer reduce tissue tension over the olecranon as well as cubital bunching of the elastomer material as the elbow ranges through flexion.

Section 2: Upper Limb

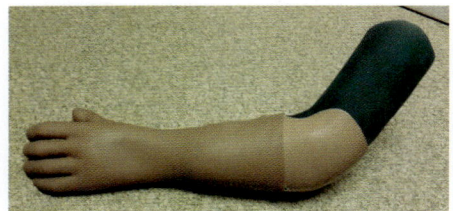

FIGURE 20 Photograph of a transradial HCR silicone socket with an integrated humeral sleeve. The sleeve will need to be reflected over the rigid socket to facilitate donning and then rolled proximally to secure a proximal seal. The resultant suction suspension obviates the need for aggressive anatomic suspension over the bony anatomy of the elbow (Photo courtesy of Phil Stevens, MEd, CPO, FAAOP.)

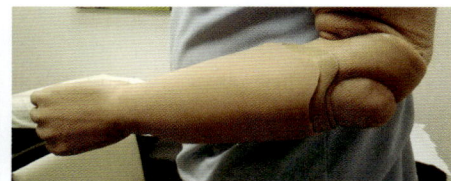

FIGURE 21 Photograph of a transradial HCR silicone socket with a floating triceps bar securing anatomic suspension over the olecranon and condyles. The flexibility of the silicone permits a high anterior trimline at the cubital fold without restricting elbow mobility. The lowered anterior trimlines of the rigid frame allow the compression and bulging of the flexible inner silicone socket during elbow flexion (Photo courtesy of Phil Stevens, MEd, CPO, FAAOP.)

extend as proximal and the apex of the condyles to provide a degree of coronal stabilization. In addition to the increased comfort afforded by these lowered proximal trimlines, this socket concept permits full sagittal range of motion at the elbow.

When the simplicity of anatomical suspension is preferred, the flexibility of the HCR silicone allows the mid-length transradial amputation to be fit with proximal trimlines approximating those of the Muenster socket while the trimlines of the rigid frame are trimmed back to those associated with the Northwestern design (**Figure 21**). The Sauter modification is frequently incorporated, resulting in a compliant triceps bar that extends medially and laterally to secure anatomic purchase over the olecranon and condyles with increased comfort and elbow range of motion.

More recently, tension wire wheel locking systems have been used to create interfaces that allow the patient to rapidly modulate interface compression and comfort (**Figure 22**). This feature may add particular benefit with myoelectric designs as compression over the myo-electrodes can be adjusted for optimal performance, even with minor volume changes within the limb that otherwise would lead to improper function of the prosthesis because of lost contact between the skin and the electrode (**Figure 23**). Patients with unilateral amputation can use the dial using only their sound limb with relative ease. The disadvantages include the added bulk of the wheel lock mechanism, the potential loss of interface stability and suspension should either the wheel lock or wire become defective, rendering the prosthesis unusable until repaired, and the added fabrication labor and maintenance involved for the prosthetist. In addition, though modifications may be made to the system for the TR bilateral patient to more readily facilitate engagement/disengagement and rotation of the wheel lock, this adds an additional burden on the patient. Careful consideration with the trade-off between the increased adjustability and the simplicity of a traditional push-in self-suspended design is warranted before using this option for the bilateral TR amputee.

Advancing Technology

Additive manufacturing, otherwise known as three-dimensional (3D) printing, combined with the use of digital 3D scanners which are readily accessible on smartphones and tablets, is providing several exciting opportunities with upper limb prosthetic designs that were not possible to consider before (**Figures 24 and 25**). Some of the advantages of additive manufacturing over other manufacturing techniques include: freedom of design, customization, repeatability of manufacture, rapid distribution potential of innovative designs, and relative low cost of materials.[29] That is not to say it does not have its share of disadvantages: readily available printers have a limited amount of materials they can work with, the size of the printer limits the size of the object which can be manufactured, and it is difficult to predict the mechanical properties as the strength of the product is dependent on numerous variables. Accuracy may be affected by material shrinkage, machine

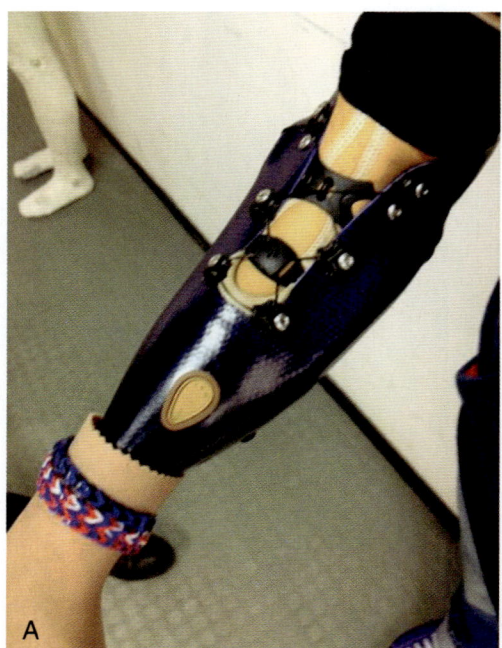
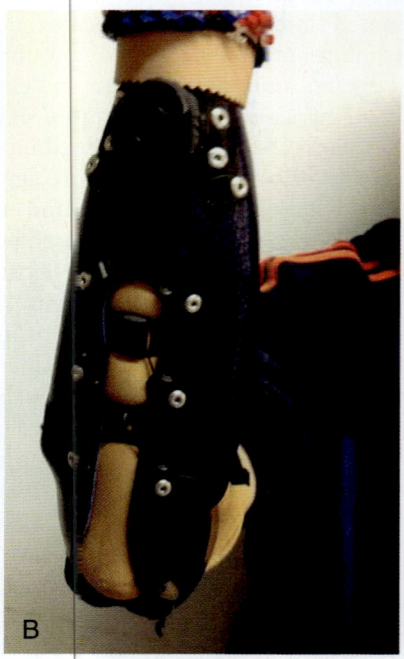

FIGURE 22 Photographs of a transradial myoelectric interface which uses an adjustable tension wire wheel-locking system which allows the patient to easily and rapidly adjust tension within the interface. **A**, Anterior view. **B**, Posterior view.

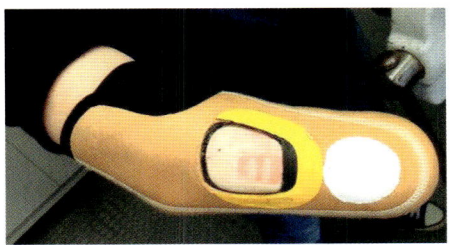

FIGURE 23 Photograph showing the residual limb after the interface from **Figure 22** is removed. The liner has been modified to include cutouts to which allow electrode contact with the skin.

parameters, the CAD/CAM software, and post processing.[29]

Applications of 3D printed upper limb devices are most commonly those for children. As a child with limb loss grows, new devices need to be created to maintain fit, suspension, and function. A major benefit of 3D printing for upper extremity prostheses is that the parts can be conveniently personalized to suit the patient's aesthetic and functional requirements. Moreover, production costs can be reduced, a major benefit for patients who struggle to access conventional options. However, the functionality of these devices is currently lacking with no valid studies on the efficacy or effectiveness of 3D printed designs.[30] Consequently, further development into this sector is required.

In addition to the technological progress in materials and production of prosthetic devices previously discussed, innovative and complex advancements in other areas promise to have a significant impact on the management of individuals with limb loss. Strategies in controlling advanced prostheses featuring increased powered degrees of freedom, the provision of sensory feedback, and securing the prosthesis to the human body continue

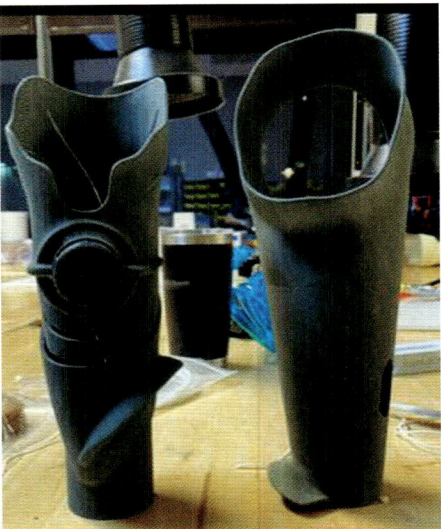

FIGURE 25 Photograph of concept bilateral (WD on the left side, TR on the right) interface frames printed out of Nylon 12, featuring oblique flares designed into the distal forearm to facilitate operation of a manual wheelchair. (Courtesy of William B. Layman CP, BOCOP, New Orleans, LA.)

their development. These burgeoning technologies include but are not limited to: research into implanted subcutaneous and intramuscular electrodes; nerve implants which receive efferent and afferent signals; artificial prosthetic skin that can sense light touch, proprioception, and temperature; haptic feedback devices; and advancements in surgical techniques such as targeted muscle reinnervation and osseointegration.[31]

The challenge for clinical professionals is to continually evolve the upper extremity prosthetics armamentarium with practical fitting solutions and protocols to keep pace with both, the pioneering hardware as it becomes available, and the expectations and needs of patients.

SUMMARY

Understanding the opportunities, challenges, and limitations associated with amputations at this level is important in developing the optimal plan of care. New materials and components allow for innovative interface designs, however designs for this cohort do best when adhering to certain proven fundamental principles that ensure

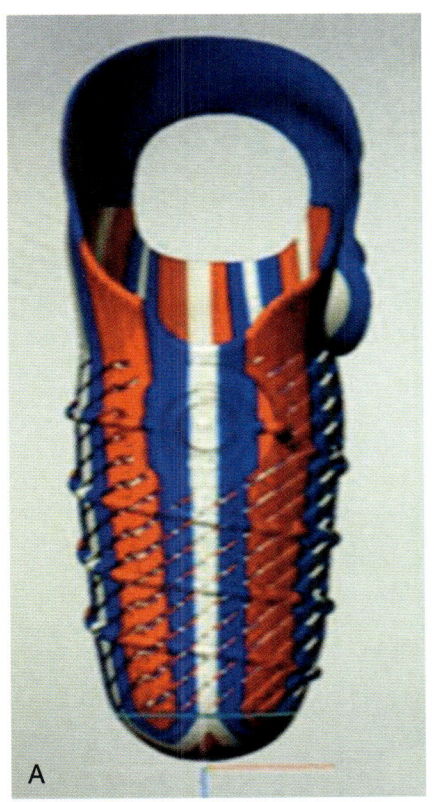
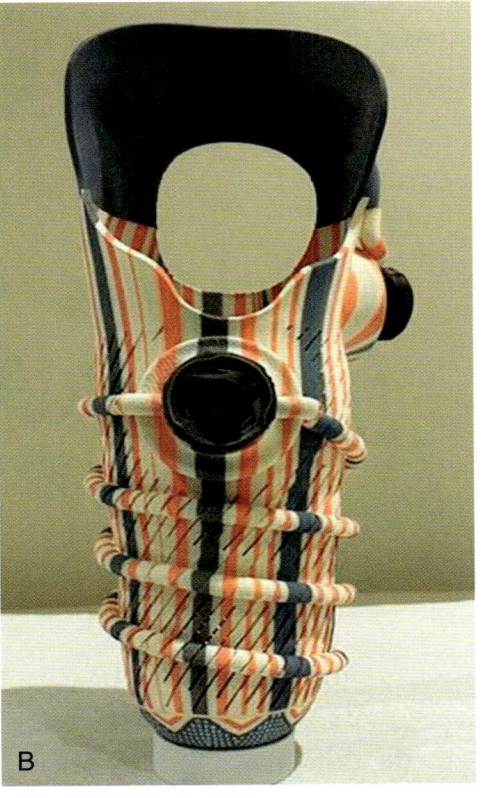

FIGURE 24 A, Photograph of a transradial concept design rendered in CAD format, featuring use of a tension wire wheel-locking system installed around an interface with a series of thin diagonal perforations. The design is intended to use the tension wire to allow a more circumferential compression force to be applied around the interface for a more global reduction in volume, rather than that of a bidirectional force from use of a lacing pattern. B, Photograph of the concept interface made of Nylon 12. (Courtesy of William B. Layman CP, BOCOP, New Orleans, LA.)

appropriate comfort, loading, counterforces, and suspension on the residual limb to provide safe, reliable, and efficient control of the prostheses. Understanding the principles of traditional self-suspending interface designs, as well as various alternate techniques, improves success when considering unique design modifications to suit a patient's needs.

Clear communication between the patient, prosthetist, therapist, and physician, relating to all appropriate options, with regard to prostheses, will provide a basis for realistic expectations and enhance the chance of a successful outcome in improving the quality of life for the upper limb amputee.

References

1. Ziegler-Graham K, MacKenzie EJ, Ephraim PL, Travison TG, Brookmeyer R: Estimating the prevalence of limb loss in the United States: 2005 to 2050. *Arch Phys Med Rehabil* 2008;89(3):422-429.
2. Nanos GP III: Wrist disarticulation and transradial amputation: Amputation surgical management, in Krajbich JI, Pinzer MS, Potter BK, Stevens PM, eds: *Atlas of Amputation and Limb Deficiencies: Surgical Prosthetic, and Rehabilitation Principles*, ed 4. American Academy of Orthopaedic Surgeons, 2016, pp 221-231.
3. Raichle KA, Hanley MA, Molton I, et al: Prosthesis use in persons with lower- and upper-limb amputation. *J Rehabil Res Dev* 2008;45(7):961-972.
4. Dudkiewicz I, Gabrielov R, Seiv-Ner I, et al: Evaluation of prosthetic usage in upper limb amputees. *Disabil Rehabil* 2004;26(1):60-63.
5. Wright TW, Hagan AD, Wood MB: Prosthetic usage in major upper extremity amputations. *J Hand Surg Am* 1995;20(4):619-622.
6. Fantini C, Yancosek K: Upper-limb prostheses: Perspectives involving the veteran population. *J Prosthet Orthot* 2017;29(4S):P51-P56.
7. Brenner CD: Wrist disarticulation and transradial amputation: Prosthetic management, in Smith DG, Bowker J, Michael J, eds: *Atlas of Amputation and Limb Deficiencies: Surgical Prosthetic, and Rehabilitation Principles*, ed 3. American Academy of Orthopaedic Surgeons, 2004, pp 223-230.
8. Zlotolow DA, Kozin SH: Advances in upper extremity prosthetics. *Hand Clin* 2012;28(4):587-593.
9. Brenner JK: Wrist disarticulation and transradial amputation: Prosthetic management, in Krajbich JI, Pinzer MS, Potter BK, Stevens PM, eds: *Atlas of Amputation and Limb Deficiencies: Surgical Prosthetic, and Rehabilitation Principles*, ed 4. American Academy of Orthopaedic Surgeons, 2016, pp 233-241.
10. U.S. department of veterans affairs/department of defense clinical practice guideline for the management of upper limb amputation rehabilitation. Version 1.0-2014 Accessed July 10, 2021. https://www.healthquality.va.gov/guidelines/Rehab/UEAR/VADoDCPGManagementofUEAR121614Corrected508.pdf
11. Miguelez J, Conyers D, Macjulian L, Gulick K: Upper extremity prosthetics, in Pasquina PF, Cooper RA, eds: *Care of the Combat Amputee*. US Department of the Army, Office of The Surgeon General, Borden Institute, 2009, pp 607-640.
12. Freeland AE, Psonak R: Traumatic below-elbow amputations. *Orthopedics* 2007;30(2):120-126.
13. Gaine WJ, Smart C, Bransby-Zachary M: Upper limb traumatic amputees. Review of prosthetic use. *J Hand Surg Br* 1997;22(1):73-76.
14. Pinzur MS, Angelats J, Light TR, Izuierdo R, Pluth T: Functional outcome following traumatic upper limb amputation and prosthetic limb fitting. *J Hand Surg Am* 1994;19(5):836-839.
15. Malone JH, Childers SJ, Underwood J, Leal JH: Immediate postsurgical management of upper-extremity amputation: Conventional, electric and myoelectric prosthesis. *Orthot Prosthet* 1981;35(2):1-9.
16. Malone JM, Fleming LL, Roberson J, et al: Immediate, early, and late postsurgical management of upper-limb amputation. *J Rehabil Res Dev* 1984;21(1):33-41.
17. Dromerick AW, Schabowsky CN, Holley RJ, Monroe B, Markotic A, Lum PS: Effect of training on upper-extremity prosthetic performance and motor learning: A single-case study. *Arch Phys Med Rehabil* 2008;89(6):1199-1204.
18. Resnik L, Meucci MR, Lieberman-Klinger S, et al: Advanced upper limb prosthetic devices: Implications for upper limb prosthetic rehabilitation. *Arch Phys Med Rehabil* 2012;93(4):710-717.
19. Smurr L, Yancosek K, Gulick K, et al: Occupational therapy for polytrauma casualty with limb loss, in Pasquina PF, Cooper RA, eds: *Care of the Combat Amputee*. US Department of the Army, Office of The Surgeon General, Borden Institute, 2009, pp 493-533.
20. Dakpa R, Heger H: Prosthetic management and training of adult upper limb amputees. *Curr Orthop* 1997;11(3):193-202.
21. Stevens PM, Highsmith MJ: Myoelectric and body power, design options for upper-limb prostheses: Introduction to the state of the science conference proceedings. *J Prosthet Orthot* 2017;29(4S):P1-P3.
22. Hess A: Upper limb body-powered components, in Krajbich JI, Pinzer MS, Potter BK, Stevens PM, eds: *Atlas of Amputation and Limb Deficiencies: Surgical Prosthetic, and Rehabilitation Principles*, ed 4. Rosemont, IL, American Academy of Orthopaedic Surgeons, 2016, pp 151-153.
23. Kay H, Cody K, Hartmann G, Casella D: *A Fabrication Manual the "Muenster-Type" Below-Elbow Prosthesis*. New York University, School of Engineering and Science Research Division, Prosthetic and Orthotic Studies, 1965.
24. Billock J: The Northwestern University Supracondylar suspension technique for below-elbow amputation, in *Selected Readings: A Review of Orthotics and Prosthetics*. American Orthotic and Prosthetic Association, 1980, pp 229-235.
25. Alley RD, Williams TW, Albuquerque MJ, Altobelli DE: Prosthetic sockets stabilized by alternating areas of tissue compression and release. *J Rehabil Res Dev* 2011;48(6):679-676.
26. Alley RD: Advancement of upper extremity prosthetic interface and frame design. *Proceedings UNB Myoelectric Controls/Powered Prosthetics Symposium*; 2002; Fredericton, Canada. Fredericton (Canada), University of New Brunswick, 2002, pp 28-32.
27. Miguelez J, Lake C, Conyers D, Zenie J: The Transradial Anatomically Contoured (TRAC) interface: Design principles and methodology. *J Prosthet Orthot* 2003;15(4):148-157.
28. Sauter WF, Nauman S, Milner M: A three-quarter type below elbow

socket for myoelectric prostheses. *Prosthet Orthot Int* 1986;10(2):79-82.

29. Ten Kate J, Smit G, Paul B: 3D-printed upper limb prostheses: A review. *Disabil Rehabil Assist Technol* 2017;12(3):300-314.

30. Diment LE, Thompson MS, Bergmann JHM: Three-dimensional printed upper limb prostheses lack randomized controlled trials: A systematic review. *Prosthet Orthot Int* 2018;42(1):7-13.

31. Bates TJ, Fergason JR, Pierre SN: Technological advances in prosthesis design and rehabilitation following upper extremity limb loss. *Curr Rev Muskuloskelet Med* 2020;13(4):485-493.

Elbow Disarticulation and Transhumeral Amputation: Surgical Management

CDR Scott M. Tintle, MD, FAAOS

ABSTRACT

The choice between elbow disarticulation and transhumeral amputation always should be considered in the context of the primary goal, which is to achieve the best functional outcome for the patient. Most upper limb amputations are necessitated by trauma, and the definitive amputation level often is determined by the injury. The condition of the soft-tissue envelope, the residual limb length, and future prosthetic suspension options all must be considered. The continued success of transhumeral osseointegration also is a key consideration that must now be factored into the surgical planning.

Keywords: amputation complications; amputation technique; elbow disarticulation; transhumeral amputation

Introduction

Amputation of an upper limb is a catastrophic event primarily performed as the result of high-energy trauma,[1,2] with approximately 90% of upper limb amputations resulting from trauma[3] (**Figure 1**). The surgeon's goal in selecting a definitive amputation level after traumatic amputation is to ensure that the residual limb has maximal length and soft-tissue coverage so that a highly functional prosthetic limb can be painlessly accepted (**Figure 2**). The amputation itself is only the first step in the patient's rehabilitation from injury and should not be considered a treatment failure. Consideration should be made toward improving prosthesis wear in amputees who reject standard prostheses through potential osseointegration at the transhumeral level.

General Surgical Considerations

As much limb length as possible should be preserved to maximize the patient's options for later prosthetic fitting. In addition, having a relatively long residual limb is useful for allowing the patient to interact with the environment when the prosthesis is not being worn.[4] The caveat in maintaining maximal limb length is that the soft tissues must be able to support the residual limb to achieve comfortable use of a prosthesis. The zone of injury is the most important factor in choosing the final limb length. Usually the most durable coverage is achieved with local skin flaps. The ultimate size, shape, durability, and appearance of the residual limb will affect a patient's satisfaction and should be considered in surgical decision-making.[4]

Distraction osteogenesis and microvascular techniques can be used to allow successful soft-tissue closure during an initial proximal transhumeral amputation.[5,6] Free tissue transfer may be indicated for preserving the shoulder joint (allowing a forequarter or shoulder disarticulation to be converted to a transhumeral amputation), the elbow joint, or bone length of more than 7 cm below the shoulder or elbow (to improve prosthetic fit and performance).[7]

Although a transhumeral amputation proximal to the deltoid insertion functions as a shoulder disarticulation, it has advantages over shoulder disarticulation. Retaining the proximal humerus preserves the contour of the shoulder, thus improving the fit of the prosthesis and cosmesis. There is greater controversy as to whether a long transhumeral amputation or an elbow disarticulation is preferable. The disarticulation offers enhanced prosthetic suspension and rotational control because the medial and lateral flares of the distal humerus are preserved. However, preserving the full length of the humerus may preclude the use of a prosthetic elbow by limiting the space available for a prosthesis; at a minimum, a bulky, nonanatomic elbow component is required. The available external hinge elbow mechanisms can be cosmetically displeasing, particularly if the patient has an unaffected contralateral upper limb. An angulation osteotomy of the distal humerus or humeral shortening proximal to the elbow can be used to improve rotational control and avoid

Dr. Tintle or an immediate family member serves as a board member, owner, officer, or committee member of Society of Military Orthopaedic Surgeons.

This chapter is adapted from Cho MS. Elbow disarticulation and transhumeral amputation: Surgical management, in Krajbich JI, Pinzur MS, Potter BK, Stevens PM, eds: *Atlas of Amputations and Limb Deficiencies: Surgical, Prosthetic, and Rehabilitation Principles*, ed 4. American Academy of Orthopaedic Surgeons, 2016, pp 249-255.

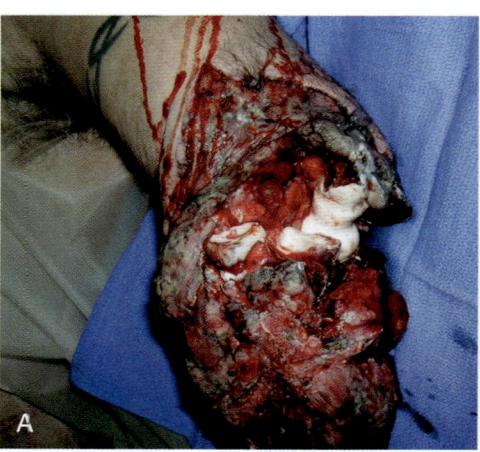
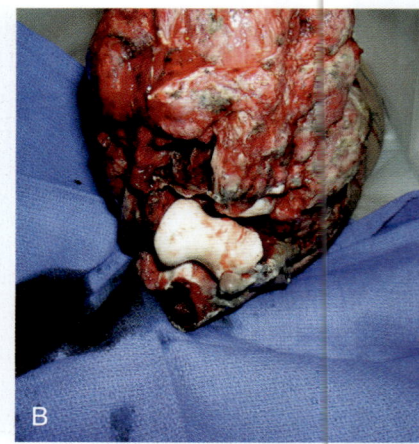

FIGURE 1 Clinical photographs of an upper limb injury sustained from the blast of an improvised explosive device. **A**, A more proximal level amputation is needed because of the loss of soft tissue and gross contamination. **B**, The limb after thorough débridement of devitalized soft tissue and bone. An elbow disarticulation was required.

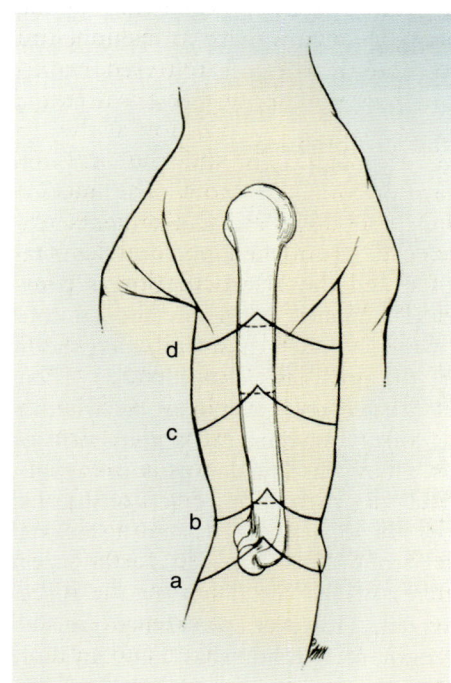

FIGURE 2 Schematic drawing showing definitive humeral amputation levels. The level of an elbow disarticulation (a), a distal humeral amputation (b), a midhumeral amputation at the level of the deltoid insertion (c), and a proximal humeral amputation proximal to the deltoid insertion (d) are shown.

limiting prosthetic elbow options.[3,8] On average, 7.6 cm of space above the center of rotation of the elbow is required so that the prosthetic elbow center is at the level of the intact elbow.[9]

Regardless of the final amputation level, proper management of the nerves and muscles of the residual limb is of paramount importance. Adequate padding of the residual bone end and prevention of postoperative neuritic pain substantially affect prosthetic wear comfort. Therefore, myoplasty or myodesis should be done to pad any bony prominence about the residual limb. One suggested consideration for dealing with the muscles that has recently begun investigation is the agonist–antagonist myoneural interface, which allows for innervated muscles that are linked together to reform normal muscle tendon agonist–antagonist relationships that have the potential to augment control of a prosthesis, preserve proprioception, and prevent limb atrophy.[10] When dealing with the peripheral nerves, historically, traction neurectomies were advocated. The armamentarium of the surgeon currently dealing with peripheral nerves in amputations, however, is substantially greater. Strong consideration should be given to addressing nerves with options that provide the nerve with direction, such as targeted muscle reinnervation or regenerative peripheral nerve interfaces, as well as improving terminal device control. In the author's experience a combination of these two techniques is frequently used.

Modern prosthetic techniques allow comfortable fitting and function in patients who have undergone amputation at almost any humeral level. However, despite improved suspension techniques and advances in bioprosthetic interfaces for myoelectric prostheses, the rejection rate of upper limb prostheses is more than 30%.[11,12] A prosthetic limb cannot replace the sensibility or dexterity of the natural hand, and, as the amputation level progresses proximally, the relative function of the prosthesis decreases. The result can be diminished wear or use by the patient. To improve the bioprosthetic interface and function of myoelectric prostheses, research efforts have focused on improving suspension, durability, degrees of freedom at the terminal device, and myoelectric control at additional intuitive input sites. In addition, reducing the weight of the prosthesis and extending its battery life are being studied.[13-15]

Elbow Disarticulation

General Considerations

Prosthetic elbow options are limited after an elbow disarticulation because of the length of the humerus, and cosmetic issues can be a concern. A proximal shortening osteotomy of the humerus, as described by Beltran et al,[3] is an attractive option that allows additional prosthetic elbow options and improved cosmesis while maintaining the advantages of rotational control and prosthetic suspension (Figure 3).

Chapter 18: Elbow Disarticulation and Transhumeral Amputation: Surgical Management

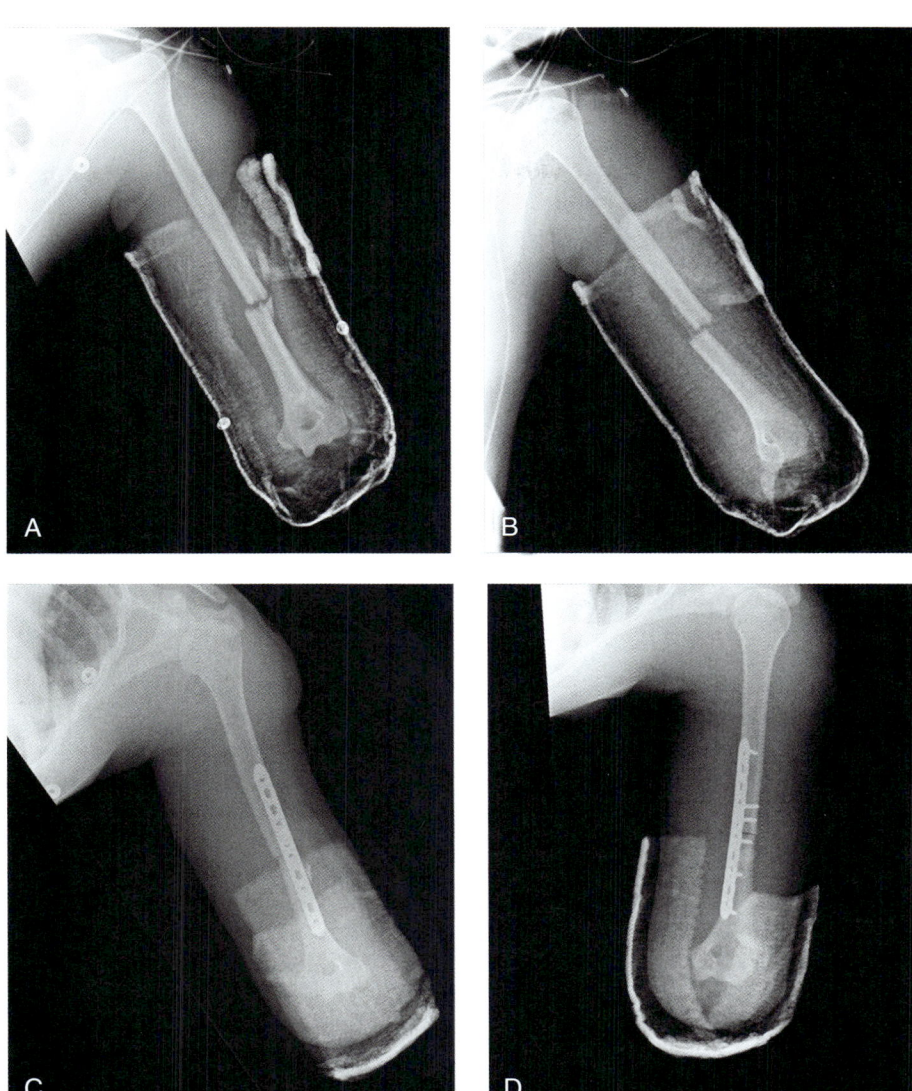

FIGURE 3 Preoperative AP (**A**) and lateral (**B**) radiographs of a transverse humeral fracture with apex lateral angulation. Postoperative AP (**C**) and lateral (**D**) radiographs of the humerus after an osteotomy and fixation with a locking compression plate. (Reproduced from Beltran MA, Kirk KL, Hsu JR: Minimally invasive shortening humeral osteotomy to salvage a through-elbow amputation. *Mil Med* 2010;175[9]:693-696, by permission of Oxford University Press.)

Surgical Technique

The patient is positioned supine, with the limb on a hand table, and a tourniquet is placed high on the brachium and inflated to 250 mm Hg after exsanguination. Equal anterior and posterior skin flaps are fashioned in a fish-mouth pattern, with the proximal extent of the flap at the level of the humeral epicondyles and the distal extent 3 cm distal to the tip of the olecranon (**Figure 4, A and B**). It is better to fashion flaps that are longer than anticipated for closure because they can always be trimmed. The use of atypical flaps may be necessary depending on the soft tissue available for closure. The lacertus fibrosus is identified and divided (**Figure 4, C**). The lateral and medial antebrachial cutaneous nerves are identified, and traction neurectomies are performed. Superficial veins are double clipped using medium or small ligating clips and cut. Larger veins, such as the medial cubital and cephalic veins, are ligated using 2-0 silk suture and cut. The flexor-pronator mass is identified, released from the medial epicondyle, and reflected distally to expose the median nerve and brachial artery adjacent to the biceps tendon (**Figure 4, D through F**). The artery is traced proximal to the elbow joint, double ligated using 2-0 silk suture, and cut. The median nerve is cut sharply using a No. 10 blade. The ulnar nerve is identified within the cubital tunnel and divided sharply in a similar manner. The biceps tendon is released from its insertion on the radius, and the brachialis is released from its insertion on the ulna and reflected proximally. The radial nerve is identified between the brachialis and brachioradialis and divided in the same manner as the median and ulnar nerves. The forearm extensor musculature is identified and divided 6 cm distal to the joint line, in a transverse fashion, and the muscle mass is reflected proximally. The posterior fascia is divided, as are the triceps insertion at the tip of the olecranon and the anterior capsule of the elbow. The medial and lateral collateral ligaments are released from their epicondylar origins, and the disarticulation is completed (**Figure 4, G**).

The articular cartilage is maintained on the distal end of the humerus. The myoplasty is done by bringing the triceps tendon anteriorly and suturing it to the brachialis and biceps muscles using size 0 polyglycolic acid absorbable suture, such as Vicryl (Ethicon). To further pad any bony prominences on the distal humerus, the forearm extensor muscle mass is brought medially and sutured to the periosteum or remnants of the flexor-pronator mass at the medial epicondyle, using size 0 polyglycolic acid suture.

Before final skin closure, the tourniquet is deflated, and meticulous hemostasis is obtained. The subcutaneous tissue is closed with 2-0 polyglycolic acid suture and with staples or monofilament suture for the skin (**Figure 5**). A bulky soft dressing is applied over the distal humerus in a figure-of-8 fashion, using a sterile, woven six-ply gauze bandage and elastic wrap, and is left in place for 3 days. A drain is frequently used.

Section 2: Upper Limb

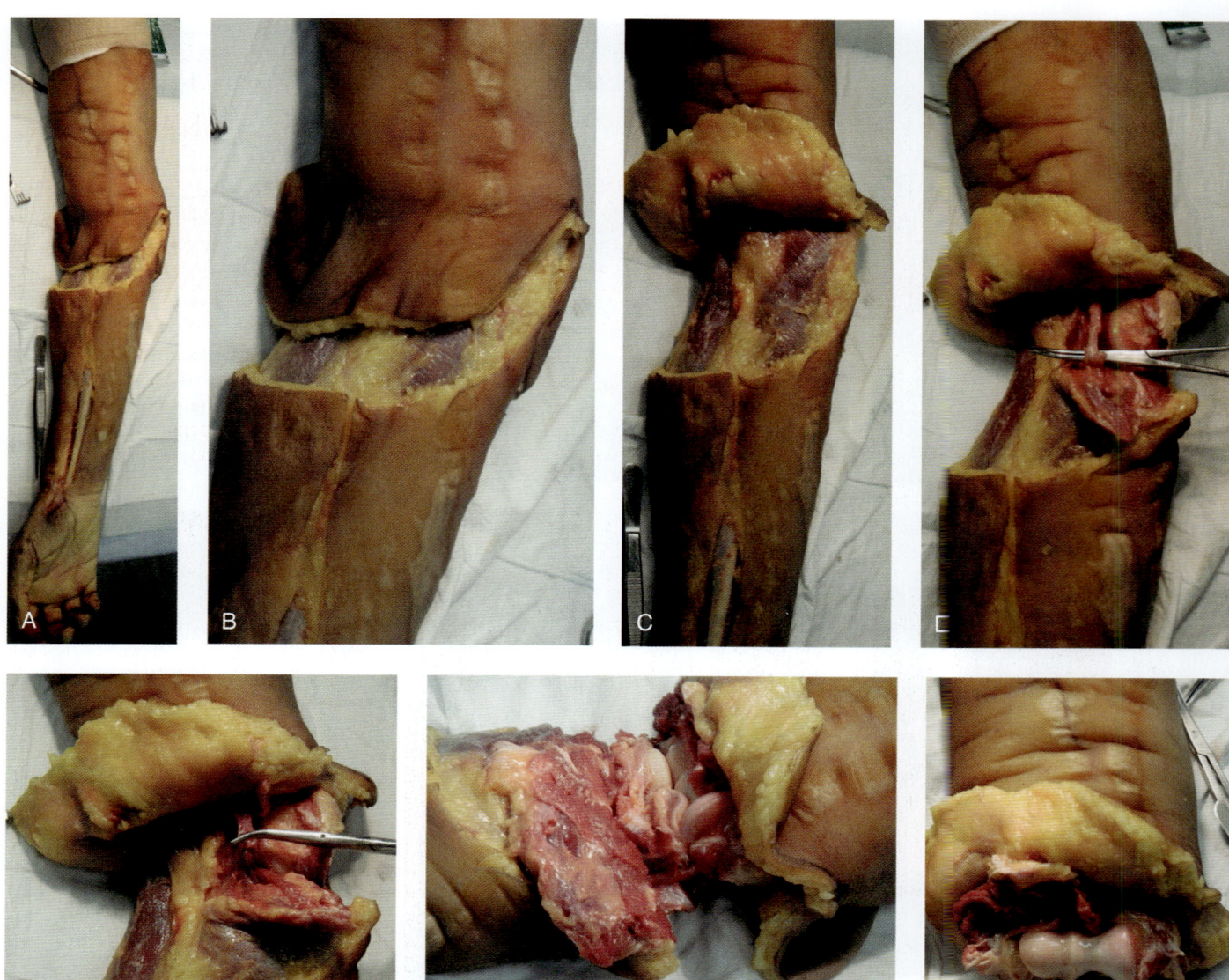

FIGURE 4 Photographs showing a cadaver elbow disarticulation. **A** and **B**, Equal anterior and posterior skin flaps are fashioned in a fish-mouth pattern, with the proximal extent of the flap at the level of the humeral epicondyles and the distal extent 3 cm distal to the tip of the olecranon. **C**, The anterior skin flap is elevated to show the lacertus fibrosus and underlying forearm musculature before division. **D**, The flexor-pronator mass is released from the medial epicondyle and reflected to expose the median nerve. **E**, The released brachial artery is shown. **F**, The released biceps, brachialis, and collateral ligaments are shown. **G**, The completed elbow disarticulation is shown.

Transhumeral Amputation

General Considerations

Every effort should be made to follow the principles of length preservation and soft-tissue management when selecting a transhumeral amputation level. If the condyles are not preserved, the ideal level of amputation should be at least 4 cm proximal to the elbow joint.[5] For long transhumeral amputations, an angulation osteotomy of the distal humerus as described by Marquardt and Neff,[8] or a modification, should be considered. The benefit of using an angulation osteotomy rather than an elbow disarticulation is to allow a wider choice of prosthetic elbow options and to eliminate limb length issues with prosthesis wear. The osteotomy also improves rotational control and suspension of the prosthesis, compared with a traditional transhumeral amputation.

It is important to ensure that an angulation osteotomy does not shorten total humeral length substantially more than intended. For the osteotomy to have maximal benefit, the starting length of the humerus must extend to the metaphyseal flare or farther (**Figure 6**). An anterior closing-wedge osteotomy is preferred, with the distal segment at least 5 cm in length. The use of a contoured 3.5-mm reconstruction plate at a 70° angle is preferred to the original Marquardt technique because the final desired angle of osteotomy is easier to obtain and maintain when a plate is used rather than a screw or Kirschner wire (**Figures 7** and **8**).

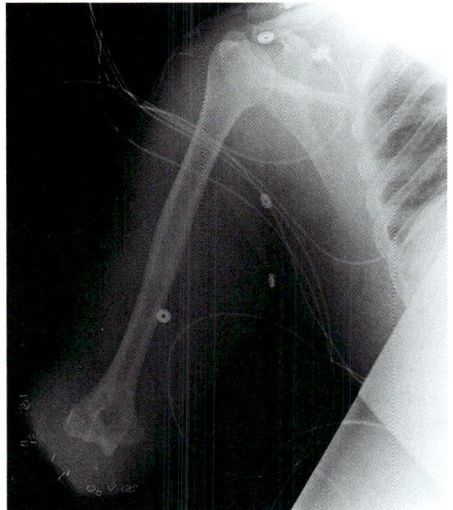

FIGURE 5 AP radiograph of a completed elbow disarticulation.

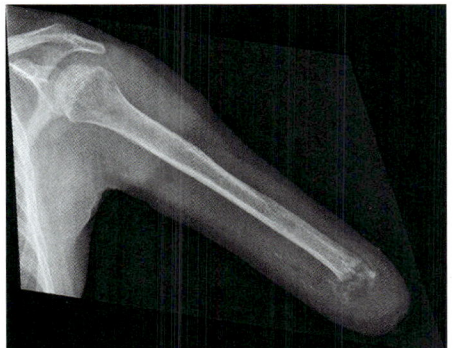

FIGURE 6 Preoperative AP radiograph of a long transhumeral amputation before an angulation osteotomy.

Surgical Technique

As in an elbow disarticulation, a sterile tourniquet should be used on the brachium if the humeral length allows. Beginning at the level of the intended bone resection, equal anterior and posterior skin flaps are made in a fish-mouth fashion. The length of the flaps should be half the diameter of the brachium at that level. The condition of the soft-tissue envelope will dictate the final configuration of the skin and muscle flaps.

The brachial artery and the brachial and cephalic veins are double ligated using 2-0 silk suture. The smaller veins and vessels can be ligated with clips or ties. Nerves should be addressed with targeted muscle reinnervation or regenerative peripheral nerve interface.

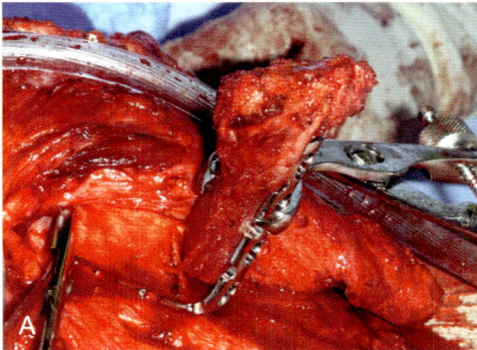 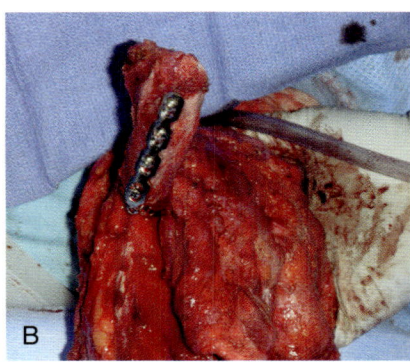

FIGURE 7 **A**, Intraoperative photograph showing provisional fixation of a closing wedge osteotomy with a 3.5-mm stainless steel reconstruction plate, which was bent to approximately 70°. Note that the osteotomy was made at least 5 cm from the end of the residual humerus to allow for an appropriate fulcrum for suspension of a prosthesis. **B**, Intraoperative photograph showing completed fixation of the osteotomy site with the reconstruction plate.

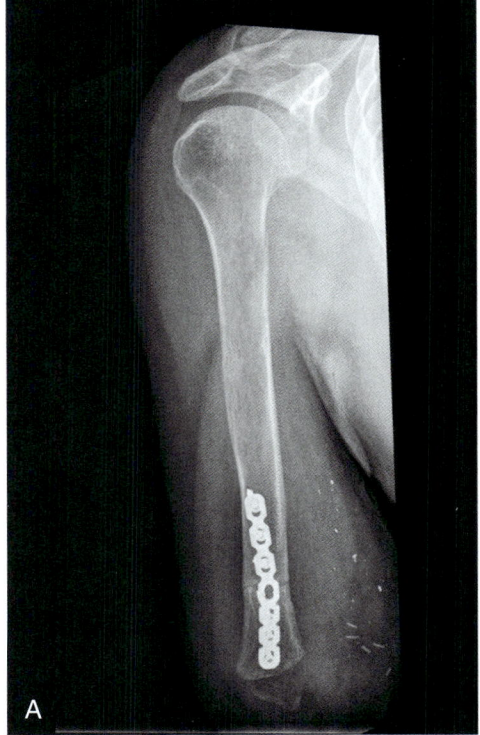 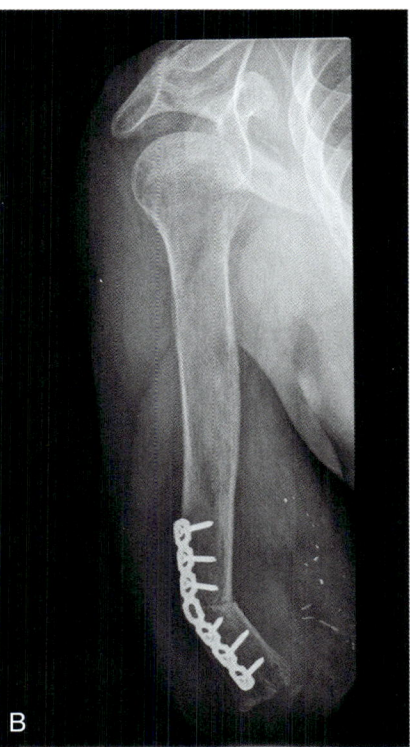

FIGURE 8 AP (**A**) and lateral (**B**) radiographs showing a humerus after an angulation osteotomy.

The muscles in the anterior compartment of the brachium should be divided at least 2 cm distal to the intended bone resection level. The insertion of the triceps tendon is freed from the olecranon; the triceps fascia and muscle are preserved. The triceps is mobilized proximal to the level of the planned bone resection. Electrocautery is used to score the periosteum circumferentially at the level of the planned bone resection. The bone is divided at this level using a sagittal power saw or Gigli manual saw. The bone ends are smoothed with a rasp or saw. Myodesis is done using two holes drilled into the anterior cortex of the humerus with a 2.0-mm drill bit just proximal to the level of the bone resection. Two No. 2 polyester nonabsorbable sutures are used to bring the triceps anteriorly over the end of the residual humerus and secure it through the drill holes. A suture anchor can be used as an alternative

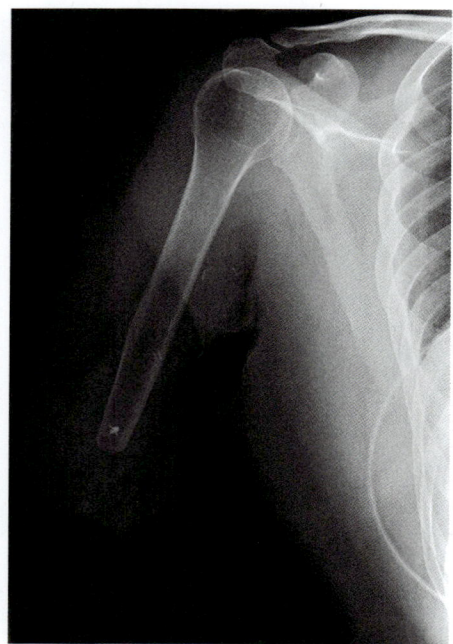

FIGURE 9 AP radiograph of a humerus after a transhumeral amputation. A metallic anchor in the distal humerus was used for myodesis.

(Figure 9). The anterior musculature is secured to the fascia of the triceps that was brought over the end of the humerus, using size 0 polyglycolic acid suture, thus securing the proximal musculature and further padding any remaining bony prominences.

Before closure, the tourniquet is deflated, and meticulous hemostasis is obtained. The skin flaps are trimmed, and subcutaneous tissue is closed using 2-0 polyglycolic acid suture and staples or monofilament suture for the skin. A bulky soft dressing is applied over the distal humerus in a figure-of-8 fashion, using a sterile, woven six-ply gauze bandage and elastic wrap, and is left in place for 3 days. A drain is frequently used.

Rehabilitation

After an elbow disarticulation or transhumeral amputation, the use of an indwelling pain catheter is recommended for control of postoperative pain. The patient typically is hospitalized 2 to 3 days for pain control. The postoperative dressing is changed before discharge, and the staples or sutures are removed at 2 weeks. At this point, a formal residual limb shrinker is applied, and by 4 weeks the patient is fitted with the initial body-powered prosthesis. It is critical for the initial fitting to take place as soon as the condition of the soft tissues allows. Wright et al[11] and Robinson et al[16] found a positive relationship between early fitting and the patient's sustained use of a prosthesis. Patients who underwent unilateral transhumeral amputation were least likely to use a prosthesis. During the early phases of prosthetic fitting and rehabilitation, it is critical for the patient to have both social and peer support for dealing with the loss of the limb.[17]

Managing Complications

Infection and wound-related complications such as dehiscence and scar sensitivity are the most common complications after definitive closure, and they necessitate additional surgical intervention. Many complications are directly related to the amount of initial traumatic contamination and energy impact on the soft tissue. The treatment for a deep infection or abscess is débridement and irrigation. Wound dehiscence or scar sensitivity can be managed by revision primary closure or excision of the painful scar, respectively.

A postoperative infection or wound complication can occur after any surgical procedure, but phantom limb pain, residual limb pain, neuroma pain, and heterotopic ossification occur relatively often in patients who have undergone amputation. More than 50% of these patients are affected by phantom limb pain at some point during the rehabilitation process.[12] Pain after upper limb amputation does not always impair functional use of a prosthesis.[4]

Discomfort while wearing a prosthesis is the most common reason for revision surgery to treat patients with neuroma pain and heterotopic ossification. Excessive pressure on sensitive neuromas or bony prominence while the limb is in the prosthetic socket may prevent the patient from wearing or using the prosthesis. Neuromas have long been considered inevitable after transection of peripheral nerves, but thoughtful treatment can reduce neuroma size, the risk of symptomatic neuromas, and the risk or severity of phantom pain.[16-24]

SUMMARY

The ultimate upper limb amputation level usually is dictated by the initial injury. In choosing a definitive amputation level, careful consideration must be given to bone length and, more importantly, the condition of the soft-tissue envelope. Modern prosthetic techniques allow the patient to be fitted with a prosthesis at any humeral amputation level. In most patients, maintaining the maximal possible humeral length is desirable. Maintaining the humeral epicondyles allows rotational control at the elbow disarticulation level and allows better suspension of the prosthesis. The disadvantages of limited elbow component options and an undesirable cosmetic appearance at the elbow disarticulation level can be overcome through humeral shortening. Another attractive option is a distal humeral angulation osteotomy that maintains the epicondyles. An amputation level at least 3 to 5 cm proximal to the native elbow center of rotation increases the number of options for elbow components and maintains the benefits of the epicondyles.

Aside from infection, discomfort related to prosthetic wear is the most common reason for revision surgery after definitive amputation. Most causes of uncomfortable prosthetic wear are related to suspension issues at the residual limb–socket interface, leading to pain from pressure spots. Painful scars, inadequately padded bony prominences, heterotopic ossification-related discomfort, and neuromas are common. Although humeral length is of paramount importance in surgical decision-making, the importance of adequate padding of distal bone ends and appropriate peripheral nerve management, regardless of the amputation level, should not be overlooked in the interest of achieving an optimal functional outcome.

References

1. Atroshi I, Rosberg HE: Epidemiology of amputations and severe injuries of the hand. *Hand Clin* 2001;17(3):343-350, vii.
2. Freeland AE, Psonak R: Traumatic below-elbow amputations. *Orthopedics* 2007;30(2):120-126.

3. Beltran MJ, Kirk KL, Hsu JR: Minimally invasive shortening humeral osteotomy to salvage a through-elbow amputation. *Mil Med* 2010;175(9):693-696.

4. Tintle SM, Baechler MF, Nanos GP III, Forsberg JA, Potter BK: Traumatic and trauma-related amputations: Part II. Upper extremity and future directions. *J Bone Joint Surg Am* 2010;92(18):2934-2945.

5. Cleveland KB: Amputations of the upper extremity, in Canale TS, Beaty JH, eds: *Campbell's Operative Orthopaedics*. Elsevier-Mosby, 2013, pp 662-664.

6. Alekberov C, Karatosun V, Baran O, Günal I: Lengthening of congenital below-elbow amputation stumps by the Ilizarov technique. *J Bone Joint Surg Br* 2000;82(2):239-241.

7. Baccarani A, Follmar KE, De Santis G, et al: Free vascularized tissue transfer to preserve upper extremity amputation levels. *Plast Reconstr Surg* 2007;120(4):971-981.

8. Marquardt E, Neff G: The angulation osteotomy of above-elbow stumps. *Clin Orthop Relat Res* 1974;104:232-238.

9. Schnur D, Meier RH III: Amputation surgery. *Phys Med Rehabil Clin N Am* 2014;25(1):35-43.

10. Carty MJ, Herr HM: The agonist-antagonist myoneural interface. *Hand Clin* 2021;37(3):435-445.

11. Wright TW, Hagen AD, Wood MB: Prosthetic usage in major upper extremity amputations. *J Hand Surg Am* 1995;20(4):619-622.

12. Tintle SM, Baechler MF, Nanos GP, Forsberg JA, Potter BK: Reoperations following combat-related upper-extremity amputations. *J Bone Joint Surg Am* 2012;94(16):e1191-e1196.

13. Hutchinson DT: The quest for the bionic arm. *J Am Acad Orthop Surg* 2014;22(6):346-351.

14. Kung TA, Bueno RA, Alkhalefah GK, Langhals NB, Urbanchek MG, Cederna PS: Innovations in prosthetic interfaces for the upper extremity. *Plast Reconstr Surg* 2013;132(6):1515-1523.

15. González-Fernández M: Development of upper limb prostheses: Current progress and areas for growth. *Arch Phys Med Rehabil* 2014;95(6):1013-1014.

16. Robinson KP, Andrews BG, Vitali M: Immediate operative fitting of upper limb prosthesis at the time of amputation. *Br J Surg* 1975;62(8):634-637.

17. Williams RM, Ehde DM, Smith DG, Czerniecki JM, Hoffman AJ, Robinson LR: A two-year longitudinal study of social support following amputation. *Disabil Rehabil* 2004;26(14-15):862-874.

18. Souza JM, Cheesborough JE, Ko JH, Cho MS, Kuiken TA, Dumanian GA: Targeted muscle reinnervation: A novel approach to postamputation neuroma pain. *Clin Orthop Relat Res* 2014;472(10):2984-2990.

19. Dumanian GA, Ko JH, O'Shaughnessy KD, Kim PS, Wilson CJ, Kuiken TA: Targeted reinnervation for transhumeral amputees: Current surgical technique and update on results. *Plast Reconstr Surg* 2009;124(3):863-869.

20. Pet MA, Ko JH, Friedly JL, Mourad PD, Smith DG: Does targeted nerve implantation reduce neuroma pain in amputees? *Clin Orthop Relat Res* 2014;472(10):2991-3001.

21. Mioton LM, Dumanian GA, Shah N, et al: Targeted muscle reinnervation improves residual limb pain, phantom limb pain, and limb function: A prospective study of 33 major limb amputees. *Clin Orthop Relat Res* 2020;478(9):2161-2167.

22. Dumanian GA, Mioton LM, Potter BK, et al: Targeted muscle reinnervation successfully treats neuroma pain and phantoms in major limb amputees: A randomized clinical trial. *Ann Surg* 2019;270(2):238-246.

23. Woo SL, Kung TA, Brown DL, Leonard JA, Kelly BM, Cederna PS: Regenerative peripheral nerve interfaces for the treatment of postamputation neuroma pain: A pilot study. *Plast Reconstr Surg Glob Open* 2016;4(12):e1038.

24. Cheesborough JE, Souza JM, Dumanian GA, Bueno RA Jr: Targeted muscle reinnervation in the initial management of traumatic upper extremity amputation injury. *Hand (N Y)* 2014;9(2):253-257.

Elbow Disarticulation and Transhumeral Amputation: Prosthetic Management and Design

Gerald E. Stark, PhD, MSEM, CPO/L, FAAOP
Christopher Fantini, MSPT, CP, BOCO

Abstract

The transhumeral prosthesis can present a number of fitting challenges for the prosthetist because of the underlying musculoskeletal anatomy of the residual limb as well as the variety of components and control options. Often, alternative socket designs are necessary to meet the needs of the individual patient. A clinical knowledge of loading characteristics, volumetric considerations, control options, postoperative management, and the fabrication of the interface is necessary to develop a comprehensive prosthetic care plan for a patient using a transhumeral prosthesis.

Keywords: amputation; arm prosthesis; elbow disarticulation; prosthetics; transhumeral

Introduction

The transhumeral socket interface presents several unique prosthetic challenges.[1] As with other levels of prosthetic interface design, it must provide adequate proximal musculoskeletal stability while managing the distal volume of the residual limb. These objectives must be accomplished even though the transhumeral prosthesis is suspended from a highly mobile proximal skeletal joint, with its own weight distracting the tissue distally. The triaxial stability and coupling of the interface to the residual limb is further influenced by the interaction of the upper limb harness design and by the choice of control system used. For example, body-powered systems with laterally mounted control cables may inadvertently pull the interface into external rotation if the socket is loose or does not have adequate posterior proximal support. In many instances, an otherwise well-made interface may not provide adequate comfort or suspension if the harness is not fitted well enough to address these functional suspension needs.

Similar to the transfemoral level, where the prosthetic socket provides volumetric containment of mobile soft tissue surrounding the relatively narrow femoral shaft, prostheses at the transhumeral level encompass the tissues surrounding the shaft of a humerus that is generally too narrow to provide the distal skeletal substructure needed to fully stabilize and maintain the position of the socket. As a result, both body-powered control activation and external loads create disruptive force couples within the socket that must be anticipated and managed.

In the sagittal plane, the interface has the tendency to be pulled into extension as loads on the forearm cause the distal socket to rotate posteriorly relative to the residual limb. This places additional localized loads on the anterior distal area of the limb. In the frontal plane, patients with a high degree of glenohumeral abduction may experience increased lateral-distal loading if the arm is not properly aligned. In the absence of adequate soft tissue, these areas can be vulnerable to painful distal socket pressures. Alternatively, when treating patients with excessive redundant tissue, management of this tissue is important because the rigid skeletal structures are deeper and more difficult to load. The various lengths of transhumeral amputation provide additional challenges, with longer amputations requiring accommodation of the humeral condyles, and proximal-level amputations requiring greater proximal loading.

The prosthetist may be further challenged by a lack of any widely accepted, consistent clinical protocols for impression taking and modification techniques. In many instances, because of the relative rarity of transhumeral amputations, the clinician may not have had sufficient experience to have a clinical reference for managing these patients successfully and may lack self-efficacy.

All of these factors combine to make the transhumeral interface design challenging to manage and may contribute to low prosthesis acceptance rates (range, 27% to 61%) in individuals treated by practitioners unfamiliar with the transhumeral fitting level.[2-5] As with other levels of upper limb involvement, ultimate acceptance of prosthetic

---

Dr. Stark or an immediate family member serves as a paid consultant to or is an employee of Ottobock. Neither Christopher Fantini nor any immediate family member has received anything of value from or has stock or stock options held in a commercial company or institution related directly or indirectly to the subject of this chapter.

Section 2: Upper Limb

use by transhumeral amputees is based on the ability to achieve their desired functional goals within their individual comfort tolerance. It is critical that prosthetists are aware of the process, components, concepts, and expected outcome for each prosthesis to ensure that their patients have the best chance of success.[6]

Related Amputation Types

Although this chapter focuses on the prosthetic management of transhumeral amputations, related amputations are also briefly described. In certain instances of limb paralysis, such as a brachial plexus injury, patients may elect transhumeral amputation and fusion of the paralyzed glenohumeral joint, with 20° abduction, 30° flexion, and 40° internal rotation.[7] In this elective amputation, all prosthetic elbow componentry can be accommodated if the humerus is amputated 100 mm (3.94 inches) proximal to the tip of the olecranon.[8,9] Although amputation offers a more functional solution than a flail arm, the decision to amputate is very difficult and amputation must be performed with great sensitivity because it involves the removal of an arm that appears normal.

An elbow disarticulation (through-elbow amputation) has several advantages, including maximizing the length of the mechanical lever arm, minimizing disruption to soft tissues, providing a load-tolerant distal end, and permitting distal supracondylar suspension.[10,11] However, the major disadvantage is that the long length of the prosthesis precludes the use of distally mounted prosthetic elbow mechanisms. Rather, this amputation level necessitates the use of elbow hinges that are laminated outside of the interface (**Figure 1**). Cosmetically, this increases the distal mediolateral dimension at the elbow joint. Functionally, it restricts the number of componentry options and shortens the prosthetic forearm.

Pediatric amputation can become problematic because of pointed bony overgrowth that may emerge from the cut end of the bone.[12] Elbow disarticulation is often used in this cohort because it reduces bony overgrowth by preserving the epiphyseal growth plates. As the child ages, growth of the ipsilateral humerus can be surgically restricted to shorten the arm over time so that the length discrepancy is not noticeable in adulthood. This creates a load-tolerant residual limb capable of self-suspension at a transhumeral limb length.

Less frequently used variants of transhumeral amputation have also been described with the intent of improving the rotational stability of the socket over the residual limb.[9,10,12,13] These include an osteotomy procedure described by de Luccia and Marino[14] in which a bony section of the diaphysis is removed to place the humeral epicondyles more proximally (**Figure 2**). In another variation, Marquardt and Neff[12] described an angulation osteotomy that fixes the distal humeral shaft length at 45° (**Figure 3**). This procedure

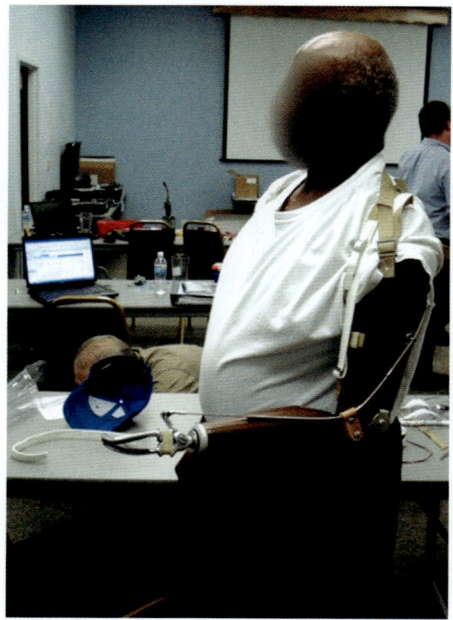

FIGURE 1 Photograph of an individual wearing a typical elbow disarticulation prosthesis with outside hinges.

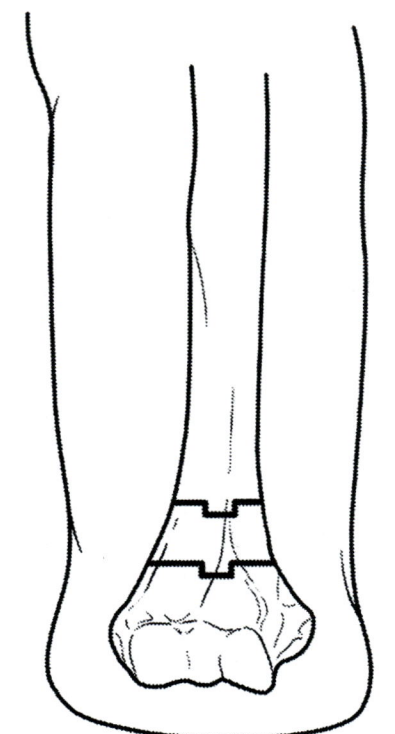 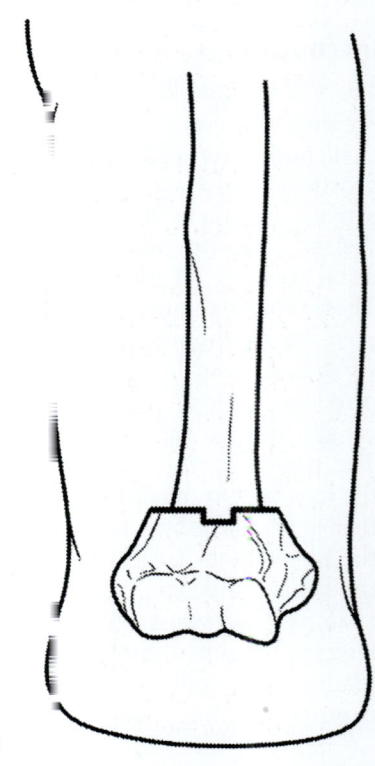

FIGURE 2 Illustrations of the de Luccia and Marino osteotomy procedure to reduce humeral length. **A**, Location of the cut lines on the humerus. **B**, Reduced length with removal of the bone segment. (Reproduced from Daly WK: Elbow disarticulation and transhumeral amputation: prosthetic management, in Smith DG, Michael JW, Bowker JH, eds: *Atlas of Amputations and Limb Deficiencies: Surgical, Prosthetic, and Rehabilitation Principles*, ed 3. American Academy of Orthopaedic Surgeons, 2004, pp 243-249.)

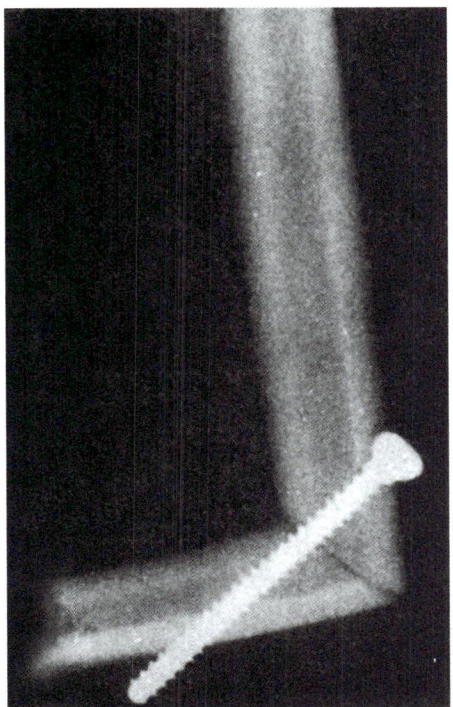

FIGURE 3 Radiograph showing a Marquardt angulation achieved with an anterior closing wedge osteotomy. (Reproduced with permission from Marquardt E, Neff G: The angulation osteotomy of above elbow stumps. *Clin Orthop Relat Res* 1974;104:232-238.)

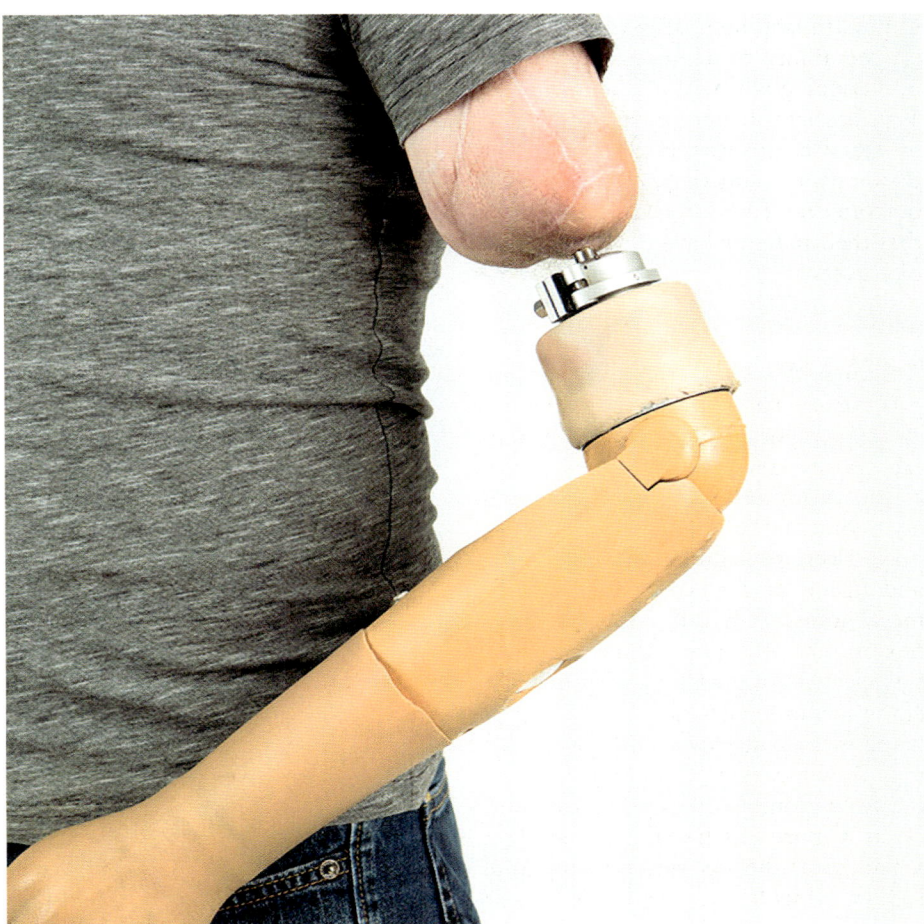

FIGURE 4 Osseointegration with transhumeral distal abutment and coupling. (Courtesy of Integrum AB, Mölndal, Sweden.)

is most often used to treat patients with bilateral amputation or those desiring a more secure coupling with the transhumeral interface.[9,10,13]

Osseointegration has begun to emerge as a possible alternative, eliminating the need for traditional prosthetic interfaces. In this surgical approach a distal titanium abutment is secured to an implant that has been screwed or press-fit in the remaining humeral diaphysis. The external prosthesis must incorporate a proximal attachment that receives the abutment. Transhumeral osseointegration eliminates the need for a harness for axial support, allowing full glenohumeral rotation and a greater range of abduction than standard prosthetic fitting methods (**Figure 4**).

Postoperative Prosthetic Management

It is commonly accepted that early prosthetic fitting results in greater acceptance of an upper limb prosthesis. The 30 days after surgery are often referred to as the golden period for prosthetic fitting.[15] It is thought that if fitting occurs beyond this period, the patient will have adapted to some degree, becoming reliant on unilateral activation strategies.[15] Early management of the amputation results in volume reduction and pain attenuation by enclosing the residual limb in a more rigid dressing or a flexible liner.[16] Early prosthetic fitting also may have a psychological benefit because the patient can begin to incorporate the proprioception or kinesthetic awareness of the prosthesis into their body image.

Elastic shrinker socks or bandages can be used to initially shape and reduce the distal soft-tissue volume. Subsequently, a basic upper limb prosthesis can be constructed of endoskeletal componentry and attached to a rigid dressing or preparatory socket to begin training in prosthesis control. After the shape and volume of the distal limb stabilize, a more definitive interface can be made (**Figure 5**). As the limb undergoes volumetric changes, the use of an adjustable harness will assist in maintaining suspension.

During the postoperative phase, the rehabilitation team should meet to establish immediate, short-term, and long-term goals.[17,18] The preparatory prosthesis allows the patient to become accustomed to the loading characteristics, control movements, weight, and operation of a prosthesis.[17,18] The prosthetist should involve the patient and their support group in all phases of prosthesis development. The patient who is informed about recommendations and who actively participates in decisions regarding their prosthesis will typically establish a greater sense of ownership and dedication to the process.[17,18]

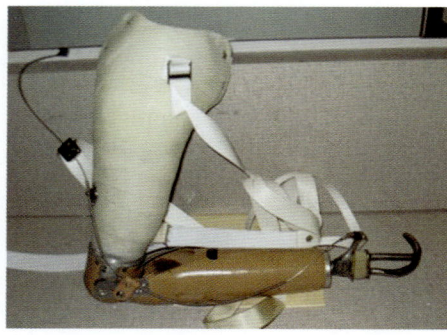

FIGURE 5 Photograph of a transhumeral immediate postoperative prosthesis, with a frame constructed of fiberglass casting tape, an adjustable cable length, a figure-of-8 harness, and a split-housing dual-control cable system.

The value of immediate psychological counseling and peer visits during the early postoperative phase should not be underestimated because the upper limb plays a vital role in function and human social interaction. A peer who has experienced upper limb loss can help the new amputee establish realistic expectations and prepare for future challenges that may aid in long-term prosthesis acceptance and use.[18]

Soft-Tissue Considerations

Most transhumeral amputations involve the use of anterior-posterior flaps for closure, with a myodesis of the biceps and triceps muscles to the distal humerus to preserve stability and maintain alignment.[10] Additional myoplasty is performed to preserve the soft-tissue padding and muscular balance of the residual limb. Myoplasty provides good distal padding, but it may make it difficult for the patient to differentiate the independent myoelectric signals during initial training.

Although the muscle bellies of the biceps and triceps are initially in the original longitudinal physiologic position, there is a tendency for them to migrate medially, which alters the position of the electromyographic (EMG) sites as the limb matures. It is important to recheck and adjust EMG sites to maintain correct positioning. If the muscle bellies release from the myodesis or myoplasty, muscle bunching may occur, with the muscle belly migrating

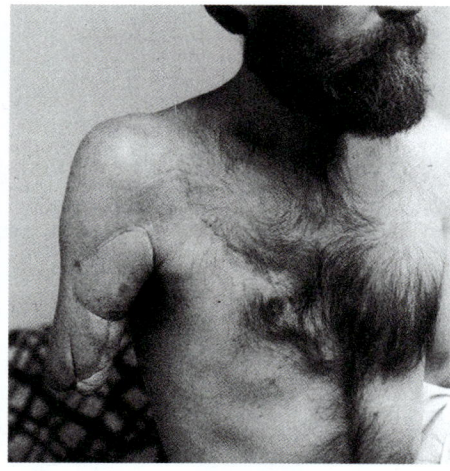

FIGURE 6 Clinical photograph of an individual who was treated with an innervated pectoralis transfer for the purpose of maintaining an active electromyographic control site for a possible future myoelectrically controlled prosthesis. (Reproduced from Andrew JT: Prosthetic principles, in Bowker JH, Michael JW, eds: *Atlas of Limb Prosthetics: Surgical, Prosthetic, and Rehabilitation Principles*, ed 2. Mosby-Year Book, 1992, pp 255-264.)

proximally and medially during contraction. This can create problems in volume management and the placement of myoelectrodes as the muscle dynamically contracts. This internal movement can also cause release of the proximal seal within suction sockets, which allows air to enter into the socket and eliminates the negative-pressure environment necessary for suspension.

Because most of the muscle structures are left intact, these concerns are less common with elbow disarticulation. However, some surgical reduction of distal soft-tissue bulk may be preferred because it allows the transverse geometry of the distal humerus to provide greater suspension and rotational control. Excessive distal redundant tissue can prevent a tight fit and impede control of the prosthesis.[8]

Muscle transfers and targeted muscle reinnervation techniques can be used to provide additional EMG sites for external power activation. Transfer of an innervated latissimus dorsi, a gracilis, or a pectoralis muscle can be used to create useful EMG sites if none are available[19-21] (**Figure 6**). Targeted muscle reinnervation repositions existing nerves to the remaining muscle groups that have been separated. Some patients who have undergone such procedures have achieved surprising levels of control complexity in combination with sophisticated pattern recognition control systems.[22]

Transhumeral Interface Considerations

Historically, transhumeral interfaces fit rather loosely about the residual limb, and heavy socks were used to increase anatomic loading.[17] After donning with a thick sock, the residual limb was simply pushed into the loose fitting socket, and few anatomic characteristics or contours were considered.[17] Subsequently, the half-and-half socket, which is characterized by an open proximolateral deltoid area and the use of a flexible band over the shoulder, offered an improvement in musculoskeletal and volumetric control.[23] The integrated saddle design, described by McLaurin et al[24] in 1969, served as a forerunner to more modern designs that use extended deltopectoral and infraspinous wings to help support the weight of the limb. The above-elbow suction socket described by Pentland and Wasireif[25] suggested that suction suspension could be used to support the transhumeral limb and minimize the need for extra harnessing.[26] The Utah Dynamic Socket, described by Andrew,[8] introduced several fitting objectives based on the anatomy of the transhumeral limb (**Figure 7**). These principles are valuable, not only for externally powered arms as originally proposed, but also for stability in body-powered systems. Although other authors have introduced design nuances, several common goals have persisted in all of the design variations.[25-27]

Prosthetic transhumeral interface fitting is influenced by the length of the humerus, the thickness and condition of the skin, underlying musculature and skeletal substructure, the resultant shape of the limb, the load tolerance of the patient and the range of motion of the glenohumeral and sternoclavicular joints.[8] The consideration of these attributes helps formulate which features of the interface design are emphasized to a greater or lesser extent.

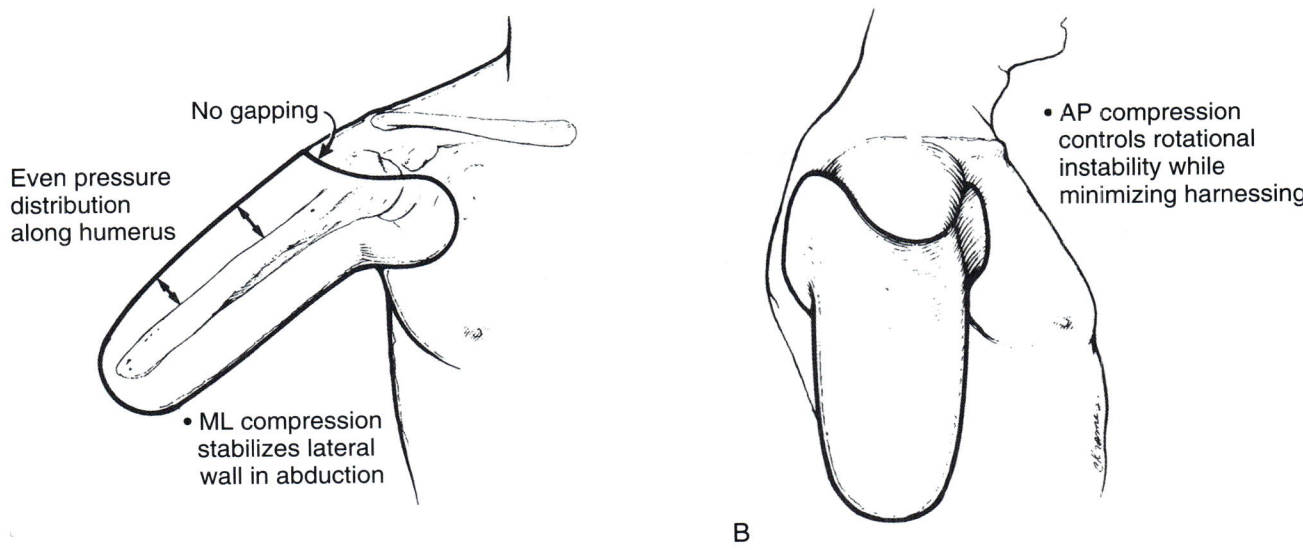

FIGURE 7 Illustrations of the Utah Dynamic Socket. **A**, The socket improves comfort by providing a better fit. **B**, AP compression controls rotational instability while minimizing harnessing. ML = mediolateral. (Reproduced from Andrew JT: Prosthetic principles, in Bowker JH, Michael JW, eds: *Atlas of Limb Prosthetics: Surgical, Prosthetic, and Rehabilitation Principles*, ed 2. Mosby-Year Book, 1992, pp 255-264.)

Limb Length

The length and condition of the humerus, which acts as the functional lever arm, determines the amount of load that the patient can support, especially during glenohumeral flexion and abduction. The condition of the cut end of the humerus is of particular importance because it is the distal point of contact in the interface. A suitable amount of distal relief will allow comfortable loading of the more proximal humeral shaft rather than the cut end. In some instances, when humeral length is short, bone-lengthening procedures have been used to increase the available gradient of loading.

Limb Volume

The volume of the distal limb can be evaluated for general compressibility and firmness. The subcutaneous tissue and overlying skin also can be assessed by lightly pinching the tissue at the midhumeral level. These qualitative measures can be used to determine the amount of tension or circumferential reductions below the anatomic measure that are necessary for a pull-in–type socket design. Typically, a greater amount of tension is necessary if the distal limb has a greater amount of compressibility and subcutaneous thickness.

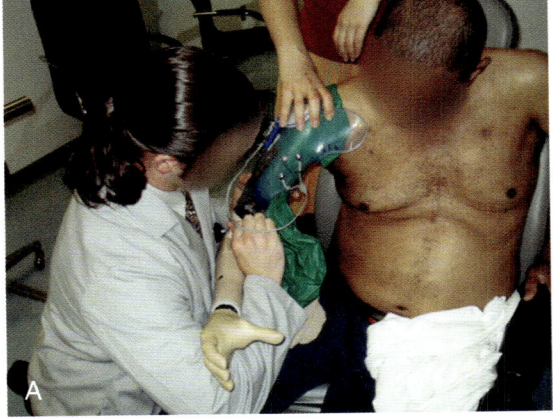 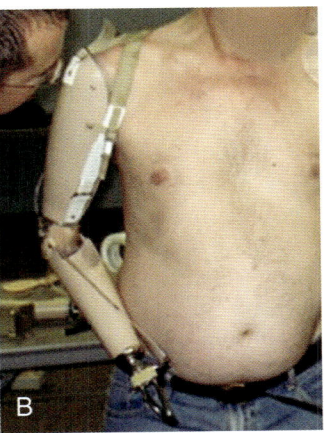

FIGURE 8 Photographs of patients wearing different socket designs. **A**, Pull-in socket design. **B**, Push-in socket design.

A major consideration in the selection of the transhumeral interface design is the choice between a pull-in or push-in design (**Figure 8**). Historically, a push-in design has been used because of its ease of construction and relatively loose fit[18] (**Figure 9**). The patient simply pushes the residual limb into the interface after donning the harness in an overhead sweater or lateral coat fashion. This is possible because the interface fits loosely over the limb with a thick wool sock.[18] Because the shape of the residual limb is not intimately captured, a substantial amount of movement, termed bell clapping, is possible within the interface. As a result, much of the excursion and movement needed for body-powered control is lost, especially with shorter residual limb lengths. However, if the push-in interface design is tightened excessively, the patient may experience proximal hammocking in which the tissue of the residual limb is pushed proximally and gathers at the top of the interface causing soft-tissue tension and pain over the distal end.[18]

Push-in designs are popular with shorter limb lengths in which the volume of the distal tissue does not need to be strictly managed. In addition, push-in designs are preferred for elbow disarticulations when the distal skeletal substructure allows for comfortable

Section 2: Upper Limb

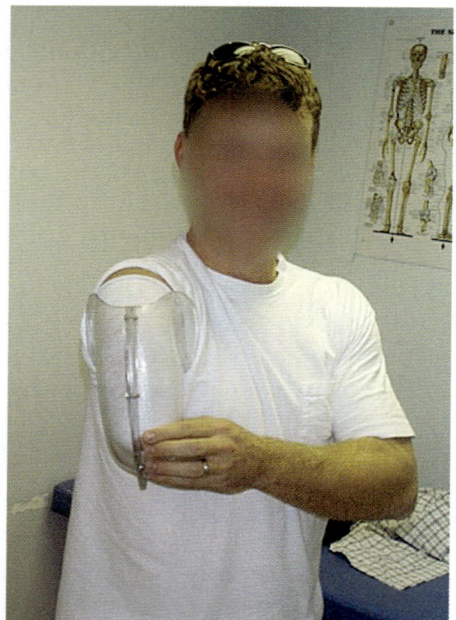

FIGURE 9 Photograph of an individual with a transhumeral prosthesis with a push-in interface design. Donning involves pushing the residual limb into the interface, usually with the aid of a prosthetic sock. The interface must be made loose to allow easy donning.

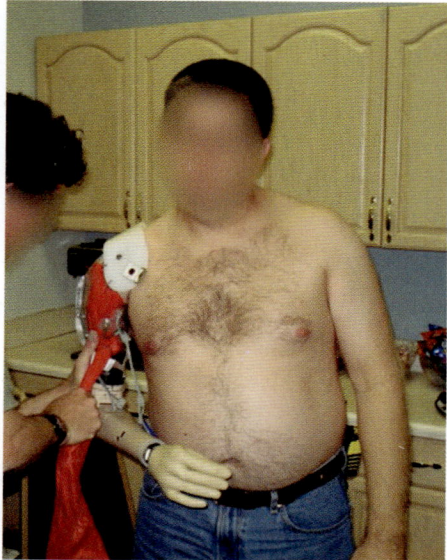

FIGURE 10 Photograph demonstrating the donning of a pull-in interface design. A sheath is used to pull the residual limb into the interface. Because the prosthetic interface has a smaller circumference than the anatomic limb, volumetric pressure is created within the donned socket.

insertion (there is not excessive redundant tissue) and distal suspension alternatives are used. Push-in designs with a tighter fit typically use an evaporative lubricant, such as a gel hand sanitizer or water-based ultrasound gel, to allow easier insertion.

Suction suspension using an inner membrane or prominence of silicone in a soft silicone interface as a sealing gasket at the midshaft area is another practical solution for elbow disarticulation suspension. This method uses a constant-leak valve to allow air to be expelled as the arm is inserted. Suction suspension makes use of characteristics of elbow disarticulation anatomy with greater distal anchoring of soft tissue, as opposed to the more pliable properties of transhumeral amputation, to allow the arm to be pushed past a fitted suction membrane or silicone bead. As the arm is inserted into the custom distal profile, the air is expelled through the valve creating negative pressure. In addition to the benefits of donning ease, lowered proximal trimlines, and reduced harnessing, this design offers direct contact with myosites for

external power. However, the disadvantages are that the membrane or silicone must be incorporated and adjusted precisely during fabrication of the socket with the appropriate amount of tension, and replaced periodically if there is wear.

With the advent of externally powered prostheses, a more intimate socket fit was needed to gain a more consistent position for the myoelectrodes over the surface of the residual limb because they detect muscle activity. The pull-in design uses the suspension techniques derived from transfemoral fitting in which the residual limb, without an interface cushioning sock, is pulled into a socket with a smaller circumference than the anatomic limb (**Figure 10**). This allows an intimate and consistent direct skin fit that is necessary for myoelectric control. This also creates a partial suction suspension when using an external suction valve that is applied after donning. Another advantage of the pull-in design is that physical movement of the residual limb is well-captured, which allows for lower proximal trim lines, greater axilla comfort, and improved range of motion. For

these reasons, some individuals who use body-powered prostheses may also benefit from the use of pull-in designs.

However, donning a pull-in prosthesis can be challenging. The patient must temporarily place and hold the prosthetic arm in a secure position (without the benefit of the harness because it has not been donned) while pulling the residual limb distally into the socket. Although a low-friction donning sheath is used to improve donning speed, assistance is often required. Pull-in designs are often used for medium to long transhumeral amputations in which the distal volume of the limb must be managed. The donning procedure can be prohibitive for patients with compromised contralateral dexterity and patients with bilateral upper limb amputation.

Limb Shape

The general shape of the transhumeral residual limb also is an important consideration. The shape of the lateral humeral shaft should be evaluated for loading ability, especially along the distal half of its bony length. Longer limb lengths are typically flatter along the humeral shaft, whereas elbow disarticulation exhibit a distal lateral concavity. Shorter limb lengths are more convex because the bony substructure is not present. Limb shape may also be affected by the subcutaneous tissue or the degree of muscular attachment, as was previously mentioned. A firm residual limb with little compressible tissue, such as an elbow disarticulation, will have a more characteristic shape, whereas a shorter limb with a more fleshy presentation will exhibit a more rounded and uncharacteristic shape.

In elbow disarticulation, the lateral and medial supracondylar ridges and condyles should be noted (generally observed as a coronal dimension that is wider than the midshaft of the humerus). The complexity of the interface design is increased because it will be necessary to make an allowance for the passage of this wider dimension into the distal interface. This may be accomplished with alternative interface designs, such as a removable medial door, a padded stovepipe liner, a spiral modification, an inflatable bladder, a clamshell, or an open design, which are discussed later in this chapter.

Carrying Angle

The way the patient holds the limb in the frontal plane, referred to as the carrying angle, should be noted. Patients with broader chests will typically hold the upper arm in a more abducted position, whereas a more adducted position will usually be favored by patients with narrower chests. This positioning may be further affected by limb length because the increased weight of a longer limb may tend to adduct the arm, whereas the absence of distal muscular attachments in shorter limbs may create a more abducted carrying angle. This positioning should be considered in the final assembly of the prosthesis (**Figure 11**). If the elbow axis is not aligned properly, based on the carrying angle, the elbow axis will not be parallel to the ground and the elbow will flex in an oblique manner.

Substructure

During the evaluation process, the underlying musculature and skeletal structure should be noted, especially in the load-bearing areas. The patient should be asked to contract the musculature of the anterior biceps and posterior triceps. The apex of each muscle belly should be evaluated for any resultant changes in shape and volume and, if indicated, for myoelectrode placement. Asking the patient to contract the biceps with simulated internal glenohumeral rotation and the triceps with external glenohumeral rotation may help identify the muscle positions at the transhumeral level.

The subsurface skeletal structures also should be examined. The locations of the clavicle and spine of the scapula should be noted because the proximal trim lines of the interface are usually placed just inferior to these pressure-sensitive areas. The position of the acromioclavicular joint is noted by palpating to the lateral edge of the posterior spine of the scapula. This position is indicative of the lateral position of the glenohumeral joint, and it is used for limb-length assessment and measurement. The lateral shaft of the humerus is marked as a load-tolerant surface area that terminates 10 mm proximal to the cut end where distal humeral relief is provided.

Load-Bearing Tolerance

As the muscular and skeletal structures are located, it is crucial to evaluate the residual limb for load-bearing tolerance and sensitivity. Proximal load bearing is often obtained through an anterior-posterior force couple comprised of the deltopectoral region (bordered by the clavicle proximally, the pectoralis medially, and the pectoralis tendon inferiorly) and the area inferior to the spine of the scapula. If sufficient anterior-posterior pressure is achieved within the interface, a degree of self-suspension can be created, which is especially important with the added weight of an externally powered prosthesis. However, the pressure of the interface against the sensitive prominences of the humeral head and the coracoid process should be considered. Often, a superior saddle fabricated from compliant materials will connect the anterior-posterior wings providing additional axial suspension (**Figure 12**).

Distally, the loading area is along the lateral shaft of the humerus and should terminate proximal to the cut end of the bone. Load bearing in this area can be compromised by scarring, wounds, internal neuromas, or a distal end of the humerus that was inadequately beveled at the time of amputation. Relief

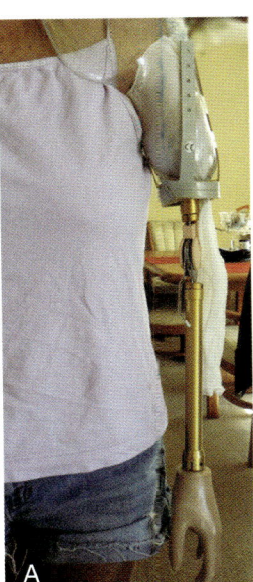
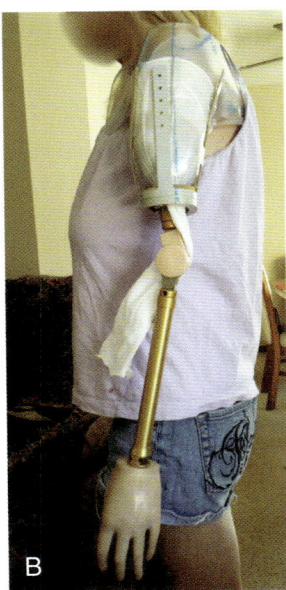
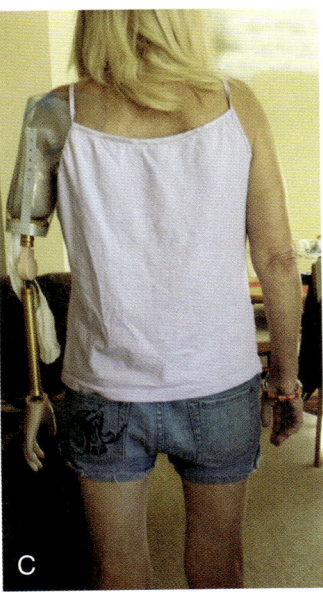

FIGURE 11 Clinical photographs of a patient demonstrating anterior (**A**), lateral (**B**), and posterior (**C**) alignment of an endoskeletal transhumeral prosthesis.

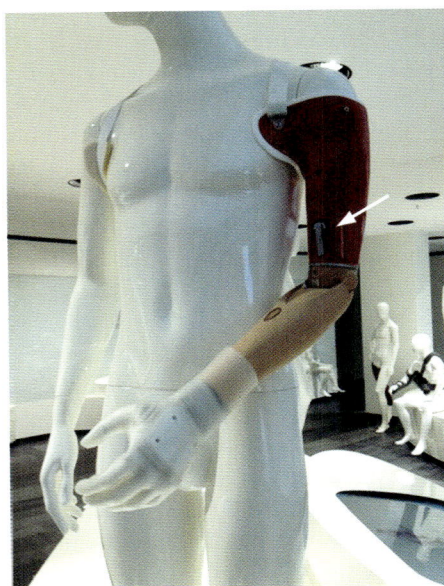

FIGURE 12 Photograph of an externally powered transhumeral prosthesis with a silicone flexible inner socket and a rigid external carbon frame. The superior saddle of the silicone socket aids in suspension of the prosthesis while the rigid frame provides rotational stability.

alone may be inadequate to off-load a tender area in this aspect of the socket. Frequently, relief must be coupled with loading just proximal to the sensitive area. In addition to managing the loads associated with the weight of the prosthesis, the distal end of the limb may experience direct distal loading when the arm is pushed distally against a table or other object. This area should be evaluated for any sensitivity that may occur if there is inadequate distal padding.

Distally, the mediolateral tension supports the carrying angle of the residual limb as well as maximizing the amount of distal coupling to the interface. A loose interface would allow excessive motion of the socket and precipitate increased impingement on the lateral distal area. Often, practitioners will pad the proximolateral area if there is a lateral gap, but this practice does not correct the position of the socket on the limb and ultimately makes the lateral distal end more prone to impingement.

Range of Motion

The range of motion of the glenohumeral and sternoclavicular joints and the mobility of the scapula should be examined with respect to movement within the interface. This range of motion, especially glenohumeral flexion and extension, is dictated by the size of the deltopectoral and infraspinous wings incorporated within the trim line. The longer the residual limb, the less prominent these wings need to be because rotation can be resisted more distally.

The mobility of the shoulder is also important when considering the control options for body or external power. Glenohumeral flexion and biscapular abduction are the most commonly used biomechanical methods for operating a body-powered prosthesis. However, smaller movements, including shoulder elevation, biscapular retraction, or biscapular depression, can be used to activate electronic switches. Internal pressure switches may be used, but the shoulder must be able to move independently within the interface to make consistent contact and apply pressure.

Taking a Transhumeral Casting Impression

When taking the impression for a transhumeral interface, it is important to consider (1) distal volume management, (2) proximal anterior-posterior musculoskeletal loading, (3) comfortable loading with the control preference, (4) ease of donning and doffing the prosthesis, and (5) maximum range of motion.

Volume Management

Management of distal limb volume can be achieved by loading the tissue circumferentially using elastic plaster distally over standard casting gauze or an elastic sock that has been tightly fitted to the patient. If the patient does not have firm musculature, the limb may be pulled into a compression sock with a cotton stockinette. This technique applies circumferential tension and pulls the tissue distally from the proximal axilla area. Because this technique will also have the effect of elongating the limb 25 mm or more, the length measurement from the axilla should be measured after the elongation has been done (**Figure 13**).

Careful measurements may include the limb length from the acromion process to the distal end, from the axilla to the distal end and circumferences at the axilla, along the midhumeral shaft, and at the apex of the distal end. Many practitioners believe that the measurements are accurately represented in the mold; however, if careful measurements are not recorded, it is difficult to attain the correct amount of compression, especially when the limb is under circumferential tension. If a compression sock is used, the circumferences should be measured after the limb has been pulled into the elastic compression sock.

Proximal Contours

Proximal musculoskeletal loading is accomplished by achieving a tight anterior-posterior dimension between the deltopectoral groove and the infraspinous area. Before taking the impression, this dimension should be measured with calipers while a comfortable level of compression is being applied. This anterior-posterior measurement should be recorded for modification and also taken over the impression during casting. To preserve this position as the negative impression is removed, the calipers can be placed into position after removal of the casting to ensure accurate dimensional control. This contour can be molded with a plaster splint running from the posterior to the anterior wing or with recurrent back-and-forth splinting over the shoulder to encapsulate the deltopectoral region and the scapula.

During casting, the index finger of the posterior hand should be placed just inferior to the spine of the scapula, and the breadth of the hand should be placed along the posterior plateau of the scapula (**Figure 14, A**). Anteriorly, the fingers should be placed around the head of the humerus in a horseshoe or a backward C-shape (**Figure 14, B**). The fingers should not make localized indention points in the impression, but rather should provide broadened and general loading by massaging the regions in a circular fashion and avoiding the bony anatomy of the spine of the scapula and humeral head.

An alternative handhold for smaller hands is to place the thenar and hypothenar areas of the posterior hand in the infraspinous area, with the

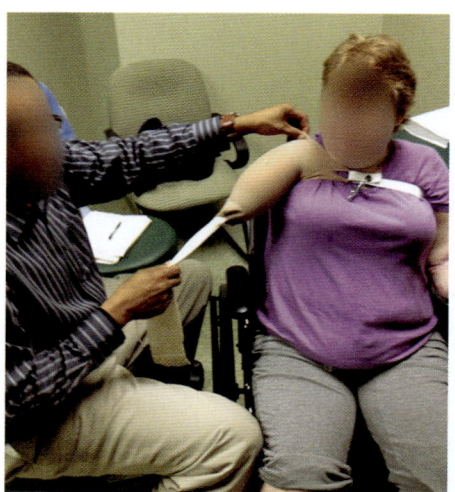

FIGURE 13 Clinical photograph of a practitioner pulling the distal tissue of the residual limb into circumferential tension (beige material) using a cotton sock (white material).

Mediolateral Compression

With this second casting strategy, the clinician should periodically squeeze the mediolateral dimension at the axilla (**Figure 14, D**). In doing so, it is important to maintain a vertical orientation of the medial hand relative to the long axis of the limb. If the fingertips of the medial hand exert an excessive push into the axilla laterally toward the humerus, a dovetailing effect can occur at the proximomedial brim, making the socket painful and difficult to doff. The lateral hand should be used to form the lateral side of the shaft of the humerus, and the distal portion of the hand should be placed proximal to the cut end of the bone. At this point, if any muscle bunching has been observed, the muscles should be repeatedly flexed and relaxed. The muscle node should be located and supported distally during the impression taking. It is important to remember that with fleshy limb shapes, the clinician should not overflatten or pancake the mediolateral dimension because this would prevent easy donning of the prosthesis.

It is important to hold the patient's arm in maximal adduction with the back of the medially positioned hand contacting the thoracic area. A common error is to inadvertently hold the limb in abduction while the impression is being taken. In such cases, the evaluation interface will appear to fit only when the arm is in abduction rather than adduction. This also can result in lateral distal pressure, especially with heavier external power componentry.

It must be remembered that as proximal anterior-posterior shaping is achieved, there will be increased proximolateral deformation, which can result in substantial gapping. As the plaster begins to harden, the depth to the tissue can be indicated with the index finger. At the time of modification, this volume of material may be removed to the indicated depth. It is not uncommon for 25 mm of material to be removed in this area during modification.

Considerations With Longer Limbs

With longer limb lengths and in elbow disarticulations, additional steps are

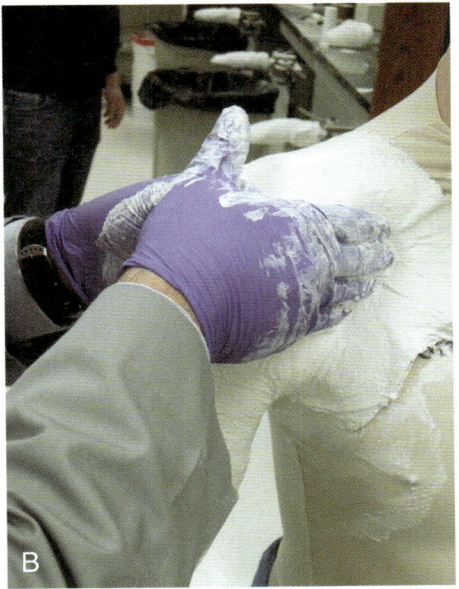
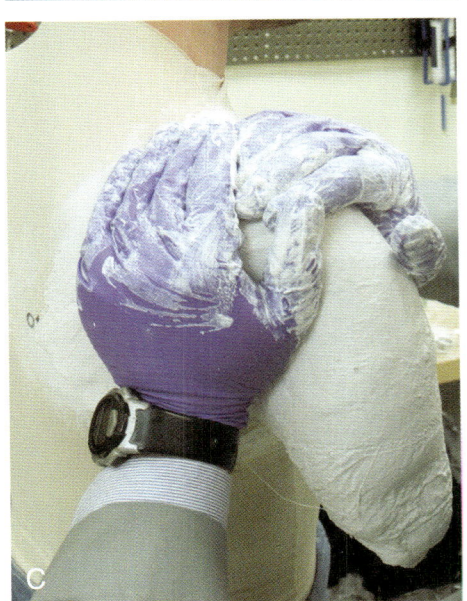
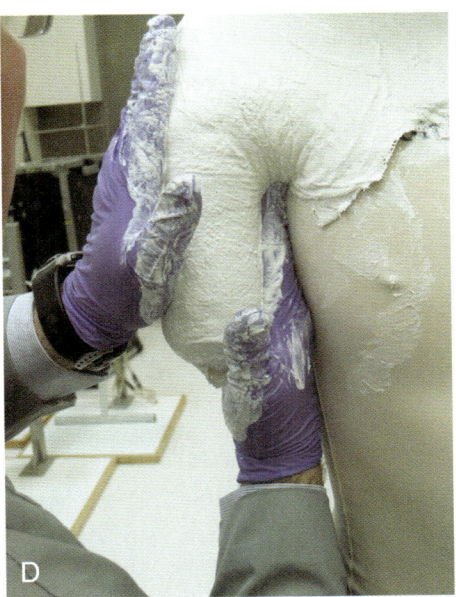

FIGURE 14 Photographs show techniques for taking a transhumeral casting impression. **A**, The posterior-proximal finger position. The index finger is inferior to the spine of the scapula in the infraspinous area. **B**, The posterior-anterior finger position. The digits form a C-shape around the head of the humerus but inferior to the clavicle. The thumb positions are crossed. **C**, An alternative proximal hand grip demonstrating use of the thenar and hypothenar eminences of both hands to apply load posteriorly and anteriorly. This hand hold is often recommended for prosthetists with smaller hands. **D**, Secondary distal hand hold. The outer hand is placed just proximal to the cut end of the humerus. The inner hand is placed against the thoracic area pushing into the axilla. Notice that the fingers are aligned perpendicular to the chest wall to avoid excessive proximal compression. Slight mediolateral pressure is applied, but not so much as to pancake the residual limb. (Courtesy of Gerald Stark, PhD, MSEM, CPO/L, FAAOP(D).)

fingers wrapping superiorly and anteriorly (**Figure 14, C**). The anterior hand is placed with the thenar and hypothenar areas encapsulating the head of the humerus. The fingers may then be clasped over the proximolateral area. With this technique, the interface creates an internal saddle that can partially load the shoulder of the involved side; this interface quality is especially important for use with externally powered components.

required distally to accommodate the wider distal mediolateral dimension. If a seamless impression is desired, a felt or foam pad can be created that spans from the medial epicondyle to the height at which the mediolateral dimension of the arm matches the mediolateral dimension of the distal condyles. This pad can be secured to the casting garment with double-sided tape before impression taking. Alternatively, the impression may be taken in a clamshell fashion.

Interface Modification and Evaluation

Using the anterior-posterior measurement taken at the time the impression was made and that of the mold, two-thirds of the difference is removed at the depth of the deltopectoral area and one-third from the infraspinous area of the scapula. Care should be taken not to impinge on the head of the humerus and to ensure that the posterior modification reflects the longitudinal, transverse, and frontal plane angles of the scapula. Distally, the reduction should be general and consistent with the firmness of the residual limb and subcutaneous tissue, with greater reductions indicated for softer tissue.

The evaluation interface can then be created with the trim lines located just inferior to the clavicle, the spine of the scapula, and the acromioclavicular joint, and the axilla proximally. Additional material may be removed from the proximal wings to allow a greater range of motion. The evaluation interface should be donned using a low-friction donning sheath, and the prosthetist should note the distal tension within the socket (especially at the axilla). As the interface is donned, the tension with the donning sheath should be firm because of the tight fit.

The evaluation interface should be checked for impingement at the clavicle and the anterior and posterior axilla, especially during glenohumeral flexion and biscapular abduction. The proximal wings should be examined for rotational stability. The posterior wall will control external rotation for body-powered devices, and the anterior wing will control internal rotation caused by heavier external control systems. If the limb was cast under compression it is not uncommon for there to be 25 mm or more gapping distally in the evaluation interface. This distal gap can be marked or packed with fitting putty and subsequent trial devices should have distal contact without end bearing when donning.

It is advisable for the evaluation interface to be set up with the externally powered or body-powered components to evaluate how the interface performs with the associated weight and displacement. This helps the practitioner evaluate how the interface reacts to harness positioning, alignment, and loading characteristics during normal use (**Figure 15**). At this point in the process, the electrode sites, trim lines, and component positioning may be refined. The typical alignment in the frontal plane is at the location where the proximal turntable of the elbow is parallel to the floor and approximately 25 mm lateral to the hip or widest part of the body. The sagittal alignment is usually at neutral, with the turntable parallel to the floor. With shorter residual limb lengths and heavier external control systems, the interface may be preflexed slightly to prevent greater concentration of a load on the anterior humerus.

Interface Construction

The transhumeral interface is created with many of the same materials as a transfemoral prosthesis, including a flexible socket with a more rigid external supportive frame. A softer interface material is chosen so that it conforms to the contours of the shoulder. This material can be soft thermoplastic, an interface liner, or custom silicone to bend with the body. Usually, an acrylic composite laminated outer frame is created over the mold of the flexible interface in the correct frontal and sagittal plane alignments as previously described. The composite materials typically consist of varying layers of fiberglass, carbon, and nylon. Between the layers, additional geometries for electrodes, batteries, and connection devices can be created as needed and are commonly located in the distal portion of the device between the end of

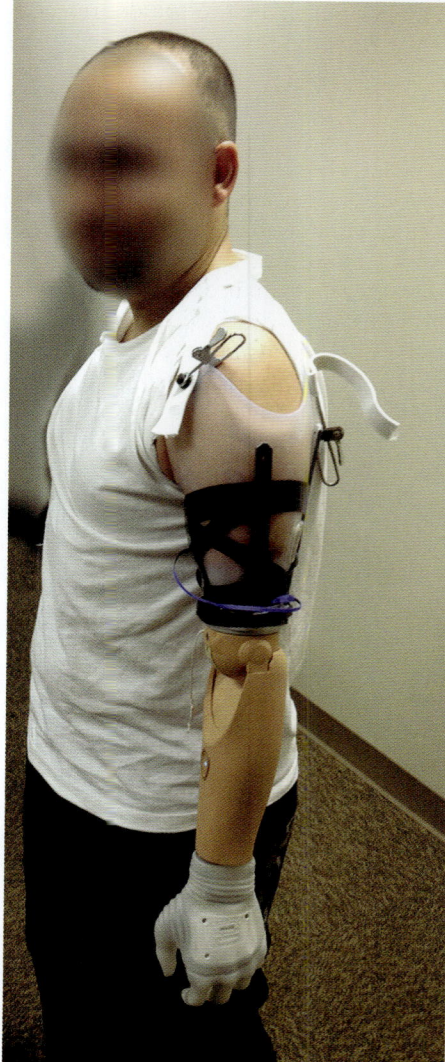

FIGURE 15 Photograph of a patient during a rough fitting of a transhumeral prosthesis to determine how the interface will perform with the selected componentry. (Courtesy of Gerald Stark, PhD, MSEM, CPO/L, FAAOP(D).)

the interface and the turntable of the elbow or posteriorly. The trim line of the frame is typically 6 to 12 mm inferior to the trim line of the interface so that it can be adjusted as necessary. It also provides the attachment points for the harness and body-powered control points. These may require special anchors and fittings to hold the straps and cable in position.

For individuals who use their prostheses for heavy-duty tasks or in inherently dusty environments, it may be desirable to use exoskeletal construction consisting of a laminated socket. This is constructed by using structural foam that is shaped to the desired cosmetic form of the interface, and then an outer, hard laminated form is created to form the exterior surface.[17] Although less adjustable, this method is typically selected for users of body-powered prostheses, when greater strength and limb stability are required. Although various skin tones are available, patients often decorate the laminated outer frame with custom colors, images, logos, tattoos, or carbon composite materials to personalize their devices.

Endoskeletal systems that are lighter and more cosmetic also can be made with an interface and frame construction, but are typically covered with a more lifelike foam shell and glove to enhance cosmetic quality.

Interface Alternatives

Socket variations are typically used when the residual limb and humeral length are longer or shorter than usual. When the residual humerus is extremely short, the shortened interface resembles the fitting for a shoulder disarticulation interface. The deltopectoral and infraspinous wings project proximally from the axilla and fit around the exposed humeral remnant. An articulating shoulder joint can be placed more inferiorly in the axilla or lateral to the residual limb, with rigid support structures; this is called birdcage construction.[27] With this style of construction, the interface is relatively open. However, the residual limb is not directly used for shoulder positioning, and the prosthesis is functionally equivalent to a shoulder disarticulation prosthesis (**Figure 16**).

Liner Suspension

Another variation is the use of a roll-on suspension liner, which is popular with patients who desire self-suspension. The liner can be custom-made, or a production liner can be chosen to match the shape and taper of the residual limb. Distally, the attachment is provided with a distal pin-catch shuttle lock or a lanyard configuration in which a narrow strap is pulled through a slot within the interface and secured

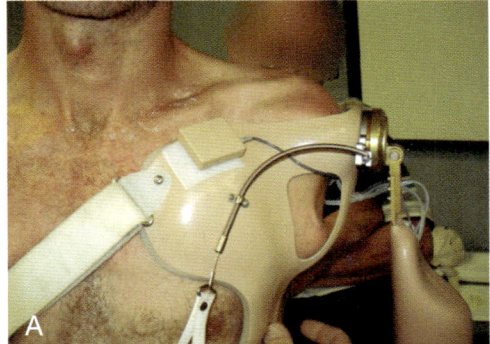 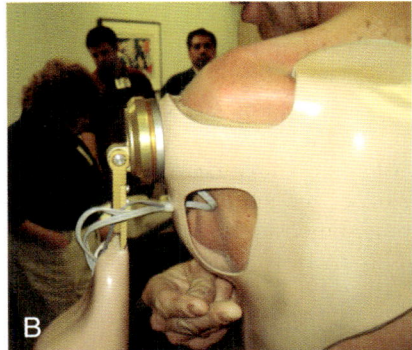

FIGURE 16 Anterior (**A**) and posterior (**B**) photographic views of a patient wearing a transhumeral prosthesis with birdcage construction.

with an external fabric hook-and-loop fastener system. The latter method is often used for longer limb lengths when the additional length of a pin lock system is not available.

The combination of a liner and external power requires consideration of how the EMG signals will be conducted through the liner to the electrodes. Holes can be cut into the liner, but issues arise if the holes in the liner are not aligned with the electrode sensors in the socket wall. The patient must be instructed on how to use anatomic landmarks to properly don the liner or the myoelectrode sensors will be blocked and control function may be compromised. Other options are electrodes that snap onto studs that are attached to the liner (**Figure 17**) or custom liners that use a conductive silicone that allows the EMG signal to be conducted through the liner to the myoelectrode mounted in the laminated frame.

Elbow Disarticulation Alternatives

Many of the alternative socket designs are used to accommodate longer limb lengths and elbow disarticulations in which the distal mediolateral dimension of the humeral epicondyles is wider than the midshaft dimension.[28] The most common method of addressing this dimensional difference is the creation of a medial door through which the medial epicondyle may pass. The opening for the medial door spans between the distal epicondyle and the proximal border where the

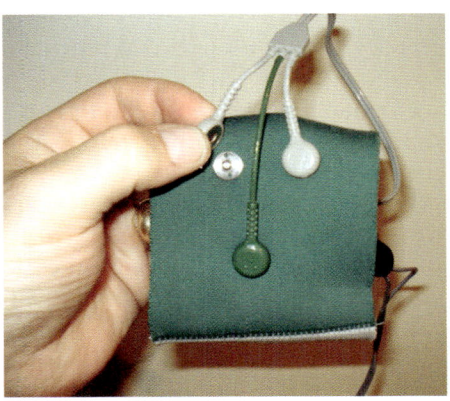

FIGURE 17 Photograph of snap-on electrodes for a humeral prosthesis liner that allow for improved conduction of electromyographic signals.

mediolateral dimension is equal to the distal dimension.

Additional options for the paneled designs can use strong flexible fabrics for the medial panel. Being porous, the fabric is prone to an odor issue, but they can be washable if they can be disconnected (**Figure 18**). Such open-paneled designs would prohibit the use of ancillary suctions suspension by applying tension distally.

The open-paneled concept can be further enhanced with the use of high-tension wire filament that can be tightened with a one-way click reel to adjust the volumetric tension that can be released (**Figure 19**, BOA®, Steamboat Springs, CO). The panels can be created in any orientation, but are frequently placed in the medial and lateral aspects. Channels for the wire filament are formed in the laminated layers and the click valve is tightened to the

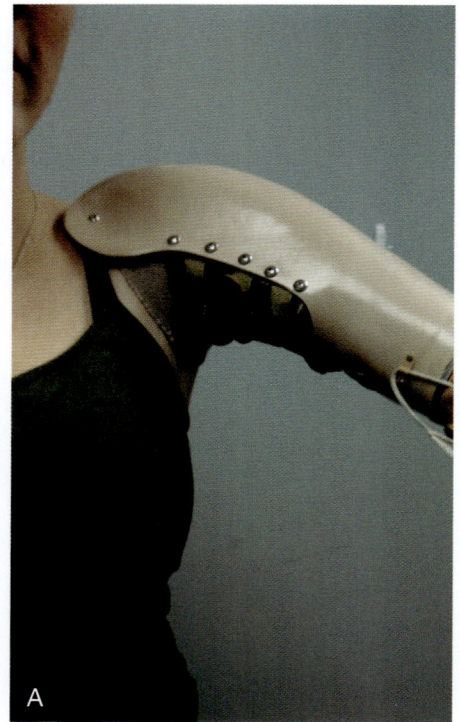
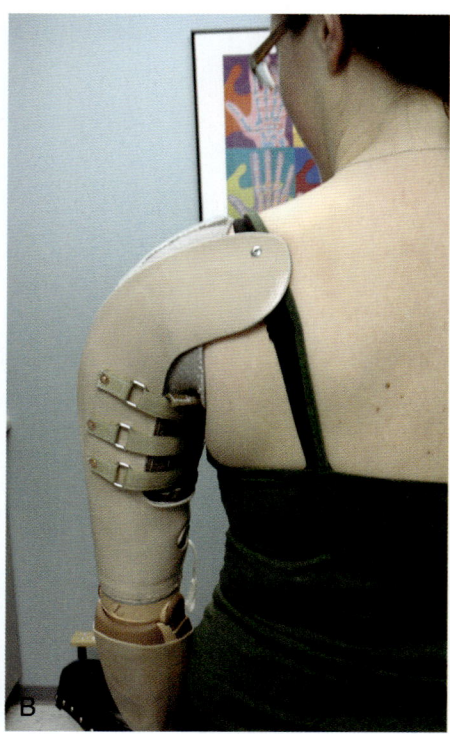

FIGURE 18 **A**, The flexible medial fabric panel design allows adjustable tissue compression. **B**, This allow greater adjustment and ROM for the transhumeral prosthetic user. (Courtesy of CJ Socket Technologies, Beverly, MA.)

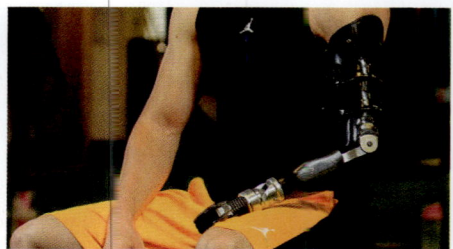

FIGURE 19 Photograph of an elbow disarticulation prosthesis where mediolateral compression is obtained through a high-tension click reel pulling upon panels. (Courtesy of Gerald Stark, PhD, MSEM, CPO, L, FAAOP(D).)

desired level of tension. By pulling up on the adjustable click reel the tension can be released. This further accentuates the viability and use of open-paneled designs for unique or bulbous limb shapes. In some cases self-suspension can be achieved; however, there should be caution when loading the medial axillary tissue, which are more sensitive when distracted distally.

Control Strategies

Because a transhumeral prosthesis represents an interconnected functional system with an interface design, control strategy, and harness, each of these factors affects the others directly and indirectly. With respect to body and external power, the type of control has a major effect on socket position. In body-powered devices, control is dependent on the movement of the residual limb. As a result, the proximal trim lines must allow adequate excursion of the arm to enable its functional use. The proximal trim lines are terminated at the deltopectoral groove, below the clavicle, and at the border of the posterior deltoid distal to the spine of the scapula. Often, they must be lowered during the initial fitting to accommodate the requirements of glenohumeral flexion and biscapular abduction. The prosthetic interface must not block the control movements, especially in glenohumeral flexion (**Figure 20**).

Typically, longer limb lengths can generate a greater amount of body-powered excursion in genohumeral flexion and biscapular abduction compared with shorter limb lengths. Because of the longer length of the effective lever arm of a longer limb, the leverage that can be applied is greater than that of a shorter limb. The loading forces felt inside the interface during cable activation are localized at the anterior distal and posterior proximal areas. A shorter limb length exhibits more localized forces at the distal end because there is less surface area and greater movement within the interface.

External power creates a different set of challenges when used for a transhumeral interface. With externally powered devices, control of the prosthesis is

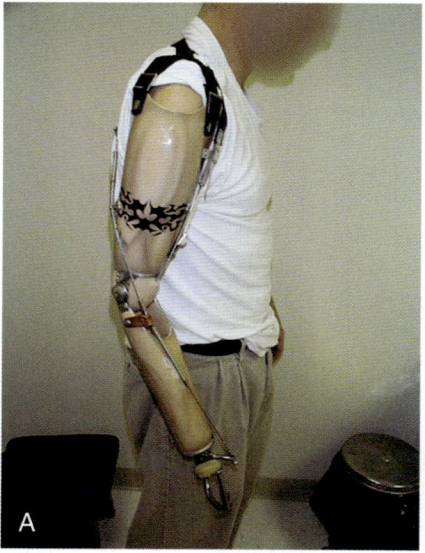
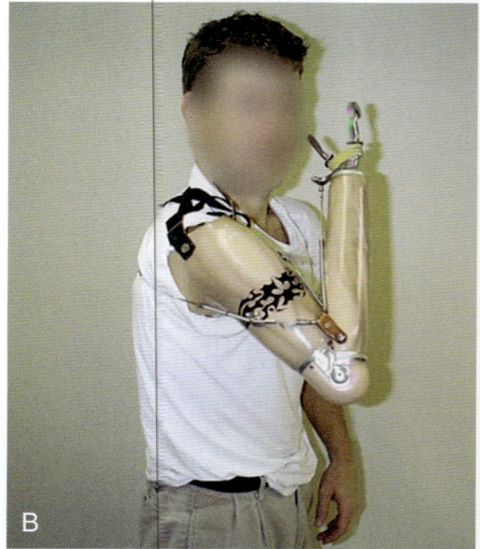

FIGURE 20 Photographs of an individual fitted with a body-powered transhumeral prosthesis. **A**, The posterior cable retainer is positioned proximal to the cut end of the humerus. **B**, The interface should not block glenohumeral flexion or biscapular abduction.

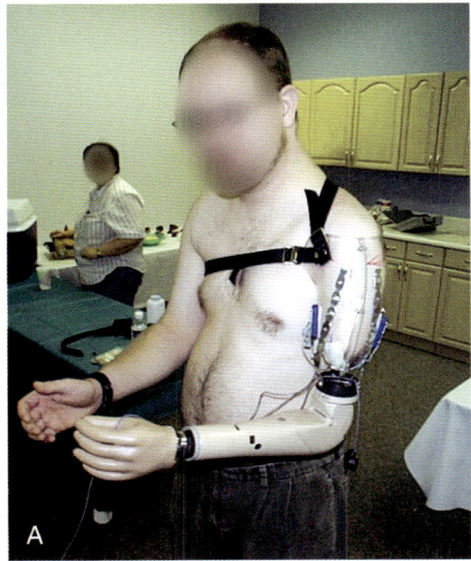 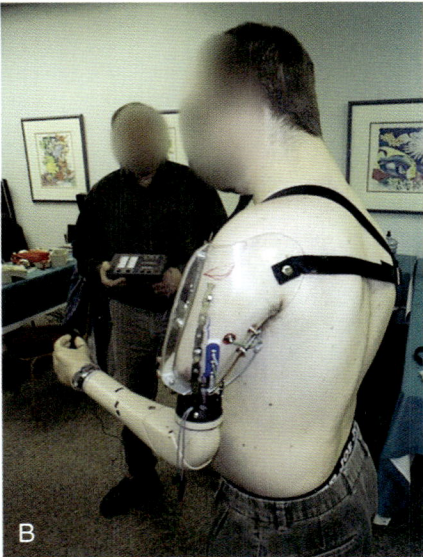

FIGURE 21 Photographs of an individual fitted with an externally powered transhumeral prosthesis. **A**, The socket of the prosthesis should help distribute the weight of the device while providing adequate suspension and resistance to movement as the forearm flexes. **B**, The proximal posterior infraspinous wing of the externally powered interface is important in resisting movement.

not dependent on gross movement, but fine contractions, so the trim lines can be extended more proximally into the deltopectoral groove and infraspinous areas to distribute the added weight of the prosthetic arm (**Figure 21**). Distally, the control electrodes must maintain intimate contact with the residual limb over the available muscle sites, such as the medial biceps and medial triceps. If the limb is especially soft, the practitioner may choose to load those areas so that the myosites can make better contact with the muscle bellies. As previously mentioned, pull-in designs are often preferable for externally powered devices because they maintain the positioning of the myoelectrodes. Alternative externally powered control strategies may include internal pressure switches, linear transducers, pull switches, and touch sensors, all of which must be appropriately located and anchored in the harness.

SUMMARY

Although the prosthetic interface at the transhumeral level presents several unique challenges, practitioners can create comfortable and functional socket designs by having a good knowledge of the process and paying careful attention to detail. It is important to listen to the patient and identify and fully understand their needs. Knowledge of the variety of socket design options and control strategies will help the practitioner meet the unique needs and challenges of a patient with a transhumeral amputation or an elbow disarticulation.

References

1. Billock J: Upper limb prosthetic terminal devices: Hands versus hooks. *Clin Prosthet Orthot* 1986;10:57-65.
2. Berger N: Studies of the upper-extremity amputee: II. The population (1953-55). *Artif Limbs* 1958;5(1):57-72.
3. Biddiss E, Chau T: Upper-limb prosthetics: Critical factors in device abandonment. *Am J Phys Med Rehabil* 2007;86(12):977-987.
4. Burrough SF, Brook JA: Patterns of acceptance and rejection of upper limb prostheses. *Orthot Prosthet* 1985;39(2):40-47.
5. Millstein SG, Heger H, Hunter GA: Prosthetic use in adult upper limb amputees: A comparison of the body powered and electrically powered prostheses. *Prosthet Orthot Int* 1986;10(1):27-34.
6. Stark G: Factor analysis of upper extremity prosthetic patient acceptance. Available at: http://www.oandp.org/publications/jop/2015/2015-01.pdf. Accessed July 1, 2015.
7. Michael J, Nunley J: Brachial plexus injuries: Surgical advances and orthotic/prosthetic management, in Bowker JH, Michael JW, eds: *Atlas of Limb Prosthetics: Surgical, Prosthetic, and Rehabilitation Principles*, ed 2. Mosby Year Book, 1992, pp 293-310.
8. Andrew JT: Prosthetic principles, in Bowker JH, Michael JW, eds: *Atlas of Limb Prosthetics: Surgical, Prosthetic, and Rehabilitation Principles*, ed 2. Mosby-Year Book, 1992, pp 255-264.
9. Daly WK: Elbow disarticulation and transhumeral amputation: Prosthetic management, in Smith DG, Michael JW, Bowker JH, eds: *Atlas of Amputations and Limb Deficiencies: Surgical, Prosthetic, and Rehabilitation Principles*, ed 3. American Academy of Orthopaedic Surgeons, 2004, pp 243-249.
10. Owens P, Ouellette EA: Elbow disarticulation and transhumeral amputation: Surgical management, in Smith DG, Michael JW, Bowker JH, eds: *Atlas of Amputations and Limb Deficiencies: Surgical, Prosthetic, and Rehabilitation Principles*, ed 3. American Academy of Orthopaedic Surgeons, 2004, pp 239-241.
11. Pinzur MS, Angelats J, Light TR, Izuierdo R, Pluth T: Functional outcome following traumatic upper limb amputation and prosthetic limb fitting. *J Hand Surg Am* 1994;19(5):836-839.
12. Marquardt E, Neff G: The angulation osteotomy of above-elbow stumps. *Clin Orthop Relat Res* 1974;104:232-238.
13. Baumgartner R: Upper extremity amputations, in DuParc J, ed: *Surgical Techniques in Orthopaedics and Traumatology*. Harcourt International, 2003.
14. de Luccia N, Marino HL: Fitting of electronic elbow on an elbow disarticulated patient by means of a new surgical technique. *Prosthet Orthot Int* 2000;24(3):247-251.
15. Malone JM, Fleming LL, Roberson J, et al: Immediate, early, and late postsurgical management of upper-limb amputation. *J Rehabil Res Dev* 1984;21(1):33-41.
16. Daly W: Clinical application of roll-on sleeves for myoelectrically controlled transradial and transhumeral prostheses. *J Prosthet Orthot* 2000;12:88-91.
17. Bray JJ: *Prosthetic Principles: Upper Extremity Amputations. Fabrication and Fitting Principles*, ed 3. Prosthetics Orthotics Education Program, University of California Press, 1989.
18. Brenner C, Brenner J: The use of preparatory/evaluation/training prostheses

in developing evidence-based practice in upper limb prosthetics. *J Prosthet Orthot* 2008;20(3):70-82.

19. Andrew S: Self-efficacy as a predictor of academic performance in science. *J Adv Nurs* 1998;27(3):596-603.

20. Maxwell GP, Manson PN, Hoopes JE: Experience with thirteen latissimus dorsi myocutaneous free flaps. *Plast Reconstr Surg* 1979;64(1):1-8.

21. Salam Y: The use of silicone suspension sleeves with myoelectric fittings. *J Prosthet Orthot* 1994;6(4):119-120.

22. Simon AM, Lock BA, Stubblefield KA: Patient training for functional use of pattern recognition-controlled prostheses. *J Prosthet Orthot* 2012;24(2):56-64.

23. Bush G: *Above-Elbow Fittings*. Hugh MacMillan Rehabilitation Center-Rehabilitation Engineering Department, 1990.

24. McLaurin CA, Sauter WF, Dolan CM, Hartmann GR: Fabrication procedures for the open-shoulder above-elbow socket. *Artif Limbs* 1969;13(2):46-54.

25. Pentland JA, Wasileif A: An above-elbow suction socket. *Orthot Prosthet* 1972;36:40.

26. Lake C: The evolution of upper limb prosthetic socket design. *J Prosthet Orthot* 2008;20(3):85-92.

27. Alley RD: *Advancement of upper extremity prosthetic interface and frame design*, in Proceedings of the 2002 MyoElectric Controls/Prosthetics Symposium August 21-23, 2002, Fredericton, New Brunswick, Canada. Available at: http://dukespace.lib.duke.edu/dspace/bitstream/handle/10161/2684/r_alley_paper01.pdf. Accessed August 5, 2015.

28. McAuliffe J: Elbow disarticulation and transhumeral amputation, in Bowker JH, Michael JW, eds: *Atlas of Limb Prosthetics: Surgical, Prosthetic, and Rehabilitation Principles*, ed 2. Mosby-Year Book, 1992, pp 251-253.

Amputations About the Shoulder: Surgical Considerations

CHAPTER 20

COL Joseph F. Alderete, MD

ABSTRACT

Proximal upper limb amputations such as those about the shoulder and chest wall are complex procedures requiring a thorough understanding of indications, surgical principles for optimal function, alternative treatments, and rehabilitation techniques to facilitate optimal outcomes. It is helpful to be aware of the limited range of reasons for performing shoulder-level limb ablation and the types of classic and modified methods for performing shoulder disarticulations and forequarter amputations. In some instances, alternative coverage and limb salvage techniques can be used to avoid shoulder-level amputations. Complications are common with these procedures.

Keywords: forequarter amputation; intercalary shoulder resection; shoulder disarticulation

Introduction

Shoulder-level amputations are rare. The typical reasons for limb ablation at the shoulder include tumor, trauma, burn (electrical), and infection.[1] With the advent of modern multiagent chemotherapy regimens and advanced surgical techniques, 90% of all neoplasia around the shoulder girdle can be managed with limb salvage.[2] Nonablative techniques for tumor resection and even limb-threatening infections are usually successful. These resections, with some modification, follow the classic Tikhoff-Linberg procedure for limb salvage. Amputations at the shoulder level involve a glenohumeral disarticulation, forequarter amputation, or ultrahigh transhumeral amputation. Many traditionally planned shoulder disarticulations can be converted to ultrahigh transhumeral amputations with a small part of the humeral head and neck remaining to preserve cosmesis and even motor function with the help of composite free tissue transfer and neuromodulation.[3,4] When tumor, trauma, and/or infection prove amenable, such amputations are vastly preferred; therefore, the surgical team contemplating proximal level amputation or advocacy for limb salvage must have in their armamentarium both neuromodulatory tools and methods for extending classic tissue coverage.[5-8] In surgical neuromodulation, advanced surgical techniques provide the elements necessary to favor coordinated nerve regeneration providing behavioral adaptation and prevention of painful stimuli.[9] These surgical neuromodulation techniques encompass the spectrum of true targeted muscle reinnervation (TMR), targeted nerve implantation, regenerative peripheral nerve interface, and guided dessication or "bridge to nowhere" where the nerve is capped and allowed to stop its axonal growth but in an organized fashion.[10] These techniques are necessary for the amputation surgeon to optimize function and are covered in more depth elsewhere in this text.

The forequarter amputation is extremely morbid in terms of body dysmorphism and function. This procedure is reserved for tumors, life-threatening trauma, or infections in which the axillary artery and the brachial plexus have been contaminated or destroyed, or when it is not prudent to leave these two structures in place because of the risk of local recurrence (**Figure 1**). Most patients treated with forequarter amputation have soft-tissue sarcoma, osteosarcoma, recurrent malignant melanoma, or epidermoid carcinoma.[11] This procedure also can be used to treat patients with large, ulcerated, or very painful metastatic carcinomas in whom the tumor often causes extreme pain from plexus radiculopathy.[5] In these patients, the entire forelimb is removed, in some instance with part of

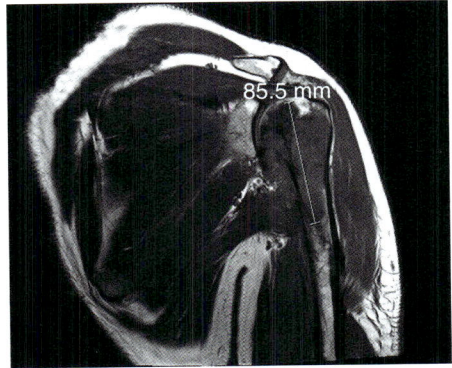

FIGURE 1 Magnetic resonance image of a large proximal humeral osteosarcoma with pathologic fracture and soft-tissue extension to the brachial artery and the brachial plexus.

Dr. Alderete or an immediate family member has received research or institutional support from Musculoskeletal Transplant Foundation and serves as a board member, owner, officer, or committee member of Musculoskeletal Transplant Foundation.

the chest wall, as well as the scapula, the humerus, and a portion of the clavicle.

Although there are classic methods for performing these two procedures, the procedure must be tailored to the patient and the corresponding pathophysiology. This often requires modifications to the classic approaches to fit the individual situation. In patients injured by high-energy trauma, amputation about the shoulder can be performed early or late, secondary to the wishes of patients with a flail limb. Early posttraumatic amputations, both shoulder disarticulation and forequarter amputation, are predicated on the amount of viable tissue that is free of contamination. If the tissue around the deltoid is viable, or if local or free tissue transfer is reasonable, an ultrahigh transhumeral amputation combined with shoulder fusion is preferable to removal of the humerus secondary to an intra-articular fracture and distal destruction.[2,12-15]

In keeping with the more classic approaches, several flaps must be maintained, and these determine the surgical technique. First, the ultrashort transhumeral amputation is based on an intact chevron region, which is the skin and muscle of the deltoid region. The ability to bias a chevron-shaped flap of skin, subcutaneous tissue, and full-thickness deltoid muscle to bone makes the ultrashort transhumeral amputation an attractive option. The true shoulder disarticulation can be performed with a lateral chevron region flap, a posterior flap, or an axillary-based flap of durable undersurface tissue. When possible, the axillary flap is preferred because there is no muscle to atrophy over the osseous structures and durable padding is provided for an articulating or a cosmetic prosthesis. The forequarter amputation can be based on a posterior periscapular flap or an anterior pectoralis flap. If neoplasm is an indication for amputation, the absolute necessity to achieve wide margin means that these classic flaps may not be available, so regional rotational or free flaps become essential. The latissimus dorsi rotational flap, either ipsilateral or contralateral, is preferred for defect coverage. Free tissue from the amputated limb is sometimes necessary for coverage if tumor irradiation has been performed.[16,17]

Alternatives to Amputation

As noted earlier, shoulder-level amputation should be a last resort because 90% of tumor resections and infections can be managed with limb salvage procedures. These limb salvage techniques involve resecting the proximal humerus, the glenoid with or without the main body of the scapula, and the entire or only part of the clavicle. This procedure, which was first described in 1928, is commonly referred to as the Tikhoff-Linberg resection and is the basis for maintaining function and movement in the distal upper limbs while allowing resection of tumor or infection in the shoulder region. The procedure was modified in 1977 by Ralph Marcove to include preservation of the uninvolved scapula despite extensive proximal humeral and glenoid resection.[18-21] In 1991, Malawar introduced the most useful classification system for shoulder-level deficits and reconstruction. When considering structural loss and replacement or the need to amputate, the author of this chapter finds Malawar's system to be most user-friendly.[18-20] The system was later modified according to a classification from the Musculoskeletal Tumor Society (**Figure 2**).

The requirements for limb salvage are a free tumor plane adjacent to the axillary neurovascular bundle, the chest wall, or the lymph nodes[22,23] or indications in palliative cases where amputation is not justified because of extensive chest wall involvement.[14] After the surgical team understands the defect, it is important to be aware of the goal of achieving a periarticular shoulder reconstruction that can provide a mobile but stable axis for elbow and wrist rotation, which allows placement of the hand in space. Reconstruction can involve the use of allograft, endoprosthesis, fibular autograft, and even pasteurized autograft or combinations of these to provide fusion or an articulating shoulder. Most surgeons who are adept with shoulder resection prefer a

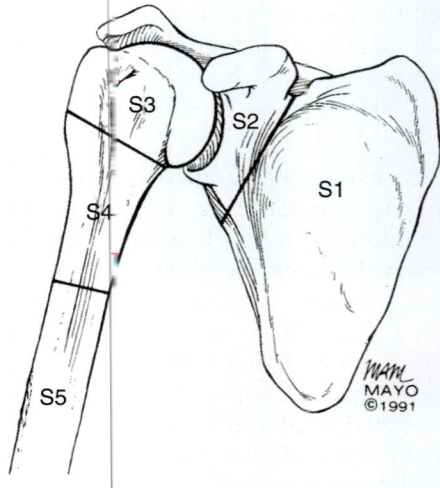

FIGURE 2 Illustration of the Musculoskeletal Tumor Society classification of skeletal resections about the shoulder girdle. At least one-half of the region must be resected to be so designated. S1 = the blade or spine of the scapula, S2 = the acromion-glenoid cavity complex (the glenoid cavity must be removed), S3 = the proximal epiphysis of the humerus, S4 = the proximal metaphysis of the humerus, and S5 = the proximal part of the diaphysis of the humerus. (Used with permission of Mayo Foundation for Education and Research, all rights reserved.)

stable fusion for a young laborer and a mobile endoprosthetic or allograft prosthetic composite for an older individual.

Forequarter or Interscapulothoracic Amputation

Indications

The indications for forequarter amputations are soft-tissue sarcoma arising in the axilla beneath the pectoral muscle or the scapula with adherence to the chest wall, osteosarcoma and high-grade chondrosarcoma with extension into the axilla and invading the brachial plexus and the great vessels, and primary tumors arising in the chest wall and involving structures of the thoracic inlet or the axilla.[12,14,22-24] Case reports of mycosis fungoides illustrate that proximal amputation can be necessary in life-threatening infections of the upper extremity. Palliation of malignant carcinoma, where plexopathy is intolerable, can also be an indication. Finally, trauma and electrical injury can produce defects and contamination so large that forequarter amputation becomes necessary.[11]

Technique

Forequarter amputation is the preferred ablative procedure for extensive tumor or infection in which invasion of the brachial plexus, the chest wall, or the axilla makes shoulder disarticulation impossible (**Figure 3**). This amputation uses anterior-based or posterior-based local flaps. If forequarter amputation is indicated, the flap often is determined by pathology, and the surgical procedure is an adaptation of both anterior-based and posterior-based flaps; however, a bias for one or the other often exists. Most forequarter amputations can be performed by fashioning a posterior skin flap, although an anterior flap is an alternative.[16,24] The surgical procedure revolves around whether ligation of the subclavian artery and the brachial plexus is managed anteriorly by osteotomy of the clavicle or posteriorly after dividing the muscles from the medial and superior scapula, which facilitates identification of the neurovascular structures through traction and allows ligation from within. The author of this chapter prefers a modification of the two approaches, whereby a posterior full-thickness skin flap is fashioned, but the subclavian vessels and the plexus are managed anteriorly. Before the procedure begins, it should be determined if there is need for free tissue rather than skin graft over viable muscle. This is necessary because the vascularity for a distal filet flap must be preserved when proximal dissection is performed, making subclavian ligation the last step performed before the limb is delivered to the back table.

The patient is positioned in the sloppy lateral decubitus position with a beanbag pliable enough to allow bias anteriorly and posteriorly (by manually tilting the patient over the bag) as the amputation proceeds. If multiple assistants are not available, a limb positioning system often is helpful in keeping the limb elevated and under tension to facilitate dissection (**Figure 4**).

Incision

Skin flaps are marked along the bony prominence of the clavicle and the scapular spine to allow elevation of the posterior flap from the glenohumeral articulation to the medial border of the scapula. The large teardrop exposure outline begins with an anterior limb that centers on the middle third of the clavicle. The posterior incision traverses the lateral acromion full thickness to fascia overlying the latissimus dorsi, the trapezius, and the infraspinatus. The two incisions meet deep in the axilla based on the patient's pathophysiology.

Deep Dissection

The sternocleidomastoid and deltoid muscles are elevated off the middle third of the clavicle, and the middle third is osteotomized with a saw. The subclavius muscle is identified and transected to reveal the subclavian artery and the brachial plexus. The subclavian artery is isolated but not ligated if distal harvesting of spare parts will be necessary; otherwise, the author of this chapter controls and quickly ligates the artery and vein and proceeds to nerve identification and transection. Nerve transection is done sharply, but the perineural ends are tagged with polydioxanone suture in the event TMR is an option and to facilitate the placement of intraoperative neural catheters. After the brachial plexus has been ligated, attention is turned to the posterior limb. From the full-thickness skin flap that was created, the medial border of the scapula is identified; an Israel retractor can pull the large posterior flap toward the midline, and a bone hook can be used to put tension on the scapula. The trapezius, rhomboid, and levator muscles are divided to reveal the subscapularis muscle covering the scapula. Next, the medial angle muscles are released from the medial scapula in the following order: the latissimus dorsi and trapezius superficially, followed by the deep rhomboid and levator scapulae muscles. This is best accomplished with a Bovie electrocautery to manage the periscapular plexus. Care is taken to identify and ligate the branches of the transverse cervical and scapular arteries coursing around the scapula. The serratus muscles are then divided by pulling the scapula posterolaterally with a bone hook to reveal the subscapularis and place the forelimb on stretch. After this is complete, there is usually only the need to ligate the suprascapular fossa and the anterior trapezius, which are ligated several centimeters away from the tumor. The axillary incisions are then connected, and the limb is delivered to the back table. The pectoral fascia is sewn to the trapezial and the rhomboid fascia after large suction drains (18 French round or pediatric chest tubes) are placed inferoaxillary and cervicoscapularly, in line with the incisions, with one under the pectoral muscles and one in line with the vertebral dissection. Incisional negative-pressure wound dressings are used, and a large, well-padded circumferential elastic compressive wrap is applied.

Posterior Vascular Isolation With an Anterior Flap

Posterior vascular isolation with an anterior flap is also known as the Littlewood technique.[15] The patient is positioned in a sloppy lateral decubitus position on a beanbag. The clavicle and the scapula are marked, and the clavicle becomes the basis for the skin incisions. First, a full-thickness skin and subcutaneous incision begins along the medial border of the scapula and runs the length of this bone along the superior margin, over the top of the accordion, and finally proceeds distally along the posterolateral acromion. The distal limb is in line with the surgical neck of the scapula and continues distally along the axillary border of the scapula to the distal angle, where the incision is curved medial to a point approximately 5 cm from the midline of the back. Next, the posterior incision is directed anteriorly to meet the anterior incision in the axilla. The anterior incision is then started along the medial border of the clavicle and runs laterally to the deltopectoral groove, where it runs just lateral but in line with this relationship. The skin incision is then curved inferiorly along the pectoral border in the axilla to meet

Section 2: Upper Limb

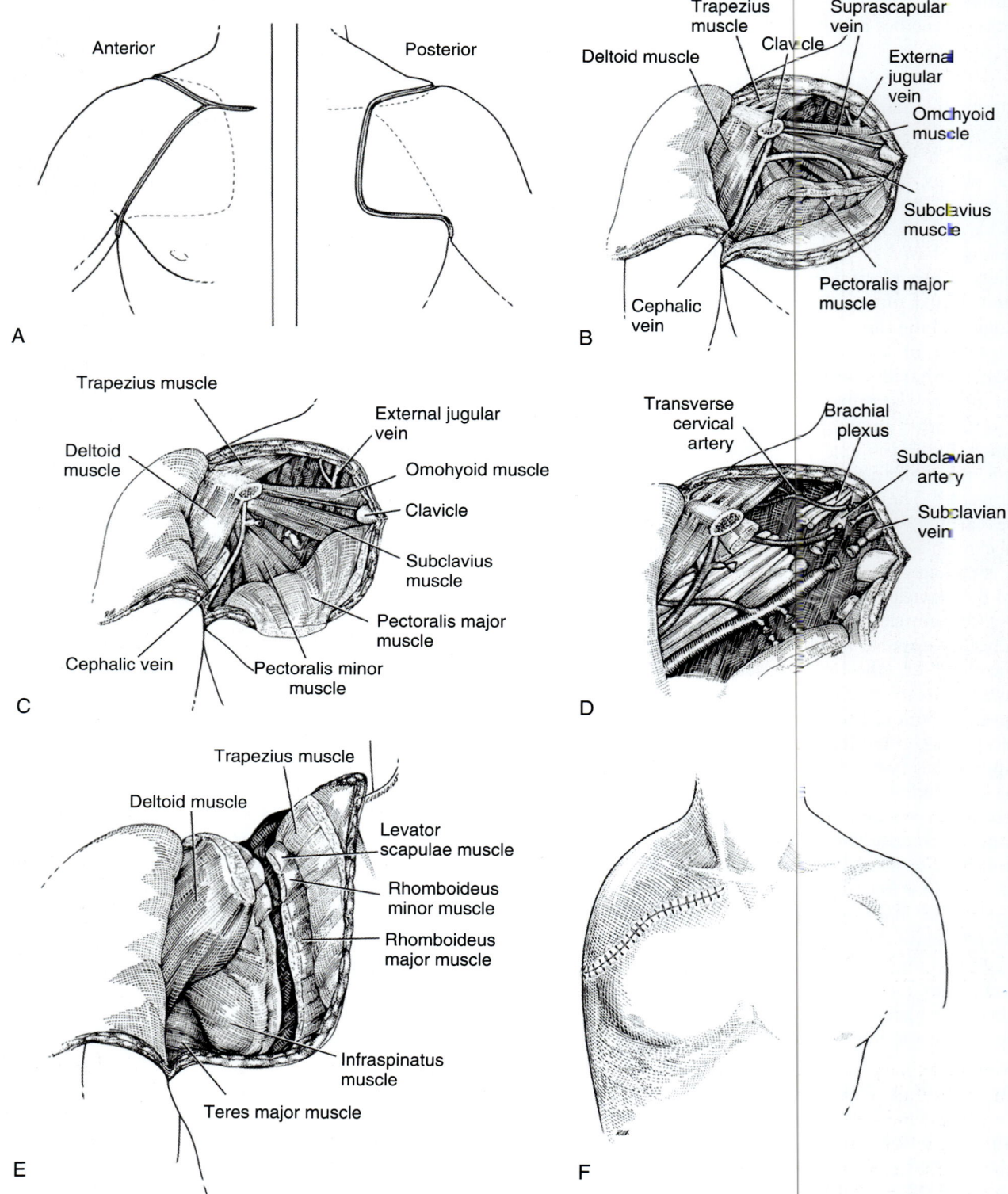

FIGURE 3 Illustrations of anterior vascular exposure with a posterior-based flap. **A**, Skin incision. **B**, Clavicle resection. **C**, Lifting the pectoralis major muscle. **D**, Section of the vessels and nerves after transecting the subclavius. **E**, Section of the medial scapular muscles. **F**, Closure. (Reproduced with permission from Tooms RE: Amputations of the upper extremity, in Crenshaw AH, ed: *Campbell's Operative Orthopaedics*, ed 8. Mosby-Year Book, 1992, pp 771-721.)

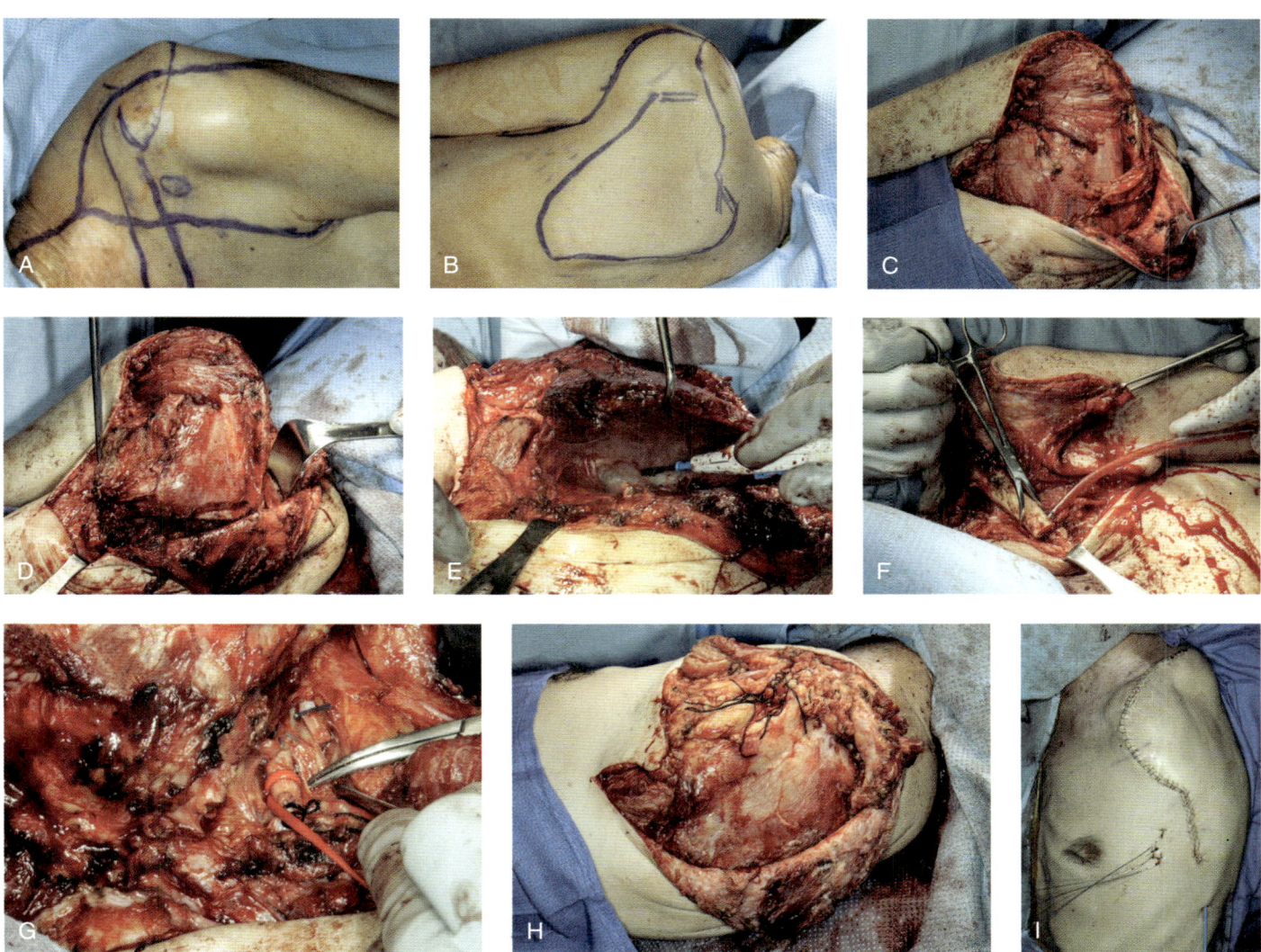

FIGURE 4 Intraoperative photographs of anterior vascular exposure with a posterior-based flap. The incisions are outlined anteriorly (**A**) and posteriorly (**B**), and dissection can proceed either medially over the middle clavicle or posteriorly over the scapular flap based on the preference of the surgeon. **C** and **D**, When the tumor is not encasing the vessels, the posterior flap is created, and posteromedial dissection is done first because this is often the most tedious part of the procedure. **E**, After the posteromedial angle has been elevated away from vertebral remnant muscles along the medial scapula, most of the scapular blood supply and the suprascapular neurovascular bundle can be visualized by pulling dorsally on the scapula. **F**, The clavicular osteotomy is performed. With most of the procedure completed and the limb still vascularized, spare parts can be harvested if required. **G**, The subclavian artery is controlled and ligated, with the plexus in view. **H**, Silk ties are placed before cleanup to help identify structures that will require nerve catheter inlay. **I**, Closure before application of the wound vacuum, with nerve catheters emanating from the skin.

the posterior axillary incision. The surgeon must carefully create a large full-thickness skin and subcutaneous flap to the fascia, which has been elevated medially off the scapular muscles to 1 cm medial of the medial border of the scapula, and a clavipectoral flap. This flap can include the pectoral muscles if the tumor is biased much posteriorly.

Release of the medial angle muscles proceeds in the manner described for a forequarter amputation, with the same technique used to divide the serratus muscles. Blunt dissection is next carried to the omohyoid and subclavius muscles, which are divided under direct visualization. Soft tissue is bluntly freed from the undersurface of the clavicle, and the forelimb is placed under tension by an anterolaterally directed moment to put the plexus and subclavian vessels on stretch.

The vessels are double ligated, and the plexus trunks are divided sharply after tagging each separately for TMR or intraoperative intraneural catheters. The pectoral muscles are then divided, and the limb is removed to the back table. The pectoral fascia is sewn to trapezial and rhomboid fascia after large suction drains are placed inferoaxillary and cervicoscapularly in line with the incisions, one under

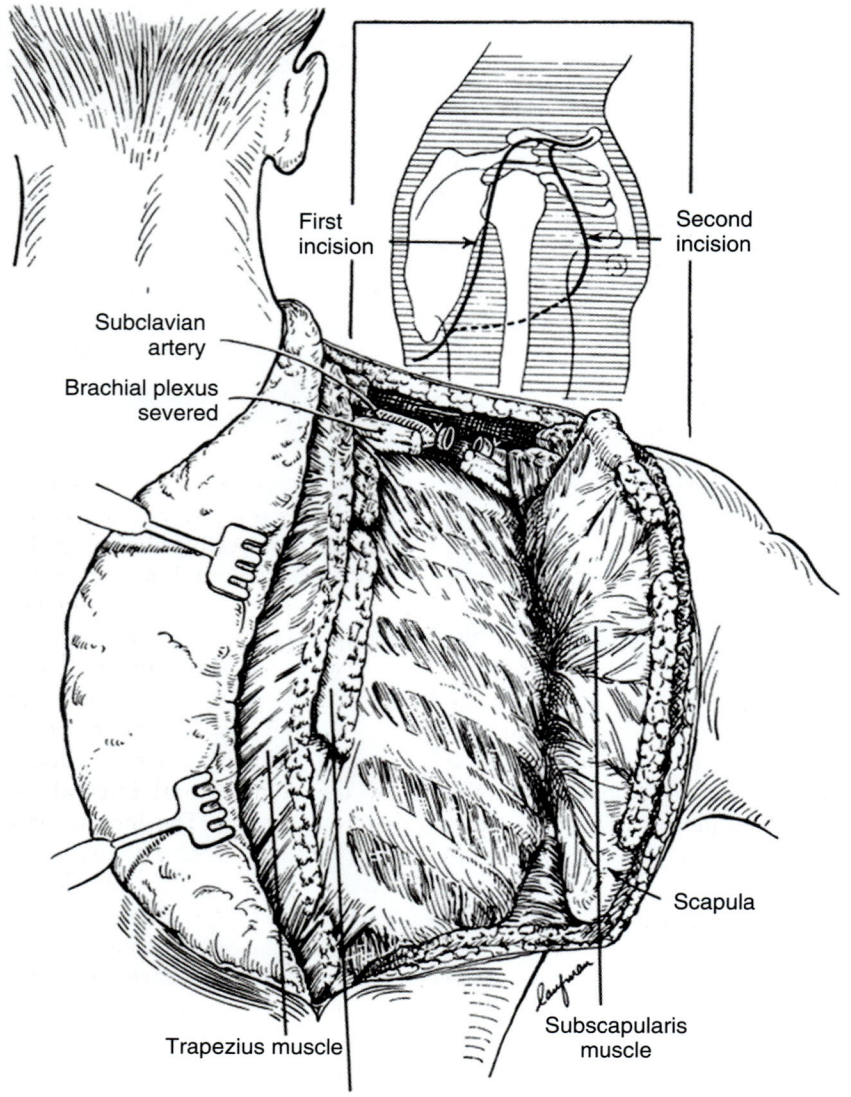

FIGURE 5 Illustration of the posterior vascular access forequarter amputation based on an anterior flap. The skin incision is brought more medial on the dorsal limb and more lateral anteriorly. The dissection proceeds posterior to anterior under the scapula while placing the arm in adduction and internal rotation to bring the scapula into chicken wing prominence. (Reproduced with permission from Tooms RE: Amputations of the upper extremity, in Crenshaw AH, ed: *Campbell's Operative Orthopaedics*, ed 8. Mosby-Year Book, 1992, pp 711-721.)

the pectoral muscles and one in line with the vertebral dissection (**Figures 5** and **6**). Patients with large, posterior high-grade sarcomas require an anterior flap. Incisional negative-pressure wound dressings are used, and a large, well-padded circumferential elastic compressive wrap is applied.

Exploration of the Anterior Cervical Triangle

Either vascular management or a skin flap swung superiorly can be used to facilitate exploration of the cervical triangle; however, it is preferable to plan a teardrop incision with a posterior flap and anterior vascular management when cervical triangle management is required. The sternocleidomastoid muscle is divided as it inserts along the clavicle and the junction between the internal jugular vein and the subclavian vein. The trunks of the brachial plexus are exposed and divided. Cervical lymph nodes are dissected, ligated, and sent to pathology to verify clear margins and to aid in deciding if brachytherapy or external beam adjuvant therapy is needed. The internal jugular vein and the common carotid artery are inspected for humeral invasion and reconstruction as necessary.[25]

En Bloc Chest Wall Excision

The thoracic entry interspace is chosen distal enough to allow cephalic mobilization and removal of tumor from structures to be preserved. Posterior ribs are divested of periosteum longitudinally, and the neuromuscular bundles are ligated beneath. Ribs are divided with a saw, rib cutters, or a Gigli saw, and the chest wall is opened wide with rib spreaders. The lung parenchyma is then inspected for pulmonary metastases. If the lung is the solitary site of metastases and the metastases are localized, they can be resected with wide local excision to preserve viable lung tissue. The surgeon should then reach as cephalad as possible around the lung with the other hand in the cervical triangle to assess for thoracic inlet metastases or to control midline bleeding in patients with traumatic injury.[14]

If a portion of the chest wall is to be removed with the forelimb, a median sternotomy is required, and the posterior chest wall dissection is thereby connected to the anterior chest wall block. Internal mammary vessels are ligated at the lowest interspace, and the sternum is split with a saw to the corresponding level. The medial clavicle is divested of remaining soft tissues superiorly because the medial clavicle will need to be removed after the sternotomy to facilitate identification of the first rib. Finally, the first rib is skeletonized with the electrocautery as it attaches to the manubrium. The strap, sternohyoid, and sternothyroid muscles are divided to expose

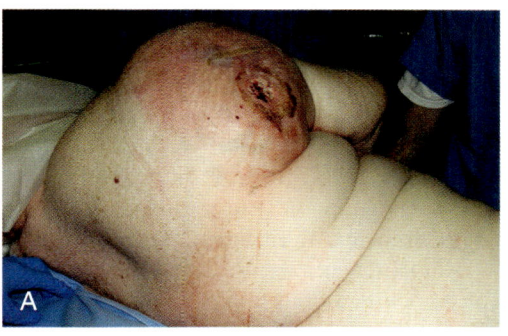 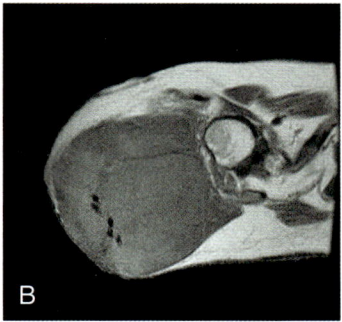 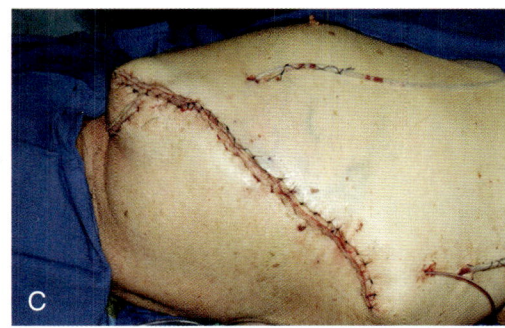

FIGURE 6 **A**, Photograph of a large, high-grade pleomorphic sarcoma of the right shoulder. Necrosis of the skin and subcutaneous tissue can be seen. **B**, T1-weighted magnetic resonance image of the tumor. Note the very large feeder vessels as the dark flow voids and the tumor comprising most of the deltoid. **C**, Photograph shows the shoulder area after closure. The patient was treated with a forequarter amputation with an anterior flap.

the innominate vein. The trunk of the subclavian artery and vein that were ligated during the forelimb ablation are traced medial to their junction with the vertebral artery and then double ligated again; this is best accomplished by dissecting the artery and the vein from within the thorax. At this point, this chapter's author prefers to leave the cords of the brachial plexus long to the trunk level for TMR, even if the chest wall is to be resected. The medial and posterior scalene muscles are then divided to complete the chest wall resection. If the tumor is on the left side, care must be taken to preserve the left vagus and phrenic nerves and ligate the thoracic duct. Chest tubes are placed. The chest wall is reconstructed with a polymethyl methacrylate polypropylene mesh plate.

Adjuncts for Coverage

Usually, substantial defects can be managed with local or regional flaps; however, large posterior exophytic tumors, radiation fibrosis, and chest wall or rib invasion preclude local coverage. Free tissue transfer is the only option in these instances. This can be accomplished in a separate procedure by elaborating the contralateral latissimus dorsi muscle and skin grafting after a rest interval with negative-pressure vacuum wound therapy. A modified, free forearm filet flap with healthy, well-vascularized, nonirradiated tissue for coverage is another option. Cordeiro et al[16] described use of the volar musculature with fasciocutaneous extensions based on the brachial artery and a single vein. In their series, the flap size averaged 25 × 30 cm, and the pedicle ranged from 10 to 15 cm, easily tying into the subclavian, innominate, or carotid arteries. Most of the amputation is performed with the subclavian vessels isolated but intact and the distal limb still perfused. Fasciocutaneous flaps are raised in the subfascial plane on the dorsum of the forearm. After the extensor carpi ulnaris is reached medially and the first dorsal compartment is reached laterally, dissection is carried to bone subperiosteally and beneath all of the flexor muscles. Distally, the median and ulnar nerves along with the radial and ulnar arteries are ligated at the wrist. Proximally, everything is divided at the elbow, and the interosseous vessel is identified and ligated as it leaves the radial artery. The brachial pedicle is dissected proximal to the flap in the utilitarian medial arm exposure, at a length dictated by the amputation. This technique is an extremely effective approach for patients with very poor soft-tissue envelopes.[16,17,26]

Modified and True Shoulder Disarticulation

Because of improved body symmetry and prosthetic fitting, the ultrashort transhumeral amputation is preferred over a true shoulder disarticulation or a forequarter amputation (**Figure 7**). A short residual limb can provide the prosthetist with the necessary surface area for fitting a device that uses voluntary motion to actuate an externally powered gripper, and it is extremely powerful when paired with TMR. Differentiation of anterior, middle, and posterior deltoid signals is possible, providing three sites for myoelectric control. When available, the chevron flap with deltoid muscle and regional skin is projected for coverage. The typical skin incisions follow the deltopectoral interval to the deltoid insertion. The incision is then curved bluntly over the lateral arm to the posterior deltoid border. The incision is then carried proximally to the deltoid-latissimus dorsi junction.

After a full-thickness incision has been made to fascia in all planes, the initial dissection proceeds in the standard deltopectoral interval, which is familiar to most surgeons. The anterior deltoid conjoined tendon with the pectoral muscles is then identified and transected, and a Bovie electrocautery is used to elaborate the broad deltoid insertion off the humerus from anterior to posterior. The latissimus dorsi is divided off the humerus, and both the latissimus dorsi and the pectoralis major are tagged for later reattachment.

Attention is then turned to the brachial vessels, which are quickly located by reaching into the proximal anterior incision and using a cautery to cut the conjoined tendon of the coracobrachialis. The author of this chapter then identifies the length of the vascular pedicle necessary to perfuse deltoid skin or provide an easy docking site for

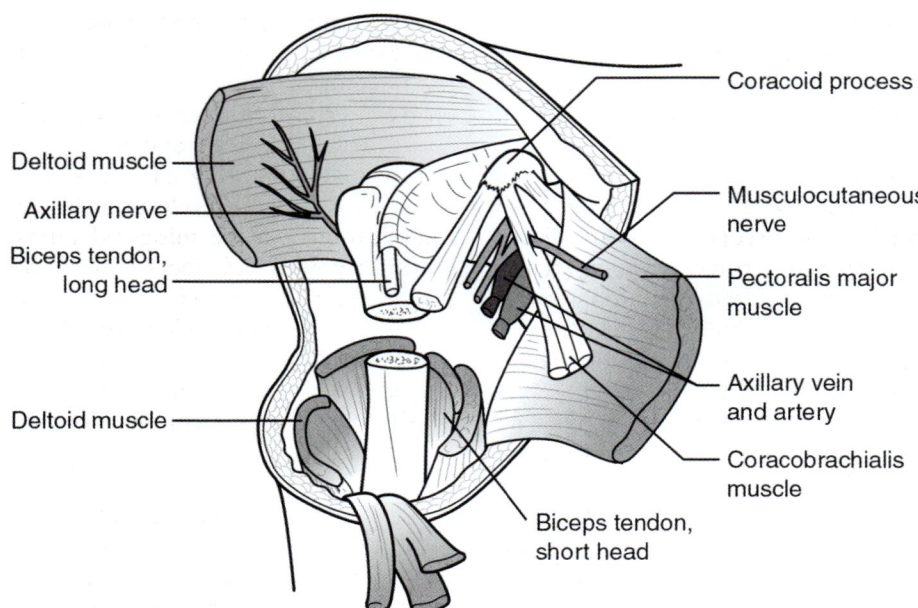

FIGURE 7 Illustration of a modified shoulder disarticulation skin incision with a traditional chevron flap. The deltoid is elevated, the rotator cuff is left intact, and the humerus is transected at the surgical neck. The latissimus dorsi and pectoralis muscles are suture imbricated into the residual humerus for balanced adduction and abduction.

a filet flap in the event of catastrophic trauma or exophytic tumor invasion of the deltoid region. The nerves of the brachial plexus are identified and cut sharply with a No. 10 blade and allowed to retract under tension after being tagged with polydioxanone suture if TMR becomes an option. The humerus is osteotomized with a saw at the level of the surgical neck. Much like the adductor myodesis of the transhumeral amputation, careful attention must be paid to reattaching the pectoral and deltoid muscles. The rotator cuff attachments on the humerus are maintained with the procedure, and the residual humerus will abduct and externally rotate. Careful balancing can be achieved by transferring and tensioning the latissimus dorsi and pectoralis muscles as well as splitting the trapezius if necessary. If the soft tissues have been stripped by traumatic injury or sacrificed because of tumor, arthrodesis with AO 7.3-mm cannulated screws into the glenoid is still preferable for contouring compared with excision of the proximal fragment. This is necessary more times than not due to the abduction and external rotation of the remnant in cases where the rotator cuff is preserved.

If it becomes necessary to perform a true shoulder disarticulation, most of the surgical procedures proceed as previously described. After the deltoid myocutaneous flap has been dissected off the lateral two-thirds of the humerus, the pectoral muscle is resected and tagged for reattachment into the glenoid. The coracobrachialis tendon is isolated with a right-angled forceps and transected to provide access to the axillary brachial artery takeoff and the brachial plexus. The axillary artery is double ligated, and the individual components of the brachial plexus are transected sharply after tagging with polydioxanone suture for later identification if TMR is an option. The shoulder capsule is placed on stretch, and the anterior joint space is entered, allowing direct inside-to-outside division of the superior, inferior, and posterior capsule to deliver the limb. The pectoralis major and latissimus dorsi are then sutured to the rotator cuff and the capsule remnants to fill the glenoid. No ablation of the glenoid cartilaginous surface is necessary, but a taut sling with remaining soft tissues is paramount to avoid a painful bursa that can develop if the envelope is mobile and floppy. Suture anchors to secure the dead space are helpful in avoiding this complication.

The deltoid fascia is secured to the axillary fascia over an anterior and posterior drain in line with the skin incisions, and an incisional negative-pressure vacuum wound dressing is applied. A compressive shoulder dressing is fashioned with either a circumferential elastic wrap or a commercially available fabric hook-and-loop fastener shoulder wrap dressing.

If the deltoid is not available for coverage, another secondary flap of the axillary skin and subcutaneous tissues is equally durable. This flap requires management of eccrine sweat glands and laser hair ablation. However, in most individuals, this added manipulation is a minor inconvenience compared with the durability of the axillary flap. If the axillary flap is used, two modifications to the ultrashort transhumeral amputation and the true shoulder disarticulation can be applied. The skin incision starts in the deltopectoral groove just under the clavicle, as in the chevron flap, and then is carried over the medial arm just over the cephalic vein. It traverses posteriorly toward the triceps at the level of the deltoid insertion and then courses superiorly along the posterior border of the deltoid and over the acromioclavicular joint to meet the deltopectoral limb. The whole deltoid is dropped inferolaterally by dissecting it along with lateral skin and likely tumor. The axillary/brachial artery is controlled as previously described, and the humerus is lifted laterally from the wound by dividing the supraspinatus and superior capsule sequentially anteriorly and posteriorly in the true shoulder disarticulation. If amenable, the humerus is osteotomized at the surgical neck. If the ultrashort transhumeral amputation is possible, which is usually unlikely if sacrifice of the deltoid is required, then the axillary soft tissues are sewn into the proximal incision. In the true shoulder disarticulation, where the deltoid is not available, the pectoralis and latissimus dorsi are brought into the gleaned fossa, and the accordion is osteotomized, as is the coracoid process if needed to contour the bony prominences. A compressive dressing is applied over an incisional negative-pressure vacuum wound dressing and suction drains.

Postoperative Management

When possible, nerve catheters are placed in the perineurium under direct visualization to facilitate postoperative regional anesthesia. Large-caliber suction drains are used to evacuate the dead space and emanate from the skin in line with incisions in the event a tumor margin is positive and requires reexcision. Gabapentin is given the morning of surgery preoperatively and continued postoperatively, titrating to a dose of 30 mg three times per day. Amitriptyline (25 mg) is started the night of surgery and titrated to 50 mg at bedtime. Patients are monitored in the intensive care unit (overnight at a minimum) because the neuromodulators often can be sedating and care must be taken to avoid oversedation. An incisional negative-pressure wound dressing is applied in the surgical suite and removed on postoperative day 5. Compressive elastic wraps are applied in a circumferential fashion to prevent hematoma or seroma. Desensitization therapy is started on postoperative day 2, and mirror therapy is added as soon as the patient is discharged to a regular monitoring protocol.

Complications

Current developments in transfusion practices, the use of local and intravenous hemostatic agents, and improvements in surgical critical care have considerably reduced the morbidity and mortality of shoulder disarticulations and forequarter amputations.[5] However, the life span of many of these patients is often short because of the disease processes that necessitated the proximal upper limb amputation. Major complications are common, and every effort should be made to prevent them. Complications can be divided into the following groups: early postoperative, near-term oncologic, and long-term body asymmetry and prosthetic.

Early complications include cardiopulmonary and wound issues. Infection at the wound site should be managed aggressively, and every effort should be made to prevent hematoma or seroma formation. The incisional negative-pressure wound dressing is removed after 5 days, but the deep suction drains should be maintained until the effluent is less than 30 mL per shift (usually 8 hours) for a 24-hour period. Skin edge and flap necrosis is always a possibility in preoperatively irradiated wounds, and perioperative hyperbaric oxygen therapy should be considered for any wound (preexisting, postoperative, or fibrosis resulting from radiation) at risk of infection.

Phantom limb sensations and nerve-related pain must be managed aggressively by an occupational therapy team experienced in caring for patients with upper limb amputations. An aggressive regional anesthesia team aids in this process. If wound complications are eminent, every effort should be made for early provision of regional or free-oxygenated tissue in the form of contralateral latissimus dorsi or rectus abdominis free flaps to expedite wound healing and enable the patient to resume chemotherapy. A chronic draining wound requires aggressive treatment, and alternative coverage is vital to prevent severe complications.

Near-term oncologic complications include local recurrence and metastases or repeat infection in a patient with a prior life-threatening infection. These complications can be mitigated intraoperatively with wide local excision of lesions. At times, when a completely clear margin is impossible to obtain or local recurrence is a substantial risk, careful consideration should be given to adjuvant treatment with brachytherapy or postoperative external beam radiation.

Late complications include high shoulder in a patient with a proximal upper limb amputation, postural scoliosis, and issues with prosthesis wear (**Figure 8**). The normal upright posture of a patient with a forequarter amputation is inhibited by a lack of scapulothoracic tension, muscle imbalance, and the lack of arm weight. The patient lists to the uninvolved side because the unopposed tension of the muscles that normally elevate the forelimb acts

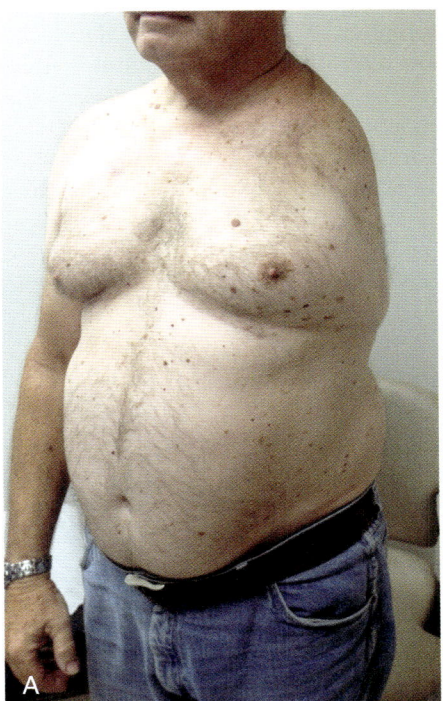
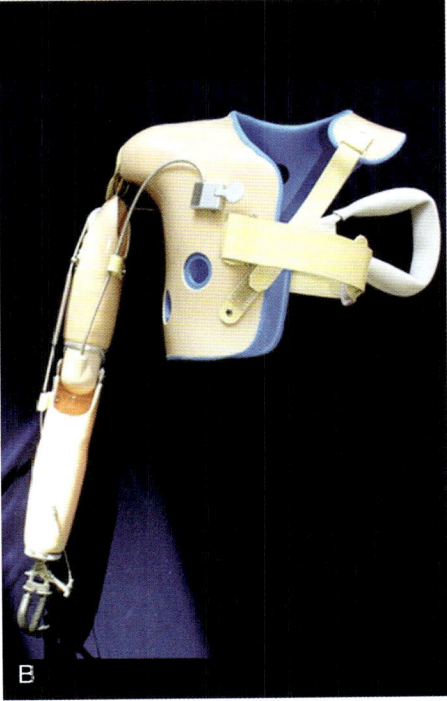

FIGURE 8 **A**, Clinical photograph of a patient with a forequarter amputation 3 years after the procedure. Slight postural scoliosis and a high shoulder can be seen. **B**, Photograph of a body-capture forequarter prosthesis. Despite the modern design, many patients elect not to use such a prosthesis because of its bulk.

against the weight of the arm.[27] For this reason, postural physical therapy is started immediately in conjunction with desensitization and mirror therapies to combat body asymmetry issues. Postural scoliosis is problematic, especially in patients with skeletal immaturity. Postural asymmetry can often lead to scoliosis and occipital headaches caused by prosthesis wear, contralateral trapezial tension, and ipsilateral unopposed shoulder elevators.[27] Every effort should be made to facilitate an early and aggressive multidisciplinary physical therapy approach.

Limb Salvage Alternatives to Shoulder-Level Disarticulation

Many limb salvage techniques avoid shoulder disarticulation;[13,15,23,28-30] however, it may be difficult to match the pathology to the indicated technique. Approximately 90% of tumors about the shoulder and the periscapular region can be managed with limb salvage.[2] In patients with infection or tumor, the risk of local recurrence should be weighed against the benefits of limb salvage. In cases of trauma, the functionality of the reconstructed limb and the patient's quality of life must be weighed against the psychological benefit of definitive amputation surgery.

Indications for limb salvage include a viable soft-tissue envelope distal to the shoulder with normal nerve function below the elbow or the ability to perform tendon transfers to augment specified functions. With modern techniques, these so-called internal amputations are extremely viable procedures and result in improved quality of life compared with amputation. In a study by Wada et al,[30] the internal amputation or shoulder resection group achieved a mean Musculoskeletal Tumor Society functional score between 68% and 72%. The limiting factor in any reconstruction after shoulder-level resection is the amount of abductor present, which is dependent on contracting the trapezius and sliding the remaining scapula over the chest wall. Distal grip is usually maintained, but limb girdle strength is substantially compromised. Several limb salvage techniques are available for the treatment of patients with catastrophic soft-tissue and osseous loss if the distal motor nerves are preserved (**Figures 9** and **10**).

Tikhoff-Linberg Resection

The en bloc upper humeral interscapulothoracic resection, also known as the Tikhoff-Linberg procedure, is the basis for limb salvage in patients with catastrophic loss of the shoulder (**Figure 11**). The Malawar classification system aids in understanding the defects and planning reconstruction. Generally, reconstruction after resection takes the form of arthrodesis, endoprosthetic replacement, osteoarticular allograft, and autogenous grafts, such as the autograft fibula or clavicle pro humeri.[31,32] The prerequisites for the procedure are that the tumor does not extend into the axillary neuromuscular bundle, the chest wall, or the lymphatic system.[22]

Patients are positioned in the sloppy lateral decubitus position, but some physicians prefer to slightly jackknife the bed with a reverse Trendelenburg position to facilitate an almost sideways beach chair posture. This position readily facilitates the Mercedes incision that is often required to better visualize tumors of the shoulder while facilitating preservation of the axillary/brachial medial arm contents and periscapular dissection. The initial limb of the incision starts longitudinally over the suprascapular fossa and branches just proximal to the acromioclavicular joint to the anterior and posterior limbs. The anterior limb approximates the deltopectoral approach to the shoulder, with the exception that the coracoid process is osteotomized early or the conjoined tendon is cut to deliver the axillary neuromuscular bundle. The anterior incision is carried distally as far as necessary to facilitate a humeral transection at least 2 cm away from the tumor. After the dissection has projected the medial arm structures, it is usually possible for the surgeon to reach laterally and anteriorly over the humerus to the

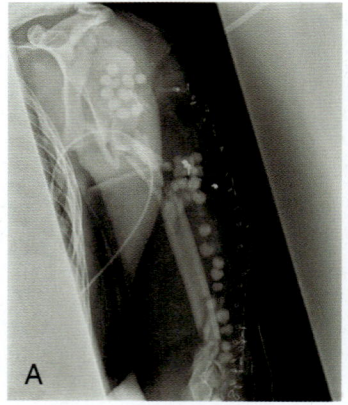 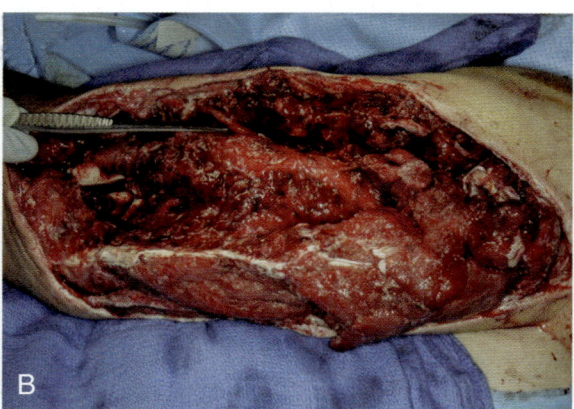 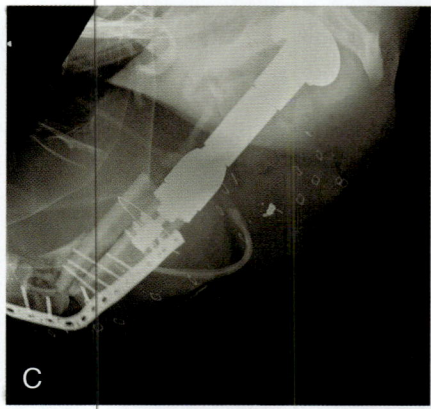

FIGURE 9 Images from a soldier who was injured by a high-velocity gunshot, resulting in massive proximal humerus, deltoid, and elbow loss. **A**, Preoperative AP radiograph of the left arm. The gunshot wound was débrided and irrigated several times during the patient's evacuation from the combat area. Antibiotic beads were placed in an effort to prevent infection and achieve limb salvage. **B**, Intraoperative photograph of the arm. Note the excellent muscle bed and attachment to major humeral fragments. The forceps is pointing to the identified and protected radial nerve. **C**, Perioperative oblique radiograph of the upper limb after reconstruction with a tumor endoprosthesis, elbow fusion, and a free innervated latissimus dorsi flap.

interval between the biceps and the brachialis to identify and protect the radial nerve.

Attention is then turned to the posterior limb of the incision, which curves posterolaterally over the surgical neck of the scapula. Through this incision, it is possible to mobilize a massive posterior soft-tissue envelope for a complete scapulectomy alone or in combination with extracapsular humeral resection (Malawar type III or VI). After the brachial artery and the plexus have been protected and the periscapular muscles have been sectioned, the deltoid and trapezius are cauterized in a manner that allows safe delivery of the tumor proximally. A partial scapulectomy usually does not need to be reconstructed. The abductors are retained; however, most of the other resections will combine proximal humeral replacement with scapular reconstruction.

If a Malawar type I or V resection is being performed, the preferred method of reconstruction is an allograft composite reverse total shoulder with glenoid allograft. Other methods include an intercalary spacer with dowel into the clavicle, endoprosthetic proximal humeral replacement with polyethylene terephthalate aortic graft to reconstruct the capsule, or osteoarticular allograft. If a total resection of both the proximal humerus and the scapula (Malawar type VI) is required, a constrained or unconstrained humeroscapular prosthesis, which can have numerous complications, must be considered. The proximal humerus also can be reconstructed with an allograft prosthetic composite coupled to a scapular prosthesis.[29,30,33]

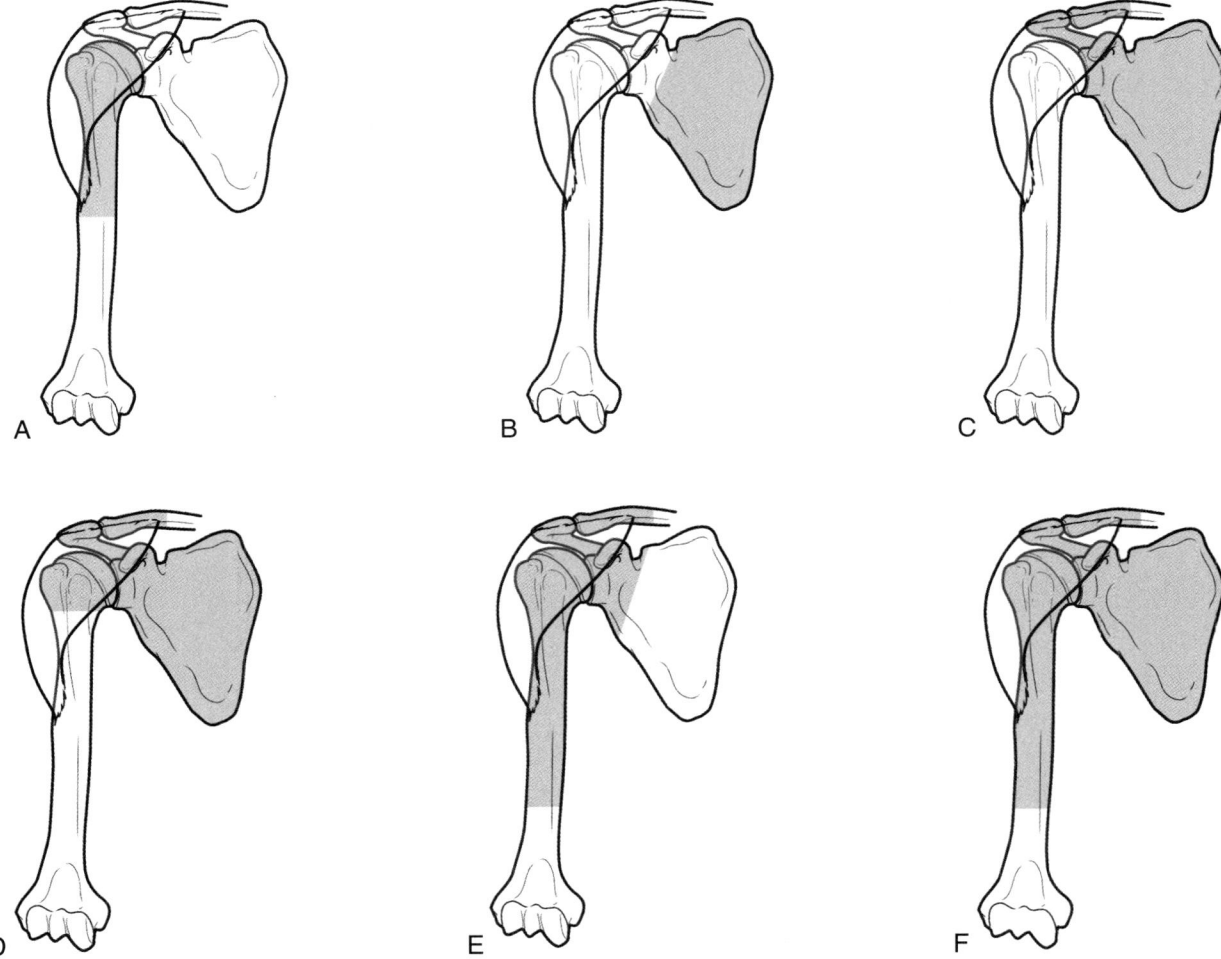

FIGURE 10 Illustrations of the Malawar classification for intercalary shoulder resections. The abductors can be retained or resected in each type of resection. **A**, Type I, intra-articular proximal humeral resection (shown, type I-A: abductors retained; not shown, type I-B: abductor resected). **B**, Type II, partial scapulectomy (shown, type II-A: abductors retained; not shown, type II-B: abductors resected). **C**, Type III, intra-articular total scapulectomy (shown, type III-A: abductors retained; not shown, type III-B: abductors resected). **D**, Type IV, extra-articular scapular and humeral head resection (shown, type IV-B: abductors resected; not shown, type IV-A: abductors retained). **E**, Type V, extra-articular humeral and glenoid resection (shown, type V-B: abductors resected; not shown, type V-A: abductors retained). **F**, Type VI, extra-articular humeral and total scapula resection (shown, type VI-B: abductors resected; not shown, type VI-A: abductors retained).

Section 2: Upper Limb

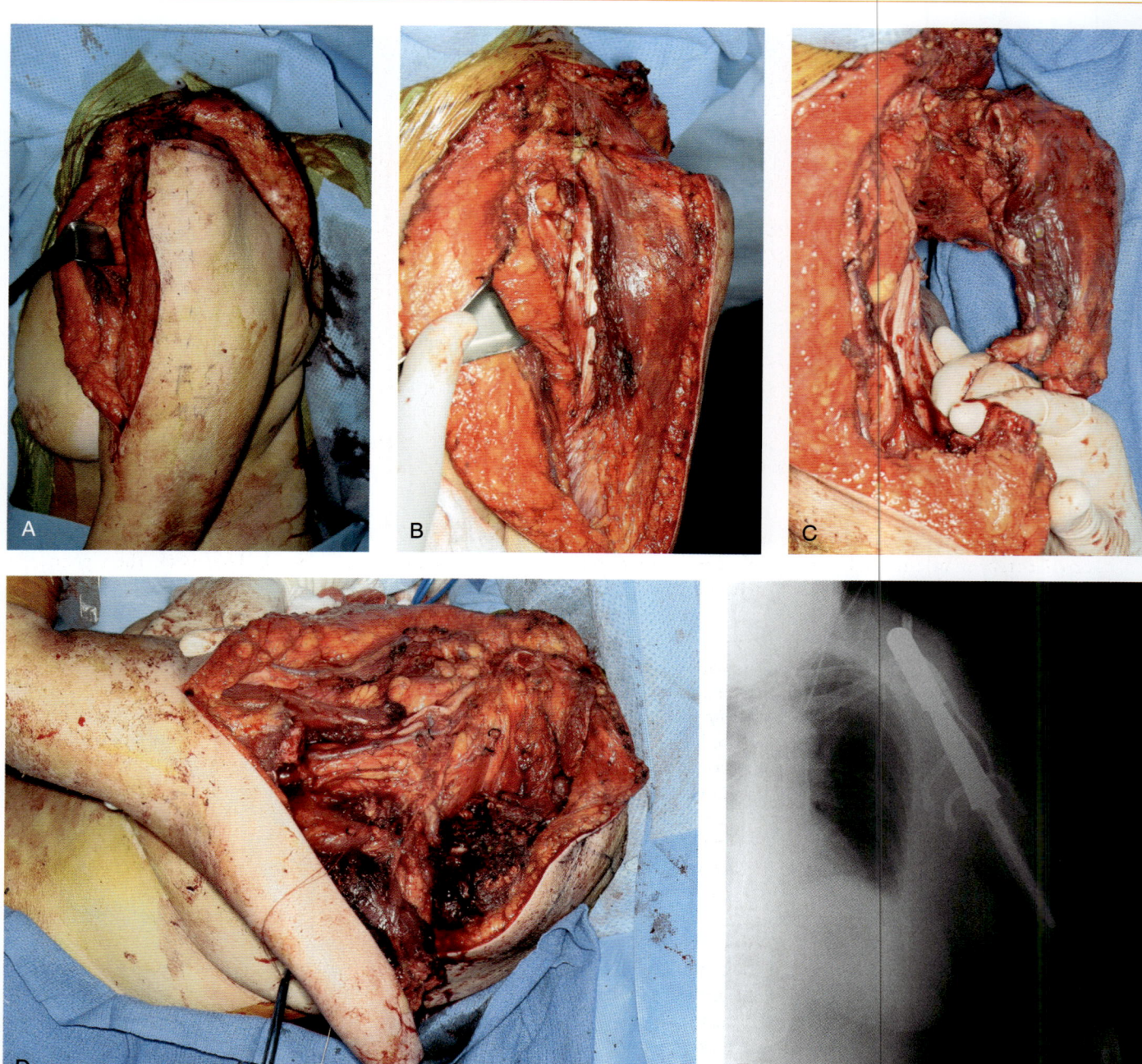

FIGURE 11 Images from a patient with dedifferentiated chondrosarcoma of the proximal humerus. **A**, Intraoperative photograph of a typical Mercedes incision for development of a Tikhoff-Linberg resection and reconstruction. The procedure involves the anterior limb for protection of the subclavian to axillary artery and brachial plexus, the posterior flap for dealing with the resection, and a longitudinal extension over the trapezius to facilitate exposure and later tension-free closure. **B**, Intraoperative photograph shows the proximal humerus and tumor contained with the deltoid. Because the tumor broke into the joint, a periscapular resection was needed. **C**, Intraoperative photograph shows exposure and osteotomy of the proximal humerus prior to resection. **D**, Posterior-superior intraoperative view of the scapular resection. **E**, Postoperative radiograph shows creation of a prosthetic pseudarthrosis, with suture tape placed through holes in the prosthesis to the chest wall for stability.

Scapulectomy

Scapulectomy is a shoulder-level resection alternative to amputation for rare indications mostly caused by a tumor involving only the scapula or infection that has so devitalized the periscapular soft tissues as to render the scapula unsalvageable. Syme[34] originally described his experience with the procedure in 1857 and discussed many of the same complications currently seen—major wound dehiscence and severe loss of strength in the shoulder girdle[25,35,36] (**Figure 12**).

The patient can be positioned either prone or lateral for this procedure; however, the author of this chapter prefers to drape the arm with the patient in

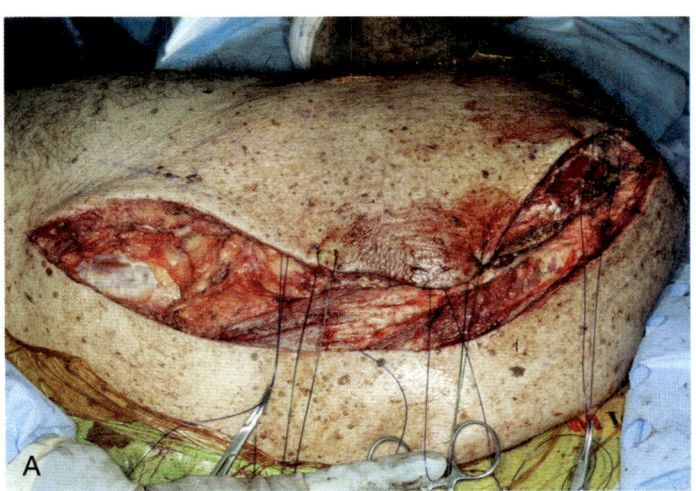 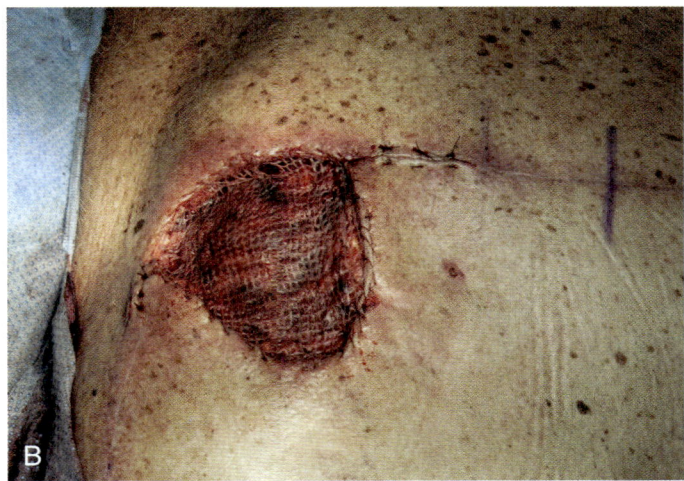

FIGURE 12 Intraoperative photographs of morbidity in a scapulectomy after radiation. Medial angle flap necrosis necessitated a contralateral latissimus dorsi flap (**A**) and a split-thickness skin graft (**B**).

a prone position to facilitate adduction and internal rotation of the limb and to bring the inferior angle of the scapula dorsally. The technique involves an incision that begins at the lateral edge of the acromion and follows in line with the Judet approach to scapular fixation.[36] The incision traverses medially to the medial angle and then courses distally to meet the inferior angle. The trapezius, rhomboid, and levator muscles are then transected, and the arm is brought into adduction and internal rotation behind the patient's back to deliver the inferior angle of the scapula. The inferior angle is then placed on tension with a bone hook, and the latissimus dorsi is transected. The dissection then continues along the subscapular space to its medial capsular extent. At this point, the supraspinatus, infraspinatus, and serratus muscles are divided, and the proximal trapezius is divided from the scapular spine and the acromion. Elevating the specimen dorsally then brings the brachial plexus and the axillary vessels into view and allows ligation of the superficial cervical, descending scapular, and suprascapular vessels and the suprascapular nerve. The acromioclavicular joint is then disarticulated, and the coracoclavicular joints are transected to allow delivery of the scapula. After the conjoined tendon is detached, the specimen is delivered to the back table. Soft-tissue remnants can then be used to stabilize the clavicle with a transosseous suture or suture anchors and, in a similar manner, stabilize the acromial remnant and create a deltoid suspension. The flaps are closed over a minimum of two drains, and the wound is covered with an incisional negative-pressure wound dressing with a compressive elastic wrap. The author of this chapter prefers to allow scar tissue to form for 7 to 14 days to minimize the risk of hematoma and seroma. Patients are asked to wear a compressive shoulder sleeve for 4 to 6 weeks.

Claviculectomy

Paratracheal, esophageal, and other neck malignancies are the usual indications for clavicular resections.[37] Occasionally, it will be necessary to perform a partial or complete resection of the clavicle for isolated chondrosarcoma of the clavicle or osteomyelitis after radiation for other neoplasms. The procedure is relatively simple, with an incision that follows the anterior border of the clavicle from the sternoclavicular joint to the acromioclavicular joint. Dissection begins medially by dividing the sternocleidomastoid muscles in a fashion that allows identification and protection of the external jugular vein. Next, the dissection proceeds laterally with transection of the trapezius and deltoid insertion on the superior clavicle. The acromioclavicular joint is then disarticulated, and the conoid and trapezoid ligaments are divided. The work then proceeds medially again under the clavicle; this is greatly facilitated by using a forceps to elevate the medial edge. This process usually brings the subclavius muscle into view, which often is resected with the tumor because the margin is usually very close along the subclavian artery and vein. The sternoclavicular joint is disarticulated, and the clavicle is removed. Dead space is mitigated by careful, layered closure over drains. No attempt is made to reconstruct the clavicular strut.[37] As with a scapulectomy, the author of this chapter prefers to allow scar tissue to form for 7 to 14 days; postural exercises are then started to emphasize rhomboid and periscapular strength to open up the thoracic outlet.

SUMMARY

Shoulder-level amputations are complex and challenging surgical procedures. To provide optimal patient care, the surgeon must understand the indications for such procedures along with limb salvage alternatives. Complications are frequent and often require creative solutions, including local or free flap coverage. Although these procedures entail loss of function and disfigurement, they offer the patient the potential for disease-free survival or recovery from a massive traumatic injury.

References

1. Ramly EP, MacFie R, Eshraghi N, Cole F, Engel D: Bowel necrosis and 3 limb amputation from high-voltage electrical injury. *J Burn Care Res* 2018;39(4):628-633.
2. O'Connor MI, Sim FH, Chao EY: Limb salvage for neoplasms of the shoulder girdle: Intermediate reconstructive and functional results. *J Bone Joint Surg Am* 1996;78(12):1872-1888.
3. Kuiken TA, Dumanian GA, Lipschutz RD, Miller LA, Stubblefield KA: The use of targeted muscle reinnervation for improved myoelectric prosthesis control in a bilateral shoulder disarticulation amputee. *Prosthet Orthot Int* 2004;28(3):245-253.
4. Flurry M, Melissinos EG, Livingston CK: Composite forearm free fillet flaps to preserve stump length following traumatic amputations of the upper extremity. *Ann Plast Surg* 2008;60(4):391-394.
5. Fanous N, Didolkar MS, Holyoke ED, Elias EG: Evaluation of forequarter amputation in malignant diseases. *Surg Gynecol Obstet* 1976;142(3):381-384.
6. Getty PJ, Peabody TD: Complications and functional outcomes of reconstruction with an osteoarticular allograft after intra-articular resection of the proximal aspect of the humerus. *J Bone Joint Surg Am* 1999;81(8):1138-1146.
7. Gibbons CL, Bell RS, Wunder JS, et al: Function after subtotal scapulectomy for neoplasm of bone and soft tissue. *J Bone Joint Surg Br* 1998;80(1):38-42.
8. Kiss J, Sztrinkai G, Antal I, Kiss J, Szendroi M: Functional results and quality of life after shoulder girdle resections in musculoskeletal tumors. *J Shoulder Elbow Surg* 2007;16(3):273-279.
9. Dumanian GA, Potter BK, Mioton LM, et al: Targeted muscle reinnervation treats neuroma and phantom pain in major limb amputees: A randomized clinical trial. *Ann Surg* 2019;270(2):238-246.
10. Alderete JF, Smith TS: Targeted muscle reinnervation in amputee care. *AAOS Now*, 2021.
11. Kuroiwa T, Kawano Y, Maeda A, et al: A case of open scapulothoracic dissociation with forequarter amputation. *JSES Int* 2021;5(5):846-849.
12. Alford WC Jr, Stephenson SE Jr: Traumatic forequarter amputation: A report of two cases. *J Trauma* 1965;5:547-553.
13. Ross AC, Wilson JN, Scales JT: Endoprosthetic replacement of the proximal humerus. *J Bone Joint Surg Br* 1987;69(4):656-661.
14. Roth JA, Sugarbaker PH, Baker AR: Radical forequarter amputation with chest wall resection. *Ann Thorac Surg* 1984;37(5):423-427.
15. Rödl RW, Gosheger G, Gebert C, Lindner N, Ozaki T, Winkelmann W: Reconstruction of the humerus after wide resection of tumours. *J Bone Joint Surg Br* 2002;84:1004-1008.
16. Cordeiro PG, Cohen S, Burt M, Brennan MF: The total volar forearm musculocutaneous free flap for reconstruction of extended forequarter amputations. *Ann Plast Surg* 1998;40(4):388-396.
17. Zachary LS, Gottlieb LJ, Simon M, Ferguson MK, Calkins E: Forequarter amputation wound coverage with an ipsilateral, lymphedematous, circumferential forearm fasciocutaneous free flap in patients undergoing palliative shoulder-girdle tumor resection. *J Reconstr Microsurg* 1993;9(2):103-107.
18. Enneking WF: A system of staging musculoskeletal neoplasms. *Clin Orthop Relat Res* 1986;204:9-24.
19. Enneking W, Dunham W, Gebhardt M, Malawar M, Pritchard D: A system for the classification of skeletal resections. *Chir Organi Mov* 1990;75(1 suppl):217-240.
20. Enneking WF, Dunham W, Gebhardt MC, Malawar M, Pritchard DJ: A system for the functional evaluation of reconstructive procedures after surgical treatment of tumors of the musculoskeletal system. *Clin Orthop Relat Res* 1993;286:241-246.
21. Kumar D, Grimer RJ, Abudu A, Carter SR, Tillman RM: Endoprosthetic replacement of the proximal humerus: Long-term results. *J Bone Joint Surg Br* 2003;85(5):717-722.
22. Marcove RC, Lewis MM, Huvos AG: En bloc upper humeral interscapulothoracic resection: The Tikhoff-Linberg procedure. *Clin Orthop Relat Res* 1977;124:219-228.
23. Voggenreiter G, Assenmacher S, Schmit-Neuerburg KP: Tikhoff-Linberg procedure for bone and soft tissue tumors of the shoulder girdle. *Arch Surg* 1999;134(3):252-257.
24. Linberg BE: Interscapulo-thoracic resection for malignant tumors of the shoulder joint region. *J Bone Joint Surg* 1928;10:344-349.
25. Nakamura S, Kusuzaki K, Murata H, et al: Clinical outcome of total scapulectomy in 10 patients with primary malignant bone and soft-tissue tumors. *J Surg Oncol* 1999;72(3):130-135.
26. Weiland AJ, Moore JR, Daniel RK: Vascularized bone autografts: Experience with 41 cases. *Clin Orthop Relat Res* 1983;174:87-95.
27. Smith DG: Amputations about the shoulder: Surgical management, in Smith DG, Michael JW, Bowker JH, eds: *Atlas of Amputations and Limb Deficiencies: Surgical, Prosthetic, and Rehabilitation Principles*, ed 3. American Academy of Orthopaedic Surgeons, 2004, pp 251-261.
28. Damron TA, Rock MG, O'Connor MI, et al: Functional laboratory assessment after oncologic shoulder joint resections. *Clin Orthop Relat Res* 1998;348:124-134.
29. De Wilde L, Sys G, Julien Y, Van Ovost E, Poffyn B, Trouilloud P: The reversed Delta shoulder prosthesis in reconstruction of the proximal humerus after tumour resection. *Acta Orthop Belg* 2003;69(6):495-500.
30. Wada T, Usui M, Isu K, Yamawakii S, Ishii S: Reconstruction and limb salvage after resection for malignant bone tumour of the proximal humerus: A sling procedure using a free vascularised fibular graft. *J Bone Joint Surg Br* 1999;81(5):808-813.
31. Capanna E, Giunti A, Biagini R, Ferruzzi A: Modular endoprosthesis for humerus and Tikhoff-Linberg resection, in Yamamuro T, ed: *New Developments for Limb Salvage in Musculoskeletal Tumors*. Springer, 1989, pp 547-555.
32. Clarke A, Dewnany G, Neumann L, Wallace WA: Glenothoracic fusion: An adjunct to radical scapulectomy. *J Bone Joint Surg Br* 2004;86(4):531-535.
33. Mankin HJ, Gebhardt MC, Jennings LC, Springfield DS, Tomford WW: Longterm results of allograft replacement in the management of bone tumors. *Clin Orthop Relat Res* 1996;324:86-97.
34. Syme J: On disarticulation of the scapula from the shoulder-joint. *Med Chir Trans* 1857;40:107-112.
35. Rodriguez JA, Craven JE, Heinrich S, Wilson S, Levine EA: Current role of scapulectomy. *Am Surg* 1999;65(12):1167-1170.
36. Das Gupta TK: Scapulectomy: Indications and technique. *Surgery* 1970;67(4):601-606.
37. Abbott LC, Lucas DB: The function of the clavicle: Its surgical significance. *Ann Surg* 1954;140(4):583-599.

Amputations About the Shoulder: Prosthetic Management

CHAPTER 21

Branden Petersen, BS, CP, LP

ABSTRACT

The complex functionality of the natural shoulder, elbow, wrist, and hand are awe inspiring, both individually and as a collective whole. The coupling of accurate, coordinated movements with sensory input provides humans with an amazing instrument to perform intricate functions. Replacing the exquisitely designed complex structure at and distal to the natural shoulder region with a mechanical prosthesis presents many challenges. The short lever arm, involvement of multiple joints, and diminished excursion capabilities create functional limitations in a prosthesis and often dictate the selection of components. There are many possible presentations of amputations in the shoulder region that require prosthetic management; some of the most common are glenohumeral disarticulation (shoulder disarticulation), and interscapulothoracic amputation.

Socket design, interface materials, suspension methods, alignment, and component considerations can affect the successful use of a prosthesis in the shoulder region and must be carefully considered. There are several approaches to prosthetic management, including no prosthesis use; protective shoulder caps; and passive, adaptive, body-powered, hybrid, and externally powered systems. All aspects of prosthetic management should be discussed with the amputee during their initial evaluation.

Keywords: forequarter; intercalary amputation; interscapulothoracic; shoulder disarticulation; Tikhoff–Linberg resection

Introduction

Amputations in the shoulder region are relatively uncommon and are generally related to malignant lesions, trauma, and congenital etiologies.[1,2] The complete loss of an upper limb is a substantial loss. Replacing the natural limb with a mechanical limb presents many challenges, including short lever arms, multiple joint involvement, and diminished excursion capabilities.[3,4] In addition, proximal amputation levels can limit componentry selection and may require the use of externally powered components for improved functional outcomes.[5] Individuals with shoulder-level amputations often reject the use of a prosthesis for a variety of reasons, including socket discomfort, lack of heat dissipation, the weight of the prosthesis, and displeasing appearance.[6-8] Based on the literature, the overall rejection rate for a high-level upper limb prosthesis ranges from 32% to 65%.[6-10] However, with advances in modern socket designs and materials, many of these rejection factors have been mitigated.

Amputations and deficiencies in the shoulder region present in a range of configurations; however, this chapter focuses on humeral neck amputation, glenohumeral (shoulder) disarticulation, and interscapulothoracic (forequarter) amputation. These levels of amputation differ in their clinical presentation but are managed prosthetically in a very similar fashion.[3]

Amputation Levels

Amputations and deficiencies about the shoulder region present differently and require different fitting considerations.[11] It is important to understand the unique clinical presentations and functional capabilities of each level of amputation when designing a prosthesis for the shoulder region.

Patients with an amputation at the level of the humeral neck have an intact glenohumeral joint and a considerably shortened residual humerus (**Figure 1**). Because the residual limb does not have the necessary length to be fitted with standard transhumeral socket designs, thoracic-style sockets are generally chosen. A glenohumeral disarticulation is an amputation through the glenohumeral joint or a disarticulation of the humeral head from the glenoid cavity (**Figure 2**). Individuals with an interscapulothoracic amputation have undergone complete removal of the shoulder girdle, including the scapula and the lateral two-thirds of the clavicle (**Figure 3**).

Evaluation

The initial stage in designing a prosthesis requires a comprehensive patient evaluation. This evaluation is essential to the development of the most

Neither Branden Petersen nor any immediate family member has received anything of value from or has stock or stock options held in a commercial company or institution related directly or indirectly to the subject of this chapter.

Section 2: Upper Limb

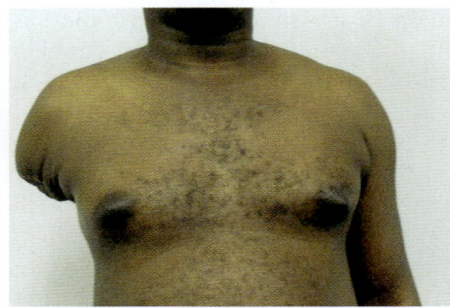

FIGURE 1 Clinical photograph of an individual with an amputation at the level of the humeral neck.

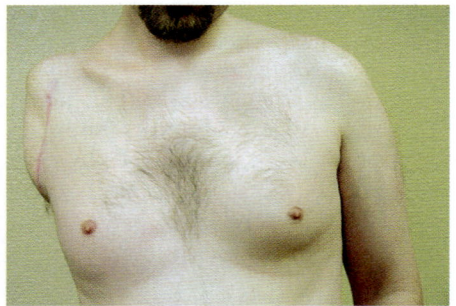

FIGURE 2 Clinical photograph of an individual with a glenohumeral disarticulation.

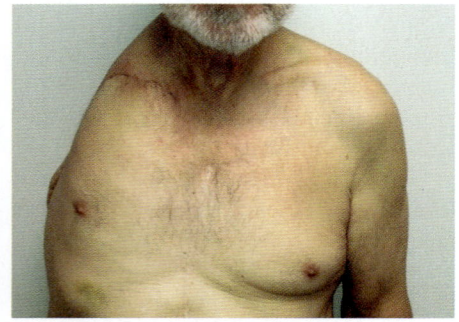

FIGURE 3 Clinical photograph of an individual with a interscapulothoracic amputation.

appropriate prosthetic prescription to meet an individual patient's psychosocial and functional needs. Prosthetic components should be matched to the patient's physical characteristics, customary activities of daily living, and vocational goals. The physical findings from the residual limb examination as well as any associated injuries must be considered.

The rehabilitation team should take great care in gathering the necessary information during the evaluation and design of the prosthesis.[12,13] Obtaining information on the amputation level, the characteristics of the residual limb, the location of scarring, preinjury hand dominance, the results of myoelectric and manual muscle testing, range of motion, and the presence of phantom pain or sensation can assist in designing the prosthesis, including component selection. Comorbidities, including diabetes, overuse symptoms, decreased functionality of the sound side, and any history of neck and back pain, provide further guidance in determining the most appropriate prosthetic approach.

A thorough understanding of the patient's work-related tasks is necessary in designing the prosthesis. In some instances, a visit to the patient's worksite may be necessary to better understand vocational requirements and to justify the components being provided. In other cases, the patient may be transitioning to a new occupation. Understanding the requirements of current and future vocational goals is an important consideration in prosthetic design.

The clinical evaluation lays the foundation for selecting the design and control of the prosthesis. During the patient evaluation process, the conceptual design of the prosthesis begins to develop. The size, shape, and features of the socket for the shoulder region become apparent based on the needs and abilities of the individual. For example, if a patient has an amputation at the humeral neck level, the use of the movable humeral head to activate force-sensitive resistors or switches is a consideration in the design of the prosthesis. Alternatively, strong, distinct muscle contractions allow for the consideration of myoelectric control strategies. Taking into account the individual's unique capabilities to control the prosthesis helps in the creation of a device that more easily permits intuitive learning.

Shoulder Region Socket Design

Socket designs for the shoulder region have substantially evolved from the original bucket-style sockets, which encompassed the entire shoulder proximally, extended 6 inches distally from the axilla, and wrapped around almost to the midline of the torso in their anterior and posterior dimensions. The contributions of many clinicians and researchers have reduced the bulk of these sockets, improved heat dissipation, enhanced suspension, incorporated advanced materials, and refined harnessing techniques.[14-16]

The prosthetic socket can be evaluated in the following five critical support areas: anterior proximal, posterior proximal, lateral wall, anterior distal, and posterior distal. A critical evaluation of these five support areas with respect to suspension, soft-tissue loading, force couples during prosthesis use, comfort, and stability will collectively provide the framework for designing the shoulder socket.

During the molding process, it is necessary to provide anterior proximal compression over the pectoralis and infraspinatus muscles (**Figure 4**). This compression creates a wedge shape that assists with suspension, axial loading, rotational stability, and maintaining electrode contact in externally powered prosthetic designs. The anterior socket trim line is typically located inferior to the clavicle for improved comfort. The posterior proximal trim line is located over the supraspinatus and is responsible for load bearing as well as reducing distal migration of the socket. The lateral wall connects the proximal and distal sockets. This area assists with the transfer of forces to the inferior aspect of the socket. The lateral wall is generally 3 to 5 inches wide, assists with

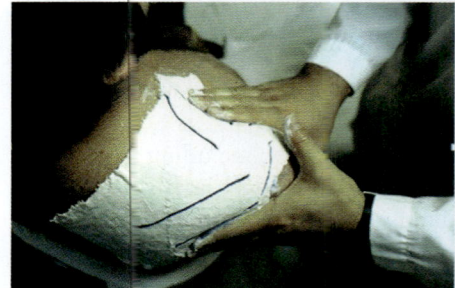

FIGURE 4 Superior photographic view of anterior proximal casting compression techniques commonly used in modern thoracic level sockets (Courtesy of J. Thomas Andrew, CP, FAAOP, Nokomis, FL.)

soft-tissue containment, and broadens the surface area of the socket for force distribution.

Socket torque increases when the shoulder or elbow joint is flexed. The resultant torque produces force couples at the anterior distal and posterior proximal aspects of the socket interface (**Figure 5**). The anterior distal and posterior proximal socket regions assist with torque stabilization and should be dynamically simulated during diagnostic socket fitting to ensure that the necessary force couple support has been achieved. In contrast, because of the predominance of the force couple previously described, the posterior distal aspect of the socket can be reduced to a smaller area of support. This area of the socket generally assists with rotational stability and is useful in activities involving shoulder and elbow extension.

Socket Material Selection

The selection of appropriate socket interface materials is a critical factor in the successful application of a prosthesis for the shoulder region. In general, socket interface materials with a higher coefficient of friction assist in maintaining the position of the socket on short residual limbs. Securing the position of the socket assists in maintaining the optimal mechanics of the prosthesis.

In the past, rigid, laminated hard sockets were commonly used; however, the low friction characteristics of the laminated surface created difficulties in maintaining socket position. With the development of frame-type sockets, the laminated sockets were largely replaced by flexible thermoplastic inner sockets. The flexible thermoplastic material provided greater stability and improved comfort compared with laminated sockets (**Figure 6**).

In recent years, there has been a shift from traditional thermoplastic socket interfaces to silicone rubber materials. A high-consistency rubber (HCR) silicone socket offers several advantages over thermoplastic materials. It can be manufactured to the desired thickness and stiffness (shore durometer), allowing the prosthetist to have localized control over the physical properties of the socket construction. The HCR silicone socket design for a shoulder disarticulation generally includes an over-the-shoulder strap that is integrated into the silicone (**Figure 7**). This strap, coupled with the high coefficient of friction of HCR silicone, helps prevent distal migration of the prosthesis. The strap fits the contour of the shoulder exactly and is soft and flexible so it moves with the patient to provide greater comfort than other strap materials used in this application. Because the HCR silicone is custom pigmented to approximate the general skin tone of the amputee and the strap is continuous with the inside surface of the socket, the cosmetic appearance is good. To provide greater comfort in the transition area from a rigid structure to a patient's body, the HCR silicone socket is made to extend farther than the composite frame to which it is attached. If there are particularly sensitive areas that require additional cushioning, silicone gel pads can be integrated into the HCR silicone to provide excellent padding for improved comfort. This feature is especially useful when a hybrid or body-powered prosthesis is used, because high forces may be needed for activation of prosthesis components.

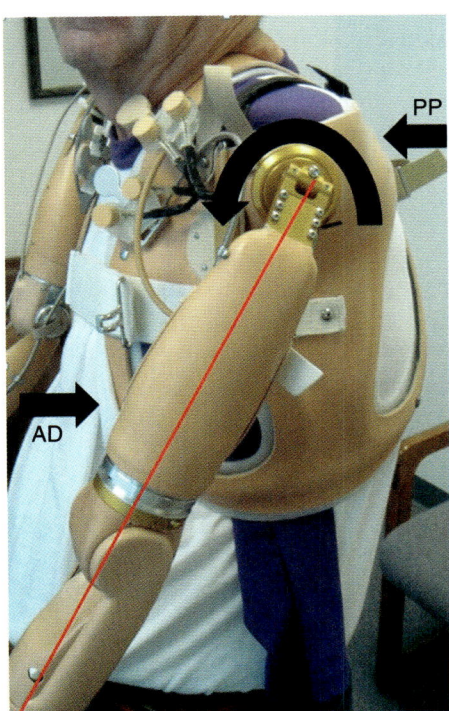

FIGURE 5 Clinical photograph of an individual demonstrating that with the shoulder joint flexed and gravity acting on the humeral section and forearm, a rotational torque is created on the socket (curved arrow). The torque force couples experienced are located in the posterior proximal (PP) and anterior distal (AD) aspects of the socket interface during flexion activities and require socket support.

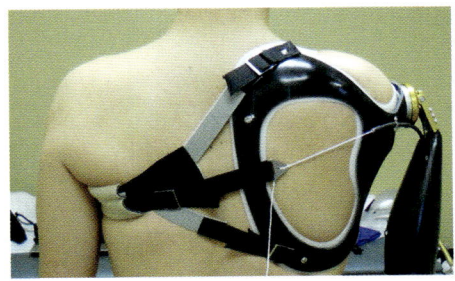

FIGURE 6 Photograph of an individual wearing a frame-type socket with a flexible inner socket material and an external laminated frame. The flexible thermoplastic inner socket material provides greater friction and improved comfort compared with laminated sockets.

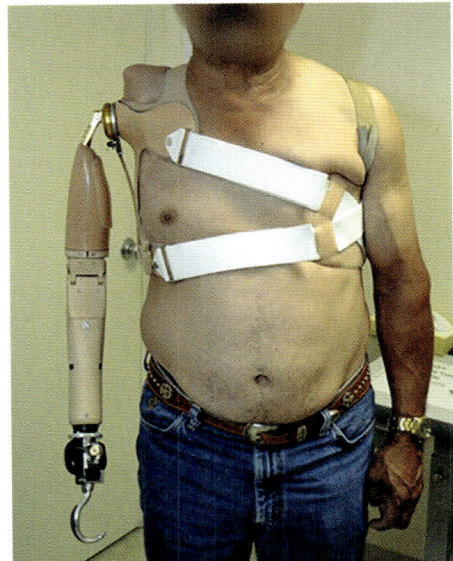

FIGURE 7 Photograph of a patient with a custom, high-consistency rubber (HCR) socket for a myoelectric shoulder disarticulation prosthesis. Note the HCR axilla padding. (Courtesy of Jack Uellendahl, CPO, Hanger Clinic, Austin, TX.)

Component Setup Considerations

Proper component selection and setup is key to the successful use of a prosthesis. When designing a prosthesis for the shoulder region, the device is essentially fabricated twice—once during an expedited provisional fitting to evaluate the function and biomechanics of the prosthesis and then a second time in the form of the definitive prosthesis. The initial provisional fitting involves evaluating the fit of the test socket, the location and alignment biomechanics of the components, the harness design, the configuration of the control inputs, and the consistency of the resultant control. After these factors are deemed satisfactory, the definitive prosthesis is fabricated based on the provisional template.

Several factors should be considered with respect to the prosthetic shoulder joint. Many individuals benefit from a shoulder joint that allows free swinging in the sagittal plane. The freeing of the shoulder joint affords improved posture and gait, decreases extraneous body motions to accomplish certain tasks, and diminishes the forces on the individual's residual limb.[17] Free-swinging shoulder joints should be aligned perpendicular to the ground and in 10° to 15° of internal rotation for improved midline positioning. For individuals with amputations at the level of the humeral neck, the prosthetic shoulder joint is sometimes placed inferior to the humeral neck. Although this placement does not provide a natural appearance, it allows the weight of the components to be situated closer to the body and reduces the torque and lateral bulk of the prosthesis.[4]

Prosthetic elbow alignment also has key considerations. The elbow joint is typically placed to approximate the center of the sound side elbow joint or slightly more proximal. The more proximal placement of the elbow joint center decreases the pendulum effect perceived by the amputee. In addition, the more proximal placement of the elbow joint allows improved seating capabilities in chairs with a side arm. These benefits must be balanced against a shorter prosthetic appearance, which is often less cosmetically acceptable.

Because a prosthesis for the shoulder region replaces several joints, it is desirable to use wrist components that have multiple positioning capabilities. For body-powered devices, flexion and spring rotation wrist units are frequently used to improve the individual's ability to place the terminal device in multiple positions during midline tasks. For externally powered devices, electric wrist rotation is a consideration in individuals with a unilateral amputation and an essential component for those with a bilateral upper limb amputation.

With respect to prosthetic suspension, there are several variations of chest strap harnesses. Harness designs for the shoulder region can be challenging and elaborate depending on functional and suspension goals. However, the chest strap is the most commonly used harness to prevent socket displacement.

Prosthetic Approaches

The seven general categories for prosthetic approaches for the shoulder region are as follows: no prosthesis; protective shoulder caps; passive oppositional restorations; adaptive, body-powered, hybrid, and externally powered prostheses. Because certain types of prostheses are contraindicated for some activities, an individual may require secondary prostheses to accomplish the many activities of daily living and work-related tasks. Secondary prostheses are essential for individuals with bilateral upper limb amputations.[9,18]

No Prosthesis

Individuals with shoulder amputations comprise a small patient cohort. In general, prostheses for the shoulder region are less functional and more likely to be abandoned when compared with prostheses for distal amputation levels. Factors that contribute to rejection of a prosthesis are decreased functional benefit, socket discomfort, weight, heat retention, loss of sensory feedback after the residual limb is covered by the socket, and appearance.[6,7] The choice of not using a prosthesis for the shoulder region should be presented as an option. However, it is also common for amputees to request a prosthesis several years after amputation because of overuse symptoms. Although overuse syndrome does not affect all amputees, this syndrome should be discussed when options for prosthesis use are presented.

Protective Shoulder Caps

Amputees often report improved security of their residual limb after it is covered and protected. A shoulder cap can protect the residual limb from environmental bumps. After a shoulder amputation, large neurovascular bundles can be sensitive to touch. Shoulder caps can assist in protecting these sensitive portions of the residual limb. Protective shoulder caps for interscapulothoracic amputations are shaped to restore the symmetry of the shoulders (**Figure 8**). The built-in shoulder shape assists in maintaining proper positioning of clothing on the body. The protective caps are lightweight; and are fabricated from a variety of materials, such as soft foam, and require a chest strap for suspension.

Passive Oppositional Restoration Prostheses

Passive devices for the shoulder region are a good option for individuals requiring a lightweight device. As the name implies, the device can be passively positioned for various activities (**Figure 9**). It is a misconception that

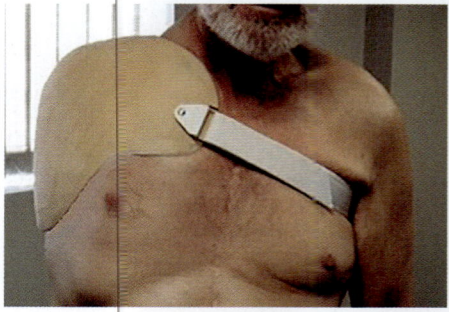

FIGURE 8 Photograph of a patient with an interscapulothoracic amputation wearing a protective shoulder cap with lightweight closed-cell cross-linked polyethylene soft foam shaping and a chest strap

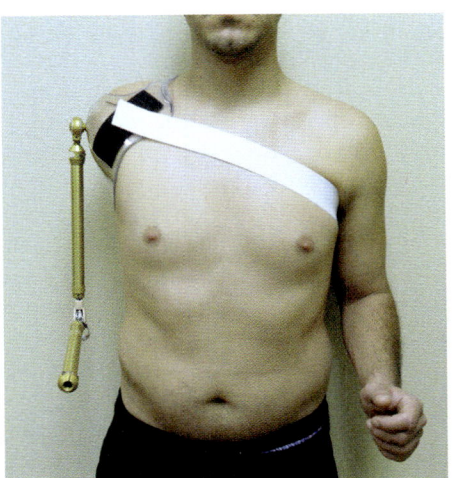

FIGURE 9 Photograph of an individual wearing a passive, oppositional prosthetic restoration during the provisional fitting stage. The prosthesis is lightweight and has passively positioned endoskeletal componentry. The reduced weight and lack of active control permit a reduced socket size.

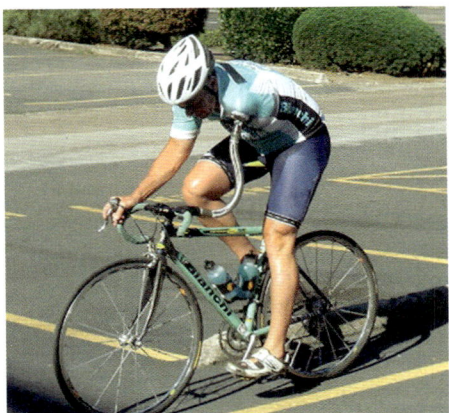

FIGURE 10 Photograph of an individual using an adaptive shoulder region prosthesis for cycling.

oppositional devices provide no functional benefits. There is some evidence that passive devices are used to perform activities of daily living as often as prostheses with active grasping capabilities.[19] These devices can restore the functional length of the limb and promote bimanual functionality. A passive prosthesis can be socially beneficial because it can assist in promoting the psychological acceptance of the amputee's impaired body image.[20] A restored body appearance can provide more confidence in work and social settings.

Endoskeletal elbow joints allow the user to position the elbow in several different positions and lock it into place. With the elbow locked in flexion, the prosthesis can assist the user in functional activities such as carrying grocery bags.

Multiple glove options are available for a passive prosthesis. Off-the-shelf production gloves are inexpensive but must be replaced frequently because of staining. Production gloves are selected based on a color swatch. Another option is silicone gloves, which do not stain as easily as vinyl gloves but lack durability and are more costly to replace. Silicone gloves have a high coefficient of friction that aids users in holding down objects for contralateral hand manipulation. In some instances, gloves are fabricated as custom silicone restoration prostheses. Custom silicone gloves better match the contralateral limb in color and other aspects of physical appearance.

Adaptive Prostheses

Designing adaptive prosthetic devices requires persistence, knowledge, and creativity. Adaptive, activity-specific devices are not commonly used for patients with amputations about the shoulder region, but they can be considered as an option to meet an individual's need to accomplish activities. In some instances, adaptive prostheses do not resemble a typical prosthesis in appearance because they are designed for a specific activity (**Figure 10**).

Adaptive terminal devices can be used on an existing passive, a body-powered, or a myoelectric prosthesis. The individual can apply the appropriate terminal device based on the activity being performed. This presents an attractive option because the prosthesis can be used for multiple purposes. Adaptive terminal devices are available for a wide range of activities.

Body-Powered Prostheses

Body-powered prostheses require that the individual be capable of generating both force and excursion through joint motion captured through a harness. The excursion required to fully flex a prosthetic elbow joint and open a terminal device is 4.5 inches. This excursion is generally captured through two body motions: glenohumeral flexion and biscapular abduction. For individuals with shoulder amputations, capturing this amount of excursion is difficult and in some cases impossible.[4] Although these amputees have biscapular abduction capabilities (except at the interscapulothoracic level), the lack of a humerus or adequate humeral bone length eliminates glenohumeral flexion as a source of excursion. In the absence of glenohumeral joint motion, an individual lacks approximately 50% of the needed excursion required to operate a body-powered prosthesis to its end range. As a result, externally powered components are often required, especially for those with interscapulothoracic-level amputations in which approximately 25% of the total required excursion is available.

Prosthetic elbow alignment and setup are critical for shoulder prostheses. Because of the compromises previously described, the body-powered prosthesis needs to be set up to capture maximum excursion. For high-level, body-powered prostheses, double lift assists can be coupled at the elbow while placing the fairlead cable slightly anterior to the elbow's axis of rotation. This placement of the fairlead cable decreases the excursion required to flex the elbow but increases the required force. The double lift assists compensate for the additional force requirements. This principle can be applied to hybrid designs as well. Using lift assists and cable positioning can improve the mechanics of the shoulder prosthesis.

Excursion amplifiers can be used to reduce the required excursion (**Figure 11**). Excursion amplifier pulleys generally decrease the excursion requirement by 50% but double the force needed to activate the component.

Other design tradeoffs can be considered for body-powered prostheses for shoulder-region amputations. Because of the limitations to available excursion, body-powered devices are often designed to dedicate cable excursion exclusively to the activation of the terminal device while allowing the elbow to be passively positioned. This allows the user to have full activation of

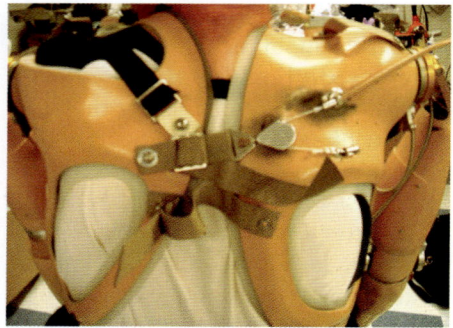

FIGURE 11 Posterior photograph of an individual with a bilateral shoulder disarticulation fitted with a prosthesis using an excursion amplifier to reduce the excursion requirements.

a hook or a hand, despite the inherently limited excursion capabilities. This mechanical tradeoff is accomplished by using a Bowden cable instead of a fairlead cable (**Figure 12**). After the elbow is passively placed in a midline position, 2.5 inches of captured scapular motion allows the user to open the terminal device for grasping.

Hybrid Prostheses

Hybrid prostheses combine various technologies and can be designed in many configurations, including externally powered elbows coupled with body-powered terminal devices and, more commonly, body-powered or passive elbows coupled with myoelectric terminal devices[14,21] (**Figures 13 and 14**). Hybrid designs offer a lighter-weight option compared with a fully externally powered system. At the humeral neck and glenohumeral levels, the individual can use biscapular motion to position the elbow through a harness and control cable and myoelectrically control the terminal device. At the interscapulothoracic level, the elbow can be passively positioned by the sound-side, preserving myoelectric sites for control of the terminal device (**Figure 14**). Socket designs for hybrid systems should provide a stable platform to ensure that the electrodes will remain in the proper position and provide consistent control. Hybrid designs also may afford proprioceptive feedback through the harness regarding elbow position.

Externally Powered Prostheses

Externally powered devices typically use a powered elbow, powered terminal device, and, in some instances, electric wrist rotation. These components can be set up and controlled in many configurations. Some of the input options for controlling an externally powered device include myoelectric surface electrodes, switches, force-sensing resistors, and linear transducers. In some instances, multiple inputs are required to gain the desired function. These devices are often programmed wirelessly using a graphic user interface and allow the selection of multiple control strategies to customize function based on the unique capabilities of the individual. A stable socket design ensures consistency of control for externally powered prostheses and offers important functionality for individuals with shoulder region amputations.[5]

Recently, targeted muscle reinnervation surgery has been associated with several advantages, including long-term neuronal pain management and improved simultaneous myoelectric control (the ability to simultaneously control movements at multiple prosthetic joints).[22-25] The latter is more fully realized when targeted muscle

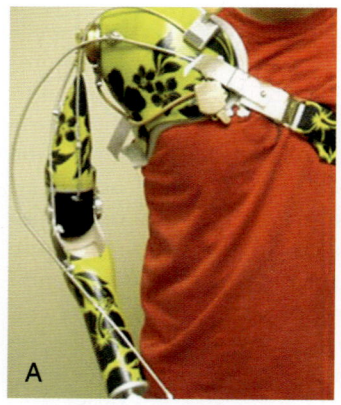
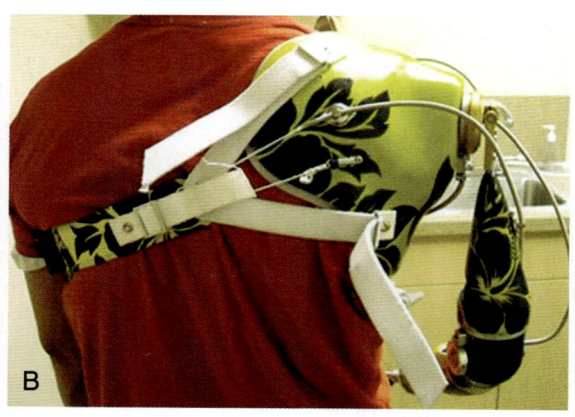

FIGURE 12 Anterior (**A**) and posterior (**B**) photographic views of an individual wearing a shoulder disarticulation body-powered exoskeletal prosthesis with an excursion amplifier and chest strap. Anterior chest expansion creates terminal device activation through a dedicated Bowden cable. Elbow flexion is controlled with biscapular abduction through a second dedicated cable. This individual can capture additional excursion for both movements by applying pressure to the chest strap as it passes through the sound-side axilla to modulate its relative position. He can reach back with his sound-side brachium and compress the chest harness against his body wall to improve excursion capture during bilateral scapular abduction. Similarly, reaching forward with his sound-side brachium and compressing the harness against his body improves cable excursion during chest expansion.

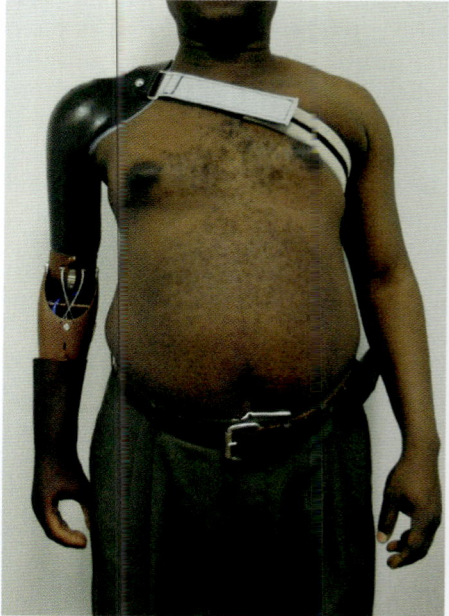

FIGURE 13 Clinical photograph of an individual wearing a humeral-neck–level hybrid prosthesis with a passive locking elbow and an externally powered hand. A Sauter half-and-half socket design uses an integrated shoulder saddle that allows the acromion and bony anatomy to exit the socket. The weight of the components is then supported by the integrated saddle. The socket footprint on these socket designs closely approximates transhumeral designs.

Chapter 21: Amputations About the Shoulder: Prosthetic Management

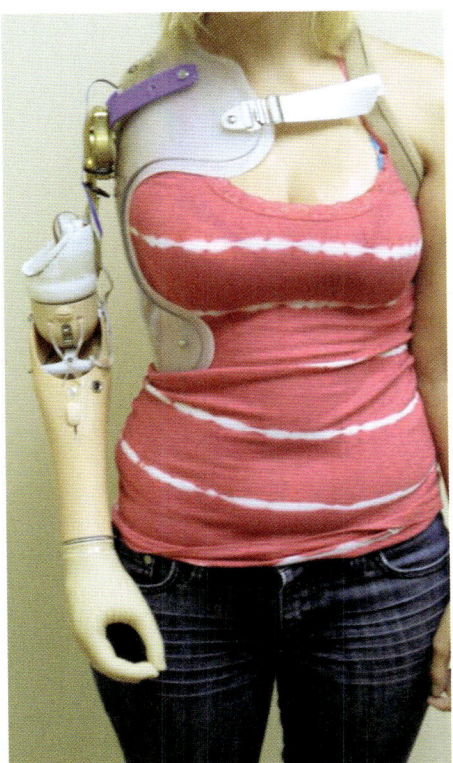

FIGURE 14 Clinical photograph of an individual with an interscapulothoracic-level amputation fitted with a provisional hybrid prosthesis with a passive elbow and an externally powered hand.

reinnervation is combined with pattern-recognition–based systems in which microprocessors recognize specific characteristics of differing myoelectric signals and classify them into desired functions. Various methods for advanced signal acquisition are currently being evaluated; however, the best method to capture information from the nerves is still being investigated.[21]

Atypical Presentations in the Shoulder Region: Tikhoff–Linberg Procedure

In malignant lesions in which the shoulder girdle must be removed but the distal humerus, forearm, and hand are uninvolved, a Tikhoff–Linberg procedure may be considered by the rehabilitation team. In contrast to a shoulder disarticulation, this procedure can preserve function in the arm and hand.[1,2] Although these cases are relatively rare, they can be treated with a prosthesis using thoracic socket design concepts. The Tikhoff–Linberg resection can be challenging to stabilize with prosthetic and orthotic devices.[3] This type of surgical resection does not lend itself to allowing the patient to carry objects of substantial weight or to position the forearm in greater than 90° of flexion for midline tasks (**Figures 15** and **16**).

Bilateral Shoulder Region Considerations

The prosthetic needs of individuals with bilateral limb loss differ greatly from those with unilateral limb loss. In bilateral shoulder amputations, the rehabilitation team must consider all options to improve functionality, including limb lengthening for amputations at the level of the humeral neck.[26] Regardless of hand dominance before amputation, in bilateral high-level amputations, the longer residual limb typically becomes the dominant limb. Component selection is critical in designing a functional prosthesis to improve the bilateral amputee's independence. A protocol for fitting bilateral shoulder amputations consists of fitting the dominant residual limb with a body-powered system and the nondominant residual limb with an externally powered system (**Figure 17**). This protocol provides some control differentiation between the bilateral prosthetic arms. Another important consideration is providing a secondary set of prostheses. This ensures that the individual has a working set of prostheses in the event that the primary set requires major repairs.

Rehabilitation Team

Using a team approach for the rehabilitation of a patient with a high-level shoulder amputations can improve both short- and long-term outcomes. This is especially true in those patients with bilateral upper limb amputations. The rehabilitation team approach should consist of a patient-centered model with access to the surgeon, the physical medicine and rehabilitation physician, the psychologist, the physical therapist, the occupational therapist, and the prosthetist. The team and patient should work together to develop the best prosthetic prescription to accomplish activities of daily living and work-related tasks.

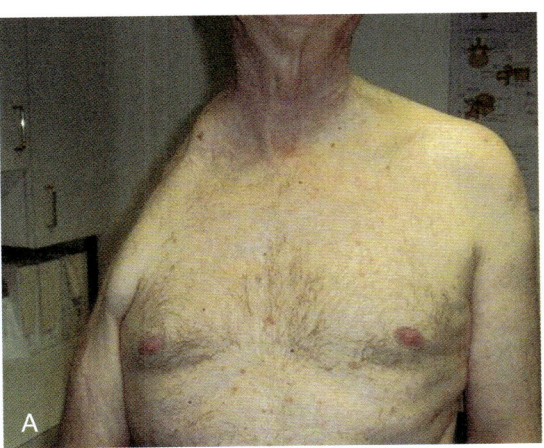 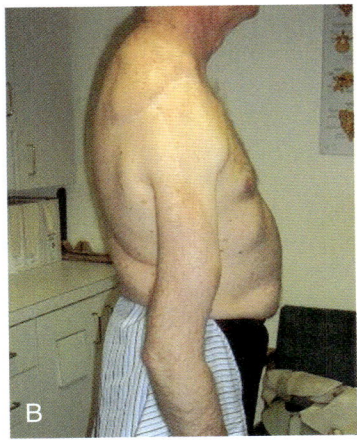 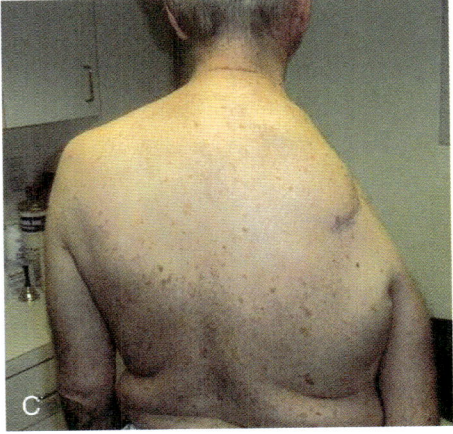

FIGURE 15 Anterior (**A**), lateral (**B**), and posterior (**C**) clinical photographs of an individual with a Tikhoff–Linberg resection. (Courtesy of John Rheinstein, CP, FAAOP, Hanger Clinic, Austin, TX.)

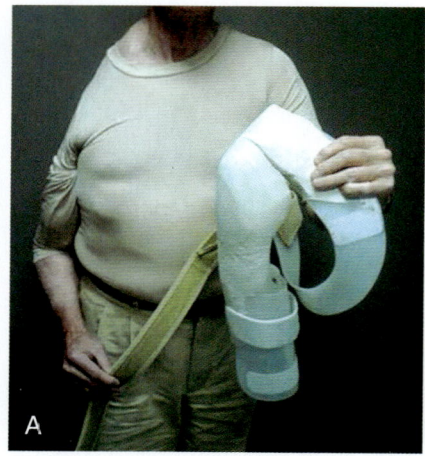
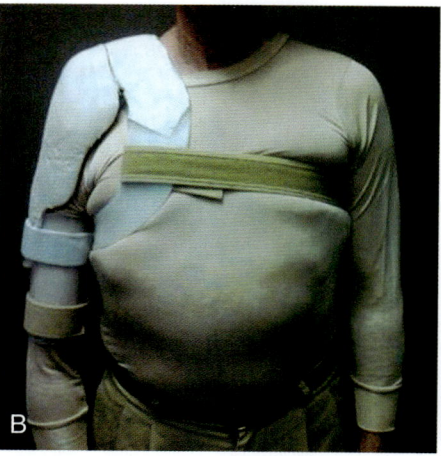
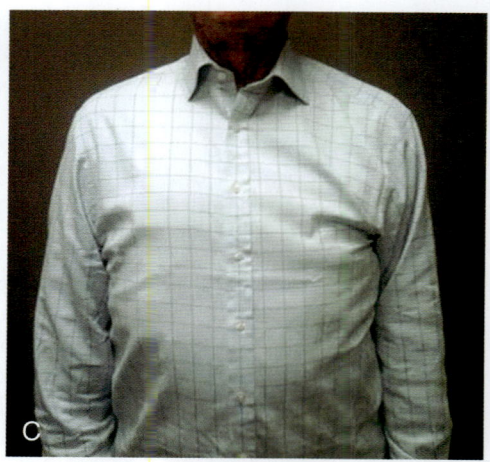

FIGURE 16 Clinical photographs of a patient who was treated with a Tikhoff-Linberg resection. **A**, Anterior view of a thoracic socket design with humeral support. **B**, Appearance of the prosthesis in place. **C**, The prosthesis affords a good cosmetic result under clothing.

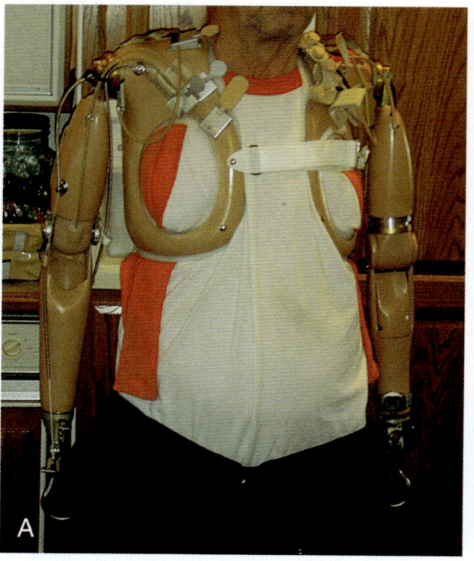
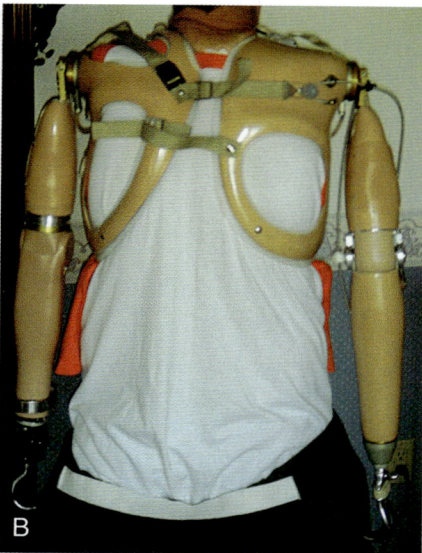

FIGURE 17 Anterior (**A**) and posterior (**B**) photographic views of an individual with a bilateral upper limb amputation with a body-powered device on the right side and an externally powered device on the left side.

Rehabilitation professionals must be acutely aware of the psychological aspects of limb loss. The process of going through an amputation has been described by many amputees as similar to going through a grieving process, and it can affect all aspects of the patient's life. Individuals experiencing amputation may also present with emotional stress related to the unknown. Educating the individual so that they understand the rehabilitation steps and the expected functional return can alleviate some of these stressors. Individuals with amputations can benefit from meeting others with a similar amputation level. This can provide renewed hope. There are many organizations, including local peer support groups that can help new amputees and their families cope with the life-changing effects of limb loss.

With the rapid advancement and improvements in the functionality of prosthetic components, comprehensive occupational therapy is required to ensure optimal functional outcomes. Occupational therapy in using prosthetic devices provides a foundation for the amputee to overcome functional challenges and live a productive life.[27] As prosthetic technologies continue to advance, it is anticipated that there will be an increasing need for therapists with experience in the latest technologies.

SUMMARY

Designing high-level upper limb prosthetic devices presents many challenges. Amputation levels need to be evaluated closely, and the prosthesis should capitalize on the remaining functional features of the individual's residual limb. It is important to understand that one socket type may not work in all prosthetic approaches. Socket design considerations in the successful use of a prosthesis for shoulder amputees include comfort, anatomic contouring, stability, heat dissipation, and suspension. Designing and selecting the appropriate prosthetic components to match the individual's activities and work-related tasks coupled with occupational therapy provide the best scenario for success. A thorough knowledge of each type of prosthesis, including features, indications, and contraindications, allows the amputee and rehabilitation team to make the best decisions. A thorough knowledge in the subtleties of component selection and alignment of the various joint segments optimizes the functional characteristics of the final prosthesis. Thorough evaluations and a patient-centered team approach by the rehabilitation team will optimize functional outcomes for those with amputations about the shoulder region.

Acknowledgments

Family members Christina, Grady, and Logan are thanked for their support during the writing of this chapter.

References

1. Marshall MB, Cooper C, Carter YM: Modified Tikhoff–Linberg procedure for posterior chest wall sarcoma. *Ann Thorac Surg* 2012;94(4):1328-1330.

2. Xie L, X D T, Yang RL, Guo W: Interscapulothoracic resection of tumours of shoulder with a note on reconstruction. *Bone Joint J* 2014;96-B(5):684-690.

3. Miguelez JM, Miguelez MD, Alley RD: Amputations about the shoulder: Prosthetic management, in Smith DG, Michael JW, Bowker JH, eds: *Atlas of Amputations and Limb Deficiencies*, ed 3. American Academy of Orthopaedic Surgeons, 2004, pp 263-273.

4. Uellendahl J: Management of the very short/humeral neck transhumeral amputee, in *MEC '05 Integrating Prosthetics and Medicine: Proceedings of the 2005 MyoElectric Controls/Powered Prosthetics Symposium* 2005. Available at: http://dukespace.lib.duke.edu/dspace/bitstream/handle/10161/2750/Uellendahl_01.pdf?sequence=3. Accessed April 8, 2015.

5. Heger H, Millstein S, Hunter GA: Electrically powered prostheses for the adult with an upper limb amputation. *J Bone Joint Surg Br* 1985;67(2):278-281.

6. Biddiss E, Chau T: Upper-limb prosthetics: Critical factors in device abandonment. *Am J Phys Med Rehabil* 2007;86(12):977-987.

7. Biddiss EA, Chau TT: Upper limb prosthesis use and abandonment: A survey of the last 25 years. *Prosthet Orthot Int* 2007;31(3):236-257.

8. Farnsworth T, Uellendahl J, Mikosz MJ, Miller L, Petersen B: Shoulder region socket considerations. *J Prosthet Orthot* 2008;20:93-106.

9. Datta D, Selvarajah K, Davey N: Functional outcome of patients with proximal upper limb deficiency: Acquired and congenital. *Clin Rehabil* 2004;18(2):172-177.

10. Wright TW, Hagen AD, Wood MB: Prosthetic usage in major upper extremity amputations. *J Hand Surg Am* 1995;20(4):619-622.

11. Lipschutz RD: Upper extremity amputations and prosthetic management, in Lusardi MM, Nielsen CC, eds: *Orthotics and Prosthetics in Rehabilitation*. Butterworth-Heinemann, 2000, pp 569-588.

12. Meier RH, Esquenazi A: Rehabilitation planning for the upper extremity amputee, in Meier RH, Atkins DJ, eds: *Functional Restoration of Adults and Children With Upper Extremity Amputation*. Demos Publishing, 2004, pp 55-61.

13. Lake C, Dodson R: Progressive upper limb prosthetics. *Phys Med Rehabil Clin N Am* 2006;17(1):49-72.

14. Lake C: The evolution of upper limb prosthetic socket design. *J Prosthet Orthot* 2008;20:85-92.

15. Miguelez JM, Miguelez MD: The microframe: The next generation of interface design for glenohumeral disarticulation and associated levels of limb deficiency. *J Prosthet Orthot* 2003;15(2):66-71.

16. Sauter WF, Naumann S, Milner M: A three-quarter type below-elbow socket for myoelectric prostheses. *Prosthet Orthot Int* 1986;10(2):79-82.

17. Bertels T, Schmalz T, Ludwigs E: Biomechanical influences of shoulder disarticulation prosthesis during standing and level walking. *Prosthet Orthot Int* 2012;36(2):165-172.

18. Datta D, Kingston J, Ronald J: Myoelectric prostheses for below-elbow amputees: The trent experience. *Int Disabil Stud* 1989;11(4):167-170.

19. Fraser CM: An evaluation of the use made of cosmetic and functional prostheses by unilateral upper limb amputees. *Prosthet Orthot Int* 1998;22(3):216-223.

20. Pillet J, Didierjean-Pillet A: Aesthetic hand prosthesis: Gadget or therapy? Presentation of a new classification. *J Hand Surg Br* 2001;26(6):523-528.

21. Hutchinson DT: The quest for the bionic arm. *J Am Acad Orthop Surg* 2014;22(6):346-351.

22. Cheesborough JE, Souza JM, Dumanian GA, Bueno RA Jr: Targeted muscle reinnervation in the initial management of traumatic upper extremity amputation injury. *Hand (N Y)* 2014;9(2):253-257.

23. Souza JM, Cheesborough JE, Ko JH, Cho MS, Kuiken TA, Dumanian GA: Targeted muscle reinnervation: A novel approach to postamputation neuroma pain. *Clin Orthop Relat Res* 2014;472(10):2984-2990.

24. Lipschutz RD, Kuiken TA, Miller LA, Dumanian GA, Stubblefield KA: Shoulder disarticulation externally powered prosthetic fitting following targeted muscle reinnervation for improved myoelectric control. *J Prosthet Orthot* 2006;18(2):28-34.

25. Simon AM, Lock BA, Stubblefield KA: Patient training for functional use of pattern recognition-controlled prostheses. *J Prosthet Orthot* 2012;24(2):56-64.

26. Schnur D, Meier RH III: Amputation surgery. *Phys Med Rehabil Clin N Am* 2014;25(1):35-43.

27. Smurr LM, Gulick K, Yancosek K, Ganz O: Managing the upper extremity amputee: A protocol for success. *J Hand Ther* 2008;21(2):160-175.

Bilateral Upper Limb Prostheses

Jack E. Uellendahl, CPO

CHAPTER 22

ABSTRACT

After a bilateral upper limb amputation, the ability to perform basic and routine tasks, such as eating and self-care, becomes difficult or impossible without assistance. The goal of prosthetic rehabilitation for a patient with a bilateral arm amputation is to enable the individual to achieve functional independence and to successfully participate in vocational and recreational pursuits. Subtle details of socket fit, control system configuration, and suspension can sometimes mean the difference between success and failure. Success relies on selecting the most appropriate components, matching those components with optimal control sources, and interfacing them with the human body in a comfortable and functional manner. Equally important is the user's dedication and motivation to succeed in the face of adversity.

Keywords: bilateral arm prostheses; bilateral upper limb amputee; body-powered prostheses; myoelectric

Introduction

Bilateral upper limb amputation is a profound loss for an individual. The ability to perform basic and routine tasks, such as eating and self-care, becomes difficult or impossible without assistance. Prostheses and other assistive devices can enable the users to regain a measure of their lost ability to manipulate objects and allow them to successfully accomplish a variety of tasks. However, replacement of the many exquisite features of the physiologic hand is not yet possible. Even simple tasks require an amazing amount of complex manipulation. For example, these words were typed using 10 fingers working in concert. Each finger performs both independent and coordinated simultaneous functions, relying on sensation and precise positioning to accurately produce the intended result. These abilities often are taken for granted until they are lost.

The goal of prosthetic rehabilitation for the bilateral arm amputee is to enable them to achieve functional independence and successfully participate in vocational and recreational pursuits. Although bilateral arm prostheses restore only a small amount of the lost functionality, users are able to perform many activities that otherwise would be impossible.[1,2] Recent data have confirmed the earlier observations that individuals with bilateral upper limb amputation are more likely to use one or more prostheses than their peers with a single upper limb amputation, with more hours of daily use. Subtle details of socket fit, control system configuration, and suspension can sometimes mean the difference between success and failure. Unlike a patient with a unilateral arm amputation, a patient with a bilateral arm amputation does not have the option of compensating for the inadequacies of a prosthesis by using their intact physiologic arm.[3] Every detail of prosthetic design should be optimally accomplished. Because of the inability to duplicate the diverse and complex functions of the human arm, prosthetic systems should be viewed as tools with different components best suited for different applications. Success relies on selecting the most appropriate components, matching those components with optimal control sources, and interfacing them with the human body in a comfortable and functional manner. Equally important is the user's dedication and motivation to succeed in the face of adversity.

Patient Evaluation

Because of the complexity of bilateral upper limb loss and the fluid nature of the early rehabilitation period, a thorough evaluation of the new bilateral arm amputee should take place over a period of time. Most individuals who sustain bilateral upper limb amputations have experienced a traumatic injury and have additional medical comorbidities beyond limb loss. Ideally, a team of experienced professionals should work together to address the many challenges facing the new amputee. The treating or consulting professionals may include an orthopaedic surgeon, a physiatrist, a prosthetist, an occupational therapist, a physical therapist, a psychologist, a nurse, and a social worker. In addition, the access to peer support is an invaluable adjunct to the care and treatment provided by medical professionals. The

---

Jack E. Uellendahl or an immediate family member serves as a paid consultant to or is an employee of Hanger Clinic and has stock or stock options held in Hanger Clinic.

Section 2: Upper Limb

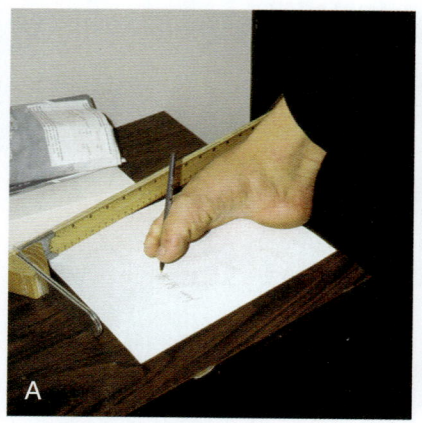
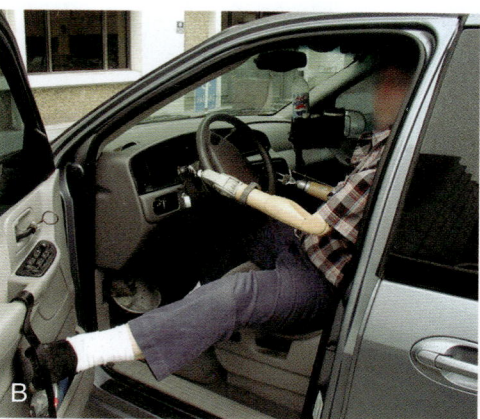

FIGURE 1 **A,** Photograph of an individual with a bilateral congenital upper limb absence who has developed remarkable dexterity and manipulative foot function. **B,** Photograph of a man with acquired bilateral upper limb loss. Adults usually do not develop remarkable foot function but may find foot use an efficient alternative to prosthetic function for tasks away from the body.

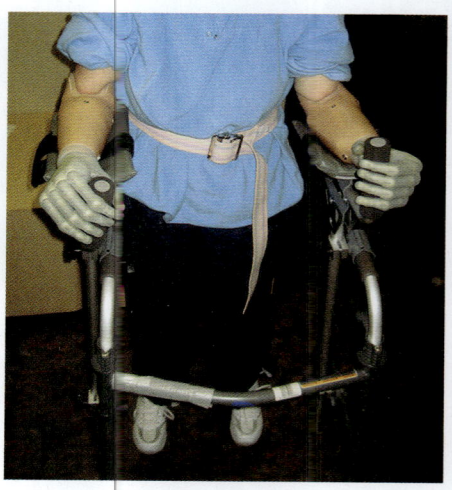

FIGURE 2 Photograph of a patient who needs an assistive device for ambulation. The design of the upper limb prosthesis should take into consideration how to best hold the assistive device and comfortably distribute the pressure of partial weight bearing through the upper limbs.

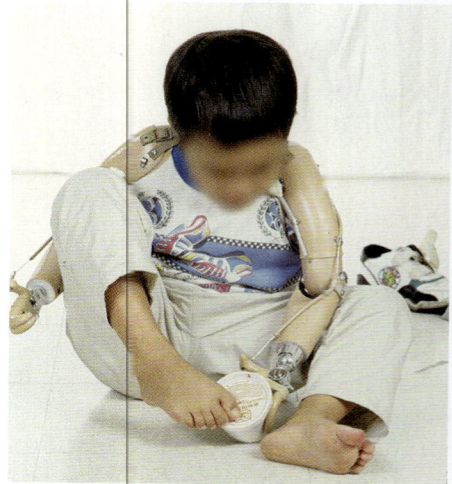

FIGURE 3 Photograph of a young boy with acquired bilateral very short transhumeral amputations demonstrating the superior manipulative function provided by his sensate feet as he stabilizes the object with his prosthesis.

patient, as the center of the team, will ultimately determine several aspects of their own care, including which type of prosthesis is preferred.

Factors that affect the selection of the prosthetic component and control scheme include cognitive level, mechanical aptitude, family life, occupation, hobbies, and self-image. Residual limb length, strength, and range of motion of the upper limbs, including scapulothoracic motion, should be evaluated. These factors have direct implications regarding the method of fitting the prosthesis. The general strength and flexibility of the lower limbs should be assessed. With more proximal amputations, foot use should be encouraged, with training dedicated to exploring and developing the manipulative capabilities of the feet (**Figure 1**). Alternatively, individuals with comorbid lower limb involvement may need to use their upper limb prostheses to hold and transfer weight through an assistive device (**Figure 2**). At the conclusion of the initial evaluation process, a defined plan should be in place regarding the prosthetic component selection and control. However, the team should also be flexible and open to change throughout the rehabilitation process. It should be expected that the prosthesis configuration will change over time in response to the changing needs and abilities of the user.

Throughout the evaluation process, the prosthetist should consider the advantages and disadvantages of various component and control options as they relate to the specific individual. To give structure to this evaluation process, it is useful to understand the attributes of the ideal prosthesis and then compare those attributes with available technologies.

The ideal prosthesis would restore the appearance and function of the lost limbs and control would be intuitive and subconscious. The ideal prosthetic prehensile device would be a lightweight, durable hand that is capable of manipulating a wide variety of objects that differ in size, shape, and texture. The characteristics of the objects would be related back to the user through a sensory feedback system. Proprioception regarding the speed of prosthetic movement, the force exerted, and the position of the prosthetic device would be inherent.

Currently available, state-of-the-art prostheses and prosthetic prehensile devices fail to meet all of these criteria. However, considering the needs and priorities of each individual and comparing these against the attributes of each prosthetic component and control scheme will help achieve optimal use of current technology.

Although this chapter primarily focuses on the treatment of adult amputees, many of the concepts may have application for the treatment of children. However, because of their small size and often immature cognitive ability, children cannot be treated as small adults. Pediatric cases are characterized by decreased force and excursion and a lower tolerance for weight and prosthesis complexity. Congenital bilateral limb deficiency is very rare, and the issues regarding prosthetic fitting can be quite different from those of adults. Children will often learn to use their feet with remarkable dexterity to augment their manipulative capabilities[4] (**Figure 3**).

Staging of Care

In all patients with an arm amputation, whether unilateral or bilateral, it is advisable to fit the prosthesis as soon as possible, preferably within the first 30 to 90 days. The period of 30 days after amputation has been referred to as the golden fitting period for upper limb prosthetic devices, leading to optimal acceptance and usage.[5] There are many advantages to early postoperative fitting, including decreased edema and pain, accelerated wound healing, improved patient rehabilitation, decreased length of hospital stay, increased prosthetic use, maintenance of some continuous type of proprioception input through the residual limb, and improved patient psychological adaptation to amputation.[5] In patients in whom other injuries or other complicating factors make fitting within the golden period infeasible, it may be necessary to delay prosthetic use. In many patients, one side may be ready to fit before the other, and it is advisable to do so. Initially, providing a prosthesis on one side only is often desirable.

Prosthetic training should begin using a component configuration and control scheme that is as simple as possible to prevent the patient from experiencing gadget overload. This is especially true at higher levels of amputation where the possibility exists for multiple dynamically positioned components on each limb. In these cases, it is advisable to introduce new components sequentially, allowing time for the user to become accustomed to each new device before increasing the overall complexity of the prosthesis.

Given the dynamic nature of prosthetic rehabilitation of the bilateral arm amputee, it is useful to develop short-term and long-term goals. As the skills of an amputee develop, their medical condition stabilizes and priorities change in response to the challenges of daily life. The optimal prosthetic device, usage pattern, and individual preferences also may change. It is reasonable to expect that this process will take 6 to 12 months, depending on the level of limb loss, the extent of other complicating factors, and the speed at which an individual adapts. A prototype prosthesis is valuable during this period because it will allow the amputee and the rehabilitation team to evaluate various prosthetic systems before deciding on a definitive prescription (**Figure 4**).

Short-term goals will generally focus on mastering use of the prosthesis for basic daily functions, including donning the prosthesis, eating, and toileting. Long-term goals may include dressing, vocational skills, and avocational pursuits. During this period of experimentation, it is recommended that the amputee spends most of their time at home, returning to the rehabilitation facility periodically for prosthetic modifications and additional training. This allows the user to determine which prosthetic configurations work best in real-life situations and identify specific problems that need attention during the next consultation with the rehabilitation team. It is reasonable to expect that complete independence will be achieved by nearly all patients, except those with the loss of both limbs at or above the transhumeral level or in patients with other limiting factors. However, even some bilateral transhumeral amputees are able to attain complete independence in accomplishing daily tasks.

Socket Design

Generally, socket designs for the bilateral amputee do not differ from unilateral designs. However, because of the absence of both hands, it is necessary to consider the donning ease and the positioning flexibility of the prosthesis. Positioning flexibility includes the range of motion of the intact physiologic joints when a prosthesis is worn and, in some instances, the ability to reposition the prosthesis in useful ways at the limb-socket interface to increase the scope of functional use (**Figure 5**).

Although the socket may not be completely self-suspending, the interface should fit snugly and work with the suspension system to provide a prosthesis that feels firmly connected to the user. This intimate fit will afford optimal positioning control of the prosthesis and minimize its perceived weight. In both body-powered and electronically controlled systems, the socket is the foundation of the prosthetic system; any shortcomings will substantially affect the successful use of the prosthesis. Ineffectual motion

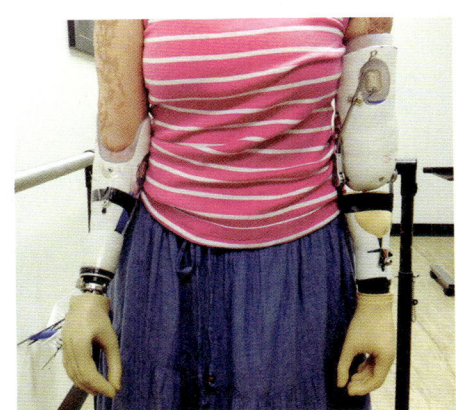

FIGURE 4 Photograph of a patient with prototype prostheses that allow her to experience the use of various components before implementation in the final design. Prosthesis alignment, length, and other parameters can be evaluated and optimized during this stage of the fitting.

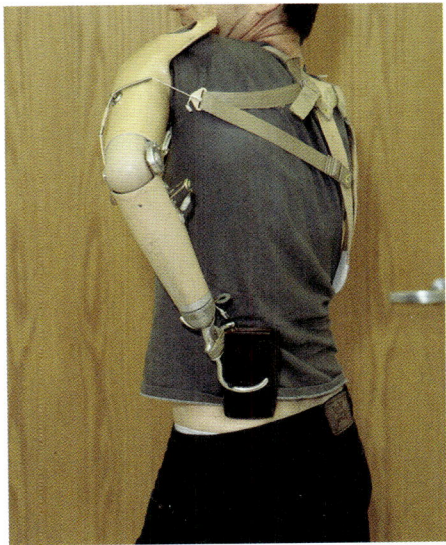

FIGURE 5 A patient's functional envelope can sometimes be expanded by repositioning the prosthesis on the limb. Photograph of a man retrieving his wallet from his back pocket, which requires operation of the prosthesis hook behind his back.

should be minimized so that when the residual limb begins to move, the prosthesis will move.

The materials used in the construction of a prosthesis are an important consideration. For example, carbon fiber and other composite materials provide a strong and lightweight prosthesis.

Custom-made silicone sockets provide improved comfort for all levels of upper limb prostheses users compared with previous construction materials. These sockets are made of high-consistency rubber (HCR) silicone, which has several advantages over the rigid and flexible plastics previously used for socket construction.[6] Because HCR silicone is very flexible and elastic, it facilitates greater range of motion as the material bends and stretches with limb movement (**Figure 6**). However, the tackiness of HCR silicone can complicate donning, and this should be taken into consideration.

Transradial Sockets

Patients with transradial amputations who use body-powered control will often benefit from flexible hinges because they allow the amputee to retain physiologic forearm rotation. When self-suspension is desired, supracondylar sockets such as those typically used for myoelectric control, and to a lesser extent, for body-powered control, are generally best donned by pushing the residual limb into the socket. The Northwestern University self-suspending socket[7] offers particular advantages for bilateral transradial fittings in which supracondylar suspension is desired because it tends to offer good range of motion at the elbow and is easily donned by pushing in. The Northwestern socket can be modified with a cutout over the olecranon, which reduces heat buildup and improves appearance, especially when the elbow is extended.[8]

Socket designs that require the limb to be pulled in are generally avoided because of the obvious difficulties presented by bilateral upper limb loss. However, in rare instances when pulling in is considered necessary, the use of a nylon donning bag has proved an effective tool and can be used independently by some patients.

Transhumeral Sockets

The socket for a transhumeral prosthesis should provide for close coupling of the residual limb and the prosthesis to maximize prosthetic function. Because the ideal socket design should cause little or no restriction of intact joint motion, open shoulder designs are preferred because they allow relatively free range of motion at the shoulder joint, especially when sufficient residual limb length remains.[9] Another option for transhumeral socket design is the half-and-half socket.[10] This socket uses a flexible silicone proximal section that is fitted over the shoulder region and is fabricated as an integral part of a distal inner flexible socket. The deltoid area is cut out laterally, providing improved flexibility and air circulation within the socket. The rigid external frame of the socket extends from the axilla level distally (**Figure 6**). Another option similar to the half-and-half socket is the flexible shoulder suspension system in which a strip of spandex-backed neoprene (or similar material) replaces the silicone saddle and is attached to the wings of the standard open shoulder socket.[3]

In contrast, closed shoulder designs are best used for short residual limbs where insufficient leverage exists to use the full range of physiologic shoulder motion. The closed shoulder socket offers good stabilization of the prosthesis on the user and a convenient and secure anchor point for the lateral suspension strap of the harness.

Shoulder Disarticulation Sockets

Designs for a shoulder disarticulation interface require sufficient surface area to effectively stabilize the prosthesis on the amputee. Because of the length of the lever arm of the prosthesis and the weight of the components, there is a strong tendency for rotation at the prosthesis-user interface, especially as the terminal device is moved away from the body. Therefore, the socket perimeter should extend sufficiently on the torso to resist these forces.[11] A frame-type socket allows for stabilization and heat dissipation while minimizing weight. If body-powered control is used, the frame should capture as much body motion as possible, particularly biscapular abduction. Any lost motion will reduce the function of the prosthesis.

If the components are controlled myoelectrically, the generation of control signals may create incidental shoulder motion that could displace the socket and

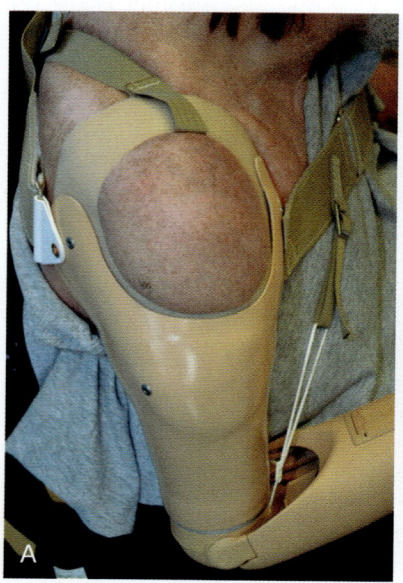
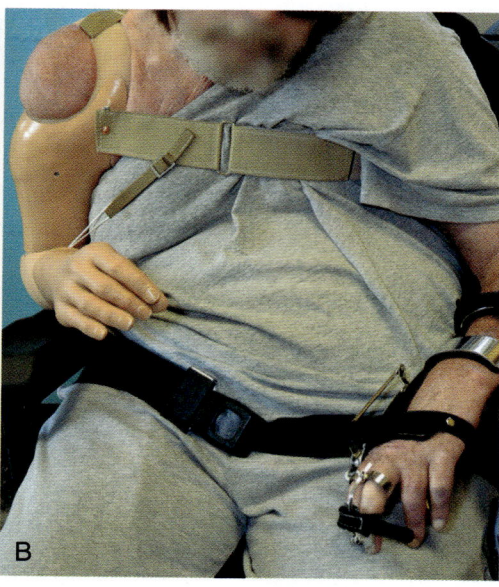

FIGURE 6 Clinical photographs of a patient wearing a shoulder saddle. **A**, A custom, high-consistency rubber silicone socket with an integrated shoulder saddle provides good suspension and socket stability. **B**, The patient, who has quadriplegia, uses a hybrid myoelectric transhumeral prosthesis with an integrated silicone shoulder saddle.

Chapter 22: Bilateral Upper Limb Prostheses

allow electrode movement. In such cases, it may be advantageous to allow the shoulder to move independently within the frame. The weight of the prosthesis can serve to anchor the frame to the user while allowing the use of shoulder motion to activate various electronic inputs.

Several shoulder disarticulation frame designs are currently used. When designing a frame for a particular individual, the prosthetist should consider control sources, harness attachments, and shoulder joint mounting as well as design objectives. These design requirements will dictate the optimal frame geometry for a particular individual.

Harnessing

Conventional harnessing serves the dual role of suspension and control of a body-powered prosthesis. In designing a harness system for the bilateral arm amputee, it may be useful for the prosthetist to consider suspension and control separately. Harness requirements are altered when electrically powered components are used or when the socket design provides suspension. Either or both of these situations can lead to a simpler harness design that can be worn less tightly, potentially making the harness more comfortable.

In situations in which bilateral prostheses are harnessed together, each prosthesis serves as the anchor point for the other. When both prostheses rely on the harness for control, inadvertent cable excursion (sometimes referred to as cross-control) becomes a potential problem. One solution to cross-control is to provide a fully body-powered prosthesis on one side and a fully electrically powered prosthesis on the other side so that the control motions affect only the intended device.

In some instances, a socket may be fitted to provide an anchor for the contralateral prosthesis (**Figure 7**). For example, in the shoulder disarticulation/transhumeral combination, the side of the shoulder disarticulation might be managed with a frame-type socket or passive prosthesis to provide a firm anchor for suspension and control of the transhumeral prosthesis. These options can be shaped to provide aesthetic shoulder symmetry.

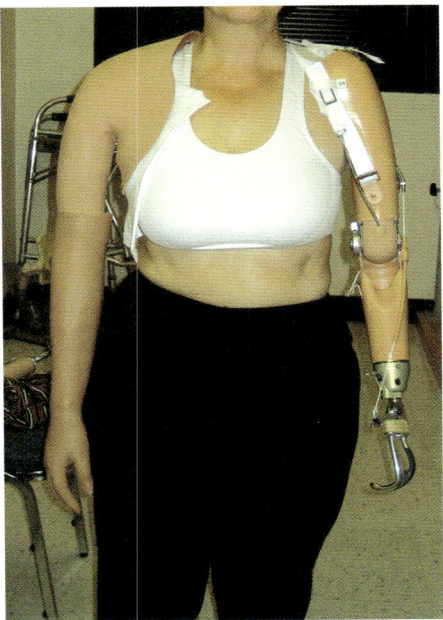

FIGURE 7 Photograph of a patient with a shoulder level and transhumeral limb absence. In some instances, the user may prefer to activate only the more dominant transhumeral prosthesis. The passive shoulder level prosthesis then serves as an anchor for the control harness.

The patient with a bilateral transradial amputation who uses body-powered control will generally be fitted with a standard figure-of-8 harness, which typically incorporates a ring at the cross point for free movement of the straps, with flexible hinges and a triceps pad. Compared with the unilateral figure-of-8 harness, the bilateral version eliminates the axilla loop, which frequently causes discomfort. This type of harness is well tolerated by almost all patients and is easy to don and doff independently. At the transradial level, bilateral myoelectrically controlled prostheses typically require no harness.

Similarly, a bilateral transhumeral amputee wearing body-powered systems will usually be fitted with a figure-of-8 harness with or without a ring. If cable excursion is limited, it is advisable to use a harness design without a ring to limit any loss of motion that may occur when the harness straps rotate on the ring during use. Either a sewn configuration or a leather pad may be beneficial to direct the control attachment straps more inferiorly on

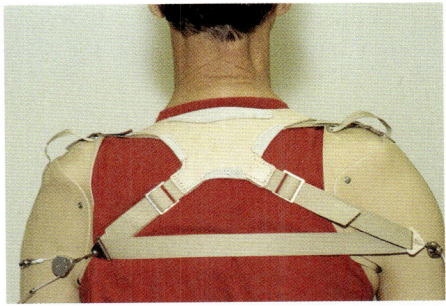

FIGURE 8 Photograph of a patient wearing a harness with a leather pad that is used to replace the cross point of the webbing harness. This design spreads the load over a larger area and helps position the control attachment straps lower on the back.

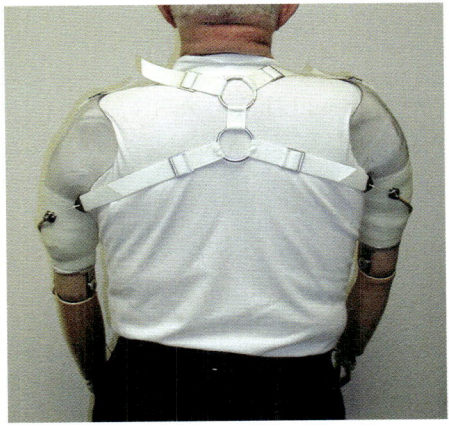

FIGURE 9 Photograph of a patient with a bilateral transhumeral amputation wearing a prosthesis with a double ring harness that increases available excursion by positioning the control attachment straps lower on the scapulae.

the scapulae and increase the available excursion (**Figure 8**). Alternatively, a cross-back strap can be used to keep the control attachment straps low on the scapulae. This also can be accomplished with a dual-ring type harness, with two rings fixed to each other by a strap, one inferior to the other (**Figure 9**). Harness configurations for mixed-level fittings must use sound principles for prosthesis stabilization, suspension, and control (**Figure 10**).

Components

Terminal Devices

The new bilateral upper limb amputee will likely express a preference to be fitted with prosthetic hands because of the assumption that available

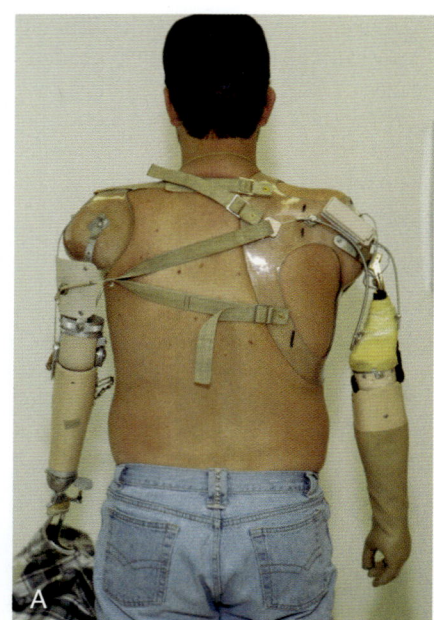
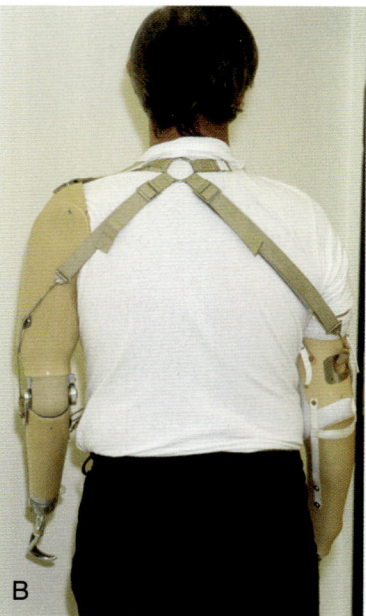
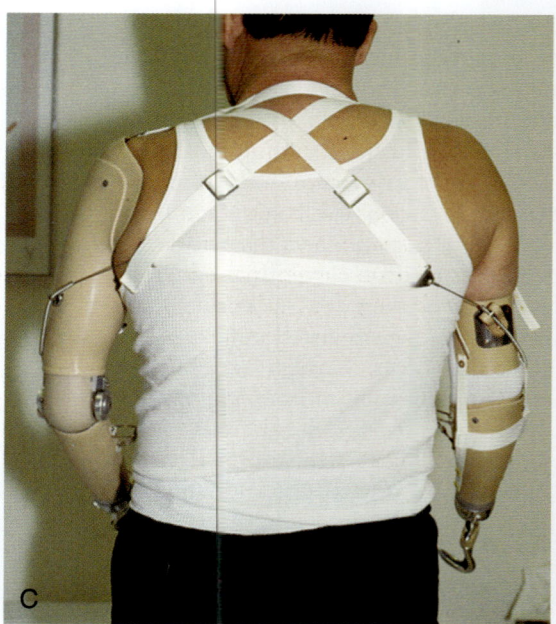

FIGURE 10 Photographs of various harness systems. **A**, A patient wearing a harness for a shoulder disarticulation/transhumeral amputation. The transhumeral prosthesis is entirely body powered and the shoulder disarticulation uses hybrid control with myoelectric control of the terminal device and body-powered control of the elbow. Anteriorly, a single chest strap allows for independent donning and doffing. **B**, A simple figure-of-8 ring harness can be used for a transhumeral/transradial amputee when sufficient excursion exists. **C**, If excursion is limited, it is advisable to use a harness with a sewn cross point and a cross-back strap to maximize excursion.

technology can replace the function and appearance of the physiologic hand. Unfortunately, most body-powered hands are mechanically inefficient and are not useful to the bilateral amputee. If hands are desired, electrically powered hands are generally indicated, although such hands provide little or no proprioceptive feedback.[12] The advantage of electrically powered prehensile devices is a high grip force that can be sustained without continued control input. Multifunctional hands offer a wider variety of grip patterns and hand postures that some bilateral prosthesis users have found useful (**Figure 11**). Most bilateral amputees fitted with electrically powered hands will also benefit from the use of interchangeable electric hook prehensile devices (**Figure 12**). This option allows the amputee to choose which device is best suited to accomplish specific tasks.

Cable-driven components, such as the split hook, offer proprioception through the cable and harness system because component movement and forces are reflected to and perceived by the controlling body part.[12] However, electrically powered devices provide prehension forces three to six times greater than those experienced by users of typical voluntary-opening split hook devices.[3]

It is generally advisable to use two different types of prehensile devices to

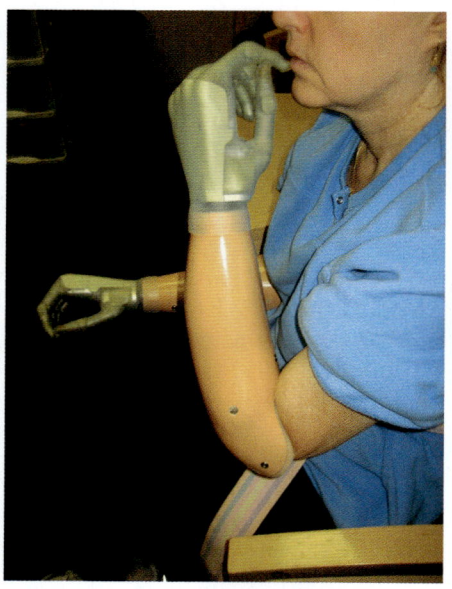

FIGURE 11 Photograph of a patient with a bilateral transradial amputation wearing prostheses with multifunctional hands. A variety of grip patterns can be selected to accomplish the activities of daily living.

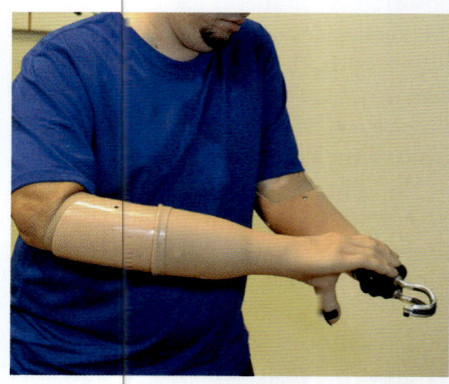

FIGURE 12 The use of multiple terminal devices is routine among bilateral prosthesis users. Photograph of a patient using a myoelectric hand to rotate his electric hook. Mixing terminal devices in this way provides the user with the ability to manipulate a wider range of objects.

provide greater grasp versatility to the bilateral upper limb amputee. A commonly used prehensile device combination is a canted approach hook on the dominant side and a lyre-shaped hook on the contralateral side. The canted hook allows good visual feedback for manipulating objects, whereas the lyre-shaped hook provides better stability for gripping large round objects.

Another successful terminal device combination uses a canted hook on the dominant side and an electrically powered prehensile device on the nondominant side. This combination, which has been particularly well accepted by the amputee with a transhumeral/shoulder disarticulation, provides the fine manipulation capabilities of a split hook and the superior gripping forces available with an electrically powered prehensile device.

Voluntary-opening hooks are primarily used because they maintain grip without the need for continued cable tension and are available in an array of shapes, sizes, and specific patterns of prehension. In contrast, voluntary-closing hooks have more limited use for the bilateral amputee because of the limited number of available designs and the requirement for either continuous cable tension or a locking mechanism to maintain grasp. However, these hooks offer both high grip strength and excellent feedback regarding prehensile forces.

Task-specific terminal devices with quick disconnect wrist components should be considered for the bilateral arm amputee. One innovative approach uses a hands-free tool exchanger that allows for automatic release and exchange of one device for another.

Wrists

Because wrist flexion is especially helpful in body-centered activities (such as feeding, dressing, oral and facial hygiene, and toileting), it should be provided at least on the dominant side, if not bilaterally. Similarly, wrist rotation is essential for effective orientation of the prehensile device.

If a cable-actuated prehensile device is used, the range of wrist rotation will be limited by the control cable that crosses the joint. When an electric rotator is used in conjunction with an electric prehensile device, the elimination of the control cable permits a rotation range greater than 360°.[3] Such continuous wrist rotation can be useful for activities such as turning a water spigot.

It is generally beneficial to use locking wrist components rather than friction designs because bilateral amputees often find it necessary to apply high forces through the prostheses to accomplish various tasks. When friction devices are used, it is often necessary to adjust the friction to a very high setting, which makes it difficult to reposition the device when needed. Positive-locking components become a rigid extension of the body that can maintain position under high loads and can be repositioned with ease when unlocked.

The four-function forearm setup is a particularly useful body-powered wrist system (**Figure 13**). This system has been used successfully on transradial, transhumeral, and shoulder disarticulation prostheses.[13] This system has a common control cable to position four different body-powered prosthetic components—the split hook, the wrist flexion unit, the wrist rotation unit, and the elbow. The simplicity of the system allows the same physiologic control motion to be used to position each of the four components, thus conserving available control sources. However, the control is sequential (only one device can be positioned at a time). Therefore, it is not possible to produce coordinated movements involving two or more components. User feedback suggests that the straightforward manner of the control and the presence of proprioceptive feedback outweigh these disadvantages.[3]

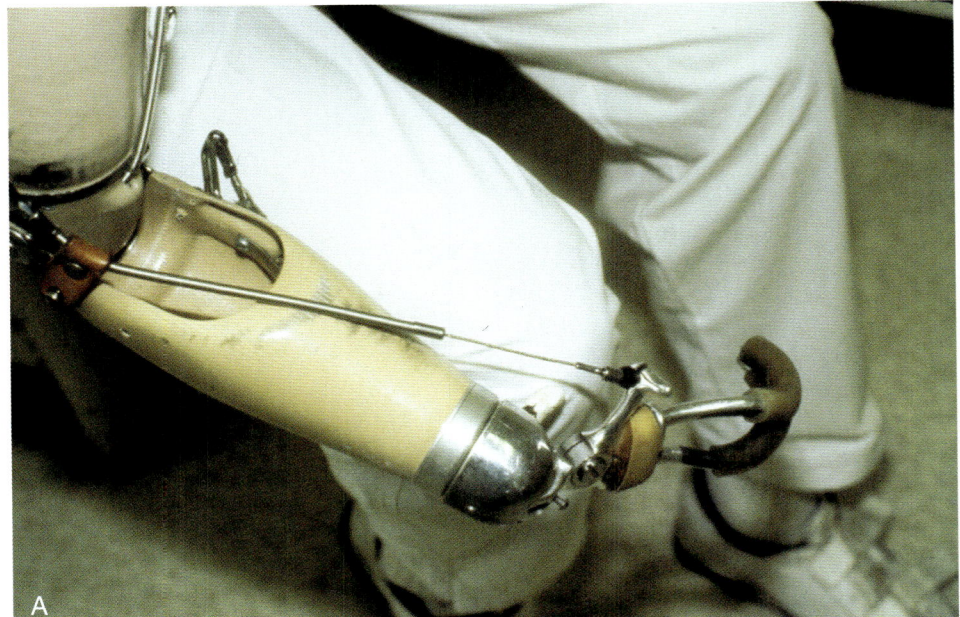
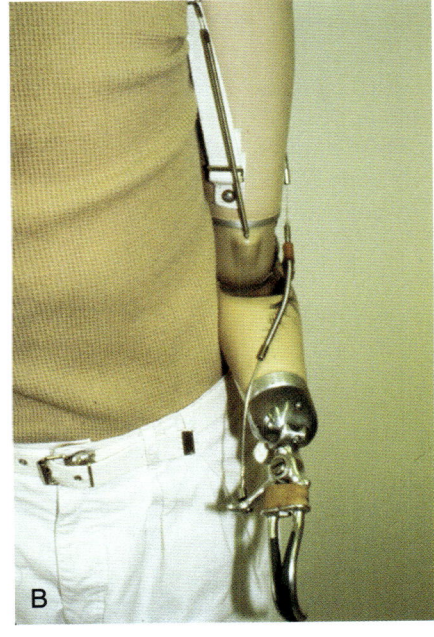

FIGURE 13 Photographs of the four-function forearm setup, which allows body-powered control of wrist flexion and rotation. **A**, The wrist flexion lock can be actuated by pulling against the knee. When unlocked, the wrist is flexed by pulling on the control cable and extended by an elastic tension band. **B**, The wrist rotation feature is unlocked by depressing a lock lever against the torso. When unlocked, cable tension causes supination while pronation is provided by an internally mounted coil spring.

Midforearm flexion offers a nonanthropomorphic solution to limited range of motion that has been particularly useful for the patient with a short or very short transradial amputation. By placing the flexion device more proximal in the prosthesis, a greater arc of motion is achieved at the terminal device. This improves the ease of midline tasks. Because of the altered line of pull, a greater amount of cable excursion is required to activate the hook in the flexed position (**Figure 14**).

Elbows

The selection of the most appropriate prosthetic elbow should include careful evaluation of weight, control options, and compatibility with the other desired components. Body-powered elbows are lighter than electrically powered units, but they provide considerably less live lift. Electrically powered elbows have greater lifting capacity but are heavier and lack the proprioceptive feedback inherent in the cable control of body-powered elbows.[3]

A spring lift assist or automatic forearm balance should be considered for all body-powered elbow fittings. These devices allow the prosthetist to optimize and balance the force/excursion requirements of a particular system with the abilities and needs of a particular user.

In patients with bilateral arm amputations who require two elbows, it is sometimes beneficial to provide one body-powered and one electrically powered elbow. The two elbows complement each other, with the electrically powered device providing greater live lift capacity and the body-powered elbow providing better positioning control.[3]

Elbow hinges are seldom indicated for bilateral transradial amputees. A rarely used but effective exception is the appropriate application of step-up hinges. The disadvantages of step-up hinges include the increased force required to flex the elbow and, depending on the residual limb length, poor forearm cosmesis when the elbow is flexed. However, these disadvantages are sometimes outweighed by the increased range of motion afforded by this option. Also, a fair-lead cable housing can be used with these hinges to supplement elbow flexion forces if there is sufficient physiologic elbow extension strength to stabilize the flexed elbow during operation of the terminal device. This same approach can be used for an individual who presents with weak elbow flexion force using standard single-pivot hinges if passive flexion range is available and there is enough extension force to resist further flexion during operation of the terminal device (**Figure 15**).

Humeral Rotation

All internal locking elbow systems routinely used in North America, both body-powered and electrically powered, are equipped with friction-moderated humeral rotation. Friction control is simple and does not require a control source for operation. However, as with the cited limitations of friction wrists, friction control of humeral rotation may compromise the usefulness of the prosthesis for certain tasks requiring high force. Therefore, locking humeral rotation may be beneficial. Locking humeral rotators may be used on body-powered as well as electrically powered elbows.[3,14] The lock is operated by a control cable that can be actuated through a control harness in parallel with the elbow lock or by a chin-actuated nudge control (**Figure 16**).

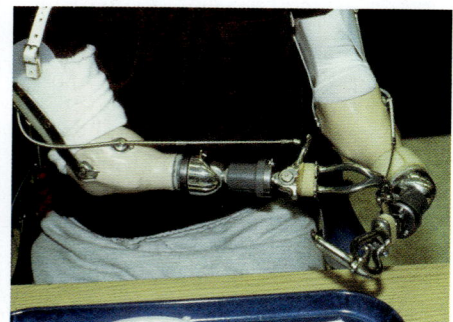

FIGURE 14 Photograph of an amputee with limited elbow range of motion. Midforearm flexion affords the necessary hook placement for midline activities for these patients.

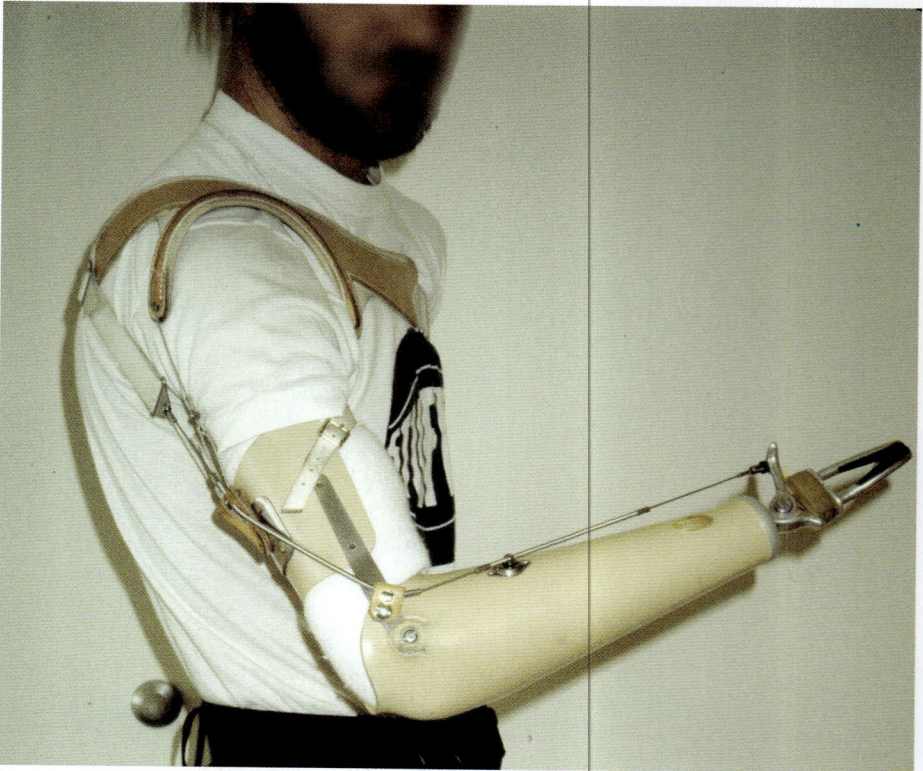

FIGURE 15 Photograph of a man with a prosthesis with a fair-lead cable, which can be used to assist elbow flexion if there is sufficient extension force to stabilize the elbow during hook operation.

Chapter 22: Bilateral Upper Limb Prostheses

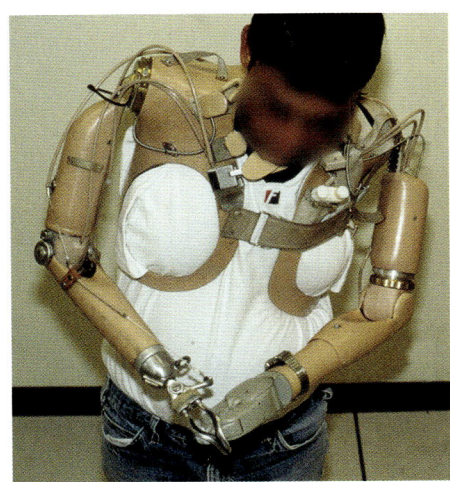

FIGURE 16 Locking humeral rotation allows easy positioning of the terminal device while providing a rigid limb as needed to resist high forces. Photograph of a man with a bilateral shoulder disarticulation who is demonstrating the ability to bring his terminal devices into contact with each other; this allows bimanual manipulation.

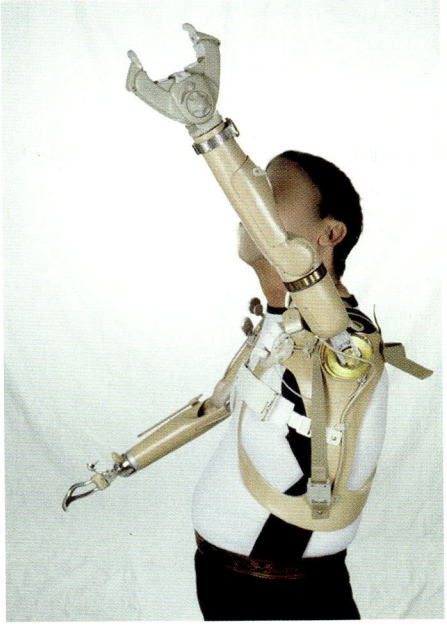

FIGURE 17 Photograph showing that a locking shoulder joint allows a patient with a bilateral shoulder disarticulation to operate the terminal device overhead. The terminal device is controlled by a linear transducer using shoulder elevation, providing reliable variable speed control.

TABLE 1 Body Position Control Sources

Primary Work Sources That Produce Good Force and Excursion
Glenohumeral flexion
Scapular/biscapular abduction
Control Sources for Mechanical Locks and Electronic Inputs
Glenohumeral extension/abduction/shoulder depression
Shoulder elevation
Chest expansion
Abdominal expansion
Chin nudge
Glenohumeral adduction
Other (any movable body part)

Shoulder Joints

The bilateral amputee who requires a prosthetic shoulder joint will benefit from a device that locks in position for similar reasons as those described for locking wrist and humeral components. The Axis Locking Shoulder Joint (College Park) provides a positive locking feature for flexion and friction for abduction control. The lock can be operated by a cable nudge control or with an electric actuator. The rigidity of the locked shoulder joint allows the amputee to use the prosthesis more effectively as an extension of the body to transmit forces through the structure of the complete prosthesis.[3] In addition, the terminal device allows overhead operation (**Figure 17**).

Control Systems

Currently, the available control options in upper limb prostheses can be divided into two basic categories—body position control and myoelectric control. Body position control refers to the use of intact body motions and the excursion and/or forces produced by those motions (**Table 1**). The most familiar of these control options are cable-operated systems, but body motions also are used to operate electric inputs such as switches, servos, transducers, and force-sensitive resistors (**Figure 18**). Alternatively, myoelectric control makes use of the electric byproducts of voluntary muscle contractions. As such, myoelectric control is generally independent of joint position.

It is necessary to understand the relationship between the available control sources and the types of components that can be most effectively controlled. Component selection should be based on a careful analysis of which devices and control options will best serve the intended function of the particular user.

Of critical importance to the bilateral amputee is the reliability of the control system. A control source is reliable if every control command results in the desired component function. Equally important, a component should function only as a result of an intentional control command. When a control command fails to consistently produce the desired result, the overall usefulness of the prosthesis is greatly compromised. Therefore, control systems that are too complicated or that rely on a marginal control source are prone to failure. Training on use of the prosthesis is often essential in maximizing the reliability of control. If training fails to produce consistently reliable control function, an alternative control method is indicated.

When controlling multiple components, control options can be further categorized as either dedicated or sequential. Sequential control means that two or more components will be controlled from a common source; simultaneous control is not possible. Dedicated control assigns separate control sources to each prosthetic component. This method provides the user with immediate access to use of a component and, in some instances, may support the simultaneous control of two components for the production of coordinated movements.[3,12] It is generally desirable to devise a control scheme that provides dedicated control whenever possible. At higher amputation levels, this poses a substantial challenge because of the increased number of prosthetic joints that require control and the limited number of available control sources. It is sometimes necessary to combine sequential and dedicated control to provide the desired functions. In these cases, the component functions that may be combined in simultaneous useful ways should be prioritized and assigned separate control sources (**Figure 19**).

Section 2: Upper Limb

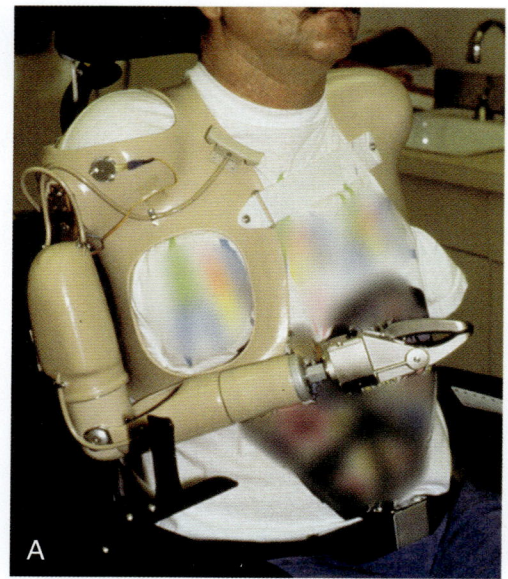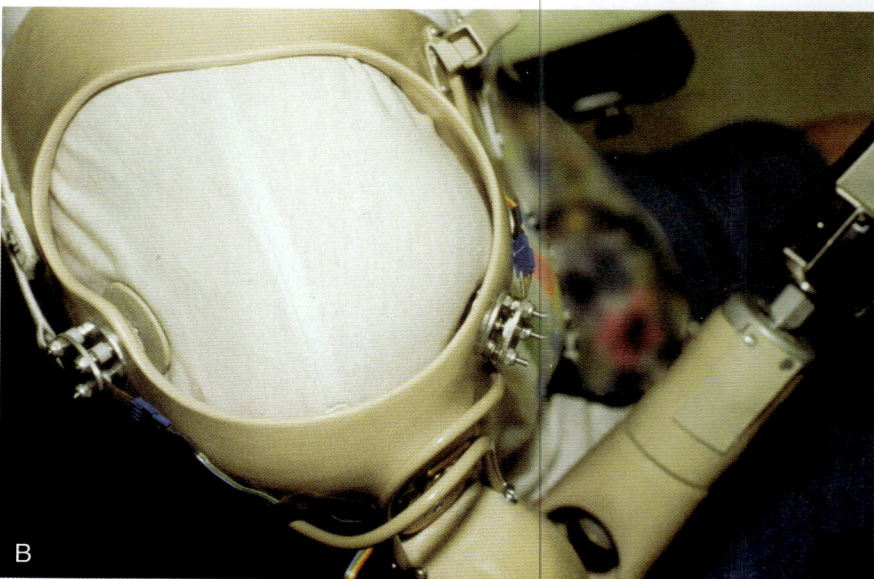

FIGURE 18 Photographs of a single multifunctional prosthesis worn by a patient with bilateral shoulder disarticulations, bilateral transtibial amputations, and paraplegia. The use of a single multifunctional prosthesis provides some independence in self-feeding and simple object manipulation. **A**, The wrist rotator, positioned at midforearm, is controlled by a chin-activated rocker switch. A wheelchair mounted bracket assists with internal and external rotation of the humeral turntable. Wrist flexion is achieved using a conventional flexion wrist. **B**, An electric elbow is operated with a pair of force-sensing resistors mounted anteriorly and posteriorly within the socket, and the terminal device is controlled using contralateral scapular abduction and a harness pull switch. Coordinated simultaneous elbow flexion and wrist rotation are possible and useful for self-feeding.

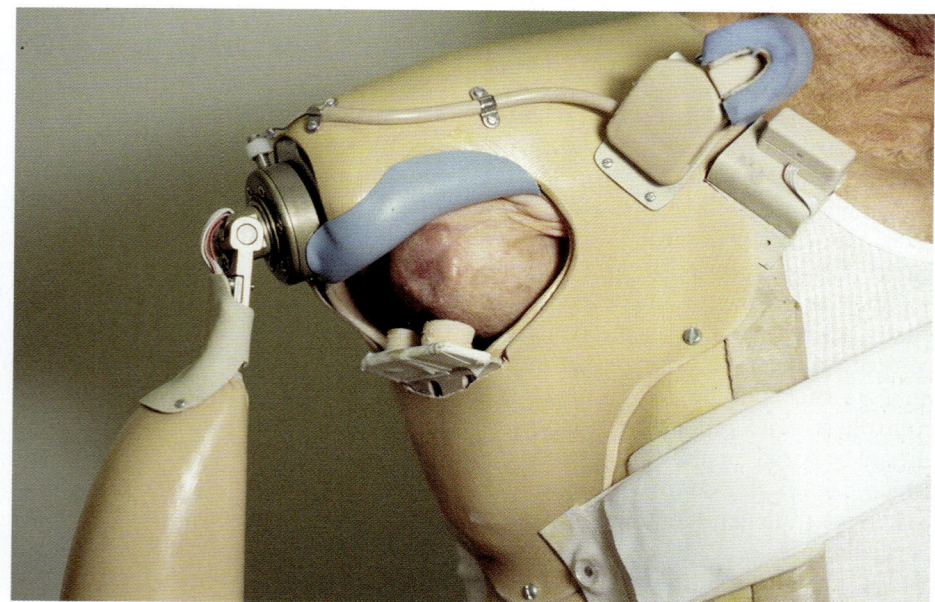

FIGURE 19 Photograph from a patient with bilateral humeral neck amputations. A mobile residual humerus provides excellent dedicated control of the electric terminal device using a pair of force-sensitive resistors.

It is often advisable to provide two or more complete sets of prostheses with different control and power sources to enable the widest variety of functional capabilities and to provide a backup when repairs are needed.

Body-Powered Control

Cable actuation of body-powered prostheses provides users with a wealth of proprioceptive feedback through the physiologic joints harnessed to the prosthetic components.[15]

Users of these devices can readily perceive the position and speed of movement of the prosthetic components.[3] Body-powered, cable-operated control offers many of the desirable characteristics of the theory of control proposed by Childress based on the work of Simpson,[16,17] which states: "The most natural and most subconscious control of a prosthesis can be achieved through use of the body's own joints as control inputs in which joint position corresponds (always in a one-to-one relationship) to prosthesis position, joint velocity corresponds to prosthesis velocity, and joint force corresponds to prosthesis force."

This type of control is referred to as extended physiologic proprioception. Although implementation of extended physiologic proprioception control is possible with electronic components,[15,18-20] it requires fast, high-performance components to produce optimal results. Currently, such a system is not commercially available.

Because of the inherent feedback provided through the cable and harness system, body-powered elbow control is well accepted and quite functional if adequate force and excursion exist. Body-powered control of an elbow affords the greatest degree of graceful and accurate positioning of the prehensile device in space. Control can become subconscious, as has been observed in bilateral transhumeral amputees who dynamically incorporate use of their prostheses by gesturing with their limbs and gracefully repositioning their elbows when speaking.

Cable efficiency is of critical importance to the success of a body-powered fitting. Careful attention should be devoted to producing the straightest line of pull using materials that offer the least amount of friction.[21]

Myoelectric Control

In contrast to control methods that require body motions of more proximal body segments, myoelectric control is a more natural-appearing system because the method of controlling the prosthesis is invisible.[12] It also represents the most physiologically natural method of controlling an electric hand. This is especially true for the transradial amputee because control is accomplished in a physiologically natural fashion, with myoelectric signals from the forearm flexors closing the hand and signals from the extensors opening the hand. At this level, the harness can be eliminated, which allows for an improved functional envelope because the position of the prosthesis and operation of the terminal device are not confined by straps. For more proximal amputation levels, the flexor and extensor patterns of more proximal muscles are associated with and well suited for the tasks of grasping and releasing objects. The transhumeral amputee would use the biceps to close the hand and the triceps to open the hand because a flexion pattern is closely associated with grasping and an extensor pattern is associated with releasing.[12] Childress[16] described this as the principle of myoprehension, which suggests that myoelectric control can be somewhat naturally connected with the control of prehension. An important disadvantage of this type of control is the lack of direct feedback from the control system to the user regarding the position, velocity, and force of the component controlled. Users of a myoelectric control system must rely primarily on visual feedback as they manipulate their environment with the prosthesis.[12]

Targeted muscle reinnervation (TMR) surgery has been successful in increasing the number of usable myoelectric control sites and directly associating them with more distal functions. With TMR, remaining nerves in the arm are transferred to residual chest or upper arm muscles that are no longer biomechanically functional because of limb loss. After reinnervation, these muscles serve as biologic amplifiers of motor commands from the transferred arm nerves and provide physiologically appropriate electromyographic signals for control of the elbow, wrist, and hand.[22] Kuiken et al[23] reported the success of TMR surgery for improving ease of control and allowing simultaneous myoelectric control in an amputee with a bilateral shoulder disarticulation.

Another promising technology for prosthesis control is the use of pattern recognition with or without TMR surgery. Pattern recognition uses multiple electrodes placed around the residual limb to record patterns of muscle activity that are then associated with corresponding prosthetic functions.[24] Pattern recognition control systems have the potential to provide more intuitive, direct control of multiple functions without the need for mode selection strategies. Pattern recognition control systems have recently become commercially available and training protocols have been suggested.[25]

Hybrid Control

The selected control arrangement should impose the minimum amount of mental stress on the user (ie, the control of the prosthesis should not be so complicated that it becomes the primary object of the user's attention).[3] Faced with the complexity of high-level bilateral fittings, one seemingly small change in the control strategy can cause a chain reaction of control source interaction.[3] Although hybrid components (electric combined with body-powered) and hybrid input devices may provide the most desirable results, these systems can be technically demanding and require that the prosthetist have a high degree of creativity and knowledge. In the experience of this chapter's author, the benefits realized by the users of hybridized systems far outweigh the technical difficulties in producing these systems. The key to optimal design of prostheses for the bilateral amputee is in the details, and each detail must be carefully considered to achieve optimal results.

Prototype Prostheses

Given the large number of component and control options available to the upper limb amputee, it is often advisable to set up a clinical trial of the proposed design using a prototype prosthesis. For a patient with a higher level arm amputation, this process can be critical to the outcome of prosthetic rehabilitation. The availability of all component options and the technical ability to mix and match components from different manufacturers are critical to the success of this approach. The foundation of the prototype prosthesis is a well-fitted interface for evaluation. A prototype prosthesis may be used for periods of time ranging from a few hours for very straightforward fittings to several months for challenging cases in which several prosthetic options must be evaluated. The use of a prototype prosthesis allows the amputee and other concerned parties to evaluate and validate the efficacy of any particular prosthetic component and control configuration before completion of the definitive prosthesis[12] (**Figure 20**).

Fitting Consideration by Level

Partial Hand

In patients with one or both limbs amputated at the partial hand level, the main prosthetic considerations are to provide effective prehension while limiting the amount of sensate area that is covered or encumbered by the device. Opposition posts (**Figure 21**),

Section 2: Upper Limb

handihooks, and myoelectric prostheses can be fitted at the partial hand level. Opposition posts are particularly useful if a movable digit(s) remains. These devices are simple, lightweight, and generally cover the least amount of area.

Body-powered options include wrist-driven designs for activation of fingers when amputated at or proximal to the metacarpophalangeal joints or finger-driven designs for partial finger amputations (**Figure 22**). The cable-actuated handihook will provide grasp and release for amputees who lack a movable digit(s) (**Figure 23, A and B**). When fitted loosely, the user can quickly doff the socket, leaving it attached by the control system, while objects are manipulated using their sensate residual hand.

Powered fingers are best suited for amputations at or proximal to the metacarpophalangeal joints. Powered fingers may be controlled with myoelectric signals or force-sensing resistors and have been successfully fitted to bilateral partial hand amputees (**Figure 23, C**). Wrist motion as well as motion of any intact fingers should be unrestricted by the prosthesis whenever possible.

Transradial Level

Body-powered hooks and myoelectric systems can be successfully fitted for a patient with a bilateral transradial amputation. Body-powered hooks offer fine manipulation and are robust and lightweight (**Figure 24, A**). Myoelectric hands offer a good appearance with acceptable manipulative abilities (**Figure 24, B**). Myoelectric hooks offer good, fine manipulation ability, and because they have no cosmetic cover, they are better suited to use for manual labor than myoelectric hands. Myoelectric systems are unconstrained by the need for a harness, increasing the work envelope. Some users find both types of prostheses useful and routinely

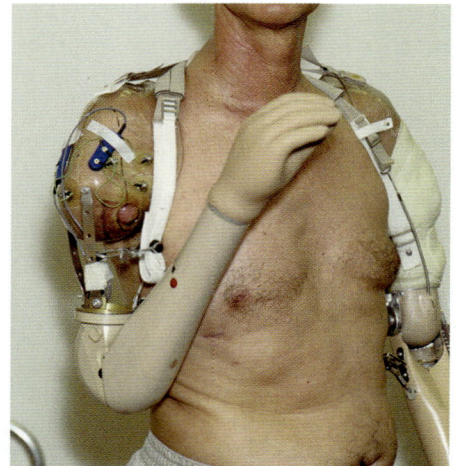

FIGURE 20 Photograph of a patient with a bilateral transhumeral amputation using a prototype prosthesis, which is a valuable tool in the development of an optimal prosthesis. The well-fitted socket serves as the foundation for the prototype, and modular construction allows for trials of various prosthetic component and control options.

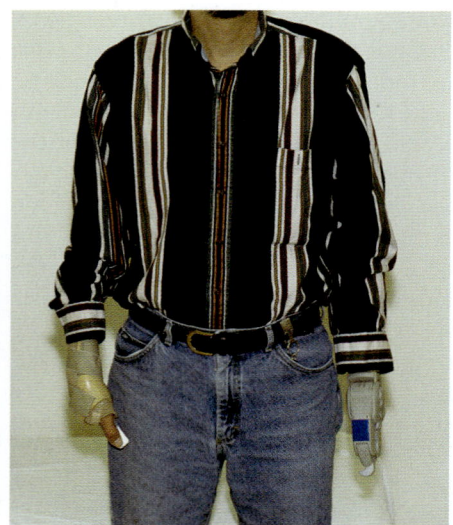

FIGURE 21 An opposition post can provide a simple and robust device to enhance the function of a partial hand amputee with one or more remaining movable digits. Photograph of a patient with transradial/partial hand amputations. He finds his partial hand side most useful for fine motor tasks primarily because of the feedback provided by his sensate thumb.

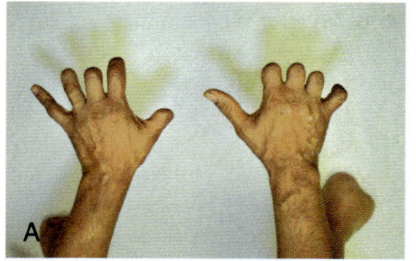
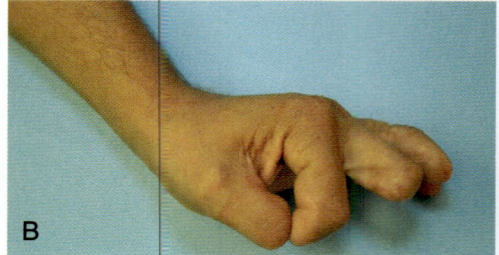
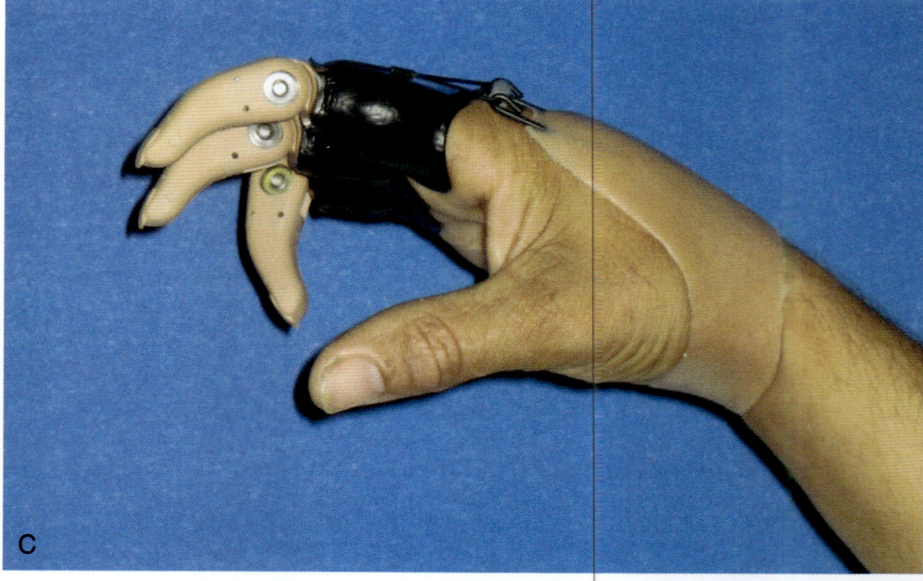

FIGURE 22 Photographs from a patient with bilateral partial finger amputations (**A**) demonstrating good function with his left hand without a prosthesis (**B**). **C**, Right hand grasp was improved with Partial M-Finger (Partial Hand Solutions) prostheses in which metacarpophalangeal flexion results in flexion of the prosthetic fingers.

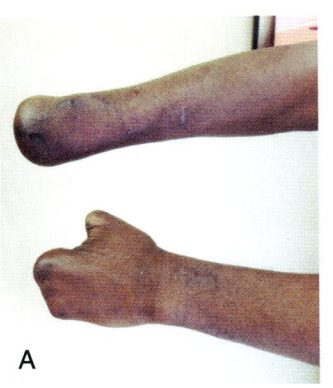 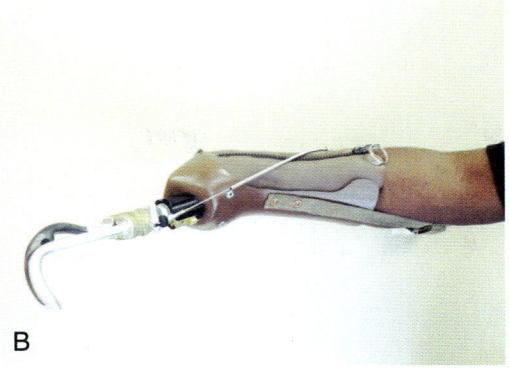 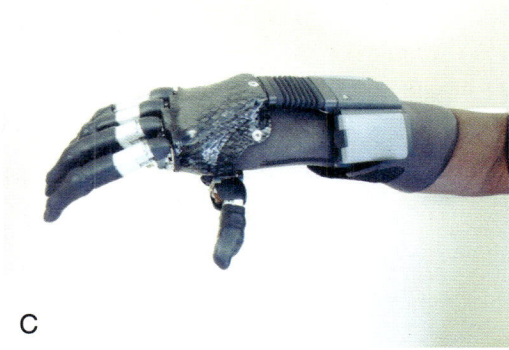

FIGURE 23 Clinical photographs from a patient with bilateral partial hand amputations. **A**, The patient relied on the sensation of his left hand but was unable to hold objects securely because of the short length of the remnant digits. His right partial hand was fitted with a body-powered handihook–type prosthesis (**B**) and a powered finger prosthesis (**C**), allowing stable grasp of a wide variety of objects.

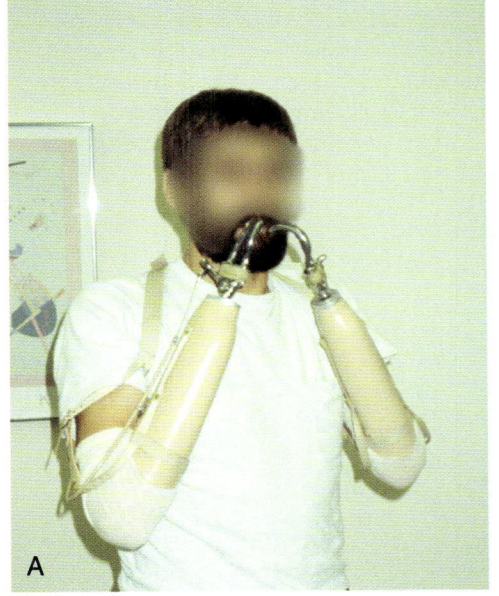 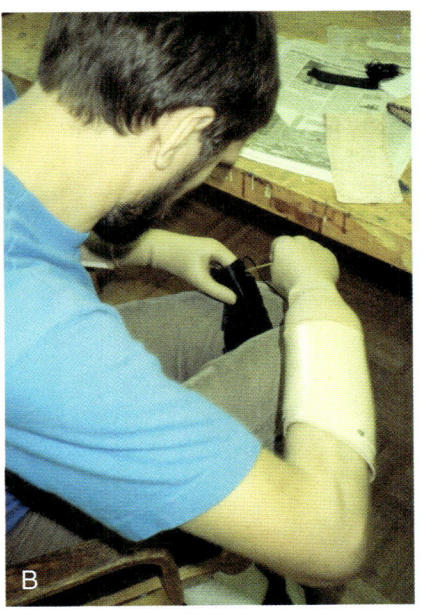 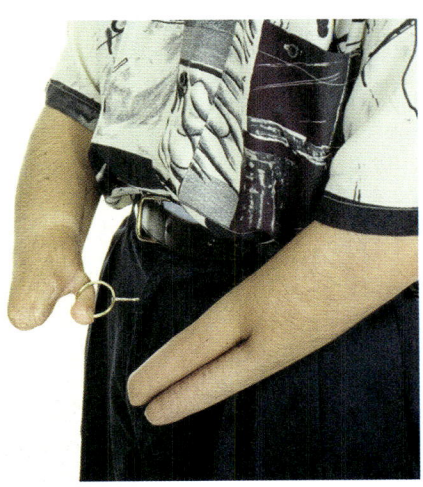

FIGURE 24 Photographs of a patient with bilateral wrist disarticulations who was fitted with both body-powered and myoelectric prostheses. **A**, Both systems allow full elbow range of motion and retain forearm rotation. **B**, Electric hands provide greater grip force and a more natural appearance than voluntary-opening split hooks. This patient finds both sets of prostheses valuable and can match the most appropriate design with a particular activity.

FIGURE 25 Photograph of a blind, bilateral transradial amputee who underwent a Krukenberg procedure on the left hand and a Vilkki procedure on the right hand. These procedures provided the patient with sensate limbs with a variety of gripping options.

switch between prostheses as required by the type of activities pursued.

Sensation is of critical concern for the transradial amputee. Exposed skin can be desirable, especially at the longer transradial and wrist disarticulation levels. For the blind bilateral transradial amputee, sensation is required for function. In these patients, surgical intervention (such as a Krukenberg procedure or a toe transfer to the forearm [Vilkki procedure]) is indicated to produce a limb with manipulative capabilities[26] (**Figure 25**).

Transhumeral Level

Body-powered systems appear to offer the best results for the patient with a bilateral transhumeral amputation. However, electric terminal devices and elbows provide greater forces and can be worn on the nondominant side to complement the function of a dominant side body-powered prosthesis. The ability to easily and securely position the prosthesis in space becomes more critical as physiologic joints are lost. Positive locking wrists and humeral rotators should be considered for these patients. Because of the loss of glenohumeral rotation in the transhumeral prosthesis, it may be beneficial for the surgeon to perform an angulation osteotomy to enhance the useful dynamic positioning of the prosthesis in space[27] (**Figure 26**). Surgical lengthening using bone allograft, which allows for improved function resulting from a longer residual limb, has been beneficial for managing short transhumeral amputations[28] (**Figure 27**).

As with a transradial prosthesis, independent donning of the transhumeral prosthesis is a primary goal. Donning independence is almost always achieved when body position control is used, but it may be

Section 2: Upper Limb

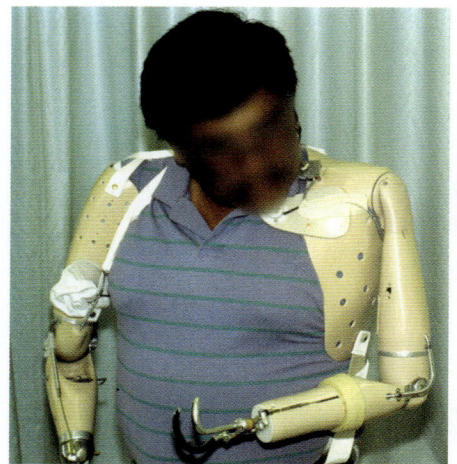
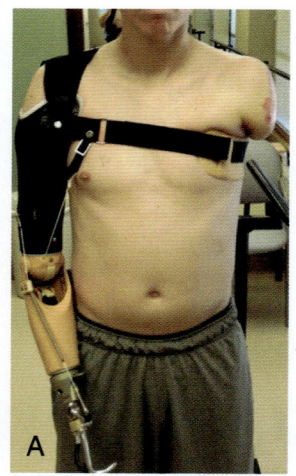
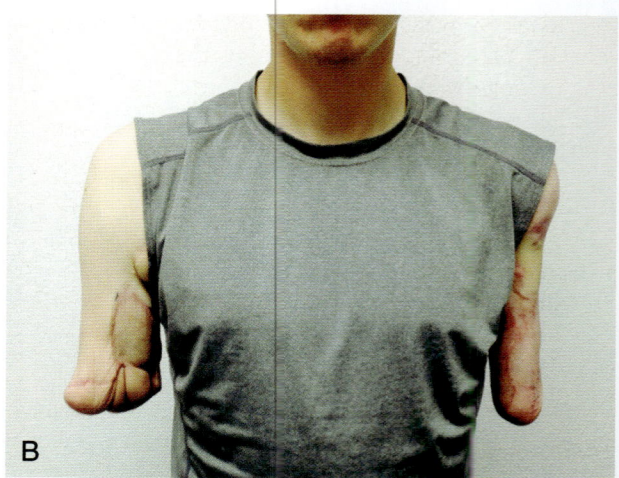

FIGURE 26 Photograph of a transhumeral/shoulder disarticulation amputee who benefited from an angulation osteotomy on his right limb that facilitates physiologic humeral rotation, which improves rotational stability and provides added positioning control of the prosthesis.

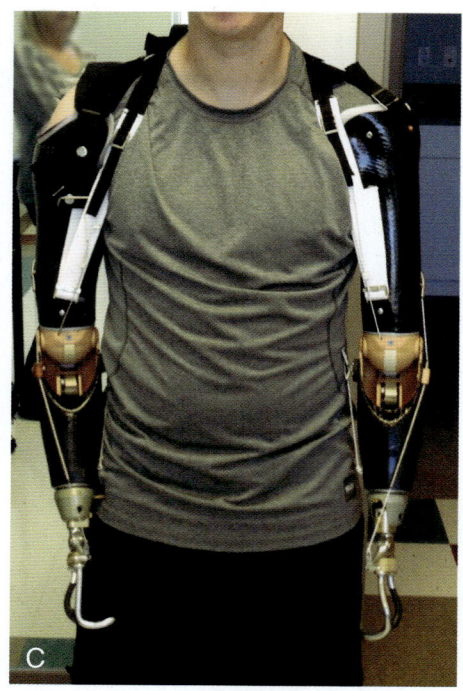

FIGURE 27 Photographs of a patient with bilateral transhumeral amputations who underwent surgical bone lengthening with allograft on his left limb to improve function by providing a longer lever to allow better prosthesis control and stability. **A**, Because the patient had a very short left residual limb, he was initially fitted with a prosthesis only on his dominant right side. Photographs show the left limb after allograft transplantation (**B**) and after fitting with bilateral body-powered prostheses (**C**).

compromised when myoelectric control is used because of the need for skin-to-electrode contact and the difficulty in donning these systems. In the experience of this chapter's author, nearly all bilateral arm amputees with one or both amputations at the transhumeral level prefer a body-powered prosthesis on the transhumeral side that incorporates a four-function forearm setup over myoelectric or other hybrid control options. Nevertheless, electric control of one or more components may be advantageous for some individuals if the requisite force and/or excursion for body-powered control are unavailable. New suspension/control systems, such as those with HCR silicone suction sockets with myoelectric interface capabilities[6] and other electrically controlled input options under development, may necessitate the incorporation of these newer technologies into bilateral fitting practice if they offer functional advantages for the user.

Shoulder Disarticulation

When fitting a patient with a bilateral shoulder disarticulation, it is advisable to start with as simple a prosthetic system as possible. Often, only the dominant side is fit initially. The complexity of the control system should be kept to a minimum, starting perhaps with only an activated terminal device and elbow. As the patient becomes familiar with the use of the prosthesis, wrist function can be added, followed by humeral rotation and a locking shoulder joint. The prosthesis for the nondominant side can be fitted after the user has gained confidence in using the dominant-side prosthesis. Complexity on the nondominant side can be staged in a similar fashion as used for the dominant-side prosthesis. In general, the dominant-side prosthesis of the bilateral pair is configured with mechanical, cable-actuated components (similar to the four-function setup), whereas the nondominant-side prosthesis incorporates either all-electric or hybrid components to provide complementary functions.[3] When possible, the electric prosthesis should use dedicated variable speed control of the prehensile device, the wrist, and the elbow.

SUMMARY

Successful rehabilitation of a patient with a bilateral arm amputation is best achieved with a team approach. Bilateral arm amputees, especially those with high-level loss, will benefit greatly from prosthetic intervention and other assistive technologies, including automobile modification, communication devices, self-care devices, and nonprosthetic manipulation devices that serve to augment the functions of the user. Each bilateral arm amputee must be treated as a unique individual. The needs, goals, and desires of the individual should be the focus of the rehabilitation team. The fitting methods and philosophies presented in this chapter should serve only as a guide for successful prosthetic rehabilitation. Variations to this approach will be required based on the particular unique presentation of the individual being treated and their expressed preferences for particular prosthetic options.

Experience has shown that careful attention to socket fitting, ease of use of the control system, and minimized prosthesis weight are critical aspects in successful rehabilitation. Proven desirable features of a successful prosthesis are comfort, aesthetics, feedback, donning independence, control reliability, variable speed control, and locking joints. Clinical fitting protocol is driven by the availability of contemporary components and the control strategies for their operation. As new components and control schemes emerge, they should be objectively evaluated. New possibilities should be explored in the light of what is possible and should not be limited by what has previously been done. Despite the many shortcomings of state-of-the-art arm prostheses, bilateral amputees often make good use of these tools as they strive to achieve functional independence.

References

1. Resnik L, Ekerholm S, Borgia M, Clark MA: A national study of Veterans with major upper limb amputation: Survey methods, participants, and summary findings. *PLoS One* 2019;14(3):e0213578.

2. Jang CH, Yang HS, Yang HE, et al: A survey on activities of daily living and occupations of upper extremity amputees. *Ann Rehabil Med* 2011;35(6):907-921.

3. Uellendahl JE, Heckathorne CW: Creative prosthetic solutions for the person with bilateral upper extremity amputations, in Atkins D, Meier R, eds: *Functional Restoration of Adults and Children With Upper Extremity Amputation*. Demos Medical Publishing, 2004, pp 225-237.

4. Uellendahl JE, Heelan JR: Prosthetic management of the upper limb deficient child, in Alexander M, Molnar G, eds: *Physical Medicine and Rehabilitation: State of the Art Reviews*. Vol 14, No 2. Hanley & Belfus, 2000, p 232.

5. Malone JM, Fleming LL, Roberson J, et al: Immediate, early, and late postsurgical management of upper-limb amputation. *J Rehabil Res Dev* 1984;21(1):33-41.

6. Uellendahl JE, Mandacina S, Ramdial S: Custom silicone sockets for myoelectric prostheses. *J Prosthet Orthot* 2006;18(2):35-40.

7. Billock JN: The Northwestern University supracondylar suspension technique for below elbow amputations. *Orthot Prosthet* 1972;26(4):16-23.

8. Sauter WF, Naumann S, Milner M: A three-quarter type below-elbow socket for myoelectric prostheses. *Prosthet Orthot Int* 1986;10(2):79-82.

9. McLaurin CA, Sauter WF, Dolan CM, Hartmann GR: Fabrication procedures for the open-shoulder above-elbow socket. *Artif Limbs* 1969;13(2):46-54.

10. Bush G: Powered upper extremity prosthetics programme: Above elbow fittings, in *Hugh MacMillan Rehabilitation Centre, Rehabilitation Engineering Department Annual Report* 1990, pp 35-37.

11. Farnsworth T, Uellendahl J, Mikosz MJ, Miller L, Petersen B: Shoulder region socket considerations. *J Prosthet Orthot* 2008;20(3):93-106.

12. Uellendahl JE: Upper extremity myoelectric prosthetics. *Phys Med Rehabil Clin N Am* 2000;11(3):639-652.

13. Uellendahl J, Heckathorne C: Prosthetic component control schemes for bilateral above-elbow prostheses, in *Proceedings of the Myoelectric Control Symposium, University of New Brunswick* 1993, pp 3-5.

14. Ivko JJ: Independence through humeral rotation in the conventional transhumeral prosthetic design. *J Prosthet Orthot* 1999;11(1):20-22.

15. Heckathorne CW: Manipulation in unstructured environments: Extended physiological proprioception, position control, and arm prostheses, in *Proceedings of the International Conference on Rehabilitation Robotics*. Institute of Electrical and Electronic Engineers, 1990, pp 25-40.

16. Childress DS: Control of limb prostheses, in Bowker JH, Michael JW, eds. *Atlas of Limb Prosthetics: Surgical, Prosthetic, and Rehabilitation Principles*. Mosby-Year Book, 1992, pp 175-198.

17. Simpson DC: The choice of control system for the multi-movement prosthesis: Extended physiological proprioception, in Herberts P, Kadefors R, Magnusson R, Petersen I, et al, eds: *The Control of Upper Extremity Prostheses and Orthoses*. Charles C Thomas Publishers, 1974, pp 146-150.

18. Doubler JA, Childress DS: Design and evaluation of a prosthesis control system based on the concept of extended physiological proprioception. *J Rehabil Res Dev* 1984;21(1):19-31.

19. Heckathorne C, Childress D, Grahn E, Strysik J, Uellendahl J: E.P.P. control of an electric hand by exteriorized forearm tendons, in *Proceedings of the Eighth World Congress of the International Society for Prosthetics and Orthotics*. Brussels, Belgium, ISPO, 1995, p 101.

20. Heckathorne CW, Uellendahl J, Childress DS: Application of a force-actuated position-servo controller 8 for electric elbows, in *Proceedings of the Seventh World Congress of the International Society for Prosthetics and Orthotics*. Brussels, Belgium, ISPO, 1992, p 315.

21. Carlson L, Veatch B, Frey D: Efficiency of prosthetic cable and housing. *J Prosthet Orthot* 1995;7(3):96-99.

22. Kuiken TA, Li G, Lock BA, et al: Targeted muscle reinnervation for real-time myoelectric control of multifunction artificial arms. *J Am Med Assoc* 2009;301(6):619-628.

23. Kuiken TA, Dumanian GA, Lipschutz RD, Miller LA, Stubblefield KA: The

use of targeted muscle reinnervation for improved myoelectric prosthesis control in a bilateral shoulder disarticulation amputee. *Prosthet Orthot Int* 2004;28(3):245-253.
24. Hudgins B, Parker P, Scott RN: A new strategy for multifunction myoelectric control. *IEEE Trans Biomed Eng* 1993;40(1):82-94.
25. Simon AM, Lock BA, Stubblefield KA: Patient training for functional use of pattern recognition-controlled prostheses. *J Prosthet Orthot* 2012;24(2):56-64.
26. Vilkki SK: Free toe transfer to the forearm stump following wrist amputation: A current alternative to the Krukenberg operation. *Handchir Mikrochir Plast Chir* 1985;17(2):92-97.
27. Marquardt E, Neff G: The angulation osteotomy of above-elbow stumps. *Clin Orthop Relat Res* 1974;104:232-238.
28. Wilkins RM, Brown WC: Allograft transplantation to lengthen transhumeral amputation limbs, in *Conference Proceedings of the 12th World Congress of International Society for Prosthetics and Orthotics.* Brussels, Belgium, ISPO, 2007, p 310.

Targeted Muscle Reinnervation for Enhanced Prosthetic Control

CHAPTER 23

Jason M. Souza, MD, FACS • Gregory A. Dumanian, MD

ABSTRACT

Targeted muscle reinnervation (TMR) is a surgical procedure whereby transected nerves are transferred to intact motor nerves within the residual limb to recapture the motor control information previously transmitted by the transected donor nerves. After neurotization, the reinnervated muscle acts as a biologic amplifier capable of generating an electromyographic signal large enough for surface detection by the prosthesis. Since it was first reported in 2004, TMR has gained widespread use as a pain management strategy, with prosthetic control often serving as a secondary indication in most cases. However, the increased prosthetic usage and enhanced function offered by direct skeletal attachment of extremity prostheses has renewed interest in efforts to optimize prosthetic control outcomes.

Keywords: nerve transfer; neuroma; prosthetic control; targeted muscle reinnervation

Introduction

Refinements in amputation techniques throughout the 20th century led to great improvements in the durability and functionality of the residual limb. Strategies for controlling the prosthesis primarily remained the responsibility of the prosthetist. However, continuing improvements in the capabilities of myoelectric prosthetic devices have led to the need for an improved control strategy. In 1995, Kuiken et al[1] found that an amputated rat nerve transferred into a nearby denervated muscle produced a transcutaneously detectable electromyographic (EMG) signal corresponding to the transferred nerve. This finding led to the use of the targeted muscle reinnervation (TMR) technique in humans. The use of TMR was reported in 2004 in a patient with a shoulder disarticulation and subsequently in patients with transhumeral amputation.[2-6] TMR was found to bridge the gap between prosthetic capability and control. The TMR surgical procedure effectively salvages and amplifies information contained in motor nerve endings that had been rendered functionless by major limb amputation.

The TMR technique is best characterized as a series of nerve transfers between the amputated brachial nerves and muscle targets within the residual limb or chest wall. After successful neurotization, the target muscles produce myoelectric activity that is easily detected by surface electrodes and can be harnessed to control the function of a prosthesis. Importantly, TMR enables intuitive pairing between a transferred nerve's myoelectric signal and prosthetic functions that correspond to the nerve's premorbid function (eg, a median nerve signal for closing the hand).

TMR represents a dramatic improvement over both body-powered and conventional myoelectric prostheses, in which control signals are provided by muscles that are at best indirectly related to the prosthetic functions they control. The intuitive pairing provided by TMR greatly reduces the duration and difficulty of a patient's early prosthetic rehabilitation.[7] By increasing the number and variety of available control signals, TMR offers the potential for simultaneous functionality of prosthetic hands, wrists, and elbows with multiple degrees of freedom. This chapter is intended to provide an update on adjuncts for optimizing upper extremity prosthetic control in conjunction with TMR, as well as to provide a technical framework for the upper extremity amputation levels where TMR is most used. There is a growing body of anatomical dissections and technical reports to augment the information provided.[8,9]

While targeted muscle reinnervation to enhance lower extremity prosthetic control has been explored,[10,11] there is an absence of literature to support a clear benefit over conventional control strategies. This is likely attributable to the difference in functional demands between the upper and lower extremities, as well as the more

---

Dr. Souza or an immediate family member serves as an unpaid consultant to Balmoral Medical, LLC, Checkpoint Surgical, Inc., and Integrum, Inc. Dr. Dumanian or an immediate family member serves as an unpaid consultant to MSi and has received nonincome support (such as equipment or services), commercially derived honoraria, or other non–research-related funding (such as paid travel) from Checkpoint Surgical.

limited degrees of freedom offered by conventional lower extremity prosthetic components. Despite the lack of functional data to support a control benefit for lower extremity TMR, widespread adoption of the procedure for the purpose of neuroma and phantom pain management or prevention presents a large cohort of patients with reinnervated residual limb musculature. It is possible that improvements in prosthetic componentry or implantable strategies for signal detection may unmask a functional benefit in these patients.

Myoelectric Control

The series of nerve transfers encompassed by TMR produces a predictable pattern of reinnervated muscles within the residual limb. However, prosthetic control is dependent on reliable detection of the electromyographic activity generated by those nerve transfers. The EMG signals are extracted by surface electrodes housed within the prosthetic liner or socket and interpreted by sophisticated control algorithms to predict and generate the intended movements. Early TMR control was mediated by a direct control strategy that paired a single EMG signal with a single degree of freedom (ie, specific prosthetic function). As such, the degrees of freedom offered by TMR were limited by the number of native and reinnervated signals detectable within the residual limb.[12] Pattern recognition algorithms enabled increased degrees of freedom by interpreting the signals from multiple electrodes as predefined movements.[13] While pattern recognition offers a greater range of intuitively controlled functions, interpretation of a pattern of EMG activity as a single function precludes simultaneous control of multiple functions, as is possible with a direct control strategy.[14] Since consistent activation patterns are required to ensure predictable prosthetic function, pattern recognition is dependent on effective training and cognitive effort. Adjunctive algorithms are being developed to improve usability and decrease the cognitive burden on the user.

Synergy With Osseointegration

While the pain benefits of TMR are largely independent of prosthesis use, the prosthetic control benefits of TMR are clearly dependent on the use of a myoelectric prosthesis. By expediting donning and doffing, enabling increased range of motion, and eliminating socket-related discomfort, osseointegration of upper extremity prostheses has proven to have a synergistic benefit when combined with TMR.[15] By decoupling prosthetic suspension from myoelectric control, osseointegration offers greater signal fidelity than can be achieved with a conventional liner and socket construct that must house the surface electrodes necessary for myoelectric control while also providing suspension and spatial control of the prosthetic. It is not uncommon for relative motion between the socket and residual limb to be perceived as electromyographic activity that prompts errant activity in the prosthesis. While the surface control band used in conjunction with osseointegration may be subject to a similar phenomenon, it is often less frequent. Optimal signal fidelity can be achieved through implantation of electrodes directly into the native and reinnervated residual limb muscles. Osseointegration offers a conduit for passage of the wired components via the percutaneous abutment, as shown in **Figure 1**. The e-OPRA (Osseointegrated Prostheses for the Rehabilitation of Amputees) system has been reported to provide improved prosthetic control and stable long-term outcomes in a small group of patients.[15] As the safety of osseointegration becomes more clearly defined and the cost of the technology becomes less prohibitive, it is likely to be more broadly used. Because osseointegration techniques involve resection of muscle distal to the residual skeleton, it is important that the TMR nerve transfer patterns anticipate potential conversion to osseointegration and avoid use of distal targets or mobilize distal muscle targets proximally. In the setting of prior TMR at the transhumeral level, the reinnervated brachialis muscle has been successfully transferred based on its donor ulnar nerve. Alternatively, the coracobrachialis muscle has served as a useful target for revision TMR in the setting of osseointegration

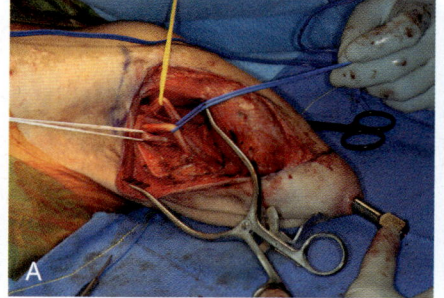
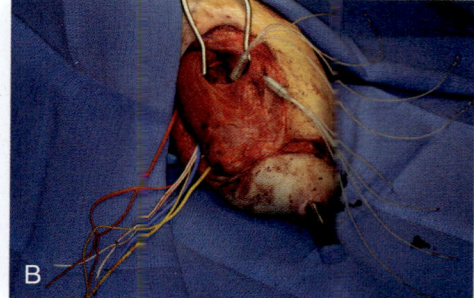
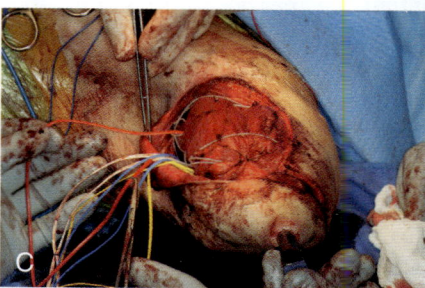

FIGURE 1 Intraoperative photographs of the e-OPRA procedure. **A**, Photograph showing medial exposure of the median (yellow), ulnar (blue), and radial (white) nerves as part of the e-OPRA procedure. The patient had previously undergone targeted muscle reinnervation and these nerves were dissected to facilitate positioning of the implanted electrodes. **B**, Photograph showing the implanted electrodes before implantation. **C**, Photograph of the implanted electrodes.

Sensory Feedback for Enhanced Control

Sensory feedback is a critical, and yet inadequately addressed, component of prosthetic control. Sensory feedback is a fundamental component of safe and efficient ambulation and is cited by upper limb amputees as one of the major gaps in the capabilities offered by commercially available prosthetics.[16-18] Tremendous effort and investigational funds have been expended in an effort to devise strategies capable of providing meaningful touch perception. Targeted sensory reinnervation offered a promising strategy to restore sensation.[19] Stimulation of the reinnervated skin results in the sensation of the patient's hand being touched, thus providing cortical feedback to the hand representation on the cortical homunculus. There is restoration of all modalities of cutaneous sensation, including pressure, vibration, and thermal sense. These patients gained an ability to discriminate gradations of force that matched that of their uninjured skin. However, the sensory reinnervation maps generated by targeted sensory reinnervation have proven less predictable than expected and commercially available prostheses are still unable to capitalize on the surface sensory information. Alternative sensory strategies have included implantable nerve interfaces, artificial skin, peripheral nerve stimulation, and the agonist–antagonist myoneural interface technique.[20] By recreating the dynamic agonist–antagonist relationship that exists between opposing muscle groups in the extremity, the agonist–antagonist myoneural interface technique offers a means to restore some degree of proprioceptive sensation.[21] The clinical impact of this technique on prosthetic function requires further exploration, and existing techniques require the distal joint anatomy to be intact at the time of amputation. TMR may prove to be a valuable means of adapting a regenerative form of the agonist–antagonist myoneural interface concept for use in those who have already experienced limb loss.

Surgical Planning for TMR in the Upper Limb

While prosthetic technology continues to advance, the general surgical framework for performing TMR for the primary purpose of motor control has remained relatively stable. The TMR procedure was designed to create control sites for the following four basic prosthetic functions in a patient with an upper limb amputation: elbow flexion, elbow extension, hand opening, and hand closing. If possible, the surgeon should create additional control sites to allow greater wrist and hand control as well as the potential benefits offered by advanced control algorithms. The number of control sites can be maximized by splitting residual limb muscles into separate segments based on neurovascular anatomy.

The most important considerations in planning a TMR procedure are the length of the amputated nerves and the availability of the residual limb or chest wall muscle targets. The amputation level is defined by the presence or absence of recipient muscle motor entry points rather than by conventional skeletal levels. All upper limb amputations can be categorized at three basic levels (transradial, transhumeral, and shoulder disarticulation), which span the six commonly described skeletal amputation levels (**Figure 2**).

Amputation at the middle to distal forearm (the transradial level) leaves remnant forearm muscles with intact median, ulnar, and radial nerve motor entry points. As a result, intuitive control of a myoelectric prosthesis is possible without the need for nerve transfers. Intrinsic ulnar and median nerve function is lost at this level but can be regained through TMR. However, the currently available commercial prostheses do not offer the digital dexterity and fine control mechanisms necessary to capitalize on the neural information salvaged through distal ulnar and median nerve transfers. Consequently, the principal indication for TMR at this level is to manage symptomatic end neuromas.

In an amputation between the proximal forearm and the proximal humerus, the forearm motor points responsible for native hand and wrist control are lost, but the upper arm motor points

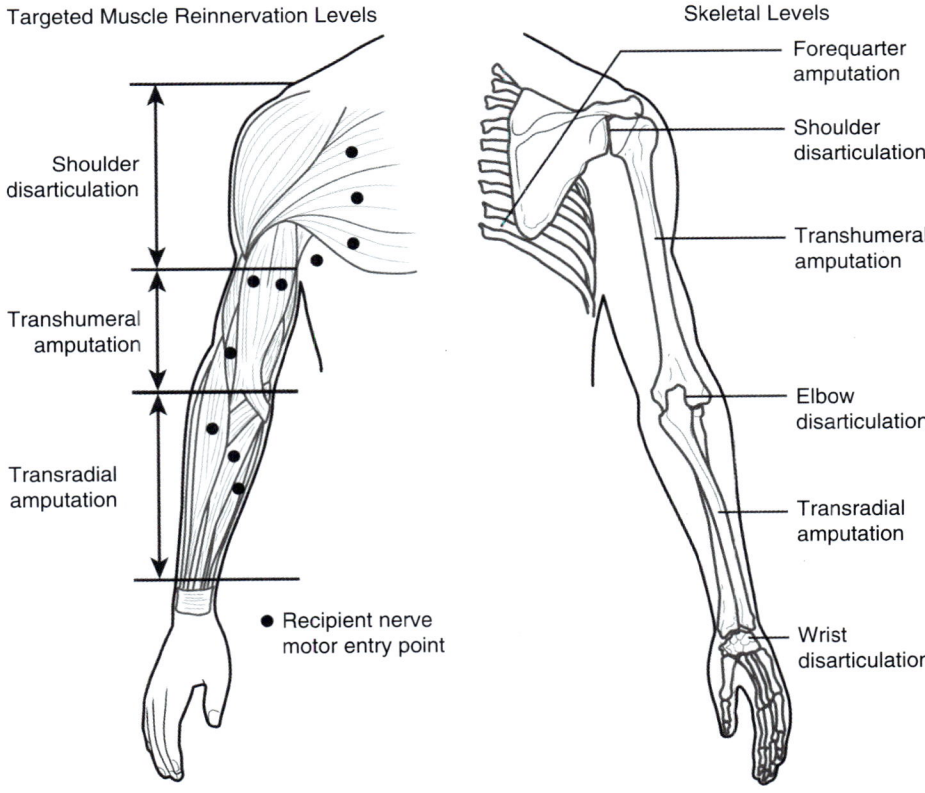

FIGURE 2 Schematic drawing comparing targeted muscle reinnervation (TMR) and skeletal amputation levels in the upper limb. The TMR level is dictated by the availability of recipient motor nerve entry points (black dots).

responsible for elbow function remain intact. TMR at this level is called transhumeral even though the elbow joint may be present and functional. Nerve transfers at the transhumeral level seek to restore functions previously controlled by the median, ulnar, and distal radial–posterior interosseous nerves, while preserving elbow function provided by the intact musculocutaneous and proximal radial nerves.

At the shoulder disarticulation level, the upper arm motor points of the musculocutaneous and radial nerves have been removed. The proximal humerus and the shoulder joint may be present, but the remnant biceps and triceps lack the potential for reinnervation. The musculocutaneous, median, radial, and ulnar nerves all should be transferred. The pectoralis major, pectoralis minor, and latissimus dorsi most commonly are used as nerve transfer recipients.

Transhumeral TMR

General Considerations

At the transhumeral level, TMR may be indicated if the patient has unsatisfactory prosthetic function with the use of a standard body-powered, myoelectric or hybrid system despite adequate training. The optimal candidate is vibrant, in good health, and has adequate capacity for nerve healing. Although there is no specific age cutoff, younger patients often have more capacity for nerve regeneration. On physical examination, the amputee has strong biceps and triceps contractions and has a long residual limb with supple soft tissue. A patient with bilateral amputation may benefit from unilateral TMR surgery to enhance dexterity, with body-powered prosthesis use retained for the contralateral limb to allow robust activity. Patients with an amputation resulting from an avulsion mechanism should be screened to rule out a brachial plexopathy, because proximal damage to potential donor nerves precludes successful reinnervation. Brachial plexopathies can be difficult to diagnose clinically if the forearm and hand have been amputated. Clinically detectable pectoralis and latissimus muscle contractions are useful markers of brachial plexus function but cannot entirely rule out the presence of a partial brachial plexus injury. TMR can be done only with transected donor nerves that retain cortical control, and this critical element is lacking if the patient has a severe proximal brachial plexopathy.

The presence of a long residual limb is important for mechanical advantage and fitting of the prosthesis. Typically, the level of the donor nerve injury is relatively distal in a long residual limb. The nerve, therefore, can be aggressively trimmed back to visualize healthy-appearing fascicles before transfer to the more proximal motor entry point. In addition, the brachialis muscle and its motor entry points frequently are preserved in a long transhumeral amputation. This muscle can be used to provide a wrist control signal after reinnervation by the ulnar nerve. In a short transhumeral bone amputation, brachialis muscle sufficient for reinnervation typically is lacking, and it is often challenging to trim and mobilize the donor nerves without creating undue tension at the coaptation site. Supple soft-tissue coverage is essential because it is difficult to obtain a wide dissection if the limb is scarred by skin grafts or heterotopic ossification.

The preoperative workup is straightforward. Radiographs should be obtained to assess limb length and the extent of heterotopic ossification. Earlier surgical reports should be obtained. On physical examination, the level and location of the median, ulnar, and radial nerves are determined by evaluating the Tinel sign relative to the residual bone. The Tinel sign is identified at or proximal to the level of nerve injury. Thus, a Tinel sign close to the end of the residual limb suggests the presence of a relatively long healthy donor nerve. Native innervation of the remnant biceps and triceps muscles is confirmed by visualization and palpation during voluntary muscle contraction. Additional nerve and vascular studies typically are not required. However, if the Tinel signs are difficult to reliably identify and the associated neuromas are not palpable, confirmatory MRI or ultrasonography evaluation can be useful to confirm the neuroma level and location.

Surgical Technique

The Tinel sign locations of the median, ulnar, and radial nerves are marked while the patient is in the preoperative holding area. The borders of the biceps and triceps muscles should be clearly outlined because it can be disorientating to operate on an upper arm in the absence of forearm and hand landmarks to delineate true anterior and posterior surfaces. The transhumeral procedure is done through two incisions, with an anterior incision oriented longitudinally along the raphe between the long and short heads of the biceps brachii muscle. The posterior incision mirrors the anterior incision and is positioned over the raphe between the long and lateral heads of the triceps. The orientation of these incisions is offset 90° from the incisions traditionally used to create anterior and posterior fish-mouth skin flaps. When TMR is done at the time of the initial transhumeral amputation, the TMR incisions should maintain their AP orientation; they can simply be extended distally to create medial and lateral skin flaps for distal limb coverage. Thin skin flaps are elevated on both sides of the incision, leaving a layer of fat on top of the deep fascia. A proximally based adipofascial flap is then elevated to reveal the raphe between the short (medial) and long (lateral) heads of the biceps brachii. Blunt digital dissection reveals the musculocutaneous nerve, which is characterized by its trifurcation into the motor nerve to the long head of the biceps, the motor nerve to the short head of the biceps, and the distal continuation of the nerve as the brachialis motor branch and lateral antebrachial cutaneous nerve. Dissection on the medial aspect of the arm is done to identify the median nerve next to the brachial artery. The medial antebrachial cutaneous nerve often can be seen early in the dissection. This nerve can be distinguished from the median or ulnar nerves by its smaller caliber and relative posterior position along the intermuscular septum. A typical anterior exposure and the median, ulnar, musculocutaneous, and medial antebrachial cutaneous nerves are shown in **Figure 3**. Because the hand is not present, the surgeon cannot stimulate the major mixed nerves to confirm their identities. Motor axon frozen section staining is possible but usually is unnecessary.

The median nerve is shortened until healthy fascicles are observed and is mobilized to the motor point of the short head of the biceps. The musculocutaneous nerve motor branch to the short head of the biceps is divided approximately 1 cm from its entry into the muscle, thus providing length sufficient for a coaptation while limiting the overall reinnervation length and, as a result, the time required for reinnervation. Under loupe magnification, a nerve coaptation is done by bringing the small motor nerve into the center of the much larger median nerve; 7-0 or 8-0 polypropylene suture is used. To guard against dehiscence, nearby epineurium is sutured to adjacent muscle epimysium using additional small-caliber polypropylene sutures. Successful neurotization of the short head after the median nerve transfer will result in an intuitive hand-close signal, and preservation of the musculocutaneous nerve innervation to the long head of the biceps is maintained as an elbow flexion signal. If the brachialis muscle is present, the ulnar nerve can be identified posterior to the median and medial antebrachial cutaneous nerves, through the same anterior approach, and it is mobilized to the motor nerve of the brachialis muscle. Because the brachialis has retained its musculocutaneous innervation, a portable nerve stimulator can be used to track the continuation of the musculocutaneous motor nerve to its entry into the brachialis. The ulnar nerve transfer is useful for control of a prosthetic wrist. Before the anterior incision is closed, the previously elevated adipofascial flap is positioned between the short and long heads of the biceps to encourage spatial differentiation of the myoelectric signals. The elevation of this flap and deeper transposition also may improve myoelectric signal conduction through the thinned overlying skin flaps and limit aberrant reinnervation.

The distal radial nerve is then transferred. Although the posterior dissection can be done with the patient supine, with the shoulder hyperextended it is much easier to reposition the patient and perform the radial nerve transfer with the patient in the prone position. A generous longitudinal incision is made between the long and lateral heads of the triceps, and a proximally based adipofascial flap is again elevated. It is helpful to begin the deep dissection relatively cephalad because the interspace is best found where the deltoid insertion overlies the proximal triceps. Elevation of the long head of the triceps typically reveals the major trunk of the radial nerve, with one or two small motor nerves branching to supply the lateral head (**Figure 4**). The radial motor branch to the long head of the triceps arises significantly more proximally and usually is not seen. This exposure is analogous to that used for radial nerve transfers intended for restoration of shoulder abduction. The radial nerve typically enlarges after the amputation and feels

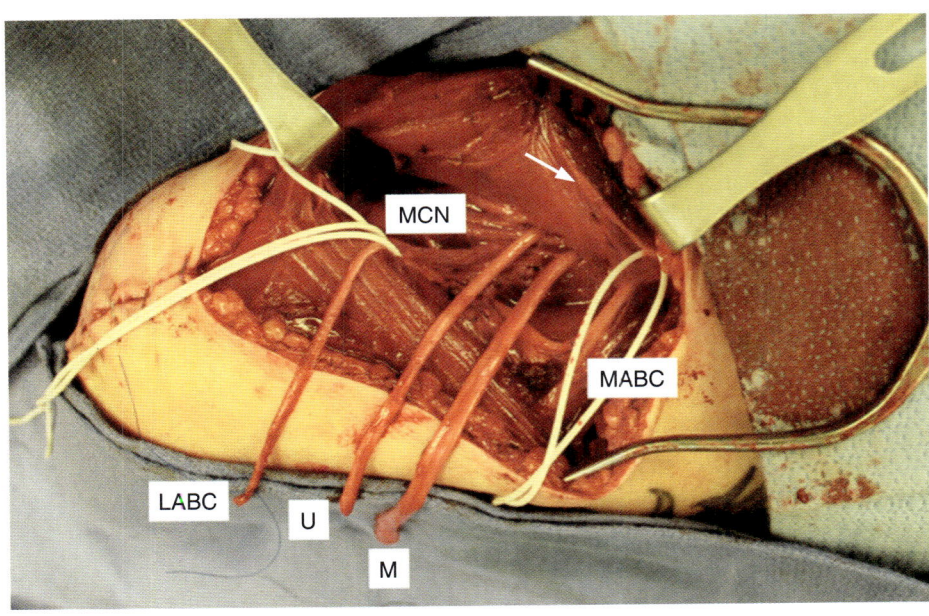

FIGURE 3 Photograph showing an anterior exposure in a patient undergoing transhumeral targeted muscle reinnervation. The medial antebrachial cutaneous (MABC), median (M), musculocutaneous (MCN), and ulnar (U) nerves are identified before nerve transfer. In this patient, the distal limb had been shortened, and a long segment of the lateral antebrachial cutaneous (LABC) nerve also is present. A recipient motor branch to the short head of the biceps (arrow) has been tagged with a vessel loop.

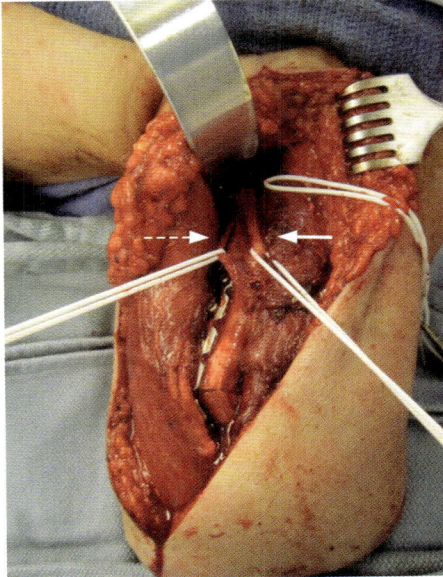

FIGURE 4 Photograph showing a posterior exposure in a patient undergoing transhumeral targeted muscle reinnervation. The radial nerve (solid arrow) and a motor branch from the radial nerve to the lateral head of the triceps (dashed arrow) have been identified. The motor branch will be transected and serve as the recipient for a coaptation with the distal radial nerve proper. The patient also was treated with an angulation osteotomy of the humerus.

relatively firm. Stimulation of the main trunk should fail to produce any muscle contraction. As with a median nerve transfer, the radial nerve is divided and coapted to the motor nerve(s) to the lateral head of the triceps close to the motor entry point. A hand-open signal will be created in the lateral head of the triceps, with preservation of the elbow extension signal mediated by proximal radial nerve innervation of the long head of the triceps. As with the anterior approach, the adipofascial flap is positioned along the raphe between the long and lateral heads of the triceps. Postoperative drains and a mildly compressing dressing are applied. Therapy to maintain shoulder motion can be initiated 2 weeks after the nerve transfer procedure.[8]

Several technical pearls have emerged from experience with the transhumeral TMR procedure. First, it is helpful to avoid a distal division of the biceps or brachialis muscle because the muscle will retract proximally and may become buried beneath the deltoid muscle; as a result, an EMG signal can be obscured by the overlying deltoid muscle. Second, it is important to widely explore the space between the target muscle bellies to identify all of the individual motor nerve branches to each muscle. To encourage reinnervation and eliminate cross-talk competition from remnant native innervation, it is critical to completely denervate the target muscle before performing the nerve transfer. The skin flap thinning that occurs as a byproduct of adipofascial flap elevation serves to improve signal detection by limiting the distance between the reinnervated muscle and cutaneous electrode. Liposuction or direct excision of the subcutaneous tissues can facilitate future signal detection at sites remote from the access incision.

Ultimately, the success of reinnervation is contingent on the ability to achieve normal fascicular architecture by sufficient proximal trimming of the donor nerve before transfer. Two factors favor successful reinnervation of the target muscle: TMR (unlike hand transplantation, in which maximal nerve length must be preserved) almost always requires coaptations at a location proximal to the site of nerve injury, and there are substantially more fascicles in the donor nerves than in the coapted recipient nerves. The second factor has been called hyperinnervation. In the experience of this chapter's authors, more than 95% of these transfers yield detectable EMG control sites, without the need for nerve wraps or fibrin glue. Theoretic failures of TMR would occur from a nonviable muscle segment after isolation, a poor donor nerve with an unsuspected higher injury, a donor nerve that does not comfortably reach the target motor nerve, and aberrant reinnervation. Over the past decade, this chapter's authors have seen each of these issues only once.

Shoulder Disarticulation TMR

General Considerations

TMR at the shoulder level is primarily indicated to improve poor prosthetic function, despite adequate rehabilitation, in a patient with a standard prosthetic device. After amputation at the shoulder level, poor function is ubiquitous with currently available prostheses. In some respects, TMR at the shoulder level has even greater potential than at the transhumeral level because of the greater loss of native innervation and the limitations of conventional prosthetic rehabilitation. The preoperative workup is similar to the workup for a patient with a transhumeral amputation, although the physical examination must particularly evaluate the function of the pectoralis major, serratus anterior, and latissimus dorsi muscles. A history of limb avulsion should heighten suspicion that the nerve endings may be too proximally located to allow tension-free transfer to the chest wall muscle targets. Although nerve grafts are not desirable, they can be used to add length to donor nerves. Alternatively, free muscle transfer has been used to bring the muscle target to short donor nerves.[22] Brachial plexopathy is the only absolute contraindication to surgery. Relative contraindications include a lack of muscle targets, a lack of distally located nerve endings, poor-quality local soft tissue, and inability of the patient to tolerate a 3- to 5-hour surgical procedure.

Surgical Technique

Access to the brachial plexus and proximal nerve branches is achieved using an infraclavicular approach through the interspace between the sternal and clavicular heads of the pectoralis major. A transverse incision is designed approximately two fingerbreadths below the clavicle (**Figure 5**). As in the transhumeral approach, a medially based adipofascial flap is elevated (**Figure 6**). In addition, the subcutaneous tissue overlying the pectoralis major muscle is thinned in an area of approximately 100 cm² extending from the sternum to the anterior axillary line and from the clavicle inferiorly toward the nipple. The motor nerve to the clavicular head usually is the first to be found in the space between the two heads of the pectoralis. This nerve enters the muscle in a vertical direction and almost always lies adjacent to the vascular pedicle to the muscle. Occasionally, a second small motor nerve innervates the muscle more laterally. Dissection proceeds inferiorly, where medial, middle, and lateral motor branches can be found innervating the sternal head. The middle branch emerges medial to the

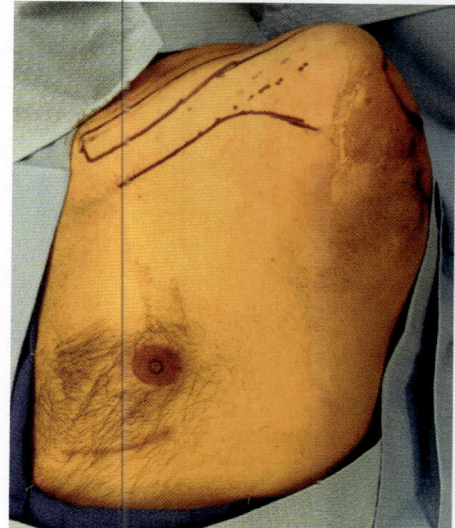

FIGURE 5 Photograph showing curved incision markings in a patient undergoing targeted muscle reinnervation after shoulder disarticulation. The clavicle has been outlined to serve as a reference point.

Chapter 23: Targeted Muscle Reinnervation for Enhanced Prosthetic Control

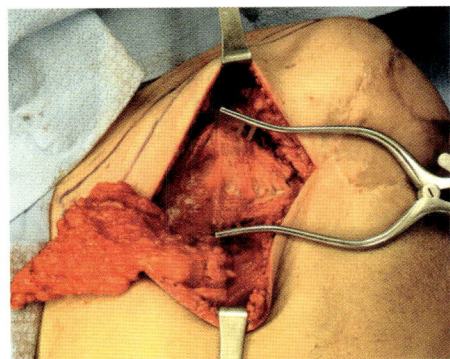

FIGURE 6 Photograph showing an infraclavicular approach for targeted muscle reinnervation in a patient with a shoulder disarticulation. A medially based adipofascial flap has been elevated and reflected medially. The space between the clavicular and sternal heads of the pectoralis major muscle has been opened and is being maintained with the use of a self-retaining retractor.

pectoralis minor tendon, and the lateral branch commonly travels through the substance of the pectoralis minor muscle. All nerve branches to the pectoralis major must be identified to ensure complete denervation of the muscle before the nerves are transferred. The exact origin of these motor nerves is not relevant because there is no reason to preserve native pectoralis function in the absence of an upper arm. Only the size and distribution of the motor entry points are pertinent to the pattern of nerve transfers. For this reason, an extensive supraclavicular approach to the brachial plexus is not justified.

After the pectoralis motor branches are identified, the donor nerves are located as they course deep to the pectoralis minor tendon (**Figure 7**). The donor nerves are differentiated by their proximal branching pattern and relative size. The radial nerve is the largest of the donor nerves. However, accurate identification of each donor nerve is not critical to the success of the procedure. The pattern of nerve transfers primarily is dictated by the inherent spatial arrangement of the donor and recipient nerves, rather than by a preplanned pattern of transfers based on intended function. The proximal thoracodorsal nerve can be found deep to the mobilized donor nerves if the latissimus dorsi muscle is to serve as an additional transfer recipient. After adequate dissection, the donor nerves are trimmed with the goal of achieving normal fascicular architecture (**Figure 8**). However, the proximal nature of the nerve injury necessitates tempering the extent of trimming to maintain length sufficient for avoiding tension at the nerve coaptation sites. Often it is possible to remove 2 to 3 cm of damaged nerve without compromising the nerve transfer. The nerve coaptation is done in a manner similar to that used for transhumeral TMR.

The most commonly used pattern of transfers primarily is based on the proximity of donor nerves to recipient sites. The musculocutaneous nerve is transferred to the motor nerve branch of the clavicular head, the median and ulnar nerves are transferred to the motor nerves innervating the sternal head, and the radial nerve is coapted to the thoracodorsal nerve (**Figure 9**). Because the radial-thoracodorsal coaptation site is relatively proximal, a relatively long time period elapses before reinnervation of the latissimus muscle control site. The serratus anterior and pectoralis minor can serve as alternative targets for reinnervation but are less desirable because of the deep position of the muscles on the chest wall. The previously elevated adipofascial flaps and/or free fat grafts are used to create separation between the pectoralis segments.

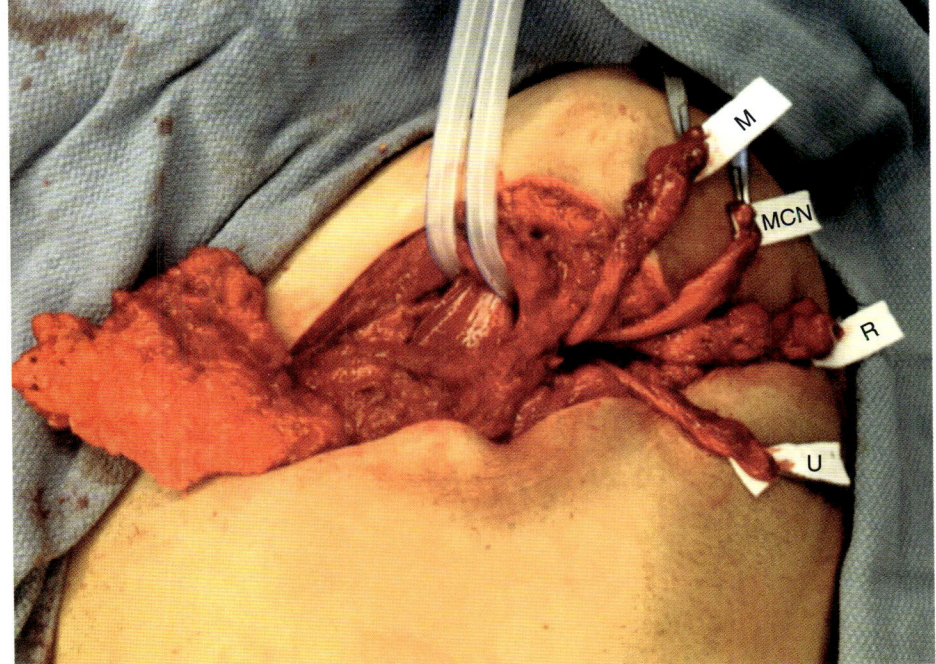

FIGURE 7 Photograph showing the median (M), musculocutaneous (MCN), radial (R), and ulnar (U) brachial donor nerves, which are identified as they run deep to the pectoralis minor tendon (retracted with a Penrose drain).

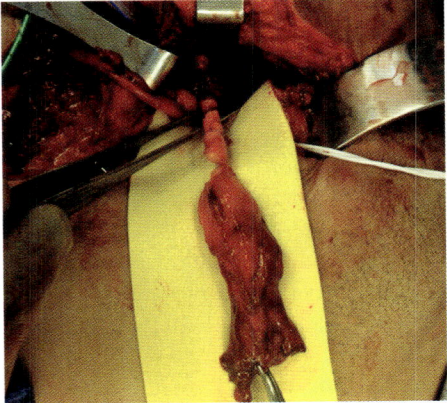

FIGURE 8 Photograph showing donor nerve trimming in a shoulder disarticulation targeted muscle reinnervation. The end neuromas are excised from the brachial donor nerves, and the nerves are trimmed proximally until healthy individual fascicles are observed.

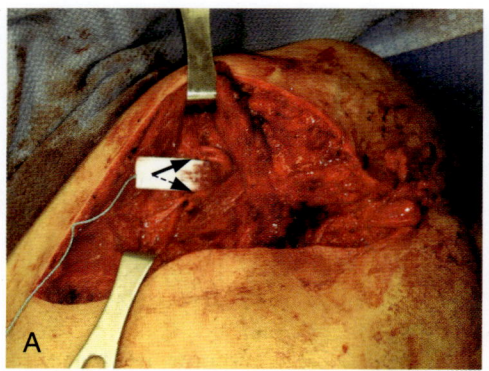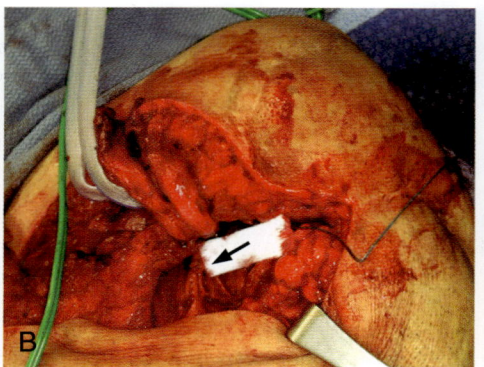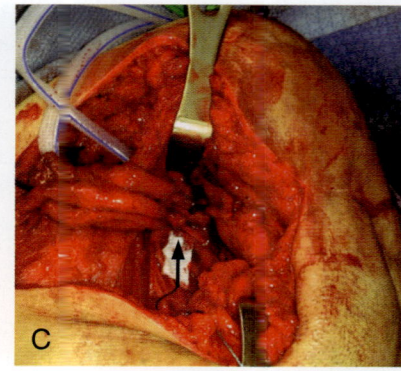

FIGURE 9 Photographs showing nerve coaptation in a shoulder disarticulation targeted muscle reinnervation. **A**, The musculocutaneous nerve has been coapted to the clavicular head motor branch (solid arrow), and the median nerve has been coapted to the medial and middle motor branches to the sternal head (dashed arrow). **B**, The ulnar nerve will be coapted to the lateral motor branch to the sternal head (arrow). **C**, The radial nerve will be coapted to the thoracodorsal nerve (arrow).

When the humeral head is removed at the time of the amputation, the pectoralis and all the associated motor nerves retract medially toward the sternum, which makes the donor nerve dissection more complicated. If a portion of the humerus is present, it should not be excised even if it is too short to serve as a lever arm for prosthetic control. Preserving the pectoralis major insertion keeps the pectoralis muscle out to length, and the broad surface area facilitates later signal acquisition. In addition, the presence of the humeral head creates a cosmetically pleasing contour under clothing. Occasionally, a small remnant of triceps remains innervated by the radial nerve and is useable for an elbow extension signal.

After quilting sutures are placed, the skin is closed over closed suction drains to reduce the risk of seroma formation after the extensive subcutaneous thinning. The patient typically resumes use of the original prosthesis 4 to 6 weeks after surgery, when postoperative swelling subsides and the wound has adequately healed. Prosthetic fitting for new control sites is done when EMG signals from the newly neurotized muscles have become robust; a minimum of 3 to 6 months usually is required. The latissimus muscle, which is most distant from the coaptation site, can take 9 to 12 months to show detectable reinnervation.

SUMMARY

TMR has been shown to reliably restore intuitive limb control in patients with upper limb amputation and is most appropriate for use for terminal device control in patients with transhumeral or more proximal amputation levels.

References

1. Kuiken TA, Childress DS, Rymer WZ: The hyper-reinnervation of rat skeletal muscle. *Brain Res* 1995;676(1):113-123.
2. Kuiken TA, Dumanian GA, Lipschutz RD, Miller LA, Stubblefield KA: The use of targeted muscle reinnervation for improved myoelectric prosthesis control in a bilateral shoulder disarticulation amputee. *Prosthet Orthot Int* 2004;28(3):245-253.
3. Hijjawi JB, Kuiken TA, Lipschutz RD, Miller LA, Stubblefield KA, Dumanian GA: Improved myoelectric prosthesis control accomplished using multiple nerve transfers. *Plast Reconstr Surg* 2006;118(7):1573-1578.
4. Kuiken TA, Li G, Lock BA, et al: Targeted muscle reinnervation for real–Time myoelectric control of multifunction artificial arms. *J Am Med Assoc* 2009;301(6):619-628.
5. Kuiken TA, Miller LA, Lipschutz RD, et al: Targeted reinnervation for enhanced prosthetic arm function in a woman with a proximal amputation: A case study. *Lancet* 2007;369(9559):371-380.
6. Dumanian GA, Ko JH, O'Shaughnessy KD, Kim PS, Wilson CJ, Kuiken TA: Targeted reinnervation for transhumeral amputees: Current surgical technique and update on results. *Plast Reconstr Surg* 2009;124(3):863-869.
7. Miller LA, Stubblefield KA, Lipschutz RD, et al: Surgical and functional outcomes of targeted muscle reinnervation, in Kuiken TA, Barlow AK, Schultz AE, eds. *Targeted Muscle Reinnervation: A Neural Interface for Artificial Limbs*. CRC Press, 2013, pp 149-164.
8. Gart MS, Souza JM, Dumanian GA: Targeted muscle reinnervation in the upper extremity amputee: A technical roadmap. *J Hand Surg Am* 2015;40(9):1877-1888.
9. Fowler TP: Targeted muscle reinnervation in the hand: A technical roadmap. *J Hand Surg Am* 2021;47(3):287.e1-287.e8.
10. Souza JM, Fey NP, Cheesborough JE, Hargrove LJ, Agnew SP, Dumanian GA: Advances in transfemoral prosthesis control: Early experience with transfemoral targeted muscle reinnervation. *Curr Surg Rep* 2014;2:1-9.
11. Hargrove LJ, Simon AM, Young AJ, et al: Robotic leg control with EMG decoding in an amputee with nerve transfers. *N Engl J Med* 2013;369(13):1237-2124.
12. Farina D, Jiang N, Rehbaum H, et al: The extraction of neural information from the surface EMG for the control of upper-limb prostheses: Emerging avenues and challenges. *IEEE Trans Neural Syst Rehabil Eng* 2014;22:797-809.
13. Hargrove LJ, Miller LA, Turner K, Kuiken TA: Myoelectric pattern recognition outperforms direct control for transhumeral amputees with targeted muscle reinnervation: A randomized clinical trial. *Sci Rep* 2017;7:1-9.

14. Mereu F, Leone F, Gentile C, Cordella F, Gruppioni E, Zollo L: Control strategies and performance assessment of upper-limb TMR prostheses: A review. *Sensors (Basel)* 2021;21(6):1953.
15. Ortiz-Catalan M, Mastinu E, Sassu P, Aszmann O, Brånemark R: Self–Contained neuromusculoskeletal arm prostheses. *N Engl J Med* 2020;382(18):1732-1738.
16. Miller WC, Speechley M, Deathe B: The prevalence and risk factors of falling and fear of falling among lower extremity amputees. *Arch Phys Med Rehabil* 2001;82:1031-1037.
17. Nolan L, Wit A, Dudziński K, Lees A, Lake M, Wychowański L: Adjustments in gait symmetry with walking speed in trans-femoral and trans-tibial amputees. *Gait Posture* 2003;17:142-151.
18. Petrini FM, Valle G, Strauss I, et al: Six–Month assessment of a hand prosthesis with intraneural tactile feedback. *Ann Neurol* 2019;85:137-154.
19. Morasco PD: Targeted sensory reinnervation. Surgical and functional outcomes of targeted muscle reinnervation, in Kuiken TA, Barlow AK, Schultz AE, eds. *Targeted Muscle Reinnervation: A Neural Interface for Artificial Limbs*. CRC Press, 2013, pp 121-148.
20. Raspopovic S, Valle G, Petrini FM: Sensory feedback for limb prostheses in amputees. *Nat Mater* 2021;20(7):925-939.
21. Carty MJ, Herr HM: The agonist–Antagonist myoneural interface. *Hand Clin* 2021;37(3):435-445.
22. Bueno RA Jr, French B, Cooney D, Neumeister MW: Targeted muscle reinnervation of a muscle-free flap for improved prosthetic control in a shoulder amputee: Case report. *J Hand Surg Am* 2011;36(5):890-893.

Advanced Nerve Management Techniques for Management and Prevention of Pain

Jason M. Souza, MD, FACS • Paul S. Cederna, MD • Amy M. Moore, MD

ABSTRACT

Postamputation pain can result from multiple etiologies; however, phantom limb pain and neurogenic pain secondary to neuroma formation are often the most debilitating and most difficult to manage. Throughout the 20th century, amputation nerve management techniques were focused on relocating, burying, ablating, or containing the transected nerve ends in a futile effort to prevent nerve regeneration and neuroma formation. A recognition of the limitations of these approaches, combined with recent advances in nerve reconstruction techniques, has fostered enthusiasm for management strategies that are intended to guide nerve regeneration rather than prevent it. By facilitating coordinated nerve regeneration, these advanced nerve management techniques have shown promise for the management and prevention of neurogenic pain after amputation in addition to their originally intended potential to improve terminal device control.

Keywords: central sensitization; neuroma; phantom limb pain; residual limb pain

Introduction

Postamputation pain is broadly categorized based on its location. Residual limb pain refers to pain that is localizable to the residuum, whereas phantom limb pain is perceived as emanating from portions of the limb that are no longer physically present. By definition, phantom pain is neurogenic in nature.[1] Conversely, residual limb pain is often attributable to nonneurogenic sources.[2] The residual limb is constantly placed under physical stress through weight bearing, ambulation, and prolonged prosthesis use. These physical factors lead to soft-tissue breakdown, bursa formation, myodesis disruption, skeletal stress, heterotopic ossification, and arthritis, which commonly cause pain in patients with either upper and/or lower limb loss.[2] End neuromas serve as the primary source of neurogenic pain within the residual limb, although people with limb loss are also susceptible to the same nerve compression syndromes that plague those with intact limbs.[3] In fact, proximal nerve compression may contribute to the symptomatology of the obligate distal nerve injury.[4]

The prevalence of postamputation pain varies based on the subpopulation studied and the methodology used, with retrospective and cross-sectional studies serving as the basis for much of the available literature. The pervasive reliance on medical record review for outcomes is particularly problematic given the diagnostic challenge of identifying a primary pain etiology in the setting of multiple potential or overt neurogenic and somatic sources. Pooled prevalence rates of lower extremity residual limb pain have been reported to be 59%, with the same study identifying a pooled prevalence of neuroma pain to be 15%.[2] Phantom limb pain has been found to be present in 64% of patients with limb loss after pooled analysis of available studies.[5] Preoperative pain, proximal level of amputation, concomitant residual limb pain, and lower limb amputation were identified as risk factors for phantom limb pain.[5]

Although it is helpful to appreciate the scope of the problem, efforts to manage and prevent postamputation pain are even more reliant on an understanding of the biologic processes that underlie neurogenic pain following amputation. Unfortunately, a limited understanding of central and peripheral pain mechanisms has proven to be the greatest obstacle to developing a rational approach to postamputation pain management. In the absence of a comprehensive understanding, clinicians must combine basic science and clinical observations with sound theory to bridge these knowledge gaps. Although unquestionably an oversimplification, a framework that differentiates peripheral and central pain mechanisms can be useful for assessing pain interventions. Likewise, an understanding of physiologic nerve regeneration can provide a template on which to design and judge reconstructive strategies for management of the divided nerves within a residual limb.

Dr. Souza or an immediate family member serves as an unpaid consultant to Balmoral Medical, LLC, Checkpoint Surgical, Inc., and Integrum, Inc. Dr. Moore or an immediate family member has received research or institutional support from Checkpoint Surgical, Inc. Neither Dr. Cederna nor any immediate family member has received anything of value from or has stock or stock options held in a commercial company or institution related directly or indirectly to the subject of this chapter.

Framework for Understanding Postamputation Pain

While recognizing the cortical role in pain perception, neuroma pain can largely be considered peripheral in origin.[6] In the absence of a regenerative target and favorable environment, axonal nerve damage induces a state of abnormal regeneration and inflammation that results in bulbous thickening of the transected nerve end.[6] An unrepaired nerve transection uniformly results in neuroma formation, although the relatively low prevalence of neuroma pain following amputation suggests that only a small number of neuromas become symptomatic.[2] If better understood, the environmental and intrinsic factors that drive this differentiation would be clear targets for intervention. When painful, the neuroma bulb is often the symptomatic focus, but the entirety of the peripheral nerve is affected, as evidenced by changes at the level of the dorsal root ganglion.[7] This recognition suggests there may be a role for proximal decompression in conjunction with end neuroma management.[8] Hyperexcitability from ion channel dysfunction results in focal sensitivity to pressure or palpation that is typical for neuroma pain. When combined with uncontrolled axonal sprouting, reduced axonal depolarization potentials, and scar tissue formation, this dysfunction drives the ectopic firing that typifies neuroma pain.[7] Neuroma formation occurs within 1 month of nerve injury and neuroma pain is typically present within 3 months of amputation, although clinical presentation can vary widely based on patient activity and neuroma location.[9]

Phantom limb pain is largely considered to be a central phenomenon, although it can exist concurrently with neuroma pain and may be exacerbated by manipulation of the residual limb.[1] Most patients with limb loss experience phantom limb sensations and/or the ability to control phantom movements. Unfortunately, most of the patients also report intense episodic pain that is often characterized as throbbing, cramping, stabbing, or burning and is thought to originate within the amputated segment.[10] Although reported rates of phantom limb pain are higher in the developed world, it is a global problem that affects nearly all patients with limb loss to some degree.[5] Although the mechanisms underlying phantom limb pain are yet to be fully elucidated, cortical reorganization is thought to be a major contributor. The cortical remapping theory suggests that the brain responds to limb loss by reorganizing its somatosensory map. No treatment has been found to be universally effective, but the reported efficacy of therapies that specifically target cortical remapping, such as mirror therapy and virtual reality, supports a central origin for phantom limb pain.[1] However, it is also known that sensitized nerve endings in the residual limb and dorsal root ganglion cells are associated with aberrant sensory afferent feedback that can produce somatosensory cortical changes.[11,12] Both the absence of physiologic input and the excess of pathophysiologic feedback appear to be drivers for pathologic cortical reorganization.

The process of central sensitization often serves to blur the distinction between central and peripheral pain processes. Central sensitization refers to neuronal hyperexcitability and reduced inhibition in the central nervous system that results from peripheral pathology.[13] Driven by increases in membrane excitability and reduced inhibition, central sensitization represents an abnormal state of responsiveness of the nociceptive system, where pain is no longer coupled to the presence, intensity, or duration of peripheral stimuli.[13] This uncoupling of the pain response from the peripheral lesion produces pain that is often refractory to peripheral pain interventions. Unfortunately, there is still much to be learned about the timeframe for sensitization and the patient and anatomic factors associated with a susceptibility to this process. In the absence of a more complete understanding, the significant therapeutic challenge posed by central sensitization can be used to justify a proactive approach to neurogenic pain management.

Strategies for Management and Prevention of Postamputation Pain

Surgical techniques to manage or prevent neurogenic pain after amputation have been classified as active and passive strategies.[14] Active strategies aim to facilitate physiologic regeneration of the transected nerve, whereas passive techniques are intended to prevent regeneration, alter the neuroma environment, or reduce physical stimulation of the nerve ending. When applying the previous framework for understanding postamputation pain, it becomes apparent that passive nerve management strategies aim solely to address the peripheral pain focus, without the ability to influence the central processes that contribute to postamputation pain. The common practice of traction neurectomy seeks simply to relocate the inevitable neuroma to an area where it is less vulnerable to direct stimulation.[15] Cap or burial techniques are passive methods that use various tissues or foreign materials to isolate the regenerating nerve end from environmental factors that encourage regeneration.[14] Similarly, implantation of the transected nerve end into innervated muscle was explicitly hypothesized to prevent neuroma formation by limiting exposure to nerve growth factor.[16] As evidenced by the high rates of neuroma recurrence and pain, these passive strategies do not address the reduced depolarization potentials, nerve hypersensitivity, and ectopic discharges that produce dysfunctional sensory afferent feedback that typifies neuroma pain, even without mechanical stimulation. In addition, these passive strategies provide no mechanism to address the central processes that underlie phantom limb pain.

By providing the substrates necessary for coordinated nerve regeneration, advanced nerve management techniques use active strategies for minimizing or preventing postamputation pain.[14] Preclinical data and a growing volume of clinical studies suggest that these approaches may be more effective than conventional passive techniques for the treatment and prevention of postamputation pain.[17,18] When used for the treatment of established postamputation pain, an ideal strategy would effectively prevent neuroma recurrence following neurectomy, while also serving to reverse any associated central pain processes. In the prophylactic setting, these strategies should aim to inhibit formation of a symptomatic neuroma in the periphery, while also preventing central sensitization of pain. The most commonly described active strategies for management or prevention of postamputation pain are nerve allograft reconstruction, regenerative peripheral nerve interface (RPNI) creation, and targeted muscle reinnervation (TMR). Allograft reconstruction provides a conduit with which to direct regenerating axons, whereas RPNI is intended to provide a denervated muscle target and associated neurotrophic signal. TMR offers the transected nerve a denervated target, a neurotrophic signal, and a pathway or conduit across which to regenerate.

Allograft Reconstruction

Background

Based on preclinical studies that suggest a regenerative limit of 40 to 60 mm, processed nerve allografts (PNAs) have been used as an active strategy to manage and prevent postamputation pain by inhibiting neuroma formation. Following nerve gap repair with a PNA, Schwann cells migrate from both the proximal and distal ends of the reconstructed nerve.[19,20] The host Schwann cells support axonal regeneration across the PNA via production of neurotropic factors, adhesion molecules, and axonal myelination.[21] However, as the graft length increases, the ability for the Schwann cells to support regeneration decreases because of cellular senescence.[21,22] Cellular senescence arises in response to telomere shortening or dysfunction from consecutive cell divisions, DNA damage, and development of oncogenes.[22] Senescent Schwann cells are characterized by irreversible arrest in proliferation and altered gene expression, with changes in the secretory profile leading to inhibitory factor release.[23] Thus, nerve regeneration is inhibited in this state and poor regeneration and function are observed.[21] Given these findings, when coapted to a transected nerve following neuroma excision or at the time of amputation, PNAs offer an ideal construct to guide regenerating axons but limit axonal growth within the construct because of Schwann cell senescence and the inhibitory microenvironment that is created.

When used for neuroma prevention, PNAs are often combined with an isolated proximal nerve crush injury intended to create a controlled axonotmetic injury proximal to the coaptation site. By disrupting the axons but preserving the enveloping endoneurium and other supporting connective tissue structures (perineurium and epineurium), the proximal crush provides a regenerative environment that is not associated with a painful expression profile at the neuron level.[24] Thus, the theoretical benefit of using a crush followed by the addition of a PNA for neuroma control is that the crush will create a proximal nerve injury that is associated with a less painful expression profile than the distal transection. The transected nerve can then regenerate into the long PNA (>5 cm) over time. Schwann cell senescence dwindles regeneration along the length of the PNA and the added length of the PNA allows relocation into a less symptomatic location.[25] Importantly, this surgical strategy is simple and can be performed by all variety of surgeons at the time of definitive limb amputation without the need of a microscope, multiple incisions, or extensive dissection. Although PNA reconstruction may reduce the pathogenic stimulation that exacerbates phantom limb pain, this technique is not intended to address the lack of physiologic feedback that serves as the foundation for the development of phantom limb pain.

Neuroma Management and Prevention

Although conceptually intriguing and supported by good preclinical data, there is a paucity of clinical outcomes data pertaining to PNA use for management of postamputation pain. A single case report outlines the use of PNAs to facilitate relocation nerve grafting following excision of multiple digital neuromas.[26] Much of the literature pertaining to PNA use for neuroma pain describes allograft reconstruction of neuromas-in-continuity, where a distal nerve segment is available to receive the graft.[27-29] The lack of clinical data may be related to significant cost of PNA, which can become prohibitive in the amputation setting because of the involvement of multiple nerves.

Targeted Muscle Reinnervation

Background

As a surgical technique, TMR has its foundation in mixed motor nerve transfers intended to repurpose residual limb muscles as bioamplifiers capable of conveying prosthetic control information.[30,31] The basic technique, which has been broadly described with various adaptations, involves mobilization of a transected donor nerve for direct end-to-end coaptation to a recipient motor branch. The choice of recipient nerve is largely based on proximity to the donor nerve and the clinical relevance of denervation of the target muscle or muscle segment. Performed for its original purpose, the TMR nerve transfers often involve a significant size mismatch between the larger donor nerve and recipient motor branch. This was thought to enhance the likelihood of effective reinnervation through a process of hyperreinnervation. This technique has enabled TMR to produce consistent reinnervation of the targeted muscles or muscle segments, as evidenced by electromyographic recording or observable contraction. This detectable motor activity was theorized to be the result of coordinated nerve regeneration, suggesting a different regenerative process than the chaotic one that underlies neuroma formation. This recognition, combined with favorable anecdotal pain outcomes, prompted preclinical investigation into the histologic effects of TMR on neuroma formation. In a rabbit model, TMR was found to yield a histomorphometric appearance more typical of a nerve repair than that of a neuroma.[32] A separate rodent model demonstrated decreased myelinated fiber counts and increased axon cross-sectional area relative to both a control neuroma group and burial into innervated muscle.[33] This encouraging nerve histology motivated clinical evaluation of the role of TMR on pain outcomes.

Neuroma Management

A retrospective review of 26 patients undergoing TMR for prosthetic control first highlighted the potential role of TMR in the management of postamputation neuroma pain.[34] This study prompted design and execution of a multicenter randomized controlled trial comparing TMR with nerve implantation for the management of neuroma and phantom limb pain after major limb amputation. Despite extensive recruitment and screening, only 28 patients consented to randomization and were included in the trial.[35] Thirty-three additional patients refused to be randomized to muscle implantation and were thus included in a separate prospective case series.[36] The 14 patients randomized to TMR demonstrated statistically and clinically significant reduction in phantom limb pain, but a nearly identical trend toward improvement in neuroma pain did not prove statistically significant because of insufficient patient numbers and study power. Overall, 72% of patients who underwent TMR were found to be free of phantom limb pain, with only 40% of those treated with muscle implantation reporting absence of phantom limb pain.[35] The 33 patients included in the prospective case series demonstrated clinically meaningful and statistically significant improvement from baseline in both residual limb pain and phantom limb pain.[36] These promising clinical findings have spurred a litany of case series and technical reports highlighting the use of TMR for management of neuroma pain throughout the body. The role of TMR for management of postamputation pain has largely been supported by this additional body of work, but robust clinical outcomes studies are still necessary to validate these early findings.

Neuroma Prevention

The enthusiasm for TMR as a treatment strategy rapidly evolved into application of the technique for prevention of postamputation pain. Outcomes from a case series of 51 patients who underwent TMR at the time of initial amputation were compared with normative data obtained from 438 amputees who did not have diabetes.[37] Whereas only 21.5% and 19% of amputees in the control group were free of phantom limb pain and residual limb pain, respectively, 45.3% and 49.2% of patients who underwent TMR were free of phantom limb pain and residual limb pain, respectively. Similarly, only 18.7% and 16.9% of patients reported phantom limb pain and residual limb pain after TMR, respectively, whereas 33.4% and 31.9% of amputees in the normative data set described severe phantom limb pain and residual limb pain, respectively. Although most of the patients who underwent TMR reported a worst pain score of 3 or less, five patients reported severe pain. On retrospective review of these outliers, all patients had a history of severe chronic pain for years preceding the amputation and TMR, supporting the importance of a proactive approach to pain management and suggesting roles for central sensitization, pain catastrophization, and early intervention before these phenomena become established. The effective use of TMR for the prevention of postamputation pain in most of the population with diabetes and dysvascular amputation has recently been demonstrated in a well-controlled study.[38] Increased ambulation rates and decreased narcotic use were observed in addition to the clear pain outcome benefits, with a dearth of major complications in this high-risk patient population.

Pearls and Pitfalls

TMR is as much a concept as it is a procedure. Therefore, the technique can vary dramatically depending on the clinical setting and indication, as well as the anatomic region where it is being applied. From a technical standpoint, TMR is comparable to other nerve transfers, in that the procedure requires identification and mobilization of both a donor and a recipient nerve, with the nerves coapted in an end-to-end fashion. However, the significant size mismatch between the donor and recipient nerves often requires an alteration in coaptation technique (**Figure 1**). If multiple recipient nerve branches are available, the donor nerve can be split into smaller fascicle groups to allow multiple coaptations with less discrepancy in cross-sectional area (**Figure 2**). Alternatively, composite techniques that combine direct nerve coaptation with implantation of the remnant nerve into denervated muscle have also been described. To accomplish these composite techniques, the donor nerve is sutured to the recipient nerve as close as possible to the recipient motor nerve

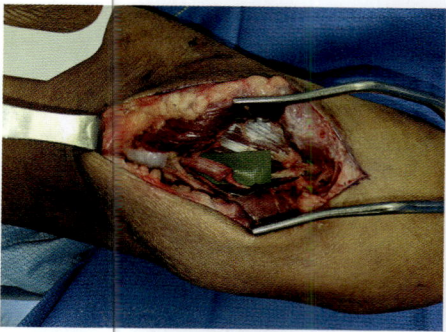

FIGURE 1 Clinical photograph depicts targeted muscle reinnervation for neuroma management. Common peroneal nerve to lateral gastrocnemius muscle branch transfer was performed. Note the size mismatch between the donor common peroneal nerve and the recipient motor branch. Often the coaptation site is reinforced with epineurial to epimysial sutures that aim to bury the coaptation within the denervated recipient muscle.

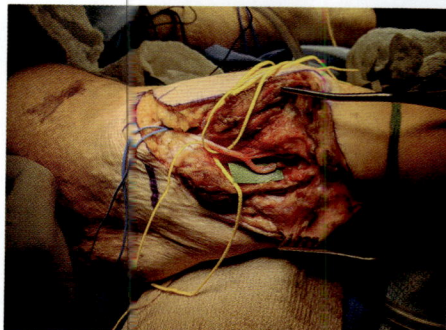

FIGURE 2 Clinical photograph depicts split targeted muscle reinnervation for neuroma management. The common peroneal nerve has been split along its fascicles to create a better size match for coaptation to the motor branch to the lateral gastrocnemius muscle.

entry point into the muscle. In this way, TMR differs from conventional nerve transfers as it violates the "donor distal, recipient proximal" mantra and relies on more extensive mobilization of the donor nerve, with relatively little mobilization of the recipient. Presented with a significant size discrepancy, a common technique is to use a small caliber (eg, 8-0), nonabsorbable suture in loose mattress fashion to centralize the smaller recipient motor branch within the larger donor nerve. The donor nerve can then be delivered into the substance of the denervated muscle target using slightly larger caliber (eg, 6-0) epineurial to epimysial sutures. A common pitfall for those inexperienced with the TMR technique is to try to compensate for the discordant nerve cross-sectional areas with excessive epineurial to epineurial sutures. The combination of excess foreign material and undirected donor nerve axons almost certainly results in neuroma recurrence.

Regenerative Peripheral Nerve Interface

Like TMR, the RPNI was originally intended as a neuroprosthetic control strategy.[39] From a postamputation pain standpoint, the RPNI is also conceptually analogous to TMR, in that it seeks to provide the regenerating axons of a transected nerve with a denervated target in the form of an autologous free skeletal muscle graft (**Figure 3**). Free skeletal muscle grafts were originally designed to be used for facial reanimation.[40] In this case, small skeletal muscle grafts were transferred to the face and directly neurotized by branches of the facial nerve. The skeletal muscles were shown to undergo a process of robust regeneration based on the activities of the muscle satellite cells. The process of muscle reinnervation through direct neurotization (implanting the nerve into the muscle) has been well established in the muscle literature.[41] All aspects of this approach for facial reanimation were based on sound physiologic principles; this technique was unfortunately not successful because the small skeletal muscle grafts did not generate sufficient force to correct facial asymmetry. However, these studies provided the foundational understanding of the biologic processes supporting the creation of RPNIs. Extensive literature has since demonstrated robust free skeletal muscle regeneration and reinnervation with adequate RPNI muscle force generation and even greater amplification of neural signals for motor control of a prosthesis.[42] In contrast to implanting a nerve into an innervated skeletal muscle, the free skeletal muscle graft is completely denervated so that every muscle fiber is available for reinnervation. Thus, the likelihood of the development of a recurrent neuroma should be reduced. In addition, because the muscle is directly neurotized, there is no possibility of the development of a neuroma-in-continuity from a large nerve size mismatch. The process of physiologic synaptogenesis within the skeletal muscle target of both TMR and RPNI is the key distinguisher of these active techniques from the passive technique of burying a residual nerve into natively innervated muscle. RPNI is contrasted to TMR by the relative simplicity of the surgical technique and the avoidance of donor muscle atrophy from motor nerve division. Any 30 mm × 15 mm × 5 mm skeletal muscle segment can be used as an RPNI graft. As a result, otherwise expendable muscle tissue (ie, muscle harvested from the amputated segment during concurrent amputation) can be used, effectively eliminating donor site morbidity. In addition, RPNI avoids the additional dissection required for TMR recipient motor nerve identification and limits the degree to which the donor nerves must be mobilized. In addition, the ease of graft harvest and the lack of a requirement for a recipient motor nerve enable multiple RPNI constructs to be created for a donor nerve with a large cross-sectional area. This circumvents concerns related to the disproportionate donor nerve to recipient nerve axon ratio that is commonly cited with TMR; however, this concern regarding TMR can be largely mitigated by attaching the donor nerve directly to muscle in addition to the recipient nerve, and a larger, vascularized muscle target is generally provided by TMR. Last, the technical ease with which the RPNI procedure can be performed makes it scalable to all surgeons, even those with no training in nerve surgery or microsurgery.

Neuroma Management

Preclinical studies have provided the foundation for use of RPNI as a strategy for managing postamputation pain. Multiple animal models have demonstrated axonal sprouting, elongation, synaptogenesis, and formation of new neuromuscular junction within the RPNI graft, suggesting that RPNI facilitates a physiologic regenerative process.[43,44] Equally important, these studies confirmed the absence of neuroma formation. This encouraging preclinical work motivated a retrospective study whereby 46 RPNIs were performed for postamputation neuroma pain treatment in 17 residual limbs (16 patients).[45] At 7.5 months follow-up, mean neuroma pain score was decreased from 8.7 preoperatively to 2.5 postoperatively ($P < 0.001$), and mean phantom pain score went from 8.0 preoperatively to 3.8 postoperatively ($P < 0.009$).

Neuroma Prevention

RPNI has also been used prophylactically to minimize postamputation pain. In a retrospective review, 45 patients who underwent RPNI at the time of primary major amputation were compared with 45 matched control subjects.[45] After a mean follow-up of approximately 1 year, none of the 45 patients who underwent RPNI at the time of primary amputation had

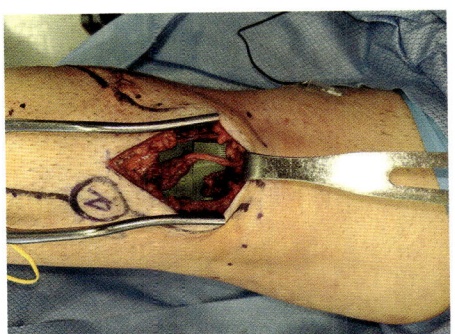

FIGURE 3 Clinical photograph shows regenerative peripheral nerve interface for neuroma management. The sural nerve has been wrapped with an approximately 20 mm × 40 mm muscle graft harvested from the medial gastrocnemius muscle.

symptomatic neuromas after major limb amputation, compared with 6 of 45 patients who underwent conventional passive nerve management techniques. There was also a significant difference in the incidence of phantom limb pain postoperatively, with the condition developing in 51.1% of patients who underwent RPNI compared with 91% of the matched control group. Of note, the high rate of phantom limb pain observed in the control population markedly exceeds the 64% pooled prevalence that was previously noted and may be explained by the liberal use of nerve ligation techniques in that cohort. The use of RPNI added an hour to the surgical time, and the control group demonstrated a greater rate of postoperative complications.

Pearls and Pitfalls

Although procedurally simplistic, there are several important technical constraints that must be adhered to in order to optimize RPNI outcomes. As with any tissue graft, revascularization of the RPNI muscle graft is at least partially dependent on adequate vascular perfusion from the wound bed. It is hypothesized that the vasa nervorum of the implanted nerve also contributes to perfusion of the central portion of the graft; however, an excessively large muscle graft or poorly vascularized wound bed will likely result in graft necrosis. The optimal size for RPNI skeletal muscle has been described to be 30 to 40 mm long, 15 to 20 mm wide, and 5 mm thick (**Figure 4**).

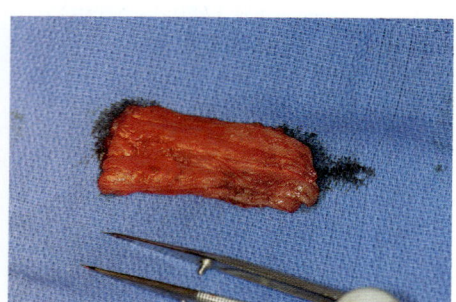

FIGURE 4 Clinical photograph shows regenerative peripheral nerve interface. The ideal muscle graft dimensions are approximately 40 mm long × 20 mm wide × 5 mm thick. The nerve is positioned within the graft so as to run lengthwise with the orientation of the muscle fibers.

Previous descriptions of the RPNI technique also suggest that the peripheral nerve end be implanted parallel to the direction of the muscle fibers. A small-caliber, nonabsorbable monofilament suture is used to secure the nerve to the central portion of the graft, after which the graft is rolled circumferentially around the nerve to encompass it entirely. Once created, the RPNI construct and donor nerve can be mobilized as needed to position both in a location that is well vascularized and has sufficient soft-tissue coverage. In addition to excessive graft size, a disproportionate ratio of donor axons to target endplates may predispose the RPNI construct to neuroma formation. As a result, it is recommended that donor nerves with large cross-sectional areas be split into multiple smaller fascicle groups and managed with multiple RPNI grafts. As an example, it is typical for three to four RPNI grafts to be used for neuroma prevention following transection of the sciatic nerve.

SUMMARY

Patients with limb loss experience severe neuroma pain, phantom limb pain, and residual limb pain, which adversely affect their functional restoration and psychosocial well-being. This effect can be so severe that it affects the patient's ability to perform simple activities of daily living and can lead to narcotic addiction. To address these issues, advanced active strategies have been developed to control nerve regeneration by providing physiologic targets for reinnervation, rather than passive strategies to stop nerve regeneration. These techniques provide a conduit or target for nerve regeneration and essentially give the axons "somewhere to go." In addition, TMR and RPNI also provide the regenerating nerves with denervated muscle fibers and empty motor endplates essentially giving the axons "something to do" (ie, reinnervate muscle). The tremendous enthusiasm for these techniques for management and prevention of postamputation pain highlights the scope and severity of the clinical challenge that postamputation pain presents, as well as the inadequacy of conventional surgical management techniques. However, much of this enthusiasm has been driven by small case series and limited preclinical studies. In the absence of a mechanistic understanding of postamputation pain or the benefit offered by these advanced nerve management techniques, it is challenging to refine or directly compare these techniques. Although additional preclinical work should focus on a better understanding of these mechanisms, future clinical studies should aim to move beyond case series and anecdotal experience by using rigorous outcomes studies that use well-matched control populations, recognizing the challenges posed by execution of these trials.

References

1. Collins KL, Russell HG, Schumacher PJ, et al: A review of current theories and treatments for phantom limb pain. *J Clin Invest* 2018;128(6):2168-2176.
2. List EF, Krijgh DD, Martin E, Coert JH: Prevalence of residual limb pain and symptomatic neuromas after lower extremity amputation: A systematic review and meta-analysis. *Pain* 2021;162(7):1906-1913.
3. Pyo J, Pasquina PF, DeMarco M, Wallace R, Teodorski E, Cooper RA: Upper limb nerve entrapment syndromes in veterans with lower limb amputations. *PM R* 2010;2(1):14-22.
4. Christopher RP: Peripheral nerve entrapment as a cause of phantom sensation and stump pain in lower extremity amputees. *Arch Phys Med Rehabil* 1963;44:631.
5. Limakatso K, Bedwell GJ, Madden VJ, Parker R: The prevalence and risk factors for phantom limb pain in people with amputations: A systematic review and meta-analysis. *PLoS One* 2020;15(10):e0240431.
6. Neumeister MW, Winters JN: Neuroma. *Clin Plast Surg* 2020;47(2) 279-283.
7. Finnerup NB, Kuner R, Jensen TS: Neuropathic pain: From mechanisms to treatment. *Physiol Rev* 2021;101(1):259-301.
8. Dellon L, Andonian E, Rosson GD: Lower extremity complex regional pain syndrome: Long-term outcome after surgical treatment of peripheral pain generators. *J Foot Ankle Surg* 2010;49(1):33-36.
9. Lee M, Guyuron B: Postoperative neuromas, in *Nerves and Nerve Injuries*. Elsevier, 2015, pp 99-112.

10. Stankevicius A, Wallwork SB, Summers SJ, Hordacre B, Stanton TR: Prevalence and incidence of phantom limb pain, phantom limb sensations and telescoping in amputees: A systematic rapid review. *Eur J Pain* 2021;25(1):23-38.
11. Makin TR, Scholz J, Henderson Slater D, Johansen-Berg H, Tracey I: Reassessing cortical reorganization in the primary sensorimotor cortex following arm amputation. *Brain* 2015;138(8):2140-2146.
12. Vaso A, Adahan H-M, Gjika A, et al: Peripheral nervous system origin of phantom limb pain. *Pain* 2014;155(7):1384-1391.
13. Latremoliere A, Woolf CJ: Central sensitization: A generator of pain hypersensitivity by central neural plasticity. *J Pain* 2009;10(9):895-926.
14. Eberlin KR, Ducic I: Surgical algorithm for neuroma management: A changing treatment paradigm. *Plast Reconstr Surg Glob Open* 2018;6(10):e1952.
15. Poyntz SA, Hacking NM, Dalal M, Fowler S: Peripheral interventions for painful stump neuromas of the lower limb: A systematic review. *Clin J Pain* 2018;34(3):285-295.
16. Dellon AL, Aszmann OC: In musculus, veritas? Nerve "in muscle" versus targeted muscle reinnervation versus regenerative peripheral nerve interface: Historical review. *Microsurgery* 2020;40(4):516-522.
17. Janes LE, Fracol ME, Dumanian GA, Ko JH: Targeted muscle reinnervation for the treatment of neuroma. *Hand Clin* 2021;37(3):345-359.
18. Ganesh Kumar N, Kung TA: Regenerative peripheral nerve interfaces for the treatment and prevention of neuromas and neuroma pain. *Hand Clin* 2021;37(3):361-371.
19. Whitlock EL, Myckatyn TM, Tong AY, et al: Dynamic quantification of host Schwann cell migration into peripheral nerve allografts. *Exp Neurol* 2010;225(2):310-319.
20. Hayashi A, Koob JW, Liu DZ, et al: A double-transgenic mouse used to track migrating Schwann cells and regenerating axons following engraftment of injured nerves. *Exp Neurol* 2007;207(1):128-138.
21. Saheb-Al-Zamani M, Yan Y, Farber SJ, et al: Limited regeneration in long acellular nerve allografts is associated with increased Schwann cell senescence. *Exp Neurol* 2013;247:165-177.
22. Campisi J, Andersen JK, Kapahi P, Melov S: Cellular senescence: A link between cancer and age-related degenerative disease? *Semin Cancer Biol* 2011;21(6):354-359.
23. Pazolli E, Stewart SA: Senescence: The good the bad and the dysfunctional. *Curr Opin Genet Dev* 2008;18(1):42-47.
24. Kenney AM, Kocsis JD: Peripheral axotomy induces long-term c-Jun amino-terminal kinase-1 activation and activator protein-1 binding activity by c-Jun and junD in adult rat dorsal root ganglia in vivo. *J Neurosci* 1998;18(4):1318-1328.
25. Pan D, Bichanich M, Wood IS, et al: Long acellular nerve allografts cap transected nerve to arrest axon regeneration and alter upstream gene expression in a rat neuroma model. *Plast Reconstr Surg* 2021;148(1):32e-41e.
26. Freniere BB, Wenzinger E, Lans J, Eberlin KR: Relocation nerve grafting: A technique for management of symptomatic digital neuromas. *J Hand Microsurg* 2019;11(suppl 1):S50-S52.
27. Souza JM, Purnell CA, Cheesborough JE, Kelikian AS, Dumanian GA: Treatment of foot and ankle neuroma pain with processed nerve allografts. *Foot Ankle Int* 2016;37(10):1098-1105.
28. Schur MD, Sochol KM, Lefebvre R, Stevanovic M: Treatment of iatrogenic saphenous neuroma after knee arthroscopy with excision and allograft reconstruction. *Plast Reconstr Surg Glob Open* 2021;9(2):e3403.
29. Ducic I, Yoon J, Eberlin KR: Treatment of neuroma-induced chronic pain and management of nerve defects with processed nerve allografts. *Plast Reconstr Surg Glob Open* 2019;7(12):e2467.
30. Kuiken TA, Li G, Lock BA, et al: Targeted muscle reinnervation for real-time myoelectric control of multifunction artificial arms. *J Am Med Assoc* 2009;301(6):619-628.
31. Vu PP, Vaskov AK, Irwin ZT, et al: A regenerative peripheral nerve interface allows real-time control of an artificial hand in upper limb amputees. *Sci Transl Med* 2020;12(533):2857.
32. Kim PS, Ko JH, O'Shaughnessy KK, Kuiken TA, Pohlmeyer EA, Dumanian GA: The effects of targeted muscle reinnervation on neuromas in a rabbit rectus abdominis flap model. *J Hand Surg* 2012;37(8):1609-1616.
33. Ko JH, Kim PS, Smith DG: Targeted muscle reinnervation as a strategy for neuroma prevention, in Kuiken TA, ed: *Targeted Muscle Reinnervation - A Neural Interface for Artificial Limbs*. Taylor & Francis, 2014, pp 45-66.
34. Souza JM, Cheesborough JE, Ko JH, Cho MS, Kuiken TA, Dumanian GA: Targeted muscle reinnervation: A novel approach to postamputation neuroma pain. *Clin Orthop Relat Res* 2014;472(10):2984-2990.
35. Dumanian GA, Potter BK, Mioton LM, et al: Targeted muscle reinnervation treats neuroma and phantom pain in major limb amputees: A randomized clinical trial. *Ann Surg* 2019;270(2):238-246.
36. Mioton LM, Dumanian GA, Shah N, et al: Targeted muscle reinnervation improves residual limb pain, phantom limb pain, and limb function: A prospective study of 33 major limb amputees. *Clin Orthop Relat Res* 2020;478(9):2161-2167.
37. Valerio IL, Dumanian GA, Jordan SW, et al: Preemptive treatment of phantom and residual limb pain with targeted muscle reinnervation at the time of major limb amputation. *J Am Coll Surg* 2019;228(3):217-226.
38. Chang BL, Mondshine J, Attinger CE, Kleiber GM: Targeted muscle reinnervation improves pain and ambulation outcomes in highly comorbid amputees. *Plast Reconstr Surg* 2021;148(2):376-386.
39. Freilinger G: A new technique to correct facial paralysis. *Plast Reconstr Surg* 1975;56(1):44-48.
40. Thompson N: A review of autogenous skeletal muscle grafts and their clinical applications. *Clin Plast Surg* 1974;1(3):349-403.
41. Ganesh Kumar N, Cederna PS, Kung TA: Regenerative peripheral nerve interfaces for advanced prosthetic control and mitigation of postamputation pain. *Tech Orthop* 2021;36(4):321-328.
42. Hu Y, Ursu DC, Sohasky RA, et al: Regenerative peripheral nerve interface free muscle graft mass and function. *Muscle Nerve* 2021;63(3):421-429.
43. Kung TA, Langhals NB, Martin DC, et al: Regenerative peripheral nerve interface viability and signal transduction with an implanted electrode. *Plast Reconstr Surg* 2014;133(6):1380-1394.
44. Woo SL, Kung TA, Brown DL, et al: Regenerative peripheral nerve interfaces for the treatment of postamputation neuroma pain: A pilot study. *Plast Reconstr Surg Glob Open* 2016;4(12):e1038.
45. Kubiak CA, Kemp SWP, Cederna PS, Kung TA: Prophylactic regenerative peripheral nerve interfaces to prevent postamputation pain. *Plast Reconstr Surg* 2019;144(3):421e-430e.

Targeted Muscle Reinnervation: Prosthetic Management

Craig Jackman, CPO, FAAOP • Brian Monroe, CPO • Ryan Sheridan, MS, CPO, FAAOP

ABSTRACT

Targeted muscle reinnervation is a surgical technique that has been developed to improve an individual's ability to control a myoelectric prosthesis and reduce postamputation pain. Prosthetists who attempt to fit individuals with powered prostheses after target muscle reinnervation must first be knowledgeable in the basic principles of fitting myoelectric devices. In addition, the prosthetist should understand the surgical procedure and the intended outcomes. The application of both traditional and advanced myoelectric control strategies can optimize function for this patient population. The incorporation of emerging technologies will benefit both the user and the prosthetist.

Keywords: antagonistic muscle action; coaptation; electromyographic (EMG) signal; mode selection; myoelectric control

Introduction

For individuals with upper limb amputation, especially at or proximal to the transhumeral level, successful operation of a prosthesis requires the performance of control motions that are rarely analogous to actions performed before the amputation. For body-powered prostheses, users must incorporate gross body movements such as glenohumeral flexion, scapular protraction, or biscapular protraction to flex the elbow and/or operate the terminal device. In myoelectrically controlled, externally powered systems, the actions for controlling a powered elbow can be more physiologic for individuals with transhumeral amputations if contraction of the biceps is used to control elbow flexion and the triceps is used to control elbow extension. Beyond this exception, for the other powered components of a transhumeral prosthesis (electronic wrists and terminal devices) and all the motors in an externally powered prosthesis for shoulder disarticulation, both the electromyographic (EMG) input signals and other physical body movements that are used as control inputs are nonphysiologic strategies. For example, strategies for using a myoelectrically controlled transhumeral prosthesis may include using the residual biceps and triceps muscles to control elbow flexion and extension, wrist supination and pronation, and terminal device prehension. Various mode selection strategies are required to allow the user to switch between these antagonistic pairs of movements. An example of mode selection may be an intentional co-contraction of the biceps and triceps muscles to switch active control inputs from one component to another (eg, elbow to hand). Other methods of mode selection could include activating a bump switch mounted on the exterior surface of the prosthetic socket or a momentary pull switch incorporated into the harness. Regardless of the method of mode selection, another action is required to direct input signals from one component to another. More importantly, the muscle signals used to control these various motors are rarely consistent with the action being performed.

Targeted muscle reinnervation (TMR) is a means by which users can operate their myoelectrically controlled prostheses in a manner that is more intuitive and physiologically consistent with the actions and thought processes that users had before their amputations.[1-8] Adding two to three physiologic electrode sites for the individual with a transhumeral prosthesis, and four to six physiologic sites for the shoulder disarticulation prosthesis, creates the potential for a more natural means of controlling the prosthesis. TMR also allows the user to control multiple motors intuitively and reduce the delays associated with mode selection for most prosthetic actions and movements.

Craig Jackman or an immediate family member serves as a paid consultant to or is an employee of Hanger Clinic. Brian Monroe or an immediate family member serves as a paid consultant to or is an employee of Hanger Clinic. Ryan Sheridan or an immediate family member serves as a paid consultant to or is an employee of Hanger Clinic.

This chapter is adapted from Lipschutz RD: Targeted muscle reinnervation: prosthetic management, in: Krajbich JI, Pinzur MS, Potter BK, Stevens PM, eds: *Atlas of Amputations and Limb Deficiencies: Surgical, Prosthetic, and Rehabilitation Principles*, ed 4. American Academy of Orthopaedic Surgeons, 2016, pp 339-350.

Since its initial application to proximal upper limb amputation levels, multiple surgical centers have performed TMR with the primary goal of improved prosthetic control.[9] However, subsequent clinical experience and observation suggested that patients who underwent TMR reported less postamputation pain and fewer instances of recurrent painful neuroma formation.[9] A retrospective multicenter study that examined the role of TMR in postamputation nerve pain confirmed the potential for reducing residual and phantom limb pain.[9] Further studies have confirmed the potential benefits of performing TMR at both the primary closure of the amputation and as a secondary procedure.[10,11]

The general principles of fitting individuals with upper limb prostheses who have undergone TMR, the challenges encountered during clinical fittings, and technologic advancements associated with TMR are discussed.

General Principles

TMR has moved from experimental case studies to the standard of care at many surgical centers in the United States for managing the transected nerves in limb amputation. Although postoperative care for an amputation with nerve treatment is the same as a non-TMR procedure, it is essential that the surgical and rehabilitation teams fully comprehend the surgical procedure, any benefits and risks associated with the process, the postoperative protocol, and prosthetic fitting principles and training.[12]

Muscle Recovery Period

After a successful TMR procedure, the patient will be asked to pay particular attention to their neuromuscular development of reinnervation, most notably what occurs when attempting to perform a muscle contraction that was absent before TMR.[13] Reinnervation will occur gradually, reaching a consistently measurable EMG level as soon as 3 to 6 months after the procedure. However, EMG signals may continue to increase in magnitude, and optimal electrode locations may reorient as further development occurs in subsequent months and years after the procedure.[14] During this period of reinnervation, the patient should be given a protocol of how to exercise both the reinnervated and natively innervated muscles. In addition to the typical practices of wound care and healing maintenance of the residual limb, overall strength and range of motion should also be pursued.[13,14]

One principle often overlooked in this transition period is prosthetic wear after TMR for individuals who had been previously fitted with prostheses. Generally, it is expected that after a brief surgical recovery period, the user will resume prosthetic wear with their legacy device. Prosthesis use may be complicated by the fact that the overall limb volume may change substantially because of the removal or movement of adipose tissue during the TMR procedure as well as transient atrophy of muscles that have been deinnervated and reinnervated. Although the repositioning of adipose tissue, termed debulking, is a benefit for signal acquisition, the removal or movement of subcutaneous fat will also alter the shape of the residual limb to the degree that either major socket modifications or socket replacement becomes necessary.

Myotesting Principles

Fitting individuals with traditional myoelectric control requires that the prosthetist follow the basic strategies for myosite testing. Signal thresholds, antagonistic muscle pairs, the appropriate alignment of the electrodes, and maintenance of electrode contact on the skin surface are essential elements of these fittings. The addition of TMR sites does not alter these strategies. Depending on the level of amputation and surgical technique performed, the patient may have five or more reinnervated muscle sites. The use of pattern recognition systems, discussed later in this chapter, as a diagnostic tool can test up to eight EMG sites simultaneously to assist this pre-prosthetic phase of rehabilitation (**Figure 1**). The site selection of antagonistic pairs of muscles, including isolation, attaining thresholds, and proportional control, can be identified with either traditional or advanced myotesting systems.

Coactivation of Signals

TMR has created an avenue for discrete EMG signals to control discrete prosthetic movements. For example, elbow flexion and extension can be controlled independently from the opening and closing of a terminal device. These individual signals are comparatively easy to attain when selecting them in isolation and testing the residual limb for control of the desired motions. However, when all the electrodes are in contact with the user's body, eliminating unintended coactivation of muscles is quite difficult. This is, in part, because following TMR distinct control muscles are part of the same synergistic pattern (elbow flexion and hand close, elbow extension and hand open). In addition to the surgical attempt to separate these muscles by means of adipofascial flaps,[8] the use of pattern recognition control can eliminate the confusion caused by the unintended coactivation of muscles as such coactivation becomes part of that recognized pattern for a given movement.

Visualization of Desired Movement

A primary goal of TMR is to enable the user to provide an intuitive neuromuscular signal that is native to the action desired from the prosthesis. For the individual with a transhumeral amputation, the native neural pattern for elbow flexion and extension signals are present both before and after TMR. However, hand and wrist movements require a rerouted neural signal from a different muscle. For the individual with a shoulder disarticulation, this rerouting occurs for all elbow, wrist, and hand signals. When motor reinnervation occurs, it is unclear as to exactly what neural information reaches its destination in the motor point of the muscle. For example, after reinnervation of the median nerve to a motor point on a targeted muscle, it is expected that the user's attempt to elicit the EMG

Chapter 25: Targeted Muscle Reinnervation: Prosthetic Management

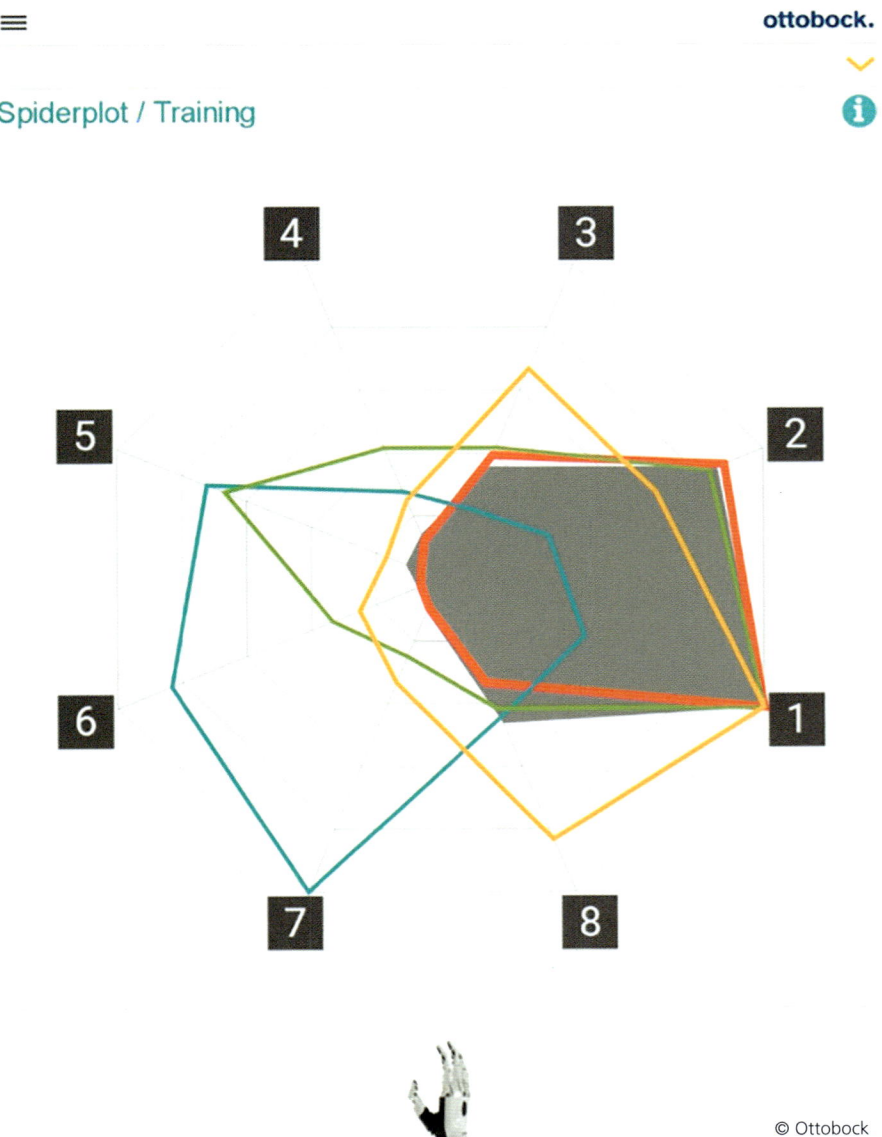

FIGURE 1 Illustration of a graphical user interface screen that allows the simultaneous viewing of multiple electromyographic channels. (Courtesy of Ottobock.)

signal for "hand close" will send the desired neural signal to contract the targeted muscle. Generally, this attempt is successful. However, some factors may necessitate slight variations to the user's visualized movement of their amputated limb to generate the proper corresponding EMG signals. First, the portion of the median nerve that reinnervated the target muscle may have been biased toward thumb movements more so than the second and third digits. In this case, the patient may have to visualize more thumb movement for "hand close" versus visualizing the entire hand closing. In other cases, the patient may think that their phantom limb cannot completely move into the desired position, again necessitating a variation of the desired visualization. Both circumstances require the patient, the prosthetist, and the occupational therapist to be flexible enough to try alternative motions that are normally innervated by the reinnervated peripheral nerve to determine what is most effective.[14,15] As in all myoelectric control, consistency in the activation patterns is the key to successful prosthetic operation.

Electrode Placement and Socket Designs

Prosthetists usually have their own preferred electrodes and socket design for myoelectric fittings that they have found successful. Such components and design concepts should remain within each prosthetist's repertoire, adding the possibility of minor modifications caused by the surgical method used, the location and number of EMG sites, and significant movement of superficial tissue during muscle contraction.[15]

Similar to prosthetists, surgeons have their own ideas of how to achieve successful results. Although TMR has somewhat standardized surgical principles, the results from TMR will depend on what is discovered both before and during the procedure. For example, a muscle transfer from another region of the body may be necessary to provide a viable site for reinnervation of the peripheral nerve. Such transfer may also be necessary to provide coverage over bony prominences, such as within an interscapulothoracic amputation. Alternatively, the originally targeted muscle may be determined as nonviable intraoperatively. In other surgical variations, the surgeon may opt to detach the origin of the muscle tendon to prevent proximal migration of the muscle during contraction. In all of these cases, it is essential for the prosthetist to review the surgical report and/or discuss the case with the surgeon to ensure that both appreciate (and understand) how to best design the socket.

Consideration should be given for the length of the residual limb and the location of usable EMG sites, which need to be contained within the socket interface. Traditional myoelectric prostheses are designed with two electrode sites. After TMR, at least four sites should be available. In these cases, greater surface coverage of the socket may be necessary to capture the reinnervated sites, while ensuring electrodes are placed distal to the remaining major joints.

It has been noted that in both transhumeral and shoulder disarticulation limbs, substantial movement occurs in particular areas of superficial tissue

Section 2: Upper Limb

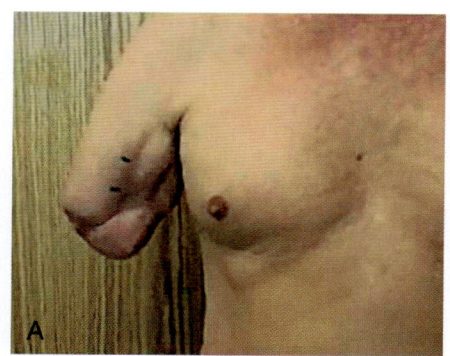 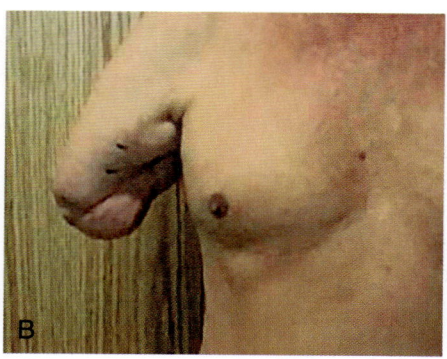 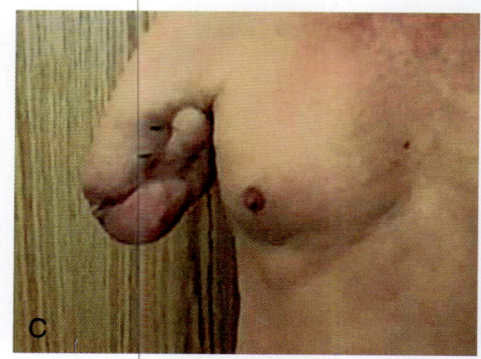

FIGURE 2 Clinical photographs of soft-tissue movements of the transhumeral residual limb associated with generating various control signals in a patient after targeted muscle reinnervation. **A**, Relaxed. **B**, Hand close. **C**, Elbow up. (Courtesy of Shirley Ryan AbilityLab, Chicago, IL.)

overlying reinnervated muscle sites[1-8] (**Figure 2**). Such movement is problematic because the electrodes must maintain surface contact with the soft tissue to prevent inadvertent movement of the prosthesis. Sockets may need to be modified for a tighter fit over these regions or, alternatively, use a flexible interface that can expand and still maintain contact with the skin surface. In addition to the movement of superficial tissues, subcutaneous muscle may shift during contraction. This may occur because the newly targeted muscle did not undergo myodesis or myoplasty during the initial amputation surgery. Alternatively, during TMR, the origin of the muscle may not have been detached, allowing for a floating muscle belly. Because this muscle with only a proximal attachment is reinnervated, a contraction makes the muscle move proximally toward its origin.[12] In these instances, it may be necessary to install the electrodes quite proximally on the socket.

Direct Control and Pattern Recognition

Traditionally, the use of a myoelectric prosthesis most commonly involves direct control from dual-site electrodes. Two surface electrodes that are built into the prosthetic socket make contact with an antagonistic muscle pair, for example, the biceps muscle and triceps muscle. From a voluntary muscle contraction, electrical activity is detected by the electrode. This EMG signal must cross the on-threshold to send a signal to the powered component. For example, a contraction of the biceps muscle that crosses the on-threshold will cause the terminal device to close. Regardless of the level of amputation, the number of powered components, and the number of usable EMG sites, with direct control the prosthetic system is limited to two electrodes. For more proximal amputations, this necessitates the additional use of external switches, linear transducers, force sensing resistors, or manually positioned components.

In the context of myoelectric prostheses, pattern recognition describes a method by which numerous EMG signals are collected and analyzed, resulting in a single decision for how the prosthesis should move (or not move). Instead of using EMG information at only two myoelectric sites, pattern recognition can use EMG information from up to 16 sites (**Figure 3**). A major benefit of pattern recognition is that the isolation of muscles is not necessary to distinguish one intended movement from another. Even for antagonistic muscle groups, coactivation of muscles may provide a distinct pattern that can be classified as a particular movement of the prosthesis. In traditional myoelectric systems, even with adjustments to thresholds, gains, and the control strategy, the prosthetic elbow might not consistently extend because the coactivation may compromise the signal output such that it is not clean enough to represent an isolated elbow extension signal. Suppose, instead, that the isolated EMG signal from the biceps was used for elbow flexion, and the combined signals from the biceps and triceps coactivation were used for elbow extension. Controlling the prosthesis

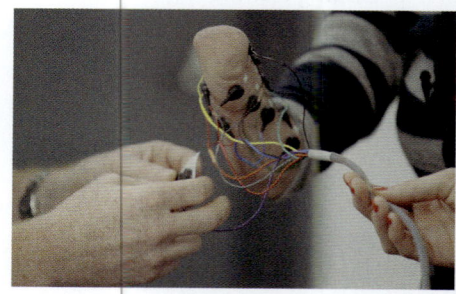

FIGURE 3 Clinical photograph of the additional myoelectric sites used in a pattern recognition system. (Courtesy of Coapt, LLC, Chicago, IL.)

in this manner is plausible when pattern recognition control is used, which substantially reduces the burden on the user to isolate distinct muscle signals.

TMR has created an increased number of EMG sites and, thus, an increased set of data from which to draw.[16] Earlier, it was explained that although the surgical procedure proved effective, prosthetic control may still be difficult because of the unintended coactivation of muscles with synergistic actions. The application of pattern recognition can help eliminate this signal confusion because it collectively examines all the signals before deciding how the prosthesis should or should not move.

One key to pattern recognition control is analogous to that of all myoelectric prostheses: consistency in signal intent and level. The user must create the same pattern and level of contraction to control the prosthesis as when these classifiers were created. An additional feature of available pattern recognition controllers is that the user can recalibrate the system whenever they think that the prosthesis is not responding to current EMG signals. Similarly, recalibration can be performed when the user wishes to add multiple classifier settings for times when the prosthesis may be used in different positions or for different tasks. With this feature, the user does not need the prosthetist to alter the settings within the graphic interface system; the user can simply recalibrate the settings by donning the prosthesis, pushing a physical or digital button, and providing signals to the prosthesis while following a predefined sequence of movements. The microprocessor within the prosthesis automatically uses the new data to redefine the user's settings to the current signal classifiers that were just provided.

Although pattern recognition has proven to be a very powerful tool in the prosthetist's arsenal, it still has some limitations. The mastery of a prosthesis with pattern recognition should involve regular training with an occupational therapist for several months. For a transradial prosthesis with fewer degrees of freedom, for example, the additional training to use pattern recognition may not yield significantly better outcomes versus a direct control system. This may be especially true for a patient who has not undergone TMR. Another limitation may be the patient's gadget tolerance of the added system. Certain pattern recognition control systems require the use of mobile phone apps, regular firmware or software updates, or more frequent prosthetic maintenance.

Prosthetic Fittings

As discussed earlier, TMR is now widely performed for neuroma prevention and pain management in both existing amputations and primary amputations. The prosthetic treatment plan for a patient who has undergone TMR should be similar to that of a non-TMR patient. If TMR surgery was performed as part of the primary amputation, normal postoperative protocols can be followed. A postoperative protective device can be used to reduce the severity of tissue damage because of a fall or bump. When the sutures are removed, a preparatory device can be used to restore basic grasp, allowing the patient to incorporate the affected limb into bimanual functional tasks as soon as possible. This promotes proximal muscle strengthening, prevents joint contracture by actively using the residual limb, and helps stabilize limb volume in preparation for the definitive prosthesis. Once residual limb volume stabilizes, the definitive prosthesis can be fitted to the patient.

TMR surgery can improve outcomes for all types of prosthetic fittings. Although the presence of additional EMG signals allows for more options when fitting an external powered prosthesis, even an individual who elects not to wear a prosthesis may experience a reduction in pain that can improve their quality of life.[17] An individual who has had TMR surgery does not necessarily require a myoelectric prosthesis to best accomplish their functional goals. A thorough evaluation of the patient and discussion between the patient, the prosthetist, and the rehabilitation team are still necessary to ensure the optimal design of the prosthesis. This includes weighing the advantages and disadvantages of operating a myoelectric prosthesis, a hybrid prosthesis, a body-powered prosthesis, an oppositional prosthesis, or not using a prosthesis at all.

In the case of a myoelectric prosthesis fitting, it is important for the rehabilitation team to access the surgical report that typically shows which nerves were coapted to which muscles. This is a helpful guide for EMG testing and visualization of the correct motor pathway. The viability and health of the nerves and muscles may dictate particular coaptations. As with any fitting of a myoelectric prosthesis, assessing comfort, range of motion, and electrode contact throughout a variety of positions and functional tasks is paramount. Loss of contact with an electrode in any plane will compromise the control and operation of the prosthesis.

Training an individual with a myoelectric prosthesis after TMR is easier if the user has not had substantial previous myoelectric experience, where the necessary substitution of nonphysiologic muscle signals was ingrained into their thought control process. Users with prior myoelectric experience will have to unlearn many of the previous strategies for controlling the various motors. After TMR, the native muscles will control their intended movements. Users should now be able to activate these movements by sending nerve signals to reinnervated muscles by means of natural thought processes.

Transradial Fittings

Multiple muscle targets are available in the transradial level amputation; therefore TMR nerve transfer standards vary between surgeons and surgical centers. The ulnar nerve is commonly transferred to the flexor carpi ulnaris, while the median nerve can be transferred to the flexor carpi radialis.[18,19] The wrist extensor and supinator functions of the radial nerve are mostly preserved at this level, but the nerve can be transferred to the brachioradialis.[18]

An individual with a transradial amputation with TMR who is a candidate for a myoelectric prosthesis will require the same considerations as a non-TMR individual regarding the design of the prosthesis. This includes the terminal device, wrist unit, socket interface, suspension method, and control strategy. A prosthesis that incorporates a multiarticulating hand with a pattern recognition system allows the patient to use direct access grip control. With direct access grip control, the individual can calibrate a distinct muscle pattern for a particular grip, allowing that grip to be easily accessed. Although this is an option for a non-TMR patient as well, multiple distinct patterns are more easily accomplished for a patient with TMR. The same is true for a powered wrist unit. A pattern recognition system allows the patient to calibrate a distinct muscle pattern for pronation and supination and/or flexion and extension. Again, multiple distinct patterns are more accessible to a patient with TMR, especially when four patterns are dedicated to the basic movements of hand open, hand close, wrist pronation, and wrist supination.

Regarding the socket interface, an individual with TMR will likely experience a higher amount of muscle movement during contraction for the reasons stated earlier. It can be beneficial to use a rolled silicone interface that allows for dynamic expansion during prosthesis use (**Figure 4**). An additional benefit of this material is ensuring appropriate contact between the electrodes and soft tissue through a variety of movements and muscle contractions. For short transradial limbs where pattern recognition control is desired, it is important to ensure that the electrode locations are distal to the elbow joint if possible. As the biceps and triceps muscles both insert distal to the elbow joint, pre-positioning the prosthesis or lifting objects may cause an inadvertent signal to be sent to a powered component.

Transhumeral Fittings

Since the first initial fittings of patients with TMR, the standard surgical procedure for TMR for individuals with a transhumeral amputation has changed to include coapting the distal radial nerve to the lateral head of the triceps[20] (**Figure 5**). This change has improved the success of the subsequent prosthetic fittings. With the natively innervated long and medial heads of the triceps available for physiologic control of elbow extension, the reinnervated lateral head of the triceps can be used for intuitive control of the hand opening signal. In addition, the ulnar nerve can be transferred to the brachialis muscle as a potential means of controlling a powered wrist rotator. Because it is necessary to locate the reinnervated pair of antagonistic muscle actions, palpating for distinct muscle contractions is imperative.

Component selection for the terminal device and wrist unit is similar for a transradial and a transhumeral prosthesis fitting. However, with multiple EMG sites already dedicated to the terminal device and wrist unit, special consideration should be given to the elbow unit selected. As with any transhumeral prosthesis fitting, a passive elbow can be used to decrease overall prosthesis weight, while requiring the use of the sound side hand for positioning, locking, and unlocking. A hybrid elbow that is cable-operated may be advantageous by eliminating the need for sound hand positioning. Additionally, certain hybrid elbows can be locked and unlocked through the use of an external switch, a co-contraction signal, or through a dedicated muscle contraction in a pattern recognition system. A powered elbow unit eliminates nearly all cabling, and when combined with a pattern recognition system can also eliminate all external mode switching mechanisms. As with any fully myoelectric prosthesis, the major disadvantage is the total weight of the prosthesis.

Transhumeral prosthetic socket fittings present unique challenges compared with a transradial prosthetic fitting. The humeral segment has a higher proportion of soft tissue to bone than the radial segment, so volume fluctuations can more easily compromise electrode contact through a variety of movements. Whereas a transradial socket often contains an element of anatomic suspension, a transhumeral prosthesis more typically relies on suction suspension and auxiliary harness suspension. Additionally, the humeral segment is most often oriented vertically, so migration of the socket because of gravity or axial loading can create distal electrode contact issues. An important assessment during the socket fitting is that all electrodes maintain appropriate skin contact through various muscle contractions, movements, and axial loads. A rolled silicone interface that allows the electrodes to move with muscle contraction can help to maintain electrode to skin contact. The use of an adjustable socket system can also be an effective means of accommodating volume fluctuations to help with prosthesis consistency (**Figure 6**), while socket windows can help minimize distal migration in an especially fleshy patient.

Shoulder Disarticulation Fittings

The main difference for shoulder disarticulation fittings compared with transhumeral or transradial fittings is that

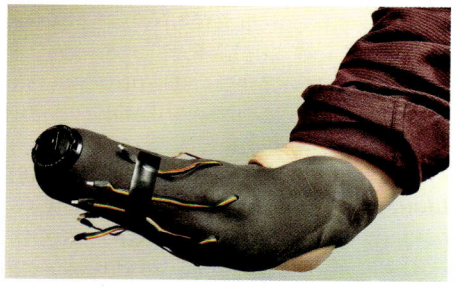

FIGURE 4 Clinical photograph of a rolled silicone interface that allows for dynamic expansion during prosthesis use while maintaining electrode–skin contact. (Courtesy of Hanger Clinic, Austin, TX.)

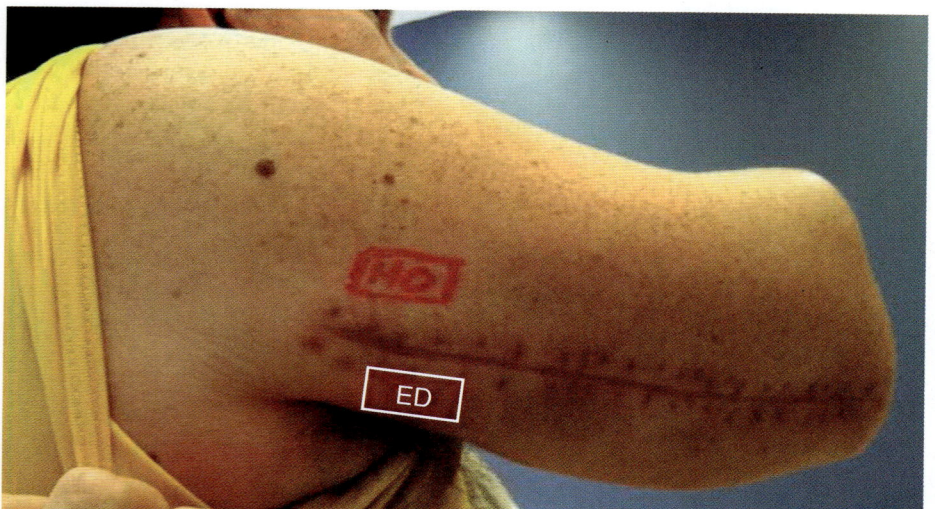

FIGURE 5 Clinical photograph of electrode placement over the lateral head of the triceps muscle, reinnervated by the distal radial nerve and used for the hand opening signal (HO) and the elbow down (ED) signal. (Courtesy of Shirley Ryan AbilityLab, Chicago, IL.)

no native muscles with physiologically analogous motions to prosthetic actions are being used. As described previously, regardless of the surgical technique, it is crucial for the prosthetist and the therapist to obtain a report that identifies the nerves that were transferred and the locations to which they were coapted.

The TMR procedure for shoulder disarticulations has also varied greatly since its inception. The most common nerves and sites for reinnervation are the musculocutaneous nerve and the median nerve to the clavicular head and sternal head (upper portion) of the pectoralis major muscle, respectively.[8] The musculocutaneous nerve/site is responsible for elbow flexion and will be located just inferior to the clavicle. Median nerve reinnervation is used for the signal to close the hand (**Figure 7**). Beyond these two coaptations, the remaining peripheral nerves of the brachial plexus may be transferred to any number of sites, depending primarily on which skeletal, muscular, and neural structures remain after amputation.

After the TMR procedure and the reinnervation period, site selection will occur in a similar, methodical procedure. Because these two muscles, and possibly others, have been reinnervated with signals that correspond to elbow, hand, and wrist control, these are the thoughts and actions that the user should be performing to contract the newly innervated sites rather than substituting nonphysiologic movements. The actions that the user is prompted to perform by the prosthetist or the therapist should begin with the basic (gross) movements of elbow flexion and extension, wrist pronation and supination, and hand opening and closing. Ultimately, the movement visualized by the user may be a variant one of these basic motions, a combined movement, or another action that is innervated by the targeted nerve/muscle location. For example, spreading the fingers may provide a more distinct and isolated signal for hand opening than a more passive hand opening attempt (**Figure 8**). As mentioned previously, consistency in the method and magnitude of muscle contractions is of utmost importance to reliable, sound, isolated prosthetic performance.

Most of the fitting principles of a shoulder disarticulation prosthesis can be applied to a patient who has undergone TMR. A closed encapsulated socket provides maximum stability and the greatest surface area for the attachment of components or harnessing. An open frame socket can provide the required stabilization, while minimizing weight and allowing for improved heat dissipation.[21] In addition to accommodations for breast tissue in females, some changes to these designs may be necessary, including adjustable socket systems to ensure that the electrodes maintain contact with the skin during contraction.[22] As with transhumeral limbs, tissue in the area of the shoulder disarticulation reinnervation can move quite substantially during muscle

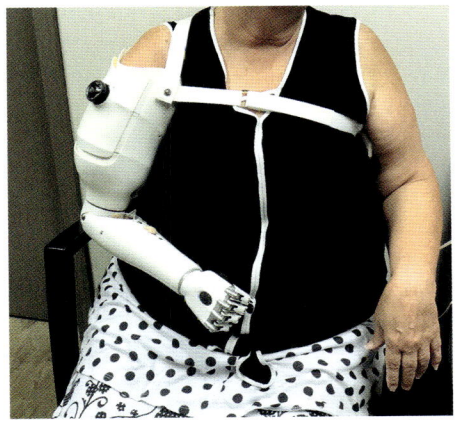

FIGURE 6 Clinical photograph of an adjustable socket system to accommodate volume fluctuation. (Courtesy of Hanger Clinic, Austin, TX.)

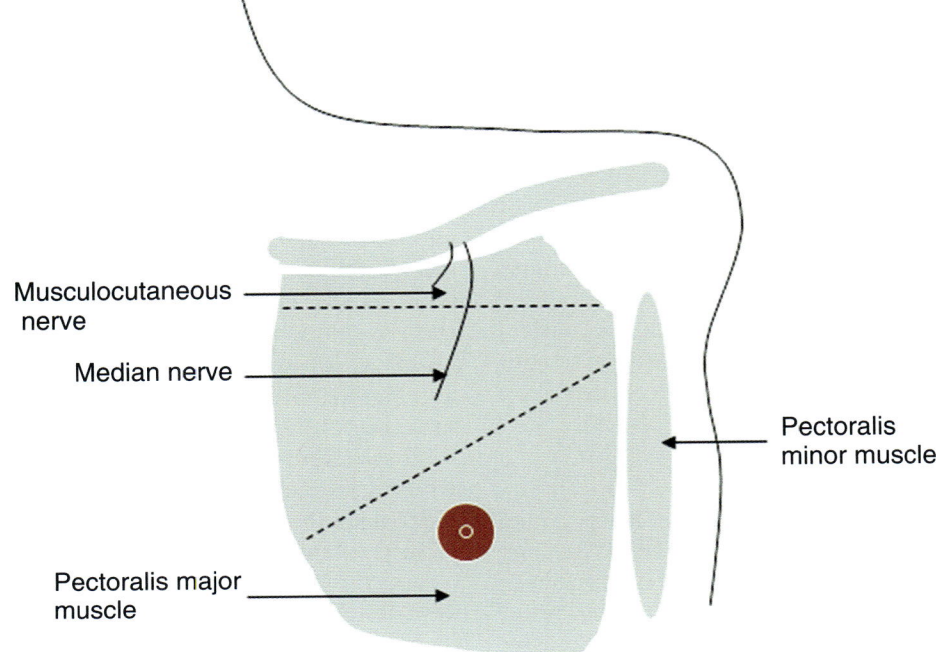

FIGURE 7 Illustration of standard nerve coaptations of the musculocutaneous and median nerves. Coaptations of the ulnar and radial nerves are more patient specific. (Courtesy of Shirley Ryan AbilityLab, Chicago, IL.)

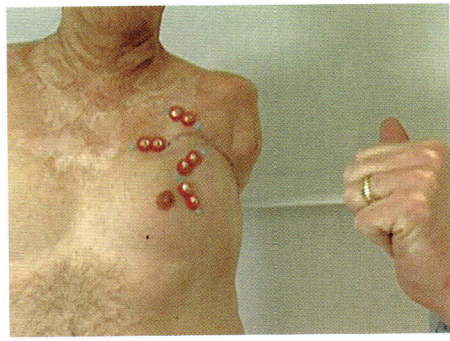

FIGURE 8 Clinical photograph of a man with a shoulder disarticulation who is generating electromyographic signals for finger movement and hand grasp in response to observed hand and finger movements being performed by the treating prosthetist. (Courtesy of Shirley Ryan AbilityLab, Chicago, IL.)

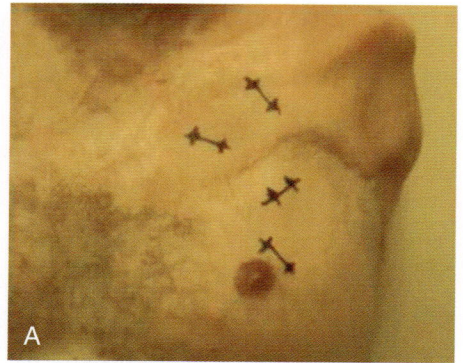 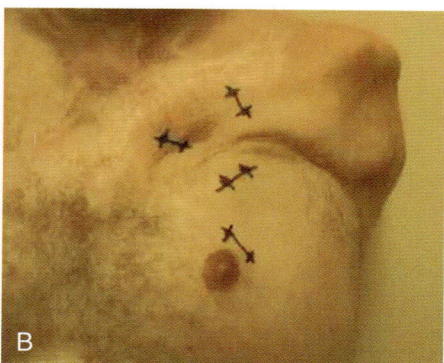 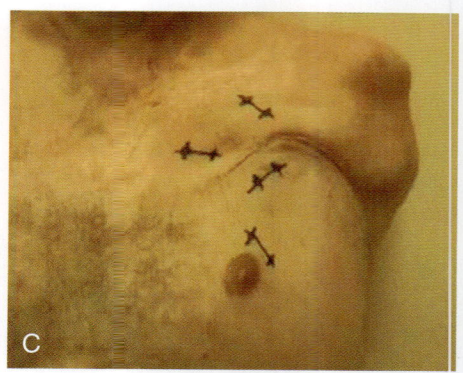

FIGURE 9 Clinical photographs of soft-tissue movements of the shoulder disarticulation residual limb associated with the generation of various control signals in a patient after targeted muscle reinnervation. Note the differences in the orientation of both the marked electromyographic sites and the skin underlying the soft tissue when the individual is relaxed (**A**), and during muscle contraction for hand opening (**B**) and hand closing (**C**). (Courtesy of Shirley Ryan AbilityLab, Chicago, IL.)

contractions[1-8] (**Figure 9**). Maintaining good skin contact is crucial for sound myoelectric control and may be even more difficult to achieve after a TMR procedure.

Flexible interfaces can serve a suspensory purpose for socket fittings in the glenohumeral region through the use of an integrated shoulder saddle. Although cable-operated elbows and terminal devices at this level can be challenging because of cable excursion requirements, careful consideration should be given to the use of passive components, cable-operated locks, and myoelectric components. If a patient with TMR is a candidate for myoelectric control, myosite selection can be similar to that in a patient without TMR. When using a single-site or dual-site myoelectric control system, electrode placement is ideally located where a strong signal is present that potentially represents more than one gross movement. If a pattern recognition system is being fitted, it is helpful to palpate muscle contractions for elbow, wrist, hand, and finger movements, and marking on the patient's anatomy where that contraction is felt. With the large surface area in this region and finite number of electrodes, this type of muscle mapping can indicate where electrodes should be placed within the socket.

Similar to the transhumeral amputation, additional inputs may be needed to control the wrist rotator or to shift power between components. After TMR, fewer, if any, native sites exist that the user must control, thus making switching more challenging. Although using reinnervated muscles for either co-contraction, quick impulses, or slow-soft/fast-hard strategies may be more difficult, they are nonetheless worth exploring. Individuals with externally powered prostheses generally prefer using EMG signals to control motors because it is much easier and more intuitive than performing gross body movements.

Application of Technologic Advancements

Since the inception of TMR, technologic advancements have continued to meet the needs of both the user and the prosthetist. Many of these changes relate to the ability to incorporate a greater number of EMG inputs and adjustments to a system. The advantages from emerging technologies such as sensory feedback combined with externally powered prosthetics have created direct benefits for TMR recipients.[23-32]

Sensory Feedback

The advent of terminal devices (and systems) that provide refined sensory feedback is another advancement in powered prosthetics that will prove highly beneficial to TMR recipients. Forms of sensory (also known as haptic) feedback to the prosthesis user have been explored for many years, but most of these applications remain confined to the research setting.[26-33] Stimuli have been applied to the residual limb or other parts of the body to relay senses of force, pressure, vibration, or simulated temperature. The difference for individuals with TMR is that, although the stimulus will still be over the residual limb, it will provide signals to the brain that the stimulus is elsewhere (eg, in the missing hand) because sensory reinnervation has spontaneously occurred in some TMR recipients.[8,32] Sensory nerves have grown to the surface of the skin in several TMR recipients and have since become a planned part of the surgery. Nerve patterns, often replicating those of normal dermatomes, have developed in the residuum. For example, in the first TMR recipient with a shoulder disarticulation and TMR to the left pectoralis region, sensory nerves grew to the surface of the patient's chest so that when certain stimuli were given, the signals were felt in the missing hand.[32] This is clearly different from previous work because now the feedback from the prosthesis is perceived in the user's hand versus pressure on the residual limb (**Figure 10**). With the refined work on tactile elements for prosthetic hands that is now occurring worldwide, the benefits for TMR recipients may be dramatic. Many in the field of prosthetics think that a direct sensory link is the missing variable for greater acceptance and use of upper limb prostheses.

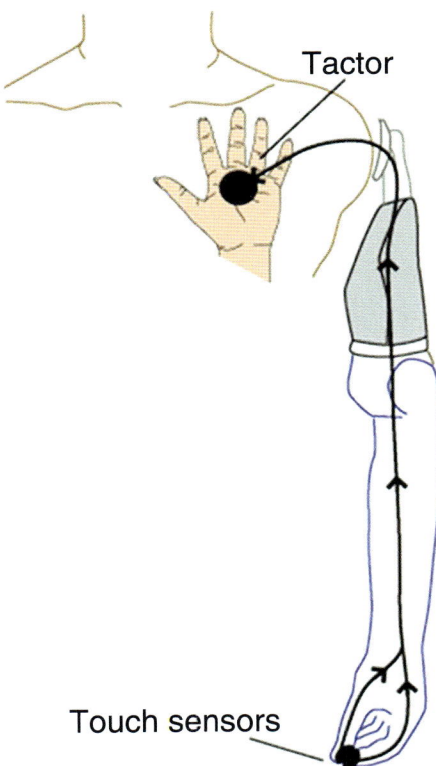

FIGURE 10 Illustration of sensory reinnervation that spontaneously arose from the motor reinnervation of the pectoralis region in a patient with a shoulder disarticulation and targeted muscle reinnervation. Sensory nerves grew to the surface of the patient's chest so that when certain stimuli were given, the signals were felt in the missing hand. (Courtesy of Shirley Ryan AbilityLab, Chicago, IL.)

Regenerative Peripheral Nerve Interfaces

Regenerative peripheral nerve interface surgery is another nerve treatment procedure where severed peripheral nerve ends are implanted into free muscle grafts. Regenerative peripheral nerve interface surgery prevents neuroma formation by providing a physiologic target for regenerating nerves deep in the residual limb.[34] Although its use with commercially available prosthetic systems is limited because of low signal amplitude, the use of percutaneous electrodes with regenerative peripheral nerve interface has been shown to improve prosthetic control and provide sensory feedback from prosthetic limbs to the patient's brain.[35]

SUMMARY

Fitting myoelectric prostheses can be challenging because of the lack of a direct correlation between the remaining EMG source(s) from the user and the actions required by the device. Additionally, residual limb pain following amputation can severely limit the functional success of the end user. The addition of a TMR procedure enables some individuals with amputations to have physiologically appropriate signals and additional data available to control the multiple motions of their prostheses. The prosthetist should have a thorough understanding of myoelectric control and the additional benefits of TMR to provide successful fittings. The prosthetist and entire rehabilitation team must be familiar with the different fitting and training strategies that can be used for TMR candidates. TMR, in conjunction with dual-site electrode and pattern recognition systems, has allowed enhanced control of powered prostheses. In the future, the development of sensory reinnervation will likely add to the benefits of this surgical procedure and improve outcomes for users of upper limb myoelectric prostheses.

References

1. Kuiken TA, Dumanian GA, Lipschutz RD, Miller LA, Stubblefield KA: The use of targeted muscle reinnervation for improved myoelectric prosthesis control in a bilateral shoulder disarticulation amputee. *Prosthet Orthot Int* 2004;28(3):245-253.
2. Kuiken T: Targeted reinnervation for improved prosthetic function. *Phys Med Rehabil Clin N Am* 2006;17(1):1-13.
3. Lipschutz R, Kuiken T, Miller LA, Dumanian GA, Stubblefield KA: Shoulder disarticulation externally powered prosthetic fitting following targeted muscle reinnervation for improved myoelectric control. *J Prosthet Orthot* 2006;18(2):28-34.
4. Hijjawi JB, Kuiken TA, Lipschutz RD, Miller LA, Stubblefield KA, Dumanian GA: Improved myoelectric prosthesis control accomplished using multiple nerve transfers. *Plast Reconstr Surg* 2006;118(7):1573-1578.
5. Miller LA, Lipschutz RD, Stubblefield KA, et al: Control of a six degree of freedom prosthetic arm after targeted muscle reinnervation surgery. *Arch Phys Med Rehabil* 2008;89(11):2057-2065.
6. Kuiken TA, Li G, Lock BA, et al: Targeted muscle reinnervation for real-time myoelectric control of multifunction artificial arms. *J Am Med Assoc* 2009;301(6):619-628.
7. Kuiken T: The scientific basis of targeted muscle reinnervation, in Kuiken T, Schultz-Feuser A, Barlow A, eds: *Targeted Muscle Reinnervation: A Neural Interface for Artificial Limbs*. CRC Press, 2013, pp 9-20.
8. Dumanian G, Souza J: Surgical techniques for targeted muscle reinnervation, in Kuiken T, Schultz-Feuser A, Barlow A, eds: *Targeted Muscle Reinnervation: A Neural Interface for Artificial Limbs*. CRC Press, 2013, pp 21-44.
9. Souza JM, Cheesborough JE, Ko JH, Cho MS, Kuiken TA, Dumanian GA: Targeted muscle reinnervation: A novel approach to postamputation neuroma pain. *Clin Orthop Relat Res* 2014;472(10):2984-2990.
10. Dumanian GA, Potter BK, Mioton LM, et al: Targeted muscle reinnervation treats neuroma and Phantom Pain in major limb amputees. *Ann Surg* 2019;270(2):238-246.
11. Valerio IL, Dumanian GA, Jordan SW, et al: Preemptive treatment of Phantom and residual limb pain with targeted muscle reinnervation at the time of major limb amputation. *J Am Coll Surg* 2019;228(3):217-226.
12. Kuiken T: Rehabilitation of the targeted muscle reinnervation patient, in Kuiken T, Schultz-Feuser A, Barlow A, eds. *Targeted Muscle Reinnervation: A Neural Interface for Artificial Limbs*. CRC Press, 2013, pp 67-76.
13. Stubblefield K, Kuiken T: Occupational therapy for the targeted muscle reinnervation patient, in Kuiken T, Schultz-Feuser A, Barlow A, eds: *Targeted Muscle Reinnervation: A Neural Interface for Artificial Limbs*. CRC Press, 2013, pp 99-120.
14. Stubblefield KA, Miller LA, Lipschutz RD, Kuiken TA: Occupational therapy protocol for amputees with targeted muscle reinnervation. *J Rehabil Res Dev* 2009;46(4):481-488.
15. Miller L, Lipschutz R: Prosthetic fitting before and after targeted muscle reinnervation, in Kuiken T, Schultz-Feuser A, Barlow A, eds: *Targeted Muscle Reinnervation: A Neural Interface for Artificial Limbs*. CRC Press, 2013, pp 77-98.

16. Hargrove L, Lock B: Future research directions, in Kuiken T, Schultz-Feuser A, Barlow A, eds: *Targeted Muscle Reinnervation: A Neural Interface for Artificial Limbs*. CRC Press, 2013, pp 165-184.
17. Ehde DM, Czerniecki JM, Smith DG, et al: Chronic phantom sensations, phantom pain, residual limb pain, and other regional pain after lower limb amputation. *Arch Phys Med Rehabil* 2000;81(8):1039-1044.
18. Johnson CC, Loeffler BJ, Gaston RG: Targeted muscle reinnervation: A paradigm shift for neuroma management and improved prosthesis control in major limb amputees. *J Am Acad Orthop Surg* 2021;29(7):288-296.
19. Kuiken TA, Barlow AK, Hargrove LJ, Dumanian GA: Targeted muscle reinnervation for the upper and lower extremity. *Tech Orthop* 2017;32(2):109-116.
20. Dumanian GA, Ko JH, O'Shaughnessy KD, Kim PS, Wilson CJ, Kuiken TA: Targeted reinnervation for transhumeral amputees: Current surgical technique and update on results. *Plast Reconstr Surg* 2009;124(3):863-869.
21. Farnsworth T, Uellendahl J, Mikosz MJ, Miller L, Petersen B: Shoulder region socket considerations. *J Prosthet Orthot* 2008;20(3):93-106.
22. Kuiken TA, Miller LA, Lipschutz RD, et al: Targeted reinnervation for enhanced prosthetic arm function in a woman with a proximal amputation: A case study. *Lancet* 2007;369(9559):371-380.
23. Englehart K, Hudgins B: A robust, real-time control scheme for multifunction myoelectric control. *IEEE Trans Biomed Eng* 2003;50(7):848-854.
24. Parker P, Englehart K, Hudgins B: Myoelectric signal processing for control of powered limb prostheses. *J Electromyogr Kinesiol* 2006;16(6):541-548.
25. Hargrove LJ, Li G, Englehart KB, Hudgins BS: Principal components analysis preprocessing for improved classification accuracies in pattern-recognition-based myoelectric control. *IEEE Trans Biomed Eng* 2009;56(5):1407-1414.
26. Wurth SM, Hargrove LJ: A real-time comparison between direct control, sequential pattern recognition control and simultaneous pattern recognition control using a Fitts' law style assessment procedure. *J Neuroeng Rehabil* 2014;11(1):91.
27. Kuiken TA, Marasco PD, Lock BA, Harden RN, Dewald JP: Redirection of cutaneous sensation from the hand to the chest skin of human amputees with targeted reinnervation. *Proc Natl Acad Sci USA* 2007;104(50):20061-20066.
28. Schultz AE, Marasco PD, Kuiken TA: Vibrotactile detection thresholds for chest skin of amputees following targeted reinnervation surgery. *Brain Res* 2009;1251:121-129.
29. Marasco PD, Schultz AE, Kuiken TA: Sensory capacity of reinnervated skin after redirection of amputated upper limb nerves to the chest. *Brain* 2009;132(6):1441-1448.
30. Sensinger JW, Schultz AE, Kuiken TA: Examination of force discrimination in human upper limb amputees with reinnervated limb sensation following peripheral nerve transfer. *IEEE Trans Neural Syst Rehabil Eng* 2009;17(5):438-444.
31. Marasco PD, Kim K, Colgate JE, Peshkin MA, Kuiken TA: Robotic touch shifts perception of embodiment to a prosthesis in targeted reinnervation amputees. *Brain* 2011;134(3):747-758.
32. Marasco P: Targeted sensory reinnervation, in Kuiken T, Schultz-Feuser A, Barlow A, eds: *Targeted Muscle Reinnervation: A Neural Interface for Artificial Limbs*. CRC Press, 2013, pp 121-148.
33. Sabolich J, Ortega G: Sense of feel for lower limb amputees: A phase-one study. *J Prosthet Orthot* 1994;6:36-41.
34. Woo SL, Kung TA, Brown DL, Leonard JA, Kelly BM, Cederna PS: Regenerative peripheral nerve interfaces for the treatment of postamputation neuroma pain. *Plastic Reconstr Surg Glob Open* 2016;4(12):e1038.
35. Urbanchek MG, Sando IC, Irwin ZT, et al: Abstract: Validation of regenerative peripheral nerve interfaces for control of a myoelectric hand by macaques and human. *Plastic Reconstr Surg Glob Open* 2016;4(9 suppl):69.

Upper Limb Prosthetic Training and Occupational Therapy

Sandra Fletchall, OTR/L, CHT, MPA, FAOTA

CHAPTER 26

ABSTRACT

To assist an individual with upper limb loss in improving functional performance and the ability to return to work, the occupational therapist should provide both preprosthetic and postprosthetic care programs. The preprosthetic program is focused on edema and pain reduction, wound care, general strengthening, and gaining specific personal care skills. The postprosthetic program begins with delivery of a device and progresses to training in activities of daily living and work skills important to a particular user.

Keywords: occupational therapy; upper limb amputation; upper limb outcomes; upper limb prosthetic training

Introduction

More than 80% of upper limb amputations in the United States are performed following a traumatic injury.[1] The remaining upper limb amputations are necessitated by a congenital deficiency or a medical condition such as end-stage renal disease or cancer. Four times as many men as women undergo upper limb amputation, and most patients are 15 to 30 years old.[2] Amputations distal to the wrist are more common that those proximal to the wrist, with three-quarters of upper limb amputations occurring at the digit level.[1,3] In such cases there is often a concerted effort to salvage at least two digits that can oppose.[4]

The loss of an upper limb at any level influences the ability to participate in tasks and other activities. According to the American Medical Association, amputation of a single digit leads to a hand impairment of 20% to 40%. The loss of an upper limb below the elbow can lead to 70% impairment, and shoulder disarticulation causes as much as 90% impairment.[5] Upper limb loss at any level, especially if it is the result of trauma, can also lead to a change in roles within the family, home, community, and work environments. A structured occupational therapy program can facilitate an individual's efforts to develop skills for returning to his or her highest level of functional independence.

Preprosthetic Therapy

Because of the traumatic nature of most upper limb amputations, it is usually not possible to plan a preoperative occupational therapy program. In those rare instances where there is a short time between the injury and amputation, patients and their families can benefit from information on the abilities and skills that can be acquired after surgery. This information should include a plan for postoperative, preprosthetic occupational therapy.

Many patients are discharged from the hospital a few days after the surgery and are able to immediately begin a preprosthetic occupational therapy program on an outpatient basis. The objectives of such a program should include psychologic support, coping techniques, wound care, edema reduction, residual limb shaping, pain reduction, scar and soft-tissue elongation and pliability, total body muscle endurance and strengthening, training in selected self-care, and changing hand dominance where appropriate.[6] In addition, some studies have identified that those with upper limb loss experience standing/dynamic balance issues,[7,8] therefore the incorporation of balance training during the preprosthetic OT program can minimize fall risk.

The duration of a therapy program is influenced by the number of limbs amputated as well as the amputation level and the patient's cognitive function, executive skills, support system, and funding source. An experienced amputee team should develop documentation to rationalize the need for the initial preprosthetic program, subsequent prosthetic training, and life-long follow-up through an amputee clinic. During the preprosthetic phase, the OT can also perform a home assessment with recommendations for durable medical equipment and/or architectural modifications.

Immediate Postoperative Considerations

Wound Care

A residual limb with wounds or a primary closure site can be cleaned with antibacterial soap and water and covered with a silver-type wound dressing. The use of a silver-type dressing can reduce the risk of wound complications, edema, or biofilm formation.[9] If a mesh skin graft or sheet graft was surgically applied to the residual limb,

Sandra Fletchall or an immediate family member has stock or stock options held in Stedman Medical.

close inspection may be required during the first 10 to 14 postoperative days to maintain the proper moisture environment for the graft to express hematoma or serous fluid as needed.

Whether the limb is closed with native tissues or skin grafts, the application of elastic compression through bandage wraps or a compressive shrinker sock will stabilize wound dressings and initiate edema reduction. Many patients with unilateral upper limb loss can be instructed in appropriate wound care and limb management in the early postoperative period. However, a caregiver may need to be trained if the patient has bilateral upper limb loss.

Edema Reduction and Residual Limb Shaping

Prolonged edema can lead to residual limb pain, poor wound healing, increased firmness of scar tissue, and a poor residual limb shape. Edema reduction can be initiated with the use of an elastic compression bandage even if wounds are still present. This is often followed with the use of compressive shrinker socks once the limb will tolerate the associated sheer forces. The application of compression can increase the pliability of scar tissue and thereby limit pain and skin irritation. Continuous compression is recommended until the scar tissue matures 12 to 18 months after wound closure. After a partial hand amputation, a self-adherent elastic wrap can be used to apply pressure (**Figure 1**). For a transradial or transhumeral amputation, a 3- or 4-inches elastic compression bandage can be used for initial edema management. After a shoulder disarticulation, initial pressure from a 4- to 6-inches elastic compression bandage encompassing the trunk is beneficial, with subsequent use of a noncustom, moisture-wicking compression garment.

Elastic bandage compression should be used until wounds are sufficiently healed to tolerate the shear forces produced when a residual limb shrinker is donned. An upper limb residual shrinker can be fabricated from tubular compressive fabrics (**Figure 2**). Both elastic compression bandages and residual limb shrinkers have been shown to reduce residual limb edema, but the skilled use of an elastic compression bandage can facilitate greater edema reduction in less time than the use of a shrinker.[10] The early application of compression also begins residual limb shaping, which can lead to easy donning of the prosthetic socket and minimize development of redundant soft tissue. A conical residual limb shape is the goal. Even after successful prosthetic fitting, continued use of a residual limb shrinker or elastic compression bandage may be required throughout the first year after the amputation whenever the prosthesis is not being worn; this will continue the process of edema reduction and limb shaping.

Pain Reduction

Ninety-five percent of individuals with upper limb loss secondary to trauma report phantom limb sensation or pain, residual limb pain, or nonamputated limb pain.[11,12] The type and level of upper limb pain should be assessed during preprosthetic treatment. In phantom limb sensation, the amputee feels that he or she is experiencing various sensations in all or part of the absent segments of the amputated limb; these sensations may include a feeling of movement of the phantom limb. Phantom limb pain includes sensations that can be described as burning, twisting, shooting, squeezing, cramping, or dull aching of the amputated body part. By contrast, residual limb pain is experienced in the remaining tissues of the limb and may be the result of the initial injury, the amputation surgery, persistent wounds, or neuromas. In addition, the contralateral, nonamputated upper limb should be assessed for pain resulting from a previously undiagnosed injury, overuse syndromes, cumulative trauma, or a repetitive stress injury.[13-15]

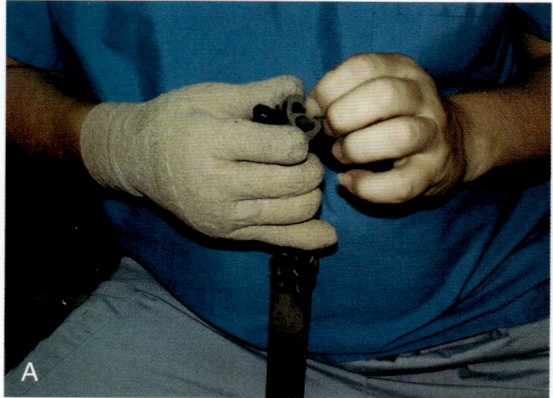
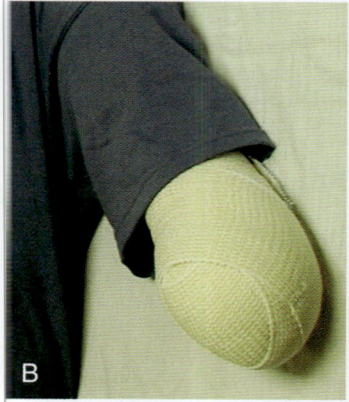

FIGURE 1 Photographs showing the use of compression for residual limb shaping and edema reduction. **A**, A self-adherent elastic wrap used after a partial hand amputation. **B**, A figure-of-8 elastic compression bandage was used after a transhumeral amputation. (Courtesy of Sandra Fletchall OTR/L, CHT, MPA, FAOTA, Firefighters Burn Center, Memphis, TN.)

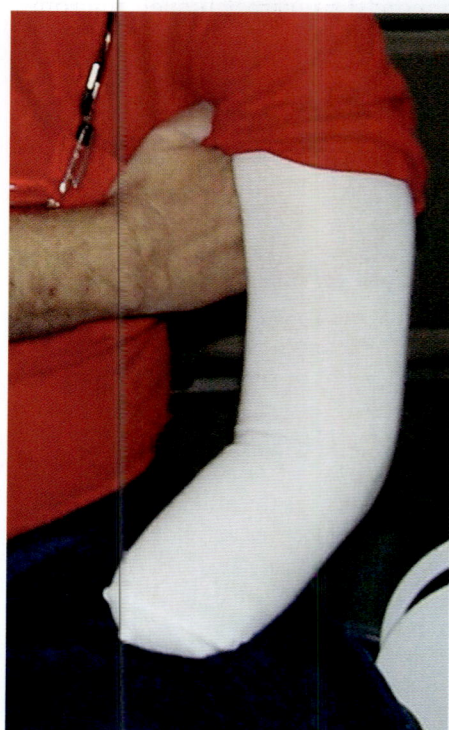

FIGURE 2 Clinical photograph of a patient with a residual limb shrinker fabricated by an occupational therapist. (Courtesy of Sandra Fletchall OTR/L, CHT, MPA, FAOTA, Firefighters Burn Center, Memphis, TN.)

Chapter 26: Upper Limb Prosthetic Training and Occupational Therapy

The early application of firm pressure, such as pressure applied with an elastic compression bandage, can reduce nerve or wound irritation, pain from edema, and sometimes phantom limb pain. The therapist also may need to use visual feedback, guided mental motor imagery, or mirror therapy to treat phantom limb sensations or phantom limb pain (**Figure 3**). Many individuals can be trained to use these techniques while in the clinic and then progress to incorporating the techniques into the home and work environments. Structured, guided visual feedback techniques can be used to reduce selected pain issues by means of cortical reorganization.[16-19] In contrast, the use of electrical modalities was found to lead to only minimal pain reduction.[20,21]

In comparison with the general population, individuals with upper limb loss are more likely to develop an overuse pain syndrome, most commonly affecting the neck, lower back, and/or shoulder.[13] Individuals with unilateral upper limb loss often exhibit lateral epicondylitis, carpal tunnel syndrome, cubital tunnel syndrome, or stenosing tenosynovitis. A simple off-the-shelf orthosis may be useful in managing some overuse syndromes in the contralateral upper limb (**Figure 4**).

Flexibility, strength, and correct body and arm mechanics can help alleviate pain. Accordingly, preprosthetic and postprosthetic occupational therapy should include an emphasis on increasing and maintaining the flexibility of the trunk and extremities. In addition, the therapy program should focus on strengthening associated muscle groups and providing instruction in appropriate body and arm mechanics and posture.

Positive coping skills related to anger and stress also are useful in managing pain. An individual with limited or poor coping skills or a tendency to depression may benefit from early integration of positive coping skills into the therapy program, with reinforcement from the individual's support system.

A medical professional who is experienced and knowledgeable in limb loss treatment can provide additional techniques for pain reduction.[22] The therapist should continue to assess the individual for overuse syndrome issues related to changes in work, avocational activities, or aging. Techniques to minimize pain and enhance a return to function should be used as needed.

Preprosthetic Program Essentials

Limb and Core Assessment and Treatment

The therapist's assessment should not be limited to the affected limb because other body areas may also require treatment. The range-of-motion assessment should include both joint and soft-tissue movements in both the limbs and the trunk. Soft-tissue limitations can be promptly treated with an aggressive elongation program focusing on increasing trunk flexibility and active movement of the upper and lower limbs. Similarly, a strengthening program can minimize abnormal trunk, back, and limb changes secondary to upper limb amputation.[23] With bilateral upper limb loss, treatment should focus on the ability to actively bring both residual upper limbs to midline to facilitate self-care tasks in the preprosthetic phase (**Figure 5**).

General age-based physical fitness assessments can be used to identify the physical condition of the individual and the general safety skills needed for the home environment.[24] Muscle strength can be assessed by manual muscle examination as needed. When there is peripheral nerve loss or atrophied muscle mass, the OT should develop a treatment program to compensate for the losses while facilitating independence in activities of daily living.

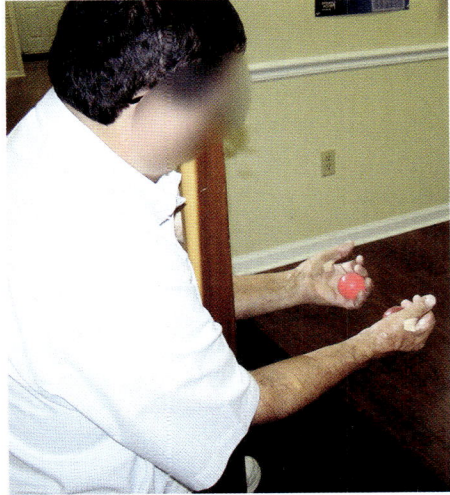

FIGURE 3 Photograph showing the use of mirror therapy to achieve pain reduction. Mirror therapy assists with decreasing the pain cycle in the amputated limb by watching the reflection of movement of the nonamputated limb in a mirror; this creates positive feedback in the motor cortex of the brain. (Courtesy of Sandra Fletchall OTR/L, CHT, MPA, FAOTA, Firefighters Burn Center, Memphis, TN.)

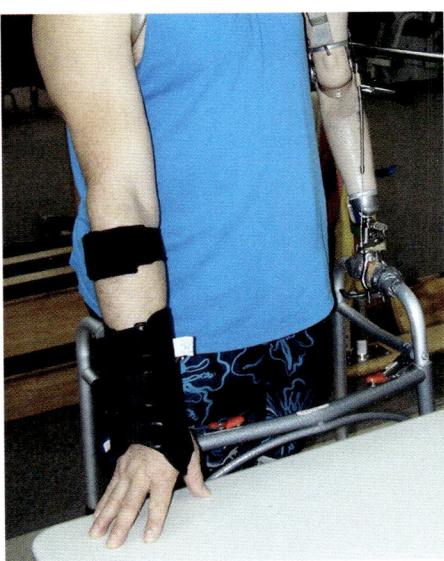

FIGURE 4 Photograph showing the use of a noncustom armband and wrist support orthosis to assist with pain reduction associated with lateral epicondylitis in the nonamputated limb. (Courtesy of Sandra Fletchall OTR/L, CHT, MPA, FAOTA, Firefighters Burn Center, Memphis, TN.)

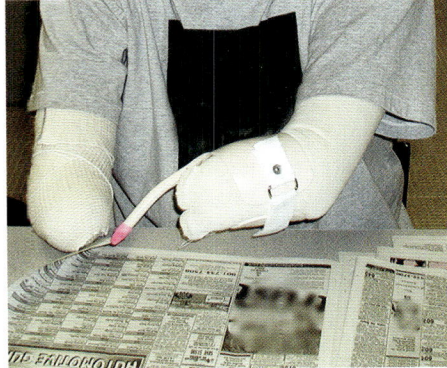

FIGURE 5 Photograph showing midline use of the residual limbs in a person with bilateral upper limb loss. The patient is using a universal cuff with a low thermoplastic pointer/turner fabricated by the occupational therapist. (Courtesy of Sandra Fletchall OTR/L, CHT, MPA, FACTA, Firefighters Burn Center, Memphis, TN.)

Section 2: Upper Limb

The preprosthetic therapy program can initiate both core and extremity endurance and strengthening tasks. Core stabilization during resistive upper limb exercises can prepare the individual for assuming the weight of the prosthesis (**Figure 6**). Good muscle strength can allow relatively rapid progression to extended periods of prosthesis use. Similarly, increasing cardiovascular endurance contributes to an improved tolerance for wearing and using an upper limb prosthesis.

Perceptual Motor Skills

Perceptual motor skills influence the ability to resume dynamic balance and change hand dominance. A brief assessment of perceptual motor skills, including hand–eye coordination, body–eye coordination, postural adjustment, and visual skills, helps the therapist determine how to provide training for new tasks and functional prosthesis use.[25]

Preprosthetic Self-Care Training

Before beginning training to use a prosthesis, an individual with unilateral upper limb loss can benefit from training that will help him or her become independent in cutting food, tying shoes, bathing, and donning upper torso garments without the aid of a prosthesis. For individuals with bilateral upper limb loss, adaptive equipment is commonly used for training in self-feeding, grooming and hygiene tasks, showering, and donning upper torso garments (**Figure 7**). The efficient performance of self-care tasks is influenced by total body endurance, strength, and flexibility. For those individuals with limited perceptual motor skills or difficulty in transferring newly learned skills to multiple tasks, repetitive training in the clinic can enhance the timeliness and efficiency of performance in preparation for using self-care skills outside of the clinic.

Home Assessment

For more complex cases, such as individuals affected by bilateral limb loss, a home assessment should be completed before prosthetic training begins. The basic home recommendations should include independence in entering and leaving the home, showering (including turning the water on and off and washing the body), toileting, removing items from the refrigerator or microwave oven, and managing internal doors and light switches. Many individuals benefit from instruction in the use of electronic technologies for managing door entrances, lights, and other items in the home. Architectural modifications may be recommended if funding allows. If architectural modifications cannot be considered, alternate recommendations can emphasize portable devices, especially for the bathroom, that can be relocated to another residence.

Support System

An individual's ability to regain function can be fostered by appropriate family, community, work, and school support systems. Each support system should be assessed to determine the feasibility of integrating it into the rehabilitation program. The therapist should understand the individual's family, community, work, and school roles in the interest of assisting in the resumption of medically, physically, and emotionally appropriate aspects of these roles. Having the ability to interact with others in previously established roles contributes to reestablishing a sense of self-worth. Shared occupational therapy treatment sessions for individuals with a similar limb loss can serve as an important additional source of support. Incorporating a certified peer visitor into the treatment program may facilitate the individual's emotional acceptance of a body change and recognition that participation in roles and activities can continue. The Amputee Coalition provides a certified peer visitor training program and can "match" a certified peer visitor with the individual with a limb loss.[1-6]

Sleep Patterns

Referral to a psychologist or the attending physician is indicated if the individual's sleep habits have changed since the amputation. A change in sleep pattern is common and may be attributable to the use of pain medication, recent surgery, reduced physical activity, or emotional responses. Often the sleep pattern improves with a structured therapist-initiated program to enhance total body endurance and strength.

Hand Dominance

If the dominant hand was part of the amputated limb, the therapist can begin hand dominance retraining activities as part of the preprosthetic program. Changing hand dominance can affect handwriting, keyboard use, and dexterity in work-related tasks and activities of daily living. Specific computer software may be useful for increasing keyboard speed and accuracy.

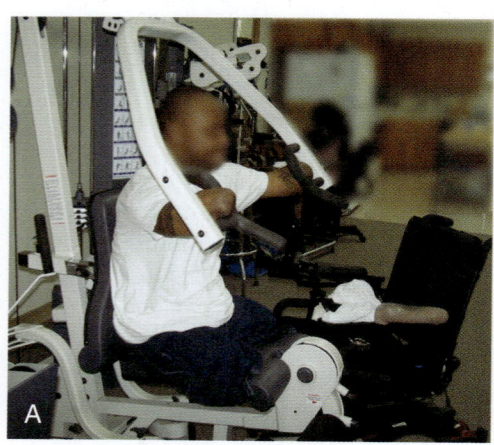
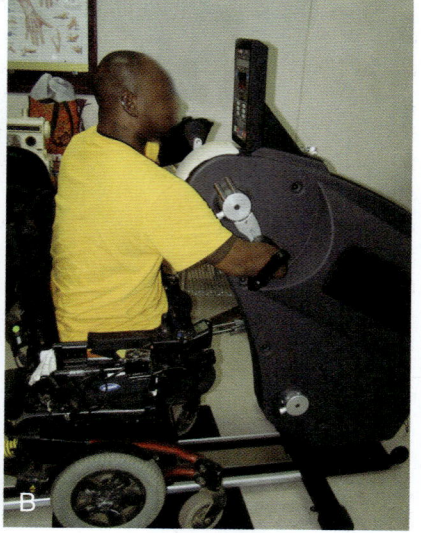

FIGURE 6 Photographs showing an individual with quadrilateral limb loss training to improve core and extremity strength (**A**) and cardiovascular endurance (**B**). (Courtesy of Sandra Fletchall OTR/L, CHT, MPA, FAOTA, Firefighters Burn Center, Memphis, TN.)

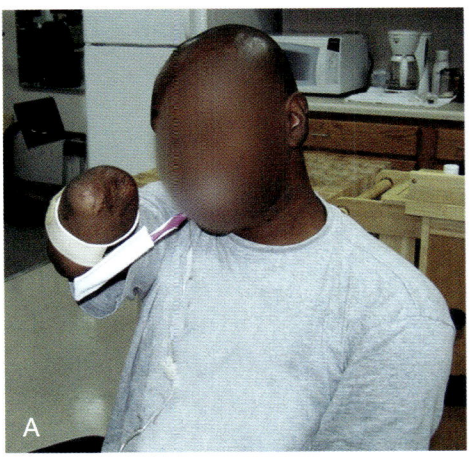
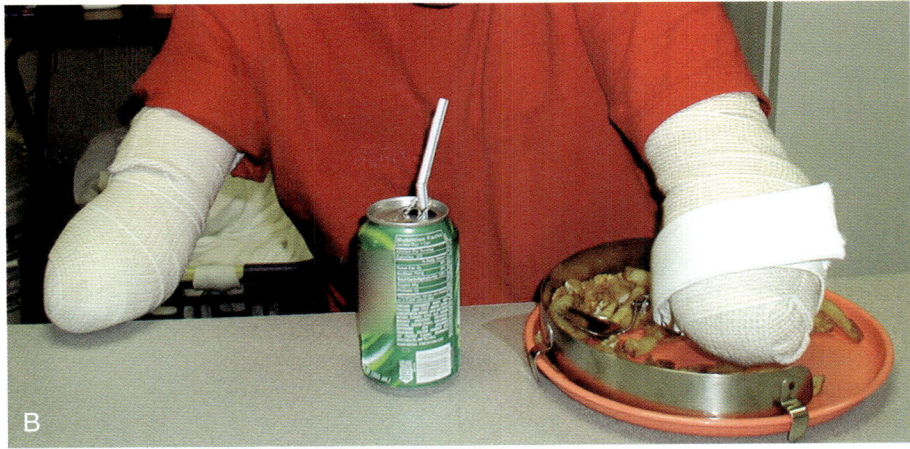

FIGURE 7 Photographs showing an individual with quadrilateral limb loss using an adaptive device for self-care (**A**) and an individual with bilateral upper limb amputation using an adaptive device for feeding (**B**). (Courtesy of Sandra Fletchall OTR/L, CHT, MPA, FAOTA, Firefighters Burn Center, Memphis TN.)

Prostheses and Prosthetic Control

The goal of preprosthetic therapy is to sufficiently increase endurance, mobility, and strength to allow multiple hours of daily prosthesis use. During the preprosthetic program, the individual can be trained in the motor skills or movement needed for operating the anticipated prosthesis. However, the style and operation of the prosthesis must be determined in consultation with a prosthetist who is knowledgeable about upper limb amputations.

Body-Powered Prosthesis

The use of a body-powered prosthesis after a transradial or transhumeral amputation requires scapular abduction training, with strengthening of the serratus anterior, pectoralis major, and pectoralis minor muscles. Scapular abduction is commonly used to create tension through a control cable that operates the terminal device. In addition, an individual with a transhumeral amputation must work on strengthening the movements of scapular depression with shoulder extension because these movements may be needed for operating the cable that will lock and unlock the elbow.

Myoelectric Prosthesis

A myoelectric prosthesis uses electromyographic signals captured through surface electrodes in the prosthetic socket. In consultation with the prosthetist, the therapist should identify one or more muscle groups appropriate for this use. Individuals with a transradial amputation often use two-site muscle control composed of forearm flexors and extensors. The therapist should provide a program to increase the endurance of the forearm muscles to allow a long period of daily myoelectric prosthesis use. The voluntary firing of the forearm muscle groups must be independent of the position of the elbow or shoulder to allow functional use of the prosthesis in multiple degrees of movement. Similarly, the user should be able to isolate the contractions of the two muscle groups to ensure clear input signals to the prosthesis.

An individual with a transhumeral amputation can often use upper arm elbow flexors and extensors to operate the terminal device and elbow. Preprosthetic training should include the general strengthening and endurance of these muscle groups as well as their discrete control in different shoulder positions. Throughout the training, the individual should be reminded to avoid using the myoelectric prosthesis in activities involving moisture, vibration, dust, or high voltage.

Hybrid Prosthesis

A hybrid prosthesis incorporates both body-powered and myoelectric elements to maximize function while reducing the overall weight and complexity of the prosthesis. Such prostheses can be used after transhumeral or shoulder level amputations. Prosthetic component operation at these proximal amputation levels can include control of a terminal device as well as wrist, forearm, elbow, and shoulder joint movement. In close consultation with the treating prosthetist, the therapist should understand the anticipated prosthetic components and their control. Armed with this understanding, they can then identify the movements and muscle functions needed for operating the proposed prosthetic components and develop a program to increase the individual's endurance in preparation for use of the prosthesis.

Targeted Muscle Reinnervation

Targeted muscle reinnervation is a surgical approach in which otherwise unused motor nerves are reinnervated to targeted muscles in an attempt to augment the number of myoelectric control sites. This allows the number of control sites to better match the degrees of freedom provided by the prosthesis. Targeted muscle reinnervation should be performed within a multidisciplinary team that has been trained in this unique treatment approach. Considerations include consultations on the design of the proposed prosthesis, training on its use, and associated follow-up. Because the reinnervation process can take several months to generate substantive muscle contractions under the newly innervated motor control, the individual should be fitted and trained with a traditional direct-controlled myoelectric or hybrid prosthesis until the muscles are fully innervated. After targeted muscle reinnervation surgery, the therapy program should focus on developing unique motor patterns for eliciting the desired muscle contractions of the amputated limb. A program of 3 to 6 months or longer may be required.

Terminal Devices

The many functions of the hand cannot be effectively reproduced by a single prosthetic terminal device. However, appropriately designed interchangeable terminal devices can serve in multiple activity-related functions. Most individuals with a body-powered prosthesis choose the functional utility of a hook-style terminal device, but a hand terminal device can be used in social environments (**Figure 8**). Those individuals with a myoelectric or hybrid prosthesis can use interchangeable terminal devices including a basic hand, a multifunctional hand, an electronic terminal device (ETD, Motion Control), or a Greifer (Ottobock) (**Figure 9**). Some terminal devices are more effective for most daily activities and should be the focus of formal training. Others may be used for specific activities, but require training in proper use and storage. The user should be instructed on which terminal devices are appropriate for strenuous activity or in the presence of moisture, dust, or vibration and which devices should be limited to light-duty and medium-duty activities.

Prosthetic Training

Following preprosthetic care, the literature supports the value of expediting prosthetic training. In one study, patients who were fitted and trained in the use of a prosthesis within 4 to 6 weeks after amputation were found to be more successful in long-term prosthesis use than those who received a later postoperative fitting and delayed training.[27] Another study found that individuals who were fitted within 6 months of amputation were likely to achieve long-term functional prosthesis use.[28]

The therapist should ensure a smooth transition from the preprosthetic program into the prosthetic skills

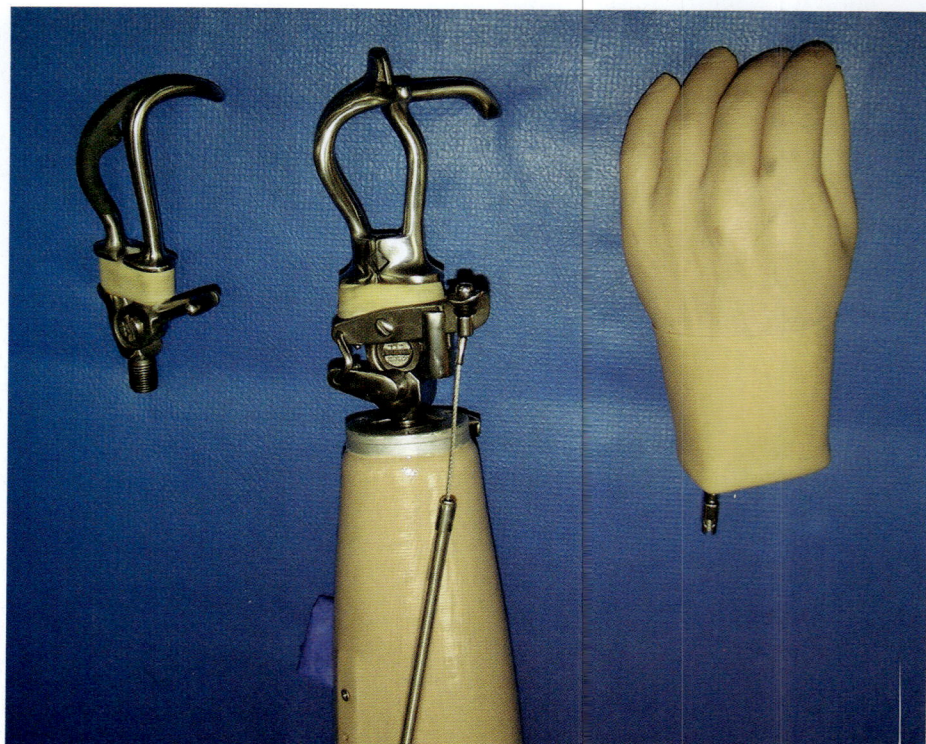

FIGURE 8 Photograph showing a body-powered prosthesis (center) with interchangeable hook and hand terminal devices (left and right, respectively). Hooks are available in various sizes and opening capabilities. (Courtesy of Sandra Fletchall OTR/L, CHT, MPA, FAOTA, Firefighters Burn Center, Memphis, TN.)

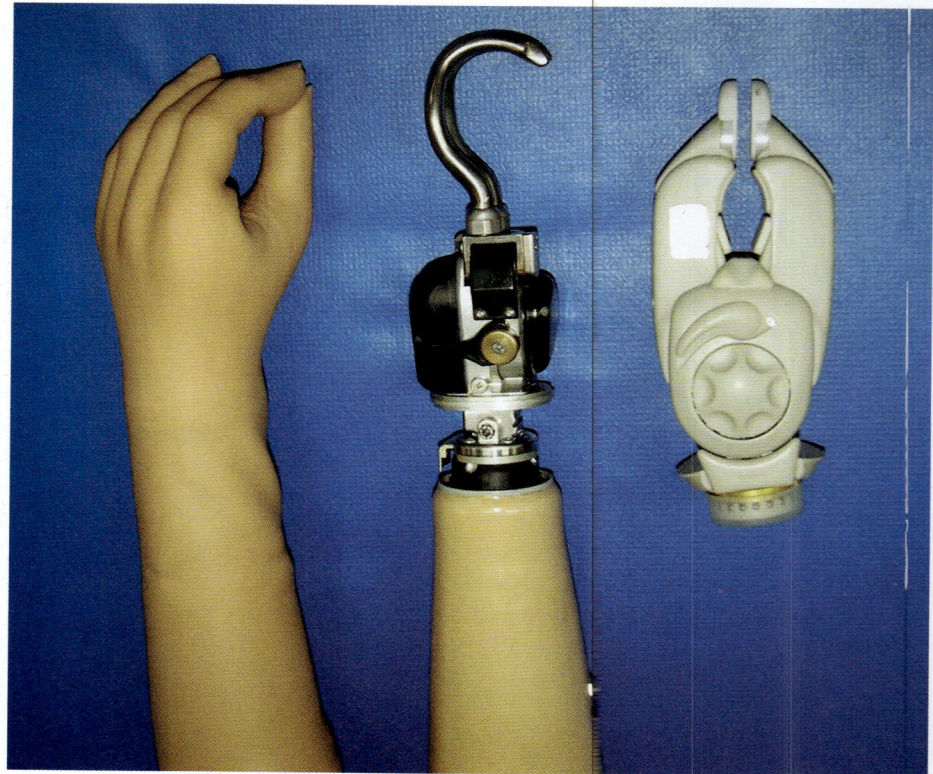

FIGURE 9 Photograph showing a myoelectric prosthesis (center) with a variety of terminal devices (left to right): an interchangeable hand, an electronic terminal device, and a Greifer (Ottobock). (Courtesy of Sandra Fletchall OTR/L, CHT, MPA, FAOTA, Firefighters Burn Center, Memphis, TN.)

training program, usually as soon as the prosthesis is delivered. Initiating prosthetic training soon after delivery of the device can assist the brain in maintaining the appropriate cortical body representation, movement, and sensation.[29,30] The length of the OT prosthetic training program is influenced by the individual's cognitive skills including their attention span, memory for new learning, and ability to transfer skills to new activities.[31]

Initial Training Sessions

Prosthetic training should begin with prosthetic terminology, component function and operation, time-efficient donning and doffing techniques, residual limb care, and general prosthesis maintenance. For many with a transhumeral or transradial amputation, the prosthesis is donned using an overhead technique (**Figure 10**). For those with a shoulder disarticulation or forequarter amputation, donning often can be accomplished in a manner similar to donning of a front-opening garment. Some individuals with bilateral upper limb loss need to use a prosthetic dressing tree, which is custom designed and fabricated based on the individual's flexibility, motor skills, and balance. The donning method ultimately is based on the individual's functional abilities, which may be influenced by the presence of other injuries as well as flexibility and muscle strength. Training in the general maintenance of the prosthesis includes topics such as application of tension bands to a body-powered hook, changing terminal devices, care and cleaning of socks and interface liners, and cleaning of inner socket and residual limb skin to decrease skin bacteria irritation.

Control Training

Control training should be done separately for each prosthetic component. As each prosthetic operation is mastered, a subsequent operation is added. Training should progress from tabletop activities to the use of the prosthesis while standing or reaching (**Figure 11**). Control training often begins with the patient manipulating unbreakable items positioned on

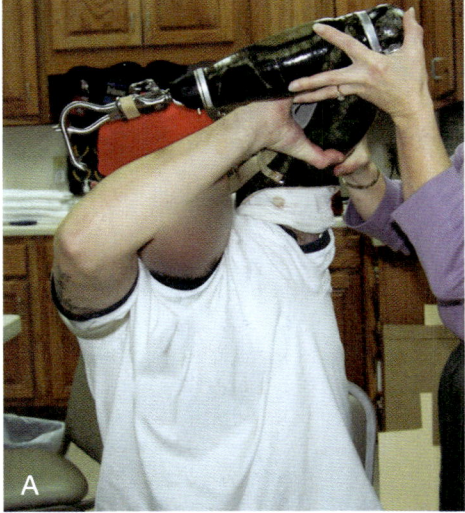
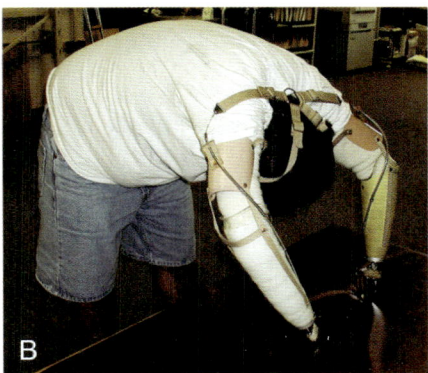

FIGURE 10 Photographs showing the use of an overhead prosthesis donning method by a person with unilateral limb loss (**A**) and a person with bilateral limb loss (**B**). (Courtesy of Sandra Fletchall OTR/L, CHT, MPA, FAOTA, Firefighters Burn Center, Memphis, TN.)

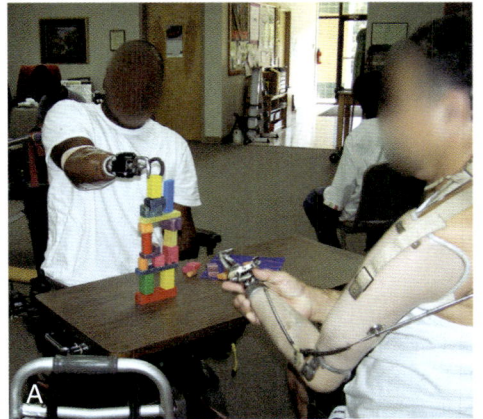
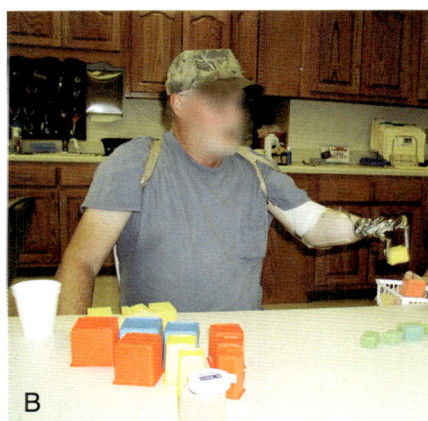
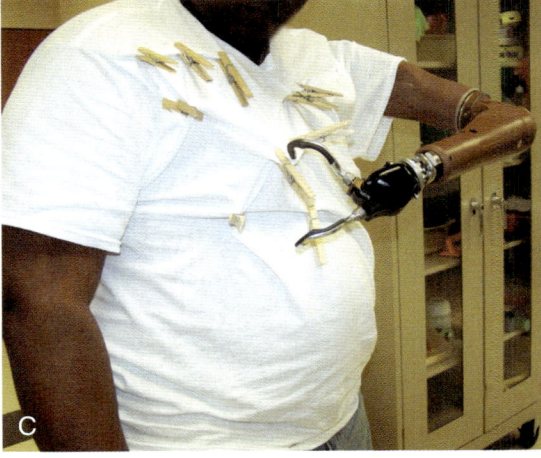
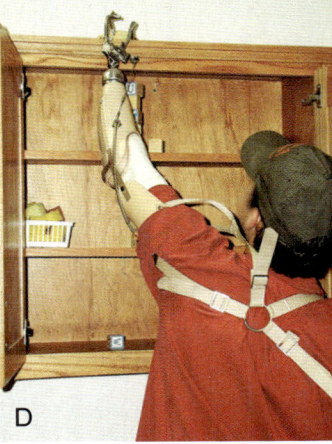

FIGURE 11 Photographs showing the progression of prosthesis and terminal device control training in individuals with upper limb loss. **A**, A tabletop-activity competition using unbreakable objects. **B**, Manipulation of fragile objects. **C**, Positioning of objects at the midline of the body. **D**, Overhead reaching. (Courtesy of Sandra Fletchall OTR/L, CHT, MPA, FAOTA, Firefighters Burn Center, Memphis, TN.)

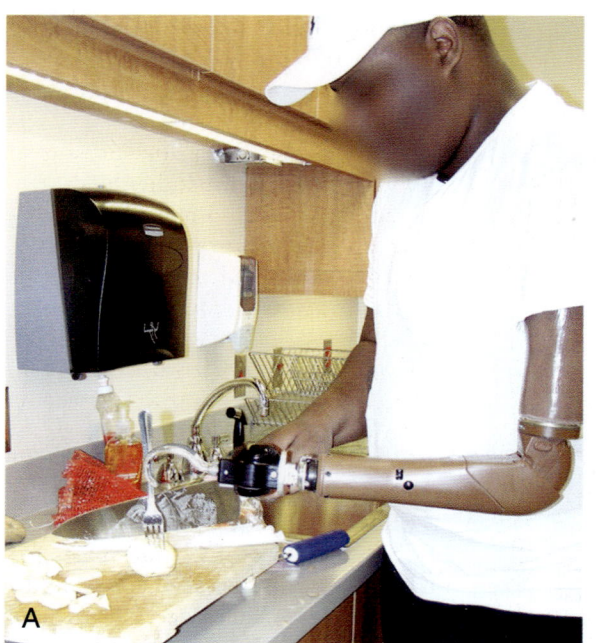
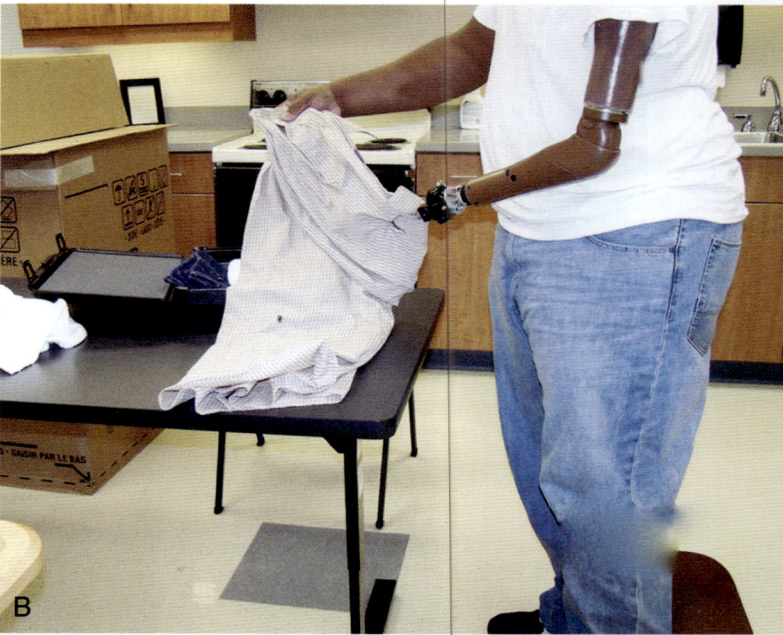

FIGURE 12 Photographs showing the use of a shoulder disarticulation prosthesis for support in meal preparation (**A**) and for functional tasks, such as packing a suitcase (**B**). (Courtesy of Sandra Fletchall OTR/L, CHT, MPA, FAOTA, Firefighters Burn Center, Memphis, TN.)

a table and progresses to fragile or crushable items. The patient should attempt to move the objects from the table to each side of the body and to the midline. Learning to open the terminal device to the specific diameter of the object being manipulated increases the efficiency of prosthetic function and minimizes the use of other body parts. The training progresses to prepositioning of the terminal device, wrist, forearm, elbow, and shoulder before engaging in an activity. Continued training leads to prosthesis use while the opposite limb or the body is in motion. Prosthesis use in coordination with other body movements can facilitate the transference of skills to complex activities.

Self-Care, Activities of Daily Living, and Work Tasks

Integration of the prosthesis into self-care tasks should begin once success with component operation has been achieved. The use of the prosthesis in these activities should be reinforced because the individual may have become independent in some tasks before receiving the prosthesis. Using the prosthesis to perform these core tasks will positively affect its overall usage rate and may minimize overuse or stress injuries to other body areas.

Training should progress to basic meal preparation tasks and skills required for independent living (**Figure 12**). Training to incorporate prosthesis use into child care may be important for some users (**Figure 13**). The individual should also learn how to safely carry items using the prosthesis (**Figure 14**). Ultimately, there should be a progression from home and community tasks to lifting, carrying, and work-related tasks. Instruction must be provided on

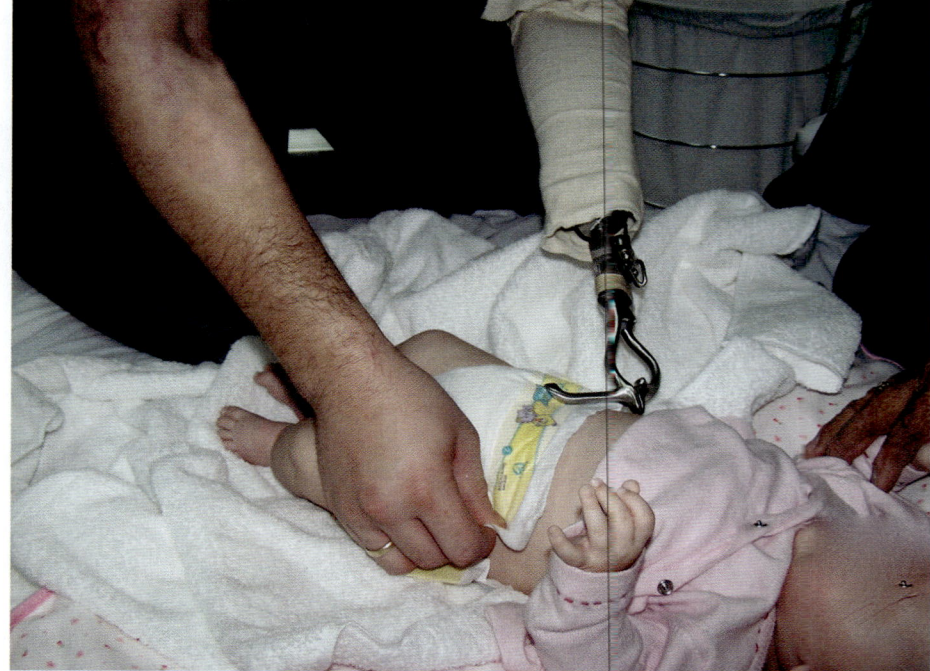

FIGURE 13 Photograph showing training for tasks related to child care. (Courtesy of Sandra Fletchall OTR/L, CHT, MPA, FAOTA, Firefighters Burn Center, Memphis, TN.)

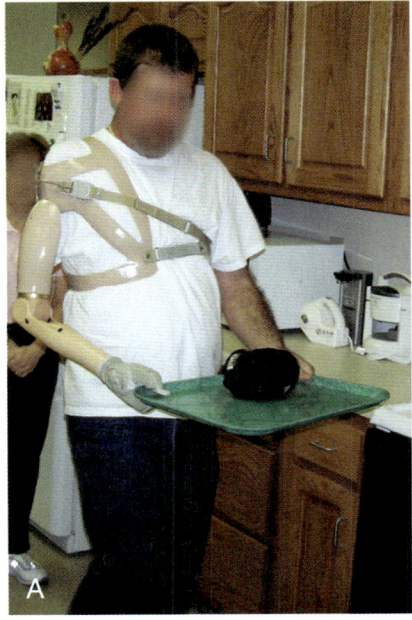 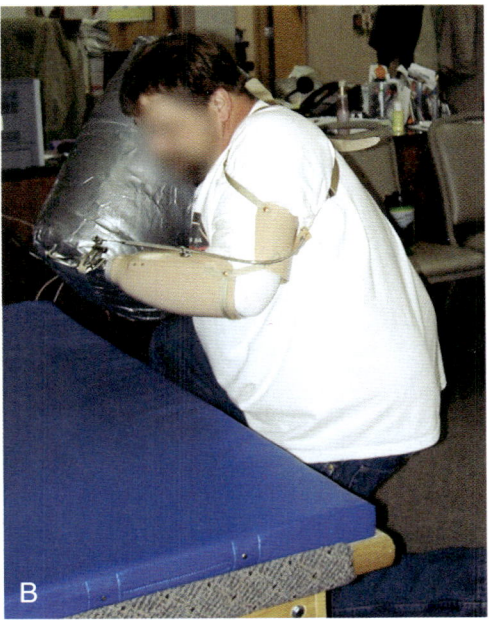

FIGURE 14 Photographs showing training in positioning and carrying a food tray (**A**) and a heavy load (**B**). (Courtesy of Sandra Fletchall OTR/L, CHT, MPA, FAOTA, Firefighters Burn Center, Memphis, TN.)

The onsite work assessment may also result in the need for changes in the prosthesis or additional occupational therapy sessions.

Assessing skills during prosthetic training can show the individual's performance growth and mastery of prosthetic operation. However, there is a shortage of validated assessments for all areas of prosthetic function including proficiency with basic component operation, self-care, activities of daily living and leisure activities, or the timing and progression from one type of prosthesis to another.[32,33] To facilitate healthcare funding, the experienced healthcare clinician/team must be knowledgeable in documentation of the rationales for prosthesis repair, replacement or additional devices, or change of prosthetic type, as there are not validated assessments to provide such information.

the dynamic and static lift abilities of the prosthetic components and should be reinforced to minimize component failure, residual-limb skin irritation, and the potential for an overuse syndrome.

Training in the use of the prosthesis in homemaking, work tasks, and leisure activities must include prepositioning of the prosthetic components and proper body and arm positioning to minimize the risk of overuse syndromes. With appropriate training, most individuals can acquire independence in self-care and selected homemaking and work activities without the need to frequently change the terminal device (**Figure 15**). A return to work may require the therapist to complete an onsite work assessment and recommend environmental modifications, assistive technologies, or ways to integrate the prosthesis into work tasks.

Leisure Activities and Mobility

Many people with a unilateral or bilateral upper limb amputation wish to resume driving an automobile and can benefit from assessment or training by a certified driver rehabilitation specialist (**Figure 16**). A therapist can help individuals seeking to regain or obtain a driver's license. The therapist's assessment of pre-injury activities can determine whether adaptations are needed for operating special equipment such as a lawn mower,

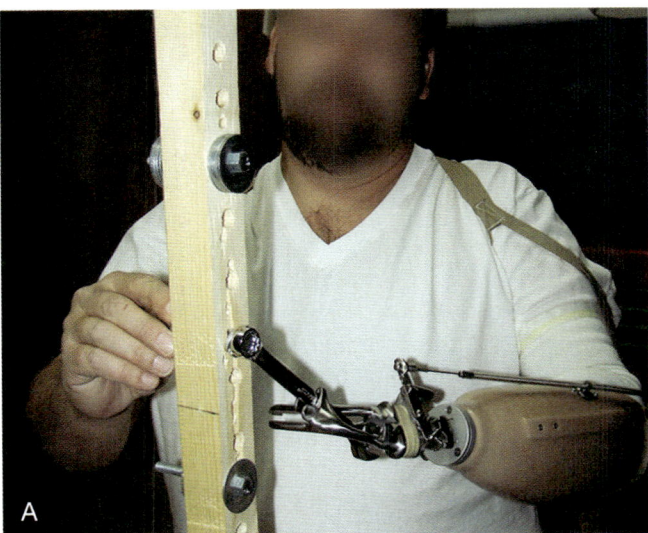 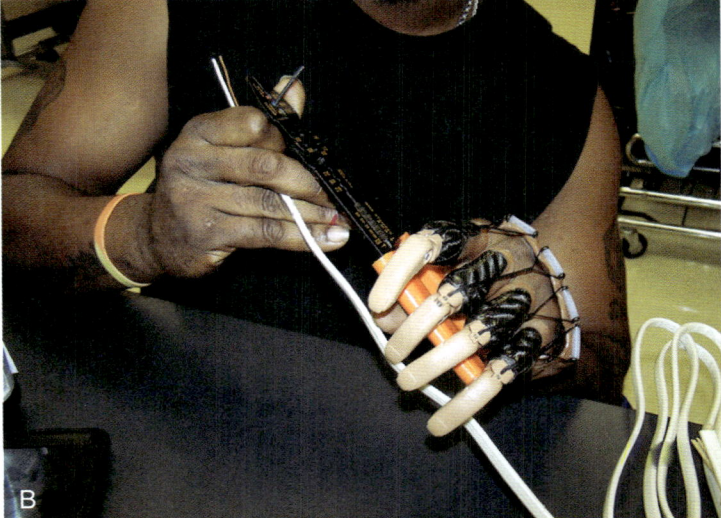

FIGURE 15 Photographs showing the use of prostheses in job tasks. **A**, A body-powered transradial prosthesis used in tool manipulation. **B**, An M-finger (Partial Hand Solutions) cable-driver prosthesis being used by an individual to accomplish a task involving electrical wiring. (Courtesy of Sandra Fletchall OTR/L, CHT, MPA, FAOTA, Firefighters Burn Center, Memphis, TN.)

Section 2: Upper Limb

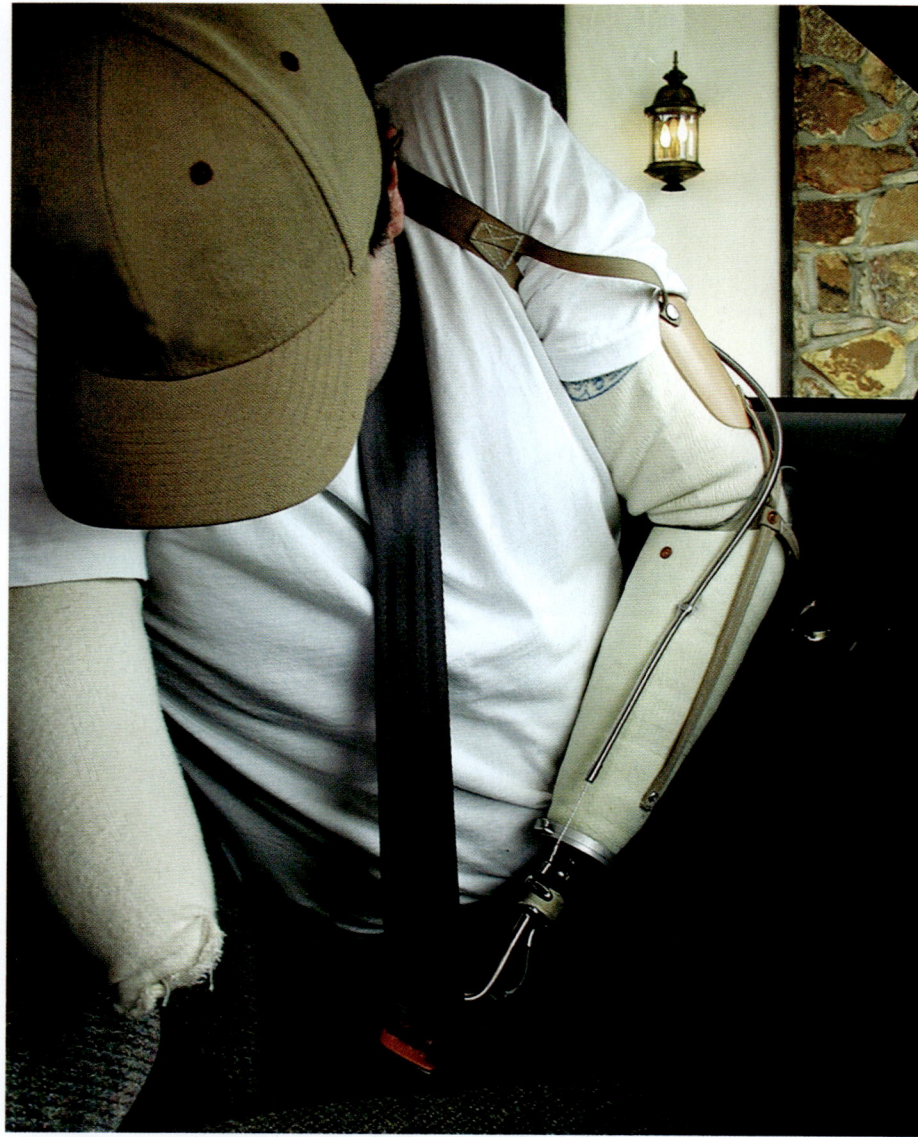

FIGURE 16 Photograph showing a person with bilateral upper limb amputation and a unilateral prosthesis buckling a seat belt. Training for driving resumption should progress from seat belt buckling to door and steering wheel manipulation. (Courtesy of Sandra Fletchall OTR/L, CHT, MPA, FAOTA, Firefighters Burn Center, Memphis, TN.)

a boat, an all-terrain vehicle, or a tractor. The therapist should inquire about leisure pursuits and provide recommendations and training to allow a return to preinjury activities. For those with a specific avocational interest, referrals to established resources or groups may be appropriate. For many individuals, a return to a preinjury activity such as hunting, fishing, golfing, or swimming can improve self-esteem and emotional outlook (**Figure 17**). Some individuals may benefit from information about or exposure to Paralympic or other competitive adaptive sports activities. Not-for-profit organizations devoted to the welfare of individuals living with an amputation may be helpful in locating local agencies.

The Effect of Prosthetic Training on Outcomes

Promoting Long-Term Use of a Prosthesis

The goal of an occupational therapy prosthetic training program is to facilitate the individual's return to preinjury activities in the home, community, school, and work environments. Sustained use of a prosthesis can be compromised if training is not provided immediately after fitting and delivery of a prosthesis. Structured sessions can have a direct, measurably positive effect on the long-term use of a prosthesis.[34-36] In a study comparing the effects of preprosthetic therapy on prosthesis use, two groups of individuals with upper limb amputation were compared. Members of the first group received early occupational therapy and preprosthetic training of an average 7.16 weeks' duration from the date of injury to the prosthetic fitting. Those in the second group received delayed prosthetic training of an average 41.04 weeks' duration from the date of injury to the prosthetic fitting. One year after completing their program, 98% of the members of the first group were using their prosthesis, and 74% had returned to work or school. Among members of the second group, the percentages were approximately 56% for both outcomes.[37] This study showed that early, aggressive preprosthetic occupational therapy training leads to improved outcomes for users of a prosthesis.

Expediting Progress Toward Prosthetic Goals

Frequent therapy sessions serve to reinforce and enhance learning and skill retention related to prosthesis use. Clinical trials have reported the benefits experienced by individuals who underwent treatment two or three times a week.[38,39] However, those who received treatment 5 days per week for 2 to 4 hours each day made more rapid progress in prosthesis use and daily wear, which led to an earlier return to work.

Individuals with difficulty in processing new information, those with amputation at a high level, or those with bilateral upper limb loss need additional time to learn and implement self-care techniques and to incorporate the movements and muscle function required for operating the prosthesis. Some individuals can achieve successful prosthetic operation within the first 15 to 20 hours of training, but others require a longer period of occupational therapy.[40]

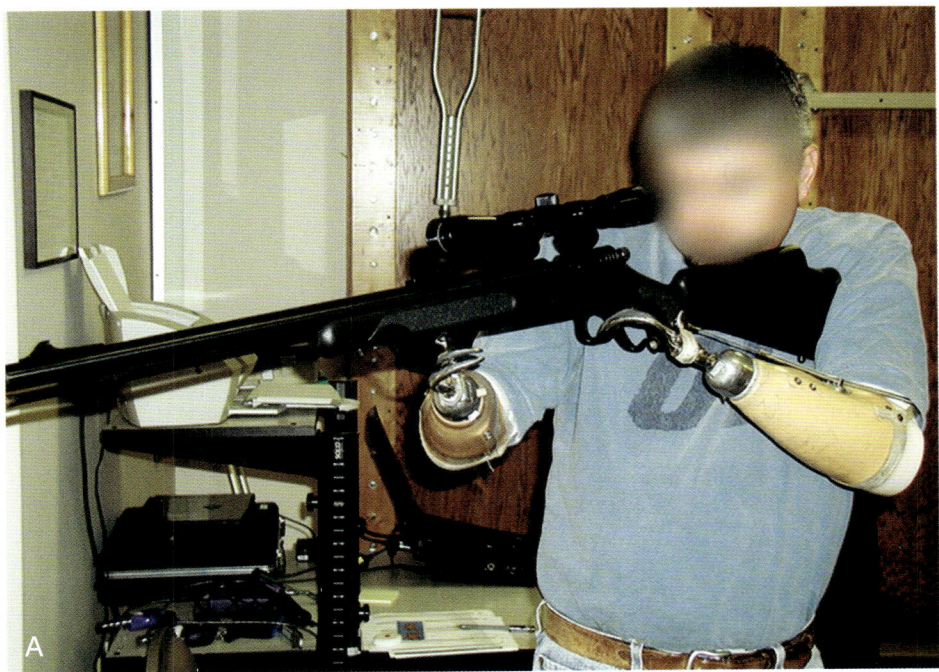
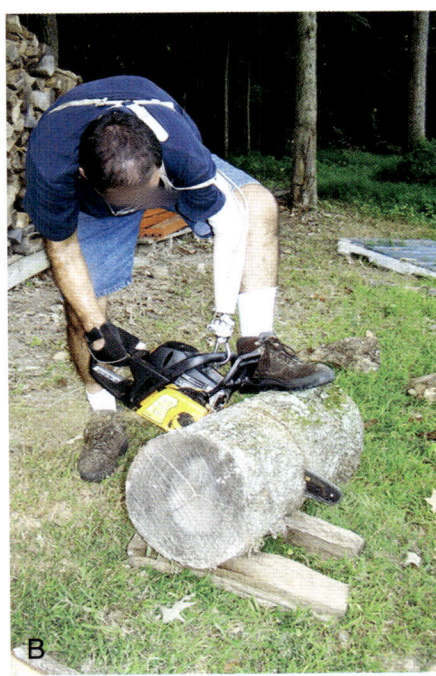

FIGURE 17 Photographs showing prosthesis use in activities that require good body–arm function and a high level of prosthetic skills. **A,** Bilateral prostheses used to operate a hunting rifle; information and training can minimize the need for changes to the gunstock. **B,** A unilateral prosthesis used to operate a power saw. (Courtesy of Sandra Fletchall OTR/L, CHT, MPA, FAOTA, Firefighters Burn Center, Memphis, TN.)

Long-Term Considerations

Individuals with a traumatic upper limb amputation are usually younger and healthier at the time of injury than those with a lower limb amputation.[1,4] After completion of an upper limb prosthetic occupational therapy program, scheduled, structured annual or semiannual follow-up visits to an amputee rehabilitation team are useful to monitor the need for prosthetic repair, replacement, or upgrade; treat skin issues; minimize pain from an overuse syndrome; and preserve functionality throughout the aging process.

Long-term atrophy of the residual limb may be exacerbated if the original amputation required soft-tissue loss and skin graft coverage. The identification of skin issues in the clinic can minimize time away from prosthesis use and may provide justification for socket replacement or a change in style or components. Individuals should be advised to contact the rehabilitation team if a neuroma, skin sensitivity, or overuse syndrome arises between appointments.

Life-Care Planning

Life-care plans are often required for individuals with a workers' compensation file or when a legal suit is being pursued. The occupational therapist's contribution to a life-care plan should be based on general knowledge of upper limb amputation and prosthetic devices and detailed knowledge of the individual's medical and emotional condition, prosthesis use, and support system. The occupational therapist should also be able to contribute to information related to potential aging of the individual with amputations. With aging, there may be changes to physiology and life interests, both of which may require different prosthetic needs or further medical intervention. This information can inform decisions related to funding for future medical, prosthesis, and training needs over the individual's lifetime.

SUMMARY

Preprosthetic and postprosthetic occupational therapy can foster a faster return to function for an individual with upper limb loss. Immediate and frequent occupational therapy after prosthesis delivery can enhance the incorporation of the device into daily activities and work tasks. Structured long-term follow-up at an amputee clinic can assist the individual with remaining functional throughout the aging process and can provide the rationale for prosthetic changes.

Acknowledgments

Hector Torres, BS IT, the author's husband, and Bill Hickerson, MD, FACS, Medical Director Amputee Clinic, Memphis, TN, are thanked for the support and encouragement they provided during the development of this chapter.

References

1. Ziegler-Graham K, MacKenzie EJ, Ephraim PL, Travison TG, Brookmeyer R: Estimating the prevalence of limb loss in the United States: 2005 to 2050. *Arch Phys Med Rehabil* 2008;89(3):422-429.
2. Sheehan TP, Gondo GC: Impact of limb loss in the United States. *Phys Med Rehabil Clin N Am* 2014;25(1):9-28.

3. Dillingham TR, Pezzin LE, MacKenzie EJ: Limb amputation and limb deficiencey: Epidemiology and recent trends in the United States. *South Med J* 2002;95(8):875-883.

4. Whelan LR, Farley J: Functional outcomes with externally powered partial hand prostheses. *J Prosthet Orthot* 2018;30(2):69-73.

5. Rondinelli RD: *AMA Guides to the Evaluation of Permanent Impairment*. ed 6. American Medical Association, 2008, pp 441-444.

6. Klarich J, Brueckner I: Amputee rehabilitation and preprosthetic care. *Phys Med Rehabil Clin N Am* 2014;25(1):75-91.

7. Major MJ, McConn SM, Zavaleta LJ, Stine R, Gard SA: Effects of upper limb loss and prosthesis use on proactive mechanisms of locomotor stability. *J Electromyogr Kinesiol* 2019;48:145-151.

8. Major MJ, Shirvaikar T, Stine R, Gard SA: Effects of upper limb loss or absence and prosthesis use on postural control of standing balance. *Am J Phys Med Rehabil* 2020;99(5):366-371.

9. Neil A: Silver wound dressings: Improving the function of advanced wound care 2012. Accessed June 22, 2014. http://medipurpose.com/blog/entry/silver-wound-dressings-improving-the--function-of-advanced-wound-care

10. Louie Wai-Shan S, Ho-Yin F, Poon Mei-Yee C, Leung Wai-Ting S, Wan Sau-Ying I, Wong Kam-Man S: Residual limb management for persons with transtibial amputation: Comparison of bandaging technique and residual limb sock. *J Prosthet Orthot* 2010;22(3):194-201.

11. Ephraim PL, Wegener ST, MacKenzie EJ, Dillingham TR, Pezzin LE: Phantom pain, residual limb pain, and back pain in amputees: Results of a national survey. *Arch Phys Med Rehabil* 2005;86(10):1910-1919.

12. Hanley MA, Ehde DM, Jensen M, Czerniecki J, Smith DG, Robinson LR: Chronic pain associated with upper-Limb loss. *Am J Phys Med Rehabil* 2009;88(9):742-751.

13. Fletchall S: Overuse syndromes in upper-limb loss: Recognizing problems and implementing change. *Acad Today* 2011;7(3):A8-A10.

14. Hsu E, Cohen SP: Postamputation pain: Epidemiology, mechanisms, and treatment. *J Pain Res* 2013;6:121-136.

15. Weeks SR, Anderson-Barnes VC, Tsao JW: Phantom limb pain: Theories and therapies. *Neurologist* 2010;16(5):277-286.

16. Moura VL, Faurot KR, Gaylord SA, et al: Mind-body interventions for treatment of phantom limb pain in persons with amputation. *Am J Phys Med Rehabil* 2012;91(8):701-714.

17. Hasanzadeh Kiabi F, Habibi MR, Soleimani A, Emami Zeydi A: Mirror therapy as an alternative treatment for phantom limb pain: A short literature review. *Korean J Pain* 2013;26(3):309-311.

18. Foell J, Bekrater-Bodmann R, Diers M, Flor H: Mirror therapy for phantom limb pain: Brain changes and the role of body representation. *Eur J Pain* 2014;18(5):729-739.

19. Hagenberg A, Carpenter C: Mirror visual feedback for phantom pain international experience on modalities and adverse effects discussed by an expert panel: A Delphi study. *PM R* 2014;6(8):708-715.

20. Pirowska A, Wloch T, Nowobilski R, Plaszewski M, Hocini A, Ménager D: Phantom phenomena and body scheme after limb amputation: A literature review. *Neurol Neurochir Pol* 2014;48(1):52-59.

21. Subedi B, Grossberg GT: Phantom limb pain: Mechanisms and treatment approaches. *Pain Res Treat* 2011;2011:864605.

22. Margalit D, Heled E, Berger C, Katzir H: Phantom fighters: Coping mechanisms of amputee patients with phantom limb pain. A longitudinal study. *Open J Orthop* 2013;3:300-305.

23. Postema SG, van der Sluis CK, Waldenlöv K, Norling Hermansson LM: Body structures and physical complaints in upper limb reduction deficiency: A 24-year follow-up study. *PLoS One* 2012;7(11):e49727.

24. Heyward VH: *Assessing Muscular Fitness in Advanced Fitness Assessment and Exercise Prescription*. 6th ed. Human Kinetics, 2010, pp 129-153.

25. Occupational therapy practice framework: Domain and process. *Am J Occup Ther* 2014. Accessed February 27, 2015. http://ajot.aota.org/article.aspx?articleid=1860439

26. *Certified peer visitor program*. Amputee Coalition Assessed July 19, 2021. https://www.amputee-coalitionorg

27. Malone JM, Fleming LL, Roberson J, et al: Immediate, early, and late postsurgical management of upper--limb amputation. *J Rehabil Res Dev* 1984;21(1):33-41.

28. Biddis EA, Chau TT: Multivariate prediction of upper limb prosthesis acceptance or rejection. *Disabil Rehabil Assist Technol* 2008;3(4):181-192.

29. Elbert T, Rockstroch B: Reorganization of human cerebral cortex: The range of changes following use and injury. *Neuroscientist* 2004;10(2):129-141.

30. Peterson JK, Prigge P: Early upper-Limb prosthetic fitting and brain development: Considerations for success. *J Prosthet Orthot* 2020;32(4):229-235.

31. Hancock L, Ahern D, Correia S, Barredo J, Resnik L: Cognitive predictors of skilled performance with an advanced upper limb multifunction prosthesis: A preliminary analysis. *Disabil Rehabil Assist Technol* 2017;12(5):504-511.

32. Hermansson LN, Turner K: Occupational therapy for prosthetic rehabilitation in adults with acquired upper-limb loss: Body-powered and myoelectric control systems. *J Prosthet Orthot* 2017;29(45):45-50.

33. Resnik L, Borgia M: Responsiveness of outcome measures for upper limb prosthetic rehabilitation. *J Prosthet Orthot* 2016;-0(1):96-108.

34. Johnson SS, Mansfield E: Prosthetic training: Upper limb. *Phys Med Rehabil Clin N Am* 2014;25(1):133-151.

35. Lake C: Effects of prosthetic training on upper-extremity prosthesis use. *J Prosthet Orthot* 1997;9(1):3-4.

36. Weeks D, Anderson D, Wallace S: The role of variability in practice structure when learning to use an upper-Extremity prosthesis. *J Prosthet Orthot* 2003;15(3):84-92.

37. Fletchall S: Managing daily activities in adults with upper-extremity amputations, in Christiansen CH, Matuska KM, eds. *Intervention Strategies to Enable Participation: Ways of Living*. ed 4. American Occupational Therapy Press, 2011, pp 327-328.

38. Fletchall S: Returning upper-extremity amputees to work. *The O&P Edge* 2005;4:28-33.

39. Smurr LM, Gulick K, Yancosek K, Ganz O: Managing the upper extremity amputee: A protocol for success. *J Hand Ther* 2008;21(2):160-176.

40. Resnik L, Meucci MR, Lieberman-Klinger S, et al: Advanced upper limb prosthetic devices: Implications for upper limb prosthetic rehabilitation *Arch Phys Med Rehabil* 2012;93(4):710-717.

Upper Limb Adaptive Prostheses for Vocation and Recreation

CHAPTER 27

Robert Radocy, MS • Debra Latour, OTD, MEd, OTR/L

ABSTRACT

Adaptive prostheses continue to evolve, expanding the choices for persons with a hand absence(s), enabling them to participate bilaterally and more competitively in challenging activities that can be vocationally, domestically, or recreationally oriented. Many adaptive prostheses and specially designed terminal devices provide multipurpose or crossover capability, offering reliable function and performance in unrelated activities. Multiple factors have created the stimulus for growth in this area of prosthetic technology, including changes in the Healthcare Common Procedure Coding System. In many cases adaptive components are more sophisticated, higher performance, nonanthropomorphic designs that emphasize function and biomechanics over appearance. Additionally, a growing variety of modern, quick-disconnect, vocationally oriented tools and domestic use implements are now available to meet patient needs. Also, a growing influence in individualized and custom designs is being created via computer-assisted design and additive manufacturing technologies leading to further innovations and more consumer-driven solutions. A broad array of sports and recreational adapters provide the opportunity for many persons with hand absence(s) to not only participate, but be competitive in activities ranging from archery to kayaking and weightlifting. Specific adaptive solutions for many activities are explored in detail.

Keywords: activity-specific; prosthesis; prosthosis; sports and recreation; vocation

Introduction

The term "activity specific" began to replace the general reference for sports and recreational prosthetic adaptations during the late 1990s.[1] Activity-specific or adaptive prostheses currently refer to a wide range of designs that serve vocational, domestic, and sports and recreation pursuits. Certain of these designs have evolved into true "crossover" devices, as consumers have successfully applied the technologies to activities beyond the original intention. The broadened "crossover" usage can help the justification for prescribing activity-specific designs. These types of devices can differ from traditional prostheses in a variety of ways. Replicating correct human hand or upper limb anatomical features is not the primary goal of these components. Rather, the design emphasis is on duplicating precise upper limb biomechanics and in many cases rigorous high-performance function. The adaptive prostheses are designed and constructed to enable the user to achieve higher levels of competency and performance in specific activities where traditional body-powered and/or myoelectric (externally powered) technologies do not perform well.

Early commercialized designs for activity-specific terminal devices such as the Hosmer Bowling Ball Adapter and Baseball Glove Adapter date back to the 1950s. Between the 1950s and the early 1980s development remained stagnant, except for a prosthetic golf TD that was built on a limited basis and sold by Robin-Aids of northern California.[2] In 1983 the TRS Super Sport Hand was introduced. Most commercially available, innovative activity-specific prosthetic adaptations were introduced in the 1990s. Around the turn of the new millennium the demand for quality, commercially built adaptive devices finally began to grow.

Published articles and educational textbooks on the topic of activity-specific–type prosthetic technology are somewhat limited but relevant literature exists.[3-11] It is not uncommon for an occupational therapist (OT) to fabricate an implement and attach it to a universal cuff to help people with upper limb absence to participate in meaningful activities. More often, the OT might collaborate with the prosthetist to help the person acquire a specific TD or adaptation to existing prosthetic technology. The activity-specific terminal device is typically static and attaches

Robert Radocy or an immediate family member serves as a paid consultant to or is an employee of Fillauer TRS Inc. Dr. Latour or an immediate family member serves as a paid consultant to or is an employee of Handspring, Liberating Technologies, Inc., and TRS Prosthetics.

to the forearm unit at the wrist. This technology often is robust, lightweight, and offers quick release. It typically does not require harnessing or cables and is low maintenance. The activity-specific prosthesis is often suspended with a pin-lock style of liner or a neoprene sleeve. This design configuration allows participation and improved performance during specific activities such as personal care tasks, cooking, woodworking and gardening, and diverse recreational activities.[10]

A multitude of forces and events have contributed to the development of adaptive prostheses. Beginning in the 1970s, individuals with physical challenges became more visible in the public and the public became more accustomed to seeing persons with prostheses taking on sports challenges such as snow skiing. The birth and growth of adaptive ski programs in the United States and abroad have significantly raised the exposure levels of those with a limb absence. Simultaneously, college educational programs began to progress in the disciplines of Physical Education, Adaptive Sports, and Therapeutic Recreation creating trained professionals with an academic focus on these topics. This influence has trended on a global level with the recommendations of the World Health Organization focusing of wellness, well-being, and preventing further disability.

In the 1980s and into the early 1990s, the entrance into the prosthetic industry by two entrepreneurs, who themselves were individuals with upper limb absence, led to the creation of viable commercialized businesses oriented toward manufacturing and selling "standardized" activity-specific prosthetic components. The designs of Therapeutic Recreation Systems (TRS Inc. now Fillauer TRS, Inc.) were primarily oriented toward adaptive sports and recreation technology, while Texas Assistive Devices (TAD) targeted the design and development of specialized hand tool attachments and domestic-use implements. These technologies were designed to enhance the functional capabilities of the prosthesis user, allowing them to be more competitive in two-handed tasks and believing that there was no need to be limited by current prosthetic technology.

In addition, the benefits and values of sports and recreation in the rehabilitation program have continued to be recognized. The healthful benefits of physical activity are well-known for persons without limb absence and seem to be even more relevant for people with limb absence. Numerous authors have associated positive self-esteem with participation in sports and other meaningful recreational pursuits. Wearing and using a prosthesis affords the person with upper limb absence the opportunity to participate in such pursuits, and to perform to their best ability. These factors directly influence one's self-identity, self-esteem, and self-concept. Murray found that to prosthesis users, the prosthesis may be more than a tool, and that with mastery, it may correlate with self-identity.[12] He suggested that the valued personal identities and the self-management of patients' ability status should be a priority for the health professionals involved in prosthesis users' medical care and personal development.

The evolution, growth, and popularity of national disabled sports organizations such as Disabled Sports USA and Adaptive Sports USA (now merged as Move United), the National Amputee Golf Association, and Physically Challenged Bowhunters of America, and many other organizations, have also fueled the interest in these adaptive prosthetic technologies. The creation of specialized competitions and "Games" for the physically challenged athlete all have contributed to the growth and interest in activity-specific prostheses. The development of the Paralympics in the late 1980s gave credence to the overall challenged athletic movement and increased interest in activity-specific or adaptive prosthetic technologies. The allowance for use of an upper extremity prosthesis in all the Paralympic sports still does not exist. Potentially, in the future, "classes" of competition will be created to eliminate this restriction for certain physically challenged athletes, allowing them to perform at even higher levels, using prosthetic technology.

Improved representation and exposure for athletes with upper limb absence and peer role models via national organizations such as the Amputee Coalition, the Challenged Athletes Foundation (CAF), and others has helped to expand information and communications between prosthetic users interested in sports pursuits and new adaptive technologies. The general explosion of communications, information, and data via the internet and social media have opened and created interest in new prosthetic technologies.

The demands placed upon the military's rehabilitation hospitals such as Walter Reed in Washington, DC, Brooks Army Medical Center (BAMC) in San Antonio, Texas, and Balboa Naval Hospital in San Diego, CA, by young, strong, but physically traumatized soldiers returning from the wars in Iraq and Afghanistan have played an important role in driving the development of new and innovative prosthetic designs. These military facilities have created state-of-the-art programs that have actively integrated sports reconditioning, for the first time, into our soldiers' comprehensive rehabilitation.

Insurance companies and vocational rehabilitation agencies have begun to realize the health values and psychological benefits of adaptive prosthetic technologies in the insured's rehabilitation scheme. Reimbursement for the provision of activity-specific or adaptive upper extremity prosthetic technology has expanded and improved but is still not adequate to meet the needs of those with limb absence. Insurance companies appear to see value in prosthetic technology that allow functional outcomes in personal care, home management, community access, and vocational activities. While many of these same companies incentivize members with access to gym clubs and weight loss programs, they do not pay for recreational devices that would enable the person to participate. Some activity-specific recreational devices offer "crossover" functions so that the user may access recreation and/or sports endeavors as well as functional tasks that require similar biomechanics. For example, a device used for bicycling may also be used to grasp the handles of a shopping cart, a stroller, lawnmower, or snow-blow, and thus enhance the functional envelope of the technology. **Table 1** depicts specific devices that offer cross over functions.

Importantly in 2009 Healthcare Common Procedure Coding System (HCPCS) revised numerous upper extremity L Codes via the Durable Medical Equipment Coding System (DMECS), creating *Code: L6704: Terminal Device, Sport/Recreational/Work Attachment. Any Material, Any Size* that provided coverage and reimbursement for terminal devices designed for specialized work and sports and recreational activities. Creating this code was an important step for HCPCS in recognizing the importance and value of activity-specific or adaptive prosthetic technology in the overall rehabilitation spectrum for persons with an upper extremity limb absence.

Another factor related to the growth and popularity of activity-specific prosthetics is cost and affordability. Bionic technology appears to have captured the attention of the media and public. However, the reality for some users of such prostheses is that their higher cost is associated with lower performance and less reliability, and they may be neither affordable nor provide practical solutions to daily demands. Bionic-electric prostheses are not capable of reliable performance in most sports pursuits or in certain vocational activities with demanding bimanual skill requirements. Activity-specific technologies are far more affordable and have a much higher level of reliable function and performance for targeted activities than electric prostheses. The adaptive prosthesis can, however, compliment and augment the capability of externally powered prostheses that might otherwise be used in inappropriate environments or for inadvisable tasks. The activity-specific prosthesis is robust and well-suited to physical, functionally demanding vocational and avocational pursuits, while the bionic or myo-electric limb can be complimentary and complete other important user functions where dexterity or appearance may be indicated.

Prosthetic Interfaces and Limb Design

Activity-specific prostheses are typically used in either high-force/stress or high-performance environments and therefore require a socket (interface) design and construction that is extremely comfortable, while providing high levels

TABLE 1 Activity-Specific Devices With Crossover Function

Device	Action	TRS Design Use	Crossover Function
Criterium series	Grasps handles with small to medium diameter Pivot allows steering, improved control	Biking (road and flat land)	Pushing/pulling Sweeping/raking Steering
Dragon	Aperture in device absorbs forces and captures cylindrical handles Loosely interacts with objects Allows freedom of movement	Martial arts	Home management Property management Climbing Steering
Helix	Molded, high-performance, polyurethane. "DNA" helical shape replicates holding action of the hand in the control of short or long cylindrical handles grips. Unique strength and flexibility "feels" like the hand and forearm with "reflexive," energy capture, storage, and release action	Especially useful in any activity-specific task that uses long handles or "sticks" like lacrosse, hockey (ice, street, field)	Vocational–avocational prosthetic device Especially useful in any activity-specific task that uses long handles, such as rakes, shovels, as well as smaller garden tools, water hose control Many undiscovered uses
ISHI and F~ISHI	Adjustable grasp Secure, stable with strap	Archery, fishing	Grooming Holding handled objects
Multi-D	Adjustable grasp Secure, stable with strap Larger More robust	Multipurpose	Home management Yard work Holding larger handled objects Fishing (salt water)
Raptor	High strength, "large *#7" shaped titanium lifting and supporting terminal device with replaceable, protective tip for cushion and nonmarring applications and greater friction control over surfaces. Unique pivot action increases versatility in lifting, supporting, climbing, etc.	Indoor and outdoor rock and gym climbing	Heavy-duty lifting and transport and loading tasks Handling/lifting veneer woods, panels, or similar
Swinger	Loosely interfaces with objects Allows freedom of movement	Gymnastics	Carrying Climbing Steering Fishing

Adapted with permission from Fillauer TRS, Inc. *TRS High Performance Prosthetics Product Catalog.* TRS Prosthetics, January 2019. https:www.trsprosthetics.com/wp-content/uploads/2019/01/Web-Catalog-JANUARY2019.pdf.

of pressure tolerance and exceptional suspension. The prosthesis is typically constructed using light-weight carbon fiber or equivalent materials and special bonding resins that provide high strength. Other chapters of this Atlas concentrate specifically on aspects of prosthetic design and fabrication. The relevant, important factors to emphasize are secure suspension, adjustable compression, residual limb comfort under both static and dynamic loads, range of motion (ROM), physical weight, structural strength, and prosthesis length and alignment.

Suspension

Depending upon the limb morphology there are currently a variety of options to achieve a secure prosthetic suspension. The prosthetic platform could start with a well-designed self-suspending socket that enhances comfort with a partial liner or custom-fabricated silicone or polymer liner which at a minimum encompasses the medial and lateral epicondyles and olecranon. Locking liners should always control for longitudinal stretch in an upper extremity socket if secure suspension is to be maintained. Suction suspension can also augment prosthetic stability and security. A short residual limb prosthesis can be enhanced for load bearing by extending the rear brim of the socket to distribute load to the back of the humerus. Socket security can be augmented with REVO-LIMB type technology that uses BOA tension system mechanisms as illustrated by two current adjustable compression socket designs (**Figures 1** and **2**). Socket design can pattern any number of proven technologies, such as TRAC,[13] ACCI,[14] HI-FI,[15] or variants thereof depending upon the patient's needs and requirements. Suspension technology continues to evolve.

Load Bearing and Comfort

The socket should be tested under both static and dynamic loads on the patient to ensure that no painful pressure "pinpoints" exist that will make the socket intolerable under dynamic load. While liners can help cushion load, they will not take the place of a properly modified socket that creates secure suspension but still provides for the movement of the olecranon and condyles throughout complete elbow–forearm flexion ROM. A professionally designed socket should provide enough comfort and security for the patient to conduct a "pull-up" or "push-up" without creating debilitating pain in the socket.

Physical Weight and Structural Strength

While lighter is not always better, a lower weight prosthesis is typically preferred provided strength is not sacrificed. Materials such as woven carbon fiber or its equivalent fabricated with appropriate, compatible high-strength resins in both the socket and forearm of the prosthesis should provide a reliable limb for use in almost any activity. Materials and resins continue to evolve to improve socket integrity. Additive manufacturing technologies are beginning to play a role in custom socket and prosthesis construction. In certain cases, these prostheses can provide a reliable outcome for certain individuals and activities. However, at this point in its history and development, this is somewhat "unknown territory," and caution is a good prescription regarding relying on such prostheses for

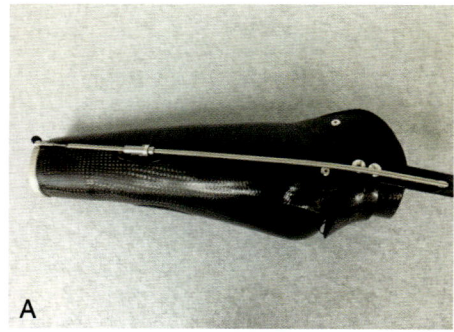
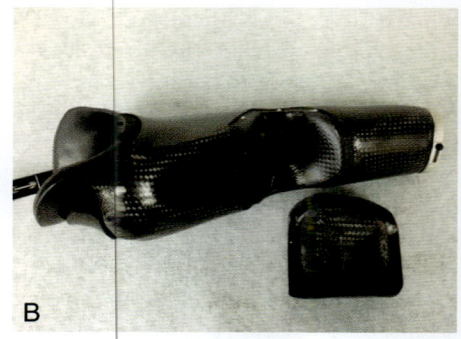

FIGURE 1 **A** and **B**, Clinical photographs of self-suspending forearm prosthesis incorporating BOA technology fabricated by Chris Baschuk, CPO, of Handspring and illustrating a removable cover and a rear compression plate that captures the olecranon. (Courtesy of Fillauer TRS, Inc.)

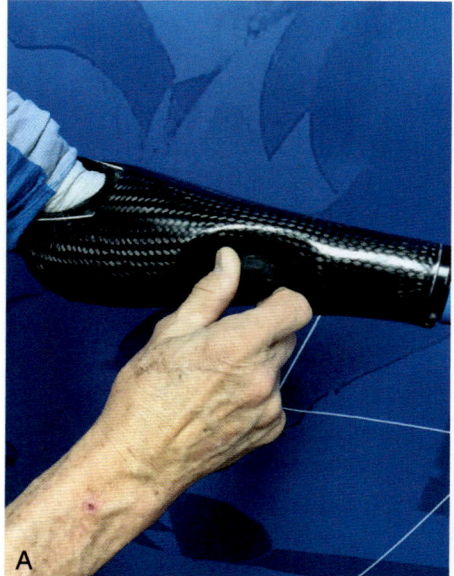
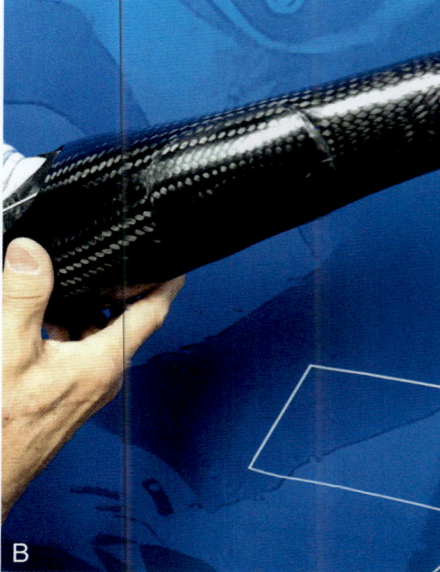

FIGURE 2 **A** and **B**, Clinical photographs of forearm prosthesis illustrating BOA technology with and without cover by Dave Rotter CPO, Dave Rotter Prosthetics, LTD, that captures the short forearm with flexible cable-controlled brims that tension together supporting the medial and lateral epicondyles. (Courtesy of Fillauer TRS, Inc.)

Chapter 27: Upper Limb Adaptive Prostheses for Vocation and Recreation

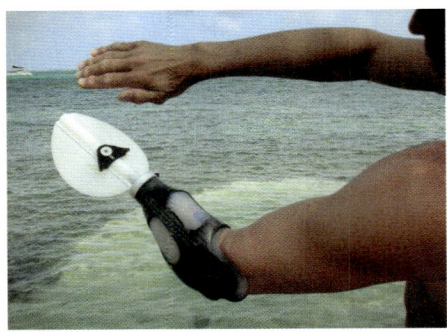

FIGURE 3 Clinical photograph of short sports swimming prosthesis using Hi-Fi technology built by Randy Alley of Biodesigns, Inc. (Courtesy of Fillauer TRS, Inc.)

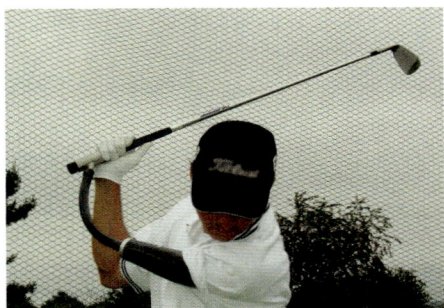

FIGURE 4 Clinical photograph of forearm prosthesis illustrating trans-humeral golf prosthesis. (Courtesy of Fillauer TRS, Inc.)

high-performance activities until the reliability and structural integrity of such materials in definitive prostheses have been substantiated. Advances in additive manufacturing and new materials technology, applied by trained, certified prosthetic professionals, may ultimately compliment or replace existing techniques and technology for fabricating prostheses.

Prosthesis Length

The length of the prosthesis may not necessarily need to conform to the normal limb. There are certain load control and biofeedback benefits to the user that can be achieved by shortening the overall length of the prosthesis and either bring the TD closer to the remnant limb as in this custom, swimming prosthesis (**Figure 3**) or using the shortened prosthesis as a more stable platform for a high-performance flexible TD connector such as this trans-humeral golf prosthesis design (**Figure 4**).

Another technique that has seen positive functional outcomes is to attach a musical instrument prosthetic accessory directly to a roll-on locking liner (**Figure 5**). The intimate fit of this type of liner magnified by its compliance enhances "sensitivity" and control over the musical instrument accessory. The musical adapter is much closer to the end of the limb in this design. The feedback and "feel" that are created are not inhibited, mitigated, or shielded by the outer shell of a prosthesis. Higher levels of sensation can be experienced between the instrument and the musician.

Alignment

Specific activities such as archery or weightlifting can dictate that prosthesis alignment be factored into the design to achieve optimal performance. End weight-bearing and balance are directly impacted by the degree to which the forearm of the prosthesis is "preflexed" from the socket. The wrist mounting angle also impacts load bearing and can impact performance. Typically, a more neutrally aligned prosthesis (minimal preflexion) should be considered for better performance in sports activities where a significant amount of gross motor motion is occurring or to help the stabilization and control of heavy loads placed upon the prosthesis, such as in weight training, archery, kayaking, etc. A more neutral socket to forearm alignment will help facilitate a greater ROM and more comfort and better control for the user.

Activity-Specific (Vocational-Domestic) Technology

Direct prosthetic tool and implement technology is far from being a new idea. In medieval periods certain well-to-do knights and royalty, who had lost a limb, were fitted with a creative prosthesis equipped with an integral dagger, sword, or eating implement.[16] In the 21st century the concept has experienced a rebirth, and the validity and viability of such designs continues to grow. TAD has engineered direct tool and implement attachment to an art form, continually expanding on the number of tool and implement options that are available (**Figures 6** and **7**). The initial inspiration in developing adaptive prosthetic components arose from a passion for cooking and frustration with being unable to adeptly handle carving knives. Voluntary opening split-hook prostheses could not capably or safely handle chef's knives and other cooking utensils and implements. In response, the field began to develop a line of highly functional adaptive tools. These devices were complimented by

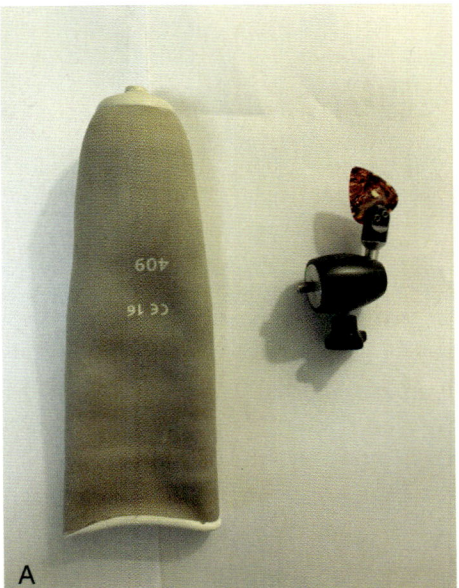 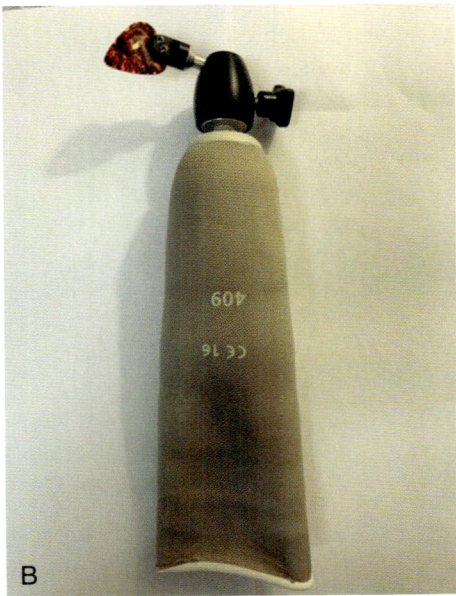

FIGURE 5 A and **B**, Clinical photographs of forearm Roll-On Locking Liner with Guitar Pick Adapter. (Courtesy of Deb Latour, Med, OTR/L.)

Section 2: Upper Limb

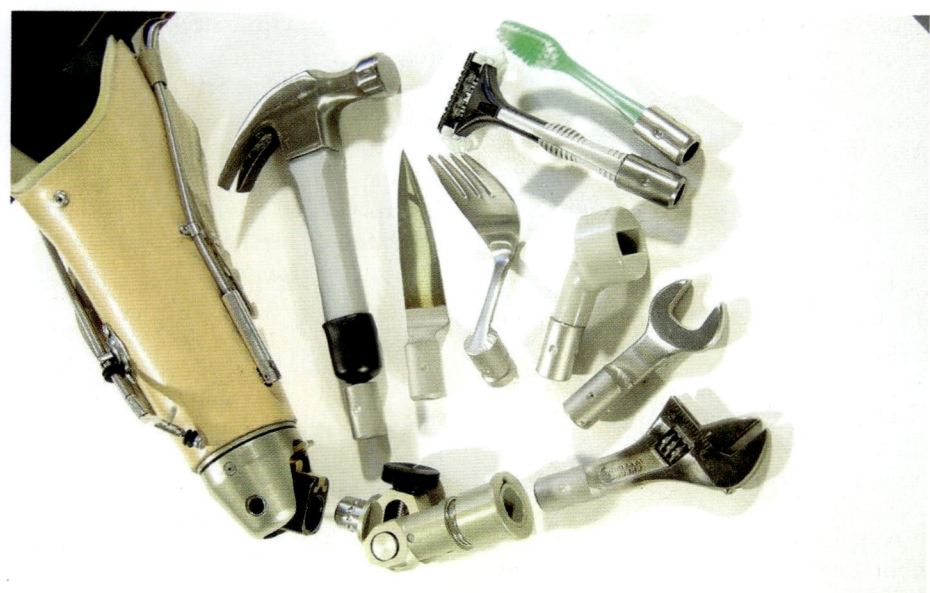

FIGURE 6 Clinical photograph of forearm prosthesis illustrating Texas Assistive Device's (TAD) working tool attachments. (Courtesy of TAD.)

the evolution of a novel product called the N-Abler, developed TAD in the early 1990s. The N-Abler was a multi-function wrist interface that connected the tools and implements into the prosthesis. The N-Abler allowed for precise flexion and rotation of the "tool" in ways not possible before. The N-Abler technology has now evolved into a family of five-function wrists. These wrist components have created the opportunity for persons to accomplish activities that they could not competently complete before. These technologies are particularly beneficial to persons missing both hands or presenting with partial hands bilaterally. The TAD adaptive components make the individual's work efforts more productive, expending less energy, and improving efficiency. The therapeutic results and benefits of these successful accomplishments include improved independence, self-esteem, and quality of life.

Activity-Specific (Avocational) Adaptive, Sports, and Recreational Technology

The interest in prosthetic sports and recreation, adaptive terminal devices has grown significantly since the beginning of the 21st century. The diverse designs provide people with hand absence better access to sports, and in many instances, a solid platform from which to compete with two-handed peers. The key to achieving competitive, high-performance capability in sports and recreation is an emphasis and focus on designing prostheses that replicate the natural biomechanics required to perform an activity. In many cases this is achieved by providing improved ROM of the forearm and wrist well beyond the single plane or biplanar motion that traditional prosthetic construction and wrist systems provide. Additionally, greater emphasis has been placed upon generating and capturing externally developed energy during the activity's execution and transferring that energy through the torso into the upper extremities and down into and through the prosthesis and terminal device. Capturing the natural "back swing" energy created by the mass and momentum of a golf club during a golf swing, or a baseball bat during a bat swing, then controlling it through the swing cycle and releasing that energy at the appropriate time not only enhances the performance of the activity but provides the prosthetic user with a continual, intimate, biofeedback that can help to improve control over the activity.

Consumer involvement in the development of activity-specific prostheses has been paramount to the success and growth of technology in this segment of the upper extremity prosthetics market and led to vast increases in persons with a hand absence using

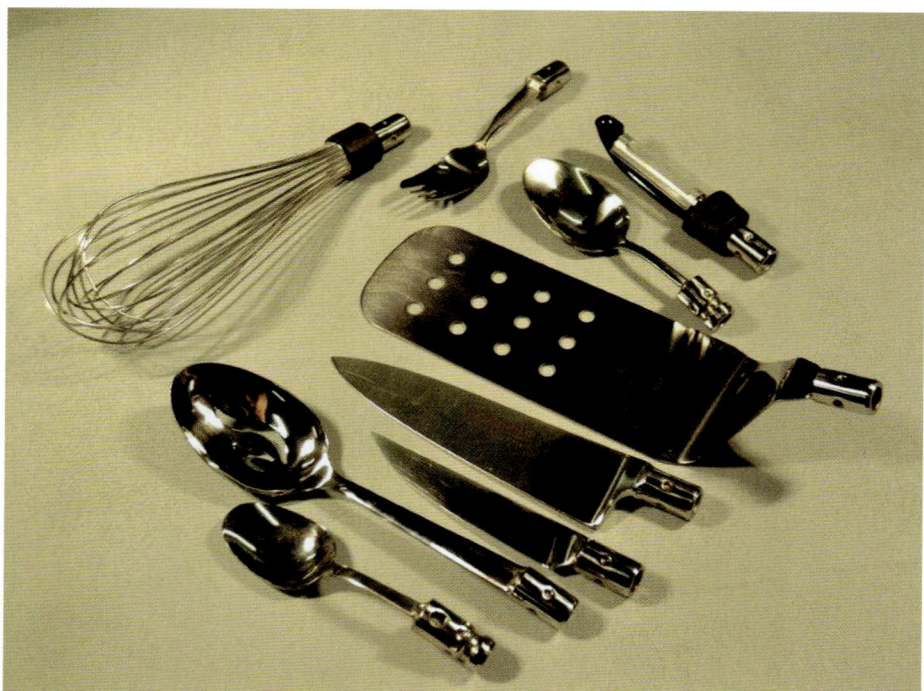

FIGURE 7 Clinical photograph illustrating Texas Assistive Device's (TAD) domestic use prosthetic adaptations. (Courtesy of TAD.)

a prosthesis in a wider range of physical challenges. The Mill's Rebound TD and Hoopster TD, both for basketball play, were both conceived by consumers. TRS took those initial concepts and refined them into producible products with standardized, reproduceable manufacturing practices. The Black Iron Master (BIM) resulted from the request of a semipro body builder,[17] who had lost his hand in an auto accident. The BIM provided the technology and generated the confidence that the individual needed to return to competitive weightlifting and win a world title in bench pressing, competing against able-bodied peers. The Swinger was designed in cooperation with a child and her father over a year timeframe, allowing her to perform inspiring feats on the uneven parallel bars, again competing with able-bodied peers. The Freestyle Swimming TD concept evolved directly from a Canadian Prosthetist's patented design. The diverse climbing TDs were codeveloped with input and testing by two well-known, one-armed climbers. The KAHUNA was requested and created for the Navy's Balboa Rehabilitation. Both the HAMMERHEAD and LAMPREY GUN TURRET were created at the request of personnel from Walter Reed Hospital. The value of such collaboration is difficult to measure but without it most likely the development of these products, that have proved so inspirational and valuable to hundreds of physically challenged athletes, may never have occurred.

Murray[18] explored factors about the social meanings of prostheses use, and particularly sought perceptions of prosthetic limb users. His findings revealed several themes such as actual prosthesis use, social rituals, user perceptions of social isolation, reactions of others, social implications of concealment or disclosure, and perceptions or experiences about social and intimate relationships. Factors that influence adjustment and successful rehabilitation were early prosthetic fitting, prosthetic satisfaction associated with increased self-esteem, increased social integration and absence of emotional challenges, and the need for individual expression including social expression, person-first language, societal acceptance, and personalizing the appearance of the prosthesis.

Preprosthetic Exercise

Preprosthetic conditioning or exercise without a prosthesis can be valuable to the person with a hand absence, especially in cases where traumatic injury or burn has created sensitive skin surfaces or scar tissue that cannot tolerate the potential shear forces created by a prosthesis. Exercise straps and elastomer exercise bands, custom harnesses supported by triceps cuff suspension techniques (**Figure 8**), or type harness systems can provide the ability to exercise in a wide ROM through most body zones, challenging atrophied muscles and stiffened joints. The CARTER CUFF is an example of one of the first commercialized exercise technologies developed specifically for those with a hand absence who are interested in higher performance resistance exercise training without a prosthesis. The TRS SWIM FIN is a kit system that does not involve a prosthesis and has been successfully applied by therapists for resistance exercise conditioning during pool therapy. Providing additional resistance to the affected limb helps improve the shoulder ROM and strengthen shoulder and arm musculature without the aggravation and load bearing of a prosthesis.

Preprosthetic exercise can help prepare an individual for the therapeutically valuable exercise that resistance training with a prosthesis can provide. Therapists and prosthetists often may collaborate to prepare the individual to tolerate wearing the prosthesis and use it independently for daily activities using prosthesis simulator technology. In this way, the individual can become accustomed to the weight and length of the device, the feeling of the socket and the harness, and the functional workings of the components.[19] TRS developed a prosthesis simulator that offers access to both body-powered and static activity-specific devices.

Specific Adaptive Sports and Recreational Technologies

Ball Sports

Ball sports can be broken down into those that require either unilateral or bilateral function and control. Baseball and softball throwing are primarily unilateral activities, while playing volleyball or basketball involves bilateral upper limb function. Simple flexible polymer terminal devices, such as the TRS SUPER SPORT and FREE FLEX technologies (**Figure 9**), simulate the volar surface of the palm providing much of the function used in controlling larger diameter balls such as volleyballs, basket

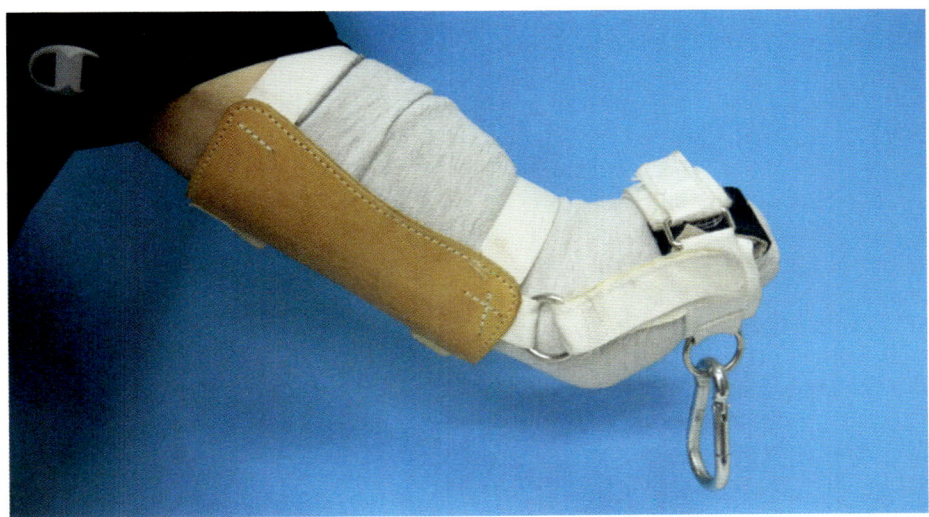

FIGURE 8 Clinical photograph illustrating trans-radial exercise harness. (Courtesy of Fillauer TRS, Inc.)

Section 2: Upper Limb

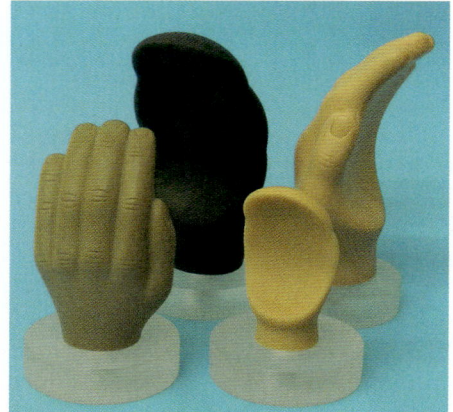

FIGURE 9 Clinical photograph illustrating SUPER SPORT and FREE FLEX TDs. (Courtesy of Fillauer TRS, Inc.)

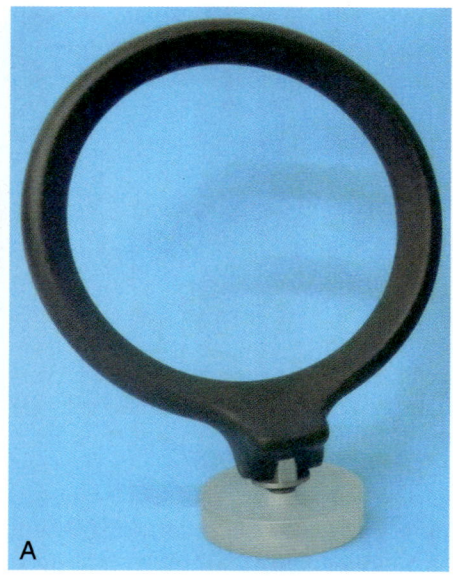
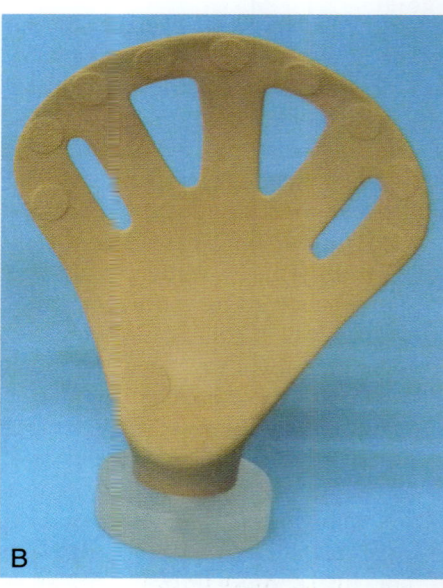

FIGURE 10 **A** and **B**, Clinical photographs illustrating REBOUND and HOOPSTER TDs. (Courtesy of Fillauer TRS, Inc.)

balls, and soccer balls, while being resilient and strong enough to support body weight for activities such as push-ups and handstands. The devices function well for both two-handed catching and ball tossing. They also provide a safe interface at the end of the prosthesis for contact sports, protecting both the user and other players from physical injury. More advanced prosthetic designs, such as the REBOUND, HOOPSTER, and BARRAGE (**Figures 10** and **11**), are very basketball and volleyball specific, inspired by designs and ideas of consumers with a hand absence. Competitive unilateral throwing of baseballs, soft balls, and similarly sized sports balls such as cricket balls with a prosthesis was not possible until 2012 when the COBRA BASEBALL (**Figure 12**) prosthetic adapter was introduced. The COBRA[5] ball throwing technology provides an adjustable, elastomer support arm and ball-capturing cup system, that has provided trans-radial amputees with the documented capability of throwing a baseball with control and accuracy at speeds over 50 mph and to distances that exceed 30 yards.

Another challenge of baseball-type ball sport involves the biomechanics and techniques of catching. Typically, pronation and supination are used while fielding and catching a ball depending upon how it enters and impacts the catcher's body zones. Fielding a ground ball (catching below the waist) usually requires forearm supination (palm forward, thumb lateral) while fielding a fly ball (catching above the waist) requires pronation (palm forward, thumb medial). Using a prosthetic adaption such as the HOSMER BASEBALL GLOVE ADAPTER[3] allows for the mounting of a traditional first baseman's glove onto an oversized, voluntary opening split hook but does not accommodate for the rapid pronation or supination required. The TRS HI FLY FIELDERs[5] were conceived in the 1990s to eliminate the traditional glove entirely and replace it with a modified lacrosse stick head and specialized oversized net. The oversized net allows for a ball to be caught either forehanded or backhanded (bidirectionally) so that the need for pronation and supination is eliminated. The HI FLY FIELDERs provide a strong, lightweight platform for catching a baseball or softball spontaneously and meets the surface size standards for legal play. The TAD DOUBLE PLAY[15] is a design like the HI FLY FIELDER but uses a standard, lacrosse netting system instead of a dual direction netting design, forcing the need to pronate and supinate the device to satisfy varying catching and fielding situations.

Golf, Baseball, and Lacrosse (Sports Requiring Swinging and Large ROM Arm Biomechanics)

Discussion about these activities has been combined because of their parallel biomechanical demands. Swinging

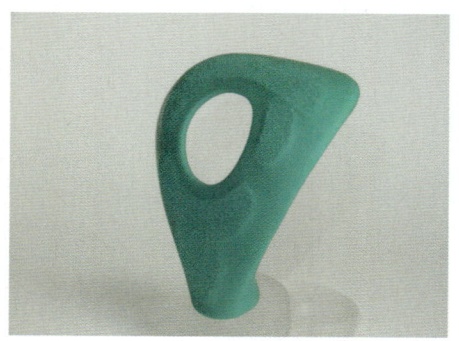

FIGURE 11 Clinical photograph illustrating BARRAGE TD. (Courtesy of Fillauer TRS, Inc.)

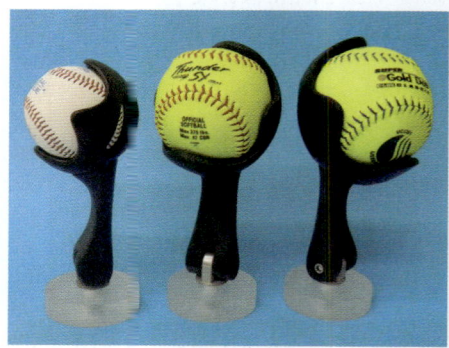

FIGURE 12 Clinical photograph illustrating COBRA Baseball and Softball TDs. (Courtesy of Fillauer TRS, Inc.)

a golf club or baseball/softball bat, and maneuvering and throwing with a lacrosse stick, all require coordinated, gross motor motions involving the torso, arms, and hands. Creating the appropriate degrees of freedom in movement and capturing the energy created in the back swing phase of these sports is essential in achieving the highest performance.

Historical designs for golf prosthesis applied ball and socket or universal joint linkages connecting the prosthetic wrist to the golf club. Contrasting designs orient around a direct, rigid golf club attachment. Neither of these extremes were successful in replicating the biomechanics of a natural two-armed swing. Modern golf club prosthetic adapters such as the TRS GOLF PRO, GOLF EAGLE, and EAGLE-FLEX (**Figure 13**) and Troppman Grip connect the prosthesis to a golf club grip engaging element using a high-strength, flexible coupling. The flexible coupling of these adapters provides unparalleled flexibility and ROM, enabling the golfer to replicate accurate, powerful, controlled "two-handed" golf swings. The basic devices are designed for the prosthetic user with a trans-radial absence, but custom, trans-humeral designs are easily accomplished that eliminate the need for a prosthetic elbow and forearm (**Figure 4**). This lightens the prosthesis significantly and creates a high-performance energy transfer system to control the golf club swing. Designs exist for persons with both right- or left-hand absence and specific models accommodate either right- or left-hand dominant swing styles.

The powerful controlled swing of a bat hitting a baseball, softball, or cricket ball requires providing the multiple degrees of freedom required to replicate the upper extremity biomechanics involved. Secondarily, engaging the bat handle with a secure but releasable grip is also advantageous. The PINCH HITTER, PINCH HITTER HD, and PINCH HITTER FLEX[5] (**Figure 14**) are designed for the leading arm prosthesis (lower grip hand), while the GRAND SLAM TD[5] (**Figure 14**) has been redesigned to provide function for

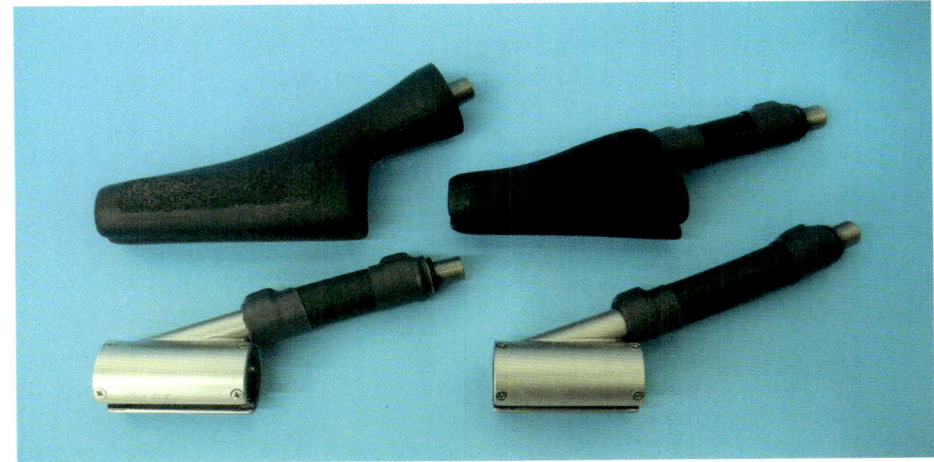

FIGURE 13 Clinical photograph illustrating TRS GOLF EAGLE, EAGLE FLEX, GOLF PRO L, and GOLF PRO R TDs. (Courtesy of Fillauer TRS, Inc.)

those with a trailing arm (upper hand grip) prosthesis. A model exists to meet the needs of both dominant right- or dominant left-handed batters. These adapters allow for the capture, storage, and release of energy. Energy is created by the bat's mass and momentum during the rear swing phase of the bat swing cycle and released through the prosthesis.

Controlling a lacrosse stick requires multiple degrees of freedom throughout the shoulders, elbow, forearm, and wrist, while additionally requiring the changing of the hand grasp position on the stick. The TRS HELIX TD (**Figure 15**), available in both right and left versions, is a unique design that functions well in satisfying these stick control challenges. The flexible polymer is a helical configuration that "sizes" down in internal diameter under torque and grasps the stick but eases and relaxes to allow for repositioning. The Helix has enough flexibility to allow the stick to be controlled throughout a wide range of body zones while "feeling" and responding with the resiliency of a human wrist.

Tumbling, Gymnastics, Floor Exercise, and Yoga

These activities require the successful transfer of body weight through the residual limb and prosthetic interface. Terminal devices such as the

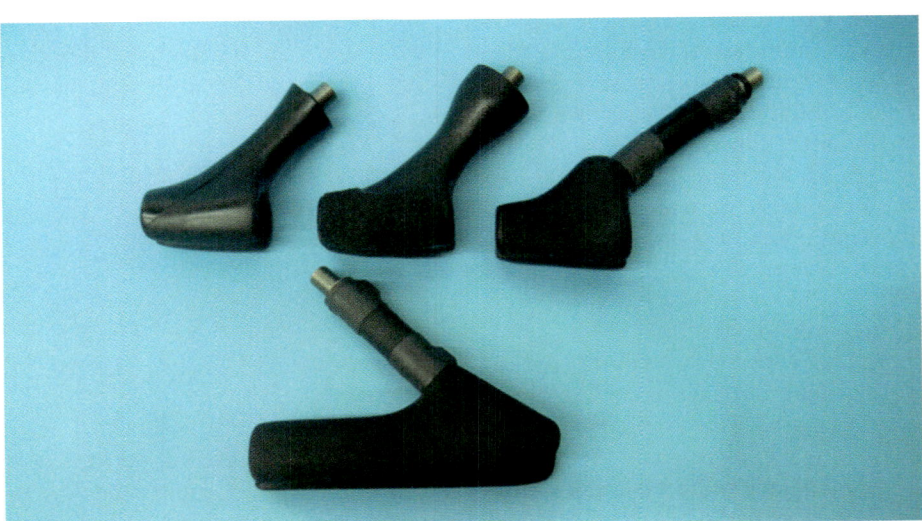

FIGURE 14 Clinical photograph illustrating TRS PINCH HITTER, PINCH HITTER HD, PINCH HITTER FLEX, and GRAND SLAM TDs. (Courtesy of Fillauer TRS, Inc.)

SUPER SPORTS AND FREE FLEX[5] (**Figure 9**) can be applied successfully to these activities but several other adaptive devices have proven to provide enhanced control. The SHROOM TUMBLER (**Figure 16**) is widely used for tumbling, floor gymnastics, and yoga because of its stability and strong, resilient, nonslip polymer surfaces and omni-directional flexion capability. No orientation of the TD is required while performing yoga postures or gymnastic challenges such as the balance beam or more rapid-fire activities such as cartwheels or back flips that are required in floor exercise routines. Interestingly, the SHROOM has also been "crossover" applied for functional use in wheelchair propulsion.

Gymnastic activities that require the capability to hang and swing are also challenging for the person with a hand absence(s). Upper extremity strength is required, and a prosthesis designed to comfortably support the user's full body weight is essential. The SWINGER (**Figure 17**) adaptive terminal device introduced in 2013 by TRS has been successfully used for performance on the uneven parallel bars and for more straightforward exercise such as pull ups. The unique design allows the practiced prosthetic wearer to capture and release the parallel bars, support their weight in a forearm press above the bar, perform 360° hip circles and then dismount. The SWINGER, because of its offset "C"-shaped design and rugged, polyurethane molded surfaces, can also be used for activities where a general, "hook" shape TD can be applied and helpful. The SWINGER TD was developed with the help, input, and testing of young women with congenital hand absence and their parents.

Swimming and Swimming Pool-Based Therapeutic Exercise

Swimming without a prosthesis is possible, but swimming with a custom swimming adapter or swimming prosthesis can improve performance, propulsion, and therapeutic value by adding resistance to the stroke. The SWIM FIN and FREESTYLE SWIMMING TD (**Figure 18**) both can assist persons wishing to achieve better swimming performance in any swimming environment. The SWIM FIN[5] is provided as a kit and is custom fabricated to fit onto the residual limb without a prosthesis. The SWIM FIN provides water resistance that can be beneficial in pool therapy situations where upper body conditioning and strengthening are goals. The FREESTYLE is an actual TD requiring

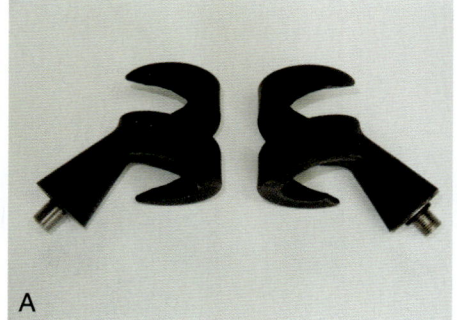
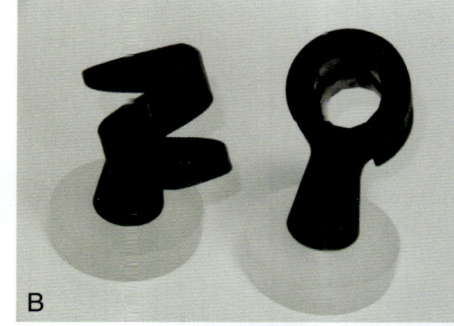

FIGURE 15 **A** and **B**, Clinical photographs illustrating TRS HELIX TD. (Courtesy of Fillauer TRS, Inc.)

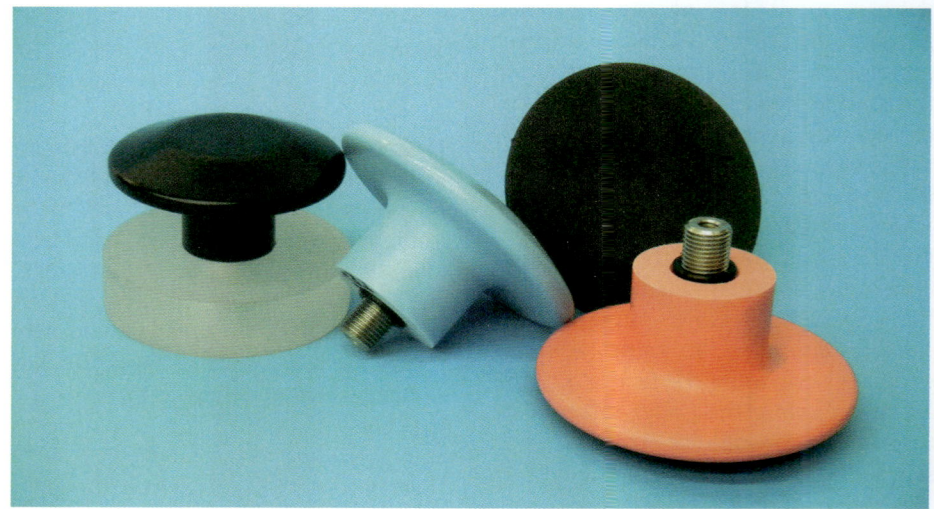

FIGURE 16 Clinical photograph illustrating MUSHROOM (SHROOM) and MINI-SHROOM TUMBLERS. (Courtesy of Fillauer TRS, Inc.)

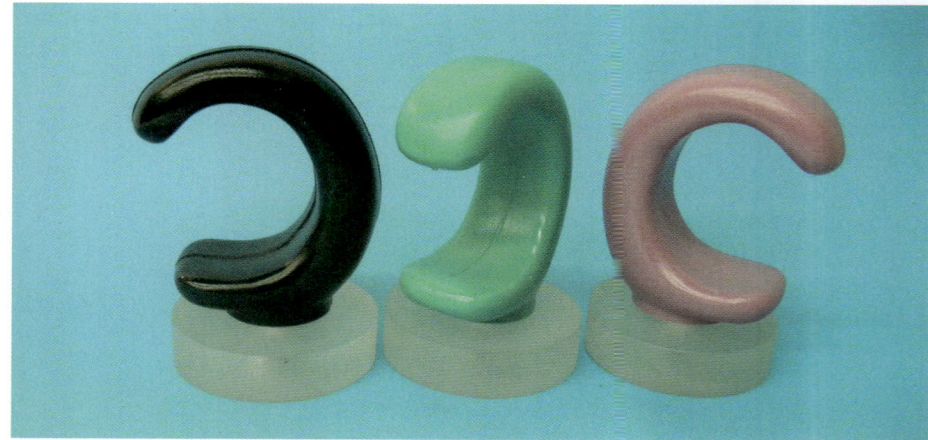

FIGURE 17 Clinical photograph illustrating SWINGER TD. (Courtesy of Fillauer TRS, Inc.)

the use of a prosthesis. A short, lightweight, custom swimming prosthesis is suggested and will improve performance, as compared with a full-length prosthesis for those with short to midlength trans-radial absence or for swimmers with trans-humeral absence. These are both simple devices that rely on a folding-fin or "butterfly" wing design to enhance swimming performance. Persons with a hand absence above the mid-radial level have no ability to pronate and supinate or "feather" a stiff, rigid paddle while swimming, resulting in potential exhaustion from wasted energy. The folding fin design eliminates the need for pronation and supination, allowing water to flow past the device during arm retrieval and then flare back open during the power stroke. This action conserves energy and improves efficiency to the swimmer's stroke, modulating resistance and improving stroke volume for increased control, propulsion, and speed in the water. Both prostheses can be modified easily to conform to the surface area and displacement of the swimmer's hand if that is a requirement for competition or a goal for therapy.

Weight Training and Conditioning

Many children born with a congenital hand absence or anomaly are faced with growing up while not being able to physically challenge their affected limb enough to stimulate balanced, upper extremity muscular and skeletal growth. With maturation to adolescence, they naturally are more self-conscious of body image, and many decide to become involved in upper extremity training regimes for strengthening and symmetry. Other individuals are challenged with traumatic hand loss and either wish to continue their pretrauma body conditioning and exercise activities or to begin exercise for therapeutic sports conditioning or body building reasons.

The weightlifting and conditioning prosthesis must have a secure, comfortable suspension, a carbon-reinforced socket and forearm and a well bonded-laminated wrist unit to ensure safe function. The prosthetist should consider a nontraditional

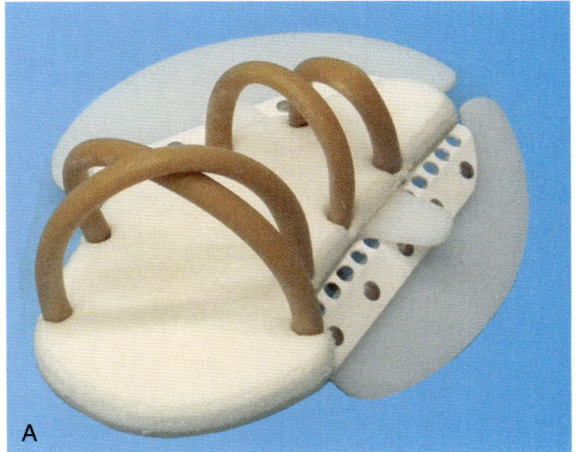 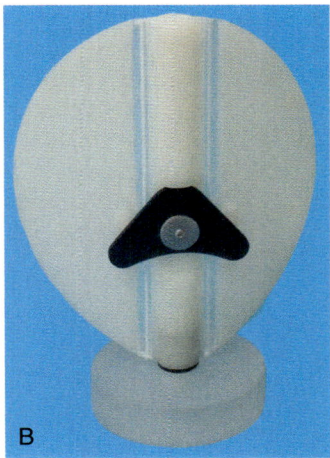

FIGURE 18 Clinical photograph illustrating FREESTYLE SWIM TD and SWIM FIN KIT. (Courtesy of Fillauer TRS, Inc.)

neutral or minimally preflexed alignment in the prosthesis to enhance control and performance for short- to medium-length trans-radial patients. A highly preflexed socket to forearm alignment will not perform well in these activities. A more neutral, less preflexed prosthesis will provide for better ROM and control over heavier weight loads. Wrist alignment should also be considered to optimize balancing heavier loads. New adjustable pressure sockets using BOA or similar socket adjustment technology can enhance the user's ability to safely perform in these activities and adjust their socket pressures to accommodate changes in their prosthetic suspension because of sweating or muscle volume changes during exercise.

There are multiple choices in prosthetic technology to help perform confidently and functionally in weightlifting, therapeutic resistance exercise training, and body building. Certain voluntary closing terminal devices such as the GRIP2S and GRIP3 (**Figure 19**) can be easily modified to be capable of locking around and onto weight machine handles, dumbbells, and barbells but they are not specifically designed for weightlifting. The GRIP 5 (**Figure 20**) combined with SURE-LOK cable locking technology also provides at lot of versatility in the gym but has limited capacity for handling heavy weights. The JAWS voluntary Opening TD (**Figure 21**) with adjustable tension also has application to many types of exercise equipment even though it was

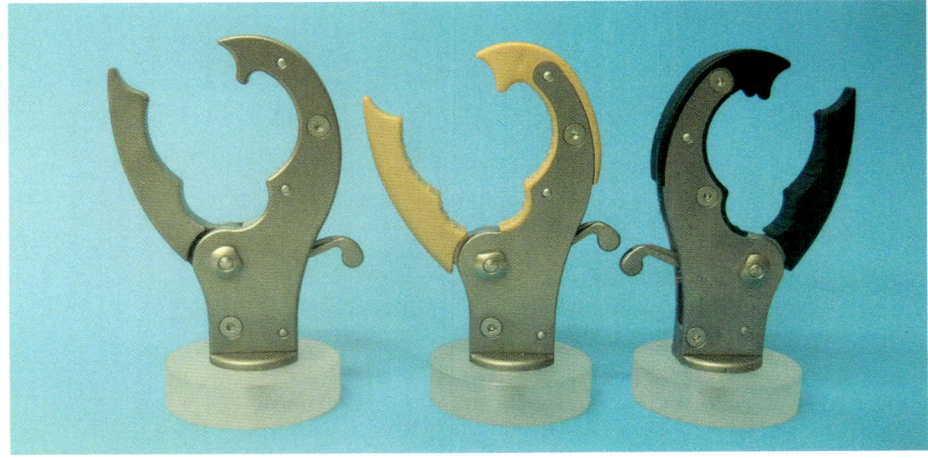

FIGURE 19 Clinical photograph illustrating GRIP 2S and GRIP 3 TDs (tan and black). (Courtesy of Fillauer TRS, Inc.)

Section 2: Upper Limb

originally designed for other activities. Devices such as the TRS BLACK IRON TRAINER or BLACK IRON MASTER (**Figure 22**) and the TAD WEIGHTLIFTING DEVICE (**Figure 23**) are specifically designed to take on the rigors of training with free weights and cable-actuated stack-weight exercise machines, as well as other types of exercise equipment. These devices provide stable platforms for controlling heavier weights through a wide range of motions and body zones. The BLACK IRON MASTER is capable of Olympic level competition and was successfully used in breaking a world bench pressing record of more than 650 lb.[17] The colorful, BLACK IRON LITE TDs (**Figure 22**) introduced in 2013 by TRS provide a sporty-looking alternative for lightweight aerobic style dumbbell conditioning and similar lightweight gym exercise. The user should work initially with a professional exercise trainer or therapist to ensure that proper and safe posture and exercise techniques are executed and maintained.

Archery and Bowhunting

Archery and bowhunting involve either using the prosthesis for drawing the string and releasing the arrow, or holding and stabilizing the bow. Two factors that will impact how the prosthesis is used are hand and eye dominance. Certain individuals can master shooting a bow with the nondominant eye, but others cannot. A person missing a left hand with right eye dominance can shoot right-handed using the prosthesis to hold the bow. The same individual with a left eye dominance must shoot like a right hander or switch to a left-handed bow and draw the string with the prosthesis. An individual with a right-hand absence and right eye dominance can shoot right-handed and draw the bow with the prosthesis or be forced to shoot left-handed holding the bow with the prosthesis and use the nondominant eye for sighting. A voluntary closing prehensor such as the GRIP 2 or GRIP 3 has the physical configuration to capture the riser-handle of virtually any bow and a simple lock pin or

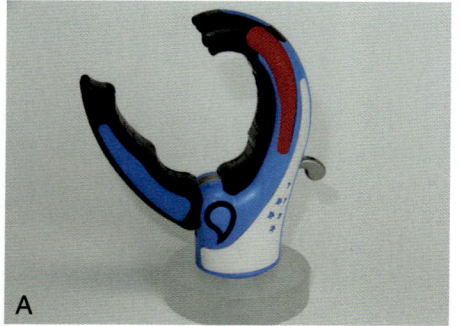
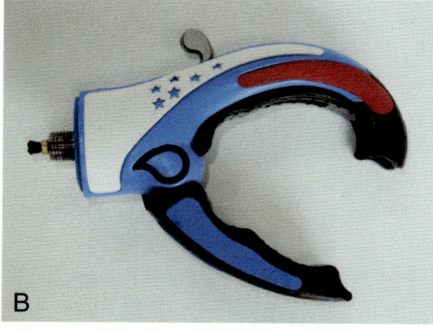

FIGURE 20 **A** and **B**, Clinical photographs illustrating GRIP 5. (Courtesy of Fillauer TRS, Inc.)

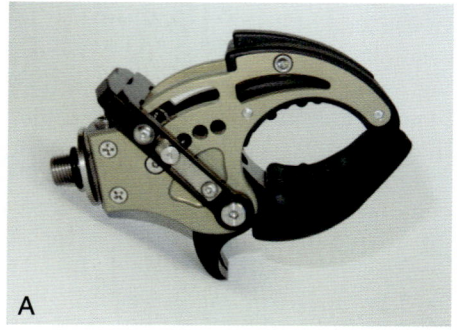
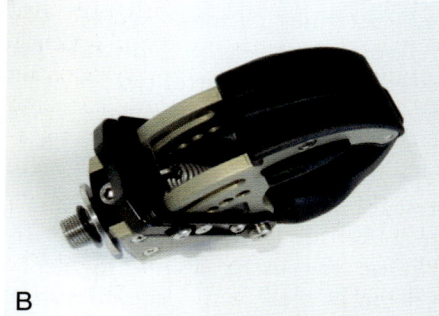

FIGURE 21 **A** and **B**, Clinical photographs illustrating JAWS. (Courtesy of Fillauer TRS, Inc.)

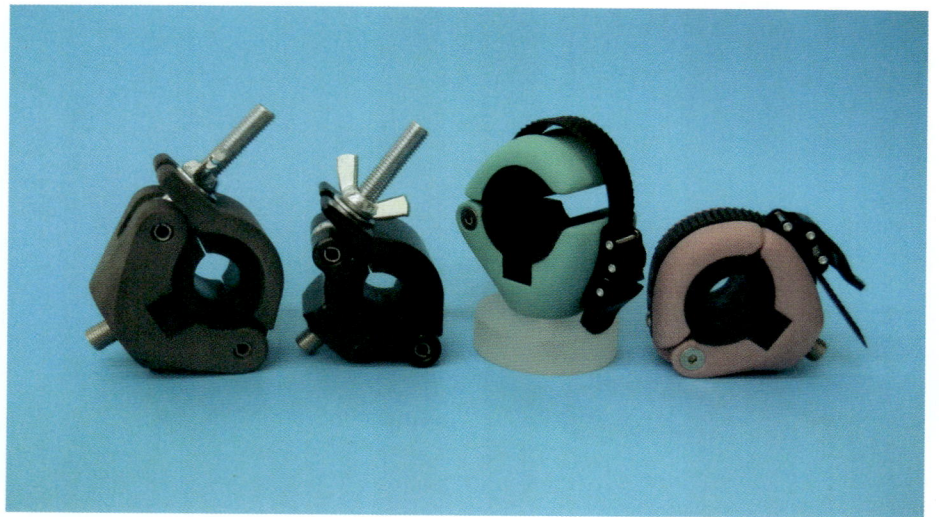

FIGURE 22 Clinical photograph illustrating BLACK IRON MASTER, BLACK IRON TRAINER, and BLACK IRON LITE (aqua and pink) TDs. (Courtesy of Fillauer TRS, Inc.)

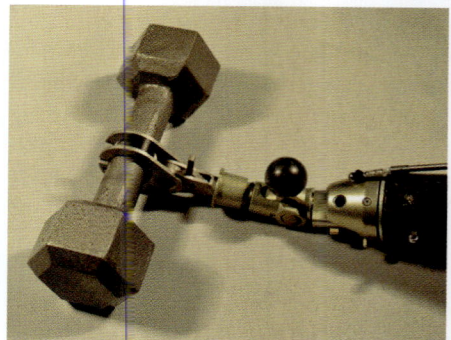

FIGURE 23 Clinical photograph of forearm prosthesis illustrating Texas Assistive Device's (TAD) WEIGHTLIFTING DEVICE. (Courtesy of TAD.)

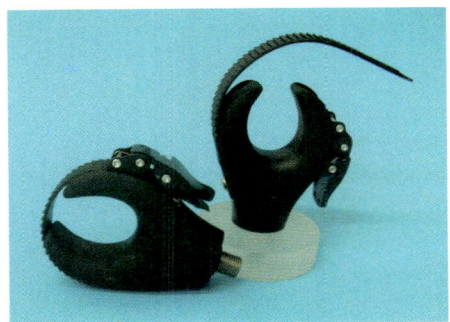

FIGURE 24 Clinical photograph illustrating TRS ISHI Archery TD. (Courtesy of Fillauer TRS, Inc.)

another more complex locking system can be used to eliminate the need for conscious, continuous, prosthetic cable tension while shooting. In most cases padding the handle with soft and durable, compressible material helps to create a better gripping platform for more accurate bow control and improved arrow flight. A tight or rigid grip on the bow is counterproductive to accurately shooting an arrow.

The ISHI ARCHERY TD (**Figure 24**) was introduced in 2013 specifically for holding and shooting a bow. The ISHI is designed for either left- or right-handed use and has a special offset aperture-receiver that helps the bow align properly in the prosthesis during the string draw phase of the shooting cycle. Two models with different strengths and flexibilities are available to meet the needs of those with different shooting needs. A ratchet strap system secures the bow to the prosthesis within two flexible, polymer "mandible-like," clasping elements, allowing the bow's handle to "center" itself for proper alignment during the string draw and release phase of shooting.

The TAD QUICK RELEASE GRIPPER (archery trigger) (**Figure 25**) is especially designed for capturing, drawing, and releasing the bow string. The adapter uses an integrated trigger that is actuated by pressing a side-mounted lever against the jaw or cheek to release the string. The design is consistent with established and reliable trigger releases widely used in the sport by two-handed archers and bowhunters.

The downside to any prosthetic device designed very narrowly to meet the needs of a specific activity such as holding a bow or bow string is that it limits the user's ability to perform other activities that might require two-handed competence. In cases where this may be a dilemma, such as bowhunting, it could be preferable to use a more versatile terminal device such as a voluntary closing (V/C) prehensor (TRS GRIP 2 or GRIP 3),[5] rather than to restrict the prosthesis function or force the user to carry and interchange additional, alternative prosthetic adapters.

Archery is one activity where an externally powered myo-electric hand prosthesis can be used. The opposed thumb and forefinger gripping configuration of a myo-electric hand prosthesis lends itself to holding a bow in a natural manner.

Fishing

Fishing, like golf, has challenges related to hand dominance and hand absence. Certain fishing reel and rod systems are designed to function with a left-hand retrieve, while others have a right-hand retrieve. Some types of reels are convertible to either right- or left-hand retrieve. The prosthesis can be used for the function of reeling with a normal reel handle if the terminal device can create enough controlled prehension (grip) throughout the reeling cycle. Split hook prostheses that are held closed by elastic bands or springs are typically not capable of reliably controlling and operating the reel handle. They tend to pry or slip off. A voluntary closing prehensor such as a TRS GRIP 2S, GRIP 3, or GRIP 5 (**Figures 19, 20, and 26**) enables the user to create enough gripping force to control reel handles of a variety of shapes and sizes. Sometimes it is valuable to reshape the reel handle or pad the handle with compressible, high-friction material to create a better surface for securely grasping and controlling the handle.

Holding the rod in the sound hand and reeling with the prosthesis is a functional and versatile way to fish because handling the rod properly is enhanced by having a functional wrist and hand. Specialized prosthetic reeling adaptations such as TAD's ALL PURPOSE CRANK ADAPTOR (**Figure 27**) are an alternative to using a standard terminal device such as the GRIP TDs mentioned above.

If the preference is to hold the rod with the prosthesis, there are a few alternatives. TRS's F~ISHI (**Figure 28**) is designed to easily grasp and clamp around a fishing rod handle. The flexible polymer body simulates a radial-ulnar

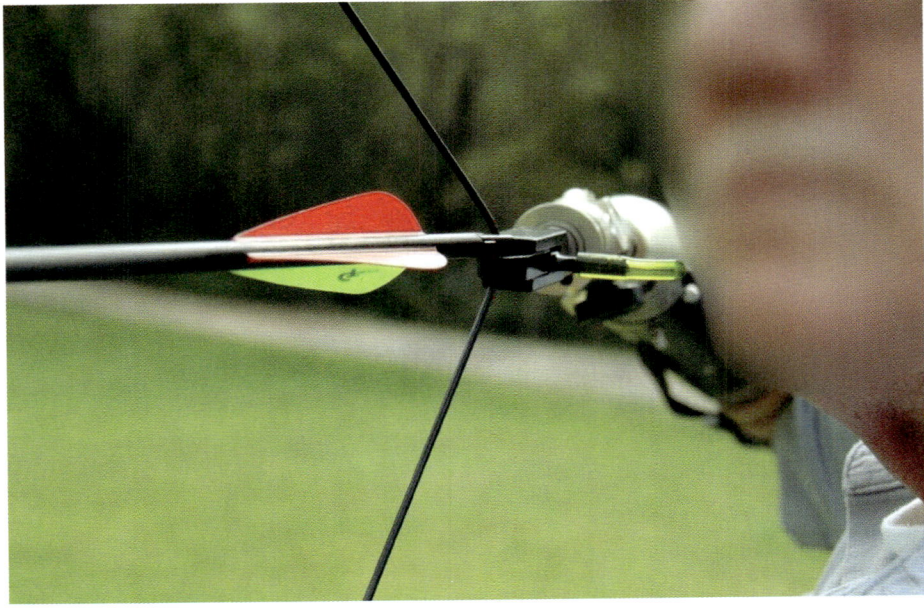

FIGURE 25 Clinical photograph of forearm prosthesis illustrating Texas Assistive Device's (TAD) ARCHERY QUICK RELEASE ADAPTER. (Courtesy of TAD.)

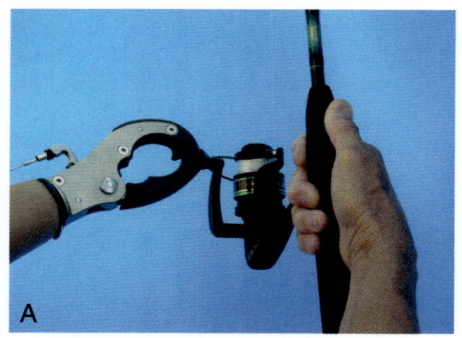
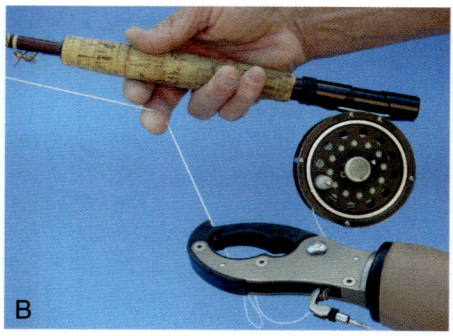
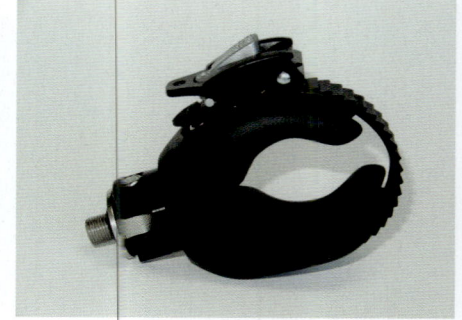

FIGURE 26 **A** and **B**, Clinical photographs of forearm prosthesis illustrating TRS GRIP 3 with spinning and fly-fishing gear. (Courtesy of Fillauer TRS, Inc.)

FIGURE 29 Clinical photograph illustrating TRS MULTI D PIVOT TD. (Courtesy of Fillauer TRS, Inc.)

type wrist action when the rod and line are "under-load," creating a "feeling" and type of feedback much like having a normal wrist. The Multi-D (**Figure 29**) is a larger, more robust version that can be used for heaver tackle and saltwater fishing. Texas Assistive Device's (TAD) prosthetic FISHING ROD is another alternative designed to allow the rod to be directly connected into the prosthesis or interim wrist component. A third option is one of TAD's UNIVERSAL HANDLE HOLDERS (**Figure 30**) that can be used to capture and support the rod near the reel.

Additive manufacturing technology is providing the ability for some anglers to create their own custom solutions. Recently, when a single-handed angler and avid fisher-lady was not satisfied with the prosthetic technology available for the rugged salt-water angling that she enjoys, she partnered up with a friend with CAD design experience and produced a custom fishing pole control system using additive manufacturing techniques that successfully meets her needs. This is an example of how additive manufacturing may augment the prosthetic needs for persons needing custom prosthetic solutions for activity-specific pursuits in the future (**Figure 31**).

Myoelectric or externally powered hands and TDs can handle a rod and reel also, but because of the water environment and chance of immersion, these types of technologies are not often used for fishing.

Fly fishing offers extra challenges to the person with a hand absence because of the complexity of handling the fly line while casting and retrieving. The rod must be controlled by the sound hand and arm for accurate casting. A prosthesis equipped with a TRS GRIP 3 (**Figure 26**) has been shown to be capable of handling the delicate line in a wet environment for line retrieval and reeling. Automatic retrieve fly reels will bring in slack line, but they are not capable of manipulating the retrieve of a wet fly or strong enough to bring in a fish without the assistance of another hand or prosthetic device like the GRIP 3. Electric retrieve fishing reels in both spinning and casting models, that have rechargeable battery packs, are available for those with more severe upper extremity involvement.

Canoeing, Kayaking, Paddling, Crew

The first commercially available prosthetic device for kayaking, the HAMMERHEAD, now HAMMERHEAD PIVOT (**Figure 32**) was developed in the mid-2000s by TRS at the request of rehabilitation personnel at Walter Reed Hospital. Walter Reed was expanding the therapy challenges for soldiers returning from wars in the Middle East. Kayaking was being pursued because of its therapeutic value for strengthening core, shoulder, and arm musculature, and helping to improve ROM, as well as for expanding the general recreational opportunities for soldiers undergoing rehabilitation.

Activities such as canoeing, kayaking, and rowing require the user to perform a wide range of gross motor upper body movements while controlling and powering an oar or paddle through the water. The Hammerhead was designed to replicate the degrees of freedom required to handle a paddle and control it efficiently, thus creating propulsion. Certain terminal devices such as TRS's GRIP 3 were capable of handling oars and paddles but the

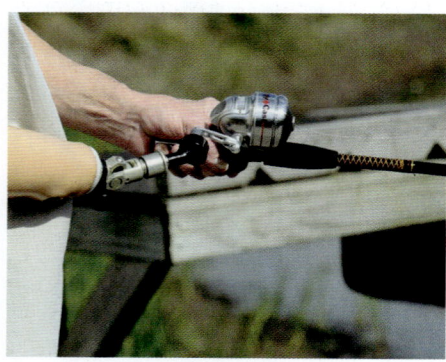
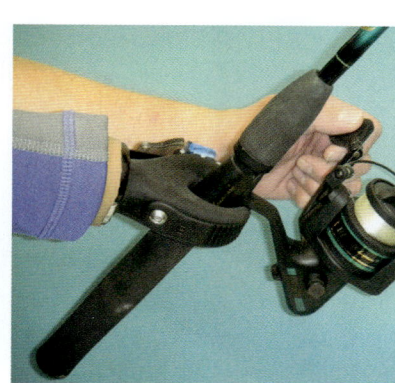

FIGURE 27 Clinical photograph of forearm prosthesis illustrating Texas Assistive Device's (TAD) ALL PURPOSE CRANK ADAPTER for fishing. (Courtesy of TAD.)

FIGURE 28 Clinical photograph of forearm prosthesis illustrating TRS F~ISHI TD Fishing device. (Courtesy of Fillauer TRS, Inc.)

Chapter 27: Upper Limb Adaptive Prostheses for Vocation and Recreation

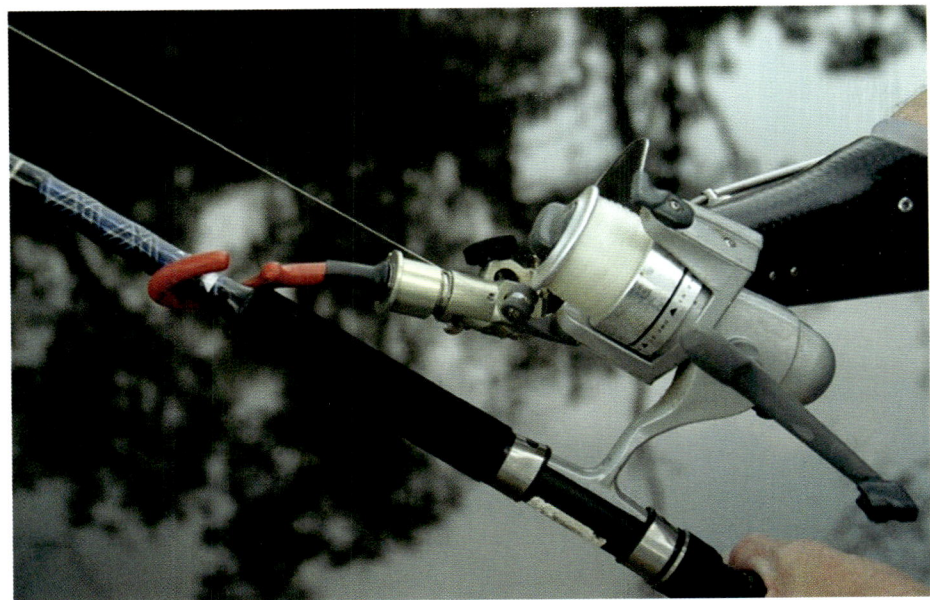

FIGURE 30 Clinical photograph of forearm prosthesis illustrating Texas Assistive Device's (TAD) UNIVERSAL HANDLE HOLDERS. (Courtesy of TAD.)

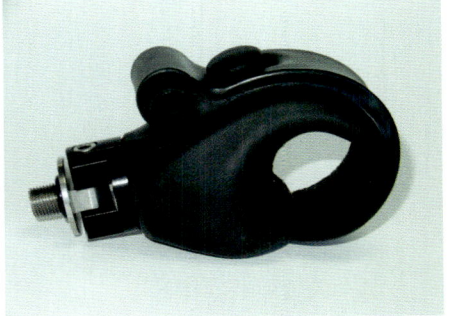

FIGURE 32 Clinical photograph illustrating TRS HAMMERHEAD PIVOT TD. (Courtesy of Fillauer TRS, Inc.)

"activity-specific" HAMMERHEAD provided improved function and enhanced performance because of its ROM and flexible energy capture and release capability, mimicking the human wrist and forearm.

Canoeing requires a unique set of paddle handle and paddle shaft grasping demands, different from kayaking, that involve alternating hands and grasp patterns to power, paddle, and propel the canoe from either the port or starboard side. The HAMMERHEAD works well for handling the shaft aspect of the paddle but does not conform to the delta-shaped handle end. It cannot be used in the traditional way of paddling a canoe but still performs the activity by capturing the shaft below the end of the paddle handle.

Crew and other rowing water sports use oars rather than paddles. Oar handles are typically larger in diameter than paddle handles and some oars have convex-curved gripping areas that can provide additional holding challenges for someone with a prosthesis. The TRS MULITI-D PIVOT adaptive device (**Figure 29**) was created to address the design challenge of these larger diameter handles. A quick-release ratchet strap system securely controls the tension of two flexible, polymer "mandibles" that wrap around and tension down on the oar handle. A variety of diameter handles for both sports and vocational activities are possible to control with this adjustable adapter. The Multi-D evolved to be another true "crossover" TD that is used for controlling a variety of shafts and tool handles, lifting light-weight dumbbells, etc.

Externally powered prostheses usually are not applied to these types of activities because of the rugged usage and surface wear that they would experience, the limited degrees of freedom they provide while holding an oar, and because of the water environment that would compromise or destroy the internal electronic elements of this type of technology.

Hockey

Hockey is a sport requiring quick reflexes combined with significant gross motor upper extremity movements and the need to control a hockey stick with precision. Rigidly attaching a stick to the prosthesis is ineffective and dangerous because of the forces involved that could easily break a prosthetic wearer's lower arm, elbow, or humerus during a fall or impact. Several adaptive prosthetic devices allow for safe and effective control of the hockey stick. The TRS SLAP SHOT devices[5] and POWER PLAY[5] (**Figure 33**) offer options for "top-handing" or "shaft-handling" the hockey stick. The SLAP SHOTS employs a high-strength, flexible coupling to allow for articulation at the wrist; while the POWER PLAY is constructed entirely from high-performance polyurethane and is a top stick design only. The HELIX TD, discussed earlier in this chapter, has also proven to function well for

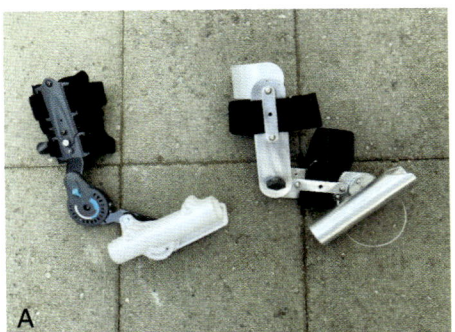
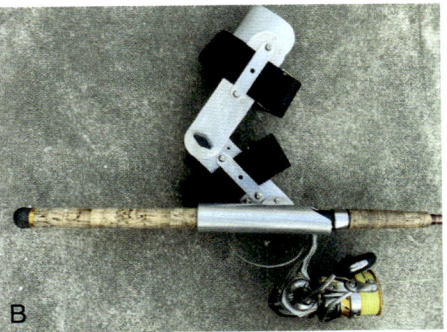

FIGURE 31 **A** and **B**, Clinical photographs of forearm hybrid prosthesis illustrating custom fishing pole control system using additive manufacturing techniques. (Courtesy of Joanne Tilley.)

Atlas of Amputations and Limb Deficiencies, Fifth Edition

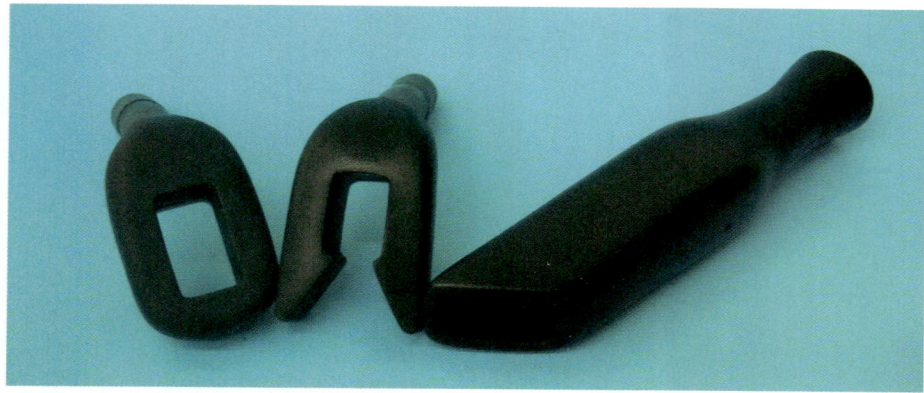

FIGURE 33 Clinical photograph illustrating TRS SLAP SHOTS AND POWER PLAY TDs. (Courtesy of Fillauer TRS, Inc.)

shaft stick handling providing a lot of control yet having enough flexibility to be used safely. A variety of custom prosthetic adapters have evolved over the years as well, with many of those designs understandably originating in Canada. CHAMP, the Canadian magazine published by The War Amps of Canada, has featured many of these unique "one-off" custom hockey adapters.

Snow Skiing, Water Skiing, and Trekking

Highly specialized activities such as downhill (Alpine) and cross-country (Nordic) skiing are challenging. A secure grasp is required on the ski pole and in Nordic skiing the upper body is highly involved for propulsion of the skier over the snow. Using a prosthesis to control a pole while downhill skiing also can aid balance and maneuvering through moguls and rough terrain or varying snow conditions. Three commercially available devices exist for snow skiing. Fillauer produces the Hosmer SKI/FISH Terminal Device or HAND (**Figure 34**) and TRS creates the SKI 2 (**Figure 35**) and the DOWNHILL RACER TD (DHR) (**Figure 36**). The devices vary in design, providing different levels of function and performance. However, the normal grip handle on the ski pole is removed for all of them.

The Hosmer SKI HAND is a one-piece, molded silicone, fist-shaped device into which the ski pole is force fit. The pole is inserted almost vertically in the SKI HAND and the flexible silicone allows for the pole to be snapped forward using its weight for momentum through a pendulum-type action initiated by the forearm and elbow.

The pole held in the SKI 2 mechanically pivots on the end of the prosthesis and can be either activated with a pendulum thrust of the arm or, more preferably, cable driven for an accurate, controlled pole "plant." The advantage of the cable excursion technology is that it eliminates needless upper body

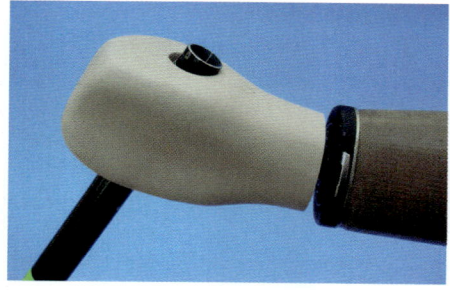

FIGURE 34 Clinical photograph of forearm prosthesis illustrating HOSMER SKI and FISH HAND with ski pole. (Courtesy of Fillauer.)

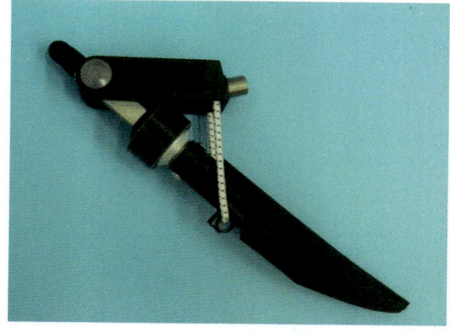

FIGURE 35 Clinical photograph illustrating TRS SKI 2 TD. (Courtesy of Fillauer TRS, Inc.)

movement allowing for improved, balanced downhill skiing form. While Nordic skiing, the cable drive provides for more efficient pole extension and placement while propelling the skier on flat terrain or while climbing. The pole remains slightly retracted to clear the snow when cable tension is relaxed. The SKI 2 system also operates well with standard hiking poles for persons wishing to hike in steeper terrain or those who just wish to engage more upper extremity involvement into their general hiking activities.

The DHR is constructed from a high-strength but flexible polymer. The ski pole snaps into and out of the DHR. The pole is covered with a protective cap. The system is designed in both right and left versions so that pole release is always away from the skier's midline off to one side or the other. The pole is held in a fixed angular position for snow clearance and has been typically used for slalom racing skiing, although it has other applications in skiing and for hiking-trekking poles.

Mountaineering and Technical Rock Climbing

Prosthetic adaptations for technical climbing, whether in natural outdoor environments or indoor gyms have traditionally been totally custom built (**Figure 37**) by TRS Inc. These designs incorporate standard technical rock-climbing hardware such as Ice Picks, Leepers, Sky Hooks, and Ficas onto a custom pedestal that mounts securely to the prosthesis. TRS has modified the GRIP 2SS, voluntary closing device, into a rock-climbing device by integrating a modified SKY HOOK (**Figure 38**) onto one side of the prehensor. This allows for almost 100% function of the prehensor, while providing a laterally mounted precision hook element for engaging and grasping rock "holds." The expanded interest in indoor and outdoor climbing has encouraged the development of the first standardized TD for climbing called the RAPTOR (**Figure 39**). The RAPTOR was developed with direct input from amputee climbers. It is a simple design with the profile of the

Chapter 27: Upper Limb Adaptive Prostheses for Vocation and Recreation

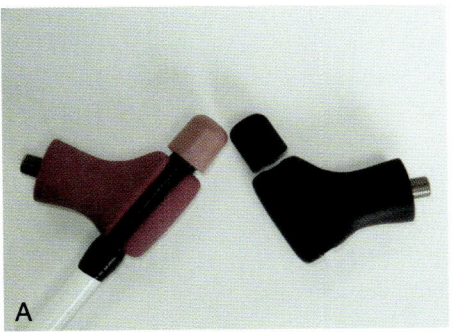
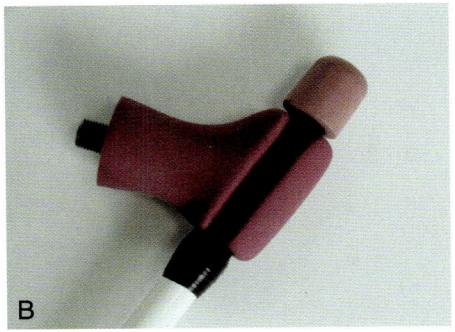

FIGURE 36 **A** and **B**, Clinical photographs illustrating DOWNHILL RACER TD (DHR) and ski pole. (Courtesy of Fillauer TRS, Inc.)

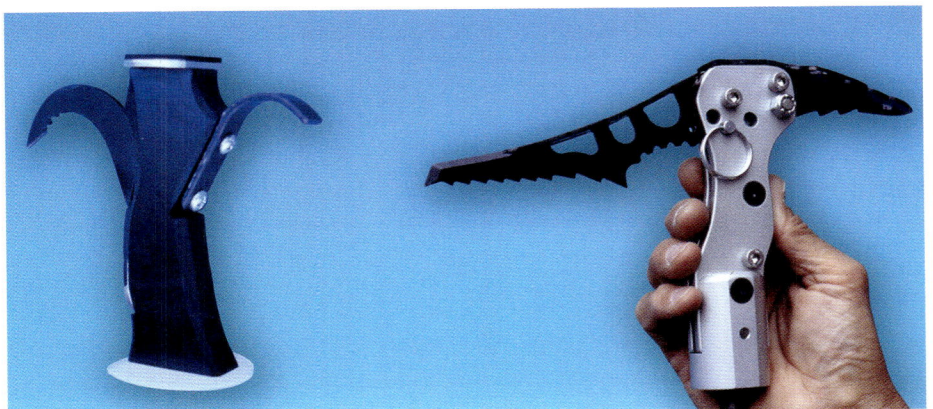

FIGURE 37 Clinical photograph illustrating TRS AR and HARD ROCK custom rock-climbing TDs. (Courtesy of Fillauer TRS, Inc.)

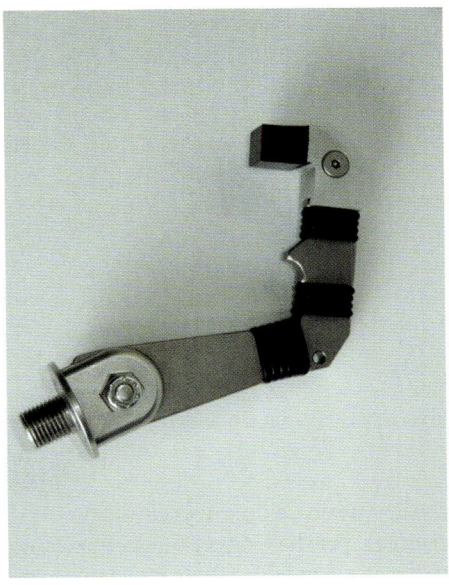

FIGURE 39 Clinical photograph illustrating RAPTOR. (Courtesy of Fillauer TRS, Inc.)

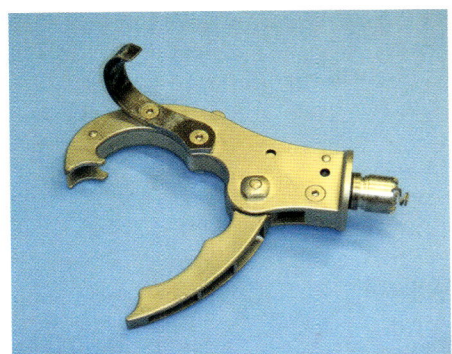

FIGURE 38 Clinical photograph illustrating TRS SKY HOOK TD. (Courtesy of Fillauer TRS, Inc.)

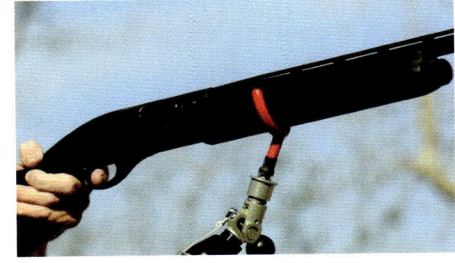

FIGURE 40 Clinical photograph of forearm prosthesis illustrating Texas Assistive Device's (TAD) Tool Cradle for firearms. (Courtesy of TAD.)

number "7" that enables grasping over ledges. Machined from titanium, the narrow profile allows for insertion into narrow cracks without sacrificing strength. The RAPTOR has available replaceable tips made of different materials to meet different climber's preferences or environmental conditions. Climbing is a dangerous activity with a high risk of injury and death and must always be approached with caution. The prosthetist must be aware of the liability and legal exposure involved when providing climbing prostheses to patient-consumers.

Firearms and Shooting

Holding, stabilizing, and firing of a rifle, shotgun, or carbine with a prosthesis is possible, and several prosthetic devices have been designed explicitly for such activity. TAD builds three variations of a rubber-coated TOOL CRADLE (**Figure 40**) that are used to support the fore end, forearm, or front stock portion of a rifle, shotgun, or crossbow. One version of the TOOL CRADLE pivots for improved firearm balance and control. TRS manufactures the LAMPREY GUN TURRET (**Figure 41**), an adapter that securely grasps the gun's stock with a flexible yoke system that is mounted to a pivoting lockable ball and socket system for versatility in bench target shooting, trap, and skeet competitions or hunting. The LAMPREY allows the shooter to swing the firearm above shoulder level without losing control over the gun. Both the TOOL CRADLE and LAMPREY GUN TURRET were designed because of requests and needs of soldiers at Walter Reed Hospital for safer, more functional, and versatile firearms-handling prosthetic adapters.

Pistol shooting can be safely accomplished using an appropriate prosthetic device such as a GRIP 3 or GRIP 5, where the shooter has conscious control over the pistol grip. Oversized rubber pistol grips can help enhance control over a

© 2024 American Academy of Orthopaedic Surgeons

Atlas of Amputations and Limb Deficiencies, Fifth Edition

357

pistol. Handling and cocking the slide on a semiautomatic pistol can be a challenge that must be practiced. Prostheses are rarely, if ever, used for pulling the trigger of any firearm because of the lack of touch and feel that is required for safe firearm operation. Revolvers are a good alternative to semiautomatic pistols because safeties and firing mechanisms are less complicated and easier to deal with using a prosthesis. It must be emphasized that handling and firing a pistol, one-handed, using just a prosthesis is not a simple technological problem and probably cannot be accomplished without combining electronic elements with mechanical controls. A proven solution to this challenge does not exist to the authors' knowledge.

Road and Mountain Bicycling

Bicyclists must be able to securely and quickly manipulate handlebars, brake levers, and gear-shift controls for performance road or mountain biking pursuits. Terminal devices such as the GRIP 3 and JAWS Prehensor have proved valuable in these applications, although they are not specifically designed for bicycling. A nonactivity-specific prehensor has the advantage of functioning for other activities such as changing punctured tires and conducting other bicycle repair functions as may be required. Modern bicycle technology and accessories for gear shifting and braking are compact and offer multiple control modalities such as thumb paddles, levers, twist grips, and even electronic shifting options to help meet the needs of a person with a hand absence or limited hand function. These technologies can be individually selected and combined to provide for optimum safe performance and control.

Specialized adaptive prosthetic technology for bicycling has been available since the early 2000s and has since evolved. The TRS CRITERIUM PIVOT is available in two size models with several options for engaging the handlebars (**Figure 42**). The devices use strong, flexible, molded, polyurethane available in two flexibilities to

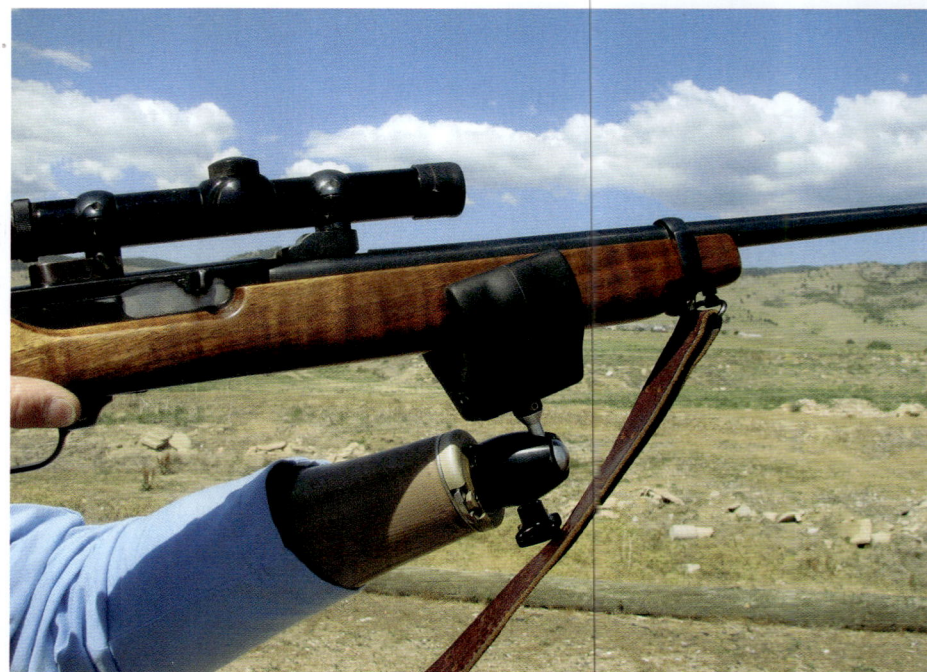

FIGURE 41 Clinical photograph of forearm prosthesis illustrating TRS LAMPREY GUN TURRET. (Courtesy of Fillauer TRS, Inc.)

create "snap on and off" handlebar components. The CRITERIUM TDs are designed primarily for road biking and will not function satisfactorily during the rigors of mountain or trail biking. The TRS MOUNTAIN MASTER (**Figure 43**) is designed specifically for mountain biking and combines a handlebar-mounted pedestal with a flexible snap-on-over TD. The system provides for shock absorption and handlebar control but still allows the TD to be pulled up and off the pedestal for dismount and safety. Other soft external features on the device aid in carrying the bike and/or balancing on the handlebars. A DUAL BIKE BRAKE LEVER system that was initially developed for tandem bicycles controls two brake cables simultaneously and is a good option for riding with a prosthesis. Additionally, new design hydraulic bike brakes are very compact and can be "ganged" together on one side and controlled with the fingers of a single hand.

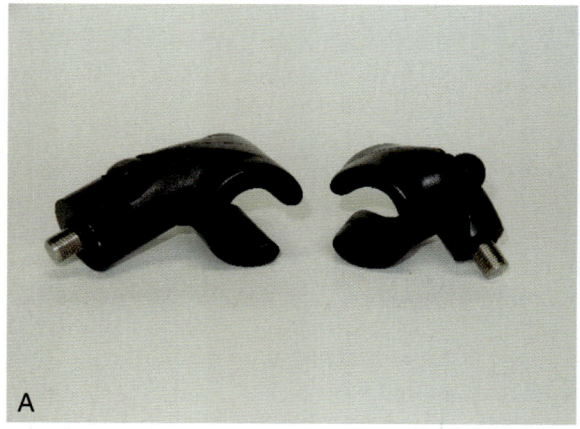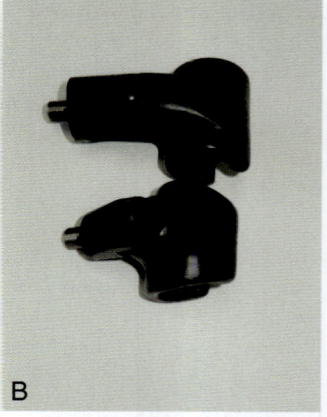

FIGURE 42 A and **B**, Clinical photographs illustrating TRS CRITERIUM PIVOT and CRITERIUM PIVOT SHORT TDs. (Courtesy of Fillauer TRS, Inc.)

Clustering all the controls to one side for operation with a sound hand simplifies bicycling. The prosthesis is then used primarily for handlebar control, balance, and steering.

Another very sophisticated, highly engineered bicycle control system is the MERT LAWILL BICYCLE RIDING HAND. This technology features a specialized ball-ended terminal device that snaps in and out of an adjustable releasable handlebar-mounted socket.

Motorcycling, Off-Highway Vehicles (OHVs), and Motor Vehicle Control

Vehicle steering, gear shifting, and overall, general, motor vehicle control requires secure gripping capability and, in many instances, quick reflexive release action. Voluntary opening split hook prostheses have proved inadequate when applied to most vehicle control circumstances because the terminal device cannot provide reliable prehension during varying vehicle control situations. Myo-electric hands and electromechanical TDs are functional for general automobile and motorcycle operation but are not as useful or reliable for off-highway and recreational vehicle control. Body-powered, voluntary closing prehensors, such as the GRIP 3 and voluntary opening JAWS Prehensor, have been proven to provide the type of reflexive grasp and release action and gripping forces necessary to handle auto-driving situations, motorcycling, bicycling, and off-road vehicle control. Typically, the brake, clutch, and gear-shifting controls need to be grouped or ganged together for single-handed or foot-assisted operation, leaving the prosthesis to be used primarily for handlebar and steering control.

Wrestling and Martial Arts

Interest and adaptations for wrestling or martial arts using a prosthesis are limited. The TRS DRAGON TD (**Figure 44**) has been developed specially to try to meet the needs of these intimate contact sports using a prosthesis. Designed to emulate the shape of a curled fist, the soft, flexible, polyurethane material absorbs the shock of

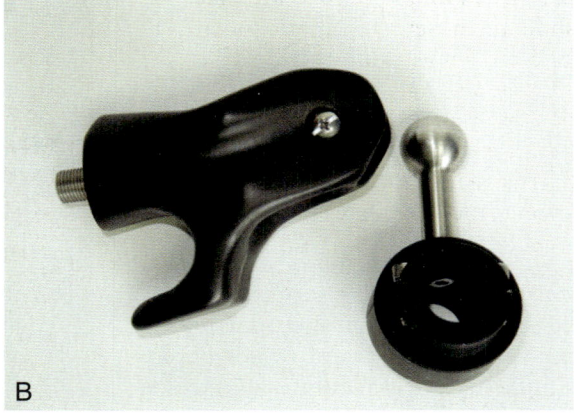

FIGURE 43 **A** and **B**, Clinical photographs illustrating MOUNTAIN MASTER. (Courtesy of Fillauer TRS, Inc.)

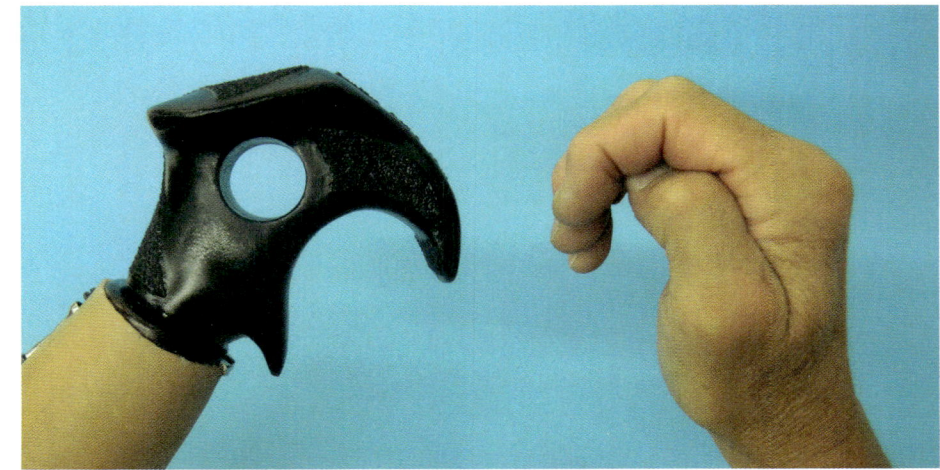

FIGURE 44 Clinical photograph of forearm prosthesis illustrating TRS DRAGON TD. (Courtesy of Fillauer TRS, Inc.)

punches and yet has a high enough friction coefficient to enhance grappling with an opponent. Interestingly, the DRAGON has evolved as a very functional tool for wheelchair propulsion because it can withstand the forces and highly abrasive contact with the wheelchair's pusher rims and wheels.

Equestrian Sports

A variety of prosthetic devices, including both voluntary opening and voluntary closing body-powered TDs and myo-electric hands, can be used for controlling reins for riding horses and other equestrian pursuits. No specific adapters have been commercialized specifically for these types of activities. TRS has built a few customized adapters specifically for "calf roping" (**Figure 45**) that are designed to capture a series of rope coils, freeing the terminal device to hold and control the reins while the sound hand is used for tossing the lasso.

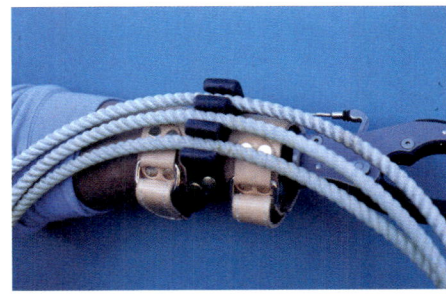

FIGURE 45 Clinical photograph of forearm prosthesis illustrating TRS custom calf roping prosthesis. (Courtesy of Fillauer TRS, Inc.)

Section 2: Upper Limb

Musical Instrument Adapters

Commercially available musical instrument prosthetic adapters such as the TRS GUITAR PICK ADAPTER, DRUMSTICK ADAPTER, and VIOLIN BOW ADAPTER (**Figure 46**) have been widely used to help initiate novices into the world of musical instruments or provide experienced musicians with the opportunity to begin regaining their instrument playing skills. These adaptive devices are simple mechanical solutions attempting to duplicate the subtle wrist and forearm biomechanical movements required to accurately play these instruments. In most instances it is advantageous to mount the terminal device as close to the end of the limb as possible for improved control and enhanced proprioceptive biofeedback. A special short prosthesis can accomplish this objective or attach the musical instrument adapter directly to a roll-on style, silicone or similar locking liner is another viable option.

Miscellaneous Specialty Prosthetic Adapters

Adaptive prostheses have also successfully solved very specialized activity needs. The TRS AMP-U-POD Camera mount, HUSTLER pool and billiards shooting TD, and ROCKY MOUNTAIN HIGH SKIP ROPE adapter system (**Figure 47**) provide answers to those with a hand absence wishing to indulge in these pursuits.

Partial Hand

Partial hand absence and/or limited hand function have always been a design challenge when fabricating prostheses. TAD (**Figure 48**) introduced the innovative, N-Abler Wrist-Hand Orthosis (WHO) in 2003 after receiving encouragement from professionals at a national occupational therapy conference. The WHO system provides a viable solution for reliably mounting adaptive prostheses to the partial or disabled hand. Tools and domestic implements or sports accessories can be readily connected and disconnected into the WHO technology. Another alternative is the TRS PROCUFF system (**Figure 49**), which is a *prosthosis* that mounts onto the forearm behind the wrist. The PROCUFF uses a BOA closure. Unlike the TAD WHO brace system it has no thumb hole and does not provide wrist support. The PROCUFF is designed to accept tools and implements as well as other adaptive sports and recreational attachments. The PROCUFF comes as a basic "platform" that the prosthetist needs to reinforce and custom fit to the user's needs and can be fit to both pediatric and adult cohorts. In similar fashion, the TRS VC-VO

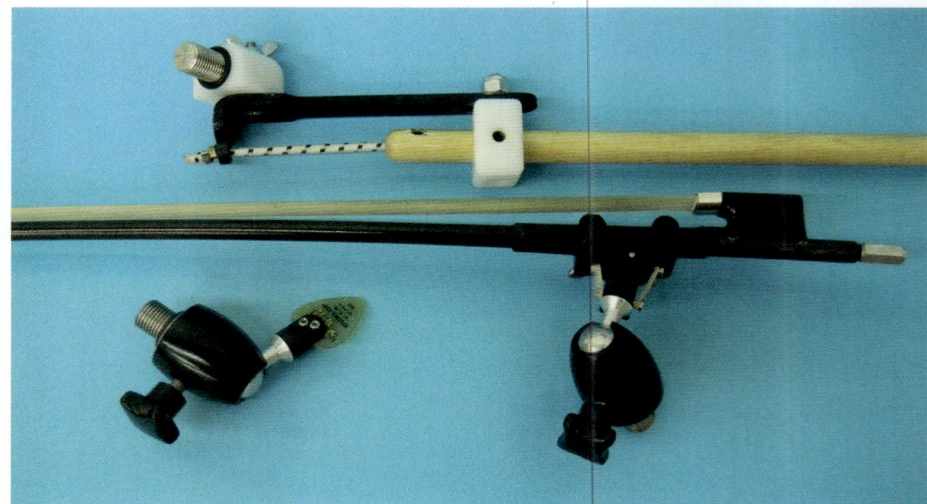

FIGURE 46 Clinical photograph illustrating TRS Drumstick, Violin Bow, and Guitar Pick adapters. (Courtesy of Fillauer TRS, Inc.)

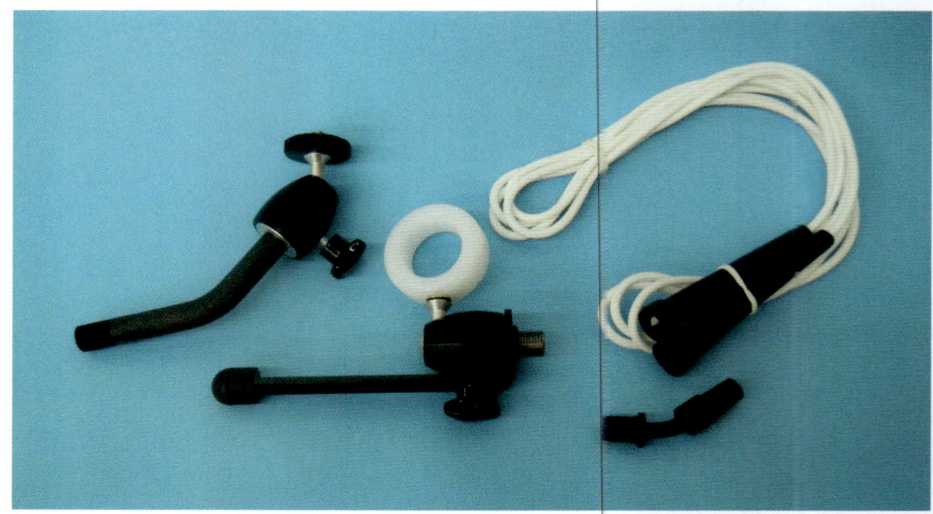

FIGURE 47 Clinical photograph illustrating TRS AMP-U-POD, HUSTLER, and ROCKY MOUNTAIN HIGH Skip Rope adapters. (Courtesy of Fillauer TRS, Inc.)

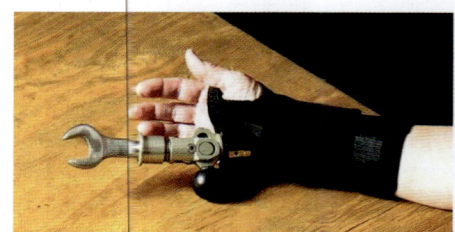

FIGURE 48 Clinical photograph of forearm hybrid prosthosis illustrating Texas Assistive Device's (TAD) N-Abler WHO prosthesis. (Courtesy of TAD.)

BODY POWERED SIMULATOR has been used to offer *prosthosis* support to a person with partial hand absence or functional loss.[20]

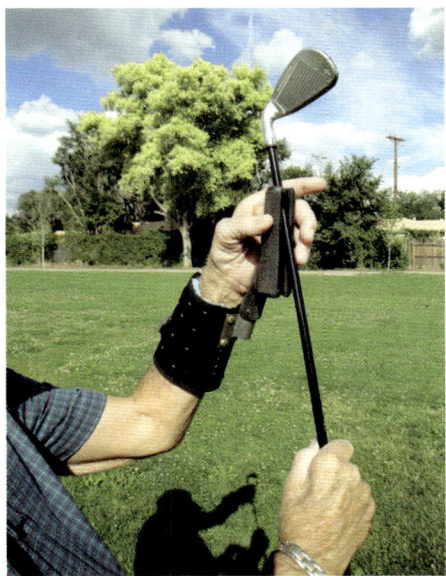

FIGURE 49 Clinical photograph illustrating TRS PRO CUFF "prosthesis." (Courtesy of Fillauer TRS, Inc.)

SUMMARY

Adaptive or activity-specific prostheses have developed in type, number, sophistication, and popularity since the 1980s. A variety of factors have influenced the growth of this segment of prosthetic technology. These influences include the contributions of specific individuals including prosthetic consumers, companies, the military, adaptive sports organizations and programs, medical and rehabilitation professionals, the media, and the general explosion of worldwide communications and consumerism via the internet. Additionally, changes made in the HCPCS and the DMECS directly impacted the justification and credibility for prescribing specialized, upper extremity adaptive prosthetic components. These adaptive prostheses can satisfy a wide range of needs including both vocational and avocational (recreational) challenges. Many devices are "crossover" technologies performing well in multiple activities spanning the gap between vocational and avocational activities and challenges. Placing a design emphasis on duplicating biomechanical function and increasing the ROM in upper extremity prostheses has significantly enhanced the ability of users to participate and compete in a variety of activities that were difficult or impossible to achieve "bilaterally" in the past. A wide variety of direct attachment tools, domestic use implements, and sports and recreational adapters are now standardized and commercially available. Adaptive solutions continue to steadily evolve. Additive manufacturing will most likely help expand the development of individualized solutions for persons with a hand absence. These evolving prosthetic technologies are enhancing prosthetic user's functional, bilateral capabilities. Adaptive prostheses improve patients' rehabilitation potential and significantly increase their performance in vocational and recreational activities that were not accessible previously. Adaptive activity-specific components are excellent compliments to externally powered "myo-electric" type prostheses. More economical adaptive components enable users to select the best, most cost-effective prostheses to employ for the task or activity at hand, extending the life of more expensive bionic prostheses. The profession should expect that the current success of adaptive prostheses will continue to drive the evolution, development, and popularity of these types of technology into the future.

Acknowledgment

The authors would like to thank and acknowledge the contributions of key individuals who have been involved in the development of activity-specific upper extremity prosthetic technology, not otherwise named in the chapter's text. These include prosthetic professionals, inventor-designers, consumers, and consumer families who include, but are not limited to, Randy Alley, Chris Baschuk, Andrew Carter, S. Crowley Family, Robert Gabourie, Ron Farquharson, N. Howard Family, Michael Hummel, Will Mills Family, Hector Picard, J. Peterson Family, John Miguelez, Aron Ralston, Dave Rotter, Johnnie Rouse, Jon Sedor, and Gerald Stark. Without their creativity, perseverance, interest, input, testing, and evaluation efforts, this technology would not exist and be readily available in the profession today.

References

1. Miguelez JM: Personal conversation with B Radocy regarding activity-specific prosthesis, 1997.
2. Sheppard J: Robin aids. *Can J Occup Ther* 1956;23(2):69-71.
3. Radocy B: Upper-extremity prosthetics: Considerations and designs for sports and recreation. *Clin Prosthet Orthot* 1987;11:131-153.
4. Radocy B: Upper-limb prosthetic adaptations for sports and recreation, in Bowker JH, Michael JW, eds: *Atlas of Limb Prosthetics: Surgical, Prosthetic, and Rehabilitation Principles*, ed 2. Academy of Orthopaedic Surgeons, 2002, pp 325-344. (Originally published by Mosby-Year Book, 1992.).
5. Radocy R: Prosthetic adaptations in competitive sports and recreation, in Smith DG, Michael JW, Bowker JH, eds: *Atlas of Amputations and Limb Deficiencies: Surgical, Prosthetic, and Rehabilitation Principles*, ed 3. Academy of Orthopaedic Surgeons, 2004, pp 327-338.
6. Radocy R: Upper limb prosthetics for sports and recreation, in Lenhart MK, ed: *Textbooks of Military Medicine: Care of the Combat Amputee*, Office of the Surgeon General. Department of the Army, 2009, pp 641-668.
7. Atkins DJ: Adult upper limb prosthetic training, in Atkins DJ, Meier RH, eds: *Comprehensive Management of the Upper-Limb Amputee*. Springer-Verlag New York Inc., 1989, pp 39-59.
8. Radocy R, Furlong A: Recreation and sports adaptations, in Meier RH, Atkins DJ, eds: *Functional Restoration of Adults and Children With Upper Extremity Amputation*. Demos Medical Publishing, Inc., 2004, pp 251-274.
9. Baumgartner R: Physiotherapie und ergotherapie, in Baumgartner R, Botta P, eds: *Amputation und Prosthesenversorgung der oberen Exremitat*. Ferdinand Enke Verlag Stuttgart, 1997, pp 249-290.
10. Latour D: Upper extremity prosthetics, in Jacobs ML, Austin N eds: *Orthotic Intervention for the Hand and Upper Extremity: Splinting Principles and Process*. Wolters Kluwer, 2021, pp 150-176.
11. Latour D, Vacek K: Upper extremity prosthetics, in Coppard B, Lohman H, eds: *Introduction to Orthotics*. Elsevier, 2019, pp 461-481.
12. Murray CD: Being like everybody else: The personal meanings of being a prosthesis user. *Disabil Rehabil* 2009;31:573-581.

13. Miguelez JM, Lake C, Conyers D, Zenie J: The Transradial Anatomically Contoured (TRAC) interface: Design principles and methodology, technologies and applied research. *J Prosthet Orthot* 2003;15(4):148-157.
14. ACCI, Anatomically Contoured and Controlled Interface: *Alley RD Exploring the Functional Performance of Interface Design*. Clinical Matter, O and P Business News June 15, 2003, pp 30-33.
15. Farley M: *High Fidelity Interface, Farley M, High-Fi Flies HIGH in New Prosthetic Interface, Tissue Compression/ Release Concept Gains Control*. The O & P EDGE, 2010, pp 38-44.
16. In pictures: Prosthetics through time 2012. Available at: http://www.bbc.co.uk/news/health-16599006. Accessed July 1, 2021.
17. Hummel M: World Class Bench Press Record. Available at: www.powerliftingwatch.com/node/9839. Accessed July 1, 2021.
18. Murray CD: The social meanings of prosthesis use. *J Health Psychol* 2005;10(3):425-441.
19. Latour D: *Impact of bilateral upper limb prosthesis simulators in pre-prosthetic training: A case study*, in Oral Presentation at the American Orthotics and Prosthetics Association (AOPA) Annual Conference September, 2016, Boston, MA. https://www.aopanet.org/wp-content/uploads/2016/07/Friday-Poster-Presentations.pdf. Accessed September 27, 2022.
20. Latour D, Delgado C: *Use of prosthesis simulator to create body-powered prosthosis for functional needs*, in Oral Presentation at the Association of Children's Prosthetic and Orthotic Clinics (ACPOC) Annual Conference May 3, 2019, Clearwater, FL. https://www.aopanet.org/education/13072-2/poster-presentations/. Accessed September 27, 2022.

Functional Aesthetic Prostheses: Upper Limb

CHAPTER 28

Matthew J. Mikosz, CP, LP • Kim Doolan, BS

ABSTRACT

A successful prosthetic outcome is best achieved by balancing the elements of form and function. For individuals with congenital or acquired upper limb difference, prostheses that incorporate active or passive function can be indicated to enhance vocational, avocational, and psychological rehabilitation. Aesthetic restorations can take the form of lifelike appearance, mimicking the lost anatomy, or pursue the opposite approach of drawing attention to the novel possession of a mechanical prosthesis as part of one's new body image.

Keywords: finger prosthesis; partial hand prosthesis; passive prosthesis; psychological considerations; upper limb prosthesis

Introduction

The importance of both the appearance and function of aesthetic prostheses are well documented, although not always consistently discussed with the individual who has an amputation or limb deficiency.[1-11] In the past, this term referred almost exclusively to custom silicone prostheses or custom silicone coverings for mechanical hands. These were made to resemble the missing part of the upper limb in size, shape, and coloring. The highest quality solutions for such lifelike aesthetic restorations continue to be made of silicone because of its versatility and compatibility with human tissue.[4,10,12,13] However, the criteria for an "aesthetic" appearance have greatly expanded over the past decade, to include surface features that in no way resemble human skin. Beauty, in this case, is truly "in the eyes of the beholder".

Recent changes have occurred in public perception and patient demand with respect to the ideal appearances of a prosthesis. Simultaneously, manufacturers have chosen to move away, at times, from making devices that "look real," to making the devices have more functional grasping abilities, and incorporating features that make no attempt to resemble human skin. Although custom silicone restorations still feature prominently in the pantheon of what are considered "aesthetic" solutions among prosthetic devices, they are now joined by devices with customized surface characteristics that draw attention to, rather than away from, the fact that the person is wearing a prosthesis. A comprehensive treatment should consider the associated aesthetic implications, focusing on a patient's ultimate acceptance and integration of their prosthesis.[12]

History

In the 1950s, French physician Jean Pillet noted that the loss of a single digit could profoundly affect an individual's body image, self-esteem, and psychological status.[8] Pillet established clinics around the world and pioneered the use of silicone prostheses that were sculpted and painted to match the characteristics of individual patients. Two decades later, Horst Buckner developed a new fabrication method to cover conventional prosthetic components, such as mechanical and electric hands, with lifelike silicone skin.[14]

As attitudes toward what defines functional aesthetic prostheses have changed, so have the materials, fabrication, and application techniques. In the 20th century, aesthetic functional prostheses were divided into two categories. The first was considered "high definition," in which a great deal of time was spent in accurately duplicating the human appearance. The second was considered "low definition," which was less costly and less realistic in appearance. Now, in the 21st century, more restoration options can be added using custom artwork, three-dimensional (3D) scanning, hydrographic films, and other technologies.

Neither of the following authors nor any immediate family member has received anything of value from or has stock or stock options held in a commercial company or institution related directly or indirectly to the subject of this chapter: Matthew J. Mikosz and Kim Doolan.

This chapter is adapted from Passero T, Doolan K: Functional aesthetic prostheses, in Krajbich JI, Pinzur MS, Potter BK, Stevens PM, eds: *Atlas of Amputations and Limb Deficiencies: Surgical, Prosthetic, and Rehabilitation Principles*, ed 4. American Academy of Orthopaedic Surgeons, 2016, pp 379-387.

Function Associated With Oppositional Prostheses

For individuals who have had an upper limb amputation, the term function is often associated with grasp. However, activities that do not require active manipulation, including static prehension, support, stabilization, pushing, pulling, transferring proprioceptive inputs, and nonverbal communication, are extremely important.[3,5,7,11,15-17]

A Dutch study divided the function of cosmesis or aesthetics into three categories: passive cosmesis (the appearance of the device), the cosmesis of wearing (the naturalness with which the individual who has had an amputation wears the device), and the cosmesis of use (the naturalness with which the individual who has had an amputation uses the device).[11] The appearance of the prosthesis carries subtle psychosocial implications. An aesthetic prosthesis balances the active and passive functional characteristics of the residual limb. For some wearers, the appearance of the sound side is duplicated; for others, the mechanical or robotic look of the prosthesis is emphasized.

Historically, the prosthetic management of finger and partial hand amputations was largely disregarded because of reduced prosthetic options resulting from space limitations. However, because the thumb and fingers comprise 90% of human arm function, the loss of one or more fingers can have a substantial effect on hand function.[15] A single aesthetic prosthesis for an index finger actively functions in prehensile activities such as writing, grasping small objects, and typing on a keyboard[7] (**Figure 1**). For a hand without a thumb or forefinger, even a nonmobile partial hand prosthesis provides opposition to the remaining fingers. For those with unilateral total hand amputation, an aesthetic, nonmobile functional hand prosthesis provides opposition to the sound hand while performing bimanual activities and aids with nonmanipulative tasks.

Individuals with more proximal upper limb amputations can take advantage of the entire surface of an oppositional prosthesis because its use is not limited to the terminal device. It is common to see a prosthesis user stabilizing a book against the forearm, sandwiching a grocery bag between their hip and the prosthesis, or pushing up from a chair by placing weight against the elbow componentry of the device. Fraser[1] noted that fewer than 25% of individuals used a terminal device for active manipulation, which can be overly emphasized as a determinant for good prosthetic use.

Psychological Considerations

Because hand use is so important to humans, people with upper limb loss or difference usually face more scrutiny from those around them than do people with lower limb loss or difference, who can easily conceal their prostheses. Just as there are variations in an individual's level of amputation, culture, vocation, avocational interests, sex, age, socioeconomic profile, and life stage, there are also varied psychologic responses to upper limb deficiency and amputation. An individual's reaction to limb loss or difference does not necessarily correlate to the level of amputation.[1] Those reactions are also very likely to change over time and, for many, follow a similar course to the feelings of grief experienced after the death of a loved one.

Most often, someone with a new amputation or parents of a child with congenital limb difference prefer a prosthesis that greatly resembles the appearance of the missing body part. These prostheses allow the wearer to blend in and use the device without being seen as "other." Within this spectrum, individuals face the phenomenon of the "uncanny valley," a term used to describe the feelings of repulsion and rejection that are elicited by devices that approach, but ultimately fall short of human-like appearance.[18] Frequently, as prosthesis users incorporate changes into an altered body image they may become more open to differently designed, less lifelike prostheses that meet other functional needs.

An alternate reaction that is becoming more common, especially in the United States, is for a person with limb loss or difference to choose a prosthesis with a mechanical or robotic appearance. This represents an opposing aesthetic need of the individual who has had an amputation recently to show that the changed state of their upper limb has become part of their new body image.

It is important to remember that the psychological considerations experienced by those affected by limb loss or difference are dynamic, with ever-changing requirements and desires. As Dr. Pillet noted, "Often the disfigurement is more pronounced in the mind of the amputee than others. However, the man who finds himself unable to take his hand from his pocket, even though it is very 'functional', may be as handicapped as if it were lost."[8]

Rehabilitation Therapy

The need for rehabilitation therapy for individuals who have had an upper limb amputation must be recognized. Individuals with passive functional upper limb devices benefit from occupational and physical therapy. These therapies can improve overall body schema, strength, and the flexibility and range of motion of nearby joints. Therapies also reduce postoperative and phantom limb pain and help with desensitization, scar management, and edema control.

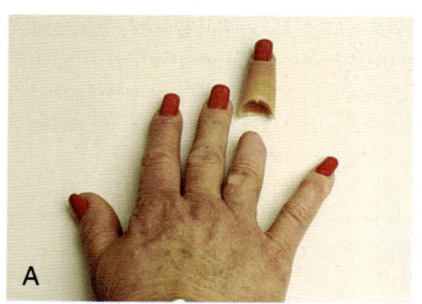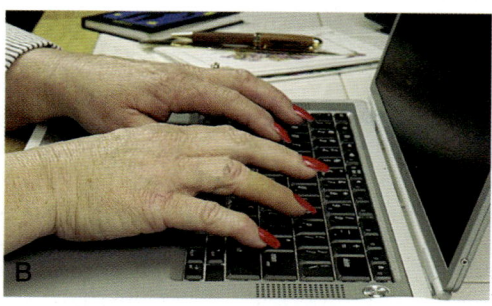

FIGURE 1 Photographs depicting a passive functional ring finger prosthesis while detached (**A**) and in use (**B**). (Courtesy of Össur.)

Often, therapy may be of greater value if the manipulation of small objects is deemphasized. Using the prosthesis in everyday situations involving supporting, stabilizing, pushing, pulling, holding, and facilitating balance can have better results.[1] Thus, training must not be limited to controlled prehension based on the erroneous assumption that fine motor activities require a terminal device. For a patient who has had a unilateral amputation, the prosthesis is typically used to assist with nondominant movements.[2]

van Lunteren et al[11] observed that many individuals who have had an amputation were taught direct grasp in clinical settings in which they used their terminal devices to pick up and hold an object. However, many users adopted indirect grasp approaches by picking up an object with their sound hand and transferring it to their terminal device. The individual who has had an amputation is best served by training protocols that teach not only targeted control of prosthetic componentry (terminal devices, wrists, elbows, and shoulders) but also the most efficient way to complete daily living, occupational, and avocational tasks (**Figure 2**).

Prosthetic Compliance

A prosthesis must be comfortable, functional, and have a pleasing appearance to be accepted and used by the individual who has had an amputation.[6] Other priorities include reduced weight, reasonable durability, ease of cleaning, and sufficient length of daily operation (up to 12 hours).[4] Individuals who have had an amputation also frequently request that the prosthesis have the correct benefit-to-burden ratio,[11] aligning the user's prosthesis with their current body image and preventing it from becoming an encumbrance.

Comprehensive prescription development should consider the importance of form and function to the patient. For most prosthetic solutions, this entails some level of compromise, trading elements of function for appearance and vice versa. Identifying the patient's priorities based on their anticipated use of the prosthetic device at home, work, and during recreational activities facilitates better understanding and, ultimately, acceptance of the necessary tradeoffs.[12]

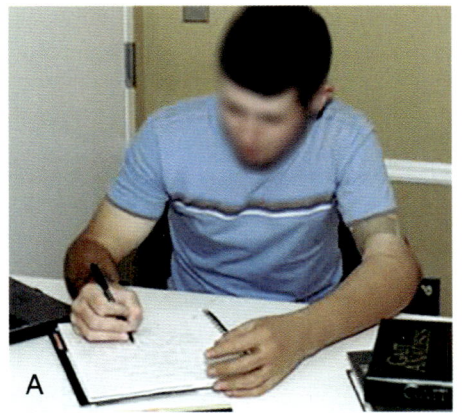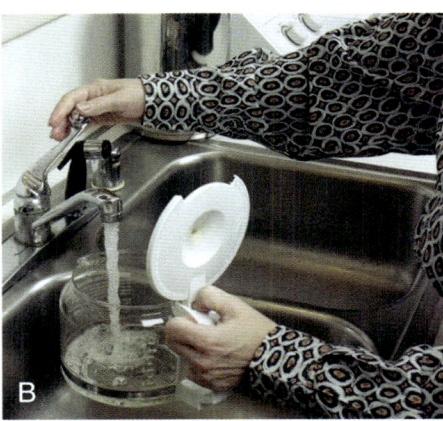

FIGURE 2 Photographs show upper limb prostheses with indirect grasp for stabilizing (**A**) and pulling (**B**).

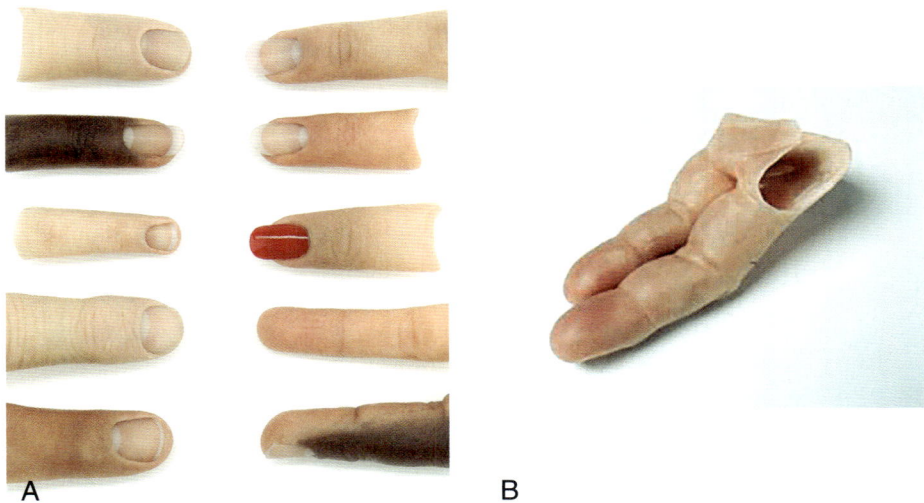

FIGURE 3 **A**, Photograph of finger prostheses for single digit loss. **B**, Photograph of a finger prosthesis for multiple digit loss. (Courtesy of Össur.)

Finger Amputation

Full and partial finger amputations are among the most frequently encountered forms of partial hand loss.[5] The benefits associated with restoration of digital amputations are well documented[7-9,19,20] and include a range of functional and psychological improvements, as well as appearance. The length of the residual finger is a primary consideration for several issues related to prosthetic design in a functional esthetic restoration. Other issues include the method of suspension (suction or mechanical), the length of the prosthesis (whether the proximal edge of the prosthesis terminates at the proximal interphalangeal or metacarpophalangeal [MCP] joint), the shape, the relative flexion of the finger joints, and the choice of a hard acrylic or soft silicone fingernail (**Figure 3, A**).

Although most digital prostheses are attached primarily using suction, osseointegration has demonstrated benefits, including increased pinch force and transfer of deep pressure sensation.[21] The risks of osseointegration include those commonly associated with other surgeries. This procedure is especially useful when the digital residuum length is insufficient to maintain acceptable retention. Additional methods of retention on short residual digits include the use of medical adhesives, incorporation of vacuum chambers in the distal portion of the prosthesis, and the use of adjacent fingers and rings to anchor the prosthesis to the hand (similar to a dental crown and bridge)[22] and of mechanical armatures (**Figure 3, B**).

Because suction is the primary means of suspension for most silicone finger prostheses, the residual digit must have sufficient length (minimum, 1.0 to 1.5 cm)[5,8] and appropriate shape (ideally, cylindric or bulbous). In contrast, a short length combined with a conical shape makes suspension unreliable, and the previously mentioned alternative retention methods can be used. If the involved hand has multiple short residual fingers, a glove design anchoring about the base of the hand may be needed to establish attachment and retention that is firm enough to withstand the force required to grasp and hold objects.

If the middle or distal phalanx of the involved digit has sufficient length and shape to adequately maintain suspension, a half-finger prosthesis is generally indicated. This prosthesis would terminate at the proximal interphalangeal joint, with a feathered proximal edge to minimize the transition between the silicone and the natural tissue and avoid limitations in joint range of motion. A full-finger prosthesis terminating at the MCP joint is recommended when the involved digit is at the level of the proximal phalanx or when the middle phalanx remains but has inadequate length. A full-finger prosthesis also can be used with a more distal level of amputation for activities that will generate substantial forces because the additional length increases leverage, providing better resistance to these forces. In either case, the termination, or transition of a full-finger prosthesis occurs at the base of the proximal phalanx or MCP joint. A ring can be used to enhance the attachment and minimize the transition line.

For distal fingertip amputations in which part of the nail/nail bed remains or the amputation is just at the base of the nail, a half-finger prosthesis is indicated. Because of the space requirements of the mounting mechanism, using an acrylic nail is often impossible; a silicone nail can be used instead. The disadvantages associated with silicone nails are that they cannot be painted and cannot be extended beyond the length of the fingertip.

Thumb Prostheses

Thumb prostheses present unique challenges because of the mobility and stability required of the prosthesis.[5] Given the presence of soft tissue in the web space between the thumb and index finger and the wide range of motion and substantial force generated during prehension, a full-length prosthesis is generally indicated to maintain adequate stability. For maximum stability, a glove-type partial hand prosthesis may be preferable. Osseointegration can be used effectively with a proximal thumb amputation (**Figure 4**).

Internal Armatures

In partial or full hand restorations, a semirigid internal armature can be incorporated into the fingers. The armatures stiffen the fingers and allow them to flex, pre-positioning them for specific tasks and providing additional functional capability. The armature adds a skeletal component to the flexible silicone of the prosthesis. The armature is often composed of braided stainless steel, but other materials can be used, provided they are durable enough to bend and rebend without breaking. The increased weight of the finished device with armatures is a consideration.

Partial Hand Prostheses

A partial hand prosthesis is indicated for acquired or congenital conditions that involve the total loss of one or more digits, either at the MCP joint or proximal to the metacarpal region.

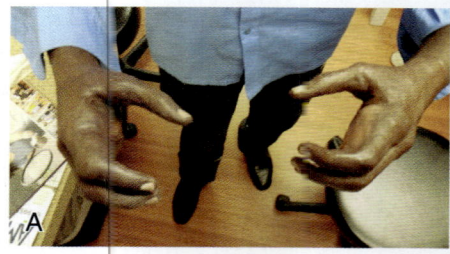

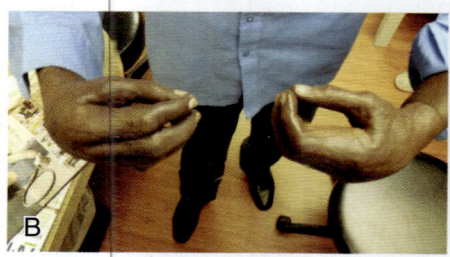

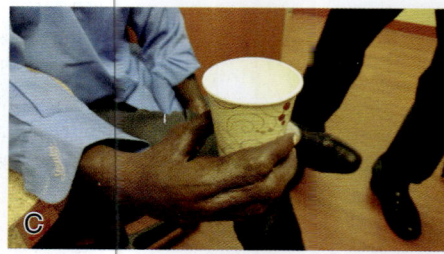

FIGURE 5 Photographs showing a novel bilateral partial hand presentation. The patient presented with bilateral preservation of a single metacarpal and full active wrist flexion. By mounting the aesthetic thumb restoration proximal to the wrist joint (**A**), wrist flexion brought the aesthetic finger restorations into functional opposition (**B**). This restored a measure of active opposition (**C**). (Courtesy of Phil Stevens, MEd, CPO, FAAOP.)

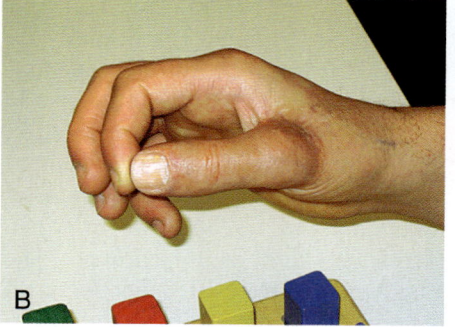

FIGURE 4 Photographs of an osseointegrated thumb prosthesis unattached (**A**) and attached (**B**). (Panel A reproduced with permission from Jönsson S, Caine-Winterberger K, Brånemark R: Osseointegration amputation prostheses on the upper limbs: Methods, prosthetics and rehabilitation. *Prosthet Orthotics Int* 2011;35[2]:190-200. © International Society for Prosthetics and Orthotics 2011. Panel B courtesy of Rickard Brånemark, MD, PhD, and Stewe Jönsson, CPO, Sweden.)

Depending on the presence of fingers or a thumb and their length and range of motion, the prosthesis is designed to maximize the active and passive functional potential of the involved hand and its appearance (**Figure 5**). The intended uses considered during the consultation phase of the process determine the eventual design. For passive silicone prostheses, proximal termination of the silicone usually occurs at an area where a watch or bracelet can be worn to minimize evidence of the transition to natural skin if it is necessary or preferred. Design options include exposing any residual digits that may be unable to oppose and grasp to preserve sensory input or containing them inside the prosthesis for improved esthetic appearance.

With the introduction of multiple mechanically and electromechanically powered fingers, active control of prosthetic finger position becomes possible (**Figure 6**). If desired, silicone skin can cover the plastic or metal digits to restore a natural appearance (**Figure 7**). Fully covering the articulating electronic finger with silicone may increase strain on the motors and gears and affect the function and range of motion of the finger. Mechanically operated fingers may be more difficult to operate if fully covered, as the silicone would provide resistance when the wearer attempts to flex the finger.

These issues should be discussed with the user before fitting so there are no unrealistic expectations of how the device will look once completed.

Full Hand Prostheses

Historically, the standard for aesthetic restoration of a full hand absence was a total oppositional silicone restoration (**Figure 8, A** and **B**). Over the past decade, roll-on suction liners with mechanical locking mechanisms have been used with increasing frequency for passive all-silicone total hand restorations.

In recent years, externally powered digits and multiarticulating total hand terminal devices have been introduced, and their use is increasing. These prostheses can be covered with thin, realistic-appearing silicone skin and can duplicate more characteristics of an intact human hand (**Figure 8, C**).

Transradial Prostheses

For a patient with a unilateral nondominant arm amputation, a passive, functional aesthetic prosthesis can provide adequate nongrasping function, acting as a helper to the intact, dominant hand. Where necessary, an endoskeletal pylon system overlaid with a contoured foam cover can span the gap between the prosthetic socket and the passive terminal device. Alternatively, aesthetic restoration is still possible when a mechanical or electromechanical hand is provided and covered with a custom silicone covering (**Figure 9**). The same technologic innovations that changed the options for individuals with partial and full hand amputations also have expanded the options for more proximal amputation levels. Smaller and more anatomically accurate shapes can now be incorporated into powered multiarticulating terminal devices that can be covered with the same type of custom silicone restoration to approach a more balanced combination of function and form.

Transhumeral and More Proximal Prostheses

A passive, transhumeral silicone prosthesis is often an acceptable option for more proximal amputations. The realistic appearance combined with the limited weight associated with this type of device make it a good alternative for individuals who have had a nondominant unilateral amputation. It is

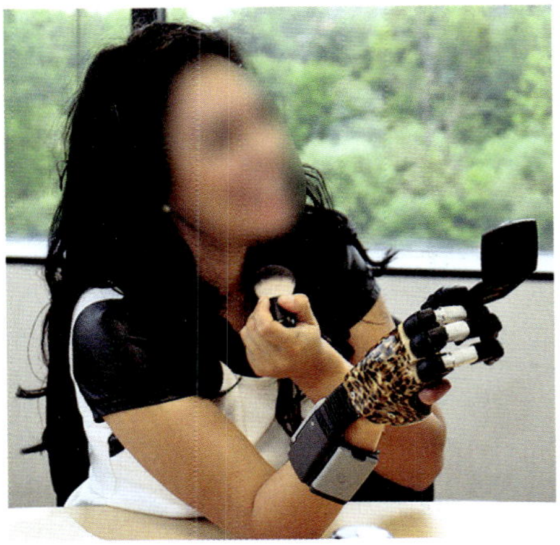

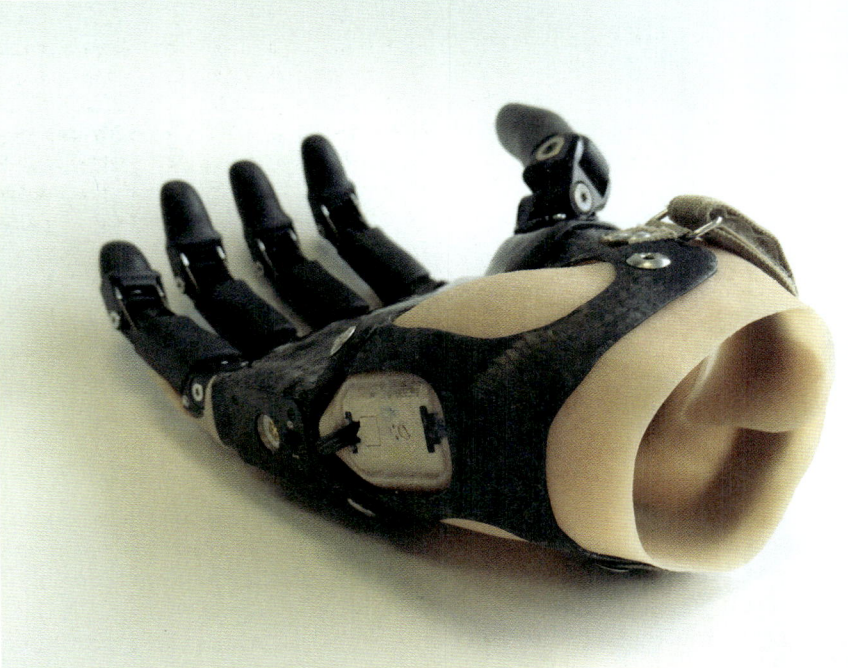

FIGURE 6 Photograph of an electromechanical prosthesis with an aesthetic appearance that is not lifelike. (Courtesy of Össur.)

FIGURE 7 Photograph of a partial hand prosthesis. (Courtesy of Pohlig, Traunstein, Germany.)

Section 2: Upper Limb

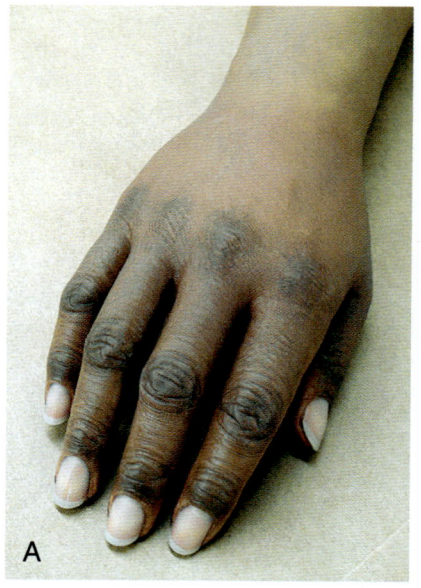
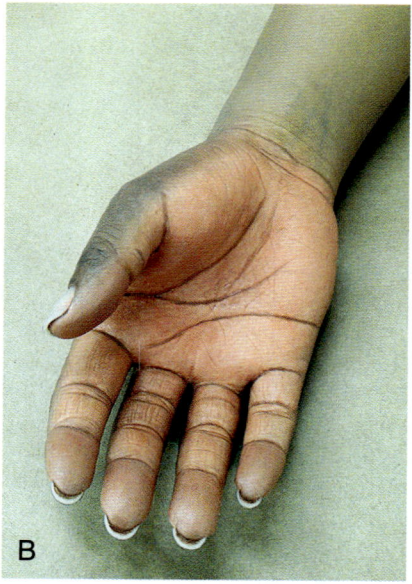
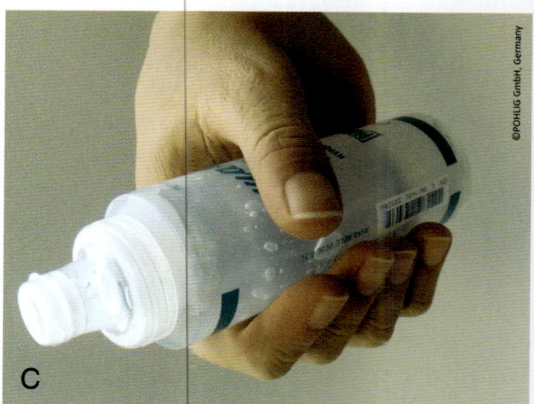

FIGURE 8 Photographs of a passive, functional full hand prosthesis with highly customized silicone restoration. **A**, Dorsal view. **B**, Palmar view. **C**, Photograph of an electromechanical full hand prosthesis with a highly customized silicone restoration. (Panels A and B courtesy of Alternative Prosthetic Services, Bridgeport, CT. Panel C, courtesy of Pohlig, Traunstein, Germany.)

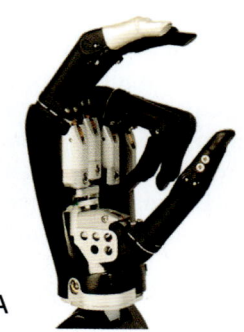
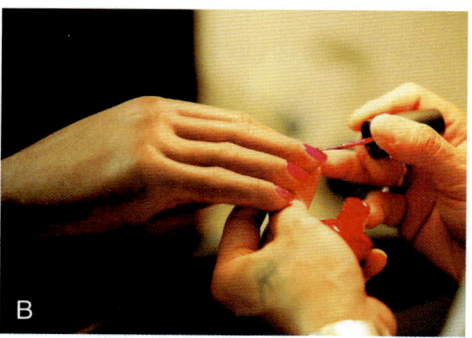

FIGURE 9 Photographs of an electromechanical hand uncovered (**A**) and with highly customized silicone restoration (**B**). (© 2023 Össur.)

not possible to cover a wrist, elbow, or shoulder joint that articulates, whether passively or otherwise, with silicone without unnatural distortion of the silicone occurring at the joint. Often, the aesthetic skin is discontinuous or terminated at the joint to minimize or eliminate this negative attribute.

Bilateral Involvement

Active unilateral or bilateral grasp can help individuals with bilateral upper limb involvement achieve a higher level of independence and supersedes the immediate need for aesthetic function. For the individual who has had a bilateral amputation, functional concerns outweigh aesthetic concerns because of substantial physical impairment, but aesthetic concerns are still important to these patients and require consideration.[8] Referring these patients to a rehabilitation team of physicians, prosthetists, occupational therapists, and psychotherapists who specialize in the treatment of bilateral upper limb amputation will help ensure the best possible outcomes while addressing aesthetic concerns.

Congenital Deficiencies

Childhood limb loss, whether congenital or acquired, is emotionally important, and coping is challenging for both the child and the child's family.[23] A child fitted with a prosthesis can appear more like other children, which can start the process of parental acceptance.[2,3,8,10] Prosthetic fitting at a young age can also encourage children to use their prostheses as they reach developmental milestones.[3]

Often, the types of prostheses fitted vary as children develop. Sometimes it is easier for infants to learn to control passive functional terminal devices. As children age, some may do better with myoelectric hands, whereas others prefer hooks or cable hands. Although prosthetic hands can limit children's activities after they begin school, they are often requested when children reach adolescence (**Figure 10**).

Enhancements

Nails

Fingernails that mimic human nails can be made from either a hard acrylic or softer, more flexible silicone material. The most realistic appearance is achieved using hard acrylic, which can be formed to match any nail in shape, length, and color, and also be painted with nail polish. Silicone or vinyl nails are soft and flexible, cannot be extended beyond the tip of the finger, and should not be painted with nail polish. Acrylic nails are most often used in finger prostheses for which the length of the residual finger is not an issue and in most partial and full hand passive functional

Chapter 28: Functional Aesthetic Prostheses: Upper Limb

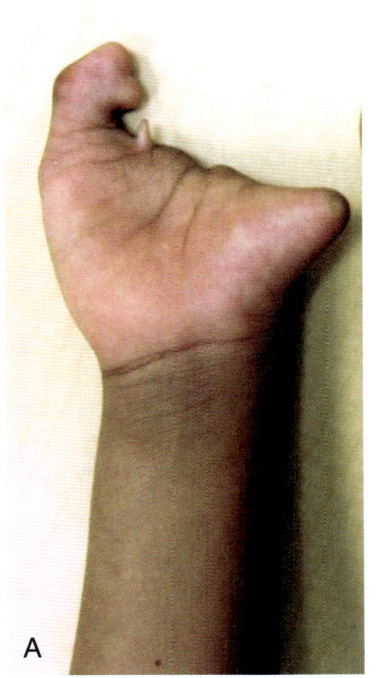 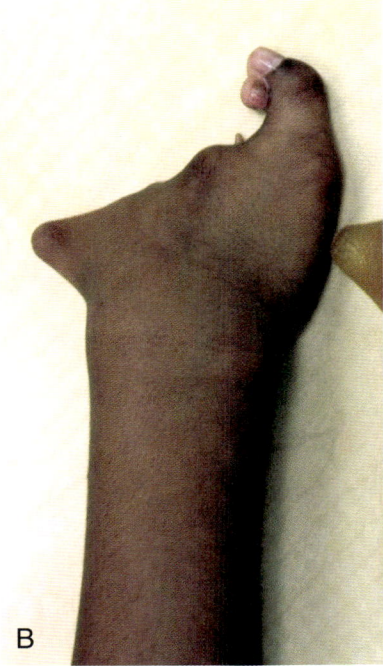 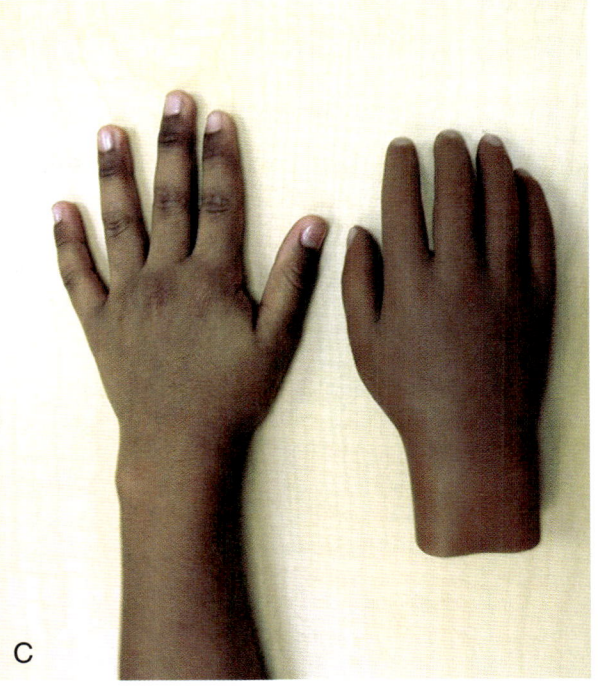

FIGURE 10 Photographs showing a congenital hand deficiency. **A**, Palmar view. **B**, Dorsal view. **C**, Photograph of a customized silicone restoration (right) and the contralateral hand (left).

restorations. For electric or mechanical devices, it may be more appropriate to exclude acrylic nails, which can become dislodged during strong grasping and/or impede fine motor grasping.

Hair and Surface Embellishments

In an individual with moderate or dense body hair, the appearance of the device may not be acceptable without an attempt to reproduce the hair, even in instances in which the color, shape, and texture of the prosthetic skin are a good match. Hair matching is accomplished by painting the illusion of hair into the silicone or by applying synthetic or human hair in/onto the skin in a pattern similar to that of the patient's skin. Tattoos, freckles, age spots, or prominent veining also can be added (**Figure 11**).

Skin Color

Human skin constantly changes colors, sometimes subtly or dramatically, and can be the result of external causes (such as sun tanning) or internal causes (such as capillary dilation). Unlike human skin, the colors of silicone and vinyl are static. When pigmented, these surfaces are carefully matched to the

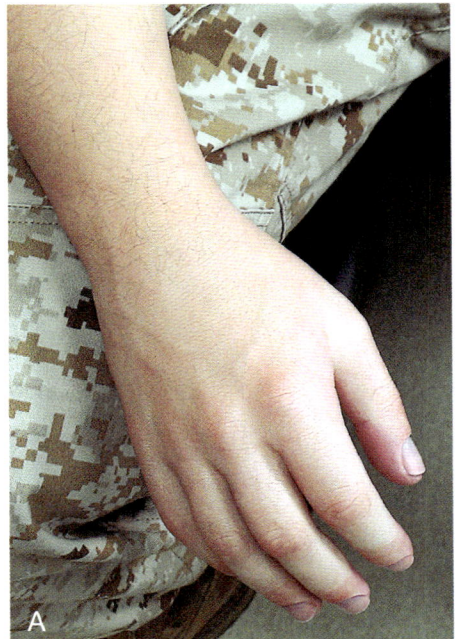 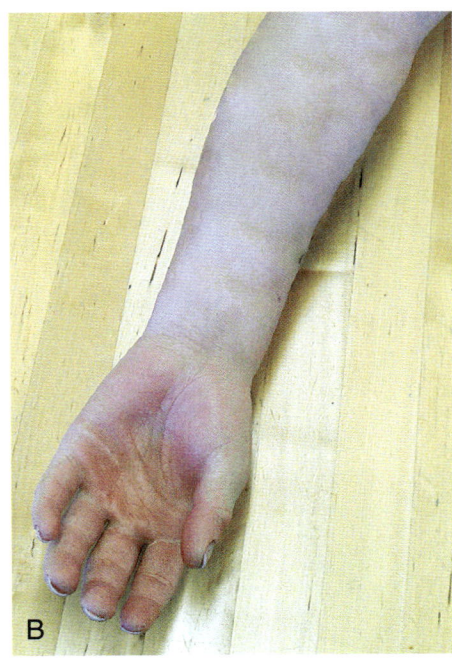

FIGURE 11 **A**, Photograph of an upper limb prosthesis with hair, veining, and acrylic nails. **B**, Photograph of an upper limb prosthesis with tattoo application. (Courtesy of Alternative Prosthetic Services, Bridgeport, CT.)

colors of the amputee's skin at the time of painting; once applied, they cannot easily be changed. Prospective users of such prostheses should fully understand this limitation. If an amputee's skin darkens substantially, the prosthesis may need to be changed to maintain an acceptable match. To address this, some providers make two devices that match the lighter and darker shades typical of the amputee's color changes. Alternatively, a surface pigment to

Section 2: Upper Limb

temporarily darken the prosthetic skin can be applied (**Figure 12**).

Alternative Restoration Options

As previously stated, many individuals at all levels of limb loss are seeking alternatives to the traditional anthropomorphic prostheses. There are many nonanthropomorphic aesthetic options that range from painting the prosthesis a favorite color to custom-painted artwork or special hydrographic films which truly personalize the prosthesis. When involved in the design and finishing of the prosthesis, the user often tends to develop a greater appreciation for the device as they have been more involved in the process of customizing it to their specifications.

Advancements in high-definition 3D scanners have also allowed for improvements in the ability to personalize a prosthesis for an individual. One option is to take an impression of the user's sound side and then scan the plaster model to create a 3D model of the sound side. The 3D model can then be mirrored to create a passive hand that is the precise size, shape, and appearance for their affected side. The 3D printed model can then be painted to either match the skin tone of the user or add films to the surface to add a different look to the hand (**Figures 13** and **14**).

Computer-aided design and advancements in lower cost laser sintering technologies have opened many

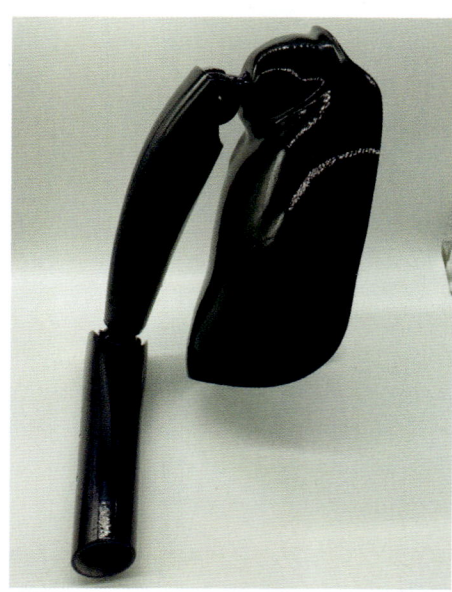

FIGURE 13 Fully custom-designed and three-dimensional printed shoulder disarticulation prosthesis in purple with a high gloss finish. (Courtesy of Partial Hand Solutions, Southington, CT.)

new opportunities for creative designs and finishing options. Using computer-aided design (CAD) along with 3D scanning provides capabilities otherwise not possible with traditional fabrication methods such as designing custom inlays in the frame of the prosthesis, decorative patterns, or novel surface coloring to add another level of detail (**Figure 15**).

As with silicone lifelike restorations, providing the user with options and allowing them to be involved in the design and finishing process has shown improvements in acceptance of the device. This then leads to increased confidence and the ability to discuss their prosthetic experience more openly. Another option that has increased patient acceptance is the use of hydrographic films and thermochromatic paint. This process involves painting the prosthesis and then applying a hydrographic radiograph followed by thermochromatic paint that changes color at a set temperature. This process would create two totally different-looking prostheses based on the air temperature (**Figures 16** and **17**).

Applying custom patterns to devices has offered children many more options

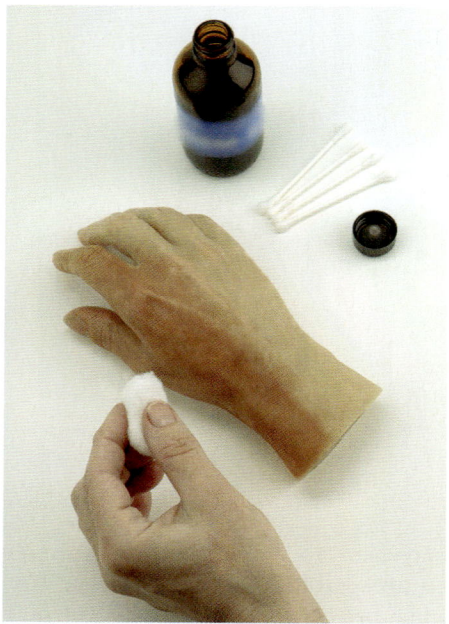

FIGURE 12 Photograph shows application of pigment stain to temporarily darken a prosthesis. (Courtesy of Össur.)

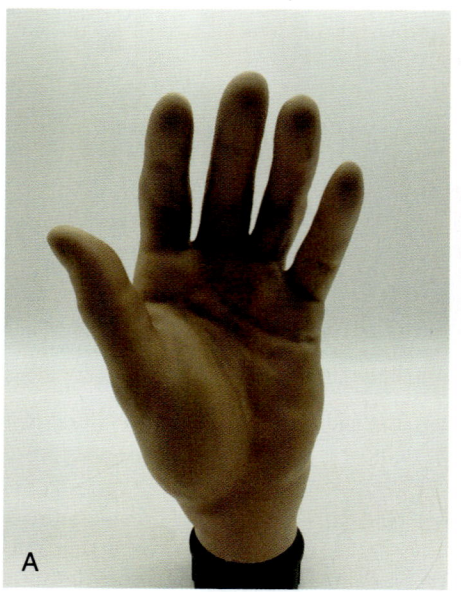

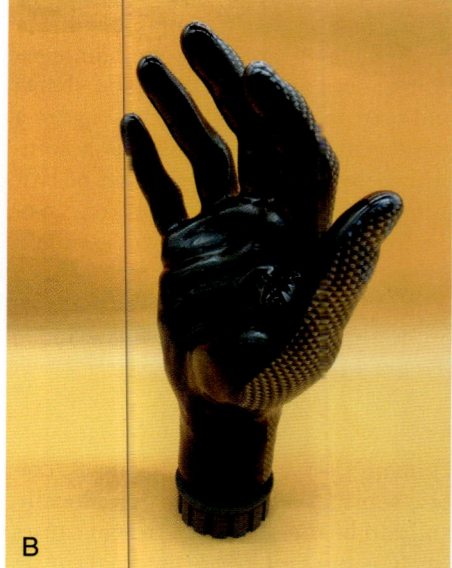

FIGURE 14 **A**, Three-dimensional printed hand from the user's sound side that was then painted to match his sound side. **B**, Three-dimensional printed hand from the user's sound side that was then painted black with a carbon fiber film applied. (Courtesy of Partial Hand Solutions, Southington, CT.)

Chapter 28: Functional Aesthetic Prostheses: Upper Limb

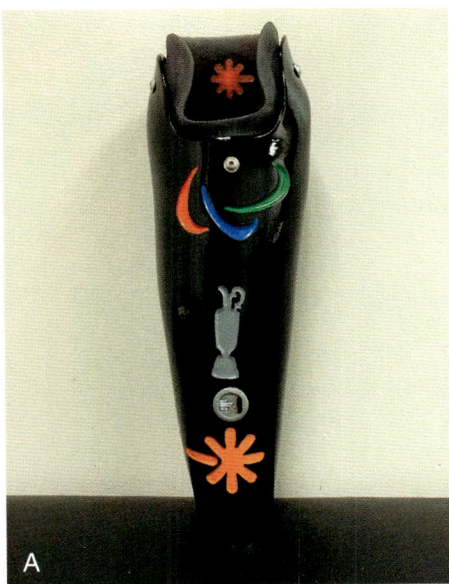 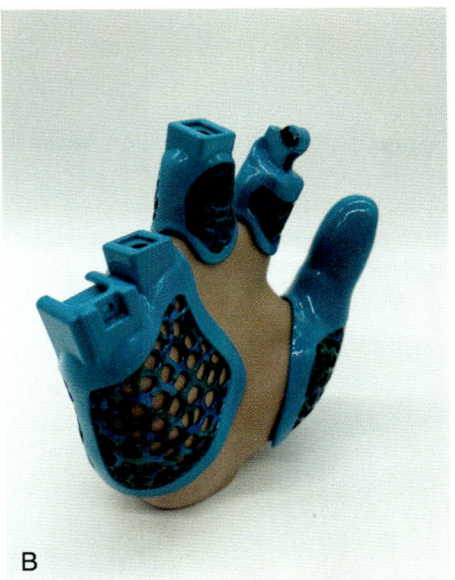 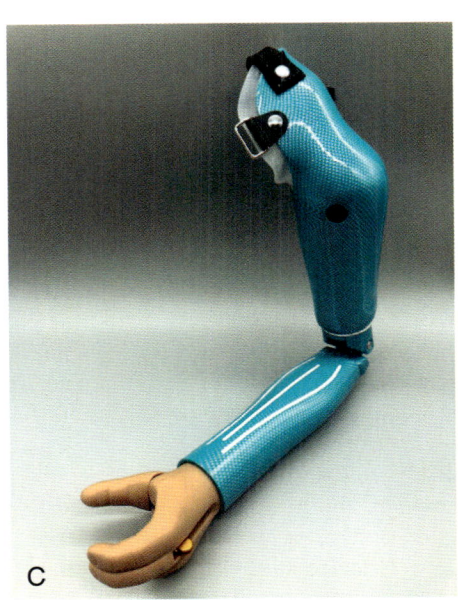

FIGURE 15 **A**, Transradial prosthesis with a three-dimensional custom-printed frame printed with inlays of various logos chosen by the user. **B**, Examples of partial hand frame designs with Voronoi patterns designed into the frame with custom paint and hydrographic film applied. **C**, Transhumeral prosthesis with three-dimensional socket with custom-made elbow and forearm shell with decorative designs in the forearm. (Panels A and C courtesy of Hanger Clinic, USA. Panel B courtesy of Partial Hand Solutions, Southington, CT.)

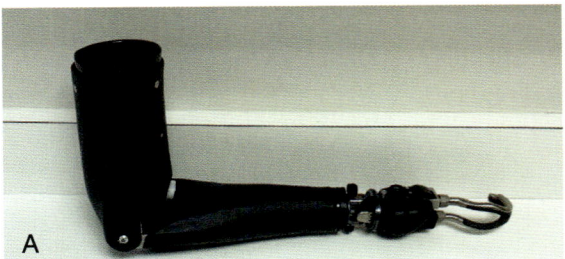 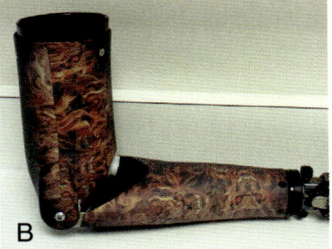

FIGURE 16 **A**, Prosthesis painted, hydrodipped, and then painted with a thermochromatic paint. **B**, The same prosthesis that was heated above 86° F, which clears the thermochromatic paint to show the design underneath. (Courtesy of Hanger Clinic, USA.)

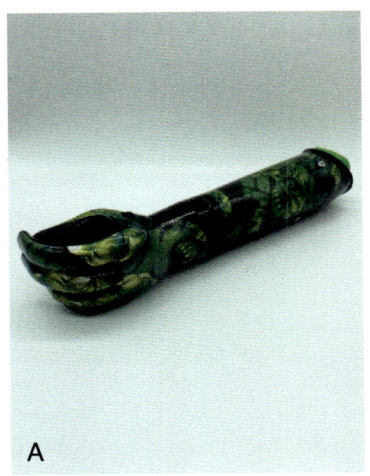 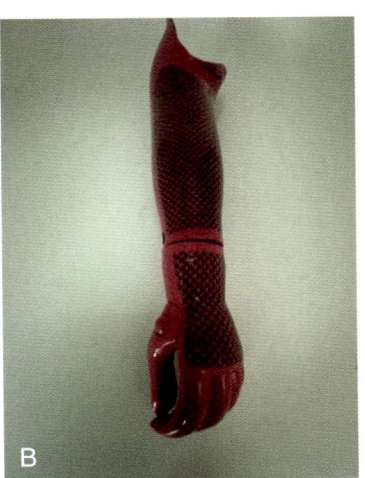 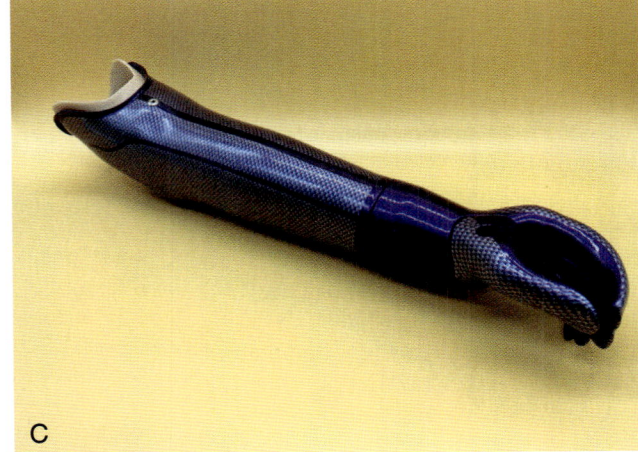

FIGURE 17 **A** through **C**, Three separate custom three-dimensional printed prostheses with different patterns applied to the surface. (Courtesy of Hanger Clinic, USA.)

© 2024 American Academy of Orthopaedic Surgeons — Atlas of Amputations and Limb Deficiencies, Fifth Edition — **371**

Section 2: Upper Limb

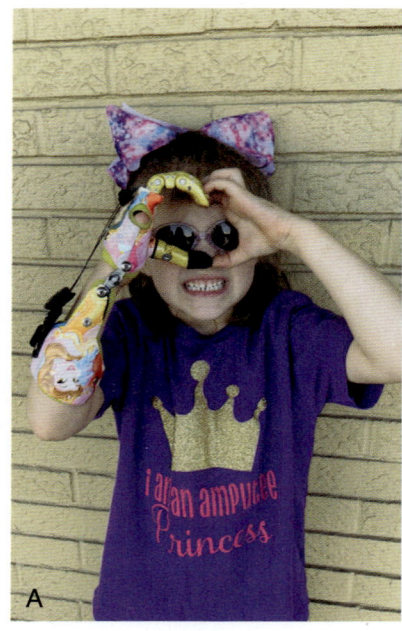 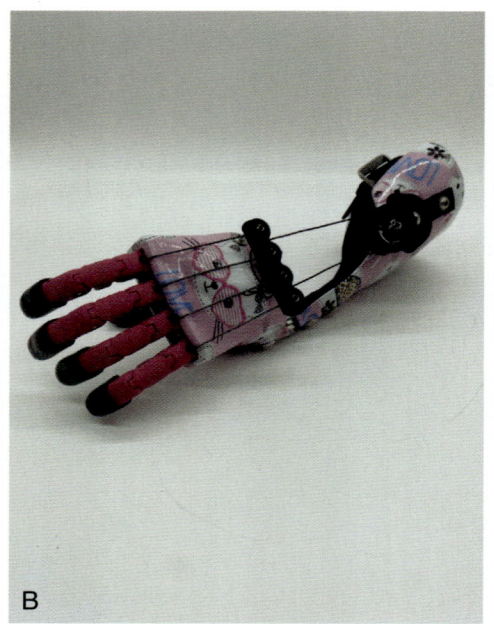 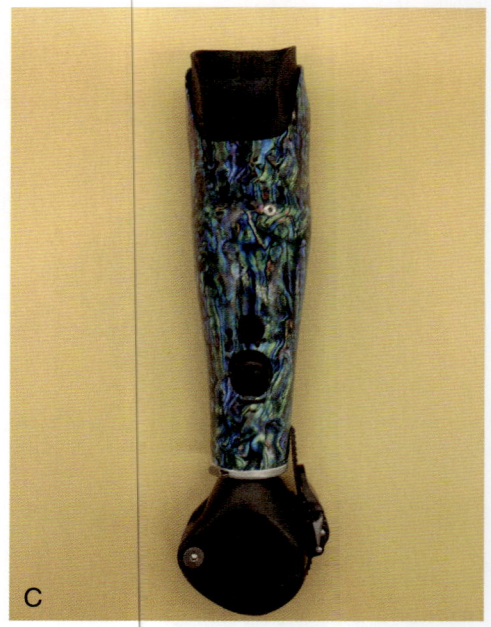

FIGURE 18 **A**, Custom three-dimensional printed prosthesis with custom princess pattern using the pediatric M-Finger from Partial Hand Solutions. **B**, Similar pediatric M-Finger from Partial Hand Solutions. **C**, Weight-lifting prosthesis with a custom pattern applied to the surface. (Courtesy of Hanger Clinic, USA.)

to choose from now to make their new device feel more a part of them. These may include favorite colors or cartoon characters (**Figure 18**).

SUMMARY

New innovations in fabrication techniques and custom finishes have created many options for customizing the resultant aesthetics of upper limb prosthetic devices. Allowing the user to have more of a participatory role in the overall appearance of their prosthesis has been shown to be effective in improving acceptance of their devices. Greater acceptance of the device can lead to increased wear time, improved function, and better outcomes.

No single prosthesis addresses the multiple deficits associated with upper limb loss. Given this, the role of aesthetics in prosthetic restoration should not be underestimated, especially in individuals with upper limb loss. Educators, case managers, and healthcare workers treating this patient cohort increasingly understand that a false distinction has been made between cosmetic and functional prostheses. The concept that a prosthesis that mimics a normal appearance is nonfunctional is obsolete. When circumstances establish a sound basis for the prescription and use of aesthetic prostheses, they should be provided either as primary prostheses or as one of a combination of prostheses that together address the cluster of functional deficits experienced by the individual who has had an amputation.

References

1. Fraser CM: An evaluation of the use made of cosmetic and functional prostheses by unilateral upper limb amputees. *Prosthet Orthot Int* 1998;22(3):216-223.
2. Hubbard S, Bush G, Naumann S: Myoelectric prostheses for the limb-deficient child. *PM R* 1991;2:847-866.
3. Hubbard SA, Kurtz I, Heim W, et al: Powered prosthetic intervention in upper extremity deficiency, in Herring JA, Birch JG, eds: *The Child With a Limb Deficiency*. American Academy of Orthopaedic Surgeons, 1998, pp 417-431.
4. Kyberd PJ, Davey JJ, Dougall Morrison J: A survey of upper-limb prosthesis users in Oxfordshire. *J Prosthet Orthot* 1998;10:85-91.
5. Michael JW, Buckner H: Options for finger prostheses. *J Prosthet Orthot* 1994;6(1):10-19.
6. Millstein SG, Heger H, Hunter GA: Prosthetic use in adult upper limb amputees: A comparison of the body powered and electrically powered prostheses. *Prosthet Orthot Int* 1986;10(1):27-34.
7. O'Farrell DA, Montella BJ, Bahor JL, Levin LS: Long-term follow-up of 50 Duke silicone prosthetic fingers. *J Hand Surg Br* 1996;21(5):696-700.
8. Pillet J, Mackin EJ: Aesthetic restoration, in Bowker JH, Michael JW, eds: *Atlas of Limb Prosthetics*. ed 2. Mosby-Year Book, 1992, pp 227-235.
9. Pilley MJ, Quinton DN: Digital prostheses for single finger amputations. *J Hand Surg Br* 1999;24(5):539-541.
10. Uellendahl JE, Riggo-Heelan J: Prosthetic management of the upper limb deficient child. *Phys Med Rehabil Clin N Am* 2000;11:221-235.
11. van Lunteren A, van Lunteren-Gerritsen GH, Stassen HG, Zuithoff MJ: A field evaluation of arm prostheses for unilateral amputees. *Prosthet Orthot Int* 1983;7(3):141-151.
12. Passero T: Devising the prosthetic prescription and typical examples. *Phys Med Rehabil Clin N Am* 2014;25(1):117-132.
13. Burkhart A, Weitz J: Oncological applications for silicone gel sheets in soft tissue contractures. *Am J Occup Ther* 1990;44(5):460-462.
14. Life-like laboratory: History. Available at: http://www.lifelikelab.com/history.html. Accessed June 2, 2015.

15. Kistenberg RS: Prosthetic choices for people with leg and arm amputations. *Phys Med Rehabil Clin N Am* 2014;25(1):93-115.
16. Ohmori S: Effectiveness of silastic sheet coverage in the treatment of scar keloid (hypertrophic scar). *Aesthetic Plast Surg* 1988;12:95-99.
17. Quinn KJ: Silicone gel in scar treatment. *Burns Incl Therm Inj* 1987;13:S33-S40.
18. Graham E, Hendricks R, Baschuk C, Atkins D: Restoring form and function of the partial hand amputee. *Hand Clinic* 2021;37(1):167-187.
19. Alison A, Mackinnon SE: Evaluation of digital prostheses. *J Hand Surg Am* 1992;17(5):923-926.
20. Beasley RW, de Beze GM: Prosthetic replacements for the thumb. *Hand Clin* 1992;8(1):63-69.
21. Manurangsee P, Isariyawut C, Chatuthong V, Mekraksawanit S: Osseointegrated finger prosthesis: An alternative method for finger reconstruction. *J Hand Surg Am* 2000;25(1):86-92.
22. Herring HW, Romerdale EH: Prosthetic finger retention: A new approach. *Orthot Prostet* 1983;37(2):28-30.
23. Kahle AL: Psychological issues in pediatric limb deficiency, in Bowker JH, Michael JW, eds: *Atlas of Limb Prosthetics*, ed 2. Mosby-Year Book, 2004, pp 801-811.

Brachial Plexus Injuries

MAJ Ean Saberski, MD

CHAPTER 29

ABSTRACT

Traumatic brachial plexus injuries present with devastating deficits of upper extremity utility. These deficits ultimately result in lifelong functional, occupational, social, and psychological consequences. Predictable injury patterns aid in the localization of traumatic lesions, but further evaluation is required for prognostication and treatment planning. Serial examination, advanced imaging, and electrodiagnostic studies all are critical elements in the evaluation of brachial plexus injuries, and with these tools the appropriate treatment is determined. In many cases, brachial plexus exploration and reconstruction with intraplexus or extraplexus nerve transfers results in excellent restoration of function. In other cases, plexus reconstruction is not feasible, and secondary reconstruction with free functional muscle transfer or amputation leads to improved upper extremity utility. In all cases, co-management of these complex patients between a multidisciplinary team optimizes outcomes and minimizes patient suffering.

Keywords: brachial plexus injuries; brachial plexus reconstruction; free-functioning muscle transfer; nerve grafting; nerve transfers

Introduction

Brachial plexus injuries (BPIs) disrupt the function of the upper extremity and result in devastating long-term disability. Patients confront a wide scope of morbid issues including loss of function, psychological distress, chronic pain and dysesthesias, and aesthetic disappointment. BPIs are common in high-energy activities and misadventures, and are globally on the rise.[1-6]

Epidemiology

Males between the ages of 15 and 25 years are the most likely demographic to sustain BPI.[6-8] BPIs most commonly result from motor vehicle accidents, and of these accidents 70% involve motorcycles or bicycles.[9] The most common injury pattern is a supraclavicular injury with at least one root avulsion, and the most common root avulsions are the lower roots.[9,10]

Both blunt and penetrating trauma can result in traumatic BPI. Closed BPI due to blunt trauma results in a traction injury between the mobile units of the neck, shoulder, arm, and torso (**Figure 1**). Penetrating injuries can result from any variety of trauma, including both high-energy and low-energy sources such as gunshot wounds and stab wounds.

Pathoanatomy

Five cervical nerve roots coalesce to form the brachial plexus, typically C5, C6, C7, C8, and T1. Contributions from C4 and T2 also have been described.[11] In the presence of a C4 or T2 contribution, the brachial plexus is termed prefixed or postfixed, with incidences of 28% to 62% and 16% to 73% in cadaver specimens, respectively. The brachial plexus has five sections: roots, trunks, divisions, cords, and terminal branches (**Figure 2**).

The dorsal and ventral nerve rootlets converge to form the spinal root as it passes through the spinal foramen. The cell bodies for motor nerves that course within the ventral rootlets originate from the anterior horn cells of the spinal cord. Conversely, the cell bodies for the sensory nerves that travel within the dorsal rootlets reside in the dorsal root ganglion (DRG), which is protected within the spinal canal and foramen (**Figure 3, A**).

The anatomic location of nerve injury in relation to the DRG has prognostic value. When the spinal rootlets are injured proximal to the DRG, a preganglionic injury has occurred (**Figure 3, B**). Preganglionic BPIs can be further differentiated into central avulsions in which the rootlets are avulsed directly off the spinal cord and intradural ruptures in which the rootlets rupture proximal to the DRG. Injuries to the brachial plexus distal to the DRG result in postganglionic injury[10] (**Figure 3, C and D**). Although the dorsal and ventral rootlets are both avulsed in most cases, either rootlet can be avulsed in isolation in as many as 10% of cases.[12-14] Distinguishing a preganglionic

---

Neither Dr. Saberski nor any immediate family member has received anything of value from or has stock or stock options held in a commercial company or institution related directly or indirectly to the subject of this chapter.

This chapter is adapted from Rhee PC, Shin AYS: Brachial plexus injuries, in Krajbich JI, Pinzur MS, Potter BK, Stevens PM, eds: *Atlas of Amputations and Limb Deficiencies: Surgical, Prosthetic, and Rehabilitation Principles*, ed 4. American Academy of Orthopaedic Surgeons, 2016, pp 389-407.

Section 2: Upper Limb

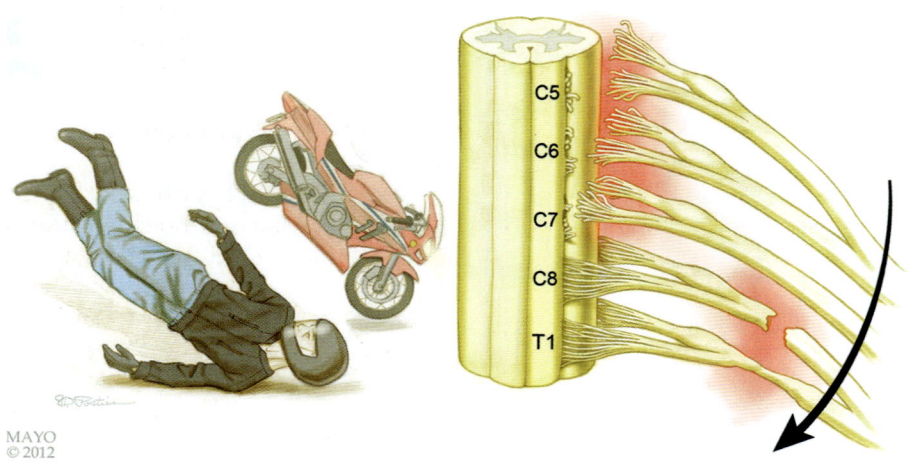

FIGURE 1 Illustration depicting one common mechanism (a fall from a motorcycle) that can result in a closed, traumatic brachial plexus injury. The arrow represents the direction of the force causing the nerve avulsions and ruptures. (Courtesy of the Mayo Foundation for Medical Education and Research, Rochester, MN.)

from a postganglionic injury is imperative because spontaneous recovery cannot occur with a preganglionic BPI. In addition, the technique for brachial plexus reconstruction is markedly different for the two types of injuries.

The roots merge to form the upper trunk (C5 and C6), middle trunk (C7), and lower trunk (C8 and T1). The site at which C5 and C6 unite (the point of Erb) marks the location where the suprascapular nerve emerges.[10] The trunks divide into anterior and posterior divisions as the brachial plexus passes beneath the clavicle (**Figure 4**). The posterior divisions coalesce to form the posterior cord; the anterior divisions of the upper and middle trunk form the lateral cord. The anterior

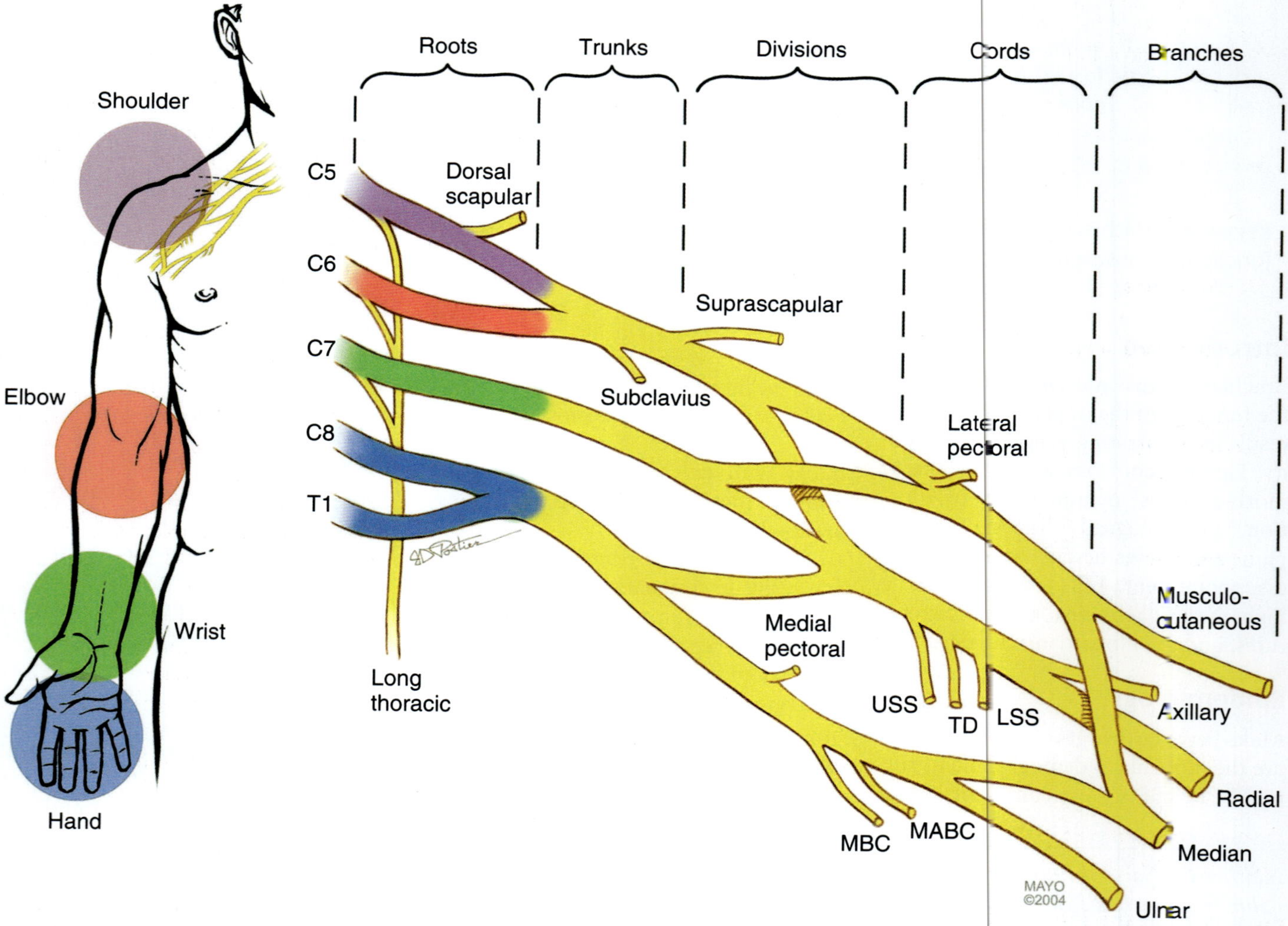

FIGURE 2 Illustration of the brachial plexus nerves. LSS = lower subscapular, MABC = medial antebrachial cutaneous, MBC = medial brachial cutaneous, TD = thoracodorsal, USS = upper subscapular. (Courtesy of the Mayo Foundation for Medical Education and Research, Rochester, MN.)

376 Atlas of Amputations and Limb Deficiencies, Fifth Edition   © 2024 American Academy of Orthopaedic Surgeons

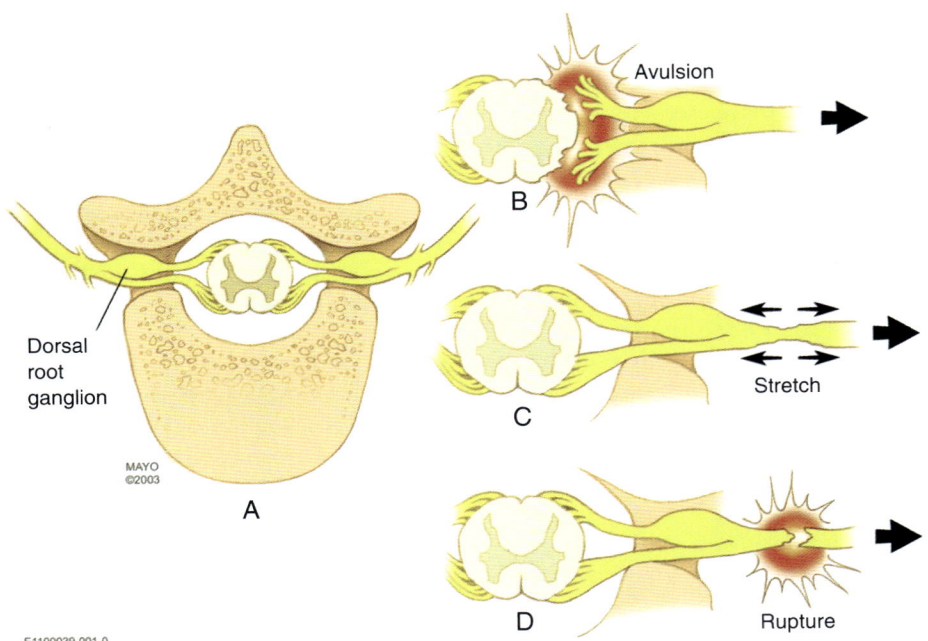

FIGURE 3 **A**, Illustration of spinal rootlets and the dorsal root ganglion within the spinal canal. Illustrations depict avulsion (**B**), stretch (**C**), and rupture (**D**) brachial plexus injuries. (Courtesy of the Mayo Foundation for Medical Education and Research, Rochester, MN.)

lateral cord contribution to the median nerve. The medial cord parts to form the ulnar nerve and the medial cord contribution to the median nerve. The posterior cord divides into the axillary and radial nerves.

Terminal branches can arise in various sites within the brachial plexus. The phrenic, dorsal scapular, and a contribution to the long thoracic nerve branches off the C5 nerve root. The suprascapular nerve and the nerve to the subclavius muscle originate from the upper trunk. The lateral pectoral nerve originates from the lateral cord; the medial pectoral, medial brachial cutaneous, and medial antebrachial cutaneous nerves form from the medial cord. The thoracodorsal and upper and lower subscapular nerves emerge from the posterior cord.

In addition to root avulsions causing BPIs, traumatic BPIs can occur when the neural elements are stretched or ruptured (**Figure 3, C and D**). Lesions that remain in continuity (stretch) have the potential for spontaneous recovery based on the degree of neural injury (neurapraxia or axonotmesis).[15] A rupture (neurotmesis) of the neural elements can occur at any site distal to the DRG to the terminal branches. Ruptures most commonly occur at the root or peripheral nerve levels.

BPIs can be described by the nerve root level involved, by the location of the injury, or in relation to the DRG. Common patterns of injury based on the neural level involved include the upper trunk, upper and middle trunk, lower trunk, and panplexus (complete) BPIs. A panplexus BPI affects all neural elements of the brachial plexus with similar or varied degrees of injury. Otherwise, the location of the BPI can be described in reference to the clavicle as supraclavicular (root and trunk), retroclavicular (division), and infraclavicular (cords and terminal branches). Similarly, the location of injury relative to the DRG can be expressed as preganglionic or postganglionic.

BPIs usually occur at sites where the nerve is relatively fixed, restrained by surrounding structures, or changes direction. Examples include the suprascapular nerve within the suprascapular

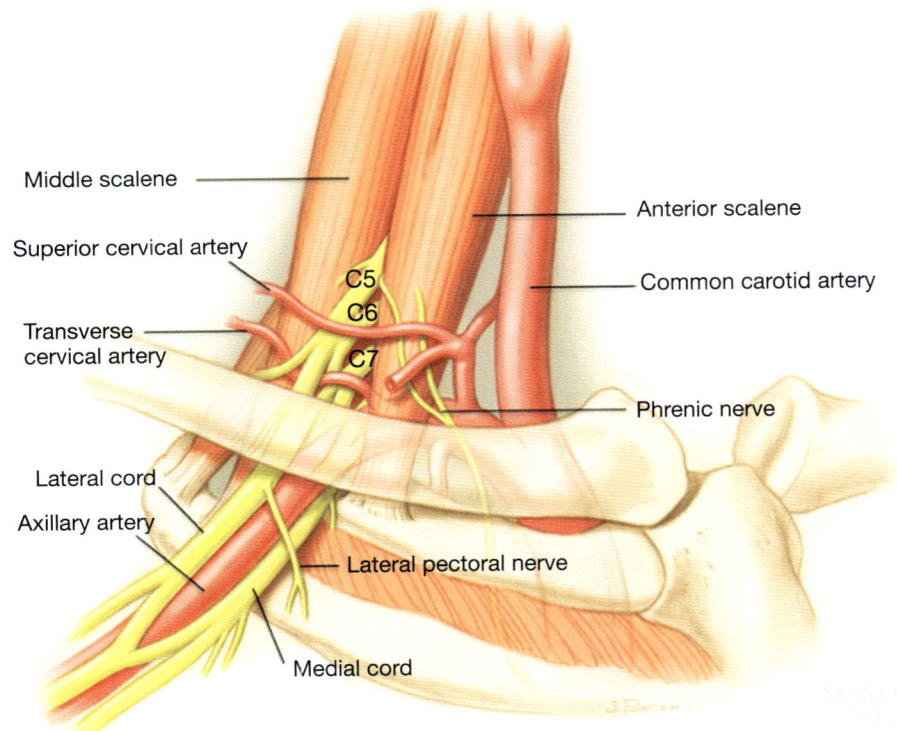

FIGURE 4 Illustration of the brachial plexus in relation to the clavicle and the axillary artery. (Courtesy of the Mayo Foundation for Medical Education and Research, Rochester, MN.)

division from the lower trunk continues as the medial cord. The cords are named based on their location relative to the axillary artery (**Figure 4**).

Many terminal branches of the brachial plexus originate from the cords (**Figure 2**). The lateral cord splits into the musculocutaneous nerve and the notch, the axillary nerve within the quadrilateral space, or the musculocutaneous nerve as it penetrates the coracobrachialis.[15] In general, supraclavicular injuries are more common than infraclavicular injuries. Of the supraclavicular injuries, a panplexus BPI is the most common injury pattern. In addition, upper trunk lesions are more common than lower trunk injuries.

Physical Examination

A thorough physical examination can aid in the accurate diagnosis of a BPI. On inspection, any traumatic or surgical wounds are noted. The resting position of the hand, wrist, elbow, and shoulder girdle can help elucidate the dysfunctional motor units. Percussion along the course of the nerve can elicit paresthesias in the distribution of the nerve root that can help distinguish between preganglionic and postganglionic injuries. Pain over a percussed nerve typically indicates a rupture, whereas lack of pain can indicate an avulsion.[10] An advancing Tinel sign suggests a recovering nerve lesion and should be serially examined over time.[13]

A systematic motor examination of the entire affected upper extremity is imperative to localize the BPI (**Figure 5**). Motor strength can be graded based on the modified British Medical Research Council system, with useful motor function defined as grade 3 or higher. To assign grade 3 strength to a muscle, the muscle unit tested needs to have motion against gravity in the full arc of passive range of motion. Grade 3 strength cannot be obtained if active motion is unequal to passive motion, no matter how strong the muscle is in the lesser arc of motion. In addition, the integrity of cranial nerve XI should be assessed with strength testing of the upper, middle, and lower trapezius, because the spinal accessory nerve can be used as a donor nerve for nerve transfers or the trapezius tendon can serve as a donor for shoulder tendon transfers.

In most cases, upper trunk injury results in a predictable loss of shoulder abduction, external rotation, and elbow flexion. Additional damage to the C7 nerve root in an upper trunk BPI can be indicated by triceps, pronator teres, and/or wrist and finger extensor muscle weakness. An isolated lower trunk injury often manifests as loss of hand function (intrinsic and extrinsic) with preserved shoulder and elbow function. In T1 nerve root avulsions, disruption of the sympathetic outflow to the head and neck can occur because of the intimate relationship of the sympathetic ganglion for T1 and the adjacent nerve root. This can be clinically evident with Horner syndrome (miosis, ptosis, and anhidrosis) (**Figure 6**). Similarly, certain findings on clinical examination can suggest a preganglionic BPI within the upper trunk (**Table 1**).

A comprehensive neurologic examination must be performed to identify a coexistent spinal cord injury (SCI). A prevalence of 12% has been reported for a concomitant SCI in patients with a BPI.[16] Patients with a combined BPI/SCI who have sustained a preganglionic injury at one or more root levels are more likely to exhibit Horner syndrome and phrenic nerve dysfunction than a patient with an isolated BPI. Theoretically, a shared mechanism of injury results in a combined SCI/BPI. Therefore, a neurologic examination of the contralateral upper limbs and bilateral lower limbs should be performed, including sensory levels and the presence of increased reflexes or pathologic reflexes.[10]

A vascular examination is performed because injury to the axillary artery is not uncommon with infraclavicular BPIs or in cases of scapulothoracic dissociation. The status of the axillary artery is also important because the thoracoacromial trunk is a common target vessel for free-functioning muscle transfers (FFMTs).

Imaging Studies

The radiographic priority in evaluating BPI is to define the bony anatomy with plain radiographs. These images will reveal associated trauma to the cervical spine, shoulder, and chest. Beyond illustrating the extent of the injury complex, the plain radiographs may give insight to the underlying brachial plexus lesion. Cervical transverse process, spinous process, and vertebral body fractures are known to have an association with root avulsions at their corresponding levels.[10] Shoulder radiographs demonstrate the competency of the shoulder joint, and loss of deltoid and rotator cuff muscle tone may be revealed by inferior subluxation of the humeral head from the glenoid.

CT is the modality of choice for detecting root avulsions. With avulsion, the dural sac can rupture and subsequently heal, producing a pseudomeningocele, which is characteristic of a preganglionic injury[15] (**Figure 7**). Fine-cut postmyelographic CT has a reported sensitivity and specificity between 80% and 90% in the detection of both pseudomeningoceles and the diagnosis of root avulsions.[12,13,17-19] However, immediately after a preganglionic BPI, a hematoma can be present within the pseudomeningocele that can displace the dye used for myelography, producing a false-negative result.[10] Therefore, CT myelography should be performed 3 to 4 weeks after BPI to allow blood clots to disperse and pseudomeningoceles to fully form. Ultimately, the invasive technical process and the inability to fully characterize brachial plexus injuries limit the clinical utility of CT myelography.

MRI demonstrates variable success in illustrating root avulsions, but it has many advantages over CT myelography when evaluating patients with a BPI.[18,20-22] MRI is particularly useful in evaluating the postganglionic plexus through multiple levels of potential plexus injury. MRI can visualize the entire brachial plexus, which allows identification of neuromas inflammation, edema, and mass lesions within or adjacent to the brachial plexus.[23]

Electrodiagnostic Studies

Electrodiagnostic studies are a critical tool in defining brachial plexus lesions. Electromyography (EMG) is commonly used for the outpatient evaluation of brachial plexus lesions. EMG studies are not useful in the immediate postinjury period because of the lag of wallerian degeneration. The first clinically revealing data are usually observed by EMG by week 4 after injury. EMG can detect nuanced

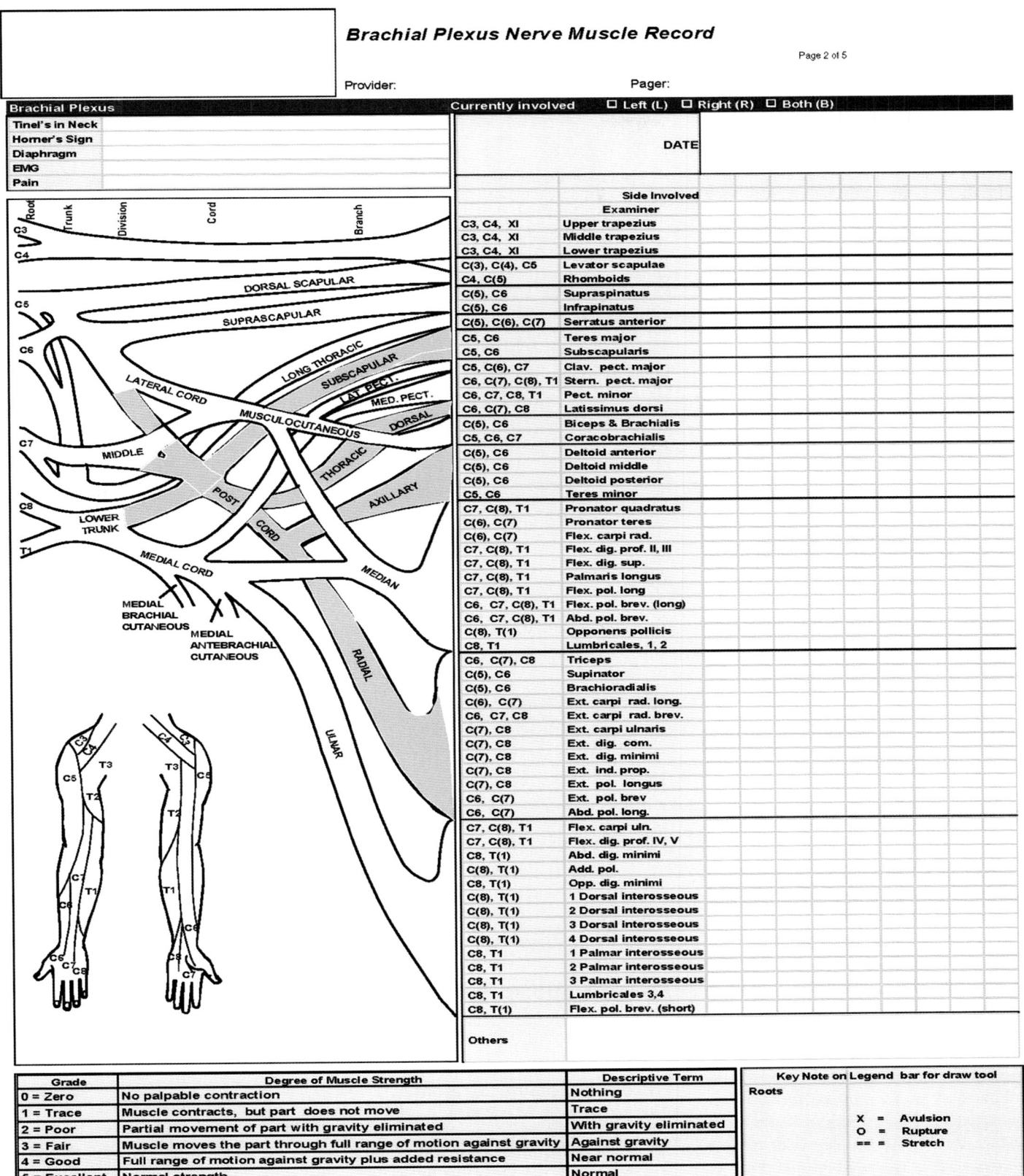

FIGURE 5 Image of the brachial plexus physical examination form. (Courtesy of the Mayo Foundation for Medical Education and Research, Rochester, MN.)

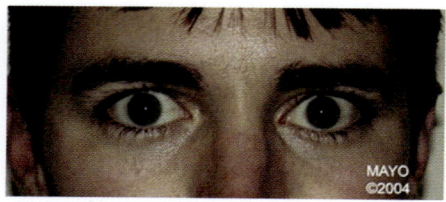

FIGURE 6 Clinical photograph of a patient with Horner syndrome, which consists of miosis, ptosis, and anhidrosis. (Courtesy of the Mayo Foundation for Medical Education and Research, Rochester, MN.)

TABLE 1 Physical Examination Findings That Suggest Preganglionic Brachial Plexus Injuries

Clinical Entity	Muscles Affected	Nerve	Spinal Level
Horner syndrome	NA	T1 sympathetic ganglia	C8-T1
Scapular winging	Serratus anterior	Long thoracic	C5-C7
NA	Levator scapulae	Dorsal scapular	C3, C4, C5
NA	Rhomboids	Dorsal scapular	C4, C5
NA	Cervical paraspinal	Dorsal rami	C4-T1

NA = not applicable

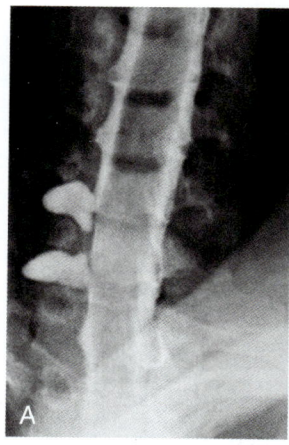
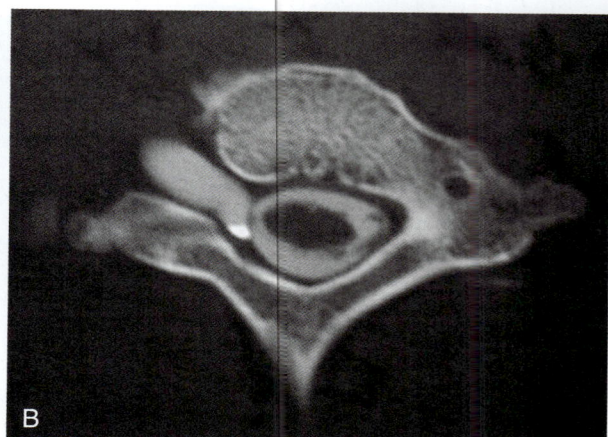

FIGURE 7 Coronal (**A**) and axial (**B**) CT myelograms of the spine show pseudomeningoceles and root avulsions. (Courtesy of the Mayo Foundation for Medical Education and Research, Rochester, MN.)

findings that allow for the determination of acutely denervated muscles. Motor unit action potentials (MUAPs) during EMG study can be used to help delineate the degree of injury. Absent MUAPs correlate with a greater degree of injury and ultimately guide toward a higher level of reconstruction. MUAPs are particularly useful for patients in whom serial examinations are required because of their qualitative and quantitative metrics (Table 2).

Sensory nerve action potentials are also critically useful. Studies showing disruption of sensory nerve action potentials suggest a postganglionic injury, and studies showing preserved sensory nerve action potentials suggest a preganglionic injury. This phenomenon is expected because of the axonal arc through the dorsal root ganglion.

Intraoperative use of electrodiagnostic studies is integral to surgical decision making. Commonly used techniques include nerve action potentials, somatosensory evoked potentials, and motor evoked potentials. The presence of a nerve action potential across a nerve lesion indicates intact (preserved or regenerating) axons and suggests that nerve recovery will occur with neurolysis alone in 90% of patients.[24] The presence of a somatosensory evoked potential or a motor evoked potential indicates an intact connection between the central and peripheral nervous system through a preserved dorsal or ventral rootlet, respectively. Therefore, both somatosensory evoked potentials and motor evoked potentials are absent in postganglionic BPIs and in combined preganglionic and postganglionic BPIs.

TABLE 2 Degree of Nerve Injury and Associated Electrodiagnostic Findings

Sunderland Classification	Fibrillations	MUAPs	Surgical Intervention
I (neurapraxia)	−	+ (normal)	None
II (axonotmesis)	+	+[a]	Initial observation, and if necessary, neurolysis
III (partial neurotmesis)	+	+[a]	Initial observation, and if necessary, neurolysis
IV (partial neurotmesis)	+	−	Nerve reconstruction
V (complete neurotmesis)	+	−	Nerve reconstruction

Reproduced with permission from Hill JR, Lanier ST, Brogan DM, Dy CJ: Management of adult brachial plexus injuries. J Hand Surg Am 2021;46(9):778-788, Table 1; adapted with permission from Ferrante MA, Wilbourn AJ: The electrodiagnostic examination with peripheral nerve injuries, in Mackinnon SE, ed: Nerve Surgery, ed 1. Thieme, 2015, Table 3.1, p 59.
[a]Early (8 to 12 weeks), collateral sprouting; late, axonal regeneration.

Fundamentals of Surgical Management for BPI

The tenets of brachial plexus reconstruction revolve around patient selection, timing of surgery, and the priority of restoring function within the upper limbs.[10] Patients are indicated for surgery in the absence of clinical or electrodiagnostic evidence of recovery on serial examinations or when recovery is impossible (root avulsions).

The timing of surgery depends largely on the mechanism of injury. In penetrating injuries with sharp transection of the brachial plexus, immediate exploration and primary repair is warranted to facilitate direct nerve coaptation before the onset of perineural scarring. Penetrating injuries from a blunt object can be treated in a subacute manner (3 to 4 weeks) to facilitate further demarcation of the neural zone of injury that can be adequately identified and resected at the time of surgery. Gunshot wounds are managed based on the projectile velocity; BPIs resulting from low-velocity gunshot wounds often cause neurapraxia, and spontaneous recovery can be expected. However, in cases of high-velocity gunshot wounds, surgical exploration is often necessary because of the magnitude of associated soft-tissue damage.[10]

For closed BPIs, the timing of surgery depends largely on the type of nerve injury. For root avulsions, early surgery is recommended at 3 to 6 weeks after injury, whereas presumed ruptures and stretch injuries should be explored at 3 to 6 months after serial examinations with demonstration of inadequate or absent reinnervation. Typically, brachial plexus exploration and reconstruction should be performed by 6 months after injury.[15] Poor outcomes can be expected in patients who undergo brachial plexus reconstruction beyond 6 to 9 months after injury because motor end plates degenerate before the regenerating nerves can reach the target muscles.[10] After 1 year, brachial plexus reconstruction is not advised because of progressive neural death and irreversible muscle atrophy.[15]

The priority of brachial plexus reconstruction is to restore elbow function, obtain shoulder abduction and stability, regain hand sensibility, provide wrist flexion and finger extension, and establish hand intrinsic function.[10] These functions can be obtained with primary and secondary brachial plexus reconstruction. Primary brachial plexus reconstruction refers to the initial surgical management to include neurolysis, direct nerve repair, nerve grafting, nerve transfers, and FFMTs. Secondary brachial plexus reconstruction is performed to improve the gains achieved with primary reconstruction or if earlier attempts at reconstruction have failed; examples include tendon/muscle transfers, FFMTs, arthrodesis, and corrective osteotomies.[10,25]

Primary Brachial Plexus Reconstruction

Brachial Plexus Exploration

Exploration of the brachial plexus represents the most direct intervention through which the scope of trauma is observed. With careful dissection, the injury pattern is defined and a coordinated plan can be determined. Surgeon preference will dictate the approach to counseling before the brachial plexus exploration. Depending on individual practice patterns, surgeons may elect to counsel patients for exploration alone or may counsel toward performing the appropriate reconstruction during the same operation.

Direct Nerve Repair

In cases where patients present acutely with penetrating trauma, a direct primary repair is often tenable and results in the best potential for recovery. Tension-free epineural repair is critical to optimize nerve recovery; however, this is often impractical with subacute presentation. Blunt trauma is rarely amenable to direct nerve repair as the mechanism of injury does not result in neural discontinuity.[15]

Neurolysis

Neurolysis using proper microsurgical optics and technique is a critical element to brachial plexus exploration and reconstruction. Neurolysis decompresses fascicles and allows for mobilization of cut nerve ends in preparation for tension-free repair. In cases where the nerve is seen in continuity but action potentials and somatosensory-evoked potentials are present, neurolysis alone optimizes the injured nerve for recovery.

Nerve Grafting

Postganglionic injuries with adequate proximal and distal targets are adequate for nerve graft reconstruction. Intraoperative assessment is imperative to determine the zone of injury and the limits of healthy fascicles. Adequate excision proximally and distally ensures that graft integration proceeds unencumbered by scar and fibrosis. Given the importance of a healthy fascicular interface, there is value in confirming the viability of graft targets with histopathologic examination and acetylcholinesterase staining.[26,27]

Nerve autografts can be harvested from a variety of donor sites, but the most common and routine is the sural nerve. Cabled sural nerve grafts match the caliber and axonal density of the plexus nice and commit the patient to little donor site morbidity. When the grafts are cabled, care is taken to reverse the proximal and distal orientation of the fascicles to limit the axonal loss because of the nature of the distal arborizing branches. Other donor sites include the cutaneous branches of the injured upper extremity such as the superficial branch of the radial, the medial brachial cutaneous, the medial antebrachial cutaneous, and the lateral antebrachial cutaneous nerves. When the C8 and T1 roots are avulsed, a vascularized ulnar nerve flap can be harvested without morbidity from the ipsilateral arm with the conceptual benefit of improved axonal regeneration.[15,28]

Nerve Transfers

Nerve transfers conceptually produce a favorable environment for recovery because the distance for functional recovery is significantly reduced. In nerve transfers, viable nerve fascicles are transferred as close to motor end plates as possible. With a shorter distance of regeneration required, the time to recovery is quickened in concert. This hastened recovery timeline offers a significant advantage over proximal nerve grafting.[15] In general, transfers can be categorized as extraplexal or intraplexal.[29]

Extraplexal transfers trace their axonal course outside of the plexus. The two most common extraplexal donors are the ipsilateral intercostal and spinal accessory nerves.[30,31] A single intercostal nerve contains approximately 1,200 to 1,300 axons, but multiple intercostal levels can be transferred as a composite bundle to maximize the axonal potential. The intercostal nerve transfer is often used to power the biceps motor branch or to power a free functional muscle to restore elbow flexion[10,15] (**Figure 8**). Similarly,

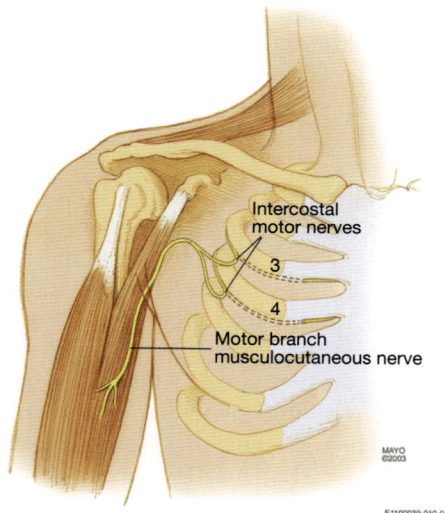

FIGURE 8 Illustration showing intercostal nerve transfers to the biceps motor branch. (Courtesy of the Mayo Foundation for Medical Education and Research, Rochester, MN.)

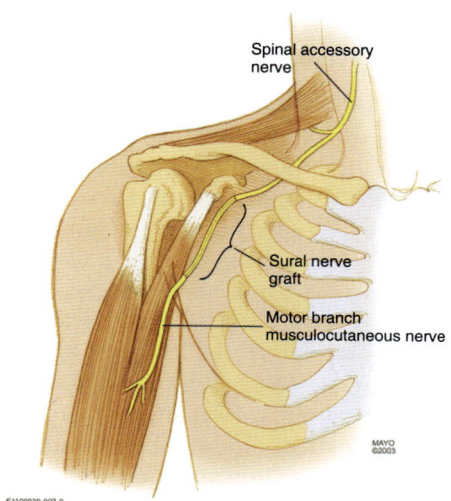

FIGURE 9 Illustration of spinal accessory nerve transfer to the biceps motor branch. (Courtesy of the Mayo Foundation for Medical Education and Research, Rochester, MN.)

the intercostal sensory nerves can be selectively transferred to restore upper limb sensibility. The spinal accessory nerve contains approximately 1,500 to 1,700 fascicles per trunk, and the distal trunk can often be harvested to sufficient length to reach the suprascapular nerve or the flap nerve from a free-functioning muscle. With the use of an interposition nerve graft, the spinal accessory can be used to power the biceps motor branch (**Figure 9**).

The phrenic nerve and the contralateral C7 nerve root are two other powerful extraplexal nerve donor sites.[32-34] The phrenic nerve contains approximately 800 myelinated fibers, which is sufficient to power the suprascapular nerve.[10] The reach of the phrenic nerve can be augmented with interposition nerve grafts to power targets such as the musculocutaneous or axillar nerves. The donor morbidity of the phrenic nerve can obviate its use in some patients. With an expected decrease of 10% in the pulmonary vital capacity, patients with chest trauma, pediatric patients, and those with underlying pulmonary disorders should not undergo phrenic harvest. The C7 root contains 27,000 to 30,000 nerve fibers and can be transferred to restore function in the shoulder, elbow, and hand.[10,15,35,36]

Intraplexal nerve transfers trace their axonal course through the ipsilateral brachial plexus. The underlying concept is to use expendable fascicles to power deficient targets. The specific utility of particular intraplexal transfers is wholly dependent on the given injury patterns.[15,37-41] The two most commonly useful intraplexal transfers are the Oberlin transfer and the Leechavengvongs transfer. The Oberlin transfer (**Figure 10**) is classically described as a transfer of flexor carpi ulnaris motor fascicles to the biceps motor nerve to restore elbow flexion. The Leechavengvongs transfer (**Figures 11** and **12**) uses the motor branch of the long head of the triceps to restore signal to the axillary nerve for shoulder abduction.[42-46] In cases of C5 and C6 avulsion, the Oberlin and Leechavengvongs transfers reliably restore M4 biceps and deltoid strength, with little impact on hand and elbow strength or utility.[15,44,45]

Free-Functioning Muscle Transfer

FFMT, also known as functional microsurgical muscle transplantation (FMMT), uses the principles of microsurgery to restore functional deficits. Donor muscles are dissected free from their insertion and origin with their microneurovascular pedicle intact and transferred to the desired recipient site for inset, coaptation, and anastomoses. A common surgical plan uses the contralateral gracilis to restore elbow flexion through anastomosing the arterial inflow to the thoracoacromial axis, the venous outflow to the cephalic, and coapting the nerve to the spinal accessory. Many combinations of FFMT exist, with various other donor muscles and recipient structures to consider (**Figure 13**).

Secondary Brachial Plexus Reconstruction of the Shoulder

Glenohumeral motor function has been categorized into three groups: the prime movers, the steering group, and the depressor group.[47] The prime movers (the deltoid and the clavicular head of the pectoralis major) provide lifting power, the steering group (the subscapularis, supraspinatus, and infraspinatus) guides humeral motion and provides additional lifting power, and the depressor group (the sternal head of the pectoralis major, latissimus dorsi, teres major, and teres minor) rotates the humeral shaft and helps achieve full overhead humeral elevation.[25] All groups must work in concert for synchronized motion of the upper limbs. With a BPI, paralysis of any of these muscles can result in an imbalance and cause painful subluxation of the glenohumeral joint.

In addition to restoring shoulder motion, correcting shoulder instability and imbalance is critical for overall upper limb function and for pain control. Shoulder stabilization can improve outcomes after brachial plexus reconstruction, specifically FFMT for elbow flexion and prehension.[48] The goals of shoulder reconstruction in the setting of a BPI are pain relief (from shoulder subluxation), stability, and restoration of forward elevation, abduction, and external rotation.[25] These goals can be obtained with soft-tissue releases, tendon transfers, derotational osteotomy of the humerus, or shoulder arthrodesis.

Shoulder Soft-Tissue Release

Supple shoulder motion is the first critical element necessary when

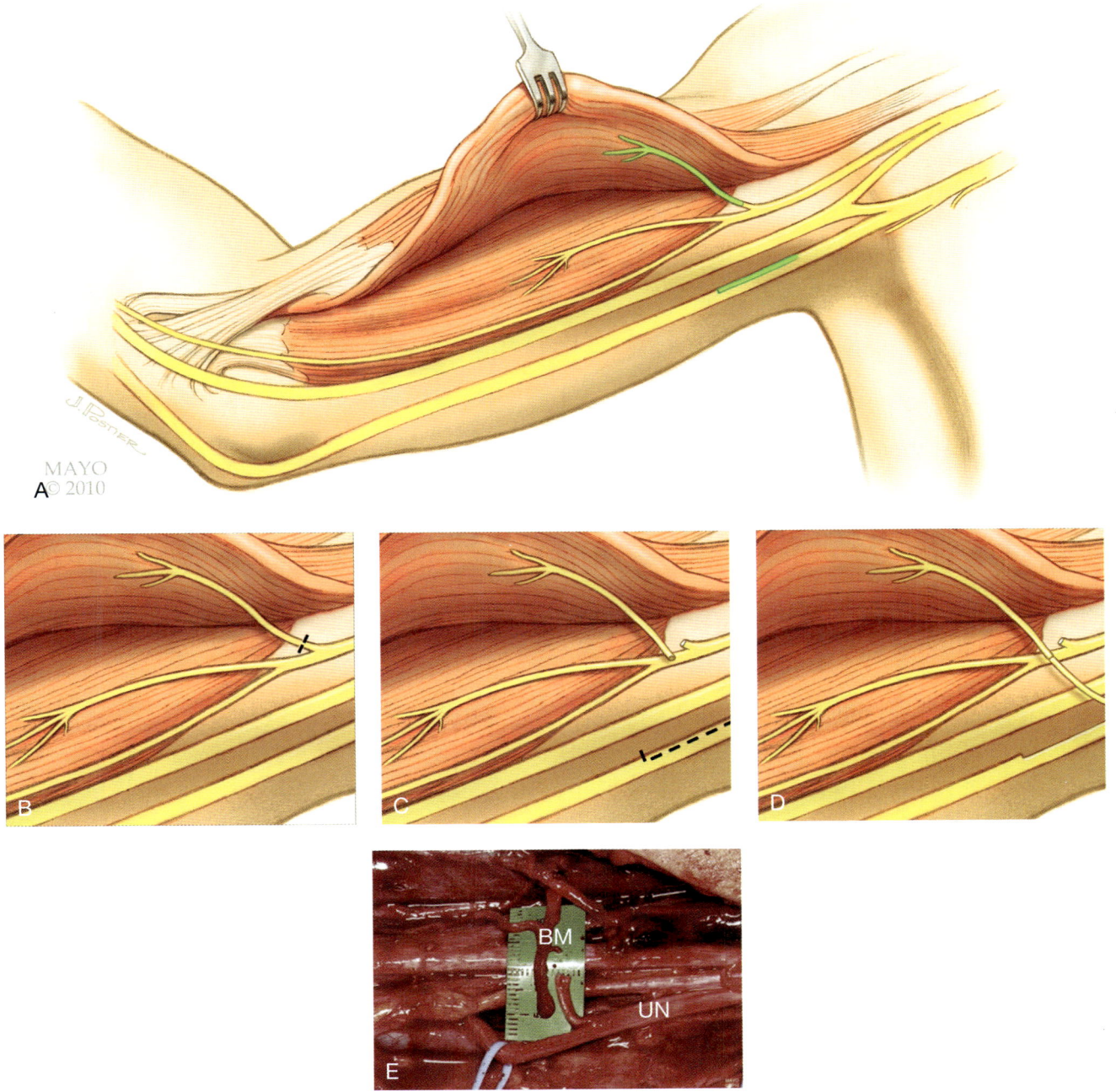

FIGURE 10 Images demonstrating the Oberlin technique of nerve transfer of the ulnar nerve (UN) fascicle to the biceps motor (BM) branch. **A**, The surgical site and the incision. **B**, The BM branch is mobilized and transected (dashed line) from the musculocutaneous nerve. **C**, The UN motor fascicle to the flexor carpi ulnaris is identified, mobilized, and transected (dashed line). **D**, The UN motor fascicle is coapted to the BM branch using microsurgical techniques. **E**, Intraoperative photograph showing the BM branch and the UN. (Courtesy of the Mayo Foundation for Medical Education and Research, Rochester, MN.)

considering any procedure to restore active motion about the shoulder. Patients with C5 and C6 lesions may present with unopposed shoulder internal rotation, which will ultimately result in an internal rotation contracture. Release of this contracture can be accomplished by releasing the subscapularis from the scapula.[49-51] Release of the pectoralis major, in addition to concomitant tendon transfer, also has been advocated.[52,53]

Shoulder Tendon Transfers

Shoulder abduction and forward flexion can be restored with various tendon transfers. Classically, the upper trapezius muscle transfer has been used to improve shoulder stability.[54-56] The initial technique entailed transfer of the bony acromial insertion of the upper trapezius to the humeral shaft (distal to the greater tuberosity).[47,57] A later modification involved medial

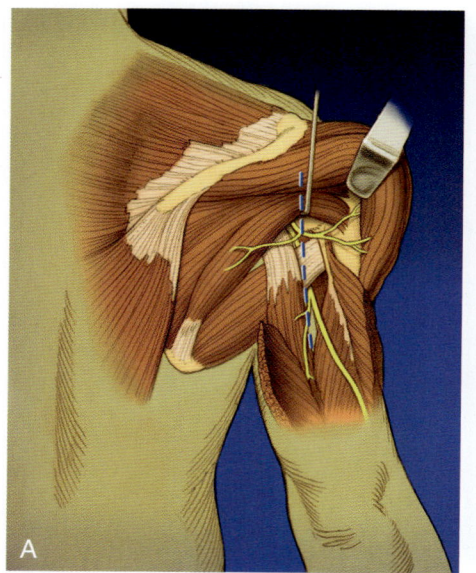 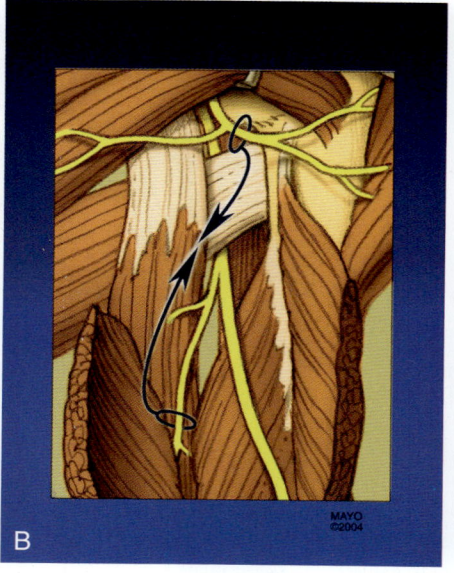 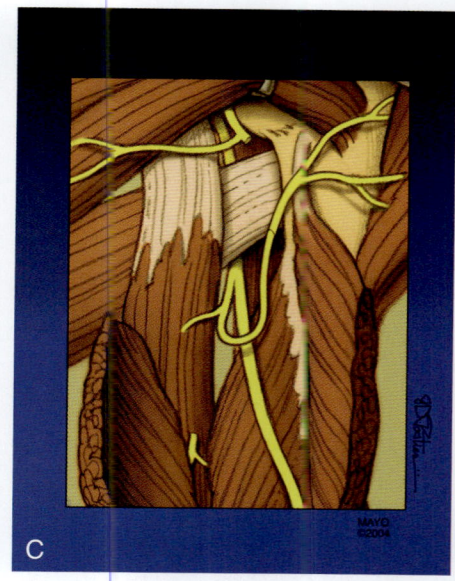

FIGURE 11 Illustrations demonstrate the Leechavengvongs nerve transfer of the triceps motor branch to the axillary nerve. **A**, Overview and overlying skin incision (dashed line). **B**, Planned nerve transfer. **C**, Completed nerve transfer. (Courtesy of the Mayo Foundation for Medical Education and Research, Rochester, MN.)

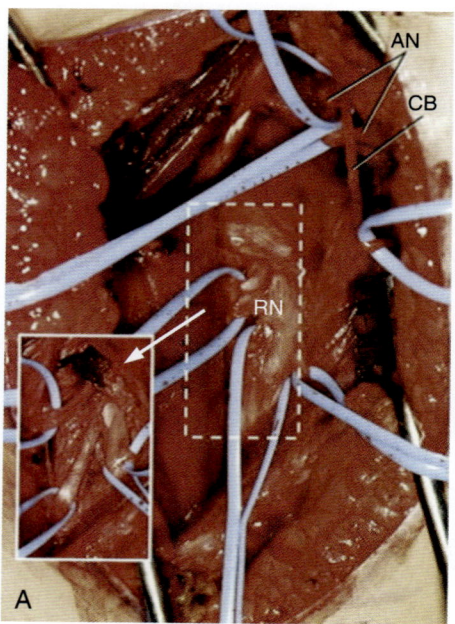 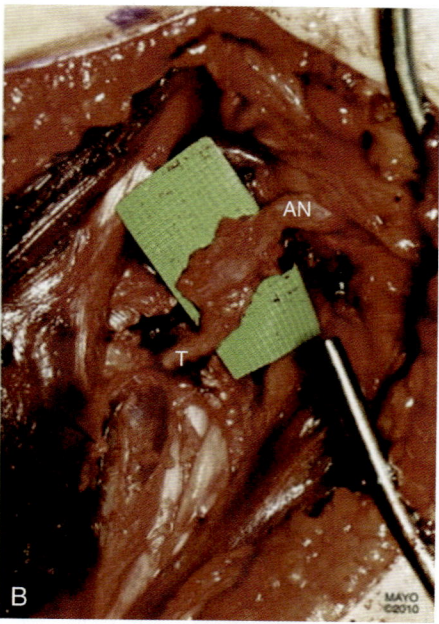

FIGURE 12 Clinical photographs obtained before (**A**) and after (**B**) the Leechavengvongs nerve transfer of the triceps motor branch (T) from the radial nerve (RN) to the axillary nerve (AN). Note the cutaneous branch (CB) of the axillary nerve. (Courtesy of the Mayo Foundation for Medical Education and Research, Rochester, MN.)

advancement of the deltoid over the transferred trapezius to improve shoulder stability.[58] Approximately 95% of the patients (70 of 74) who underwent trapezius transfer in one series were satisfied with shoulder stability and function.[55] Mean shoulder abduction after trapezius transfer ranged from 39° to 116°.[55,56,59-62] Other tendon transfers about the shoulder have been described, including transfer of the latissimus dorsi (with or without the teres major) and pectoralis major.[63-67]

Based on anatomic feasibility studies, the author of this chapter have expanded the role of tendon transfers in the paralytic shoulder. Isolated transfer of the lower trapezius to the infraspinatus can be performed directly to restore active shoulder external rotation if the glenohumeral joint remains reduced with adequate passive range of motion and minimal degenerative change[68] (**Figure 14**). In complete BPIs, complex shoulder reconstruction can be performed with transfers of the upper and middle trapezius to the deltoid, the levator scapulae to the supraspinatus, the lower trapezius to the infraspinatus, and the upper serratus to the subscapularis, provided that all donor muscles exhibit a minimal M4 level strength.[47,69-71]

Derotational Humeral Osteotomy

Derotational osteotomy of the humerus corrects hand and forearm malpositioning, which can improve upper limb function. The procedure can be performed as an alternative to shoulder tendon transfers to enable external rotation or as a salvage procedure if primary brachial plexus reconstruction or tendon transfers (latissimus dorsi or teres major) fail.[72-75] If a glenohumeral internal rotation contracture exists even with restoration of elbow flexion, the patient's forearm can limit elbow flexion by striking the chest.[55] The osteotomy is performed just proximal

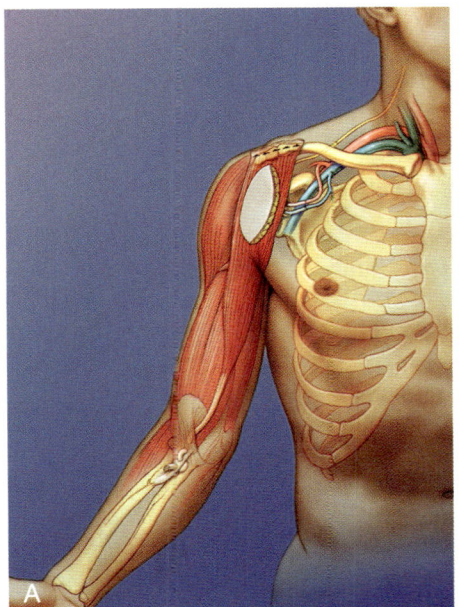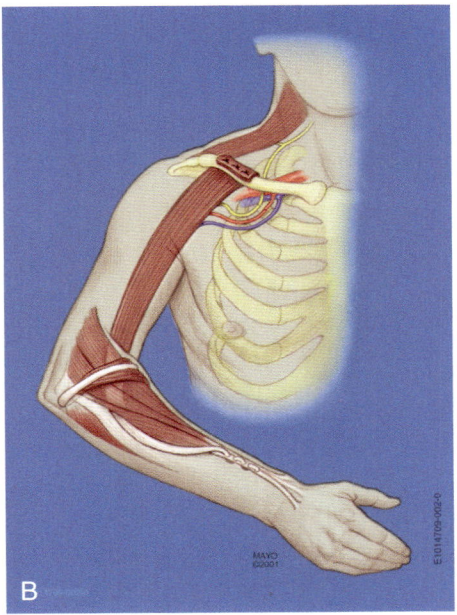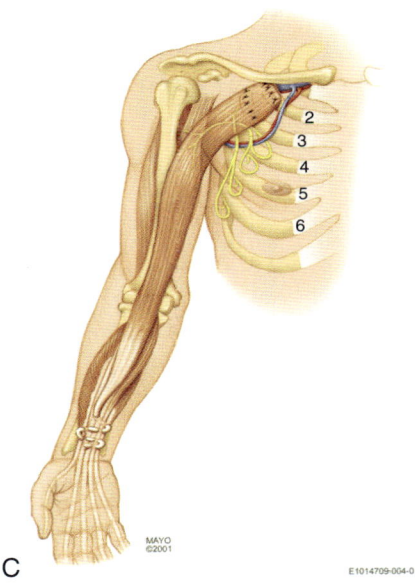

FIGURE 13 Illustrations of free-functioning muscle transfers for elbow flexion (**A**), elbow flexion and wrist extension (**B**), or elbow and finger flexion (**C**). (Courtesy of the Mayo Foundation for Medical Education and Research, Rochester, MN.)

to the deltoid insertion, and approximately 30° of external rotation is introduced to the distal segment.[72] In one series, humeral derotational osteotomy yielded a mean correction of external rotation to 27°.[62]

Shoulder Arthrodesis

The goal of glenohumeral arthrodesis is to provide a stable foundation within the upper limb kinetic chain, focusing all brachial plexus reconstruction efforts on restoring elbow and hand function. A flail shoulder can result in painful inferior glenohumeral subluxation and inability to position the hand in space. If the trapezius and levator scapulae remain intact after BPI, useful scapulothoracic motion can be achieved after glenohumeral arthrodesis.[76] Preserved serratus anterior function can even allow forward flexion of the upper limb through scapular rotation while persistent pectoralis major function permits brachiothoracic grasp.[76,77] Many factors affect outcomes after glenohumeral arthrodesis, including position of the fusion, particularly in internal rotation, continued pain, and residual hand function.[76,78-81] However, glenohumeral arthrodesis has been shown to improve function in patients with complete BPIs,

with restored elbow flexion despite poor hand function.[77]

Recent advances in nerve grafting and transfer have limited the role of primary glenohumeral arthrodesis because patients prefer voluntary shoulder abduction if it can be achieved.[10,48] Functional outcomes of brachial plexus reconstruction to restore shoulder function are less predictable than for restoration of elbow function; thus, glenohumeral arthrodesis can be considered a salvage procedure.[77,82-85] Rouholamin et al[76] reported on 13 patients with BPIs (4 complete, 7 upper trunk, and 2 lower trunk) who underwent glenohumeral arthrodesis in 30° of abduction, 30° of flexion, and 20° of internal rotation, with mean postoperative active abduction of 56° (range, 50° to 80°). Ten patients had excellent pain relief from preoperative levels and 12 perceived an improvement in postoperative limb function. For complete and partial BPIs, Atlan et al[86] observed respective mean active abduction of 57° and 62° and respective mean active arc of rotation of 50° and 46°. Chammas et al[77] noted improved hand excursion and strength of shoulder adduction and external rotation if the inferior head of the pectoralis major had at least M3

strength, and improved active shoulder range of motion and strength of adduction and internal rotation if the superior head of the pectoralis major had at least M3 strength.

Secondary Brachial Plexus Reconstruction of the Hand and Wrist: Wrist, Thumb Interphalangeal, and Trapeziometacarpal Arthrodesis

Hand utility is not solely dependent on intentional positioning in space. The function of the hand is also dependent on the ability to use the hand to grasp and release objects.[10,87,88] The biomechanics of the carpus and hand require a careful balance of forces to achieve a composite grip that functions well. Reconstruction of the brachial plexus only restores select motor functions, which will reliably result in unbalanced forces and ultimately less function about the wrist and hand. Selective arthrodesis of joints in the wrist and hand can improve hand function after brachial plexus reconstruction by rebalancing forces about functional joints. Examples of this principle are best demonstrated in hand reanimation

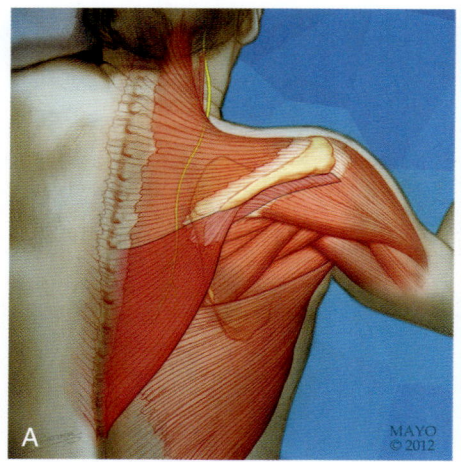
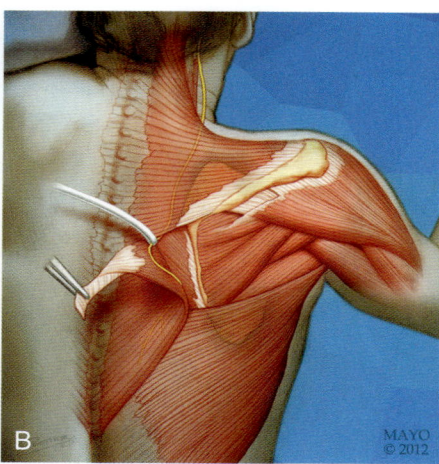
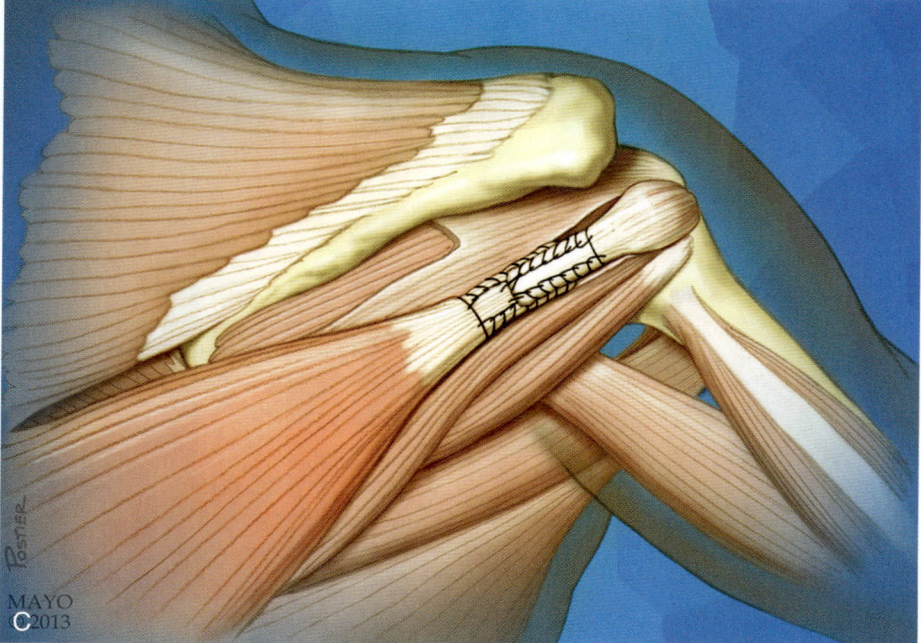

FIGURE 14 Images demonstrating ipsilateral lower trapezius transfer to the infraspinatus. **A**, Normal position of the lower trapezius. **B**, Elevation of the lower trapezius to the uninjured spinal accessory nerve. **C**, Transfer to the infraspinatus tendon. (Courtesy of the Mayo Foundation for Medical Education and Research, Rochester, MN.)

with FFMT, wherein wrist arthrodesis improves mechanics about the thumb and fingers for grasping and pinching.[89] Beyond the potential for improved mechanics, wrist arthrodesis results in a stable and painless joint that is useful in even a static position.[55,89-92]

The Role of Amputation in BPIs

Isolated Transradial Amputation

Patients with lower trunk BPIs and patients in whom reconstruction fails to reanimate the hand may consider transradial amputation. Historically, transradial amputation was considered an extreme management option and was resolved solely for patients with recurrent trauma and infection of the insensate and flail hand. However, with advances in myoneural interfacing and in myoelectric prosthetic technology, the calculus for the risks and benefits of transradial amputations is shifting. Advanced and emerging surgical techniques such as targeted muscle reinnervation and regenerative peripheral nerve interfaces allow for improved translation of cortical signal to motor signal and in turn myoelectric device control.

Isolated Transhumeral Amputation

Similar to transradial amputations, transhumeral amputations are historically considered extreme in BPI. However, studies examining BPI patient performance following amputation are outdated and do not evaluate the modern techniques available.[93] Given the advances in both surgical management of transhumeral amputations and myoelectric technology, the expectation is that patients with BPI who are undergoing transhumeral amputation today would outperform historical controls.

Combined Transhumeral Amputation and Glenohumeral Arthrodesis

The combination of transhumeral amputation and glenohumeral arthrodesis uniquely optimizes some patients for the use of a prosthetic limb.[94] This approach was first widely advocated in the 1960s by Yeoman and Seddon,[95] and their work demonstrated a faster return to function in patients treated with this approach. Further studies generally continued to validate these original findings, rooting combined transhumeral amputation and glenohumeral arthrodesis as a treatment option for BPI.[96-106] For patients with the loss of the dominant upper extremity, transhumeral amputation and glenohumeral arthrodesis can provide the most expeditious route to functional recovery (**Table 3**).

Author's Current Treatment Algorithm

The centerpiece of the chapter author's practice is the multidisciplinary Peripheral Nerve Clinic. This clinic is staffed by the Plastic and Reconstructive Surgery, Neurosurgery, Orthopaedic Surgery, Neurology, and Physical Medicine and Rehabilitation teams. Patients who sustain penetrating trauma are typically brought to the operating room for immediate

TABLE 3 Indications and Contraindications for Glenohumeral Arthrodesis, Transhumeral Amputation, and Early Prosthetic Fitting

Indications	Severe brachial plexus injury (flaccid shoulder, elbow, hand) with a poor prognosis for additional recovery (preganglionic)
	Failed primary brachial plexus reconstruction for a complete brachial plexus injury
	Patient dissatisfaction with lack of usefulness and/or discomfort of the flail limb
	Patient willing to attempt prosthetic use
	Shoulder pain or discomfort secondary to inferior glenohumeral subluxation
	Recurrent infections or injuries to the insensate arm
Contraindications	Paralysis of the scapulothoracic muscles (trapezius, levator scapulae, latissimus dorsi, serratus anterior, or rhomboids)
	Active infection in the proximal humerus or glenohumeral joint
	Earlier glenohumeral arthrodesis on the contralateral side

brachial plexus exploration and primary nerve repair or plexus reconstruction as necessary. Patients who sustain closed injury are evaluated clinically and with electrodiagnostic studies between 4 and 8 weeks after their injury to document their initial presentation. Imaging typically includes MRI in addition to other cross-section and plain radiography studies as necessary for the given trauma. Patients return for serial examinations to monitor evidence of recovery. In the absence of recovery, reconstruction is undertaken. Patients indicated for surgery are counseled about the various approaches to reconstruction, and the options are tailored to meet individual patient goals. If possible, intraplexal transfers are undertaken in concert with other reconstructive efforts to maximize the potential for functional recovery. Amputation is highlighted as a measure that may ultimately produce the most functional recovery, but attempts at primary and secondary reconstruction are typically advised before undergoing an amputation at any level.

SUMMARY

BPIs result in significant morbidity and devastating deficits in upper extremity recovery. Different patterns of injury have different treatment options available and ultimately different expectations for recovery. Primary and secondary reconstruction of the brachial plexus can result in adequate functional recovery in some patients. However, many patients cannot achieve functional recovery through reconstructive means. In these patients, amputation is a critically important consideration to weigh, as it may allow for the greatest and most expeditious return of function for the patient.

References

1. Allieu Y, Cenac P: Is surgical intervention justifiable for total paralysis secondary to multiple avulsion injuries of the brachial plexus? *Hand Clin* 1988;4(4):609-618.
2. Azze RJ, Mattar Júnior J, Ferreira MC, Starck R, Canedo AC: Extraplexual neurotization of brachial plexus. *Microsurgery* 1994;15(1):28-32.
3. Brandt KE, Mackinnon SE: A technique for maximizing biceps recovery in brachial plexus reconstruction. *J Hand Surg Am* 1993;18(4):726-733.
4. Brunelli G, Monini L: Direct muscular neurotization. *J Hand Surg Am* 1985;10(6):993-997.
5. Doi K, Kuwata N, Muramatsu K, Hottori Y, Kawai S: Double muscle transfer for upper extremity reconstruction following complete avulsion of the brachial plexus. *Hand Clin* 1999;15(4):757-767.
6. Doi K, Muramatsu K, Hattori Y, et al: Restoration of prehension with the double free muscle technique following complete avulsion of the brachial plexus: Indications and long-term results. *J Bone Joint Surg Am* 2000;82(5):652-666.
7. Malone JM, Leal JM, Underwood J, Childers SJ: Brachial plexus injury management through upper extremity amputation with immediate postoperative prostheses. *Arch Phys Med Rehabil* 1982;63(2):89-91.
8. Allieu Y: Evolution of our indications for neurotization: Our concept of functional restoration of the upper limb after brachial plexus injuries. *Chir Main* 1999;18(2):165-166.
9. Narakas AO: The treatment of brachial plexus injuries. *Int Orthop* 1985;9(1):29-36.
10. Shin AY, Spinner RJ, Steinmann SP, Bishop AT: Adult traumatic brachial plexus injuries. *J Am Acad Orthop Surg* 2005;13(6):382-396.
11. Kerr A: The brachial plexus of nerves in man, the variations in its formation and branches. *Am J Anat* 1918;23:285-395.
12. Carvalho GA, Nikkhah G, Matthies C, Penkert G, Samii M: Diagnosis of root avulsions in traumatic brachial plexus injuries: Value of computerized tomography myelography and magnetic resonance imaging. *J Neurosurg* 1997;86(1):69-76.
13. Hashimoto T, Mitomo M, Hirabuki N, et al: Nerve root avulsion of birth palsy: Comparison of myelography with CT myelography and somatosensory evoked potential. *Radiology* 1991;178(3):841-845.
14. Oberle J, Antoniadis G, Rath SA, et al: Radiological investigations and intra-operative evoked potentials for the diagnosis of nerve root avulsion: Evaluation of both modalities by intradural root inspection. *Acta Neurochir* 1998;140(6):527-531.
15. Spinner RJ, Shin AY, Bishop AT: Update on brachial plexus surgery in adults. *Tech Hand Up Extrem Surg* 2005;9(4):220-232.
16. Rhee PC, Pirola E, Hébert-Blouin MN, et al: Concomitant traumatic spinal cord and brachial plexus injuries in adult patients. *J Bone Joint Surg Am* 2011;93(24):2271-2277.
17. Hashimoto T, Mitomo M, Hirabuki N, et al: Myelography for nerve root avulsion in birth palsy [Japanese]. *Nihon Igaku Hoshasen Gakkai Zasshi* 1990;50(4):367-374.
18. Doi K, Otsuka K, Okamoto Y, Fujii H, Hattori Y, Baliarsing AS: Cervical nerve

root avulsion in brachial plexus injuries: Magnetic resonance imaging classification and comparison with myelography and computerized tomography myelography. *J Neurosurg* 2002;96(3, suppl):277-284.

19. Walker AT, Chaloupka JC, de Lotbiniere AC, Wolfe SW, Goldman R, Kier EL: Detection of nerve rootlet avulsion on CT myelography in patients with birth palsy and brachial plexus injury after trauma. *Am J Roentgenol* 1996;167(5):1283-1287.

20. Gupta RK, Mehta VS, Banerji AK, Jain RK: MR evaluation of brachial plexus injuries. *Neuroradiology* 1989;31(5):377-381.

21. Nakamura T, Yabe Y, Horiuchi Y, Takayama S: Magnetic resonance myelography in brachial plexus injury. *J Bone Joint Surg Br* 1997;79(5):764-769.

22. Wade RG, Takwoingi Y, Wormald JCR, et al: MRI for detecting root avulsions in traumatic adult brachial plexus injuries: A systematic review and meta-analysis of diagnostic accuracy. *Radiology* 2019;293(1):125-133.

23. Holzgrefe RE, Wagner ER, Singer AD, Daly CA: Imaging of the peripheral nerve: Concepts and future direction of magnetic resonance neurography and ultrasound. *J Hand Surg Am* 2019;44(12):1066-1079.

24. Tiel RL, Happel LT Jr, Kline DG: Nerve action potential recording method and equipment. *Neurosurgery* 1996;39(1):103-109.

25. Carlsen BT, Bishop AT, Shin AY: Late reconstruction for brachial plexus injury. *Neurosurg Clin N Am* 2009;20(1):51-64, vi.

26. Malessy MJ, van Duinen SG, Feirabend HK, Thomeer RT: Correlation between histopathological findings in C-5 and C-6 nerve stumps and motor recovery following nerve grafting for repair of brachial plexus injury. *J Neurosurg* 1999;91(4):636-644.

27. Hattori Y, Doi K, Fukushima S, Kaneko K: The diagnostic value of intraoperative measurement of choline acetyltransferase activity during brachial plexus surgery. *J Hand Surg Br* 2000;25(5):509-511.

28. Potter SM, Ferris SI: Reliability of functioning free muscle transfer and vascularized ulnar nerve grafting for elbow flexion in complete brachial plexus palsy. *J Hand Surg Eur Vol* 2017;42(7):693-699.

29. Hardcastle N, Texakalidis P, Nagarajan P, Tora MS, Boulis NM: Recovery of shoulder abduction in traumatic brachial plexus palsy: A systematic review and meta-analysis of nerve transfer versus nerve graft. *Neurosurg Rev* 2020;43(3):951-956.

30. Kovachevich R, Kircher MF, Wood CM, Spinner RJ, Bishop AT, Shin AY: Complications of intercostal nerve transfer for brachial plexus reconstruction. *J Hand Surg Am* 2010;35(12):1995-2000.

31. Songcharoen P, Mahaisavariya B, Chotigavanich C: Spinal accessory neurotization for restoration of elbow flexion in avulsion injuries of the brachial plexus. *J Hand Surg Am* 1996;21(3):387-390.

32. Gu YD, Zhang GM, Chen DS, Yan JG, Cheng XM, Chen L: Seventh cervical nerve root transfer from the contralateral healthy side for treatment of brachial plexus root avulsion. *J Hand Surg Br* 1992;17(5):518-521.

33. Songcharoen P, Wongtrakul S, Mahaisavariya B, Spinner RJ: Hemi-contralateral C7 transfer to median nerve in the treatment of root avulsion brachial plexus injury. *J Hand Surg Am* 2001;26(6):1058-1064.

34. Socolovsky M, Malessy M, Bonilla G, Di Masi G, Conti ME, Lovaglio A: Phrenic to musculocutaneous nerve transfer for traumatic brachial plexus injury: Analyzing respiratory effects on elbow flexion control. *J Neurosurg* 2019;131(1):165-174.

35. Chuang DC, Wei FC, Noordhoff MS: Cross-chest C7 nerve grafting followed by free muscle transplantations for the treatment of total avulsed brachial plexus injuries: A preliminary report. *Plast Reconstr Surg* 1993;92(4):717-725.

36. Gu YD, Chen DS, Zhang GM, et al: Long-term functional results of contralateral C7 transfer. *J Reconstr Microsurg* 1998;14(1):57-59.

37. Cho AB, Paulos RG, de Resende MR, et al: Median nerve fascicle transfer versus ULNAR nerve fascicle transfer to the biceps motor branch in C5-C6 and C5-C7 brachial plexus injuries: Nonrandomized prospective study of 23 consecutive patients. *Microsurgery* 2014;34(7):511-515.

38. Al-Qattan MM, Al-Kharfy TM: Median nerve to biceps nerve transfer to restore elbow flexion in obstetric brachial plexus palsy. *Biomed Res Int* 2014;2014:854084.

39. Sungpet A, Suphachatwong C, Kawinwonggowit V: One-fascicle median nerve transfer to biceps muscle in C5 and C6 root avulsions of brachial plexus injury. *Microsurgery* 2003;23(1):10-13.

40. Vernadakis AJ, Humphreys DB, Mackinnon SE: Distal anterior interosseous nerve in the recurrent motor branch graft for reconstruction of a median nerve neuroma-in-continuity. *J Reconstr Microsurg* 2004;20(1):7-11.

41. Novak CB, Mackinnon SE: Distal anterior interosseous nerve transfer to the deep motor branch of the ulnar nerve for reconstruction of high ulnar nerve injuries. *J Reconstr Microsurg* 2002;18(6):459-464.

42. Oberlin C, Ameur NE, Teboul F, Beaulieu JY, Vacher C: Restoration of elbow flexion in brachial plexus injury by transfer of ulnar nerve fascicles to the nerve to the biceps muscle. *Tech Hand Up Extrem Surg* 2002;6(2):86-90.

43. Oberlin C, Béal D, Leechavengvongs S, Salon A, Dauge MC, Sarcy JJ: Nerve transfer to biceps muscle using a part of ulnar nerve for C5-C6 avulsion of the brachial plexus: Anatomical study and report of four cases. *J Hand Surg Am* 1994;19(2):232-237.

44. Leechavengvongs S, Witoonchart K, Uerpairojkit C, Thuvasethakul P, Ketmalasiri W: Nerve transfer to biceps muscle using a part of the ulnar nerve in brachial plexus injury (upper arm type): A report of 32 cases. *J Hand Surg Am* 1998;23(4):711-716.

45. Leechavengvongs S, Witoonchart K, Uerpairojkit C, Thuvasethakul P: Nerve transfer to deltoid muscle using the nerve to the long head of the triceps: Part II. A report of 7 cases. *J Hand Surg Am* 2003;28(4):633-638.

46. Witoonchart K, Leechavengvongs S, Uerpairojkit C, Thuvasethakul P, Wongnopsuwan V: Nerve transfer to deltoid muscle using the nerve to the long head of the triceps: Part I. An anatomic feasibility study. *J Hand Surg Am* 2003;28(4):628-632.

47. Saha A: Surgery of the paralyzed and flail shoulder. *Acta Orthop Scand* 1967;97:5-90.

48. Doi K, Hattori Y, Ikeda K, Dhawan V: Significance of shoulder function in the reconstruction of prehension with double free-muscle transfer after complete paralysis of the brachial plexus. *Plast Reconstr Surg* 2003;112(6) 1596-1603.

49. Gilbert A, Brockman R, Carlioz H: Surgical treatment of brachial plexus birth palsy. *Clin Orthop Relat Res* 1991;264:39-47.

50. Gilbert A, Razaboni R, Amar-Khodja S: Indications and results of brachial plexus surgery in obstetrical palsy. *Orthop Clin North Am* 1988;19(1):91-105.
51. Gilbert A, Romana C, Ayatti R: Tendon transfers for shoulder paralysis in children. *Hand Clin* 1988;4(4):633-642.
52. Hoffer MM, Wickenden R, Roper B: Brachial plexus birth palsies: Results of tendon transfers to the rotator cuff. *J Bone Joint Surg Am* 1978;60(5):691-695.
53. Phipps GJ, Hoffer MM: Latissimus dorsi and teres major transfer to rotator cuff for Erb's palsy. *J Shoulder Elbow Surg* 1995;4(2):124-129.
54. Karev A: Trapezius transfer for paralysis of the deltoid. *J Hand Surg Br* 1986;11(1):81-83.
55. Rühmann O, Schmolke S, Bohnsack M, Carls J, Flamme C, Wirth CJ: Reconstructive operations for the upper limb after brachial plexus palsy. *Am J Orthop (Belle Mead NJ)* 2004;33(7):351-362.
56. Aziz W, Singer RM, Wolff TW: Transfer of the trapezius for flail shoulder after brachial plexus injury. *J Bone Joint Surg Br* 1990;72(4):701-704.
57. Mayer L: Transplantation of the trapezius for paralysis of the abductors of the arm. *J Bone Joint Surg* 1927;9:412-420.
58. Rühmann O, Schmolke S, Bohnsack M, Carls J, Wirth CJ: Trapezius transfer in brachial plexus palsy: Correlation of the outcome with muscle power and operative technique. *J Bone Joint Surg Br* 2005;87(2):184-190.
59. Singh K, Karki D: Modified trapezius transfer technique for restoration of shoulder abduction in brachial plexus injury. *Indian J Plast Surg* 2007;40(1):39-46.
60. Kotwal PP, Mittal R, Malhotra R: Trapezius transfer for deltoid paralysis. *J Bone Joint Surg Br* 1998;80(1):114-116.
61. Monreal R, Paredes L, Diaz H, Leon P: Trapezius transfer to treat flail shoulder after brachial plexus palsy. *J Brachial Plex Peripher Nerve Inj* 2007;2:2.
62. Terzis JK, Barmpitsioti A: Secondary shoulder reconstruction in patients with brachial plexus injuries. *J Plast Reconstr Aesthet Surg* 2011;64(7):843-853.
63. Waters PM: Update on management of pediatric brachial plexus palsy. *J Pediatr Orthop* 2005;25(1):116-126.
64. Itoh Y, Sasaki T, Ishiguro T, Uchinishi K, Yabe Y, Fukuda H: Transfer of latissimus dorsi to replace a paralysed anterior deltoid: A new technique using an inverted pedicled graft. *J Bone Joint Surg Br* 1987;69(4):647-651.
65. De Smet L: The latissimus dorsi flap for reconstruction of a paralysed deltoid. *Acta Chir Belg* 2004;104(3):328-329.
66. Hou CL, Tai YH: Transfer of upper pectoralis major flap for functional reconstruction of deltoid muscle. *Chin Med J (Engl)* 1991;104(9):753-757.
67. Lin H, Hou C, Xu Z: Transfer of the superior portion of the pectoralis major flap for restoration of shoulder abduction. *J Reconstr Microsurg* 2009;25(4):255-260.
68. Elhassan B: Lower trapezius transfer for shoulder external rotation in patients with paralytic shoulder. *J Hand Surg Am* 2014;39(3):556-562.
69. Narakas A: Muscle transposition in the shoulder and upper arm for sequelae of brachial plexus palsy. *Clin Neurol Neurosurg* 1993;95:89-91.
70. Elhassan B, Bishop AT, Hartzler RU, Shin AY, Spinner RJ: Tendon transfer options about the shoulder in patients with brachial plexus injury. *J Bone Joint Surg Am* 2012;94(15):1391-1398.
71. Elhassan B, Bishop A, Shin A, Spinner R: Shoulder tendon transfer options for adult patients with brachial plexus injury. *J Hand Surg Am* 2010;35(7):1211-1219.
72. Friedman AH, Nunley JA II, Goldner RD, Oakes WJ, Goldner JL, Urbaniak JR: Nerve transposition for the restoration of elbow flexion following brachial plexus avulsion injuries. *J Neurosurg* 1990;72(1):59-64.
73. Anderson KA, O'Dell MA, James MA: Shoulder external rotation tendon transfers for brachial plexus birth palsy. *Tech Hand Up Extrem Surg* 2006;10(2):60-67.
74. Goddard NJ, Fixsen JA: Rotation osteotomy of the humerus for birth injuries of the brachial plexus. *J Bone Joint Surg Br* 1984;66(2):257-259.
75. Waters PM, Peljovich AE: Shoulder reconstruction in patients with chronic brachial plexus birth palsy: A case control study. *Clin Orthop Relat Res* 1999;364:144-152.
76. Rouholamin E, Wootton JR, Jamieson AM: Arthrodesis of the shoulder following brachial plexus injury. *Injury* 1991;22(4):271-274.
77. Chammas M, Goubier JN, Coulet B, Reckendorf GM, Picot MC, Allieu Y: Glenohumeral arthrodesis in upper and total brachial plexus palsy: A comparison of functional results. *J Bone Joint Surg Br* 2004;86(5):692-695.
78. Richards RR, Waddell JP, Hudson AR: Shoulder arthrodesis for the treatment of brachial plexus palsy. *Clin Orthop Relat Res* 1985;198:250-258.
79. Richards RR, Beaton D, Hudson AR: Shoulder arthrodesis with plate fixation: Functional outcome analysis. *J Shoulder Elbow Surg* 1993;2(5):225-239.
80. Nagano A, Okinaga S, Ochiai N, Kurokawa T: Shoulder arthrodesis by external fixation. *Clin Orthop Relat Res* 1989;247:97-100.
81. Allieu Y, Triki F, de Godebout J: Total paralysis of the brachial plexus: Value of the preservation of the limb and the restoration of active flexion of the elbow [French]. *Rev Chir Orthop Reparatrice Appar Mot* 1987;73(8):665-673.
82. Alnot JY, Daunois O, Oberlin C, Bleton R: Total paralysis of the brachial plexus caused by supra-clavicular lesions [French]. *Rev Chir Orthop Reparatrice Appar Mot* 1992;78(8):495-504.
83. Hentz VR, Narakas A: The results of microneurosurgical reconstruction in complete brachial plexus palsy: Assessing outcome and predicting results. *Orthop Clin North Am* 1988;19(1):107-114.
84. Merrell GA, Barrie KA, Katz DL, Wolfe SW: Results of nerve transfer techniques for restoration of shoulder and elbow function in the context of a meta-analysis of the English literature. *J Hand Surg Am* 2001;26(2):303-314.
85. Sedel L: The results of surgical repair of brachial plexus injuries. *J Bone Joint Surg Br* 1982;64(1):54-66.
86. Atlan F, Durand S, Fox M, Levy P, Belkheyar Z, Oberlin C: Functional outcome of glenohumeral fusion in brachial plexus palsy: A report of 54 cases. *J Hand Surg Am* 2012;37(4):683-688.
87. Bishop AT: Functioning free-muscle transfer for brachial plexus injury. *Hand Clin* 2005;21(1):91-102.
88. Giuffre JL, Kakar S, Bishop AT, Spinner RJ, Shin AY: Current concepts of the treatment of adult brachial plexus injuries. *J Hand Surg Am* 2010;35(4):678-688.
89. Addosooki A, Doi K, Hattori Y, Wahegaonkar A: Wrist arthrodesis after double free-muscle transfer in traumatic total brachial plexus palsy. *Tech Hand Up Extrem Surg* 2007;11(1):29-36.
90. Giuffre JL, Bishop AT, Spinner RJ, Kircher MF, Shin AY: Wrist, first carpometacarpal joint, and thumb interphalangeal joint arthrodesis in patients with brachial plexus injuries. *J Hand Surg Am* 2012;37(12):2557-2563.e1.
91. Terzis JK, Barmpitsioti A: Wrist fusion in posttraumatic brachial plexus palsy.

Plast Reconstr Surg 2009;124(6):2027-2039.
92. Van Heest AE, Strothman D: Wrist arthrodesis in cerebral palsy. J Hand Surg Am 2009;34(7):1216-1224.
93. Rorabeck CH: The management of the flail upper extremity in brachial plexus injuries. J Trauma 1980;20(6):491-493.
94. Parry CB: Thoughts on the rehabilitation of patients with brachial plexus lesions. Hand Clin 1995;11(4):657-675.
95. Seddon HJ, Yeoman PM: Brachial plexus injuries: Treatment of the flail arm. J Bone Joint Surg Br 1961;43(3):493-500.
96. Parry CB: The management of injuries to the brachial plexus. Proc R Soc Med 1974;67(6 pt 1):488-490.
97. Ransford AO, Hughes SP: Complete brachial plexus lesions: A ten-year follow-up of twenty cases. J Bone Joint Surg Br 1977;59(4):417-420.
98. Malone JM, Fleming LL, Roberson J, et al: Immediate, early, and late postsurgical management of upper-limb amputation. J Rehabil Res Dev 1984;21(1):33-41.
99. Thyberg M, Johansen PB: Prosthetic rehabilitation in unilateral high above-elbow amputation and brachial plexus lesion: Case report. Arch Phys Med Rehabil 1986;67(4):260-262.
100. Bedi A, Miller B, Jebson PJ: Combined glenohumeral arthrodesis and above-elbow amputation for the flail limb following a complete posttraumatic brachial plexus injury. Tech Hand Up Extrem Surg 2005;9(2):113-119.
101. Terzis JK, Vekris MD, Soucacos PN: Brachial plexus root avulsions. World J Surg 2001;25(8):1049-1061.
102. Clare DJ, Wirth MA, Groh GI, Rockwood CA Jr: Shoulder arthrodesis. J Bone Joint Surg Am 2001;83(4):593-600.
103. Cofield RH, Briggs BT: Glenohumeral arthrodesis: Operative and long-term functional results. J Bone Joint Surg Am 1979;61(5):668-677.
104. Richards RR, Sherman RM, Hudson AR, Waddell JP: Shoulder arthrodesis using a pelvic-reconstruction plate: A report of eleven cases. J Bone Joint Surg Am 1988;70(3):416-421.
105. Wilkinson MC, Birch R, Bonney G: Brachial plexus injury: When to amputate? Injury 1993;24(9):603-605.
106. Yeoman PM: Traction injuries of the brachial plexus. Nurs Mirror Midwives J 1971;132(4):26-27.

Hand Transplantation

CDR Scott M. Tintle, MD, FAAOS • Jaimie T. Shores, MD, FACS • L. Scott Levin, MD, FAAOS, FACS

CHAPTER 30

ABSTRACT

Because hand loss affects nearly every activity of daily living and results in substantial disability, vascularized composite allotransplantation offers an alternative to prosthesis use and can be considered a restorative option for carefully selected patients. Because the outcome of a hand transplant is greatly dependent on the participation, cooperation, and patient compliance with hand therapy, medications, and follow-up screening appointments, careful evaluation of transplantation candidates is mandatory. Evaluation factors should include a patient's behavior, social support, financial security, and psychiatric and psychological health. If hand transplantation is elected, the surgeon must be familiar with donor procurement procedures, surgical techniques for transplantation at various levels, postoperative care requirements, possible complications, and the lifelong need of immunotherapy for the patient.

Keywords: amputation; hand transplant; nerve transfer; restorative surgery; vascularized composite allotransplantation

Introduction

Although vascularized composite allotransplantation (VCA) remains a controversial topic in upper limb amputations, hand transplantation remains an important restorative surgery that can currently be provided for upper limb amputations. Hand loss is a devastating event that affects nearly every activity of daily living and leaves patients with substantial disability.[1,2] The effect on a patient of losing both sensibility and prehension often results in despondency, and its adverse consequences cannot be overstated. Despite promising technologic advances in upper limb prostheses, the available literature still demonstrates high prosthesis rejection rates for upper limb amputations. These findings suggest that prostheses cannot replicate the complex prehensile and sensory functions of the native hand and arm in a reliably comfortable and useful form.[3-11] Residual limb discomfort, prosthesis weight, and limited usefulness remain the most commonly cited reasons for the rejection of upper limb prosthetics.[3,12,13]

Hand transplant pioneers surmised that prosthetic devices would never completely satisfy an individual with an upper limb amputation. Even if dexterity and prehensile function of the human hand could be restored, these would do little to restore highly coveted body image or hand sensibility. Rather, they postulated that these functions could be replaced only with "like" human tissue and full neural reintegration.[14] The VCA field has grown from this desire to fully restore the functional and emotional aspects of the human hand (**Figure 1**).

History

The world's first hand transplant, likely inspired by the solid organ transplantation community's rapid growth, was performed in South America in 1964.[1,15,16] Unfortunately, because of relatively primitive immunosuppression techniques as well as a lack of basic science preparation, acute rejection predictably occurred, and the transplanted limb was amputated less than 1 month later.[12,17] This failure, or the realization that the hand surgery community had reached too far, too fast, resulted

---

Dr. Tintle or an immediate family member serves as a board member, owner, officer, or committee member of Society of Military Orthopaedic Surgeons. Dr. Shores or an immediate family member has received research or institutional support from Axogen, Inc. and Neuraptive Therapeutics and serves as a board member, owner, officer, or committee member of American Association for Hand Surgery, American Society for Surgery of the Hand, and American Society of Transplantation. Dr. Levin or an immediate family member serves as a paid consultant to or is an employee of MMI SpA; has received research or institutional support from AxoGen, Inc. and Polyganics; and serves as a board member, owner, officer, or committee member of American College of Surgeons, American Society for Reconstructive Microsurgery, American Society for Surgery of the Hand, Vascularized Composite Allograft Transplantation Committee, and World Society for Reconstructive Microsurgery.

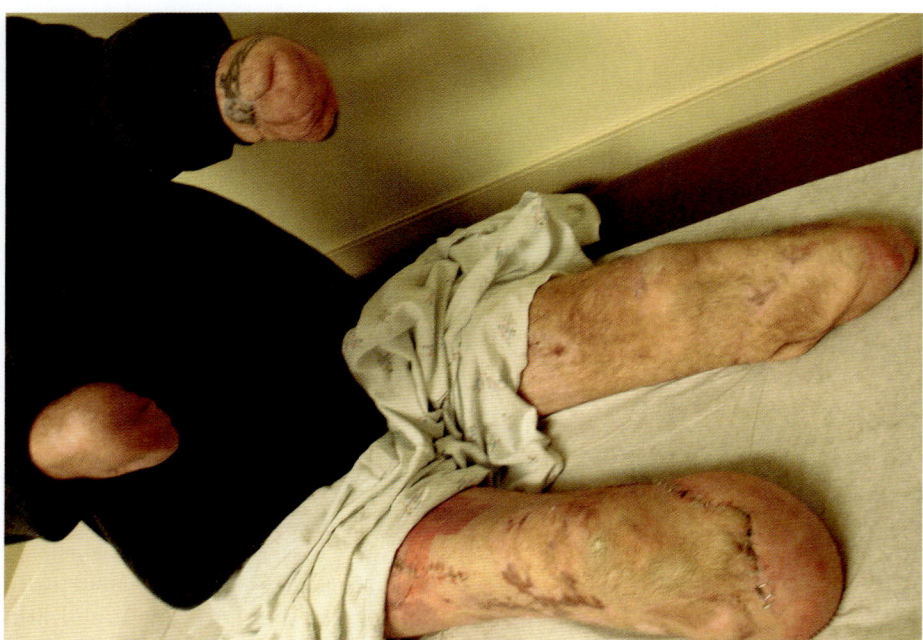

FIGURE 1 Clinical photograph of an ideal candidate for bilateral hand transplantation based on the patient's quadrimembral amputations. Ultimately, a multidisciplinary approach led this patient and the surgeon to determine that prosthetic function was too good for the risk involved with hand transplantation. (Copyright L. Scott Levin, MD, FAAOS, FACS, Philadelphia, PA.)

in a long interval before the next hand transplant attempt in Lyon, France, in 1998.[12,18,19] Technically, this procedure succeeded; however, the technical success was unsustainable because the patient did not adapt psychologically to the new hand and discontinued immunosuppressive medications. The limb was eventually amputated because of chronic rejection and lack of function.[1] Dr. Warren Breidenbach performed the first truly successful hand transplant in the United States in 1999. The patient still has the transplanted hand currently—nearly 16 years later—with excellent function, even returning to work afterward.[12,13,20]

Advances in solid organ transplantation made possible the early success in hand transplantation in the late 1990s. New medications, such as tacrolimus and mycophenolate mofetil, decreased the likelihood of rejection. Animal models of VCA have provided the basic and translational science evidence that successful allotransplantation without rejection is possible with these medications.[12,21-23] Since then, the VCA field has grown dramatically. Worldwide, estimates are that more than 130 hand transplants have been performed to date.

Indications and Ethical Considerations

Primum non nocere—first do no harm—must be the paramount principle as the VCA field progresses. Cooney et al[24] echoed this sentiment in their 2002 American Society for Surgery of the Hand position statement, when they recommended "great caution and a measured approach to the patient requesting limb transplant." This caution has, appropriately, slowed the growth of VCA compared with growth in solid organ transplantation. Because the patient considering hand transplantation is not faced with a life-or-death situation, hand transplantation is very different from most solid organ transplantations.[25] Developing widely accepted indications for subjecting a physiologically healthy person to the risks of lifelong immunosuppression remains the preeminent challenge for the allotransplantation community.[26]

In 2009, Hollenbeck et al[14] indicated that well-defined indications do not exist for hand or face transplants. Unfortunately, this statement currently remains relatively accurate, and the indications remain open to interpretation by individual VCA centers.[27,28] Having recognized the need for more refined indications for hand transplantation, the allotransplantation community founded the American Society for Reconstructive Transplantation in 2008, whose goal is to provide a platform for advancing composite tissue allotransplantation as relevant to reconstructive and transplant surgery. The society published guidelines for medical necessity determination for transplanting the hand and/or an upper limb. Despite this comprehensive and admirable attempt at defining indications, further refinement is necessary to ensure the safe advancement of the field.[12]

Screening for VCA

Hand allotransplantation represents a lifelong commitment by a surgeon, the patient, the patient's family, and, ultimately, the healthcare system. Without the commitment of each entity, the true lifelong success of transplantation will not be realized. For this reason, screening for VCA is expensive and laborious, but vitally important. Every aspect of the life of the transplant candidate must be reviewed. Medical screening should include primary care, cardiology, infectious disease, and transplant medicine. In-depth evaluations of a patient's behavior, social support, financial security, and psychiatric and psychological health are necessary and may ultimately disqualify a patient for transplant if possible risk factors that could lead to failure are identified. The outcome of a hand transplant is very much dependent on patient participation, cooperation, and compliance with hand therapy, medications, and follow-up screening appointments. Every preoperative screening is critical because these screenings may both predict patient compliance and identify other medical risk factors for failure. Literature specific to the VCA psychosocial screening is unfortunately limited, but Department of Defense–funded research is currently ongoing to hopefully add to this paucity of evidence.

The psychological assessment is likely the most critical component of transplant screening, and most patients have been found to have at least one psychological disorder.[29] The success of a kidney, liver, or heart transplant depends only on a patient's compliance with medications, but relatively high rates of medication noncompliance occur among patients who depend on the transplant(s) for life.[30,31] Among a combined heart and heart/lung transplant population, the only risk factor for graft loss between 6 and 12 months was being unmarried or not living in a stable relationship. The social support for an individual candidate must be identified, and a transplant should not occur if the surgeon is not comfortable with a patient's support system.[13] In one unique study by Kinsley et al,[32] the authors queried hand transplant recipients from the International Registry on Hand and Composite Tissue Transplantation and suggested that anxiety, depression, posttraumatic stress disorder, participation in occupational therapy, expectations for posttransplant function, and family support are associated with postsurgical transplant status.

Preferred Surgical Technique of This Chapter's Authors

Donor Procurement

Procurement is performed on donors with brain death declarations whose families have consented to donation. Donor activation and procurement specifics have been reported in more detail elsewhere and are briefly summarized here.[33] Hand procurement is performed in a coordinated fashion with all other organ procurement teams (eg, kidney, liver, heart, and lungs). The hand(s) may be procured before solid organ procurement or during solid organ procurement, although they must be perfused with preservation solution after procurement. Organ donation patients receive heparin before aorta crossclamping. For a transplant at the hand/wrist/distal forearm level, procurement by means of elbow disarticulation is rapid and provides ample tissue. For procurements at the midforearm level, an elbow disarticulation also may suffice; however, if concerns for adequate vessel or nerve length or the quality of the soft-tissue envelope are present, a supracondylar humerus procurement provides extra tissue as necessary. For proximal forearm transplants, a lower to middle humerus procurement is performed (**Figure 2**). For supracondylar to midhumerus transplantation, procurement is performed as high on the humerus as possible to obtain adequate blood vessel, nerve, and soft tissue.

Procurement is typically performed under tourniquet control, and a guillotine incision is made medially to expose the brachial vessels, which are controlled with proximal clips or ligatures. Distal to the ligatures, an arteriotomy is made, and a cannula is inserted to allow perfusion. After the cannula is in place, the superficial and deep veins are divided, and perfusion with the desired preservation solution is performed. Clinical examination of the vessels determines the dominance of the deep versus superficial venous system for outflow drainage. The soft tissues, including the nerves, are sharply divided. For disarticulations, the elbow joint is sharply opened and separated. For transhumeral procurement, a saw is used for the humeral osteotomy.

To improve coordination among all organ procurement teams, the limb can be rapidly removed and perfused on the back table in the surgical suite or it can be perfused immediately before amputation. The limb is wrapped in moist gauze and then placed into a sealed plastic bag. This bag is placed into another sealed bag, immersed in an ice and water slurry bath in a third bag, placed in a cooler, and then transported immediately. The residual limb is closed after all organ and tissue donation has ceased. A cosmetic prosthesis that is skin tone matched is then applied to the donor residual limb to permit postmortem family viewing and open casket burial, if desired.

Transplantation

The recipient is prepared by anesthesia with arterial and large central venous access. Peripheral large-bore

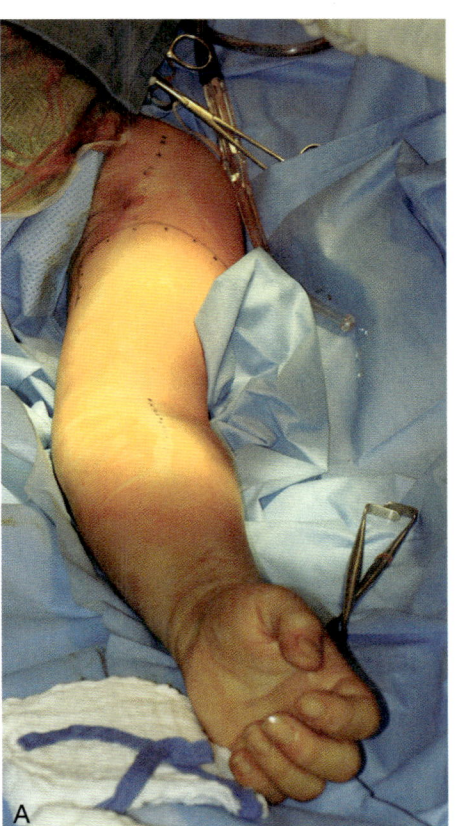
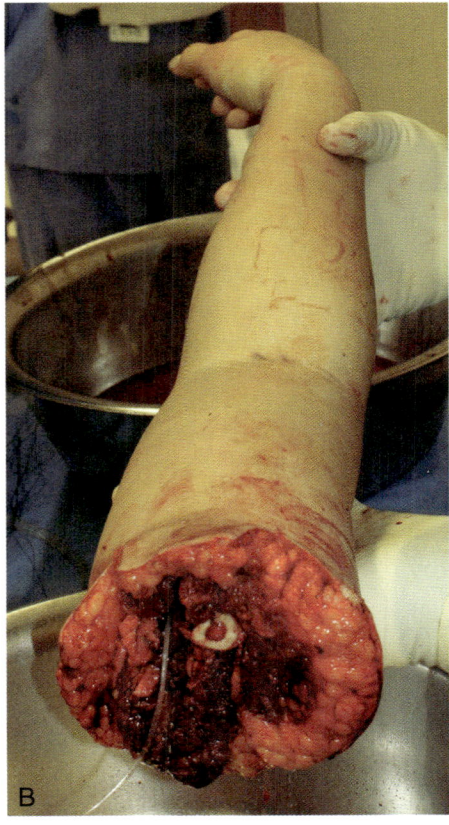

FIGURE 2 Intraoperative photographs of the setup for procurement of a donor limb at the proximal level (**A**) and the amputated donor limb being perfused with preservation solution (**B**). (Copyright Jaimie T. Shores, MD, FACS, Baltimore, MD.)

venous access is obtained, if possible. Premedication is administered using immunologic induction therapy. Peripheral block nerve catheters may be placed but should not be dosed with medication during the initial surgery.[34]

Surgery commences with the arrival and inspection of the donor limbs. One surgical team per recipient and one surgical team per donor limb are used. Simultaneous dissection of the donor and recipient limbs is performed with skin flap elevation 90° opposite one another (volar dorsal skin flaps on one limb, radial ulnar skin flaps on another limb), with each tendon, muscle, nerve, vein, and artery on each limb being tagged. Hybrid forearm lengths are determined based on the contralateral limb or a projected normal, which is symmetric in the case of bilateral transplants. All dissection on the donor limbs is performed on sterile ice with towels between the tissue and ice to keep the limb cool during the surgery right up until the arterial clamps are removed to initiate reperfusion.[35,36]

Distal Forearm Level

Radial and ulnar skin flaps are elevated on the donor limb using a carpal tunnel incision with zigzag extension across the wrist creases and midaxis incision down the forearm. The dorsal incision is midaxis as well. All veins are tagged and preserved if possible. The radial and ulnar arteries are not overdissected, and their perforators are left intact within the septae to the skin flaps. All structures are tagged (**Figure 3**). The radius and the ulna are preplated in neutral forearm rotation. The authors of this chapter have used long, locking distal radius plates as well as locking distal ulna plates for fixation.[35-37]

The recipient residual limb is dissected under sterile tourniquet with volar and dorsal skin flaps using a radial-to-ulnar fish-mouth incision and elevated skin flaps. Radial and ulnar artery perforators are preserved where possible. Tendons are identified based on position and tagged, as are vessels and nerves. Bones are débrided to healthy levels and then measured. The total forearm length is determined,

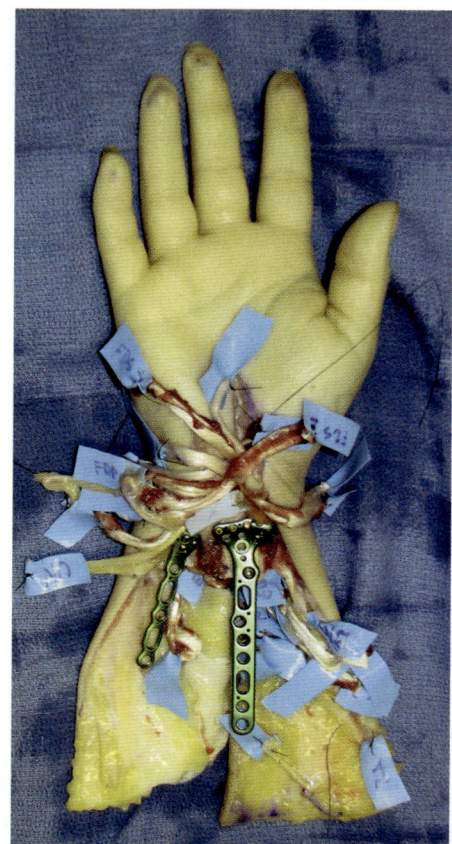

FIGURE 3 Intraoperative photograph of a distal-level donor hand that has been dissected, tagged, and preplated for transplantation. (Copyright Jaimie T. Shores, MD, FACS, Baltimore, MD.)

and corresponding osteotomies for the donor limb are marked. After this dissection is completed, the tourniquet is removed.[35,36]

The donor limb plates are removed, and osteotomies are performed. An oblique ulnar osteotomy may be used, and the plates are replaced. The osteosynthesis and condensation of two teams to one is then performed. Again, the surgery continues with sterile ice packed beneath the donor limb under sterile towels. After the osteosynthesis is complete, a Pulvertaft weave reconstruction of all extensors is typically performed, first pulling the metacarpophalangeal joints into hyperextension with the wrist in neutral position. Then the flexor tendons are reconstructed with Pulvertaft weaves, pulling the digits into a standard flexed cascade.

After the tendons are completed, a microscope is brought in, and either the arteries or the nerves may be coapted next. The benefit of the nerve-next sequence is the benefit of performing nerve coaptations in a bloodless field, which can be more rapid and accurate. If individual motor and sensory groups are identified within the median and ulnar nerves, these can be repaired individually. The superficial radial nerve also is repaired. Depending on preference and availability, the antebrachial cutaneous nerves may or may not be repaired.

The arteries are then repaired, usually in end-to-end fashion. The anterior interosseous artery also may be repaired if it appears especially large. The vena comitantes may be repaired at this time as well. The superficial veins are left open. At this time, the ice is removed, the clamps are left on all repaired veins, the clamps are removed from the repaired arteries, and reperfusion is initiated. The authors of this chapter typically give a bolus of heparin and steroids systemically for this step for ischemia-reperfusion injury. Egress of blood, which can be collected for washing/purification and autotransfusion, if desired, is allowed into a basin. Allogeneic blood transfusion is usually required before and during this step, with leukoreduced and irradiated packed red blood cells. In addition, fresh frozen plasma should be given in a 1:1 or 2:1 ratio of packed red blood cells to fresh frozen plasma.[34] After the egressing blood becomes a more normal bright red color, the clamps can be removed from the repaired veins to allow normal venous return with anesthesia on standby for metabolic derangements. The remaining superficial and deep veins are repaired. Any remaining tendons, such as the flexor carpi radialis or flexor carpi ulnaris that may have obscured the vessels previously, are now repaired. Hemostasis is achieved, and the interdigitating skin flaps are assessed for perfusion and inset over closed suction drains. The wrist is splinted in neutral position with the digits left free to begin immediate active and passive motion therapy, if this can be tolerated based on the quality of the tendon repair.[35,36]

Midforearm Level

The same skin incisions and procedures described for transplantation at the distal forearm level are performed for the midforearm level (Figure 4). The key differences are the lack of tendon for Pulvertaft-type tendon repairs or reconstructions, more proximal neurorrhaphies, and more proximal bone fixation. Osteosynthesis is performed with 3.5-mm forearm plates on the radius and 2.4- to 3.5-mm plates on the ulna, as indicated. A technique using an oblique osteotomy of the ulna and an ulnar shortening plate for osteosynthesis has been described.[38] Muscle-tendon unit repairs are typically within the muscle substance and fascia and are performed with multiple woven synthetic sutures. These may be reinforced with overlaid or woven tendon or fascial grafts as desired or necessary. Vascular reconstructions and nerve reconstructions are performed as described previously. The skin flaps are trimmed and inset, as allowed by their postreperfusion patterns, over closed suction drains. The forearm and wrist are splinted in neutral flexion and extension. The digits may be left free or splinted in the intrinsic-plus position as desired.

Proximal Forearm Level

For transplantation at the proximal forearm level, the recipient limb skin flaps are made volar/dorsal, and the donor skin flaps are made radial/ulnar. The donor flexor/pronator origin and extensor origins are dissected off the medial and lateral epicondyles and the radiocapitellar joint after a longitudinal incision down the subcutaneous border of the ulna. The volar muscle mass does not require much dissection, which is left for later and performed only as much as necessary for brachial artery and median nerve reconstruction. This sleeve of muscle is elevated off the supracondylar humerus procurement level donor arm and elevated distally on the dorsal side past the point of desired osteotomy to allow for adequate plate placement. Both plates are placed through this dorsal approach. The volar muscle attachments to the forearm bones distal to the osteotomy are undisturbed. Great care is taken to prevent injury to the posterior interosseous nerve or its branches during the dissection. Individual branches of the radial nerve into the superficial radial nerve, posterior interosseous nerve, and extensor carpi radialis brevis branch may be identified and tagged. After the position of osteotomy has been decided (and if helpful), the forearm bones may be temporarily locked into the desired position of rotation with Kirschner wires on both the donor and recipient to aid in osteosynthesis. The authors of this chapter use the ulnar shortening osteotomy plate technique for osteosynthesis of the ulna along the subcutaneous border and a 3.5-mm metaphyseal locking compression plate for the radius dorsally, again taking care to not damage the posterior interosseous nerve on either the donor or recipient sides.[38] The residual volar/dorsal muscle masses of the recipient proximal forearm are left in place. The donor flexor/pronator and extensor muscle masses are draped over the recipient muscle masses and anchored into the medial and lateral epicondyles with suture anchors and reinforced with fascia-to-fascia suture repairs.[39]

Nerve transfers are then performed by denervating the recipient native forearm muscles and transferring the divided nerves into the donor nerves with direct coaptations. The posterior interosseous nerve, the superficial radial nerve, and the extensor carpi radialis brevis branch of the radial nerve are repaired individually. The superficial head of the pronator teres may require division for the median nerve repair at the level of the first motor branch to the pronator teres. The ulnar nerve is transposed anteriorly before muscle mass anchoring, and a hybrid level of subcutaneous versus intramuscular transposition is achieved. The nerve is repaired at the level of its first motor branch. The brachial artery may be repaired either end to end or end to side. The benefit of end-to-side anastomosis is that some direct perfusion to the now denervated recipient muscle mass and the proximal radius and ulna can be maintained. All available veins (superficial and deep) are anastomosed. Hemostasis is achieved, and interdigitating skin flaps are closed over drains. The elbow is splinted in 90° of flexion with neutral forearm rotation and neutral wrist flexion and extension. The digits are left free.

Transhumeral Level

Most transhumeral transplants have used the recipient's own elbow flexors and extensors to power the elbow, and procurement is performed at the middle to upper humerus level. Anterior and posterior skin flaps are elevated on the recipient, and medial-lateral skin flaps are elevated on the donor without extending the incisions down to the olecranon. The recipient brachialis, biceps, and triceps muscles are dissected. Keeping some amount of scar on the distal muscle and all possible tendon is helpful.[40] The donor muscles are dissected, and if adequate muscle length is present on the recipient side, the muscle tissue can be removed from the donor leaving only the biceps tendon, the brachialis fascia, and the triceps tendon and fascia. However, if adequate muscle length is not present, some amount of muscle may be left on the donor. The recipient humerus is shortened back to fresh, healthy bone, and the donor humerus osteotomy is planned to re-create symmetric upper arm length. A single 4.5- or 3.5-mm metaphyseal locking compression plate may be used for osteosynthesis, with

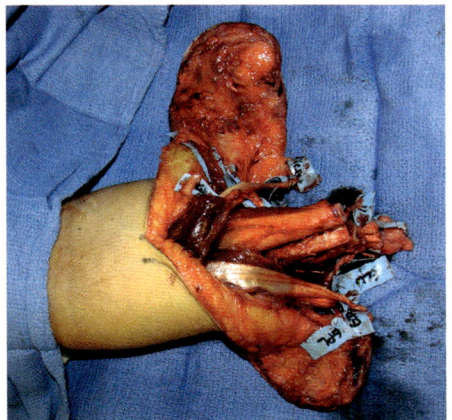

FIGURE 4 Intraoperative photograph of a recipient's limb that has been dissected and tagged and is ready to receive a midforearm level transplant. (Copyright Jaimie T. Shores, MD, FACS, Baltimore, MD.)

an anterolateral approach through the brachialis/brachioradialis interval. The donor limb may be preplated. Plate removal and osteotomy are then performed. The plate is replaced so that osteosynthesis can commence. Muscle repair or reconstruction is then performed. Muscle/scar to muscle or muscle/scar to tendon/fascia repairs are performed, depending on the level. Fascial or tendon autografts or allografts may be used for weaves or onlay reinforcement if desired. The triceps should be repaired first, followed by the elbow flexors, the radial nerve, the median nerve, and the ulnar nerve after anterior transposition. All tendons and nerves should be coapted as distally as possible. The brachial artery and veins are then repaired. It is important to make sure that there is no substantial redundancy in the brachial artery to prevent kinking of the artery during elbow flexion.[37] All superficial and deep veins available are anastomosed. Hemostasis is then obtained, and skin flap closure is performed over drains. The elbow is splinted in 90° of flexion with neutral forearm rotation and the wrist in neutral flexion and extension. Elbow motion is prevented for 6 weeks. Wrist and digit passive motion may begin immediately.

Postoperative Care

The surgical or transplant intensive care unit is used for initial postoperative management. Various monitoring devices may be used to assess perfusion, including, for example, clinical assessment of color and capillary refill, pulse oximetry probes placed on both the radial and ulnar digits compared between hands or another reference point on the body to assess both waveform and saturation, handheld Doppler monitors, and implanted venous or arterial Doppler devices. Dressings are typically changed on postoperative day 2 or 3, and therapy commences at this time. The indwelling peripheral nerve catheters are bolused with local anesthetic in the operating room after the microvascular surgery is completed and are used for postoperative pain control combined with multimodal analgesia that is managed by the acute pain management team. Specialists in transplant infectious diseases help manage necessary postoperative antibiotics. No casts or circumferential rigid binding is placed because swelling can be substantial in the first week. After the surgical team is confident that intensive-level monitoring is no longer necessary, the patient can be moved to a standard transplant floor for continued recuperation.

Immunotherapy

Currently, there is no agreement at transplant centers on a standard immunotherapy protocol, but patients should expect to be placed on lifelong immunosuppression of some sort.[41] Most immunotherapy protocols are adapted from solid organ transplantation, with, at least initially, a polyclonal or monoclonal antibody induction therapy followed by traditional triple drug combinations of corticosteroids, tacrolimus, and mycophenolate mofetil for maintenance therapy. Some centers, on a patient-by-patient basis, have weaned patients from steroids and may later attempt a slow conversion from tacrolimus to sirolimus to mitigate long-term renal toxicity. In addition, a cell-based immunotherapy protocol using donor bone marrow combined with monoclonal antibody induction and tacrolimus monotherapy has been successfully used and reported.[37] Rejection is typically first identified in the skin and is a very dynamic process, usually presenting as an erythematous maculopapular rash, with or without swelling. It can progress to coalescent patches of erythema and even blisters and ulceration. Skin biopsy is the standard diagnostic tool for acute rejection using the classification criteria created in Banff, Canada.[42-44] Transplant vasculopathy also has been described; however, it is not apparent if this is chronic rejection that is cell mediated or antibody mediated against alloantigens or stimulated by mechanical trauma during vessel dissection, which is more nonspecific. High-resolution ultrasonography can be used for noninvasive monitoring of vessel wall thickening and narrowing of the luminal diameter.[45,46] All transplant patients will experience rejection episodes that can be treated topically at the skin level (with topical tacrolimus and steroid creams) and/or systemically.

Complications

Complications can be related to (1) the transplant itself, including surgical complications (eg, bleeding, hematoma, tissue necrosis, or immediate limb loss caused by vascular complications), subacute complications in the limbs (wound healing complications, nonunions, or chronic pain), and chronic complications (eg, poor functional outcomes, poor motor or sensory recovery, rejection, or limb loss); (2) the overall procedure of transplantation (eg, heart attack, stroke, death, blood clots, thromboembolism, pneumonia); or (3) the effects of the immunomodulatory medications (eg, renal injury, malignancy, opportunistic or higher susceptibility to serious and life-threatening infections, rejection, hypertension, diabetes mellitus, leukopenia, osteonecrosis, Cushing syndrome, or serum sickness).[37,41,47,48] All patients should be monitored closely by experienced transplant physicians for the rest of their lives for both surveillance and management. For these reasons, many centers worldwide are developing or have already implemented novel immunotherapy protocols to mitigate these risks. It should be noted that all of these complications have been reported in hand transplant patients.

Outcomes

Outcomes are difficult to assess because of a lack of standardization in the measurement of outcomes, the nature of differing functionality expected by differing levels of amputation, the unique anatomic features of each limb loss and the subsequent transplant, and the overall low numbers of transplants performed. In the worldwide experience, at least 107 hand or upper limb transplants have been performed on 72 patients (with at least 3 patients and 4 limbs transplanted that are known to this chapter's authors but not yet reported).[41] In patients with reported outcomes for isolated hand or upper limb transplantation in China, Europe, and North America, one patient has died, resulting in a 99% patient survival rate. However, at least four cases of combined face plus hand or hand plus leg transplantation have been performed in France, the United States, and Turkey. Three of the four patients died, resulting in a 75% mortality rate for multisite (unilateral or bilateral upper limb plus another body region) VCAs.[49,50] The one patient who survived ultimately lost both transplanted hands but had survival of the face transplant after an immediate postoperative episode of septic shock. Although at least 7 of 12 patients in the Chinese experience had transplanted hand loss because of a lack of access to immunosuppressive medications and/or compliance, the Western European, Australian, and US experiences have shown more encouraging results.[41] In the United States, 21 patients have undergone isolated unilateral or bilateral hand or upper limb transplantation, with more patients known to the authors of this chapter but not yet reported. Of those reported, 8 were bilateral, and 13 were unilateral, with 2 transhumeral transplants. Of these 21 patients, only 1 patient sustained an immediate transplant loss (during the initial hospitalization). A second patient experienced partial graft losses with some fingertip necrosis but overall survival of the transplanted hands. Long-term follow-up of the remaining 20 patients has demonstrated delayed graft loss in 3 patients (at 9 months after the transplant resulting from aggressive vasculopathy of unknown origin, at 2 years resulting from noncompliance and advanced rejection, and at 4 years resulting from noncompliance and advanced rejection). In the Western European and Australian experiences, 30 patients have been reported to receive 47 hand or upper limb (17 bilateral, 13 unilateral) transplants in isolation. There has been one immediate postoperative loss and one long-term loss resulting from noncompliance and uncontrolled rejection.

With regard to functional outcomes, it may take several years before maximal improvement is observed in motor recovery for more proximal transplants; sensation continues to improve year by year in the transplant. Therefore, reported data may be only a snapshot of a dynamic functional recovery that patients experience. In addition, no single validated instrument for functional measurement for hand transplants exists; thus, the Hand Transplant Scoring System was developed. In addition, most centers report Disabilities of the Arm, Shoulder and Hand scores and other functional tests in an individual, center-by-center manner.[47,48]

A single repository exists at some participating centers, which is managed by the International Registry on Hand and Composite Tissue Transplantation.[47,48,51,52] This registry has published summative functional outcome results of early transplant patients in the years 2005, 2007, 2008, 2010, and 2011. Most of the data are for transplants at the distal and middle forearm levels; few proximal level transplants are included. The registry summarized 39 patients with 57 upper limb transplants with follow-ups ranging from 6 months to 3 years in the most recent publication.[47] The registry demonstrated that, at the least, protective sensation developed in all of the patients within the first year after transplantation, and tactile or discriminative sensibility developed in 90% of the patients as time progressed.[48] The Hand Transplant Scoring System result, which is a measure of function after a hand transplant, demonstrated substantial improvement within the first 2 years and continued improvement over time in those with bilateral transplants, with a more gradual improvement in those with a unilateral transplant. The Disabilities of the Arm, Shoulder and Hand score demonstrated the most substantial improvement in patients with bilateral transplants, with the most significant decrease in disability within the first 2 years. More than 75% of the patients also reported improvement in their quality of life after transplantation.[48]

Evolving Issues and the Future of VCA

Hand transplantation has seen success, and the future holds remarkable promise for this restorative treatment option. Orthopaedic and plastic surgeons must, however, reevaluate what has and has not worked and continuously reevaluate the current public and medical field acceptance of allotransplantation. Many obstacles remain, including funding, immunology, candidate selection, and the long-term assessment of outcomes. The future of VCA must be approached with cautious optimism, and physicians must continue to evaluate all they do with bench science, the peer review of clinical outcomes (both good and bad), and the ethical treatment of their patients.[13]

In select cases, VCA is an alternative to prosthesis use and must be considered as a restorative option for some patients with upper limb loss. Although true success in hand transplant has been achieved in many cases, the field is at a crossroads and funding is the critical key component, which must be solved to establish the longevity of this procedure.

SUMMARY

Although successful transplantations have been performed at the hand and other upper limb levels, the future of VCA is unclear. This modality holds incredible promise, but functional outcomes need to be more adequately defined in the literature to allow comparison with more traditional treatments of upper limb loss. Screening protocols for VCA require optimization based on collective reporting of experiences throughout the world. With minimization of immunosuppressive regimens, VCA will potentially expand to include partial hand transplants, digit transplants, vascularized joint transfers (such as the elbow or wrist), and pediatric hand transplants. In select patients, VCA is an alternative to prosthesis use and should be considered as a restorative option for some patients with upper limb loss.

References

1. Errico M, Metcalfe NH, Platt A: History and ethics of hand transplants. *JRSM Short Rep* 2012;3(10):74.
2. Grob M, Papadopulos NA, Zimmermann A, Biemer E, Kovacs L: The psychological impact of severe hand injury. *J Hand Surg Eur Vol* 2008;33(3):358-362.
3. Wright TW, Hagen AD, Wood MB: Prosthetic usage in major upper extremity amputations. *J Hand Surg Am* 1995;20(4):619-622.
4. Pinzur MS, Angelats J, Light TR, Izuierdo R, Pluth T: Functional outcome following traumatic upper limb amputation and prosthetic limb fitting. *J Hand Surg Am* 1994;19(5):836-839.
5. Stürup J, Thyregod HC, Jensen JS, et al: Traumatic amputation of the upper limb: The use of body-powered prostheses and employment consequences. *Prosthet Orthot Int* 1988;12(1):50-52.
6. Millstein SG, Heger H, Hunter GA: Prosthetic use in adult upper limb amputees: A comparison of the body powered and electrically powered prostheses. *Prosthet Orthot Int* 1986;10(1):27-34.
7. Bhaskaranand K, Bhat AK, Acharya KN: Prosthetic rehabilitation in traumatic upper limb amputees (an Indian perspective). *Arch Orthop Trauma Surg* 2003;123(7):363-366.
8. Raichle KA, Hanley MA, Molton I, et al: Prosthesis use in persons with lower- and upper-limb amputation. *J Rehabil Res Dev* 2008;45(7):961-972.
9. Dudkiewicz I, Gabrielov R, Seiv-Ner I, Zelig G, Heim M: Evaluation of prosthetic usage in upper limb amputees. *Disabil Rehabil* 2004;26(1):60-63.
10. Tintle SM, Baechler MF, Nanos GP, Forsberg JA, Potter BK: Reoperations following combat-related upper-extremity amputations. *J Bone Joint Surg Am* 2012;94(16):e1191-e1196.
11. McFarland LV, Hubbard Winkler SL, Heinemann AW, Jones M, Esquenazi A: Unilateral upper-limb loss: Satisfaction and prosthetic-device use in Veterans and servicemembers from Vietnam and OIF/OEF conflicts. *J Rehabil Res Dev* 2010;47(4):299-316.
12. Foroohar A, Elliott RM, Kim TW, Breidenbach W, Shaked A, Levin LS: The history and evolution of hand transplantation. *Hand Clin* 2011;27(4):405-409, vii.
13. Tintle SM, Potter BK, Elliott RM, Levin LS: Hand transplantation. *JBJS Rev* 2014;21(1):e1.
14. Hollenbeck ST, Erdmann D, Levin LS: Current indications for hand and face allotransplantation. *Transplant Proc* 2009;41(2):495-498.
15. Gilbert R: Transplant is successful with a cadaver forearm. *Med Trib Med News* 1964;5:20.
16. Goldwyn RM, Joseph E, Murray MD: Nobelist: Some personal thoughts. *Plast Reconstr Surg* 2013;131(4):918-920.
17. Dubernard JM, Petruzzo P, Lanzetta M, et al: Functional results of the first human double-hand transplantation. *Ann Surg* 2003;238(1):128-136.
18. Dubernard JM, Owen E, Lefrançois N, et al: First human hand transplantation: Case report. *Transpl Int* 2000;13(suppl 1):S521-S524.
19. Jones JW, Gruber SA, Barker JH, Breidenbach WC: Louisville hand transplant team: Successful hand transplantation one-year follow-up. *N Engl J Med* 2000;343(7):468-473.
20. Breidenbach WC, Gonzales NR, Kaufman CL, Klapheke M, Tobin GR, Gorantla VS: Outcomes of the first 2 American hand transplants at 8 and 6 years posttransplant. *J Hand Surg Am* 2008;33(7):1039-1047.
21. Benhaim P, Anthony JP, Lin LY, McCalmont TH, Mathes SJ: A long-term study of allogeneic rat hindlimb transplants immunosuppressed with RS-61443. *Transplantation* 1993;56(4):911-917.
22. Ustüner ET, Zdichavsky M, Ren X, et al: Long-term composite tissue allograft survival in a porcine model with cyclosporine/mycophenolate mofetil therapy. *Transplantation* 1998;66(12):1581-1587.
23. Jones JW Jr, Ustüner ET, Zdichavsky M, et al: Long-term survival of an extremity composite tissue allograft with FK506-mycophenolate mofetil therapy. *Surgery* 1999;126(2):384-388.
24. Cooney WP, Hentz VR, American Society for Surgery of the Hand: Hand transplantation–primum non nocere. *J Hand Surg Am* 2002;27(1):165-168.
25. Chang J, Mathes DW: Ethical, financial, and policy considerations in hand transplantation. *Hand Clin* 2011;27(4):553-560, xi.
26. Brandacher G, Gorantla VS, Lee WP: Hand allotransplantation. *Semin Plast Surg* 2010;24(1):11-17.
27. Chung KC, Oda T, Saddawi-Konefka D, Shauver MJ: An economic analysis of hand transplantation in the United States. *Plast Reconstr Surg* 2010;125(2):589-598.
28. Marske P: The sound of one hand clapping. *J Hand Surg Am* 2008;33(7):1037-1038.
29. Melcer T, Walker GJ, Galarneau M, Belnap B, Konoske P: Midterm health and personnel outcomes of recent combat amputees. *Mil Med* 2010;175(3):147-154.
30. Shores JT: Recipient screening and selection: Who is the right candidate for hand transplantation. *Hand Clin* 2011;27(4):539-543, x.
31. Dobbels F, Vanhaecke J, Dupont L, et al: Pretransplant predictors of posttransplant adherence and clinical outcome: An evidence base for pretransplant psychosocial screening. *Transplantation* 2009;87(10):1497-1504.
32. Kinsley SE, Song S, Petruzzo P, Sardu C, Lesina E, Talbot SG: Psychosocial predictors of upper extremity transplantation outcomes: A review of the international registry 1998-2016. *Plast Reconstr Surg Glob Open* 2020;8(9):e3133.
33. Hausen O, Swanson EW, Abraham JA, et al: Surgical and logistical aspects of donor limb procurement in hand and upper extremity transplantation. *VCA* 2014;2(1-2):31-41.
34. Lang RS, Gorantla VS, Esper S, et al: Anesthetic management in upper extremity transplantation: The Pittsburgh experience. *Anesth Analg* 2012;115(3):678-688.
35. Azari KK, Imbriglia JE, Goitz RJ, et al: Technical aspects of the recipient operation in hand transplantation. *J Reconstr Microsurg* 2012;28(1):27-34.
36. Hartzell TL, Benhaim P, Imbriglia JE, et al: Surgical and technical aspects of hand transplantation: Is it just another replant? *Hand Clin* 2011;27(4):521-530, x.
37. Schneeberger S, Gorantla VS, Brandacher G, et al: Upper-extremity transplantation using a cell-based protocol to minimize immunosuppression. *Ann Surg* 2013;257(2):345-351.
38. Higgins JP, Shores JT, Katz RD, Lee WP, Wolock BS: Forearm transplantation osteosynthesis using modified ulnar shortening osteotomy technique. *J Hand Surg Am* 2014;39(1):134-142.
39. Haddock NT, Chang B, Bozentka DJ, Steinberg DR, Levin LS: Technical implications in proximal forearm transplantation. *Tech Hand Up Extrem Surg* 2013;17(4):228-231.
40. Shores JT, Higgins JP, Lee WP: Above-elbow (supracondylar) arm transplantation: Clinical considerations and

surgical technique. *Tech Hand Up Extrem Surg* 2013;17(4):221-227.

41. Shores JT, Brandacher G, Lee WP: Hand and upper extremity transplantation: An update of outcomes in the worldwide experience. *Plast Reconstr Surg* 2015;135(2):351e-360e.

42. Haas M, Sis B, Racusen LC, et al: Banff meeting report writing committee: Banff 2013 meeting report–inclusion of c4d-negative antibody-mediated rejection and antibody-associated arterial lesions. *Am J Transplant* 2014;14(2):272-283.

43. Mengel M, Sis B, Haas M, et al: Banff Meeting Report Writing Committee: Banff 2011 meeting report new concepts in antibody-mediated rejection. *Am J Transplant* 2012;12(3):563-570.

44. Cendales LC, Kanitakis J, Schneeberger S, et al: The Banff 2007 working classification of skin-containing composite tissue allograft pathology. *Am J Transplant* 2008;8(7):1396-1400.

45. Kaufman CL, Ouseph R, Blair B, et al: Graft vasculopathy in clinical hand transplantation. *Am J Transplant* 2012;12(4):1004-1016.

46. Małecki R, Gacka M, Boratyńska M, et al: Assessment of vascular function of hand allografts. *Ann Transplant* 2014;19:621-628.

47. Petruzzo P, Dubernard JM: The international registry on hand and composite tissue allotransplantation. *Clin Transpl* 2011:247-253.

48. Petruzzo P, Lanzetta M, Dubernard JM, et al: The international registry on hand and composite tissue transplantation. *Transplantation* 2010;90(12):1590-1594.

49. Carty MJ, Hivelin M, Dumontier C, et al: Lessons learned from simultaneous face and bilateral hand allotransplantation. *Plast Reconstr Surg* 2013;132(2):423-432.

50. Shores JT, Lee WP, Brandacher G: Discussion: Lessons learned from simultaneous face and bilateral hand allotransplantation. *Plast Reconstr Surg* 2013;132(2):433-434.

51. Petruzzo P, Lanzetta M, Dubernard JM, et al: The international registry on hand and composite tissue transplantation. *Transplantation* 2008;86(4):487-492.

52. Lanzetta M, Petruzzo P, Dubernard J-M, et al: Second report (1998-2006) of the international registry of hand and composite tissue transplantation. *Transpl Immunol* 2007;18(1):1-6.

Outcome Measures in Upper Limb Prosthetics

CHAPTER 31

Laura A. Miller, PhD, CP • Linda Resnik, PT, PhD, FAPTA

ABSTRACT

Upper limb prosthetic outcome measures are needed for clinical care and research in upper limb amputation. However, the field of amputation rehabilitation has yet to reach consensus on a recommended suite, or toolbox, of measures for routine use. It is important to provide a brief overview of measurement properties to consider when selecting an outcome measure and to highlight outcome measures that have been recommended for use in upper limb amputation rehabilitation, along with emerging measures and important constructs that may be relevant to upper limb amputation rehabilitation. The clinician should be aware of barriers to implementing outcome measures and select strategies to improve adoption.

Keywords: disability evaluation; outcome measures; upper limb prosthetics

Introduction

An outcome measure is a means of systematically collecting data through a testing procedure that has emerged through a formal development process, which includes an evaluation of psychometric (ie, measurement) properties.[1,2] Outcome measures are essential clinical tools that can be used to evaluate patient status and assess change over time, provide data to identify patient needs, and help establish treatment priorities.[3] Outcome measures can also be used to gauge effectiveness of a treatment during usual care delivery and are often used in research to describe populations and to assess effectiveness or efficacy. Collections of standardized outcome measures across practices or systems of care can be used to evaluate and improve quality.[4]

Outcome measures can be generic, population specific, or patient specific. Generic measures are designed for use in a broad variety of patient populations. However, condition-specific measures are designed for use in specific patient populations (eg, conditions, diseases), such as patients who are prosthesis users, or persons with upper limb conditions. As such, condition-specific measures are designed to target content areas that are most relevant to the disease or condition. Because of this they may be more responsive to change compared with generic instruments. Finally, patient-specific measures are used to assess activities and participation and goals that are identified and valued by the individual.

Some outcome measures assess performance (performance-based measures) and are administered and scored by a tester. Other outcome measures, particularly those that assess aspects of the client/patient experience, are self-reported and can be administered by an interviewer or self-administered. All outcome measures have formal scoring rules, some measures are scored with a single summary score, and other measures are scored via multiple subscales and/or component scores. Developing, refining, and testing a psychometrically strong outcome measure is a rigorous process that can take 10 to 15 years.

Researchers and clinicians have many choices for outcome measures. The best outcome measures must demonstrate reliability, validity, and responsiveness to change. Reliability means that outcome results are consistent and relatively free from errors. Validity means that a measure is gauging the concepts that it intends to measure. Responsiveness is the ability of a measure to detect meaningful change over time. More details about these key psychometric attributes of measures are provided later and in **Table 1**. Standards for evaluating the sufficiency of these psychometric properties have been described in detail in the scientific literature, and will not be summarized in this chapter. Because the psychometric properties of outcome measures are not fixed, measures must be studied in their intended population because measures may be reliable or valid in one patient population, but not in another.

Historically, it has been common for those working in upper limb amputation research and clinical care to create their own outcome measures for patient evaluation, either by adapting an existing measure and/or using

---

Dr. Miller or an immediate family member serves as a board member, owner, officer, or committee member of US Chapter of the International Society of Prosthetics and Orthotics. Neither Dr. Resnik nor any immediate family member has received anything of value from or has stock or stock options held in a commercial company or institution related directly or indirectly to the subject of this chapter.

Section 2: Upper Limb

TABLE 1 Key Psychometric Attributes of Measures

Psychometric Attribute	Methodologic Requirements
Reliability	
Internal consistency	Internal consistency is a measure based on the correlation between items of a measure. It measures whether separate items are similar enough that they are capturing the same general construct.
Test-retest reliability	Test-retest reliability (or repeatability) is a measure of stability of a test over time, under the same conditions.
Interrater reliability	Interrater reliability is the repeatability of a test when administered by more than one rater.
Intrarater reliability	Intrarater reliability is the degree of agreement among repeated measurements by a single rater.
Validity	
Face validity	Face validity is a subjective determination of how well the content of the measures covers the target construct and whether the test is intuitively meaningful to the tester and patient.
Content validity	Content validity is similar to face validity and is typically established by expert evaluation.
Criterion validity	Criterion validity is a measure of good agreement between test scores and scores of a current gold standard. Gold standards are not available for most rehabilitation measures.
Predictive validity	Predictive validity is a measure's ability to predict outcomes or scores of another measure or significant event at a future point in time.
Construct validity	Construct validity is the degree to which a measure assesses what it intends to be measuring. There are several ways to demonstrate construct validity including the known-groups method, hypotheses testing, factor analysis, and contemporary measurement methods such as Rasch analysis.
Concurrent/discriminant validity	Concurrent and discriminant validity assess how much a measure correlates with other validated measures of similar or different constructs.
Minimal detectable change (MDC)	The MDC is the minimal amount of change in a measure's score that exceeds measurement error. The MDC can be used to help interpret change scores in repeated measures.
Responsiveness evaluation	Responsiveness is the ability of a measure to detect change that is meaningful to the patient over time.
Examination of scale difficulty	A good measure should be well targeted to its intended population. If it is too difficult or easy, then it will be difficult to determine if decline or improvement has occurred. Scale difficulty can be examined, in part by evaluating floor and ceiling effects. These refer to the lower and upper bounds of a measurement past which the measure cannot be considered accurate or reliable.

selected portions of a measure in an attempt to tailor it to a specific question or clientele. However, this practice may threaten a measure's reliability and validity and is generally frowned upon. Although there may be a need for new, revised, and innovative measures in the field, their use should be supported by psychometric evaluation, which is generally outside the scope of clinical care and most research projects. There is also widespread recognition of the value of using standardized outcome measures with strong psychometric properties within the patient/target population whenever possible. Use of such standardized measures makes tracking progress or comparing outcomes across patients and groups possible. Collection of standardized data can enable pooling of outcomes across research studies in future systematic reviews and maximize usefulness of research findings in development of clinical practice guidelines.

There are many standardized measures available for use in upper limb amputation rehabilitation. Although strong evidence of reliability, validity, and responsiveness is key, it is also critical that users of outcome measures select those that address the constructs (eg, activity performance, prosthesis satisfaction) and questions that are most important to patients, clinicians, and payers. The choice of measures is also contingent on other factors related to the measure's utility, for example, the time it takes to administer the measure (administrative burden), the need for and availability of specialized testing equipment, the need for special training for the test administrator, as well as the ease of scoring and interpretation of the scores.

Using Outcomes in Prosthetics

As mentioned previously, there are multiple reasons that a researcher or clinician might want to use outcome measures. The goal of using outcome measures may be to evaluate and improve quality of care, to predict or detect change over time within patients or between groups, or to distinguish between types of devices. Measures may be used to understand the breadth of function, application to activities, use in daily life, and quality of life (QOL). To measure multiple domains, a suite or toolkit of measures will be required.

When choosing outcome measures, it is important to carefully consider whether the measure provides the most useful information to address specific questions of interest or targets of treatment. For example, data from a measure that focuses on general QOL may not be able to detect the differences between the function of two different prosthetic hands.

Various groups of researchers and clinicians continue to work to evaluate the psychometric properties of measures and categorize their content. Although there is no current consensus, a variety of efforts have been made to help guide the selection measures that should be used in routine clinical care and/or research. Given the small population of users of upper limb prosthetic devices, the use of a core set of measures could also provide a larger, uniform pool of data for the profession to help advance the field of research in upper limb prosthetics.

Efforts to Evaluate and Categorize Upper Limb Outcomes Measures

Over nearly 20 years, a variety of groups have worked to categorize and evaluate outcome measures for upper limb amputation rehabilitation. The framework of the World Health Organization

International Classification of Functioning, Disability and Health (ICF) model has been used to describe the content of outcome measures used in upper limb prosthetics. The ICF framework describes the relationships between a health condition and the associated effects on the components of Function, Activity, and Participation, as well as Environmental and Personal Factors, and presents a taxonomy for defining each of these components of functioning and health.[5,6] **Table 2** shows how the broad taxonomy of the ICF may be useful in selecting outcome measures to answer specific questions.

The Upper Limb Prosthetic Outcome Measures group formed at the Myoelectric Controls Symposium[6] endeavored to critically evaluate outcome measures routinely used by clinicians and researchers. The purpose, clinical utility, and psychometric properties of each measure were documented.[5,6] A State of the Science Conference (SSC), sponsored by the American Academy of Orthotists and Prosthetists, combined work of the Upper Limb Prosthetic Outcome Measures group[5] with an evidence-based review of the literature on outcome measures[7] and proposed an early toolbox of recommended and to-be-considered outcome measures.[8] These outcome measures were categorized by stakeholder questions, the ICF domain they addressed, and the field of application (development, clinical research, or patient care).

Another review of upper limb outcome measures focusing only on the domain of physical function was published by the US Department of Veterans Affairs as part of a clinical practice guideline for the management of upper extremity amputation rehabilitation.[9] The measures in this review were specific to adult users of upper limb prostheses. Tables in the Guidelines summarized the ease of use and content of the physical function measures and rated the strength of evidence supporting the psychometric properties of the measures in persons with upper limb amputation. Additionally, the tables summarized the minimal detectable change for those measures in which it had been reported.

Two additional systematic reviews of measures for persons with upper limb trauma and amputation have been completed.[10,11] One review addressed measures of impairment and activity limitation and the other addressed community integration/participation in life roles. These two reviews identified measures with the strongest psychometric properties and classified the content of each measure using ICF categories of body function, activity, and participation.

Summary of Highlighted Outcome Measures

Outcome measures that were recommended by the Academy's SSC (indicated as SSC),[8] were considered strong measures in the 2014 Veterans Administration/Department of Defense clinical practice guidelines (indicated as VA),[9] or were used in upper limb amputation population and rated highly in either of the two systematic reviews described previously (indicated as SystRev1[11] or SystRev2[10]) are described. **Table 3** provides a synopsis of the content of the subset of measures that have application to adults. **Table 4** provides a list of known minimal detectable change values for the outcome measures shown in **Table 3**.

Performance Measures

Activities Measure for Upper Limb Amputees: VA and SystRev1

The Activities Measure for Upper Limb Amputees (AM-ULA) is a performance-based measure of activity.[12] It includes 18 self-care and activity of daily living tasks, such as pouring from a can, tying a shoe, zipping a jacket, and buttoning a shirt. Every item is scored between 0 and 4, based on a scoring rubric that takes into account task completion, speed, movement quality, and skillfulness of prosthesis use.

Assessment of Capacity for Myoelectric Control: SSC and VA

The Assessment of Capacity for Myoelectric Control (ACMC and ACMC 2.0) is a performance-based measure that uses observational analysis, typically from video, of an adult or pediatric patient with an upper limb prosthesis during functional bimanual activities.[13-15] A 4-point scale is used to evaluate 30 aspects of myoelectric prosthesis use (eg, the ability to hold an object over the course of a task, with or without support; coordination with both hands; and the ability to adjust grip force, with or without visual feedback). Any bimanual task can be evaluated provided it allows all aspects of use to be observed. ACMC 2.0 reduced the aspects of control scored from 30 to 22 and clarified item definition. Final scores are calculated via the ACMC website, which uses a Rasch analysis. Originally, raw scores were converted into a logit scale. The ACMC version 3.0 manual updated the scoring to transform the logit scale to a range of 0 to 100, with higher scores indicating improved capacity.[16] Raters are required to complete a training course to obtain certification.

Box and Blocks: SSC, VA, and SystRev1

The Box and Blocks (BB) is a performance-based measure that evaluates gross manual dexterity.[17,18] Individuals are asked to transfer as many 1-inch wooden blocks as possible over a divider from one side of a box to another, within 1 minute (**Figure 1**). The number of blocks represents the score. No specialized training is required to administer the test, and the necessary equipment can be purchased or constructed.

Jebsen-Taylor Hand Function Test: SSC and SystRev1

The Jebsen-Taylor Hand Function Test (JTHF) is a seven-part timed dexterity test.[19] The tasks include writing, flipping index cards, picking up small objects, spooning beans into a jar, stacking checkers, and moving light and heavy cans (**Figure 2**). The time to complete each task is recorded, and each of the activities is scored separately. Recent work on the Jebsen-Taylor Hand Function Test (specific to prosthetics) resulted in modification to the scoring method of the original measure.[17] The prosthesis-specific scoring involves counting the number of items completed (eg, checkers stacked,

Section 2: Upper Limb

TABLE 2 Questions of Interest in Upper Limb Outcomes[a]

Question	ICF Category — B. Body Functions			ICF Category — D. Activities and Participation						Other			
	Sensation of Pain (B280)	b7. Neuromuscular and Movement-Related Functions	d4. Mobility[b]	Self-care (d5)	Domestic Life (d6)	Interpersonal Interactions and Relationships (d7)	Major Life Areas (d8)	Community, Social, and Civic (d9)	Unspecified Activities (Patient Selected)	Quality of Life	Goals	Satisfaction	Prosthesis Use Measures
What is the effectiveness of prosthetic or occupational treatment for improving...	—	—	—	—	—	—	—	—	—	—	—	—	—
How does the choice of prosthetic componentry affect...	—	—	—	—	—	—	—	—	—	—	—	—	—
How do my patients or my patient care compare to benchmarks for...	—	—	—	—	—	—	—	—	—	—	—	—	—
Movement control?	—	X	X	—	—	—	—	—	—	—	—	—	—
Activity performance?	—	—	X	X	X	X	X	X	X	—	—	—	—
Hours of use?	—	—	—	—	—	—	—	—	—	—	—	—	X
Prosthesis adoption?	—	—	—	—	—	—	—	—	—	—	—	—	X
Satisfaction with device?	—	—	—	—	—	—	—	—	—	—	—	X	—
Quality of life?	—	—	—	—	—	—	—	—	—	X	—	—	—
Pain?	X	—	—	—	—	—	—	—	—	—	—	—	—
How well does an individual control their prosthesis?	—	—	X	—	—	—	—	—	—	—	—	—	—
Are there areas of control/function that could be improved?	—	X	X	—	—	—	—	—	—	—	—	—	—
Is one type of prosthesis control better than another type of control?	—	X	X	—	—	—	—	—	—	—	—	—	—
What level of control/function should a prosthetic user expect?	—	X	—	—	—	—	—	—	—	—	—	—	—
Are users satisfied with the device?	—	—	—	—	—	—	—	—	—	—	—	X	—
How well does amputation rehabilitation help clients achieve their goals?	—	—	—	—	—	—	—	—	X	—	X	—	—
What is the quality of life for an individual with upper limb loss/deficiency?	—	—	—	—	—	—	—	—	—	X	—	—	—
With how much difficulty and how often does the individual use their upper limb prosthesis in everyday activities?	—	—	—	X	X	X	X	X	X	—	—	—	—
Is the upper limb prosthesis useful to the individual for specific tasks?	—	—	—	X	X	—	X	X	X	—	X	—	—
What is the physical function for an individual with upper limb loss/deficiency not using a prosthesis?	—	X	X	—	—	—	—	—	—	—	—	—	—

[a] Table shows what ICF categories are included in many of the clinical and research questions of interest when evaluating upper limb prosthetic devices. (Only B and D ICF categories listed here.) An X indicates that the question addresses the ICF category or 'other' category. A dash indicates that the question does not directly address the category.

[b] d4 Mobility examples: fine motor tasks (d440), hand and arm use gross motor (d445), carrying and handling objects (d430-d439), using transportation (d470)

cards flipped) as well as the time it takes to complete the test. The score is calculated by dividing the number of items completed by the number of seconds required to complete. Because of the difficulty of some tasks for persons using prostheses, the time allowed for each task is capped at 2 minutes. No specialized training is required to administer the outcome measure, and the necessary equipment can be purchased or made.

Patient-Reported Measures

Disabilities of the Arm, Shoulder and Hand: SystRev1

The Disabilities of the Arm, Shoulder and Hand (DASH) is a self-report measure that assesses symptoms and disability in individuals with upper limb musculoskeletal disorders (disease or injury).[20] It consists of 30 questions covering function, symptoms, and social/role functioning. Total scores range from 0 to 100, with higher scores indicating greater disability. There are two optional modules for sports/performing arts and work.

QuickDASH: SystRev1

The QuickDASH is a shorter version of the DASH questionnaire. It is a self-report survey designed for persons with upper limb impairments.[21] The QuickDASH, which has been validated in persons with upper limb amputation, contains 11 items assessing functioning and systems in musculoskeletal disorders of the upper limb.[22] The QuickDASH also includes two optional scales for work activities and sports or playing an instrument.

Trinity Amputation and Prosthesis Experience Scales: SSC and SystRev2

Trinity Amputation and Prosthesis Experience Scales (TAPES) is a self-report measure originally designed to assess a user's adaptation to lower limb amputation and prosthesis use.[23] Desmond and MacLachlan used items from the TAPES in a study of persons with upper limb amputation and proposed a different scoring approach.[24] The result, the TAPES-ULA, has four psychosocial adjustment scales: General Adjustment, Social Adjustment, Adjustment to Limitation, and the Optimal Adjustment scale reflecting the development of an optimistic outlook and the positive appraisal of life despite the trauma associated with amputation and the use of an artificial limb. There are four activity restriction scales: athletic activity restriction reflecting the limitation of activities that involve more dynamic physical effort, for instance, sport and recreation and running for a bus; social restriction that addresses limitation of social activities such as visiting friends and working on hobbies; mobility restriction that address physical function and mobility; and a new occupational restriction scale relating to restrictions in occupational performance.

The TAPES-ULA has a single 10-item device satisfaction scale consisting of 10 items reflecting satisfaction with the appearance of the prosthesis, satisfaction with weight of the prosthesis, and satisfaction with the functionality of the prosthesis.

Sickness Impact Profile Psychosocial Domain: SystRev2

The Sickness Impact Profile (SIP) is a generic self-report measure assessing 12 areas: ambulation, mobility, body care and movement, social interaction, alertness behavior, emotional behavior, communication, sleep and rest, recreation and pastimes, eating, work, and home management.[25] There are a total of 136 items and two-dimension scores can be calculated. The psychosocial domain of the Sickness Impact Profile was identified in the systematic review of communication reintegration measures as having strong psychometric properties in samples of persons with amputation and limb trauma.[10] The psychosocial domain includes 48 items within 4 categories of psychosocial function: social interaction (addressing relationships with others—20 items), alertness (addressing alertness and ability to concentrate—10 items), emotional behavior (addressing emotional well-being—9 items), and communication (related to speaking and ability to communicate—9 items).

Goal Attainment Scale: SSC

The Goal Attainment Scale (GAS) is a self-report measure, originally developed for use in mental health settings.[26] It uses goal selection and goal scaling that is standardized by the use of a mathematical formula calculating the extent to which a person's goals are met. As part of the process, five outcome levels are set for each goal at the beginning of treatment and are reassessed at predetermined times to determine progress toward achieving the goal.

Canadian Occupational Performance Measure: SSC

The Canadian Occupational Performance Measure (COPM) is a self-report measure designed for use by occupational therapists to evaluate self-perception of performance in personally identified personal tasks, over time.[27] Through semistructured discussion with the occupational therapist, the user identifies five goals in areas of self-care, productivity, and leisure, which are rated on a scale from 0 to 10 in terms of importance, user perception of performance, and satisfaction with performance. The Canadian Occupational Performance Measure is copyrighted and the manual and measure must be purchased.

36-Item Short Form Health Survey (Role-Emotional, Role-Physical, Social Function): SystRev2

The 36-Item Short Form Health Survey (SF-36) is a widely used, generic self-report measure of health-related QOL.[28,29] The items on the SF-36, the Medical Outcomes Study 36, and Rand 36-item healthy survey 1.0 are the same. The VR-36, a freely available Veterans version of the measure, has been used in studies of persons with upper limb amputation. Higher scores on these measures indicate more favorable health-related QOL. The questions can be scored on eight separate scales (physical functioning, role physical, bodily pain, general health, vitality, social functioning, role emotional, and mental health). The results can also be combined into two summary measures

Section 2: Upper Limb

TABLE 3 Content Analysis of Recommended Measures for Adults[a]

Measure	Age Group[c]	Target Population[d]	B. Body Function — b7. Neuromuscular and Movement-Related Functions					Communication (d3)	D. Activities and Participation — d4. Mobility			
			Sleep Functions (b134)	Sensation of Pain (B280)	Mobility of Joint Functions: Stiffness (b710)	Strength: Muscle Power Functions (b 73)	Unspecified or Patient-Selected Functions		Fine Motor Tasks (d440)	Hand and Arm Use (d445)	Carrying and Handling Objects (d430-d439)	Walking and Moving d450-469
ACMC/ACMC2[b]	P/A	A	—	—	—	—	—	—	X	X	x	—
AM-ULA	A	A	—	—	—	—	—	—	x	x	X	—
BB	P/A	UL	—	—	—	—	—	—	X	—	X	—
COPM	P/A	G	—	—	—	—	—	—	—	—	—	—
DASH	A	UL	X	X	X	—	—	—	x	x	X	—
GAS[b]	P/A	G	—	—	—	—	X	—	—	—	—	—
JTHF	A	UL	—	—	—	—	—	—	X	X	X	—
QuickDASH	A	UL	X	X	X	—	—	—	x	x	X	—
SIIP psychosocial	A	G	—	—	—	—	—	X	—	—	—	—
SF-36 role-emotional	A	G	—	—	—	—	—	—	—	—	—	—
SF-36 role-physical	A	G	—	—	—	—	—	—	—	—	—	—
SF-36 social function	A	G	—	—	—	—	—	—	—	—	—	—
TAPES ALL	A	A	—	X	—	—	—	—	—	—	—	X
TAPES social restriction	A	A	—	—	—	—	—	—	—	—	—	—
TAPES adjustment to limitations	A	A	—	—	—	—	—	—	—	—	—	—
UNB Skill	P/A	A	—	—	—	—	—	—	x	X	X	—
UNB Spontaneity	P/A	A	—	—	—	—	—	—	x	X	X	—
WHOQOL BREF	A	G	X	X	—	—	—	—	—	—	—	X

[a]See text for expansion of abbreviations. The X indicates content from the ICF or 'Other' category is included as part of the outcome measure. The dash indicates that the measure does not directly address the category.
[b]ACMC2, COPM, and GAS content of these measures may vary depending upon tasks selected.
[c]Age group: pediatric (P), adult (A), pediatric and adult (P/A).
[d]Target population: generic (G), upper limb specific (UL), amputation specific (A).

TABLE 3 Content Analysis of Recommended Measures for Adults[a] (Continued)

Using Transportation (d470)	Self-care (d5)	Domestic Life (d6)	Interpersonal Interactions and Relationships (d7)	Major Life Areas (d8)	Community, Social and Civic (d9)	Unspecified Activities (or Patient-Selected Priorities)	Autonomy	Adjustment	General Health	Quality of Life	Prosthesis Satisfaction	Goals
—	—	—	—	—	—	X	—	—	—	—	—	—
—	X	X	—	—	—	—	—	—	—	—	—	—
—	—	—	—	—	—	—	—	—	—	—	—	—
—	—	—	—	—	—	X	—	—	—	—	—	—
X	X	X	X	X	X	—	—	—	—	—	—	—
—	—	—	—	—	—	X	—	—	—	—	—	X
—	X	—	—	—	—	—	—	—	—	—	—	—
—	X	X	X	X	X	—	—	—	—	—	—	—
—	—	—	X	—	X	—	—	—	—	X	—	—
—	—	—	—	X	—	X	—	—	—	X	—	—
—	—	—	—	X	—	X	—	—	—	X	—	—
—	—	—	X	—	X	—	—	—	—	X	—	—
—	—	—	X	X	X	—	—	X	X	X	X	—
—	—	—	—	X	X	—	—	—	—	—	X	—
—	—	—	X	X	—	—	X	X	—	—	—	—
—	X	X	—	—	—	—	—	—	—	—	—	—
—	X	X	—	—	—	—	—	—	—	—	—	—
X	X	—	X	X	X	—	—	—	X	X	—	—

TABLE 4 Minimal Detectable Change in Samples of Adults With Upper Limb Amputation[a]

Measure	MDC 90	MDC 95
ACMC2	Unknown	0.55-0.69 logits or 2.5-3.1 points[b]
AM-ULA	3.7	4.4
BB	6.49	7.77
COPM	Unknown	Unknown
DASH	Unknown	Unknown
GAS	Unknown	Unknown
JTHF (tasks scored separately)	—	—
Writing	0.18	0.21
Page turning	0.11	0.14
Small items	0.09	0.1
Feeding	0.1	0.11
Checkers	0.11	0.13
Light cans	0.15	0.17
Heavy cans	0.13	0.16
PUFI	Unknown	Unknown
QuickDASH	13.9	17.4
SIP psychosocial	Unknown	Unknown
SF-36 role-emotional	Unknown	Unknown
SF-36 role-physical	Unknown	Unknown
SF-36 social function	Unknown	Unknown
TAPES satisfaction	0.78	0.08
TAPES social restriction	Unknown	Unknown
TAPES adjustment to limitations	Unknown	Unknown
UNB Skill	0.7	0.8
UNB Spontaneity	0.7	0.9

[a]See text for expansion of abbreviations.
[b]ACMC minimal detectable change range is indicated for intrarater assessment and interrater assessment.

Data from Lindner HY, Langius-Eklof A, Hermansson LM: Test-retest reliability and rater agreements of assessment of capacity for myoelectric control version 2.0. J Rehabil Res Dev 2014;51(4):635-644; Hermansson LN, Lindner H, Hill W: Assessment of Capacity for Myoelectric Control v3.0 Manual. Liselotte Norling Hermansson, 2015; Resnik L, Adams L, Borgia M, et al: Development and evaluation of the activities measure for upper limb amputees. Arch Phys Med Rehabil 2013;94(3):488-494.e484; Resnik L, Borgia M. Reliability and validity of outcome measures for upper limb amputation. J Prosthet Orthot. 2012;24(4):192-212; Resnik L, Borgia M. Reliability, validity, and responsiveness of the QuickDASH in patients with upper limb amputation. Arch Phys Med Rehabil 2015;96(9):1676-1683; and Resnik L, Baxter K, Borgia M, Mathewson K: Is the UNB test reliable and valid for use with adults with upper limb amputation? J Hand Ther 2013;26(4):353-359; quiz 359.

(physical component summary and mental component summary). The role physical, role emotional, and social functional subscales of the SF-36 were rated highly in the systematic review of community reintegration measures. Later versions of the SF-36 are copyrighted with scoring changed to norm-based T-scores with the population norm set to 50 and the population SD set to 10.[30]

World Health Organization Quality of Life Assessment: SSC

The World Health Organization Quality of Life Assessment: Brief Version (WHOQOL-BREF) is a 26-item self-report survey.[31] It is a shorter Field Trial Version of the WHOQOL-100, developed to look at domain level profiles, which assess QOL.[32] The WHO-BREF produces four domain scores: physical, psychological, social relationships, and environment. Two additional items are examined separately that ask about an individual's overall perception of QOL and about an individual's overall perception of their health. Domain scores are scaled in a positive direction (ie, higher scores denote higher QOL).

Pediatric Performance Measures

University of New Brunswick Test of Prosthetic Function (UNB Skill and UNB Spontaneity): SSC, VA, SystRev1

The UNB Test of Prosthetic Function is a performance-based measure that was specifically developed to evaluate prosthesis use in children with a unilateral upper limb amputation.[33] This observational function test contains two separate scales, Skill and Spontaneity. These scales assess the method/skill and the spontaneity of prosthesis use using two 5-point rating scales. The UNB is suitable for use in children aged 2 to 13 years; four age-based modules are designed to be developmentally appropriate for children within a 3-year age range. The module for older children has been used with adults.[34] No specific training is required to use this test, and the tasks require only easy-to-obtain items.

Assisting Hand Assessment: SSC

The Assisting Hand Assessment is a performance-based assessment of hand use developed for pediatric use.[35,36] It is designed to evaluate how a child with unilateral upper limb involvement uses the noninvolved hand during bimanual play activities. Training is required to learn the rating system. Raters score 22 actions from video and rate them on a 4-point effectiveness of performance rating scale.

Pediatric Self-Reported or Proxy-Reported Measures

Prosthetic Upper Extremity Functional Index: SSC

The Prosthetic Upper Extremity Functional Index (PUFI) is a prosthesis-specific self-report measure designed for children. Versions exist for younger children (parent report) or older children (parent report and child report).[37] For each task, the child (or parent) indicates if the child does the activity and how they usually do the activity on a six-point scale (hand used actively, prosthesis used passively, with assistance of residual limb, nonprosthetic hand alone, with

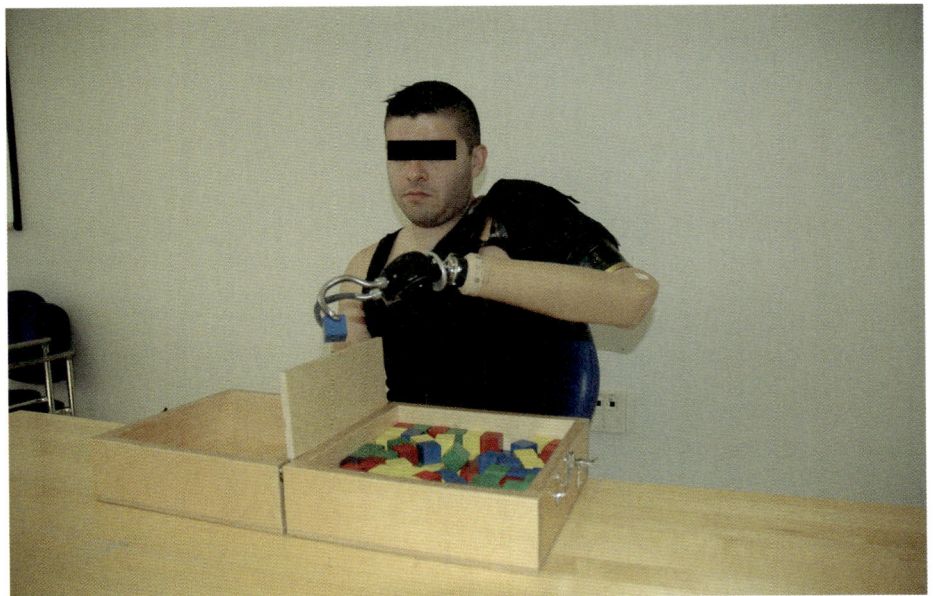

FIGURE 1 Photograph showing a man with a transhumeral upper limb prosthesis performing the box and block test.

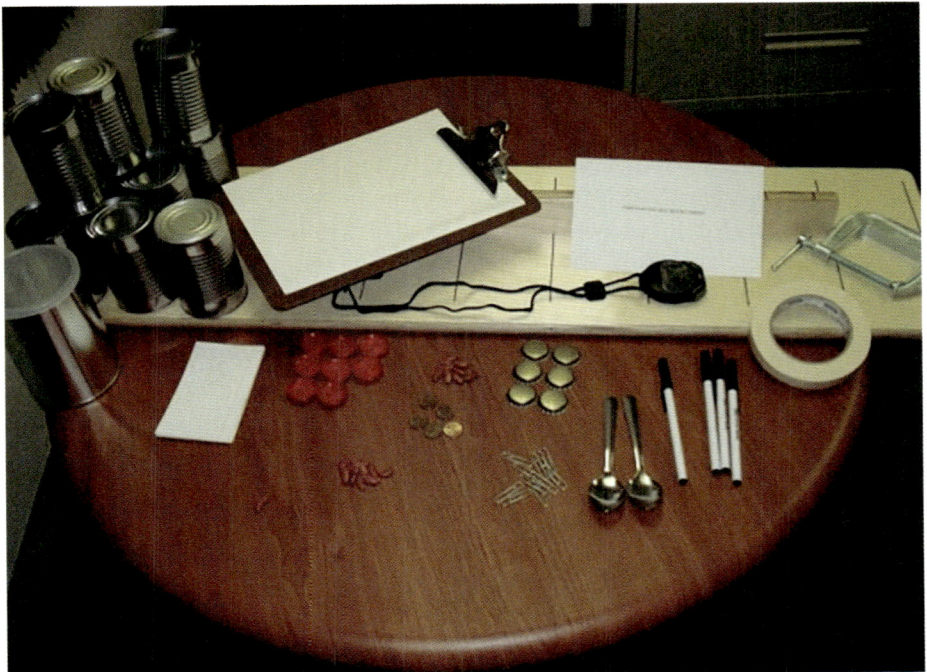

FIGURE 2 Photograph of the equipment needed for Jebsen-Taylor Hand Function Test tasks: writing, flipping index cards, picking up small objects, spooning beans into a jar, stacking checkers, and moving light and heavy cans. Items, from left to right, include empty and filled cans, 3 × 5 inch index cards, clipboard and paper, checkers, beans, coins, paperclips, bottle caps, spoon, pens, timer, and board with clamp and tape, for labeling positions.

assistance from others, another way). They then evaluate the comparative ease of task performance with and without the prosthesis (each scored on a five-point ordinal scale) and its perceived usefulness, scored on a five-point ordinal scale. Higher scores represent more ease of performance and higher usefulness of the prostheses. Within each of the response sets, the scores from the individual items are summed and then expressed as a percentage. Higher scores represent greater comparative ease of task performance with and without the prosthesis and its perceived usefulness.

DISABKIDS: SSC

DISABKIDS Chronic Generic Measure is a child/adolescent or parent-proxy self-report measure of health-related QOL. The original instrument[38] was updated to a 37-item version for ages 8 to 12 years[39] that addresses six dimensions (Independence, Physical Limitation, Emotion, Social Inclusion, Social Exclusion, and Treatment). Seven condition-specific modules have been developed (asthma, juvenile idiopathic arthritis, atopic dermatitis, cerebral palsy, cystic fibrosis, diabetes, and epilepsy). There is no specific module for amputation/prosthetics.

Pediatric Quality of Life Inventory: SSC

The Pediatric Quality of Life Inventory is a pediatric health-related QOL questionnaire.[40,41] The Generic Core Scale consists of 23 questions designed to assess five domains of health (physical functioning, emotional functioning, psychosocial functioning, social functioning, and school functioning). There are also disease-specific and condition-specific modules, though not for upper limb loss. Designed for ages 2 to 18 years, there are specific child and parent-proxy versions with language and terms adapted for various age groups.

Pediatric Orthopaedic Data Collection Outcomes Instrument: SSC

This is a self-report measure that was designed for use in patients with musculoskeletal conditions.[42,43] It assesses ability to participate in daily activities and sports. It has four main functional scales (basic mobility and transfers, sport and physical functioning, upper extremity function, and pain/comfort) and additional items that assess pain/comfort, treatment expectations, happiness, and satisfaction with health. Each scale has a possible range from 0 to 100, with higher scores representing greater function.

Other Measures of Interest

The measures described previously and contained in **Tables 3** and **4** are those that met recommendation criteria or were rated highly in specific reference documents. There are other measures currently in use or recently developed that may have application to amputation rehabilitation, but may still require additional study to evaluate their psychometric properties in the upper limb amputation/limb deficiency population. Several of these measures are highlighted in the following sections.

Community Reintegration of Injured Service Members

The Community Reintegration of Injured Service Members is a self-report measure designed to assess elements of the nine ICF chapters of activity and participation in Veterans.[44] It consists of three scales that are scored separately. Extent of participation asks respondents to indicate how often they experience or participate in specific activities. Items are coded on a seven-point frequency scale ("Never" to "More than Once per Day," or "Not at All" to "Always"). Perceived limitations scale asks respondents to rate their perceived limitations in participation. Responses are coded on a seven-point agreement scale ("Completely Disagree" to "Completely Agree"). Last, the satisfaction with participation scale asks respondents to indicate the degree of satisfaction with different aspects of participation. Responses are coded on a seven-point scale ("Very Unhappy" to "Very Happy"). Higher scores on these scales indicate better community integration. Prior research suggests that the Community Reintegration of Injured Service Members scales are reliable and valid for use in a population with severe limb trauma including amputation. A briefer, computer-adaptive test version of the measure is also available.[45]

Southampton Hand Assessment Procedure

The Southampton Hand Assessment Procedure (SHAP) was originally developed to evaluate hand function of multifunction prosthetic hands.[46] The SHAP tasks evaluate manipulation of 8 light or heavy objects (abstract tasks) and 14 simulated activities of daily living. All tasks are self-timed by the user. The SHAP tasks are scored using a proprietary scoring algorithm, which produces an overall Index of Functionality as well as separate Prehensile Pattern Scores. No specialized rater training is required, but the equipment must be rented or purchased from the University of Southampton, England to access the proprietary scoring database. This measure has been widely used in prosthetic research. Recent work has further evaluated the SHAP and explored new methods for scoring without using the SHAP database.[47,48] A recent study has also identified a briefer version of the test, which includes fewer tasks.[48]

Socket Comfort Score

Socket comfort has the potential to affect fitting and prosthesis acceptance. A measure of socket comfort may be useful in evaluating new socket technology, socket interfaces, or socket designs in a clinical or research setting. Although the TAPES-ULA prosthesis satisfaction scale and OPUS Client Satisfaction with Device[49] contain items related to prosthesis comfort and fit, they do not specifically address the comfort of the socket and this item is not typically evaluated by itself. In contrast, the Socket Comfort Score is a single item, self-report measure in which users rate the comfort of their socket on a scale from 0 to 10, representing the most uncomfortable and the most comfortable socket imaginable.[50] The Socket Comfort Score has not been evaluated with upper limb prosthetic users, though limited psychometric data is available for lower limb prosthesis users.[51]

Patient-Reported Outcomes Measurement Information System

An additional resource for rehabilitation outcome measures is the Patient-Reported Outcomes Measurement Information System (PROMIS) program. PROMIS is a National Institutes of Health–funded initiative to develop and validate generic patient-reported outcomes in areas such as pain, fatigue, physical functioning, emotional distress, and social role participation that have a major effect on QOL across a variety of chronic diseases. To date, there is limited research on the PROMIS measures and their appropriateness for persons with upper limb loss.[52] However, it is likely that these measures will be studied, and eventually may be adopted into clinical care and research with or without refinement.

Other Constructs of Interest

Other areas, not specifically addressed in the measures described previously, may be of interest to clinicians and researchers working within the field. A few of these key areas are pain, usage, prosthesis embodiment, body image, and self-efficacy.

Measures of pain are often needed in prosthetic fitting and care of individuals with an amputation and are often collected in research. Although well-established approaches to pain measurement exist, for example, the visual analog scale[53] and numeric rating scales, these do not specifically address the various types of pain (neck, back, residual limb, phantom limb, etc) and the intensity and type of sensations of pain, such as shooting, throbbing, etc. time dependence of this pain (morning, evening, etc), or impact on sleep and function. There are a variety of pain-specific measures such as the McGill pain questionnaire,[54] Brief Pain Inventory,[55,56] or the PROMIS Pain Interference measure[57] that may be needed.

Improving use of the prosthesis is often a target of research and clinical care. Self-report surveys may ask about prosthesis use, but they have limitations because of potential recall bias and may not accurately quantify how much the device is used, how it is used, and in what situations. To better understand prosthesis usage, additional tools may be required. Motion capture systems may be beneficial and has been used to document and compare kinematics in certain tasks with different devices[58-60] and actigraphs[61,62] and other sensors have the potential to track usage in real-world environments.

Prosthesis embodiment has also been proposed as a key factor in prosthetic acceptance[63] and a target of new technologies to enable sensorized prostheses[64] and osseointegrated devices.[65] Although a variety of definitions of the construct of embodiment exist,[56] most definitions include aspects of agency and sense of ownership of the prosthesis in terms of its incorporation of the device into the body representation. Several experiments have been developed to assess embodiment, and some measures of embodiment have been used in research.[67-69] However, further research is needed to examine the psychometric properties of these measures.

Body image, or the perception of how an individual feels about their body, may affect the psychological reaction to an amputation and prosthetic fitting, and may also affect eventual prosthetic acceptance. To date, there are no measures of body image developed specifically for persons with upper limb amputation/limb deficiency that have strong evidence of reliability and validity. However, there is a measure, the Amputee Body Image Scale, which has been used for persons with lower limb amputation,[70] and a scale within the Patient Experience Measure targeted at body image.[68]

Most recognize that one of the primary goals of therapy is to enhance patient self-efficacy, that is, ability and confidence in their abilities and in managing their own health. Studied in other fields with generic measures of self-efficacy,[71] there is clearly a need for self-efficacy measures in amputee rehabilitation where patients need to have confidence in their functional abilities, as well as problem solving and condition management skills to handle minor technical issues and problems such as skin breakdown. The Patient Experience Measure contains a self-efficacy scale that was designed to assess confidence in upper limb function.[68] Additional research is needed to examine the psychometric properties of self-efficacy measures in persons with upper limb amputation.

Discussion

A variety of outcome measures have been recommended for use in upper limb amputation rehabilitation, and some emerging measures and important constructs that may be relevant to upper limb amputation rehabilitation are pointed out. The number of outcome measures with strong evidence of reliability, validity, and responsiveness in this population will continue to expand as additional research provides data on the psychometric properties of new and existing measures.

The analysis of outcome measures in this chapter focused mainly on their content relative to the ICF taxonomy; however, when selecting outcome measures, it is also important to consider that measures whose items fall into the same ICF domain/chapter may assess differing aspects or dimensions and it is important to choose measures that assess those dimensions that are deemed most important or informative. The measures described in this chapter assess a wide range of dimensions including speed of task performance, quality of movement, ability to complete tasks, skillfulness of prosthesis use, frequency of activity, difficulty with activity, need for assistance, impact of difficulty, and/or satisfaction with function, prosthesis satisfaction, and QOL.

Given the many important outcome domains involved in amputation rehabilitation and research on prosthetics and amputation care, it is clear that no single outcome measure would be appropriate for all uses. Rather, it is likely that a toolbox or core set of measures will be needed to capture critical domains. The field of upper limb amputation rehabilitation would benefit from the use of a standardized core set that addresses those domains that are most important to patients and clinical decision making is indicated for clinical care and lifetime management. Although no widespread consensus exists at this time, several large systems, including the Department of Veterans Affairs, the Department of Defense, and some large prosthetic practices, have adopted such sets of standardized measures.

A core set of measures for research might be different than a core set for clinical care, and the selection of measures would likely vary depending on the nature of the research. For example, studies to develop and test new prosthetic hardware and control methods might require measures of body function (eg, fine motor tasks, handling and carrying objects) during the early stages of development, and then incorporate measures of activities and participation (eg, self-care, domestic activities) and prosthesis satisfaction and QOL when examining outcomes of research on longer term device use.

The field of measurement in upper limb prosthetics/amputation rehabilitation is relatively young and there is a continuing need for research on existing outcome measures as well as the development of new, targeted measures with sufficient sensitivity to important change. This is especially true, given the advances in prosthesis technology, controls and user interfaces, and the unique, expected benefits from these advances, which may not be captured by existing measures.

One of the greatest barriers to implementation of outcome measures in clinical settings is the feasibility of their use. To be maximally useful, outcome measures must be able to be administered during routine clinical practice without creating excessive administrative burden. Some measures are lengthy to administer, require specialized training or certification to administer and score, and may require special equipment. These factors may be a barrier to use. The collection of standardized measures in amputation rehabilitation may require a redesign of clinical practice with greater multidisciplinary involvement and sharing of outcome scores, so that time-intensive performance measures could be administered by physical and occupational therapists and summary scores shared with prosthetists and physicians. Such a team approach is likely to improve overall outcomes and enhance the benefit to patients.

Another barrier to implementation of standardized outcome measures is the ease of scoring and the interpretability of scores. Clinicians and researchers need to understand how their patient or research population compares to population norms to be able to understand the degree of impairment or limitation. Some early work has provided normative values for some outcome measures, with values provided by amputation level and device type.[72] Although there are exceptions, most normative data and evaluation of outcomes have been conducted with individuals with unilateral transradial amputation. Additional research is needed to be certain that measures are appropriate for a variety of amputation levels as well as for individuals with bilateral upper limb amputations. Users of outcome measures must also understand what amount of change in a score is meaningful and is clinically important to use outcome measures in clinical decision making. Although some data on minimal detectable change of some currently available outcome measures is available[12,13,16,17,22,34] (Table 4), more research is needed to quantify the magnitude of clinically meaningful change. Efforts to develop convenient dashboards and clinical decision support tools for summarizing and visualizing outcomes over time; data may facilitate ease of use and provide easily accessible guidance on scoring and interpretation.

Although patient status and clinical change must be evaluated using the standardized scoring method for each measure, clinicians and researchers will sometimes want to examine item by item scoring of assessments with multiple items/tasks. Evaluating the performance of specific items can provide a deeper understanding of the elements that have contributed to the total score, and that information may be useful for targeting intervention or directing research activities.

SUMMARY

It is becoming increasingly necessary for clinicians to use outcome measures to more accurately track progress and compare outcomes across patients and groups. Outcome measures should be selected from those known to be reliable, valid, and responsive to change in persons with an upper limb amputation. Outcomes selected will likely vary depending upon the reason for use, and multiple measures may be required to evaluate the domains of interest. The field of amputation rehabilitation has yet to reach consensus on a recommended suite, or toolbox, of measures for clinical care or research.

References

1. Roach KE: Measurement of health outcomes: Reliability, validity, and responsiveness. *J Prosthet Orthot* 2006;18(6 Proceedings):P8-P12.
2. Wade DT: Assessment, measurement and data collection tools. *Clin Rehabil* 2004;18(3):233-237.
3. Wright V: Measurement of functional outcome with individuals who use upper extremity prosthetic devices: Current and future directions. *J Prosthet Orthot* 2006;18(2):46-56.
4. Salive ME, Mayfield JA, Weissman NW: Patient outcomes research teams and the agency for health care policy and research. *Health Serv Res* 1990;25(5):697-708.
5. Hill W, Stavdahl O, Hermansson LN, Kyberd P, Swanson S, Hubbard S: Functional outcomes in the WHO-ICF Model: Establishment of the upper limb prosthetic outcome measures group. *J Prosthet Orthot* 2009;21(2):115-119.
6. Hill WB, Kyberd PP, Norling Hermansson LP, et al: Upper Limb Prosthetic Outcome Measures (ULPOM): A working group and their findings. *J Prosthet Orthot* 2009;21(9):P69-P82.
7. Wright V: Prosthetic outcome measures for use with upper limb amputees: A systematic review of the peer-reviewed literature, 1970 to 2009. *J Prosthet Orthot* 2009;21(9):P3-P63.
8. Miller LA, Swanson S: Summary and recommendations of the academy's state of the science conference on upper limb prosthetic outcome measures. *J Prosthet Orthot* 2009;21(9):P83-P89.
9. Management of Upper Extremity Amputation Rehabilitation WorkingGroup: *VA/DoD Clinical Practice Guideline for the Management of Upper Extremity Amputation Rehabilitation*. Department of Veterans Affairs, Department of Defense; 2014.
10. Resnik L, Borgia M, Silver B: Measuring community integration in persons with limb trauma and amputation: A systematic review. *Arch Phys Med Rehabil* 2017;98(3):561-580.e8.
11. Resnik L, Borgia M, Silver B, Cancio J: Systematic review of measures of impairment and activity limitation for persons with upper limb trauma and amputation. *Arch Phys Med Rehabil* 2017;98(9):1863-1892.e14.
12. Resnik L, Adams L, Borgia M, et al: Development and evaluation of the activities measure for upper limb amputees. *Arch Phys Med Rehabil* 2013;94(3):488-494.e4.
13. Lindner HY, Langius-Eklof A, Hermansson LN: Test-retest reliability and rater agreements of assessment of capacity for myoelectric control version 2.0. *J Rehabil Res Dev* 2014;51(4):635-644.
14. Hermansson LN, Fisher AG, Bernspang B, Eliasson AC: Assessment of capacity for myoelectric control: A new Rasch-built measure of prosthetic hand control. *J Rehabil Med* 2005;37(3):166-171.
15. Hermansson LN, Bodin L, Eliasson AC: Intra- and inter-rater reliability of the assessment of capacity for myoelectric control. *J Rehabil Med* 2006;38(2):118-123.
16. Hermansson LN, Lindner HY, Hill W: *Assessment of Capacity for Myoelectric Control v3.0 Manual*, 2015.
17. Resnik L, Borgia M: Reliability and validity of outcome measures for upper limb amputation. *J Prosthet Orthot* 2012;24:192-201.
18. Mathiowetz V, Volland G, Kashman N, Weber K: Adult norms for the box and blocks test of manual dexterity. *Am J Occup Ther* 1985;39(6):386-391.
19. Jebsen RH, Taylor N, Trieschmann RB, Trotter MJ, Howard LA: An objective and standardized test of hand function. *Arch Phys Med Rehabil* 1969;50(6):311-319.
20. Beaton DE, Katz JN, Fossel AH, Wright JG, Tarasuk V, Bombardier C: Measuring the whole or the parts? Validity, reliability, and responsiveness of the disabilities of the arm, shoulder and hand outcome measure in different regions of the upper extremity. *J Hand Ther* 2001;14(2):128-146.
21. Gummesson C, Ward MM, Atroshi I: The shortened disabilities of the arm, shoulder and hand questionnaire (Quick DASH): Validity and reliability based on responses within the full-length DASH. *BMC Muscoskelet Disord* 2006;7(1):44.
22. Resnik L, Borgia M: Reliability, validity, and responsiveness of the QuickDASH in patients with upper limb amputation. *Arch Phys Med Rehabil* 2015;96(9):1676-1683.
23. Gallagher P, Franchignoni F, Giordano A, Maclachlan M: Trinity amputation and prosthesis experience scales: A psychometric assessment using classical test theory and Rasch analysis. *Am J Phys Med Rehabil* 2010;89(6):487-496.
24. Desmond DM, MacLachlan M: Factor structure of the Trinity Amputation and Prosthesis Experience Scales (TAPES) with individuals with acquired upper

limb amputations. *Am J Phys Med Rehabil* 2005;84(7):506-513.

25. Bergner M, Bobbitt RA, Carter WB, Gilson BS: The sickness impact profile: Development and final revision of a health status measure. *Med Care* 1981;19(8):787-805.

26. Ottenbacher KJ, Cusick A: Goal attainment scaling as a method of clinical service evaluation. *Am J Occup Ther* 1990;44(6):519-525.

27. Law M, Baptiste S, McColl M, Opzoomer A, Polatajko H, Pollock N: The Canadian occupational performance measure: An outcome measure for occupational therapy. *Can J Occup Ther* 1990;57(2):82-87.

28. Ware JE Jr, Sherbourne CD: The MOS 36-item short-form health survey (SF-36). I. Conceptual framework and item selection. *Med Care* 1992;30(6):473-483.

29. Ware J, Snow K, Kosinski M, Gandek B: *SF-36 Health Survey: Manual and Interpretation Guide*. The Health Institute, New England Medical Center, 1993.

30. Ware JE Jr: SF-36 health survey update. *Spine* 2000;25(24):3130-3139.

31. Skevington SM, Lotfy M, O'Connell KA: The World Health Organization's WHOQOL-BREF quality of life assessment: Psychometric properties and results of the international field trial. A report from the WHOQOL group. *Qual Life Res* 2004;13(2):299-310.

32. Group W: Development of the World Health Organization WHOQOL-BREF quality of life assessment. *Psychol Med* 1998;28(3):551-558.

33. Sanderson ER, Scott RN: *UNB Test of Prosthetics Function, a Test for Unilateral Upper Extremity Amputees, Ages 2-13*. University of New Brunswick, Bio-engineering Institute, 1985.

34. Resnik L, Baxter K, Borgia M, Mathewson K: Is the UNB test reliable and valid for use with adults with upper limb amputation? *J Hand Ther* 2013;26(4):353-359.

35. Krumlinde-Sundholm L, Holmefur M, Kottorp A, Eliasson AC: The assisting hand assessment: Current evidence of validity, reliability, and responsiveness to change. *Dev Med Child Neurol* 2007;49(4):259-264.

36. Krumlinde-Sundholm L, Eliasson A: Development of the assisting hand assessment: A Rasch-built measure intended for children with unilateral upper limb impairments. *Scand J Occup Ther* 2003;10:16-26.

37. Wright FV, Hubbard S, Jutai J, Naumann S: The prosthetic upper extremity functional index: Development and reliability testing of a new functional status questionnaire for children who use upper extremity prostheses. *J Hand Ther* 2001;14(2):91-104.

38. Petersen C, Schmidt S, Power M, Bullinger M: Development and pilot-testing of a health-related quality of life chronic generic module for children and adolescents with chronic health conditions: A European perspective. *Qual Life Res* 2005;14(4):1065-1077.

39. Simeoni MC, Schmidt S, Muehlan H, Debensason D, Bullinger M: Field testing of a European quality of life instrument for children and adolescents with chronic conditions: The 37-item DISABKIDS Chronic Generic Module. *Qual Life Res* 2007;16(5):881-893.

40. Varni JW, Seid M, Rode CA: The PedsQL: Measurement model for the pediatric quality of life inventory. *Med Care* 1999;37(2):126-139.

41. Varni JW, Limbers CA: The pediatric quality of life inventory: Measuring pediatric health-related quality of life from the perspective of children and their parents. *Pediatr Clin North Am* 2009;56(4):843-863.

42. Lerman JA, Sullivan E, Barnes DA, Haynes RJ: The Pediatric Outcomes Data Collection Instrument (PODCI) and functional assessment of patients with unilateral upper extremity deficiencies. *J Pediatr Orthop* 2005;25(3):405-407.

43. Daltroy LH, Liang MH, Fossel AH, Goldberg MJ: The POSNA pediatric musculoskeletal functional health questionnaire: Report on reliability, validity, and sensitivity to change. Pediatric Outcomes Instrument Development Group. Pediatric Orthopaedic Society of North America. *J Pediatr Orthop* 1998;18(5):561-571.

44. Resnik L, Plow M, Jette A: Development of CRIS: Measure of community reintegration of injured service members. *J Rehabil Res Dev* 2009;46(4):469.

45. Resnik L, Borgia M, Ni P, Pirraglia PA, Jette A: Reliability, validity and administrative burden of the community reintegration of injured service members computer adaptive test (CRIS-CAT). *BMC Med Res Methodol* 2012;12(1):1-17.

46. Light CM, Chappell PH, Kyberd PJ: Establishing a standardized clinical assessment tool of pathologic and prosthetic hand function: Normative data, reliability, and validity. *Arch Phys Med Rehabil* 2002;83(6):776-783.

47. Burgerhof JG, Vasluian E, Dijkstra PU, Bongers RM, van der Sluis CK: The Southampton hand assessment procedure revisited: A transparent linear scoring system, applied to data of experienced prosthetic users. *J Hand Ther* 2017;30(1):49-57.

48. Resnik L, Borgia M, Cancio JM, Delikat J, Ni P: Psychometric evaluation of the Southampton Hand Assessment Procedure (SHAP) in a sample of upper limb prosthesis users. *J Hand Ther* 2021; August 13 [Epub ahead of print].

49. Heinemann AW, Bode RK, O'Reilly C: Development and measurement properties of the Orthotics and Prosthetics Users' Survey (OPUS): A comprehensive set of clinical outcome instruments. *Prosthet Orthot Int* 2003;27(3):191-206.

50. Hanspal R, Fisher K, Nieveen R: Prosthetic socket fit comfort score. *Disabil Rehabil* 2003;25(22):1278-1280.

51. Hafner BJ, Morgan SJ, Askew RL, Salem R: Psychometric evaluation of self-report outcome measures for prosthetic applications. *J Rehabil Res Dev* 2016;53(6):797-812.

52. England DL, Miller TA, Stevens PM, Campbell JH, Wurdeman SR: Assessment of a nine-item patient-reported outcomes measurement information system upper extremity instrument among individuals with upper limb amputation. *Am J Phys Med Rehabil* 2021;100(2):130-137.

53. Carlsson AM: Assessment of chronic pain. I. Aspects of the reliability and validity of the visual analogue scale. *Pain* 1983;16(1):87-101.

54. Melzack R: The short-form McGill pain questionnaire. *Pain* 1987;30(2):191-197.

55. Cleeland CS, Ryan KM: Pain assessment: Global use of the brief pain inventory. *Ann Acad Med Singap* 1994;23(2):129-138.

56. Cleeland CS, Ryan K: *The Brief Pain Inventory*. Pain Research Group, 1991, pp 143-147.

57. Amtmann D, Cook KF, Jensen MP, et al: Development of a PROMIS item bank to measure pain interference. *Pain* 2010;150(1):173-182.

58. Carey SL, Dubey RV, Bauer GS, Highsmith MJ: Kinematic comparison of myoelectric and body powered prostheses while performing common activities. *Prosthet Orthot Int* 2009;33(2):179-186.

59. Carey SL, Jason Highsmith M, Maitland ME, Dubey RV: Compensatory movements of transradial prosthesis users during common tasks. *Clin Biomech (Bristol, Avon)* 2008;23(9):1128-1135.

60. Cowley J, Resnik L, Wilken J, Smurr Walters L, Gates D: Movement quality of conventional prostheses and the DEKA arm during everyday tasks. *Prosthet Orthot Int* 2017;41(1):33-40.

61. Chadwell A, Kenney L, Granat MH, et al: Upper limb activity in myoelectric prosthesis users is biased towards the intact limb and appears unrelated to goal-directed task performance. *Sci Rep* 2018;8(1):11084.

62. Chadwell A, Kenney L, Granat M, Thies S, Galpin A, Head J: Upper limb activity of twenty myoelectric prosthesis users and twenty healthy anatomically intact adults. *Sci Data* 2019;6(1):199.

63. Bekrater-Bodmann R: Factors associated with prosthesis embodiment and its importance for prosthetic satisfaction in lower limb amputees. *Front Neurorobot* 2021;14:604376.

64. Marasco PD: Using proprioception to get a better grasp on embodiment. *J Physiol* 2018;596(2):133-134.

65. Lundberg M, Hagberg K, Bullington J: My prosthesis as a part of me: A qualitative analysis of living with an osseointegrated prosthetic limb. *Prosthet Orthot Int* 2011;35(2):207-214.

66. Jan Z, Eva L, Max O-C: Prosthetic embodiment: Review and perspective on definitions, measures, and experimental paradigms. *TechRxiv*. Preprint. 2021.

67. Graczyk EL, Resnik L, Schiefer MA, Schmitt MS, Tyler DJ: Home use of a neural-connected sensory prosthesis provides the functional and psychosocial experience of having a hand again. *Sci Rep* 2018;8(1):9866.

68. Resnik L, Graczyk E, Tyler D: Measuring user experience of a sensory enabled limb prosthesis. Paper presented at: MEC17: Myoelectric Controls and Upper Limb Prosthetics Symposium 2017, Fredericton, New Brunswick, Canada.

69. Imaizumi S, Asai T, Koyama S: Embodied prosthetic arm stabilizes body posture, while unembodied one perturbs it. *Conscious Cogn* 2016;45:75-88.

70. Gallagher P, Horgan O, Franchignoni F, Giordano A, MacLachlan M: Body image in people with lower-limb amputation: A Rasch analysis of the amputee body image scale. *Am J Phys Med Rehabil* 2007;86(3):205-215.

71. Dixon G, Thornton EW, Young CA: Perceptions of self-efficacy and rehabilitation among neurologically disabled adults. *Clin Rehabil* 2007;21(3):230-240.

72. Resnik L, Borgia M, Cancio J, et al: Dexterity, activity performance, disability, quality of life, and independence in upper limb Veteran prosthesis users: A normative study. *Disabil Rehabil* 2020;44(11):2470-2481.

SECTION 3

Lower Limb

Prosthetic Foot and Ankle Mechanisms

Matthew J. Major, PhD • Phillip M. Stevens, MEd, CPO, FAAOP

CHAPTER 32

ABSTRACT

The purpose of prosthetic foot and ankle mechanisms is to simulate the functions of the absent foot and ankle during standing, walking, and transfers while modulating the impacts of ground reaction forces at the interface of the residual limb and the prosthesis. For passive-elastic prosthetic feet, this is accomplished through the consideration and manipulation of mechanical stiffness, dampening characteristics, and energy efficiency. Localized movement can be facilitated through mechanical joints with the extent of that movement modulated by elastomeric bumpers or fluid resistance. Fluid resistance can be regulated in real time in microprocessor-controlled feet. The field continues to explore the benefits and realization of powered propulsion in prosthetic foot and ankle mechanisms.

Keywords: dynamic response; foot; hydraulic ankle-foot; lower limb prosthesis; microprocessor foot

Introduction

Modern prosthetic foot mechanisms are often characterized in terms of their mechanical stiffness. The level of prosthetic foot stiffness will affect the user's walking experience and their mobility outcomes, as stiffer feet will deform less under the same load. In general, compliant materials are used in prosthetic feet designed for more reserved walkers, whereas stiffer materials with greater energy storage potential are preferred by more dynamic walkers. Localized movement can be facilitated at mechanical ankle joints and can be modulated by compressible elements or fluid resistance. In the case of the latter, onboard sensors can inform a centralized microprocessor of the need to modulate ankle joint stiffness in real time according to environmental cues. Externally powered ankle mechanisms are now commercially available with ongoing efforts to identify ideal programming parameters, means of actuation, and patient candidates.

Passive-Elastic Prosthetic Foot Concepts

In the effort to restore the lost function provided by the anatomic foot and ankle, the primary role of a prosthetic foot-ankle mechanism (referred to as simply foot through the balance of this chapter) is to support a patient user during weight-bearing activities such as standing, walking, and transitioning. For standing, the prosthesis must adequately support some or all of a user's body weight while providing an adequate base of support to accommodate fluctuations in the plantar center-of-pressure position during postural sway. For walking, the principal objectives of the prosthesis are to (1) accommodate energy absorption during load acceptance in early stance, (2) adapt to the ground surface by achieving a stable foot position following initial contact, (3) provide close-to-normal shank kinematics during center-of-pressure progression by replicating the loaded rollover geometry of the anatomic ankle-foot complex, and (4) contribute to late stance push-off and facilitating limb transition into the swing phase.[1] As required during transitions from standing to walking or seated to standing and vice versa, the prosthetic foot provides a structural element to transfer ground forces to the proximal components. Consequently, the user experience and mobility outcomes will be intimately linked to the inherent mechanical function of a prosthetic foot.[1,2]

For a passive-elastic prosthetic foot, the function is dictated by its mechanical properties, namely stiffness and damping.[3] The amount of deformation that a prosthesis experiences under load is a function of its stiffness, which for modern feet will vary throughout the structure and is typically nonlinear.[1] Therefore, the deformation of the prosthetic foot is dependent on the region (eg, heel, keel) being loaded, and the orientation and magnitude of the applied force. By association, because of their passive-elastic nature, the same factors will also determine the amount of both the energy stored and the energy dissipated by a prosthetic foot. Importantly, as with any passive-elastic

Neither of the following authors nor any immediate family member has received anything of value from or has stock or stock options held in a commercial company or institution related directly or indirectly to the subject of this chapter: Dr. Major and Phillip M. Stevens.

spring, the amount of energy return will not exceed the energy stored and is ultimately dependent on the unloading of the prosthesis. Consequently, although a prosthetic foot may possess excellent energy efficiency, meaning it returns a relatively high percentage of the energy stored, that energy return may not be provided in full or at the right moment in the gait cycle because of a user's unique gait dynamics or the design of the foot. Advancements in materials science have played a pivotal role in the evolution of prosthetic feet, in which passive-elastic materials can range from foams to carbon fiber–reinforced plastics and fiberglass composites. These materials offer tremendous flexibility to prosthesis design and their corresponding mechanical properties, thereby accommodating a wide range of users with different activity levels and lifestyles.

Regarding design, the passive-elastic structures in prosthetic feet can assume different shapes. Although heels and keels of prosthetic feet can often be considered cantilever springs, integrated (**Figure 1**) or modular pylons (**Figures 2 and 3**) are akin to linear or rotational springs. Their mechanical properties and hence loaded behavior are then a function of structural design details, including geometry, attachment, and preloading. The decision to incorporate passive-elastic structures as opposed to rigid, noncompliant materials within a design will dictate where the prosthesis deforms and by how much. One way to increase localized degree-of-freedom range of motion is to incorporate articulations or prosthetic joints such as an ankle pivot (**Figure 4**). Ankle joints can serve to increase sagittal and/or coronal plane range of motion, whereas certain pylon adaptors can increase axial absorption and transverse plane torsional range of motion. Although these articulated prostheses may seem distinct from their nonarticulated counterparts, it is important to acknowledge that the mechanical behavior of articulations is still dependent on passive-elastic principles. Normally these articulations are not simply free hinges, but their range of motion is often controlled through

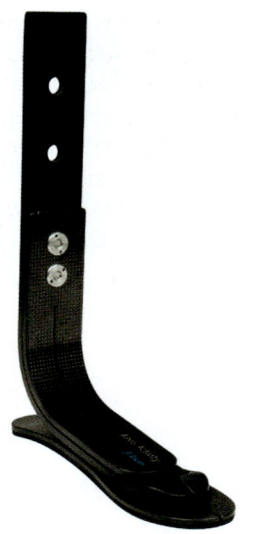

FIGURE 1 Photograph of a carbon fiber dynamic elastic response foot with an integrated carbon pylon. The split keel enables multiaxial compliance. (Courtesy of Fillauer, Chattanooga, TN.)

viscoelastic elements, such as bumpers (**Figure 4**). Loaded deformation in any anatomic plane can be achieved through either articulations or continuous structures of solid composite materials. Strategic cutouts in continuous structures can further increase range

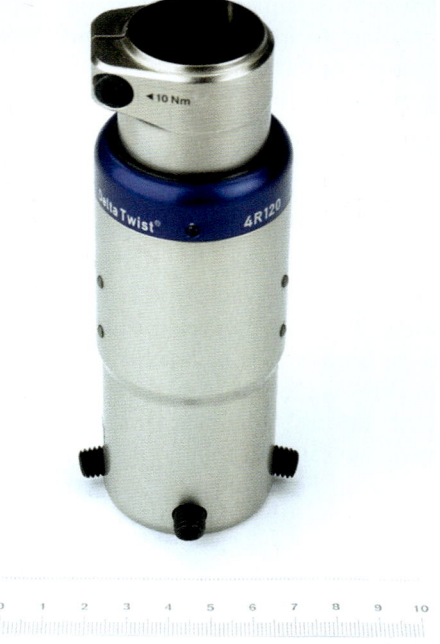

FIGURE 2 Photograph of an endoskeletal shock-absorbing pylon. (Courtesy of Ottobock.)

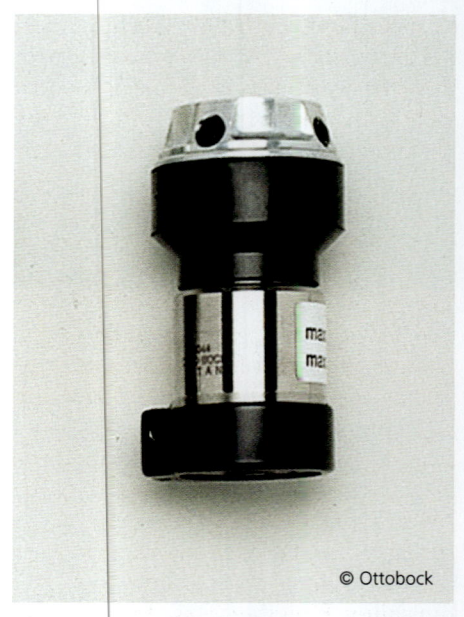

FIGURE 3 Photograph of an endoskeletal torsion adaptor. (Courtesy of Ottobock.)

of motion (**Figure 1**). Therefore, based on structural design, prostheses that incorporate articulations can behave similarly to those without such articulations. Thus, their user-independent mechanical function is more relevant to a patient's experience than their inherent design details. For instance, keel or heel deformation, whether through compression of a solid composite or articulation, can simulate dorsiflexion and plantar flexion, respectively.

Nonarticulated Dynamic Response Prosthetic Feet

The design and function of nonarticulated prosthetic feet have benefited greatly from advancements in material

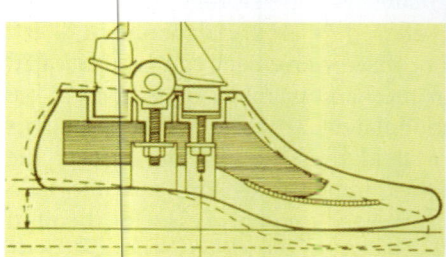

FIGURE 4 Schematic illustration of a cross-section view of a single-axis ankle-foot with a mechanical ankle axis allowing movement in the sagittal plane. Compressible bumpers positioned anterior and posterior to the ankle axis regulate the rate and amount of movement.

science. The Solid Ankle Cushion Heel (SACH) foot is the earliest version of these types of feet and perhaps the most well known given its history and the widespread use of its design concepts. As the name implies, the SACH foot is designed with a compliant heel that deforms with load at initial contact to store and dissipate energy (**Figure 5**). The heel typically occupies a third of the plantar surface and is often made from an open-cell foam. The user transitions from the heel as they advance over the prosthetic limb onto a rigid keel and eventually a compliant toe section to facilitate late stance rollover. These types of feet remain relevant in resource-limited environments because of their simple design, low cost, and durability. However, these features also make this design applicable as a basic prosthesis for individuals with limited mobility. The compressible heel can facilitate load acceptance following limb collision, and the relatively rigid keel[4] can act to limit prosthesis keel deformation to aid in stability during standing and walking. Because there is a rapidly expanding selection of prosthetic feet, modern prostheses tend not to incorporate this type of foot and so their use is becoming more limited.

A now more common nonarticulated, passive-elastic prosthetic foot of which there are many different designs is the dynamic (elastic) response foot, also known as flexible keel (**Figure 6**) or energy storage and return feet (**Figures 1** and **7**). A caveat here is that all passive-elastic prosthetic feet, even including the SACH foot, will store

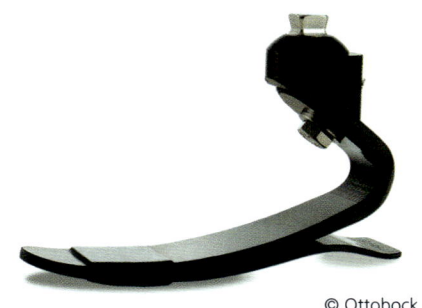

FIGURE 7 Photograph of a carbon fiber, dynamic elastic response foot. (Courtesy of Ottobock.)

and return some amounts of energy given the viscoelastic properties of the materials used to construct these prostheses and their constituent parts.[4] The combined elastic and viscous characteristics dictate the amount of energy stored and returned when loaded and unloaded at a given rate, thereby generating the characteristic hysteresis curve of instantaneous force versus displacement that describes features of stiffness and energy efficiency (**Figure 8**).

Although the design specifics, including structural elements, materials, and geometry, might vary across dynamic response feet, they are typically composed of keel and heel cantilever elements (blades) of a material with relatively high levels of strength and energy efficiency (eg, carbon fiber–reinforced plastics and fiberglass composites) (**Figures 1** and **7**). One primary advantage of using these

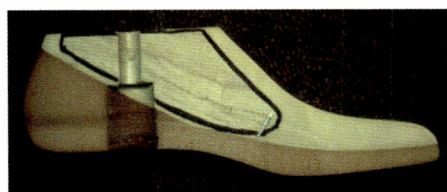

FIGURE 5 Photograph showing a cross-section view of a Solid Ankle Cushion Heel foot with its compressible foam heel and rigid wooden keel.

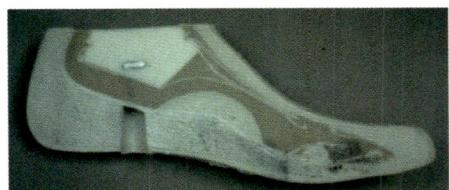

FIGURE 6 Photograph showing a cross-section view of the solid ankle flexible keel foot.

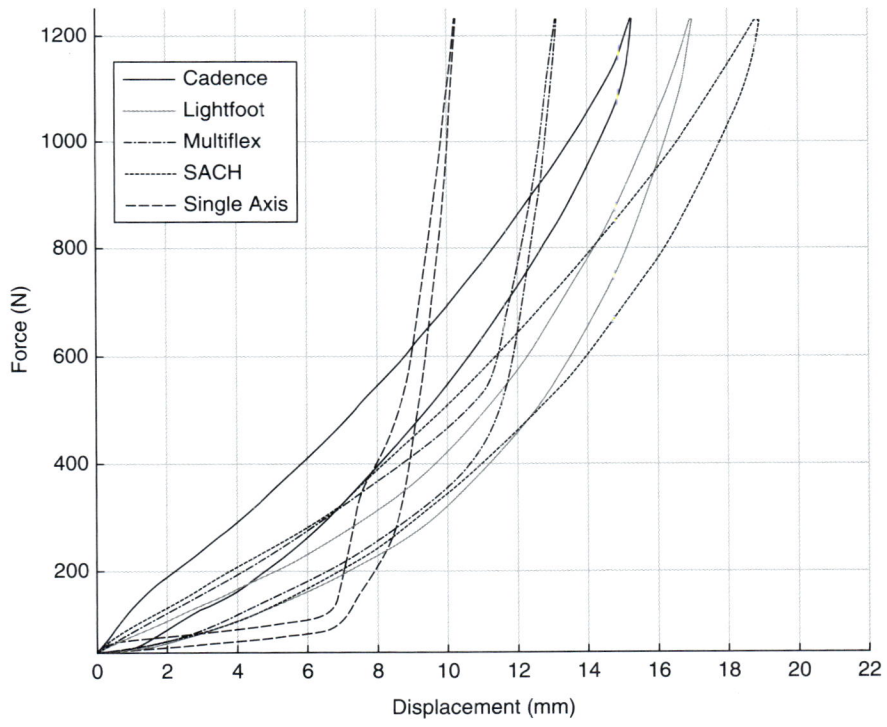

FIGURE 8 Representative hysteresis curves of five prosthetic foot designs loaded with a materials test system at the heel region. The area within each closed-loop curve represents the foot's energy efficiency (energy return relative to energy stored). Of note is the clear difference in loaded behavior of each foot design. Although the nonarticulated feet demonstrate a smooth curve during loading, there is an inflection point for the articulated feet denoting when the foot has rotated relative to the pylon to achieve foot flat resulting in increased foot stiffness. (Reprinted from Major MJ, Scham J, Orendurff M: The effects of common footwear on stance-phase mechanical properties of the prosthetic foot-shoe system. *Prosthet Orthot Int* 2018;42[2]:198-207.)

materials is that the prosthesis can store and return greater amounts of energy upon unloading, which would theoretically be advantageous for assisting with prosthetic limb push-off. However, again, this push-off assistance would be dependent on returning energy at the correct time. The material flexibility and structural design, and hence mechanical properties, of such blades allow these feet to accommodate a wide range of users according to their stature, weight, and activity level. Regarding the structural design of keel blades, they can either be of a solid element (**Figure 7**) or split toe (**Figure 1**) to increase coronal plane compliance and hence range of motion to accommodate movement in that plane. Furthermore, although traditional dynamic response feet have only one keel blade, embodiments exist that have included multiple stacked blades that engage after some load threshold to increase stiffness (**Figure 9**).

Physical principles dictate that given the opportunity for greater deformation the energy storage capacity of a keel shares a positive relationship with its length. In other words, a longer keel with greater build-height can potentially store more energy than a low-profile design of the same material. The first generation of energy-storing feet was characterized by shorter build-heights (referred to by some as flex-walk systems) and continue to find application where special constraints preclude the use of taller feet[5] (**Figure 7**). Second-generation energy-storing feet elongated their build-heights with longer springs that acted as integrated pylons to enable additional deformation and associated energy storage (referred to by some as flex foot systems) (**Figure 1**). In subsequent development efforts, the integrated pylon segments of such feet have been engineered to allow vertical deflection (referred to by some as a shank foot system with vertical loading pylon) (**Figure 10**). In response to external policy influences, vertical deflection has been increasingly localized to discrete shock-absorption mechanisms (**Figure 11**).

Given the flexibility in design afforded with dynamic response feet, the crossover foot is a relatively new type of foot meant to accommodate both walking and running for higher activity users (**Figure 12**). This particular foot type incorporates design elements of running-specific feet, including a carbon fiber keel blade that extends to the socket, and elements of dynamic response feet for walking, including a heel element for initial contact of the limb. These combined features enhance utility of these feet by offering energy storage and return for running through their keel design while providing a heel to support heel-to-toe rollover during walking and a stable base of support for standing. Consequently, this design can offer users access to a single foot for engaging in a range of ambulatory activities without the cost and burden of swapping between feet.

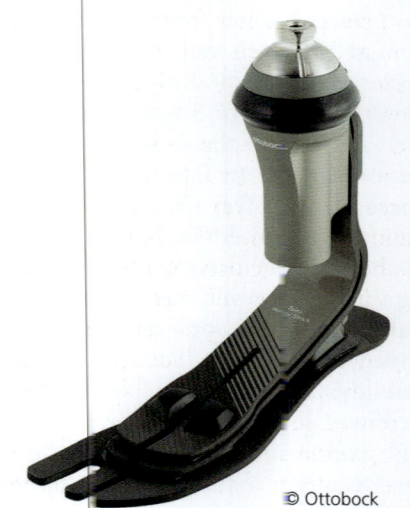

FIGURE 11 Photograph of a carbon fiber dynamic elastic response foot with a discrete mechanism engineered for axial torsion and vertical shock absorption. (Courtesy of Ottobock.)

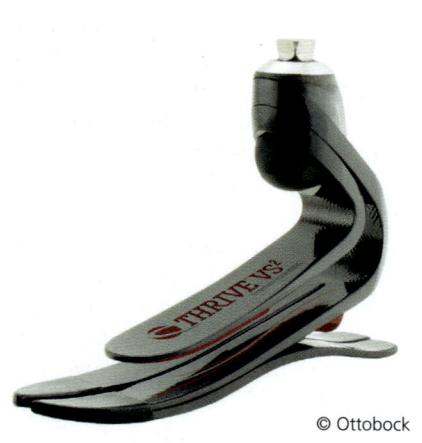

FIGURE 9 Photograph of a carbon fiber dynamic elastic response foot with dual keel design where the primary keel engages with a secondary upper keel when loaded to a certain threshold to increase foot stiffness. (Courtesy of Ottobock.)

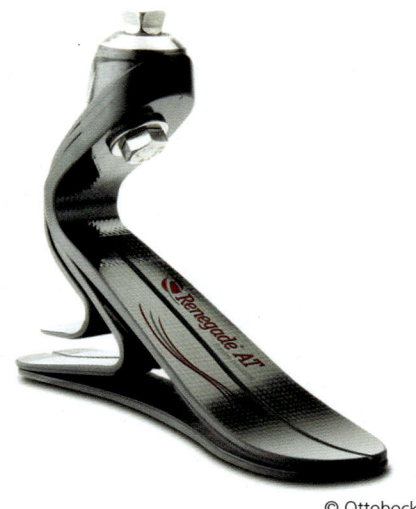

FIGURE 10 Photograph of a carbon fiber dynamic elastic response foot engineered with multiaxial compliance and vertical shock absorption. (Courtesy of Ottobock.)

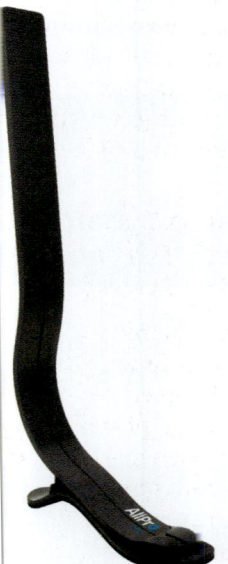

FIGURE 12 Photograph of a crossover carbon fiber dynamic elastic response foot combining elements of a running-specific foot with a long carbon blade extending to the socket, and the heel element of a more traditional foot. (Courtesy of Fillauer, Chattanooga, TN.)

Evidence suggests that these feet are preferred over traditional dynamic response feet by moderate to active ambulators, who also demonstrated improvements in mobility, balance confidence, and satisfaction with these designs.[6]

Evidence from classic comparative studies has suggested improved clinical outcomes when walking with dynamic response feet compared to the SACH foot design. These outcomes include increased walking velocity,[7,8] increased stride/step length,[8-10] increased step length symmetry,[10] improved rollover and shank progression control,[11,12] lower sound limb loading,[8,9] and increased push-off power at faster walking speeds.[10,13,14] Notably, there has been inconclusive evidence regarding differences in metabolic energy demands during self-selected walking on level ground, but some suggest that dynamic response feet display improved outcomes at higher walking speeds and gradients.[7,12,15] More recently, there has been some limited evidence to suggest that users may demonstrate greater walking speed, stride/step length, prosthesis power generation, and prosthesis-related quality of life when using a fiberglass dynamic response foot compared with carbon fiber.[16] Given these superior outcomes, improved designs, and now vast selection of dynamic response feet to accommodate a range of users, SACH foot designs are less commonly used in modern prostheses.

Articulated Dynamic Response Prosthetic Feet and Shock-Absorbing Pylons

Although dynamic response prosthetic feet with continuous structures can be cleverly designed to provide varying levels of range of motion when under load, the incorporation of articulations is a common design technique to strategically increase regional motion. The single-axis prosthetic foot design includes an ankle joint articulation to provide additional sagittal plane rotation, or effectively plantar flexion and dorsiflexion (Figure 4). In commercial single-axis feet, the motion provided by the ankle joint is typically regulated through viscoelastic bumpers that act as springs to resist rotation. One primary function of this joint is that it allows the entire foot structure distal to the articulation to rotate into plantar flexion at initial contact to achieve foot flat akin to anatomic function. Nonarticulated feet will still achieve some level of foot flat because of heel compression and/or the shank deformation, but the single-axis foot will in most cases display quick rotation of the foot at initial contact[17] to allow the forefoot structure to meet with the ground.[18] In this way, the ground reaction force vector, and hence center of pressure, quickly progresses anteriorly from initial contact as opposed to stalling at the posterior end in nonarticulated feet because of heel deformation. As tibial progression continues, the ankle can enter into dorsiflexion that is limited by another bumper element to further advance the ground reaction force vector toward the keel end, thereby sustaining an increasing knee extension moment. Overall, these features may be advantageous for users who lack sufficient stance stability and could benefit from early foot flat and knee control. However, a noted disadvantage of this design is that although the center of pressure is able to advance quickly following initial contact, it may stall near the ankle joint until the tibia advances to allow for dorsiflexion. The seemingly less constrained ankle motion and unique progression of the center of pressure during stance could work to disrupt a user's forward advancement.[18]

An extension of the single-axis foot design is the multiaxial ankle-foot, which through a universal ankle joint increases regional rotation in the sagittal, coronal, and transverse planes. This joint is designed to allow limited rotational range of motion in all three planes for accommodating ground surface gradients and uneven terrain, as well as transverse plane rotations of the socket relative to the foot. Consequently, this foot allows more of the plantar foot surface to maintain contact with the ground when traversing irregular surfaces, during either community ambulation or recreational activities. Such ground compliance can not only facilitate a larger base of support for stance stability but also minimize rotational moments applied to the socket that can cause user discomfort.

Although their articulations are not intended to act dynamically in gait, several prosthetic foot designs are commercially available to accommodate different heel heights and hence different footwear. The ability to accommodate different footwear is important for prosthesis users who may desire to don various shoe types according to their occupation, lifestyle, and daily activities, and this is especially relevant to women.[19,20] One version of accommodating feet that does not possess an articulation is the modified SACH foot, which is available in different geometries that can accommodate heel heights up to 3.5 inches. Although the SACH feet can accommodate shoes of different heel heights, their geometry is fixed, so a user would require multiple feet to fit a selection of shoes. However, modern heel-height adjustable prosthetic feet offer a more convenient solution in which an ankle articulation permits small adjustments in the sagittal-plane angle of the foot relative to the pylon. These adjustable feet allow the user to make these alignment changes, often through activating a button that locks and unlocks the articulation, and can accommodate up to a 2-inch heel rise.[19] As opposed to the SACH feet, these heel-height adjustable feet often include a carbon fiber keel and can behave similar to dynamic response feet[21] (Figure 13). A limitation of adjustable feet, however, is that although the sagittal-plane alignment can be adjusted, the plantar insole geometry remains fixed. Recent advancements in prosthetic foot design have begun to address this issue by adopting the fixed geometry approach of the SACH foot but using different three-dimensional printed feet that can be swapped and attached to a modular ankle unit.[22]

There is evidence to suggest that for low-mobility users, walking with articulated prosthetic feet can demonstrate improved clinical outcomes

Section 3: Lower Limb

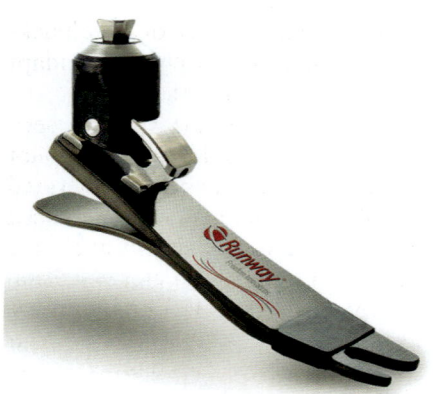

FIGURE 13 Photograph of a carbon fiber dynamic elastic response foot with an adjustable heel height. (Courtesy of Ottobock.)

compared with nonarticulated feet. Compared with the SACH foot, low-mobility users walking with a multiaxial prosthetic foot demonstrated improved energy cost of walking, self-selected walking speed, perceived walking effort, satisfaction, functional balance, and mobility capability.[23,24] Furthermore, when multiaxial ankle units were added to the nonarticulated prostheses of persons with bilateral transtibial amputation to increase simulated ankle range-of-motion, users expressed that walking was smoother and that it was easier to traverse uneven ground. Users also displayed a base of support and roll-over shape that was closer to able-bodied individuals.[25,26] However, for low-mobility users, it is critical to tune the bumper stiffness according to their weight and mobility level so adequate motion control is provided for stability.

Dynamic Pylons

A technique to increase axial and transverse plane (rotational) motion is to incorporate a shock-absorbing/attenuating, or dynamic, pylon. These pylons can either be modular components that are added to compatible prosthetic feet to augment their function (**Figures 2** and **3**) or are integrated as part of the foot design as described earlier in the chapter (**Figure 11**). Modern shock-absorbing pylons are often designed to accommodate both longitudinal and transverse plane motion. These motions are controlled through passive-elastic elements, such as viscoelastic bumpers or metal springs, and they can be tuned for each user to limit their range of motion. Axial motion is normally achieved through a telescoping action, and its mechanical behavior has been modeled as a viscoelastic system.[27,28] As the design name implies, these pylons can absorb some linear/rotational motion and hence energy within the prosthetic system distal to the socket to limit their transfer to the residual anatomy. The original intention and perhaps long held impression of these components is to attenuate impact force transients when the limb collides with the ground and experiences rapid deceleration. However, evidence on clinical outcomes regarding inclusion of shock-absorbing pylons has been mixed. Compared with rigid pylons, shock-absorbing pylons have not demonstrated effective reductions in either vertical ground reaction forces[29-31] or shank accelerations[31,32] during either walking or running, but evidence suggests that this may be due to stiffness and damping of the residuum tissue that dominates the residuum-prosthesis system dynamics.[27,33] There is also the possibility that other prosthesis structures, including footwear,[4] may contribute to force attenuation[34] and therefore make these pylons redundant. However, these devices remain popular as encouraged by subjective feedback from users who prefer them to rigid pylons, including indication that the prosthesis feels less stiff.[30,35] To this effect, there is some evidence that increasing axial compliance through shock-absorbing pylons can allow the prosthesis to store more energy during weight acceptance[33] and amplify the prosthesis damping effect,[34] as well as reduce metabolic demands at faster walking speeds.[35] Regarding the limited transverse motion, such additional compliance may be better suited for specific activities that involve considerable body rotations, such as golf, that may otherwise be assumed by the socket-residuum coupling interface.[36]

Hydraulic Ankle Feet/Microprocessor Feet

Although limited by the rudimentary design of an articulation controlled through passive-elastic bumpers, single-axis feet have demonstrated the benefit of restricted movement about a mechanical ankle joint. An alternate mechanism of controlling ankle joint motion through hydraulic resistance was reported as early as 1981.[37] In contrast to the resistance to motion directed by the relatively static viscoelastic properties of solid materials, hydraulic resistance is guided by the laws of fluid dynamics, which is the resistance to liquid volume flow through pipes and valves. This feature provides clinicians with an added measure of adjustability for fine-tuning the relative resistance to dorsiflexion and plantar flexion motion according to the needs of the individual user. In addition, the immediate rebound of solid bumper materials in single-axis feet is not present. Rather, once a hydraulic ankle joint is moved into relative dorsiflexion in late stance, the ankle will retain some degree of that relative alignment until the ground reaction forces of heel strike bring the ankle into plantar flexion. Large-scale market availability of such feet began with the release of the Blatchford Echelon in 2009 (**Figure 14**). Since that time, a

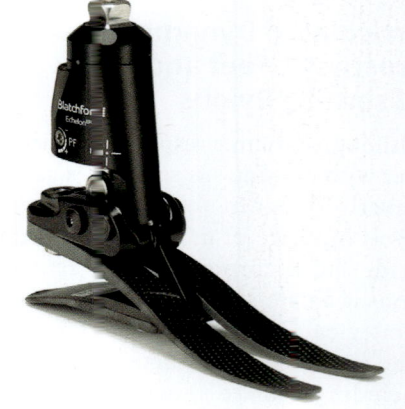

FIGURE 14 Photograph of a carbon fiber foot with an adjustable hydraulic ankle mechanism. (Courtesy of Blatchford, Miamisburg, Ohio.)

number of hydraulic ankle feet (HAF) have become commercially available and widely used.

Concurrent with the development of widely used HAF has been the inception of microprocessor-controlled feet (MPF). For most MPF the purpose of the microprocessor is to dynamically regulate the passive hydraulic resistance of the joint across gait speeds and walking environments (**Figure 15**), similar to the more historically established functionality of microprocessor knees. An exception to this model is observed in the Össur Proprio Foot that provides active swing phase dorsiflexion (**Figure 16**).

Although HAF and MPF are associated with elevated build-heights and modest increases in weight, recent literature has explored a number of potential benefits associated with these foot types, including increased foot clearance in swing, decreased localized socket pressures, increased walking velocity, improved interlimb symmetry, increased environmental mobility, and decreased energy consumption.

The concept of minimum foot clearance, or the minimum vertical distance between the foot and the floor during gait, originated in studies of fall prevention among the geriatric community. However, the simple variable of minimum toe clearance (MTC) has since been applied to users of lower limb prostheses given its relationship to foot catch with the ground and potential for stumbling and trip-related falls. Early studies confirmed that compared with able-bodied ambulation, MTC values are reduced among users of nonarticulated prosthetic feet, and unlike observations in able-bodied control patients, MTC values do not increase with increased gait speed. Consistent with the mechanical properties described earlier, pilot data have suggested a modest increase in MTC values with the use of HAF because of their ability to retain some amount of dorsiflexion through swing from loading during late stance. An even more pronounced reduction has been associated with the active dorsiflexion of the Proprio MPF.[38] Subsequent studies of HAF and MPF have reported increased MTC values and decreased MTC variability during slope negotiation compared with nonarticulated prosthetic feet, with these values being more pronounced among MPF. Such findings are important as reduced MTC values have correlated with prospective stumble and fall risk among users of lower limb prostheses.[39]

Additional safety benefits specific to transfemoral prosthesis users have been suggested through improved stability of the prosthetic knee during slope descent (ie, reduced risk of knee buckling) as these ankle mechanisms adapt to declined standing surfaces.[40]

With respect to pressures experienced in the transtibial socket, pilot data have suggested that the elevated knee flexion moments experienced during slope and stair decent apply the highest level of localized anterior distal pressures on the residual limb.[41] These peak stresses and loading rates appear to be significantly reduced with the use of HAF,[42] though this relationship has not been universally reported. Pilot data suggest the ability of both HAF and MPF to absorb loadbearing forces as they adopt a plantarflexed alignment during slope descent, thereby reducing the negative work required from the knee joint of the affected extremity. The ability of such feet to reduce the external moments acting on the prosthesis and the associated peak stresses experienced by the limb appears to contribute to the increased socket comfort reported by users of MPF compared with nonarticulated feet.

The reductions in residuum-socket interface pressures associated with HAF and MPF may help facilitate additional benefits. The use of HAF has been associated with improvements in interlimb temporal symmetry through increased stance time on the prosthetic limb.[43] Additionally, the reduction of socket pressures combined with the reduced braking effect experienced during loading response may facilitate the frequently observed increase in walking speed with HAF.[44] Finally, the ability of such feet to adapt across a range of walking surfaces and to reduce the energy costs of ambulation across a range of gait speeds and gradients[44] may begin to explain the increased prosthetic mobility scores reported by users of both HAF and MPF relative to nonarticulated dynamic response feet.

Propulsive Microprocessor Feet

In addition to their thoughtful manipulation of both passive energy absorption, storage and dynamic return capabilities, developers of foot-ankle

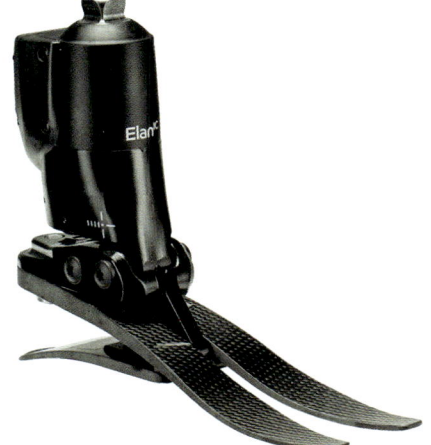

FIGURE 15 Photograph of a passive microprocessor-controlled foot-ankle mechanism designed to regulate the passive hydraulic resistance of the ankle across gait speeds and walking environments. (Courtesy of Blatchford, Miamisburg, Ohio.)

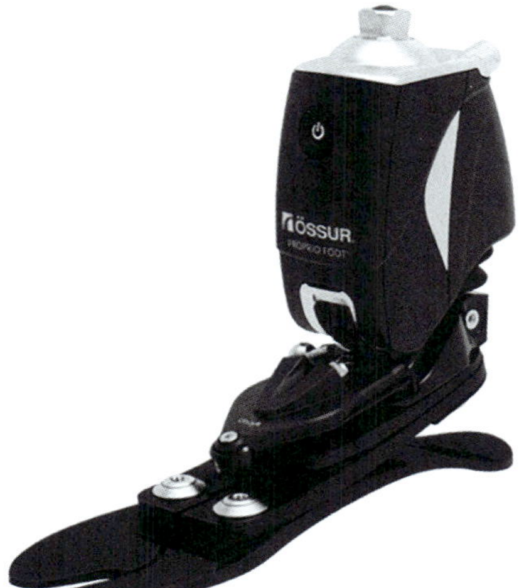

FIGURE 16 Photograph of an active, nonpropulsive microprocessor foot-ankle mechanism designed to provide active ankle dorsiflexion in swing phase. (Courtesy of Össur.)

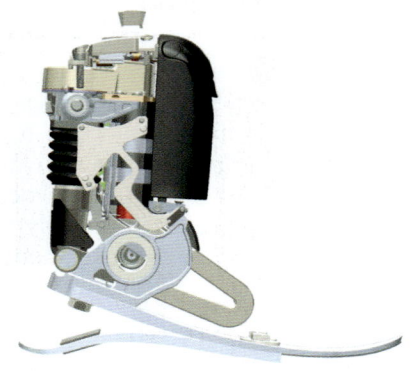

FIGURE 17 Photograph of an active, propulsive microprocessor-controlled foot-ankle mechanism designed to provide positive power during the transition from late stance into swing phase. (Courtesy of Ottobock.)

prostheses have been challenged to further address the propulsive deficits encountered in the absence of concentric contractions across the major joints of the lower limbs. Most of the propulsion of the able-bodied lower limb is derived from the concentric activity of the plantar flexors during late stance. Given that the ankle generates 3 to 5 times the energy it absorbs during walking on level ground,[45,46] this deficit can be only partially addressed by passive-elastic prosthetic feet.[47,48]

Several approaches are being explored to provide propulsive movement at the prosthetic ankle joint. In the first commercially available, externally powered, propulsive MPF, the BiOM foot (now called Empower), battery-powered electronic drive motors are coupled with parallel, mechanical springs to mimic the push-off behavior of the intact plantar flexors (**Figure 17**).

Early clinical reports on propulsive MPF were promising and included increases in peak ankle power generation in late stance of more than 50%, reductions in oxygen consumption values of 8%, and increased self-selected walking speeds approaching 25%.[47,48] These observations were followed by early reports of considerable reductions in the peak ground reaction forces, loading rates, and external knee moments acting on the users' sound side limb.[49,50] These favorable results were consistent with early patient reports of reduced walking effort and a sparing of the loads experienced by the sound side limb during weight acceptance.

Subsequent clinical reports have remained positive but have been less consistent in their findings. Contradictory data have been reported on the extent of the effect of propulsive MPF on metabolic demands during level ground and slope ascent,[51-54] preferred walking speeds,[53,54] and the protective influence of MPF on the sound side limb.[51] Although the reasons behind these inconsistencies are not fully understood, patient selection criteria and the programming of the technology with respect to the timing and magnitude of its power bursts appear to be influential.[51-53,55]

As this technology is further developed, future clinical studies will likely provide additional evidence regarding the influence of these powered MPF with propulsive capabilities on clinically relevant outcomes. Although most are not yet commercially available, there have been several alternative approaches to this type of prosthetic foot that have been explored to date.[56] The various design solutions to driving propulsion include pneumatic actuators, hydraulic actuators, or electric motors with different transmission assemblies. The weight and build-height of these prosthetic feet remain a function of the unique methods selected for actuating and powering the device, but they are subject to change as that technology develops and miniaturizes.

Mechanical Characterization and Taxonomy

The loaded mechanical function, or stance-phase properties (stiffness, damping, rollover geometry), of a prosthetic foot will have a direct effect on clinically relevant user outcomes.[1,3] This relationship is evidenced from classic comparison studies,[57] but results of studies using experimental prosthetic devices have emphasized that changes in specific properties (ie, the bench) can influence performance outcomes, metabolic energy expenditure, gait stability, walking dynamics, and limb loading (ie, the bedside).[3,33] User preference may be driven by the mechanical function of the prosthesis during walking where even small differences in properties can be detected.[58] A prosthesis is clinically optimized by way of selecting and mechanically tuning prosthetic components based on manufacturer recommendations according to user characteristics and activity level, and then alignment adjustments to fulfil clinical and individual user objectives.[3] The modern clinical design process of a prosthesis is a function of practitioner experience, clinical practice guidelines, and objectives shared between the patient user and their rehabilitation team. However, although the relationship between prosthesis mechanical properties and user outcomes is recognized, knowledge of those properties to help drive clinical decisions is not widely available to practitioners.[59]

Various bench test methods have been proposed to characterize the mechanical function of socket-distal transtibial prosthetic components under different and realistic loading conditions (orientations, magnitude, rate).[1,2,60,61] It is important to emphasize that these bench test methods measure mechanical function independent of the user because individual gait mechanics will load a prosthesis in different ways to produce a unique response and hence user experience. Although there currently is no standardized method for characterizing user-independent mechanical properties that have been broadly adopted by the orthotics and prosthetics field, these bench test methods generally aim to measure the viscoelastic properties of prosthetic feet during stance. A common test method is to load and unload the prosthesis in different orientations reflective of critical points during stance (initial contact, midstance, terminal stance) using universal material testing systems or bespoke test rigs to generate hysteresis curves (**Figure 8**) that reveal information on stiffness and energy storage, return, and efficiency (**Figure 18**). Using these outcomes, the mechanical behaviors of prosthetic feet have been modeled as physical systems, using either

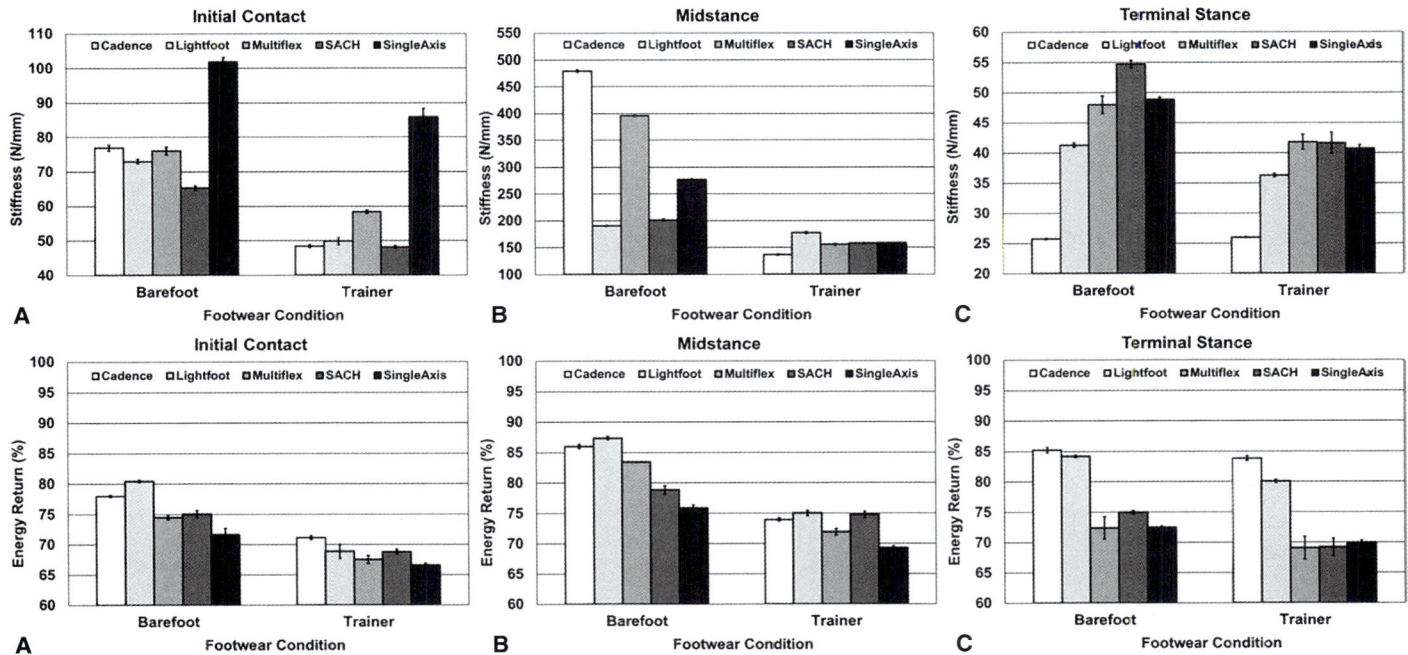

FIGURE 18 Approximated linear stiffness (top) and percent energy return (bottom) of five different prosthetic foot designs at regions of (**A**) initial contact, (**B**) midstance, and (**C**) terminal stance while barefoot and wearing a trainer shoe. Notice the effect footwear can have on regional properties of a prosthetic foot and that linear stiffness may not fully capture the nonlinear behavior of feet displayed in the hysteresis curves of Figure 8. (Data from Major MJ, Scham J, Orendurff M: The effects of common footwear on stance-phase mechanical properties of the prosthetic foot-shoe system. *Prosthet Orthot Int* 2018;42[2]:198-207.)

spring-damper models or rollover shape[1,2,62] (**Figure 19**).

Two key findings have been generated from this characterization work. First, with well-defined methodology, these characterization methods can have high levels of precision.[4,61,63] This result encourages the development of standardized methods to establish a more universal language of communicating prosthesis properties, and The International Organization for Standardization has begun to develop methods for this purpose.[64] Second, prostheses can express similar mechanical function when measured independent of the user despite their different design elements.[4,60] Moreover, although prosthesis mechanical function is clinically optimized through selection and tuning of assembled prosthetic components, footwear worn outside of the clinic can substantially affect mechanical properties in important ways.[4]

The clinical relevance of these key findings is that although design classifications such as SACH, dynamic response, and single/multiaxial may accurately describe the design features of a given prosthesis, they do not define its mechanical function that ultimately matters to the user experience. Therefore, a taxonomy based on outcomes from a standardized procedure for measuring user-independent mechanical function of a prosthesis can offer a more clinically relevant and reliable classification scheme. The American Orthotic & Prosthetic Association proposed such a taxonomy and associated methodology in 2011, known as the Prosthetic Foot Project, where prosthetic feet were classified, and hence assigned L-Codes, by design according to their measured mechanical function, such as the amount of heel deformation or keel energy return.[63,65] Although not a full departure from the use of design classifications, this work represents a first attempt at defining feet according to their mechanical properties rather than superficial factors.

Ultimately, the purpose of enhancing prosthetic foot classification schemes with well-defined functional information is to improve the process of matching patients to the most appropriate prosthesis. This process embodies the concept of personalized rehabilitation interventions, where prosthetic systems and their corresponding mechanical behavior are optimized to maximize and support long-term user outcomes. Selecting a prosthetic foot for a given user is dependent on several factors, including their stature, body mass, activity level, mobility capacity, and motivation. In the United States, the Medicare Functional Classification (K-)Level classification scheme is often used to categorize patients according to their mobility capacity for helping decide which types of prosthetic feet are most appropriate, and for third-party reimbursement agencies which devices and features (labeled by L-code) may be considered medically necessary. Consequently, a K-level assignment can then restrict patients to certain prosthesis designs. Practitioners have reported consideration of many different patient factors to assign K-level, including outcomes from performance measures.[66] Importantly, however, the process of

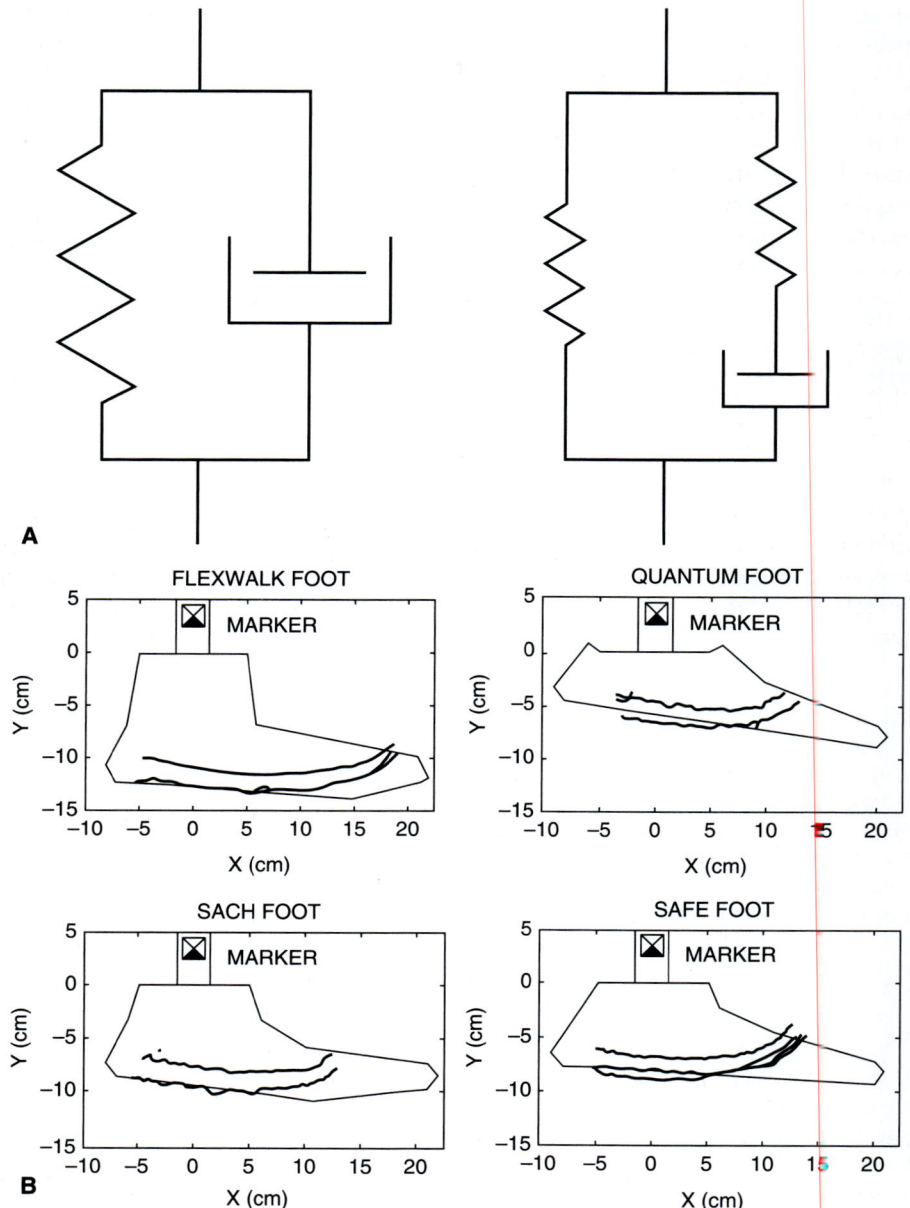

FIGURE 19 **A**, Two example arrangements of spring and damper elements for modeling viscoelastic behavior. **B**, Example of measured foot deformation in a foot-based reference frame superimposed on a foot profile to visualize rollover shape for several prosthesis designs with (solid lines) and without (dashed lines) shoes. (Panel A reprinted from Major MJ, Kenney LPJ, Twiste M, Howard D: Stance phase mechanical characterization of transtibial prostheses distal to the socket: A review. *J Rehabil Res Dev* 2012;49[6]:815-830. Panel B reprinted from Hansen AH, Childress DS, Knox EH: Prosthetic foot roll-over shapes with implications for alignment of trans-tibial prostheses. *Prosthet Orthot Int* 2000;24[3]:205-215.)

matching a user with a prosthesis that supports their full rehabilitation potential is a shared-decision among the intended user and their clinical rehabilitation team. Furthermore, several of these deciding factors may change as a user progresses through their rehabilitation journey, so longitudinal evaluation of a user may suggest the prosthesis selection should be updated accordingly.[3] Even limiting a patient initially to prosthesis designs that primarily support low-mobility activities may delay or ultimately stall rehabilitation progress. Therefore, clinical practice guidelines that are built and updated according to current evidence exist to suggest interventions and management pathways to help practitioners support a patient's rehabilitation.[67]

SUMMARY

Driven by advances in material science and robotics, prosthetic foot and ankle mechanisms have evolved considerably since their early conceptual designs. In general, prosthetic feet can be considered in terms of how their behavior is governed, either passively and therefore dictated exclusively through user loading, or actively modulated through microprocessor control that interacts with user dynamics. Passive dynamic prosthetic feet of various types are now widely used, and their effects on mobility outcomes are linked to their inherent mechanical properties. Efforts are underway to standardize measurement of foot mechanical properties (stiffness and damping) to inform device classification and better understand their effect on rehabilitation outcomes. Ankle articulations are readily incorporated in prosthetic feet with their behavior modulated through either elastomeric bumpers or fluid resistance, such as in the widely used HAF. Prosthetic feet providing late stance propulsion continue to be developed with different methods of actuation and tested to identify their influence on clinically relevant outcomes for a range of users.

References

1. Major MJ, Kenney LPJ, Twiste M, Howard D: Stance phase mechanical characterization of transtibial prostheses distal to the socket: A review. *J Rehabil Res Dev* 2012;49(6):815-829.
2. Major MJ, Twiste M, Kenney LPJ, Howard D: Amputee independent prosthesis properties – A new model for description and measurement. *J Biomech* 2011;44(14):2572-2575.
3. Major MJ, Fey NP: Considering passive mechanical properties and patient user motor performance in lower limb prosthesis design optimization to enhance rehabilitation outcomes. *Phys Ther Rev* 2017;22(3-4):202-216.
4. Major MJ, Scham J, Orendurff M: The effects of common footwear on stance-phase mechanical properties of the prosthetic foot-shoe system. *Prosthet Orthot Int* 2018;42(2):198-207.
5. Hafner BJ, Sanders J, Czerniecki JM, Fergason J: Transtibial energy-storage and return prosthetic devices: A review of energy concepts and a proposed nomenclature. *J Rehabil Res Dev* 2002;39(1):1-11.
6. Morgan SJ, McDonald CL, Halsne EG, et al: Laboratory- and community-based health outcomes in people with transtibial amputation using crossover and energy-storing prosthetic feet: A randomized crossover trial. *PLoS One* 2018;13(2):e0189652.
7. Nielsen DH, Shurr DG, Golden JC, Meier K: Comparison of energy cost and gait efficiency during ambulation in below-knee amputees using different prosthetic feet – A preliminary report. *J Prosthet Orthot* 1988;1(1):24-31.
8. Snyder RD, Powers CM, Fontaine C, Perry J: The effect of five prosthetic feet on the gait and loading of the sound limb in dysvascular below-knee amputees. *J Rehabil Res Dev* 1995;32(4):309-315.
9. Powers C, Torburn L, Perry J, Ayyappa E: Influence of prosthetic foot design on sound limb loading in adults with unilateral below-knee amputations. *Arch Phys Med Rehabil* 1994;75(7):825-829.
10. Houdijk H, Wezenberg D, Hak L, Cutti AG: Energy storing and return prosthetic feet improve step length symmetry while preserving margins of stability in persons with transtibial amputation. *J Neuroeng Rehabil* 2018;15(suppl 1):76.
11. Torburn L, Schweiger GP, Perry J, Powers CM: Below-knee amputee gait in stair ambulation. A comparison of stride characteristics using five different prosthetic feet. *Clin Orthop Relat Res* 1994;303:185-192.
12. Lehmann JF, Price R, Boswell-Bessette S, Dralle A, Questad K, deLateur BJ: Comprehensive analysis of energy storing prosthetic feet: Flex foot and Seattle foot versus standard SACH foot. *Arch Phys Med Rehabil* 1993;74(11):1225-1231.
13. Müller R, Tronicke L, Abel R, Lechler K: Prosthetic push-off power in transtibial amputee level ground walking: A systematic review. *PLoS One* 2019;14(11):e0225032.
14. Wezenberg D, Cutti AG, Bruno A, Houdijk H: Differentiation between solid-ankle cushioned heel and energy storage and return prosthetic foot based on step-to-step transition cost. *J Rehabil Res Dev* 2014;51(10):1579-1590.
15. Gardiner J, Bari AZ, Howard D, Kenney L: Transtibial amputee gait efficiency: Energy storage and return versus solid ankle cushioned heel prosthetic feet. *J Rehabil Res Dev* 2016;53(6):1133-1138.
16. Kaufman KR, Bernhardt K: Functional performance differences between carbon fiber and fiberglass prosthetic feet. *Prosthet Orthot Int* 2021;45(3):205-213.
17. Rao SS, Boyd LA, Mulroy SJ, Bontrager EL, Gronley JK, Perry J: Segment velocities in normal and transtibial amputees: Prosthetic design implications. *IEEE Trans Rehabil Eng* 1998;6(2):219-226.
18. Perry J, Boyd LA, Rao SS, Mulroy SJ: Prosthetic weight acceptance mechanics in transtibial amputees wearing the single axis, seattle lite, and flex foot. *IEEE Trans Rehabil Eng* 1997;5(4):283-289.
19. Major MJ, Hansen AH, Russell Esposito E: Focusing research efforts on the unique needs of women prosthesis users. *J Prosthet Orthot* 2021;34(1):e37-e43.
20. Russell Esposito E, Slater B, Muschler K, et al, eds: *Perceived Footwear Limitations in Women Prosthesis Users and Their Impact on Patient Reported Outcomes.* American Academy of Orthotists & Prosthetists 47th Academy Annual Meeting & Scientific Symposium, 2021.
21. Quinlan J, Hansen AH, Russel Esposito E, Major MJ, eds: *Stance-Phase Mechanical Properties of Women-Specific Adjustable Heel-Height Prosthetic Feet and Footwear.* American Academy of Orthotists & Prosthetists 47th Annual Meeting & Scientific Symposium, 2021.
22. Nickel E, Voss G, Slater B, Mueller E, Hansen AH, eds: *Improving Footwear Options for Persons With Lower Limb Amputations.* 2020 Design of Medical Devices Conference, 2020.
23. Delussu AS, Paradisi F, Brunelli S, Pellegrini R, Zenardi D, Traballesi M: Comparison between SACH foot and a new multiaxial prosthetic foot during walking in hypomobile transtibial amputees: Physiological responses and functional assessment. *Eur J Phys Rehabil Med* 2016;52(3):304-309.
24. Paradisi F, Delussu AS, Brunelli S, et al: The conventional non-articulated SACH or a multiaxial prosthetic foot for hypomobile transtibial amputees? A clinical comparison on mobility, balance, and quality of life. *Sci World J* 2015;2015:261801.
25. Su PF, Gard SA, Lipschutz RD, Kuiken TA: The effects of increased prosthetic ankle motions on the gait of persons with bilateral transtibial amputations. *Am J Phys Med Rehabil* 2010;89(1):34-47.
26. Gard SA, Su PF, Lipschutz RD, Hansen AH: Effect of prosthetic ankle units on roll-over shape characteristics during walking in persons with bilateral transtibial amputations. *J Rehabil Res Dev* 2011;48(9):1037-1048.
27. Boutwell E, Stine R, Gard S: Impact testing of the residual limb: System response to changes in prosthetic stiffness. *J Rehabil Res Dev* 2016;53(3):369-378.

28. Berge JS, Klute GK, Czerniecki JM: Mechanical properties of shock-absorbing pylons used in trans-tibial prostheses. *J Biomech Eng* 2004;126(1):120-122.

29. Boutwell E, Stine R, Gard S: Shock absorption during transtibial amputee gait: Does longitudinal prosthetic stiffness play a role? *Prosthet Orthot Int* 2017;41(2):178-185.

30. Gard SA, Konz RJ: The effect of a shock-absorbing pylon on the gait of persons with unilateral transtibial amputation. *J Rehabil Res Dev* 2003;40(2):109-124.

31. Berge JS, Czerniecki JM, Klute GK: Efficacy of shock-absorbing versus rigid pylons for impact reduction in transtibial amputees based on laboratory, field, and outcome metrics. *J Rehabil Res Dev* 2005;42(6):795-808.

32. Adderson JA, Parker KE, Macleod DA, Kirby RL, McPhail C: Effect of a shock-absorbing pylon on transmission of heel strike forces during the gait of people with unilateral trans-tibial amputations: A pilot study. *Prosthet Orthot Int* 2007;31(4):384-393.

33. Major MJ, Zavaleta JL, Gard SA: Does decreasing below-knee prosthesis pylon longitudinal stiffness increase prosthetic limb collision and push-off work during gait? *J Appl Biomech* 2019;35(5):312-319.

34. Maun JA, Gard SA, Major MJ, Takahashi KZ: Reducing stiffness of shock-absorbing pylon amplifies prosthesis energy loss and redistributes joint mechanical work during walking. *J Neuroeng Rehabil* 2021;18(1):143.

35. Buckley JG, Jones SF, Birch KM: Oxygen consumption during ambulation: Comparison of using a prosthesis fitted with and without a tele-torsion device. *Arch Phys Med Rehabil* 2002;83(4):576-580.

36. Rogers JP, Strike SC, Wallace ES: The effect of prosthetic torsional stiffness on the golf swing kinematics of a left and a right-sided trans-tibial amputee. *Prosthet Orthot Int* 2004;28(2):121-131.

37. Sowell TT: A preliminary clinical evaluation of the Mauch hydraulic foot-ankle system. *Prosthet Orthot Int* 1981;5(2):87-91.

38. Rosenblatt NJ, Bauer A, Rotter D, Grabiner MD: Active dorsiflexing prostheses may reduce trip-related fall risk in people with transtibial amputation. *J Rehabil Res Dev* 2014;51(8):1229-1242.

39. Rosenblatt NJ, Bauer A, Grabiner MD: Relating minimum toe clearance to prospective, self-reported, trip-related stumbles in the community. *Prosthet Orthot Int* 2017;41(4):387-392.

40. Bai X, Ewins D, Crocombe AD, Xu W: A biomechanical assessment of hydraulic ankle-foot devices with and without micro-processor control during slope ambulation in trans-femoral amputees. *PLoS One* 2018;13(10):e0205093.

41. Portnoy S, van Haare J, Geers RP, et al: Real-time subject-specific analyses of dynamic internal tissue loads in the residual limb of transtibial amputees. *Med Eng Phys* 2010;32(4):312-323.

42. Portnoy S, Kristal A, Gefen A, Siev-Ner I: Outdoor dynamic subject-specific evaluation of internal stresses in the residual limb: Hydraulic energy-stored prosthetic foot compared to conventional energy-stored prosthetic feet. *Gait Posture* 2012;35(1):121-125.

43. Moore R: Effect on stance phase timing asymmetry in individuals with amputation using hydraulic ankle units. *J Prosthet Orthot* 2016;28(1):44-48.

44. Askew GN, McFarlane LA, Minetti AE, Buckley JG: Energy cost of ambulation in trans-tibial amputees using a dynamic-response foot with hydraulic versus rigid 'ankle': Insights from body centre of mass dynamics. *J Neuroeng Rehabil* 2019;16(1):39.

45. Winter DA: Energy generation and absorption at the ankle and knee during fast, natural, and slow cadences. *Clin Orthop Relat Res* 1983;175:147-154.

46. DeVita P, Helseth J, Hortobagyi T: Muscles do more positive than negative work in human locomotion. *J Exp Biol* 2007;210(pt 19):3361-3373.

47. Mancinelli C, Patritti BL, Tropea P, et al: Comparing a passive-elastic and a powered prosthesis in transtibial amputees. *Annu Int Conf IEEE Eng Med Biol Soc* 2011;2011:8255-8258.

48. Herr HM, Grabowski AM: Bionic ankle-foot prosthesis normalizes walking gait for persons with leg amputation. *Proc Biol Sci* 2012;279(1728):457-464.

49. Grabowski AM, D'Andrea S: Effects of a powered ankle-foot prosthesis on kinetic loading of the unaffected leg during level-ground walking. *J Neuroeng Rehabil* 2013;10:49.

50. Russell Esposito E, Wilken JM: Biomechanical risk factors for knee osteoarthritis when using passive and powered ankle-foot prostheses. *Clin Biomech* 2014;29(10):1186-1192.

51. Quesada RE, Caputo JM, Collins SH: Increasing ankle push-off work with a powered prosthesis does not necessarily reduce metabolic rate for transtibial amputees. *J Biomech* 2016;49(14):3452-3459.

52. Russell Esposito E, Aldridge Whitehead JM, Wilken JM: Step-to-step transition work during level and inclined walking using passive and powered ankle-foot prostheses. *Prosthet Orthot Int* 2016;40(3):311-319.

53. Gardinier ES, Kelly BM, Wensman J, Gates DH: A controlled clinical trial of a clinically-tuned powered ankle prosthesis in people with transtibial amputation. *Clin Rehabil* 2018;32(3):319-329.

54. Kim J, Wensman J, Colabianchi N, Gates DH: The influence of powered prostheses on user perspectives, metabolics, and activity: A randomized crossover trial. *J Neuroeng Rehabil* 2021;18(1):49.

55. Malcolm P, Quesada RE, Caputo JM, Collins SH: The influence of push-off timing in a robotic ankle-foot prosthesis on the energetics and mechanics of walking. *J Neuroeng Rehabil* 2015;12:21.

56. Liu J, Abu Osman NA, Al Kouzbary M, et al: Classification and comparison of mechanical design of powered ankle-foot prostheses for transtibial amputees developed in the 21st century: A systematic review. *J Med Dev* 2021;15(1):010801.

57. Linde HVD, Hofstad CJ, Geurts ACH: A systematic literature review of the effect of different prosthetic components on human functioning with a lower limb prosthesis. *J Rehabil Res Dev* 2004;41(4):555-570.

58. Shepherd MK, Azocar AF, Major MJ, Rouse EJ: Amputee perception of prosthetic ankle stiffness during locomotion. *J Neuroeng Rehabil* 2018;15(1):99.

59. Klute GK, Kallfelz CF, Czerniecki JM: Mechanical properties of prosthetic limbs: Adapting to the patient. *J Rehabil Res Dev* 2001;38(3):299-307.

60. Womac ND, Neptune RR, Klute GK: Stiffness and energy storage characteristics of energy storage and return prosthetic feet. *Prosthet Orthot Int* 2019;43(3):266-275.

61. Webber CM, Kaufman K: Instantaneous stiffness and hysteresis of dynamic elastic response prosthetic feet. *Prosthet Orthot Int* 2017;41(5):463-468.

62. Hansen AH, Childress DS, Knox EH: Prosthetic foot roll-over shapes with

implications for alignment of trans-tibial prostheses. *Prosthet Orthot Int* 2000;24(3):205-215.

63. Major MJ, Johnson WB, Gard SA: Inter-rater reliability of mechanical tests for functional classification of prosthetic components. *J Rehabil Res Dev* 2015;52(4):467-476.

64. International Organization for Standardization: *ISO/TS 16955:2016. Prosthetics—Quantification of Physical Parameters of Ankle Foot Devices and Foot Units*. International Organization for Standardization, 2016.

65. Dodson K, McTernan J: *AOPA'S Prosthetic Foot Project: What It Is, What It Is Not, and What Patient Care Facility Providers/Practitioners Need to Know...*. American Orthotic and Prosthetic Association, 2010.

66. Borrenpohl D, Kaluf B, Major MJ: Survey of US practitioners on the validity of the medicare functional classification level system and utility of clinical outcome measures for aiding K-level assignment. *Arch Phys Med Rehabil* 2016;97(7):1053-1063.

67. Stevens PM, Rheinstein J, Wurdeman SR: Prosthetic foot selection for individuals with lower-limb amputation: A clinical practice guideline. *J Prosthet Orthot* 2018;30(4):175-180.

Prosthetic Knee Mechanisms

Matthew J. Major, PhD • Phillip M. Stevens, MEd, CPO, FAAOP

ABSTRACT

The purpose of prosthetic knee mechanisms is to simulate the functions of the absent knee joint during standing, walking, and transfers. Safe, efficient ambulation is accomplished by facilitating stability when the limb is loaded and achieving adequate and timely ground clearance of the prosthesis during swing. For mechanically passive prosthetic knees, stance limb stability is accomplished through mechanical locks and geometric designs that aid in generating knee extension moments. For single-speed walkers, swing phase knee resistance is limited to simple friction-based mechanisms. For walkers capable of variable speed ambulation, the use of hydraulic resistance permits a range of knee resistance values that adapt to different walking speeds. Microprocessors regulate knee flexion resistance in both swing and stance, with resultant benefits of safety, stability, and reduced cognitive loads of ambulation. The field continues to explore the benefits and realization of powered prosthetic knees that generate knee extension and/or flexion through either automatic means or direct muscle control.

Keywords: knee; lower limb prosthesis; microprocessor-controlled knee; stance control; swing control

Introduction

Modern prosthetic knee mechanisms are often characterized in terms of their joint configuration, their means of mechanical stability in stance, and their means of swing phase flexion/extension resistance. Joint configurations are characterized as either single axis or polycentric. Mechanical stance stability occurs through various locking mechanisms or geometrically favorable joint designs. This mechanical stability can be supplemented by yielding hydraulic resistance mechanisms. Swing phase flexion/extension resistance occurs through simple constrained frictional elements or more adaptive hydraulic resistance. Microprocessors are now able to govern knee resistance values in both stance and swing.

Knee selection is based on the needs of the user with respect to their ability to actively stabilize the knee in stance and their capacity to walk at variable speeds. Users with relatively short limb length, reduced hip extensor strength, or limited experience with prosthetic ambulation are more reliant on the mechanical stability afforded by certain mechanisms. Users capable of ambulation across a range of walking speeds benefit from the added cost and weight of knee designs with hydraulic cylinders, whereas those confined to a single walking speed in household environments may be well served by lighter, simpler knees. Microprocessors capable of adapting knee resistance values in both stance and swing are increasingly recognized for the added safety and stability they provide during prosthetic mobility.

Prosthetic Knee Concepts

The prosthetic knee mechanism serves to restore the lost functions of the anatomic knee joint and is responsible for facilitating safe and smooth ambulation for individuals with limb absence at or proximal to the knee. During standing, the knee mechanism is meant to provide adequate support and resist collapsing when loaded. Safety during walking is more involved as optimal knee flexion resistance values cycle with the cadence of ambulation. During stance, the knee must maintain limb stability to prevent buckling and, ideally, permit the initiation of knee flexion in preswing to prepare for the transition into the swing phase. During swing, knee flexion characteristics are designed to avoid collisions between the prosthetic foot and the ground to prevent stumbles and trips. Furthermore, knee resistance values must be low enough in terminal swing to permit full knee extension in preparation for the transition into the stance phase.

These goals are opposed with respect to optimizing the sagittal alignment of

---

Neither of the following authors nor any immediate family member has received anything of value from or has stock or stock options held in a commercial company or institution related directly or indirectly to the subject of this chapter: Dr. Major and Phillip M. Stevens.

the knee beneath the socket. In consideration of the demands placed on the user in controlling their prosthetic limb, a more posterior alignment facilitates stance stability but compromises the ease of initiating swing phase flexion. By contrast, a more anterior alignment facilitates an easier initiation of swing phase flexion but reduces stance phase knee stability. Thus, alignment decisions must balance the divergent needs of a given patient while considering the mechanical performance characteristics of a given knee mechanism.

To achieve the stance phase goal of stability, prosthetic knee users must manage the flexor-extensor moments of the knee mechanism. The knee moment is a function of the magnitude of the ground reaction force vector and its line of action relative to the prosthetic knee center of rotation in the sagittal plane (ie, lever arm).[1,2] The optimal position of the prosthetic knee relative to the residual hip joint is defined by the design of the knee mechanism and optimized by a prosthetist during clinical fitting of the prosthetic knee-ankle-foot system.[1] For knees with greater inherent stability, such as certain polycentric knees or microprocessor knees (MPKs), more dynamic alignments can be considered. In the absence of inherent prosthetic knee stability, safer alignments with the knee positioned more posteriorly beneath the socket must be considered. The biomechanical phenomenon of controlled knee flexion in early stance is pursued by some users of certain prosthetic knee joints that permit this feature and will be discussed later in the chapter.

During early stance, prosthetic knee users must prevent knee buckling and facilitate limb stability by maintaining a knee extension moment. This knee extension moment is achieved by positioning the ground reaction force vector anterior to the knee center of rotation.[1,3-5] The user must then smoothly transition from an extension moment to a flexor moment to initiate knee flexion during preswing.[2] Importantly, the position and orientation of the ground reaction force vector changes as the user advances over the prosthetic foot and is influenced by the foot's mechanical properties, prosthesis alignment, and selected footwear.[2]

To achieve swing phase goals, prosthetic knee users must carefully control the swing mechanics of the prosthetic limb to manage its global position and timing through a smooth arc of motion. Specifically, the effective length of the prosthetic limb must be shortened to provide adequate foot clearance and avoid contact of the heel or toe with the ground, and then it should be lengthened during terminal swing into full extension to prepare the limb for ground collision at stance phase initial contact.[6] The action of leg shortening is a function of the prosthetic knee joint design, the prosthetic ankle-foot mechanism and alignment, and volitional control of linear and angular position of the hip joint.[6-10] Given its relatively large range of motion, knee joint flexion is the primary contributor to limb shortening and providing sufficient foot clearance through midswing.[6,7] Thus, the prosthetic knee mechanism and its knee flexion/extension resistance values are critical to consistent swing phase clearance. These values will directly influence both angular positions and rates of change of the prosthetic shank at the knee, and hence the type and magnitude of compensatory dynamics employed by the user.

To accomplish these subtasks of stance and swing, a prosthetic knee user will directly modulate knee moments through compensation strategies. In stance these include their control of the trunk position and regulation of extensor and flexor moments of the residual hip joint.[1,3-5,11] In swing this may entail some combination of prosthetic limb circumduction, contralateral limb vaulting, ipsilateral hip hiking, and residual hip control.[9,10,12,13] Successful prosthetic knee control is therefore dependent on appropriately timed and sufficiently strong hip moments and would be affected by walking speed.[4,11,14] Given these varied compensation strategies, evidence suggests that prosthetic knee users exhibit greater demands on the sound limb relative to persons with transtibial level limb loss,[5,14,15] which could place them at greater risk of overuse injury and secondary musculoskeletal trauma of the sound limb.[16]

The amount of active control and compensation required by the user to ambulate with a prosthetic knee is highly dependent on their physical capacity for ambulation, their anticipated walking environments and activities, and the mechanical design of the knee mechanism itself.

Mechanically Passive Knee Joints

Knee Resistance Mechanisms: Friction Versus Fluid

Although variations in prosthetic knee options abound, the provision of resistance to knee motion is obtained through two common approaches. The simplest method of delivering resistance is constant friction. With constant-friction knees, the clinician can often easily adjust the friction resistance acting about the joint within the clinic. A limitation of constant-friction knees is that, once set by the clinician, the level of resistance is optimized for a single, generally slower gait speed. Walking faster will create excessive knee flexion in swing phase, prolonging this phase of gait because the user must wait for the knee to reach full extension in terminal stance. Walking slower will reduce the momentum of the knee into swing phase flexion and create quick, halting steps.[17] Accordingly, constant-friction knees are generally reserved for limited walkers who ambulate at a single, relatively slow speed and who are not functionally constrained by the performance limitations of the knee unit.

In contrast, fluid-controlled knees are capable of providing variable resistance across a modest range of walking speeds. Fluid-controlled knees use pneumatic or hydraulic cylinder configurations to dampen knee motion. With over half a century of regular use in prosthetic rehabilitation, it is well established that fluid-controlled knees provide a smoother, more normal swing phase movement than knees with mechanical friction.[17-19] Because of the nature of hydraulic resistance in which greater external forces are met with greater resistance, fluid control will automatically adapt knee resistance levels according to changes in the user's walking speeds. For that reason, they are indicated for those capable of walking at different speeds.

Choosing between pneumatic and hydraulic fluid control begins with an understanding of their compressibility. Gases are readily compressible, whereas liquids are not. The compressibility of the gases in a pneumatic knee requires a specific cylinder volume to provide adequate swing phase resistance through this medium. By contrast, the incompressibility of hydraulic fluids means that a smaller volume is needed to provide effective swing phase control. As a result, hydraulic knees can be both smaller and lighter than their pneumatic equivalents. In addition, their incompressibility allows hydraulic cylinders to accommodate a broader range of gait speeds.

Finally, pneumatic control is unable to deliver adequate knee flexion resistance to provide stance phase stability. Only the incompressibility of hydraulic fluid is capable of providing sufficient stance control to prevent limb collapse, typically in the form of a slowly yielding resistance to sudden knee flexion, as pioneered by Mauch in the 1950s,[20] which can aid stumble recovery. That the Mauch knee concept is still widely used and copied in modern prosthetic rehabilitation supports the clinical effectiveness of fluid-controlled prosthetic knee mechanisms (**Figure 1**).

Single-Axis Constant-Friction Knee

Consistent with its name, the single-axis constant-friction knee represents a basic hinge design that allows the knee joint to bend during the swing phase of gait. Various design mechanisms provide an adjustable friction-based dampening of knee flexion, commonly through a turn screw. Because of their relative mechanical simplicity, such knees represent a lightweight, low-cost, durable knee option. However, as described previously, these joints are generally reserved for users who walk at a single, reduced, fixed cadence (**Figure 2**). Although the adjustable friction

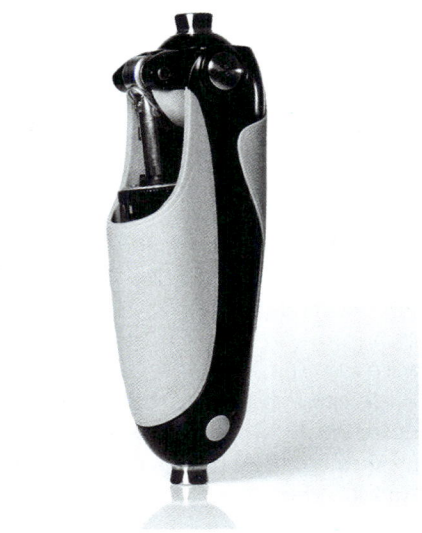

FIGURE 1 Photograph of a single-axis knee where both stance and swing knee resistance values are regulated by a hydraulic cylinder. (Courtesy of Össur.)

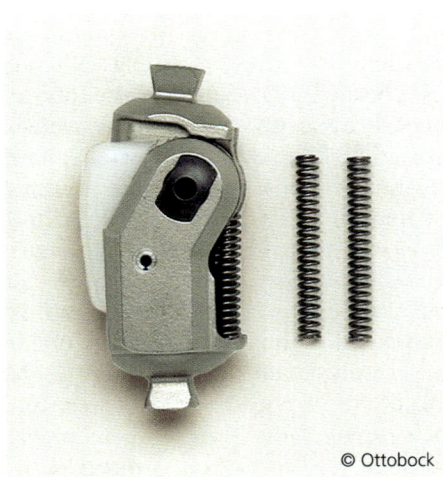

FIGURE 2 Photograph of a single-axis constant-friction knee. (Courtesy of Ottobock.)

provides a measure of customizability to the swing characteristics of the knee, the shank of the prosthesis largely functions as a passive pendulum with a swing rate determined by its length.[21] The slower walking speeds mandated by this knee can be frustrating to those users otherwise capable of faster, variable cadences. In addition, recent data have suggested that, although higher swing phase knee flexion resistance can generate earlier swing phase knee extension and improve swing time symmetry, it does so at the cost of smaller and earlier minimum toe clearance. Thus, improvements in swing symmetry are accompanied by an increased risk of insufficient toe clearance in swing.[6] In the United States, Medicare recognizes the single-axis constant-friction knee as the most basic prosthetic knee option, suitable for individuals with limited walking abilities. Exceptions to this standard application may be found in settings where the knee is chosen because of extreme financial constraints, the knee is preferred because of its simple durability, or in limited pediatric applications when size restrictions preclude the use of alternatives.

Importantly, although constant friction provides a measure of resistance to swing phase knee flexion, it provides no restriction to stance phase knee flexion. In the absence of any inherent knee stability as found in most alternative knee mechanisms, every step must be carefully controlled through the user's active hip extension. Although contradictory to their indication for more limited ambulators, management of these knees may be unrealistic for prosthesis users who lack the necessary strength and control of their hip extensors, such as frail walkers. Applying a relatively posterior alignment of this knee joint beneath the socket will provide a measure of knee stability through encouraging an external knee extension moment, but it increases the hip flexion demand to initiate knee flexion in late stance to transition into prosthetic swing phase.

Weight-Activated Stance Control

One solution to the lack of inherent knee stability attributed to single-axis constant-friction knees has been engineered in the form of weight-activated stance control (WASC). In such systems, a friction brake mechanism is applied to the prosthesis during stance to augment knee stability (**Figure 3**). When engaged, this adjustable supplemental friction prevents knee flexion and eliminates the risk of knee buckling during standing and walking. This knee mechanism is sometimes considered for use in the initial prosthesis of a patient with limited ambulatory potential.

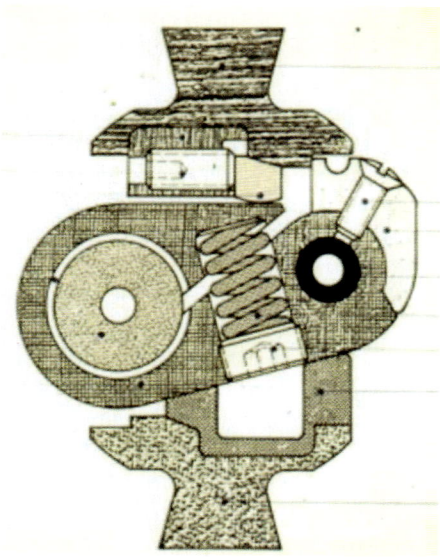

FIGURE 3 Schematic illustration of a cross-section view of a weight-activated stance-control knee. Weight bearing compresses the spring and causes the knee to clamp against the cylindric brake bushing. Unweighting the prosthesis allows the spring to open the clamping mechanism so that the lower leg can swing freely. (Reproduced from Michael JW: Prosthetic suspensions and components, in Smith DG, Michael JW, Bowker JH, eds: *Atlas of Amputations and Limb Deficiencies: Surgical, Prosthetic, and Rehabilitation Principles*, ed 3. American Academy of Orthopaedic Surgeons, 2004, pp 409-428.)

However, the typical weight-activated friction brake is associated with an important biomechanical limitation. Specifically, the knee does not release to allow flexion until the prosthesis is fully unloaded. This condition is problematic because it precludes the normal knee flexion that should occur during the preswing phase of gait and appears to reduce walking speed relative to other alternatives.[22] This limitation also renders the traditional WASC knee unusable in bilateral applications because the user is unable to fully offload both knee units to flex the knees and obtain a seated posture. As a result, this component is largely reserved for users of unilateral transfemoral prostheses with a slow, shuffling gait.

More recently, limited variants of the traditional WASC knee have been designed to release their friction braking mechanism under weight-bearing loads when the knee reaches full extension. The automatic stance phase lock knee joint represents another alternative of comparative simplicity, cost, and durability. Unlike traditional WASC knee units, the automatic stance phase lock is unlocked by the loading of the forefoot in terminal stance, allowing earlier knee break to prepare for transitioning into swinging the limb forward.[23,24]

Polycentric Knees

Polycentric knees are readily differentiated from simpler single-axis knees by their multiple points of articulation. Among these, the four-bar design is most common, characterized by four articulations connected by four linkage bars (**Figure 4**). Polycentric knees offer several biomechanical advantages over both single-axis constant-friction and WASC knees, and as a result, they have become increasingly popular. In contrast to the friction breaking mechanisms of the WASC knee, the inherent stability of polycentric knees is found in the geometry of their variable instantaneous center of rotation (ICOR). The ICOR represents the functional center of rotation of the knee at a given knee flexion angle. Unlike the single-axis knee, where the center of rotation can only be positioned at the knee axis, in polycentric configurations the ICOR is often located outside the knee mechanism itself. Specifically, when the polycentric joint is straight or nearly straight, the ICOR is positioned proximal and posterior to the joint itself (**Figure 5**).

The net effect to the user of a polycentric knee positioned in extension is the mechanical advantage of an articulation experienced closer and relatively posterior to the hip joint. This feature reduces the hip extensor strength (ie, the extension moment) required to maintain a knee extension moment to prevent buckling. As the knee flexes, the ICOR moves both anteriorly and distally in a curved pathway described as the centrode. With modest flexion, the ICOR is translated anterior to the hip joint, reducing the effort required of the hip flexors to dynamically flex the knee.

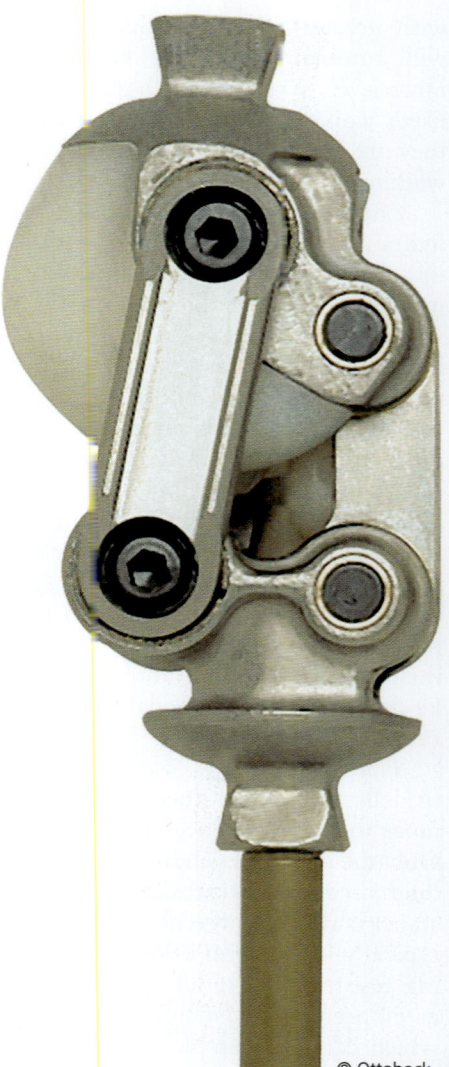

FIGURE 4 Photograph of a four-bar, polycentric knee. (Courtesy of Ottobock.)

This culminates in inherent knee extension stability in early stance with easily initiated knee flexion in late stance. These combined benefits have found broad clinical acceptance.

Critically, although some polycentric knees are designed to provide the biomechanical advantages previously described, the mechanical behavior and clinical benefits of a given polycentric knee are dependent on its design. Some polycentric designs act to shorten the relative length between the proximal attachment of the knee mechanism and foot during knee flexion, providing increased toe clearance at midswing compared with

Chapter 33: Prosthetic Knee Mechanisms

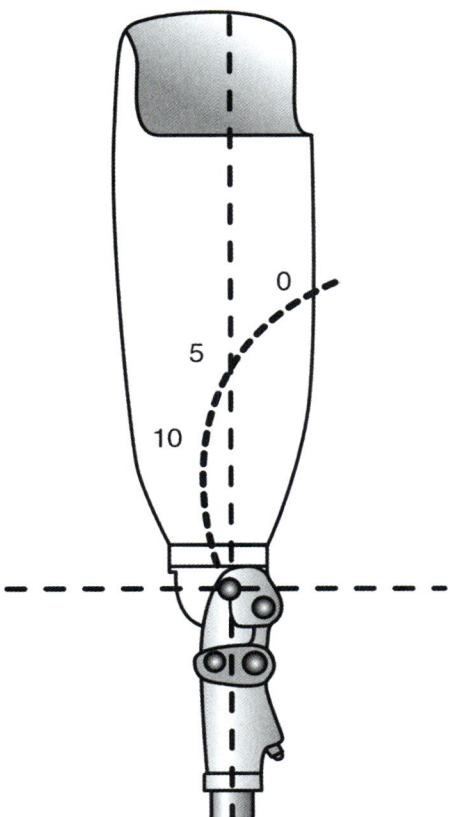

FIGURE 5 Illustration of the initial instantaneous center of rotation (ICOR) for polycentric knees that typically falls proximal and posterior to the mechanical axes when the knee is at or near full extension. As the knee is flexed, the ICOR usually moves in an anterior and distal direction, as shown here, along a characteristic arc.

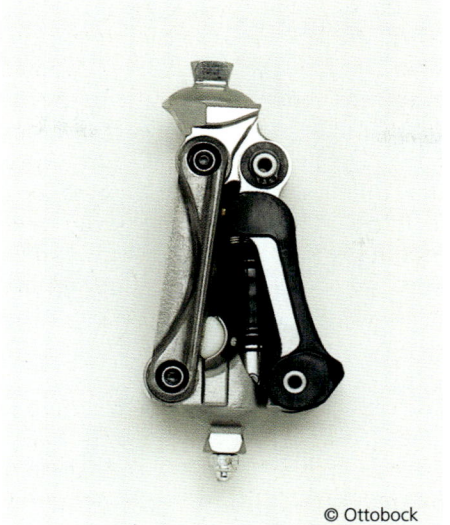

FIGURE 6 Photograph of a polycentric knee designed for use in knee disarticulation prostheses, where it folds under the socket to minimize protrusion of the knee distal to the socket in sitting. (Courtesy of Ottobock.)

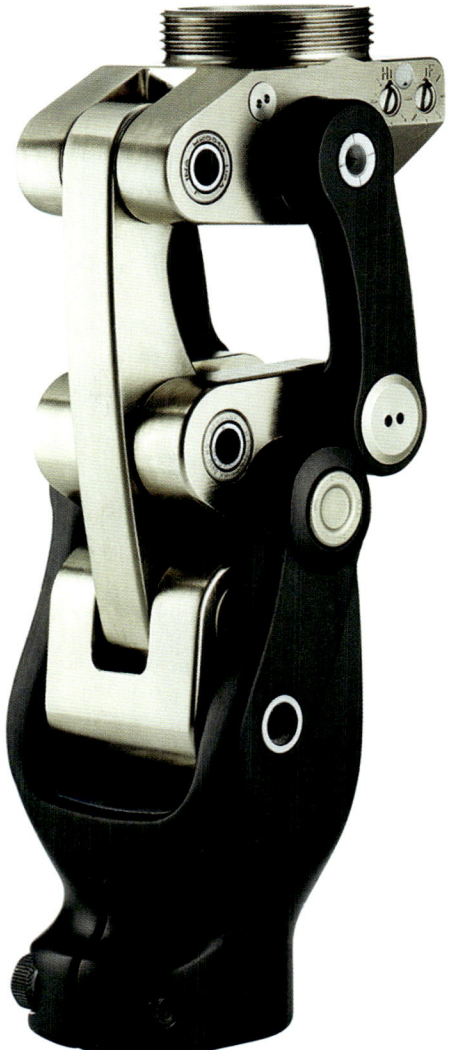

FIGURE 7 Photograph of a multiple linkage polycentric knee with a geometric lock feature that engages during loading response. (Courtesy of Össur.)

single-axis knee designs.[7] With this increased toe clearance, users may then be less reliant on compensatory mechanisms such as ipsilateral hip hiking, contralateral vaulting, or circumduction of the ipsilateral hip to avoid prosthetic limb collision with the ground during swing. Alternately, other polycentric knees are designed to accommodate longer residual limb lengths by positioning the knee joint posterior to the bent knee rather than anterior to it (**Figure 6**). Notably, because such knees are intended for longer residual limb lengths, these users are generally capable of enhanced volitional control of their residual femur and are therefore less reliant upon the stability inherent to other polycentric designs. Moreover, a recent bench study to simulate transfemoral prosthetic leg swing identified a large variation in lower leg shortening and ground clearance values across 11 different polycentric knee designs when statically aligned according to manufacturer recommendations.[8] Clinicians should cautiously appraise available polycentric knees to ensure they possess the indicated benefits for a given prosthetic treatment plan.

Polycentric Stance Flexion Features

Subsequent iterations of the polycentric knee joint have culminated in more complex linkage mechanisms including five-bar and six-bar variations. With their added build height, weight, and complexities, these knees can offer additional biomechanical benefits beyond the inherent stability of ICOR considerations. These designs generally include various approaches to the provision of stance flexion or a modest amount of controlled, resisted knee flexion during the loading response of the prosthetic step[25,26] (**Figures 7** and **8**). The level of stance flexion resistance is often adjustable and provided through other interchangeable compressive elastic bumpers or some mechanism of fluid resistance. The role of this design feature is to mimic the physiologic stance flexion that occurs in the early part of the stance phase to absorb the ground reaction forces associated with initial weight acceptance. Pilot data have revealed faster walking speeds and more normalized ground reaction forces with early stance flexion mechanical design[25] but have emphasized the importance of foot selection to derive the most benefit from this design element.[26]

Section 3: Lower Limb

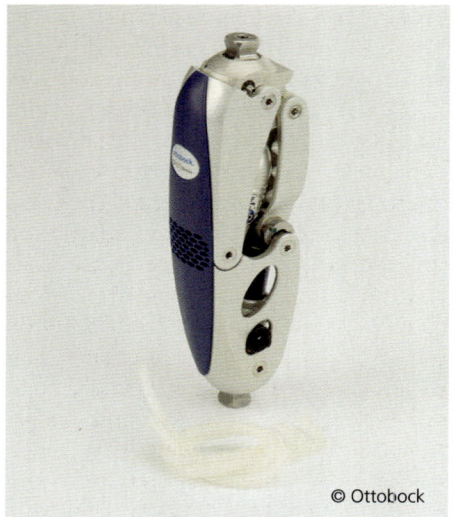

FIGURE 8 Photograph of a multiple linkage polycentric knee that provides a limited range of knee flexion during loading response through the adjustable compression of a bumper. (Courtesy of Ottobock.)

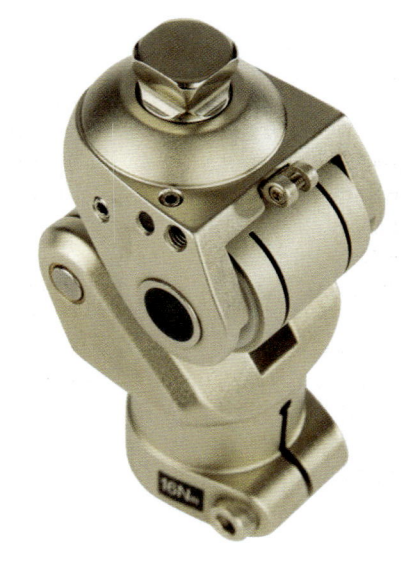

A

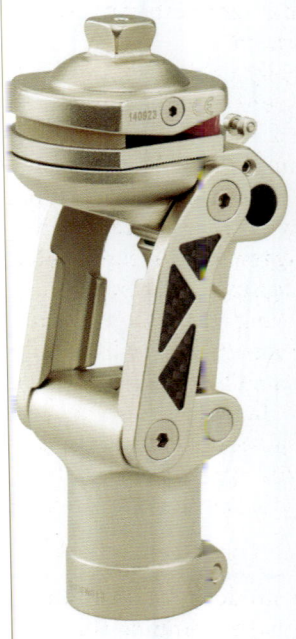

B

FIGURE 9 Photographs of hybrid knee mechanisms with convertible mechanical locking features that can be used as locking knees during early rehabilitation and/or mechanical articulating knees with optional locking functions as user mobilization increases. **A,** Polycentric. **B,** Stance control. (Courtesy of Össur.)

Manual Lock Feature

Many of the knee types described to this point are available with the option of a manual locking feature. As the name implies, this feature allows the user to manually lock the knee into full extension throughout the gait cycle. Locked extension is activated through engaging a lever on the body of the knee mechanism or manipulating a cable mechanism mounted to the proximal aspect of the transfemoral socket. With a manual lock engaged, the prosthesis cannot shorten via knee flexion in swing phase. As a result, the user will need to compensate for the added functional length of the prosthesis through some combination of ipsilateral hip hiking, contralateral vaulting, or circumduction of the ipsilateral hip.

In modern prosthetic applications, most manual locks are a supplemental feature available on hybrid polycentric and stance-control knees (**Figure 9**). Used in this capacity, the manual locking feature can be engaged situationally, such as during the early phases of gait training and ambulation, or during the navigation of unfamiliar or irregular walking environments. The knee otherwise remains unlocked with the user benefiting from the alternate means of knee stability described previously without the need for sustained gait compensations and pronounced irregularities.

Less frequently, individuals can be treated with a true manual locking knee that has no additional means of providing knee stability and is intended to be unlocked for sitting purposes only. In such applications, the gait compensations required to obtain swing phase clearance can be somewhat mitigated by shortening the prosthesis approximately 1 to 2 cm. The trade-off to this concession is that the patient may feel as though they are stepping into a hole during prosthetic stance phase and will present with an asymmetric standing posture. Moreover, evidence suggests that walking with a locked prosthetic knee compared with an unlocked knee can encourage unnatural compensatory motions of the pelvis and lumbar spine that could increase risk for low back pain.[27]

In its traditional design, the manual locking knee is rightly viewed as a knee of last resort. Patients with the potential to ambulate with an articulating knee joint are better serviced through the provision of hybrid polycentric knees with manual locking features that can be progressively disengaged through supervised gait training activities. An exception to this guideline is observed in the bilateral use of locking knees as part of the graduated length protocols associated with bilateral transfemoral stubby prostheses. This allows the prostheses to flex for sitting as the user experiences progressively longer prostheses before transitioning to more functional knee alternatives.[28]

Pilot evidence from 20 years ago observed that manual locking knees may be preferred by less-experienced elderly prosthesis users as they enable them to walk with greater confidence and speed than with free swinging knees.[29] However, more recent data have suggested that this patient group may benefit from the enhanced security features of microprocessor knees, which will be discussed later in the chapter. If funding limitations or the weight of such units preclude their use, hybrid locking knees can provide added security for older individuals situationally while allowing the user to progress toward a more efficient swing-through gait pattern.

Finally, although convention has long asserted that locking knees should be used for toddlers and small children until they have developed sufficient motor control and balance to walk with a free knee, recent evidence has suggested this care philosophy to be misguided. When managed with nonlocking knee options during the development of crawling and cruising, younger children can readily master the use of their prosthesis and appear to develop more mature gait patterns at an earlier age than those who transition from a locked to an unlocked knee.[30,31]

Hybrid Mechanical Knees

Many modern knee mechanisms for active users combine the features and benefits of the various knee designs described to this point in the chapter. For example, the dynamic benefits of fluid control can be experienced in the durable design of single-axis mechanisms (**Figure 1**) as well as the more stable polycentric variations (**Figures 7 and 8**). These fluid control mechanisms have been engineered to allow discrete adjustability to the varying needs of the different phases of gait. Thus, the knee flexion resistance of early swing phase and the knee extension resistance of late swing phase are tuned separately to meet the individual needs of the user. Similarly, the yielding resistance values of stance phase fluid-resisted knee flexion are independent of those values associated with swing phase dynamics. This function permits the calibration of stance phase knee flexion resistance for activities such as stair and ramp descent where the user rides the yielding hydraulic resistance.

Stance flexion mechanisms have become ubiquitous in modern knee mechanisms, combining this measure of shock absorption during loading response with both mechanical friction resistance and fluid control. These mechanisms can occur through either interchangeable/adjustable bumpers or adjustable fluid resistance and can be physically positioned either above or below the axis of the knee joint.

Although originally designed within mechanical knee devices, weight-activated stance resistance has since been coupled with fluid-based swing resistance. Similarly, whereas originally designed for simple mechanical knee units, mechanical locking mechanisms can be found in both single-axis and polycentric designs as well as both mechanical friction and fluid-controlled knee units. The prevalence of this feature acknowledges the broad spectrum of prostheses users who have found benefit in the ability to situationally lock out their prosthetic knee units for unfamiliar or unpredictable walking environments.

Microprocessor Knees

As described earlier, hydraulic knee units were originally engineered to control the resistance of the knee during swing phase, stance phase, or both.[20,32] The relative passive knee resistance characteristics of such knees are tuned by the prosthetist to match the needs of individual patients according to their limb strength and preferred walking speed. However, these resistance levels can only be optimized within a modest range of walking speeds. Thus, mirroring the limitations described earlier for mechanical friction knees, if an individual walks significantly faster than the gait speed used when the resistance parameters for the knee were set, these values may be experienced as inadequate, allowing excessive heel rise in swing phase and causing the individual to wait on the prosthesis. In contrast, if an individual is walking significantly slower, the amount of resistance could be experienced as excessive, creating a relatively stiff knee.

In the first application of microprocessors to prosthetic knees,[33,34] the level of knee resistance during swing phase could be programmed by the prosthetist to those values appropriate for the user's self-selected, fast, and slow walking speeds. Sensors within the knee unit recorded the speed of knee flexion during gait, allowing an onboard microprocessor to adjust the swing resistance to the most appropriate preset knee flexion resistance values. This adaptation was performed in real time to best match the user's gait speed.

Second-generation MPKs, beginning with the C-leg (Ottobock), expanded the role of the onboard microprocessors, monitoring the need and allowing for real-time adaptation to both swing and stance phase knee resistance levels according to environmental inputs (**Figure 10**). In addition to adapting the knee resistance values to variable walking speeds, these second-generation MPKs could recognize aberrant movements that might suggest a stumble or misstep and modulate the resistance to knee flexion accordingly to prevent limb buckling. In practice, this generally equates to a rapid real-time increase in knee flexion resistance to allow the user to catch themselves before a trip or stumble equates to a fall.

Early research inquiries on MPKs tended to focus on questions of energy consumption and efficiency.[4,33] Results from that work led to the erroneous impression that the benefits of MPKs could only be experienced by young and active amputees.[3] Fortunately, subsequent research efforts focused on other clinically relevant outcomes including

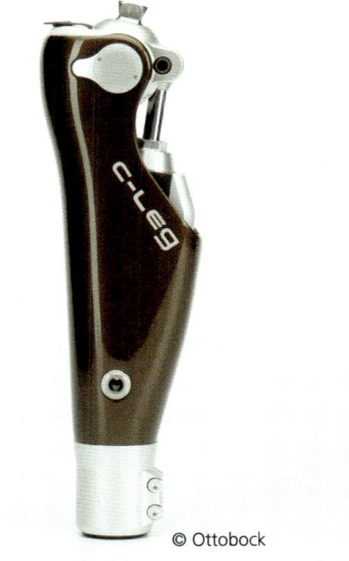

FIGURE 10 Photograph of the C-leg, a passive microprocessor-controlled knee mechanism. (Courtesy of Ottobock.)

balance, walking confidence, stumbles, falls, cognitive loads during ambulation, and the negotiation of environmental obstacles.[35,36] With this shift in focus, it has become increasingly clear that many of the benefits associated with the use of MPKs could also be experienced by older or lower activity level patients who may not initially present with the ability to ambulate at elevated walking speeds. The literature has recently witnessed a flurry of such research.[37-39] The observed benefits of MPKs within this patient group include increased walking velocity, especially over uneven terrain,[37] decreased uncontrolled falls and fear of falling,[37,38] increased physical and perceived balance,[37,39] increased physical activity levels,[38] and improved satisfaction and quality of life.[39]

There are now more than 2.5 decades of research on MPKs with the bulk of that research conducted on the product offerings of Ottobock. In aggregate, this research suggests that the greatest values of these devices to end users may be observed in a reduction in the number of stumbles and falls, lower perceived cognitive burden during ambulation, and increased self-reported mobility and well-being.[35,36] Notably, as the number and maturity of commercially available MPKs have increased, there are now a range of approaches to microprocessor-enabled dynamic adaptation during gait. Some MPKs rely entirely on hydraulic pistons, whereas others use varying combinations of hydraulics and pneumatics to achieve controlled knee flexion and extension.[40] Still others rely on an entirely different mechanical control system incorporating a magnetorheological fluid chamber to control knee flexion and extension.[40] Recent studies have begun to explore the comparative efficacy of different MPK designs, suggesting that some of the assumed benefits associated with MPKs are observed more frequently with certain designs.[41]

A related area of recent study has been in the field of health care economics. The RAND organization completed a 10-year simulation model examining the economic effect of MPKs.[42] Modeling the economic effects associated with anticipated reductions in both major and minor injurious falls, this effort determined that the initial cost of the more expensive MPK technology is largely offset by reductions in subsequent direct health care costs. For example, a subsequent study suggested that across a small cohort of transfemoral prosthesis users, medical costs associated with falls are similar to those seen in the elderly, with the 6-month cost for individuals requiring hospitalization estimated at $25,652.[43] When the mitigated differential in cost was considered against the consistent reports of increased quality of life with the use of an MPK, the model culminated in a favorable incremental cost-effectiveness ratio of $11,606 per quality-adjusted life years with the investment of an MPK.[42] Notably, a second modeling exercise was independently conducted by European economists and concluded with similar findings for individuals with and without comorbid diabetes.[44]

Microprocessor Knee-Ankle-Foot Mechanisms

Microprocessors are used in lower limb prostheses to adapt to environmental stimuli such as changes in walking velocity and surface gradient or the perception of a trip or stumble. As microprocessor feet and MPKs have gained increasing acceptance in the field, they have largely been paired with nonmicroprocessor components. Having two microprocessors aligned in series within a transfemoral prosthesis could create a clinical scenario in which both components respond to an environmental stimulus in different ways, potentially undermining the adaptation of the other component. To mitigate this risk, the field has begun to see the emergence of integrated microprocessor prostheses in which a single control system regulates the adaptations of the microprocessor knee and foot, so both components communicate with each other to enhance overall function of the prosthetic system (**Figure 11**). Although this

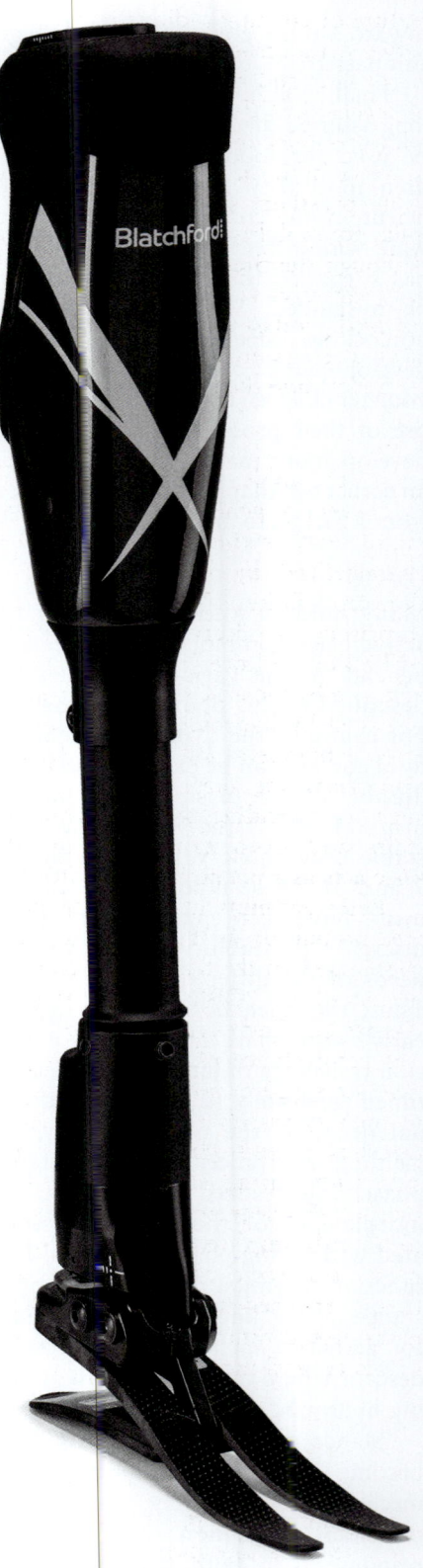

FIGURE 11 Photograph of a microprocessor-regulated knee and ankle, both regulated by a single control system. (Courtesy of Blatchford, Inc., England)

feature of creating a direct connection between the prosthetic knee and foot is not new and has been implemented in mechanical designs,[45] this function addresses the concept described earlier in which both the knee and foot acting as the prosthetic system will ultimately influence mobility safety and efficiency. Although the premise of such systems is intuitively viable and they have received good early clinical acceptance, additional research is indicated to better understand their benefits to the user.

Propulsive Microprocessor Knees

Unlike the ankle, which acts primarily as an energy generator during walking on level ground, the knee is better characterized by its energy absorption capabilities.[46] Therefore it is not surprising to observe that prosthetic replication of knee joint function has historically focused on the resistance provided by hydraulic cylinders, elastomeric bumpers, and mechanical friction. However, during certain tasks, such as ascending sloped terrain or stairs and sit-to-stand transfers, the knee acts as a net power generator.[46]

Early attempts at providing powered propulsion at the knee joint have been based on the battery-driven drive motors of the POWER KNEE (Össur) (**Figure 12**). Early evidence on the clinical performance of this knee is limited but suggests potential advantages in limb symmetry during sit-to-stand transfers[47,48] and sparing of the sound side limb during step-over-step stair ascent.[49] Subsequent research has yet to identify improved physical performance in activities that would normally require and benefit from positive knee work such as ramp and stair ascent and distanced walking.[50]

Propulsive Microprocessor Knee-Ankle-Feet

In addition to the current efforts to provide propulsive power at the ankle and the knee separately, an approach has been described in which a powered knee and powered ankle are coupled together within the same prosthesis with a common power source and control system.[51,52] Again, this coupling speaks to a reasonable approach of addressing

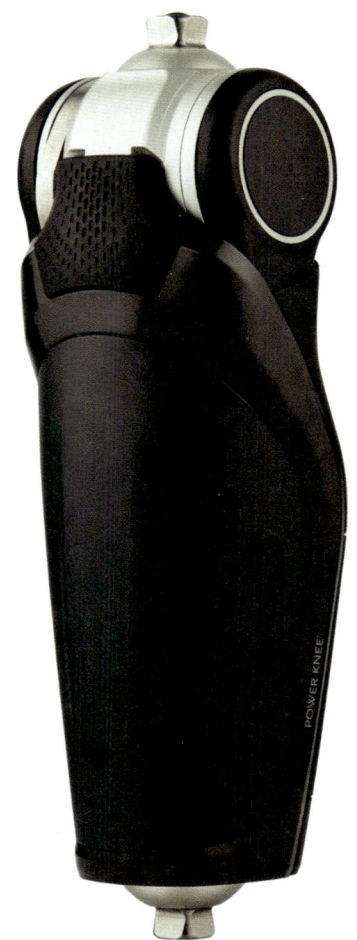

FIGURE 12 Photograph of the POWER KNEE, an active propulsive microprocessor-controlled knee mechanism. (Courtesy of Össur.)

the prosthetic system as a whole to provide full benefit of the intervention. Extensively described within the literature, prototypes of the Vanderbilt knee (developed by Vanderbilt University in Nashville, TN) suggest a substantial increase in self-selected walking velocity, decreased energy cost of walking, and improved biomechanics during the negotiation of stairs and ramps[52-54] (**Figure 13**). To date, these encouraging pilot studies have yet to culminate in a commercially available component offering.

Myoelectric Control of Propulsive Microprocessor Components

Modern microprocessor knees and ankle-feet currently rely on input gathered from sensors embedded with the

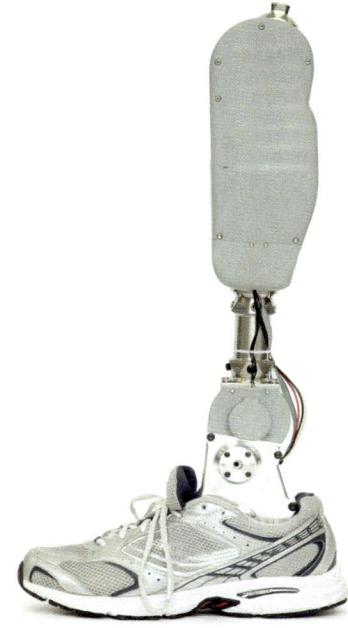

FIGURE 13 Photograph of an active propulsive microprocessor-controlled knee-ankle-foot mechanism. (Courtesy of Brian Lawson.)

components themselves. Using angular velocities measured at the mechanical joints or load sensors positioned within the prosthesis, various microprocessor mechanisms integrate and interpret this feedback to infer the needs of the end user and adapt the passive or propulsive characteristics of the prosthesis accordingly.

Absent from this current standard of practice is a direct means of neuromuscular control. One of the most established means of directly conveying the user's intent to their prosthesis is through the mechanism of electromyography, a common input signal that has been successfully implemented in upper limb prosthetic rehabilitation for over 50 years and has demonstrated considerable benefit to users. By comparison, direct control of lower limb devices has been underexplored. Reasons for the lack of research and development in this control concept may be due to the historic absence of powered lower limb prosthetic components, the sufficient performance of noncontrolled microprocessor-directed systems, and the propensity of the muscles of the residual lower limb to generate unintended control signals during ambulation.

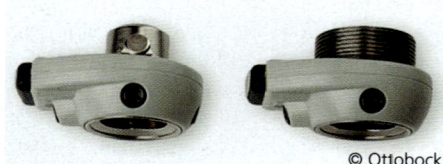

FIGURE 14 Photographs of locking positional rotators. (Courtesy of Ottobock.)

However, prosthesis users with transfemoral-level amputation have now demonstrated successful myoelectric control of both virtual prosthetic devices[55,56] and powered prostheses during both overground walking[57] and stair ascent.[58] Surgical procedures have and continue to be explored that offer potential for increased myoelectric control signals[59] and greater motor control of residual muscles[60] that can be used for commanding actuated, myoelectric-controlled prostheses. Given these promising approaches, the field can expect to see further development in the area of myoelectric control of prosthetic components.

Locking Positional Rotators

Although not as complex as the mechanical elements of swing or stance phase knee control, components that permit the user to rotate and lock their knee position can greatly reduce the difficulty associated with certain activities of daily living. Positional rotators are generally incorporated immediately above the prosthetic knee joint and permit passive positioning of the knee and prosthetic shank into both internal and external rotation (**Figure 14**). This functionality facilitates easier dressing of the prosthesis and entering and exiting confined spaces such as an automobile.

SUMMARY

Prosthetic knee mechanisms range from the comparatively simple to those of increasing complexity and sophistication characterized by microprocessor regulation and external power. In general, prosthetic knees can be considered in terms of their joint type (single axis or polycentric), their mechanisms of stance resistance (mechanical locks, geometric locks, and/or yielding fluid resistance), and their mechanisms of swing resistance (constant friction versus fluid resistance). These considerations are further supplemented in terms of control (mechanical versus microprocessor) and power (passive, adaptive, or propulsive). The selection and subsequent alignment of the prosthetic knee should reflect the user's need for stance phase stability as well as their capacity for variable speed ambulation. Factors such as residual limb length, hip extensor strength, and experience with a prosthesis must also be taken into account. Although MPKs were once reserved for more active walkers, available research continues to suggest that their associated safety benefits may be most impactful among more limited walkers.

References

1. Radcliffe CW: Four-bar linkage prosthetic knee mechanisms: Kinematics, alignment and prescription criteria. *Prosthet Orthot Int* 1994;18(3):159-173.
2. Pace A, Howard D, Gard SA, Major MJ: Using a simple walking model to optimize transfemoral prostheses for prosthetic limb stability-a preliminary study. *IEEE Trans Neural Syst Rehabil Eng* 2020;28(12):3005-3012.
3. Johansson JL, Sherrill DM, Riley PO, Bonato P, Herr H: A clinical comparison of variable-damping and mechanically passive prosthetic knee devices. *Am J Phys Med Rehabil* 2005;84(8):563-575.
4. Schmalz T, Blumentritt S, Jarasch R: Energy expenditure and biomechanical characteristics of lower limb amputee gait: The influence of prosthetic alignment and different prosthetic components. *Gait Posture* 2002;16(3):255-263.
5. Seroussi RE, Gitter A, Czerniecki JM, Weaver K: Mechanical work adaptations of above-knee amputee ambulation. *Arch Phys Med Rehabil* 1996;77(11):1209-1214.
6. Kent JA, Arelekatti VNM, Petelina NT, et al: Knee swing phase flexion resistance affects several key features of leg swing important to safe transfemoral prosthetic gait. *IEEE Trans Neural Syst Rehabil Eng* 2021;29:965-973.
7. Sensinger JW, Intawachirarat N, Gard SA: Contribution of prosthetic knee and ankle mechanisms to swing-phase foot clearance. *IEEE Trans Neural Syst Rehabil Eng* 2013;21(1):74-80.
8. Köhler TM, Bellmann M, Blumentritt S: Polycentric exoprosthetic knee joints–extent of shortening during swing phase. *Canadian Prosthet Orthot J* 2020;3(1):1-9.
9. Michaud SB, Gard SA, Childress DS: A preliminary investigation of pelvic obliquity patterns during gait in persons with transtibial and transfemoral amputation. *J Rehabil Res Dev* 2000;37(1):1-10.
10. Armannsdottir A, Tranberg R, Halldorsdottir G, Brien K: Frontal plane pelvis and hip kinematics of transfemoral amputee gait. Effect of a prosthetic foot with active ankle dorsiflexion and individualized training – A case study. *Disabil Rehabil Assist Technol* 2018;13(4):388-393.
11. Jaegers SM, Arendzen JH, de Jongh HJ: Prosthetic gait of unilateral transfemoral amputees: A kinematic study. *Arch Phys Med Rehabil* 1995;76(8):736-743.
12. Villa C, Drevelle X, Bonnet X, et al: Evolution of vaulting strategy during locomotion of individuals with transfemoral amputation on slopes and cross-slopes compared to level walking. *Clin Biomech* 2015;30(6):623-628.
13. Vrieling AH, van Keeken HG, Schoppen T, et al: Obstacle crossing in lower limb amputees. *Gait Posture* 2007;26(4):587-594.
14. Bonnet X, Villa C, Fode P, Lavaste F, Pillet H: Mechanical work performed by individual limbs of transfemoral amputees during step-to-step transitions: Effect of walking velocity. *Proc Inst Mech Eng H* 2014;228(1):60-66.
15. Nolan L, Lees A: The functional demands on the intact limb during walking for active trans-femoral and trans-tibial amputees. *Prosthet Orthot Int* 2000;24(2):117-125.
16. Gailey R, Allen K, Castles J, Kucharik J, Roeder M: Review of secondary physical conditions associated with lower-limb amputation and long-term prosthesis use. *J Rehabil Res Dev* 2008;45(1):15-29.
17. Murray MP, Mollinger LA, Sepic SB, Gardner GM, Linder MT: Gait patterns in above-knee amputee patients: Hydraulic swing control vs constant-friction knee components. *Arch Phys Med Rehabil* 1983;64(8):339-345.
18. Safaeepour Z, Eshraghi A, Geil M: The effect of damping in prosthetic ankle and knee joints on the biomechanical

18. outcomes: A literature review. *Prosthet Orthot Int* 2017;41(4):336-344.
19. Volatile TB, Roberson JR, Whitesides TE Jr: The Mauch hydraulic knee unit for above knee amputation. *Orthopedics* 1985;8(2):229-230.
20. Mauch H: Stance control for above-knee artificial legs-design considerations in the SNS knee. *Bull Prosthet Res* 1968;10:61-72.
21. Hicks R, Tashman S, Cary JM, Altman RF, Gage JR: Swing phase control with knee friction in juvenile amputees. *J Orthop Res* 1985;3(2):198-201.
22. Taheri A, Karimi MT: Evaluation of the gait performance of above-knee amputees while walking with 3R20 and 3R15 knee joints. *J Res Med Sci* 2012;17(3):258-263.
23. Andrysek J, García D, Rozbaczylo C, et al: Biomechanical responses of young adults with unilateral transfemoral amputation using two types of mechanical stance control prosthetic knee joints. *Prosthet Orthot Int* 2020;44(5):314-322.
24. Andrysek J, Wright FV, Rotter K, et al: Long-term clinical evaluation of the automatic stance-phase lock-controlled prosthetic knee joint in young adults with unilateral above-knee amputation. *Disabil Rehabil Assist Technol* 2017;12(4):378-384.
25. Sutherland JL, Sutherland DH, Kaufman KR, Teel M: Gait Comparison of two prosthetic knee units. *J Prosthet Orthot* 1997;9(4):168-173.
26. Blumentritt S, Scherer HW, Wellershaus U, Michael JW: Design principles, biomechanical data and clinical experience with a polycentric knee offering controlled stance phase knee flexion: A preliminary report. *J Prosthet Orthot* 1997;9(1):18-24.
27. Sloth W, Fabricius J, Pedersen AR: Compensatory gait strategies in persons with transfemoral amputations walking with a locked prosthetic knee joint compared with an unlocked knee joint: A crossover trial. *J Prosthet Orthot* 2022;34(3):159-164.
28. Irolla C, Rheinstein J, Richardson R, Simpson C, Carroll K: Evaluation of a graduated length prosthetic protocol for bilateral transfemoral amputee prosthetic rehabilitation. *J Prosthet Orthot* 2013;25(2):84-88.
29. Devlin M, Sinclair LB, Colman D, Parsons J, Nizio H, Campbell JE: Patient preference and gait efficiency in a geriatric population with transfemoral amputation using a free-swinging versus a locked prosthetic knee joint. *Arch Phys Med Rehabil* 2002;83(2):246-249.
30. Geil M, Coulter C: Analysis of locomotor adaptations in young children with limb loss in an early prosthetic knee prescription protocol. *Prosthet Orthot Int* 2014;38(1):54-61.
31. Geil MD, Safaeepour Z, Giavedoni B, Coulter CP: Walking kinematics in young children with limb loss using early versus traditional prosthetic knee prescription protocols. *PLoS One* 2020;15(4):e0231401.
32. Staros A: The principles of swing-phase control: The advantages of fluid mechanisms. *Prostheses Brace Tech Aides* 1964;13:11-16.
33. Kirker S, Keymer S, Talbot J, Lachmann S: An assessment of the intelligent knee prosthesis. *Clin Rehabil* 1996;10(3):267-273.
34. Buckley JG, Spence WD, Solomonidis SE: Energy cost of walking: Comparison of "intelligent prosthesis" with conventional mechanism. *Arch Phys Med Rehabil* 1997;78(3):330-333.
35. Stevens PM, Wurdeman SR: Prosthetic knee selection for individuals with unilateral transfemoral amputation: A clinical practice guideline. *J Prosthet Orthot* 2019;31(1):2-8.
36. Sawers AB, Hafner BJ: Outcomes associated with the use of microprocessor-controlled prosthetic knees among individuals with unilateral transfemoral limb loss: A systematic review. *J Rehabil Res Dev* 2013;50(3):273-314.
37. Kannenberg A, Zacharias B, Pröbsting E: Benefits of microprocessor-controlled prosthetic knees to limited community ambulators: Systematic review. *J Rehabil Res Dev* 2014;51(10):1469-1496.
38. Kaufman KR, Bernhardt KA, Symms K: Functional assessment and satisfaction of transfemoral amputees with low mobility (FASTK2): A clinical trial of microprocessor-controlled vs. non-microprocessor-controlled knees. *Clin Biomech* 2018;58:116-122.
39. Lansade C, Vicaut E, Paysant J, et al: Mobility and satisfaction with a microprocessor-controlled knee in moderately active amputees: A multicentric randomized crossover trial. *Ann Phys Rehabil Med* 2018;61(5):278-285.
40. Thiele J, Schöllig C, Bellmann M, Kraft M: Designs and performance of three new microprocessor-controlled knee joints. *Biomed Tech* 2019;64(1):119-126.
41. Campbell JH, Stevens PM, Wurdeman SR: OASIS 1: Retrospective analysis of four different microprocessor knee types. *J Rehabil Assist Technol Eng* 2020;7:2055668320968476.
42. Chen C, Hanson M, Chaturvedi R, Mattke S, Hillestad R, Liu HH: Economic benefits of microprocessor controlled prosthetic knees: A modeling study. *J Neuroeng Rehabil* 2018;15(suppl 1):62.
43. Mundell B, Maradit Kremers H, Visscher S, Hoppe K, Kaufman K: Direct medical costs of accidental falls for adults with transfemoral amputations. *Prosthet Orthot Int* 2017;41(6):564-570.
44. Kuhlmann A, Krüger H, Seidinger S, Hahn A: Cost-effectiveness and budget impact of the microprocessor-controlled knee C-Leg in transfemoral amputees with and without diabetes mellitus. *Eur J Health Econ* 2020;21(3):437-449.
45. Sapin E, Goujon H, de Almeida F, Fodé P, Lavaste F: Functional gait analysis of trans-femoral amputees using two different single-axis prosthetic knees with hydraulic swing-phase control: Kinematic and kinetic comparison of two prosthetic knees. *Prosthet Orthot Int* 2008;32(2):201-218.
46. DeVita P, Helseth J, Hortobagyi T: Muscles do more positive than negative work in human locomotion. *J Exp Biol* 2007;210(pt 19):3361-3373.
47. Highsmith MJ, Kahle JT, Carey SL, et al: Kinetic asymmetry in transfemoral amputees while performing sit to stand and stand to sit movements. *Gait Posture* 2011;34(1):86-91.
48. Wolf EJ, Everding VQ, Linberg AA, Czerniecki JM, Gambel JM: Comparison of the power knee and C-Leg during step-up and sit-to-stand tasks. *Gait Posture* 2013;38(3):397-402.
49. Wolf EJ, Everding VQ, Linberg AL, Schnall BL, Czerniecki JM, Gambel JM: Assessment of transfemoral amputees using C-Leg and Power Knee for ascending and descending inclines and steps. *J Rehabil Res Dev* 2012;49(6):831-842.
50. Hafner BJ, Askew RL: Physical performance and self-report outcomes associated with use of passive, adaptive, and active prosthetic knees in persons with unilateral, transfemoral amputation: Randomized crossover trial. *J Rehabil Res Dev* 2015;52(6):677-700.
51. Sup F, Bohara A, Goldfarb M: Design and control of a powered transfemoral prosthesis. *Int J Rob Res* 2008;27(2):263-273.
52. Sup F, Varol HA, Mitchell J, Withrow TJ, Goldfarb M: Self-contained

powered knee and ankle prosthesis: Initial evaluation on a transfemoral amputee. *IEEE Int Conf Rehabil Robot* 2009;2009:638-644.

53. Lawson BE, Varol HA, Goldfarb M: Standing stability enhancement with an intelligent powered transfemoral prosthesis. *IEEE Trans Biomed Eng* 2011;58(9):2617-2624.

54. Lawson BE, Varol HA, Huff A, Erdemir E, Goldfarb M: Control of stair ascent and descent with a powered transfemoral prosthesis. *IEEE Trans Neural Syst Rehabil Eng* 2013;21(3):466-473.

55. Ha KH, Varol HA, Goldfarb M: Volitional control of a prosthetic knee using surface electromyography. *IEEE Trans Biomed Eng* 2011;58(1):144-151.

56. Hargrove LJ, Simon AM, Lipschutz RD, Finucane SB, Kuiken TA: Real-time myoelectric control of knee and ankle motions for transfemoral amputees. *J Am Med Assoc* 2011;305(15):1542-1544.

57. Hoover CD, Fulk GD, Fite KB: The design and initial experimental validation of an active myoelectric transfemoral prosthesis. *J Med Dev* 2012;6(1):011005.

58. Hoover CD, Fulk GD, Fite KB: Stair ascent with a powered transfemoral prosthesis under direct myoelectric control. *IEEE ASME Trans Mechatron* 2013;18(3):1191-1200.

59. Kuiken T: Targeted reinnervation for improved prosthetic function. *Phys Med Rehabil Clin N Am* 2006;17(1):1-13.

60. Srinivasan SS, Gutierrez-Arango S, Teng AC, et al: Neural interfacing architecture enables enhanced motor control and residual limb functionality postamputation. *Proc Natl Acad Sci USA* 2021;118(9):e2019555118.

Partial Foot Amputations and Disarticulations: Surgical Management

Terrence M. Philbin, DO • Benjamin D. Umbel, DO

ABSTRACT

In the correct clinical scenario, partial foot amputation can be an appropriate and beneficial procedure. These amputations can provide a functional weight-bearing limb while decreasing patient morbidity and mortality. Potential benefits include increased independence and decreased energy expenditure when compared with more proximal amputations. Before surgery, it is important to select the most appropriate amputation level. Soft-tissue balancing becomes a critical component of the surgery with a more proximal partial foot amputation. In addition to patient selection and surgical technique, proper fitting, patient education, and use of an orthosis or prosthesis help to minimize the risk of complications, with the goal of providing good outcomes and maintain patients' daily needs.

Keywords: boyd amputation; chopart disarticulation; lisfranc disarticulation; ray resection; syme ankle disarticulation; transmetatarsal amputation

Introduction

The need for an amputation at any level is a life-changing event, increasing patient morbidity and ability to perform their activities of daily living. In the United States, amputation most commonly is necessitated by vascular insufficiency, a diabetes-related complication, trauma, or congenital deficiency.[1] Patients with diabetes are 10 times more likely to require an amputation at some level during their lifetime than the general population.[1] According to the Centers for Disease Control and Prevention, in 2010 there were 73,000 nontraumatic lower limb amputations in people with diabetes who were 20 years or older.[2] In 2016, about 131 million people worldwide had diabetes-related lower extremity complications, including 6.8 million amputations, according to the Global Burden of Diseases, Injuries, and Risk Factors Study.[3]

More than 60% of nontraumatic amputations occur in patients with diabetes.[2,4] After transtibial amputation, the 1-year mortality rate is 20.8% to 35.5%, and the 5-year mortality rate is 65%.[5] A 2021 study found that for both patients with diabetes and without diabetes, 30-day mortality rate following lower extremity amputation was also significantly increased, with rates as high as 34% and 29%, respectively.[3] One study interviewing 605 patients found that the Mental and Physical component summary scores of the Short Form health survey were found to be significantly lower for amputees when compared with those for the general population.[6]

Although it is unclear whether these poor outcomes are related to the amputation level or the underlying disease process, a more distal amputation is preferable to a transtibial amputation. If possible, foot and ankle surgeons use partial foot amputation as a salvage procedure, so that the patient can retain a functional weight-bearing residual limb.[4] Compared with transtibial amputation, partial foot amputation requires less energy expenditure for ambulation and may allow the patient to retain greater independence.[4,5] Transmetatarsal amputation has a lower mortality rate 1 and 3 years

---

Dr. Philbin or an immediate family member has received royalties from Arthrex, Inc., Crossroads, Fusion, IN 2 Bones, and Medline; is a member of a speakers' bureau or has made paid presentations on behalf of Arthrex, Inc., Crossroads, IN 2 Bones, Medline, and Medshape; serves as a paid consultant to or is an employee of Artelon, Arthrex, Inc., Crossroads, IN 2 Bones, Medline, and Medshape; has stock or stock options held in Artelon, Crossroads, Medshape, and Tissue Tech; has received research or institutional support from Biomimetic, DJ Orthopaedics, and Zimmer; and serves as a board member, owner, officer, or committee member of AOAO Board of Directors. Neither Dr. Umbel nor any immediate family member has received anything of value from or has stock or stock options held in a commercial company or institution related directly or indirectly to the subject of this chapter.

This chapter is adapted from Philbin TM, Riley AJ: Partial foot amputations and disarticulations: surgical management, in Krajbich JI, Pinzur MS, Potter BK, Stevens PM, eds: *Atlas of Amputations and Limb Deficiencies: Surgical, Prosthetic, and Rehabilitation Principles*, ed 4. American Academy of Orthopaedic Surgeons, 2016, pp 453-461.

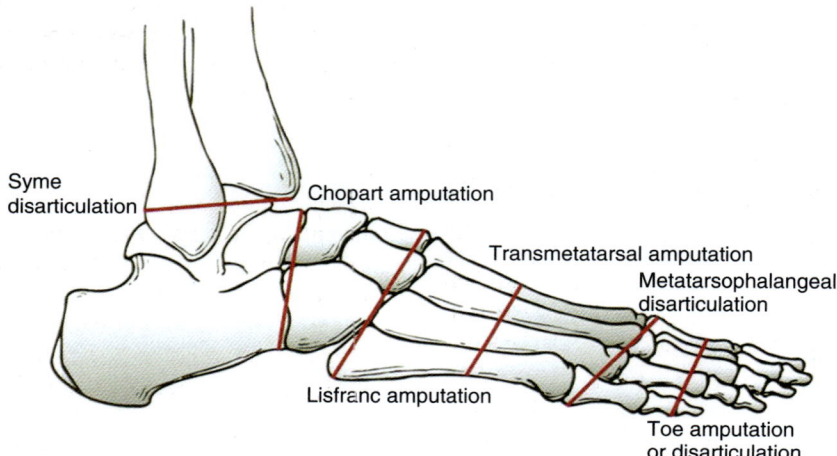

FIGURE 1 Schematic drawing showing some of the levels of partial foot amputation or disarticulation. (Adapted from Witt BL, Philbin TM: Midfoot amputations, in Flatow E, Colvin EC, eds: *Atlas of Essential Orthopaedic Procedures.* American Academy of Orthopaedic Surgeons, 2013, pp 551-556.)

after surgery, compared with transtibial amputation.[5] Because a salvage partial foot amputation greatly reduces the area of weight bearing on the foot, proper fitting and use of an orthosis or prosthesis are essential. This factor is even more critical if the patient has impaired sensation.[7] When deciding on the level of partial foot amputation, options include ray resection, transmetatarsal, Lisfranc tarsometatarsal, and hindfoot (Chopart, Boyd, and Pirogoff) amputation (**Figure 1**).

Preoperative Evaluation

A thorough preoperative patient assessment is critical in evaluating patients who may require surgical intervention for limb salvage. This assessment begins with a comprehensive current and past medical history, particularly in patients with diabetes, who may have other risk factors for peripheral arterial disease. Peripheral arterial disease in itself may predispose patients to foot ulcers and compromise the ability for healing of more distal partial foot amputations. Physical examination and evaluation of limb perfusion are useful in determining whether a patient can benefit from a partial foot amputation rather than amputation at a more proximal level.[5,8,9] The level of amputation most commonly is determined by the location of necrotic tissue, the distal extent of the viable soft-tissue envelope, and the potential ambulatory status of the patient.[10,11] The goal of a partial foot amputation is to salvage the foot at a level at which the soft-tissue envelope will heal, without concern for further breakdown during the patient's lifetime.[7]

Limb Perfusion Assessment

Limb perfusion can be noninvasively assessed using transcutaneous oxygen tension, the ankle-brachial index (ABI), arterial Doppler ultrasound studies, toe systolic blood pressures, and toe brachial indices.[7,12,13] An ABI lower than 0.9 is considered abnormal, and the likelihood of healing is poor if the ABI is lower than 0.45;[7,8,14] however, the ABI may be inaccurate in a patient with calcification of the blood vessels.[15] ABIs have a moderate predictive value in diagnosing peripheral arterial disease.[16] However, when planning surgical intervention in these patients, ABI can be combined with advanced imaging (Doppler ultrasound or peripheral CT angiogram) to better characterize the underlying arterial disease.[16] Toe brachial indices and toe systolic blood pressures appear to be more accurate than the ABI in patients with diabetes or peripheral vessel calcifications because the digital arteries are less commonly affected by calcifications when compared with larger arteries about the ankle and remain compressible for obtaining accurate pressure readings.[15,17] The toe brachial indices and toe systolic blood pressures are obtained by inflating a cuff on the toe. These tests may not be feasible when very distal toe necrosis or toe ulceration is present in an area where the cuff would be placed.[17,18]

When assessing for level of adequate perfusion, arterial Doppler ultrasound is the most useful initial screening test to determine if vascular consultation or arteriogram is indicated.[19] Biphasic or triphasic signal on arterial Doppler ultrasound indicates a healthy vessel, but monophasic signal indicates a diseased artery. The likelihood of a successful distal amputation often can be increased by preamputation use of endovascular methods or surgical revascularization of the lower limb; therefore consultation with a critical limb or vascular surgery service may be helpful for preoperative planning. At least 72 hours should elapse between the revascularization and the amputation.[14] However, although a thorough preamputation assessment with diagnostic imaging and specialty consultation is important in assessing patients with peripheral vascular disease, one study found that these interventions did not necessarily lead to more limb-saving revascularizations in patients with chronic kidney disease. This highlights the issue that more effective preventive therapies are still needed to reduce amputation in at-risk populations.[20]

Evaluating for distal healing potential can best be done with transcutaneous tissue oxygen tension, which is a measurement of the amount of oxygen that has diffused across capillaries to the epidermis.[19] This test can reliably and easily be used in all patients.[13,15,21] A tension measurement higher than 30 mm Hg suggests adequate healing potential; a measurement lower than 20 mm Hg is predictive of wound-healing failure.[7,8,13,14,22] Position of the limb during this assessment is important. Yang et al[2] assessed 61 patients with diabetes with foot ulcers and measured their transcutaneous oxygen pressure

(TcPO$_2$). They found that in the supine position, a TcPO$_2$ > 25 mm Hg was the most predictive cut-off point for healing of diabetic foot ulcers, with all wounds healing when the TcPO$_2$ was >40 mm Hg. Because this test does not rely on the mechanical compression of arteries, it is well suited to patients with diabetes or arterial calcification.[15] Andrews et al[13] recommended using both this test and those previously described in deciding on an amputation level. In a study of 261 patients with diabetes, Faglia et al[18] found that transcutaneous tissue oxygen tension was a more reliable test than ankle or toe pressures and that it could be used independently in risk stratification for limb ischemia. The primary disadvantage to the use of this test is the time needed to calibrate and equilibrate the machine after attachment to the patient and before measurements are obtained.[13] In addition, the measurements can be inaccurate in the presence of infection or peripheral edema.[24]

Imaging

Three radiographic views of the foot and ankle should be obtained, and they should be weight bearing if possible.[8] Additional imaging studies sometimes are useful for further delineating the extent of soft-tissue or bony involvement and deciding on the amputation level. MRI can best depict soft-tissue masses, fluid collections, or osteomyelitis. CT can show subtle osseous changes such as fractures, periosteal reactions, or sequestra. Indium-111–labeled white blood cell scans can detect focal areas of infection, such as osteomyelitis, and can differentiate an infectious from a noninfectious process.[22]

Metabolic and Nutritional Status

Maximizing the patient's metabolic and nutritional status is an important part of preoperative optimization of wound-healing potential. Proper control of blood glucose levels in a patient with diabetes is essential for lowering the risk of infection and improving the healing ability of surgical wounds.[7-10] Partial foot amputation is less likely to succeed in a patient with a hemoglobin A1c level higher than 8.0%.[5] A serum albumin level higher than 3.0 g/dL, total serum protein level greater than 6.0 g/dL, or hemoglobin levels greater than 11.0 g/dL are values that likely represent adequate nutritional status needed for wound healing.[7,9,19] Additionally, greater preoperative albumin levels have been shown to be statistically significant in predicting clean surgical margins in partial foot amputations in patients with diabetic foot osteomyelitis.[25] Historically, a lymphocyte count higher than 1,500 cells/µL was considered to indicate high wound-healing capacity, but Pinzur et al[26] found that this measurement was not prognostic.

General Surgical Considerations

The patient is positioned supine on the operating table with a bump underneath the ipsilateral hip to limit external rotation of the lower limb.[8,27-29] Planned skin incisions are marked to indicate the position of future skin flaps. In an amputation necessitated by infection, exsanguination of the limb historically has been avoided because of the theoretic risk of spreading the infection proximally.[12] However, this practice is not known to be supported by research. It is acceptable to use a tourniquet to limit blood loss when infection is present, but exsanguination of the limb is not recommended before inflation of the tourniquet. Placement of the tourniquet over an area of vascular bypass grafts or stents should be avoided because of the theoretic risk of injury, although this recommendation is also historical and not supported by known studies.[12] Alternatively, an Esmarch bandage can be used as an ankle tourniquet in a distal procedure.[12,30]

As a general surgical principle, obtaining intraoperative proximal surgical margins free of infection should always be the goal when performing partial foot amputations. In a prospective study of 72 patients, proximal margins deemed clean by postoperative histopathologic analysis resulted in improved patient outcomes and lower postoperative complication rate. The authors noted that postoperative wound dehiscence, re-ulceration, and need for re-amputation were decreased in patients where a clean margin was successfully obtained.[25]

Ray Resection

Outcome Considerations

In an appropriate patient, ray resection can be more durable and functional than a transmetatarsal amputation.[12,28] Depending on the functional status of the patient, a single ray resection, particularly of the lateral column, may allow for ambulation with normal shoe wear and only minor insole modifications. Ray resection is used only if necrosis and soft-tissue loss are limited and is most successful if no more than two rays are resected.[8,12,28] Resection of the lateral rays best maintains the foot balance needed for ambulation.[8] Partial resection of the medial forefoot tends to increase stress at the lateral border of the foot, which can lead to transfer lesions throughout the forefoot.[31] Resection of the first ray leads to loss of the anterior tibial tendon insertion, which decreases the dorsiflexion power of the ankle and increases pronation of the forefoot. Resection of the first ray also leads to instability of the medial column during the terminal stance phase of gait because of the loss of the flexor hallucis brevis and flexor hallucis longus insertions.[32] If the entire fifth metatarsal is resected, including the base, the peroneus brevis insertion is lost, causing loss of eversion strength and contributing to varus deformity of the hindfoot unless it is reattached to a surrounding structure.[8,28] Patients should be informed that claw toes may develop after ray resection because of loss of balance of the intrinsic musculature. A 2019 retrospective study of 185 patients found that ray resection is a viable option after proper patient selection. An overall failure rate (requiring further major amputation) of 11.9% and overall revision rate of 38.4% were noted. Additionally, postoperative re-ulceration was significantly associated with revision surgery and occurred at, on average, 19.5 months from the time of the index ray resection.[31] Therefore, the authors concluded that prevention

Section 3: Lower Limb

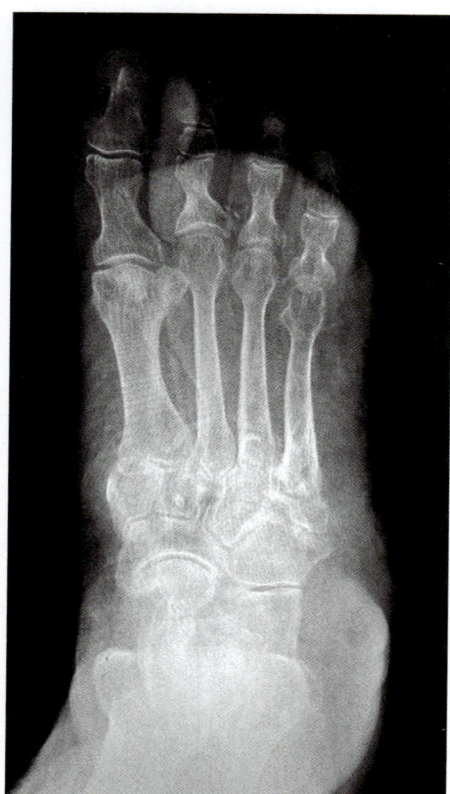

FIGURE 2 AP radiograph showing resection of the entire fifth ray with transfer of the peroneus brevis insertion to the cuboid.

of ulcer recurrence was paramount in preventing further revision surgery.[31]

Figure 2 shows a radiograph of an entire fifth-ray resection in which the peroneus brevis insertion was transferred to the cuboid.

Surgical Technique

A dorsal longitudinal skin incision is made along the affected metatarsal. At the level of the metatarsophalangeal joint, the skin incision is continued through the adjacent web space to the plantar aspect of the foot.[28] The sensory nerves are identified just deep to the skin incision, gentle traction is applied, and the nerve is transected sharply with the scalpel and allowed to retract proximally. The extensor tendon is identified and transversely incised at the level of the tarsometatarsal joint. Proximally, the lumbrical and interosseous muscles are identified and transversely incised. At this point, the base of the metatarsal is identified. If possible, the metatarsal distal to the base should be resected to preserve the tarsometatarsal joint and the transverse metatarsal arch.[8,28] An oscillating saw is used to make a transverse cut in the proximal metatarsal. If any of the metatarsal remains, the distal end is beveled at roughly 30° to 45°, from dorsal-distal to plantar-proximal, to prevent soft-tissue irritation on the residual plantar foot during the late stance phase of ambulation.[33] If the entire metatarsal is to be resected, however, a disarticulation of the tarsometatarsal joint is substituted. The proximal aspect of the metatarsal is lifted out of the wound, and the soft tissues deep to the metatarsal are identified. The flexor tendon is transected transversely, and all soft-tissue attachments to the metatarsal are carefully removed in a proximal-to-distal fashion.[28] The metatarsal can then be removed.

After the metatarsal is removed, the remaining adjacent metatarsophalangeal joint capsules are anchored together using 0 nonabsorbable suture.[28] This step is intended to hold the adjacent metatarsal heads in proximity as the soft tissue heals. A small drain can be placed into the void between the remaining metatarsals, if desired. The subcutaneous tissue is approximated using 3-0 absorbable suture, and the skin is approximated using 3-0 nylon suture. A well-padded posterior splint is placed onto the limb with mild compression to hold the metatarsal heads in proximity.[28]

Transmetatarsal Amputation

Outcome Considerations

If soft-tissue or bony involvement precludes an isolated ray resection, transmetatarsal amputation historically has led to excellent long-term function and ambulation as well as decreased energy expenditure and risk of mortality.[5,8,9,11,27] Transmetatarsal amputation first was described in 1949 by McKittrick, and approximately 10,000 of these procedures are performed in the United States each year.[8,9,12] The benefits of a transmetatarsal amputation over a more proximal resection include maintenance of the anterior tibial and peroneus brevis insertions, which helps maintain power of ankle motion, ankle stability, and forefoot balance.[8,11,34] Younger et al[35] found that the most important predictor of success in transmetatarsal amputations was a hemoglobin A1c level lower than 10%. To avoid wound-healing complications, a patient's diabetes should be well-controlled before surgery. The surgeon should assess for an Achilles tendon contracture and, if necessary, should lengthen the tendon during the index surgery to avoid equinus positioning of the residual limb.[8,11,27,35] Careful attention should be given to the metatarsal cuts to maintain a balanced cascade because the tarsometatarsal joint is more proximal as it progresses from medial to lateral. A poorly resected cascade is a major cause of wound complication or recurrent ulceration after transmetatarsal amputation.[7,19] Despite proper patient selection and surgical technique, one systematic review found revision to major amputation to be as high as 33.2% following the index procedure.[36] Harris and Fang[37] found in their retrospective review that neuropathy and a positive metatarsal bone margin following surgery significantly affected transmetatarsal wound healing.

A relatively long plantar flap is key to the soft-tissue closure, with the goal of reducing high shear forces and pressure on the shortened forefoot during the late stance phase of gait.[7,29,38] However, soft-tissue involvement is often significant, and a plantar flap of adequate length is unable to be achieved. This presents considerable concern for successful wound healing of the amputation site. Holloway et al describe a novel approach for limb salvage transmetatarsal amputation in patients without a viable plantar flap.[39] In their study, 27 patients underwent open guillotine transmetatarsal amputation for nonviable plantar flap because of either extensive tissue loss on initial presentation or secondary transmetatarsal amputation flap necrosis. Negative-pressure wound therapy was used at the conclusion of the index procedure for coverage of the amputation wound, which was continued until the wound granulated over. Wound closure was obtained by either the application of a split-thickness skin graft or through continued negative-pressure wound therapy allowing the wound to heal by secondary intention. Nineteen patients (70%) went on to heal the distal wound by a median time of 82 days.[39] This novel attempt at wound closure for transmetatarsal amputation without a viable plantar flap presents a potential option for patients who would otherwise require more proximal amputation.

Surgical Technique

The goal of the transmetatarsal amputation is to preserve as much metatarsal length and viable plantar skin as possible so that the resulting residual limb will have a long enough lever arm for forward progression during ambulation.[38] The initial, dorsal transverse skin incision extends from the midshaft level of the first metatarsal to the midshaft of the fifth metatarsal.[9,12] A longitudinal incision is made from the medial aspect of the dorsal skin incision down to the level of the first metatarsal head and laterally from the dorsal skin incision down to the level of the fifth metatarsal head. A plantar transverse skin incision is made along the metatarsal heads to complete the skin incisions. The dissection continues sharply through the subcutaneous tissue and intrinsic muscles deep to the skin incisions until the metatarsals are encountered. Vascular structures such as the dorsalis pedis and branches of the posterior tibial artery are identified and ligated. Neurologic structures, including the superficial and deep peroneal nerves and branches of the tibial nerve, are transected sharply with a scalpel after applying gentle traction, and they are allowed to retract proximally.[9,29] Flexor and extensor tendons also are transected and allowed to retract (**Figure 3, A**). It is important to maintain the insertions of the anterior tibial tendon, peroneus longus, and peroneus brevis to preserve foot balance for ambulation.

The metatarsals are resected following a gentle cascade, using a small oscillating saw at the level of the dorsal skin incision (**Figure 3, B**). The distal end of each bone is cut at a 30° dorsal-distal to plantar-proximal angle.[8,29] The ends of each bone are smoothed with a rasp

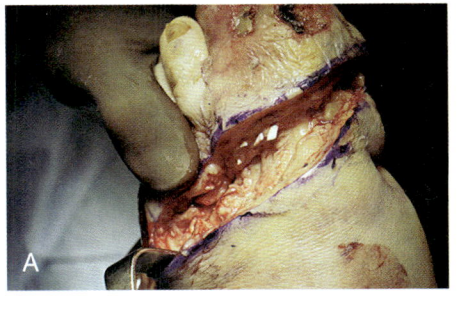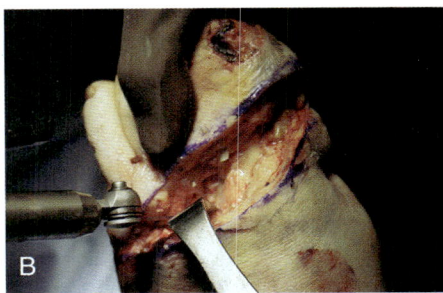
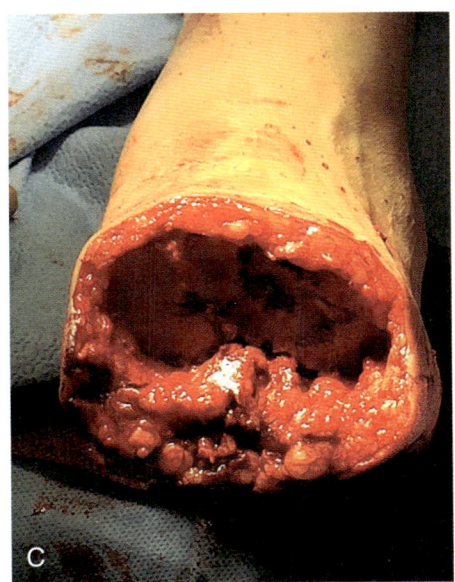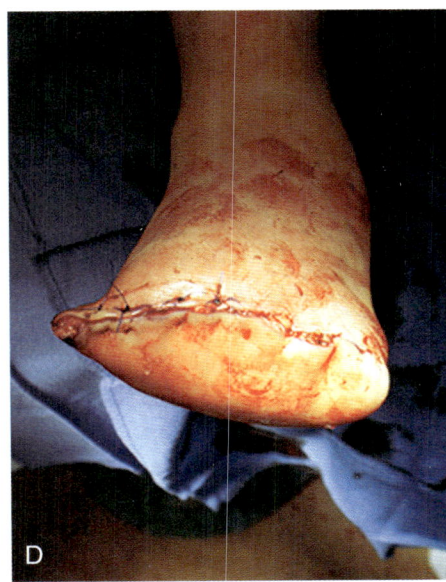

FIGURE 3 Photographs showing a transmetatarsal amputation. **A**, The transverse incision is made at the midmetatarsal level. Extensor tendons have been transected and allowed to retract. **B**, A small oscillating saw is used to transect the metatarsals at the level of the dorsal skin incision. Cuts are made in a dorsal-distal to plantar-proximal direction. **C**, The plantar flap. **D**, The skin closure.

to remove any sharp bony prominences that could cause skin ulceration.[12] Improved midfoot balance can be achieved when all five metatarsal bases are ideally preserved, which is particularly important to prevent further midfoot breakdown in patients with neuropathy.[19] The wound is thoroughly irrigated with sterile saline to remove any bone particles. If a tourniquet is being used, it is deflated, and hemostasis is obtained by cauterizing or ligating all bleeding vessels.

The plantar skin flap is debulked if necessary to allow adequate flap coverage of the wound with no excess soft tissue.[12,29] The plantar flap may also be secured with suture to the metatarsals via drill holes.[40] A small drain can be placed into the distal aspect of the wound. The plantar flap is brought up and over the ends of the remaining metatarsals (**Figure 3, C**). The deep fascia is approximated using 0 absorbable suture. The subcutaneous closure is done with 3-0 absorbable suture, and the skin is approximated using 3-0 nylon suture or staples (**Figure 3, D**). If the foot cannot be passively dorsiflexed past neutral, an Achilles tendon–lengthening procedure should be done (and possibly posterior ankle or subtalar joint capsulotomies) at this time to maintain the ankle in a neutral dorsiflexion position.[8,9,19,41] The limb is placed into a well-padded short leg cast if an Achilles tendon–lengthening procedure was done. Otherwise, a well-padded posterior splint will suffice. The patient is not allowed to bear weight for approximately 3 to 4 weeks, until all wounds have completely healed.

Tarsometatarsal (Lisfranc) Disarticulation

Outcome Considerations

The tarsometatarsal amputation first was described by Lisfranc de St. Martin during the 1800s.[12] This procedure is a disarticulation between the tarsal and metatarsal bones.[12,29] The primary indication for a Lisfranc disarticulation is soft-tissue loss in the forefoot that precludes a successful transmetatarsal amputation.[8,27,42] The insertion of extensor hallucis longus, tibialis anterior, peroneus longus, and peroneus brevis tendons are all compromised with this procedure.[43] Therefore, soft-tissue balancing by appropriate tendon transfers is the key to preventing wound complications and contracture with a tarsometatarsal amputation. The lever arm resulting from a more proximal foot amputation is shorter than that from a more distal foot amputation, and equinus contracture is common because of inability to balance the overpull of the Achilles tendon.[8] For this reason, an Achilles tendon–lengthening procedure almost always is necessary with a tarsometatarsal amputation.[8,9,24,41] The base of the fifth metatarsal should be left intact or shelled out subperiosteally and advanced to the cuboid to preserve the peroneus brevis insertion. The peroneus longus tendon may also be transferred to the proximal and lateral aspect of the cuboid through drill holes.[43] If the insertion is resected, the foot will fall into equinovarus because of the unopposed pull of the posterior tibial tendon. To counteract the pull of the Achilles tendon complex, tibialis anterior tendon transfer is often performed to maintain a more plantigrade foot.[19,43] Greene and Bibbo[43] describe a technique that transfers extensor hallucis longus tendon to the lateral cuneiform while preserving the attachment of tibialis anterior to the medial cuneiform. The authors believed that this technique produced a more plantigrade foot with more balanced range of motion.[43]

Surgical Technique

A transverse dorsal skin incision is made across the foot at the proximal-third level of the metatarsals.[29] From the medial aspect of this incision, a longitudinal incision is made down to the level of the first metatarsal neck. Laterally, a longitudinal incision is made down to the fifth metatarsal neck. A transverse plantar skin incision completes the superficial dissection at the level of the metatarsal necks. As the dissection is carried deep through the subcutaneous tissue, branches of the superficial and deep peroneal nerves as well as sensory nerves are identified and transected sharply with the scalpel after applying gentle traction. The dorsalis pedis is encountered in the first intermetatarsal space and must be ligated, as are the medial and lateral plantar arteries as they are encountered. Flexor and extensor tendons are transected sharply after applying mild traction and are allowed to retract proximally. Those tendons planned to be transferred later for soft-tissue balancing purposes are tagged.[43] At this point, the tarsometatarsal joints can be seen. The disarticulation of the joints begins medially at the first tarsometatarsal joint. The base of the second metatarsal is left intact to preserve the Lisfranc joint.[8,22] A small oscillating saw is used to cut the second metatarsal flush with the medial and lateral cuneiforms.[29,44] The third and fourth metatarsals are disarticulated from the lateral cuneiform and cuboid, respectively. When the fifth metatarsal is encountered, a small oscillating saw is used to cut through the metaphysis, distal to the peroneus brevis insertion. Alternatively, a subperiosteal dissection of the fifth metatarsal base can be done, with complete removal of the metatarsal, followed by advancement of the periosteum with peroneus brevis insertion to the cuboid.[8] All bony prominences are smoothed down with a rasp or rongeur. The remaining tendon transfers are then performed. The tourniquet is released, and meticulous hemostasis is obtained. Debulking of the plantar flap is performed if necessary. A small drain can be placed into the deep aspect of the wound. The deep fascial layers are approximated using 0 absorbable suture; 3-0 absorbable suture is used on the subcutaneous tissues, and 3-0 nylon suture or staples are used for skin closure. An Achilles tendon–lengthening procedure is done in almost all procedures because of the high risk of equinus contracture, even if dorsiflexion past neutral can be obtained in the operating room.[8,9,41] A well-padded posterior splint or short leg cast is placed onto the limb. Casting is recommended for any patient with a foot-based amputation who also undergoes an Achilles tendon–lengthening procedure.

Hindfoot-Level Amputations

Transtarsal (Chopart) Disarticulation

Outcome Considerations

The Chopart disarticulation, first described in 1792, is a disarticulation of the talonavicular and the calcaneocuboid joints.[5,8] This salvage procedure is indicated if the condition of the soft tissues does not allow a more distal resection but a weight-bearing residual limb is desirable.[8] An extremely active patient may not tolerate a Chopart disarticulation because of the decrease in push-off power and stability.[42] This procedure nonetheless is a reasonable option, especially in patients with diabetes, patients who have minimal ambulation but would benefit from having a stable limb for standing during transfers, and patients who have limited access to prostheses.[8,11,27] Brown et al[5] found that the mortality rate for a transtarsal amputation was similar to that for a transtibial amputation but that the transtarsal amputation had better functional results. An advantage of a transtarsal disarticulation over transtibial amputation is that the thick plantar heel skin may be preserved to better prevent wound issues with weight bearing long term.[19] Krause et al[45] found that patients had better function after a transtarsal amputation than after a Syme disarticulation or transtibial amputation because ankle motion and limb length were maintained, leading to better sensory perception and a larger weight-bearing surface. Additionally, for a Chopart disarticulation, patients may be fitted for an ankle-foot-orthosis postoperatively rather than knee-high prosthesis used form Syme or transtibial amputations.[19]

The Chopart disarticulation does not change the overall leg length, and it can be a better option than a more proximal amputation in a correctly selected patient.[46] After a transtarsal amputation, patients were found to have a normal gait while wearing appropriate braces.[4] The key to a successful outcome is correct soft-tissue balancing, which will avoid the most common equinovarus deformity.[10] Anterior tibial and peroneal tendon insertions must be preserved, most commonly by reattachment through drill holes in the neck of the talus.[10] The peroneus longus tendon alternatively can be transferred to the cuboid, or a tenotomy of the posterior tibial tendon can be performed to balance its pull.[11] Achilles tendon lengthening also is recommended to allow adequate dorsiflexion and prevent contracture that would lead to wound-healing difficulty.[8,10,12,42,46] Achilles tenectomy (excision of 2 to 3 cm of tendon) has also been described.[19] Given the potential complications that arise from postoperative equinus contracture, Greene et al[47] recommend performing a gastrocnemius-soleus recession in addition to an Achilles tenotomy. From the same report, the authors endorse transfer of the tibialis anterior, extensor hallucis longus, and extensor digitorum longus tendons to the talar neck from dorsal to plantar through three separate bone tunnels.[47] This technique may be technically challenging given the risk of talar neck fracture; however, the authors believe this improves dorsiflexion of the residual limb to improve function and combat residual equinus contracture.[47]

A modification of the Chopart disarticulation that has been described is to perform arthrodesis of the subtalar and ankle joints using a hindfoot fusion nail.[48] The ultimate goal of this technique is to provide greater stability against equinus contracture postoperatively.

Surgical Technique
A transverse dorsal skin incision is begun medially at the level of the navicular tuberosity and continued laterally to a point halfway between the base of the fifth metatarsal and the lateral malleolus.[9,27,41] Medial and lateral longitudinal incisions are made along the first and fifth metatarsal shafts, respectively.[29] At the midshaft metatarsal level, a transverse skin incision is made across the plantar aspect of the foot.[8,9,29,41] All major branches of nerves are transected, and all major arteries are ligated. Flexor and extensor tendons are transected and allowed to retract. The posterior tibial, anterior tibial, and peroneus brevis tendons are carefully dissected and preserved for later attachment. At this point, the talonavicular and calcaneocuboid joints are identified. Procedures to lengthen the Achilles can be performed at this step or earlier in the surgery. If Achilles tenectomy is selected, a separate posteromedial incision is required.[19] Circumferential capsulotomies are done at each joint to allow disarticulation. The talus and calcaneus are left intact with the hindfoot.[8,29] A prominent dorsal talar head or anterior process of the calcaneus can be smoothed down with a rasp or rongeur. The articular cartilage is removed from the distal talus and calcaneus to improve the soft-tissue flap adherence.[12,41] Tendon transfers are completed to balance the soft tissues of the residual limb. The anterior tibial tendon is anchored through an oblique drill hole in the talar neck, from dorsolateral to plantarmedial.[29] If multiple drill holes are used (for transfer of more than one tendon), adequate spacing of at least 5 mm is paramount to prevent fracture of the bone bridge.[47] Additionally, sequential drilling with large drill bits or curettes are used to enlarge bone tunnels to facilitate safe tendon passage.[47] The posterior tibial tendon can be allowed to retract proximally or alternatively can be transferred to the dorsum of the foot to augment dorsiflexion. For the transfer, the posterior tibial tendon is routed through the interosseous membrane to the dorsal talar neck and secured with a suture anchor or through a drill hole. The peroneus brevis is transferred to the remaining anterior process of the calcaneus.[9,12,41] Transferring the posterior and anterior tibial tendons and the peroneus brevis tendons not only augments dorsiflexion but also helps resist the pull of the hindfoot into equinus and can prevent contracture.[9,12,29,41] The plantar flap is brought up over the bony prominences, and the deep fascia is approximated with a 0 absorbable suture. A small drain can be placed into the deep wound if desired. The subcutaneous layer is closed with 3-0 absorbable suture, and 3-0 nylon suture or staples are used to approximate the skin.[12,29] The limb is placed into a well-padded cast if an Achilles tendon–lengthening procedure was done or otherwise into a posterior splint in as much dorsiflexion as possible.[29]

Transcalcaneal (Boyd) Amputation
Outcome Considerations
Transcalcaneal amputations first were described in 1939 to encompass a talectomy with a primary tibiocalcaneal arthrodesis.[49] This amputation is considered to be an alternative to the Syme ankle disarticulation and a last resort for a length-preserving foot amputation before transtibial amputation becomes necessary. The goal of transcalcaneal amputations is to produce a full weight-bearing residual limb with stable soft-tissue coverage and maintenance of plantar heel pad sensation.[50] Patency of the posterior tibial artery should be assessed preoperatively either by examination or by advanced imaging as indicated. Only patients who have the ability to be ambulatory are appropriate candidates. The use of the weight-bearing residual limb with almost its entire limb length remaining requires only a minimal increase in energy expenditure compared with the use of a normal limb.[49] Compared with a Syme disarticulation, a transcalcaneal amputation has the disadvantages of relying on the tibiocalcaneal union and precluding the use of an energy-storing prosthesis; its advantages include less heel pad migration, decreased risk of equinus contracture, and greater leg length with less widening at the distal residual limb.[49,51] For these reasons, the transcalcaneal amputation may be preferable to a Syme ankle disarticulation for an ambulatory patient with limited access to modern prostheses.

Weight-bearing protocols following these procedures may vary by surgeon, but patients may be required to avoid full weight bearing while awaiting tibiocalcaneal fusion.

The Boyd and Pirogoff amputations are two types of transcalcaneal amputations described in literature.[51] Both procedures involve a talectomy and rely on tibiocalcaneal fusion, but they differ in the calcaneal osteotomy. The Pirogoff amputation uses a calcaneal osteotomy in the coronal plane that retains the posterior aspect of the calcaneus, which is rotated 90° to meet the distal tibia. The Boyd amputation involves a horizontal osteotomy of the calcaneus that leaves the inferior aspect of the calcaneus to meet the distal tibia.

Although transcalcaneal amputations are reported to have fairly high complication rates, there is a paucity of literature regarding patient outcome, function, and residual limb survivorship. Andronic et al[50] performed a systematic review including 123 transcalcaneal amputations (including modified Pirogoff and Boyd procedures) with a mean follow-up of 45 months. Although there was heterogeneity in the functional outcome assessments from the included studies, 69% of patients were reported to have a very good or good functional outcome score at a mean of 45 months follow-up.[50] Average leg length discrepancy was reported in five studies (65 patients) and was 2.5 cm.[50] The mean time to ambulation in a prosthesis was 12.7 weeks and mean tibiocalcaneal union occurred at 17.2 weeks.[50] Last, the authors noted a mean residual limb survivorship (no further proximal amputation) of 77% from their review.[50]

Surgical Technique

A transverse dorsal skin incision is made at the level of the ankle joint.[52] A transverse plantar incision is made at the distal aspect of the heel pad. The incisions are connected medially and laterally approximately 1 cm distal to the medial and lateral malleoli, respectively. All major blood vessels are identified and ligated. With the foot in maximal plantar flexion, dorsal nerves and extensor tendons are transected and allowed to retract proximally. Flexor tendons are transected and allowed to retract. The tibiotalar joint is carefully released anteriorly. The anterior talofibular ligament is transected laterally, and the deltoid ligament is transected medially. The posterior tibial artery and tibial nerve are protected and left intact. A bone hook or skin rake can be used for pulling the talar dome anteriorly to expose the posterior joint capsule and allow release. The talus is excised after all talocalcaneal attachments have been removed. If excision is difficult, an osteotome can be used to divide the talus into smaller pieces for removal in more than one piece.[49] An oscillating saw is used to remove the distal tibial articular surface until cancellous bone is seen.[49,52] The oscillating saw also is used to remove the anterior process and superior articular surface of the calcaneus. The calcaneus and tibia are then approximated and provisionally held in place with Kirschner wires.[52] Two partially threaded 6.5-mm cancellous screws are placed across the tibiocalcaneal articulation from distal to proximal.[49] The plantar flap is brought anterior, and the deep fascial layers are approximated with 0 absorbable suture. A small drain can be placed into the deep aspect of the wound if desired. The subcutaneous tissue is approximated using a 3-0 absorbable suture, and the skin is closed with 3-0 nylon suture or staples. The limb is placed into a well-padded posterior splint.

Rehabilitation

In general, a benefit of a partial foot amputation at any level is the decreased need for extensive postoperative rehabilitation. The patient is left with a weight-bearing residual limb, and after fitting with the proper prosthesis, orthosis, or modified shoe, the patient's gait energy expenditure is almost normal.[4,49] Pinzur et al[53] found a relatively linear increase in metabolic demands with increasing amputation levels and concluded that after amputation necessitated by peripheral vascular insufficiency, functional walking capacity was related to the level of amputation.

It is important that the patient does not bear weight until all skin incisions are fully healed and, after a Boyd amputation, until osseous union has occured.[8,12,38] When the skin has healed, the patient can be fitted for a molded foot orthosis or prosthesis.[8,12,27] The goal of the device is to allow ambulation with the smallest possible increase in energy expenditure while minimizing stress at the interface of the prosthesis and the residual limb.[27,46]

Complications

Roukis et al[38] identified several risk factors for unsuccessful partial amputation, which were categorized as host factors, noncompliance, and poor soft-tissue balancing. Most postoperative complications are related to wound healing.[8,9,11,38] Many patients who require an amputation have diabetes or abnormal vascular flow and are at risk for wound-healing complications. The risk increases if neuropathy is present and the patient cannot feel friction-related pain at the end of the residual limb.[8,9,11] Wound-healing complications may require further surgical intervention in the form of irrigation and débridement or more proximal amputations. Seckin et al[54] reviewed several potential risk factors for reamputation in patients with diabetic foot wounds. Hypoalbuminemia, smoking, hypertension, duration of diabetes, number of débridements required after index surgery, and a long hospitalization were found to be risk factors for reamputation. They also noted that more distal index amputations were more likely to require reamputation.[54]

Patient adherence to postoperative weight-bearing restrictions is a key factor in preventing complications after a partial foot amputation. Usually the patient must avoid weight bearing until the skin and soft tissues are fully healed.[12,38] After a transcalcaneal amputation, patients must not bear weight until osseous union occurs at the tibiocalcaneal interface.[49]

Soft-tissue balancing is the key to surgical success at most levels of partial foot amputation.[8,9,12,29,41] Ray resections are the least difficult for maintaining the balance of the foot, but as the amputation becomes more proximal, tendon transfer and/or lengthening becomes more essential to maintaining the balance of the foot. A unique complication of ray resection is postoperative clawing or drifting of the remaining digits toward the residual digits, which may require further surgical intervention.[19] As the lever arm of the foot shortens, it is more difficult for the foot to overcome the pull of the gastrocnemius complex. If the foot remains in a plantarflexed position, the Achilles tendon will tighten, and an equinus contracture will result. The equinus contracture causes stress at the distal wound and interferes with incision healing. If the skin incisions have healed, the equinus contracture can lead to new areas of pressure ulceration. An equinovarus contracture of the foot can result if the hindfoot balance is disturbed because of detachment of the anterior tibial and peroneus brevis tendons with the posterior tibial tendon left intact. The contracture not only limits the opportunity for a plantigrade foot during weight bearing but also makes prosthesis or orthosis wear difficult and leads to pressure ulcerations. The unfortunate consequence of wound-healing complications, pressure ulcerations, and the resulting infections or soft-tissue deficits is the need for a subsequent, more proximal amputation that can cause the loss of independent ambulation.

SUMMARY

Partial foot amputation is a reasonable alternative to a more proximal transtibial amputation in appropriately selected patients. Patients for whom a primary partial foot amputation is preferred to a more proximal amputation usually are of relatively advanced age and have limited ambulatory demands. Partial foot amputation preserves a weight-bearing residual limb that minimizes the increase in energy expenditure, allows the patient to maintain independent ambulation and overall function, and decreases the risk of mortality. Preoperative evaluation of soft-tissue involvement, limb perfusion, and medical comorbidities is essential. Meticulous surgical technique in the creation of long plantar flaps and soft-tissue balancing is essential. Postoperative attention to soft-tissue healing and prevention of ulceration recurrence, patient compliance, and treatment by a knowledgeable prosthetist all facilitate improved outcomes and minimize the risk of complications.

References

1. Varma P, Stineman MG, Dillingham TR: Epidemiology of limb loss. *Phys Med Rehabil Clin N Am* 2014;25(1):1-8.
2. Centers for Disease Control and Prevention: *National Diabetes Statistics Report: 2014.* http://www.cdc.gov/diabetes/data/statistics/2014StatisticsReport.html. Accessed November 26, 2014.
3. Walicka M, Raczyńska M, Marcinkowska K, et al: Amputations of lower limb in subjects with diabetes mellitus: Reasons and 30-day mortality. *J Diabetes Res* 2021;2021:8866126.
4. Schade VL, Roukis TS, Yan JL: Factors associated with successful Chopart amputation in patients with diabetes: A systematic review. *Foot Ankle Spec* 2010;3(5):278-284.
5. Brown ML, Tang W, Patel A, Baumhauer JF: Partial foot amputation in patients with diabetic foot ulcers. *Foot Ankle Int* 2012;33(9):707-716.
6. Sinha R, van den Heuvel WJ, Arokiasamy P: Factors affecting quality of life in lower limb amputees. *Prosthet Orthot Int* 2011;35(1):90-96.
7. Sullivan JP: Complications of pedal amputations. *Clin Podiatr Med Surg* 2005;22(3):469-484.
8. Philbin TM, Berlet GC, Lee TH: Lower-extremity amputations in association with diabetes mellitus. *Foot Ankle Clin* 2006;11(4):791-804.
9. Sanders LJ: Transmetatarsal and midfoot amputations. *Clin Podiatr Med Surg* 1997;14(4):741-762.
10. Baima J, Trovato M, Hopkins M, Delateur B: Achieving functional ambulation in a patient with Chopart amputation. *Am J Phys Med Rehabil* 2008;87(6):510-513.
11. Boffeli TJ, Thompson JC: Partial foot amputations for salvage of the diabetic lower extremity. *Clin Podiatr Med Surg* 2014;31(1):103-126.
12. Philbin T, Witt B: Midfoot amputations, in Flatow E, Colvin AC, eds: *Atlas of Essential Orthopaedic Procedures.* American Academy of Orthopaedic Surgeons, 2013, pp 551-556.
13. Andrews KL, Dib MY, Shives TC, Hoskin TL, Liedl DA, Boon AJ: Noninvasive arterial studies including transcutaneous oxygen pressure measurements with the limbs elevated or dependent to predict healing after partial foot amputation. *Am J Phys Med Rehabil* 2013;92(5):385-392.
14. Wallace GF: Indications for amputations. *Clin Podiatr Med Surg* 2005;22(3):315-328.
15. Redlich U, Xiong YY, Pech M, et al: Superiority of transcutaneous oxygen tension measurements in predicting limb salvage after below-the-knee angioplasty: A prospective trial in diabetic patients with critical limb ischemia. *Cardiovasc Intervent Radiol* 2011;34(2):271-279.
16. Alagha M, Aherne TM, Hassanin A, et al: Diagnostic performance of ankle-brachial pressure index in lower extremity arterial disease. *Surg J (N Y)* 2021;7(3):e132-e137.
17. Bonham PA: Get the LEAD out: Noninvasive assessment for lower extremity arterial disease using ankle brachial index and toe brachial index measurements. *J Wound Ostomy Continence Nurs* 2006;33(1):30-41.
18. Faglia E, Clerici G, Caminiti M, Quarantiello A, Curci V, Somalvico F: Evaluation of feasibility of ankle pressure and foot oximetry values for the detection of critical limb ischemia in diabetic patients. *Vasc Endovascular Surg* 2010;44(3):184-189.
19. Brodsky JW, Saltzman CL: Amputations of the foot and ankle, in Coughlin MJ, Saltman CL, Anderson RB, eds: *Mann's Surgery of the Foot and Ankle*, ed 9. Elsevier Saunders, 2014, pp 1481-1506.
20. Subramanian N, Han J, Leeper NJ, Ross EG, Montez-Rath ME, Chang TI: Comparison of pre-amputation evaluation in patients with and without chronic kidney disease. *Am J Nephrol* 2021;52(5):388-395.
21. Sonter J, Sadler S, Chuter V: Inter-rater reliability of automated devices for measurement of toe systolic blood pressure and the toe brachial index. *Blood Press Monit* 2015;20(1):47-51.
22. Cook KD: Perioperative management of pedal amputations. *Clin Podiatr Med Surg* 2005;22(3):329-341.
23. Yang C, Weng H, Chen L, et al: Transcutaneous oxygen pressure measurement in diabetic foot ulcers: Mean values and cut-point for wound healing. *J Wound Ostomy Continence Nurs* 2013;40(6):585-589.

24. Stuck RM, Sage R, Pinzur M, Osterman H: Amputations in the diabetic foot. *Clin Podiatr Med Surg* 1995;12(1):141-155.
25. Schmidt BM, McHugh JB, Patel RM, Wrobel JS: Prospective analysis of surgical bone margins after partial foot amputation in diabetic patients admitted with moderate to severe foot infections. *Foot Ankle Spec* 2019;12(2):131-137.
26. Pinzur MS, Stuck RM, Sage R, Hunt N, Rabinovich Z: Syme ankle disarticulation in patients with diabetes. *J Bone Joint Surg Am* 2003;85(9):1667-1672.
27. Philbin TM, Leyes M, Sferra JJ, Donley BG: Orthotic and prosthetic devices in partial foot amputations. *Foot Ankle Clin* 2001;6(2):215-228.
28. Chou L, Temple T, Ho Y, Malawer M: Foot and ankle amputations: Ray resections, in Weisel S, ed. *Operative Techniques in Orthopaedic Surgery*. Lippincott Williams & Wilkins, 2011, pp 2047-2052.
29. Chou L, Temple T, Ho Y, Malawer M: Foot and ankle amputations: Lisfranc/Chopart, in Weisel S, ed: *Operative Techniques in Orthopaedic Surgery*. Lippincott Williams & Wilkins, 2011, pp 2072-2080.
30. Brodsky J: Amputations in the foot and ankle, in Coughlin M, Mann R, Saltzman E, eds: *Surgery of the Foot and Ankle*, ed 8. Mosby-Elsevier, 2007, pp 1369-1398.
31. Häller TV, Kaiser P, Kaiser D, Berli MC, Uçkay I, Waibel FWA: Outcome of ray resection as definitive treatment in forefoot infection or ischemia: A cohort study. *J Foot Ankle Surg* 2020;59(1):27-30.
32. Pinzur M: Amputations in trauma, in Browner B, ed: *Skeletal Trauma: Basic Science, Management, and Reconstruction*. Elsevier Health Sciences, 2009, pp 2863-2881.
33. Grimm P, Potter B: *Amputation Surgeries for the Lower Limb*. Elsevier, 2020, pp 471-503.
34. Reyzelman AM, Hadi S, Armstrong DG: Limb salvage with Chopart's amputation and tendon balancing. *J Am Podiatr Med Assoc* 1999;89(2):100-103.
35. Younger AS, Awwad MA, Kalla TP, de Vries G: Risk factors for failure of transmetatarsal amputation in diabetic patients: A cohort study. *Foot Ankle Int* 2009;30(12):1177-1182.
36. Thorud JC, Jupiter DC, Lorenzana J, Nguyen TT, Shibuya N: Reoperation and reamputation after transmetatarsal amputation: A systematic review and meta-analysis. *J Foot Ankle Surg* 2016;55(5):1007-1012.
37. Harris RC, Fang W: Transmetatarsal amputation outcomes when utilized to address foot gangrene and infection: A retrospective chart review. *J Foot Ankle Surg* 2021;60(2):269-275.
38. Roukis TS, Singh N, Andersen CA: Preserving functional capacity as opposed to tissue preservation in the diabetic patient: A single institution experience. *Foot Ankle Spec* 2010;3(4):177-183.
39. Holloway JJ, Lauer K, Kansal N, Bongard F, Miller A: A novel approach to limb salvage: Healing transmetatarsal amputations without a viable plantar flap. *Ann Vasc Surg* 2021;70:51-55.
40. Canales MB, Heurich ME, Mandela AM, Razzante MC: An approach to transmetatarsal amputation to encourage immediate weightbearing in diabetic patients. *J Foot Ankle Surg* 2017;56(3):609-612.
41. DeCotiis MA: Lisfranc and Chopart amputations. *Clin Podiatr Med Surg* 2005;22(3):385-393.
42. Marks RM, Long JT, Exten EL: Gait abnormality following amputation in diabetic patients. *Foot Ankle Clin* 2010;15(3):501-507.
43. Greene CJ, Bibbo C: The lisfranc amputation: A more reliable level of amputation with proper intraoperative tendon balancing. *J Foot Ankle Surg* 2017;56(4):824-826.
44. Bowker J: Partial foot amputations and disarticulations: Surgical aspects. *J Prosthet Orthot* 2007;19(3 suppl):62-76.
45. Krause FG, Pfander G, Henning J, Shafighi M, Weber M: Ankle dorsiflexion arthrodesis to salvage Chopart's amputation with anterior skin insufficiency. *Foot Ankle Int* 2013;34(11):1560-1568.
46. Yondas P, O'Donnell CJ: Prosthetic management of the partial foot amputee. *Clin Podiatr Med Surg* 2005;22(3):485-502.
47. Greene CJ, Bibbo C, McArdle A, Knight C: A functional chopart's amputation with tendon transfers. *J Foot Ankle Surg* 2021;60(1):213-217.
48. DeGere MW, Grady JF: A modification of Chopart's amputation with ankle and subtalar arthrodesis by using an intramedullary nail. *J Foot Ankle Surg* 2005;44(4):281-286.
49. Tosun B, Buluc L, Gok U, Unal C: Boyd amputation in adults. *Foot Ankle Int* 2011;32(11):1063-1068.
50. Andronic O, Boeni T, Burkhard MD, Kaiser D, Berli MC, Waibel FWA: Modifications of the pirogoff amputation technique in adults: A retrospective analysis of 123 cases. *J Orthop* 2020;18:5-12.
51. Ng V, Berlet G: Amputations of the foot and ankle, in Parekh S, ed: *Foot and Ankle Surgery*. JP Medical, 2012, pp 377-388.
52. Scaduto A, Bernstein R: Syme and Boyd amputations for fibular deficiency, in Weisel S, ed: *Operative Techniques in Orthopaedic Surgery*. Lippincott Williams & Wilkins, 2011, pp 1295-1303.
53. Pinzur MS, Gold J, Schwartz D, Gross N: Energy demands for walking in dysvascular amputees as related to the level of amputation. *Orthopedics* 1992;15(9):1033-1036.
54. Seçkin MF, Özcan Ç, Çamur S, Polat Ö, Batar S: Predictive factors and amputation level for reamputation in patients with diabetic foot: A retrospective case-control study. *J Foot Ankle Surg* 2021;61(1):43-47.

Partial Foot Amputation: Prosthetic Management

CHAPTER 35

Michael P. Dillon, PhD, BPO(Hons) • Stefania Fatone, PhD, BPO(Hons)

ABSTRACT

Partial foot amputation is the most common amputation surgery and typically affects the toe(s) and/or metatarsals. Partial foot amputation is often performed in people with advanced peripheral arterial disease when extensive efforts to heal recalcitrant wounds have been unsuccessful. Although many people perceive that partial foot amputation will resolve long-standing issues with poor wound healing, a large proportion of people will experience serious complications such as infection, wound breakdown, or reamputation on the same limb in the months and years that follow. Although there is good evidence describing the surgical outcomes following partial foot amputation, research focused on other outcomes such as community mobility, health-related quality of life, or psychosocial outcomes is limited. Similarly, there is little evidence comparing the effectiveness of different types of prosthetic and orthotic interventions, which makes it difficult to determine which interventions most reduce the risk of complications and reamputation. An introduction to partial foot amputation and common prosthetic and orthotic interventions is provided, and current knowledge about the effect of different prosthetic and orthotic interventions is summarized. The clinical and research implications are also discussed with a view to addressing the wide range of challenges faced by those living with partial foot amputation.

Keywords: amputation; partial foot; prosthetics; orthotics; outcomes

Introduction

Partial foot amputation (PFA) is perhaps the most common amputation surgery with an annual incidence rate of 4.0 per 100,000 general population (95% confidence interval 3.8 to 4.2).[1] However, significant complexity belies such simple statistics. For example, the incidence rate is about fourfold higher in studies that only include people older than 30 years, which might better describe the population at risk.[1] Similarly, the incidence rate is about 25 times higher in cohorts with diabetes compared with those without.[1] Studies that exclude people with toe amputation or repeat amputations underestimate the incidence rate. These illustrative examples highlight how minor variations in the design of epidemiologic research can have a profound effect on the calculated incidence rate, which adds significantly to the challenge of accurately describing the number of amputation procedures each year.

Given these sorts of variations in the design of epidemiologic research, there is also uncertainty about whether the incidence rate of PFA has changed over time.[1] For example, many time-series investigations are too short to allow small changes in the annual incidence rate—typically less than 1% to 2% per annum—to become large enough to be statistically significant.[1] Similarly, studies of individual health services often have small participant numbers that make them susceptible to chance variations from year to year that tend to dwarf the small, cumulative, changes in the incidence rate over time.[1]

Although there is some uncertainty about whether the incidence of PFA has changed over time, public health initiatives designed to curb the incidence of limb loss, such as early assessment at specialist high-risk foot clinics or better management of diabetes at a community level,[2-6] may mean that the number of people at risk because of diabetes[7,8] are presenting with less severe vascular disease that may help avoid the need for amputation surgery in their lifetime.

About three-quarters of all PFAs affect one or more toes, with comparatively few ray resections, transmetatarsal, tarsometatarsal (Lisfranc), or transtarsal (Chopart) amputations[9-12] (**Figure 1**). The proportion of PFA affecting the toes may seem unusually high to prosthetists/orthotists given that they tend to only see people with more proximal amputation. A large proportion of people with amputation of the toe(s) may receive follow-up care through high-risk foot clinics rather than prosthetic and orthotic centers.

Dr. Dillon or an immediate family member serves as a board member, owner, officer, or committee member of the International Society for Prosthetics and Orthotics. Dr. Fatone or an immediate family member serves as a board member, owner, officer, or committee member of the American Academy of Orthotists and Prosthetists, the American Orthotic and Prosthetic Association, and the International Society for Prosthetics and Orthotics.

© 2024 American Academy of Orthopaedic Surgeons

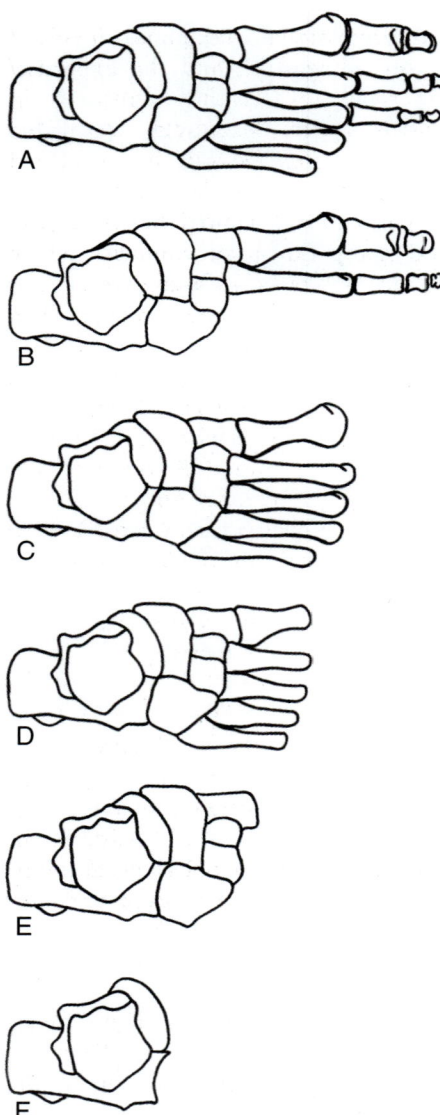

FIGURE 1 Schematic representation of common levels of partial foot amputation. **A**, Amputation of the fourth and fifth toes. **B**, Resection of the third, fourth, and fifth metatarsals and toes (rays). **C**, Disarticulation at the metatarsophalangeal joint. **D**, Transmetatarsal amputation. **E**, Tarsometatarsal (Lisfranc) amputation. **F**, Transtarsal (Chopart) amputation (sometimes also referred to as midtarsal).

Over recent years, a greater appreciation of the complications experienced by people living with PFA has developed. Between 30% and 50% of people with PFA experience complications such as dehiscence, ulceration, and wound failure.[13] To some extent, these complications may be attributable to the complexities of predicting which amputation levels will heal best; particularly in people with serious vascular compromise and complex comorbidities (eg, end-stage renal disease, hypertension, diabetes).[13,14] There are longer term challenges: managing progressive equinovarus contractures[15-18] and moderating higher forefoot plantar pressures relative to the contralateral limb or appropriately matched control subjects.[19-21] These sorts of complications likely contribute to the fact that half of all initial PFA require secondary amputation on the same limb within 5 years; a rate not appreciably different between levels of PFA.[13] These rates of complications are often not markedly better in people without diabetes, making it difficult to conclude that the high rate of complications are merely a reflection of advanced systemic disease.[13]

Recognizing these challenges, researchers have recently developed shared decision-making resources to help patients engage in more meaningful conversations about amputation surgery,[22,23] as well as decision support tools that allow health professionals to accurately predict the likely success of different amputation procedures based on individualized patient demographic, laboratory, and health-related factors.[14,24,25] Common to these resources is the desire to help facilitate more meaningful communication between patients and health care clinicians, as well as provide accurate information about the likely outcomes and risks. In this way, patients can make more informed decisions about amputation surgery and exercise greater control over their health care.[22,23]

For those living with PFA, a wide variety of prostheses and orthoses are provided to help minimize complications and restore premorbid function,[26-28] thus facilitating self-care and participation in activities that bring joy and meaning to life. The types of devices provided to meet these treatment goals have changed little over time: toe fillers, insoles, silicone cosmetic prostheses, ankle-foot orthoses (AFOs), and above-ankle prostheses are still commonly used.

Although the types of devices may have changed little over time, emerging research challenges long-held views about how effectively current prosthetic and orthotic interventions can meet the needs of people with PFA.[29] For example, although prostheses and orthoses can be designed to restore the effective foot length,[30,31] it is unclear whether normalizing gait is important to return people to their premorbid level of community mobility. There is little knowledge about which interventions significantly reduce the rates of complications and reamputation. Similarly, it is uncertain whether different interventions affect health-related quality of life (HR-QoL) or facilitate participation in activities that bring joy and meaning to life. These emerging insights continue to guide efforts to better understand how prosthetic and orthotic interventions can be of benefit to people living with PFA.

Current knowledge about PFA and the effect of prosthetic and orthotic interventions are summarised in this chapter. The following sections briefly describe common categories of prostheses and orthoses currently provided to meet the needs of people living with PFA. The emerging evidence, and implications for clinical practice and research, are also discussed.

Interventions

A wide variety of custom prosthetic, orthotic, and footwear interventions are provided to people living with PFA.[26-28,32,33] These interventions are often categorized as below-ankle or above-ankle depending on whether the device crosses the ankle joint.[16,27] Common below-ankle interventions include toe fillers, insoles, and silicone cosmetic prostheses; common above-ankle interventions include AFOs and above-ankle prostheses. Some investigators have recently tried to incorporate elements of the two by embedding supramalleolar or short AFOs inside silicone prostheses.[34,35]

These interventions may fulfil several different treatment goals. For example, devices may be provided to minimize interface pressures on the distal end of the residuum and prevent equinovarus contracture with the expectation that they reduce the risk of ulceration and skin breakdown that often leads to more proximal

Chapter 35: Partial Foot Amputation: Prosthetic Management

amputation.[27,32,36,37] Devices may be provided to make standing and walking more comfortable or restore premorbid mobility.[26,27,32,38-41] Other devices provide a high degree of cosmetic restoration.[26,27,32] Devices may also be used in combination to achieve multiple treatment goals. For example, a carbon-fiber, anterior shell AFO might be used with an insole and toe filler (**Figure 2**) to restore the effective foot length and normalize gait, as well as distribute pressure away from the distal end of the residuum to provide protection and improve comfort during standing and walking.

As a generalization, people with more proximal amputations tend to be provided with more substantial devices. A person with amputation disarticulating the metatarsophalangeal joints might be provided with an insole and/or toe filler (**Figure 3**). By comparison, someone with a Chopart (transtarsal) amputation might be provided with an above-ankle prosthesis that encloses the residuum and leg in a solid plastic shell (**Figure 4**). Those with amputations through the midfoot (eg, transmetatarsal amputation or ray resections) tend to be provided with a much wider variety of interventions varying from insoles, silicone cosmetic prostheses, and/or AFOs.

The types of interventions provided to people with PFA vary across countries and health jurisdictions depending on the stipulations of funding bodies,

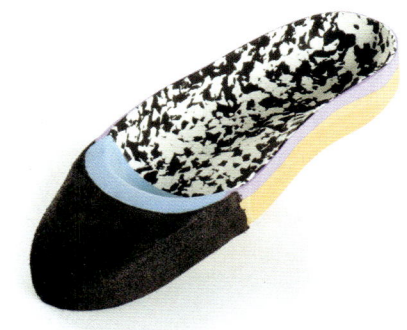

FIGURE 3 Photograph of an insole and toe filler for a transmetatarsal residuum. Ethylene-vinyl acetate sole supporting the hindfoot and arch. Poron, an open-cell polyurethane foam, has been used to protect the sensitive distal/inferior end of the residuum. The toe filler is made from Plastazote, an expanded low-density polyethylene closed-cell foam. (Courtesy of Prosthetics and Orthotics Department, Royal Melbourne Hospital, Melbourne, Australia.)

the professional disciplines involved in providing care, and the expertise/experience of treating clinicians. In Australia, for example, pedorthic approaches (eg, custom or customized footwear) seem to be less common than in parts of the United States, Japan, and many European countries where the formal training and expertise of pedorthotists are better recognized in healthcare practice.

It is beyond the scope of this chapter to comprehensively describe the wide variety of devices provided to people living with PFA. As such, the following subsections aim to characterize the most common categories of prosthetic and orthotic interventions in terms of their application to different amputation levels, design variations, and treatment objectives.

Toe Fillers and Insoles

Toe fillers and insoles (**Figure 3**) are common interventions for people with distal forefoot amputations such as amputation of the toe(s), disarticulation at the metatarsophalangeal joints, or ray resections. However, it is not uncommon for people with transmetatarsal amputation to also be provided with toe fillers and insoles.

Toe fillers are used to fill the cavity in normal length footwear. They can be used alone or attached to an insole. Insoles serve as a bed for the remnant foot and can be designed with the intention to maintain the alignment of the residuum and redistribute pressure away from the sensitive distal end with a view to minimizing the likelihood of skin breakdown.[42] Both toe fillers and insoles are designed to be worn as part of footwear. Given that they do not encompass the residuum, they rely on the shoe to maintain their position with respect to the remaining foot (ie, a form of suspension). Extra-depth footwear or low-top boots may be provided to accommodate the orthoses and provide adequate suspension.

Toe fillers and insoles are often made from closed-cell foams that resist compression and therefore thinning (eg, ethylene-vinyl acetate) but may incorporate materials with different mechanical properties based on

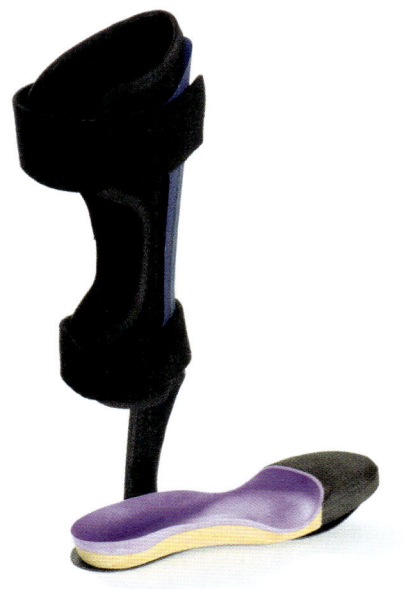

FIGURE 2 Photograph of a Blue Rocker ToeOff ankle-foot orthoses combined with an ethylene-vinyl acetate insole. (Courtesy of Prosthetics and Orthotics Department, Royal Melbourne Hospital, Melbourne, Australia.)

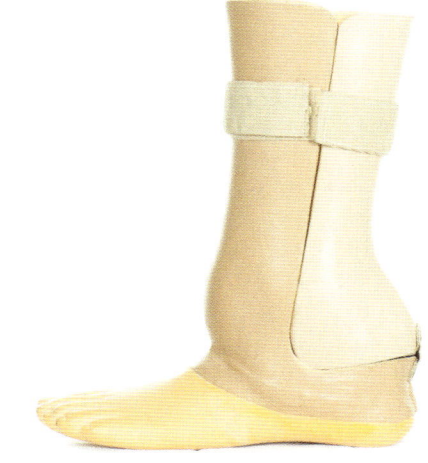

FIGURE 4 Photograph of a bivalved above-ankle prosthesis for a Chopart residuum (sometimes referred to as a clamshell prosthesis). The laminated socket is made of a resin and glass-fiber composite and includes a closed-cell polyethylene foam liner. (Courtesy of Prosthetics and Orthotics Department, Royal Melbourne Hospital, Melbourne, Australia.)

the defined treatment goals. For example, closed-cell polyethylene foam might be used under the heel and arch to correct foot alignment, whereas a low-density material might be used to protect the distal end of the residuum against shear forces (**Figure 3**). Some toe fillers incorporate vertical cuts through the dorsum, much like the Shape&Roll prosthetic foot,[30,43] with a view to reducing the stiffness of the filler and facilitating bending when rolling over the forefoot during walking. Some devices take the opposite approach and include a carbon-fiber foot plate to help prevent buckling of the orthoses across the distal end of the residuum when loaded. Unfortunately, the efficacy of these approaches has not been evidenced by research.

Silicone Cosmetic Prostheses

Silicone cosmetic prostheses (**Figure 5**) provide the most cosmetic restoration of the partially amputated foot given that it is possible to match the shape and alignment of the toes and nails, and skin color variations, to that of the contralateral limb. These devices are usually, but not exclusively, provided to people with amputation at or distal to the midfoot.

The design of the prosthesis depends on the remnant foot: a prosthesis for someone with transmetatarsal amputation might take the form of a slipper socket that encompasses the entire residuum (**Figure 5, A**), whereas a prosthesis for someone with a lateral ray resection would require a distal opening for the medial rays/toes to protrude through the end of the prosthesis (**Figure 5, B**).

Silicone prostheses are made to intimately fit the residuum, requiring water-based lubricant and a shoehorn for donning. This intimacy of fit provides suction suspension enabling the prosthesis to be worn with flip flops or sandals. Although silicone prostheses may be worn without footwear, providers usually recommend wearing footwear outdoors to prolong the life of the prosthesis.

More recently, investigators have sought to improve the function of

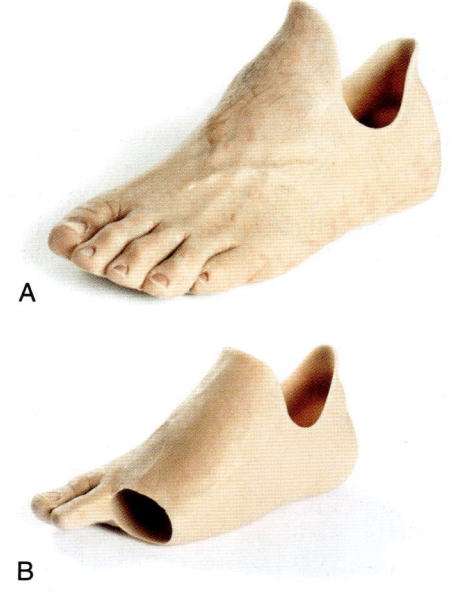

FIGURE 5 Photographs of two silicone cosmetic prostheses. **A**, Prosthesis for a transmetatarsal residuum complete with color matching, hair and nails. **B**, Prosthesis for a medial ray resection. The third, fourth, and fifth toes protrude through the lateral opening at the distal end of the prosthesis. (Courtesy of APC Prosthetics, Sydney, Australia.)

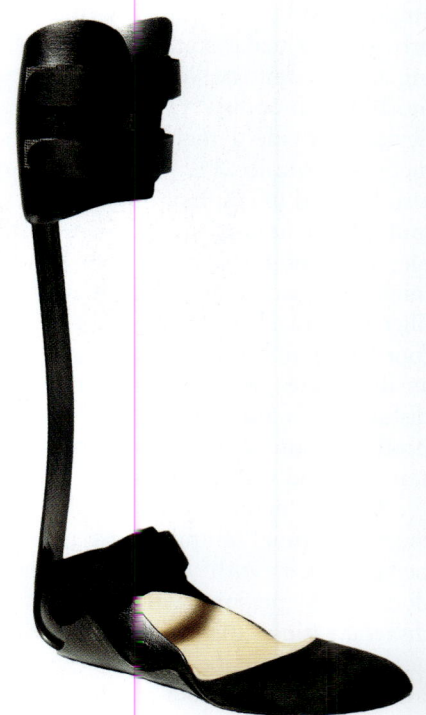

FIGURE 6 Photograph of a carbon-fiber ankle-foot orthosis with custom-made toe filler. (Courtesy of Tillges Technologies, Maplewood, MN.)

silicone prostheses. For example, silicone prostheses can be designed with different durometers based on individual pressure measurements to reduce localized areas of high pressure.[37,44] Other examples attempt to embed short AFOs,[34] supramalleolar orthoses,[35] or foot plates into the silicone prostheses[45] to restore the foot lever with the intent to normalize gait.

Ankle-Foot Orthoses

AFOs encompass the whole or part of the foot and extend proximal to the ankle. AFOs of varying designs are often provided for people with transmetatarsal and Lisfranc (tarsometatarsal) amputation (**Figures 2, 6, and 7**).

Given that AFOs can be designed of different materials, foot plate lengths, trim lines, and articulation (or not) at the ankle, AFOs can serve different mechanical functions and fulfil different treatment goals. For example, an AFO that incorporates a weight-bearing brim may help reduce plantar pressure on the remnant foot by allowing a proportion of body weight to be borne by the brim as well as control progression of the leg over the stance foot (**Figure 7**). Similarly complex treatment goals may also be achieved when AFOs are used in conjunction with other interventions. For example, an insole that aligns the residuum and distributes pressure away from the sensitive distal end of the residuum could be used in combination with an anterior shell AFO to control progression of the leg over the stance foot (**Figure 2**). Recently, custom-made, carbon-fiber, dynamic AFOs with toe filler were used in conjunction with individualized physiotherapy training that focused on gait and activity performance for a person with bilateral transmetatarsal amputations.[4] Training was required to learn to load and deflect the posterior strut of the AFO during various activities[41] which suggests that people living with PFA may also benefit from specific gait retraining as is

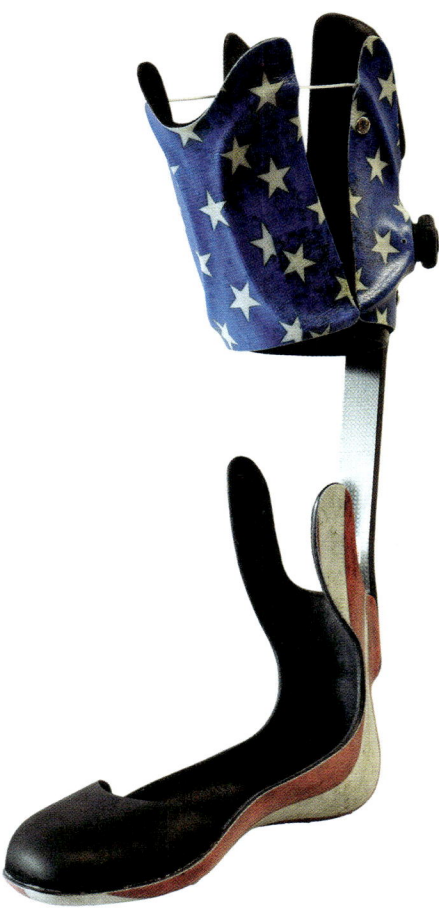

FIGURE 7 Photograph of a carbon-fiber ankle-foot orthosis with weight-bearing brim, posterior carbon-fiber strut, and rigid foot plate. (Courtesy of Tillges Technologies, Maplewood, MN.)

commonplace for people living with above-ankle amputation.

Above-Ankle Prostheses

Above-ankle prostheses are usually only provided to people with proximal forefoot amputation (eg, Chopart amputation). These devices typically enclose the residuum and leg segment in a rigid socket, eliminating ankle motion (**Figure 4**). The socket is often bivalved to facilitate donning given the narrow dimension of the leg just proximal to the ankle, and the relatively bulbous distal residuum. Other design variants include a medial opening window or a built-up liner. The shape of the residuum and leg makes mechanical self-suspension of the prosthesis relatively simple.

Given the limited build height beneath the socket, a conventional prosthetic forefoot or a carbon-fiber foot plate is usually bonded directly to the socket to replace the missing forefoot. These foot plates are specific to prostheses for Chopart amputation given the difficulties creating a foot plate that is stiff enough to support body weight, and bonding it to the socket such that it will not fail under the large external moments applied during the late stance phase of walking.

As illustrated by a recent case series, the anterior shell of the socket can be designed to distribute a portion of the individual's weight away from the residuum and onto the leg.[36] This is often necessary given the small surface area of the remnant foot over which interface pressures can be comfortably distributed.[46]

Despite being able to restore the prosthetic forefoot lever during level ground walking,[38,46] clamshell-style above-ankle prostheses are not often favored by people with PFA[47] as it is difficult to obtain a slim and cosmetic prosthesis that easily fits into conventional footwear. It also may disrupt other activities such as stair climbing.[39] For many practitioners and prosthesis users, elimination of ankle motion by the socket seems counterproductive to the retention of the anatomic ankle joint. Prosthetic design variations that allow ankle motion (eg, separate foot and leg shells with external ankle joints) may be provided, acknowledging that there must be some mechanism to control ankle dorsiflexion during mid-to-late stance if the device is to also restore the effective foot length.[30]

Effectiveness

Increasing interest in the effectiveness of interventions for people living with PFA has led to a greater understanding of their benefits and limitations. Research in this area is best characterized as emerging, with much of the literature comprising small-scale, descriptive studies of what is observed when people with PFA wear various devices.[48] Although studies of this type are an important step toward experiments designed to demonstrate what these devices do, evidence gaps remain. Fortunately, these evidence gaps are increasingly the focus of research efforts, with some progress in recent years. This section aims to characterize the current evidence about interventions for people living with PFA, including what is currently known about gait, balance, plantar pressure, energy expenditure, community mobility, and HR-QoL. Areas that should become the focus of future research efforts are also highlighted.

Characterization of Gait, Balance, Energy Expenditure, and Plantar Pressure

Most of the research regarding function in people living with PFA has focused on laboratory-based measures of gait, balance, energy expenditure, and plantar pressure.

Regardless of the cause of amputation, people living with PFA present with a number of well-characterized gait anomalies[48] including reduced center of pressure (CoP) excursion beneath the residuum,[30,31,46,47,49] reduced ankle power on the amputated side,[49-52] and increased power generation at the affected and/or unaffected hips.[49] However, people with PFA secondary to diabetes and/or peripheral vascular disease walk at about two-thirds the velocity of their healthy counterparts.[48,53-57] Given that this reduction in walking speed is not observed in people with traumatic PFA,[31,49,58] it seems that the underlying systemic disease may dictate an individuals' walking speed. Although there do not seem to be any marked differences in walking speed between different levels of PFA, nor between different prosthetic and orthotic interventions,[48,49,59,60] there is a need for further research to confirm this understanding as most studies were not specifically designed to address these issues.

Retention of the metatarsal heads appears to be essential to generate ankle power (ie, push-off) in late stance.[49-52] Once the metatarsal heads are compromised, power generation at the ankle during gait is virtually negligible, regardless of residuum length or the type of prosthetic and orthotic intervention provided.[49,52,60-62] It has been hypothesized that the lack of ankle power generation may serve as a useful adaptation to avoid localized pressure on the distal end of the residuum or to reduce shear forces caused by ankle plantar flexor contraction.[49] Increased power at either or both hips is used to compensate for the lack of ankle power generation and contributes to a gait pattern that bears many similarities to that of persons with transtibial amputation (TTA).[29,48,63] This is true for level walking[38] and also likely for other activities such as stair ascent.[39]

Observational studies suggest that devices such as toe fillers, insoles, and slipper sockets do not allow the CoP to progress beyond the end of the residuum until after weight is shifted to the unaffected limb at contralateral heel contact.[31,49] However, devices that extend above the ankle, such as above-ankle prostheses or a BlueRocker ToeOff AFO, have been shown to normalize CoP excursion.[30,31,49] It has been hypothesized that the ability of a device to restore the effective foot length requires the following three design features: (1) a suitably stiff forefoot capable of supporting body mass, (2) a socket or anterior leg shell capable of comfortably distributing to the leg and remaining foot the interface pressures caused by loading the toe lever, and (3) a relatively stiff connection between the foot and leg segment to help moderate the moments caused by loading the toe lever.[46] Either a rigid ankle, a free joint with a dorsiflexion stop, or the sort of stiffness inherent in a BlueRocker ToeOff AFO may be appropriate to normalize CoP excursion.[30,31,47,48]

Few studies report on balance in people with PFA,[41,47,64] which limits confidence in the conflicting observations that have been drawn. One study reported that PFA compromised standing balance more than diabetic neuropathy alone, and to the same degree as TTA and diabetic foot ulceration.[64] This was based on an assessment of anterior-posterior CoP excursion and attributed to loss of ankle control. No changes were observed in medio-lateral CoP excursion, which is controlled primarily by the hip. Given that the risk of falling increases with diabetic neuropathy, and that balance was further compromised by PFA, balance training for people with PFA was recommended.[64] Another study reported no difference in dynamic balance during walking with below-ankle and above-ankle devices,[47] whereas another suggested improved balance confidence with bilateral custom carbon-fiber dynamic AFOs and device-specific training compared with toe fillers and cushioned shoes.[41]

Based on classic research showing a reduction in oxygen cost with decreasing levels of amputation,[65,66] it is often assumed that walking with a PFA is less energy expensive than walking with higher levels of lower limb amputation.[67-71] Although limited, the available evidence does not support this understanding, suggesting that energy expenditure is likely to be comparable in people with PFA and TTA.[53,59,72] This is not an unreasonable assertion given that, unlike groups with higher levels of amputation (ie, hip disarticulation, transfemoral and transtibial amputation), the mechanics of walking do not appreciably differ between people with TTA and PFA once the metatarsal heads have been compromised.[29] Assuming that people with different levels of PFA modify their walking speed to keep the rate of oxygen uptake within normal limits, like other groups with amputation, and given that walking speed is comparable between persons with PFA and TTA, net oxygen cost is also likely to be similar.[29]

In terms of plantar pressures, there is some indirect evidence that devices can redistribute pressure away from the distal end of the residuum to other parts of the foot or leg.[31,36,48,73] This is an important evidence gap given the high rate of complications in people with PFA.[29] There are similar evidence gaps describing which prosthetic and orthotic interventions are effective at minimizing the rate of complications, surgical revision, or more proximal amputation. Perhaps other factors, such as systemic health, vascular supply, and/or diabetic control, are more important to minimizing complications than any device that might be provided; or perhaps devices can be designed in the future that effectively mitigate these problems.

Community Mobility

Although the preceding evidence summary suggests that some understanding about the effect of PFA and prosthetic/orthotic intervention on gait, balance, energy expenditure, and plantar pressure has developed, it is not yet known whether these laboratory-based measures are important to the sorts of real-world outcomes that matter most to people with PFA.

The extent to which people living with PFA can achieve independent community mobility may arguably be important to prosthesis users. In studies that have monitored changes in community mobility over time, it was observed that only about one-third of people with PFA regained their pre-morbid level of community mobility 12 months after amputation.[74,75] For most people, the decline in mobility was akin to transitioning from independent walking to walking with a gait aid. Given these observations were similar between people with PFA and TTA, it seems reasonable to expect similar changes in community mobility between people with different levels of PFA.

Health-Related Quality of Life

A handful of studies have quantified HR-QoL in people living in the community with PFA.[76-79] Although these studies were not explicitly designed to illuminate differences in HR-QoL between cohorts living with different levels of PFA or different types of prosthetic/orthotic intervention, they suggest that neither amputation level nor prosthesis use explained significant variation in HR-QoL. The factors that seem to most influence HR-QoL reflect a broad range of demographic, health-related, and amputation-related factors such as older age, time living with diabetes, time since amputation, physical function, as well as the presence of depression, anxiety, fatigue, and altered sensation or pain interference.[76,77] There were complex interactions between many of these factors that influenced HR-QoL.[76] For example, although more frequent feelings of depression had a significant and negative effect on HR-QoL, the effect of depression was exacerbated in people who also experienced more frequent feelings of fatigue or anxiety.[14]

Clinical and Research Implications

As knowledge about PFA and the influence of prosthetic and orthotic interventions grows, many long-held beliefs become less certain. For example, PFA has long been viewed by health care professionals as a preferential surgical intervention compared with more proximal amputation given the belief that, if successful, PFA will lead to better outcomes.[80-82] However, the emerging evidence suggests that PFA leads to very similar outcomes compared with TTA—similar gait pattern, energy expenditure, community mobility, and HR-QoL—yet has a higher rate of serious complications, surgical revision, or more proximal amputation.[13] Additionally, for those people who experience reamputation on the same limb, the lived experience can be very difficult given that the foot complications that led to the initial PFA often endured until after TTA, where participants reported finally being able to get on with their lives.[83]

Innovations in prosthetic and orthotic interventions are needed to improve device effectiveness. By coupling the ability to innovate device design with the issues important to people living with PFA, it may be possible to arrive at more effective orthotic and prosthetic interventions as exemplified by the following two studies. For example, a case study of PFA due to trauma suggested that the use of a nonarticulated above-ankle prosthesis with vacuum-assisted suspension may be viable for improving comfort, function, and residual limb health.[84] It has also been proposed that indirect additive manufacturing can be used to improve the fabrication process for a customized silicone partial foot prosthesis.[85]

As knowledge about the effects of prosthetic and orthotic interventions grows, it is becoming clearer which aspects of gait can be normalised by different interventions. However, it is not clear whether normalizing gait is important to peoples' ability to mobilize in the community, participate in recreation and vocational pursuits, or restore premorbid HR-QoL. Similarly, there is little evidence describing whether the high rates of complications and reamputation can be affected through prosthetic and orthotic intervention.

Minimizing the high rates of complications and reamputation could be considered particularly important from both a personal and health-economic perspective. As an illustrative example of the personal impact, people with PFA describe a persistent and pervasive fear about the prospect of further amputation that was not reported for people living with other levels of lower limb amputation.[86] This experience may be a contributor to the depression and anxiety reported by people living with PFA.[86] From a health-economic perspective, the burden is staggering when considering that only around half of all PFA heal adequately[71,87] and that efforts to achieve wound healing after PFA occur over many months and cost between USD$27,000 to $36,000 per person.[88] As an illustrative example, it is estimated that in the United States the cost of providing wound care following PFA exceeds USD$600 million per annum based on a modest incidence rate and the proportion of people requiring secondary amputation.[1,13] When the cost of secondary amputation surgery is included,[89] this figure would exceed USD$1 billion per annum.

Although research focused on minimizing the rates of complications and reamputation may seem self-evident, there is a compelling need to understand the problems that are most important to people living with PFA. Collaborating with people who have a lived experience of PFA might help to address the most important problems. For example, many researchers and clinicians focused on device effectiveness might intuitively look to evaluate which prosthetic/orthotic interventions are most effective at minimizing the risk of complications and reamputation. However, a more thoughtful approach grounded in interviews with people living with PFA, highlight opportunities to address system-level barriers such as the ability to get a timely and convenient appointment with a knowledgeable specialist, or provide access to inexpensive transport that does not consume a whole day to attend an appointment.[90] Weighing up the merit of these different avenues of research is a real challenge if the desire is to have the greatest impact for those living with PFA. Hence why it is so important to increasingly look to collaborate with end users in the design of future research.

SUMMARY

As knowledge about PFA and the effect of prosthetic and orthotic intervention grows, it is becoming clearer what clinicians can expect from current treatments, and which evidence gaps require further research. With a greater understanding of the needs of people living with PFA, it will be easier to focus innovations and research efforts to ensure that prosthetic and orthotic interventions can effectively meet the needs of those living with PFA.

Acknowledgments

The authors acknowledge and thank the following clinical services that provided images of the devices included in this chapter: APC Prosthetics, Sydney, Australia; the Prosthetics and Orthotics Department, Royal Melbourne Hospital, Melbourne, Australia; Tillges Technologies, Maplewood, USA; and Hanger Clinic, Texas, USA.

References

1. Dillon MP, Quigley M, Fatone S: A systematic review describing incidence rate and prevalence of dysvascular partial foot amputation; how both have changed over time and compare to transtibial amputation. *Syst Rev* 2017;6:230.
2. van Battum P, Schaper N, Prompers L, et al: Differences in minor amputation rate in diabetic foot disease throughout Europe are in part explained by differences in disease severity at presentation. *Diabet Med* 2011;28:199-205.

3. Griffiths GD, Wieman TJ: Meticulous attention to foot care improves the prognosis in diabetic ulceration of the foot. *Surg Gynecol Obstet* 1992;174:49-51.
4. Kuo S, Fleming BB, Gittings NS, et al: Trends in care practices and outcomes among medicare beneficiaries with diabetes. *Am J Prev Med* 2005;29:396-403.
5. Hinchliffe R, Andros G, Apelqvist J, et al: A systematic review of the effectiveness of revascularization of the ulcerated foot in patients with diabetes and peripheral arterial disease. *Diabetes Metab Res Rev* 2012;28:179-217.
6. Larsson J, Apelqvist J, Agardh C, et al: Decreasing incidence of major amputation in diabetic patients: A consequence of a multidisciplinary foot care team approach? *Diabet Med* 1995;12:770-776.
7. Mobasseri M, Shirmohammadi M, Amiri T, et al: Prevalence and incidence of type 1 diabetes in the world: A systematic review and meta-analysis. *Health Promot Perspect* 2020;10:98-115.
8. Magliano DJ, Islam RM, Barr ELM, et al: Trends in incidence of total or type 2 diabetes: Systematic review. *Br Med J* 2019;366:l5003.
9. Dillon MP, Kohler F, Peever V: Incidence of lower extremity amputation in Australian hospitals from 2000-2010. *Prosthet Orthot Int* 2014;38:122-132.
10. van Houtum WH, Rauwerda JA, Ruwaard D, et al: Reduction in diabetes-related lower-extremity amputations in the Netherlands: 1991-2000. *Diabetes Care* 2004;27:1042-1046.
11. Driver VR, Madsen J, Goodman RA: Reducing amputation rates in patients with diabetes at a military medical centre: The limb preservation model. *Diabetes Care* 2005;28:248-253.
12. Tseng C, Rajan M, Miller DR, et al: Trends in initial lower extremity amputation rates among Veterans Health Administration Health Care system users from 2000-2004. *Diabetes Care* 2011;34:1157-1163.
13. Dillon MP, Quigley M, Fatone S: Outcomes of dysvascular partial foot amputation and how these compare to transtibial amputation: A systematic review for the development of shared decision-making resources. *Syst Rev* 2017;6:54.
14. Czerniecki JM, Turner AP, Williams RM, et al: The development and validation of the AMPREDICT model for predicting mobility outcome after dysvascular lower extremity amputation. *J Vasc Surg* 2017;65:162-171.e3.
15. Bowker J: Partial foot amputations and disarticulations: Surgical aspects. *J Prosthet Orthot* 2007;19:P62-P76.
16. Tang P, Ravji K, Key JJ, et al: Let then walk! Current prosthesis options for leg and foot amputees. *J Am Coll Surg* 2008;206:548-560.
17. Barry D, Sabacinski K, Habershaw G, et al: Tendo Achillis procedures for chronic ulcerations in diabetic patients with transmetatarsal amputations. *J Am Podiatr Med Assoc* 1993;83:96-100.
18. Sage R: Biomechanics of ampulation after partial foot amputation: Prevention and management of reulceration. *J Prosthet Orthot* 2007;19:77-79.
19. Armstrong DG, Lavery LA: Plantar pressures are higher in diabetic patients following partial foot amputation. *Ostomy Wound Manage* 1998;44:30-32.
20. Lavery LA, Lavery DC, Quebedeax-Farnham TL: Increased foot pressures after great toe amputation in diabetes. *Diabetes Care* 1995;18:1460-1462.
21. Mueller MJ, Strube MJ, Allen BT: Therapeutic footwear can reduce plantar pressures in patients with diabetes and transmetatarsal amputation. *Diabetes Care* 1997;20:637-641.
22. Quigley M, Dillon MP, Fatone S: Development of shared decision-making resources to help inform difficult healthcare decisions: An example focused on dysvascular partial foot and transtibial amputations. *Prosthet Orthot Int* 2018;42:378-386.
23. Dillon MP, Fatone S, Quigley M, et al: *Amputation Decision Aid* 2021. https://www.amputationdecisionaid.com. Accessed October 9, 2021.
24. Norvell DC, Suckow BD, Webster JB, et al: The development and usability of the AMPREDICT decision support tool: A mixed methods study. *Eur J Vasc Endovasc Surg* 2021;62:304-311.
25. Centre for Limb Loss and Mobility: AMPREDICT – decision support tool 2021. Accessed September 4, 2021. https://www.ampredict.org/
26. Soderberg B, Wykman A, Schaarschuch R, et al: *Partial Foot Amputations: Guidelines to Prosthetic and Surgical Techniques*, ed 2. Centre for Partial Foot Amputees, 2001.
27. Berke G, Rheinstein J, Michael J, et al: Biomechanics of ambulation following partial foot amputation: A prosthetic perspective. *J Prosthet Orthot* 2007;19:85-88.
28. Moore JW: Prostheses, orthoses, and shoes for partial foot amputees. *Clin Podiatr Med Surg* 1997;14:775-783.
29. Dillon MP, Fatone S: Deliberations about the functional benefits and complications of partial foot amputation: Do we pay heed to the purported benefits at the expense of minimizing complications? *Arch Phys Med Rehabil* 2013;94:1429-1435.
30. Dillon MP, Fatone S, Hansen AH: Effect of prosthetic design on centre of pressure excursion in partial foot prostheses. *J Rehabil Res Dev* 2011;48:161-178.
31. Wilson E, Dillon MP: Restoring centre of pressure excursion using toe-off orthoses in a single partial foot amputee, in Dillon MP, Hodge MC, eds. *Annual Scientific Meeting of ISPO Australia*. Carlton Crest Hotel, Sydney, DCConferences, 2005, pp 31-32.
32. Yonclas PP, O'Donnell CJ: Prosthetic management of the partial foot amputee. *Clin Podiatr Med Surg* 2005;22:485-502.
33. Crowe CS, Impastato KA, Donaghy AC, et al: Prosthetic and orthotic options for lower extremity amputation and reconstruction. *Plast Aesthetic Res* 2019;6:4.
34. Sahu SK, Behera M, Sumithra K: Integrated Ankle Foot Orthosis (AFO) with silicone foot prosthesis in the management of partial foot amputation-a case study. *Int J Health Sci Res* 2020;10:383-387.
35. Janarthani P, Panda CS, Behura SK: Prosthetic management of partial foot amputation (Trans-metatarsal foot)-a case study. *Int J Health Sci Res* 2020;10:320-323.
36. Kaib T, Block J, Heitzmann D, et al: O 012—A biomechanical approach to estimate the moment distributed to the shank by partial foot prosthesis with a ventral leg shell. *Gait Posture* 2018;65:21-22.
37. Zarezadeh F, Arazpour M, Bahramizadeh M, et al: Design and construction of a new partial foot prosthesis based on high-pressure points in a patient with diabetes with transmetatarsal amputation: A technical note. *J Prosthet Orthot* 2018;30:108-113.
38. Kaib T, Block J, Heitzmann D, et al: Prosthetic restoration of the forefoot lever after Chopart amputation and its consequences onto the limb during gait. *Gait Posture* 2019;73:1-7.
39. Kaib T, Schäfer J, Block J, et al: Biomechanical analysis of stair ascent in persons with Chopart amputation. *Prosthet Orthot Int* 2020;44:164-171.
40. Young J: Impact of orthotic prescription in pediatric partial foot amputation: A case study. *J Prosthet Orthot* 2019;31:76-80.

41. Anderson KM, Evans RE, Connerly CE, et al: Custom dynamic orthoses and physical therapist intervention for bilateral midfoot amputation: A case report. *Phys Ther* 2021;101:pzab028.
42. Guo J-C, Wang L-Z, Chen W, et al: Parametric study of orthopedic insole of valgus foot on partial foot amputation. *Comput Methods Biomech Biomed Eng* 2016;19:894-900.
43. Sam M, Childress D, Hansen A, et al: The Shape&Roll prosthetic foot (part 1): Design and development of appropriate technology for low-income coutries. *Med Confl Surviv* 2004;20:294-306.
44. Zarezadeh F, Arazpour M, Bahramizadeh M, et al: Comparing the effect of new silicone foot prosthesis and conventional foot prosthesis on plantar pressure in diabetic patients with transmetatarsal amputation. *Arch Rehabil* 2019;20:124-135.
45. Khaghani A, Takamjani IE, Layeghi F: Tehran silicon partial foot prosthesis new method of making silicon partial foot prosthesis. *Int J Adv Biotechnol Res* 2016;7:2045-2057.
46. Dillon MP, Barker TM: Can partial foot prostheses effectively restore foot length? *Prosthet Orthot Int* 2006;30:17-23.
47. Spaulding SE, Chen T, Chou LS: Selection of an above or below-ankle orthosis for individuals with neuropathic partial foot amputation: A pilot study. *Prosthet Orthot Int* 2012;36:217-224.
48. Dillon MP, Fatone S, Hodge MC: Biomechanics of ambulation after partial foot amputation: A systematic literature review. *J Prosthet Orthot* 2007;19:2-61.
49. Dillon MP, Barker T: Comparison of gait of persons with partial foot amputation wearing prosthesis to matched control group: An observational study. *J Rehabil Res Dev* 2008;45:1335-1342.
50. Dillon MP, Barker TM: Preservation of residual foot length in partial foot amputation: A biomechanical analysis. *Foot Ankle Int* 2006;27:110-116.
51. Mueller MJ, Salsich GB, Bastian AJ: Differences in the gait characteristics of people with diabetes and transmetatarsal amputation compared with age-matched controls. *Gait Posture* 1998;7:200-206.
52. Tang SFT, Chen CPC, Chen MJL, et al: Transmetatarsal amputation prosthesis with carbon-fiber plate: Enhanced gait function. *Am J Phys Med Rehabil* 2004;83:124-130.
53. Kanade RV, van Deursen RWM, Harding K, et al: Walking performance in people with diabetic neuropathy: Benefits and threats. *Diabetologia* 2006;49:1747-1754.
54. Mueller MJ, Salsich GB, Strube MJ: Functional limitations in patients with diabetes and transmetatarsal amputations. *Phys Ther* 1997;77:937-943.
55. Boyd LA, Rao SS, Burnfield JM, et al: Forefoot rocker mechanisms in individuals with partial foot amputation, in *Gait and Clinical Movement Analysis*. Gait and Posture, 1999, p 144.
56. Burnfield JM, Boyd LA, Rao SS, et al: The effect of partial foot amputation on sound limb loading force during barefoot walking, in *Gait and Clinical Movement Analysis*. Gait and Posture, 1998, pp 178-179.
57. Kelly VE, Mueller MJ, Sinacore DR: Timing of peak plantar pressure during the stance phase of walking: A study of patients with diabetes mellitus and transmetatarsal amputation. *J Am Podiatr Med Assoc* 2000;90:18-23.
58. Greene WB, Cary JM: Partial foot amputations in children. A comparison of several types with the Syme amputation. *J Bone Joint Surg Am* 1982;64:438-443.
59. Pinzur MS, Gold J, Schwartz D, et al: Energy demands for walking in dysvascular amputees as related to the level of amputation. *Orthopedics* 1992;15:1033-1036.
60. Burger H, Erzar D, Maver T, et al: Biomechanics of walking with silicone prosthesis after midtarsal (Chopart) disarticulation. *Clin Biomech (Bristol, Avon)* 2009;24:510-516.
61. Brown M, Tang W, Patel A, et al: Partial foot amputation in patients with diabetic foot ulcers. *Foot Ankle Int* 2012;33:707-717.
62. Rubin G: Indications for variants of the partial foot prosthesis. *Orthop Rev* 1985;14:688-695.
63. Dillon M, Fatone S, Morris M: Partial foot amputation may not always be worth the risk of complications. *Med J Aust* 2014;200:252-253.
64. Kanade R, Van Deursen R, Harding K, et al: Invesigation of standing balance in patients with diabetic neuropathy at different stages of foot complications. *Clin Biomech (Bristol, Avon)* 2008;23:1183-1191.
65. Waters RL, Mulroy S: The energy expenditure of normal and pathological gait. *Gait Posture* 1999;9:207-231.
66. Waters RL, Perry J, Antonelli D, et al: Energy cost of walking of amputees: The influence of level of amputation. *J Bone Joint Surg* 1976;58:42-46.
67. Elsharawy MA: Outcome of midfoot amputations in diabetic gengrene. *Ann Vasc Surg* 2011;25:778-782.
68. Wallace GF, Stapleton JJ: Transmetatarsal amputations. *Clin Podiatr Med Surg* 2005;22:365-384.
69. Geertzen JHB, Jutte P, Rompen C, et al: Calcanectomy, an alternative amputation? Two case reports. *Prosthet Orthot Int* 2009;33:78-81.
70. Sobel E, Japour CJ, Giorgini RJ, et al: Use of prostheses and footwear in 110 inner-city partial-foot amputees. *J Am Podiatr Med Assoc* 2001;91:34-49.
71. Pollard J, Hamilton GA, Rush SM, et al: Mortality and morbidity after transmetatarsal amputation: Retrospective review of 101 cases. *J Foot Ankle Surg* 2006;45:91-97.
72. Goktepe AS, Cakir B, Yilmaz B, et al: Energy expenditure of walking with prostheses: Comparison of three amputation levels. *Prosthet Orthot Int* 2010;34:31-36.
73. El-Hilaly R, Elshazly O, Amer A: The role of a total contact insole in diminishing foot pressures following partial first ray amputation in diabetic patients. *Foot* 2013;23:6-10.
74. Czerniecki J, Turner A, Williams R, et al: Mobility changes in individuals with dysvascular amputation from the presurgical period to 12 months postamputation. *Arch Phys Med Rehabil* 2012;93:1766-1773.
75. Norvell D, Turner A, Williams R, et al: Defining successful mobility after lower extremity amputation for complications of peripheral vascular disease and diabetes. *J Vasc Surg* 2011;54:412-419.
76. Dillon MP, Quigley M, Stevens P, et al: Factors associated with health-related quality of life in people living with partial foot or transtibial amputation. *Arch Phys Med Rehabil* 2020;101:1711-1719.
77. Quigley M, Dillon M, Duke E: Comparison of quality of life in people with partial foot and transtibial amputation: A pilot study. *Prosthet Orthot Int* 2016;40:467-474.
78. Boutoille D, Feraille A, Maulaz D, et al: Quality of life with diabetes-associated foot complications: Comparison between lower-limb amputation and chronic foot ulceration. *Foot Ankle Int* 2008;29:1074-1078.
79. Peters EJ, Childs MR, Wunderlich RP, et al: Functional status of persons with diabetes-related lower-extremity amputations. *Diabetes Care* 2001;24:1799-1804.
80. Landry GJ, Silverman DA, Liem TK, et al: Predictors of healing and functional outcome following transmetatarsal amputation. *Arch Surg* 2011;146:1005-1009.

81. Dudkiewicz I, Schwarz O, Heim M, et al: Trans-metatarsal amputation in patients with diabetic foot: Reviewing 10 years experience. *Foot* 2009;19:201-204.

82. McCallum R, Tagoe M: Transmetatarsal amputation: A case series and review of literature. *J Aging Res* 2012;2012:797218.

83. Dillon MP, Anderson SP, Duke EJ, et al: The lived experience of sequential partial foot and transtibial amputation. *Disabil Rehabil* 2020;42:2106-2114.

84. Arndt B, Caldwell R, Fatone S: Use of a partial foot prosthesis with vacuum-assisted suspension: A case study. *J Prosthet Orthot* 2011;23:82-88.

85. Abdelaal O, Darwish S, Abd Elmougoud K, et al: A new methodology for design and manufacturing of a customized silicone partial foot prosthesis using indirect additive manufacturing. *Int J Artif Organs* 2019;42:645-657.

86. Livingstone W, Mortel TF, Taylor B: A path of perpetual resilience: Exploring the experience of a diabetes-related amputation through grounded theory. *Contemp Nurse* 2011;39:20-30.

87. Stone PA, Back MR, Armstrong PA, et al: Midfoot amputations expand limb salvage rates for diabetic foot infections. *Ann Vasc Surg* 2005;19:805-811.

88. Apelqvist J, Armstrong DG, Lavery LA, et al: Resource utilization and economic cost of case based on a randomized trial of vacuum-assisted closure therapy in the treatment of diabetic foot wounds. *Am J Surg* 2008;195:782-788.

89. Ragnarson Tennvall G, Apelqvist J: Health-economic consequences of diabetic foot lesions. *Clin Infect Dis* 2004;39:S132-S139.

90. Littman AJ, Young J, Moldestad M, et al: How patients interpret early signs of foot problems and reasons for delays in care: Findings from interviews with patients who have undergone toe amputations. *PLoS One* 2021;16:e0248310.

Ankle Disarticulation and Variants: Surgical Management

CHAPTER 36

LTC Tobin Thomas Eckel, MD, FAAOS • Scott B. Shawen, MD

ABSTRACT

Advancements in transtibial amputation techniques and prostheses have led to decreased use of ankle disarticulation. However, these distal amputations are still a viable option in select circumstances. They are most commonly used in diabetic infection, nonhealing ulcers, deformity, and trauma. Advantages include earlier weight bearing, decreased dependence on prosthetics, and decreased energy expenditure with ambulation. Common complications include delayed wound healing, infection, and heel pad migration.

Keywords: ankle disarticulation; Boyd amputation; Pirogoff amputation; Syme amputation

Introduction

With recent advancements in transtibial prostheses and the concern for wound healing with more distal amputations, the ankle disarticulation has fallen somewhat out of favor, but still remains a viable option in select patients. The ankle disarticulation is commonly referred to as a Syme amputation, as James Syme is credited with first describing this amputation in 1843.[1,2] Transtibial amputations account for nearly 25% of all lower extremity amputations, whereas only 10% of all lower extremity amputations are performed about the foot and ankle.[3]

At the time Syme described his novel amputation, he stated the advantages of his described disarticulation were: "the risk of life will be smaller, that a more comfortable stump will be afforded, and that the limb will be more seemly and useful for progressive motion."[4] These claims remain largely unchallenged today. The mortality rate with ankle disarticulation has been reported as 33% at 5 years compared with 33% at 2 years with transtibial amputation.[5] Some have attributed the decreased mortality to decreased blood loss and the ability to perform under regional anesthesia.[6] This decreased mortality must be tempered by the high failure rate of ankle disarticulation, with revision rates ranging between 20% and 50%.[7]

The Syme amputation is considered to be more comfortable because the heel pad is preserved. The heel pad contains fat cells enclosed by dense fibrous septae, which allows for direct weight bearing. The preservation of the heel pad therefore affords end weight bearing without a prosthetic.[1,3-5] Although the ability to bear direct weight without a prosthetic is a significant advantage, it is important to realize that the weight is absorbed by a single bony surface, compared with an entire foot that consists of a multitude of joints and surrounding musculature that is specialized to bear weight and adapt to uneven surfaces. For these reasons, weight bearing without a prosthetic is typically limited to very short distances.[2,8] Nonetheless, the ability to end weightbear and simplicity of prosthetic fitting can lead to decreased length of rehabilitation and negate the need for long-term inpatient care following amputation.[9] Furthermore, the ability to end weightbear is very important when considering prosthetic design. The Syme amputation allows for sockets to function in suspension, whereas transtibial sockets bear weight by indirect load transfer, and thus with any volume changes in the residual limb, the socket would need to be revised to prevent any tissue breakdown.[2]

Last, Syme's claim was "that the limb would be more seemly and useful for progressive motion." Many would argue against an ankle disarticulation being a cosmetically pleasing amputation, as the residual limb tends to be bulbous and early prostheses were considered unsightly.[10] The malleoli are

---

Dr. Shawen or an immediate family member has received royalties from CrossRoads and Medline and serves as a paid consultant to or is an employee of CrossRoads, KCI, Medline, Panther Orthopaedics, and Restore 3D/Kinos. Neither Dr. Eckel nor any immediate family member has received anything of value from or has stock or stock options held in a commercial company or institution related directly or indirectly to the subject of this chapter.

This chapter is adapted from Eckel TT, Chi BB, Shawen SB. Ankle disarticulation and variants: surgical management. In: Krajbich JI, Pinzur MS, Potter BK, Stevens PM, eds. *Atlas of Amputations and Limb Deficiencies: Surgical, Prosthetic, and Rehabilitation Principles*. 4th ed. American Academy of Orthopaedic Surgeons, 2016, pp 473-477.

trimmed to help decrease the size of the residual limb both for cosmetic reasons as well as to facilitate prosthetic fitting.[8] Nonetheless, this amputation is more useful for locomotion, as there is an increased mechanical efficiency, which leads to a decreased metabolic cost of ambulation. The mechanical benefit is a result of a full-length prosthetic foot that provides a normal lever arm for push-off. The use of an energy storage and return prosthetic foot can further improve gait and walking speed while decreasing metabolic demand.[2,11] The decrease in energy expenditure to ambulate is particularly advantageous in patients with diabetes, who generally have poorer baseline health and would be less likely to ambulate with a transtibial prosthesis.[3]

Indications

The indications for ankle disarticulation are diabetic infection, trauma, nonhealing diabetic and/or dysvascular ulcers, Charcot arthropathy, crush injury, frostbite, and congenital malformations, with the most common being diabetic infection. This results in two distinct patient populations: children with congenital anomalies and adults with vascular and/or immune compromise.[12] Approximately 7% of the US population has diabetes, and the incidence of amputation is increased 10-fold in these patients. In fact, patients with diabetes account for over two-thirds of all lower extremity amputations. Of course, the prerequisite for ankle disarticulation in all the aforementioned etiologies is a preserved heel pad with adequate blood flow. Therefore, the only absolute contraindication to an ankle disarticulation is a compromised heel pad, which may be the result of inadequate blood flow, infection, or soft-tissue loss.[1,5]

Unfortunately, this patient population often has decreased perfusion, and a major challenge is determining which patients have enough arterial flow to be able to heal an amputation at such a distal level. Many of these patients lack a palpable posterior tibial pulse, in which case the ankle-brachial index can be measured. Typically an ankle-brachial index of 0.5 or greater would indicate adequate flow, although patients with diabetes often have calcified arteries that may falsely elevate the ankle-brachial index. Another perhaps more accurate assessment of perfusion is measuring the transcutaneous partial pressure of oxygen, with values between 20 and 30 mm Hg indicative of adequate perfusion necessary for tissue healing.[1,3] Other laboratory tests have long been used to help predict tissue healing capacity, including a serum albumin of at least 2.5 g/dL, and a total lymphocyte count of greater than 1,500 mm^3. Although healing rates have been reported as low as 50%, studies have shown that when all the aforementioned criteria are met, healing rates can be as high as 88%.[13,14] Ultimately, if concerns about blood flow persist, a vascular surgery consult is warranted with options to include angioplasty or even bypass to increase perfusion. Others advocate for ankle disarticulation as a staged amputation before definitive transtibial amputation. Particularly in diabetic foot infection, a staged approach allows for source control of the infection and appropriate resuscitation before definitive amputation. This approach has been shown to decrease the risk of revision transfemoral amputation when compared with single-stage amputation[15] (**Figures 1** and **2**).

Surgical Technique

The patient is placed supine with a thigh tourniquet. An anterior fishmouth incision is made with the apices located at the anterior midpoints of the malleoli. The incision is carried sharply to bone, although any peroneal or saphenous nerve branches should be cut under tension to allow retraction and prevent symptomatic neuroma formation at the level of the incision. Next subperiosteal dissection and removal of the talus and calcaneus is performed, with care not to violate the posterior skin or the heel pad, or damage the posterior tibial vasculature, which is essential for heel pad perfusion. Dissection can be facilitated by use of a large bone hook on the talus and subsequently calcaneus to forcefully plantarflex the foot and put the soft tissues on stretch.[2,5,14] A traction bow can also be used with a

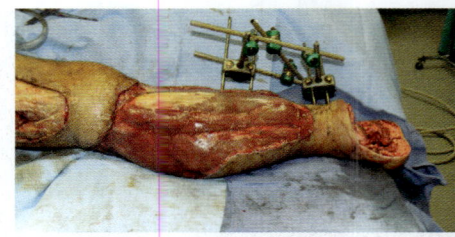

FIGURE 1 Clinical photograph from a patient who sustained severe lower extremity injury from an explosion. The severity of the injury in the midfoot and forefoot prevented salvage. To preserve the optimal length of the residual limb and provide stable soft-tissue coverage, a Syme amputation was planned. The distal fishmouth incision with removal of the talus and calcaneus has been performed at this stage.

pin through the talus, with the advantage over a bone hook of not requiring manual traction and perhaps improving surgical visualization.[16]

Next, the malleolar flares are removed at the level of the tibial articular surface. This narrows the residual limb, making less bulbous and more cosmetically pleasing, and it also provides a broad surface of metaphyseal bone for the soft tissues to adhere to, helping to secure the flap.[8] The heel pad is then secured to the anterior tibia through drill holes to help prevent heel pad migration. It has also been described to secure the Achilles tendon to the posterior tibia as well to help secure the heel pad in place. Additional techniques to prevent heel pad migration, particularly varus migration, include tenodesis of the peroneal tendons to the lateral heel pad, or securing the lateral band of the plantar fascia to the lateral aspect of the tibia.[2,6,14,17] Suction drains are optional before closure and cast application. Interval casting is continued until the wound is healed and the residual limb volume has stabilized.[5,14] (**Figures 3** through **5**).

Outcomes

Historically, outcomes after ankle disarticulation were poor, particularly in patients with diabetes, often with failure requiring revision within the first year ranging from 20% to 50% of patients.[7,18] However, the level of the amputation, whether it be an ankle

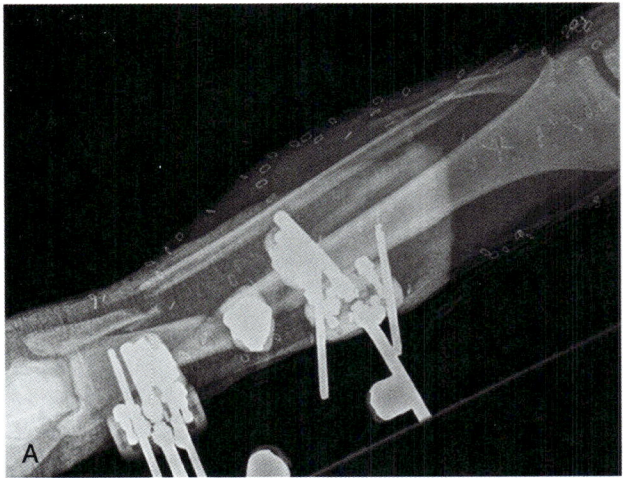
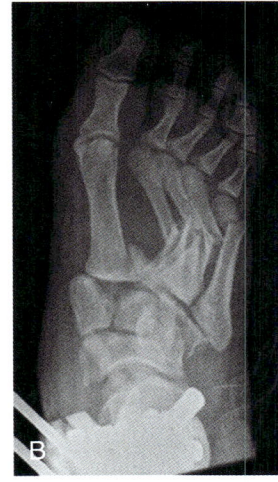

FIGURE 2 Initial AP radiographs of tibia/fibula (**A**) and foot (**B**) from the patient depicted in **Figure 1**. The severity of the injury is reflected in the segmental comminution and the multiple fractures and dislocations in the midfoot and forefoot. The soft tissue surrounding the mid was severely compromised and ultimately nonviable, precluding salvage. Large soft-tissue and skin defects over the mid and proximal tibia prevented a primary transtibial amputation.

disarticulation or an amputation more distal in the limb, does not affect the reamputation or revision rates to a higher level.[18] Many patients undergoing this irreversible operation have multiple comorbidities and conditions that influence these outcomes.

More recent data refute the previous finding and outcomes and highlight the success of this procedure now and in the past. In a 2003 retrospective review by Pinzur et al,[14] a 90% success rate was reported after Syme amputation in patients with diabetes. These improved outcomes are likely due to more careful patient selection, ensuring adequate arterial flow and sufficient nutrition parameters before surgery. Another study from the same surgeon demonstrated success across not only patient population with diabetes but also trauma and oncologic patients without diabetes, with low revision rates to higher levels of amputation. These patients also required less rehabilitation and achieved improved levels of functional independence as demonstrated by multiple indices.[9] Multiple modifications over the years as mentioned previously have resulted in improved outcomes. Through these modifications, some authors conclude that ankle disarticulation is an excellent procedure in multiple patient populations.[19]

In the pediatric population, the condition of fibular hemimelia, a congenital disorder characterized by the partial or complete absence of the fibula, tibial growth inhibition, and foot and ankle deformity and deficiency, is the most common deficiency of long bones. Ankle disarticulation is a common treatment among this population. In studies comparing Syme amputation with limb reconstruction or bracing techniques, Syme amputation was found to be either noninferior or superior to other treatments.[20,21] Also, in this population it was found that limb length discrepancy, or a shorter amputated limb, had a positive effect on outcomes because of ease of prosthetic fitting and function. The ability to ambulate without a prosthetic in this group was more dependent on the type of flooring (softer), but decreases with advancing age.[22]

The most common early complication is delayed wound healing or infection, which occurs around 25% of the time, but can most often be managed with local wound care. Heel pad migration is the most common late complication, occurring in approximately 30% of patients.[2,14]

Complications vary based on patient population. In children, the most common complications are heel pad migration and bone overgrowth. In adults, however, the most common complications include infection, phantom limb pain, and revision amputation. Nearly 100% of children are fitted with a prosthesis, compared with

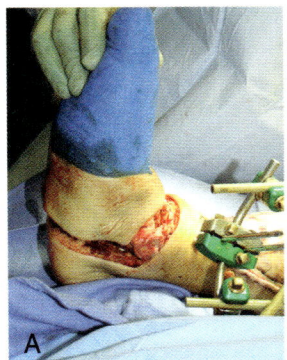
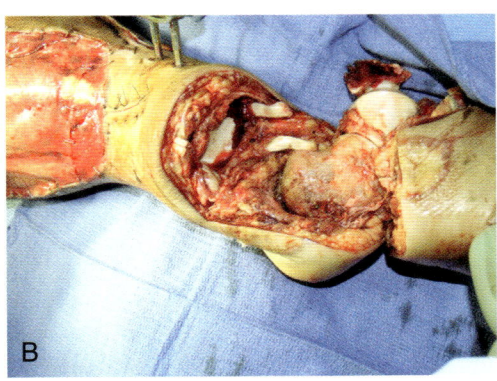
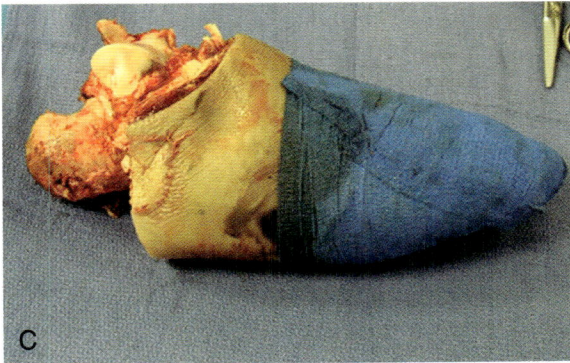

FIGURE 3 Intraoperative photographs showing that disarticulation can be performed sharply under tourniquet. Incision of skin and fascia is carried straight through to the capsule. Major vessels are ligated with suture ties. Traction neurectomy of major identified nerves is performed while the talus is disarticulated and calcaneus removed. The final disarticulated foot. **A**, Skin incision. **B**, Completion of the amputation, and **C**, disarticulated foot.

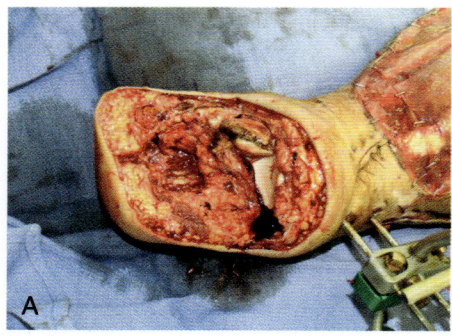
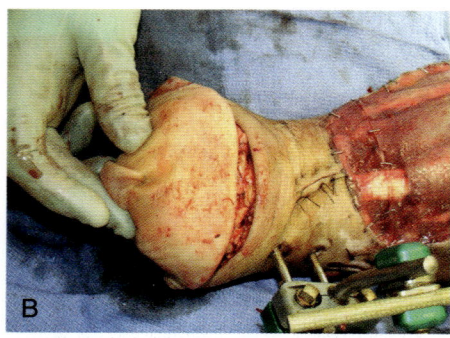

FIGURE 4 Intraoperative photographs demonstrating planned soft-tissue coverage. The talus and calcaneus have been removed. Tibial articular cartilage can be seen at the distal end. The lateral malleolus is seen here but will be resected to provide an even surface for weight bearing. The proposed position of closure allows viable fat pad of the heel to provide a cushioned surface. **A**, Posterior flap exposed. **B**, Planned skin closure.

68% of adults, and only 40% of adults reported being able to end weightbear on their residual limb. In contrast, all children reported being able to end weightbear.[12] There is a paucity of long-term outcome data in this patient population secondary to the high mortality rate. For patients with diabetes undergoing transtibial amputation, the two-year mortality rate is reported around 30%. Similar rates have been reported in patients with diabetes undergoing Syme amputation, with 4-year mortality increasing to around 50%.[12]

Ankle disarticulation still affords several advantages over higher amputation levels to include earlier weight bearing; minimal prosthetic gait training; improved gait velocity, cadence, and stride length; and less energy expenditure and cardiovascular demand with ambulation. These patients also have a decreased 5-year mortality rate compared with transtibial and transfemoral amputees.[3,13] Another commonly cited advantage with the Syme amputation is the ability to end weightbear without a prosthetic. Although this in fact may only be for short distances, as many as 70% of all ankle disarticulations are able to end weightbear at home[7] (**Figure 6**).

Alternate Hindfoot Amputations

Previously described methods of ankle disarticulation refer to a soft-tissue procedure. In methods such as the Boyd or Pirogoff modifications, calcaneal bone stock is retained and fused to the distal tibial residual limb. This method provides several advantages over ankle disarticulation without osteoplasty. Preservation of calcaneal bone preserves greater length and prevents subluxation of the heel pad if osseous union is obtained.[23] In low-demand patients, this allows for the use of very rudimentary prostheses. Although the Boyd amputation was originally described in the adult population, it is increasingly used in children. These amputations provide more heel pad stabilization, improved proprioception, better prosthetic fitting, and increased end weight bearing, which are all critical in the pediatric population.[24]

The technique of the osteoplasty modification is only slightly different from the traditional Syme. In the Boyd modification, the talus and anterior calcaneus is removed, as well as the calcaneal surface of the subtalar joint. Tibiofibular and tibiocalcaneal fusion is then performed.[25] The Pirogoff modification excises the anterior two-thirds of the calcaneus, and the residual calcaneal fragment, with the Achilles tendon attached, is rotated and fixed distally to the tibia. The advantage of calcaneal rotation is that limb length is preserved.[23,26] Fixation of the bone and heel pad fragment has been described in several different modalities including Ilizarov-type frames and internal fixation with compression screws in a crossed configuration.[27]

Indications for use of the Boyd or Pirogoff remain the same as the Syme. However, use of this method requires healthy osseous and soft tissue at the calcaneus. Clinical results are dependent on union of the calcaneal and tibial fragments. Outcomes following use of these modifications have borne out worse rates of union and healing in those performed for vascular disease and diabetes than those performed for trauma. It is therefore recommended that thorough assessment of the overall[23] clinical status of the patient be undertaken before proceeding. The most common reported complications include wound dehiscence, infection, and tibiocalcaneal nonunion.[24]

Postoperatively, these techniques are treated the same as a Syme but allow for fitting of an elephant boot to allow distal weight bearing with minimal loss of leg length. In areas where more sophisticated shoe prosthesis may not be available, this provides a viable alternative.

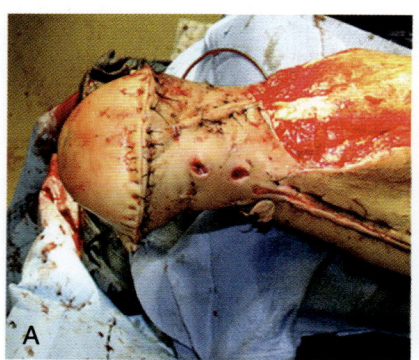
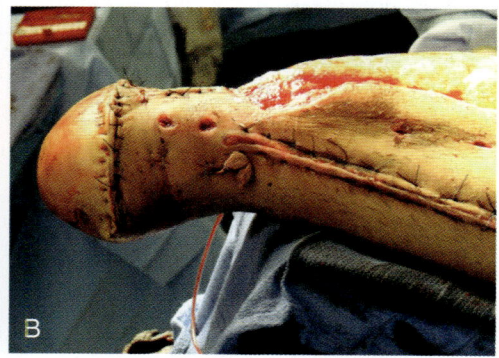

FIGURE 5 Intraoperative photographs showing the completed closure, with a vacuum-sealed drain. Tension-free closure and dead-space minimalization prevents wound complications. With time and prosthetic fitting, atrophy of the distal soft tissues will result in a well-formed, stable amputation. **A**, Anterior photograph of final closure. **B**, Lateral photograph of final closure.

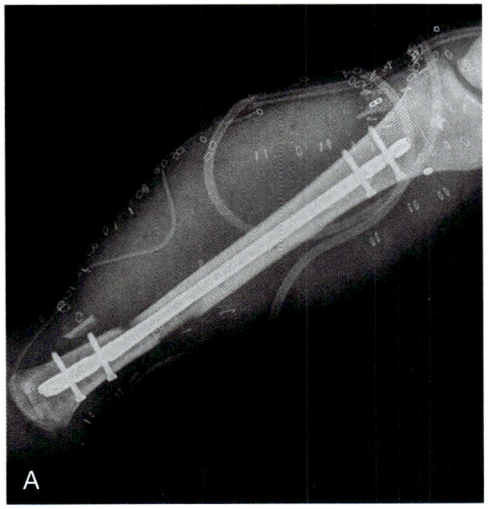
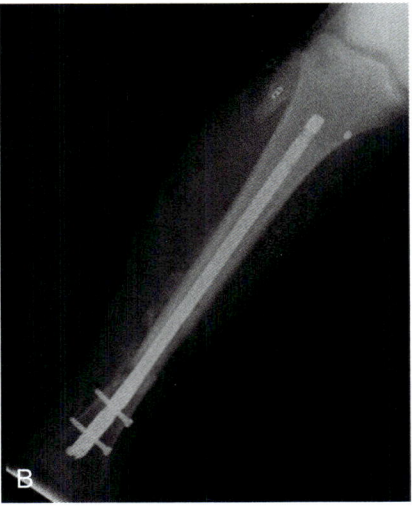

FIGURE 6 Immediate postoperative AP radiographs and follow-up depicting the interval healing of the residual limb. Additional procedures during the Syme amputation included fibulectomy, proximal tibiofibular fixation, and retrograde intramedullary nailing. The patient progressed to weight bearing in a shoe prosthesis. **A**, Immediate postoperative AP radiograph. **B**, Six-week postoperative AP radiograph.

SUMMARY

Ankle disarticulation remains a viable option for lower extremity amputation. Early complications can be mitigated with careful screening and medical optimization before surgery. The advantages of end weight bearing and the decreased metabolic demand of ambulation cannot be overstated in a patient population that often has many medical comorbidities and little functional reserve.

References

1. Philbin TM, Berlet GC, Lee TH: Lower–Extremity amputations in association with diabetes mellitus. *Foot Ankle Clin* 2006;11:791-804.
2. Pinzur MS: Syme's ankle disarticulation. *Foot Ankle Clin* 2010;15:487-494.
3. Smith DG: Amputation. Preoperative assessment and lower extremity surgical techniques. *Foot Ankle Clin* 2001;6:271-296.
4. Harris RI: Syme's amputation; the technical details essential for success. *J Bone Joint Surg Br* 1956;38-B:614-632.
5. Philbin TM, DeLuccia DM, Nitsch RF, Maurus PB: Syme amputation and prosthetic fitting challenges. *Tech Foot Ankle Surg* 2007;6:147-155.
6. Bibbo C: Modification of the Syme amputation to prevent postoperative heel pad migration. *J Foot Ankle Surg* 2013;52:766-770.
7. Gaine WJ, McCreath SW: Syme's amputation revisited: A review of 46 cases. *J Bone Joint Surg Br* 1996;78:461-467.
8. Fergason J, Keeling JJ, Bluman EM: Recent advances in lower extremity amputations and prosthetics for the combat injured patient. *Foot Ankle Clin* 2010;15:151-174.
9. Finkler ES, Marchwiany DA, Schiff AP, Pinzur MS: Long-term outcomes following Syme's amputation. *Foot Ankle Int* 2017;38:732-735.
10. Diveley RL, Kiene RH: An improved prosthesis for a syme amputation: Rex L. Diveley MD (1893-1980), Richard H. Kiene MD. *Clin Orthop Relat Res* 2008;466:127-129.
11. Mulder IA, Holtslag HR, Beersma LF, Koopman BF: Keep moving forward: A new energy returning prosthetic device with low installation height after Syme or Pirogoff amputation. *Prosthet Orthot Int* 2014;38:12-20.
12. Braaksma R, Dijkstra PU, Geertzen JHB: Syme amputation: A systematic review. *Foot Ankle Int* 2018;39:284-291.
13. Frykberg RG, Abraham S, Tierney E, Hall J: Syme amputation for limb salvage: Early experience with 26 cases. *J Foot Ankle Surg* 2007;46:93-100.
14. Pinzur MS, Stuck RM, Sage R, Hunt N, Rabinovich Z: Syme ankle disarticulation in patients with diabetes. *J Bone Joint Surg Am* 2003;85:1667-1672.
15. Carroll PJ, Ragothaman K, Mayer A, Kennedy CJ, Attinger CE, Steinberg JS: Ankle Disarticulation: An underutilized approach to staged below knee amputation – Case series and surgical technique. *J Foot Ankle Surg* 2020;59:869-872.
16. Öznur A: Syme ankle disarticulation: A simplified technique. *Foot Ank Int* 2001;22:484-485.
17. Smith NC, Stuck R, Carlson RM, et al: Correction of varus heel pad in patients with Syme's amputations. *J Foot Ankle Surg* 2012;51:394-397.
18. Ermutlu C, Akesen S: Level of surgery does not affect the reamputation rates in patients with diabetic foot ulcers requiring amputation of the ankle or foot. *Ann Med Res* 2020;27:1637-1640.
19. Saini UC, Rawat SS, Dhillon MS: Syme's amputation: Do we need it in 2020. *J Foot Ankle Surg* 2021;8:87-90.
20. Birch JG, Paley D, Herzenberg JE, et al: Amputation versus staged reconstruction for severe fibular hemimelia: Assessment of psychosocial and quality-of-life status and physical functioning in childhood. *JBJS Open Access* 2019;4(2):e0053.
21. Calder P, Shaw S, Roberts A, et al: A comparison of functional outcome between amputation and extension prosthesis in the treatment of congenital absence of the fibula with severe limb deformity. *J Child Orthop* 2017;11:318-325.
22. Morrison SG, Thomson P, Lenze U, Donnan LT: Syme amputation: Function, satisfaction, and prostheses. *J Pediatr Orthop* 2020;40:e532-e536.
23. Taniguchi A, Tanaka Y, Kadono K, et al: Pirogoff ankle disarticulation as an option for ankle disarticulation. *Clin Orthop Relat Res* 2003;414:322-238.
24. Westberry DE, Davids JR, Pugh LI: The Boyd amputation in children: Indications and outcomes. *J Pediatr Orthop* 2014;34:86-91.
25. Tosun B, Buluc L, Gok U, Unal C: Boyd amputation in adults. *Foot Ank Int* 2011;32:1063-1068.
26. Langeveld ARJ, Meuffels DE, Oostenbroek RJ, et al: The Pirogoff amputation for necrosis of the forefoot: Surgical technique. *J Bone Joint Surg Am* 2011;93(suppl 1):21-29.
27. Gessmann J, Citak M, Fehmer T, Schildhauer TA, Seybold D: Ilizarov external frame technique for Pirogoff amputations with ankle disarticulation and tibiocalcaneal fusion. *Foot Ankle Int* 2013;34:856-864.

Ankle Disarticulation and Variants: Prosthetic Management

CHAPTER 37

Phillip M. Stevens, MEd, CPO, FAAOP • David J. Baty, CPO, LPO

ABSTRACT

Syme ankle disarticulation has been suggested as the most functional amputation level of the lower limb, yet it is increasingly rarely encountered in clinical practice. The procedure typically allows for a functional gait pattern because of the preservation of a long residual limb and good muscle strength in the hip and knee proximal to the amputation. However, prosthetic fittings can be challenging because of the long and bulbous shape of the residual limb, which can result in less than optimal cosmesis and limitations to options for prosthetic componentry and feet.

Keywords: lower limb prosthesis; prosthetic design; Syme ankle disarticulation; through-ankle disarticulation

Introduction

An amputation through the ankle joint was originally described by Syme[1] in 1843 and has colloquially retained his name ever since. Although Syme's initial surgical technique has undergone changes and refinements over time, it remains an ankle disarticulation in which the distal heel tissue is reattached to the limb to allow direct weight bearing through its distal end (**Figure 1**). Although an ankle disarticulation has been suggested by some as the most functional amputation level,[2] certified prosthetists in the United States report spending only 4% of their time working with patients who have undergone a Syme ankle disarticulation.[3] These divergent observations are the result of the striking advantages and disadvantages associated with this amputation level. The inherent advantages include full distal weight bearing in most cases, a long lever arm with a large surface area for load distribution, anatomic suspension with innate rotational stability of the socket over the limb, and minimal disturbance to growth plates in pediatric applications. The disadvantages are the difficulty in creating a cosmetically acceptable prosthesis and the reduced space available for modern prosthetic foot options. The anticipated outcomes associated with an ankle disarticulation amputation along with its inherent advantages and disadvantages are reviewed. Variations in socket and suspension designs as well as component considerations are discussed.

Anticipated Outcomes

Ankle disarticulation may be indicated for several different adult patient populations including those with vascular compromise, diabetes mellitus with gangrenous tissue, severe Charcot foot arthropathy, nonhealing dysvascular ulcers, severe diabetic ulcers, trauma, crush injuries, severe frostbite, and malignancy.[4,5] Although recent literature has been silent with respect to the functional outcomes associated with this amputation level, legacy publications suggest that these outcomes will vary with the underlying etiology and overall health and well-being of the patient.

Siev-Ner et al[5] reported on the results of ankle disarticulations in 70 patients. The procedure was performed in 51 of the patients because of diabetic vascular disease. A successful outcome was defined as one in which revision amputation was not needed in the first year postoperatively, and the patient successfully received a prosthesis and completed prosthetic gait training. Using these criteria, success rates of 94% were reported for the 19 patients without vascular disease and 49% for those with vascular disease. Further classification based on age in those with vascular disease showed the success rate was 68% for patients younger than 65 years, 31% for those 65 to 69 years, and 14% for those older than 70 years.

Yu et al[4] reported on a cohort of individuals with ankle disarticulation of mixed etiology, including Charcot

---

David J. Baty or an immediate family member serves as a paid consultant to or is an employee of Össur. Neither Phillip M. Stevens nor any immediate family member has received anything of value from or has stock or stock options held in a commercial company or institution related directly or indirectly to the subject of this chapter.

This chapter is adapted from Kanas JL, Stevens PM: Ankle disarticulation and variants: Prosthetic management, in Krajbich JI, Pinzur MS, Potter BK, Stevens PM, eds: *Atlas of Amputations and Limb Deficiencies: Surgical, Prosthetic, and Rehabilitation Principles*, ed 4. American Academy of Orthopaedic Surgeons, 2016, pp 479-484.

Section 3: Lower Limb

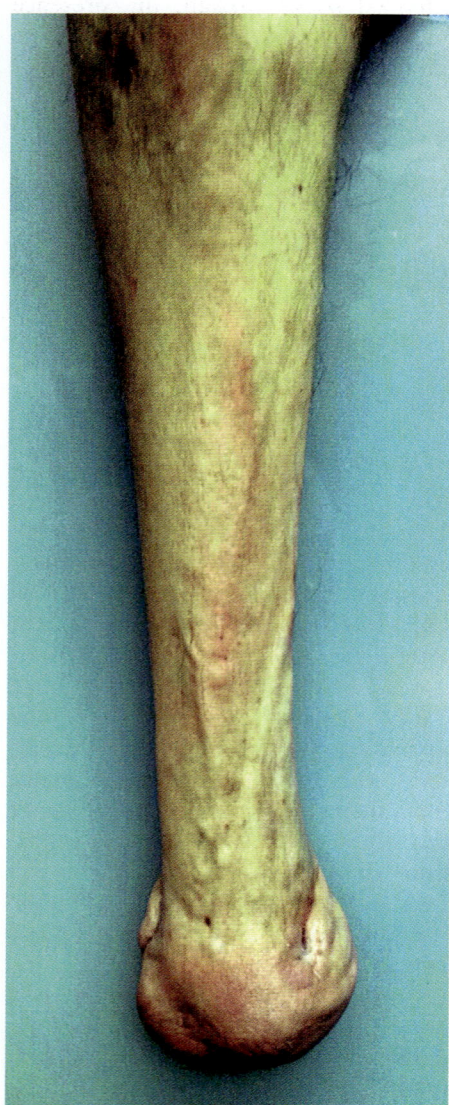

FIGURE 1 Photograph of the limb of a patient after a right ankle disarticulation.

arthropathy, osteomyelitis, crush injury, and elective amputation of severe clubfoot. Nine of 10 patients achieved ambulation with a prosthesis by 4 to 6 months after amputation, and 7 patients reported improved quality of life and return to activities of daily living.

In a retrospective study of patients treated with a Syme ankle disarticulation, Pinzur et al[6] evaluated 97 patients with diabetes mellitus with a mean age of 53 years and at least 2 years of follow-up. Of 82 patients whose wounds healed, 80 were able to use a prosthesis, a higher rate than that generally observed among patients with diabetes who have more proximal amputations.

Of these, 50% were classified as household walkers and 50% as community walkers.

A relatively recent subsequent retrospective long-term analysis of 51 patients treated by the same primary author included 33 patients with diabetes mellitus and 18 patients with nonvascular etiologies.[7] The average age at amputation for the first group was 62 years, whereas the average age of the second group was 38 years. Four of those patients with diabetes (12%) had eventually gone on to transtibial amputation because of wound failure or infection, compared with one patient (5.5%) among the cohort without diabetes. Half of the cohort with diabetes were deceased at the time of review, with an average of 4.6 years between their amputation and death. The long-term function and mobility of 11 patients who could be contacted were assessed. Although scores were higher for patients without diabetes, outcome scores were favorable for both cohorts.

Frykberg et al[8] reported on a cohort of 26 patients who underwent a Syme ankle disarticulation. Before surgery, these patients had an infection and/or substantial peripheral arterial disease and 92% had diabetes. Even with prior recommendation for transtibial or transfemoral amputation in all patients and a high rate of postoperative complications, including dehiscence, recurrent osteomyelitis, infection, and pressure ulcers, 65% of the patients successfully attained initial ambulation with a prosthesis. However, several of the patients required more proximal amputations at a mean period of 28 weeks after the ankle disarticulation because of progressive sepsis or recurrent ulcers. Ultimately, 46% of the patients were functioning well with an ankle disarticulation prosthesis approximately 1 year postoperatively. The preoperative patient criteria were less strict than in other published standards and may have resulted in the comparatively high failure rate, but several patients who would have been excluded using stricter criteria went on to ambulate successfully with a prosthesis after ankle disarticulation.

Thus, the success of prosthetic ambulation after ankle disarticulation varies, depending on the causative etiology and other medical considerations. Patients with traumatic amputation appear to do quite well, whereas the success of amputees with vascular comorbidities is more varied.

Clinical Considerations

A few unique clinical considerations differentiate ankle disarticulation from the more common transtibial amputation. These include the defined benefits and drawbacks of the associated shape and length of the residual limb, the preservation of the distal heel pad with the associated ability to bear weight distally, and the cosmetic challenges associated with the disarticulation prosthesis.

Residual Limb Shape and Length

After ankle disarticulation, the residual limb is characterized by an often pronounced bulbous contour secondary to the shape of the distal tibia and fibula. In addition, the heel pad is spared from the abated foot during surgery and reattached distal to the tibia and fibula. Proponents of ankle disarticulation cite several associated benefits of this characteristic limb shape and length. Because of the absence of any transected long bones, coupled with the preservation of the heel pad of the foot, the residual limb often has the potential to provide distal end bearing with increased proprioception following ankle disarticulation. In addition, by preserving the entire length of the tibia and fibula, one of the most important and unique advantages of ankle disarticulation is that it permits limited ambulation without a prosthesis, albeit with a considerable limb-length discrepancy. Although this limb-length discrepancy and the stability of the distal heel pad preclude ambulation over extended distances, limited direct end bearing can be useful for short-distance ambulation in the home (eg, for a nightly bathroom visit) or at a swimming pool.

In addition, the extended length of the residual limb after ankle disarticulation provides a long lever arm for control of a prosthesis. When the limb can tolerate full distal weight bearing, the proximal trimlines of the prosthesis can be lowered relative to those used in transtibial applications. Anteriorly this trimline can be lowered to the tibial tubercle or lower. However, consideration needs to be given to the shape of the anterior proximal edge of the socket because the dynamic forces experienced in late stance will tend to load the anterior tibial crest.

When the position or stability of the distal heel pad is compromised and distal weight bearing is poorly tolerated, a transtibial patellar tending brim can be used to help distribute the axial forces across the proximal aspects of the limb as in transtibial applications. In addition, the extended length of the residual limb provides a large surface area over which these proximal weight-bearing forces can be distributed. The bulbous shape of the ankle disarticulation also provides the ability to self-suspend the prosthesis.

These benefits notwithstanding, several clear disadvantages are associated with the prosthetic management of a patient after an ankle disarticulation. The extended length of the residual limb can limit prosthetic component options. In an adult treated with ankle disarticulation, the available space is inadequate to fit a higher profile prosthetic foot capable of energy storage and return and shock absorption. Similarly, space is limited for modular components that can be used in more proximal limb prostheses for alignment adjustability. Finally, providing a cosmetically acceptable ankle disarticulation prosthesis can be challenging, especially for an individual with a more bulbous residual limb.

Heel Pad

The heel pad is optimally positioned in line with the long bones of the lower leg to provide a physiologic cushion at the distal end of the residual limb. Depending on the surgical procedure used, the heel pad can become unstable, migrating from the preferred position. If a displaced heel pad remains mobile, a well-fitted prosthesis can maintain its position at the distal aspect of the limb. The integrity and stability of the heel pad largely affect the patient's ability to bear weight through the distal aspect of the limb. For individuals who are unable to tolerate full distal weight bearing, the principles of transtibial prosthetic management can be used to provide proximal load-bearing surfaces in the ankle disarticulation prosthesis.

Cosmesis

Depending on the width of the residual malleoli and the socket type used, obtaining acceptable cosmesis for the ankle disarticulation prosthesis can be challenging. The wall thickness of the socket itself and any additional interfaces augment the bulkiness of the prosthesis (**Figure 2**). This is especially noticeable at the distal aspect of the socket where it attaches to the prosthetic foot. This additional bulk, combined with the common need to align the foot in a relatively outset alignment, can make fitting the prosthesis into certain shoe types difficult and result in aesthetic concerns for the patient.

Primary Socket-Suspension Approaches

A well-fitted socket is a key component to a successful prosthetic outcome. This begins with effective measurement of the limb's shape and volume, which is most commonly obtained by applying an external wrap cast using plaster of Paris or synthetic fiberglass. Alternative measuring techniques include alginate molding and digital scanning approaches. The treating clinician's intended socket design, the presence and characteristics of any interface material used, and the patient's ability to tolerate distal weight bearing should be assessed and integrated into the treatment plan before limb capture because each consideration affects the measuring technique. An external wrap cast can be used in a weight-bearing, semi–weight-bearing, or non–weight-bearing position according to the planned distal socket shape. In addition, the clinician can preload certain areas of the limb during the casting procedure if proximal weight bearing is intended. Several socket-suspension design approaches are commonly used in the prosthetic management of ankle disarticulations, including the liner-based stovepipe socket, the medial window, the posterior window, and the expandable wall socket.

Stovepipe Socket

The aptly named stovepipe socket relies on a custom-designed flexible interface to fill the space between the characteristic contours of the residual limb and an outer rigid socket of generally uniform diameter across its length (the stovepipe shape) (**Figure 3**). Both historically and in current practice, this interface is commonly composed

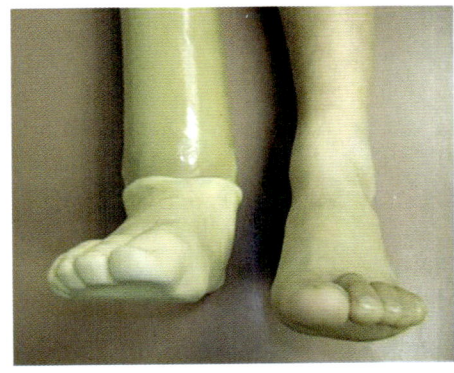

FIGURE 2 Photograph of an ankle disarticulation prosthesis shown with the unaffected limb. The bulbous nature of the residual limb creates aesthetic challenges in prosthetic design.

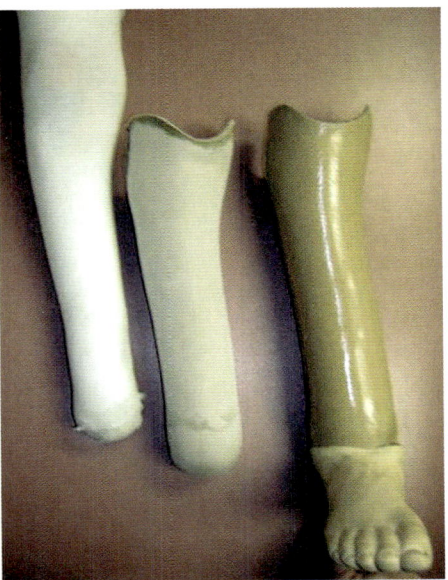

FIGURE 3 Photograph of a stovepipe ankle disarticulation prosthesis (right) with custom foam insert (center) and the residual limb covered by a thin fitting sock (left).

of medium-density foam. Constructed over a positive model of the residual limb, the thinnest wall of the liner is over the distal bulbous aspect of the limb; its thickest wall is in the comparatively narrow supramalleolar region. In such systems, the patient dons the flexible foam liner over the residual limb and interface sock, relying on the compliance of the material to allow the distal end of the limb through the hourglass-shaped inner contours of the liner. If necessary, a vertical slit can be made along the posterior long axis of the liner to allow additional foam displacement. An additional fitting sock is applied over the liner, which allows air to wick out of the system as the rigid outer socket is donned. The rigid outer socket prevents any distortion of the inner foam liner, and an anatomic suspension is obtained over the malleoli of the residual limb.[9] In addition, the stovepipe socket can be used to unload the distal aspect of the limb through proximal load bearing. As with other socket applications, additional fitting socks can be used to accommodate reductions in limb volume.

In recent years, this concept has also been used with alternative liner materials, including silicones and thermoplastic elastomers. Given the comparative flexibility and tackiness of these elastic liners, they must be rolled rather than pulled over the limb. A bonded external fabric cover or external fitting sock is generally used to allow the outer socket to pass over the exterior of the tacky liner material. Alternatively, a noncovered liner or a covered liner accompanied by a hypobaric sealing ring can be used with a socket that has a distal one-way expulsion valve to allow air removal from the system (**Figure 4**). The tackiness of such systems can be briefly overcome with liquid lubricating agents, allowing the limb to seat within the socket. This creates an airtight seal of the liner against the inner socket wall, providing both anatomic and suction suspension. Although noncustom liners have been successfully used with this technique, custom liners are often indicated to accommodate the unique contours of the residual limb.

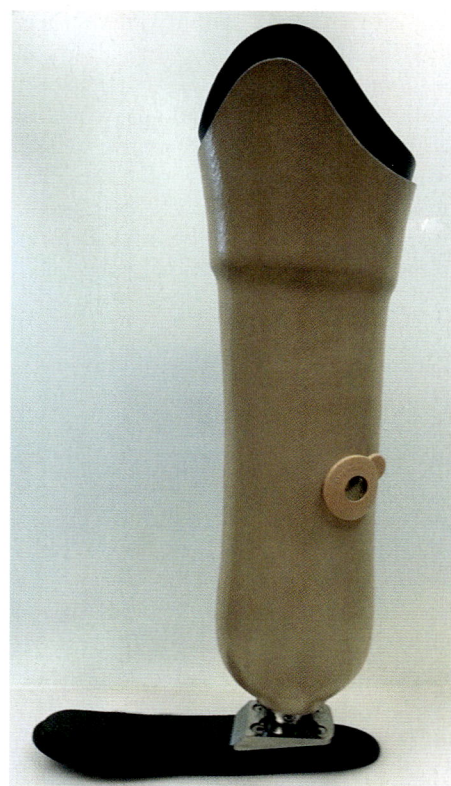

FIGURE 4 Photograph of an ankle disarticulation prosthesis with a one-way air expulsion valve.

Notably, given the offset in the limb circumferences, these custom liners can be both thick and heavy as they fill the area superior to the malleoli. As such liners increase in thickness, they become progressively more difficult to don. Finally, in applications of distal weight bearing, elastomeric liners may experience premature wear at their plantar surfaces because of the disproportionate loading in this area of the socket.

Medial Window Socket

The medial window socket design is another technique for obtaining anatomic suspension (**Figure 5**). In this design, the rigid socket matches the contours of the residual limb. However, to allow the distal ball of the limb through the narrow channel in the supramalleolar region of the socket, a medial opening is cut out, creating a removable custom panel. The height of both the opening and accompanying panel is determined by the width of the malleoli. The distal edge of the opening is located at the apex of the medial contour of the ankle and extends proximally to the point in the socket with a coronal width equal to that of the distal opening. If the proximal height of the opening is inadequate, the residual limb will not fit through the socket to the depth of the medial window and the patient will be unable to don the prosthesis. After the limb is fully seated into the socket, the medial panel is secured over the medial window to provide anatomic suspension of the prosthesis over the malleoli.

This socket approach preserves the capacity for proximal socket modifications to unload the distal end of the socket. Care must be given to the radiuses of the corners of the cutout as tighter radiuses will result in higher localized forces. This is especially relevant at the posterior distal aspect of the cutout as this becomes an area of extremely high stress in terminal stance and can be prone to material failure. Larger radiuses will better distribute these forces.

Posterior Window Socket

A posterior window socket design may be indicated in cases in which the shape of the residual limb is characterized by a particularly large differential between its smallest and largest circumference.[9] In this application, a large posterior cutout allows the passage of the distal end of the limb in both the sagittal and coronal planes (**Figure 6**). However, the size of the posterior cutout may compromise the strength of the prosthesis and its resilience to forces in the sagittal plane. As a result, increased wall thickness is often advised to increase the structural durability of the socket system. In addition, the large surface area of the posterior cutout precludes the use of proximal loading forces to offload the distal aspect of the limb.

Modified Posterior Window Socket

Similar to the posterior window socket, this modified approach is fabricated over a flexible inner socket to facilitate simple donning with anatomic

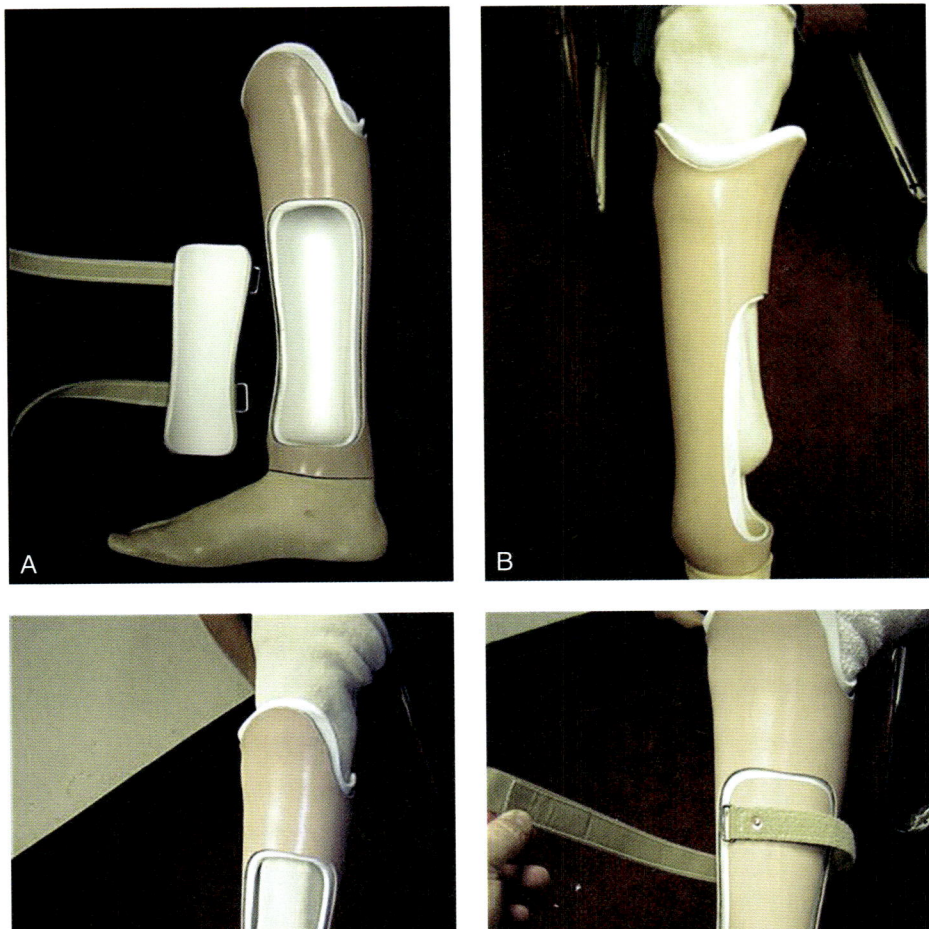

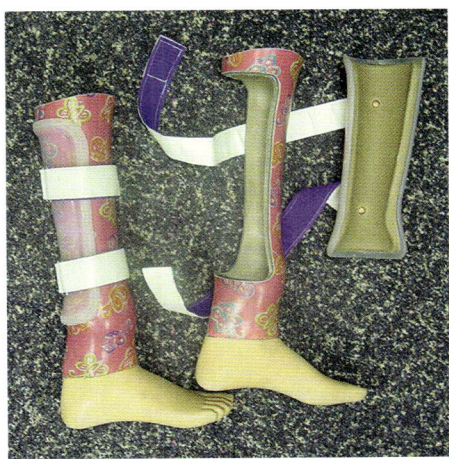

FIGURE 6 Photograph of prostheses with bilateral posterior window sockets.

FIGURE 5 Photographs of an ankle disarticulation prosthesis with a medial window socket design. **A**, The window is removed. **B** and **C**, The limb is inserted into the socket. **D**, The window is replaced to secure anatomic suspension.

suspension. An interior slit in the inner socket permits donning of the flexible material over the limb and fitting sock. The rigid prosthesis with an aggressive posterior cutout is donned over the flexible inner socket where it is secured with straps. The intimate contour of the flexible socket, secured by the strapping system, provides secure suspension in applications where the patient can comfortably tolerate full distal load bearing. This system works well on bony limbs because there is no rigid material over the bony malleoli, reducing the likelihood of localized pressure in this potentially troublesome area of the socket (**Figure 7**).

Expandable Wall Socket

Less commonly used, the expandable wall socket is similar to the stovepipe design in that the outer socket is column-like and continuous, with no holes or windows. However, instead of a custom-molded liner interface, an internal air bladder permits the passage of the residual limb into the socket and then conforms around the shape of the limb to maintain anatomic suspension.[9] Although this design also permits off-loading of the distal limb, it is complex to fabricate and maintain and is rarely used.

Component and Alignment Considerations

In adult ankle disarticulations, little space remains for distal componentry. The choice of a prosthetic foot is limited to low-profile designs (**Figures 8 and 9**). Although the use of low-profile carbon fiber feet has allowed for a dynamic solution within the limited space beneath the socket, the resultant gait mechanics have their limitations. The relatively stiff heel of the carbon plate tends to create an aggressive knee flexion moment at initial contact followed by an abrupt transition to foot flat. As the weight line progresses forward, there is often an aggressive knee extension moment in late stance as the short, stiff keel of the foot, required for structural integrity and longevity, resists elastic deformation.

Exceptions to this observation are found in adolescent and adult patients who sustained their amputations in childhood and in whom a reduced residual limb length progressively developed (**Figure 10**).

Alignment adjustability is also compromised by the available space at this disarticulation level. Although the use of a conventional pyramid adaptor is sometimes possible (**Figure 8**),

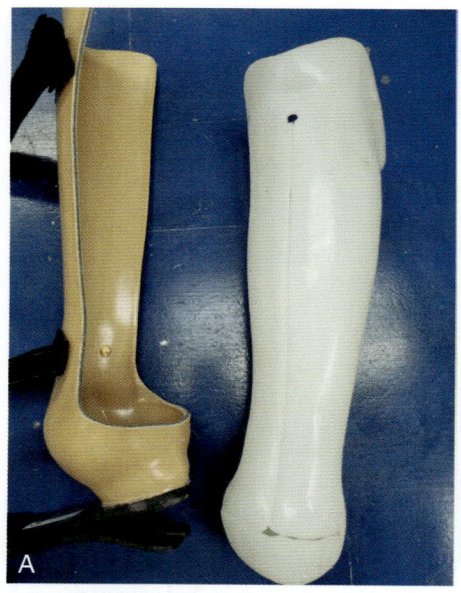 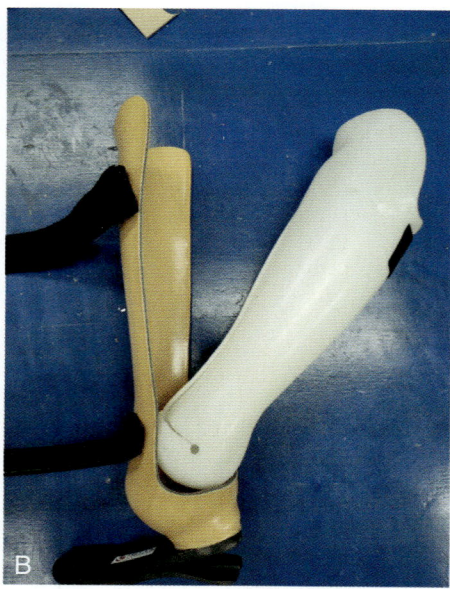 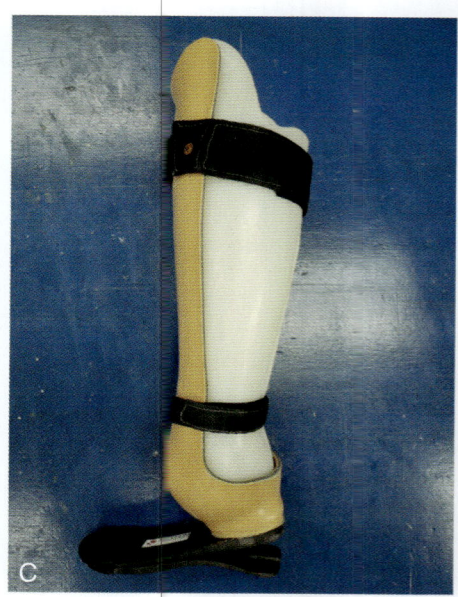

FIGURE 7 Photographs of a modified posterior wall socket. **A**, Prior to donning. **B**, During donning. **C**, Fully donned and secure. Similar to the posterior window socket, but fabricated over a flexible inner socket to facilitate simple donning while preserving anatomic suspension.

in many instances, the socket attaches directly to the foot with no endoskeletal adjustment adaptors. Therefore, the dynamic alignment during the test socket phase is crucial in managing the ankle disarticulation. As with partial foot amputations, it is often necessary to outset the position of the prosthetic foot laterally to provide adequate coronal stability (**Figure 11**). The lateral outset further compromises both the aesthetics of the prosthesis and the ability to fit it into certain shoe designs.

In recent years, clinicians have disrupted this long-held space limitation by mounting long carbon fiber feet to the posterior proximal aspect of the Syme socket to allow this population to benefit from the energy return associated with the greater carbon deflection. Anecdotal reports include an increased smoothness in gait with this adaptation. However, such feet

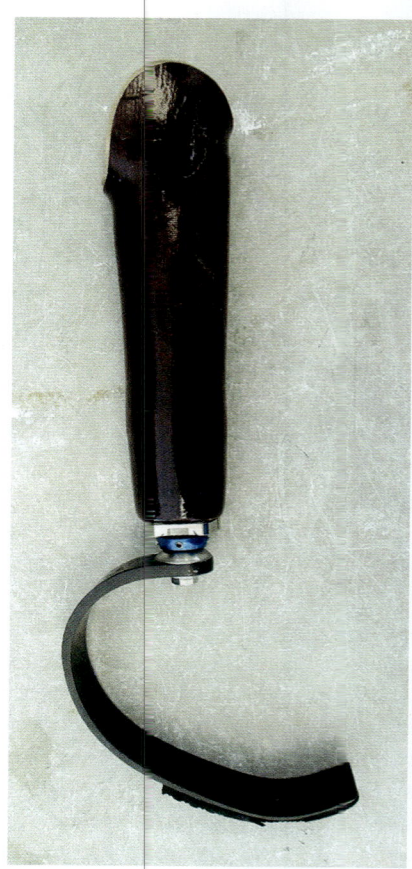

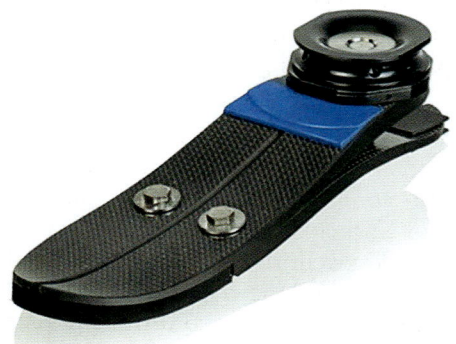

FIGURE 8 Photograph of a low-profile prosthetic foot that allows adequate space to retain a pyramid adaptor for alignment.

FIGURE 9 Photograph of a low-profile ankle disarticulation foot prosthesis.

FIGURE 10 Photograph of a high-profile prosthetic foot that allows energy storage and return. This type of prosthesis is permitted by the limb-length discrepancy that commonly occurs in patients who underwent ankle disarticulation as children.

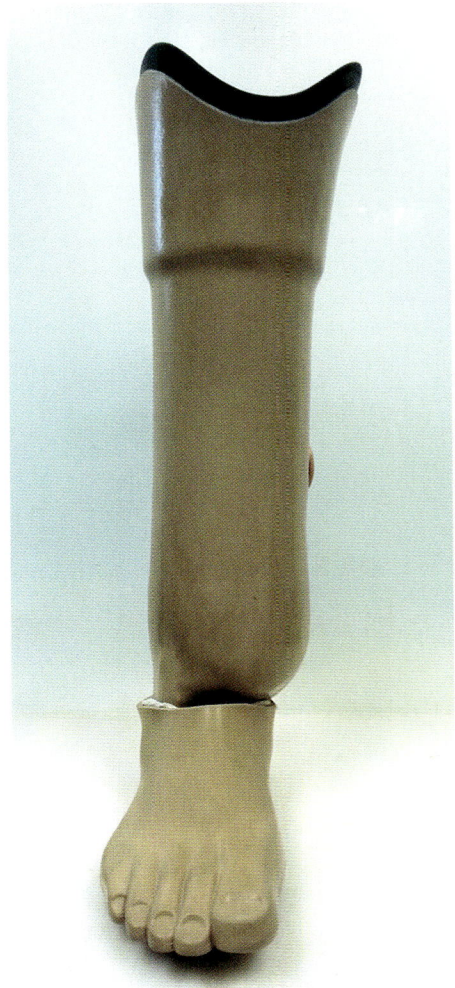

FIGURE 11 Photograph shows lateral outset of a prosthetic foot beneath the ankle disarticulation prosthetic socket.

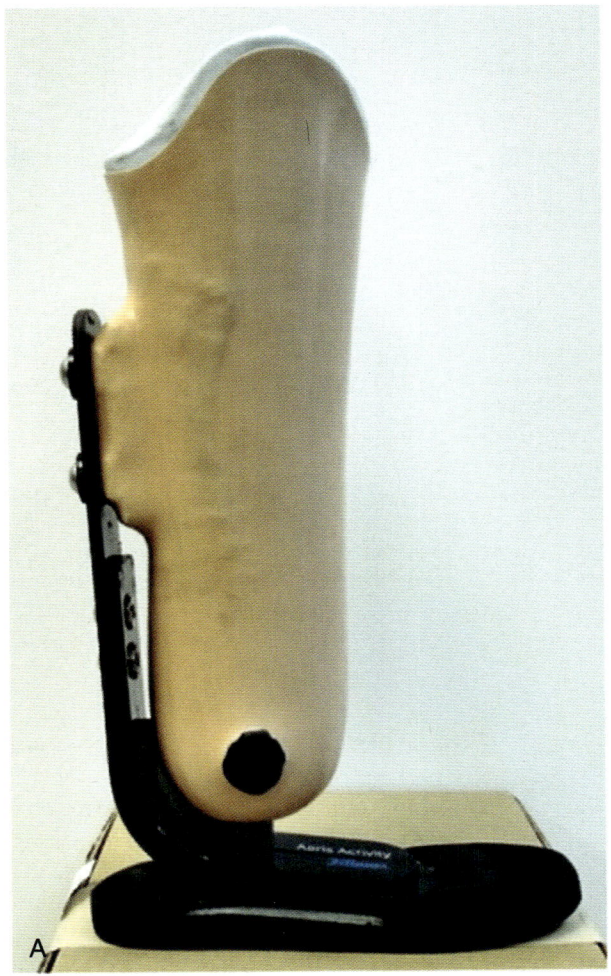
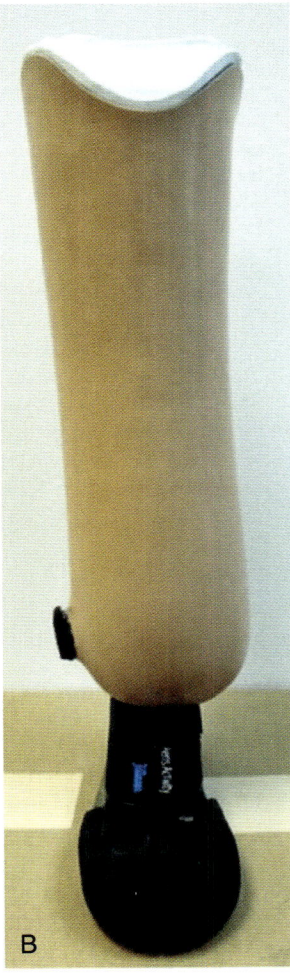

FIGURE 12 Photographs showing (**A**) lateral and (**B**) anterior view of a Syme prosthesis with a long, posterior-mounted prosthetic foot. This technique requires that such feet be aligned with enough posterior clearance to allow for carbon deflection without contacting the socket.

must be aligned with enough posterior clearance to allow for carbon deflection without contacting the socket. As much as 2 inches can be required to accommodate the phenomenon (**Figure 12**).

Gait

In 1976, Waters et al[10] reported greater gait velocity, cadence, stride length, and preserved function in individuals with ankle disarticulations compared with those with transtibial and transfemoral amputations. Similarly, energy expenditure and cardiovascular demand are reduced at the ankle disarticulation level relative to more proximal amputation levels. Although not proved in the laboratory, it is generally accepted that a distal end bearing provides improved proprioception and, thus, stability during gait.[11] Patients generally require minimal prosthetic gait training after an ankle disarticulation, reducing outpatient rehabilitation costs.[5,8,11]

SUMMARY

Syme ankle disarticulation is characterized by well-described advantages and disadvantages. The ability to bear weight distally and ambulate limited distances without a prosthesis is tempered by limitations to prosthetic foot options and alignment considerations as well as cosmetic finishing challenges. The expected outcomes associated with this disarticulation level vary with the underlying etiology. Socket suspension is often obtained anatomically, securing its purchase proximal to the malleoli. This can be attained using several socket designs. Component options are limited by the available space beneath the residual limb, and alignment components are often excluded by this limitation. Thus, dynamic alignment during the test socket phase of prosthetic fitting is particularly important in individuals with an ankle disarticulation. After appropriate alignment is obtained, patients usually ambulate with relatively normal spatiotemporal parameters and energy costs. Gait training and outpatient rehabilitation are generally minimal in this population.

References

1. Syme J: On amputation at the ankle joint. *Lond Edinb Mon J Med Sci* 1843;26:93-96.
2. Berk GM: Lower limb prosthetics, in Coughlin MJ, Saltzman CL, Mann RA, eds: *Mann's Surgery of the Foot and Ankle*, ed 9. Elsevier, 2014, pp 1508-1533.
3. James H: Practice analysis of certified practitioners in the disciplines of orthotics and prosthetics: Prosthetic practice areas and devices. The American Board for Certification in Orthotics, Prosthetics & Pedorthics. Available at: https://www.abcop.org/publication/section/practitioner-practice-analysis/prosthetic-practice-areas-and-devices. Accessed March 17, 2021.
4. Yu GV, Schinke TL, Meszaros A: Syme's amputation: A retrospective review of 10 cases. *Clin Podiatr Med Surg* 2005;22(3):395-427.
5. Siev-Ner I, Heim M, Warshavski M, Daich A, Tamir E, Dudkiewicz I: A review of the aetiological factors and results of trans-ankle (Syme) disarticulations. *Disabil Rehabil* 2006;28(4):239-242.
6. Pinzur MS, Stuck RM, Sage R, Hunt N, Rabinovich Z: Syme ankle disarticulation in patients with diabetes. *J Bone Joint Surg Am* 2003;85(9):1667-1672.
7. Finkler ES, Marchwiany DA, Schiff AP, Pinzur MS: Long-term outcomes following Syme's amputation. *Foot Ankle Int* 2017;38(7):732-735.
8. Frykberg FG, Abraham S, Tierney E, Hall J: Syme amputation for limb salvage: Early experience with 26 cases. *J Foot Ankle Surg* 2007;46(2):93-100.
9. Philbin TM, DeLuccia DM, Nitsch RF, Maurus PB: Syme amputation and prosthetic fitting challenges. *Tech Foot Ankle Surg* 2007;6(3):147-155.
10. Waters RL, Perry J, Antonelli D, Hislop H: Energy cost of walking of amputees: The influence of level of amputation. *J Bone Joint Surg Am* 1976;58(1):42-46.
11. Pinzur MS: Syme's ankle disarticulation. *Foot Ankle Clin* 2010;15(3):487-494.

Transtibial Amputation

CHAPTER 38

James Robert Ficke, MD, FAAOS, FACS

ABSTRACT

Transtibial level amputation (previously referred to as below-knee amputation) is very commonly performed for trauma, vascular injury, and gangrene, and has undergone many modifications and technical improvements over the great span of surgical history. This level, while not the most difficult technically, has many risks and complications that can render a patient nonambulatory or dysfunctional. This chapter outlines the historical context, literature supporting three useful techniques, and common complications and approaches to avoid and/or manage these complications. The essential principles of débridement, hemorrhage control, and soft-tissue balancing, including addressing adequate coverage and cushioning of the terminal bone surfaces (myodesis or myoplasty), are described. Additionally, resection of the fibula as described by Bruckner and bridging of the distal tibia and fibula as described by Ertl with literature supporting modifications are also described in detail.

Keywords: below-knee amputation; Ertl; myodesis; trans-tibial amputation

Introduction

Surgical amputation has been recorded in archeologic specimens since Hippocrates,[1] and was first described as a last resort primarily to control infection. Transtibial level amputation has been described in texts for reducing mortality because of limb trauma since the invention of gunpowder,[2] yet continues to have wide variation in technique. This chapter provides an overview of indications, available evidence to support various aspects of the procedure, the author's preferred technique, based upon available evidence, and common complications. One of the most important considerations is that this level of limb loss is a watershed for function: distal to the tibia, most patients retain a large degree of activities, often without extensive prosthetic requirements. Proximal to the tibia, ambulation becomes a substantially higher energy and typically less vigorous function. Indications for transtibial amputation include uncontrollable sepsis, malignancy in which limb salvage is not an acceptable option, unsalvageable trauma, and chronic pain unresolved with traditional methods.

Outcome Considerations

Patients who require transtibial amputation can be grouped into nonischemic or dysvascular causes. Nonischemic indications generally include trauma, tumor, infection, or congenital deformities. These patients are typically younger and healthier, with fewer comorbid conditions. Patients with dysvascular limbs likely have additional comorbidities that need to be assessed before surgical intervention. Successful wound healing in the setting of vascular compromise can be dramatically improved through appropriate surgical technique using a long posterior flap as described by Burgess et al.[3,4] A recent Cochrane Database analysis demonstrated no significant differences between a variety of incisions to include skew flap, sagittal flap, and long posterior techniques.[5]

When possible, preoperative assessment of healing potential should be performed. Ideally, patients undergoing a transtibial amputation should have an ankle-brachial index greater than 0.5, transcutaneous oxygen saturation on room air greater than 20 to 30 mm Hg, an albumin level greater than 2.5 g/dL, and an absolute lymphocyte count greater than 1,500 per μL.[6]

Indications

General indications for a transtibial amputation include high-energy trauma in which limb salvage is not initially possible;[7] nonreconstructible dysvascular extremity;[8-10] uncontrolled infection in the setting of general sepsis; tumor when limb salvage is not possible or chosen after informed consent; certain congenital deformities/deficiencies, and chronic pain when less ablative options have been exhausted. The ultimate goal of an amputation should be lifesaving or as a reconstructive option among other alternatives when function is likely to be better with removal of the terminal limb. Specific indications in trauma still are gradually

---

Dr. Ficke or an immediate family member serves as a board member, owner, officer, or committee member of American Academy of Orthopaedic Surgeons, American College of Surgeons, and Orthopaedic Research and Education Foundation.

Section 3: Lower Limb

becoming better defined, while older reports demonstrate equivalent function for amputations and limb salvage. This will be further discussed in other chapters, but a few specific concepts merit comment. Evidence is available that loss of plantar sensation should not be considered an indication in the early-trauma patient[11] and complications requiring ankle arthrodesis, severe destructive foot injuries and free tissue transfer to the foot may have improved outcomes with early amputation.[12]

Contraindications

Patients with vascular compromise who are not in extremis but require amputation should undergo optimization before limb removal at a transtibial level or consideration of amputation at a higher level. In the setting of trauma, initial limb salvage affords a dialogue with the patient and possibly their family regarding expectations and outcomes and affords opportunity for the patient to participate in the decision-making process. This is not a contraindication, per se, rather a delay to include the patient in decisions. An insensate foot is not considered a reliable indicator of function and therefore is not an indication for amputation.[11] Finally, ascending infection proximal to the knee is a contraindication for this level.

Procedure (Author's Preferred Surgical Technique)

The patient is positioned in the supine with a bump under the buttocks to position the patella in a direct anterior position. A well-padded thigh tourniquet is often placed, however exsanguination should not be performed with malignancy or active infection. The ideal length of the residual limb is at least 12 cm distal to the knee joint line, and at least 2.5 cm above the plantar heel pad at a level where sufficient gastrocnemius muscle can effectively serve as padding by way of a myodesis. The positioning below the knee allows optimal residual lever arm, while the position from the floor allows for optimum prosthesis components and adequate distal padding.

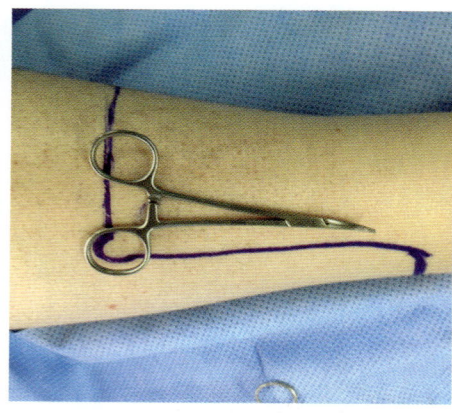

FIGURE 1 Photograph showing an outline of the hemostat handle drawn proximal to the transverse incision line. This permits resection of redundant "dog ear" tissue.

A standard posterior flap, as described by Burgess, is drawn circumferentially. The transverse skin incision should be 1 to 2 cm below the proposed tibial transection line and should extend from 1 cm posterior to the posterior medial border of the tibia laterally to the fibula. The handle of a hemostat can be used to outline a curve at each border medially and laterally (**Figure 1**). The incision extends distally in longitudinal fashion following the posterior medial border of the tibia medially, posterior to the fibula laterally, and is carried completely around the posterior aspect of the distal calf. The length of this flap should be roughly twice that of the transverse arm or twice the diameter of the calf. Additional skin can later be resected. In certain trauma situations the extended posterior flap has been described as being emplaced onto the anterior tibial fascia proximal to the tibial bevel. Tisi and Than[5] performed a detailed Cochrane review of various skin incisions and noted no difference in wound healing, but the ability to wear a prosthesis appears to be optimal when the scar is not over the weight-bearing end of the residual limb.

Following the circumferential skin marking of anticipated incision, the limb is exsanguinated and the tourniquet elevated and the entire skin incision performed down to the fascia. If an osteoperiosteal flap is to be raised, care should be taken on the anteromedial border to preserve the tibial periosteum, tibial periosteum proximally, which in bone bridge cases should be separately elevated. Following complete skin and fascial incision, the anterior and lateral muscular compartments are transected. It is helpful to carry out the transection proximally into the anterior and lateral compartments as these compartments add nothing to a myodesis and often add tension to the fascia and skin in wound closure. The anterior tibial artery is identified before transection and is doubly ligated. The deep and superficial peroneal nerves can be identified and injected before transection with 1% lidocaine. Similarly, on the medial side the saphenous vein is identified and ligated and the saphenous nerve is transected following injection. It is equally important to perform traction neurectomy for the sural remnant in the posterior flap so as to avoid incisional neuromata.[13]

Subperiosteal dissection around the posterior tibia using a Cobb elevator enables exposure of the intermuscular septum, the tibial shaft, and the fibula. This tibial shaft bone cut can be made by a oscillating saw or Gigli saw with care taken to ensure perpendicular cut in both the AP and lateral plane. One can avoid splintering a posterior bone spike by ensuring support of the foot during the cut. Next the fibula is cut no more than 1 cm proximal to the tibia and performed in a contoured position from proximal lateral to distal medial. Sharp bone edges can be rounded using a hand rasp or power saw. An anterior bevel is essential for prosthesis comfort, and deserves additional comments. If a bevel is begun within the medullary canal, later reabsorption of the bone can result in two medial and lateral prominent points and therefore the bevel should be clearly outside the medullary canal and fully intracortical (**Figure 2**). The bevel is made at a 30° to 45° angle, with care taken to preserve the proximal periosteum for myodesis or myoplasty.

Following tibial and fibular osteotomies, a long amputation knife is best used to optimize the contour of the gastrocnemius fascia. This knife, using long

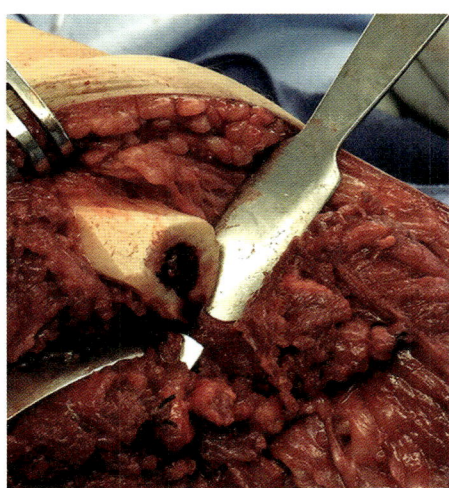

FIGURE 2 Photograph illustrating the long posterior flap showing generous anterior cortical bevel which does not violate the inner margin of cortex and rounded outer edges of the tibial cut.

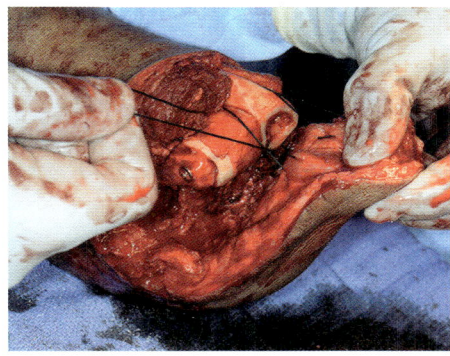

FIGURE 3 Bone-bridge photograph demonstrating secure periosteal sleeve and external stabilization while the bridge ossifies. (Reproduced with permission from Philip Stahel, MD, Asheville, NC.)

sweeping strokes, permits resection of the posterior tibial muscle; transection of the neurovascular bundle distal to the bone ends; and a tapered resection of the soleus followed by transection of the gastrocnemius fascia at the most distal aspect. Completing a circumferential skin incision initially prevents inadvertent buttonhole or irregular skin edges. The foot is passed off the field and attention is turned to the neurovascular bundle. Proximal dissection and removal of the posterior tibialis muscle belly permit exposure of the tibial neurovascular bundle where the artery is doubly tied with a suture ligature and the veins are separately ligated. The tibial nerve is separately dissected from the vessels to prevent pulsatile irritation. This nerve is similarly injected proximally and gentle traction neurotomy, or more advanced nerve management technique as discussed in later chapters, is performed above the level of the tibial bone cut. At this point the tourniquet should be released, hemostasis can be fully obtained, and an assessment of the gastrocnemius fascia for myodesis or myoplasty performed.

When a myodesis is performed, it is best to avoid a central core style of suture as these can create sterile abscesses. A large #5 braided suture is used to perform a Krackow style locking stitch with four strands.[14] A 2 to 3 mm drill bit is used when creating a formal myodesis and the drill hole should be proximal to the bevel to facilitate complete coverage of the distal tibia (**Figure 3**). If a myoplasty is performed, the terminal end of the gastrocnemius fascia is simply secured to the anterior tibial periosteum and fascia; it is worth noting that, because the gastrocnemius-soleus complex is not stabilized to a truly dynamic, opposing muscle group, this technique of myoplasty technically is a form of myodesis. Even in vascular patients, security of the gastrocnemius over the distal tibial cut is important for future prostheses wear. Following meticulous hemostasis, myodesis is secured and fascial closure is performed in layers. While the decision for draining is individual, there is little scientific evidence to support routine placement of drains. Meticulous hemostasis before closure is the best practice for avoiding postoperative hematomas or wound healing problems. The skin is closed in layers, and the dressing of choice applied. A postoperative splint protecting the distal residual limb prevents wound complications in postoperative falls. There is some risk for the patient to forget in the early phases and depend on the now-absent limb. Falls on the residual limb can be devastating.

European (Bruckner) Technique: Fibulectomy

In the 1980s, a German surgeon, Dr. L. Brückner, published a series of vascular occlusive patients who underwent a modification of the Burgess technique.[15,16] He performed a complete fibulectomy and complete resection of the anterior and lateral muscular compartments. He reported this in the English literature in 1992, and Stahel et al[9] reproduced his successful findings in 2006 (**Figure 4**). This method is described because it lessens the likelihood for migration of the proximal fibula, ischemia of the often tenuous anterior or lateral muscular compartments, and permits a relatively lower tension myoplasty for the retained gastrocnemius-soleus complex (**Figure 5**).

Ertl Technique

Although the specific patient cohort that would most benefit from the bone-bridge synostosis has not been defined in the literature, available data do allow some generalizations. Gwinn et al[17] performed a retrospective analysis of 37 patients who underwent bone-bridge transtibial amputations in 42 extremities for lower extremity trauma to identify perioperative differences between those undergoing bone-bridge and non-bone–bridge amputations. Their results demonstrated increased surgical times in those undergoing bone bridging (179 versus 112 minutes, $P < 0.0005$) and increased tourniquet times (115 versus 71 minutes, $P < 0.0005$). Although they argue that the longer surgical and tourniquet times should not be considered a contraindication to performing a bone-bridge transtibial amputation in a young, healthy patient, these factors have been associated with increased complications in those undergoing other lower extremity surgery.[18]

Because of the increased surgical and tourniquet times associated with the bone-bridge synostosis technique,[17] this technique is best reserved for young, healthy, active individuals. In addition, those with fibular instability or disruption of the interosseous membrane may benefit from this technique as a primary or revision amputation.[19]

When a decision is made to perform an osteoperiosteal flap as described by Dr. Janos Ertl,[20] this is best done using a single bevel wide chisel before the tibial bone transection (**Figure 6**). It

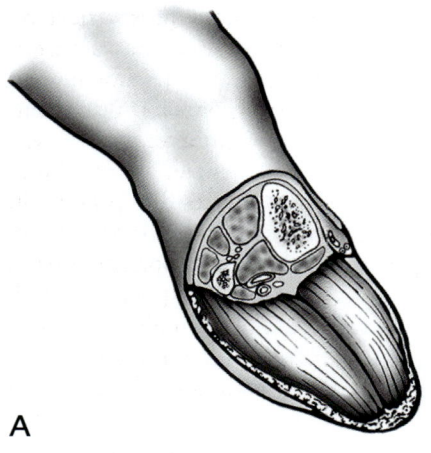 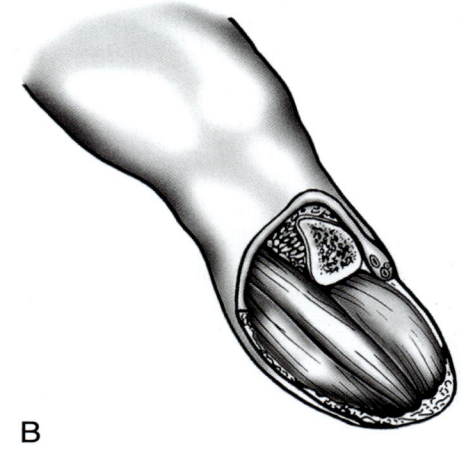 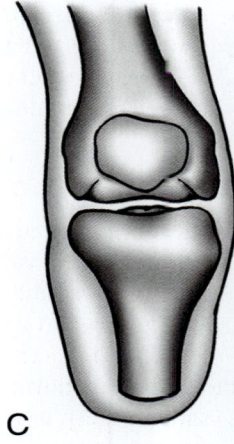

FIGURE 4 Drawing of the Bruckner description for anterior and lateral compartment resection with fibulectomy. (Reproduced with permission from Philip Stahel, MD, Lakewood, CO.)

is important to measure the distance between the tibia and fibula and develop the osteoperiosteal flap that will extend onto the lateral fibula. Any widening of this distance, and excessive narrowing is not well tolerated. Additional points to this procedure include fibular resection at the level of the tibia with or without a periosteally perfused bone spacer. Similarly, a variety of fixation methods for this bone bridge have been described using screws, suture-washer constructs, simple sutures, or only the periosteum.[19,21,22] None have been shown to be superior, but Gwinn et al demonstrated increased surgical time blood transfusion requirements and additional subsequent procedures to be associated with the bone-bridge procedure, regardless of technique. Tucker et al[23] demonstrated using cineradiography in successful Ertl prostheses users that the limb did not actually make direct contact, and therefore was not a critical factor in improving clinical outcomes. Similarly, outcomes of the long posterior flap standard amputation versus the bone bridge have not been shown in prospective trials to make significant difference in outcomes.[24] Nonetheless, the procedure is popular among elite athletes and high-performance, combat warriors. Additional outcomes study and comparative effectiveness are required to answer this question.

Rehabilitation

Detailed description of limb loss rehabilitation is covered fully in subsequent chapters, but consideration to early therapy is essential. Immediate postoperative prostheses have been described and used; however, comparative effectiveness evidence is lacking. It is better to permit healing of a stable wound closure, with soft-tissue equilibrium, than to attempt to expedite premature ambulation in a prosthesis. Experience with recent conflicts has demonstrated that early preprosthetic rehabilitation in conjunction with comprehensive peer-mentor–based group approaches to rehabilitation are quite effective.[25-27] Therefore, whenever possible, amputee rehabilitation in centers where the patient is among others going through similar experiences, or among peers who have previously experienced loss and successful recovery, is the best practice. The Military Extremity Trauma-Amputation versus Limb Salvage Study (METALS) recently demonstrated that in a rehabilitation-focused environment amputees function better, regain higher vigorous activity, have lower markers for posttraumatic stress disorder, and lower rates of depression than limb salvage.[12] This study was conducted at a period during the Iraq and Afghanistan conflicts in which every US service-member with limb loss underwent intensive, often long-term, rehabilitation in centers of excellence where all social, family, and financial support

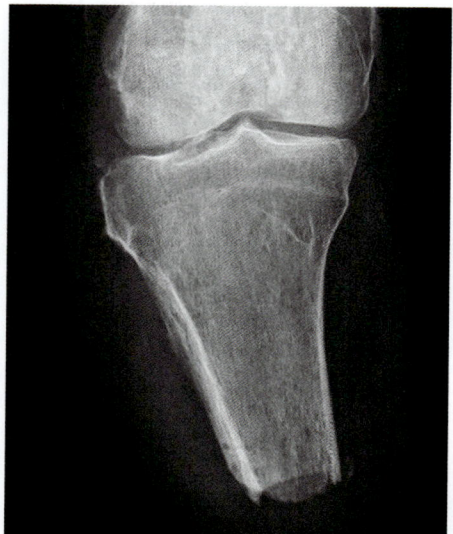

FIGURE 5 Radiograph of patient with Bruckner technique demonstrating absent fibula and stable soft tissue envelope and no evidence of lateral instability.

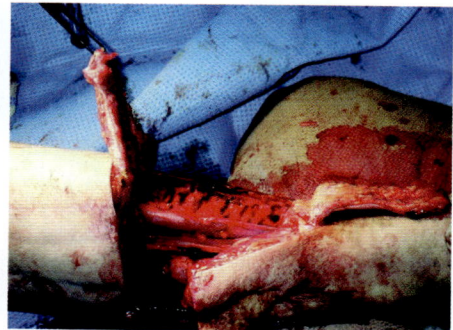

FIGURE 6 Photograph of formal elevation of Ertl osteoperiosteal sleeve from anteromedial tibia distally and prior to tibial transection.

systems were mature and fully engaged in a comprehensive network of care. Such systems did not necessarily exist for limb salvage patients nor are widely available to civilian amputees.

Level-Specific Complications

Complications related to the transtibial amputation level can be categorized as acute, and include systemic and local effects; or chronic, and generally are considered mechanical or functional. While a transtibial amputation is a major surgery, and extensive blood loss, fluid shifts, and systemic stress is common, most acute complications are neither regionally specific nor peculiar to the level. Tourniquet use has been shown to be safe and effective in traumatic, neoplastic and dysvascular patients undergoing amputations, all showing similar healing rates.[28] The use of tourniquets has made amputations vastly more survivable, yet may be a cause for other instigation, such as neuritis and complex regional pain syndrome. The most common complications regarding the long posterior flap include acute infection and wound dehiscence, hematoma formation or bleeding complications, painful neuromata, and loss of motion.[29,30] More recently, Low et al reported 2,879 patients who underwent trauma-related major lower limb amputation who were recorded in the U.S. National Trauma Database.[31] The transtibial level accounted for 46% of all, with transfemoral at 37% and partial foot representing the third most common at 7.6%. They discovered that 41.8% of the total required at least one revision, leading to an average increase in hospital length of stay more than 5.5 days. Also of note, Black or African Americans experienced a 49% higher rate of postsurgical complication, with an additional 2.5 day increase in length of stay. In the traumatic amputee, preservation of length can result in salvage of critical joint function, and Gordon et al[32] demonstrated an extremely high rate of early infection, but long-term resolution and length salvage when they stabilized fractures present proximal to the lowest viable level of soft tissue, and they consequently recommended early bone stabilization and retention of the lowest viable level without regard for "classic" named amputation levels. Recently, Katikar et al[33] reported a randomized controlled trial comparing primary versus delayed primary closure in trauma patients undergoing lower limb amputation. They studied 63 lower extremity amputations in 56 patients with mean age 34 years, where 66% of the patients sustained road traffic injuries. While this is the only prospective study specifically looking at traumatic amputees and randomizing closure, the authors reported no significant differences in length of stay, revision surgeries, or surgical site infections. However, with relatively low numbers it is possible the study was underpowered. Regardless of indication for the amputation, venous thrombo-embolism is a significant risk, and has been associated with the highest mortality among orthopaedic surgery procedures.[34] Risk factors for venous thrombo-embolism in amputees include advanced age, sedentary lifestyle, and Virchow's triad to include long-standing arterial disease and potential for hypercoagulability and low flow state. While no specific methods have been shown to be most effective, chemoprophylaxis may be most feasible in light of the limb loss. In a recent Cochrane review (updated in 2020 without new findings) of all amputation studies, no one method was more effective, but no increase in wound complications was noted either.[35] Complications and prolonged surgical case length have been reported with the Ertl bone-bridge, but they have not shown lower rates of return to function nor prosthesis usage.[17,24,36] Mechanical failure can occur because of the formation of heterotopic ossification, myodesis/myoplasty failure, or painful symptomatic neuroma. Surgical resection of symptomatic heterotopic ossification is ideally deferred until mature and no longer growing, but no current data have shown higher recurrence rates when resected early. When prosthesis[37-40] wear is significantly impeded, or progressive neurovascular functional decline is noted, judicious resection should be considered. The myodesis, when stabilized to bone, has been found most effective, and with a braided noncore suture.[41] Finally, multimodal pain management in the acute setting, including continuous regional pain catheters, has made substantial improvements in long-term outcomes.[42] Pain can present in many forms in this patient cohort. In addition to typical postoperative pain, patients can experience phantom limb pain, complex regional pain syndrome, or localized residual limb pain from prominent neuromata, limb–socket interface problems, or insufficient soft-tissue coverage. With well-documented advances in upper limb function and improvement of postoperative neuroma pain through application of targeted muscle reinnervation,[43] some leading centers have begun exploring targeted muscle reinnervation use in lower limb amputations.

Rehabilitation

A complete discussion of amputee rehabilitation is beyond the scope of this chapter, but several aspects regarding acute inpatient postoperative recovery warrant discussion. Inpatient preprosthetic conditioning can begin the first postoperative day with assisted transfers. A durable cover for the residual limb, either molded plastic or splint material, is protective in the event the patient rises and for the first several weeks does not typically realize they no longer have the leg and subsequently mis-step. One of the first goals in the initial postoperative period is edema control because edema can have a profound effect on wound healing. This is typically done with elevation, rigid dressings with soft compression, and eventual progression to elastic prosthetic shrinkers.

Following a transtibial amputation, knee flexion contractures must be prevented. Rigid dressings with the knee in extension help to prevent contractures. In addition, early prone positioning can help prevent hip flexion contractures before patient mobilizing. Wound breakdown is more common in patients with vascular disease and diabetes but it can occur in any patient. Optimizing preoperative nutrition, ensuring meticulous intraoperative hemostasis, and initiating postoperative edema control should all be undertaken to minimize this risk.

SUMMARY

The most common level for major limb amputation is at the transtibial level, and this is a watershed between the requirement for prosthetic use or potential orthosis with a shoe filler. The tibial end of the residual limb affords a functional interface with a well-fitting prosthesis when surgical considerations and principles such as respectful soft-tissue handling, meticulous hemostasis, and tension neurotomies for all five major nerves is performed. A transverse tibial cut with appropriate anterior tapered bevel and then muscle coverage for the bone renders the terminal leg suitable for prosthesis wear once the wounds are healed. Alternative methods such as the Bruckner resection of fibula and anterior and lateral compartments, or the extended posterior flap show promise in appropriate situations, and the Ertl bone bridge, while over 85 years old, has little objective evidence of its comparative effectiveness. It is most important to approach all amputations as major reconstructive efforts, and to be aware of the many complications possible, including wound breakdown and infections, myodesis failure, and neuroma or heterotopic ossification setting back essential rehabilitation. Prophylaxis of infection, venous thromboembolism, and contracture are equally important to long-term outcomes. Finally, rehabilitation, involving peer-mentors, family, and the patient's own engagement, is critical.

References

1. Kirk NT: The development of amputation. *Bull Med Libr Assoc* 1944;32(2):132-163.
2. Kirkup J: Perceptions of amputation before and after gunpowder. *Vesalius* 1995;1(2):51-58.
3. Allcock PA, Jain AS: Revisiting transtibial amputation with the long posterior flap. *Br J Surg* 2001;88(5):683-686.
4. Assal M, Blanck R, Smith DG: Extended posterior flap for transtibial amputation. *Orthopedics* 2005;28(6):542-546.
5. Tisi PV, Than MM: Type of incision for below knee amputation. *Cochrane Database Syst Rev* 2014;4:CD003749.
6. Dickhaut SC, DeLee JC, Page CP: Nutritional status: Importance in predicting wound-healing after amputation. *J Bone Joint Surg Am* 1984;66(1):71-75.
7. MacKenzie EJ, Bosse MJ, Kellam JF, et al: Factors influencing the decision to amputate or reconstruct after high-energy lower extremity trauma. *J Trauma* 2002;52(4):641-649.
8. Befroy DE, Kibbey RG, Perry R, Petersen KF, Rothman DL, Shulman GI: Response to burgess. *Nat Med* 2015;21(2):109-110.
9. Stahel PF, Oberholzer A, Morgan SJ, Heyde CE: Concepts of transtibial amputation: Burgess technique versus modified Bruckner procedure. *ANZ J Surg* 2006;76(10):942-946.
10. Yurttas Y, Kürklü M, Demiralp B, Atesalp AS: A novel technique for transtibial amputation in chronic occlusive arterial disease: Modified Burgess procedure. *Prosthet Orthot Int* 2009;33(1):25-32.
11. Bosse MJ, McCarthy ML, Jones AL, et al: The insensate foot following severe lower extremity trauma: An indication for amputation? *J Bone Joint Surg Am* 2005;87(12):2601-2608.
12. Doukas WC, Hayda RA, Frisch HM, et al: The Military Extremity Trauma Amputation/Limb Salvage (METALS) study: Outcomes of amputation versus limb salvage following major lower-extremity trauma. *J Bone Joint Surg Am* 2013;95(2):138-145.
13. Tintle SM, Donohue MA, Shawen S, Forsberg JA, Potter BK: Proximal sural traction neurectomy during transtibial amputations. *J Orthop Trauma* 2012;26(2):123-126.
14. Krackow KA, Thomas SC, Jones LC: Ligament-tendon fixation: Analysis of a new stitch and comparison with standard techniques. *Orthopedics* 1988;11(6):909-917.
15. Brückner L: A standardised trans-tibial amputation method following chronic occlusive arterial disease. *Prosthet Orthot Int* 1992;16(3):157-162.
16. Brückner L: Standardized amputation of the lower leg in chronic arterial occlusive disease (IV). *Beitr Orthop Traumatol* 1986;33(4):182-187.
17. Gwinn DE, Keeling J, Froehner JW, McGuigan FX, Andersen R: Perioperative differences between bone bridging and non-bone bridging transtibial amputations for wartime lower extremity trauma. *Foot Ankle Int* 2008;29(8):787-793.
18. Horlocker TT, Hebl JR, Gali B, et al: Anesthetic, patient, and surgical risk factors for neurologic complications after prolonged total tourniquet time during total knee arthroplasty. *Anesth Analg* 2006;102(3):950-955.
19. Pinzur M, Pinto MA, Saltzman M, Batista F, Gottschalk F, Juknelis D: Health-related quality of life in patients with transtibial amputation and reconstruction with bone bridging of the distal tibia and fibula. *Foot Ankle Int* 2006;27(11):907-912.
20. Ertl J: Über amputationsstumpfe. *Chirurg* 1949;20:218-224.
21. Berlet GC, Pokabla C, Serynek P: An alternative technique for the Ertl osteomyoplasty. *Foot Ankle Int* 2009;30(5):443-446.
22. Lewandowski LR, Tintle SM, D'Alleyrand JC, Potter BK: The utilization of a suture bridge construct for tibiofibular instability during transtibial amputation without distal bridge synostosis creation. *J Orthop Trauma* 2013;27(10):e239-e242.
23. Tucker CJ, Wilken JM, Stinner PD, Kirk KL: A comparison of limb-socket kinematics of bone-bridging and non-bone-bridging wartime transtibial amputations. *J Bone Joint Surg Am* 2012;94(10):924-930.
24. Keeling JJ, Shawen SB, Forsberg JA, et al: Comparison of functional outcomes following bridge synostosis with non-bone-bridging transtibial combat-related amputations. *J Bone Joint Surg Am* 2013;95(10):888-893.
25. Ebrahimzadeh MH, Hariri S: Long-term outcomes of unilateral transtibial amputations. *Mil Med* 2009;174(6):593-597.
26. Stinner DJ, Burns TC, Kirk KL, Ficke JR: Return to duty rate of amputee soldiers in the current conflicts in Afghanistan and Iraq. *J Trauma* 2010;68(6):1476-1479.
27. Zhou J, Bates BE, Kurichi JE, Kwong PL, Xie D, Stineman MG: Factors influencing receipt of outpatient rehabilitation services among veterans following lower extremity amputation. *Arch Phys Med Rehabil* 2011;92(9):1455-1461.
28. Wolthuis AM, Whitehead E, Ridler BM, Cowan AR, Campbell WB, Thompson JF: Use of a pneumatic tourniquet improves outcome following transtibial amputation. *Eur J Vasc Endovasc Surg* 2006;31(6):642-645.

29. Harris AM, Althausen PL, Kellam J, et al: Complications following limb-threatening lower extremity trauma. *J Orthop Trauma* 2009;23(1):1-6.
30. Stone PA, Flaherty SK, Aburahma AF, et al: Factors affecting perioperative mortality and wound-related complications following major lower extremity amputations. *Ann Vasc Surg* 2006;20(2):209-216.
31. Low EE, Inkellis E, Morshed S: Complications and revision amputation following trauma-related lower limb loss. *Injury* 2017;48(2):364-370.
32. Gordon WT, O'Brien FP, Strauss JE, Andersen RC, Potter BK: Outcomes associated with the internal fixation of long-bone fractures proximal to traumatic amputations. *J Bone Joint Surg Am* 2010;92(13):2312-2318.
33. Katiyar AK, Agarwal H, Priyadarshini P, et al: Primary vs delayed primary closure in patients undergoing lower limb amputation following trauma: A randomised control study. *Int Wound J* 2020;17(2):419-428.
34. Lapidus LJ, Ponzer S, Pettersson H, de Bri E: Symptomatic venous thromboembolism and mortality in orthopaedic surgery - An observational study of 45 968 consecutive procedures. *BMC Musculoskelet Disord* 2013;14:177.
35. Herlihy DR, Thomas M, Tran QH, Puttaswamy V: Primary prophylaxis for venous thromboembolism in people undergoing major amputation of the lower extremity. *Cochrane Database Syst Rev* 2020;7(7):CD010525.
36. Dougherty PJ: Transtibial amputees from the Vietnam War. Twenty-eight-year follow-up. *J Bone Joint Surg Am* 2001;83(3):383-389.
37. Forsberg JA, Pepek JM, Wagner S, et al: Heterotopic ossification in high-energy wartime extremity injuries: Prevalence and risk factors. *J Bone Joint Surg Am* 2009;91(5):1084-1091.
38. Forsberg JA, Potter BK, Polfer EM, Safford SD, Elster EA: Do inflammatory markers portend heterotopic ossification and wound failure in combat wounds? *Clin Orthop Relat Res* 2014;472(9):2845-2854.
39. Polfer EM, Forsberg JA, Fleming ME, Potter BK: Neurovascular entrapment due to combat-related heterotopic ossification in the lower extremity. *J Bone Joint Surg Am* 2013;95(24):e195(1-6).
40. Potter BK, Burns TC, Lacap AP, Granville RR, Gajewski DA: Heterotopic ossification following traumatic and combat-related amputations. Prevalence, risk factors, and preliminary results of excision. *J Bone Joint Surg Am* 2007;89(3):476-486.
41. Mack AW, Freedman BA, Shawen SB, Gajewski DA, Kalasinsky VF, Lewin-Smith MR: Wound complications following the use of FiberWire in lower-extremity traumatic amputations: A case series. *J Bone Joint Surg Am* 2009;91(3):680-685.
42. Ayling OGS, Montbriand J, Jiang J, et al: Continuous regional anaesthesia provides effective pain management and reduces opioid requirement following major lower limb amputation. *Eur J Vasc Endovasc Surg* 2014;48(5):559-564.
43. Dumanian GA, Potter BK, Mioton LM, et al: Targeted muscle reinnervation treats neuroma and phantom pain in major limb amputees: A randomized clinical trial. *Ann Surg* 2019;270(2):238-246.

Transtibial Amputation: Prosthetic Management

CHAPTER 39

W. Lee Childers, PhD, CP • Shane R. Wurdeman, PhD, CP, FAAOP(D)

ABSTRACT

A transtibial amputation presents serious challenges to ambulation that may be overcome, in part, by using a prosthetic limb. Understanding the basic principles for socket, suspension designs, and alignment will allow informed decisions regarding transtibial prosthetic design. When selecting a prosthetic device, factors to consider include the following: (1) the importance of user-centered prosthetic design to ensure device acceptance, (2) different interfaces between the residual limb and prosthetic sockets, (3) various suspension methods, (4) prosthetic socket design options, (5) prosthetic socket/foot alignment principles, and (6) potential future transtibial prosthetic technologies. The large number of available technologies can make a decision challenging, while also allowing for design optimization to make the prosthesis unique to the individual using it and their needs.

Keywords: amputee; gait, patient-centered care; prosthetic design; transtibial amputation

Introduction

A transtibial amputation constitutes a major insult to the neural, muscular, and skeletal systems (eg, loss of the ankle joint and distal tibia, transected muscle bodies, and altered peripheral nerves) and presents serious physical challenges to ambulation. These challenges may be overcome, in part, by using a transtibial prosthetic limb. A transtibial prosthesis has five major parts: (1) an interface between the residual limb and the device, (2) a method to suspend or secure the device to the residual limb, (3) a socket (receptacle for the residual limb), (4) a pylon or shin connector, and (5) a prosthetic foot/ankle system (**Figure 1**).

It is important to define the basic principles for socket/suspension designs and alignment to enable informed decisions regarding transtibial prosthetic design. The following are to be discussed: (1) the importance of user-centered prosthetic design to ensure device acceptance, (2) different interfaces between the residual limb and prosthetic sockets, (3) various suspension methods, (4) prosthetic socket design options, (5) prosthetic socket/foot alignment principles, and (6) potential future transtibial prosthetic technologies.

A transtibial prosthesis should be designed with a focus on the user and requires an understanding of factors important for each individual user. The usefulness of a transtibial prosthesis depends on how well the device benefits the user relative to the burdens associated with its use. Patient satisfaction with the prosthesis will influence prosthesis use. Factors driving satisfaction are the amount of daily prosthesis use, patient-perceived physical function, prosthesis utility, psychological distress, clinical recovery, and the ability to return to work.[1] Prosthesis disuse is commonly associated with the patient's perception of the prosthesis being too heavy or too bulky, the socket not fitting well, or they are experiencing pain in their residual limb (which may or may not be related to the prosthesis).[2,3] Patient-reported outcome measures suggest that prosthetic function is slightly more important to users than aesthetics, and that these factors are more important than the weight of the prosthesis.[4] Prosthesis use and satisfaction are positively correlated with reduced time to the first prosthesis fitting after an amputation.[5,6] Older age and a compromised health status (such as the presence of comorbidities) are negatively correlated with prosthesis use.[5,6] The general relationship between prosthesis satisfaction and the patient's measured functional performance is currently not clear. Increases in self-selected walking speed did correlate with satisfaction in a blended cohort of people with amputation and limb salvage,[1] yet walking speed and Timed Up and Go tests did not correlate with satisfaction in another blended cohort of people with transtibial and transfemoral amputation.[3] Prosthesis users also do not report minimization of energetic cost as a pertinent factor.[2,4] Although physical performance with a prosthesis

---

Dr. Wurdeman or an immediate family member serves as a board member, owner, officer, or committee member of American Orthotic and Prosthetic Association. Neither Dr. Childers nor any immediate family member has received anything of value from or has stock or stock options held in a commercial company or institution related directly or indirectly to the subject of this chapter.

Section 3: Lower Limb

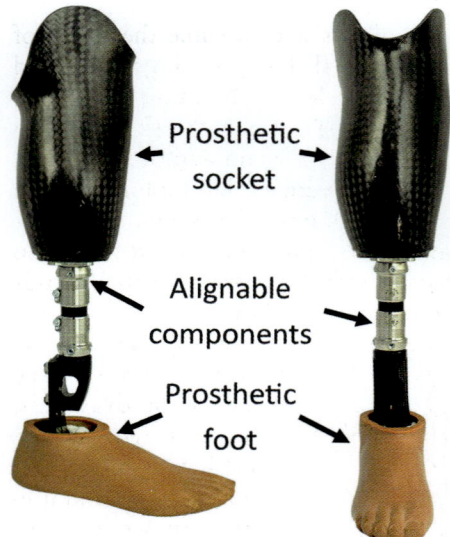

FIGURE 1 Photograph of a transtibial prosthesis consisting of a prosthetic socket, a prosthetic foot, and a method to attach and align the socket and foot. Prosthetic suspension (not shown) is the method to hold the prosthesis onto the residual limb and will occur through an interface (not shown) that will be in contact with the skin of the residual limb.

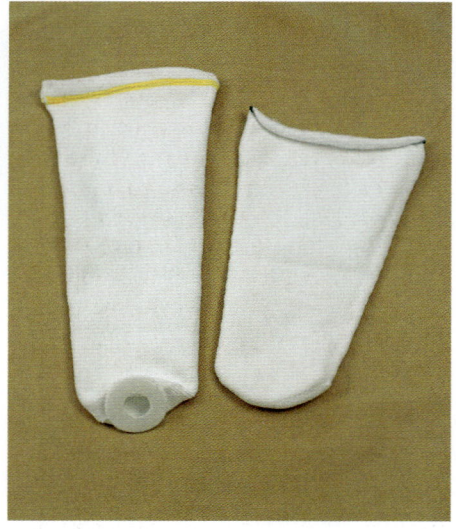

FIGURE 2 Photograph of prosthetic socks. Prosthetic socks provide a cloth-based interface. These socks come in different thickness, circumferences, and lengths to fit the residual limb. Some socks are made with a distal hole (left) to be used with pin and shuttle lock suspension systems whereas others have a closed distal end (right).

is certainly an important factor, the patient's perception of prosthetic function and utility seems to have a strong association with use. This often persists even in the absence of a measurable difference in a performance outcome.[3]

The ability to optimize prosthetic design and implement a care plan that includes building, fitting, and adjusting the prosthetic socket to achieve user comfort has been highlighted as a major factor in prosthetic usefulness and user satisfaction.[2,6] Similarly, the ability to consider the user's needs, functional abilities, and aesthetic desires play a vital role in prosthesis acceptance.

Socket Insert Design

The socket insert fits between the residual limb and the prosthetic socket. Socket inserts are broadly categorized as socks, foam inserts, and gel liners (sock-shaped inserts made of a rubber-like gel that is rolled onto the residual limb) (**Figures 2** through **4**). They provide the interface between the delicate skin of the residual limb and the hard surface of the prosthetic socket. The interface may contribute to volume management, cushioning, and/or suspension. For example, socks of different thicknesses allow the prosthesis user to change from thinner to thicker socks when the residual limb loses volume. With respect to cushioning, although an interface may diminish forces applied to delicate residual limb tissues, excessive cushioning can reduce these forces to a point where proprioceptive feedback from the residual limb is affected, thereby compromising the user's mechanical control of the prosthesis. The socket insert should provide a minimum amount of cushioning that allows for patient comfort and limb protection while maximizing prosthetic control. The socket insert may also be part of the suspension design.

Prosthetic Socks

The prosthetic sock is a traditional socket insert design for transtibial prostheses (**Figure 2**). Socks were originally used as the primary interface between the skin and the prosthetic socket and can provide volume management and cushioning. Prosthetic socks (alternatively known as stump socks) are now manufactured from wool and synthetic blends. Prosthetic socks come in various thicknesses typically referred to as the ply of the sock (eg, 1-ply, 3-ply, etc.). However, it should be noted that adding sock ply does not always increase sock thickness in an equal amount. For example, a 1-ply cotton has a measured thickness of ~0.45 mm and a 5-ply cotton sock has a measured thickness of ~1.48 mm,[7] much less than five 1-ply socks stacked together (~2.25 m). This is because the number of ply refers to the number of yarns that were woven together to create the sock and this is different than adding those same yarns on top of each other.

In some instances, the individual may need to increase or decrease sock thickness to accommodate residual limb volume fluctuations that occur throughout the day. Generally, if the patient experiences pain on the distal portion of their residuum, and/or their patella has sunken into the socket, it is an indication that they need to add a prosthetic sock to compensate for volume loss. Conversely, if they are having difficulty donning the prosthesis, and/or feel general tightness around the residuum and/or the femoral condyles, the patient should remove prosthetic socks. Prosthetic socks provide an accessible way to compensate for volume fluctuations, but there are strategies to maintain volume that do not require the use of socks. More recent research has suggested that an effective strategy to regain volume loss is to doff the prosthesis when the person will be sitting for 30 minutes.[8,9] Over longer periods of time (weeks to months), a prosthesis user may start using progressively thicker socks to achieve a comfortable fit as their residual limb continues to atrophy. The use of prosthetic socks to accommodate for residual limb volume loss will eventually compromise socket fit as residual limb volume loss is disproportional at the distal region relative to the proximal region of the limb where much of the underlying tissue is tibia and femur bone. A total volume loss of approximately 10% represents a general guideline for the point where socket replacement should be considered versus continued addition of prosthetic socks.[10] This represents a sock thickness of greater than 2.1 mm, or a sheath count of 10.[7] A prosthesis may be designed to be used with thicker socks to provide extra cushioning and potentially compensate for swelling if they are undergoing dialysis treatments. However, the use of prosthetic socks for cushioning is an older practice that has been increasingly replaced by newer materials with improved cushioning and greater comfort.[11,12]

Thermoformable Foam Inserts

Thermoformable foam inserts (**Figure 3**) generally offer increased cushioning compared with prosthetic socks. Foam inserts are composed of various closed-cell foams (such as pelite and kemblo) designed to increase cushioning and prosthetic control.[13] The foam form replicates the shape of the residual limb on the inside and the prosthetic socket on the outside, thereby providing an intimate fit. An advantage of foam inserts is the ability to vary insert thickness to provide additional cushioning where needed, creating a more uniform outer shape. Socks can only facilitate global changes in limb volume, whereas foam inserts allow localized changes to accommodate load or relieve targeted areas of the limb as needed. In some cases, foam inserts can be designed to provide anatomic suspension (discussed later in the chapter). In addition, foam inserts do not typically provide as much insulation as newer socket interface materials (discussed in the next section) and thus may be cooler for the patient. Also, foam inserts may be an alternative for prosthetic users with sensitive skin who could not tolerate newer socket interface materials without irritation. Finally, the low initial cost of a foam insert may seem advantageous, but damage or excessive wear may require the need to manufacture an entirely new socket as foam inserts are difficult to retrofit.

Prosthetic Gel Liners

The prosthetic gel liner (**Figure 4**) represented a technologic advancement beginning in the early 1980s.[11] For prosthetic liners, the term gel is synonymous with silicone, thermoplastic elastomer, and polyurethane. Gel liners have higher coefficients of friction compared with foam inserts, allowing them to protect the limb differently.[13] Specifically, the compliance of the gel liner allows it to assume the shape of the residual limb, creating a sealed layer intended to minimize movement between the gel and the skin. The gel liner now acts as an additional dermal layer, protecting the biological skin from breakdown, irritation, and abrasion.[14] This additional protection also comes with the cost of thermally insulating the residuum.[15]

Sanders et al[16] reported that silicone, thermoplastic elastomer, and urethane all have advantages and disadvantages. Thermoplastic elastomer tends to be the softest gel, behaving most similarly to soft tissue, whereas silicone and urethane tend to be stiffer under compression. When dry, none of the materials have a coefficient of friction low enough to induce slipping against the skin. Shear stiffness is similar to compression stiffness; thermoplastic elastomer is the softest, silicone is the stiffest, and urethane is similar to silicone. Using these results, the authors suggested that thermoplastic elastomer liners may be best suited for patients with bony anatomy and limited soft tissue in the residual limb. Patients with abundant soft tissue may benefit more from the stability provided by the increased stiffness of silicone or urethane. However, material properties testing does not always translate perfectly to human outcomes, and recommendations provided based on material properties should be cautiously considered.[12]

Gel liners are available in different thicknesses and profiles (such as uniform thickness or tapered from thicker to thinner more proximally). Gel liners are manufactured in numerous sizes to fit various common residual limb sizes and shapes. Liners that are custom-made based on either a scan or mold of the residual limb are also possible for those with uniquely shaped residual limbs or requiring additional cushioning in specific areas. These liners can have a fabric covering, which eases sliding of the residual limb into a socket and provides controlled stretching and stability to the entire liner. The fabric can be manufactured to reduce longitudinal stretch while allowing circumferential stretch. The liners can also have a rigid, threaded nut attached

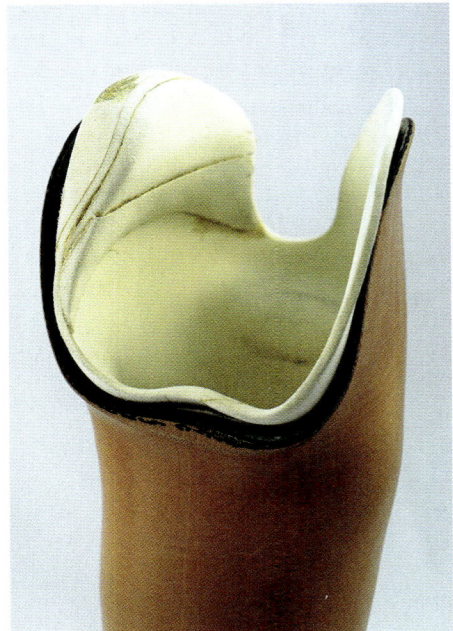

FIGURE 3 Photograph of an example of a pelite liner inside of a transtibial prosthetic socket designed with supracondylar suspension. The thickened portion on the left (medial) proximal portion of the socket will fit over and suspend the prosthesis from the femoral condyle.

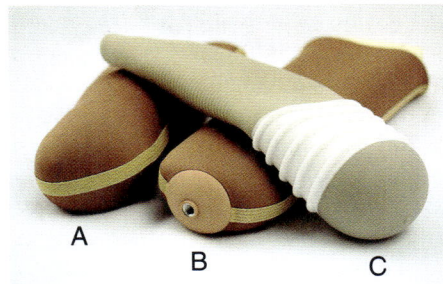

FIGURE 4 Photographs of prosthetic gel liners. Prosthetic gel liners come in many different designs. Cushion liners (A) are used with suction or elevated vacuum suspension systems. Locking liners (B) have a threaded insert to accept the pin portion of the pin-and-shuttle lock suspension. The rubber-like sealing rings of a seal-in liner (C) are used with suction suspension and allow for the socket to be sealed without using a knee sleeve.

to the distal end to allow pin-locking suspension.

A disadvantage of gel liners is thermal insulation, which has the highest insulative properties of any of the materials between the skin and the outside air.[15,17] In the presence of increased limb temperature, patients may experience excessive perspiration, dermatitis, or skin maceration. Liners made from silicone gel have the greatest measured thermal conductivity (TC)[15] and may be best suited for transferring heat away from the residual limb, yet it remains unclear if the difference in TC among liners is enough to elicit a noticeable change with the user.[18] To address this problem, researchers are now focusing on the TC of materials used for liners and sockets to help draw heat away from the residual limb. Phase-changing materials capable of absorbing and storing body heat have been tested with transtibial prosthesis users while exercising and demonstrated only a 0.2°C improvement with a large amount of variability (~2°C) compared with a placebo liner.[19] A change of 1° to 2°C may be necessary for the intervention to be clinically relevant,[18] meaning that the change of only 0.2°C in the group mean with large variability indicates a clinically relevant benefit to some, but not all, individuals.[19] A larger clinical trial is underway that may enable recommendations as to the efficacy of using phase-change materials for prosthetic liners.[20] Another creative method to minimize skin issues related to gel liners is to perforate the liner with small holes.[21] The evidence to support this use is positive yet limited to clinical case studies and a small trial using patient-reported outcome measures.[21,22] There are several active research projects currently ongoing in this area that may yield broader conclusions. Until then, caution should be used when contemplating prescription of a perforated liner. For example, it is not clear how well the liners can be cleaned to remove sweat and microbes in the perforations, the optimal size and number of perforations per square inch is not established (too large a perforation may expose the skin directly to a negative-pressure environment), and the effect on objective physiological measures of limb health is not available. Ultimately, individuals may reject gel liners because of increased limb temperature and skin problems associated with gel liners. However, the advantages of cushioning, the ability to conform to bony prominences, and the facilitation of suspension within some systems typically outweigh the disadvantages of gel liners.

Suspension Design

Prosthetic suspension, the method of securing the prosthesis to the residual limb, is an important factor in function, aesthetics, weight, and ultimately, prosthesis use. Prosthetic suspension systems attempt to minimize residual limb motion within the socket. Vertical movement within the socket is commonly referred to as pistoning because it resembles the up-and-down motion of a piston inside a cylinder. Most pistoning occurs during the swing phase of ambulation when the prosthesis and residual limb try to separate.[23] Pistoning during the swing phase will generate issues with floor clearance and the perceived weight of the prosthesis and should be minimized. The selected suspension system should also control (and ideally minimize) in-socket movement to help minimize shear forces linked to the development of abrasive skin ulcers.[24] These shear forces can be exacerbated through external movement of the socket interface moving relative to the skin or internally via the impact of the amputated bone pushing against limb tissues.[24] Therefore, minimizing limb-socket movement is considered a primary goal of prosthetic suspension systems.[25] Traditional suspension methods involve some anatomic, mechanical, or atmospheric method to secure the prosthetic socket over the soft tissues of the residual limb. These suspension systems range in complexity from designs that involve simply shaping the socket over the femoral condyles to those that involve a microprocessor-controlled pump that creates negative pressure (a vacuum) to hold the socket onto the residual limb. The benefits and drawbacks to these systems and how they fit the needs of the patient determine their usefulness.

Anatomic and Strap Suspension Systems

Anatomic suspension systems involve securing the prosthetic socket over some portion of the anatomy (typically, the femoral condyles of the distal thigh), either using socket contours or attached strapping techniques. These types of suspension systems have a long history in prosthesis use, are cost effective to produce, can be durable, and are still used in the early stages of rehabilitation or when access to prosthetic care is less reliable (eg, rural areas, populations with low socioeconomic conditions, and developing countries). However, anatomic and strap suspension systems are not commonly used in modern prosthetic practice because of the advantages of many mechanical and atmospheric-pressure–based systems that better minimize limb and socket movement.[25]

Waist Belt and Fork Strap Suspension

A waist belt and fork strap suspension (**Figure 5**) involves a belt worn around the waist with an elastic strap coming down the anterior portion of the thigh and connected to an inverted Y-strap via a buckle. The inverted Y-strap is then connected to either side of the socket and holds the prosthesis up when the foot is off the ground. The advantages of this suspension method are its simplicity and low production cost. However, the waist belt can be uncomfortable, and because the elastic strap crosses the hip and knee joints, it may not always maintain adequate tension in different limb configurations or through different motions. Therefore, its use has largely been confined to postoperative and early-stage prosthetic fittings

Cuff Strap Suspension

Cuff strap suspension (**Figure 6**) consists of a strap that wraps around the thigh just proximal to the patella and femoral condyles, which then splits, wraps around the anterior portion of the prosthesis, and connects to the medial and lateral sides of the socket. This is a simple and inexpensive

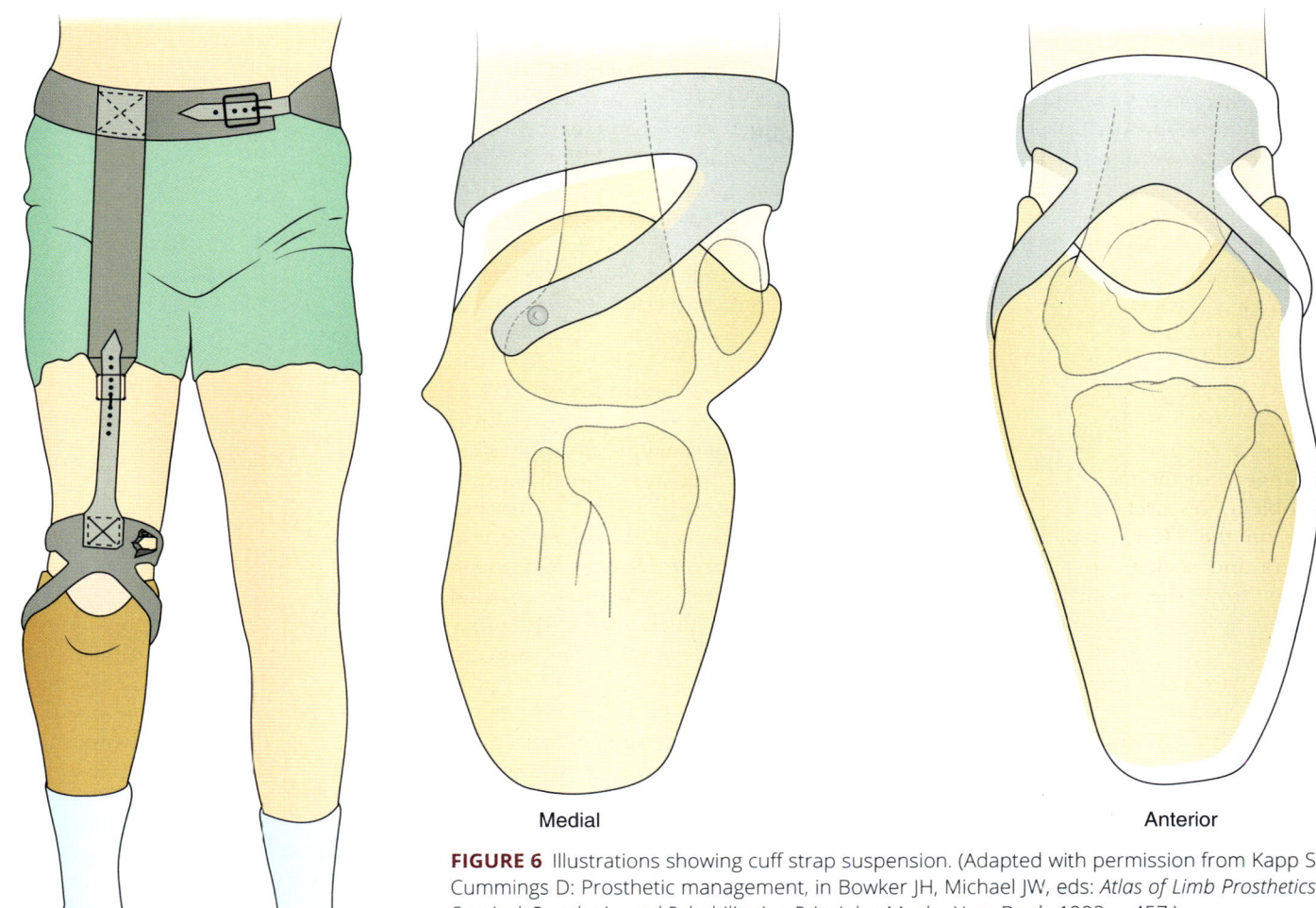

FIGURE 6 Illustrations showing cuff strap suspension. (Adapted with permission from Kapp S, Cummings D: Prosthetic management, in Bowker JH, Michael JW, eds: *Atlas of Limb Prosthetics: Surgical, Prosthetic, and Rehabilitation Principles.* Mosby-Year Book, 1992, p 457.)

FIGURE 5 Illustration of a waist belt and fork strap suspension. (Adapted with permission from Kapp S, Cummings D: Prosthetic management, in Bowker JH, Michael JW, eds: *Atlas of Limb Prosthetics: Surgical, Prosthetic, and Rehabilitation Principles.* Mosby-Year Book, 1992, p 462.)

suspension method. Fitting the cuff strap requires skill to find the correct pivot points for the strap on the prosthesis to allow for maximal knee range of motion while maintaining suspension of the prosthesis over the patella. The disadvantages of cuff suspension include reduced effectiveness at minimizing limb–socket motion relative to more modern systems and cosmetic concerns because the strap is visible through the user's pants.[26,27] Also, this suspension does not work well if there is substantial adipose tissue around the knee.

Supracondylar Suspension

Supracondylar suspension is a simple, durable, and cost-effective suspension system that secures the prosthesis by extending the medial and lateral trimlines over the femoral condyles (**Figure 3**). The proximal trimline is contoured deeper into the soft tissue, overall reducing the medial-lateral dimension proximal to the medial-lateral dimension of the femoral condyles. This creates medial-lateral support for the knee and prevents the prosthesis from slipping downward because of the condyles being unable to slip proximally past the more narrow proximal trimlines. Because the supracondylar suspension design requires an opening narrower than the width of the knee joint, donning and doffing are more complicated, and a skilled clinician is required to shape and fit the prosthesis. The most common solution for donning a socket with supracondylar suspension is to first don a foam insert that will expand over the condyles, followed by the hard socket. The opening may also be shaped in such a way as to allow the user to "twist" into the socket; alternatively, a portion of the brim or interface can be made removable. The removable brim or wedge designs allow the opening to be made wide enough to slip the limb into the socket before reestablishing a secure hold over the femoral condyles. The simplicity, durability, and cost-effectiveness of supracondylar suspension make it a good choice for users who have limited access to prosthetic care. The drawbacks include poor cosmesis when sitting, the need for increased clinical skill to shape the trimlines and socket, and poor compatibility with gel liners because the liner thickness increases the bulk around the femoral condyles. Note that recent clinical practice guidelines reported both supracondylar and cuff suspensions as yielding higher levels of pistoning compared with newer suspension approaches.[28]

Mechanical Suspension Systems

Knee Sleeve Suspension

Knee sleeve suspension, not to be confused with atmospheric pressure suspension described later, is a simple and aesthetically appealing method to suspend the prosthesis (**Figure 7**) using a neoprene, elastic fabric, or gel sleeve rolled distally over the prosthetic socket and proximally over the thigh. It suspends the prosthesis by means of mechanical contact and the resulting friction between the inside of the sleeve and outer socket wall distally and the skin of the thigh proximally. This suspension does not inhibit tissue movement relative to the bones in the thigh or residual limb and can allow some movement of the prosthesis relative to the skin via fabric stretching or movement of the sleeve relative to the socket. Knee sleeve suspension stays very close to the skin and socket, which improves aesthetics. Additionally, it is cost-effective and can be retrofitted to most prosthetic designs. Knee sleeve suspension is commonly used by older, less active prosthesis users because of ease of donning, as well as active prosthesis users in need of additional suspension. However, the thickness and stiffness of the sleeve can restrict knee joint range of motion, which is disadvantageous for some users. Also, knee sleeve suspension relies on friction between the socket and the sleeve, which can become problematic as the sleeve wears out from use and begins to slip on the socket. Last, the resultant increase in covering along the thigh can also be a deterrent for some individuals in warmer climates because of increased insulation.

Locking Liner Suspension

Locking liner suspension involves a gel liner interface worn between the residual limb and the prosthesis, with one of several mechanical methods used to attach the gel liner to the socket. This mechanical connection can be achieved with a pin-and-shuttle lock (**Figure 8**), a lanyard (**Figure 9**), or a magnetic system. In most cases, these locking suspensions involve securing the distal end of the gel liner to a receiver in the distal end of the socket.

Currently, the pin-and-shuttle lock suspension system (**Figure 8**) is one of the most commonly used systems. This system typically has a serrated pin screwed into the distal end of the gel liner that locks into a shuttle lock in the socket. A click may be audible as each serration on the pin slides through the locking mechanism, informing the user that the prosthesis has been secured. This can be advantageous to the visually impaired prosthesis user. The prosthesis is removed by depressing a button that disengages the lock. The ease of donning and doffing the prosthesis allows the user to quickly add or remove prosthetic socks to manage changes in residual limb volume. A disadvantage of this system is that the user must align the pin properly before donning the prosthesis. In addition, prosthetic socks must have a hole for the pin to allow clean insertion into the lock without pushing sock material into the locking mechanism. If this happens, the locking mechanism will likely bind and the user will be unable to remove the prosthesis without professional assistance. Active patients have reported a "milking" effect using pin-and-lock systems because the limb is predominantly suspended by the distal end. This distal suspension causes increased liner deformation more distally than

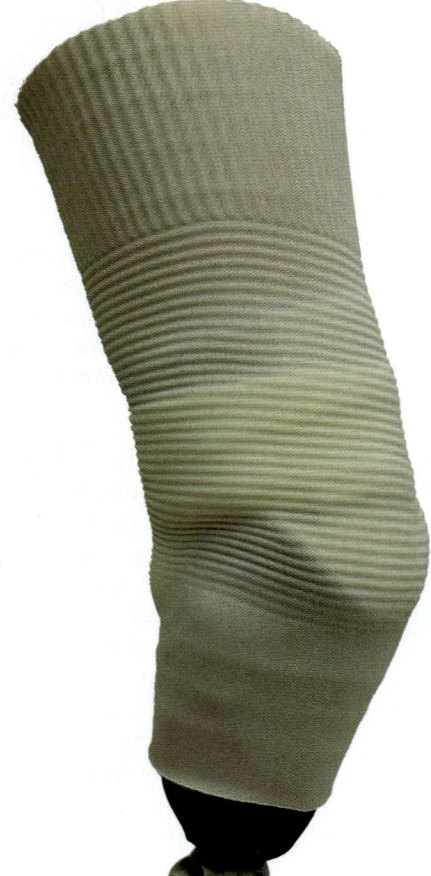

FIGURE 7 Photograph of a knee sleeve suspension system that covers the socket, knee, and thigh.

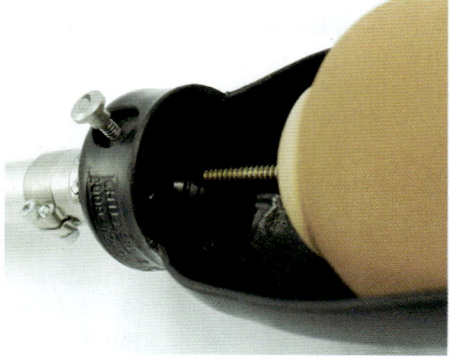

FIGURE 8 Photograph of a pin-and-shuttle lock suspension that has a pin screwed into a specially designed gel liner and this is inserted into a locking mechanism in the bottom of the socket. The prosthetic user may release the system by simply depressing the button on the side.

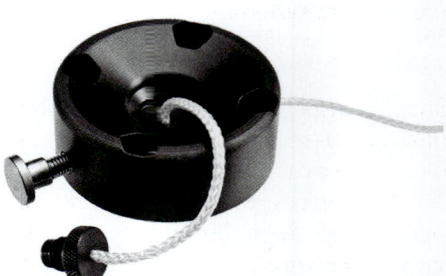

FIGURE 9 Photograph of a lanyard suspension using a cord that comes out of a locking mechanism in the bottom of the socket. The prosthetic user screws in the threaded portion into a locking style gel liner. The user then pulls on the other side of the lanyard to pull the residuum into the socket. The button on the left is to release the system. (Courtesy of Prosthetic Design, Inc.)

proximally, thereby applying a distal-to-proximal pressure gradient on the residual limb. An understanding of the possible negative health consequences of this system is limited but is of concern to some users of this type of transtibial prosthesis. A solution to reducing the additional loads on the distal end of the socket from pin suspension is to use a pin system in combination with a knee sleeve. This combination will also reduce the angular range of motion of the residuum moving in the prosthetic socket.[29]

Lanyard systems (**Figure 9**) have been developed to solve the problem of aligning a mechanical pin with a shuttle lock. A cord is attached to the gel liner and pulled through a lock mechanism in the distal end of the socket, allowing the user to pull the residual limb into the socket. A drawback to the lanyard systems is the need for sufficient hand dexterity to attach the straps and thread them through their respective components.

Atmospheric Pressure Suspension Systems

Atmospheric pressure suspension systems involve some method of sealing the space between the gel liner and the prosthetic socket. The major disadvantage to any suction-based suspension system is maintaining an airtight seal at the limb–socket interface. The durability of the sealing system and the prosthetic user's cognitive ability to understand how to use and maintain the seal are key factors in the successful use of these systems.

Suction Suspension

Suction suspension refers to the sealing of the limb–socket interface and the use of a one-way valve in the socket (**Figure 10**). Suction suspension can be achieved by sealing the limb–socket interface with a gel knee sleeve or using specifically designed liners that have a sealing gasket on the gel liner. The one-way valve combined with the cyclic pumping movement of the limb in the socket during gait gradually expels the air between the limb–socket interface and ultimately limits the movement between the residual limb and the socket.[13] During the swing phase, as gravitational

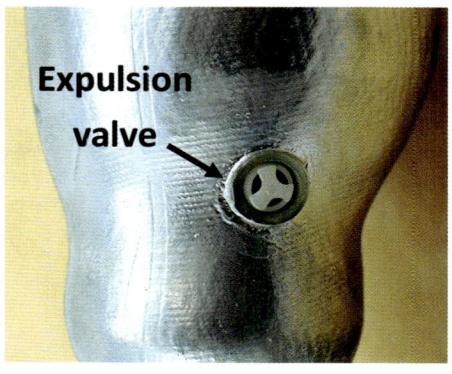

FIGURE 10 Photograph of a suction suspension that uses a method to seal the space between the residuum and the prosthetic socket via a knee sleeve (Figure 8) or a seal-in liner (Figure 5). Then a one-way expulsion valve (arrow) expels air with each step and maintains negative pressure within the residuum/socket space relative to the atmosphere.

and inertial forces pull the prosthesis away from the limb, the inability to draw air into the limb–socket interface increases the negative pressure that holds the prosthesis in place. The magnitude of displacement is related to the weight of the prosthesis and the volume of potential space between the limb and socket; as the volume of space increases, there is a resultant increase in negative atmospheric pressure countering further displacement of the prosthesis.[30] Note, however, that the system will only reach negative atmospheric pressure once the volume of space expands. As a result, the pressure between the limb and socket fluctuates between negative and positive concurrent with the swing and stance phases of gait, respectively.

Elevated Vacuum Suspension

Elevated vacuum systems have a vacuum pump to further reduce the negative pressure between the limb–socket interface relative to suction suspension. In contrast to suction suspension, which can only achieve negative pressure relative to the displacement of the prosthesis, elevated vacuum systems can obtain negative pressure as high as 80 kPa.[30] The vacuum pump can be powered mechanically by incorporating the pump into the pylon (**Figure 11**), the prosthetic foot (**Figure 12**), or using a microprocessor-controlled electric motor. The microprocessor-controlled

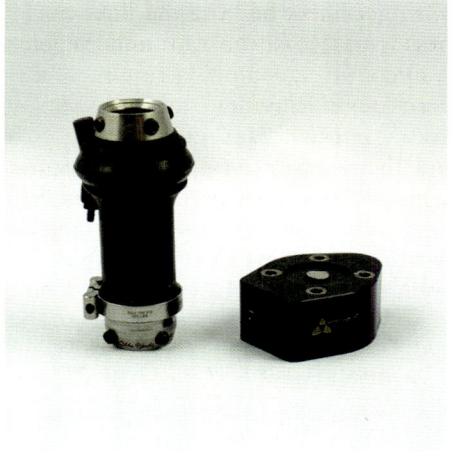

FIGURE 11 Photograph of elevated vacuum suspension systems that use a pump to remove the air from the space between the residuum and prosthetic socket. This may be done with a mechanical pump incorporated into the pylon (left) or a microprocessor-controlled electric pump (right) placed just distal to the socket.

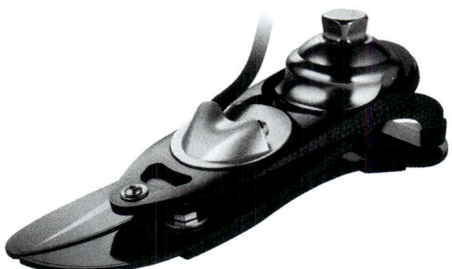

FIGURE 12 Photograph of a vacuum pump that may also be integrated to the design of the prosthetic foot. This system has a lever that actuates the pump during initial contact of each gait cycle on the amputated side. (Courtesy of Össur.)

pumps can continuously monitor and adjust vacuum pressure, whereas mechanical pumps are advantageous because they do not use a battery that must be recharged. It has been widely acknowledged that elevated vacuum systems result in the least amount of pistoning among any suspension techniques.[28] However, the added cost, complexity, and bulk of elevated vacuum systems should be taken into consideration.

Suspension System Performance

Research on transtibial suspension systems is limited, in part because of the difficulties associated with measurement.

Quantitative measures of suspension performance have traditionally been based on minimizing limb–socket movement. This movement is difficult to measure because the socket covers the residual limb being observed. This challenge has been overcome in static, simulated gait environments using radiographic techniques,[31,32] with motion-capture systems assessing markers outside the socket,[33] and markers viewed through a clear socket.[34] Creative methods to obtain these measurements in locomotion have analyzed vertical displacements in gait,[26,35] sagittal plane translation and angulation during cycling,[27] and three-dimensional analysis during gait.[29,34]

Söderberg et al[32] compared pistoning between supracondylar, pin-and-shuttle lock, cuff strap, and suction suspensions using roentgen stereophotogrammetry in a series of quasistatic positions intended to simulate gait. The results demonstrated that suction suspension was slightly better than pin-and-shuttle lock suspension, but both outperformed supracondylar and cuff strap suspension by a factor of three. Additional observations corroborate the ability of suction suspensions to minimize pistoning relative to pin-and-shuttle lock systems.[32,35] However, pin-and-shuttle lock suspension reduces pistoning and angular displacements during gait compared with cuff strap suspension.[31] Knee sleeve suspension without suction minimized pistoning relative to supracondylar and cuff strap suspensions and reduced sagittal angular movement of the residual limb within the socket more than a pin-and-shuttle lock system during gait.[26,29] Angular and translational movements can be minimized further by using a combined knee sleeve and pin suspension during gait.[29] Finally, elevated vacuum systems have minimized pistoning when compared with pin-and-shuttle lock[33] or suction suspension.[30]

To date, the methods used in research preclude direct comparisons between suspension systems across studies. However, a general theme has emerged that allows within-study comparisons. Pistoning is best minimized using approaches that involve suction and elevated vacuum systems and dual suspension (such as knee sleeve and pin). Pin-and-shuttle lock systems appear to allow modest increases in pistoning compared with atmospheric-based suspensions, but outperform more traditional anatomic suspension techniques.

Socket Design

The transtibial socket design has constantly evolved and will likely continue to change as new methodologies and material technologies are discovered. The socket provides three principal functions, the first of which is a rigid attachment to distal components such as a prosthetic foot. The other two functions are analogous to the human skeletal system in that the socket serves to facilitate energy transfer between the patient and the action point (such as the ground) and protect the residual limb from damaging pressures and impact forces.

Irrespective of the final socket design, the initial step in fabricating a transtibial prosthetic socket is to replicate the shape of the residual limb. Traditionally, plaster molding is used for this, although progress has been made in the clinical use of computer-aided design and computer-aided manufacturing techniques,[36] including MRI.[37] After shape capture using plaster or computer software, the positive model is modified according to one of three primary load designs: a patellar tendon-bearing socket design, a total surface-bearing socket design, or a hybrid design using elements of both.

Patellar Tendon-Bearing Socket

Patellar tendon-bearing (PTB) socket designs are a more traditional design, originally developed after World War II[38,39] (**Figure 13**). PTB designs are based on the principle that regions of the transtibial residual limb are inherently more capable of tolerating increased pressures without discomfort—the patellar tendon is one of these regions. There is conflicting evidence as to whether the loading of the patellar tendon effectively reduces pressure at other sites.[39,40] When modifying the positive model, regions that

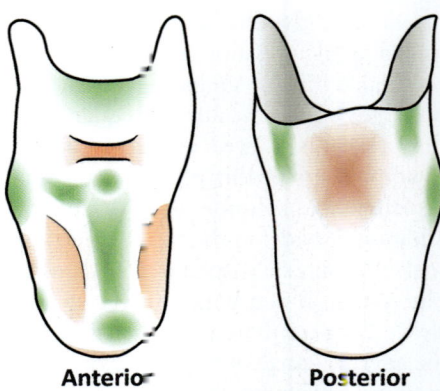

FIGURE 13 Illustration of patellar tendon-bearing prosthetic socket designs rely on contouring the socket to squeeze pressure-tolerant tissues (red) while relieving pressure-intolerant tissues (green).

are capable of increased load are carved out to increase pressure while pressure-intolerant regions are relieved with plaster or digital buildups. The patellar tendon-bearing socket design was initially used with sock interfaces, followed by foam interfaces, and most recently used with gel liner interfaces. The carved-out areas and buildups may provide improved rotational stability, but research to support this assumption is limited.

PTB sockets are best suited for patients who have long-standing history with the design. Beyond that, the drawbacks of using a traditional patellar tendon-bearing PTB design should be considered. PTB designs create regions of very high localized pressure that can induce adverse limb changes such as callus formation and skin breakdown,[41] whereas other regions are subjected to pressure levels far below their tolerances. This creates large, unnecessary pressure differentials across the limb. In-socket pressures have been reported as high as 220 to 400 kPa.[41,42] By contrast, Goh et al[43] reported peak pressures of less than 70 kPa for a total surface-bearing socket.

Total Surface-Bearing Socket

The total surface-bearing (TSB) design offers a distinctly different philosophy for socket design compared with the PTB design. TSB sockets evolved with the advent of gel liner interfaces in an effort to fully maximize load-bearing by applying uniform pressure across

Chapter 39: Transtibial Amputation: Prosthetic Management

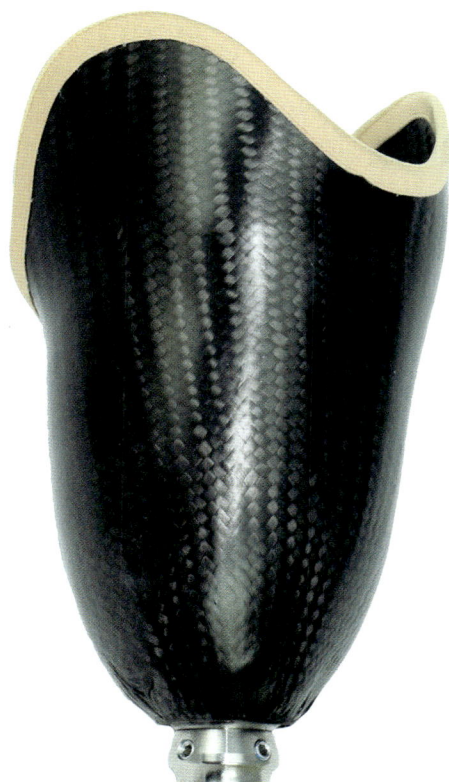

FIGURE 14 Photograph of a total surface-bearing prosthetic socket design that features less contouring, giving it a more rounded shape.

the entire surface area of the limb[44] (**Figure 14**). The TSB design therefore applies constant pressure to the gel liner, deforming it to accommodate the underlying anatomy of the residual limb. This requires global reduction of the positive model according to the residual limb's overall tissue density with increased reduction for softer tissues. Computer-aided design/computer-aided manufacturing is beneficial with this socket design, especially in cases of digital shape capture, because clinicians can easily and accurately apply global reductions via templates.

Hybrid Designs

Hybrid designs incorporate the collective advantages of both PTB and TSB designs as neither socket style is clearly indicated over the other. Recall that the PTB's philosophy to apply more pressure on pressure-tolerant regions creates large pressure differentials across the limb. Although TSB designs reduce pressure differentials, gel liners are limited in effectively reducing localized loads on certain areas of the residual limb, such as the anterior distal tibia and the fibular head. Despite these differences in design, evidence to support one socket design over another remains unclear,[45] likely because of patient variability and sensitivity of the outcome measures deployed. There were no differences in patient-reported satisfaction between PTB and TSB designs using the validated Prosthetic Evaluation Questionnaire,[46] yet another study indicated a preference for the TSB socket using an ad hoc questionnaire[47] among users who were already recommended for that design by their healthcare clinician. Gait speed comparing the two socket designs has also produced conflicting results whereby, in one study,[46] there were no changes in gait parameters while another study demonstrated a 12.9% increase in self-selected walking speed when using the TSB design.[48] The inherent variability in patient activities, demographics, amputation etiology, and patient expectations has yet to be thoroughly addressed to determine how each may contribute to an optimal socket design.

Clinicians may also consider a hybrid socket which merges prosthetic concepts from PTB and TSB designs by combining global reductions with modest localized reductions and buildups in load-tolerant and load-intolerant regions, respectively. In addition to equalizing pressures across the entire residual limb, such hybrid designs may provide some of the potential rotational control associated with PTB designs. Hybrid designs enable the clinician to adapt the socket design to the individual limb characteristics of each patient and tend to be used more ubiquitously across modern clinical practice rather than a "pure" TSB or PTB design. A notable exception is the use of elevated vacuum suspension in which the negative pressure generated by the pump pulls tissue into any relief or buildup made in a PTB or hybrid design and results in skin breakdown. For this reason, TSB designs are generally recommended by the manufacturers of elevated vacuum systems. Otherwise, socket design (PTB, TSB, or hybrid) should continue to be based on the clinical judgment of the prosthetist collaborating with the patient and the healthcare team.

Transtibial Alignment

Transtibial alignment refers to the location of the prosthetic foot relative to the prosthetic socket (**Figure 15**). Modern prosthetic components (**Figure 16**) facilitate many ways to align the foot relative to the socket that include angular (**Figure 17**) and linear adjustments in the coronal and sagittal planes along with toe in/toe out of the foot in the transverse plane. The position of the foot relative to the socket combined with the stiffness of the prosthetic foot and componentry sets up the mechanical interaction between the residual limb and the prosthesis (**Figure 18**). Prosthetic alignment is optimized based on typical movements performed by the user. The prosthesis can be used for more than just ambulation (eg, standing for long periods, running, turning, working in tight spaces, and cycling); therefore, the specific alignment should be adjusted based on feedback from the individual user to minimize discomfort and maximize stability.

Prosthetic alignment can be categorized into two types: static and dynamic. Static alignment is the initial or baseline alignment the prosthetist selects before working with the user of the prosthesis. This alignment varies based on the prosthetic foot and the recommendations of the manufacturer. Prosthetic feet are produced with different stiffness properties, and the manufacturer suggests baseline measurements that optimize alignments based on these properties and gait performance over level terrain. Static alignments represent a "best first guess" and allow room for the prosthetist to make changes to optimize outcomes based on the user's concerns and abilities.

Dynamic alignment requires the prosthetist and patient to work together to arrive at an optimal alignment based on the patient's movements and preferences. When gait is analyzed, the prosthetist should first assess the sagittal plane followed by the coronal plane to minimize the interactive effect of the coronal plane

Section 3: Lower Limb

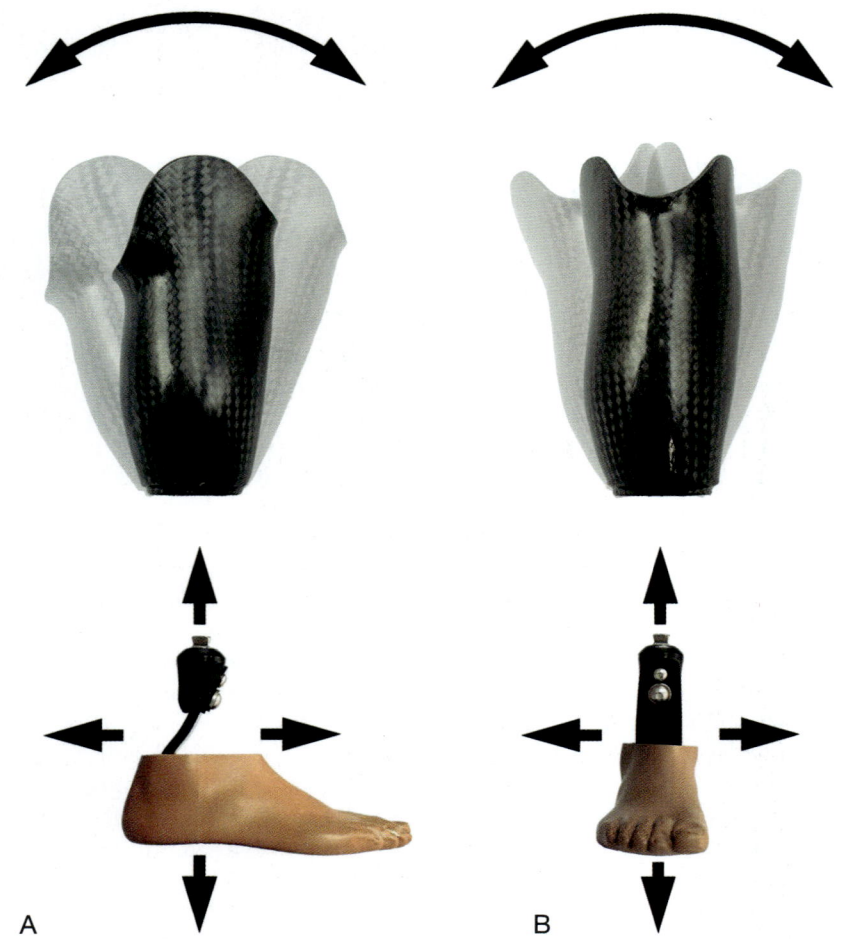

FIGURE 15 Lateral (A) and AP (B) photographic views show endoskeletal components that allow for many options to position the prosthetic foot relative to the socket, including angular and translational movements about all axes.

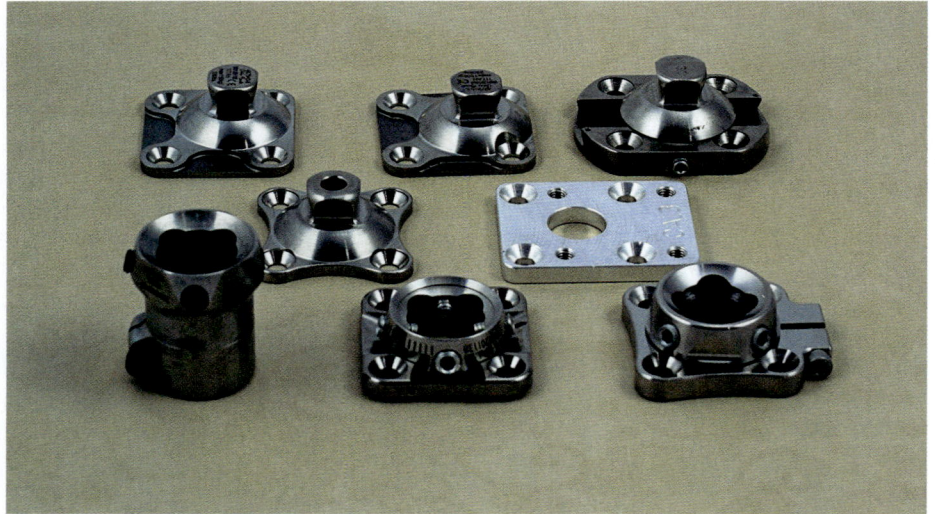

FIGURE 16 Photograph of modern prosthetic components that are modular and interchangeable, offering enormous alignment opportunities. The specially designed male pyramid (middle row, left, and top row) has angled sides and fits into a female receiver (bottom row) that has four set screws. Angular alignment changes can be made by loosening screw and tightening the opposite side. Components can be used with different offsets (middle row, right, and top row) to allow for translational adjustments. Transverse plane rotational adjustments may also be made (bottom row).

on the sagittal plane.[49] The prosthetist performs alignment changes based on visual gait analysis and the user's subjective feedback.[50] This iterative process has drawbacks. The subjective nature of the prosthetic user's ability to perceive alignment changes is good for angular adjustments, but not as good for translational adjustments.[51] In addition, the function of a prosthesis is based in large part on the mechanical forces being assisted or resisted at the interface between the residual limb and prosthesis; this cannot be seen through observational gait analysis. Recent advances in prosthetic technology have seen the advent of load cells mounted between the socket and pylon to allow forces and moments to be calculated at this interface, which can then be used to optimize alignments.[49,52] Although these technologies have the potential to improve clinical outcomes, they have not yet superseded the traditional method of observational gait analysis in normal clinical practice.

Emerging Technologies: Enhanced Socket Fit

The fit of a prosthesis changes because the residual limb volume fluctuates throughout the day while the socket shape remains fixed. This greatly impacts socket comfort, prosthesis usability, and ultimately, residual limb health. Thus, a prosthetic socket or liner system combined with some method to compensate for volume changes could be advantageous. Early volume control designs have used inflation or deflation of pneumatic[53] or hydraulic bladders[23] embedded in the liner. These methods have demonstrated limited success and have not been used as part of mainstream care. More common are systems equipped with a user-controlled cable and ratchet mechanism that allow modifiable compression of pressure-tolerant regions throughout the day to compensate for volume changes (**Figure 19**). Current designs are expected to continue improving as researchers develop better materials and creative solutions to control these systems.

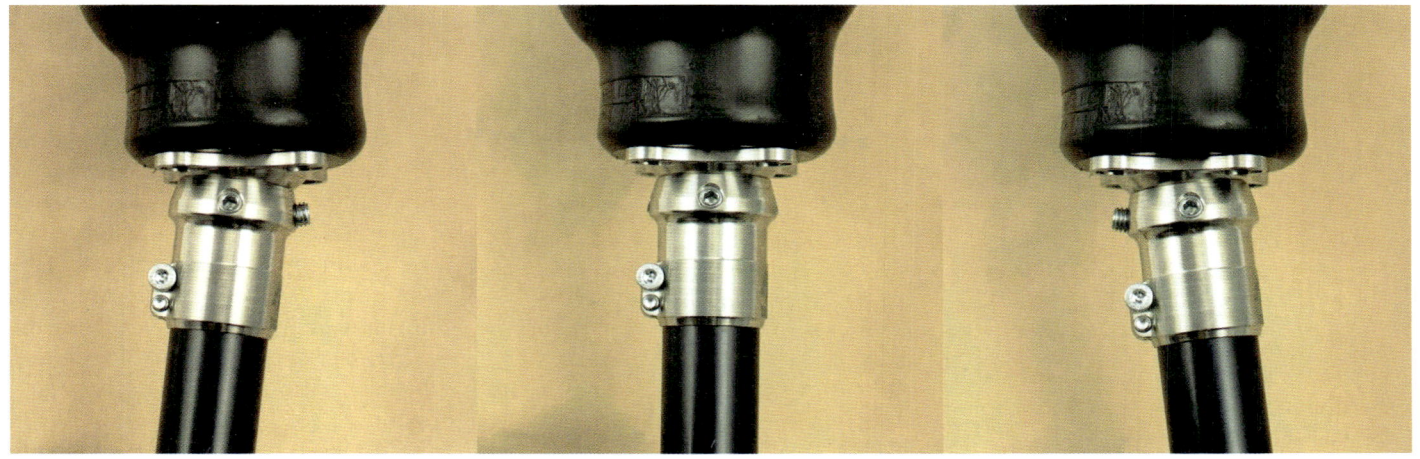

FIGURE 17 Photographs showing angular alignment changes that can be made by loosening the screw and tightening the opposite side.

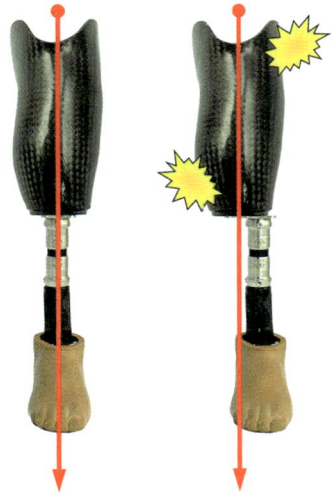

FIGURE 18 Illustration showing that alignment will affect how forces are applied to the residuum through the interface. The red arrow indicates the body weight of a person if all their weight is distributed over the center of their prosthesis. If the foot is perfectly centered under the weight line (right), loads on the residuum are minimized. As the foot is moved medially (right), loads on the proximal/medial and distal/lateral sides are increased (indicated by starbursts) because there is a moment created in the frontal plane trying to rotate the prosthesis counterclockwise and this must be resisted by a clockwise moment between the residuum and prosthesis.

Socket Design and Manufacturing

Traditional socket design relies on the skill of the prosthetist to understand the anatomy of the residual limb and the intended use of the prosthesis. Traditional manufacturing techniques are labor-intensive and require a skilled technician for fabrication by hand. New techniques are being developed that use residual limb shape capture via topographic scanning and, to an extent, MRI, that may minimize fabrication times while improving shape consistencies. MRI provides a detailed three-dimensional image of the residual limb with information about the surface and underlying anatomy. This method of limb shape capture has been explored for creating sockets with stiffness that varies based on the underlying anatomy.[37] Selective-laser sintering has also been used to not only fabricate sockets that include compliant and stiffer regions, but also to develop novel prosthetic foot prototypes. This technology relies on a high-power laser that fuses a powdered medium at specific points corresponding to a three-dimensional shape designed using a computer-aided design program.[36,54]

Methods to rapidly produce prosthetic sockets are also evolving. Three-dimensional printing technology has seen rapid growth, but has not yet been put into everyday clinical practice. As the cost of three-dimensional printing drops and the quality of printed materials improves, there is an expected increased reliance on these manufacturing techniques

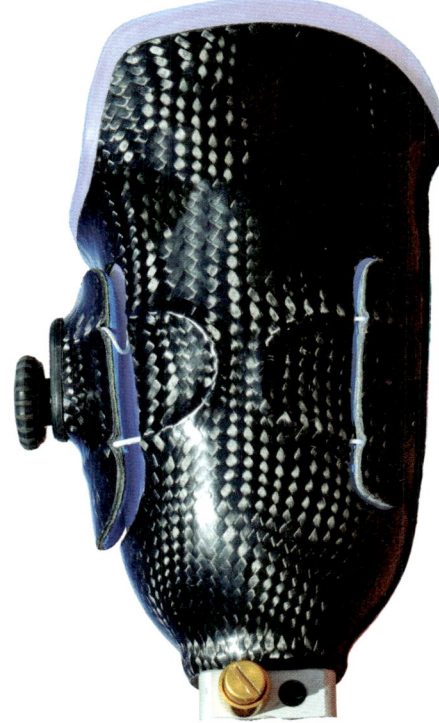

FIGURE 19 The RevoFit® utilizes socket cutouts combined with a high tension cable and dial system to allow the prosthetic user to compensate for volume changes. The cut-out portions will move in to compress and expand the limb or compensate for volume changes as the user turns the dial system. This mechanical system allows the prosthetic user to control the socket tightness but the added bulk, necessary skill to fabricate, and potential durability issues associated with cable-actuated mechanical system provide some drawbacks. (Courtesy of Click Medical LLC.)

Section 3: Lower Limb

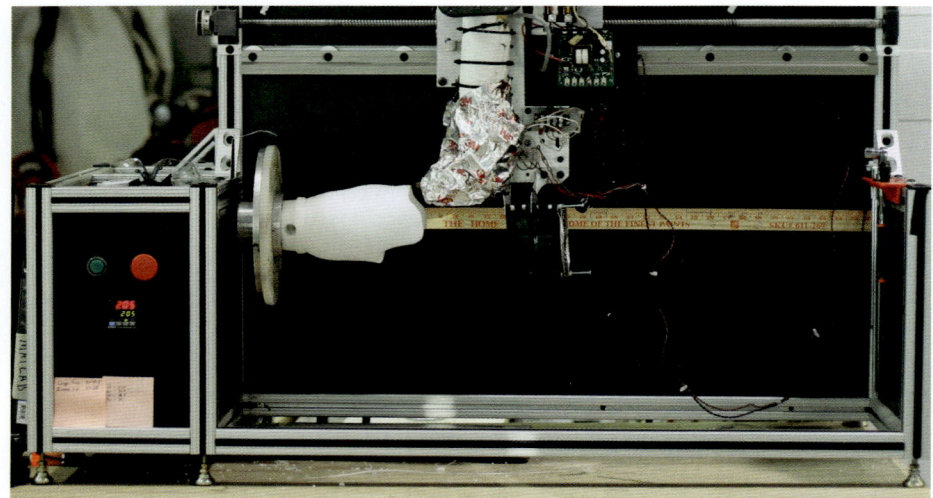

FIGURE 20 Photograph of rapid prosthetic manufacturing being demonstrated by a fused deposition modeling machine produced by Prosthetic Design Inc. that can produce sockets in less than three hours at a fraction of the traditional fabrication cost. This equipment has been producing sockets for clinical practice since 2012. (Courtesy of Prosthetic Design, Inc.)

within prosthetic care. Fused deposition modeling is another form of rapid manufacturing originally applied to prosthetic sockets in the early 1990s.[55] A machine was designed to extrude a bead of semimolten polypropylene on the head of a computer-controlled milling machine in a continuous spiral that gradually formed the contours of a socket, eliminating the need for a positive model. In the early 2000s, grant funding for that project ended. Development was continued by another company in 2002 (**Figure 20**), resulting in considerable refinement and further development. Sockets can now be manufactured, cooled, and ready for patient use in less than 3 hours. This new machine has actively produced prosthetic sockets since 2012 and represents the first successful implementation of rapid manufacturing technologies into daily clinical practice. Such setups can now be found in multiple fabrication labs across the world.

Moisture Management at the Prosthetic Interface

Gel liner interface systems are able to better protect the skin on the residual limb from pressure and shear force than foam interfaces, but have the disadvantage of high thermal insulation, resulting in subsequent sweating and potential problems with skin maceration. In addition to the heat-absorbing and perforated liners described earlier, systems under development can actively cool the limb using airflow or by pumping chilled fluid through the interface.

Many of the more sophisticated devices and concepts are still in the early phases of research or commercialization. Unfortunately, many devices that show initial promise ultimately prove too complicated or cumbersome for prosthesis users. Successful clinical implementation will take time because long-term testing is needed.

SUMMARY

Many of the prosthetic interfaces, sockets, and suspension systems currently available have been discussed and the alignment principles and potential new technologies have been reviewed. The number of available technologies may seem overwhelming, but these options exist to provide optimal customization and ensure the prosthesis is as unique as the individual using it. Through collaboration with the patient and other members of the rehabilitation team, the prosthetist should ensure that each aspect of the prosthetic design is patient-centered. Prosthetic technologies should be focused on the person using the device to optimize benefits and minimize drawbacks based on the individual's functional need and daily routine. The role of the prosthetist is to use their knowledge to enhance the patient's life during the initial rehabilitation process and to remain aware of evolving technology so that new methods can be adapted to provide optimal prosthetic care throughout the user's lifetime.

References

1. O'Toole RV, Castillo RC, Pollak AN, MacKenzie EJ, Bosse MJ, LEAP Study Group: Determinants of patient satisfaction after severe lower-extremity injuries. *J Bone Joint Surg Am* 2008;90(6):1206-1211.
2. Legro MW, Reiber G, del Aguila M, et al: Issues of importance reported by persons with lower limb amputations and prostheses. *J Rehabil Res Dev* 1999;36(3):155-163.
3. Kark L, Simmons A: Patient satisfaction following lower-limb amputation: The role of gait deviation. *Prosthet Orthot Int* 2011;35(2):225-233.
4. Gallagher P, MacLachlan M: Development and psychometric evaluation of the Trinity Amputation and Prosthesis Experience Scales (TAPES). *Rehabil Psychol* 2000;45(2):130-154.
5. Gauthier-Gagnon C, Grise M-C, Potvin D: Predisposing factors related to prosthetic use by people with a transtibial and transfemoral amputation. *J Prosthet Orthot* 1998;10(4):99-109.
6. Pezzin LE, Dillingham TR, MacKenzie EJ, Ephraim P, Rossbach P: Use and satisfaction with prosthetic limb devices and related services. *Arch Phys Med Rehabil* 2004;85(5):723-729.
7. Sanders JE, Cagle JC, Harrison DS, Karchin A: Amputee socks: How does sock ply relate to sock thickness? *Prosthet Orthot Int* 2012;36(1):77-86.
8. Sanders JE, Hartley TL, Phillips RH, et al: Does temporary socket removal affect residual limb fluid volume of trans-tibial amputees? *Prosthet Orthot Int* 2016;40(3):320-328.
9. Sanders JE, Youngblood RT, Hafner BJ, et al: Residual limb fluid volume change and volume accommodation: Relationship to activity and self-report outcomes in people with trans-tibial

amputation. *Prosthet Orthot Int* 2018;42(4):415-427.

10. Fernie GR, Holliday PJ: Volume fluctuations in the residual limbs of lower limb amputees. *Arch Phys Med Rehabil* 1982;63(4):162-165.

11. Kristinsson Ö: The ICEROSS concept: A discussion of a philosophy. *Prosthet Orthot Int* 1993;17(1):49-55.

12. Klute GK, Glaister BC, Berge JS: Prosthetic liners for lower limb amputees: A review of the literature. *Prosthet Orthot Int* 2010;34(2):146-153.

13. Sanders JE, Greve JM, Mitchell SB, Zachariah SG: Material properties of commonly-used interface materials and their static coefficients of friction with skin and socks. *J Rehabil Res Dev* 1998;35:161-176.

14. Baars ECT, Geertzen J: Literature review of the possible advantages of silicon liner socket use in transtibial prostheses. *Prosthet Orthot Int* 2005;29(1):27-37.

15. Klute GK, Rowe GI, Mamishev AV, Ledoux WR: The thermal conductivity of prosthetic sockets and liners. *Prosthet Orthot Int* 2007;31(3):292-299.

16. Sanders JE, Nicholson BS, Zachariah SG, Cassisi DV, Karchin A, Fergason JR: Testing of elastomeric liners used in limb prosthetics: Classification of 15 products by mechanical performance. *J Rehabil Res Dev* 2004;41(2):175-186.

17. Williams RJ, Washington ED, Miodownik M, Holloway C: The effect of liner design and materials selection on prosthesis interface heat dissipation. *Prosthet Orthot Int* 2018;42(3):275-279.

18. Peery JT, Ledoux WR, Klute GK: Residual-limb skin temperature in transtibial sockets. *J Rehabil Res Dev* 2005;42(2):147-154.

19. Wernke MM, Schroeder RM, Kelley CT, Denune JA, Colvin JM: SmartTemp prosthetic liner significantly reduces residual limb temperature and perspiration. *J Prosthet Orthot* 2015;27(4):134-139.

20. Fiedler G, Singh A, Zhang X: Effect of temperature-control liner materials on long-term outcomes of lower limb prosthesis use: A randomized controlled trial protocol. *Trials* 2020;21(1):1-11.

21. Caldwell R, Fatone S: Technique for perforating a prosthetic liner to expel sweat. *J Prosthet Orthot* 2017;29(3):145-147.

22. Davies KC, McGrath M, Stenson A, Savage Z, Moser D, Zahedi S: Using perforated liners to combat the detrimental effects of excessive sweating in lower limb prosthesis users. *Canadian Prosthet Orthot J* 2020;3(2):1.

23. Sanders J, Jacobsen A, Fergason J: Effects of fluid insert volume changes on socket pressures and shear stresses: Case studies from two trans-tibial amputee subjects. *Prosthet Orthot Int* 2006;30(3):257-269.

24. Mak AF, Zhang M, Tam EW: Biomechanics of pressure ulcer in body tissues interacting with external forces during locomotion. *Annu Rev Biomed Eng* 2010;12:29-53.

25. Gholizadeh H, Abu Osman NA, Eshraghi A, Ali S, Razak NA: Transtibial prosthesis suspension systems: Systematic review of literature. *Clin Biomech* 2014;29(1):87-97.

26. Wirta RW, Golbranson FL, Mason R, Calvo K: Analysis of below-knee suspension systems: Effect on gait. *J Rehabil Res Dev* 1990;27(4):385-396.

27. Childers WL, Perell-Gerson KL, Gregor RJ: Measurement of motion between the residual limb and the prosthetic socket during cycling. *J Prosthet Orthot* 2012;24(1):19-24.

28. Stevens PM, DePalma RR, Wurdeman SR: Transtibial socket design, interface, and suspension: A clinical practice guideline. *J Prosthet Orthot* 2019;31(3):172-178.

29. Childers WL, Siebert S: Marker-based method to measure movement between the residual limb and a transtibial prosthetic socket. *Prosthet Orthot Int* 2016;40(6):720-728.

30. Board W, Street G, Caspers C: A comparison of trans-tibial amputee suction and vacuum socket conditions. *Prosthet Orthot Int* 2001;25(3):202-209.

31. Narita H, Yokogushi K, Shi S, Kakizawa M, Nosaka T: Suspension effect and dynamic evaluation of the total surface bearing (TSB) trans-tibial prosthesis: A comparison with the patellar tendon bearing (PTB) trans-tibial prosthesis. *Prosthet Orthot Int* 1997;21(3):175-178.

32. Söderberg B, Ryd L, Persson BM: Roentgen stereophotogrammetric analysis of motion between the bone and the socket in a transtibial amputation prosthesis: A case study. *J Prosthet Orthot* 2003;15(3):95-99.

33. Klute GK, Berge JS, Biggs W, Pongnumkul S, Popovic Z, Curless B: Vacuum-assisted socket suspension compared with pin suspension for lower extremity amputees: effect on fit, activity, and limb volume. *Arch Phys Med Rehabil* 2011;92(10):1570-1575.

34. Lenz AL, Johnson KA, Bush TR: A new method to quantify liner deformation within a prosthetic socket for below knee amputees. *J Biomech* 2018;74:213-219.

35. Gholizadeh H, Osman NAA, Eshraghi A, et al: Transtibial prosthetic suspension: Less pistoning versus easy donning and doffing. *J Rehabil Res Dev* 2012;49(9):1321-1330.

36. Faustini MC, Neptune RR, Crawford RH, Rogers WE, Bosker G: An experimental and theoretical framework for manufacturing prosthetic sockets for transtibial amputees. *IEEE Trans Neural Syst Rehabil Eng* 2006;14(3):304-310.

37. Sengeh DM, Herr H: A variable-impedance prosthetic socket for a transtibial amputee designed from magnetic resonance imaging data. *J Prosthet Orthot* 2013;25(3):129-137.

38. Radcliffe CW: *The Patellar-Tendon-Bearing Below-Knee Prosthesis*. Biomechanics Laboratory, 1961.

39. Abu Osman NA, Spence WD, Solomonidis SE, Paul JP, Weir AM: The patellar tendon bar! Is it a necessary feature? *Med Eng Phys* 2010;32(7):760-765.

40. Kim WD, Lim D, Hong KS: An evaluation of the effectiveness of the patellar tendon bar in the trans-tibial patellar-tendon-bearing prosthesis socket. *Prosthet Orthot Int* 2003;27(1):23-35.

41. Mak AF, Zhang M, Boone DA: State-of-the-art research in lower-limb prosthetic biomechanics. *J Rehabil Res Dev* 2001;38(2-6):161-174.

42. Meier R III, Meeks E Jr, Herman R: Stump-socket fit of below-knee prostheses: Comparison of three methods of measurement. *Arch Phys Med Rehabil* 1973;54(12):553-558.

43. Goh J, Lee P, Chong S: Stump/socket pressure profiles of the pressure cast prosthetic socket. *Clin Biomech (Bristol, Avon)* 2003;18(3):237-243.

44. Staats TB, Lundt J: The UCLA total surface bearing suction below-knee prosthesis. *Clin Prosthet Orthot* 1987;11(2):118-130.

45. Safari R, Meier MR: Systematic review of effects of current transtibial prosthetic socket designs—Part 1: Qualitative outcomes. *J Rehabil Res Dev* 2015;52(5):491-508.

46. Selles RW, Janssens PJ, Jongenengel CD, Bussmann JB: A randomized controlled trial comparing functional outcome and cost efficiency of a total surface-bearing socket versus a conventional patellar tendon-bearing socket in transtibial

amputees. *Arch Phys Med Rehabil* 2005;86(1):154-161.

47. Hachisuka K, Dozono K, Ogata H, Ohmine S, Shitama H, Shinkoda K: Total surface bearing below-knee prosthesis: advantages, disadvantages, and clinical implications. *Arch Phys Med Rehabil* 1998;79(7):783-789.

48. Yiğiter K, Şener G, Bayar K: Comparison of the effects of patellar tendon bearing and total surface bearing sockets on prosthetic fitting and rehabilitation. *Prosthet Orthot Int* 2002;26(3):206-212.

49. Kobayashi T, Orendurff MS, Zhang M, Boone DA: Effect of transtibial prosthesis alignment changes on out-of-plane socket reaction moments during walking in amputees. *J Biomech* 2012;45(15):2603-2609.

50. Chow DHK, Holmes AD, Lee CKL, Sin SW: The effect of prosthesis alignment on the symmetry of gait in subjects with unilateral transtibial amputation. *Prosthet Orthot Int* 2006;30(2):114-128.

51. Boone DA, Kobayashi T, Chou TG, et al: Perception of socket alignment perturbations in amputees with transtibial prostheses. *J Rehabil Res Dev* 2012;49(6):843-853.

52. Fiedler G, Slavens B, Smith RO, Briggs D, Hafner BJ: Criterion and construct validity of prosthesis-integrated measurement of joint moment data in persons with transtibial amputation. *J Appl Biomech* 2014;30(3):431-438.

53. Greenwald RM, Dean RC, Board WJ: Volume management: Smart Variable Geometry Socket (SVGS) technology for lower-limb prostheses. *J Prosthet Orthot* 2003;15(3):107-112.

54. Rogers B, Bosker GW, Crawford RH, et al: Advanced trans-tibial socket fabrication using selective laser sintering. *Prosthet Orthot Int* 2007;31(1):88-100.

55. Rovick J, Childress J, Chan D: An additive fabrication technique for the computer-aided manufacturing of sockets, in *7th World Congress of the International Society for Prosthetics and Orthotics*. Chicago, IL, International Society for Prosthetics and Orthotics, 1992.

Knee Disarticulation: Surgical Management

Michael S. Pinzur, MD, FAAOS • COL Benjamin Kyle Potter, MD, FAAOS, FACS

ABSTRACT

In the preanesthetic era, knee disarticulations were popular because they allowed surgical efficiency and limited blood loss. Because of poor distal soft-tissue coverage, limited prosthetic options, and poor functional outcomes, this type of amputation fell out of favor in the early 1900s. Prosthetic advances and modifications in surgical technique in the last 25 years of the 20th century resulted in resurgent interest in knee disarticulation. Currently, knee disarticulation can provide excellent functional outcomes in a select subset of patients with a traumatic injury and those with oncologic conditions or infection who have a viable gastrocnemius muscle and require amputation about or proximal to the knee joint but in whom transtibial salvage amputation is not feasible. Similarly, satisfactory outcomes can be achieved in many patients with diabetes and vascular dysfunction who have low functional demands and limited ambulatory potential.

| **Keywords:** amputation; knee disarticulation

Introduction

Historically, knee disarticulation was advocated in the preanesthetic era because of the efficiency of the procedure, the limited associated bleeding, and because the technique does not violate the medullary canal.[1,2] Various skin flaps, including equal AP, long anterior or posterior, and sagittal flaps have been described and used;[3] however, each of these flaps consisted only of skin and subcutaneous tissue and lacked adequate padding to permit routine end bearing on the terminal residual limb, limiting the ability of the patient to successfully use a prosthesis.

The retention of the full femoral length represents both the principal disadvantage and advantage of amputation at this level. The distal residual limb can be bulky and some degree of knee-level discrepancy is generally inevitable, but a stable, potentially end-bearing terminal residual limb is created with a long lever arm and an intact native insertion for the adductor magnus. Numerous revisions and modifications to the procedure have been proposed to address its limitations while preserving at least some of the advantages. Stokes[4] advocated supracondylar amputation with retention of the adductor insertion and fixation of the patella to the distal femur. Mazet and Hennessy[5] advocated trimming the medial, lateral, and posterior condyles and removing the patella to decrease bulkiness; Burgess[6] advocated removing the distal 1.5 cm of the condyles and the patella. Bowker[7] combined the latter two techniques, effectively achieving a long residual femur following transfemoral amputation. Although each technique has its merits, none has gained widespread use, potentially because each compromises the end-bearing and socket suspension advantages of knee disarticulation without fully addressing the shortcomings.

One prosthetic advancement and one surgical advancement in the late 20th century resulted in a renewed interest in knee disarticulation as a common, or even preferred, amputation level for many patients. Lyquist[8] introduced the Orthopaedic Hospital of Copenhagen prosthesis, which featured a four-bar linkage polycentric knee joint that provided excellent stability while reducing cosmetic mismatch and knee height discrepancy because the shank folded under the socket when seated. Modernized versions on this knee design are currently popular. Wagner[9] described the use of gastrocnemius muscle belly with sagittal skin flaps as terminal padding to improve end-bearing comfort. Klaes and Eigler,[10] as translated by Bowker et al,[11] first reported the use of a posterior myofasciocutaneous flap incorporating the gastrocnemius muscles and leaving the perforating circulation to the skin flap intact. Thus, knee disarticulation has been rediscovered by modern, outcomes-oriented amputation surgeons for its capability to restore stable, functional ambulation for many patients after trauma or tumor resection.

Outcome Considerations

By retaining the weight-bearing femoral condyles and providing adequate distal padding, the modern knee disarticulation allows residual limb weight bearing

---

Dr. Pinzur or an immediate family member is a member of a speakers' bureau or has made paid presentations on behalf of Orthofix, Inc. and Stryker. Dr. Potter or an immediate family member serves as an unpaid consultant to Biomet and serves as a board member, owner, officer, or committee member of the Society of Military Orthopaedic Surgeons.

without discomfort. The somewhat bulky nature of the terminal residual limb facilitates enhanced socket fit and suspension, improving sitting comfort by allowing the proximal socket trim lines to be kept out of the groin and distal to the ischium. In addition, the intact adductor magnus insertion obviates concerns about myodesis performance, stability, and resulting adductor strength in those with amputation at the transfemoral level. The physiologic cost of walking with a knee disarticulation is midway between that of transfemoral and transtibial amputation levels.[12-14] Good results have been reported in many ambulatory patients after knee disarticulation, with potentially decreased phantom sensation and residual limb pain, as well as lower risk of revision surgery for complications such as heterotopic ossification after high-energy trauma.[15-17] Although worse Sickness Impact Profile disability scores were reported in the Lower Extremity Assessment Project (LEAP) study for knee disarticulations versus transfemoral amputations,[18] 12 of the 17 patients with knee disarticulation in that study did not have viable gastrocnemius muscle, and the authors of this chapter do not advocate knee disarticulation in such patients. A more recent comparative study of 10 military unilateral knee disarticulation patients and 18 patients with transfemoral amputation found no differences in multiple patient-reported functional outcome measures.[19]

In addition, knee disarticulation improves the ability to transfer from bed to chair and optimizes seating balance for low-demand or nonambulatory patients with vascular pathology, diabetes, or other severe comorbidities. From a biomechanical perspective, direct load transfer, or end bearing, is more natural than in transfemoral or transtibial amputations, allowing potentially enhanced feedback and proprioception during upright activities[11,20,21] (**Figure 1**).

Prosthetic fitting of a patient with a knee disarticulation can take advantage of the four-bar linkage polycentric knee joint that provides intrinsic knee joint stability, decreasing the risk of stumbling and falling while minimizing

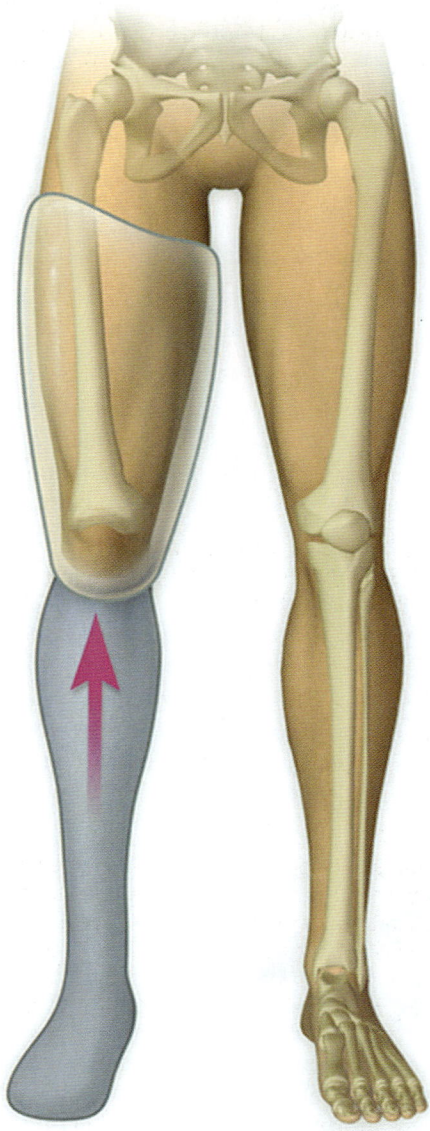

FIGURE 1 Illustration demonstrating weight bearing after knee disarticulation accomplished through direct load transfer (end-bearing load transfer; red arrow) between the residual limb and the prosthesis. A knee disarticulation allows more normal proprioceptive feedback compared with the transosseous (transtibial or transfemoral) amputation levels. Prosthetic socket fit at this level is not crucial because the shearing forces that occur in transosseous amputation levels are avoided.

knee-level discrepancies[22-25] (**Figure 2**). This enhanced intrinsic knee joint stability becomes important when the minimally ambulatory patient with unilateral transtibial amputation requires contralateral amputation. Such patients generally have limited prosthetic goals, making stability during walking even more crucial. When knee disarticulation is performed on the contralateral limb, these individuals demonstrate enhanced stability on that limb without an apparent loss of walking propulsion.[21] Despite the obligatory knee-level discrepancy with regard to shank length and sitting prominence, many higher functioning amputees perform quite well with newer, microprocessor knees.

Knee disarticulation has a valuable role in the treatment of patients with diabetes or a high body mass index who have renal failure and residual limb volume fluctuations caused by venous insufficiency and/or neuropathic swelling. Volume fluctuations make it difficult to achieve a successful prosthetic fitting after transtibial amputation. The end-bearing capacity of a knee disarticulation allows a less intimate prosthetic socket fit, with a volume-adaptable socket to allow functional ambulation (**Figure 3**). Wound complications associated with transtibial amputation in this cohort can be as high as 15% to 30%.[26] In addition, the shear forces applied to the healing residual limb from transtibial amputation can be avoided by the end-bearing load transfer of knee disarticulation.

Despite the beneficial rehabilitation potential of knee disarticulation, many patients are not suitable candidates for the procedure after trauma, tumor, or infection. In many cases, salvage at the preferred transtibial level is practicable; in others, the native gastrocnemius muscles are compromised or absent, and/or the disease process involves the knee joint or distal femur, and more proximal transfemoral amputation is required. Knee disarticulation is commonly indicated in the patient with diabetes and vascular dysfunction who has the biologic potential to heal after amputation at the proximal transtibial level, but who will be unlikely to achieve walking independence with a prosthetic limb. Knee disarticulation avoids the commonly observed knee flexion contracture associated with the nonambulatory transtibial amputee and hip flexion–adduction contracture observed in the nonambulatory transfemoral amputee. Functionally, the amputee with a knee disarticulation who primarily sits in a wheelchair has a greatly improved platform for sitting and a longer, more functional lever arm for transferring from bed to wheelchair compared with the transfemoral amputee (**Figure 4**).

Preferred Surgical Technique of This Chapter's Authors

Wagner[9] reestablished a modern role for knee disarticulation using sagittal flaps to preserve vascular supply, with the use of relatively short flaps in patients with dysvascular conditions. Although this was a reasonable intellectual concept, the flap construct resulted in a substantial incidence of skin necrosis caused by separation of the muscle and skin layers of the soft-tissue envelope. A practical solution was achieved by using the traditional posterior gastrocnemius myofasciocutaneous flap popularized by Burgess after World War II, a technique that was familiar to amputation surgeons.[6,27]

A thigh tourniquet is advocated and generally inflated to 100 mm Hg above the systolic pressure to avoid excessive bleeding and improve speed and visualization. The anterior incision is placed midway between the inferior pole of the patella and the tibial tubercle. The length of the posterior flap is equal to the diameter of the limb at the level of the knee joint, plus at least 1 cm; this flap can be shortened at the time of closure if it is too long or redundant. In transtibial amputation, the width of the flap varies based on the size of the patient and the diameter of the limb. Initially using a flap that is too wide

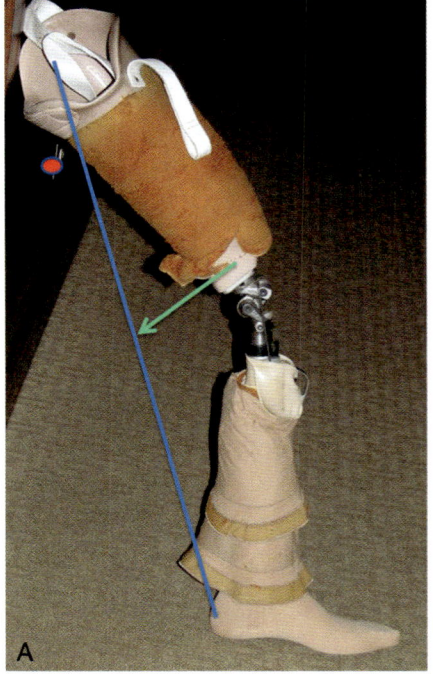
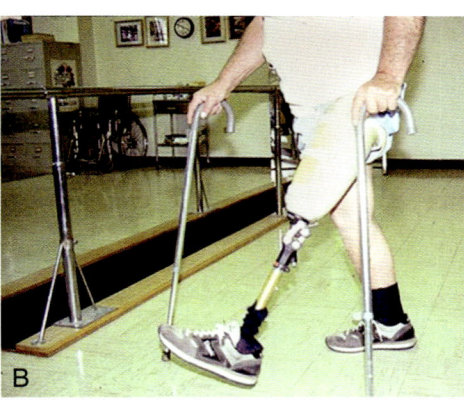

FIGURE 2 Photograph demonstrating the walking stability of a prosthetic knee joint with a polycentric four-bar linkage. **A**, The virtual knee center of the prosthetic joint (red circle) is located at a point that virtually ensures positioning weight bearing (blue line) anterior to this axis, thus creating intrinsic knee joint stability. The force vector attempting to buckle/flex the knee joint (green arrow) remains anterior to the virtual knee axis, creating intrinsic knee joint stability. **B**, Photograph demonstrating knee joint stability during preparatory prosthetic fitting and early gait training.

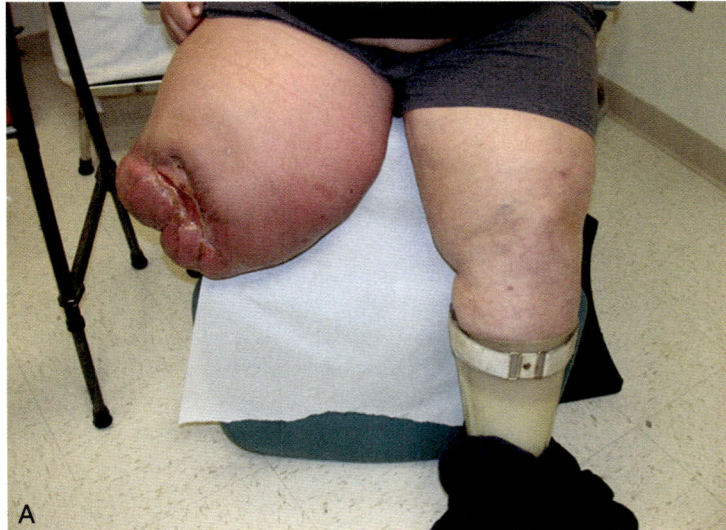
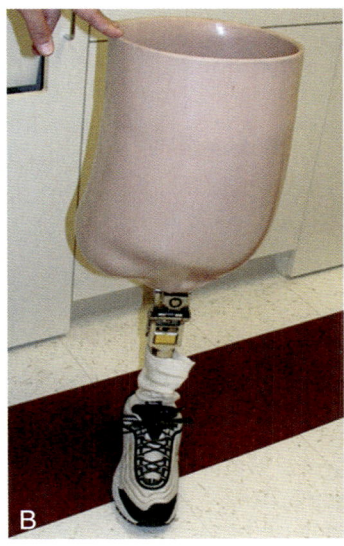
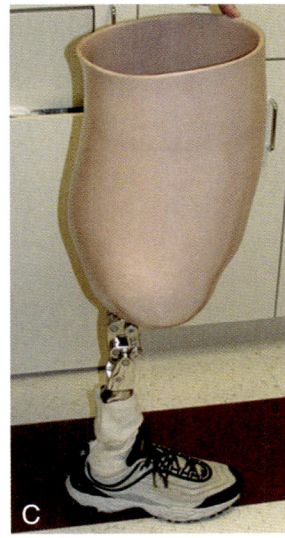

FIGURE 3 A, Photograph of the residual limb of a patient with morbid obesity after a knee disarticulation. The patient had renal failure that resulted in substantial volume fluctuations during the day. Anterior (**B**) and lateral (**C**) photographic views of a volume-adaptable prosthetic socket that allows direct load transfer and functional weight bearing.

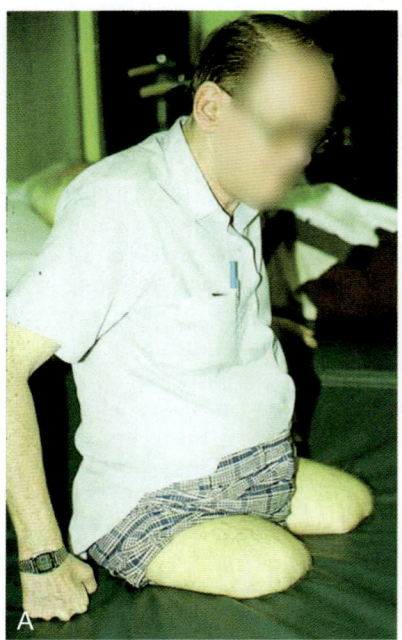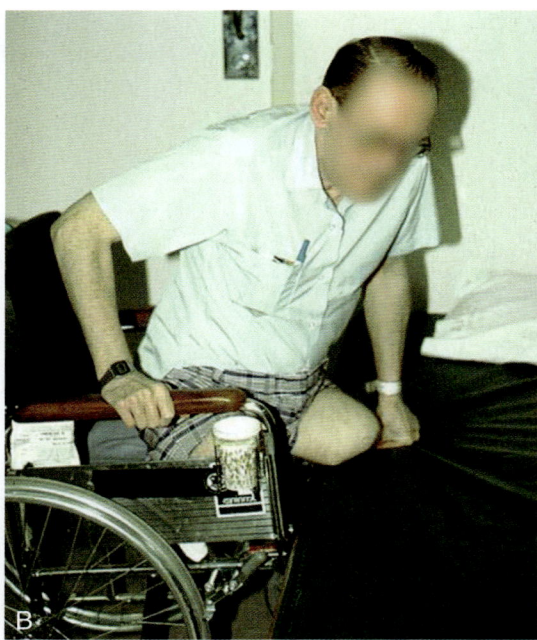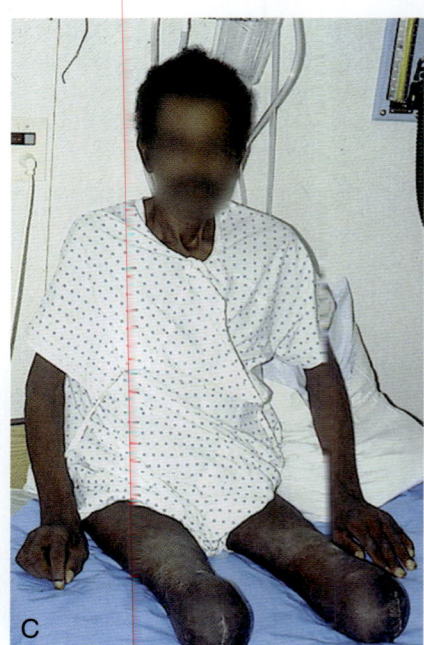

FIGURE 4 Photographs of a patient after a bilateral transfemoral amputation demonstrating a small platform for sitting in a chair (**A**) and an inefficient lever arm for transferring from a bed to a chair (**B**). **C**, Photograph of a patient after bilateral knee disarticulation showing a balanced sitting platform and an improved lever arm for bed-to-chair transfer. (Panel C courtesy of John H. Bowker, MD.)

is preferred because trimming at the conclusion of the procedure is simple and avoids an inadequate amount of tissue or a closure that is too tight. The incision is carried down to the level of the fascia circumferentially, the saphenous vein is ligated, and a traction neurectomy of the saphenous nerve is performed.

Medial and lateral incisions are then made along the patellar tendon from the tibial tubercle proximal to the inferior pole of the patella. The patellar tendon is sharply detached from the tibial tubercle, retaining as much length as possible for the reconstruction. The knee joint retinaculum is transected circumferentially with a scalpel for approximately 50% of the circumference of the knee joint. The anterior cruciate ligament is sharply detached from its tibial insertion, allowing subluxation of the anterior tibia, facilitating completion of the capsular release. The posterior cruciate ligament is then detached from the tibia.

A flap can easily be created with blunt dissection between the gastrocnemius and soleus muscles, which allows isolation and provisional clamping of the popliteal artery and veins, distal to the sural blood supply to the medial and lateral gastrocnemius muscle bellies. The amputation is completed before the tourniquet is released. The artery is double-ligated with a suture ligature and a simple ligature. A suture ligature is used to prevent arterial pulsation from dislodging the ligature; the veins are ligated with simple ligatures. The tibial and common peroneal nerves are identified and isolated, and proximal traction neurectomy is performed with gentle tension and a fresh scalpel blade, cushioning the resulting neuromas between the hamstring musculature in the proximal popliteal fossa away from the terminal residual limb. The medial sural cutaneous nerve is identified within the fascia of the posterior flap, and a more aggressive mobilization and proximal traction neurectomy are performed. This allows the nerve to retract into the popliteal fossa. This technique prevents neuromas from causing symptoms near the incision line (if no neurectomy is performed) or over the terminal residual limb's weight-bearing cushion of the gastrocnemius muscle (if a more standard, gentle neurectomy is performed). Alternatively, targeted muscle reinnervation or regenerative peripheral nerve interface creation are performed, both discussed elsewhere within this text, again with attention to performing or docking the nerves within the popliteal fossa away from the terminal limb.

The patella can be removed or retained at the discretion of the surgeon, but the authors of this chapter generally retain it to improve sagittal prosthetic suspension and stability and to avoid creating further dead space within the nascent residual limb. With adequate distal patellar tendon stabilization at closure, excessive motion and symptomatic patellofemoral arthrosis are uncommon, and formal patellofemoral arthrodesis is unnecessary.[7,8] Short medial and lateral splits along the medial and lateral extensor retinaculum facilitate suprapatellar synovectomy. Anecdotally, this eliminates the continued production of synovial fluid and accelerates the scarring of the quadriceps, patella, and patellar tendon.

After tourniquet release, hemostasis is achieved with electrocautery and/or with suture ligatures as necessary, and the wound is irrigated. Closure is initiated by repairing the patellar tendon to the residual ends of the cruciate ligaments with a double row of heavy nonabsorbable suture (**Figure 5**). The medial and lateral hamstring tendons

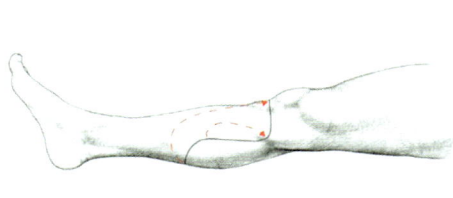 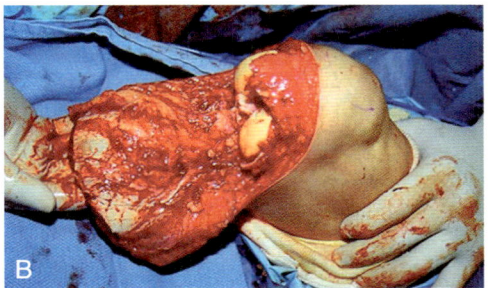 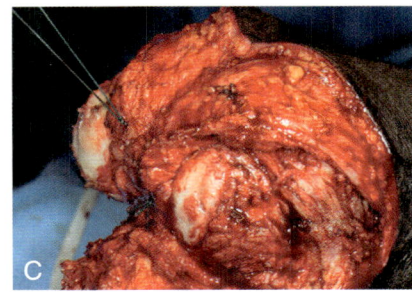

FIGURE 5 **A**, Illustration of a posterior myocutaneous soft-tissue flap in a knee disarticulation, which is similar to the commonly used transtibial amputation flap. The anterior incision is made midway between the inferior pole of the patella and the tibial tubercle. The flap length is equal to the diameter of the limb at the knee joint plus 1 cm. **B**, Intraoperative photograph showing knee disarticulation before wound closure. **C**, Photograph demonstrating the patellar tendon secured to the residual ends of the cruciate ligaments with heavy nonabsorbable suture.

may be tacked to an adjacent joint capsule or the gastrocnemius tendons proximally. Surgical drains, if indicated or preferred, may be placed within the suprapatellar pouch and/or deep to the gastrocnemius muscles over the distal femur.

Subcutaneous drains are not necessary or indicated; anterior and posterior skin flap separation from the extensor retinaculum and gastrocnemius, respectively, should be avoided. A buried, heavy nonabsorbable suture is then passed from the midline of the posterior gastrocnemius fascia to the proximal patellar tendon to anchor the terminal padding. The posterior gastrocnemius fascia is then repaired to the anterior knee joint retinaculum (which was transected at the beginning of the procedure) with figure-of-8 stitches and heavy absorbable suture. Skin closure is accomplished with nylon sutures, with or without small, buried absorbable dermal sutures.[11] The goal is a robust, viable closure providing ample stable distal residual limb padding for early end bearing. The initial bulkiness of the construct will decrease quickly with time as both edema resolution and atrophy ensue.

Alternative Surgical Technique

One valuable lesson learned from the LEAP study was that poor results occur after knee disarticulation when the amputation is performed within the zone of injury and the soft-tissue envelope created does not have viable gastrocnemius muscle to act as a cushion.[18] Orthopaedic techniques that focus on damage control emphasize

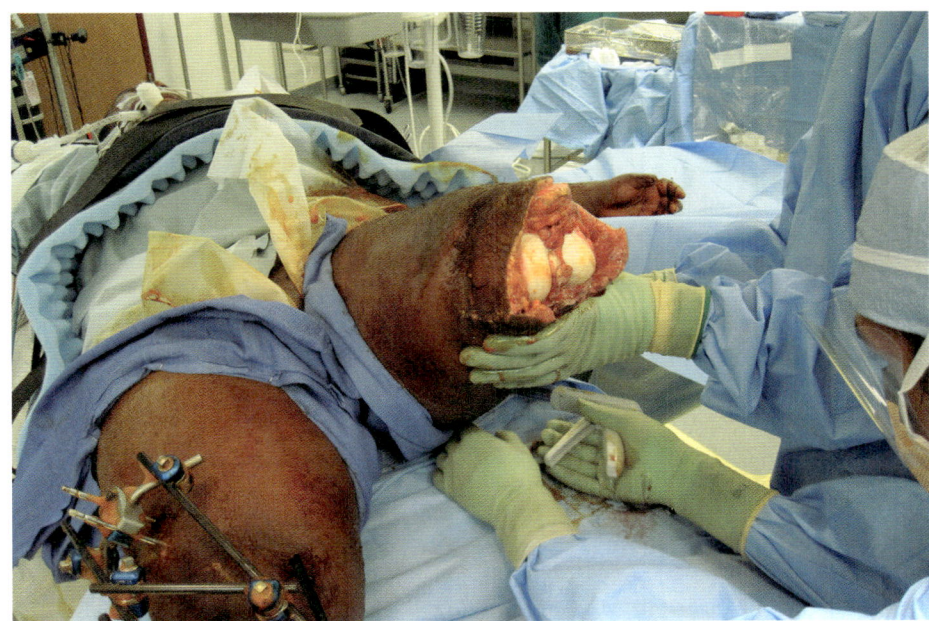

FIGURE 6 Intraoperative photograph showing a trauma patient without adequate remaining gastrocnemius muscle to provide a weight-bearing end pad for a functional knee disarticulation. This patient would be better treated with transfemoral amputation.

delaying further insult to a traumatized limb until the zone of injury has fully declared itself and stabilized. In amputation surgery, creation of a definitive soft-tissue envelope should be delayed until the zone of injury recovers. In the dysvascular limb of a patient with diabetes, best results are achieved when sufficient viable muscle exists to create a functional soft-tissue envelope.

Débridement of nonviable tissue should be the first step in creating a viable, functional residual limb. After débridement, the surgeon may be left with nontraditional soft-tissue flaps for the creation of the soft-tissue envelope. After definitive amputation, the

residual limb should have a durable myocutaneous soft-tissue flap if the goal is prosthetic fitting and functional ambulation. Although exceptions and creative modifications are possible, the authors of this chapter generally do not advocate knee disarticulation as the definitive amputation level for patients lacking a viable gastrocnemius muscle and overlying skin adequate for terminal padding (**Figure 6**). Such patients may be better served with a transfemoral or Gritti-Stokes amputation. After a well-performed transfemoral amputation with suitable and sufficient tissue to create the soft-tissue envelope, the residual limb will be more functional than after a knee disarticulation in which there is no muscle to provide a robust, cushioned soft-tissue envelope.

For patients with a viable gastrocnemius muscle in whom knee disarticulation is contemplated but for whom, because of high functional potential, concerns about knee-level mismatch and shank length are a concern, a supracondylar shortening osteotomy can be performed (**Figure 7, A**). Briefly, a retrograde intramedullary nail is reamed through the exposed distal femur. Next, 9 to 10 cm of bone is removed from the distal metaphysis, retaining the periosteum, through a lateral incision which may or may not extend from the proximal surgical incision. The retrograde nail is placed, ensuring appropriate countersinking, and compressed for immediate stability. Rapid healing occurs because of the well-vascularized bone, cortical contact, and redundant periosteum, and no postoperative weight bearing or activity restrictions are necessary after initial soft-tissue healing. Adductor magnus weakness because of loss of length is not a concern, as the shape of the distal femur facilitates continued centering of the bone along both its mechanical and anatomic axes within the soft-tissue envelope and the muscle predictably shortens and contracts over time. This technique should be used with caution for patients in whom the indication for the knee disarticulation was infection-related. The same end result can be achieved, over time, for pediatric patients (discussed in detail elsewhere in this text) with skeletal growth remaining via distal femoral physeal arrest at the time of knee disarticulation (**Figure 7, B**).

Rehabilitation

A compression dressing or rigid plaster dressing can be used, depending on the experience and preference of the surgeon. The authors of this chapter generally prefer soft compression dressings, transitioning to a shrinker stocking as soon as any drains are removed; there is no distal joint to protect from contracture following knee disarticulation, obviating many of the purported benefits of rigid plaster dressings, but the standard risks of pressure necrosis and eschar formation despite diligent padding persist. As with all lower extremity amputations, mobilization, core strengthening, and aerobic conditioning should commence postoperatively as soon as the patient's condition permits. Early ambulation without a prosthetic limb allows easy transition to weight bearing when permitted by wound healing. Because shearing forces are avoided, preparatory prosthetic limb fitting can be initiated as soon as the soft-tissue envelope and surgical wound appear to be secure. Based on the viability of the soft-tissue envelope, a safe practice is to initiate preparatory prosthetic limb fitting with a volume-adaptable socket as early as 2 weeks after surgery.[29] Full weight bearing can be achieved as early as 4 weeks postoperatively for previously healthy patients who underwent surgery for tumor or trauma, whereas the rehabilitation progress of patients with diabetes and vascular dysfunction tends to proceed more slowly.

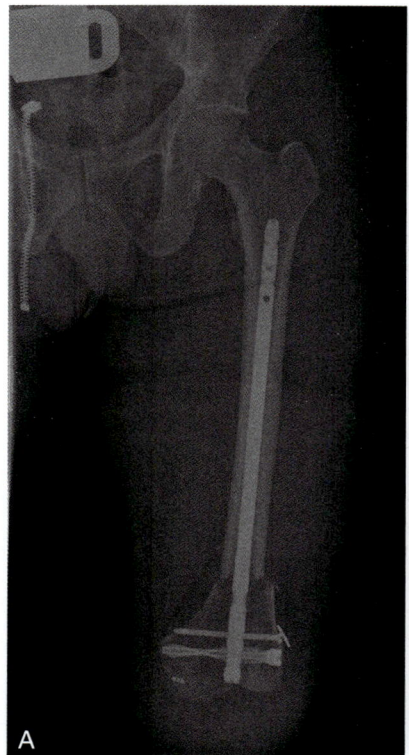 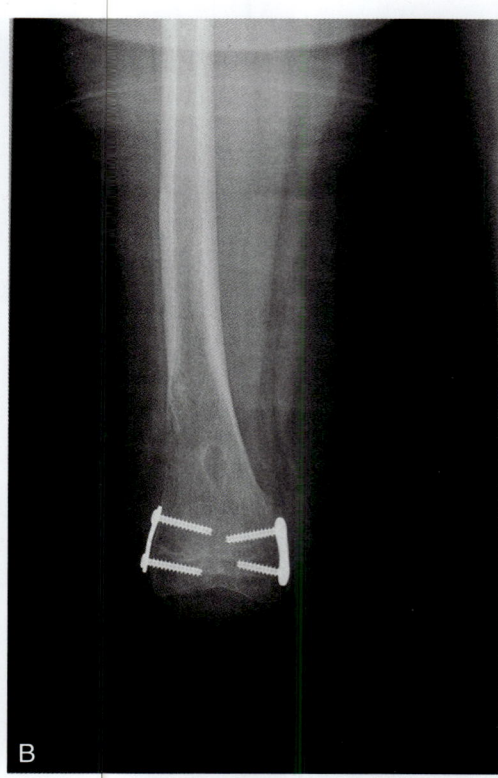

FIGURE 7 A, AP postoperative radiograph of the left femur of a skeletally mature patient in whom a supracondylar shortening osteotomy with retrograde intramedullary stabilization has been performed in conjunction with a knee disarticulation amputation. **B**, An AP radiograph of the distal femur of a pediatric patient in whom physeal arrest has been performed at the time of a knee disarticulation. These techniques solve the problem of knee-level mismatch, acutely and over time, respectively, while retaining the end-bearing benefits of this amputation level.

Managing Complications

Wound infections should be managed with early débridement. Vacuum-assisted wound closure and secondary wound closure are reasonable options. The key to success is the viability of the muscle flap and adequate skin coverage. Coverage of wounds with split-thickness skin grafts is generally avoided because of the poor durability of the resultant residual limb, but it can be successful over viable muscle. Skin grafts performed over exposed fascia, tendon, or periosteum are susceptible to frequent breakdown and should prompt consideration for more proximal revision. In certain circumstances, modern silicone sleeves can act as an interface to allow weight bearing in areas with suboptimal soft-tissue coverage. Heterotopic ossification and symptomatic neuromata are usually less problematic after successful knee disarticulations in appropriately selected patients.

SUMMARY

Knee disarticulation is an accepted surgical option in appropriately selected patients. A successful knee disarticulation can provide excellent healing, resulting in a durable, functional residual limb in both young, active patients and older, sedentary patients. Modern sockets and newer prostheses, including those with modern four-bar linkage, microprocessor-controlled components, and power knees, have improved functional outcomes and decreased cosmetic concerns regarding knee-level discrepancy for most patients. Patient selection and the viability of the gastrocnemius-based posterior myofasciocutaneous flap are crucial to the success of the procedure and, indeed, the authors of this chapter do not advocate attempted knee disarticulation in patients without a viable myofasciocutaneous flap.

References

1. Smith N: Amputation at the knee-joint. *Am Med Rev* 1825;2:370.
2. Velpeau A: Memoire sur l'amputation de la jambe dans l'articulation du genou, et description d'un nouveau procede pour pratiquer cette operation. *Arch Gen Med* 1830;24:44-60.
3. Rogers SP: Amputation at the knee joint. *J Bone Joint Surg* 1940;22:973-979.
4. Stokes W: On supracondylar amputation of the thigh. *Proc Roy Med Chir Soc London* 1870;6:289.
5. Mazet R Jr, Hennessy CA: Knee disarticulation: A new technique and a new knee-joint mechanism. *J Bone Joint Surg Am* 1966;48:126-139.
6. Burgess EM: Disarticulation of the knee: A modified technique. *Arch Surg* 1977;112(10):1250-1255.
7. Bowker JH: Abstract: Reduction osteoplasty of the distal femur to enhance prosthetic fitting in knee disarticulation, in *Proceedings of the Seventh World Congress of the International Society for Prosthetics and Orthotics*. International Society for Prosthetics and Orthotics, 1992, p 267.
8. Lyquist E: The OHC knee-disarticulation prosthesis. *Orthot Prosthet* 1976;30:27-28.
9. Wagner FW Jr: Management of the diabetic-neurotrophic foot: Part II. A classification and treatment program for diabetic, neuropathic, and dysvascular foot problems. *Instr Course Lect* 1979;28:143-165.
10. Klaes W, Eigler FW: Eine neue technik der transgenikulären amputation [German]. *Chirurg* 1985;56(11):735-740.
11. Bowker JH, San Giovanni TP, Pinzur MS: North American experience with knee disarticulation with use of a posterior myofasciocutaneous flap: Healing rate and functional results in seventy-seven patients. *J Bone Joint Surg Am* 2000;82(11):1571-1574.
12. Fisher SV, Gullickson G Jr: Energy cost of ambulation in health and disability: A literature review. *Arch Phys Med Rehabil* 1978;59(3):124-133.
13. Waters RL, Perry J, Antonelli D, Hislop H: Energy cost of walking of amputees: The influence of level of amputation. *J Bone Joint Surg Am* 1976;58(1):42-46.
14. Pinzur MS, Gold J, Schwartz D, Gross N: Energy demands for walking in dysvascular amputees as related to the level of amputation. *Orthopedics* 1992;15(9):1033-1036.
15. Pinzur MS, Bowker JH: Knee disarticulation. *Clin Orthop Relat Res* 1999;361:23-28.
16. Behr J, Friedly J, Molton I, Morgenroth D, Jensen MP, Smith DG: Pain and pain-related interference in adults with lower-limb amputation: Comparison of knee-disarticulation, transtibial, and transfemoral surgical sites. *J Rehabil Res Dev* 2009;46(7):963-972.
17. Tintle SM, Shawen SB, Forsberg JA, et al: Reoperation after combat-related major lower extremity amputations. *J Orthop Trauma* 2014;28(4):232-237.
18. Bosse MJ, MacKenzie EJ, Kellam JF, et al: An analysis of outcomes of reconstruction or amputation after leg-threatening injuries. *N Engl J Med* 2002;347(24):1924-1931.
19. Polfer EM, Hoyt BW, Bevevino AJ, Forsberg JA, Potter BK: Knee disarticulations versus transfemoral amputations: Functional outcomes. *J Orthop Trauma* 2019;33(6):308-311.
20. Pinzur MS, Smith DG, Daluga DJ, Osterman H: Selection of patients for through-the-knee amputation. *J Bone Joint Surg Am* 1988;70(5):746-750.
21. Pinzur MS, Smith D, Tornow D, Meade K, Patwardhan A: Gait analysis of dysvascular below-knee and contralateral through-knee bilateral amputees: A preliminary report. *Orthopedics* 1993;16(8):875-879.
22. Pinzur MS: New concepts in lower-limb amputation and prosthetic management. *Instr Course Lect* 1990;39:361-366.
23. Pinzur MS, Bowker JH, Smith DG, Gottschalk F: Amputation surgery in peripheral vascular disease. *Instr Course Lect* 1999;48:687-691.
24. Pinzur MS, Pinto MA, Schon LC, Smith DG: Controversies in amputation surgery. *Instr Course Lect* 2003;52:445-451.
25. Pinzur MS, Gottschalk FA, Pinto MA, Smith DG: Controversies in lower-extremity amputation. *J Bone Joint Surg Am* 2007;89(5):1118-1127.
26. Pinzur MS, Gottschalk F, Smith D, et al: Functional outcome of below-knee amputation in peripheral vascular insufficiency: A multicenter review. *Clin Orthop Relat Res* 1993;286:247-249.
27. Burgess EM, Romano RL, Zettl JH: *The Management of Lower Extremity Amputations*. US Government Printing Office, 1969. Bulletin TR 10-6.
28. Duerksen F, Rogalsky RJ, Cochrane IW: Knee disarticulation with intercondylar patellofemoral arthrodesis: An improved technique. *Clin Orthop Relat Res* 1990;256:50-57.
29. *Official Proceedings of the Sixth State-of-the-Science Conference: Outcome Measures in Lower Limb Prosthetics*. American Academy of Orthotists & Prosthetists, 2006.

Knee Disarticulation: Prosthetic Management

Phillip M. Stevens, MEd, CPO, FAAOP • David J. Baty, CPO, LPO

ABSTRACT

Knee disarticulation represents a relatively small percentage of lower limb amputations. Although the amputation level preserves femoral length and key muscle insertion points, the added length compromises the clinician's ability to match the anatomic knee center position of the sound side limb. Specialized knee joint designs have been developed to partially address this challenge. Knee disarticulation is most successful when there is adequate soft-tissue coverage over the residual limb and both load-bearing capability and rotational control can be provided. Socket designs, prosthetic alignment, and rehabilitation are generally closely linked to the presence or absence of these characteristics.

Keywords: knee disarticulation; lower limb prosthesis; prosthetic design; through-knee disarticulation

Introduction

It is estimated that patients with a knee disarticulation (through-knee amputation) represent 2% or less of the overall amputee cohort in the United States.[1,2] However, in other countries, the knee disarticulation cohort may be as high as 24%.[3] This amputation level is characterized by distinct advantages and disadvantages relative to the more commonly performed, more proximal transfemoral amputation levels.[4] The residual limb is subjected to fewer bony and muscular disruptions, yielding more balanced muscular control at the hip and a limb that is generally capable of load bearing at the distal end. In addition, the distal bony contours often lend themselves to anatomic suspension of the prosthesis. However, the length of the residual limb precludes the ability to match the knee center of the prosthesis to the anatomic knee center, creating both functional and aesthetic considerations.

Anticipated Outcomes

As with most amputation levels, the outcomes associated with through-knee amputation vary with the amputation etiology and comorbid health considerations. Polfer et al[5] reported on a small convenience sample of 10 individuals seen at US military trauma centers with knee disarticulation with an average age of 23 years at the time of amputation. These individuals were matched to a separate cohort of individuals with transfemoral amputations based on time since amputation, preinjury activity levels, and comorbid injury to the sound side extremity. The authors found no significant differences between the two cohorts with respect to outcomes of general health, satisfaction, perceived disability, activity, or participation.

By contrast, Nijmeijer et al[6] recently reported on 153 knee disarticulation amputations in 138 patients with peripheral arterial disease (98%) and diabetes mellitus (63%) at a mean age of 74 years. Survival rates at 1, 6, and 12 months were reported at 86%, 65%, and 55%, respectively. Only 10% of these primary amputations were ultimately revised to transfemoral amputations. Seventy-one percent of the patients expressed a preoperative intent to ambulate with a prosthesis, and 91% of this contingent were successfully fit with a prosthesis. Of these, 35% walked without the help of others.

Clinical Considerations

A presurgical consultation with the treating prosthetist should be considered whenever possible. Although there are clear functional benefits associated with this amputation level, they come at the expense of cosmetic appearance and functional convenience in certain sitting environments. Patients should anticipate the functional and cosmetic implications of the distally positioned prosthetic knee center that are inherent to this amputation level before

---

David J. Baty or an immediate family member serves as a paid consultant to or is an employee of Össur. Neither Phillip M. Stevens nor any immediate family member has received anything of value from or has stock or stock options held in a commercial company or institution related directly or indirectly to the subject of this chapter.

This chapter is adapted from Cummings DR, Stevens PM: Knee disarticulation: Prosthetic management, in Krajbich JI, Pinzur MS, Potter BK, Stevens PM, eds: *Atlas of Amputations and Limb Deficiencies: Surgical, Prosthetic, and Rehabilitation Principles*, ed 4. American Academy of Orthopaedic Surgeons, 2016, pp 517-524.

fabricating the prosthesis, and if possible, before the amputation. Given the opportunity to engage in this decision, some patients may elect a transfemoral amputation to afford a more cosmetically acceptable prosthetic appearance.

Knee disarticulation amputation has some distinct advantages over a transfemoral amputation. In the disarticulation, the femoral condyles typically provide the weight-bearing surface within the prosthesis. This provides the ipsilateral hip adductors a stable platform to act upon during single limb stance. As a result, rather than pulling the distal femur laterally, as is generally seen with transfemoral amputation, the hip abductors are able to stabilize the pelvis in the coronal plane, keeping the contralateral hip from dropping during swing. This maintenance of the femoral adduction angle may limit or even eliminate the need for a compensatory Trendelenburg gait during single-limb support. Additional advantages include the bulbous shape of the distal femur, which enables an anatomic suspension of the prosthesis (**Figure 1**), as well as the ability to bear weight on the limb without a prosthesis in a kneeling position. This latter consideration is particularly important for an individual with a bilateral lower limb amputation who can benefit greatly if either or both residual limbs provide improved sitting balance, assist with transfers, and enable limited knee-walking without prostheses.

In general, the individual using a knee disarticulation prosthesis should have function similar to or better than that of an individual wearing a transfemoral prosthesis.[7] Walking speed may be faster, oxygen consumption lower, and donning the prosthesis a bit easier.[8] Patients who are healthy enough to run can often do so with the appropriate prosthesis, training, and practice.

Disadvantages of knee disarticulation prostheses are generally associated with the bulbous nature of the femoral condyles. This can result in a bulky appearance of the thigh segment of the prosthesis. In addition, and often of greater concern, the full length of the ipsilateral femur, coupled with even the lowest profile prosthetic componentry will displace the prosthetic knee center distally (**Figure 2**). This creates an asymmetry in swing phase as the shortened prosthetic shank creates a smaller knee flexion arc. Further, the shortened tibial length fails to reach the ground on many sitting surfaces, which often creates a fulcrum point at the edge of the chair, placing pressure along the posterior proximal aspect of the socket. The abnormally long femoral segment can prove extremely disruptive in tight seating environments with limited legroom. Other reasons for rejection can be a painful patella, or pain or skin breakdown over bony areas.[9]

Many of the benefits associated with knee disarticulation are lost if the distal end of the limb is not tolerant of load-bearing forces. To ensure a stable, well-padded distal end, surgeons have recommended that, when possible, the gastrocnemius muscle bellies and overlying posterior skin should be used to close a knee disarticulation.[10] Regardless of the surgical technique, it is not possible to predict all complications, and the ability of the residual limb to tolerate the forces of ambulation may be compromised by poor wound healing. An imperfect soft-tissue envelope may be somewhat mitigated in the prosthesis by the use of gel interfaces and end padding. However, thicker liners will adversely affect the overall length of the femoral section of the prosthesis and increase the knee center discrepancy described earlier. In some instances, if the residual limb is not able to provide end weight bearing, revision to a higher level may be indicated.[11]

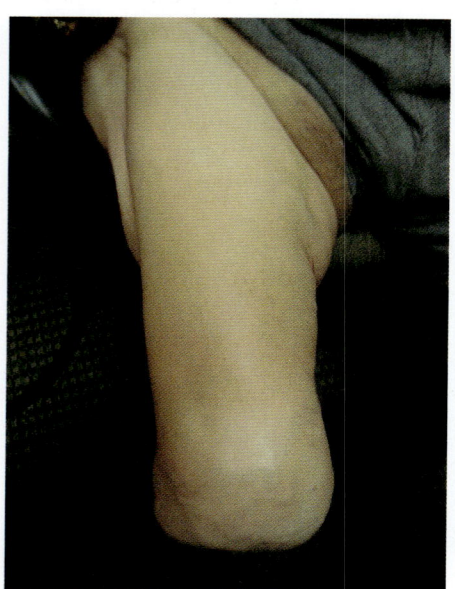

FIGURE 1 Photograph of a knee disarticulation with the characteristic bulbous distal shape.

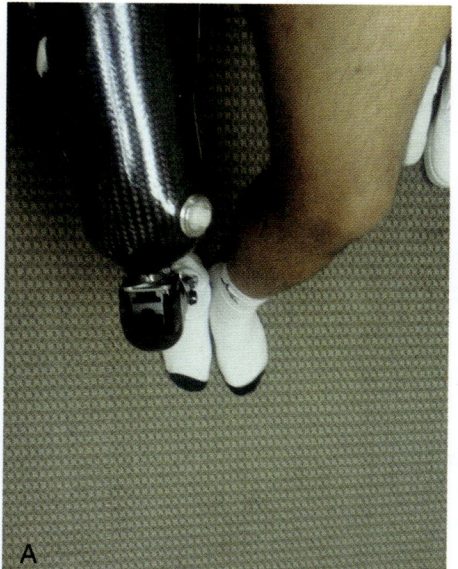 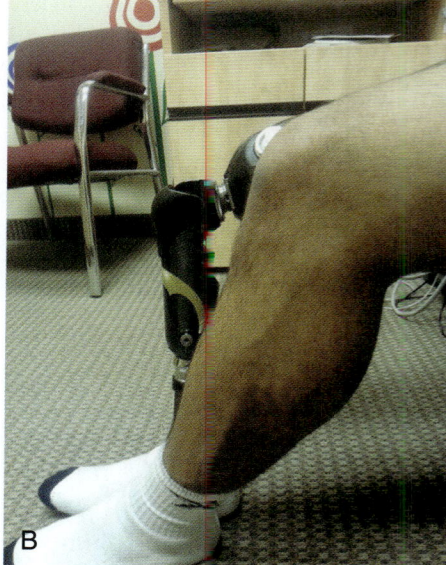

FIGURE 2 Anterior (**A**) and lateral (**B**) photographic views showing the relatively longer thigh segment and a lower prosthetic knee joint commonly seen in an individual with a knee disarticulation prosthesis. In this case, the user's active lifestyle warranted a durable hydraulic cylinder that was chosen by the patient despite the resultant asymmetries in limb lengths.

Socket Considerations

Most of the prosthetic benefits of this amputation level depend on the intact bony anatomy of the femur and the presence of a well-healed, scar-free, soft-tissue envelope surrounding the distal femur. When these conditions exist, it is possible for the prosthetic socket brim to be located below the level of the ischial tuberosity (**Figure 3**). With the ischium free of the socket, sitting comfort and freedom of hip motion can be improved. This characteristic is particularly beneficial to individuals with bilateral amputations.

The caveat of this design is that such sockets need to maintain a tight mediolateral dimension throughout their length to control the amount of side-to-side shifting that can occur at heel strike and throughout stance. A loose mediolateral dimension will lead to poor prosthetic control, a higher risk of falls, and increased energy expenditure as users attempt to control the coronal position of the prosthesis. In an associated concern, proximal tissues must be monitored and contained as necessary to prevent the progressive development of proximal tissue bunching (**Figure 4**).

In instances where the residual limb is intolerant to distal load-bearing forces, the prosthesis may require a proximal brim similar to that used in transfemoral socket designs to provide proximal weight bearing and offload the distal end of the femur (**Figure 5**). As weight bearing is moved to the proximal brim of the socket, the biomechanical benefits of distal load bearing described earlier are reduced.

Primary Socket and Suspension Approaches

When a patient presents with a knee disarticulation that is healed and ready for prosthetic fitting, the prosthetist will assess the load-bearing tolerance of the limb along with all other pertinent medical information. An assessment of the limb shape, tissue mass, and muscle density should be noted. The presence or absence of the patella should be noted, because the area may require relief or protection from excess pressure in the socket. Finally, patient hand strength, vision, and cognitive acuity all are important when deciding which socket design and suspension method will be used.

Although socket designs for a knee disarticulation level may be as unlimited as the imagination of the designer, there are several basic socket and suspension approaches that are commonly used by prosthetists. When distal loading capacity and a preference for anatomic suspension above the femoral condyles are present, there are a number of common socket and suspension types. Although anatomic suspension has historically been associated with this amputation level, recent years have seen the increasing utilization of suction suspension techniques to reduce pistoning of the limb within the socket.

A common, inexpensive method of anatomic suspension is the use of a soft, closed-cell foam inner socket. Such systems are relatively easy to fabricate, readily modifiable, and easily reparable, increasing their longevity. This system can be used if the medial/lateral difference between the femoral condyles and that of the distal thigh is at least one-half inch (12 mm). The liner is fabricated over a rectified mold where the disparity between the condylar mediolateral width and the proximal mediolateral width is filled with additional foam until a tube shape is achieved with uniform outer diameters throughout its length. A rigid socket is then fabricated over the foam.

The foam inner liner is donned over a limb interface such as prosthetic socks. If the medial buildup is too thick to allow the bulbous distal limb to pass through the narrowed neck of the liner, a slit might have to be made

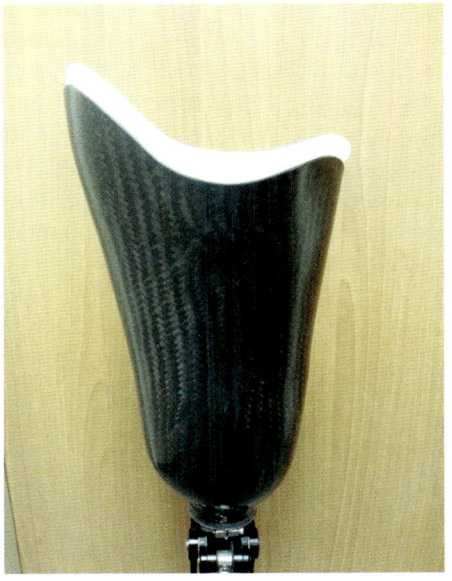

FIGURE 5 Posterior photographic view of a left knee disarticulation socket for a patient who was incapable of full distal end load bearing. The transfemoral brim shape provides some degree of proximal weight bearing.

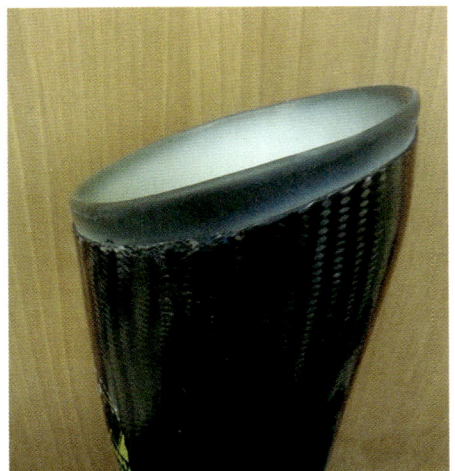

FIGURE 3 Photograph of the proximal aspect of a knee disarticulation prosthesis with characteristically lowered proximal trim lines ending well distal to the ischial tuberosity.

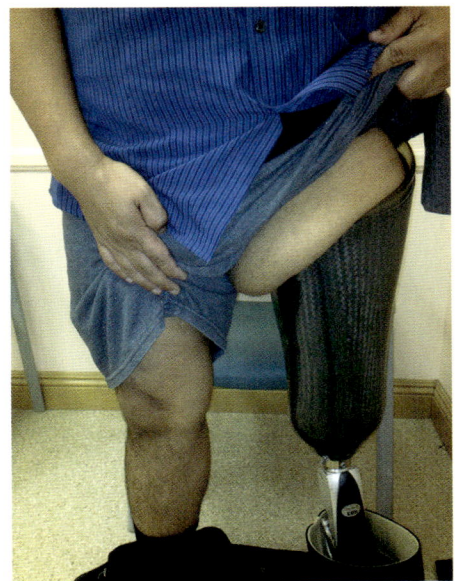

FIGURE 4 Photograph of a knee disarticulation socket in which the proximal medial tissues have been poorly managed and contained, resulting in localized tissue bunching. (Courtesy of Kevin Carroll, MS, CP, FAAOP, Orlando, FL.)

on its lateral aspect. Once the liner is fully donned onto the limb, the entire system is pushed into the rigid socket, where the inner socket is no longer able to deform its shape, creating an anatomically suspended socket. Doffing is accomplished through pulling the limb and liner proximally as the rigid outer socket is held in place.

A similar, lower profile design with similar effect is the fabrication of a closed-cell foam sleeve that is formed around the medial, posterior, and lateral aspects of the patient mold leaving the anterior section open. The sleeve is tapered at its edges and is only as thick and as long as needed to create a limb shape of uniform outer diameter. The sleeve is applied to the limb over an interface such as prosthetic socks. To hold the sleeve in place, another thin sock or nylon is then applied. The entire system is then slipped into the rigid socket to achieve a self-suspending system.

Both the full liner and reduced sleeve systems can be modified easily if there are limb maturation and volume loss that require the addition of more material to maintain a proper fit. The full-length foam liner system provides padding around the entire limb and works well with bony limbs. However, there is an increase of material under the condyles, which adds to the knee center discrepancy. The sleeve approach reduces both the length and bulk of the final socket, but it provides less cushion to the residual limb.

In a related technique, rigid, anatomically contoured sockets can be fabricated with removable panels that can be opened to allow passage of the condyles during donning, and then closed to create suspension. The opening is usually located medially, where it is more cosmetic and easier for the patient to reach, but it could be positioned on either side of the socket. When the finished plate is fastened snugly, the prosthesis suspends above the femoral condyles. One advantage of this design is that it can more closely match the sound side without added bulk. However, an associated challenge is securing the panels in place with enough force to prevent pistoning in the socket. This style of socket works best for mature and stable residual limbs with prominent femoral condyles.[12]

The challenge of obtaining adequate panel closure has recently been approached through rotary closure mechanisms that progressively tighten lacing materials about a central axis. These dials are designed so that minimal hand strength is needed to fully tighten the windows in place. When the lacing material is released from the dial of the closure mechanism, the panels loosen and expand outward, allowing donning or doffing to occur. These panel systems provide two functions. First, they provide a tight medial/lateral dimension proximal to the femoral condyles without the bulk of similar anatomical suspension systems. Second, as the limb matures and the volume decreases, the panels can be tightened to maintain a proper socket fit. When necessary these panels can also be padded on their inner surface to accommodate for additional limb maturation and volume loss.

The anterior lacing leather socket is now used only rarely in the United States, but it remains common in other settings (**Figure 6**). It is particularly

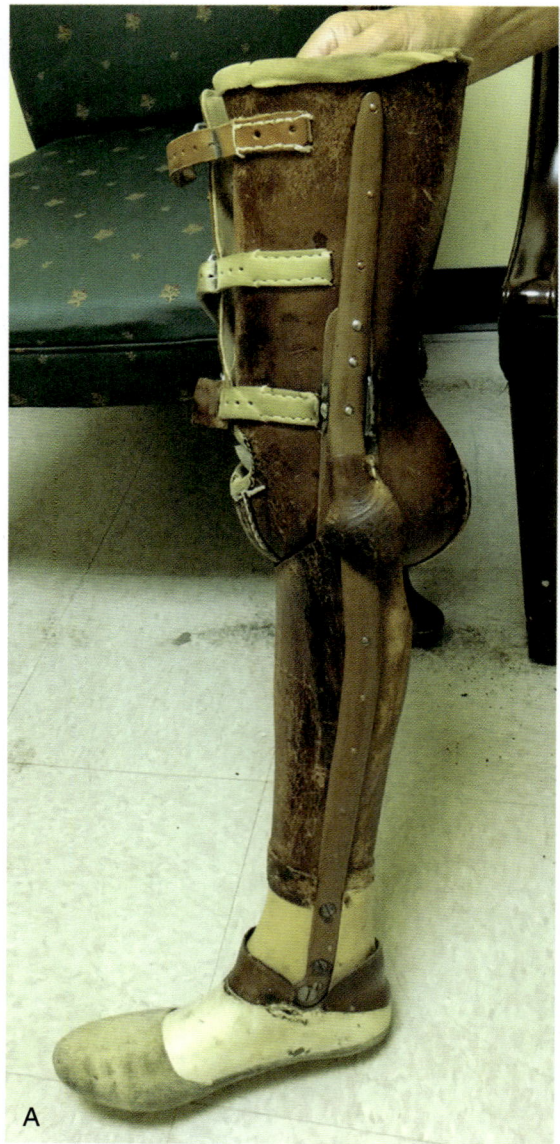
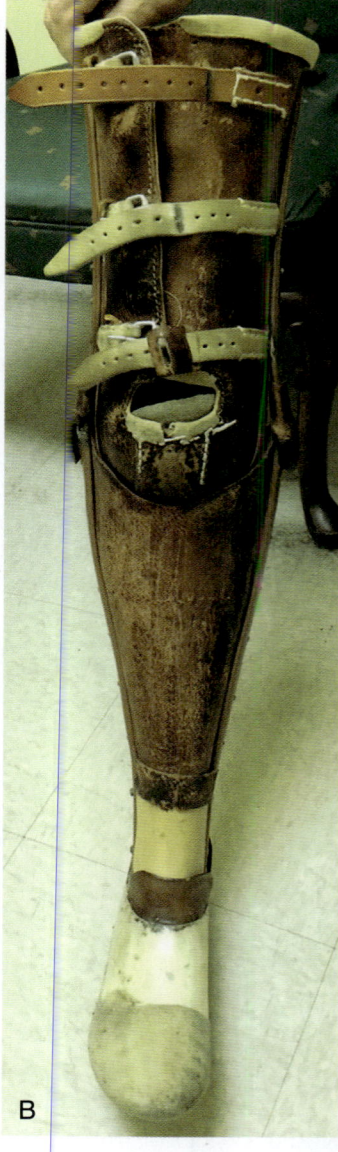

FIGURE 6 Lateral (**A**) and anterior (**B**) photographic views of an anterior-lacing, leather, corset-style socket with single-axis outside metal hinges. (Courtesy of Kevin Carroll, MS, CP, FAAOP, Orlando, FL.)

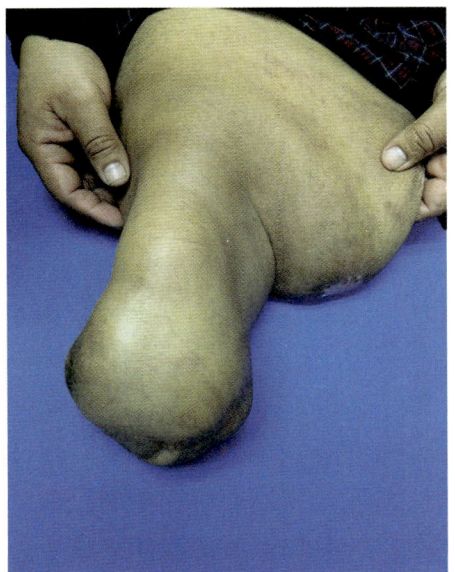

FIGURE 7 Photograph of a knee disarticulation residual limb that has experienced progressive localized atrophy proximal to the femoral condyles over time. (Courtesy of Kevin Carroll, MS, CP, FAAOP, Orlando, FL.)

useful when other materials are limited or there is local familiarity with the technique. The overall effectiveness of the design is still worthy of consideration. The leather corset suspends the prosthesis through an anterior lacing mechanism that creates a smaller dimension just proximal to the femoral condyles. However, sustained use of this technique and its associated compression can lead to localized atrophy of the residual limb (**Figure 7**).

Suction Suspension Options and Considerations

The use of liner-based suction suspension techniques will generally improve the suspension of the prosthesis and reduce the associated cyclical impact trauma upon the limb. In addition, suction suspension requires less localized pressure. Accordingly, the use of suction has become increasingly preferred by prosthetists and patients.

Well accepted as a means of suspension in transfemoral fittings, liner-based suction using fixed or movable sealing rings has begun to be explored in knee disarticulation sockets. As with all suction suspension environments, a continuous, fully sealed system must be

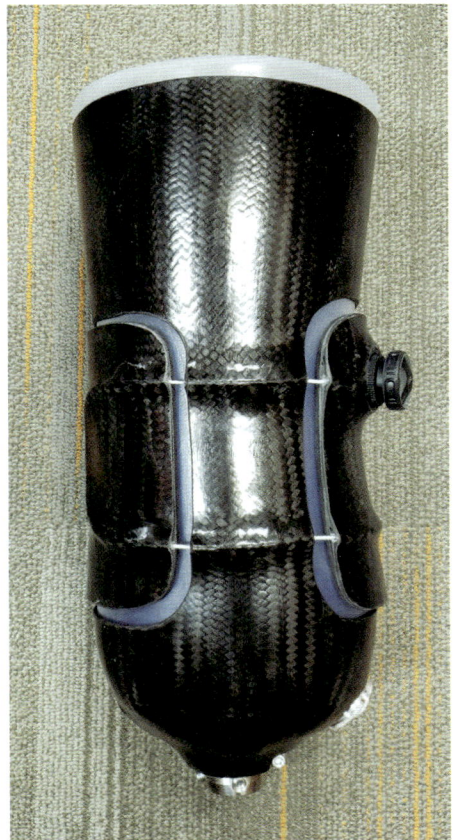

FIGURE 8 Photograph of a knee disarticulation socket with a flexible inner socket that yields sufficiently to allow the bulbous distal end of the residual limb to pass through the narrowed midshaft of the socket. Removable windows are loosened during donning and doffing to allow this material deformation. Once the socket is donned, a rotary closure system is used to secure medial and lateral panels into position to define the anatomic contours of the socket. A circumferential sealing gasket positioned over the interface liner creates the proximal seal for the system.

maintained. Inner sockets made from flexible plastics that can briefly stretch and displace when coupled with a rigid outer socket with strategically sized and positioned windows will allow passage of the bulbous residual limb through the necessarily narrowed neck of the socket. In this construct, a gasket-based sealing liner can seal against the inner flexible socket material to create a suction suspension environment. The height of the gasket seal should be distal to the distal edge of any windows in the rigid socket to maintain a suction seal. Alternately, the use of adjustable panels can ensure that the flexible socket materials do not stretch or displace in a manner that might compromise the suction environment once the limb is fully seated in the socket (**Figure 8**).

An additional variant is observed with the use of custom gel or silicone liners where sufficient liner material is added to the narrowed midshaft of its shape to provide reasonably uniform outer diameters. In this application, a sock-based gasket can be worn over the liner to create the suction seal against the inner surface of the rigid socket (**Figure 9**). However, the added thickness of these liners through their midshaft makes them more difficult to don and adds weight to the system. Thus, this approach should be reserved for presentations with only a modest differential between the medial/lateral dimensions of the femoral condyles and distal shaft of the thigh (**Figure 9**).

With a larger limb that does not have any large discrepancies in its mediolateral dimensions, an off-the-shelf transfemoral liner can be used, and no special padding or design is required. An alternate means of securing a proximal seal can be obtained when a covered liner is reflected over the proximal brim of the socket where a sealing sleeve, worn against the outer surface of the socket, is rolled proximally over the reflected liner (**Figure 10**).

As a general rule, any suspension system that adds significant length to the femoral section of the prosthesis should be avoided because this would only increase the disparity between the anatomical knee center and the lower prosthetic knee center. These include pin-locking systems and many lanyard-type systems that require a distal buildup.

Component Considerations

Although all categories of knee mechanisms may be used with knee disarticulation prostheses, only a few polycentric knees are designed specifically to address the issue of a long thigh (**Figure 11**). The long and bulky residual limb often means that knee options are limited, unless a lower knee center on the prosthesis is seen as an acceptable trade-off for a specific knee mechanism (**Figure 2**). One recent publication determined that the extent of

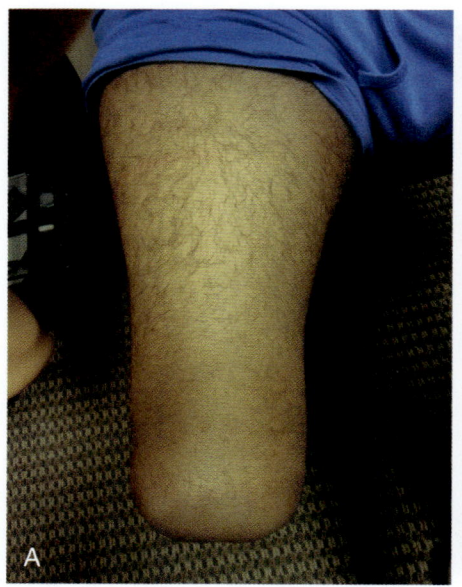 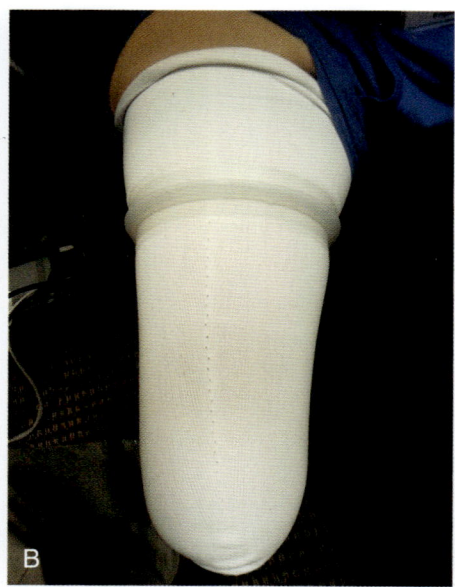 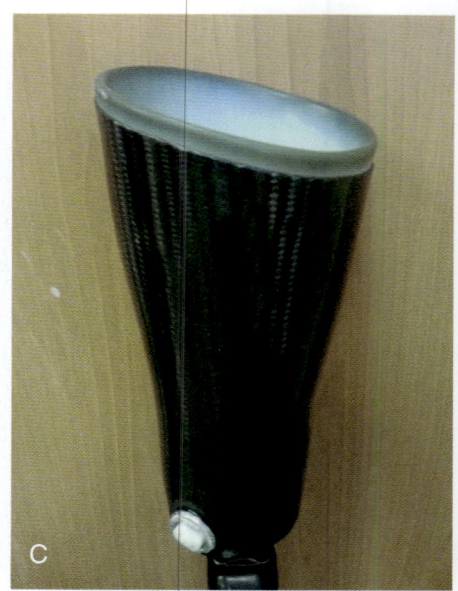

FIGURE 9 Photographs of a knee disarticulation and liner and suspension options. **A,** Residual limb after knee disarticulation. **B,** The residual limb with a noncovered silicone cushion liner and a sealing sock with a silicone sealing ring. The sealing ring engages against the inner surface of the socket, creating a proximal air seal. **C,** A distal one-way air valve allows air to exit the system, creating suction suspension.

this lengthening of the prosthetic thigh segment will range between 2.5 and 9.0 cm using modern prosthetic knee mechanisms, with shorter distances enabled by polycentric knees with specifically designed knee disarticulation socket anchors (**Figure 11**) and the largest discrepancies associated with single-axis knees with standard prosthetic anchors[13] (**Figure 2**). The prosthetist and clinic team should assess the patient's capacity for walking at variable cadence, traversing uneven ground, hiking, jogging, and running. The knee that will best match functional requirements and will create the smallest knee center discrepancy can be selected.

Single-axis knees offer multiple control options, including hydraulic, pneumatic, friction, and microprocessor control. Most manufacturers offer a specific adapter to enable their knee joint to be used with a long transfemoral amputation; however, with knee disarticulation the use of these adapters will still result in a knee center that is lower on the prosthetic side. In many instances, because of the increased function enabled by certain single-axis knee designs, the resultant discrepancy may be acceptable to the patient. In general, knees used for this long amputation level allow only limited adjustability, and there is not enough space for any optional components (such as rotation adapters) between the socket and the prosthetic knee.

Polycentric prosthetic knees are widely used for individuals with knee disarticulations. Because the instant axis of rotation in these knees is usually located above and behind the end of the residual limb, polycentric knees offer greater stability than a simple single-axis knee. However, stability is not a common problem for individuals with knee disarticulation because the long lever arm and intact thigh musculature usually mean the user will have good strength and active control of the prosthetic knee joint. Polycentric knees specifically designed for the knee disarticulations are preferred not so much for their stability, but because they match knee centers more closely, add only minimal length to the thigh, and allow the shin of the prosthesis to fold beneath the distal socket and behind the thigh when the individual sits (**Figure 11**).

Single-axis outside metal hinges can also be used with the knee disarticulation prosthesis (**Figure 6**). Although this option can be aligned to match the anatomic knee center height, these hinges do not have friction settings, nor do they permit fluid control for active patients who might benefit from hydraulic resistance. They are also bulky, noisy, and require frequent maintenance. Such hinges require a stout posterior check-strap (often made of leather and a synthetic polyester fabric). This is fastened between the thigh and shin to decelerate the knee during terminal swing phase, to spare the extension stops of the joints from excessive cyclical loading, and to reduce the noise created from full engagement of the metal joint stops. Unchecked, the hinges will wear quickly, gradually hyperextend, and eventually break.

As with other amputation levels, the prosthetic foot should be matched to the individual's activity level, size, weight, and goals. There is no contraindication for using hydraulic ankle, adjustable heel height, or microprocessor-controlled ankle units.

Cosmetic finishing of a knee disarticulation prosthesis can be challenging. The already bulky socket may mean that soft foam covers are often so thin around the thigh that they are

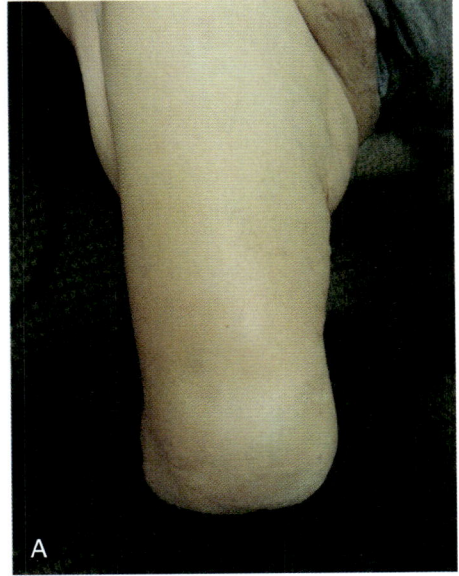
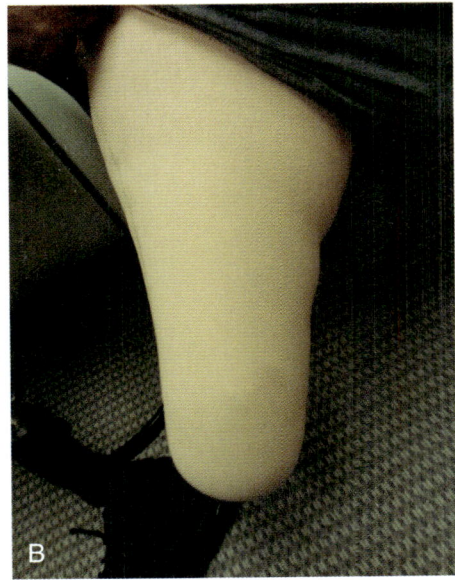
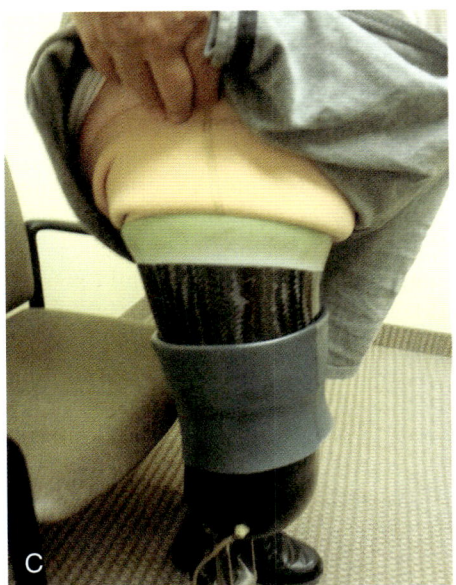
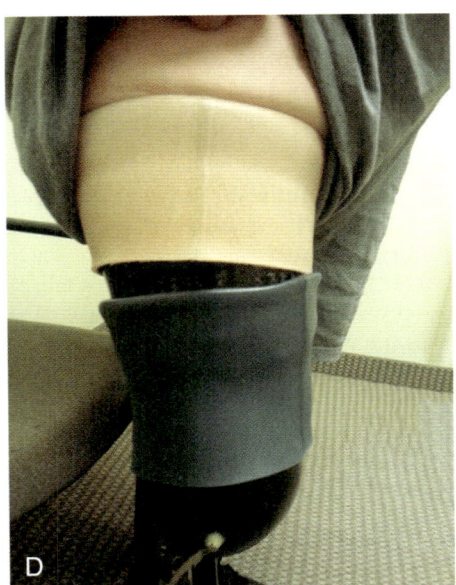
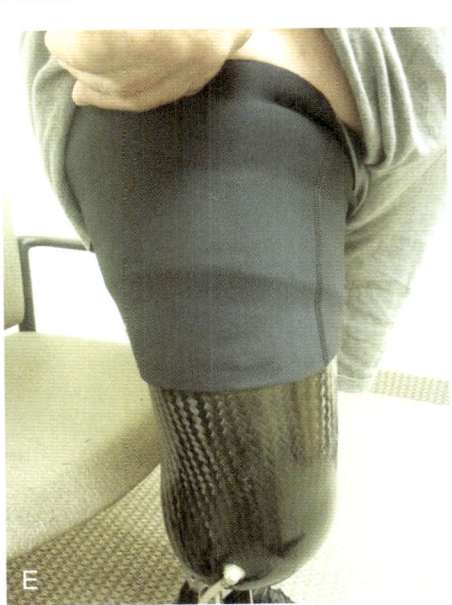

FIGURE 10 Photographs of knee disarticulation liner and suspension options. **A**, Residual limb after knee disarticulation. **B**, The residual limb with a covered thermoplastic elastomer cushion liner. **C**, The limb is inserted in a socket with a remote distal one-way air valve. **D**, The proximal aspect of the liner is reflected over the proximal brim of the socket. **E**, A sealing sleeve is rolled over the reflected liner, creating the proximal seal of the suction suspension.

very difficult to attach and have poor durability. Polycentric knees, in particular those with four-bar linkages designed for this level, often will cause the shin section to shorten during knee flexion. This may aid toe clearance during the swing phase, but it can be a cosmetic drawback when the patient is seated because the prosthetic shin will appear to be shorter than the sound side. A popular option is to cover the tibia areas up to the knee so that the prosthesis looks realistic in pants and dresses.

Alignment Considerations

Prosthetic alignment for knee disarticulation prostheses is quite similar to alignment of transfemoral prostheses, but with a few pertinent considerations. In patients with knee disarticulations, the load is generally applied to a great degree through their distal femoral condyles when standing or ambulating. In contrast, a patient with a transfemoral amputation cannot tolerate loading through the distal transected femur, which requires forces to be concentrated proximally and medially under the ischial tuberosity of the pelvis. In those with a knee disarticulation, the fulcrum of the residual limb–socket interface is

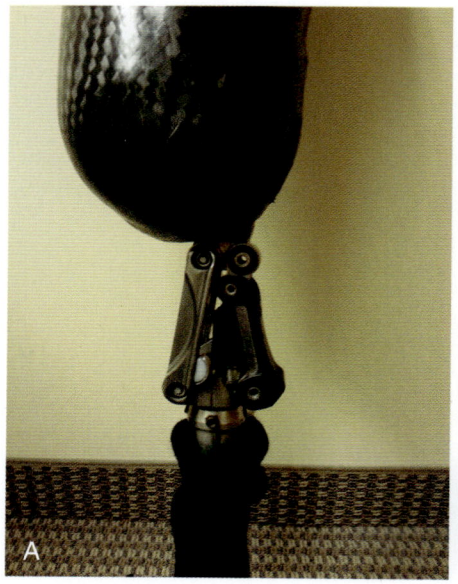 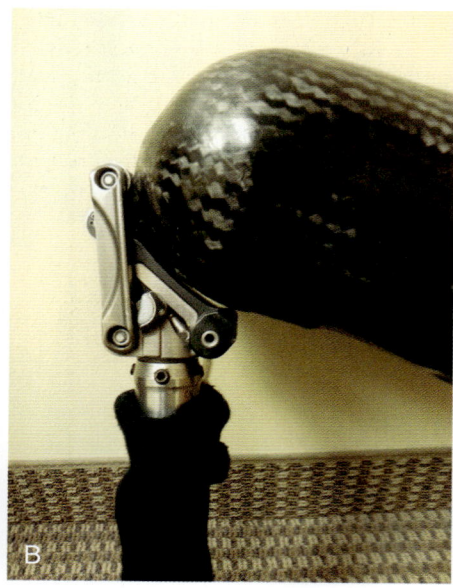

FIGURE 11 Extended (**A**) and flexed (**B**) photographs of a polycentric knee designed for a knee disarticulation prosthesis. This knee adds only minimal length to the thigh and allows the shin of the prosthesis to fold beneath the distal socket and behind the thigh when the patient sits.

located more distally and laterally.[14] This is particularly apparent (in the coronal plane) during single limb stance on the prosthesis when the forces transferred through the socket are concentrated on the medial aspect of the patient's upper thigh and distal lateral femoral condyle. For this reason, the proximal medial brim of the knee disarticulation socket should be designed with gentle flares, flexible material, or some other means of comfortably and evenly distributing forces in this area (**Figure 12**). If the medial brim is uncomfortable, the prosthesis can be aligned with relative outset of the supporting prosthetic foot. With this caveat, users of a knee disarticulation prosthesis can generally tolerate a more anatomic design, including normal femoral adduction and relative inset of the foot.

Patients with knee disarticulations generally have good hip strength, so their prosthetic knee center does not need to be extremely stable. Although rare, the presence of hip flexion contracture (or a contracture in any plane) is much more difficult to accommodate at this level without it being very apparent and negatively affecting cosmesis. The longer limb and tolerance of distal pressure may mean that the contracture can be reduced more easily over time through physical therapy and prosthesis use.

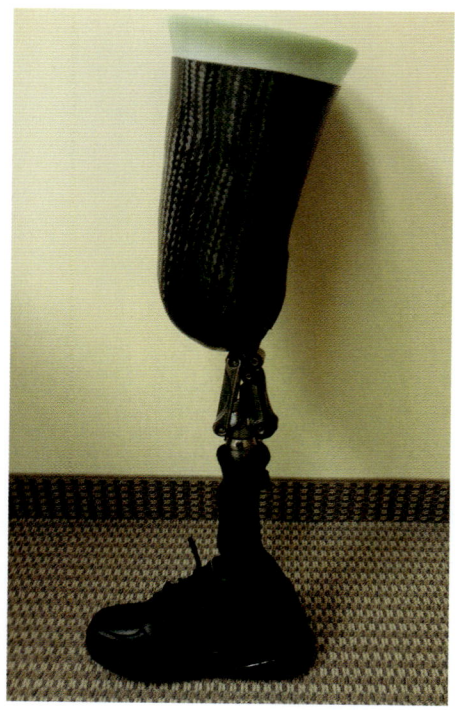

FIGURE 12 Photograph of a knee disarticulation socket with a comparatively wide flexible brim that reduces the localized forces that would otherwise be experienced at the proximal medial brim.

SUMMARY

Knee disarticulation can offer outstanding results when a well-padded, sensate, and nonscarred soft-tissue envelope is present. Prosthetic fitting challenges at this level are generally related to the bulbous femoral condyles and long length of the residual limb. Prosthetic advantages of this level include suspension over the femoral condyles and distal loading along with increased prosthetic control.

References

1. Lim S, Javorski MJ, Halandras PM, Aulivola B, Crisostomo PR: Through-knee amputation is a feasible alternative to above knee amputation. *J Vasc Surg* 2018;68(1):197-203.
2. Jackson AJ, Coburn G, Morrison D, Mrozinski S, Reidy J: Through-knee amputation in peripheral vascular disease. *Br J Diabetes Vasc Dis* 2012;12(1):26-32.
3. Pernot HF, Winnubst GM, Cluitmans JJ, De Witte LP: Amputees in Limburg: Incidence, morbidity and mortality, prosthetic supply, care utilisation and functional level after one year. *Prosthet Orthot Int* 2000;24:90-96.
4. Behr J, Friedly J, Molton I, Morgenroth D, Jensen MP, Smith DG: Pain and pain-related interference in adults with lower-limb amputation: Comparison of knee-disarticulation, transtibial, and transfemoral surgical sites. *J Rehabil Res Dev* 2009;46(7):963-972.
5. Polfer EM, Hoyt BW, Bevevino AJ, Forsberg JA, Potter BK: Knee disarticulations versus transfemoral amputations: Functional outcomes. *J Orthop Trauma* 2019;33(6):308-311.
6. Nijmeijer R, Voesten HG, Geertzen JH, Dijkstra PU: Disarticulation of the knee: Analysis of an extended database on survival, wound healing, and ambulation. *J Vasc Surg* 2017;66(3):866-874.
7. Smith D: The knee disarticulation: It's better when it's better and it's not when it's not. *Motion* 2004;14(1):56-62.
8. Pinzur M: Knee disarticulation: Surgical procedures, in Bowker JH, Michael JW, eds: *Atlas of Limb Prosthetics: Surgical, Prosthetic, and Rehabilitation Principles*, ed 2. Mosby-Year Book, 1992, pp 479-486.
9. Botta P, Baumgartner R: Socket design and manufacturing technique for through-knee stumps. *Prosthet Orthot Int* 1983;7(2):100-103.

10. Bowker JH, San Giovanni TP, Pinzur MS: North American experience with knee disarticulation with use of a posterior myofasciocutaneous flap: Healing rate and functional results in seventy-seven patients. *J Bone Joint Surg Am* 2000;82(11):1571-1574.

11. Ten Duis K, Bosmans JC, Voesten HG, Geertzen JH, Dijkstra PU: Knee disarticulation: Survival, wound healing and ambulation. A historic cohort study. *Prosthet Orthot Int* 2009;33(1):52-60.

12. Hughes J: Biomechanics of the through-knee prosthesis. *Prosthet Orthot Int* 1983;7(2):96-99.

13. de Laat FA, van der Pluijm MJ, van Kuijk AA, Geertzen JH, Roorda LD: Cosmetic effect of knee joint in a knee disarticulation prosthesis. *J Rehabil Res Dev* 2014;51(10):1545-1554.

14. Stark G: Overview of knee disarticulation. *J Prosthet Orthot* 2004;16(4):130-137.

# Transfemoral Amputation: Surgical Management

CHAPTER 42

Frank A. Gottschalk, MD* • COL Benjamin Kyle Potter, MD, FAAOS, FACS

ABSTRACT

To maintain femoral alignment that is close to normal, it is necessary to consider the biomechanics and surgical technique of transfemoral amputation. Muscle preservation and myodesis of the adductor magnus muscle is necessary for maintaining muscle tension to hold the femur in its anatomically adducted position. Adductor magnus and quadriceps muscle myodesis over the end of the femur also provides an adequate soft-tissue end pad to reduce discomfort and improve the likelihood of successful prosthesis use. Developing appropriate soft-tissue flaps allows uncompromised wound healing and early mobilization of the patient. Various wound care options help reduce healing problems.

Keywords: biomechanics; indications; postoperative management; surgical technique; transfemoral amputation

Introduction

Transfemoral amputation often is necessary in patients who have nonreconstructible peripheral vascular disease, diabetic foot infection, severe lower limb trauma, or, less commonly, a massive infection or a tumor that cannot be managed with intercalary resection. In these patients, amputation at a level below the femur is unlikely to heal. The incidence of lower limb amputation, including transfemoral amputation, remained unchanged in the Netherlands during the 2 decades leading up to 2004.[1] Patients with diabetes mellitus, especially those older than 45 years, were at greater risk for amputation than the general population.

Most patients with transfemoral amputation must expend at least 65% more energy than normal to walk at a self-selected speed on a level surface.[2,3] This limitation can be compounded by the patient's underlying medical condition; for example, many patients with a dysvascular disorder lack the physical reserve necessary for functional walking with a transfemoral prosthesis or are otherwise unsuccessful in becoming ambulatory with a prosthesis.[4] Regardless of concomitant medical conditions, patients with a lower limb amputation were found to be unable to achieve normal gait in terms of velocity, cadence, or walking economy.[1,5] Patients whose transfemoral amputation was necessitated by a nonvascular cause required increased energy expenditure for walking and had limited ambulation and difficulties related to prosthesis use.[6] Children with transfemoral amputation walked more slowly and with an increased energy cost compared with unaffected children.[7]

Although many improvements have been made in prosthesis design and fabrication, even the best prosthesis cannot adequately replace the limb in the absence of a proper residual limb. Too often, the surgical procedure is done without consideration of biomechanical principles or preservation of muscle function. A major goal of amputation surgery is primary wound healing, but the biomechanical principles of lower limb function should not be sacrificed to achieve this goal. Appropriate muscle anchorage and stabilization can improve wound healing potential by limiting shear force, tension, and motion at the terminal skin interface.

During a transfemoral amputation procedure, it is important to maintain a residual limb with as much length as possible. The longer the remaining femur is, the easier it will be to suspend and align a prosthesis. In addition, leaving the longest possible residual limb will provide the patient with optimal functional ability because the long lever arm can help with transfers and sitting balance.[8] A long residual limb also reduces the potential for bone erosion through the soft tissues (**Figure 1**). Bone protrusion through soft tissue can occur as the adductors and quadriceps retract from the end of the femur after inadequate stabilization of the muscles. In a long amputation, there is less abduction force because of the remaining counterforce in the adductor muscles. A study of military patients with transfemoral amputation found that those with a longer residual limb

---

Dr. Potter or an immediate family member serves as an unpaid consultant to Biomet and serves as a board member, owner, officer, or committee member of the Society of Military Orthopaedic Surgeons.

*Deceased.

Section 3: Lower Limb

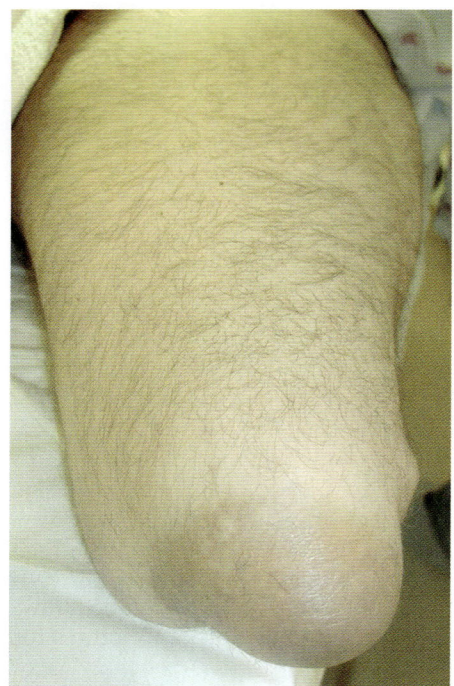

FIGURE 1 Photograph shows a transfemoral amputation with distal soft-tissue loss, bony prominence, and discoloration of skin.

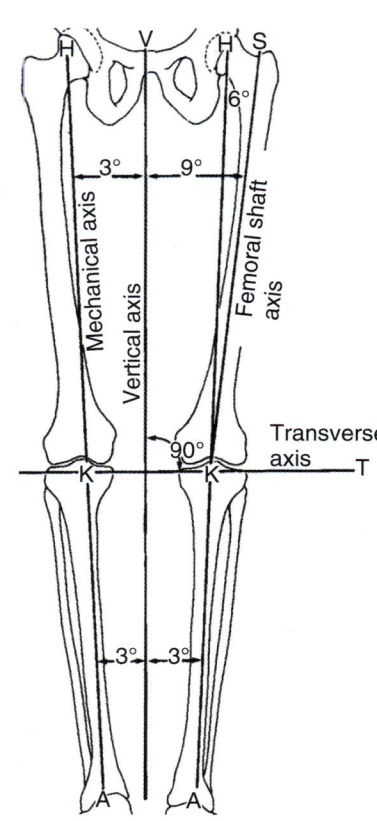

FIGURE 2 Schematic drawing shows the mechanical and anatomic axes of normal lower limbs. A = ankle, H = hip, K = knee, S = shaft axis, T = transverse axis, V = vertical axis. (Reproduced with permission from Gottschalk FA, Kourosh S, Stills M, McClellan B, Roberts J: Does socket configuration influence the position of the femur in above-knee amputation? *J Prosthet Orthot* 1989;2[1]:94-102. © 1989 American Academy of Orthotists.)

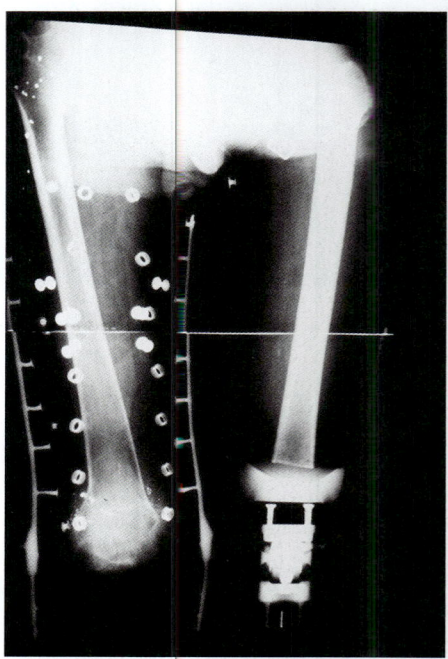

FIGURE 3 AP radiograph of the lower extremity of a patient shows a knee disarticulation with the femur in normal mechanical and femoral shaft axis alignment. The left femur has undergone a transfemoral amputation after adductor magnus myodesis with the femur in adduction and nearly normal alignment.

achieved greater self-selected walking velocity.[5] The study did not determine whether residual limb length or femoral orientation affected the energy expenditure.

In some patients, the prevailing local pathology may require a proximal transfemoral amputation. If possible, a small portion of the femur should be left at the trochanteric level to provide additional contouring for fitting of a prosthesis. A patient with less than 5 cm of bone distal to the lesser trochanter ultimately may be fitted with a prosthesis designed for a hip disarticulation.

Biomechanics

Normal Alignment

The normal anatomic and mechanical alignment of the lower limb has been well defined[9-11] (**Figure 2**). The mechanical axis of the lower limb runs from the center of the femoral head through the center of the knee to the midpoint of the ankle. In a normal two-legged stance, this axis is 3° from vertical, and the femoral shaft axis is 9° from vertical. The normal anatomic alignment of the femur is in adduction. This alignment allows the hip stabilizers (the gluteus medius and gluteus minimus) and abductors (the gluteus medius and tensor fasciae latae) to function normally and reduce the lateral motion of the center of mass of the body, thus producing a smooth and energy-efficient gait pattern.

In most patients with a transfemoral amputation, mechanical and anatomic alignment is disrupted because the femur no longer is in its natural anatomic alignment. The standard anterior-posterior soft-tissue flaps disengage the adductors of the femur and allow the unopposed abductors to displace the femur in an abducted position, compared with the contralateral limb.[12] In a conventional transfemoral amputation, most of the adductor muscle insertion is lost. Particularly affected is the adductor magnus, which has an insertion on the adductor tubercle at the distal medial femur as well as the posterior aspect of the femur on the linea aspera. Femoral alignment is maintained in a knee disarticulation because the adductor mechanism is not disrupted; in addition, the contour of the distal residual limb and soft-tissue envelope constrains the distal femur within the socket (**Figure 3**).

Conventional surgery results in the loss of the distal third of the attachment of the adductor magnus, and the femur drifts into abduction because of the relatively unopposed action of the abductor system.[8,12] The surgeon sutures the residual adductors and the other muscles around the femur with the residual femur in an abducted and flexed position. This abducted position leads to a side lurch and increased energy consumption during ambulation. Because the original insertions of the adductor muscles are lost, the effective moment arm of these muscles becomes shorter. The remaining

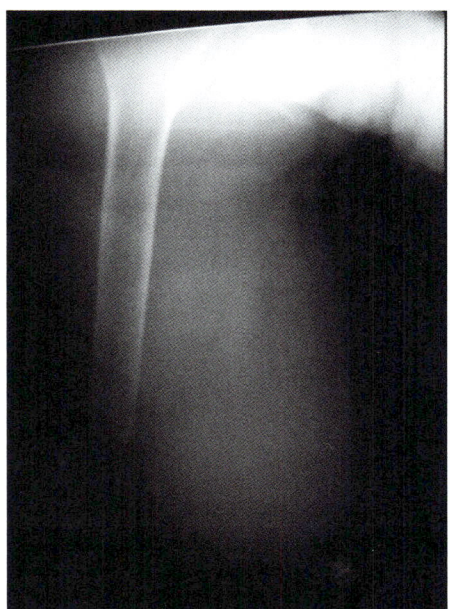

FIGURE 4 AP radiograph shows abduction of a residual femur resulting from inadequate muscle stabilization.

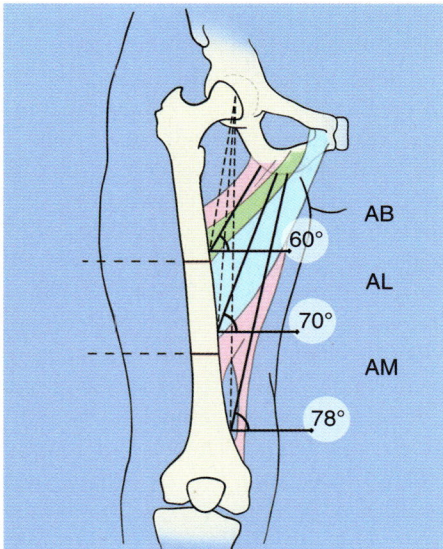

FIGURE 5 Schematic drawing shows the moment arms of the three adductor muscles in a normal limb. Loss of the distal attachment of the adductor magnus results in a 70% loss of adductor strength. The vertical dashed lines show moment arms of the adductor brevis, adductor longus, and adductor magnus muscles. The solid lines are the resultant forces of the respective muscles. The dashed horizontal lines show the levels of proposed amputation. AB = adductor brevis, AL = adductor longus, AM = adductor magnus

smaller mass of adductor muscle is unable to generate the greater force needed to hold the femur in its normal position, and an abducted position results[8,13] (**Figure 4**).

Prosthetists recognize that residual femoral abduction compromises function. Several prosthetic socket designs represent an attempt to hold the residual femur in a more adducted position by adjusting the socket shape or using the ischium as a fulcrum.[14,15] A radiologic study, however, revealed that the position of the residual femur after transfemoral amputation cannot be controlled by the socket shape or alignment.[16] Attempting to stabilize the soft tissues in adduction within the socket does not influence the position of the femur.

Of the three adductor muscles (the adductor magnus, adductor longus, and adductor brevis), the adductor magnus has the moment arm with the best mechanical advantage.[12,16,17] **Figure 5** shows the directions of the components of force of the adductor muscles, with the lines of force joining the points of attachment of the muscles. The adductor magnus is three to four times larger in cross-sectional area and volume than the adductor longus and adductor brevis combined. Transection of the adductor magnus at the time of amputation leads to a major loss of muscle cross-sectional area, a reduction in the effective moment arm, and a loss of as much as 70% of the adductor pull.[16,17] The result is overall weakness in the adductor force of the thigh and subsequent abduction of the residual femur. In addition, loss of the extensor portion of the adductor magnus leads to a decrease in hip extension power and an increased likelihood of a flexion contracture.

Muscle Atrophy

A reduction in muscle mass at amputation combined with inadequate mechanical fixation of muscles and atrophy of the remaining musculature was the most important factor responsible for the decrease in muscle strength detected after transfemoral amputation.[18] Decreased strength was most noticeable in the flexor, extensor, abductor, and adductor muscles of the hip and was correlated with inadequate muscle stabilization.[19]

Jaegers et al[20,21] documented muscle atrophy in 12 healthy patients after transfemoral amputation. Three-dimensional MRI reconstruction showed atrophy of 40% to 60% in hip muscles that had been sectioned. In the intact muscles, which included the iliopsoas, gluteus medius, and gluteus minimus, the atrophy ranged from zero to 30%. The amount of atrophy of the intact muscles was related to the length of the residual limb; there was less atrophy in longer residual limbs. Despite the presence of muscle atrophy, fatty degeneration was not noted. The iliotibial tract was not reattached in an attempt to avoid abduction contracture of the hip. This strategy, however, led to hip flexion contractures for the following reasons: (1) the action of the iliopsoas muscle was unopposed, and (2) the large insertion of the gluteus maximus into the gluteal fascia, which continues into the iliotibial tract, meant that leaving the iliotibial tract unattached weakened the extensor mechanism. The extent of atrophy of the adductor muscles also depended on the level of amputation. In none of the patients was the adductor magnus adequately reanchored. Amputations that were relatively proximal without adequate muscle stabilization led to more muscle atrophy and were more likely to lead to an abduction contracture and atrophy of the gluteus muscles. The gluteus maximus was found to be atrophied in all 12 of the patients. A lack of hamstring fixation led to as much as 70% atrophy. Changes in muscle morphology after amputation are the result of changes in volume and geometry (size and mass). Additional study findings included reduced bone density, cortical atrophy, and increased volume of the femoral medullary cavity.[20]

Electromyographic Activity

Electromyographic studies reveal adductor magnus activity during normal gait at both the beginning and end of the stance phase and into the early swing phase.[22,23] In an electromyographic study of transfemoral amputations by Jaegers et al[21] the intact muscles maintained the same sequence of activity as that found in a normal limb, but the activity extended over a longer period. The activity of sectioned muscles depended on the level of amputation and whether the muscles had been reanchored. Muscles that were correctly reanchored remained functional in locomotion, especially in distal transfemoral amputations. Alterations in muscle activity during walking probably were related to the altered morphology of once-biarticular hip muscles, the passive elements of the prosthesis, and the patient's changed gait pattern. The extent to which the gait was asymmetric was related to the length of the residual limb. The greater the atrophy of the hip-stabilizing muscles was, the greater was the lateral bending of the trunk to the amputation side.[24]

Surgical Principles

The goal of transfemoral amputation surgery should be the creation of a dynamically balanced residual limb with good motor control and sensation. Preservation of the adductor magnus helps maintain muscle balance between the adductors and abductors by allowing the adductor magnus to maintain close-to-normal muscle power and a mechanical advantage for holding the femur in the normal anatomic position. A residual limb with dynamically balanced function allows the patient to perform at a relatively normal level and to use a prosthesis with greater ease. Several experts recommend transecting the muscles through the muscle belly at a length equivalent to one-half the diameter of the thigh at the level of amputation.[25-28] Muscle stabilization after transection also has been recommended as a means of controlling the femur, but usually it cannot be achieved because the remaining muscle mass had retracted before the transection[8] (**Figure 4**). Reestablishing the normal muscle tension, as is customarily recommended, becomes difficult. Many surgeons have attempted muscle stabilization by myoplasty over the end of the femur or myodesis to the femur just proximal to the end of the bone.[8,21-24] Baumgartner[8] described using coronal flaps and placing the tissue under tension while transecting the soft tissue and muscles before the femoral osteotomy. Myoplasty, in which the agonist and antagonist groups of muscles are sutured to each other over the bone end, does not restore normal muscle tension or allow adequate muscle control of the femur. The residual femur moves in the muscle envelope, producing pain and occasionally penetrating the soft-tissue envelope. Often, a bursa develops at the end of the cut femur. The loss of muscle tension leads to a loss of control and reduced muscle strength in the residual limb. The soft-tissue envelope around the distal end of the residual limb is unstable and may compromise prosthetic fitting. Instead of myoplasty, a muscle-preserving myodesis technique in which the distal insertions of the muscles are detached from their bony insertion and reattached to the residual femur under close-to-normal muscle tension is preferred. After the myodesis is completed, any redundant tissue can be excised.[12]

Indications

Vascular Disease and Diabetes Mellitus

Vascular disease, often associated with diabetes, is the most common reason for transfemoral amputation in developed countries (**Figure 6**). Most patients who require a transfemoral amputation for vascular disease have widespread, systemic manifestations of the disease with several postoperative implications. The disease may compromise the patient's rehabilitation. The patient's physical reserve often is insufficient to allow use of a prosthesis. Acute ischemia of the lower limb can be the result of thrombosis or embolism, and it may be difficult to determine which of these two conditions is causing the ischemia. Although embolism is the more likely diagnosis in patients of relatively advanced age, both systemic and local causes must be considered.[29] Chronic ischemia necessitating amputation usually involves gangrene of the foot as a

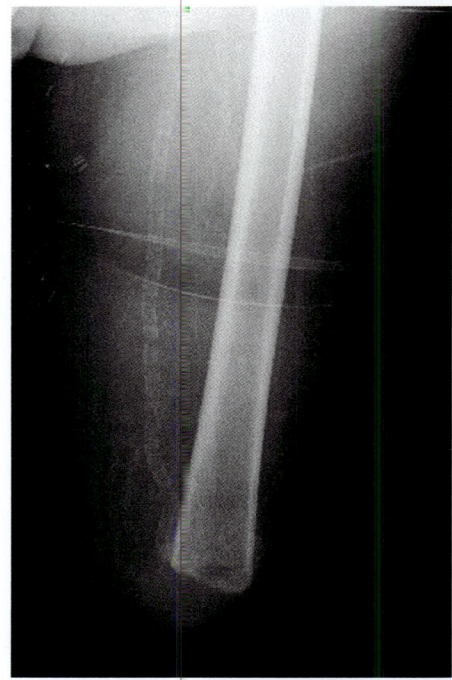

FIGURE 6 AP radiograph of a transfemoral amputation with a calcified femoral artery in a patient with diabetes mellitus.

consequence of severe atherosclerosis. Van Niekerk et al[30] reported an association between unsuccessful bypass surgery and proximal-level amputations. Successful vascular bypass surgery improves the rate of limb survival in patients with critical ischemia, but unsuccessful vascular bypass surgery leads to increased rates of transfemoral amputation and residual limb complications. Infectious gangrene requiring amputation is most common in patients with diabetes mellitus. Patients with vascular disease associated with diabetes mellitus are, on average, 10 years younger at the time of amputation than other patients with vascular disease.[31] Patients with purely vascular disease are more likely to require transfemoral amputation than patients with diabetes mellitus; however, patients with diabetes mellitus were found to be at a higher relative risk for amputation than those without diabetes mellitus.[1,32]

Patients with peripheral vascular disease and diabetes mellitus may have multiple comorbidities, including hypertension, chronic obstructive pulmonary disease, and renal disease.[33]

These patients have a 30% incidence of transfemoral amputation, with a 24-month survival rate of only 70%.

Trauma

Patients who require a transfemoral amputation as a result of trauma usually are younger than those requiring amputation because of disease.[34] The indication for surgical amputation is a complete or near-complete traumatic amputation or a combination of soft-tissue, vascular, neurologic, and bone damage so severe as to preclude satisfactory limb salvage or subsequent function. Foreign material embedded in the bone and soft tissues may require meticulous and often serial débridement.

Injuries from a land mine blast or other high-velocity penetrating source can cause extensive tissue damage because of energy transfer to the tissues.[35] Complex high-energy injury to a lower limb often necessitates a high transfemoral amputation. A patient with a bullet wound treated more than 24 hours after injury is four times more likely to require a transfemoral amputation than a transtibial amputation.[36] Any delay in treatment increases the risk of a proximal amputation because of infection and increasing soft-tissue damage. Depending on the severity of the initial injury, early intervention can minimize the risk of amputation or permit amputation at a lower level. Although the greatest possible limb length should be preserved, it also is important to secure a good soft-tissue envelope and avoid a split-thickness skin graft over bone. A multistage procedure or multiple procedures in which the wounds initially are left open to avoid wound infection and allow additional débridement as necessary may be required.[10,34] All viable tissue should be preserved until definitive wound closure. On occasion, split-thickness skin grafts can be used on muscle to help preserve length. Revision surgery may be necessary and may require secondary skin expansion. A fracture of the femur should be appropriately stabilized rather than treated by amputation through a proximal fracture site. The orientation of skin flaps is not critical, but closure must be without tension.

Infection

Amputation for severe soft-tissue infection or osteomyelitis should be done in two or more stages with appropriate antibiotic coverage. Placement of antibiotic-impregnated polymethyl methacrylate beads or absorbable antibiotic-impregnated substances sometimes is useful for controlling local infection. All infected tissue must be excised before definitive closure. There has been an increase in the number of amputations done after a knee arthroplasty becoming unsalvageable because of infection; in these patients, the soft tissue has severe fibrosis and is nonfunctioning, and insufficient bone is available for a tibiofemoral fusion (**Figure 7**).

Tumor

The level of amputation required to excise a tumor often is determined by the type, size, and location of the tumor. The principles of tumor eradication (particularly the need to obtain wide margins) must be observed, but the preserved residual limb should be as long as possible so that maximal function can be maintained.

Surgical Technique

Beginning with anesthesia induction, femoral nerve and sciatic nerve blocks are used for postoperative pain management. A femoral nerve catheter can be placed for several days. Peripheral nerve blocks were found to have advantages in amputations.[37,38]

Proper positioning of the patient on the surgical table facilitates the surgery. The patient should be supine. The buttock on the side of the leg to be amputated should be elevated with folded sheets or blankets to allow hip extension and adduction during the procedure.

A tourniquet is not used for most transfemoral amputations necessitated by vascular disease but may be used if there is a different indication. If used, a sterile tourniquet should be placed as high on the thigh as possible after the leg has been cleaned and draped. The tourniquet is released before setting muscle tensions and to allow adequate hemostasis. Skin flaps should be marked before the skin incision is made (**Figure 8**). A long medial flap in the sagittal plane is recommended.[12] The flap is developed as a myofasciocutaneous flap and sutured to the shorter lateral flap. In an amputation necessitated by trauma or tumor, however, any flap configuration is acceptable if it allows the longest feasible residual limb to be retained. Anterior skin flaps should not be longer than posterior flaps unless a long medial flap is not feasible. If anterior-posterior flaps are used, care should be taken to minimize the amount of subcutaneous tissue dissection to avoid damaging the perforating fascial vessels. The use of equal-size anterior-posterior skin

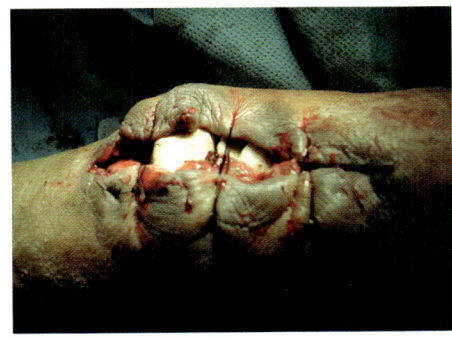

FIGURE 7 Photograph shows soft-tissue dehiscence and an antibiotic spacer in an infected knee arthroplasty. Transfemoral amputation was required.

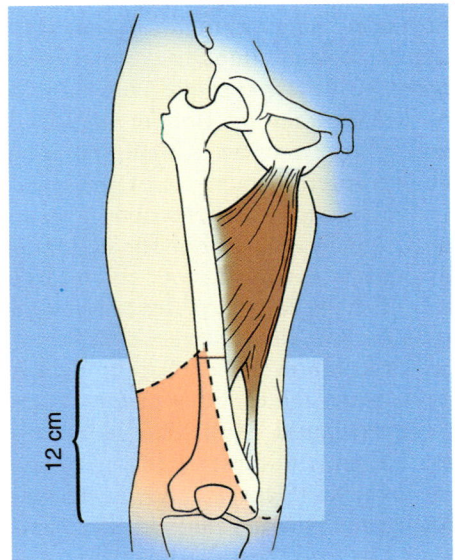

FIGURE 8 Schematic drawing shows proposed skin flaps (dashed lines) and the level of bone section (solid line) as marked before a transfemoral amputation.

flaps is recommended by some experts but may be unsatisfactory because a suture line under the end of the residual limb can lead to difficulty with use of a prosthesis.[8] However, equal-size flaps can increase skin tension at the wound closure if the amount of soft tissue needed for closure was underestimated. The skin flaps should be made longer than the initial estimated measurement to avoid having to shorten the bone more than otherwise necessary if the skin that is available for closure proves insufficient.

After the medial skin flap is created, the adductor magnus tendon attachment to the adductor tubercle of the femur is identified[12,39] (**Figure 9**). The tendon is detached by sharp dissection, marked with a suture, and reflected proximally to expose the adductor (Hunter) canal. The femoral artery and vein are identified. The major vessels are isolated and separated, and each is ligated with nonabsorbable silk suture and cut at the proposed level of bone section. The major nerves should be dissected at least 4 cm proximal to the proposed bone cut and sectioned with a new, sharp blade. The central vessel of the sciatic nerve should be lightly cauterized but should not be ligated to avoid producing neuropathic pain.[40] Local anesthetic infiltration of bupivacaine through a small catheter placed into the nerve is thought to decrease the severity of postoperative pain.[41]

Muscles should not be sectioned until they have been identified. The quadriceps is detached just proximal to the patella, with retention of some of its tendinous portion. The adductor magnus is detached from the adductor tubercle by sharp dissection and reflected medially to expose the femoral shaft. It may be necessary to detach 2 to 3 cm of the adductor magnus from the linea aspera to increase its mobility. The smaller muscles, including the sartorius and gracilis, and the medial hamstring muscles should be transected at least 2 to 2.5 cm below the proposed bone cut to facilitate their inclusion and anchorage. The biceps femoris is transected at the level of the bone cut.

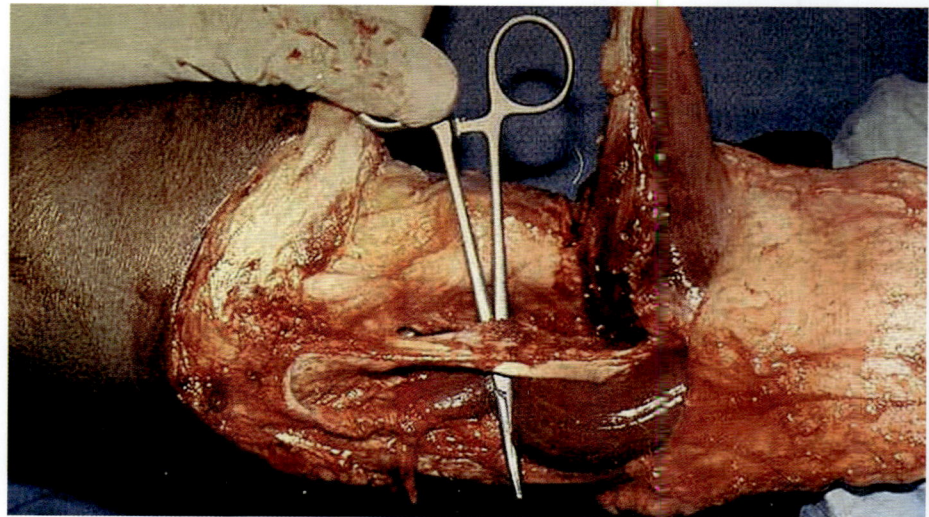

FIGURE 9 Intraoperative photograph shows isolation of the adductor tendon before detachment from the adductor tubercle. The quadriceps tendon has been cut proximal to the patella. (Courtesy of John Bowker, MD.)

The femur is exposed just above the condylar level and transected approximately 12 to 14 cm above the knee joint line with an oscillating power saw. This level is recommended because it allows sufficient space for placement of the prosthetic knee joint with robust distal padding facilitated by the quadriceps apron. The location of the cut varies, however, especially if the indication is traumatic. The blade should be cooled with saline. Two or three small drill holes for anchoring sutures are made on the lateral cortex of the distal end of the femur 1 to 1.5 cm from the cut end. Additional cortical holes are drilled anteriorly and posteriorly at a similar distance.[30,33] The femur is held in maximal adduction while the adductor magnus is brought across the cut end of the femur with its tension maintained. The adductor magnus tendon is sutured through the drill holes to the lateral aspect of the residual femur, using nonabsorbable or long-lasting absorbable suture (**Figure 10**). Additional anterior and posterior sutures are placed to prevent the muscle from sliding forward or backward on the end of the bone.

With the hip in extension to avoid creating a hip flexion contracture, the quadriceps muscle is sutured to the posterior aspect of the femur through the posterior drill holes (**Figure 11**).

These sutures also can be passed through the adductor magnus tendon. The remaining hamstrings are anchored to the posterior area of the adductor magnus or the quadriceps. The investing fascia of the thigh is sutured as dictated by the skin flaps. An adequate number of subcutaneous sutures to minimize skin tension may be used to approximate the skin edges. An absorbable thin monofilament is used for a continuous subcuticular suture if contamination is not a concern. Fine nylon sutures (3-0 or 4-0) or skin staples can be used instead to close the skin but should be placed no closer than 1 cm apart, especially if the patient has vascular disease.[12] The use of forceps on the skin edges is discouraged.

An anesthetic mixture of ropivacaine, morphine, ketorolac, and epinephrine is infiltrated into the tissues at the time of closure. A negative-pressure incisional wound dressing is applied over the suture line and kept at −75 to −125 mm Hg for 3 to 4 days[42,43] (**Figure 12**). The residual limb is then wrapped with an elastic bandage or residual limb shrinker. **Figures 13** and **14** are postoperative radiographs that show a femur held in adduction by the adductor myodesis muscle. **Figure 15** shows a healed transfemoral amputation with a long medial flap.

Chapter 42: Transfemoral Amputation: Surgical Management

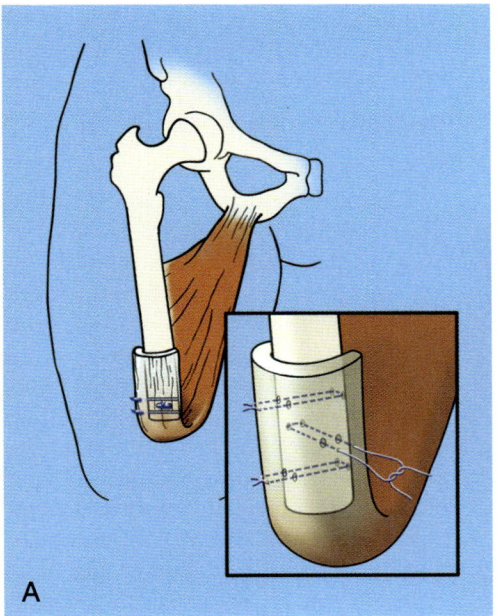

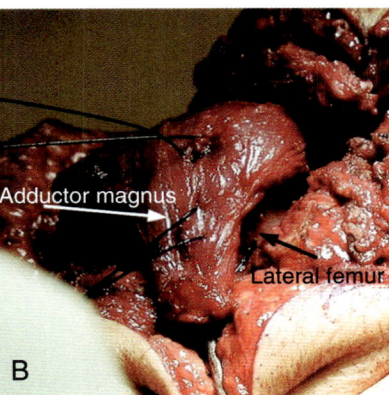

FIGURE 10 **A**, Schematic drawing shows the method of attaching the adductor magnus to the residual lateral femur. **B**, Intraoperative photograph shows the adductor magnus tendon attached with sutures through drill holes on the residual lateral femur.

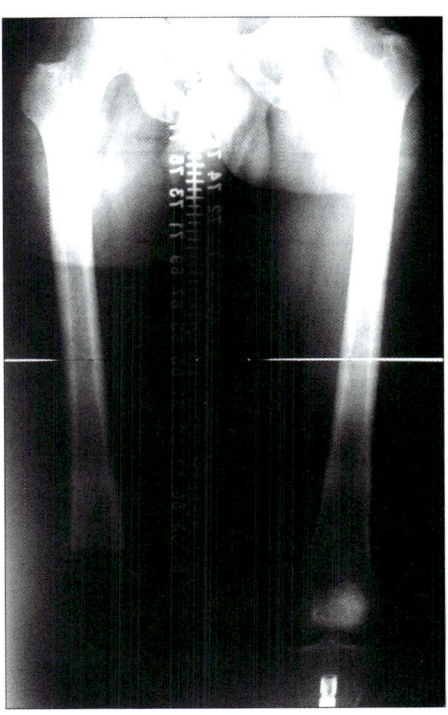

FIGURE 13 AP radiograph shows a residual femur held in normal anatomic alignment after adductor myodesis.

Alternative Techniques

Modified Adductor Myodesis

A modification of the adductor myodesis technique was used to treat 20 elderly men and 13 women (mean age, 69 years) with vascular disease.[44] In the Dundee technique, the skin incision is made 8 cm distal to the proposed bone osteotomy using equal anterior and posterior skin flaps. All muscles are sectioned at the level of the skin cuts. Bone edges are smoothed, and two 2-mm drill holes (anteromedial and anterolateral) are made at the distal end of the cut femur. The adductor muscles and medial hamstring muscles are anchored to the anteromedial hole, and the vastus lateralis and lateral hamstring muscles are sutured laterally (**Figure 16**). The quadriceps tendon and muscle are brought over the end of the femur and attached to the hamstrings. Appropriate tension of all the muscles is ensured. All 33 patients had wound healing, although one had delayed healing. Fourteen patients were fitted with a prosthesis, but the remaining 19 were not considered suitable for prosthetic fitting because of a major comorbidity (especially respiratory), inadequate progress through rehabilitation, or, in 1 patient, bilateral amputation.

This technique for myodesis was found to help restore femoral alignment. Displacement of the femur in conventional amputation was found to lead to prosthetic fitting difficulty. The technique can lead to wound-healing complications, however, because disruption of the perforating vessels to the skin can create a tissue plane between the subcutaneous tissue and the muscle and fascia layers.

Gritti-Stokes Amputation

In 1857, Italian surgeon Rocco Gritti described what he termed a through-the-knee amputation (the femur transected at the upper level of the epiphyseal line) that preserves the patella over the end of the femur to provide an end-bearing residual limb.

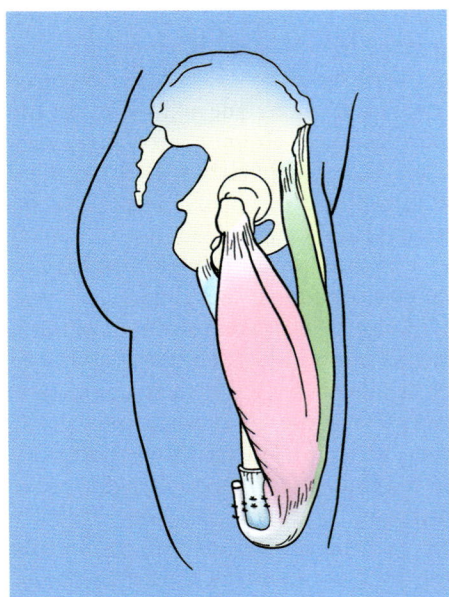

FIGURE 11 Schematic drawing shows the method of attaching the quadriceps over the adductor magnus on the residual femur.

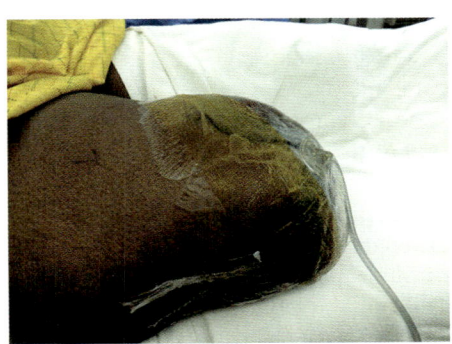

FIGURE 12 Photograph of a negative-pressure wound dressing applied after a transfemoral amputation.

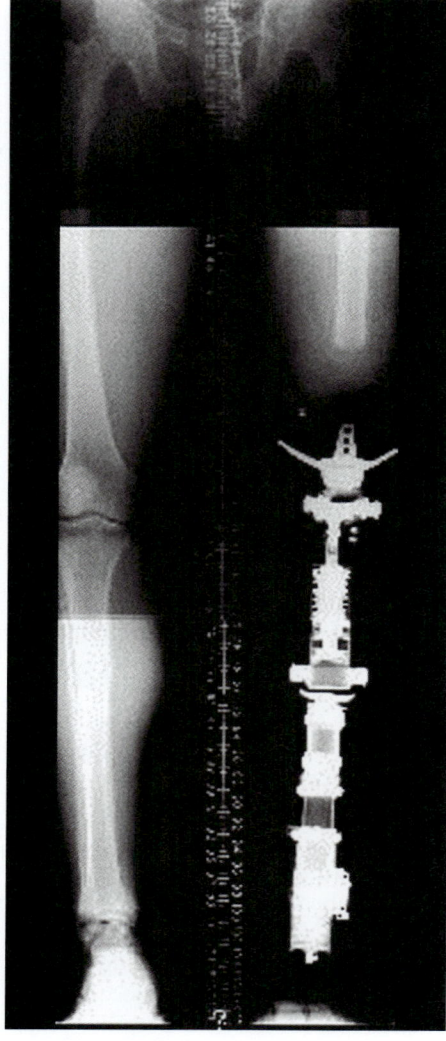

FIGURE 14 Weight-bearing AP radiograph of a patient wearing a transfemoral prosthesis to show alignment of the residual femur.

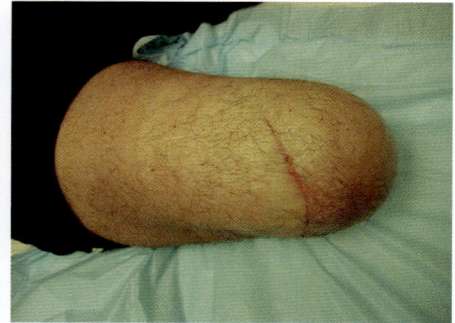

FIGURE 15 Photograph of a healed transfemoral amputation. The suture line is lateral and proximal to the end of the residual limb.

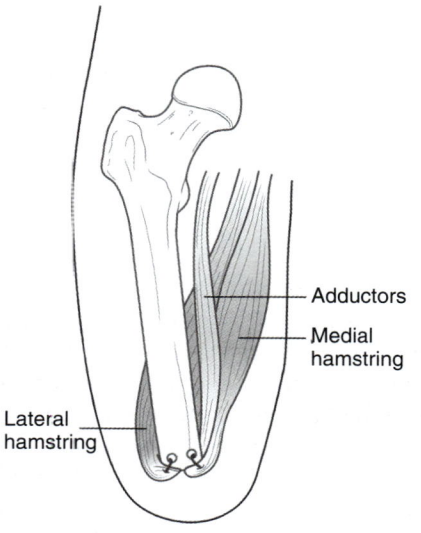

FIGURE 16 Schematic drawing shows the Dundee adductor myodesis technique.

Minor modification of this procedure has led to acceptance of femoral transection distal to the adductor tubercle that provides a large cancellous surface for the patella.[45] Recently, the Gritti-Stokes amputation with modifications has been recommended for patients with traumatic injury.[46]

A retrospective study found that trauma patients who underwent a Gritti-Stokes amputation had better scores on the Sickness Impact Profile than patients who underwent a transfemoral amputation.[46] The modified Gritti-Stokes technique was performed, as described by Beacock et al.[47] An asymmetric large anterior flap and small posterior flap are used, with the medial and lateral apices level with the femoral condyles. Hamstring tendons are sharply detached from distal insertions. There is no posterior muscle transection. The posterior half of the patella is transected, and a synovectomy is done. Femoral transection is done at the supracondylar level distal to the adductor tubercle so that there is a cancellous surface to match the patella.

The femoral osteotomy is at a 15° angle proximal-posterior to distal-anterior (**Figure 17**) to provide resistance against late patellar displacement. The patella is fixed using large nonabsorbable sutures passed through 2-mm drill holes (**Figure 18**). Hamstring tendons are sutured to the patellar tendon and deep anterior fascia. Closure is in layers over a deep drain kept in place for 48 hours. Baumgartner[8] noted that amputation through cancellous bone at the condylar level is equivalent to a knee disarticulation.

Postoperative Care

After surgery, a negative-pressure (75 to 125 mm Hg) incisional wound dressing is applied.[42,43] After 3 to 4 days, an absorbent surgical wound dressing impregnated with silver is placed over the incision site. A residual limb shrinker or elastic bandage is placed over the dressing. Although rigid dressings control edema and residual limb position better than soft dressings, they are cumbersome to apply, do not offer a substantial long-term advantage after transfemoral amputation, and have several disadvantages. The rigid hip spica cast restricts hip mobility, increases the risk of pressure sores over bony prominences, and increases the difficulty of postoperative management. The use of rigid dressings for transfemoral amputations has been abandoned by many centers. A well-applied elastic bandage will not slip off the residual limb but may become loose and should be removed and reapplied at least once a day, with careful skin inspection.

Another method of controlling swelling and reducing discomfort is to apply an elastic shrinker with a waist belt. The shrinker is made of a one-way or two-way stretch material that applies even pressure distally to proximally. The waist belt helps prevent the shrinker from slipping off the residual limb. The shrinker may be applied at the first dressing change, 72 to 96 hours after surgery. The use of elastomer or thermoplastic liners also may be helpful for controlling edema.

Phantom limb pain is common immediately after surgery and can be reduced by infiltrating the sectioned nerve with bupivacaine at the time of surgery. Local anesthetic can be administered directly to the nerve through a peripheral nerve catheter, continuously or intermittently for 3 to 4 days. Two studies found that using this method can offer immediate relief of postoperative pain and allow the amount of postoperative narcotic analgesic agents

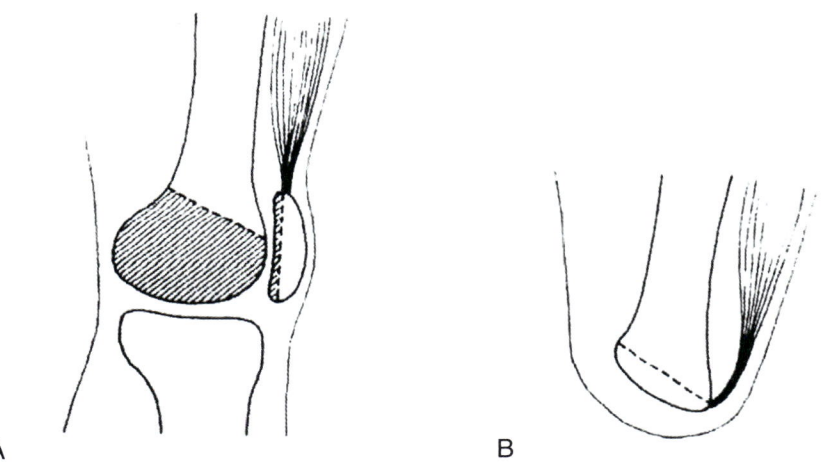

FIGURE 17 Schematic drawings show a distal femur resection in the Gritti-Stokes procedure. **A**, The dashed line shows the bone cuts on the femur and patella, with the shaded area indicating the bone to be removed. **B**, The patella placed at the end of the femur. (Reproduced with permission from Beacock CJ, Doran J, Hopkinson BR, Makin GS: A modified Gritti-Stokes amputation: Its place in the management of peripheral vascular disease. *Ann R Coll Surg Engl* 1983;65[2]:90-92.)

to be reduced;[41,48] however, neither study was randomized or controlled. Continuous infusion does not prevent long-term residual or phantom limb pain, and long-standing preoperative pain does not appear to be influenced substantially by any form of analgesic management. The use of perineural infusion does not prevent residual or phantom limb pain in patients who have had a lower limb amputation.

While the wound is healing, the patient should be mobilized in a wheelchair and on the parallel bars, and upper body exercises should be started. The goal is for the patient to have sufficient upper body strength to use crutches or a walker. Flexion contractures should be prevented by correctly positioning the patient in bed and initiating muscle-strengthening exercises. In addition, conditioning of the contralateral leg is necessary. Sutures or staples usually can be removed 2 weeks after a traumatic amputation or 3 to 4 weeks after amputation for vascular disease. During this time, the patient should wrap the residual limb or use a shrinker. After suture removal, a temporary adjustable plastic prosthesis can be fitted, and gait training is started.

With the use of aggressive rehabilitation techniques, a motivated, physically able patient can quickly return to walking. A patient who does not have the physical or mental ability to participate in a rehabilitation program oriented to the use of a prosthesis may function best using a wheelchair. Transfer training is important for these patients. The decision whether to provide the patient with a wheelchair should be made early in the postoperative period.

The overall rehabilitation of a patient with a transfemoral amputation begins at the time of surgery and continues until the patient has achieved their maximal functional independence. Appropriate surgical techniques allow easier fitting of a prosthesis, facilitate physical therapy, and help the patient achieve their goals, which have been determined in collaboration with the treating team.

Complications

The commonly described complications of transfemoral amputation include infection, heterotopic ossification, phantom sensation and pain, wound breakdown, failure to heal, and neuroma formation. None of these complications is unique to transfemoral amputations. Abductor drift is an avoidable complication of transfemoral amputation and can be mitigated by good surgical technique and methods described in this chapter.

SUMMARY

Myodesis of the adductor magnus muscle followed by the quadriceps muscle over the anchored adductor magnus (with the thigh held in adduction and extension) is crucial to maintaining the tension of these muscles. Understanding the biomechanics of the lower extremity is the basis for the correct performance of a transfemoral amputation. Recognizing normal femoral adduction and the mechanical axis of the leg allows for an understanding of the function of the adductor magnus muscle in stabilizing the femur during the stance and swing phases of gait. Developing appropriate soft-tissue flaps that minimize skin tension at the time of skin closure helps reduce the risk of wound breakdown. The application of negative-pressure wound dressings and an elastic compression bandage aids in reducing postoperative edema in the residual limb.

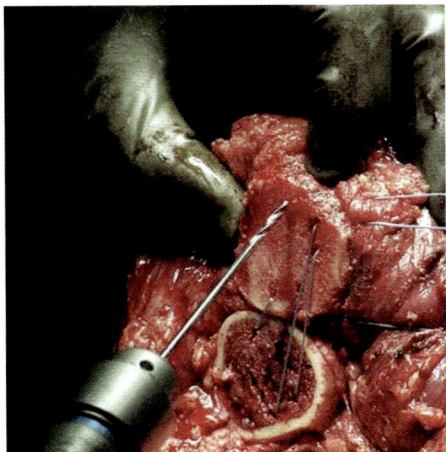

FIGURE 18 Intraoperative photograph of a patella resection and placement of drill holes during surgery using the Gritti-Stokes technique. (Reproduced with permission from Taylor BC, Poka A, French BG, Fowler TT, Mehta S: Gritti-Stokes amputations in the trauma patient: Clinical comparisons and subjective outcomes. *J Bone Joint Surg Am* 2012;94[7]:602-608.)

References

1. Fortington LV, Rommers GM, Postema K, van Netten JJ, Geertzen JH, Dijkstra PU: Lower limb amputation in Northern Netherlands: Unchanged incidence from 1991-1992 to 2003-2004. *Prosthet Orthot Int* 2013;37(4):305-310.
2. Hagberg K, Brånemark R: Consequences of non-vascular trans-femoral amputation: A survey of quality of life, prosthetic use and problems. *Prosthet Orthot Int* 2001;25(3):186-194.
3. Volpicelli LJ, Chambers RB, Wagner FW Jr: Ambulation levels of bilateral lower-extremity amputees: Analysis of one hundred and three cases. *J Bone Joint Surg Am* 1983;65(5):599-605.
4. Gonzalez EG, Corcoran PJ, Reyes RL: Energy expenditure in below-knee amputees: Correlation with stump length. *Arch Phys Med Rehabil* 1974;55(3):111-119.
5. Bell JC, Wolf EJ, Schnall BL, Tis JE, Potter BK: Transfemoral amputations: The effect of residual limb length and orientation on gait analysis outcome measures. *J Bone Joint Surg Am* 2013;95:408-414.
6. Waters RL, Perry J, Antonelli D, Hislop H: Energy cost of walking of amputees: The influence of level of amputation. *J Bone Joint Surg Am* 1976;58(1):42-46.
7. Jeans KA, Browne RH, Karol LA: Effect of amputation level on energy expenditure during overground walking by children with an amputation. *J Bone Joint Surg Am* 2011;93(1):49-56.
8. Baumgartner R: Upper leg amputation: Transfemoral amputation [German]. *Oper Orthop Traumatol* 2011;23(4):296-305.
9. Freeman MA: The surgical anatomy and pathology of the arthritic knee, in Freeman MA, ed: *Arthritis of the Knee*. Springer-Verlag, 1980, pp 31-56.
10. Hungerford DS, Krackow KA, Kenna RV, eds: *Total Knee Arthroplasty: A Comprehensive Approach*. Williams & Wilkins, 1984, pp 34-39.
11. Maquet PG, ed: *Biomechanics of the Knee*. Springer-Verlag, 1976, p 22.
12. Gottschalk F: Transfemoral amputation: Biomechanics and surgery. *Clin Orthop Relat Res* 1999;361:15-22.
13. Tintle SM, Keeling JJ, Shawen SB, Forsberg JA, Potter BK: Traumatic and trauma-related amputations: Part I. General principles and lower-extremity amputations. *J Bone Joint Surg Am* 2010;92(17):2852-2868.
14. Long IA: Normal shape-normal alignment (NSNA) above-knee prosthesis. *Clin Prosthet Orthot* 1985;9:9-14.
15. Sabolich J: Contoured adducted trochanteric-controlled alignment method (CAT-CAM): Introduction and basic principles. *Clin Prosthet Orthot* 1985;9:15-26.
16. Gottschalk FA, Kourosh S, Stills M, McClellan B, Roberts J: Does socket configuration influence the position of the femur in above-knee amputation? *J Prosthet Orthot* 1989;2:94-102.
17. Gottschalk FA, Stills M: The biomechanics of trans-femoral amputation. *Prosthet Orthot Int* 1994;18(1):12-17.
18. Thiele B, James U, Stålberg E: Neurophysiological studies on muscle function in the stump of above-knee amputees. *Scand J Rehabil Med* 1973;5(2):67-70.
19. James U: Maximal isometric muscle strength in healthy active male unilateral above-knee amputees, with special regard to the hip joint. *Scand J Rehabil Med* 1973;5(2):55-66.
20. Jaegers SM, Arendzen JH, de Jongh HJ: Changes in hip muscles after above-knee amputation. *Clin Orthop Relat Res* 1995;319:276-284.
21. Jaegers SM, Arendzen JH, de Jongh HJ: An electromyographic study of the hip muscles of transfemoral amputees in walking. *Clin Orthop Relat Res* 1996;328:119-128.
22. Green DL, Morris JM: Role of adductor longus and adductor magnus in postural movements and in ambulation. *Am J Phys Med* 1970;49(4):223-240.
23. Inman VT, Ralston HJ, Todd F, eds: *Human Walking*. Williams & Wilkins, 1981, pp 102-117.
24. Jaegers SM, Arendzen JH, de Jongh HJ: Prosthetic gait of unilateral transfemoral amputees: A kinematic study. *Arch Phys Med Rehabil* 1995;76(8):736-743.
25. Bohne WH, ed: *Atlas of Amputation Surgery*. Thieme Medical Publishers, 1987, pp 79-112.
26. Burgess EM: Knee disarticulation and above-knee amputation, in Moore WS, Malone JM, eds: *Lower Extremity Amputation*. WB Saunders, 1989, pp 132-146.
27. Harris WR: Principles of amputation surgery, in Kostuik JP, Gillespie R, eds: *Amputation Surgery and Rehabilitation: The Toronto Experience*. Churchill Livingstone, 1981, pp 37-49.
28. Barnes RW, Cox B: *Amputations: An Illustrated Manual*. Hanley and Belfus, 2000, pp 103-117.
29. Goodney PP: Patient clinical evaluation and preparation for amputation, in Cronenwett JL, Johnston KW, eds: *Rutherford's Vascular Surgery*, ed 8. WB Saunders, 2014, pp 202-213.
30. Van Niekerk LJ, Stewart CP, Jain AS: Major lower limb amputation following failed infrainguinal vascular bypass surgery: A prospective study on amputation levels and stump complications. *Prosthet Orthot Int* 2001;25(1):29-33.
31. Jensen JS, Mandrup-Poulsen T, Krasnik M: Wound healing complications following major amputations of the lower limb. *Prosthet Orthot Int* 1982;6(2):105-107.
32. Christensen KS, Falstie-Jensen N, Christensen ES, Brøchner-Mortensen J: Results of amputation for gangrene in diabetic and non-diabetic patients: Selection of amputation level using photoelectric measurements of skin-perfusion pressure. *J Bone Joint Surg Am* 1988;70(10):1514-1519.
33. Shah SK, Bena JF, Allemang MT, et al: Lower extremity amputations: Factors associated with mortality or contralateral amputation. *Vasc Endovascular Surg* 2013;47(8):608-613.
34. Gottschalk F: Traumatic amputations, in Bucholz RW, Heckman JD, eds: *Rockwood and Green's Fractures in Adults*, ed 5. Lippincott Williams & Wilkins, 2001, pp 391-414.
35. Andersen RC, Fleming M, Forsberg JA, et al: Dismounted complex blast injury. *J Surg Orthop Adv* 2012;21(1):2-7.
36. Molde A: Victims of war: Surgical principles must not be forgotten (again)! *Acta Orthop Scand* 1998;281:54-57.
37. Helayel PE, da Conceição DB, Feix C, Boos GL, Nascimento BS, de Oliveira Filho GR: Ultrasound-guided sciatic-femoral block for revision of the amputation stump: Case report. *Rev Bras Anestesiol* 2008;58(5):482-484, 480-482.
38. van Geffen GJ, Bruhn J, Gielen MJ, Scheffer GJ: Pain relief in amputee patients by ultrasound-guided nerve blocks. *Eur J Anaesthesiol* 2008;25(5):424-425.
39. Gottschalk F: Above-knee amputation, in Murdoch G, Jacobs NA, Wilson AB, eds: *Report of ISPO Consensus Conference on Amputation Surgery*. International Society for Prosthetics and Orthotics, 1992, pp 60-65.
40. Rasmussen S, Kehlet H: Management of nerves during leg amputation: A neglected area in our understanding of the pathogenesis of phantom limb pain. *Acta Anaesthesiol Scand* 2007;51(8):1115-1116.
41. Malawer MM, Buch R, Khurana JS, Garvey T, Rice L: Postoperative infusional continuous regional analgesia:

A technique for relief of postoperative pain following major extremity surgery. *Clin Orthop Relat Res* 1991;266:227-237.

42. Karlakki S, Brem M, Giannini S, Khanduja V, Stannard J, Martin R: Negative pressure wound therapy for management of the surgical incision in orthopaedic surgery: A review of evidence and mechanisms for an emerging indication. *Bone Joint Res* 2013;2(12):276-284.

43. Brem MH, Bail HJ, Biber R: Value of incisional negative pressure wound therapy in orthopaedic surgery. *Int Wound J* 2014;11(suppl 1):3-5.

44. Konduru S, Jain AS: Trans-femoral amputation in elderly dysvascular patients: Reliable results with a technique of myodesis. *Prosthet Orthot Int* 2007;31(1):45-50.

45. Middleton MD, Webster CU: Clinical review of the Gritti-Stokes amputation. *Br Med J* 1962;2(5304):574-576.

46. Taylor BC, Poka A, French BG, Fowler TT, Mehta S: Gritti-Stokes amputations in the trauma patient: Clinical comparisons and subjective outcomes. *J Bone Joint Surg Am* 2012;94(7):602-608.

47. Beacock CJ, Doran J, Hopkinson BR, Makin GS: A modified Gritti-Stokes amputation: Its place in the management of peripheral vascular disease. *Ann R Coll Surg Engl* 1983;65(2):90-92.

48. Pinzur MS, Garla PG, Pluth T, Vrbos L: Continuous postoperative infusion of a regional anesthetic after an amputation of the lower extremity: A randomized clinical trial. *J Bone Joint Surg Am* 1996;78(10):1501-1505.

Transfemoral Amputation: Prosthetic Management

Mark David Muller, CPO, MS, FAAOP

CHAPTER 43

ABSTRACT

Clinicians have long strived to create optimal transfemoral prosthetic designs that will not only enhance the user's ability to ambulate but also will be a functional element of the individual's life. Although there have been many advancements in materials, socket designs, and components, there still is little research to help quantify how the individuals that use these prosthetics devices can best be served. It is helpful to explore clinical considerations and anticipated outcomes when creating transfemoral prosthetic devices. Prosthesis use is affected by many factors, including energy expenditure, body image, voluntary control within a transfemoral prosthetic system, socket fit and design, component selection, and alignment.

Keywords: prosthetics; transfemoral; transfemoral alignment; transfemoral prosthetic socket; transfemoral prosthetic suspension; transfemoral interface

Introduction

Amputations at the transfemoral level account for approximately 19% of the approximately 1.6 million individuals in the United States who are currently living with an amputation.[1-3] Statistics from 2004 reported that 31% of all major amputations were performed at the transfemoral level,[4,5] with new evidence showing a decrease in the number of transfemoral amputations performed each year both nationally and internationally.[2] There also is evidence that individuals who have undergone amputation are living longer and will require prosthetics services throughout their lives.[1,6] In 2015, certified prosthetic practitioners spent more than 25% of their time caring for patients with a transfemoral amputation.[7]

Those in the field of prosthetics have a long history of involvement with transfemoral prosthetic socket design and construction, with the first patents awarded in England in 1790 and the first US patent for a transfemoral artificial limb given in 1846.[8-12] However, prosthetists still do not have universal clinical standards of practice for device creation, fit, suspension, and alignment. Throughout history, transfemoral design and fabrication techniques have been passed down from mentors to protégés, with no formal instructional courses available in the United States until 1949 when the University of California at Berkeley introduced a short course in transfemoral design of a suction socket. In the 1950s, several universities began formal education programs in prosthetics, with each school creating their own laboratory manuals and design iterations.[13] The prevalent design at that time was the German transfemoral quadrilateral socket, which used skin suction suspension.[14,15] In the 1980s, the first ischial containment manual emerged and was quickly adapted by other institutions, although each institution implemented design iterations. As of 2021, there were 13 accredited institutions offering master level education for prosthetic and orthotic practitioners in the United States, with each institution offering differing theories and practical implementation of both traditional and digital fabrication techniques for transfemoral socket design, suspension, and clinical application.

One rationale for the differing designs may be the variability observed in the anatomy, size, and length of transfemoral residual limbs, as well as the level of voluntary control the individual possesses. It is accepted that no single design is appropriate for every individual with a transfemoral amputation. Accordingly, variations in the clinical applications of formalized training have led numerous practitioners to create unique styles and techniques.[9,10,16,17] These variations provide practitioners with the ability to adapt a transfemoral socket to best meet the needs and goals of an individual patient.

The common clinical goals and considerations that guide rehabilitation professionals through this patient-specific process are discussed along with an overview of current transfemoral socket designs and the implications of suspension, alignment, and biomechanical considerations in evaluating, fabricating, and fitting transfemoral prostheses.

Clinical Considerations and Anticipated Outcomes

Although prosthetic devices will never truly replace a missing limb, certain clinical considerations must be addressed,

---

Neither Mark David Muller nor any immediate family member has received anything of value from or has stock or stock options held in a commercial company or institution related directly or indirectly to the subject of this chapter.

irrespective of which socket or suspension design is chosen. The transfemoral prosthetic system must balance function, comfort, and appearance both dynamically and statically.[8,11,12] To create the most appropriate plan, the treating team must consider energy expenditure, body image, the user's level of voluntary control, and the fit of the prosthetic socket. In implementing the treatment plan, the team must determine socket construction and design, the degree and complexity of the suspension system, the appropriate components, alignment considerations, and outcome measures.

Energy Expenditure

Energy expenditure for a transfemoral amputee is of great concern. The effort required to ambulate with a prosthetic device at this level is dependent on the weight of the device, the quality of fit, the degree of suspension, the accuracy of alignment, and functional characteristics of the chosen components.[17-21] If any one of these factors is not properly addressed, the individual using a transfemoral prosthesis will exhibit higher levels of energy expenditure during ambulation than are necessary, increased loading on the sound limb, and increased spinal loading.[19,21] Increased energy expenditure is accompanied by an increase in the rate of oxygen consumption and an associated elevation in heart rate. An elevated heart rate can, in turn, lower the user's self-selected walking speed and reduce gait efficiency.[22] For elderly individuals with a transfemoral prosthesis, the physical burden of ambulating with a prosthetic device may exceed their abilities, leading to a lower rate of prosthetic use.[20,23] Knowing that ambulation with transfemoral prosthetic devices requires high levels of energy, practitioners must create treatment plans that meet the individual's needs and goals with an acceptable burden level.

Fall Risk

Recent systematic review has confirmed an elevated fall risk among community ambulating users of transfemoral prostheses relative to transtibial prosthesis users.[24] This is significant as falling events can represent substantial medical expenses[25] and can limit future prosthetic mobility and activity levels. A growing body of evidence has suggested that this fall risk can be mitigated through the use of certain microprocessor knees.[26,27] Targeted exercise programs may also reduce fall risk in this population.[28]

Body Image

Body image and appearance when using a transfemoral prosthesis are complex considerations and should be addressed within the treatment plan. Satisfaction with body image, psychosocial adjustment, lack of activity restriction, and satisfaction with the function of one's prosthesis are positively associated with the cognitive performance of transfemoral amputees.[29] It is important to realize that appearance and self-image can be a cosmetic as well as a functional concern. An acceptable appearance and the ability of the user to integrate with peers play a large role in an individual's positive adaptation to their altered body image and psychosocial adjustment.[29] Body image anxiety increases depression, reduces perceived quality of life, lowers self-esteem, reduces participation in physical activity, and lowers overall satisfaction.[30,31] The prosthetist must create a device to maximize the confidence of the user through optimal fit, suspension, function, and alignment symmetry, as well as an acceptable energy expenditure.[32] There is a growing trend toward user participation in aesthetic choices, including realistic silicone covers, water transfers, or 3D printed covers. These choices may help the user feel more involved with the creation of their prosthesis and thus increase device acceptance.[29]

Effect of Voluntary Control

Functional ambulatory goals will be defined by the individual's ability or potential to control the transfemoral prosthetic device. This is commonly known as the level of voluntary control.[9,10,14,33] Because the user will not have direct musculoskeletal control of the prosthetic knee and foot, a determination of their potential voluntary control is an important consideration in determining the socket style, interface, suspension, and components used. Factors that determine the degree of voluntary control include residual limb length, positional awareness in space, active range of motion, muscle strength, and the ultimate ability to manipulate the limb in a controlled and deliberate manner. When voluntary control is limited, the rehabilitation team should design prosthetic systems that focus on prosthetic support and patient safety rather than function and performance. In contrast, enhanced voluntary control allows for the design of a more dynamic prosthesis. The degree of voluntary control also plays an integral role in component choice and alignment considerations.

Fit of the Prosthetic Socket

The ideal goal for any prosthetic device is for the user to feel that the device is part of their body. Irrespective of the socket design, materials used, or fabrication method, an optimal fit should be intimate to the contours of the residual limb and assist the user in controlling the prosthesis. Beyond these basic criteria, an optimal fit of a transfemoral prosthetic socket is poorly defined and has not been standardized. However, if users do not feel that they have control of the socket, they likely will not fully integrate their prosthetic device into their daily lives.[14]

The Transfemoral Socket

Radcliffe[14] suggested that the primary goals of a transfemoral prosthesis are to achieve comfort in weight bearing, provide a narrow base of support in standing and walking, and accomplish the swing phase of gait in a manner that is as close to normal as possible. The fit and orientation of the socket are paramount in achieving these goals. The socket must be donned in the correct orientation with respect to the user's line of progression, must match the volume of the residual limb, and must create an environment of total contact without causing impingement or discomfort. Paramount is the ability of the socket to provide adequate stability in the sagittal, coronal, and transverse planes throughout the gait cycle.

Importance of Orientation

When donning the socket, the orientation of the socket must match the user's residual limb and adjacent bony structures in a consistent rotational alignment. If the socket is malaligned, the device will cause undue pressure on the limb or the pelvis and compromise the rotational alignment of the distal prosthetic components. To properly integrate the limb within the socket, the individual should be instructed regarding socket orientation as it relates to their anatomy. This anatomic reference differs for the varying socket designs but must be addressed, especially in the initial and subsequent fittings of the device.

Importance of Total Contact Socket Fit

There are various techniques and outcome measures to assess whether the volume of the socket matches the volume of the residual limb.[35] Most clinical techniques rely on a combination of visual verification through a clear diagnostic interface and a determination of internal socket pressure through visual examination, tactile probes, or electronic pressure sensors.[36] Irrespective of the socket design, it is imperative that pressures are balanced and can be tolerated by the user.[16,37] The prosthetist should ensure that all areas within the socket make contact because lack of contact with the residual limb may result in edema, socket migration, and compromised control of the prosthesis.

The tissues proximal to the trim lines must be free from impingement throughout gait and while seated. Tissue bulging over the proximal trim lines can lead to skin breakdown, edema, subdermal cysts, blisters, irritation, and discomfort.[38] Similarly, there must be adequate relief for the bony structures within the socket. Pressure on the ischial tuberosity, ascending pubic ramus, adductor longus tendon, greater trochanter, or distal femur can lead to socket rotation, pain, gait deviations, or rejection of the prosthetic device.[39]

Socket Stability

Stability of the transfemoral prosthetic socket on the limb is vital to the control of the device. The prosthetist will make a clinical determination on the type of socket design based on the individual's level of voluntary control and the stability required. Individuals with greater levels of voluntary control are less dependent on socket modification, component choice, and alignment accommodations to control unwanted socket displacement during ambulation. Excessive motion of the transfemoral prosthetic socket on the residual limb in the sagittal, coronal, and transverse planes can lead to increased energy expenditure, gait deviations, and dissatisfaction with the prosthesis.[23,40,41]

Sagittal Plane

The principles of prosthetic control in the sagittal plane are best considered in the early stance phase of the gait cycle. As the prosthetic foot contacts the floor, the ground reaction force quickly moves posterior to the mechanical knee joint center and creates an external knee flexion moment that will cause the prosthetic knee to buckle if it is not adequately controlled by the user. The ipsilateral hip extensor musculature of the individual must fire, pulling the residual femur and the prosthetic socket posteriorly to create a counterextension moment and stabilize the mechanical knee.[42] Importantly, the residual femur must be adequately stabilized within the socket before the actions of the hip extensors can be translated through the prosthesis to act on the ground. In the absence of such femoral stabilization, the contractions of the hip extensor muscles are less effective, and the ability to control the prosthetic knee is compromised, causing the individual to compensate with a reduction in step length, a slower cadence, or an anterior shift in body weight. All of these compensatory actions increase energy expenditure.

Prosthetic control in the sagittal plane should also be considered in late stance. During this phase of the gait cycle, the individual must engage the hip flexors to drive the prosthetic socket anteriorly. This hip flexion action creates prosthetic knee flexion, thereby lifting the overall prosthesis off the ground to initiate the swing phase. Inadequate femoral stabilization may delay the execution of this action, resulting in a loss of control of the prosthetic knee and potential compromise of its function. The individual will likely display a shortened step length, reduced speed of ambulation, and a lack of confidence with the prosthetic device.[34,35]

Coronal Plane

In the coronal plane, prosthetic control is critical in limiting the movement of the torso laterally over the prosthetic device during the single-limb support phase of the gait cycle. This compensatory lateral movement over the prosthesis is one of the most common prosthetic gait deviations seen in the user of a transfemoral prosthesis and has been at the root of controversy as to whether the socket design should contain the ischial tuberosity or not.[43-45] Unless a hip abduction contracture is present, the residual femur should be placed in an adducted position equal to the contralateral femur. This position ensures the efficient firing of the hip abductor muscles on the amputated side, which limits contralateral pelvic drop and associated lateral trunk bending. This is accomplished by fitting a flattened lateral socket wall that is countered by a sufficiently high medial socket wall aligned in the correct angle of femoral adduction.[14,33,46]

During the initial fitting of a transfemoral socket, the proximal coronal instability of the socket can be easily determined by performing the lateral and the medial displacement tests. For both of these assessments, the prosthesis user must be standing safely within parallel bars. To perform the lateral displacement test, the prosthetist places one hand on the proximal lateral brim of the transfemoral socket while the other hand is placed on the prosthesis user's ipsilateral iliac crest. Gently but firmly, the prosthetist then pushes medially on the iliac crest while also pulling laterally on the proximal brim of the socket. If the socket displaces more than 0.5 inch (1.27 cm) from the residual limb during this static test, the socket may also displace laterally during single-limb stance in gait. This lateral displacement often suggests coronal instability in the socket, and it can cause the individual to experience excessive proximal medial pressures on their residual limb. A compensatory lateral shift of the torso may be adopted to restore coronal stability and reduce these pressures (**Figure 1**).

The medial displacement test is performed with simultaneous medially directed compression of the proximolateral aspect of the socket and the greater trochanter of the contralateral limb. If the socket displaces more than 0.5 inch (1.27 cm) medially, it may suggest that either the mediolateral dimension of the transfemoral socket or its overall volume is too large. Alternatively, the prosthesis user may not possess enough voluntary control to resist the lateral forces created during single-limb support[33,45,47] (**Figure 2**).

Transverse Plane

Transverse stability, observed in the swing and early stance phases of gait, is also dependent on both the level of the individual's voluntary control and the optimal fit of the transfemoral socket. During the evaluation of the residual limb, the strength of its subcutaneous tissue and musculature should be assessed to help determine if the individual can control the normal transverse plane motions of gait, including internal rotational motions during the swing phase and external rotations during early stance. If either the muscle or the underlying connective tissues are found to be inadequate, the individual will not be able to voluntarily control these forces, and the socket may rotate

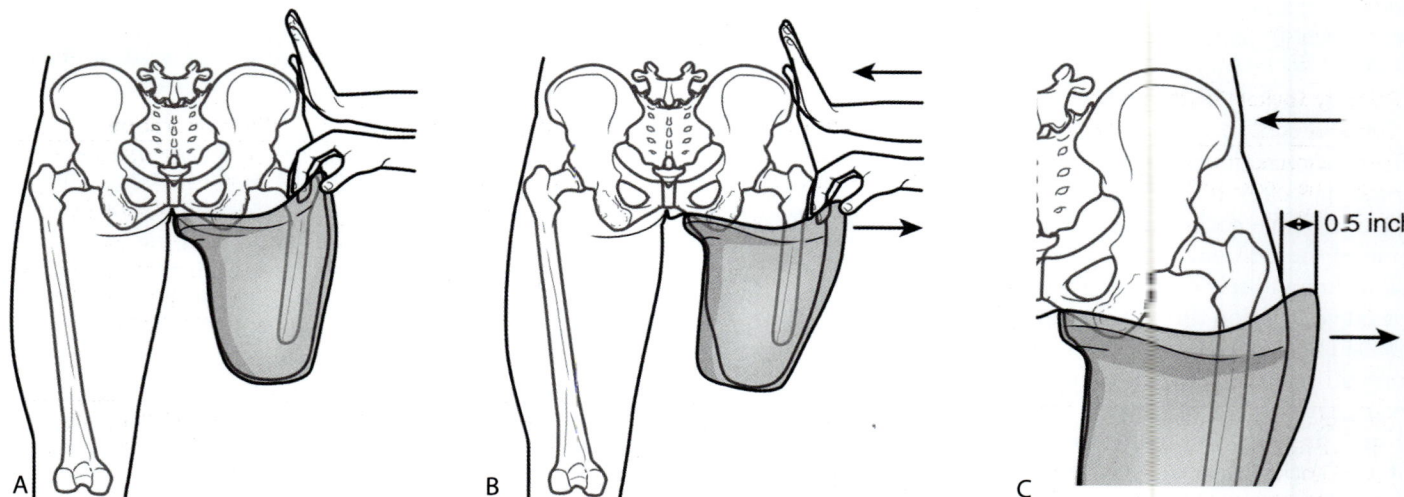

FIGURE 1 Illustrations of the steps in the lateral displacement test. After donning, the socket is aligned with the line of progression and checked to ensure a total contact fit and a level pelvis. The prosthetist then can test for lateral displacement of the socket on the limb. **A**, One hand is used to grasp the proximal edge of the socket while the other hand is placed on the ipsilateral iliac crest to provide a counterforce and stabilization. **B**, The proximal socket is pulled laterally until displacement stops. **C**, The ideal amount of displacement is 0.5 inch (1.27 cm) measured from the skin to the socket wall. If the displacement is greater than 0.5 inch (1.27 cm), the transfemoral socket likely will be unstable in the coronal plane during single-limb support.

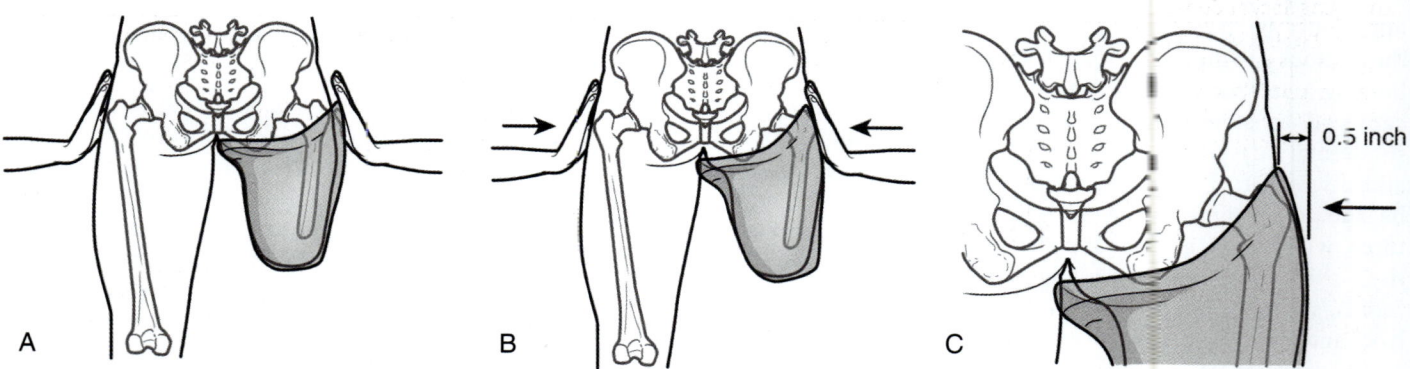

FIGURE 2 Illustrations of the steps in the medial displacement test. After donning, the socket is aligned with the line of progression and checked to ensure a total contact fit and a level pelvis. The prosthetist then can test for medial displacement of the socket on the limb. **A**, One hand is placed over the proximal lateral aspect of the socket and the other hand is placed over the greater trochanter on the contralateral side. **B** Both hands are used for medial compression until socket displacement ceases. **C**, The ideal amount of displacement is 0.5 inch (1.27 cm) from the starting point. If the displacement is greater than 0.5 inch (1.27 cm), the transfemoral socket likely will be unstable for the user in the coronal plane during single-limb support.

on the limb. In such cases, targeted socket modifications or external components are needed to aid in controlling transverse rotation.

If the individual has adequate voluntary control but still demonstrates whip-type gait deviations or excessive socket rotation, these problems may be caused by a suboptimal socket fit, with volumetric incongruences exerting the largest influence on rotational control. To reduce transverse rotation, socket fit must be optimized to match the individual's limb volume or accommodations must be made for muscle contractions.

Socket Construction

The hard socket and the flexible inner socket with a rigid frame are the two general classifications of socket construction for transfemoral prostheses. The flexible inner socket has two variations that are gaining in popularity: the flexible inner socket with dynamic panels and the flexible socket with an embedded rigid frame. The strut framed sockets are gaining popularity and may use an inner flexible socket or a roll-on elastic liner to create a total contact fit with the residual limb (**Table 1**).

Hard Sockets

Transfemoral sockets are typically constructed around a positive model or use a digital representation of the prosthesis user's limb. A hard socket is a single-walled, static socket that is designed to be in direct contact with either the user's skin or an interface such as a roll-on gel liner or prosthetic sock. The advantages of a hard socket

TABLE 1 Transfemoral Socket Construction

Primary Socket Construction

Construction	Example	Primary Indication	Major Advantages	Chief Limitations
Hard socket (integrated rigid inner socket and outer frame)		Mature limbs Firm limbs Situations that allow for reduced trim line height Minimal wall thickness	Simple design Durability Easy to clean Solid construction that will not alter over time	Comfort with rigid proximal trim lines Hard surface when sitting Adhered tissue, invaginations, or sensitive bony areas may not be accommodated
Removable flexible inner socket; rigid outer frame (flexible inner socket can be removed from outer frame)		Any limb shape Flexibility in design Dynamic muscle movement Relief areas for sensitive tissue Proximal soft-tissue support	Adjustable Allows for dynamic muscle movement and relief for sensitive tissue while maintaining a total contact fit Comfort in sitting Fenestrations can be created while retaining socket strength	Inner socket may change shape over time Durability

Emerging Socket Construction

Construction	Example	Primary Indication	Major Advantages	Chief Limitations
Removable, flexible inner socket; rigid outer frame; dynamic panels (panels are adjustable to change compression on inner flexible socket)		Volume fluctuations Progressive pressure in specific areas User adjustability	Dynamically alters inner socket shape and compression felt on limb in specific areas Compression from panels is user adjustable	Lengthy fabrication process More maintenance
Flexible socket; embedded rigid frame (rigid frame is laminated between layers of flexible material)		Mature limbs High levels of voluntary control Dynamic muscle movement	Flexible interface Soft proximal brim Comfort in sitting Soft outer surface Rigid embedded frame supports socket with minimal surface area	Lengthy fabrication process Fragile Limited adjustability Heavier than other construction types

include its simplicity, thin-walled construction, durability, and ability to be easily cleaned and maintained. Because this socket option offers little padding or accommodative flexibility and cannot absorb the shear forces generated between the limb and the socket walls, it is intended for limbs with stable volume, firm tissue, and fair to good skin sensation. This socket construction is generally contraindicated in individuals with adhered scar tissue, invaginations, and sensitive bony prominences; these prosthesis users require a more forgiving design.[38]

A transfemoral hard socket is typically fabricated from a carbon fiber or a rigid thermoplastic material with no fenestrations or cutouts. This socket construction does not readily allow for fluctuations in residual limb size, so an optimal initial fit is crucial. Similarly, the prosthesis user with a hard socket must be diligent in volume management to maintain a total contact fit.

Flexible Inner Sockets

The second type of socket construction incorporates a flexible inner socket capable of elastic movements and a rigid outer frame for stability. This design can be in direct contact with the user's skin or an interface such as a roll-on gel liner or a prosthetic sock. The main advantage of this design is that the inner flexible socket, which is made from an elastic thermoplastic or a silicone-based material, allows for both volumetric and localized fitting accommodations. In addition, when the proximal trim lines of the rigid frame are lowered, the flexibility of the proximal inner socket dramatically increases the user's comfort. The brim of the inner socket contains the proximal tissue, but it allows for elastic movement around sensitive bony areas such as the ischial tuberosity, the ascending pubic ramus, and the anterior superior iliac spine while sitting. The flexible inner socket also allows for increased proprioceptive feedback when the rigid outer frame is cut away in strategic areas. When the rigid frame is fenestrated, the compliant material of the inner flexible socket is exposed to allow an individual to feel the surface they are sitting on or to have room for residual musculature to expand during ambulation. Even with the frame cut away, the inner flexible socket contains the soft tissue and maintains the benefits of hydrostatic weight bearing. In the absence of the inner flexible socket, such fenestrations would allow the individual's skin to protrude from the openings, compromising both hydrostatic loading and pressure distribution during weight bearing and leading to localized window edema and skin breakdown.

One variation of a flexible inner socket with a rigid outer frame uses dynamic panels that can be adjusted to help regulate pressures within the socket. In this variation, instead of using open cutouts, the outer rigid frame is fabricated with free-floating panels that are connected by tensioning cords. In the fabrication process, hollow tubes are laminated into the frame in strategic locations. After the panels are cut out of the frame, the hollow tubes are exposed, allowing tensioning cords to be fed through the tubes in both the panels and the rigid frame. The cords can be tightened as needed to move the panels closer to the inner flexible socket, thereby increasing the overall compression felt by the user. The main advantage of this system is the ability of the user to change the shape and volume of the socket. When necessary, the dynamic panels can be loosened to allow bulbous limbs to enter the socket, and then compressed to create a total contact fit. The panels also can be adjusted on an activity-specific basis, such as relieving tension while sitting or kneeling or increasing compression for strenuous activities such as running.

An alternative design is a flexible socket with an embedded rigid frame. This design is the result of advances in materials and fabrication techniques. Similar to prosthetic systems popular before World War II in which a metal frame was housed within a flexible leather socket,[8] this modern variation uses rigid frames laminated within an otherwise flexible socket. This socket construction option has been successfully used in upper limb prosthetic applications and is now beginning to be used with transfemoral prostheses.[6] The major advantages of this socket construction include its overall flexibility, reported comfort, minimal trim lines, and perceived improved control of the prosthesis.[49] Although this socket is heavier, more difficult to fabricate, and less durable than other types of sockets, the final product offers a very flexible system with confined, rigid support. Alternatives to this design include sockets created using additive manufacturing (3D printing) and selective laser sintering of materials such as Nylon 12 to create single-walled sockets with both rigid and flexible elements.

Another alternative socket design uses a frame of longitudinal struts. These sockets can be modular systems purchased from a manufacturer or custom creations with areas of compression and release around the residual limb. The longitudinal struts create an open frame design where total contact with the residual limb can be obtained with an inner flexible socket or a roll-on elastic liner. The strut designs are proving to be comparable in function to other socket designs and can be cost effective for selective use.[44,50-53]

Socket Designs

The two primary socket designs for transfemoral prostheses are the ischial ramal containment and the subischial designs. Two subcategories of the ischial ramal containment design are the ischial containment and the ramal containment designs. Variations of the subischial design include the quadrilateral design and those designs that may incorporate the use of subatmospheric-assisted vacuum suspension (**Table 2**).

Ischial Containment Designs

In current practice, the ischial containment socket is the most commonly used design, with numerous iterations in both teaching and clinical practice. All variations of the ischial containment socket have the common goal of providing mediolateral stability in single-limb support. This goal is achieved by using an intimately fitted socket with a narrow

Chapter 43: Transfemoral Amputation: Prosthetic Management

TABLE 2 Transfemoral Socket Designs

Design	Example	Primary Indication	Major Advantages	Chief Limitations
Ischial/ramal containment (the ischial-ramal complex is contained within the socket to provide stability in the coronal plane during single-limb support)	Ischial containment	When enhanced coronal stability is requested; User presents with lower levels of voluntary control; Shorter residual limbs	Enhanced coronal stability with support from bony structure; Proximal tissue contained inside of socket; Amount of containment can be adjusted; Potential for ischial weight bearing	Clinical experience required to create optimal fit; High proximal trim line; May inhibit hip range of motion
	Ramal containment	Enhanced coronal stability with minimal trim lines	Enhanced coronal stability with support from bony structure; Proximal tissue outside of socket; Reduced proximal trim lines; Enhanced hip range of motion with maintenance of coronal stability	Clinical experience required to create optimal fit; Discomfort unless optimal fit around ascending ischial ramus is achieved; Lengthy fitting process
Subischial (the ischium is not contained within the socket; coronal stability during single-limb support is obtained by soft-tissue compression)	Quadrilateral	Longer residual limbs; User presents with higher levels of voluntary control; Previous user	Ischial weight bearing	Clinical experience required to create optimal fit; Minimal coronal stability; Narrow anterior-posterior dimension; Predetermined rectangular socket shape
	Subischial, vacuum-assisted suspension	Longer residual limbs; High voluntary control; High gadget tolerance; Uses hydrostatic weight bearing	Reduced trim lines; Excellent suspension that may enhance coronal stability issues because of intimate fit; Amount of assisted vacuum suspension force can be regulated; Hip range of motion not limited	Clinical experience required to create optimal fit; Tissue proximal to the brim may be stressed; Multistage donning process; May be a bulky design

mediolateral dimension while encasing the medial aspect of the ischial tuberosity and ramus within the socket.[33] Most ischial containment design variations use hydrostatic weight bearing rather than direct ischial weight bearing. In contrast to the quadrilateral socket, the medial ischial containment wall is angled to match the ischial ramus angle of the prosthesis user rather than the line of progression. The ischial containment socket can help minimize the lateral thrust of the socket during single-limb support by buttressing against bony aspects of the pelvis. If the orientation of the ischial containment wall angle does not match the anatomic angle of the ischium and ascending ischial ramus, the prosthesis user will likely feel undo pressure and discomfort with this socket design. Similarly, whereas the medial containment of such sockets is generally well tolerated, socket impingement against the distal aspect of the ramus is poorly tolerated and must be avoided in individual socket fittings.

The amount of ischial containment is variable, with most designs initially containing the ischium from 1 to 1.75 inches (2.54 to 4.45 cm) proximal to its distal aspect.[33,47] This amount of containment gives adequate mediolateral control while allowing for tissue around the ischium and ascending ischial ramus to aid in padding the sensitive bone.[54] Sockets that incorporate more proximal degrees of ischial containment typically have more proximal gluteal containment as well.

Some ischial containment designs, such as the Marlo Anatomical Socket (Ortiz International), suggest that coronal stabilization can be achieved by limiting bony containment to the ascending ischial ramus and lowering the other proximal trim lines of the socket.[55] This ramal containment socket design allows greater range of motion about the hip and decreases some metabolic costs.[18,20,55] However, this type of design is difficult to fit and may be rejected because of localized pressures on the medial ramus. Volume fluctuations can be particularly disruptive within these socket designs as an absence of hydrostatic loading results in localized proximal medial socket pressure. Achieving an optimal fit requires the prosthetist to have an elevated level of clinical skills.

Given the proximal intrusions of ischial containment designs into perineum and bony elements of the pelvis, the common challenge of ischial containment designs is determining the amount of actual bony support that can be tolerated by the individual user. Ischial containment designs tend to work well for individuals with shorter residual limbs or those who lack voluntary control of their adductor muscles. For individuals with longer residual limbs and high degrees of voluntary control, aggressive ischial containment may be unnecessary, and a subischial design might be more appropriate.[19,56,57]

Subischial Designs

The quadrilateral socket is a subischial design that uses ischial weight bearing on its posterior brim with some degree of additional hydrostatic loading of the residual limb to support the individual's weight.[14] The ischium rests on the posteromedial aspect of the socket brim where it is held in place through anterior-posterior socket compression. In contrast to ischial containment socket designs, this anterior-posterior tightness requires an increased mediolateral dimension to allow proximal soft tissue to enter the socket. However, this increased mediolateral dimension can create a lack of coronal support, leading to pressure on the perineum and common gait deviations such as lateral trunk flexion and a wide base of support. Also common with the quadrilateral design is difficulty in achieving adequate lateral support for the femoral shaft, which often leads to the reduced effectiveness of the gluteus medius to stabilize the pelvis in single-limb support. This lack of femoral support was reported by Long[26,39] in the 1980s and led to the initiation of early ischial containment designs.[10,54]

As the quadrilateral socket has declined in popularity, there has been growing interest in a subischial design that uses hydrostatic weight bearing as does the ischial containment socket but does not incorporate the ischium into the socket. This design was introduced in the 1960s by Redhead.[16] Although his work contributed to a better understanding of hydrostatic weight bearing, the design did not achieve widespread acceptance.

Current subischial socket designs are based on the original concepts described by Redhead,[16] but they also incorporate a roll-on gel liner interface and assisted vacuum suspension. These subischial sockets may be preferred over ischial containment designs because of their lowered proximal trim lines.[49,56] In addition, there are suggested advantages of increased limb health, volume stabilization, reduced perspiration, and increased comfort.[58] Studies are needed to objectively prove these suggested advantages for varying limb lengths and levels of voluntary control, but the design appears to be a viable choice at this time.[44,53]

Suspension Systems

Total contact socket fit and adequate suspension throughout the entire gait cycle is necessary to ensure the confident use of a transfemoral prosthesis. During the stance phase of gait, total contact is maintained by the user's weight. During the swing phase, the inertia and weight of the prosthesis will displace the socket from the residual limb if the suspension system is inadequate. On taking the next step, the user will force the limb back into the socket, creating a piston-type motion. This displacement or pistoning of the limb within the socket, even if it is a few millimeters, can lead to loss of prosthetic control, skin irritation, overall socket discomfort, distal residual limb edema, and gait deviations.[11,38]

Because of the large amount of remaining compliant soft tissue, general residual limb shape, and minimal bony femoral anatomy, suspension is often quite difficult to achieve for an individual using a transfemoral prosthesis. Various forms of suspension have been attempted to minimize transfemoral socket displacement. Although all of these variations have merit, there is no evidence that supports a clinical standard for a single suspension system.[38] Therefore, it is imperative for the prosthetist to have a working knowledge of the various systems available and take into consideration the unique goals and characteristics of each transfemoral prosthesis user.

Current suspension systems being used at the transfemoral level are generally classified as either subatmospheric, negative-pressure systems or belt-type systems. Subatmospheric systems use some level of negative atmospheric pressure combined with surface tension to maintain the transfemoral socket on the residual limb. Subcategories of subatmospheric designs include skin-fit suction, roll-on liners with various locking mechanisms, roll-on liners with a hypobaric sealing membrane, and vacuum-assisted suspension. Belt-type systems use positive, superiorly directed forces created by a strapping system secured around the pelvis. Subcategories of belt systems include the Silesian belt, elastic belt suspension, and hip joint and pelvic belt suspension (**Table 3**).

Subatmospheric Suspension

Subatmospheric suspension provided by skin suction or a roll-on gel liner is the most prevalent type of suspension design.[38] These systems work by combining friction with a negative pressure differential within the socket to maintain suspension of the prosthesis on the

Chapter 43: Transfemoral Amputation: Prosthetic Management

TABLE 3 Transfemoral Suspension

Suspension Type	Example	Primary Indication	Major Advantage	Chief Limitations
Subatmospheric, negative pressure (primary means of suspension used with most transfemoral prosthetic systems)	Skin-fit suction	Whenever clinically feasible Mature limb	Increased proprioception between limb and prosthesis	Susceptible to volume changes Difficult to don Limited absorption of shear and impact forces felt on limb
	Roll-on gel liner with pin lock, lanyard, or magnet locking mechanism	Firm limb Expect volume changes	Easy to don Secure suspension Allows for volume changes Absorption of shear and impact forces	Distal distraction can lead to edema Hand strength and dexterity required to apply liner Alignment and build height considerations
	Roll-on gel liner with hypobaric seal	Firm limb Expect volume changes	Easy to don Can allow for volume changes Minimal distal distraction Absorption of shear and impact forces	Hand strength and dexterity required to apply liner
	Roll-on gel liner, vacuum-assisted suspension	Mature limb Active Minimal socket displacement	Excellent suspension increases proprioception and control Minimal socket displacement decreases daily trauma to limb	Bulky Difficult to don Gel liner is fragile Gadget tolerance needed Maintenance
Belts (typically used as secondary or auxiliary suspension; primary suspension only when negative atmospheric pressure cannot be used)	Silesian	Limit socket rotation Volume changes Auxiliary suspension	Firm belt for secure feel Adjustable Can be removable	Minimal suspension Hand strength and dexterity to don Pressure around the pelvis Difficult to clean

(Continued)

TABLE 3 Transfemoral Suspension (Continued)

Suspension Type	Example	Primary Indication	Major Advantage	Chief Limitations
Elastic suspension		Reduce socket rotation Volume changes Auxiliary suspension	Flexible Adjustable Removable	Minimal suspension Elastic suspension Hand strength and dexterity to don Warm around the pelvis Difficult to clean
Hip joint and pelvic belt		Short residual limbs Weak hip abductors Low levels of voluntary control	Maximum coronal support	Belt may be uncomfortable Migrates when sitting Minimal suspension Difficult to clean

residual limb. In the literature, the term suction is used synonymously with the term vacuum when discussing transfemoral suspension systems. A suction system has been defined as a subclass of subatmospheric socket systems that allows air to be expelled from a sealed socket while preventing air from entering the socket. However, in contrast to the vacuum-assisted suspension that will be described shortly, the internal pressure of a suction socket environment is not actively regulated.[59]

The suction necessary for these suspension systems can be created between the skin and the hard socket, between the skin and a roll-on gel liner, and between the gel liner and the socket. The negative pressure within a socket can be measured with a typical vacuum gauge in inches of mercury (inHg), where normal atmospheric pressure is 0 inHg. In discussing transfemoral suspension, the larger the negative number, the greater is the suspension force (−30 inHg represents an absolute vacuum).

The original transfemoral suction suspension designs were used within a skin-fit socket where the suction was created simply between the skin and the inner socket wall.[60] Basic suction suspension systems are characterized as low, negative-pressure systems, with readings in the 0 to −8 inHg range. During weight bearing, these systems have a vacuum reading of 0 inHg. During ambulation, the vacuum reading increases in value through swing phase as the momentum of the advancing limb and weight of the prosthesis attempt to distract the prosthesis from the limb. The greater the inertial forces generated in swing, the greater are these distractive forces, thus requiring higher negative pressures to hold the socket in place.

Suction Suspension: Skin-Fit

Skin-fit suction suspension has the benefit of direct skin contact with the socket, allowing high levels of proprioceptive feedback to the user. The skin moves with the socket, allowing the user to quickly perceive and react to small changes in socket position. Proximal, circumferential socket reductions create a seal against the skin that prevents air from entering the socket, thereby permitting suction to occur during swing phase. The skin also creates surface tension along the inner socket walls that further resists some of the distraction forces felt during swing. Typically, a one-way expulsion valve is located distally on the transfemoral socket that permits air to escape during weight bearing while preventing air from entering during swing phase.

For skin-fit suction suspension systems, the internal pressure clinical readings have been found to be approximately −8 inHg during the swing phase.[42,56,58]

The individual generally dons the prosthesis by initially applying a donning sleeve over the residual limb and feeding the loose end of the sleeve through the open distal valve hole. The sleeve breaks the surface tension between the socket and the skin, allowing the individual to seat the limb inside the socket while pulling proximal soft tissue into the socket.[39] The sleeve is progressively and fully extracted from the socket. With the limb fully seated, the one-way air valve is installed in place.

The disadvantages of skin-fit suction suspension systems include difficulties with donning, comparatively poor mitigation of shear forces, and poor accommodation of residual limb volume fluctuations. Successful donning of a skin-fit suction suspension system requires strength and balance because the soft tissue needs to be pulled into the socket using a donning sleeve; this may be difficult for some users to manage. Scar tissue and invaginations represent other potential contraindications because shear forces are typically not well tolerated by these clinical presentations, and there is potential for skin breakdown if the skin is not well protected and/or padded. Because skin-fit suction requires the maintenance of a proximal, air-tight seal against the skin, even small changes in limb size caused by a change in weight or edema can compromise suspension.

Suction Suspension: Roll-On Gel Liners and Locking Mechanisms

Roll-on gel liners, when used as an interface, absorb shear and impact forces acting on the limb, stabilize soft tissue, and accommodate volume fluctuations. As with skin-fit suspension systems, liners are held in place by a combination of suction and surface tension and may also be used as a means of suspension with the attachment of a distal locking mechanism such as a pin, lanyard, or magnet.

To don these systems, the user rolls on the liner, inserts their limb into the socket, and engages a locking mechanism that is typically embedded in the distal aspect of the socket. Locking mechanisms include pins, lanyards, or magnets. The donning of such systems is generally much quicker compared with skin-fit suction suspension systems. In addition, socks can be worn over the liner to accommodate volume changes without a loss of suspension.

Disadvantages of using roll-on liners in a transfemoral prosthesis include a minimum level of hand strength and dexterity for correct donning, the potential for tearing the somewhat fragile liners because of improper handling and sustained use, and the need for liner replacement if damage occurs. Roll-on liners also require consistently good hygiene to reduce odor and maintain cleanliness.

Roll-On Gel Liners: Hypobaric and Vacuum-Assisted Suspension

Suction suspension with roll-on liners can be accomplished by direct contact with the liner against the socket wall (similar to skin-fit suspension) or with the use of hypobaric sealing membranes. Roll-on liners that use suction for suspension tend to have less distal distraction and minimized socket rotation compared with those that use a distal locking mechanism.

As is the case with skin-fit suction, these roll-on liner systems use negative pressure and surface tension to maintain suspension. To fully seat the residual limb and liner into the socket, the surface tension must be reduced, typically with the use of isopropyl alcohol in lieu of a donning sleeve. The liner is rolled on over the residual limb, alcohol is sprayed on the liner, and the limb and liner are slipped into the socket and engage against the inner socket wall as the alcohol quickly evaporates. The resultant seal maintains the pressure differential within the socket.

This variation in roll-on liner use can be incorporated with either simple suction or vacuum-assisted suspension. The two suspension methods differ in the internal socket pressure while standing. In simple suction suspension, the internal socket pressure is 0 inHg, whereas socket pressure with vacuum-assisted suspension is less than 0 inHg, and it can be as low as −25 inHg. Both systems use an expulsion valve to maintain the pressure differential, with vacuum-assisted suspension also using an external mechanism to draw air from the socket. Although suction systems have a negative-pressure environment in swing only, vacuum-assisted systems have a continual negative-pressure environment through stance and swing.

Although vacuum-assisted suspension has been shown to reduce falls and increase confidence with prosthetic users,[61] it has been slow to gain acceptance in transfemoral applications. This may be the result of complicated fabrication and donning processes and difficulties in maintaining a proximal vacuum seal. However, modern material advances, creative techniques, and design variations are making vacuum-assisted suspension a more viable choice for transfemoral applications. Anecdotal reports indicate that these systems work well for individuals with longer residual limbs and high voluntary control.[58]

The three basic subischial socket designs that incorporate vacuum-assisted suspension are the single-wall internal sealing system, the single-wall external sealing system, and the double-wall internal sealing system (Table 4). Although these three designs each have advantages and limitations, all use a roll-on gel liner as an interface and use the creation of high levels of vacuum-assisted suspension between the liner and the socket rather than the skin. Although skin is compatible with basic suction suspension, it is porous and irregular in shape, making it a poor surface for maintaining elevated levels of negative pressure. Gel liners have a smooth, flexible, nonporous surface that allows for a vacuum seal to be maintained throughout ambulation, while sitting, and during participation in activities of daily living.

All three subischial socket design systems also use a wick in the form of a sock or fabric liner cover. The wick begins at the distal aspect of the liner and terminates distal to the vacuum seal, allowing for the transfer of air molecules between the socket and the liner. This facilitates uniform internal socket pressures between −5 and −25 inHg; typical prosthesis users prefer approximately −15 inHg. The greater the negative pressure, the greater is the suspension force; however, high vacuum levels may be difficult to maintain over time.

The single-wall internal sealing design works with a hypobaric seal that is either integrated into the roll-on liner or applied over the liner. A wick is used distal to the seal, and air is drawn out of the system either manually with a hand pump or actively by with an electronic or integrated weight-activated pump. This suspension system is simple in design, fabrication, and donning and also allows for any variation of proximal trim lines. Its main limitation is the limited surface area over which a vacuum seal can be achieved, which can be an issue for individuals with shorter residual limbs.

The single-wall, external sealing design overcomes this issue with the use of a longer roll-on liner that is reflected over the proximal brim and sealed distally on the outside of the socket using a sealing sleeve. This design requires that the proximal trim lines be reduced to allow the liner to be reflected. Although the system has the benefit of lower trim lines, the

TABLE 4 Transfemoral Socket Design, Subischial Variations, Vacuum-assisted Suspension

Subischial Variation	Example	Major Advantages	Chief Limitations
Subischial, single-wall, internal sealing system (roll-on gel liner with a hypobaric seal inside of socket, wick below the seal, external vacuum pump)		Reduced bulk when compared with other subischial designs Minimal donning process More proximal trim lines may enhance coronal stability	Limited area to achieve suspension because of the height of the vacuum seal inside of the socket Shorter residual limbs
Subischial, single-wall system, outer sealing sleeve (long roll-on gel liner, wicking sock, reflected liner over brim of socket, seal on outside of socket, external vacuum pump)		Suspension over the entire socket Reduced trim lines Option for shorter limbs	Bulky Liner susceptible to tears at brim Lengthy donning process Exposed liner may adhere to clothing
Subischial, double-wall system, sealed internal socket (roll-on gel liner and wicking sock; rigid internal socket affixed to liner by a sealing sleeve; internal socket connects to outer frame; external vacuum pump)		Inner suspension seal is protected by outer frame More proximal trim lines may enhance coronal stability	Bulky Lengthy donning process Lengthy fabrication and fitting process Short residual limbs

exposed liner is subject to wear from the environment and is prone to failure because of the formation of holes. It also is bulkier than the internal sealing system.

The double-wall socket uses an internal socket to create vacuum suspension and an external socket to provide the proximal brim and distal attachment of the prosthesis. A roll-on liner is donned, followed by a wicking sock. The internal hard socket, typically half the length of the residual limb, is then applied over the liner. A vacuum seal is created when a sealing sleeve is applied over both the outer wall of the internal socket and the liner, as is often seen in transtibial systems. Negative pressures are drawn between the liner and the socket through a one-way expulsion valve. The internal socket is then inserted into the external socket where it is affixed by various forms of locking mechanisms. The major limitations of this design are its bulk, weight, and complicated donning and fabrication processes.

Belt-Type or Auxiliary Suspension

Belt-type suspension offers convenience over performance. These systems are easy to don but offer minimal primary suspension. Belt-type suspension systems are primarily used to provide secondary or auxiliary suspension and aid in control of the device. The three main types of belt-type suspension systems are the Silesian belt, elastic suspension, and the hip joint and pelvic belt (**Table 3**). Silesian and elastic systems are soft belt systems that can be attached to the socket to help reduce rotation and provide minimal suspension. For individuals who ambulate at a minimal cadence and require a socket system that is both easy to don and allows for free movement of air, these suspension systems may be an adequate primary suspension option. Alternatively, for individuals who require greater coronal stabilization because of a short residual limb or lack of abductor muscle control, a hip joint and pelvic belt can be used. This system provides maximal stability against lateral socket motion but provides minimal suspension.

Component Considerations

Prosthetic Knee Considerations

Because an individual with a transfemoral prosthesis has no direct musculoskeletal connection to the prosthetic knee or foot, the most optimal components must be selected. If the prosthetic knee unit is to simulate the function of the anatomic knee, it must provide stability in early stance, allow for shock

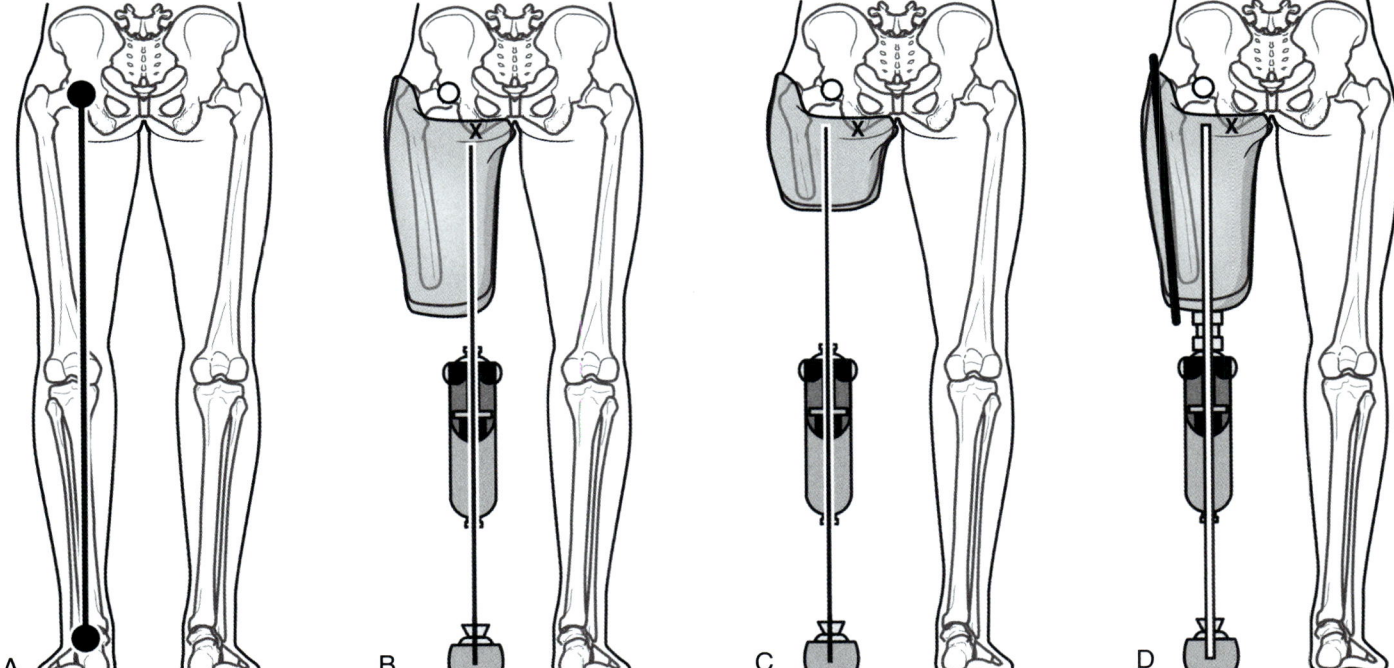

FIGURE 3 Illustrations show the process of initial coronal alignment for placement of the prosthetic knee and foot. **A**, Posterior view of anatomic alignment in the coronal plane. The hip joint aligns over the knee joint and the ankle joint. **B**, Because the hip joint is difficult to represent in transfemoral alignment, the location of the ischium (X) is used instead. For longer residual limbs, the coronal alignment line begins 1 inch (2.54 cm) lateral to the ischium; then it continues distally through the posterior bisection of the prosthetic knee and the posterior bisection of the prosthetic foot. **C**, For shorter residual limbs or individuals with lower levels of voluntary control, the coronal alignment line is shifted laterally, closer to the bisection of the prosthetic socket, but never more lateral than the bisection of the socket. **D**, A completed transfemoral alignment with the socket set at the initial adduction angle (heavy black line) and the connecting pylons attached to the socket, knee, and foot.

absorption while maintaining a lowered center of mass through midstance, provide stability through terminal stance, allow a smooth transition into swing phase, limit initial swing-phase flexion across a range of cadences, advance the limb through midswing, and smoothly decelerate at terminal swing.[22]

The first concern in knee component selection should be stability in early stance. If the individual has limited voluntary control, the knee unit must have inherent stability, which can be variously achieved through mechanical linkages, breaking mechanisms, or hydraulic dampening control. For several decades, the addition of sensors and microprocessor control units has demonstrated an increased ability to allow safe ambulation, reduced cognitive dedication to controlling the knee unit, increased gait efficiency, and increased overall user confidence with the prosthesis.[62]

Another concern in knee component selection is the ability of the knee to transition from stance to swing phase. The methodology varies by which the prosthetic knee knows when to transition from stable load bearing in stance phase to less restricted motion that will allow swing-phase flexion. Mechanically controlled knee units typically rely on a transfer of load or the mechanical knee angle to initiate this transition. In contrast, microprocessor-controlled knee units use algorithms based on input received from load sensors, accelerometers, gyroscopes, and joint angles. Because of this nuanced level of regulation, microprocessor-controlled knee units allow for more controlled prosthetic ambulation, enabling the user to confidently address changes in the environment, such as walking down slopes or ramps, movements in confined spaces, descending or ascending stairs, and walking backward. These situations illustrate scenarios in which mechanically controlled knees often fail to provide consistent support and which require the prosthesis user to be cognizant of environmental changes.

Prosthetic Foot Considerations

When selecting a prosthetic foot for an individual with a transfemoral amputation, an initial concern is the influence of the foot on the knee flexion moment in early stance. If the individual has limited voluntary control, the prosthetic foot should reduce the knee flexion moment. This can be accomplished with a soft heel component in the prosthetic foot itself or by altering the alignment of the foot relative to the socket. The next concern is the transition from stance to swing phase where the foot should generally enhance late stance stability to allow the user to take an adequate step with the contralateral limb. The length, stiffness, and design of the keel, along with alternations in alignment, will affect stability in this late stance phase.

Additional Component Considerations

With the anatomic knee and foot absent, users of transfemoral devices are missing elements of rotation, shock absorption, and stance-phase knee flexion. Additional components of transfemoral prostheses can address these missing anatomic elements. Positional rotation units allow the prosthesis user to spin the prosthetic components distal to an adaptor. The function of these units is optimized when they are applied on the distal aspect of the socket and proximal to the knee. This allows the user to cross their legs, more easily tie shoes, don pants, and enter the front seat of a car. Torque absorption units can be combined with shock absorbers to reduce the shear and impact forces felt on the residual limb. Although these components are effective, they add weight, cost, and spatial considerations to the overall design of the prosthesis.

Stance flexion, the 15° to 20° of knee flexion necessary for optimized gait, is achieved during loading response,[22] and it is often a desired feature when creating transfemoral prosthetic devices. However, this amount of knee flexion in early stance can induce a sensation of instability for many individuals with a transfemoral amputation. Prosthetic stance flexion is variously obtained through the design of the knee frame, compressive bumpers, and hydraulic cylinders.

Alignment Considerations

The principles of transfemoral prosthesis alignment have altered little over time. In 1955 Radcliffe[14] addressed transfemoral alignment considerations in his statement that the artificial limb "... must provide both adequate support and a natural-appearing gait with as modest consumption of energy as possible." These standards have not appreciably changed. Prosthetists attempt to create a stable and effective transfemoral gait pattern with proper socket fit, effective suspension, and diligence in bench, static, and dynamic alignments.

Before it is fitted to a patient, the prosthesis is set up in bench alignment, which reflects the individual's hip flexion, adduction attitude, and transverse limb orientation. The socket is generally set in a flexion angle 5° greater than the individual's maximum hip extension. This added hip flexion permits the user to take an adequate step with the contralateral limb and puts a mild stretch on the hip extensor muscles to allow them to be more efficient in early stance.[14,33,42,46,63]

The transfemoral socket is also set to match the individual's recorded adduction orientation. This will align the femur under the hip joint and put a mild stretch on the gluteus medius, increasing efficiency during single-limb support.[64] Setting the proper amount of socket adduction also reduces the tendency for proximal lateral gapping of the socket and helps to maintain a narrow base of support.[33] Transverse orientation is determined by the user's line of progression and the necessity to minimize transverse plane gait deviations. This orientation is especially important for proper fitting of ischial containment sockets.

With the socket in the proper orientation, the focus is on the placement of the prosthetic knee and foot. In able-bodied individuals, coronal alignment of the hip joint is typically directly over the knee and ankle joints (**Figure 3**, A). For initial bench alignment of the transfemoral prosthesis, the actual hip joint cannot be used as a reference point because it cannot be located on the prosthetic socket. However, locating a point on the socket brim that is 1 inch (2.54 cm) lateral to the location of the ischium will provide a reasonable approximation. The prosthetic knee and ankle joints are placed directly below this identified point. The initial coronal bench alignment allows for stability in double-limb stance, induces a modest lateral thrust in single-limb stance, and achieves a narrow 2-inches (5.08-cm) base of support (**Figure 3**, B). The prosthetic knee and ankle should be placed more laterally under the socket for shorter residual limbs or in individuals with compromised voluntary control (**Figure 3**, C). However, this necessary accommodation will increase energy expenditure by inducing a wider base of support.

In able-bodied individuals, the sagittal plane alignment of the ground reactive force is posterior to the hip joint and anterior to the knee and ankle (**Figure 4**, A). This anatomic alignment allows the prosthesis user to stand with minimal energy expenditure. Because the anatomic hip joint cannot be used as a point of reference on the prosthetic socket, the apex of the greater trochanter is used. For bench sagittal plane alignment, a simulated reference line is used to create a stable prosthetic alignment. This line is called the trochanter-knee-ankle line. To understand the use of the trochanter-knee-ankle reference line, a single-axis knee and single-axis foot will be assumed, because these components have very little inherent stability and require that the stability of the overall prosthetic system be derived by the alignment of the socket relative to the knee and ankle components.

The trochanter-knee-ankle line begins by determining a reference point for the trochanter and approximating the position of the hip joint. This point can be reasonably estimated by bisecting the socket in the sagittal plane at its most proximal aspect (**Figure 4**, B). This is followed by the placement of the prosthetic ankle joint, a reference point that differs for every prosthetic foot and is identified within individual manufacturer's guidelines. When the trochanter and prosthetic ankle reference points are vertically aligned (**Figure 4**, B), the prosthetic knee is set at its proper height and located according to the manufacturer's recommendation for the knee center's sagittal reference point. This point may be posterior, through, or anterior to the trochanter-ankle line (**Figure 4**, C through F). Placing knee center posterior to the line creates a safe alignment, because the individual's weight and the ground reaction force keep the knee locked in extension. This also can be described as an involuntary alignment because no voluntary control is required to keep the knee in extension (**Figure 4**, D). In contrast, placing knee center anterior to the trochanter-ankle line creates an alignment in which the individual has to voluntarily control the sagittal stability of the knee. This alignment is also

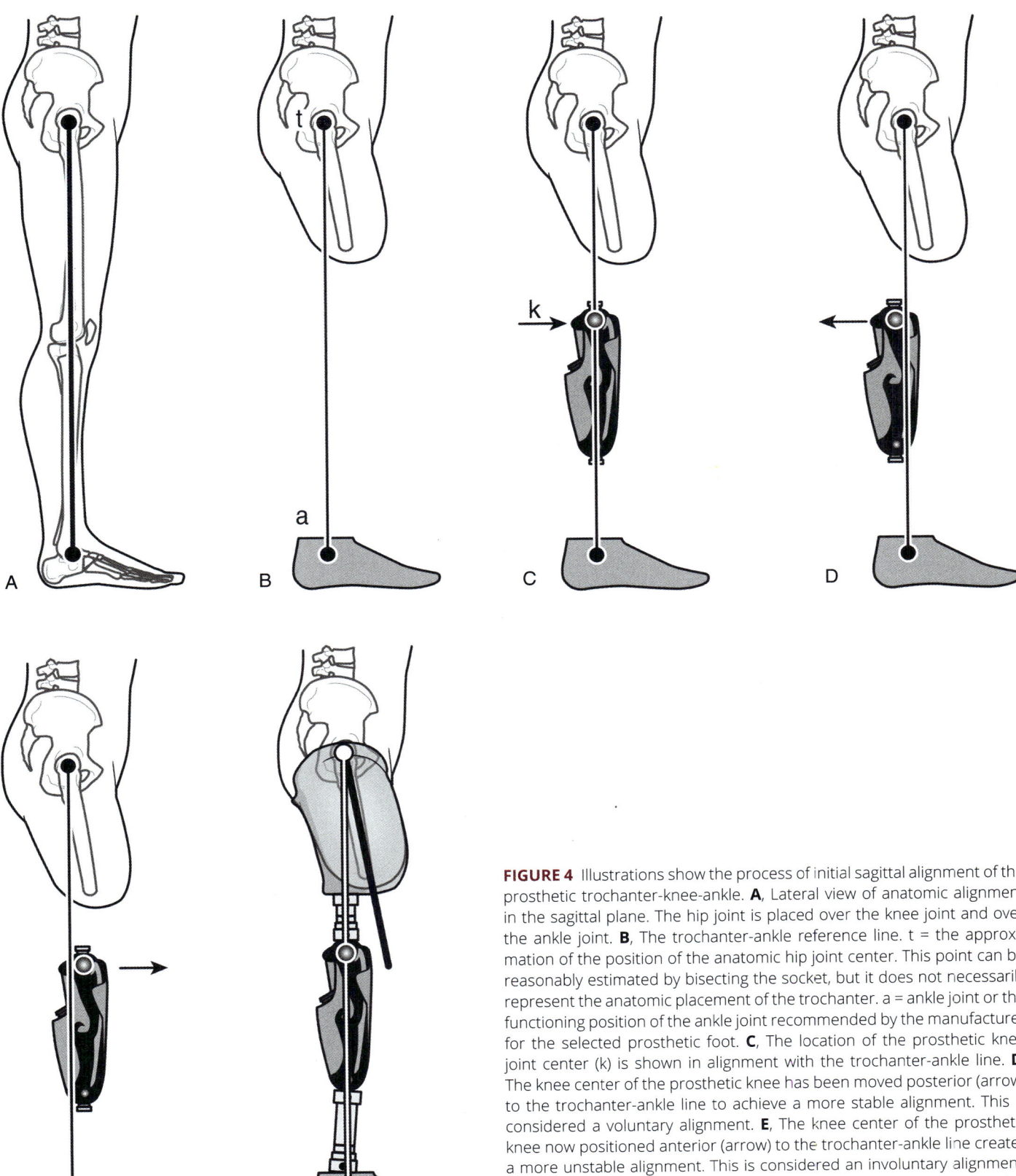

FIGURE 4 Illustrations show the process of initial sagittal alignment of the prosthetic trochanter-knee-ankle. **A**, Lateral view of anatomic alignment in the sagittal plane. The hip joint is placed over the knee joint and over the ankle joint. **B**, The trochanter-ankle reference line. t = the approximation of the position of the anatomic hip joint center. This point can be reasonably estimated by bisecting the socket, but it does not necessarily represent the anatomic placement of the trochanter. a = ankle joint or the functioning position of the ankle joint recommended by the manufacturer for the selected prosthetic foot. **C**, The location of the prosthetic knee joint center (k) is shown in alignment with the trochanter-ankle line. **D**, The knee center of the prosthetic knee has been moved posterior (arrow) to the trochanter-ankle line to achieve a more stable alignment. This is considered a voluntary alignment. **E**, The knee center of the prosthetic knee now positioned anterior (arrow) to the trochanter-ankle line creates a more unstable alignment. This is considered an involuntary alignment. **F**, A completed transfemoral alignment is shown with the initial socket flexion angle (black line) and the connecting pylons from the socket to the knee to the foot.

seen with knee units possessing inherent stability because it facilitates early stance flexion and permits easier initiation of swing-phase knee flexion in late stance (**Figure 4**, E). If the knee center point is directly on the trochanter-ankle line, it is considered to be on trigger, where the system may be in voluntary or involuntary alignment depending on the placement of the prosthetic foot with each step (**Figure 4**, F).

In the transverse plane, the prosthetic knee is externally rotated 5° to compensate for the natural 5° of internal socket rotation that will occur during swing phase. This rotation ensures that the knee will flex in the line of progression during swing. For individuals who walk faster, the amount of internal rotation will increase, and the initial external knee rotation should be larger.

When bench alignment is complete, the prosthesis is donned and static or standing alignment is assessed. The foot should be flat on the floor with 2 to 4 inches (5.08 to 10.16 cm) of base support. The knee should be extended and safe with socket flexion, adduction and rotation matching the individual's limb orientation. Generally, if bench alignment conditions were observed, minimal adjustments will need to be made to achieve a proper static fit. Any accommodative changes in flexion or adduction will change the position of the socket over the knee and foot, which will alter the stability of the system. In such instances, the proper trochanter-knee-ankle alignment should be reestablished before ambulation begins.

Because every prosthetic knee and foot has different triggers to transition from stance to swing control, the prosthesis user must be made aware of how each component functions before ambulation is attempted. The prosthesis user should be observed and instructed on proper techniques while functions such as sitting, bending the knee, and advancing the limb are practiced in a safe environment (such as with parallel bar support before ambulation). During dynamic alignment, the prosthetist will work to optimize gait and minimize energy expenditure by making incremental changes to the alignment and working with a therapist to focus on enhancing muscle strength and range of motion.[24]

SUMMARY

Great technologic advances have been made in transfemoral prosthetic sockets, components, and suspension systems in recent years. However, it must be understood that there is no single socket design, alignment, or prosthetic system that will be optimal for all individuals with transfemoral amputation. There is a need for prosthetists to continually develop their clinical and technical skills to provide the most appropriate device and the best fit for each patient.

When creating treatment plans for persons with transfemoral amputations the rehabilitation team must address issues of energy expenditure, body image, levels of voluntary control, and socket fit, and they should have an intimate knowledge of appropriate sockets designs, suspension systems, components, and alignment considerations. Clinical experience, knowledge of evolving clinical standards, the use of available evidence, and the incorporation of appropriate outcome measures also will assist the rehabilitation team in providing optimal care to their patients.

References

1. Ziegler-Graham K, MacKenzie EJ, Ephraim PL, Travison TG, Brookmeyer R: Estimating the prevalence of limb loss in the United States: 2005 to 2050. *Arch Phys Med Rehabil* 2008;89(3):422-429.
2. Belatti DA, Phisitkul P: Declines in lower extremity amputation in the US Medicare population, 2000-2010. *Foot Ankle Int* 2013;34(7):923-931.
3. National Center for Health Statistics: Health, United States: With Chartbook on Trends in the Health of Americans. 2004. Available at: http://www.cdc.gov/nchs/data/hus/hus04.pdf. Accessed May 1, 2015.
4. Newhall K, Spangler E, Dzebisashvili N, Goodman DC, Goodney P: Amputation rates for patients with diabetes and peripheral arterial disease: The effects of race and region. *Ann Vasc Surg* 2016;30:292-298.e1.
5. Cai M, Xie Y, Bowe B, et al: Temporal trends in incidence rates of lower extremity amputation and associated risk factors among patients using veterans health administration services from 2008 to 2018. *JAMA Netw Open* 2021;4(1):e2033953.
6. Dodson A, El-Gamil A, Shimer M, DaVanzo J: *Retrospective Cohort Study of the Economic Value of Orthotic and Prosthetic Services Among Medicare Beneficiaries: Final Report.* Dobson DaVanzo & Associates, 2013, pp 20-24. Available at: http://www.amputee-coalition.org/content/documents/dobson-davanzo-report.pdf. Accessed May 1, 2015
7. *Practice Analysis of Certified Practitioners in the Disciplines of Orthotics and Prosthetics.* American Board for Certification in Orthotics, Prosthetics & Pedorthics, 2015, p 37. Available at: https://www.abcop.org/docs/default-source/publications/practitioner-practice-analysis.pdf?sfvrsn=47455412_1. Accessed October 9, 2021.
8. Marks AA: *A Treatise on Artificial Limbs With Rubber Hands and Feet.* AA Marks, 1901.
9. Canty TJ, Ware RM: Suction socket for above knee prosthesis. *U S Nav Med Bull* 1949;49(2):216-233.
10. Pritham CH: Workshop on teaching materials for above-knee socket variants. *J Prosthet Orthot* 1988;1(1):50-67.
11. Gholizadeh H, Abu Osman NA, Eshraghi A, Ali S: Transfemoral prosthesis suspension systems: A systematic review of the literature. *Am J Phys Med Rehabil* 2014;93(9):809-823.
12. Palmar BF: inventor. Artificial leg. US patent 4834,846.
13. Anderson MH: Professional education: A nine-year report. *Orthop Prosthet Appl J* 1961;2:123-135.
14. Radcliffe CW: Functional considerations in the fitting of above-knee prostheses. *Artif Limbs* 1955;2(1):35-60.
15. Anderson MH, Sollars RE: *Manual of Above-Knee Prosthetics for Prosthetists.* UCLA Prosthetics Education Program, 1956.
16. Redhead RG: Total surface bearing self suspending above-knee sockets. *Prosthet Orthot Int* 1979;3(3):126-136.
17. Lusardi MM, Jorge M, Nielsen CC: *Orthotics and Prosthetics in Rehabilitation.* Elsevier, 2013, pp 652-678.
18. Van Schaik L, Geertzen JHB, Dijkstra PU, Dekker R: Metabolic costs of activities of daily living in persons with a lower limb amputation: A systematic review and meta-analysis. *PLoS One* 2019;14(3):e0213256.

19. Russell Esposito E, Rábago CA, Wilken J: The influence of traumatic transfemoral amputation on metabolic cost across walking speeds. *Prosthet Orthot Int* 2018;42(2):214-222.
20. Russell Esposito E, Whitehead JMA, Wilken JM: Sound limb loading in individuals with unilateral transfemoral amputation across a range of walking velocities. *Clin Biomech* 2015;30(10):1049-1055.
21. Shojaei I, Hendershot BD, Wolf EJ, Bazrgari B: Persons with unilateral transfemoral amputation experience larger spinal loads during level-ground walking compared to able-bodied individuals. *Clin Biomech* 2015;32:157-163.
22. Perry J: *Gait Analysis: Normal and Pathological Function*. SLACK, 2010.
23. Deans SA, McFadyen AK, Rowe PJ: Physical activity and quality of life: A study of a lower-limb amputee population. *Prosthet Orthot Int* 2008;32(2):186-200.
24. Hunter SW, Batchelor F, Hill KD, Hill AM, Mackintosh S, Payne M: Risk factors for falls in people with a lower limb amputation: a systematic review. *PM R* 2017;9(2):170-180.
25. Mundell B, Maradit Kremers H, Visscher S, Hoppe K, Kaufman K: Direct medical costs of accidental falls for adults with transfemoral amputations. *Prosthet Orthot Int* 2017;41(6):564-570.
26. Stevens PM, Wurdeman SR: Prosthetic knee selection for individuals with unilateral transfemoral amputation: A clinical practice guideline. *J Prosthet Orthot* 2019;31(1):2.
27. Campbell JH, Stevens PM, Wurdeman SR: OASIS 1: Retrospective analysis of four different microprocessor knee types. *J Rehabil Assist Technol Eng* 2020;7:2055668320968476.
28. Schafer ZA, Perry JL, Vanicek N: A personalised exercise programme for individuals with lower limb amputation reduces falls and improves gait biomechanics: A block randomised controlled trial. *Gait Posture* 2018;63:282-289.
29. Gozaydinoglu S, Hosbay Z, Durmaz H: Body image perception, compliance with a prosthesis and cognitive performance in transfemoral amputees. *Acta Orthop Traumatol Turc* 2019;53(3):221-225.
30. Schoppen T, Boonstra A, Groothoff JW, de Vries J, Göeken LN, Eisma WH: Physical, mental, and social predictors of functional outcome in unilateral lower-limb amputees. *Arch Phys Med Rehabil* 2003;84(6):803-811.
31. Gallagher P, Horgan O, Franchignoni F, Giordano A, MacLachlan M: Body image in people with lower-limb amputation: A Rasch analysis of the Amputee Body Image Scale. *Am J Phys Med Rehabil* 2007;86(3):205-215.
32. Ephraim PL, MacKenzie EJ, Wegener ST, Dillingham TR, Pezzin LE: Environmental barriers experienced by amputees: The Craig Hospital inventory of environmental factors. Short form. *Arch Phys Med Rehabil* 2006;87(3):328-333.
33. Muller MD: *Transfemoral Ischial Containment (IC) Laboratory Manual*. California State University Dominguez Hills Orthotics and Prosthetics Program, 2018.
34. Kamali M, Karimi MT, Eshraghi A, Omar H: Influential factors in stability of lower-limb amputees. *Am J Phys Med Rehabil* 2013;92(12):1110-1118.
35. Gailey R, Kristal A, Lucarevic J, Harris S, Applegate B, Gaunaurd I: The development and internal consistency of the comprehensive lower limb amputee socket survey in active lower limb amputees. *Prosthet Orthot Int* 2019;43(1):80-87.
36. Ko ST, Asplund F, Zeybek B: A scoping review of pressure measurements in prosthetic sockets of transfemoral amputees during ambulation: key considerations for sensor design. *Sensors* 2021;21(15):5016.
37. Staat T, Lundt J: The UCLA total surface bearing suction below-knee prosthesis. *Clin Prosthet Orthot* 1987;11(3):118-138.
38. Highsmith JT, Highsmith MJ: Common skin pathologies in LE prosthesis users: Review article. *JAAPA* 2007;20(11):33-36, 47.
39. Pasquina PF, Cooper RA, eds: *Care of the Combat Amputee*. Office of the Surgeon General, Borden Institute, 2009, pp 553-580.
40. Siriwardena GJ, Bertrand PV: Factors influencing rehabilitation of arteriosclerotic lower limb amputees. *J Rehabil Res Dev* 1991;28(3):35-44.
41. Munin MC, Espejo-De Guzman MC, Boninger ML, Fitzgerald SG, Penrod LE, Singh J: Predictive factors for successful early prosthetic ambulation among lower-limb amputees. *J Rehabil Res Dev* 2001;38(4):379-384.
42. Radcliffe CW: The Knud Jansen lecture: Above-knee prosthetics. *Prosthet Orthot Int* 1977;1(3):146-160.
43. *Practice Analysis of Certified Practitioners in the Disciplines of Orthotics and Prosthetics*. American Board for Certification in Orthotics, Prosthetics & Pedorthics, 2000, p 45.
44. Kahle J, Miro RM, Ho LT, et al: The effect of the transfemoral prosthetic socket interface designs on skeletal motion and socket comfort: A randomized clinical trial. *Prosthet Orthot Int* 2020;44(3):145-154.
45. Fatone S, Caldwell R, Angelico J, et al: Comparison of ischial containment and subischial sockets on comfort, function, quality of life, and satisfaction with device in persons with unilateral transfemoral amputation: A randomized crossover trial. *Arch Phys Med Rehabil* 2021;102(11):2063-2073.e2.
46. Dillon M: *Ischial Containment Socket for Transfemoral Amputees: A Manual for Assessment, Casting, Modification and Fitting*. National Centre for Prosthetics and Orthotics La Trobe University, 2006.
47. Neumann ES, Wong JS, Drollinger RL: Concepts of pressure in an ischial containment socket: Measurement. *J Prosthet Orthot* 2005;17:2-11.
48. Moran CW: Revolutionizing prosthetics 2009 modular prosthetic limb-body interface: Overview of the prosthetic socket development. Available at: http://techdigest.jhuapl.edu/TD/td3003/30_3-Moran.pdf. Accessed May 1, 2015.
49. Fatone S, Caldwell R, Major M, et al: Development of sub-ischial prosthetic sockets with vacuum-assisted suspension for highly active persons with transfemoral amputations. 2013. Available at: http://www.nupoc.northwestern.edu/research/projects/lower-limb/dev_subischial.html. Accessed May 1, 2015.
50. Kahle JT, Klenow TD, Highsmith MJ: Comparative effectiveness of an adjustable transfemoral prosthetic interface accommodating volume fluctuation: Case study. *Technol Innovat* 2016;18(2):175-183.
51. Klenow TD, Schulz J: Adjustable-volume prosthetic sockets: Market overview and value propositions. *Canadian Prosthet Orthot J* 2021;4(2):17.
52. Mitton K, Kulkarni J, Dunn KW, Ung AH: Fluctuating residual limb volume accommodated with an adjustable, modular socket design: A novel case report. *Prosthet Orthot Int* 2017;41(5):527-531.
53. Maikos JT, Chomack JM, Loan JP, Bradley KM, D'Andrea SE: Effects of

prosthetic socket design on residual femur motion using dynamic Stereo X-Ray – A preliminary analysis. *Front Bioeng Biotechnol* 2021;9:697651.

54. Sabolich J: Contoured adducted trochanteric-controlled alignment method (CAT-CAM): Introduction and basic principles. *Clin Prosthet Orthot* 1985;9:15-26.

55. Traballesi M, Delussu AS, Averna T, Pellegrini R, Paradisi F, Brunelli S: Energy cost of walking in transfemoral amputees: Comparison between Marlo anatomical socket and ischial containment socket. *Gait Posture* 2011;34(2):270-274.

56. Kahle JT, Highsmith MJ: Transfemoral sockets with vacuum-assisted suspension comparison of hip kinematics, socket position, contact pressure, and preference: Ischial containment versus brimless. *J Rehabil Res Dev* 2013;50(9):1241-1252.

57. Strachan E, Davis A, Wontorcik L: Stride-to-stride temporal-spatial gait variability and vacuum pressure deviation of trans-femoral amputees ambulating with sub-ischial prostheses. 2011. Available at: http://www.oandp.org/publications/jop/2011/2011-07.pdf. Accessed May 1, 2015.

58. Kahle JT, Orriola JJ, Johnston W, Highsmith M: The effects of vacuum-assisted suspension on residual limb physiology, wound healing, and function: A systematic review. *Technol Innov* 2014;15(4):333-341.

59. American Academy of Orthotist and Prosthetist Lower Limb Prosthetic Society Sub-Atmospheric Technology Group: Definition of terms. Available at: http://aaop-llps.ning.com/group/SATG/page/definition-of-terms-sub-atmospheric-technology. Accessed August 1, 2014.

60. Haddan CC, Thomas A: Status of the above-knee suction socket in the United States. *Artif Limbs* 1954;12:29-39.

61. Rosenblatt NJ, Ehrhardt T: The effect of vacuum assisted socket suspension on prospective, community-based falls by users of lower limb prostheses. *Gait Posture* 2017;55:100-104.

62. Highsmith M, Kahle JT, Bongiorni DR, Sutton BS, Groer S, Kaufman KR: Safety, energy efficiency, and cost efficacy of the C-Leg for transfemoral amputees: A review of the literature. *Prosthet Orthot Int* 2010;34(4):362-377.

63. Zhang T, Bai X, Liu F, Ji R, Fan Y: The effect of prosthetic alignment on hip and knee joint kinetics in individuals with transfemoral amputation. *Gait Posture* 2020;76:85-91.

64. Gottschalk FA, Kourosh S, Stills M, et al: Does socket configuration influence the position of the femur in above-knee amputation? *J Prosthet Orthot* 1989;2:94-102.

Hip Disarticulation and Transpelvic Amputation: Surgical Management

CHAPTER 44

Sheila A. Conway, MD, FAAOS, FAOA • Motasem A. Al Maaieh, MD

ABSTRACT

Hip disarticulation and hemipelvectomy are viable—sometimes necessary—alternatives to limb salvage procedures in patients with extensive pathology or trauma of the upper thigh, buttock, and pelvis. Both procedures are technically demanding, require detailed preoperative planning, and occasionally necessitate involvement from a multispecialty surgical team. Systemic and local complications are frequent and occasionally life-threatening and their management and rehabilitation are complex.

Keywords: hemipelvectomy; hip disarticulation; transpelvic amputation

Introduction

Amputations through the hip joint and the pelvis are useful surgical options for managing various, generally severe, pathologies of the upper thigh, buttock, and pelvis.[1-3] Neoplasm, including primary bone and soft-tissue sarcomas and metastatic disease, is a common indication for these high-level amputations. The oncologic goal of surgery is local disease control; however, palliative amputations may be indicated in fungating tumors or locally invasive disease when negative margins cannot be achieved. Nonneoplastic indications include severe trauma and crushing injuries, end-stage vascular disease with a functionless or gangrenous limb, and extensive bone and soft-tissue infection such as necrotizing fasciitis.[4,5] The optimal level of amputation must be determined based on the proximal extent of disease or injury and the viability of the surrounding soft tissues to ensure adequate soft-tissue coverage.[5,6]

This chapter reviews the surgical management of hip disarticulation and transpelvic amputation, with an emphasis on preoperative planning, surgical technique, postoperative care, and complications. Because these surgical procedures are highly challenging, surgical proficiency is critical to optimize outcomes and minimize complications.

Indications

A variety of pathologies may require hip disarticulation or hemipelvectomy. One of the most common indications is neoplasm, including soft-tissue sarcomas, primary bone sarcomas, and metastatic disease. Primary malignancies of the proximal thigh and recurrent tumors after a transfemoral amputation are common neoplastic indications for hip disarticulation, whereas primary and metastatic disease in the pelvis may necessitate hemipelvectomy. Extensive tumor fungation in the thigh and associated pathologic femoral fractures may result in extensive soft-tissue contamination, which may preclude limb salvage or distal-level amputations. Pediatric neoplasms of the proximal femur may necessitate high-level amputations when physeal tumor involvement or skip lesions preclude viable limb reconstruction for definitive local control.

Other indications for hip disarticulation or hemipelvectomy are severe soft-tissue infections with or without systemic sepsis, such as in a patient with diabetes and necrotizing fasciitis, which requires immediate surgical intervention, systemic antibiotics, and aggressive critical care management. Mortality rates in such patients may be as high as 50%.[7-10] Periprosthetic joint infections represent an increasing indication for hip disarticulation.[11] Severe trauma associated with extensive crush or high-energy injuries may require hip disarticulation or hemipelvectomy, either in an urgent setting or as a salvage procedure for failed lower-level amputations or limb salvage.[5,10] Ischemia, including peripheral vascular disease and prior revascularizations, is another indication for surgery and associated with high mortality rates for hip disarticulation.[10,11]

Determining the salvageability of a limb may be challenging and requires consideration of the following: tumor behavior and sensitivity to adjuvant therapies, acceptable surgical margins, neurovascular involvement, the location and degree of bone resection, the anticipated function of the residual limb, and patient factors. When definitive local control of malignant disease

---

Dr. Conway or an immediate family member serves as an unpaid consultant to DePuy, a Johnson & Johnson Company. Dr. Al Maaieh or an immediate family member is a member of a speakers' bureau or has made paid presentations on behalf of Silony Medical; serves as a paid consultant to or is an employee of Daichii Sankyo and Medtronic; and has stock or stock options held in Medtronic.

is the primary goal, careful preoperative assessment with three-dimensional imaging is essential to determine if adequate margins can be achieved with limb salvage techniques. Neoadjuvant chemotherapy or radiation therapy may help achieve limb salvage in patients with highly sensitive tumors. A similar approach to extensive infections is important to ensure adequate resection of contaminated or nonviable soft tissue and areas of chronic osteomyelitis. Estimating the functionality of the residual limb is equally critical in the decision-making process; if both the sciatic and femoral nerves are involved, a functional limb is highly unlikely. Extensive muscular disease in the thigh or large osseous resections can make a functional limb unsalvageable, even when preservation of either the sciatic or femoral nerves is possible.[10,11]

Contributing patient factors include overall health, nutritional status, comorbid disease, and patient acceptance. Nutritional status and comorbidities such as diabetes and peripheral vascular disease can affect wound healing and influence the optimal amputation level. A patient's emotional acceptance of amputation must be carefully assessed and proactively managed. When time permits, preoperative consultation with a psychiatrist, physiatrician, prosthetist, and support groups should be considered to optimize patient education and acceptance and establish realistic expectations. Given the high morbidity and mortality of both hip disarticulation and hemipelvectomy, surgical candidates with poor anticipated survivability may be better treated with a palliative, nonsurgical approach.

Preoperative Planning

Extensive preoperative assessment and surgical planning should be completed. Three-dimensional imaging, with either CT or MRI, is essential to determine the extent of both soft-tissue and bone resections. Medical optimization should be completed, and adequate blood products should be available. Consultation with a general surgeon and a plastic surgeon should be considered in cases where intrapelvic disease extension exists or traditional flaps may not be adequate. If excessive bleeding is anticipated, angiography and preoperative embolization are useful modalities in both oncologic and nonneoplastic patients. The ideal level of amputation is generally guided by the extent of disease, the viability of the soft-tissue envelope, and functional expectations and goals. The amputation level has a major effect on level of disability, prosthetic use, and walking aids—with more proximal amputation levels associated with poorer functional scores.[12]

Hip Disarticulation

Surgical Technique

Hip disarticulation accounts for only 0.5% of lower limb amputations in the United States.[13] The patient is positioned in a lateral decubitus position on a well-padded beanbag or in a semisupine position with a support under the pelvis. Split drapes or U-shaped drapes allow for wide exposure to the anterior and posterior hip and buttocks. Prepping should include the abdomen, the groin, the buttock, and the entire lower limb. Current practice is based on the technique described by Boyd[14] and uses a racquet-shaped incision that begins just medial and inferior to the anterior superior iliac spine and descends parallel to the inguinal ligament down to approximately 5 cm distal to the ischial tuberosity and the gluteal crease. The other limb of the incision runs obliquely on the anterior thigh, curving posteriorly approximately 8 cm from the greater trochanter to meet the medial incision (**Figure 1**). Deep dissection typically begins anteriorly with exposure of the femoral triangle, identification and isolation of the femoral vessels, and meticulous suture ligation and division. The femoral nerve is gently transected under tension and allowed to retract into the pelvis. Following neurovascular control, the muscles are transected in a sequential manner. The sartorius and rectus femoris are detached from their proximal origins, and the pectineus is divided close to the pubis. The external rotators of the hip and the iliopsoas are transected. The obturator vessels should be identified and suture ligated, followed by division of the adductor and the gracilis muscles and a gentle

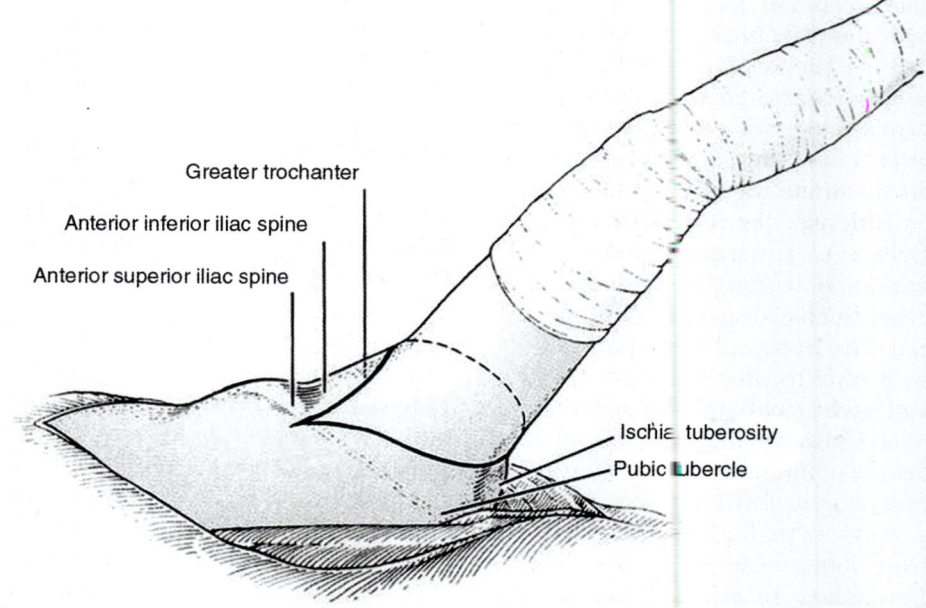

FIGURE 1 Illustration of the typical racquet-shaped incision used for hip disarticulation. The incision is centered over the femoral triangle, and the femoral vessels are ligated and transected early in the procedure. (Reprinted by permission from Springer Nature: Malawer MM, Sugarbaker PH: Hip disarticulations, in Malawer MM, Sugarbaker PH, eds: *Musculoskeletal Cancer Surgery: Treatment of Sarcomas and Allied Diseases*. Kluwer Academic Publishers, 2001, p 340.)

traction neurectomy of the obturator nerve. Posteriorly, the gluteal muscles are sequentially transected as distally as the disease process will allow to ensure a substantial myocutaneous flap. The sciatic nerve should be transected with a sharp scalpel under tension to minimize symptomatic neuroma formation; when possible, the nerve is either allowed to retract or manually placed inside the pelvis through the sciatic notch. The external rotators of the hip are released from their femoral insertions and the hamstrings from their proximal origins. The hip capsule is released around the acetabulum, the ligamentum teres is transected, and the limb is removed. The muscles of the buttock together with iliopsoas and the obturator externus thus remain attached to the pelvis.

After the limb is removed, the acetabulum is covered by approximating the preserved muscle groups, most frequently the quadratus femoris to the iliopsoas and the obturator externus to the gluteus medius. Deep drains are recommended, followed by closure of the posterior gluteus maximus fascia to the inguinal ligament. This surgical technique allows methodical dissection, avoids weight bearing over the suture lines, divides muscles at their origins or insertions, and provides a viable muscle flap as a weight-bearing surface for sitting and/or prosthetic use. Postoperative care should include strict decubitus ulcer precautions, perioperative antibiotics, and thromboprophylaxis.

Although the previously described approach is most commonly used, alternative surgical approaches may be recommended according to surgeon preference or disease location. One such modification uses a lateral approach[15] and may be more familiar to orthopaedic surgeons. A total adductor myocutaneous flap also has been described when disease precludes using more traditional anterior or posterior flaps.[16] Frey et al[17] described an alternative quadriceps muscle flap, consisting of skin, subcutaneous fat, and the quadriceps muscle. This flap receives its blood supply from the muscular branches of the superficial femoral artery and can cover defects up to the level of the posterior superior iliac spine. Infrequently, when local flaps are not available, free flap or pedicle-based augmentation flaps may be considered.

Complications

Hip disarticulation has been associated with high morbidity and mortality rates, which are more common in patients with severe infections, crushing injuries, and peripheral vascular disease. Postoperative complications occur in up to 75% of patients, with the most common being wound infections. Other local morbidities include wound dehiscence, skin necrosis, seromas, painful neuromas, and phantom pain. Mortality rates after hip disarticulation vary considerably in the literature, ranging from zero to 47% depending on patient factors, comorbid disease, and the indication for amputation.[10,17-22]

Hemipelvectomy

Transpelvic amputation involves resection of all (complete or classic hemipelvectomy) or part (modified hemipelvectomy) of the hemipelvis, with either retention of the ipsilateral lower limb (internal hemipelvectomy) or removal of the lower limb (external hemipelvectomy). The ability to preserve the lower limb depends on multiple factors, most paramount being the salvageability of an adequate neurovascular supply to the retained limb and resultant anticipated function. This factor is influenced by both the extent of the resection and whether a functional pelvic reconstruction is achievable or advisable.

Surgical Technique

The approach to surgery begins by positioning the patient in a lateral position, with the ability to modify (as needed) the patient's position intraoperatively to a more supine or prone inclination, which is commonly described as a "sloppy lateral" position. Such positioning is best achieved with a well-padded beanbag because it allows intraoperative position modifications while simultaneously ensuring adequate patient stability. An axillary roll should be placed beneath the chest wall to avoid pressure or traction on the brachial plexus. All bony prominences must be well padded because the length of the surgical procedure can predispose patients to compressive neuropathy. Prepping the leg into the surgical field allows for easy intraoperative alterations in positioning and is strongly advocated. Hip and knee flexion with hip adduction allows for enhanced exposure posteriorly (**Figure 2, A**), whereas hip and knee extension with hip external rotation and abduction allow for full anterior exposure (**Figure 2, B**). A Foley catheter is necessary to monitor fluid balance and facilitate urethra identification and bladder decompression. Preoperative ureteric catheterization and bowel preparations are often advisable to ease the intraoperative identification (or repair in the event of accidental transection) of the ureters and decompress the bowels, which is an important consideration because genitourinary injury and enterotomy are inherent risks of these procedures. When bowel or bladder involvement require visceral resection, a procedure described as a compound hemipelvectomy, including a diverting colostomy and/or ileostomy, is recommended.[23,24]

When applying surgical drapes, it is critical to ensure adequate access to the anterior viscera and the posterior structures, including the sacrum. Split drapes are recommended with the limbs of the drapes extending beyond the midline both anteriorly and posteriorly.

The extent of pelvic resection will be determined by the distribution of disease or injury, whether tumor, infection, ischemia, or trauma. The classic hemipelvectomy involves resecting the entire hemipelvis from the pubic symphysis to the sacroiliac joint. An extended hemipelvectomy involves resecting the entire hemipelvis plus a portion of the sacrum and is required for tumors extending across the sacroiliac joint or a mangled pelvis and limb with an associated ipsilateral sacral fracture. Internal hemipelvectomy defects are described according to the classification system by Enneking and Dunham.[25] A type 1 resection involves the ilium from the sacroiliac joint to

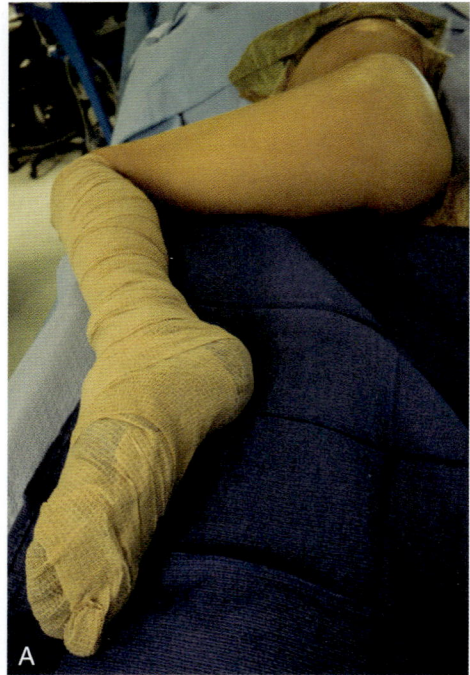
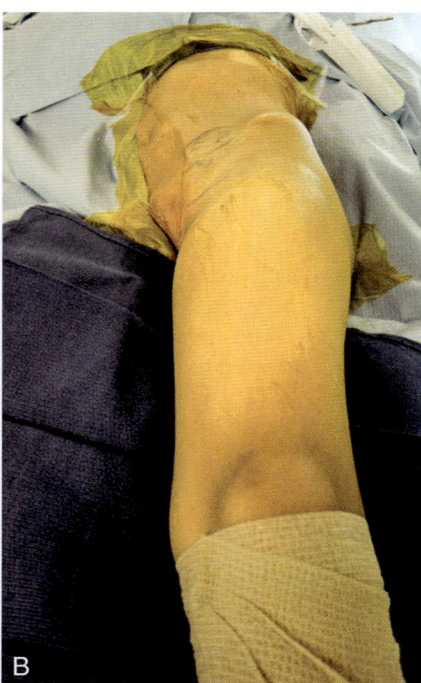

FIGURE 2 Intraoperative photographs of the lateral positioning and draping for hemipelvectomy demonstrate the leg included in the sterile field, allowing adequate access to the posterior elements with hip and knee flexion (**A**) and the anterior elements with hip and knee extension and external rotation (**B**). Drapes are applied to expose beyond the midline both anteriorly and posteriorly.

the neck of the ilium. A type 2 resection involves the acetabulum and may extend from the neck of the ilium to the lateral portion of the pubic rami. A type 3 resection involves the area from the pubic symphysis to the lateral margin of the obturator foramen, with preservation of the hip joint. A type 4 resection requires removal of the ilium plus part or all of the sacrum. When the resection involves more than one zone, the descriptors may be combined. For example, combined type 1 and 2 resections indicate removal of all or a portion of the ilium and the acetabulum.

The standard posterior flap, based on the inferior gluteal artery, is used whenever possible because the gluteal musculature affords a thick soft-tissue envelope. An anterior flap, based on the quadriceps musculature and the femoral artery, is recommended when the posterior flap is compromised, such as with trauma or tumor involvement. Flaps that are more creative have been used when neither anterior nor posterior flaps are available, including the total thigh fillet flap and various free flaps.[5,16-21] The anatomic source and blood supply for these flaps must be considered during the preoperative plan and accommodated during the positioning and prepping phase.

The most traditional (utilitarian) surgical approach begins anteriorly through an ilioinguinal incision spanning from the symphysis pubis, along the inguinal ligament, and toward either the anterior superior or anterior inferior iliac spine. This incision is extended along the posterior crest to the sacrum, particularly for classic or extended hemipelvectomies.

The posterior incision intersects with the posterior extent of the anterior incision and extends down the leg on the anterior border of the greater trochanter. The incision then curves transversely across the top of the posterior thigh, distal to the gluteal crease, and joins the most midline extent of the anterior incision (**Figure 3**). The length of the posterior limb will determine the length of the posterior flap and should be extended to ensure adequate coverage anteriorly and allow definitive closure without tension. When feasible, the gluteal muscles and fascia should be included with the posterior skin flap because this decreases the risk of flap necrosis.[23]

In select cases of internal hemipelvectomy, the anterior limb alone may be sufficient for resection. A modification of the described posterior limb is particularly useful for resections involving the posterior ilium, the sacrum, and the proximal femur. The incision is vertically oriented, originates laterally along the anterior incision, and extends vertically down the thigh along the posterior border of the greater trochanter (**Figure 4**), with the specific origin of the incision varied to accommodate the specific resection type. Multiple variants on this vertical incision have been described and are frequently referred to as the T incision or the reverse-Y incision.[23,24]

The anterior limb of the incision is further developed by releasing the rectus abdominis muscle and the inguinal ligament, which are retracted proximally to expose the retropubic space, the iliac vessels, and the spermatic cord or round ligament. The bladder is identified just posterior to the retropubic space and gently retracted away from the pubic symphysis. The inferior epigastric vessels are identified and suture ligated. At this point, it is wise to identify and protect critical intrapelvic structures, such as the ureters and the bowel, to avoid inadvertent injury. Depending on the extent of the tumor, the psoas muscle is separated from the iliacus muscle, which often remains attached to the inner table of the ilium as a neoplastic margin in tumor cases (**Figure 5, A**).

The external iliac vessel and the femoral nerve are identified and ligated in an external hemipelvectomy or protected with a vessel loop in an internal hemipelvectomy. If more proximal vascular control is required, such as a classic external hemipelvectomy, the external iliac vessel should be traced proximally to define the common iliac vessels, and the ligation occurs at this level. It is important to note that ligation of the common iliac vessels is a predictor of posterior flap necrosis, so

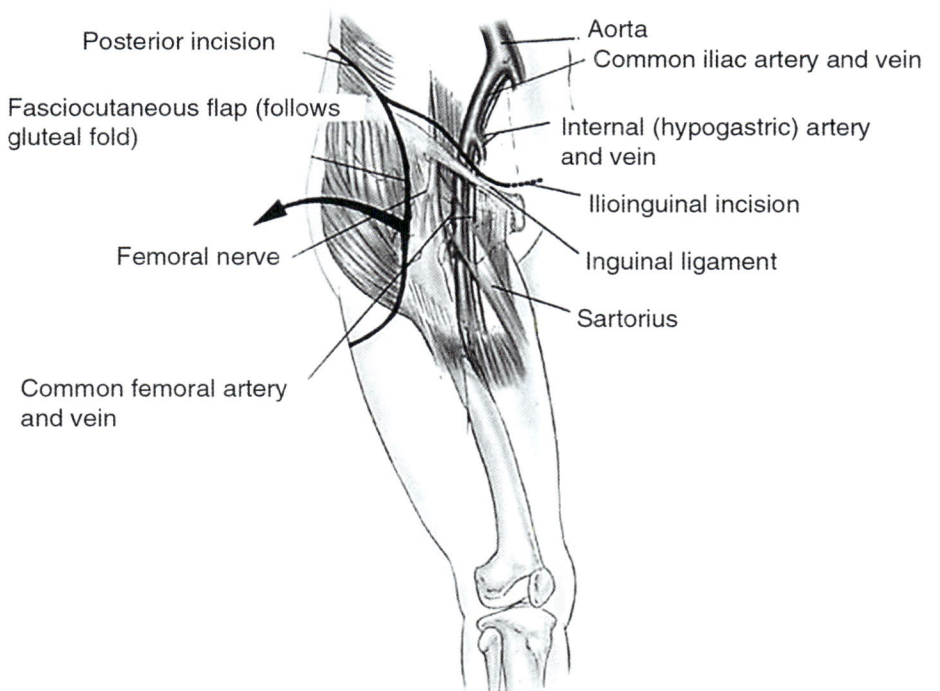

FIGURE 3 Illustration of the utilitarian incision for pelvic resection or transpelvic amputation, which begins at the pubic tubercle and extends along the inguinal ligament and the iliac crest. Depending on the surgeon's preference, the incision is directed inferiorly somewhere between the anterior superior iliac spine and the posterior superior iliac spine. For transpelvic amputation, the incision is extended posteriorly behind the thigh and then along the inferior pubic ramus to the pubic tubercle. (Reprinted by permission from Springer Nature: Bickels J, Malawer MM: Overview of pelvic resections: surgical considerations and classifications, in Malawer MM, Sugarbaker PH, eds: *Musculoskeletal Cancer Surgery: Treatment of Sarcomas and Allied Diseases.* Kluwer Academic Publishers, 2001, p 213.)

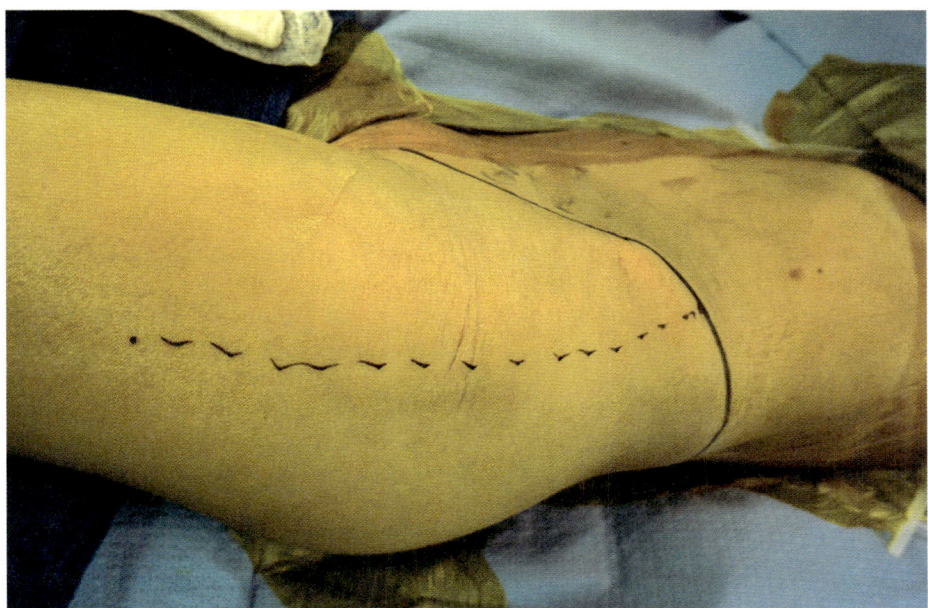

FIGURE 4 Intraoperative photograph of the common approach for hemipelvectomy demonstrates the ilioinguinal incision (solid line), which runs from the pubic symphysis, along the iliac crest, to the sacrum posteriorly. The vertical incision (dashed line) can be used to improve exposure when needed. Its origin along the ilioinguinal incision can be varied slightly according to the needs of the case and then runs vertically along the lateral thigh.

retention of the internal iliac vessels is advocated whenever possible.[23] In an internal hemipelvectomy, care must be taken to preserve the blood supply to the planned soft-tissue flap, the inferior gluteal vessel in the posterior flap, and the femoral vessel in the anterior flap. Following vascular control and ligation, the remaining anterior muscular attachments to the pelvis are sequentially released, including the abdominal wall musculature, the sartorius, the tensor fascia lata, and the iliotibial band.

The posterior incision is further developed by sequentially releasing the posterior musculature of the pelvis, including the adductors, the hamstrings, and the external rotators. The sciatic nerve should be identified and preserved in an internal hemipelvectomy and ligated and cut under tension in an external hemipelvectomy. Final resection through the pubic symphysis and the sacroiliac joint will complete the hemipelvic resection. During an internal hemipelvectomy, the location of bone resection is determined by the preoperative plan and completed with either a sagittal saw or a Gigli saw; alternatively, osteotomes with or without image guidance can be used.

The most appropriate reconstruction after an internal hemipelvectomy is controversial. Reconstruction options range from simple soft-tissue reconstruction (resection arthroplasty) to complex pelvic reconstructions that aim to restore the pelvic ring. Reconstruction techniques include resection arthroplasty; femoral transposition; iliofemoral fusion; autograft; autoclaved, diseased, resected pelvic bone; massive pelvic allograft; allograft-prosthetic composite; modular megaprostheses; and other custom prostheses. Those who prefer pelvic ring reconstruction cite superior function and quality of life and use these techniques most frequently in type 2 resections to restore a functional hip joint. Criticisms of complex reconstruction include complication rates as high as 50% and the substantial morbidity associated with failed reconstructions. The high rate of major complications, particularly deep infection, allograft fracture, hardware failure, and hip

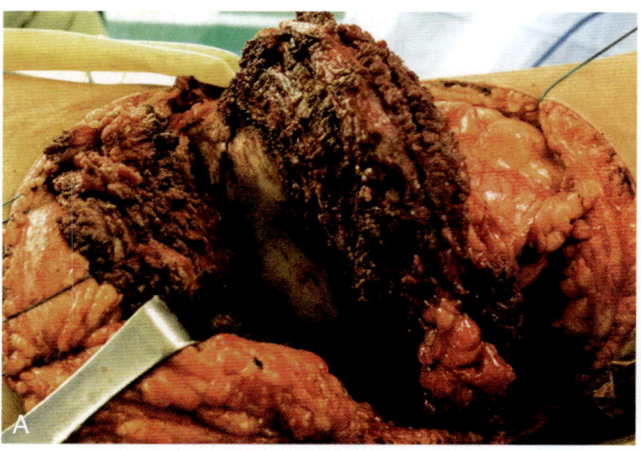
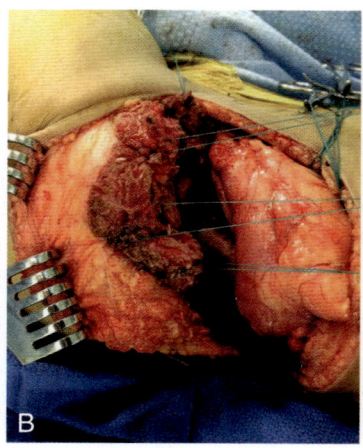
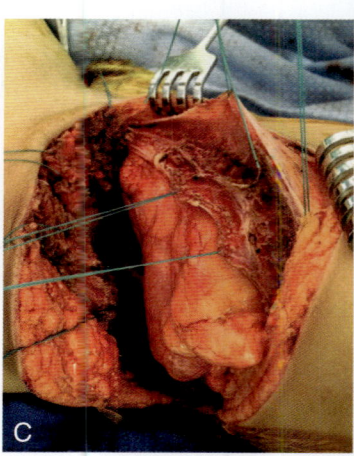
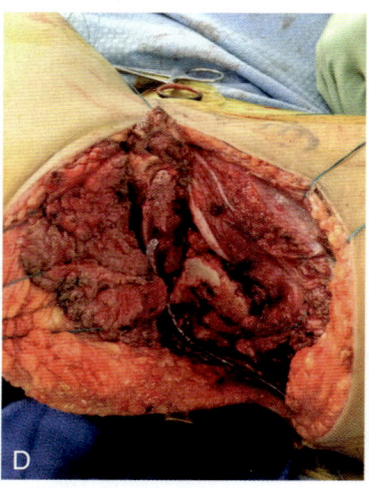
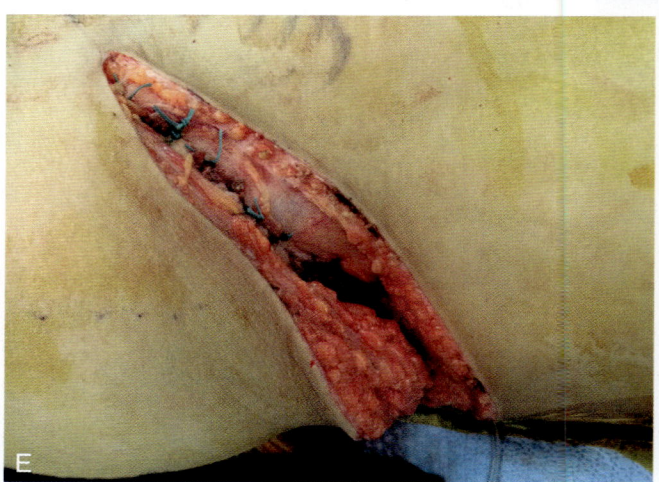

FIGURE 5 Intraoperative photographs of a hemipelvectomy. **A**, Dissection for a type I hemipelvectomy before final osseous cuts. The iliac crest is visualized inferiorly with soft tissue covering the iliac wing, in the region of the soft-tissue mass. The iliacus muscle creates a muscle margin for the intrapelvic extension of tumor. **B**, The osseous defect is created by removing the iliac crest and highlights the lack of a barrier between the posterior/gluteal flap and the retroperitoneal structures. **C**, The deep and superficial abdominal fascia. **D**, Containment of the retroperitoneum is achieved by securing the deep abdominal fascia. **E**, Final closure of the gluteal fascia to the superficial abdominal fascia completes the layered closure.

instability, diminish enthusiasm for complex reconstructions. These serious complications often necessitate removal or revision of the reconstruction or conversion to an external hemipelvectomy for definitive management.[24-46]

The recent implementation of navigation in pelvic surgery has improved the precision of surgical margins and the technology has been used in conjunction with reconstructive modalities to design a custom prosthesis. Other reported advantages of navigation-assisted techniques include improved local control and trends toward better function.[47-51]

Meticulous surgical closure is critical in pelvic surgery. Sufficient deep closure to contain the intra-abdominal contents is essential to avoid hernias; however, this can be challenging because of the loss of adequate bone and soft-tissue anatomy to serve as anchors for such a reconstruction. When possible, the deep abdominal fascia should be secured to contain the intra-abdominal organs, and the gluteal fascia should be repaired securely to the deep abdominal fascia (**Figure 5, B** through **D**). In the absence of sufficient bone or soft-tissue anatomy, mesh is widely used for soft-tissue reconstruction. Deep drains should be placed, with the postoperative output monitored closely. Closure in layers without tension is critical (**Figure 5, E**) because wound necrosis and deep infections are common complications in both external and internal hemipelvectomies.[23,36,38]

Postoperative Care

In the postoperative period, strict decubitus ulcer precautions should be instituted. Ideal weight-bearing status varies and is influenced by the degree of resection, the type of soft-tissue or pelvic ring reconstruction, and a variety of patient factors.[38] Prophylaxis for deep vein thrombosis is recommended and must be balanced against the risk of bleeding, particularly because hemipelvectomy often necessitates large-volume transfusion, which may be associated with life-threatening coagulopathy.[31] Prophylactic antibiotics are routinely administered, although the ideal duration has not been determined. Antibiotics are frequently administered until drain use is discontinued; however, shorter and longer durations have been described, and no compelling evidence exists for or against any particular regimen.

Complications

Complication rates after hemipelvectomy range from 20% to 61%, with infections being the most common postoperative complication. Skin necrosis and superficial infection are frequently and successfully managed with local wound care and antibiotics, whereas deep infections require formal surgical débridement. Neurologic complications associated with sciatic and/or femoral nerve are quite common and highlight the importance of gentle intraoperative handling of the nerves. Genitourinary and bowel injuries require both intraoperative management and specialized postoperative care. Symptomatic hernias may require revision surgery, so they are best managed with prevention by means of meticulous closure. Combat-related hemipelvectomies demonstrate very high levels of concomitant injury, particularly genitourinary and contralateral amputation injuries, which require multispecialty team management and multistaged surgeries.[5] Systemic complications may be severe and life threatening, including acute respiratory distress syndrome, coagulopathy, deep vein thrombosis, pulmonary embolism, and acute cardiac arrest.[5,33,45,52-55]

Rehabilitation

Following hip disarticulation or hemipelvectomy, prosthetic training and use are challenging because of the energy expenditure associated with successful amputation and the difficulties with adequate prosthetic fit. Patients with proximal amputation levels have lower utilization of prosthetic devices, higher reliance on walking aids, and report poorer levels of physical functioning including difficulties with activities of daily living.[12,19,56-62]

SUMMARY

Hip disarticulation and hemipelvectomy are technically challenging procedures that require skilled surgical expertise and intensive perioperative medical management. Familiarity with the anatomy, surgical techniques, and known complications will enable surgeons to definitively care for patients with proximal thigh and pelvic neoplasia, infection, trauma, and vascular disease processes to ensure optimal patient outcomes and recovery from these morbid procedures.

References

1. Karakousis CP: The technique of major amputations for malignant tumors. *J Surg Oncol* 1983;23(1):43-55.
2. Westbury G: Hindquarter and hip amputation. *Ann R Coll Surg Engl* 1967;40(4):226-234.
3. Rougraff BT, Simon MA, Kneisl JS, Greenberg DB, Mankin HJ: Limb salvage compared with amputation for osteosarcoma of the distal end of the femur: A long-term oncological, functional, and quality-of-life study. *J Bone Joint Surg Am* 1994;76(5):649-656.
4. Zalavras CG, Rigopoulos N, Ahlmann E, Patzakis MJ: Hip disarticulation for severe lower extremity infections. *Clin Orthop Relat Res* 2009;467(7):1721-1726.
5. D'Alleyrand JG, Lewandowski LR, Forsberg JA, et al: Combat-related hemipelvectomy: 14 cases, a review of the literature and lesson learned. *J Orthop Trauma* 2015;29(12):e493-e498.
6. McKenna RJ, Schwinn CD, Soong KY, Higinbotham NL: Sarcomata of the osteogenic series: An analysis of 552 cases. *J Bone Joint Surg Am* 1966;48:1-26.
7. Brandt MM, Corpron CA, Wahl WL: Necrotizing soft tissue infections: A surgical disease. *Am Surg* 2000;66(10):967-970.
8. Elliott DC, Kufera JA, Myers RA: Necrotizing soft tissue infections: Risk factors for mortality and strategies for management. *Ann Surg* 1996;224(5):672-683.
9. Francis KR, Lamaute HR, Davis JM, Pizzi WF: Implications of risk factors in necrotizing fasciitis. *Am Surg* 1993;59(5):304-308.
10. Tanner RM, Joels CS, Fisher DF, Bhattachary SD: Hip disarticulation: Retrospective review of a single surgeons's outcomes over 15 years. *Am Surg* 2021;87(11):1829-1830.
11. Schwartz AJ, Trask DJ, Bews KA, Hanson KT, Etzioni DA, Habermann EB: Hip disarticulation for periprosthetic joint infection: Frequency, outcome and risk factors. *J Arthroplasty* 2020;35:3269-3273.
12. Furtado S, Grimer RJ, Cool P, et al: Physical functioning, pain and quality of life after amputation for musculoskeletal tumours. *Bone Joint J* 2015;97-B(9):1284-1290.
13. Dillingham TR, Pezzin LE, MacKenzie EJ: Limb amputation and limb deficiency: Epidemiology and recent trends in the United States. *South Med J* 2002;95(8):875-883.
14. Boyd HB: Anatomic disarticulation of the hip. *Surg Gynecol Obstet* 1947;84(3):346-349.
15. Lackman RD, Quartararo LG, Farrell ED, Scopp JM: Hip disarticulation using the lateral approach: A new technique. *Clin Orthop Relat Res* 2001;392:372-376.
16. Dormans JP, Vives M: Wound coverage after modified hip disarticulation using a total adductor myocutaneous flap. *Clin Orthop Relat Res* 1997;335:218-223.
17. Frey C, Matthews LS, Benjamin H, Fidler WJ: A new technique for hemipelvectomy. *Surg Gynecol Obstet* 1976;143(5):753-756.
18. Unruh T, Fisher DF Jr, Unruh TA, et al: Hip disarticulation: An 11-year experience. *Arch Surg* 1990;125(6):791-793.
19. Endean ED, Schwarcz TH, Barker DE, Munfakh NA, Wilson-Neely R, Hyde GL: Hip disarticulation: Factors affecting outcome. *J Vasc Surg* 1991;14(3):398-404.
20. Pack GT: Major exarticulations for malignant neoplasms of the extremities: Interscapulothoracic amputation, hip-joint disarticulation, and interilioabdominal amputation; a report of end results in 228 cases. *J Bone Joint Surg Am* 1956;38(2):249-262.
21. Fenelon GC, Von Foerster G, Engelbrecht E: Disarticulation of the hip as a result of failed arthroplasty: A series of 11 cases. *J Bone Joint Surg Br* 1980;62(4):441-446.
22. Moura DL, Grruco A: Hip disarticulation- case series analysis and literature review. *Rev Bras Ortop* 2017;52(2):154-158.

23. Senchenkov A, Moran SL, Petty PM, et al: Predictors of complications and outcomes of external hemipelvectomy wounds: Account of 160 consecutive cases. *Ann Surg Oncol* 2008;15(1):355-363.

24. Wirbel RJ, Schulte M, Mutschler WE: Surgical treatment of pelvic sarcomas: Oncologic and functional outcome. *Clin Orthop Relat Res* 2001;390:190-205.

25. Enneking WF, Dunham WK: Resection and reconstruction for primary neoplasms involving the innominate bone. *J Bone Joint Surg Am* 1978;60(6):731-746.

26. Ross DA, Lohman RF, Kroll SS, et al: Soft tissue reconstruction following hemipelvectomy. *Am J Surg* 1998;176(1):25-29.

27. Karakousis CP: Abdominoinguinal incision and other incisions in the resection of pelvic tumors. *Surg Oncol* 2000;9(2):83-90.

28. Lackman RD, Crawford EA, Hosalkar HS, King JJ, Ogilvie CM: Internal hemipelvectomy for pelvic sarcomas using a T-incision surgical approach. *Clin Orthop Relat Res* 2009;467(10):2677-2684.

29. Aljassir F, Beadel GP, Turcotte RE, et al: Outcome after pelvic sarcoma resection reconstructed with saddle prosthesis. *Clin Orthop Relat Res* 2005;438:36-41.

30. Angelini A, Drago G, Trovarelli G, Calabrò T, Ruggieri P: Infection after surgical resection for pelvic bone tumors: An analysis of 270 patients from one institution. *Clin Orthop Relat Res* 2014;472(1):349-359.

31. Bell RS, Davis AM, Wunder JS, Buconjic T, McGoveran B, Gross AE: Allograft reconstruction of the acetabulum after resection of stage-IIB sarcoma: Intermediate-term results. *J Bone Joint Surg Am* 1997;79(11):1663-1674.

32. Biau DJ, Thévenin F, Dumaine V, Babinet A, Tomeno B, Anract P: Ipsilateral femoral autograft reconstruction after resection of a pelvic tumor. *J Bone Joint Surg Am* 2009;91(1):142-151.

33. Chao AH, Neimanis SA, Chang DW, Lewis VO, Hanasono MM: Reconstruction after internal hemipelvectomy: Outcomes and reconstructive algorithm. *Ann Plast Surg* 2015;74(3):342-349.

34. Delloye C, Banse X, Brichard B, Docquier PL, Cornu O: Pelvic reconstruction with a structural pelvic allograft after resection of a malignant bone tumor. *J Bone Joint Surg Am* 2007;89(3):579-587.

35. Gebert C, Wessling M, Hoffmann C, et al: Hip transposition as a limb salvage procedure following the resection of periacetabular tumors. *J Surg Oncol* 2011;103(3):269-275.

36. Ham SJ, Schraffordt Koops H, Veth RP, van Horn JR, Molenaar WM, Hoekstra HJ: Limb salvage surgery for primary bone sarcoma of the lower extremities: Long-term consequences of endoprosthetic reconstructions. *Ann Surg Oncol* 1998;5(5):423-436.

37. Harrington KD: The use of hemipelvic allografts or autoclaved grafts for reconstruction after wide resections of malignant tumors of the pelvis. *J Bone Joint Surg Am* 1992;74(3):331-341.

38. Hillmann A, Hoffmann C, Gosheger G, Rödl R, Winkelmann W, Ozaki T: Tumors of the pelvis: Complications after reconstruction. *Arch Orthop Trauma Surg* 2003;123(7):340-344.

39. Karim SM, Colman MW, Lozano-Calderón SA, Raskin KA, Schwab JH, Hornicek FJ: What are the functional results and complications from allograft reconstruction after partial hemipelvectomy of the pubis? *Clin Orthop Relat Res* 2015;473(4):1442-1448.

40. Kollender Y, Shabat S, Bickels J, et al: Internal hemipelvectomy for bone sarcomas in children and young adults: Surgical considerations. *Eur J Surg Oncol* 2000;26(4):398-404.

41. Langlais F, Lambotte JC, Thomazeau H: Long-term results of hemipelvis reconstruction with allografts. *Clin Orthop Relat Res* 2001;388:178-186.

42. Ozaki T, Hoffmann C, Hillmann A, Gosheger G, Lindner N, Winkelmann W: Implantation of hemipelvic prosthesis after resection of sarcoma. *Clin Orthop Relat Res* 2002;396:197-205.

43. Satcher RL Jr, O'Donnell RJ, Johnston JO: Reconstruction of the pelvis after resection of tumors about the acetabulum. *Clin Orthop Relat Res* 2003;409:209-217.

44. Witte D, Bernd L, Bruns J, et al: Limb-salvage reconstruction with MUTARS hemipelvic endoprosthesis: A prospective multicenter study. *Eur J Surg Oncol* 2009;35(12):1318-1325.

45. Zeifang F, Buchner M, Zahlten-Hinguranage A, Bernd L, Sabo D: Complications following operative treatment of primary malignant bone tumours in the pelvis. *Eur J Surg Oncol* 2004;30:893-899.

46. Campanacci D, Chacon S, Mondanelli N, et al: Pelvic massive allograft reconstruction after bone tumour resection. *Int Orthop* 2012;36:2529-2536.

47. Abraham JA, Kenneally B, Amer K, Geller DS: Can navigation-assisted surgery help achieve negative margins in resection of pelvic and sacral tumors? *Clin Orthop Relat Res* 2018;476:499-508.

48. Fujiwara T, Kaneuchi Y, Stevenson J, et al: Navigation-assisted pelvic resections and reconstruction for periacetabular chondrosarcomas. *Eur J Surg Oncol* 2021;47:416-423.

49. Sun W, Li J, Li Q, Li G, Cai Z: Clinical effectiveness of hemipelvic reconstruction using computer-aided custom-made prostheses after resection of malignant pelvic tumors. *J Arthroplasty* 2011;26(8):1508-1513.

50. Dai KR, Yan MN, Zhu ZA, Sun YH: Computer-aided custom-made hemipelvic prosthesis used in extensive pelvic lesions. *J Arthroplasty* 2007;22(7):981-986.

51. Sternheim A, Daly M, Qiu J, et al: Navigated pelvic osteotomy and tumor resection: A study assessing the accuracy and reproducibility of resection planes in Sawbones and cadavers. *J Bone Joint Surg Am* 2015;97(1):40-46.

52. Angelini A, Calabrò T, Pala E, Trovarelli G, Maraldi M, Ruggieri P: Resection and reconstruction of pelvic bone tumors. *Orthopedics* 2015;38(2):87-93.

53. Shao QD, Yan X, Sun JY, Xu TM: Internal hemipelvectomy with reconstruction for primary pelvic neoplasm: A systematic review. *ANZ J Surg* 2015;85(7-8):553-560.

54. Apffelstaedt JP, Driscoll DL, Karakousis CP: Partial and complete internal hemipelvectomy: Complications and long-term follow-up. *J Am Coll Surg* 1995;181(1):43-48.

55. Benatto MT, Hussein AM, Gava NF, Maranho DA, Engel EE: Complications and cost analysis of hemipelvectomy for the treatment of pelvic tumors. *Acta Orthop Bras* 2019;27(2):104-107.

56. Kralovec ME, Houdek MT, Andrews KL, Shives TC, Rose PS, Sim FH: Prosthetic rehabilitation after hip disarticulation or hemipelvectomy. *Am J Phys Med Rehabil* 2015;94(12):1035-1040.

57. Yari P, Dijkstra PU, Geertzen JH: Functional outcome of hip disarticulation and hemipelvectomy: A cross-sectional national descriptive study in the Netherlands. *Clin Rehabil* 2008;22(12):1127-1133.

58. Schnall BL, Baum BS, Andrews AM: Gait characteristics of a soldier with a

traumatic hip disarticulation. *Phys Ther* 2008;88(12):1568-1577.
59. Marshal C, Stansby G: Amputation and rehabilitation. *Vasc Surg II* 2010;28:284-287.
60. Fisher SV, Gullickson G Jr: Energy cost of ambulation in health and disability: A literature review. *Arch Phys Med Rehabil* 1978;59(3):124-133.
61. Chin T, Oyabu H, Maeda Y, Takase I, Machida K: Energy consumption during prosthetic walking and wheelchair locomotion by elderly hip disarticulation amputees. *Am J Phys Med Rehabil* 2009;88(5):399-403.
62. Nowroozi F, Salvanelli ML, Gerber LH: Energy expenditure in hip disarticulation and hemipelvectomy amputees. *Arch Phys Med Rehabil* 1983;64(7):300-303.

Hip Disarticulation: Prosthetic Management

Phillip M. Stevens, MEd, CPO, FAAOP • David J. Baty, CPO, LPO

CHAPTER 45

ABSTRACT

Hip disarticulation and hemipelvectomy represent extremely uncommon amputation levels that are infrequently encountered in clinical practice. In the absence of a residual limb, the user has no direct control over the affected extremity. Rather, movement and stabilization of the prosthesis can only occur through movements of the pelvis and lumbar spine. Prostheses for these amputation levels require aggressive tissue containment and unique alignment considerations with the hip joint positioned on the anterior surface of the socket and the knee joint aligned posterior to the user's center of mass. Prostheses are characterized by unique componentry considerations and gait biomechanics.

Keywords: hemipelvectomy; hip disarticulation; lower limb prosthesis; prosthetic design

Introduction

Because less than 2% of all amputations are at the hip disarticulation level,[1] the typical physiatrist, therapist, or prosthetist may not be familiar with the associated general fitting considerations and biomechanical requirements necessary for optimal gait. In the absence of direct volitional control over the major joint segments of the lower extremity, the choice and alignment of prosthetic componentry constitute critical considerations. In the absence of a residual extremity, active control of such prostheses is limited to movements of the pelvis and lumbar spine. This poses challenges to prosthetic gait training and mastery. Even with thoughtful prosthetic design and fabrication, the wear time of prostheses in this cohort is often reduced.

Anticipated Outcomes

Prostheses at these amputation levels often have higher rejection rates because of their increased energy requirements, weight, and greater coverage of the body. Available evidence is limited, but suggests that successful long-term acceptance of prostheses at these proximal amputation levels ranges between 35% and 76%.[2,3]

The ability of the user to control the prosthesis through muscular activity is greatly reduced at this amputation level, with control movements limited to motions of the pelvis and lumbar spine. As a result, middle-aged individuals with hip disarticulation walk approximately 40% slower and expend approximately 80% more energy than able-bodied individuals.[4] Energy requirements at this amputation level are considerably higher for elderly amputees.[5] However, in their report on seven elderly individuals with hip disarticulation amputation, Chin et al[6] reported on five subjects with adequate physical fitness to attain and maintain community ambulation with their prostheses. Subsequent case studies have continued to report on successful prosthetic outcomes observed among elderly users of hip disarticulation prostheses.[7,8]

Although technologic advances such as lighter componentry, more dynamic designs, and softer interface materials have resulted in improved prostheses, acceptance and optimal prosthesis use remain challenging. For many individuals who regularly use a prosthesis, the reduced energy requirements and increased speed of alternative forms of mobility preclude complete daily reliance on prosthetic ambulation. For example, elderly amputees can move twice as fast with a wheelchair and expend only 25% as much energy compared with their use of a hip disarticulation prosthesis.[5] Similarly, among a small cohort of established users of hemipelvectomy prostheses, the mean time to walk 400 m was 43% longer

---

David J. Baty or an immediate family member serves as a paid consultant to or is an employee of Össur. Neither Phillip M. Stevens nor any immediate family member has received anything of value from or has stock or stock options held in a commercial company or institution related directly or indirectly to the subject of this chapter.

This chapter is adapted from Edwards M, Stevens PM: Knee disarticulation: prosthetic management, in Krajbich JI, Pinzur MS, Potter BK, Stevens PM, eds: *Atlas of Amputations and Limb Deficiencies: Surgical, Prosthetic, and Rehabilitation Principles*, ed 4, vol 2. American Academy of Orthopaedic Surgeons, 2016, pp 565-573.

with the prosthesis compared with walking with crutches and no prosthesis.[9] It is understandable that even successful prosthesis users may limit their wear time to an average of 6 hours per day.[10] However, the recent development of new technologies specifically designed for hip disarticulation devices is transforming challenges into opportunities for improved outcomes.

Clinical Considerations

The successful fitting of a hip disarticulation prosthesis relies on the appropriate evaluation of the patient's motivation, balance, core strength, and load-bearing tolerance, along with the prosthetist's ability to capture and translate movements of the pelvis into prosthetic motion during swing while providing a secure, stable platform during stance. Greater motivation is generally required for successful ambulation with a prosthesis at this amputation level compared with that needed by most patients with a transfemoral or transtibial amputation. The possibility of successful prosthesis use can only be properly assessed when the patient has been given an accurate portrayal of the benefits, challenges, and limitations specific to a hip disarticulation prosthesis. Unrealistic expectations regarding the ease and energy costs of ambulation may result in early rejection of the prosthesis. After the patient has been given a reasonable understanding of the challenges inherent in the use of a hip disarticulation prosthesis, they can have a realistic discussion with the rehabilitation team to determine if there is sufficient motivation to proceed with a prosthetic fitting.

Superior balance on one leg is a strong positive indicator for prosthesis use because such balance is needed to successfully don and ambulate with a hip disarticulation prosthesis using minimal assistive aids.[11] As such, the demonstration of adequate single-leg balance is a prerequisite for any consideration of prosthetic management.

The strength of the core abdominal muscles should be assessed. Strength is demonstrated by creating a posterior pelvic tilt and should be evaluated because it is the main biomechanical motion used to initiate hip and knee flexion during gait and is needed for efficient ambulation. The patient should be able to demonstrate active pelvic tilt motions using the muscles of the lower back and abdomen. As a related consideration, the most successful prosthesis users are also able to maintain a lower body weight so that the full range of pelvic tilt may be captured within the prosthesis. The presence of any redundant or fleshy tissue should be noted because it must be contained and shaped to create reaction surfaces for proper prosthetic function. Further, excessive redundant tissues distal to the ischium necessitate a more distal placement of the hip joint, compromising its efficiency.

The distal aspect of the ischial tuberosity should be evaluated with respect to its load-bearing tolerance. Available gluteal tissue should be assessed for its ability to supplement axial loading. The bony prominences of the pubis and iliac crests and, in some instances, the residual femoral head should also be noted because they will require relief within the interface. If ischial weight bearing will be poorly tolerated, an alternative socket design must be considered to distribute weight-bearing loads more broadly through total surface bearing principles.

The prosthetic socket is a crucial connection between the patient and their prosthesis and must facilitate comfortable axial support, efficient ambulation, and consistent suspension. Appropriate socket designs create abdominal compression to contain soft tissue and adequately capture the control movements of the underlying pelvic anatomy. Similarly, anatomic contouring in the lumbar region is used to create a volumetrically tight and accurate anterior-posterior fit between the sacrum and lower abdomen. Compressive mediolateral dimensions are also necessary to preserve coronal stability during gait. Specifically, mediolateral measurements should be recorded over the iliac crests and between the trochanter and the iliac crests, and they should be reflected in the prosthetic socket.

Hip Disarticulation Socket

The hip disarticulation interface must serve four purposes: adequate coronal support, sagittal capture of pelvic movements, secure suspension, and appropriate weight-bearing surfaces and contours. New thermoplastic materials have been developed that greatly increase patient tolerance of the hip disarticulation sockets. Rigid laminated frames can be coupled with flexible thermoplastic inner sockets to provide both proximal flexibility and comfort at the edges of the socket as well as adequate rigidity at the attachment site of the hip joint and over the iliac crests (Figure 1). Although thermoforming offers a variety of flexible materials and ease of fabrication, it constitutes a thicker construction and represents a heavier alternative to rigid sockets.

Traditional hip disarticulation socket designs encompass the affected pelvis, contain the gluteal tissue and ischial tuberosity, and provide mediolateral stability by compressing the contralateral pelvis toward the affected side through the design of the interface. Suspension is accomplished by compression over one or both iliac crests, and an anterior closure is normally used.

Novel socket design configurations include the creative use of suction or vacuum designs with reduced contralateral trim lines (Figure 2), interface designs that use separate iliac crest attachments, flexible liners and frames, and other unique shapes that attempt to maintain appropriate stability and suspension but provide greater comfort and range of motion around the pelvis (Figure 3). However, little research has been done on hip disarticulation socket design and the variety of configurations currently used.

Impression techniques vary based on patient presentation and the preferences of the treating prosthetist. Weight-bearing impression techniques are often preferred at the hip disarticulation level because they allow the patient to have some distal end bearing while creating the impression. These approaches capture a socket shape

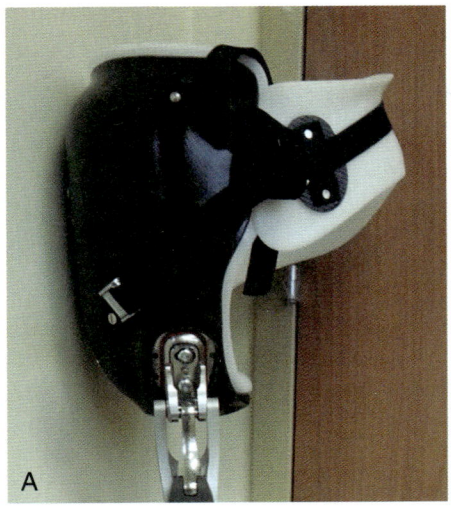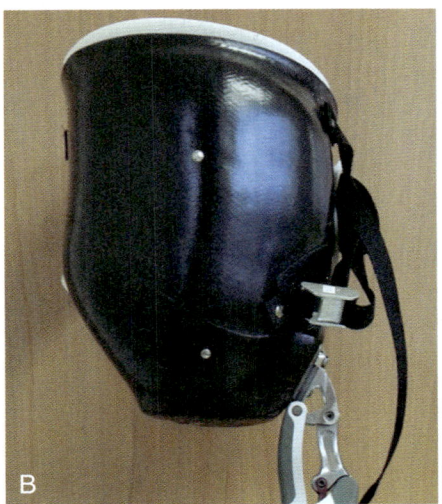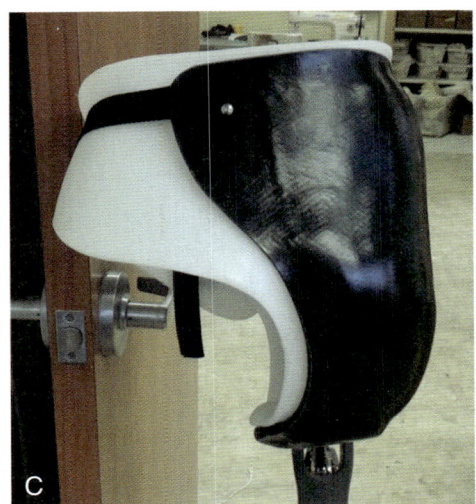

FIGURE 1 Anterior (**A**), lateral (**B**), and posterior (**C**) photographic views of a hip disarticulation socket with a flexible inner socket supported by a rigid laminated frame to provide proximal flexibility and comfort with adequate coronal support and suspension over the iliac crests. (Courtesy of Phillip M. Stevens, MEd, CPO, FAAOP, Salt Lake City, UT.)

conducive to skeletal loading. Houdek et al[12] advocated the use of deformable materials beneath the patient to assist in defining the primary weight-bearing skeletal structure during the impression capture. Wedges or forms are often used to compress the anterior-posterior dimension to better capture pelvic motion when using the prosthesis (**Figure 4**). Care must be taken to prevent excessive mediolateral tissue displacement during this procedure.

An alternative technique that is gaining popularity can be characterized as static compression. In this approach, the patient is not actively bearing weight while the impression is taken. Rather, the tissues of the residual limb are precompressed using plastic film or stout tape. The patient then remains standing on the sound side limb while the impression is obtained with casting or digital scanning techniques.

Hemipelvectomy Socket

When designing the socket for an individual using a hemipelvectomy prosthesis, in the absence of pelvic anatomy for weight bearing, care must be taken to create additional soft-tissue compression and containment. Prosthesis design for this level of amputation can be very challenging for many reasons, including the limited weight-bearing area and restrictive trim lines leading to a loss of range of motion and comfort. Providing abdominal pressure and compressing the soft tissue on the amputated side in a diagonal fashion will aid in weight bearing (**Figure 5**). Additional support may be gained from the costal margins and sound side ischium if needed (**Figure 5**).

In contrast to the skeletal loading that occurs with weight-bearing impressions, suspension casting techniques can be used during the impression capture of hemipelvectomy sockets to compress and contain the soft tissues of the residual body surface and create a more hydrostatic loading environment. This process can identify concentrated pressure-tolerant areas within the suspension sling that can be enhanced to further distribute weight-bearing forces and limit the pistoning that can occur in the absence of adequate precompression.[12] In these approaches, the patient is harnessed from a suspension apparatus to lift the pelvis off the casting surface as the impression is obtained.

However, such compression techniques are compromised by the absence of the ipsilateral iliac crest, meaning that ability to contain tissues superiorly is limited. As a result, excessive compression can ultimately lead to distal

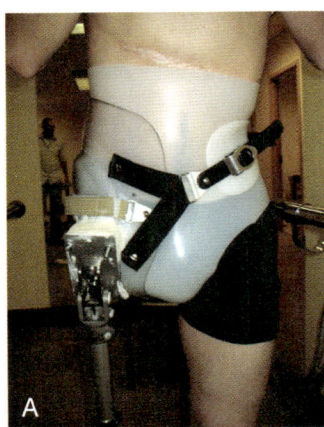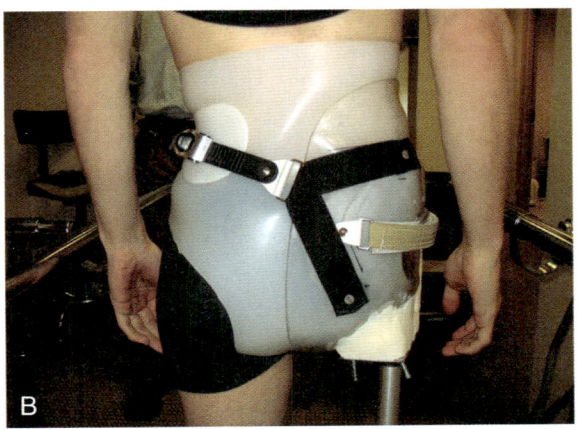

FIGURE 2 Anterior (**A**) and posterior (**B**) photographic views of a patient wearing a hip disarticulation socket in which the rigid frame is secured to a silicone interface undergarment using a combination of suction suspension and lanyard attachment. This design allows for reduced rigid trim lines. (Courtesy of Phillip M. Stevens, MEd, CPO, FAAOP, Salt Lake City, UT.)

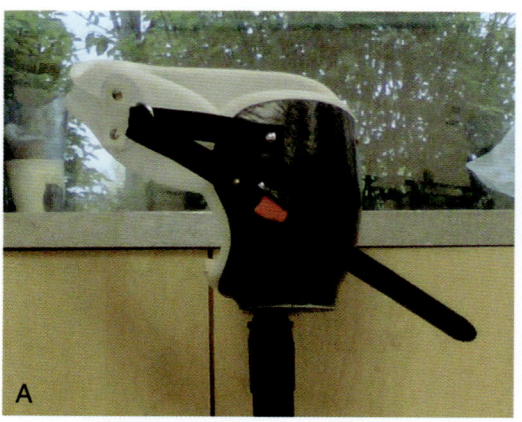
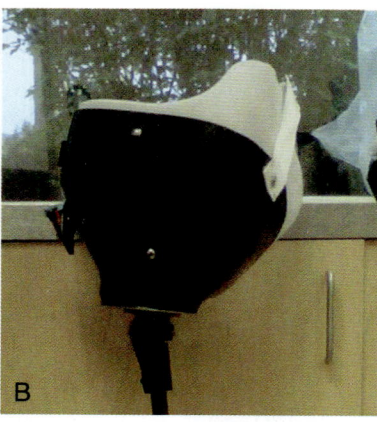

FIGURE 3 Anterior (**A**) and posterior (**B**) photographic views of a low-profile hip disarticulation socket in which the reduced rigid socket trim lines fail to capture the ipsilateral iliac crest. Suspension relies on the oblique compression created as the flexible inner socket passes over the contralateral iliac crest. (Courtesy of Phillip M. Stevens, MEd, CPO, FAAOP, Salt Lake City, UT.)

displacement of the socket in swing phase. One common means of providing superior containment of the soft tissues in the hemipelvectomy socket is to include a soft tissue lock in the area where the ilium used to be by mimicking the contour of the iliac crest roll on the sound side (**Figure 5**). This assists in suspension and compression while also giving the socket a more anatomic look and assisting in the suspension of clothing. Alternately, authors have suggested the use of a shoulder strap to provide superior containment within the socket and the prevention of excessive distal migration.[12] This technique may be preferable for patients who are intolerant to extreme compressive forces in hemipelvectomy socket.

Component and Alignment Considerations

Using endoskeletal or modular componentry is standard clinical practice for hip disarticulation prostheses because of their light weight and alignment adjustability. As with any level of amputation, assessing the patient's functional capabilities and potential are critical to appropriate componentry selection.

Hips

With a few recent exceptions, the design of hip joints has remained substantially unchanged over the years. Originally, the hip joint was mounted laterally, near the anatomic hip joint center. These joints were locked for standing and walking, then unlocked for sitting.[13] In 1954, researcher Colin McLaurin introduced the principles of the Canadian hip disarticulation prosthesis. His design, which is still in use, has an anteriorly mounted hip joint that is passively stabilized during stance by means of the posterior position of the patient's center of gravity relative to the hip joint[10,14] (**Figure 6**).

There is limited variety among a small group of Canadian-type hip joints with regard to their attachments and functions. Newer, modular systems have more compact designs and low-profile attachments that make sitting easier. These joints are mounted anteriorly to flat or dished attachment plates on the socket that are specific to the individual hip joints (**Figure 7**). Internal adjustable spring mechanisms, which provide a hip extension assist, are common to all endoskeletal hip joints. Although alignment adjustments are limited, a slight amount of abduction/adduction and flexion/extension adjustment is available. These adjustments should be identified and performed during the test socket phase to ensure the appropriate socket angle and joint stability in the definitive prosthesis. This common design is also offered in a pediatric size (**Figure 8**) and in a variation that allows the user to lock and unlock their hip joint (**Figure 9**).

The latest technology in hip joints is characterized by a helical design and hydraulic control (**Figure 10**). This joint has unique features specifically designed to address the gait deviations often seen in users of hip-level prostheses. The Helix 3D hip joint system (Ottobock) has hydraulic control of hip flexion in the swing phase and hydraulic control of hip extension in the stance phase. This allows the user to vary their cadence and regulate the speed at which the hip joint comes into full extension in late stance. The geometry of the joint also provides transverse plane rotation to compensate for the internal rotation of the pelvis in the swing phase. Specifically, the joint will externally rotate with hip flexion to keep the prosthesis tracking smoothly in the swing phase. The Helix 3D also incorporates hip flexion bands to assist the joint into flexion for better toe clearance in

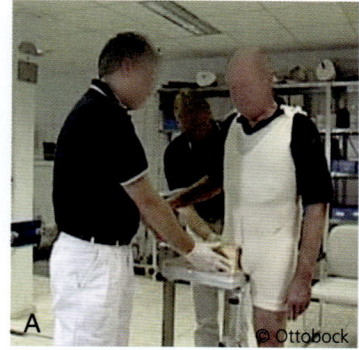
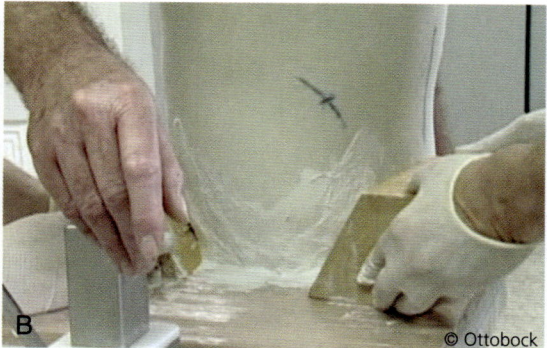

FIGURE 4 Photographs demonstrate an overview (**A**) and close-up view (**B**) of a weight-bearing impression technique that is often preferred at the hip disarticulation level because it allows the patient to have some distal end bearing during the impression capture. Anterior and posterior wedges are used to create a socket shape that best captures pelvic motion. (Courtesy of Ottobock.)

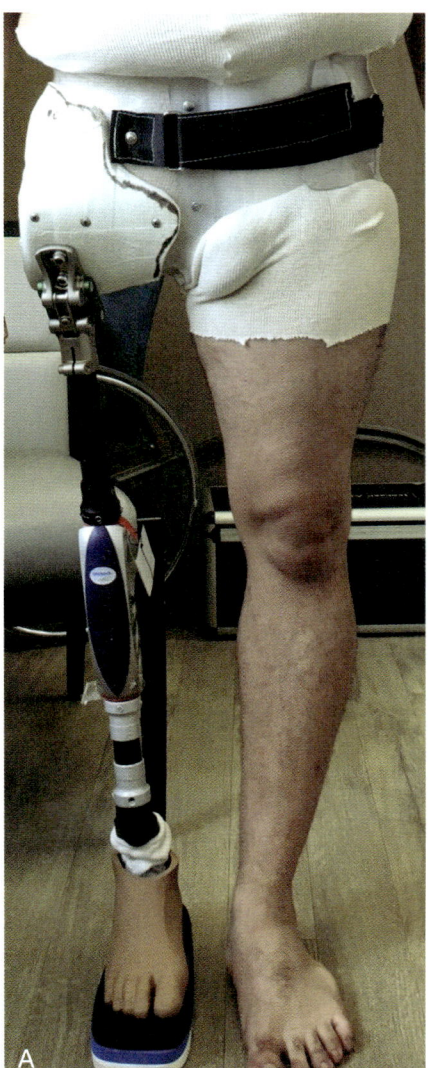 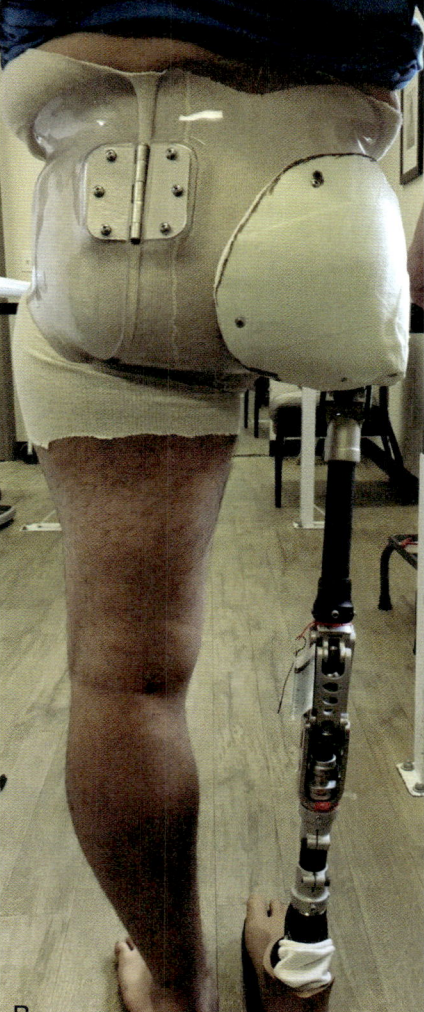 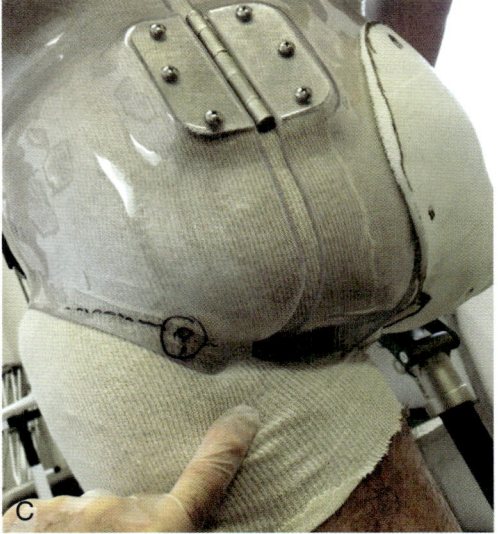

FIGURE 5 Photographs of a diagnostic hemipelvectomy socket. **A**, Anterior view and (**B**) posterior view illustrating the aggressive tissue containment with higher socket trimlines and diagonal compression against the iliac crest of the sound side. Mimicking the contour of the iliac crest roll on the affected side, even in the absence of the ipsilateral ilium provides a degree of superior tissue containment to prevent distal displacement of the socket and provides a waist groove to assist in the suspension of clothing. **C**, Inferior view illustrates the loading of the sound side ischial tuberosity within the hemipelvectomy socket. (Courtesy of Jesse Mitrani, CP(L), RFO(L) and Addam Griner, CPO(L).)

the swing phase. Although research has demonstrated some clear improvements in gait biomechanics and performance of activities of daily living using this system compared with traditional mechanical single-axis hip joints,[13-15] the joint adds substantial weight to the prosthesis and must be carefully considered for users with reduced body weight or general weakness.

Knees

Single-axis knees were the predominant choice for a hip disarticulation prosthesis because of their relatively light weight and adequacy for ambulation at a single cadence speed. However, single-axis knees with weight-activated stance control are generally contraindicated because the downward thrust that occurs when the pelvis tilts posteriorly to initiate knee flexion during gait can inadvertently engage the stance control brake of the knee and impede normal knee flexion at terminal stance. Because the sagittal stability of the knee within a hip disarticulation prosthesis is generally provided through the correct alignment of the hip and knee, added mechanical stability features are usually not necessary for individuals who walk only on level surfaces.

Many active users, however, may prefer knees with inherent stability features that enable the safer negotiation of uneven terrains, descending stairs or going down ramps, changing directions, and other related activities. Polycentric knees are often chosen for moderately active individuals who can tolerate their increased weight, desire stability across a broader range of walking surfaces, and benefit from swing clearance features. For individuals who desire the ability to ambulate

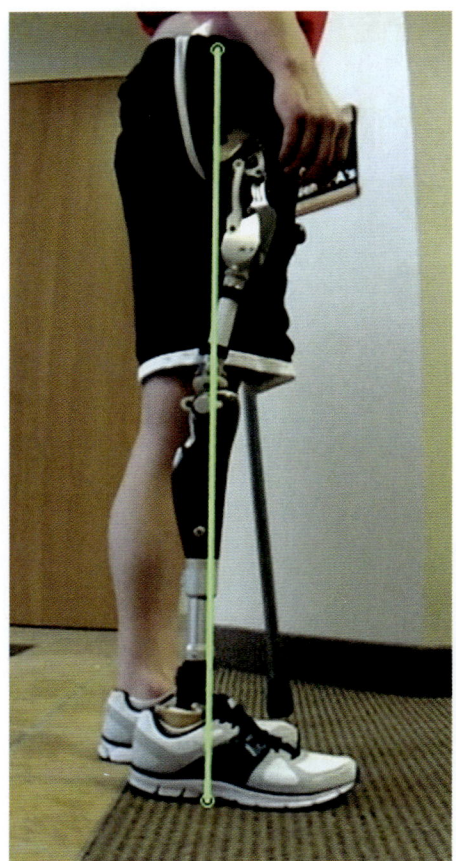

FIGURE 6 Photograph of a prosthesis that uses modern application of the principles of the Canadian hip disarticulation prosthesis. Alignment is illustrated by the sagittal plumb line (green line) from the sagittal socket bisector running posterior to the hip, anterior to the knee, and anterior to the ankle. This alignment positions the socket safely over the prosthetic knee axis and prosthetic foot to provide biomechanical stability for the user.

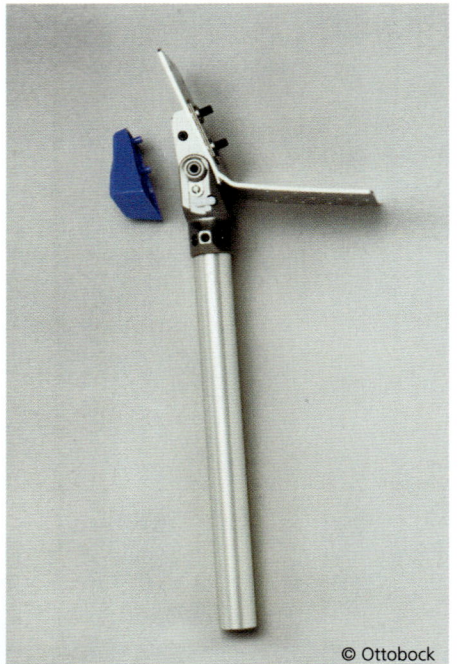

FIGURE 7 Photograph of an endoskeletal hip joint with an anterior attachment bracket. (Courtesy of Ottobock.)

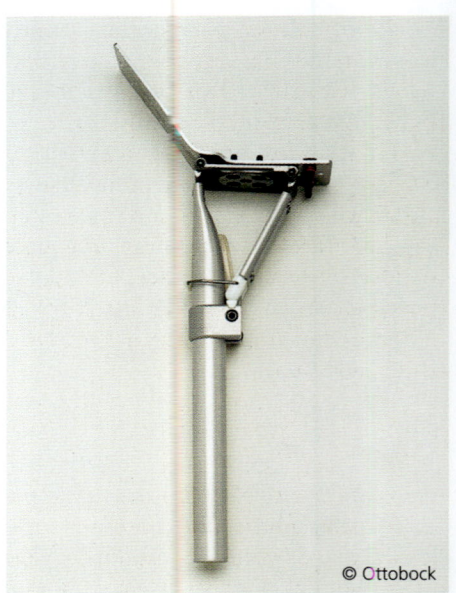

FIGURE 9 Photograph of an endoskeletal hip joint with a manual lock feature. (Courtesy of Ottobock.)

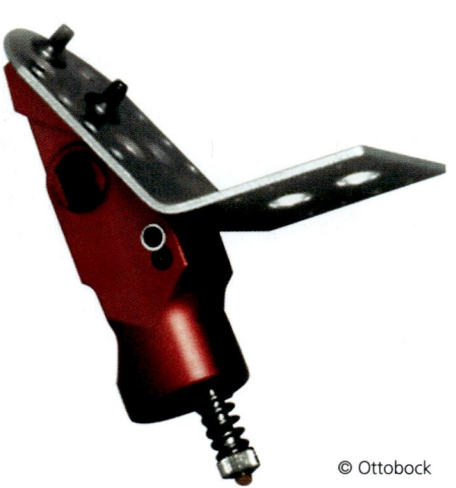

FIGURE 8 Photograph of a pediatric endoskeletal hip joint. (Courtesy of Ottobock.)

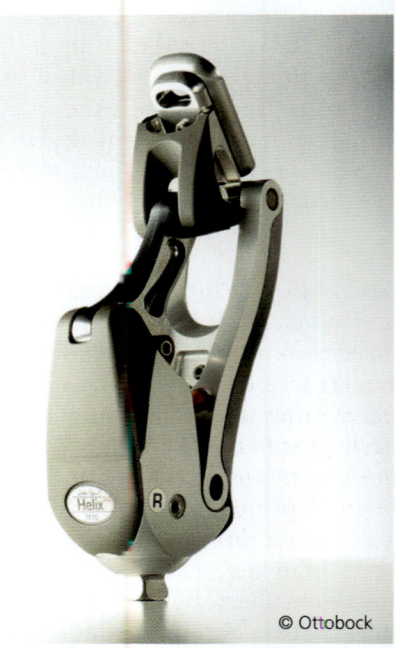

FIGURE 10 Photograph of the recently developed Helix 3D, an endoskeletal hip joint with a unique helical geometry that couples transverse rotation with sagittal hip motion and offers hydraulic control of hip flexion in the swing phase of gait and hip extension in the stance phase of gait. (Courtesy of Ottobock.)

at elevated walking speeds, polycentric knees with hydraulic swing control are commonly used. However, these knees are heavier, and their use should be limited to individuals who are capable of ambulation across variable cadences.

For those who desire even greater levels of activity and/or security, microprocessor-controlled knees are an option. These knees reduce the force required to initiate knee flexion at terminal stance and enable real-time adjustments to stance control properties, allowing the user to safely engage in the negotiation of environmental obstacles, stairs, and inclines across a range of gait speeds.[13,15]

Feet

Although single-axis and multiaxial feet can increase knee stability, they can add substantial weight to the distal end of the prosthesis. Dynamic response feet are commonly preferred at the hip disarticulation level because of their lightweight design. Because of the slower self-selected walking speeds of most users of hip disarticulation prostheses, the additional benefits of energy storage and return associated with these feet are only observed in more active users. However, a lightweight carbon fiber foot allows a smoother transition from loading response to terminal stance, with attendant benefits to the user's gait pattern. The full-length toe lever of such feet provides an extension moment at the knee in terminal stance, allowing a normal sound side step length. In the absence of an adequate toe lever in terminal stance, early knee flexion can occur, creating instability in terminal stance and force a shortened sound side step.

Height Considerations

When using traditional mechanical hip joints, there is no hip flexion in the early swing phase and minimal knee flexion at midswing. These limitations affect the ability of the user to obtain swing phase ground clearance. As a consequence, the hip disarticulation prosthesis often feels "long" and must be made slightly shorter than the anatomic leg to ensure toe clearance in the swing phase. This results in an inefficient gait pattern. Even with a shorter prosthetic build height, the user will often vault on the sound leg or hike the hip of the residual limb to further ensure toe clearance.[16]

Prosthetic Alignment

Stability of the hip disarticulation prosthesis relies primarily on the alignment of the components in relation to the socket in the sagittal plane. The alignment principles of the 1950s Canadian-style prosthesis are still used today and involve the projection of a line in the sagittal plane from the prosthetic hip joint center through the prosthetic knee axis. This reference line should fall somewhat posterior to the heel of the shoe. This sagittal reference line is still in current use (**Figure 11**).

More contemporary sagittal alignments will use a plumb line from the sagittal socket bisector. This alignment will position the socket over the prosthetic knee axis and prosthetic foot to provide biomechanical stability for the user (**Figure 6**). In the frontal plane, the hip joint approximates the bisection of the socket with 5° to 10° of external rotation to match anatomic lower limb rotation (**Figure 1, A**). As discussed earlier, in most traditional hip

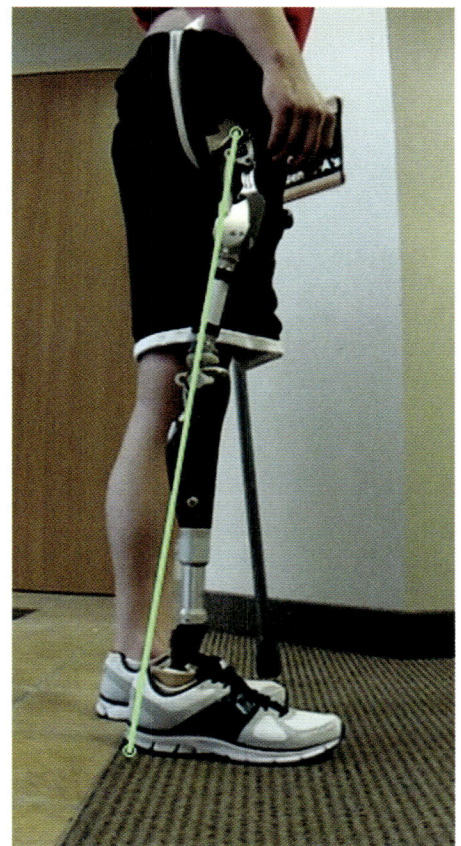

FIGURE 11 Photograph demonstrating the Canadian hip disarticulation sagittal reference line (green line). A line is projected from the prosthetic hip joint center through the prosthetic knee axis. This reference line should fall somewhat posterior to the heel of the shoe, although this will also depend on the inherent stability of the knee, with the line more posterior in less stable knees. (Courtesy of Phillip M. Stevens, MEd, CPO, FAAOP, Salt Lake City, UT.)

disarticulation designs, the length of the prosthesis is made slightly shorter than the sound side.

Gait Biomechanics and Physical Therapy

To properly align, adjust, and train the user of a hip disarticulation prosthesis, it is helpful to have knowledge of prosthetic function during the phases of gait. Training patients to properly weight shift, balance, and use their pelvic muscles are key factors in achieving successful ambulation. During initial contact, maintaining an erect posture and proper heel contact or stride is important to begin ambulating. During

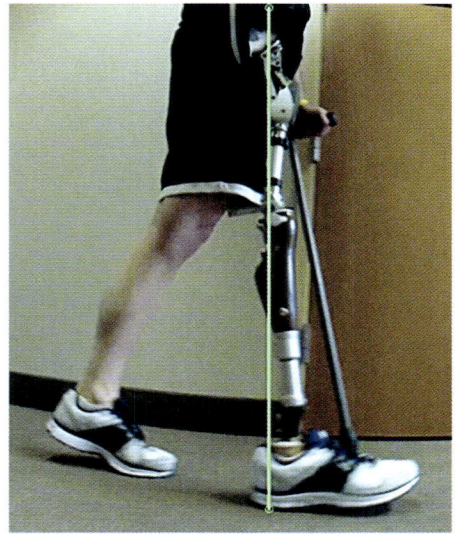

FIGURE 12 Photograph demonstrating the initial contact phase of gait in a patient with a hip disarticulation prosthesis. The ground reaction force (green line) passes posterior to the ankle of the prosthetic foot. Its position relative to the knee joint will depend on the inherent stability of the knee. Unstable knees require a posterior knee position, whereas more stable knees allow a more anterior knee position. (Courtesy of Phillip M. Stevens, MEd, CPO, FAAOP, Salt Lake City, UT.)

this phase of gait, the ground reaction force passes posterior to the ankle of the prosthetic foot and is slightly anterior to the mechanical knee center (**Figure 12**). The posterior position of the ground reaction force relative to the ankle joint causes a plantar flexion moment. In most instances, it is important that a soft heel allows this motion to occur. A firm heel may produce a resultant flexion moment at the knee, causing instability. However, when knee componentry is designed to allow stance flexion, it is also important to allow this motion to occur in the early stance phase. Stance flexion is normal in walking mechanics and provides a natural shock-absorbing feature for the user.

During the phase of loading response, the center of mass remains posterior to the ground reaction line, causing slight rotation of the socket toward extension. In single-axis hip joints, the hip bumper comes into contact with the socket, allowing the user to move forward over the foot (**Figure 13**).

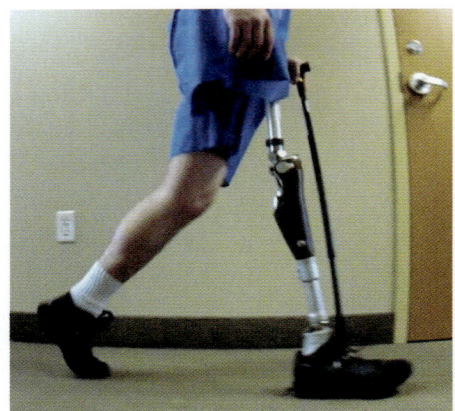

FIGURE 13 Photograph demonstrating the loading response phase of gait in a patient with a hip disarticulation prosthesis. In single-axis hip joints, the hip bumper comes into contact with the socket, allowing the user to move forward over the prosthetic foot. (Courtesy of Phillip M. Stevens, MEd, CPO, FAAOP, Salt Lake City, UT.)

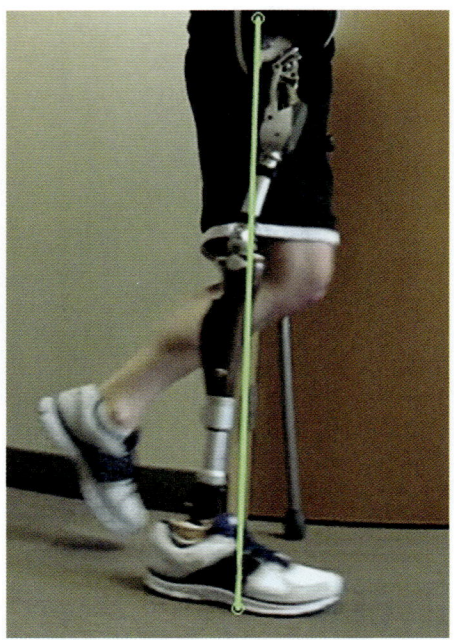

FIGURE 14 Photograph demonstrating the midstance phase of gait in a patient with a hip disarticulation prosthesis. The ground reaction force (green line) moves anterior to the ankle joint, anterior to the knee joint, and continues to pass posterior to the hip joint, creating a stable alignment. (Courtesy of Phillip M. Stevens, MEd, CPO, FAAOP, Salt Lake City, UT.)

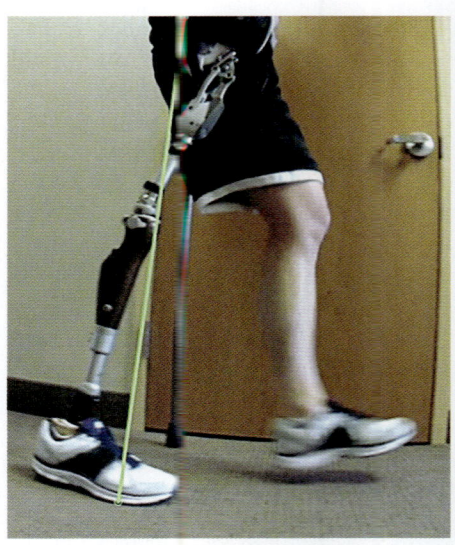

FIGURE 15 Photograph demonstrating the terminal stance phase of gait in a patient with a hip disarticulation prosthesis. The ground reaction force (green line) begins at the forefoot of the prosthesis, passing anterior to the ankle, slightly anterior to the mechanical knee axis, and well posterior to the hip joint axis. (Courtesy of Phillip M. Stevens, MEd, CPO, FAAOP, Salt Lake City, UT.)

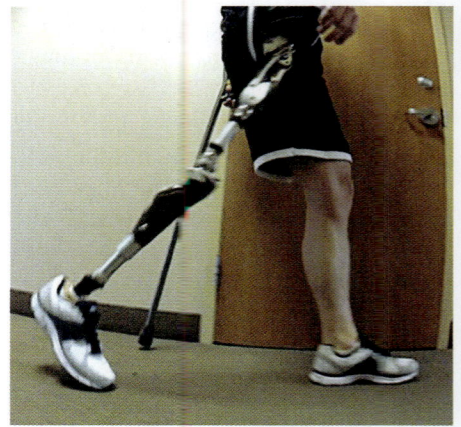

FIGURE 16 Photograph demonstrating the preswing phase of gait in a patient with a hip disarticulation prosthesis. Torque produced at the hip joint combined with controlled posterior tilting of the pelvis causes knee flexion during preswing. An intimately fitted socket in the lumbar region and compression of the abdominal region anteriorly contribute to controlling knee flexion to initiate the swing phase. (Courtesy of Phillip M. Stevens, MEd, CPO, FAAOP, Salt Lake City, UT.)

The timing and magnitude of this impact are important as an early or abrupt impact into full hip extension can trigger a flexion moment at the knee in early stance before the weight line moves anterior to the knee joint. In hip joints that have hydraulic damping of extension, this damping function provides a smoother progression over the leg and decreases the impact load through the socket.

When the user comes to the midstance phase of gait, the ground reaction line moves anterior to the ankle joint, anterior to the knee joint, and continues to pass posterior to the hip joint (**Figure 14**). The hip bumper is now in full contact, and the knee is stabilized. At this point, the user is in single-limb support and the socket must provide coronal stability through the pelvis to prevent instability. During midstance, the path of the center of mass of the body is dictated by the shape of the foot and compression of the tissues in the socket. The stability of the prosthesis results from gravity locking all three joints. Therefore, it is safe to allow full weight bearing on the prosthesis and swing through of the sound side leg. Momentum or inertia then causes the body to move forward over the prosthesis.

During terminal stance, the body must maintain an erect, upright position. The ground reaction force passes anterior from the forefoot of the prosthesis, slightly anterior to the mechanical knee axis, and well posterior to the hip joint axis (**Figure 15**).

With the body held erect, torque produced at the hip joint with the hip extension stop combined with controlled posterior tilting of the pelvis causes knee flexion during preswing (**Figure 16**). An intimately fitted socket in the lumbar region and compression of the abdominal region anteriorly contribute to controlling knee flexion to initiate the swing phase. Use of the core abdominal muscles aids in allowing the user to walk efficiently and control knee flexion for the swing phase. This is why the socket fit is so important, and proper training of this motion is necessary.

During the phase of initial swing, suspension becomes very important. The hip extension stop is engaged, the thigh is nearly vertical, and the internal knee extension spring of the knee joint prevents excessive heel rise and initiates extension of the shank (**Figure 17**).

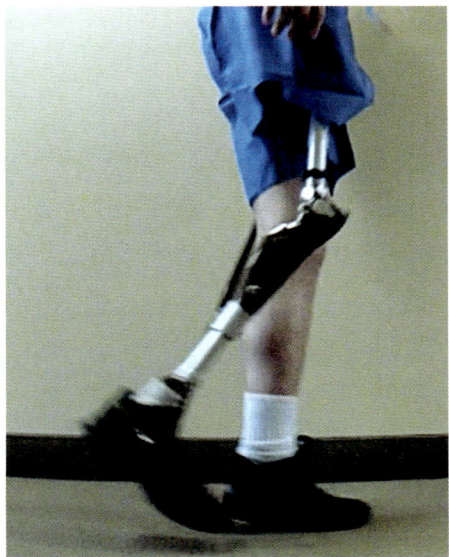

FIGURE 17 Photograph demonstrating the initial swing phase of gait in a patient with a hip disarticulation prosthesis. With the hip extension stop engaged, the thigh is nearly vertical and the extension assist of the knee joint prevents excessive heel rise and initiates extension of the shank. (Courtesy of Phillip M. Stevens, MEd, CPO, FAAOP, Salt Lake City, UT.)

During midswing, the knee comes to full extension. In normal human ambulation, swing through is the period of greatest knee angulation (approximating 65°), with the hip joint in 25° of flexion and the ankle joint in a neutral position to shorten the limb for adequate floor clearance. This is not true of a hip disarticulation prosthesis. The hip joint flexes only after the shank section has reached full knee extension and, therefore, is at its greatest length at midswing (**Figure 18**). Because of this, the prosthesis must be made slightly shorter. Adequate clearance is also obtained by keeping the trunk vertical so that the hip joint is kept forward and as high as possible. Newer hip joints have the ability to initiate hip flexion while the knee is still in flexion, thus reducing the amount of pelvic tilt needed and allowing the prosthesis to be made full length. It is still necessary for the prosthesis to maintain its position on the pelvis and not lose its suspension component. Inadequate suspension may produce gait deviations, such as hip-hiking on the amputated side and vaulting on the sound side.

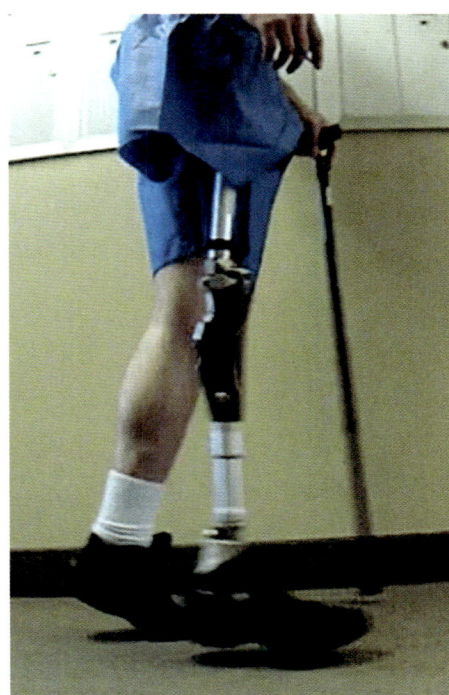

FIGURE 18 Photograph demonstrating the midswing phase of gait in a patient with a hip disarticulation prosthesis. The prosthetic knee reaches full length at midstance. Swing phase clearance is obtained by means of a shortened prosthetic build height, hip hiking, circumduction, vaulting (shown), or a combination of these accommodations. (Courtesy of Phillip M. Stevens, MEd, CPO, FAAOP, Salt Lake City, UT.)

SUMMARY

A team approach, which includes the patient, the physician, the prosthetist, and the physical therapist, will aid an individual with a hip disarticulation or hemipelvectomy prosthesis in achieving successful use. It is important that a patient with a proximal lower limb amputation understands and is provided with full information regarding the high physical and emotional demands of walking. When developing the prosthesis, the treatment team should understand the patient's wishes, physical condition, motivation, and functional activities so that the prosthesis will meet the needs of that patient. Advanced materials and technology, along with dedicated gait training, will aid the patient in reaching their goals.

References

1. Carroll KM: Hip disarticulation and transpelvic amputation: Prosthetic management, in Smith DG, Michael JW, Bowker JH, eds: *Atlas of Amputations and Limb Deficiencies: Surgical, Prosthetic, and Rehabilitation Principles*, ed 3. American Academy of Orthopaedic Surgeons, 2004, pp 565-573.
2. Yari P, Dijkstra PU, Geertzen JH: Functional outcome of hip disarticulation and hemipelvectomy: A cross-sectional national descriptive study in the Netherlands. *Clin Rehabil* 2008;22(12):1127-1133.
3. Fernández A, Formigo J: Are Canadian prostheses used? A long-term experience. *Prosthet Orthot Int* 2005;29(2):177-181.
4. Nowroozi F, Salvanelli ML, Gerber LH: Energy expenditure in hip disarticulation and hemipelvectomy amputees. *Arch Phys Med Rehabil* 1983;64(7):300-303.
5. Chin T, Oyabu H, Maeda Y, Takase I, Machida K: Energy consumption during prosthetic walking and wheelchair locomotion by elderly hip disarticulation amputees. *Am J Phys Med Rehabil* 2009;88(5):399-403.
6. Chin T, Kuroda R, Akisue T, Iguchi T, Kurosaka M: Energy consumption during prosthetic walking and physical fitness in older hip disarticulation amputees. *J Rehabil Res Dev* 2012;49(8):1255-1260.
7. Yoshikawa K, Mutsuzaki H, Sano A, et al: A case of an elderly hip disarticulation amputee with rheumatoid arthritis who regained the ability to walk using a hip prosthesis. *J Phys Ther Sci* 2019;31(4):366-370.
8. Iwasa S, Uchiyama Y, Kodama N, Koyama T, Domen K: Regaining gait using an early postoperative hip prosthesis: A case report of an elderly woman. *Prog Rehabil Med* 2021;6:20210011.
9. Houdek MT, Andrews K, Kralovec ME, et al: Functional outcome measures of patients following hemipelvectomy. *Prosthet Orthot Int* 2016;40(5):566-572.
10. Kralovec ME, Houdek MT, Andrews KL, Shives TC, Rose PS, Sim FH: Prosthetic rehabilitation after hip disarticulation or hemipelvectomy. *Am J Phys Med Rehabil* 2015;94(12):1035-1040.
11. Radcliffe CW: The biomechanics of the Canadian-type hip-disarticulation prosthesis. *Artif Limbs* 1957;4(2):29-38.

12. Houdek MT, Kralovec ME, Andrews KL: Hemipelvectomy: High-level amputation surgery and prosthetic rehabilitation. *Am J Phys Med Rehabil* 2014;93(7):600-608.

13. Nelson LM, Carbone NT: Functional outcome measurements of a veteran with a hip disarticulation using a Helix 3D hip joint: A case report. *J Prosthet Orthot* 2011;23(1):21-26.

14. Ludwig E, Bellmann M, Schmalz T, Blumentritt S: Biomechanical differences between two exoprosthetic hip joint systems during level walking. *Prosthet Orthot Int* 2010;34(4):449-460.

15. Gailledrat E, Moineau B, Seetha V, et al: Does the new Helix 3D hip joint improve walking of hip disarticulated amputees? *Ann Phys Rehabil Med* 2013;56(5):411-418.

16. Faiz M, Lassade C, Chiesa G: Gait analysis of amputee patients walking with a Canadian prosthesis. *Ann Phys Rehabil Med* 2018;61:e375.

Bilateral Lower Limb Amputation: Prosthetic Management

CHAPTER 46

Michael K. Carroll, PhD, CPO, FAAOP(D) • Kevin Carroll, MS, CP, FAAOP(D) • John Rheinstein, CP, FAAOP(D)

ABSTRACT

Recent improvements in prosthetic technology and rehabilitation techniques have made useful function and independence possible for those with bilateral lower limb amputation. Use of the graduated length prosthetic protocol is essential for individuals with bilateral transfemoral amputation to ensure long-term prosthetic use. Goal setting, high expectations, and peer support are crucial for successful rehabilitation.

Because of the enhanced stability and reduced energy expenditure provided, microprocessor-controlled knees should be considered the medically necessary standard of care for bilateral transfemoral amputees who have the ability or potential to progress beyond indoor walking on level ground.

Keywords: bilateral amputation; bilateral prostheses; bilateral transfemoral amputation; bilateral transtibial amputation; graduated length prosthetic protocol; microprocessor knees

Introduction

Individuals with bilateral lower limb loss, and their rehabilitation teams, face a unique set of challenges which are much greater than those of patients with unilateral amputations.[1] Despite these challenges, recent advances in prosthetic technology and rehabilitation protocols have raised expectations for positive functional outcomes for many of these individuals. Improved outcomes include ambulation for many activities of daily living, stair navigation, hill descent, and running (**Figures 1** through **3**). Each person presents differently because of their amputation levels, medical history, physical capabilities, and personality traits. Bilateral transfemoral and more proximal amputations require extensive prosthetic management and physical therapy for the person to regain mobility and independent function. If the knee joint can be preserved in at least one leg, better function and a shorter period of rehabilitation can be expected, however these cases still require close collaboration and planning within the rehabilitation team.[2] To maximize the likelihood of a successful outcome, a customized treatment plan must be developed for each patient's specific needs and circumstances.

This chapter discusses the specific needs of patients with bilateral lower limb amputations, including postoperative care, identifying candidates for prosthetic use, appropriate prosthetic management, and effective protocols for successful rehabilitation. In addition,

Dr. Michael K. Carroll or an immediate family member serves as a paid consultant to or is an employee of Hanger; has stock or stock options held in Hanger; and serves as a board member, owner, officer, or committee member of the American Academy of Orthotists and Prosthetists and the National Commission on Orthotic and Prosthetic Education. Kevin Carroll or an immediate family member serves as a paid consultant to or is an employee of Hanger; has stock or stock options held in Hanger; and serves as a board member, owner, officer, or committee member of the American Academy of Orthotists and Prosthetists and the National Commission on Orthotic and Prosthetic Education. John Rheinstein or an immediate family member serves as a paid consultant to or is an employee of Hanger Clinic; has stock or stock options held in Abbott and Zimmer; and serves as a board member, owner, officer, or committee member of American Academy of Orthotists and Prosthetists.

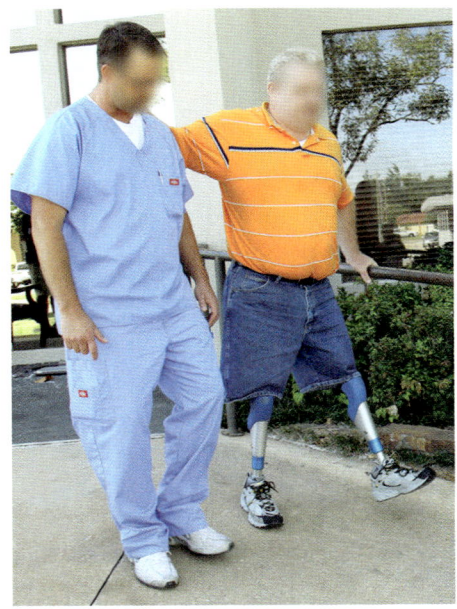

FIGURE 1 Photograph demonstrating learning to walk down a ramp with bilateral transfemoral prostheses. (Courtesy of Hanger Clinic, Austin, TX.)

This chapter is adapted from Carroll K, Rheinstein J, Richardson RW: Bilateral lower limb amputation: prosthetic management, in Krajbich JI, Pinzur MS, Potter BK, Stevens PM, eds: *Atlas of Amputations and Limb Deficiencies: Surgical, Prosthetic, and Rehabilitation Principles*, ed 4. American Academy of Orthopaedic Surgeons, 2016, pp 631-643.

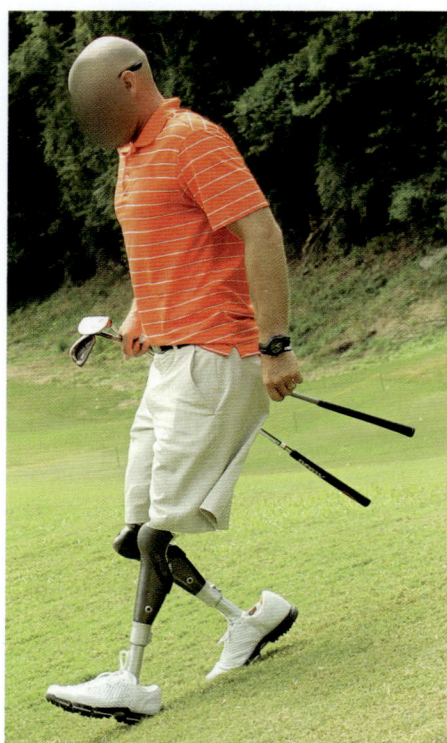

FIGURE 2 Photograph demonstrating walking downhill using bilateral transfemoral prostheses. (Courtesy of Hanger Clinic, Austin, TX.)

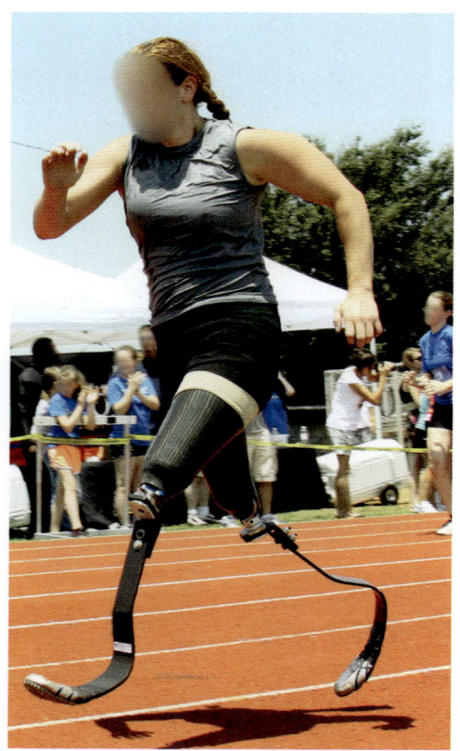

FIGURE 3 Photograph demonstrating running using bilateral transfemoral prostheses without knee joints. (Courtesy of Hanger Clinic, Austin, TX.)

factors that may affect progress, including motivation, peer support, and preparation for prosthetic use, are discussed. Most attention is given to treatment of those with bilateral **transfemoral** amputations because of their greater complexity when compared with more distal levels of amputation. Despite the small number of patients with bilateral lower limb loss relative to all amputations, there is an increasing amount of evidence and useful information available to guide clinical practice.[3,4]

Causes of Bilateral Amputation

Most bilateral amputations are the result of medical complications from diabetes and peripheral vascular disease.[5] Commonly, an individual experiences a series of lifesaving amputations, beginning with the loss of part or all of one foot. As the disease progresses, they may lose the contralateral foot after growing accustomed to ambulating with one amputated limb.[6] A high likelihood of bilateral amputation and mortality exists in this cohort.[6]

Experience with a unilateral prosthesis is a good predictor of success as a bilateral prosthetic user despite the additional emotional distress.[7] In our clinical experience, individuals facing the loss of their contralateral foot are best served when the second amputation is performed directly at the transtibial level to reduce the likelihood that multiple partial foot amputations will be needed. This approach allows patients to proceed with definitive rehabilitation rather than requiring recurrent hospitalization and rehabilitation admissions.

Bilateral amputations can also result from trauma, primarily war-related blast injuries.[8] Advances in battlefield medicine have saved many lives, but survivors often have severe injuries, including multiple limb amputations.[9] Heterotopic ossification is a difficult complication of traumatic injuries which makes prosthetic fitting challenging because of severe pain and frequent anatomical changes to the residual limb.[10] Phantom pain, residual limb pain, and lower back pain are also widely reported.[11,12]

Diseases and septic infections such as strep, meningococcal septicemia, and necrotizing fasciitis are also causes of bilateral lower limb loss and may be accompanied by upper limb loss. These patients can be difficult to fit with prostheses because of challenges related to their residual limbs. To maintain maximal residual limb length in the face of a rapidly progressing disease, the shape of residual limbs is often irregular because of the removal of necrotic tissue. Large areas of skin graft and poor distal tissue coverage are common. The skin is often fragile and prone to breakdown and ulceration, even from normal forces generated by prostheses use. Multiple revision procedures and prosthetic sockets may be required until the residual limbs are stable. This is especially the case with children.[13] Despite these challenges, patients who survive these devastating infections and diseases can lead functional productive lives[14] (**Figure 4**).

Clinical Consideration

Effective treatment of individuals with bilateral lower limb amputation begins with a thorough physical, cognitive, and psychological assessment, setting goals, developing a plan, and frequent communication between members of the rehabilitation team. The team should include, but not be limited to, physiatrists, surgeons, physical therapists, prosthetists, social workers, caregivers, and payers. Patients and caregivers alike should be connected to peer support from others who have either undergone multiple lower limb loss or cared for someone who has experienced such loss. Goals are established considering each patient's needs, future potential, and aspirations. Their motivation and determination to reach these goals are significant predictors of success.

Wound Care and Early Function

Irrespective of the level of amputation, surgical wounds must be managed with great care. Initial concerns are pain, wound healing, edema, contractures, and protection of the residual limb from falls or other impacts. Removable rigid dressings are the preferred method of

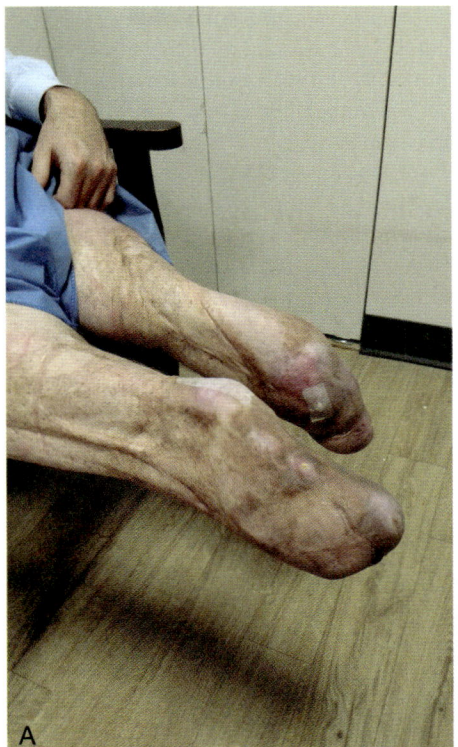 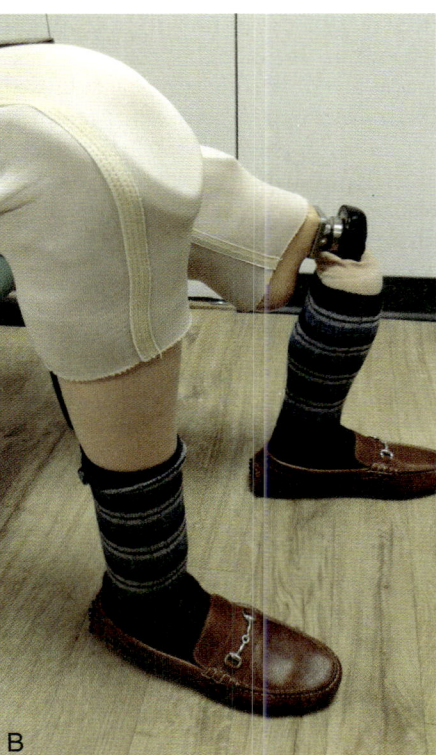 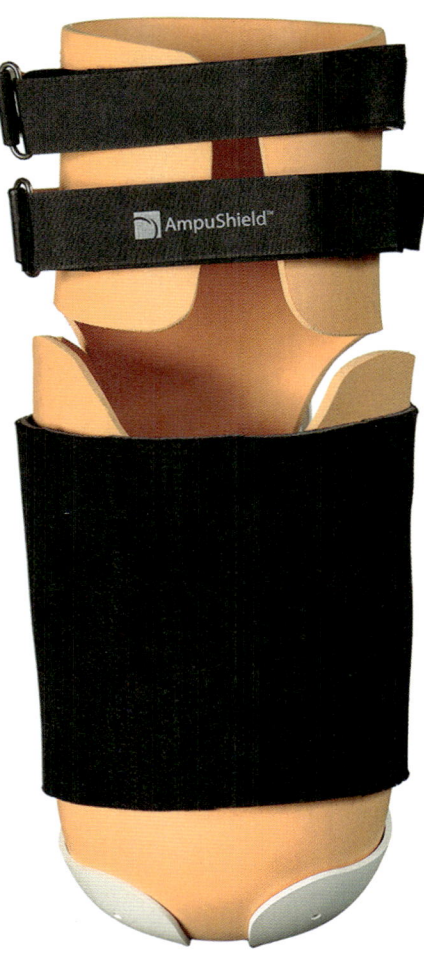

FIGURE 4 **A**, Photograph of the lower limbs of a patient with a bilateral transtibial amputation secondary to meningococcemia. **B**, Photograph of the patient fitted with prostheses. Because the left knee is fixed at 45°, the prosthetic knee was placed under the patient's residual limb to improve gait and sitting comfort. The patient is fully functional at work and in activities of daily living despite fragile skin.

FIGURE 5 Photograph of the AmpuShield (Hanger) postoperative protective removable rigid dressing. (Courtesy of Hanger Clinic, Austin, TX.)

addressing these concerns and result in earlier prosthetic fitting and shortened acute hospital stays[12,15,16] (**Figure 5**). Removable rigid dressings also provide patients with early experience managing a prosthetic device and learning self-care. Elastic compression garments can be used in conjunction with a removable rigid dressing to help control postoperative edema. Though ace wraps may be more readily available, use of shrinker socks or tubular elastic bandages are recommended as these decrease the likelihood of inconsistent pressure being applied to the limb.

Weight bearing should be restricted in patients with bilateral surgical wounds because they cannot offload either limb to achieve partial weight bearing. In patients with a recent amputation on one side and a functioning prosthesis on the other, partial weight bearing to the newly amputated side can be introduced based on the condition of the wound. If a newly performed amputation is at, or distal to, the transtibial level, the patient may be permitted to kneel with supervision during therapy. Kneeling allows the patient to assume an upright position for stretching, balance, and overall health.

The bilateral amputee may be unprepared for the change in their capabilities after the loss of the second limb. The individual's ability to transfer to and from a wheelchair, and in and out of a car will be substantially reduced by the loss of a sound leg previously used for stabilization, pivoting, and balance. Physical therapy during the initial postoperative period should focus on performing safe transfer techniques to help maintain patient independence and prevent falls.[17,18] Developing strength and flexibility in the upper body is necessary for bilateral lower limb amputees, irrespective of prosthetic use. Those who intend to use prostheses also benefit from engaging the lower extremities, which may require an adaptive training program.[19]

Patients should be advised that even after therapy sessions are complete, their fitness program should continue for the rest of their lives. A daily exercise program that includes stretching, cardiovascular endurance, core strength, and balance is a crucial component of continued long-term success.[20,21] It is especially important for individuals to maintain a healthy weight and blood glucose control. A person who is overweight will find it much more difficult to ambulate with bilateral prostheses, and weight fluctuations can adversely affect both prosthetic socket fit as well as prosthetic alignment. An effective weight control program should be instituted as early as possible to adjust diet for metabolic changes which follow amputation. Working with a dietitian is encouraged for both users and nonusers of prostheses.

Wheelchair Selection

Most bilateral amputees initially require an appropriate wheelchair after surgery; some will need one for the rest of their lives. After becoming proficient with their prostheses, many patients can be rehabilitated to function with little to no use of a wheelchair.[22] The authors currently care for many strong, active patients with bilateral transfemoral amputations, including some who are also missing arms, who are totally independent of a wheelchair.

Although a wheelchair-free life may be the preferred outcome, even individuals who achieve full-time prosthetic use may keep a wheelchair available for nighttime use, mobility over long distances, and times when they cannot wear their prostheses because of fitting or mechanical issues. Individuals who lack the strength, balance, cardiac reserve, endurance, or cognitive ability for full-time prosthetic use will need a wheelchair for some or most of their activities of daily living.[23,24] Those who use a manual wheelchair may benefit from a power-assist device that supplements their manual propulsion. The use of fully powered wheelchairs, however, should be discouraged unless necessary because they often result in deconditioning and weight gain.

After bilateral amputation, an individual's center of mass when seated in a wheelchair shifts substantially. This shift is more pronounced at more proximal levels of amputation. Such individuals should be managed with wheelchairs that have specifically designed antitipping devices, with larger wheels placed more posterior to the seat area of the chair, reducing the potential for tipping over. The authors have seen many lower limb amputees with serious head and neck injuries, as well as damage to their healing residual limbs, caused when their standard wheelchairs tipped over backward. These severe but preventable occurrences are common. In one study of 18 patients with amputation, 14 experienced falls from their wheelchairs.[25] Patients should also be taught early in their rehabilitation how to transfer to a wheelchair from the floor.

While the Americans with Disabilities Act provides and enforces standards for wheelchair accessibility in the United States, in practice, access to certain establishments, nightclubs, or restaurants may still be inconvenient. In such situations, lower limb prosthetics allow access to those venues without the need for special services and attention. In other countries, the argument for choosing prostheses over a wheelchair is even more forceful. Many attractions worldwide are not wheelchair accessible. Cobblestone streets make wheelchair navigation uncomfortable, if not impossible.

Although ambulation with bilateral lower limb prostheses is challenging, the human spirit is capable of remarkable achievements under the most adverse conditions, and the challenges facing multiple-limb amputees are not insurmountable. Patients respond well to high expectations set by the rehabilitation team and by the example of other successful prosthesis users. Recent improvements in prosthetic technology, including advanced microprocessor knees (MPKs), allow the user to function in environments previously considered impossible, including oceans and swimming pools. In the future, further improvements in the capabilities of bilateral lower limb amputees are expected as technologic advances continue. These advances will be driven by researchers and clinicians who have an expansive vision of patients' potential.

Prosthetic Care

Identifying Candidates for Prostheses

Determining suitability for prosthetic use is based on a thorough understanding of each patient's physical condition, cardiac fitness, goals, level of motivation, environmental conditions, as well as their cognitive ability.[26,27] Although bilateral prosthetic use demands higher energy expenditure than that required by able-bodied individuals (150% to 188%) or those with a unilateral prosthesis (130% to 160%), every bilateral amputee should be evaluated to determine the potential for prosthetic care.[28-30] Prosthetic use should only initially be ruled out for patients with severe irreversible medical conditions or profound cognitive deficits. More than one evaluation may be indicated because a patient's conditions can change. For example, patients who are weak as a result of disease, surgery, or extended sitting because of protracted nonsurgical treatment to preserve a diseased limb, often gain strength and progress to prosthetic use with regular physical therapy.

Patients who may not show initial potential for prosthetic use can be challenged to achieve milestones for strength, flexibility, and endurance. Once improvement is shown, preparatory prostheses can be provided. The ability to kneel in an upright position on both knees is a positive indicator for prosthesis use among patients following bilateral transtibial amputation. The Amputee Mobility Predictor (AMPNoPro), an assessment tool designed to evaluate the skills required for successful prosthetic ambulation, can be used to help determine potential functional capabilities.[4]

The rate of recovery and level of independence achieved depend largely on each individual, their unique physical and psychological makeup, as well as environmental factors such as family support and living arrangements.[31] Patients generally can be classified into one of four groups: nonusers, who do not use a functional prosthesis at all; partial users, who have one or two prostheses for transfers or wheelchair propulsion; mixed users, who use both prostheses and a wheelchair (wheelchairs are used for long distances); and full-time users independent of a wheelchair (younger, healthier individuals who are expected to progress rapidly unless there are physical or cognitive comorbidities).[32]

Prosthesis Nonusers

In most cases, patients with irreversible medical complications, insufficient cardiac reserves, severe weakness, or nonhealing wounds, as well as those who lack motivation or cognitive ability, are not candidates for prostheses.[27] Some bilateral amputees immediately recognize that they cannot benefit from prostheses. Others may be highly motivated, but have comorbidities that preclude prosthesis use. Some may be investigating the possibility of using prostheses because of pressure or encouragement from their families.

The team of rehabilitation professionals must deliver an honest but often unwelcome negative assessment when prostheses should not be provided. The negative assessment may relieve some tension and pressure for the patient and the family, allowing them to take a different approach to how the patient will live their life. It is unethical to mislead an unqualified prosthesis candidate by encouraging them to get prostheses when there is little or no potential benefit. These patients should be advised instead about the options for living a full life with wheelchair-assisted mobility and safety as a priority.

There is still a great need for rehabilitation of the individual who is not a candidate for prostheses. Conversations during the evaluation of prosthetic potential should be kind, encouraging, and honest. Patients who are not candidates for a prosthesis need proper adaptive equipment and training by a physical therapist for transfers, bathing, and toileting. A home visit from an occupational therapist with recommendations for environmental modifications can be beneficial to the patient. The patient should be encouraged to think positively, plan, and pursue opportunities to enjoy life by participating in family and community activities.

Partial Prosthesis Users

Bilateral amputees with limited physical capabilities who may not become active walkers can derive great benefit from having a prosthesis for one or both limbs. Prosthesis intervention will make daily tasks such as transfers, dressing, and transportation easier and safer. Prostheses also provide individuals more independence and options for activities in their community. A bilateral amputee can use even one transtibial prosthesis for propelling a wheelchair or transferring to a toilet. This can make the life-changing difference between an individual continuing to live at home and requiring placement in a nursing facility.[33]

Mixed and Full-Time Users

Motivation

A critical determinant of success for patients with bilateral lower limb amputations is the degree of motivation and willingness to persevere through hardship. Success does not depend on a patient's age. For example, the authors treated a 91-year-old man who was told that he was not a prosthesis candidate because of his age. Comprehensive evaluation revealed that he was motivated, strong, and agile enough to roll, slide, move around on the floor, and climb in and out of his wheelchair unassisted. He subsequently did very well with prostheses. This case underscores the importance of a thorough, unbiased evaluation of all candidates with bilateral lower limb amputation.

Some patients simply need to find or be reminded of motivating factors. One elderly man treated by the authors achieved successful use of his prostheses because of his determination to care for his invalid wife at home; another patient was motivated by his lifelong plan to take a trip to Alaska. Many people are inspired by the accomplishments of others in similar circumstances; others thrive with competition. Helping find the factors that motivate a patient and building on that inspiration are a critical aspect of successful rehabilitation.

Gender-Based Issues

In the pursuit of prosthesis success, there is no sex gap. Every individual should be encouraged to pursue their ambulation goals with an equal level of commitment and hard work. However, sex differences are evident in anatomy and toileting needs. Prosthetic sockets need to be adjusted so the wearer can perform toileting functions in a safe, hygienic manner without worry. At the transfemoral and more proximal levels, prosthetic sockets for female patients should be designed and trimmed to avoid urinary contamination. Socket trim lines should not pinch or impinge the genitals. Males often benefit from tight brief-style underwear with a pouch as this can help lift the genitals away from the sockets. Fecal contamination, which can affect both sexes, must be discussed even though it may be an uncomfortable topic. Clinicians should be sensitive to the fact that some patients may prefer to discuss these issues with a clinician of the same sex.

Balancing Support and Independence

For bilateral amputees to achieve maximal independence, family members and the rehabilitation team need to appropriately withdraw their assistance so that patients learn to perform many of their activities of daily living independently. This requires sensitivity and flexibility to each patient's fluctuating needs and emotions. Having a prior set of agreed-upon goals provides justification when requests for help are appropriately declined.

Family and friends are naturally concerned for the patient's welfare. They typically want to be accommodating and often find it difficult to identify at what point in the healing process it is appropriate to be less helpful. Performing small physical tasks for recovering surgical patients to spare them unnecessary effort or discomfort may be preferable during the initial period of homecoming and convalescence. However, family members and caregivers should be advised that continuing such services as the patient heals and grows stronger will only increase their dependence on others and decrease their motivation to achieve an independent lifestyle. Patients should gradually increase the number of things they do for themselves. The ability to transfer without assistance is especially important, as well as donning and doffing prostheses.

The following 12 suggestions were compiled for overly helpful family members and caregivers at a recent annual training and support "boot camp," attended by more than 40 bilateral transfemoral amputees: (1) do not feel guilty, (2) learn to say no, (3) offer positive reinforcement, (4) provide tough love, (5) help raise goals progressively, (6) set a good example, (7) provide more space and freedom, (8) be patient, (9) suggest more options, (10) track progress, (11) never be satisfied with progress, and (12) build confidence.

The rehabilitation team also should strike a balance between pushing patients to become stronger and proficient with familiar tasks and obstacles while not overwhelming or outpacing their capabilities to perform and learn skills.

Psychological Considerations

Loss of any part of the body is traumatic both physically and emotionally, irrespective of the cause or the amputation level. All healthcare professionals and family members should be reminded never to trivialize any amputation. Bilateral amputation can be especially difficult to deal with because of loss of a substantial portion of the body and changes in body image. Patients who thought the initial amputation was going to put an end to their difficulties may find it particularly hard to face the loss of a second leg. The more proximal the amputation, the more radical are the changes in the body and the body image.

Peer support is helpful for most patients after they first undergo amputation and as they progress through rehabilitation. Organizations such as AMPOWER and the Amputee Coalition have online peer support networks and extensive informational resources. Meeting a well-functioning person during recovery frequently expands a patient's view of what is possible and can be life changing. Participating in adaptive sports programs can also be particularly helpful following limb loss. Both the receiver and the provider of peer support benefit. Professional counseling is indicated if an individual is having trouble adjusting to their new body shape or is experiencing depression. Focusing on what patients can do, rather than on what they no longer can do, helps them achieve a healthy "new normal" view of their circumstances.[34] Mastering the new skills required for daily living can be empowering and may replace a sense of loss.

Following an amputation, most focus naturally shifts to the patient. While the loss of limbs has a significant impact on the individual, it can also have a disruptive impact on their intimate and familial relationships. Caregivers and family members should be encouraged to participate in peer support programs as well as professional counseling when needed. Both AMPOWER and Amputee Coalition have resources specifically for amputees' family members. For children that endure amputations, participating in camps like Camp No Limits that involve the whole family may help pediatric amputees, parents, and siblings adapt to their new reality.

Graduated Length Prosthetic Protocol at the Bilateral Transfemoral Level

Independence and effective walking on full-length prosthetic legs are much more likely when bilateral transfemoral amputees begin therapy on very short prosthetic legs without knees, known as graduated length prosthetic protocol (GLPP).[22] It is often difficult for patients to accept the physical and psychological challenges of being very short. However, the ultimate success with prostheses depends on the skills and function developed while following the protocol. The authors have seen many patients who tried full-length prostheses without going through the GLPP and who failed to achieve their desired function and independence because they did not achieve the foundational skills which come from walking on short prostheses.

With the GLPP, the starting prosthetic height is the minimum distance between the distal end of the sockets and the "stubbie" feet (small, flat, plastic oval pads with rubber soles, approximately 4.0 inches long × 3.5 inches wide, centered on the pylon) or the connection adapter for those with osseointegration) (**Figure 6**). This lowers the center of gravity, the consequences of inevitable falls, and the ambulatory energy costs.[35,36] The short length also allows patients to learn balance, build their core and body strength, stretch their hip muscles, and increase their confidence at a safe height. Patients learn how to reach over and touch the floor all around them. They learn how to fall, how to get up from the floor, and how to use short canes and crutches for support. While the GLPP reduces some of the barriers to ambulating with prostheses, it is important that patients are aware of their limitations and do not overexert themselves or irritate their residual limbs. Users should be instructed to begin by wearing their prostheses for 1 hour of daily

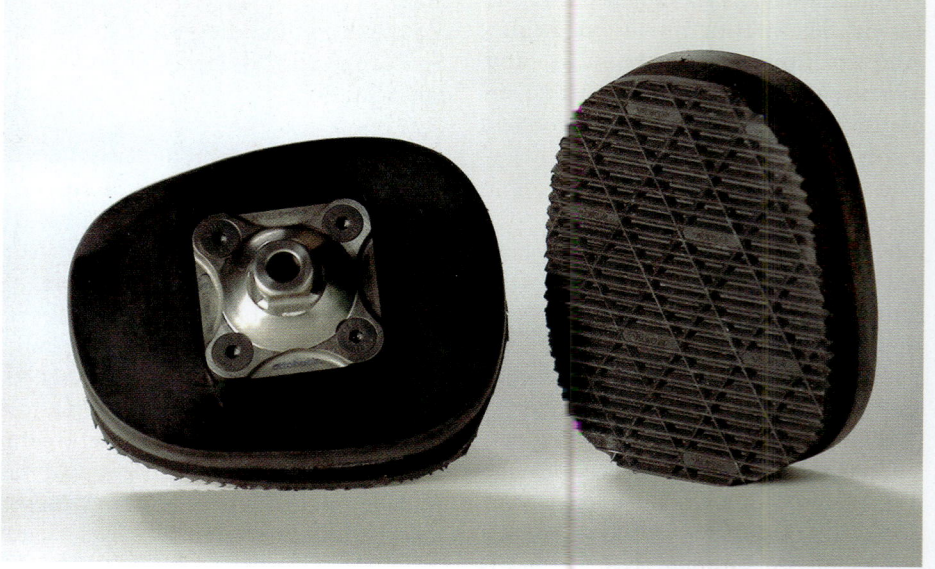

FIGURE 6 Photograph of "stubbie" feet prostheses used with the graduated length prosthetic protocol. (Courtesy of Hanger Clinic, Austin, TX.)

activity, doffing the prostheses periodically to check for any skin irritation, and redonning their prostheses. The period of activity should be increased by 1 hour daily until they are able to use their prostheses for 4 hours without skin irritation or pain. Patients should be advised to contact their prosthetist if skin irritation develops. After achieving 4 hours of use without issue, they should be able to progress to wearing the prostheses full-time, donning in the morning and doffing in the evening. Although full-time prosthetic wear is desirable, wear time is not the only determinant of success.

Careful attention should be paid to the size of the small stubbie feet described above. While larger sized pads provide more stability, they are not recommended because they make it more difficult for the wearers to walk and limit their functional progression over time. Rocker-bottom platforms that extend posteriorly from the attachment point of the pylon, and standard prosthetic feet that have been rotated backward, also give the prosthesis user too much stability. In the case of the latter, this may cause mental distress because of the unnatural appearance. Too much stability prevents the development of the dynamic balance needed to successfully transition to independent use of full-length prosthetic legs. As a user progresses to full-length prostheses, the authors generally prefer pylons without transverse torsion adapters. Fixed pylons are more stable and weigh less; however, torsion adapters may be useful if rotational forces against the residual limbs are not well tolerated by the user, or when there is a need to increase step length by allowing additional forward pelvic rotation.

As confidence, balance, core and limb strength, and the ability to fall safely increases, the prostheses are periodically made taller in 1-inch increments, based on the individual's functional progress. Small prosthetic knees that lock for standing and walking, and unlock for sitting or entering and exiting a car, are added underneath the prosthetic sockets after the pylon length becomes difficult to manage. Over time, as the individual learns to fall safely, their confidence improves. After the fear of falling is mastered, the likelihood of falling diminishes.[37]

To prepare patients for their definitive prostheses, adding weight to the short devices to simulate the weight of fully functional prosthetic knees is also helpful. Ankle weights can be secured to the pylons with fabric hook-and-loop fasteners. A small amount of weight is then added each time the length is increased until the weight of the final set of initial prostheses is the same, if not heavier, than the definitive MPKs (approximately 3.5 lb each).

Many bilateral transfemoral amputees become disappointed when the GLPP process is described because their full height is not immediately restored. This is a natural reaction, reflecting one of the stages of grief felt for the lost limbs.[38] Rather than responding negatively to their anger, clinicians should try to refocus patients' energy toward walking and gaining independence. Patients should be informed of the ultimate benefit and success of this protocol. It is important to have another person who has completed the GLPP meet with the patient to provide mentoring and encouragement to follow the protocol (**Figure 7**). It is especially helpful if the mentor demonstrates their ability to use both short and full-height prostheses.

Another benefit of the GLPP is its cost effectiveness. In addition to a high rate of success (68% of patients had success with short prostheses), it also allows the rehabilitation team to assess patients' abilities and potential before more costly prosthetic components are prescribed.[22]

There are differing views on the length of time a patient should remain in short prosthetic legs. Some clinicians fit a patient in short training prostheses for several weeks and then transition quickly to full-length prostheses for the remainder of therapy. The authors recommend gradual transitions based on achievement of functional milestones rather than a predetermined amount of time. Patients should be encouraged to become full-time users of the short prostheses, negotiating obstacles such as stairs, ramps, curbs, grass, gravel, and hills in all their daily activities, as well as walking long distances before advancing to full-height prostheses with functional knees.

Active, bilateral transfemoral prosthesis users will often find that short prostheses with stubbie feet are the preferred option for some activities (**Figure 8**). The low center of gravity and lack of articulating knees are more efficient for activities such as snowboarding, stream fishing, water park activities, mountain climbing, gardening, farming, and hunting. After

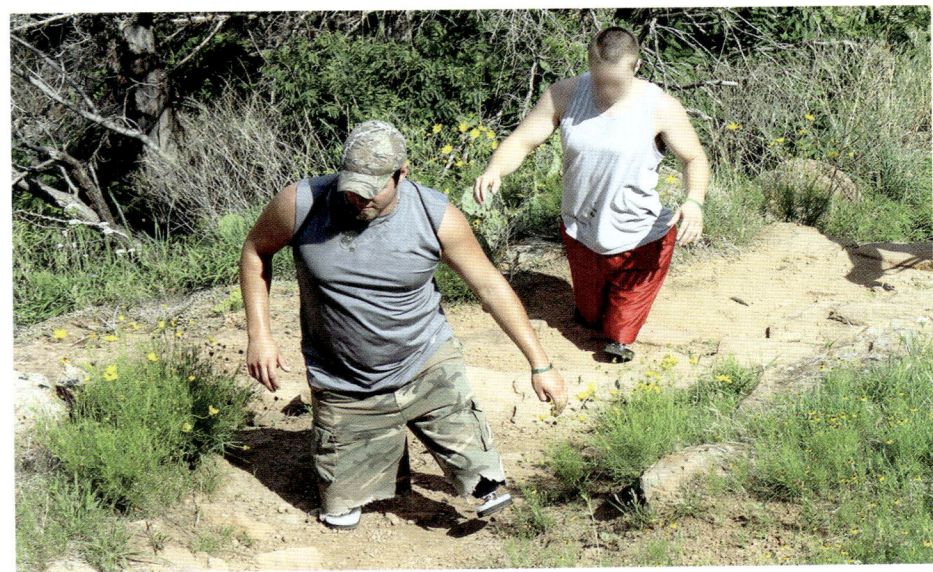

FIGURE 7 Photograph of walking using bilateral transfemoral short prostheses with a peer mentor. (Courtesy of Hanger Clinic, Austin, TX.)

Section 3: Lower Limb

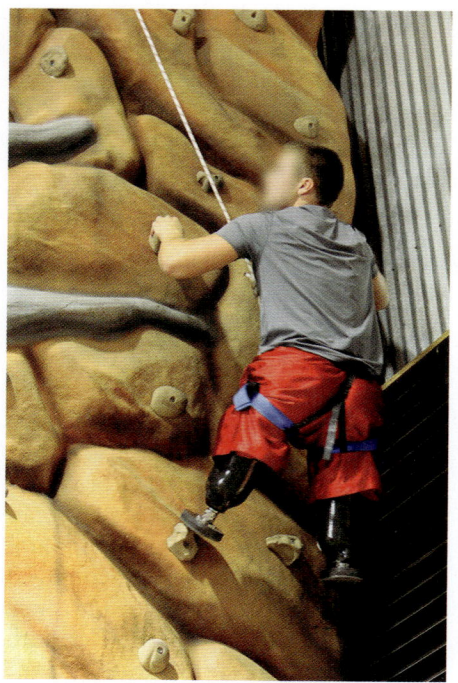

FIGURE 8 Photograph of climbing using bilateral transfemoral short prostheses. (Courtesy of Hanger Clinic, Austin, TX.)

obtaining full-height prostheses, most patients retain their short prostheses.

Slipper Prostheses

Those who have the ability to bear weight on the distal end of their residual limbs will often use protective slippers in addition to their standard prosthesis (**Figure 9, A**). These slippers can be quickly donned and doffed and are held in place with slight friction and muscle grasp. The plantar surface should be made of a high-quality rubber sole that is both durable and has good grip (**Figure 9, B**). The slippers offer protection to the limbs and allow the user to be more active without having to put on their full prosthetic sockets. Slippers are typically used indoors but sometimes, especially with children, they may be used outside, which requires that they be more rugged (**Figure 9, C**). Though they are similar to stubbies in that they allow the user to ambulate close to the ground, the trimlines of the slippers are more distal and provide less containment of proximal tissues, allowing more pressure to be applied to the distal aspect of the residual limbs (**Figure 9, D**).

Hip Disarticulation With Transfemoral Amputation

Hip disarticulation amputation is most commonly a result of combat-related injuries, but also occurs because of a traumatic motor vehicle crash or workplace injury. Those who have endured this combination of lower limb amputations also benefit from the GLPP. When following the GLPP for patients with hip disarticulation amputation, it may be best to initially use a locking prosthetic hip joint to provide increased stability for the ipsilateral hip disarticulation side. As the user's abilities improve and prosthesis length increases, the prosthetist may recommend a hip joint that closely replicates natural biomechanics.

Transtibial Amputation

Patients with bilateral transtibial amputation may initially benefit from prostheses that are somewhat shorter than full height, but not so short that it is difficult to rise from a chair. As a patient gains balance and confidence, the prostheses can be lengthened so that they are at, or close to, the patient's preamputation height. Some patients may ask to be taller than they were before their amputations. This is not recommended because the added height makes balance more difficult and places more force on the residual limbs.

Component Consideration

Selecting and Fitting the Definitive Knees

In recent years, there have been substantial advances in MPK technology (**Figure 10**), resulting in great success for users of bilateral transfemoral prostheses. Without a sound leg to depend on, patients with bilateral transfemoral amputation require the highest degree of safety and energy efficiency that only MPKs provide.[39] Patients with MPKs fall less often than those using mechanical knees.[40] A patient who falls repeatedly increases their risk of injury, loses confidence in the mechanical knees, and is less likely to become an effective prosthesis user. For bilateral amputees with the ability or potential to progress beyond fixed cadence indoor walking on level ground, MPKs should be considered the medically necessary standard of care. Higher functioning individuals with MPKs can develop the ability to walk confidently, independent of assistive devices on any terrain during activities of daily living. With training and practice, users can climb and descend stairs, walk down hills and ramps, and step-off of curbs.[41,42] Under the widely used Centers for Medicare and Medicaid Services guidelines, assessment of a patient's ability and future potential determines the selection of prosthetic technology for definitive prostheses. However, the policy states that bilateral amputees are not to be bound to the functional level classifications.[43] Documented justification for technology selection from patients' physicians and prosthetists is an important element of patient care. Assessments from physical therapists are also helpful in deciding on the most appropriate prosthetic design for each individual.

When selecting MPKs, the following design features should be considered as they specifically benefit the bilateral prosthesis user. Microprocessor-regulated hydraulic swing and stance provides consistent support when descending hills, ramps, curbs, stairs, and during sitting. MPKs that encourage stance flexion at heel strike provide biomechanical advantages over previous designs. This feature reduces the impact on patients' residual limbs and lower back, and can also decrease energy consumption[39,44] (**Figure 11**). Knees with stance extension damping provide a smooth midstance gait pattern.[44] MPKs with several additional programmable modes for specific functions allow the advanced bilateral user to pursue certain activities such as driving a car and playing sports without additional adaptations. Also preferred are smartphone apps that allow the user to change modes and to fine tune the gait characteristics of the knees.

When learning to use MPKs, patients should be provided with prostheses that are as short as possible. As patients become acclimated and more confident, their height can be increased over time. Function should outweigh body proportion considerations when

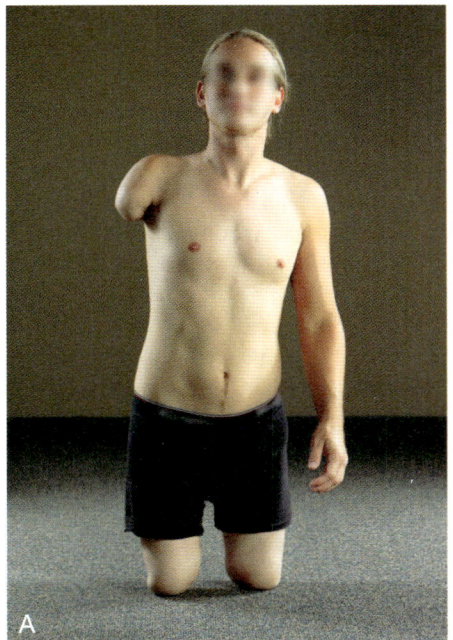 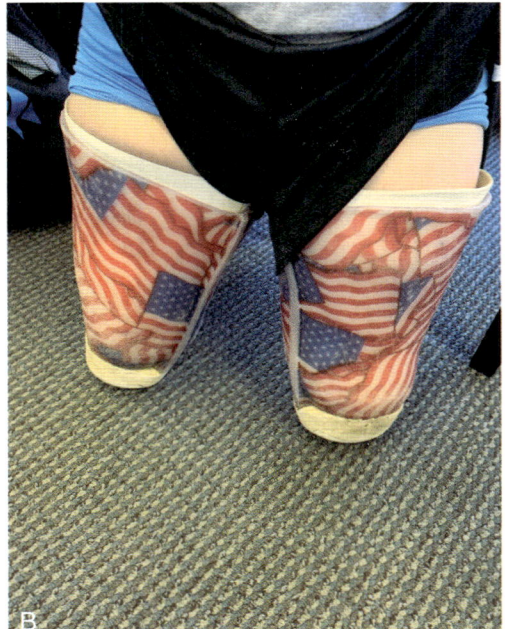 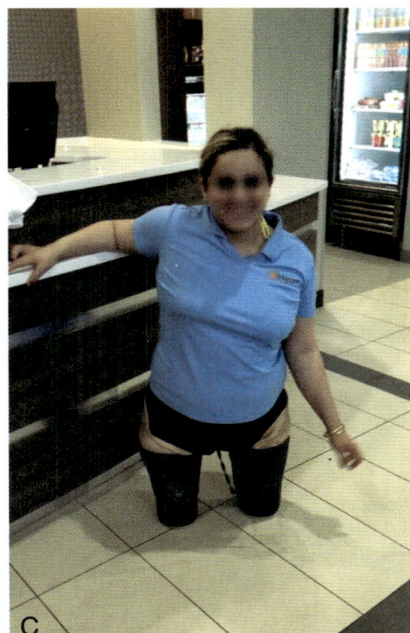
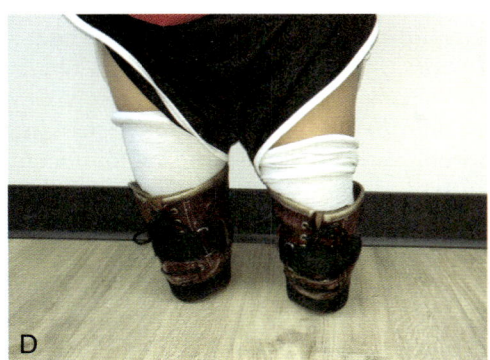

FIGURE 9 **A**, Photograph of a bilateral transfemoral amputee standing on the distal aspect of his residual limbs. **B**, Photograph of slipper prostheses showing lower trimlines and durable distal soling. **C**, Photograph of a bilateral transfemoral amputee standing inside using slipper prostheses. **D**, Photograph of leather slipper prostheses demonstrating low trimlines. (Courtesy of Hanger Clinic, Austin, TX.)

the final height of the definitive prosthesis is selected.

Because of the complexity and ongoing advances of microprocessor technology, it is best if patients choose a prosthetist who has experience in fitting and programming MPKs, and who has worked successfully with numerous transfemoral bilateral prosthesis users. Multiple interrelated variables, including height, weight, activity level, prosthetic alignment, foot selection, and general health, can affect the design of the prostheses and programming of an individual's knees. Prosthetists must avoid shortcuts by replicating their approach from one patient to another. An individualized custom approach is needed for each patient.

Positioning of Prosthetic Knee Joints

When designing the prostheses, care should be taken to position the knee joints as close as possible to the distal ends of the residual limbs. This position makes it easier and safer for rising from a chair. However, if there is a large difference in the length of the two limbs, or if both limbs are extremely short, cosmetic and comfort concerns may allow placement of one or both knees more distally from the socket. AP placement of the knees relative to the sockets is based on each patient's need for stability and range of motion at the hips. Effective alignment helps the patient achieve a balanced posture (**Figure 12**).

Selecting and Fitting the Definitive Feet and Shoes

The authors typically provide prosthetic feet that are one to three sizes smaller than a patient's previous foot size. This makes forward progression over the end of the foot easier during the toe-off phase of ambulation and allows for greater freedom of movement in tight spaces, which can be particularly difficult for these users.[45]

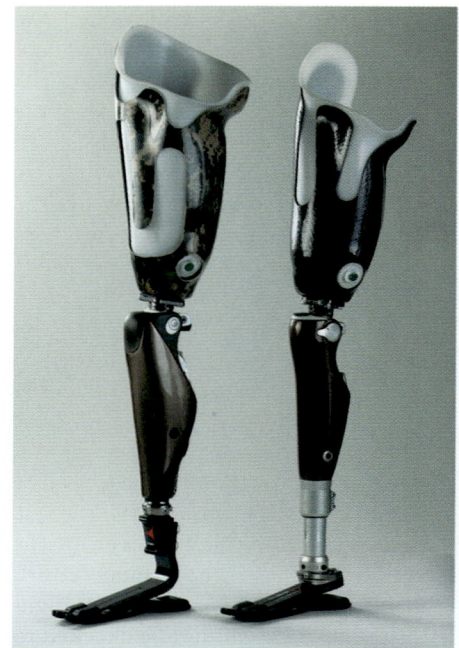

FIGURE 10 Photograph of transfemoral prostheses with microprocessor knees. (Courtesy of Hanger Clinic, Austin, TX.)

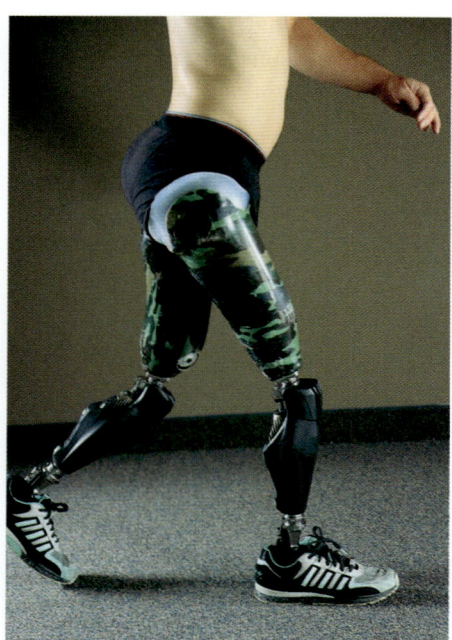

FIGURE 11 Photograph demonstrating stance flexion of the right knee using bilateral transfemoral prostheses. (Courtesy of Hanger Clinic, Austin, TX.)

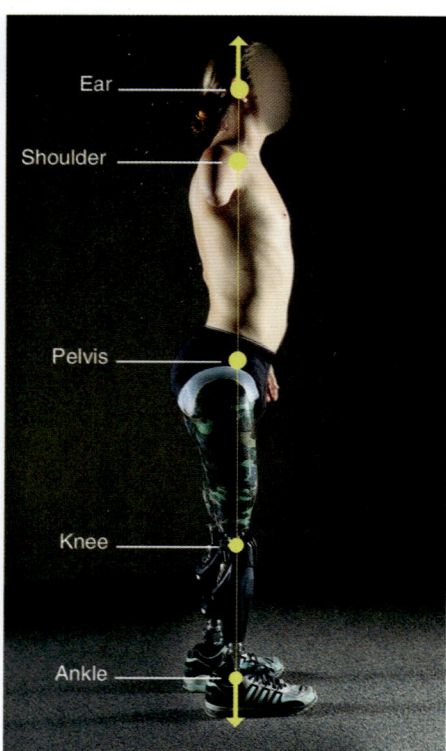

FIGURE 12 Photograph demonstrating balanced posture using bilateral transfemoral prostheses. (Courtesy of Hanger Clinic, Austin, TX.)

is relatively low. The heel allows the patient to pivot their feet over steps when descending, and it can lock onto a step during stair ascent. A soft rubber heel works better than a hard leather heel by providing force absorption at heel strike.

Microprocessor-controlled feet offer significant functional benefits, including: ground compliance, stability, reduced socket forces, and improved functional mobility on ramps and hills.[46] Some designs also provide powered plantarflexion, which supplies forward propulsion at toe-off. The drawbacks to microprocessor-controlled feet are their additional weight, limited battery life, and limited resistance to water. The capabilities of prosthetic feet and knees are expected to continue to improve as scientific discoveries are commercialized and new technologies are introduced.

Socket Design

Socket design principles are the same for unilateral and bilateral prosthesis users. However, bilateral users require greater control over their prostheses as they spend more time in double-limb support during gait and because they cannot compensate for socket issues with increased reliance on a sound limb.[45] Precisely fitting and carefully contouring the sockets around the residual limb muscles and underlying anatomy will improve stability and help prevent socket rotation. Flexible sockets with rigid outer frames are the standard of care and favored by most users.[47] Socket design must also take into account contact between the two prostheses. The added support commonly achieved in a unilateral prosthesis (by extending socket trim lines more proximally for ischial containment) may not be possible at the bilateral transfemoral level since the sockets may contact, impinging on the user's soft tissue. The gender-based observations described earlier remain key considerations in brim height and contours for these patients. Lower cut sockets can work well, as can trimming each socket at different heights to avoid contact between them. If one residual limb is longer, that side can be trimmed lower. If tolerated, subischial sockets may be indicated.[48] When this design is used, it is critical that the socket intimately contours to the residual limbs as there is reduced skeletal anatomy that would otherwise help control unwanted rotation of the prosthesis. The method of donning and doffing the prostheses also needs to be considered when designing sockets. Anatomic changes to the residual limbs are normal and expected over time because of atrophy, hypertrophy, or body weight changes. When these changes occur replacement sockets are indicated to maintain proper fit.

Suspension Options

Suspension should be selected to maximize the patient's ability to control the prostheses and improve proprioception. Secure suspension results in the most effective, efficient gait and increases the user's confidence in the stability of the prostheses. In our clinical experience,

In most cases, both feet provided are the same in terms of type and weight/activity level. Shoe choice should also be considered. It is important to have a heel on the shoe, even if it

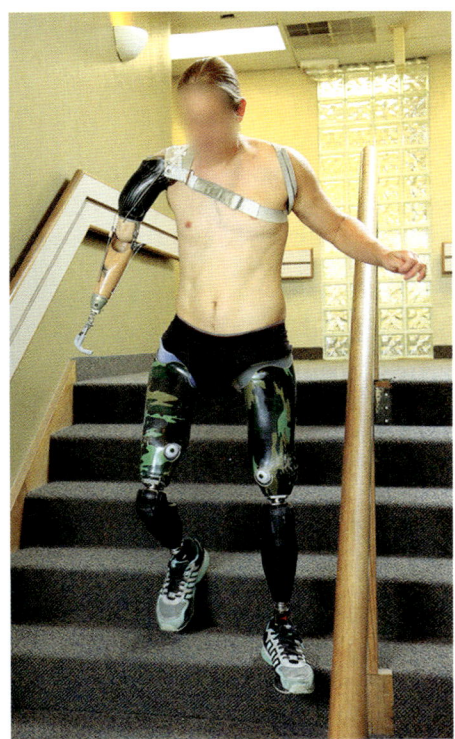

FIGURE 13 Photograph demonstrating suction fit providing secure suspension for descending stairs using bilateral transfemoral prostheses. (Courtesy of Hanger Clinic, Austin, TX.)

direct skin fit suction suspension without the use of liners is a highly effective method for bilateral transfemoral prostheses, especially for active users with mature residual limbs (**Figure 13**). Gel liners when used with suction or elevated vacuum also provide very secure suspension. Patients who present with problems such as invaginations, skin grafts, or heterotopic ossification require soft gel liners which can be customized with added padding and soft durometers. Strap and pin attachments provide less positive suspension and control than suction and vacuum, and extend the distal length of the sockets adding overall height to the prostheses. However, these may be necessary when patients cannot manage donning a suction system. If the prostheses are being used by a patient who does a minimal amount of walking and standing, straps or pins may be the easiest option. With strap and pin suspension systems, socks can also be added or removed to adjust for volume fluctuations. Some users find it difficult to position the pins into the locks. While some amputees may require caregiver assistance, it is preferred that the user be able to don and doff the prosthesis with minimal to no help from others. Upper limb amputation or impairment should be considered before selecting a suspension option. Upper limb deficits may initially add challenges that can often be overcome with training and practice. Suspension considerations for patients with bilateral transtibial amputations are the same as for unilateral prosthetic users at this amputation level.

Donning Bilateral Prostheses

A patient's ability to don the prostheses substantially enhances their independence. Patients who are missing both arms above the elbows have learned to don liners and prostheses successfully without assistance. However, donning prostheses can be ineffective and cumbersome without a clear understanding and mastery of the process. A physical or occupational therapist can teach effective donning techniques. It is generally safer for the patient, and for those nearby, to don prostheses from the floor. Patients only obtain full suspension when weight is applied through the sockets. Therefore, donning prostheses from a wheelchair can be less effective and secure. For those who cannot get to the floor, the prostheses should be retightened or redonned after a standing position is attained.

Direct Suction Systems

While sitting on the floor, preferably on a carpet, the patient applies slick donning aids (known as pull bags) onto their residual limbs (**Figure 14, A**). The patient orients the prostheses correctly and pushes the residual limbs into the sockets, making sure that undergarments will not be drawn into the sockets, unless preferred. The pull bags are fed through the valves on both sides (**Figure 14, B**). When both prosthetic legs are in place, the individual lifts the preferred leg over the other and turns around 180° with a relatively quick movement, raising up onto hands and knees, and then into a kneeling position on the prostheses (**Figure 14, C**). Using a chair for support if needed, the patient draws the pull bag out of one socket and then the other, pulling the residual limbs all the way in so there is no air remaining. The valves are inserted and locked into the sockets (**Figure 14, D**). Before standing up, the patient is advised to walk on bent knees for a few steps to allow them to feel if the prostheses are secure and in place. The patient can then rise to a standing position, using the support of a chair if needed. Standing is done by extending the stronger leg to a straight position and then powering up with arms and upper torso onto the other leg (**Figure 14, E**). After this technique is learned, the patient will be able to power up to a standing position without much effort. When standing, the rotational alignment of the knees should be checked to make sure they are in the correct positions. If not, the donning process needs to begin again.

Gel Suspension Systems

If a gel liner is used for suspension, the patient also begins the donning process on the floor or in a chair, and follows the same procedure to rise to standing. If a suction seal is used, lubricant may be applied to the seal before donning. Some patients benefit from a small amount of lotion around the proximal edge of the sockets to prevent chafing.

Osseointegrated Prostheses

Some amputees with particularly complex amputations have undergone osseointegration when all other attempts at using prostheses have failed, and no contraindications are present.[49] For multilimb amputees, osseointegration may be performed at just one site or at multiple sites, depending on the specific needs of the patient.[50] Bilateral lower limb amputees who have had osseointegration benefit from following the GLPP, and are encouraged to use stubbies at the beginning stages of the rehabilitation process.[50] Prosthetists treating these patients must work closely with the surgical team as well as the manufacturer of the osseointegration implant to minimize any risk to patient safety, and to ensure compliance with manufacturer guidelines.

Section 3: Lower Limb

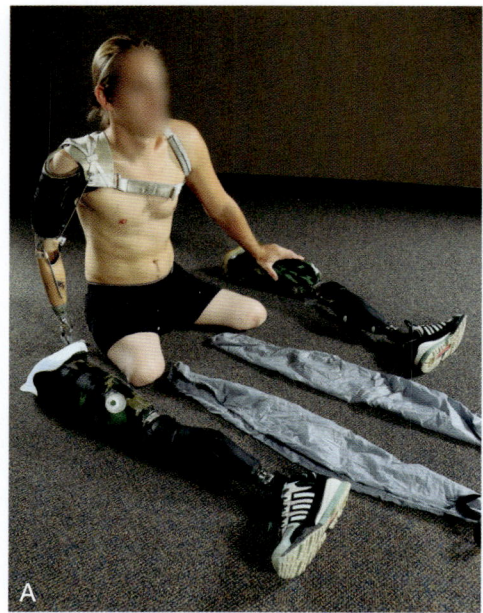
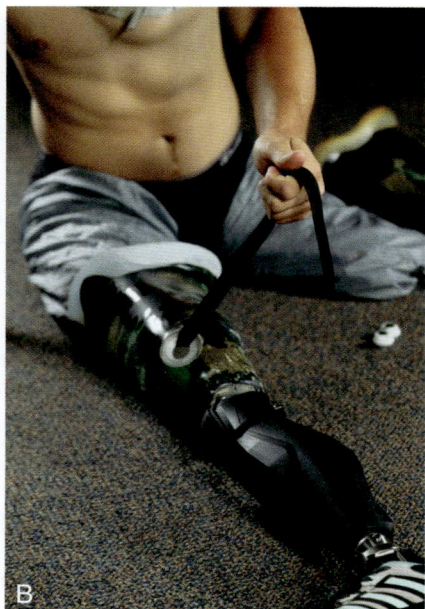
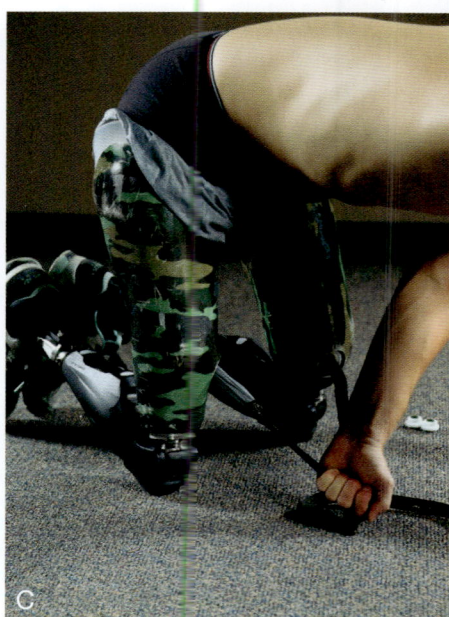
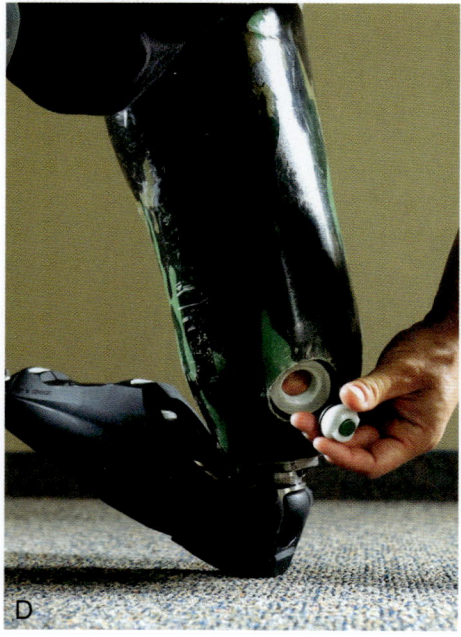
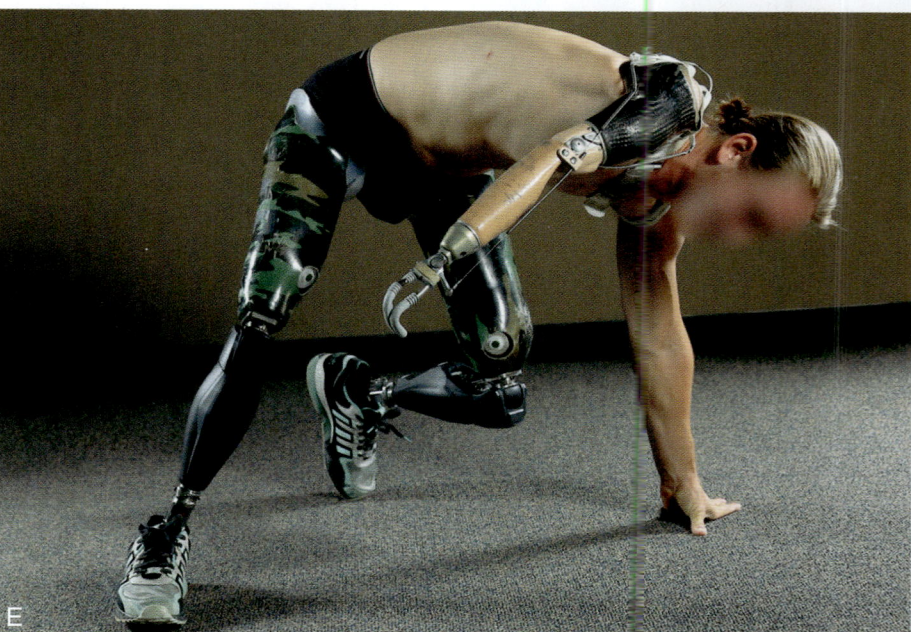

FIGURE 14 Photographs demonstrating donning bilateral transfemoral prostheses with suction sockets. **A**, The individual sits on the floor with pull bags and prostheses. **B**, The pull bags are fed through valve holes. **C**, The individual rises to a kneeling position. **D**, The suction valve is inserted. **E**, The individual rises to standing. (Courtesy of Hanger Clinic, Austin, TX.)

SUMMARY

Despite the difficult challenges faced by individuals with bilateral limb amputation, successful functional outcomes can be achieved. By combining appropriate technology with a positive mindset and continuous effort, patients can attain substantial improvements in function and quality of life. Prosthetists and other members of the rehabilitation team have an ongoing responsibility to these patients, whose independence and access to the world hinges on the ability of their healthcare team to understand their needs and continually develop innovative solutions for successful rehabilitation. Ongoing research and outcomes studies on this cohort are needed to advance technology and demonstrate the value of prosthetic care.

Acknowledgments

The authors wish to acknowledge Randall W. Richardson, ABC-CPA, RPA, for his valuable contributions to a previous edition of this chapter.

The authors would also like to thank Laura Rheinstein for her editorial assistance on this chapter and the previous edition of this chapter.

References

1. Akarsu S, Tekin L, Safaz I, Göktepe AS, Yazıcıoğlu K: Quality of life and functionality after lower limb amputations: Comparison between uni- vs. bilateral amputee patients. *Prosthet Orthot Int* 2012;37(1):9-13.

2. Li WS, Chan SY, Chau WW, Law S-W, Chan KM: Mobility, prosthesis use and health-related quality of life of bilateral lower limb amputees from the 2008 Sichuan earthquake. *Prosthet Orthot Int* 2019;43(1):104-111.

3. Stevens PM: Barriers to the implementation of evidence-based practice in orthotics and prosthetics. *J Prosthet Orthot* 2011;23(1):34-39.

4. Raya MA, Gailey RS, Gaunaurd IA, et al: Amputee mobility predictor-bilateral: A performance-based measure of mobility for people with bilateral lower-limb loss. *J Rehabil Res Dev* 2013;50(7):961-968.

5. Varma P, Stineman MG, Dillingham TR: Epidemiology of limb loss. *Phys Med Rehabil Clin N Am* 2014;25(1):1-8.

6. Izumi Y, Satterfield K, Lee S, Harkless LB: Risk of reamputation in diabetic patients stratified by limb and level of amputation: A 10-year observation. *Diabetes Care* 2006;29(3):566-570.

7. Inderbitzi R, Büttiker M, Pfluger D, Nachbur B: The fate of bilateral lower limb amputees in end-stage vascular disease. *Eur J Vasc Surg* 1992;6(3):321-326.

8. Penn-Barwell JG, Bennett PM, Kay A, Sargeant ID: Acute bilateral leg amputation following combat injury in UK servicemen. *Injury* 2014;45(7):1105-1110.

9. Gordon W, Talbot M, Fleming M, Shero J, Potter B, Stockinger ZT: High bilateral amputations and Dismounted Complex Blast Injury (DCBI). *Mil Med* 2018;183(suppl 2):118-122.

10. Potter BK, Forsberg JA, Davis TA, et al: Heterotopic ossification following combat-related trauma. *J Bone Joint Surg Am* 2010;92(suppl 2):74-89.

11. Rayegani SM, Aryanmehr A, Soroosh MR, Baghbani M: Phantom pain, phantom sensation, and spine pain in bilateral lower limb amputees: Results of a National Survey of Iraq-Iran War Victims' health status. *J Prosthet Orthot* 2010;22(3):162-165.

12. Oosterhoff M, Geertzen JHB, Dijkstra PU: More than half of persons with lower limb amputation suffer from chronic back pain or residual limb pain: A systematic review with meta-analysis. *Disabil Rehabil* 2020;44(6):835-855.

13. Canavese F, Krajbich JI, LaFleur BJ: Orthopaedic sequelae of childhood meningococcemia: Management considerations and outcome. *J Bone Joint Surg Am* 2010;92(12):2196-2203.

14. Allport T, Read L, Nadel S, Levin M: Critical illness and amputation in meningococcal septicemia: Is life worth saving? *Pediatrics* 2008;122(3):629-632.

15. Sumpio B, Shine SR, Mahler D, Sumpio BE: A comparison of immediate postoperative rigid and soft dressings for below-knee amputations. *Ann Vasc Surg* 2013;27(6):774-780.

16. Rheinstein J, Carroll K, Stevens P: Prosthetic care for the mangled extremity, in Pensy RA, Ingari JV, eds. *The Mangled Extremity: Evaluation and Management*. Springer International Publishing, 2021, pp 257-283.

17. Pauley T, Devlin M, Heslin K: Falls sustained during inpatient rehabilitation after lower limb amputation: Prevalence and predictors. *Am J Phys Med Rehabil* 2006;85(6):521-532.

18. Latlief G, Elnitsky C, Hart-Hughes S, et al: Patient safety in the rehabilitation of the adult with an amputation. *Phys Med Rehabil Clin N Am* 2012;23(2):377-392.

19. Kimble SL: Acute inpatient rehabilitation interventions and outcomes for a person with quadrilateral amputation. *Phys Ther* 2016;97(2):161-166.

20. Darter BJ, Nielsen DH, Yack HJ, Janz KF: Home-based treadmill training to improve gait performance in persons with a chronic transfemoral amputation. *Arch Phys Med Rehabil* 2013;94(12):2440-2447.

21. Lin SJ, Winston KD, Mitchell J, Girlinghouse J, Crochet K: Physical activity, functional capacity, and step variability during walking in people with lower-limb amputation. *Gait Posture* 2014;40(1):140-144.

22. Irolla C, Rheinstein J, Richardson R, Simpson C, Carroll K: Evaluation of a graduated length prosthetic protocol for bilateral transfemoral amputee prosthetic rehabilitation. *J Prosthet Orthot* 2013;25(2):84-88.

23. Wu YJ, Chen SY, Lin MC, Lan C, Lai JS, Lien IN: Energy expenditure of wheeling and walking during prosthetic rehabilitation in a woman with bilateral transfemoral amputations. *Arch Phys Med Rehabil* 2001;82(2):265-269.

24. Bilodeau S, Hébert R, Desrosiers J: Lower limb prosthesis utilisation by elderly amputees. *Prosthet Orthot Int* 2000;24(2):126-132.

25. Dyer D, Bouman B, Davey M, Ismond KP: An intervention program to reduce falls for adult in-patients following major lower limb amputation. *Healthc Q* 2008;11(3 Spec No.):117-121.

26. Coffey L, O'Keeffe F, Gallagher P, Desmond D, Lombard-Vance R: Cognitive functioning in persons with lower limb amputations: A review. *Disabil Rehabil* 2012;34(23):1950-1964.

27. Kahle JT, Highsmith MJ, Schaepper H, Johannesson A, Orendurff MS, Kaufman K: Predicting walking ability following lower limb amputation: An updated systematic literature review. *Technol Innov* 2016;18(2-3):125-137.

28. Ladlow P, Nightingale TE, McGuigan MP, Bennett AN, Phillip RD, Bilzon JLJ: Predicting ambulatory energy expenditure in lower limb amputees using multi-sensor methods. *PLoS One* 2019;14(1):e0209249.

29. Jarvis HL, Bennett AN, Twiste M, Phillip RD, Etherington J, Baker R: Temporal spatial and metabolic measures of walking in highly functional individuals with lower limb amputations. *Arch Phys Med Rehabil* 2017;98(7):1389-1399.

30. Hoffman MD, Sheldahl LM, Buley KJ, Sandford PR: Physiological comparison of walking among bilateral above-knee amputee and able-bodied subjects, and a model to account for the differences in metabolic cost. *Arch Phys Med Rehabil* 1997;78(4):385-392.

31. Batten H, Lamont R, Kuys S, McPhail S, Mandrusiak A: What are the barriers and enablers that people with a lower limb amputation experience when walking in the community? *Disabil Rehabil* 2020;42(24):3481-3487.

32. Collin C, Wade DT, Cochrane GM: Functional outcome of lower limb amputees with peripheral vascular disease. *Clin Rehabil* 1992;6(1):13-21.

33. Inderbitzi R, Buettiker M, Enzler M: The long-term mobility and mortality of patients with peripheral arterial disease following bilateral amputation. *Eur J Vasc Endovasc Surg* 2003;26(1):59-64.

34. Belon HP, Vigoda DF: Emotional adaptation to limb loss. *Phys Med Rehabil Clin N Am* 2014;25(1):53-74.

35. Kulkarni J, Wright S, Toole C, Morris J, Hirons R: Falls in patients with lower limb amputations: Prevalence and contributing factors. *Physiotherapy* 1996;82(2):130-136.

36. Perry J, Burnfield JM, Newsam CJ, Conley P: Energy expenditure and gait characteristics of a bilateral amputee walking with C-leg prostheses compared with stubby and conventional articulating prostheses. *Arch Phys Med Rehabil* 2004;85(10):1711-1717.

37. Miller WC, Deathe AB, Speechley M, Koval J: The influence of falling, fear of falling, and balance confidence on prosthetic mobility and social activity among individuals with a lower extremity amputation. *Arch Phys Med Rehabil* 2001;82(9):1238-1244.

38. Morris S: The psychological aspects of amputation, in *First Step 2003*. Amputee Coalition of America, 2003.

39. Highsmith MJ, Kahle JT, Bongiorni DR, Sutton BS, Groer S, Kaufman KR: Safety, energy efficiency, and cost efficacy of the C-Leg for transfemoral amputees: A review of the literature. *Prosthet Orthot Int* 2010;34(4):362-377.

40. Highsmith MJ, Kahle JT, Shepard NT, Kaufman KR: The effect of the C-Leg knee prosthesis on sensory dependency and falls during sensory organization testing. *Technol Innov* 2014;2013(4):343-347.

41. Aldridge Whitehead JM, Wolf EJ, Scoville CR, Wilken JM: Does a microprocessor-controlled prosthetic knee affect stair ascent strategies in persons with transfemoral amputation? *Clin Orthop Relat Res* 2014;472(10):3093-3101.

42. Burnfield JM, Eberly VJ, Gronely JK, Perry J, Yule WJ, Mulroy SJ: Impact of stance phase microprocessor-controlled knee prosthesis on ramp negotiation and community walking function in K2 level transfemoral amputees. *Prosthet Orthot Int* 2012;36(1):95-104.

43. Centers for Medicare & Medicaid Services: *LCD – Lower Limb Prostheses (L33787)*. Centers for Medicare & Medicaid Services, 2020. Accessed September 2, 2021. https://www.cms.gov/medicare-coverage-database/view/lcd.aspx?LCDId=33787

44. Thiele J, Westebbe B, Bellmann M, Kraft M: Designs and performance of microprocessor-controlled knee joints. *Biomed Tech* 2014;59(1):65-77.

45. Carroll MK, Carroll KM, Rheinstein J, Highsmith MJ: Functional differences of bilateral transfemoral amputees using full-length and stubby-length prostheses. *Technol Innov* 2018;20(1-2):75-83.

46. Wurdeman SR, Stevens PM, Campbell JH: Mobility analysis of AmpuTees (MAAT 5): Impact of five common prosthetic ankle-foot categories for individuals with diabetic/dysvascular amputation. *J Rehabil Assist Technol Eng* 2019;6:2055668318820784.

47. Gholizadeh H, Abu Osman NA, Eshraghi A, et al: Transtibial prosthetic suspension: Less pistoning versus easy donning and doffing. *J Rehabil Res Dev* 2012;49(9):1321-1330.

48. Fatone S, Caldwell R, Angelico J, et al: Comparison of ischial containment and subischial sockets on comfort, function, quality of life, and satisfaction with device in persons with unilateral transfemoral amputation: A randomized crossover trial. *Arch Phys Med Rehabil* 2021;102(11):2063-2073.e2.

49. McMenemy L, Ramasamy A, Sherman K, et al: Direct skeletal fixation in bilateral above knee amputees following blast: 2 year follow up results from the initial cohort of UK service personnel. *Injury* 2020;51(3):735-743.

50. Hagberg K: Bone-anchored prostheses in patients with traumatic bilateral transfemoral amputations: Rehabilitation description and outcome in 12 cases treated with the OPRA implant system. *Disabil Rehabil Assist Technol* 2019;14(4):346-353.

Osseointegration: Surgical Management

CHAPTER 47

Munjed Al Muderis, MB ChB, FRACS, FAOrthA, DMedSc
Jonathan A. Forsberg, MD, PhD, FAAOS

ABSTRACT

The interface between native tissue and the prosthetic limb presents the greatest challenge to amputee rehabilitation. Skin–socket interface problems, mobility and fit, and lack of proprioception are common obstacles which contribute to the failure of traditional socket-based prostheses in selected patients. Osseointegration for amputees is a revolutionary technique that involves anchoring a metal implant directly to a patient's skeleton, then permanently passing it through the patient's skin, which is connected to a prosthetic limb. By doing this, the weight of the prosthesis is borne by the patient's skeleton and is directly powered by muscles, leading to a lighter and more natural experience. The skin is no longer compressed and traumatized, eliminating the aforementioned issues. This procedure can improve the lives of appropriately selected patients who cannot tolerate traditional, socket-based prostheses. Osseointegration should be viewed as a combined surgical and rehabilitation program that requires close collaboration between surgeons, rehabilitation specialists, physical therapists, and prosthetists. The requirements to achieve long-term success include good surgical technique to minimize motion at the skin–implant interface and controlled rehabilitation with graded loading. Over the past decade, osseointegration for amputees has become more widely accepted as a valid rehabilitation option for amputees rather than being a novel procedure, and it is anticipated that it may become the benchmark for the management of amputees.

Keywords: amputation; osseointegration; skin–implant interface; trauma

Dr. Al Muderis or an immediate family member has received royalties from Medacta International SA and Osseointegration International Pty Ltd; serves as a paid consultant to or is an employee of Mobius Medical, Osseointegration International Pty Ltd, and Specifica Pty Ltd; serves as an unpaid consultant to Aesculap/B.Braun; has stock or stock options held in Osseointegration International Pty Ltd; and serves as a board member, owner, officer, or committee member of NeuRA Neuroscience Research Australia. Dr. Forsberg or an immediate family member serves as a paid consultant to or is an employee of Solsidan Group, LLC; serves as an unpaid consultant to Zimmer; and has stock or stock options held in Prognostix AB.

This chapter is adapted from Brånemark R: Osseointegration: Surgical management, in Krajbich JI, Pinzur MS, Potter BK, Stevens PM, eds: *Atlas of Amputations and Limb Deficiencies: Surgical, Prosthetic, and Rehabilitation Principles*, ed 4. American Academy of Orthopaedic Surgeons, 2016, pp 575-582.

Introduction

The first documented successful implementation of a transcutaneous skeletal device may have been Malgaigne's double-sided hook. Designed in 1840, this construct penetrated the patient's skin and clamped the superior and inferior poles of the patella, providing compression through a fracture. In 1843, Malgaigne[1] developed an early type of external fixation by applying a transdermal implant to fix a fracture, in which metal penetrated both skin and bone. Later, a more recognizable external fixation instrumentation was described by Codivilla and Steinmann between 1903 and 1910.[2-6] External fixation is an accepted form of treatment of some fractures, as well as a mainstay in the field of deformity correction and limb lengthening, albeit for a temporary period of time. The problem is not necessarily the bone–implant interface, which remains stable after true osseointegration occurs. Rather, difficulties remain with the soft tissue–implant interface, particularly if excessive motion exists between them.

Background and Outcomes

As reviewed by Murphy,[7] experimental work on bone fixation of external limb prostheses in the past has been sporadic and performed on a small scale. The first documented skeletally linked transcutaneous prosthetic attempts were likely the pilot studies performed by Cutler and Blodgett[8] as early as 1942 at Harvard University. These surgeons tested stainless steel and vitallium screws inserted

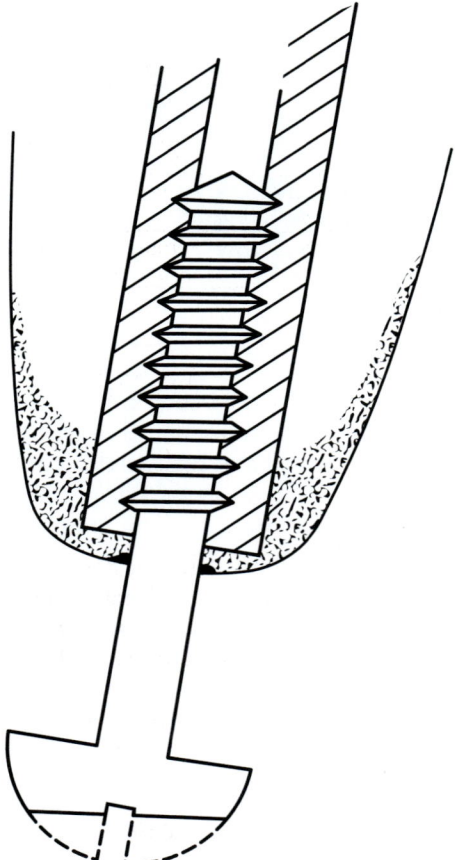

FIGURE 1 Schematic illustration of an osseointegration implant used experimentally in dogs.

into the intramedullary canal of 18 dogs (**Figure 1**). Vitallium retained better stability, and the researchers determined that the implant must remain motionless relative to the bone to prevent loosening.[7,8] By 1949, the United States Veterans Administration felt the surgical challenges for success in humans were too great and suspended further investigation.

In 1946, Dümmer in Pinneberg, Germany,[7] studied metal-implanted limb extensions in sheep and extended the study to human patients, four of whom had prostheses attached to metal implants. When one implant became infected, the study was discontinued, and all the implants were removed.

In the United States, Mooney et al[9] fitted a prosthesis to the humerus of an individual in 1967 who had three amputations. The implant was removed around 8 months later, after signs of deep infection developed. Esslinger[10] performed a further study of penetrating implants in dogs; Hall,[11] and Hall et al[12] achieved considerable success with penetrating implants that were inserted into the hindlimbs of Spanish goats. In 20 goats, only two implants failed over 14 months, during which time the animals were very active.

These data provided little encouragement for further studies until an unrelated observation by Brånemark[13] suggested the possibility of long-term tolerance of a transdermal metal implant. Brånemark[13] was studying the microcirculation within bone, which involved the insertion of an observation tube into the bone marrow of the tibia of a rabbit. The optical device was made of titanium and was found to be almost impossible to remove after several weeks of study because the titanium appeared to have "integrated" with the bone. This was a breakthrough discovery in the material science of osseointegration, which led to extensive studies involving a team of researchers led by Brånemark in Gothenburg, Sweden, in association with the Department of Orthopaedics at the University of Gothenburg showing that commercially pure titanium was well tolerated within living bone and relatively resistant to infection.[14-17] Titanium forms a resistant surface oxide layer, which in living tissue can be augmented by a peroxide layer. This peroxide layer is thought to be a hydrated titanium peroxy matrix that does not tolerate surface pathogenic activity, does not inhibit endothelial cells or osteocytes, but inhibits macrophages. This characteristic allows the material to be tolerated in living bone without the interposition of a fibrous tissue layer, so, according to Brånemark et al[14] and Linder et al,[18] this close contact has been termed osseointegration with the implanted material.

Another important property to achieve osseointegration is the implant surface roughness divided into three levels depending on the scale of the features.[19,20] Macrolevel roughness is related to the implant geometry which is essential for early mechanical stability. Microlevel roughness maximizes the interlocking between mineralized bone and the surface of the implant. At the nano-scale, the more textured surface increases surface energy, which increases osteoclastic cell proliferation, differentiation, and adherence.

Based on the abovementioned characteristics, two different implant systems were established; both systems share the microlevel and nano-scale features but differ in the macrostructures. Early in the 1980s, a screw-fixation device was used for dental implants, and the same structure was implanted in 1990 into the femoral residuum of an amputee. The osseointegrated prostheses for the rehabilitation of amputees (OPRA) screw fixation implant system remains the oldest commercially available osseointegration device to date. On the other hand, hip arthroplasty uses a press-fit implant design in the femoral shaft relying on a specific macrostructure geometry that allows early axial and rotational stability of the implant. This led to the development of the osseointegrated prosthetic limb (OPL) implant system in Australia in 2010, which is the most widely used osseointegration implant to date worldwide. These are the predominant design philosophies of the most widely used osseointegration implants.

The optimal transcutaneous implant surface coating is another area of ongoing research. While current work is focusing on the significance of bioresponsive, endogenously triggered, surface additives to reduce infection risk at the intramedullary implant interface, the abutment–soft tissue interface is an important area of focus considering that most infections occur at this interface. Though published work to date has not yet revealed any important benefit from surface coating or treatment at the intramedullary implant level, the OPL system introduced a highly polished surface with a titanium niobium oxynitride coating to provide bacteria-repellant properties at the abutment–soft tissue interface.[21]

The skin–implant interface has been the greatest challenge for osseointegration. Numerous studies have been conducted at the interface between the skin and the penetrating metal. Two divergent philosophies have been tested, one attempting to provide a full seal of the skin–implant interface,[22] and the other recognizing the development of the long-term stoma, or skin penetration site. To seal the implant–tissue interface, several techniques have been used including acrylate adhesives which provided only temporary attachment to the metal surface, and titanium gauze and textile meshes of various polymers which provided a degree of cellular invasion into mesh materials, with no success. A porous titanium transdermal surface has also been used but was later abandoned because of poor results.[22] None of these techniques has yet provided any clinical advantage over the simple skin perforation of surgically stabilized soft tissues over a smooth abutment[23] used in both the OPRA and OPL systems.

In a recent evaluation of 51 patient with transfemoral amputation who were treated with the OPRA (Integrum) implant system and followed for a minimum of 2 years, before-and-after assessments demonstrated statistically significant improvements in prosthetic use, mobility, and functional status—plus fewer problems—compared with their previous socket-based prostheses.[24] As expected, superficial infections were the most frequent complications. Twenty-eight of the 51 patients (55%) had one or more superficial infections that, without further complications, were successfully treated with antibiotics. Deep infections developed in four patients (8%), and in one of these patients, the infection loosened the fixture. However, in the remaining three patients, the fixtures were retained. In three of four patients, aseptic loosening was the reason for implant loosening. Most of the femurs demonstrated some degree of radiographic bone resorption. However, no periprosthetic fractures occurred, and no correlation to impaired rehabilitation results or implant loosening could be found. Instead, in accordance with previous experiences from oral applications, radiographic bone resorption seemed to diminish with time.

In another study, Al Muderis et al[25] reported on 86 patients (91 implants) using the pressfit system with a minimum 2-year follow-up examining the safety of osseointegrated implants for transfemoral amputees which demonstrated 36% uneventful course without complications, 34% one or more infections, and 30% had other complications but no infection. Hence a grading system for the classification of infection was devised, graded as 1 to 4 in severity, and categories A to C in recommended management (Table 1). The results show grade 1A in 27% of patients which is regarded as 87% of all infections, grades 1B and 1C in one patient each (1% of patients individually), and 5% grade 2C infection. There were no grade 3 or 4 infections. Other complications were described as stoma hypergranulation (20%), redundant soft tissues (16%), periprosthetic fractures (3%), hardware breakage (2%), and failure of osseointegration requiring revision (1%). A smaller retrospective study of 22 patients who received the OPL implant showed a significant improvement in short-term clinical outcomes in postoperative quality-of-life and function, with low associated risk of severe adverse events.[26]

There are three design paradigms for currently relevant osseointegration implants: a threaded screw, a press-fit intramedullary stem, and a spring-loaded platform inducing constant compression.[27] The key design and surgical features of each are described below and summarized in Table 2.

Engineering alone is insufficient to mitigate all complications related to the use of a surgical device, and careful attention to the surgical technique is arguably as important. Given that the OPRA system by Brånemark and the OPL system by Al Muderis have well-defined protocols, outcomes, and published data, the focus will be on these two systems.

Threaded Screw Implant—The OPRA System

The OPRA system has been extensively used for dental prosthetics, maxillofacial reconstructions, prosthetic ears, and hearing aids. In the field of limb prosthetics, phalangeal and metacarpal implants have been used for patients with digital (finger and toe) amputations and have been particularly effective for thumb prostheses. Radial and ulnar implants have been used for patients with forearm amputations, with humeral implants being used for patients with upper arm amputations. All of these patients were treated with custom-designed implant systems.

In the lower limb, implants in the residual femur for patients with transfemoral amputations represent most of the patients treated, and the OPRA system (Figure 2) is available on an off-the-shelf basis for this amputation level (it is not currently available for other lower limb levels). Because of the high loading imposed by lower limb prosthetic use, load is slowly and progressively applied. From commencement of loading to the unrestricted use of a prosthesis without aids may take 6 to

TABLE 1 Comparison of Osseointegration Implant Systems

	OPRA	ILP	OPL	Compress
Material	Titanium	Cobalt chrome molybdenum	Titanium	Titanium
Retention	Threaded	Press fit	Press fit	Cross pin
Anatomic suitability	Long bones, digits	Long bones	Long bones, pelvis	Humerus, femur
Bone-implant interface	Laser etch	Czech hedgehog 1.5 mm	Plasma spray up to 0.5 mm	Porous coat, axial compression
Skin–implant interface	Polished	Polished	Polished	Polished
Surgical stages	2	1	1	1
Months from implantation to full weight bearing	3-18	2-3	2-3	Unspecified

ILP = integral leg prosthesis, OPL = osseointegrated prosthetic limb, OPRA = osseointegrated prostheses for the rehabilitation of amputees

TABLE 2 Classification of Infection

Level of Severity	Symptoms and Signs	Treatment	Grade
Low-grade soft-tissue infection	Cellulitis with signs of inflammation (redness, swelling, warmth, stinging, pain, pain that increases on loading, tense)		1
		Oral antibiotics	1A
		Parenteral antibiotics	1B
		Surgical intervention	1C
High-grade soft-tissue infection	Pus collection, purulent discharge, raised level of C-reactive protein		2
		Oral antibiotics	2A
		Parenteral antibiotics	2B
		Surgical intervention	2C
Bone infection	Radiographic evidence of osteitis (periosteal bone reaction), radiographic evidence of osteomyelitis (sequestrum and involucrum)		3
		Oral antibiotics	3A
		Parenteral antibiotics	3B
		Surgical intervention	3C
Implant failure	Radiographic evidence of loosening	Parenteral antibiotics, explantation	4

The fixture, or implant, that is inserted into the medullary cavity of the residual long bone consists of a tubular component with a self-tapping thread on its surface to engage the endosteal cortex. The fixture serves as the connecting point for the abutment, which penetrates the skin of the residual limb and protrudes to permit attachment of the artificial limb.

The abutment is located in the lower end of the implant in a hexagonal recess and retained by a long retaining bolt, passing through the abutment, to engage an internal threaded section in the lower portion of the implant. When in place, the head of the retaining bolt forms the lowest point of the protruding abutment. This arrangement enables the abutment to be changed, from time to time, without disturbing the implant itself. A damaged abutment can be replaced in an outpatient setting, without anesthetic. If use of the system has to be discontinued, the abutment alone can be removed, and the penetration site heals rapidly.

Achieving osseointegration, that is, the direct attachment of bone to the titanium fixture, is critical to the success of any implant based on the OPRA system. The time needed for bone ingrowth to develop is currently 3 to 6 months in the residual femur, 3 months in a humerus or a digit, and even less time in a dental implant. This particular implant requires a two-stage surgical procedure to establish the system in the affected limb. During the first stage, the implant is placed within the bone, and the skin and soft tissues are closed. During the second stage, the scar is reopened, the skin penetration site is carefully prepared, and the abutment is placed in readiness for attachment of the training aids that precede use of the limb prosthesis.

Clinical Management

The management and rehabilitation of patients with a transfemoral amputation treated with osseointegration in the United Kingdom have been described by Sullivan et al.[30] Their system, with minor variations, has now been used in several countries around the world.

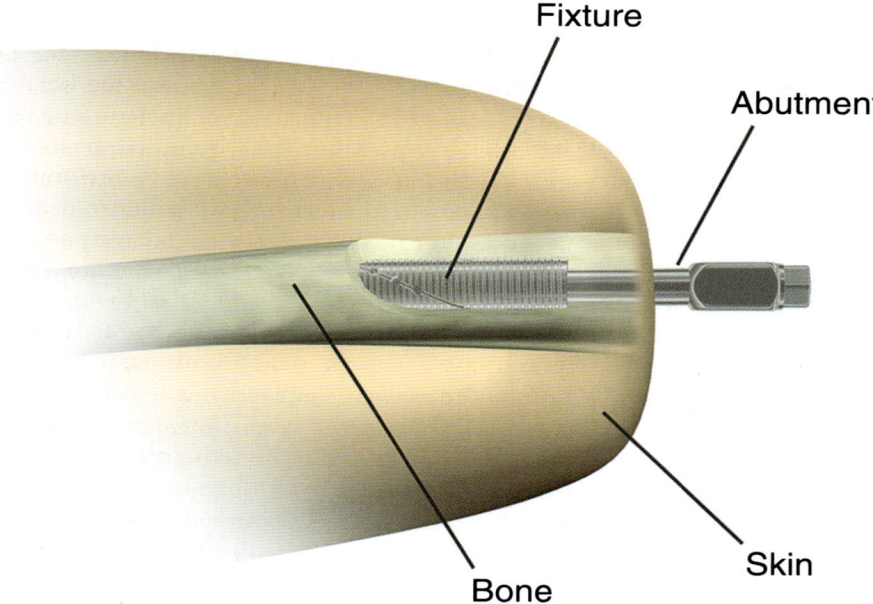

FIGURE 2 Illustration of the OPRA™ Implant System with the titanium threaded fixture, the skin-penetrating abutment, and the retaining screw. (Courtesy of Integrum, Mölndal, Sweden.)

12 months, depending on the patient's body weight and initial bone quality.

All the implant components were originally fabricated from commercially pure titanium to avoid any potential electrolytic effects or effects from the alloy; for this reason, stronger titanium alloys were not used in the system. The instruments used to handle these components also were manufactured from the same titanium. More recently, based on basic research[28] and clinical practice over the past 10 years, stronger alloys are being used. In 2011, laser etching surface finishing was added to improve osseointegration.[29]

The most current information is provided to each potential patient in a pamphlet and with preliminary clinic consultation. Then each patient's medical advisors should be consulted to obtain their approval and referral. A further consultation and discussion is performed to decide if the patient should proceed to a residential assessment, in which each member of the multidisciplinary team can contribute to the assessment so that the patient can obtain all the available information on which to make their decision to take part in the clinical study. An extensive network of patients treated with the OPRA system allows each prospective patient to visit with an individual who has undergone osseointegration, which is an important factor in ensuring that realistic expectations are maintained. Because the clinical and rehabilitation program is approximately 18 months in duration, the patient must be certain that the benefits will outweigh the risks and financial difficulties, particularly because employment may not be possible during the training period after the second stage of the procedure.

In general, patients who have factors that interfere with bone and soft-tissue healing should be excluded from the clinical study. Medications such as steroids, immunosuppressants, and chemotherapy regimens serve as criteria for exclusion. In addition, age older than 70 years, together with adverse factors such as heavy smoking, a body mass index greater than 30 kg/m^2, and personality or psychiatric disorders that might lead to failure to accept or follow the treatment protocol are also contraindications. Local factors in the residual limb must be considered, including poor bone quality or atrophy, residual and/or chronic osteomyelitis, metabolic bone disease, inadequate residual bone length to contain the fixture, degenerative hip or shoulder joint disease, and/or fixed flexion deformity of the hip.

Patients who will particularly benefit from osseointegration are those who are unable to tolerate a conventional socket prosthesis. Those with short residual limbs and bilateral transfemoral amputations are good candidates. A survey of individuals with transfemoral amputations has shown that many accept discomfort and poor function from their socket prostheses.[31] With further experience with the technique, the positive indications for the OPRA system may widen, particularly in the setting of oncologic diagnoses.

Preoperative Preparation

Before the first surgical procedure, CT is used to evaluate the skeleton of the residual femur or humerus. The spiral CT scan on a skeletal setting is set for 1-mm cuts across the entire length of the site of the implant and 3-mm cuts for the remainder of the femur. The limb must be securely immobilized during the entire scan, and the axis must be maintained constantly at 90° to the plane of the cuts. Three-dimensional reconstructions may be helpful in the case of abnormal bones.

The implant is placed where it has the optimum contact with the compact cortical bone of the femoral shaft, where the self-tapping screw thread engages to a depth of 1.5 mm over the maximum surface area of the implant. The usual diameter in a male transfemoral patient is approximately 16 to 20 mm. For the male transhumeral patient, a typical diameter is 13 to 15 mm at the mid-diaphyseal level. The optimal length of the femur or the humerus is determined from radiographs. Any shortening necessary will be performed during the first stage; if possible, at least 18 cm will be needed from the end of the residual bone to the level of the opposite knee joint line for the attachment components.

The surgical preparation is similar to that of any major orthopaedic procedure in which a prosthesis is to be implanted. The preoperative laboratory evaluation should include a complete blood count and coagulation studies. Other measures of indolent infection, such as the C-reactive protein level or the erythrocyte sedimentation rate are not routinely obtained. Low-molecular-weight heparin prophylaxis is generally used, and perioperative intravenous antibiotics are given as per institutional guidelines. The patient's blood group should be known, and an on-site transfusion facility should be used; however, transfusion is rarely required.

Surgical Procedure

First Stage

Either epidural or general anesthesia is satisfactory; however, the preference is not to use neuraxial anesthesia because of a somewhat increased risk of urinary tract infections, so general anesthesia is often used. The patient is positioned prone on the operating table with a bump under the ipsilateral hip. The limb is prepped and draped free in the typical sterile fashion. The table should permit image intensifier imaging of the surgical limb. Monopolar and bipolar electrocautery are used, and saline irrigation with suction is used as needed. Whenever possible, gravity irrigation is preferable to pulse lavage methods. Specimen containers to collect the reamings (bone graft material) should be available.

In most patients, the scar from the definitive amputation is excised, and the original full-thickness skin flaps are raised. The muscle near the bone end is cleared to reveal the bone end. The femur or the humerus is resected at the optimal length. No further soft-tissue refashioning is performed at this stage, unless absolutely necessary; such refashioning is typically addressed during the second-stage procedure.

The bone end is exposed, the femoral medullary cavity is identified, and the muscles are split proximally to expose the femoral shaft 5 to 6 cm above the bone end. In this area, the clamp of the introducer jig is applied when a provisional alignment with the bone end is fixed. Using the jig, the femoral canal is entered, and alignment is checked with the image intensifier. With this alignment, the femoral canal medullary cavity is bored with hand reamers to the diameter planned from the CT scan. With slow rotation and frequent saline irrigation, bone heating is carefully avoided. The hazard of bone damage from heating has been documented.[32] Alignment is checked using biplanar fluoroscopy until the implant is ready to be received.

The implant is mounted on its introducer, which is then placed onto the guide used for the reaming process. The introducer acts as a shaft to drive the implant mounted on the proximal end powered by the "T" handle at the other end. Some skill and strength are required to screw the implant into its planned position; if the rotation is stopped, the implant may bind despite lubrication with blood and saline. The rate of rotation is slow to minimize the chance of bone damage by heating. When the implant is in place, the position is checked again, with the image intensifier images recorded for future reference.

The fixture has a central boring that is closed by a central screw tightened to 80 N-cm using a special torque wrench. The distal lumen of the implant is thoroughly cleansed with saline irrigation before the healing screw and cylinder are inserted from below to close the lower part of the lumen of the implant and preserve the internal thread and later to accept the abutment-retaining bolt. Bone graft is placed directly under the bone graft screw and washer. The displaced muscle and soft tissue are sutured into place using absorbable suture, and the skin is closed with suction drainage. A normal residual limb compression dressing is applied in a herringbone fashion.

The patient usually makes a rapid recovery; the residual limb remains in a resting position until the suction drain is removed after 24 hours. At this time, full activity is resumed. Most patients have been unable to use an artificial limb and recommence crutch walking until postoperative swelling has subsided, normally within 4 to 6 weeks. At that time, a conventional artificial limb can be worn if this was possible before the procedure. However, it is of prime importance that hip flexion contracture does not develop, so a supervised exercise program should be started, and so-called bottoming out within the prosthetic socket is to be avoided to protect the bone graft washer and screw. Early activity and discharge from the hospital are encouraged.

In the 3 to 6 months that pass before the second-stage procedure is performed, patients are encouraged to maintain a high level of physical fitness.

Weight gain must be avoided, and anything that compromises bone healing is discouraged, including smoking, substance abuse, and excess alcohol consumption. A normal mixed diet is recommended, with calcium and vitamin D supplementation. The use of NSAIDs is not recommended during the healing process.

Second Stage
The preoperative management for the second stage is the same as for the first-stage procedure, with antibiotic prophylaxis and anticoagulant administration.

The previous surgical scar is excised or reopened to allow full-thickness skin and subcutaneous tissue flaps to be raised. The estimated site for the penetration of the abutment will be carefully marked when the final myofascial cutaneous flaps are created. Important considerations include the need for healthy normal skin with adequate blood supply, without compromise from previous scars.[33] To ensure adequate blood supply for the flap or flaps, excessive or extensive mobilization or tissue separation should be avoided. The dissection is carried to the bone end, and the graft screw is revealed.

If the first-stage procedure did not produce an effective myoplasty or myodesis, one must be created to retain the function of the residual muscles, particularly those responsible for adduction.[34] Redundant soft tissue is trimmed, and muscle is strongly sutured to the distal periosteum and the opposing muscle to effect a strong myoplasty located at but not covering the bone end. In early cases, a true myodesis was performed using multiple small drill holes at the bone end, but this proved to impair healing at the transdermal site. The bone end should be flat, smooth, and clear of periosteum, with rounded edges to produce a maximum area of living bone for adhesion to the skin at the penetration site.

The position of the penetration mark is checked when the flap is reduced over residual bone. Next, the inside of the flap at this site is thinned over an area corresponding with the bone end in the manner of a

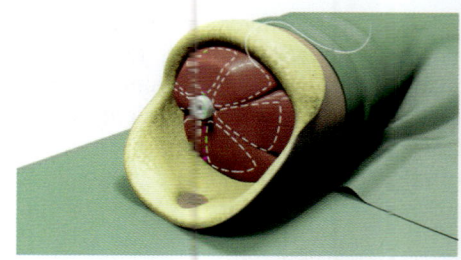

FIGURE 3 Schematic illustration of the second-stage soft-tissue procedure Note that in the area where penetration is to be created, the subcutaneous fat was removed until the follicles were just visible.

full-thickness skin graft. The edge of a glass slide is an effective scraper for achieving this thinning. Subcutaneous fat is removed from the undersurface until the follicles are just visible (**Figure 3**). The graft screw and healing cylinder are removed, and the selected abutment is checked for size and fit. In some cases, considerable cleansing and irrigation are required to clear the lumen of the lower implant. The penetration site is made using an 8-mm dermatology punch biopsy to accommodate the 11-mm abutment in the femur, and a 6-mm punch is used to accommodate a 10-mm abutment in the humerus (**Figure 4**). Considerable care is needed to attach soft tissue to residual bone, which is done to prevent motion or tension at the skin–implant interface while not impeding the necessary blood flow to ensure healing of the dermis to the underlying bone.[35] Interrupted, subcuticular stitches composed of 2-0 (femur) and 2-0 or 3-0 synthetic monofilament absorbable suture are used to suture the skin in two concentric circles around the penetration site. Each circle is lightly sutured to locate the flap without any tension on the penetration site. Buttonholing is strictly avoided. The sutures are placed so the prepared skin hole is centered on the hole in the bone. The abutment is passed through the penetration in the skin flap and seated in the hexagonal socket at the lower end of the implant. The abutment retaining bolt is then introduced into the lower end of the abutment and advanced to engage the threaded part of the lumen of the implant, and it is screwed finger-tight at this stage.

For the incision, skin closure is performed in a layered fashion, as previously done, with suction drainage. It should be remembered that a

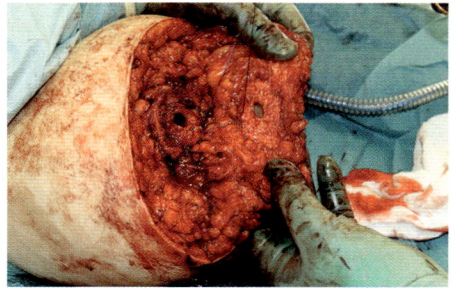

FIGURE 4 Intraoperative photograph showing the penetration site, which is made just before suturing the skin penetration site to the residual bone. Note that the penetration site is made using an 8-mm dermatology punch biopsy to accommodate an 11-mm abutment in the femur in lower limb procedures and a 6-mm punch to accommodate a 10-mm abutment in the humerus in upper limb procedures.

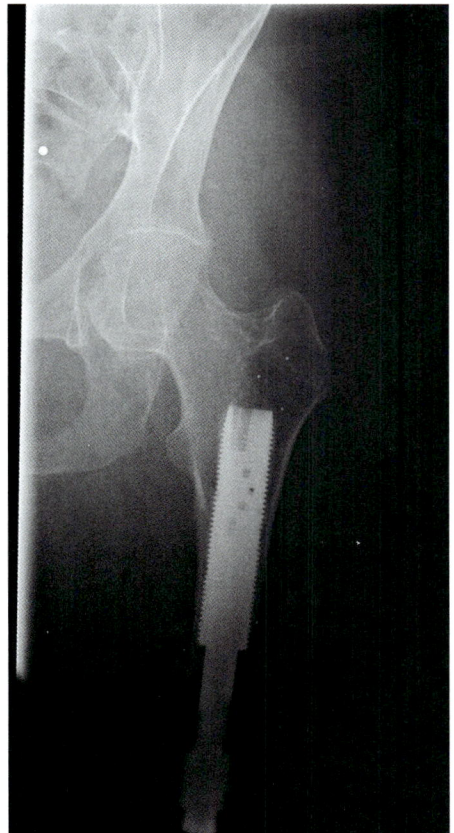

FIGURE 5 AP radiograph of the distal femur demonstrating a well-fixed OPRA implant consisting of a fixture, an abutment, and an abutment screw.

hematoma could compromise the viability of the skin at the penetration site. Furthermore, the suction effect of the drainage might help to keep the skin in contact with the bone. The abutment bolt is tightened to a torque value of 12 Nm. The penetration site is dressed with paraffin gauze, and the residual limb is dressed with a fluffed gauze, light-pressure bandage. A dressing cylinder is provided to fit on the stem of the abutment and retain the penetration dressing. This 10-cm diameter cylinder is secured by a slide to the abutment shaft, which allows it to be easily removed for dressing change. It is important to monitor the pressure exerted by the dressing to avoid skin necrosis at the penetration site. Radiography can be used to ensure that the abutment remains collinear with the fixture and that there is no change in fixture position or alignment in relation to the cortex (**Figure 5**).

After the procedure, close supervision is required to ensure rapid healing with adhesion of skin to the bone end. Close approximation of the skin to the abutment shaft and stable healing of the skin onto the bone end appear to give the best chance of a trouble-free penetration. However, daily hygiene also is essential, and the patient is instructed in the care of the penetration. Each day the site should be wiped with sterile saline and any crusting or discharge removed. After the first week, no dressing is required, but a polyethylene foam disk or a twist of dry gauze is recommended. Ventilation and cleanliness are needed to achieve a stable skin–implant interface (**Figure 6**).

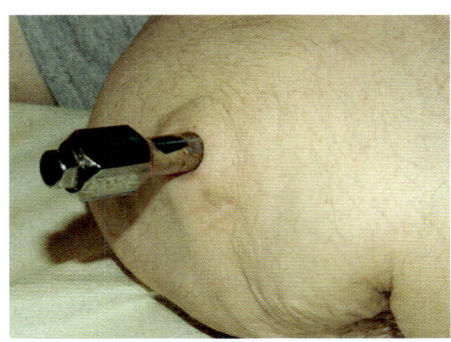

FIGURE 6 Clinical close-up photograph of a stable femoral skin-penetration site. Note that the shape of the distal femur can be seen with adherent, overlying skin.

Postoperative Management

The patient is discharged home between 10 and 14 days after the second-stage procedure, when the skin surrounding the penetration is satisfactory and all tissue reaction to the surgery has resolved. A gentle exercise program is started without resisted movements and avoiding rotational movements; the prevention of hip flexion contracture is of great importance. The patient is reviewed at 3 weeks for suture removal and again at 6 weeks when the training program begins.

A short training prosthesis is provided to facilitate the exercise program and apply measured force to the abutment and thus to the implant. The torque of the abutment-retaining bolt is checked at regular intervals, and some tightening may be required to regain 12-Nm torque. Any loosening at the abutment–implant interface will result in micromotion, with black discharge of titanium oxide particles and wear of the components.

The short training prosthesis is a 10- to 25-cm tubular extension that is clamped to the abutment. It is measured to correspond with the length of the opposite femur and is measured from the opposite knee joint line. It is fitted with a platform end on which the patient can apply measured loads—initially 20 kg vertically by pressing onto traditional spring-type bathroom scales that provide continuous analog output. The axial weight load is increased by 10 kg each week. After 3 weeks, the load is applied for 10 to 15 minutes each day. When 40-kg weight bearing is achieved, resistance exercises are started, with 1-kg weights attached to the end of the short training prosthesis. Patients may then proceed to prone kneeling. When 60-kg loading is achieved, upright kneeling can be started. If at any stage the residual limb becomes painful, the loading program is postponed until the pain has resolved. In most cases, full weight bearing should be achieved between 3 and 6 months after the second-stage procedure, at which point the patient can be supplied with a full-length temporary prosthesis containing a knee and foot mechanism.

Standing weight bearing is commenced between parallel bars, with a progressive increase in load until at 6 weeks partial weight bearing allows progression to walking with crutches. Further progress is walking with canes until unrestricted walking is possible. The patient learns to recognize that pain near the implant represents overloading, which resolves by reducing the load; persistent pain must be investigated to exclude the onset of loosening or deep infection. The time required for the overstress pain to resolve will normally take a few days, but it may take several weeks, and this effect may determine the time that it takes for full weight bearing and activity to be achieved. Current experience suggests that the patient should be prepared for the loading program to require up to 1 year after the second-stage procedure, especially in the case of poorer bone quality.

Press-Fit Intramedullary Stem—OPL System

The OPL system has been extensively used in lower limb amputees including both transfemoral and transtibial patients, as off-the-shelf implants. The standard OPL implant is designed to accommodate a custom joint arthroplasty prosthesis, and has been anchored to hip[36] and knee[37] replacement implants. On a custom implant design basis, it also has been used for hip disarticulations with a transpelvic implant,[38] and for upper limb amputees with transhumeral, radial, and ulnar implants. It also can accommodate extensions for periprosthetic fracture management and neck-of-femur screws.

The OPL system is an evolution of the Integral Leg Prosthesis (ILP) system.[27] The underlying material properties of the cast cobalt alloy (CoCrMo) used in the construction of the ILP design, while biologically inert, is inherently stiff, and often leads to issues such as stress-shielding and subsequent bone resorption at the distal end of the implant. The OPL implant is fabricated from titanium alloy (Ti_6Al_4V) which is more biocompatible. The components of the systems are divided into the intramedullary implant which is inserted in the bone cavity, the dual cone adaptor connecting the implant to the external components, the internal locking screw which secures the dual cone to the implant, the taper sleeve and the bushing which provide a failsafe mechanism and are secured at the distal end of the dual cone, the distal locking screw which secures the taper sleeve and bushing to the dual cone, and the connector that attaches the implant system to the prosthetic limb **Figure 7**). The external part of the implant system has a highly polished smooth surface and is coated with TiNb which has antibacterial and corrosion-resistance properties.[21] The dual cone adaptor can be replaced in an outpatient setting by a prosthetist, without anesthetic.

The implant is designed as a cylindrical rod that is curved to match the femoral radius of curvature. The distal half of the implant is coated with porous Ti plasma spray that is designed to facilitate rapid osseointegration. The proximal half of the implant has 10 sharp longitudinal fins, 1 mm in height, creating grooves inside the inner cortex during implantation, to provide immediate rotational stability (**Figure 8**).

To address the distal bone resorption, the distal half of the implant is 1

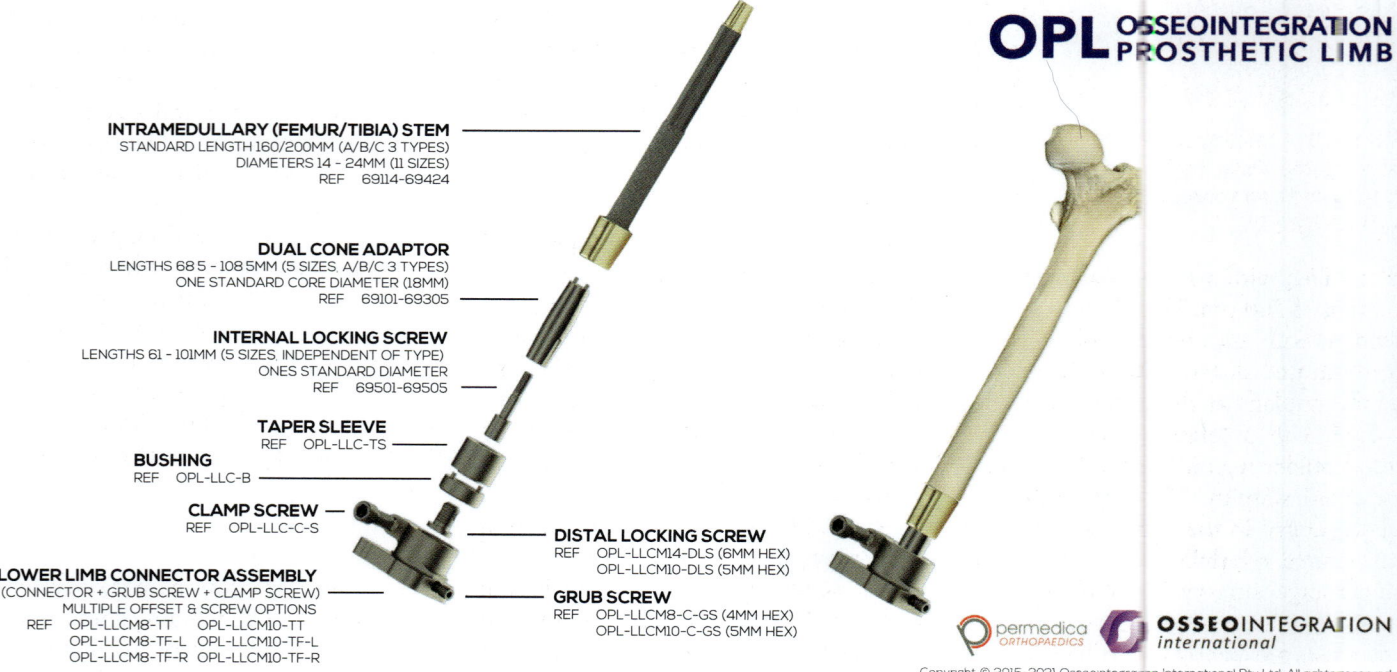

FIGURE 7 A schematic illustration showing the overview of the Osseointegration Prosthetic Limb (OPL) implant. Designed in Australia and manufactured by both Osseointegration International Pty Ltd in Australia and Permedica S.p.a. in Italy. (Reproduced with permission from Osseointegration International Pty Ltd in Australia and Permedica S.P.A. in Italy.)

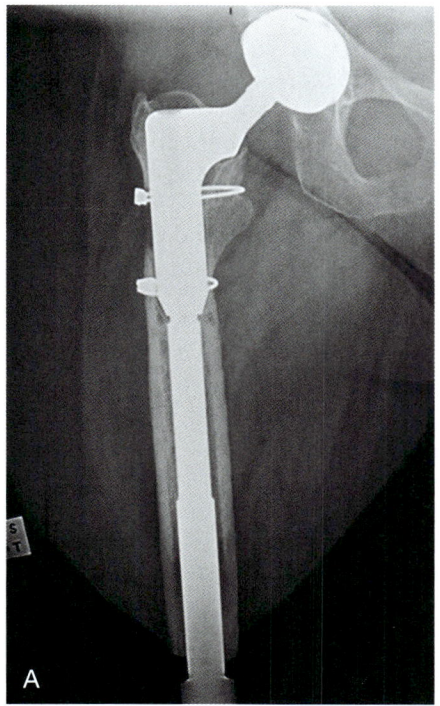
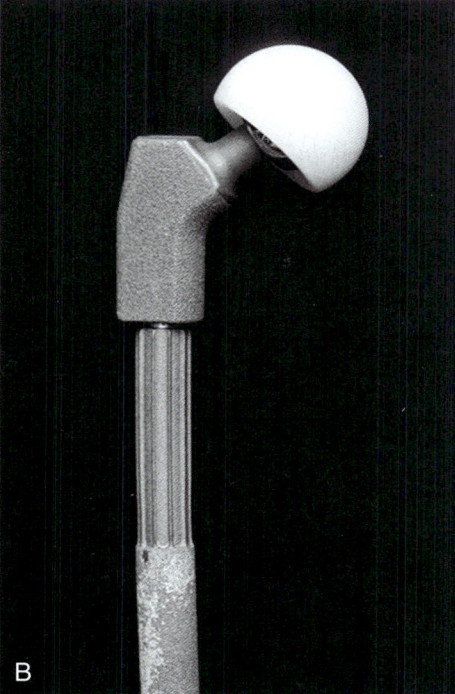

FIGURE 8 **A**, Radiographic image of the proximal attachment of a modular hip arthroplasty stem to a (**B**) photographic image of OPL implant.

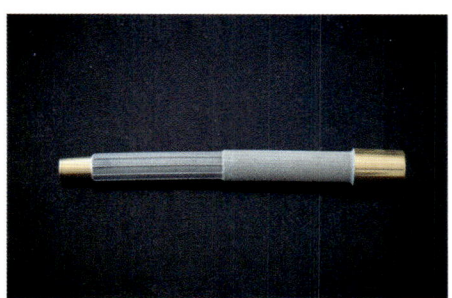

FIGURE 9 A photograph of the OPL implant showing the distal half with coarse porous coating and a narrow proximal half with longitudinal sharp fins.

mm wider, with a much coarser porous coating of 500 μm. This allows the osseointegration and bone loading to be concentrated distally. The collared part of the implant at the distal end is also coated with Ti plasma spray all along the shoulder region to provide immediate axial stability. These features were implemented in the design to enable an accelerated rehabilitation protocol and single-stage surgery. Additionally, considering that a significant portion of amputees are elderly and will eventually develop arthritic changes in the hip joint, a proximal taper has been added to the implant that can attach to a modular hip arthroplasty stem (**Figure 9**).

Considering the abovementioned features of the OPL system, osseointegration can occur after between 6 weeks to 3 months in the lower limb. During this period, the patient can be fitted with a trial prosthesis as early as 2 weeks after single-stage surgery. This is on par with patient rehabilitation from hip and knee joint arthroplasty, thereby reducing the recovery time down to 3 to 6 weeks.[39]

Clinical Management

The OGAP-2 accelerated protocol describes the guidelines of perioperative assessment, patient selection, and postoperative management for patients undergoing osseointegration using the OPL system.[39] This protocol has been adopted in many centers around the world, including the United States, on a custom implant use basis.

Patients who are considering osseointegration are assessed by a multidisciplinary team including orthopaedic surgeons, rehabilitation specialists, clinical psychologist, pain management specialist, prosthetists, physiotherapists, and a limb reconstruction nurse educator during their initial consultation. On occasion, there may be involvement from a plastic surgeon or vascular surgeon. Patients undergo a clinical, radiological, pain, and psychological assessment with objective and subjective measures taken by a dedicated OGAP researcher. Their functional outcomes are assessed using a Six-Minute Walk Test, Timed Up and Go, and Medicare Functional Classification Levels. Patients fill out subjective patient-reported quality-of-life outcomes with Questionnaire for Persons with a Transfemoral Amputation and the Short Form Health Survey (SF-36). A thorough examination is performed to assess gait, range of motion including joint contractures, skeletal alignment, length of residuum, soft-tissue coverage including previous scars and skin integrity, and presence of neuromas and location of any phantom limb pain that may necessitate concurrent targeted muscle reinnervation. Patients undergo an EOS scan, weight-bearing imaging of the affected limb with a prosthesis on (for those patients who use a socket-based prosthesis), dual-energy X-ray absorptiometry scan, and high-resolution 0.5 mm slice CT scan, which are then segmented by the Osseointegration International engineers using Materialise Mimics Software and the implant is then templated using Materialise 3-matic Software to allow patient-specific selection of implant type and size for preoperative templating. The exclusion criteria include skeletal immaturity, psychological instability, irradiated bone, active bone infection, pregnancy, patients receiving chemotherapy, and organ transplant patients on immunosuppression medication. Smoking, diabetes, and dysvascular patients are no longer regarded as exclusion criteria. There is no upper limit for the patient's age as long as the patient is independent.[39]

Preoperative Preparation

Patients undergo routine perioperative medical screening including a review by an anesthetist and medical physician, and chest radiograph and routine blood tests are performed including full blood count, baseline inflammatory markers including erythrocyte sedimentation

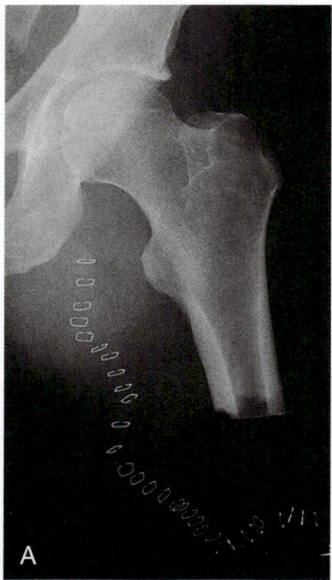 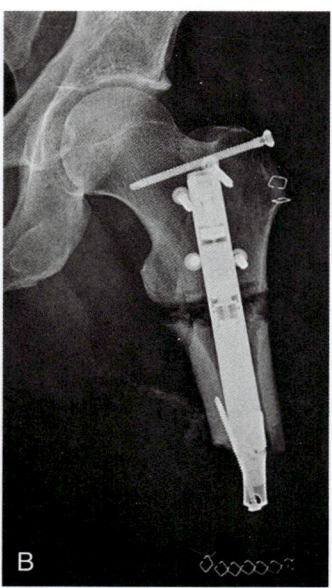 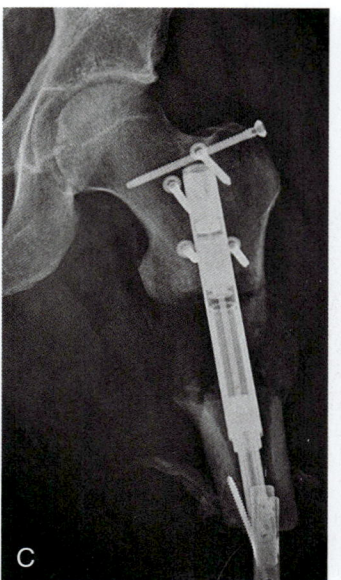 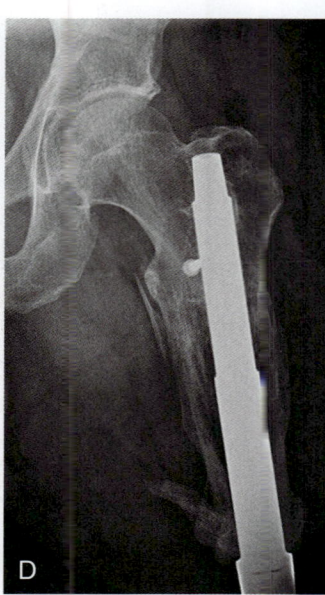

FIGURE 10 Radiographic images (**A** through **C**) sequential residual bone lengthening followed by (**D**) osseointegration using a standard implant.

rate and C-reactive protein, and liver function tests. Blood group and hold are also recorded, however blood transfusions are rarely required.

Bony residuum can vary in length. For an above-knee amputee, the minimum required resection is 150 mm above the contralateral knee joint to provide sufficient space for prosthetic fit without compromising knee height. For a standard off-the-shelf implant, 160 mm of residual bone is required from the greater trochanter. If the residual bone is shorter, then consideration is made for using a shorter custom-made implant or, alternatively, the patient undergoes a residual lengthening procedure[40] followed by implanting of a standard off-the-shelf OPL implant (**Figure 10**).

Surgical Procedure

The osseointegration procedure is performed as a single-stage surgery with the OPL system.[39,41] The patient undergoes either spinal or epidural anesthesia and is positioned supine on the orthopaedic table. An elliptical or fish-mouth incision is performed into the distal end of the residuum. Depending on the size of the tissue redundancy, skin and subcutaneous tissue fat are removed down to the muscle layer. A horizontal incision is made in the muscle layer down to the bursa covering the distal end of the residual bone. The bursa is excised completely, along with the distal end of the bone, to a healthy margin where there is good cortical thickness (minimum 2.5 mm). Meticulous care is taken to avoid stripping of the periosteum of the distal end of the bone, which maintains vascularity and is crucial to avoiding bony infection. The periosteum is incised sharply distal to the bony resection level, and repaired at the end of the procedure to cover the bone distally. The distal end of the bone is physically and radiologically inspected, and it is reshaped using an end-cutting reamer tool (face reamer) to be perpendicular to the longitudinal canal allowing maximum bony contact with the shoulder of the implant collar.

The intramedullary canal is then prepared by sequential reaming using flexible reamers over a guidewire which is positioned optimally in the AP and lateral radiographs to ensure reaming is not eccentric, while harvesting the bone that is obtained in the process for bone grafting (**Figure 11**). Broaching then takes place using the designated OPL broaches. These broaches are the same shape as the implant. They have sharp cutting fins in the proximal 80 mm of the broach and have cylindrical impaction rasps in the distal 80 mm to impact the bone in that area. Sequential broaching is performed until the broach

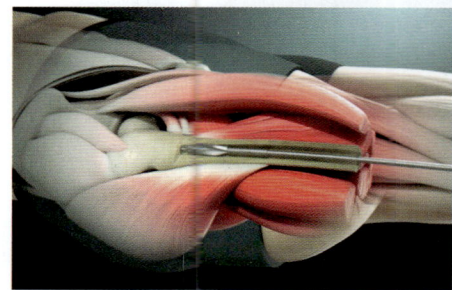

FIGURE 11 Schematic illustration showing preparation of the intramedullary canal with flexible reamers.

faces resistance to further impaction with a mallet and is rotationally stable on torsional testing. The bone that is harvested is then reimplanted into the canal and impacted using a smaller sized broach. The definitive implant is press-fit into the bone under the guidance of an image intensifier, with careful attention to gentle insertion to avoid a fracture. The soft tissue is addressed and the nerves are identified, including the sciatic (with its two branches) and the saphenous nerves. Targeted muscle reinnervation is then performed.

The next step is to address the muscle groups. The deepest layer of muscles is sutured into the periosteum. The periosteum is always left longer than the bone to allow later suturing with the muscles. The deep layer is sutured to the bone from all angles around the collar of the implant, and then the fascia of the more superficial muscle layers is sutured around the collar of the implant on both sides, at the 3 o'clock and 9 o'clock positions. The flexors are reanchored to the extensors using their fascia and around the collar of the bone to provide a myodesis around the distal end of the implant. The subcutaneous fat is then thinned, without compromising the circulation to the overlying skin. The subcutaneous tissue is closed from both sides of the wound in a firm fashion to prevent any redundancy, by excising the redundant tissues sequentially as the closure progresses.

Depending on the shape of the distal end of the residuum, there are two methods for closing the skin. One is by forming a skin flap over the implant collar and closing the wound completely, then coring the skin using a special coring device over the tip of the implant. This allows the implant collar to protrude through the opening and away from the wound closure. If there is insufficient skin to form a flap, then the skin is closed around the base of the collar allowing the implant to protrude through the wound. To date, there is no consensus as to which is the better approach. Although making a separate core hole in the skin as a skin flap would provide a more cosmetic healing wound, it increases the risk of the development of skin necrosis of the area on the edge of the flap, therefore there are pros and cons to each approach. Regardless of the approach, the principle of firm closure to minimize soft-tissue movement is essential. The skin is sutured using absorbable sutures and no drain is left in situ. The dual cone is then attached to the implant with the internal locking screw, using a handheld special device to limit rotation, along with the taper sleeve, the bushing, and the distal locking screw. The external components will often require retightening by a prosthetist before prosthetic limb attachment using a special device to prevent rotation. These patients commence rehabilitation immediately from day one postoperatively, and the wound is dressed with dry gauze, Webril cotton, and crepe bandage dressings. The initial dressings are debulked after 24 hours, followed by 3 days of an island dressing which is removed by day 4/5 and the wound is left exposed. The patient is allowed to wash the wound in the shower thereafter, with warm water and a mild soap. Thorough drying of the wound is encouraged by dabbing the wound without any abrasive wiping to reduce skin abrasion.

The abovementioned technique provided a description of transfemoral osseointegration surgery performed using the OPL implant; however, there was a deficiency in bone-anchored prosthesis applicability to the more challenging, yet more prevalent transtibial amputees.[41] Once OGA reached considerable numbers with transfemoral surgery, the decision was made to embark on extending these techniques to persons with transtibial amputations.

Anatomical challenges arose considering the cross-section of the tibia is triangular in shape, while proximally at the metaphysis, the cancellous bone widens substantially. These anatomical features mandated a change in design of the implant to provide initial stability and later osseointegration. The shorter length and larger diameter of the tibial implants allow greater stability in the cancellous bone of the proximal tibia. The skin and subcutaneous tissue below the knee are closely adherent to the bone anteriorly and medially, while there is significant bulk of soft tissue (both muscle and subcutaneous fat) in the calf. This anatomical change in soft-tissue bulk necessitated a shift in surgical management when compared with the approach with transfemoral amputees, especially given the presence of the fibula. Furthermore, it has been established that vascularity to the lower limb decreases distally, which results in problems with healing and an increased chance of surgical failure.

The surgery is performed by making a horizontal incision over the distal end of the tibia. Care must be taken to preserve the periosteum, as the tibia anteriorly and medially lies just under the skin. The only separating tissue between the skin and the bone is a thin bursa, while posteriorly in the calf there is an abundance of muscle tissue. This soft-tissue arrangement makes wound closure around the implant more challenging. A larger posterior flap is created to provide sufficient coverage for later closure.

A long guidewire is inserted into the center of the canal, which is located radiographically with the help of an image intensifier. The aim is to position the implant centrally in the tibia on AP and lateral views, considering that because of the pyramidal shape of the proximal tibia, it is possible to malposition the implant in varus or valgus malalignment. Care must be taken during the reaming and broaching steps to ensure accurate positioning of the instruments using frequent image-intensifier guidance. Furthermore, there is a significant discrepancy in the cortical thickness of the proximal tibia, as the bone is very thick anteriorly relative to posteriorly and laterally. This makes reaming and broaching more challenging as the bone can be excessively thinned posterolaterally, while remaining thick anteriorly. Often, rasping the anterior cortex is required to balance the cortical thickness. Once the intramedullary canal is prepared in a symmetric fashion, the implant is press-fit in a similar fashion to transfemoral osseointegration surgery. The bulk of the calf muscle is removed and the distal end of the fibula is resected 5 cm proximal to the amputation level to ensure it is shorter than the residual tibia, facilitating proper wound closure. Targeted muscle reinnervation is performed locally at the residuum. The muscles are reattached posteriorly and laterally around the tibia by suturing them to the periosteum. The wound is then closed using a posterior flap over the distal end of the implant with the remaining steps being similar to that of a transfemoral osseointegration surgery. The skin–implant interface seals over time, therefore it is important to maintain good hygiene with regular use of soap and water (**Figure 12**).

Postoperative Management

In most areas of orthopaedic surgery, the rehabilitation strategies receive far less attention than aspects the surgeon is more directly overseeing. The goal of rehabilitation is to facilitate the patient's

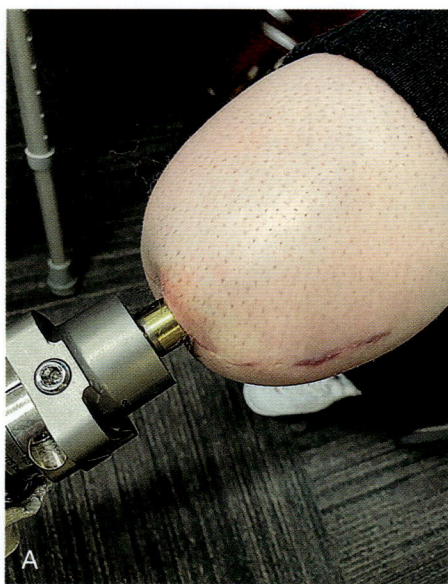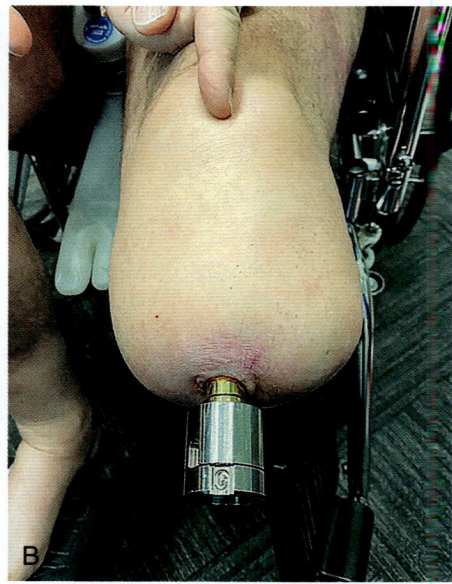

FIGURE 12 Clinical photographs of (**A**) the shape of standard transfemoral residuum and (**B**) transtibial residuum showing the skin-implant interface.

ability to gain independence as fast as possible without compromising outcomes, with gradual loading as permitted by pain, until the patient achieves a 50 kg loading, or half their body weight. The rehabilitation is divided into two groups, depending on their preoperative assessment, and intraoperative findings of bone and soft-tissue quality: fast loaders and slow loaders.[41] The fast loading protocol is carried out over 2 weeks, for patients with good bone quality and a healthy soft-tissue envelope. The slow loading protocol is reserved for osteoporotic patients and those with a suboptimal soft-tissue envelope. The phases of rehabilitation are outlined in **Table 3**. Immediately postoperatively, patients commence graduated loading as per the prescribed protocol, modulating the weight bearing using bathroom scales to achieve the optimal level of loading. Once the desired loading weight is achieved, the patient is upgraded to the second phase of the trial prosthesis, which spans a few weeks using a lightweight prosthesis and parallel bars to retrain balance, gait, and proprioception. Once they are safe to mobilize with their trial prosthesis using two crutches, they upgrade to a definitive prosthesis. The overall aim is 6 weeks mobility with two crutches, 6 weeks with one crutch in the opposite upper limb, and then unaided thereafter. Most rehabilitation is conducted on an outpatient basis, and the patient can often be discharged home 4 days postoperatively.

The rehabilitation for bilateral lower limb amputees, whether transfemoral, transtibial, or mixed, uses the same principles as mentioned above, with some modification such as using a hoist to assist with balance and facilitate gradual loading on bilateral lower limbs. A hoist is used for patients who cannot use their upper limbs for support.

Spring Loaded Constant Compression Implant

The Compress (Zimmer Biomet, Warsaw, Indiana, USA) was developed during the 1990s[42] and has been used surgically since 2000[43] as an arthroplasty megaprosthesis in situations such as bone tumor resection. It was later modified to accommodate a transcutaneous implant, with patient trials beginning in 2012.[42] The Compress is made of titanium, featuring a porous distal bone end platform. A thin intramedullary pin is coupled to this platform and anchored to proximal bone by smooth cross-pins. Turning a nut in the pin mechanism leads to progressive force applied to the bone by the platform via a Belleville disk washer spring mechanism. The theory is that an immediate and constant force applied to the bone end should promote bone integration, regardless of the patient's actual weight bearing.[42,44] A smooth transcutaneous adapter interfaces with the prosthetic limb. The Compress is not commercially available; its FDA trial is currently in the planning stages.[45]

SUMMARY

Osseointegration provides a direct skeletal attachment of prostheses; however, osseointegration should not be considered as merely a surgical solution; it is more appropriately a combined surgical and rehabilitation program that requires close coordination between orthopaedic surgeons, rehabilitation specialists, and prosthetists. For implants such as the OPRA implant that require bone ingrowth over a large surface area, a two-stage procedure is necessary to safely achieve stable osseointegration. For the OPL implant, a one-stage procedure is used to achieve stable osseointegration. The long-term success of the device requires a considerable amount of attention at the transdermal or skin penetration site to ensure a tension-free closure and minimize motion at the skin–implant interface. When applied in a diligent and conscientious manner in appropriately selected patients, the technology can dramatically improve the lives of patients with amputations who cannot tolerate traditional, socket-based prostheses.

TABLE 3 Phases of Rehabilitation

Phase	Prosthetist	PT Goals and Frequency	Hands-On Treatment	Exercises	Self-Care
1: Exposure Fit patients with strong bone can be fast (0-2 wk) Others slow (0-6 wk)	1. Choose prosthetic option 2. Measure and template a training leg	1. Load 50% BW, good alignment, minimal pain 2. Control swelling 3. Intact leg SL balance 4. Full ROM exercises 5. Fitting with training leg	1. Gentle residual limb massage and lymphatic drainage 2. Desensitizing therapy 3. Muscle release of gluteals, rectus femoris, adductors as required	1. Static axial loading 5 kg, 20 min twice daily 2. Increase 5 kg per day until 50 kg or 50% BW	1. Prone lying 2. Showering 3. Incision remains uncovered 4. Moderate sun exposure can promote dryness and bacterial control 5. Start salt baths week 2
2: Dependence Patients introduced to skills but require high supervision	1. Fitting and adaptor education 2. Adjustment for alignment	1. No unsupervised walking or prosthesis wear for 2 wk (prevent falls) 2. Supervised 2 FC walking 3. Balancing with training leg 4. Independent don/doff 5. Independence with HEP with prosthetic leg	1. 2 × FC for 6 wk after prosthesis fit 2. Flat indoor walking 3. No turns/pivots 4. 5-10 min sessions ×3 with rest 5. Stairs: Step-to GAS/SAG 6. Video and mirror feedback	1. PT 5-6 d weekly, 2-3× sessions daily for gait training	1. Daily HEP: Strength and stretching 2. Ice and compression pre/post PT 3. Daily salt baths 4. Weekend rest 5. Wear prosthetic limb for rehab walking and exercise only
3: Transition Patients begin early independence	1. Alignment review 2. Weekly increases in prosthetic height 3. Consider increasing knee resistance	1. Independent 2 × FC walking 2. Improve balance and strength 3. Ramp training	1. Mostly learning to "ride the knee" 2. Ramp training	1. Taper gait training PT to 3-4/wk	1. Wear prosthesis at meals, rehab walking, and exercise only 2. Daily strength and stretching
4: Development Patients develop their routines and preferences guided by clinicians	1. Fortnightly increase in knee resistance 2. Achieve even leg length 3. Optional: Introduce microprocessor knee	1. Start alternate crutch gait 2. Increase prosthesis wear to near full-day 3. Begin uneven ground and outdoor walking	1. Alternate crutch training 2. Ramp training 3. Hard ground outdoor walking 4. Controlled simulated uneven ground walking 5. Weaving and tight space walking	1. Taper gait training PT to 2-3/wk	1. Improve independence
5: Maturation Patients begin to determine and assess goals	1. Permanent full-weight prosthesis	1. Single FC without gait pattern regression 2. Improve distance endurance 3. Progress uneven ground stability with single FC 4. Begin stair mode practice (microprocessor knee)	1. Obstacle and decision challenges 2. Grass and uneven outdoor mobility 3. Fall training	1. Taper gait training PT to 1-2/wk	1. Wear leg entire day
6: Maintenance Nearly all patients achieve independence by 3-6 mo	As required only	1. Taper to cane/unaided per patient skills/goals 2. Independence with upstairs mode (microprocessor controlled knees)	1. Progress obstacle, decision, surface challenges	1. Taper gait training to as needed only	1. Patient becomes self-directed "expert" in prosthesis use

BW = body weight, FC = forearm crutches, GAS/SAG = order of gait when training stairs: good-affected-stick (up) then stick-affected-good (down), HEP = home exercise program, PT = physiotherapy, SL = single leg

References

1. Malgaigne J-F: *Manuel de médecine opératoire: fondée sur l'anatomie normale et l'anatomie pathologique*. G. Ballière, 1853.
2. Codivilla A: Sulla correzione della deformita de frattura del femore. *Bull Sci Med* 1903;3:246-249.
3. Peltier LF: The role of Alessandro Codivilla in the development of skeletal traction. *J Bone Joint Surg Am* 1969;51(7):1433.
4. Brand RA: Advances in limb lengthening and reconstruction: Alessandro Codivilla, MD, 1861-1912. *Clin Orthop Relat Res* 2008;466(12):2901-2902.
5. Steinmann F: *Eine neue Extensionsmethode in der Frakturbehandlung*. Korrespondenzbl. f. Schweiz Ärzte, 1908.
6. Steinmann F, Chir Z: Zur Autoschaft der Nagelextension. *Zentralbl Chir* 1910;37:153-156.
7. Murphy EF: History and philosophy of attachment of prostheses to the musculo-skeletal system and of passage

7. through the skin with inert materials. *J Biomed Mater Res* 1973;7(3):275-295.
8. Cutler E, Blodgett J: *Skeletal Attachment of Prostheses for the Leg*. Committee on Medical Research, 1945.
9. Mooney V, Predecki P, Renning J, Gray J: Skeletal extension of limb prosthetic attachment problems in tissue reaction. *J Biomed Mater Res* 1971;5:143-159.
10. Esslinger JO: A basic study in semi-buried implants and osseous attachments for application to amputation prosthetic fitting. *Bull Prosthet Res* 1970;10(13):219-225.
11. Hall CW: A future prosthetic limb device. *J Rehabil Res Dev* 1985;22(3):99-102.
12. Hall CW, Mallow WA, Hoese FO: *Permanently Attached Artificial Limb*. Google Patents, 1979.
13. Brånemark PI: Vital microscopy of bone marrow in rabbit. *Scand J Clin Lab Invest* 1959;11(supp 38):1-82.
14. Brånemark PI, Hansson BO, Adell R, et al: Osseointegrated implants in the treatment of the edentulous jaw. Experience from a 10-year period. *Scand J Plast Reconstr Surg Suppl* 1977;16:1-132.
15. Albrektsson T, Brånemark PI, Hansson HA, Lindström J: Osseointegrated titanium implants. Requirements for ensuring a long-lasting, direct bone-to-implant anchorage in man. *Acta Orthop Scand* 1981;52(2):155-170.
16. Brånemark PI: Osseointegration and its experimental background. *J Prosthet Dent* 1983;50(3):399-410.
17. Brånemark R, Brånemark PI, Rydevik B, Myers RR: Osseointegration in skeletal reconstruction and rehabilitation: A review. *J Rehabil Res Dev* 2001;38(2):175-181.
18. Linder L, Albrektsson T, Brånemark PI, et al: Electron microscopic analysis of the bone-titanium interface. *Acta Orthop Scand* 1983;54(1):45-52.
19. Kumar PS, Ks SK, Grandhi VV, Gupta V: The effects of titanium implant surface topography on osseointegration: Literature review. *JMIR Biomed Eng* 2019;4(1):e13237.
20. Barfeie A, Wilson J, Rees J: Implant surface characteristics and their effect on osseointegration. *Br Dent J* 2015;218(5):E9.
21. Du JK, Chao CY, Chiu KY, et al: Antibacterial properties and corrosion resistance of the newly developed biomaterial, Ti–12Nb–1Ag alloy. *Metals* 2017;7(12):566.
22. Pendegrass CJ, Goodship AE, Blunn GW: Development of a soft tissue seal around bone-anchored transcutaneous amputation prostheses. *Biomaterials* 2006;27(23):4183-4191.
23. Aschoff HH, Kennon RE, Keggi JM, Rubin LE: Transcutaneous, distal femoral, intramedullary attachment for above-the-knee prostheses: An endo-exo device. *J Bone Joint Surg Am* 2010;92(suppl 2):180-186.
24. Brånemark R, Berlin O, Hagberg K, Bergh P, Gunterberg B, Rydevik B: A novel osseointegrated percutaneous prosthetic system for the treatment of patients with transfemoral amputation: A prospective study of 51 patients. *Bone Joint J* 2014;96-B(1):106-113.
25. Al Muderis M, Khemka A, Lord SJ, Van de Meent H, Frölke JP: Safety of osseointegrated implants for transfemoral amputees: A two-center prospective cohort study. *J Bone Joint Surg Am* 2016;98(11):900-909.
26. Al Muderis M, Lu W, Li JJ: Osseointegrated prosthetic limb for the treatment of lower limb amputations: Experience and outcomes. *Unfallchirurg* 2017;120(4):306-311.
27. Hoellwarth JS, Tetsworth K, Rozbruch SR, Handal MB, Coughlan A, Al Muderis M: Osseointegration for amputees: Current implants, techniques, and future directions. *JBJS Rev* 2020;8(3):e0043.
28. Palmquist A, Lindberg F, Emanuelsson L, Brånemark R, Engqvist H, Thomsen P: Morphological studies on machined implants of commercially pure titanium and titanium alloy (Ti6Al4V) in the rabbit. *J Biomed Mater Res B Appl Biomater* 2009;91(1):309-319.
29. Brånemark R, Emanuelsson L, Palmquist A, Thomsen P: Bone response to laser-induced micro- and nano-size titanium surface features. *Nanomedicine* 2011;7(2):220-227.
30. Sullivan J, Uden M, Robinson KP, Sooriakumaran S: Rehabilitation of the trans-femoral amputee with an osseointegrated prosthesis: The United Kingdom experience. *Prosthet Orthot Int* 2003;27(2):114-120.
31. Hagberg K, Brånemark R: Consequences of non-vascular trans-femoral amputation: A survey of quality of life, prosthetic use and problems. *Prosthet Orthot Int* 2001;25(3):186-194.
32. Krause WR, Bradbury DW, Kelly JE, Lunceford EM: Temperature elevations in orthopaedic cutting operations. *J Biomech* 1982;15(4):267-275.
33. Eriksson E, Brånemark PI: Osseointegration from the perspective of the plastic surgeon. *Plast Reconstr Surg* 1994;93(3):626-637.
34. Gottschalk FA, Stills M: The biomechanics of trans-femoral amputation. *Prosthet Orthot Int* 1994;18(1):12-17.
35. Hansson HA, Albrektsson T, Brånemark PI: Structural aspects of the interface between tissue and titanium implants. *J Prosthet Dent* 1983;50(1):108-113.
36. Khemka A, FarajAllah CI, Lord SJ, Bosley B, Al Muderis M: Osseointegrated total hip replacement connected to a lower limb prosthesis: A proof-of-concept study with three cases. *J Orthop Surg Res* 2016;11(1):13.
37. Khemka A, Frossard L, Lord SJ, Bosley B, Al Muderis M: Osseointegrated total knee replacement connected to a lower limb prosthesis: 4 cases. *Acta Orthop* 2015;86(6):740-744.
38. Hoellwarth JS, Tetsworth K, Al-Maawi Q, Tarbosh AM, Roberts C, Al Muderis M: Pelvic osseointegration for unilateral hip disarticulation: A case report. *JBJS Case Connect* 2021;11(2):e20.00105.
39. Al Muderis M, Lu W, Tetsworth K, Bosley B, Li JJ: Single-stage osseointegrated reconstruction and rehabilitation of lower limb amputees: The Osseointegration Group of Australia Accelerated Protocol-2 (OGAAP-2) for a prospective cohort study. *BMJ Open* 2017;7(3):e013508.
40. Hoellwarth JS, Tetsworth K, Al-Jawazneh SS, Al Muderis M: Motorized internal lengthening of long bones: residual limb lengthening. *Tech Orthop* 2020;35(3):209-213.
41. Haque R, Al-Jawazneh S, Hoellwarth J, et al: Osseointegrated reconstruction and rehabilitation of transtibial amputees: The Osseointegration Group of Australia surgical technique and protocol for a prospective cohort study. *BMJ Open* 2020;10(10):e038346.
42. McGough RL, Goodman MA, Randall RL, Forsberg JA, Potter BK, Lindsey B: The Compress® transcutaneous implant for rehabilitation following limb amputation. *Unfallchirurg* 2017;120(4):300-305.
43. Bini SA, Johnston JO, Martin DL: Compliant prestress fixation in tumor prostheses: Interface retrieval data. *Orthopedics* 2000;23(7):707-711.
44. Kramer MJ, Tanner BJ, Horvai AE, O'Donnell RJ: Compressive osseointegration promotes viable bone at the endoprosthetic interface: Retrieval study of compress implants. *Int Orthop* 2008;32(5):567-571.
45. Zaid MB, O'Donnell RJ, Potter BK, Forsberg JA: Orthopaedic osseointegration: State of the art. *J Am Acad Orthop Surg* 2019;27(22):e977-e985.

Prosthetic Management of Osseointegration

CHAPTER 48

Phillip M. Stevens, MEd, CPO, FAAOP • Mark David Beachler, CP

ABSTRACT

Many patients who have undergone lower limb amputation experience skin ulcers, excessive perspiration, and both general and acute discomfort with the use of traditional socket prostheses. Prevalent and persistent shortcomings of the traditional interface between the residual limb and the external prosthesis have driven the continued pursuit of percutaneous osseointegration as a means of prosthetic attachment. Successful approaches to osseointegrated prostheses began with the translation of threaded implants from dental applications. A number of press-fit implants have also been introduced and widely adopted. Although the principles of prosthetic management have similarities across the various implant designs, each implant approach is associated with distinct rehabilitation pathways and prosthetic adaptors.

Keywords: amputation; implant; osseointegration; prosthesis; transfemoral

Introduction

According to one recent narrative literature review, up to three-fourths of patients who have undergone a lower limb amputation experience skin ulcers, excessive perspiration, or socket-fit issues because of fluctuations in the volume of their residual limb.[1] The surgical application of bone-anchored implants to facilitate the secure fixation of external prostheses in upper and lower limb amputees, once largely confined to research, has begun to shift toward broad commercial availability. Various approaches to percutaneous osseointegration (OI) have been developed, including both threaded and press-fit bone interface designs. Differences in bone interfacing approaches have necessitated differences in postimplantation rehabilitation, prosthetic management, and the inclusion or exclusion of a fail-safe device.

Osseointegrated Prosthesis for the Rehabilitation of Amputees

OI was first developed in 1965 by Dr. P.I. Brånemark for use in securing dental implants to the underlying bone via a titanium fixture. This technique allowed a foreign external device to be anchored directly to the bone and has since become firmly established in the field of dental implant technology.

These principles were first modified and applied to transfemoral amputees in Sweden by Dr. Rickard Brånemark in 1990. After further development the Osseointegrated Prosthesis for the Rehabilitation of Amputees (OPRA) device and treatment protocol were implemented in Sweden in 1998 by Dr. Rickard Brånemark and his research team.[2] Globally, the OPRA™ implant by Integrum has since been used in transfemoral, transtibial, transhumeral, transradial, and partial finger amputees. After more than a decade of proven history, the transfemoral OPRA™ implant system was introduced in the United States in 2015 under an FDA humanitarian device exemption. It became the first fully approved FDA implant for transfemoral amputees in 2020.

Stage 1 Surgery

Currently the OPRA™ implant system (**Figure 1**) requires two surgeries. Stage 1 surgery involves the intramedullary implantation of a threaded and self-tapping titanium fixture into the residual femur accompanied by closure of the soft tissue and skin. Once skin and soft tissue have recovered and healed, at approximately 4 to 6 weeks after surgery, a traditional socket prosthesis may be used for increased mobility. Although a socketed prosthesis is allowed at this time, very few choose this option. If this option is pursued, distal contact in the socket should be kept at a minimum to protect the fixture and encourage healthy bone integration.[3,4] A distal gel pad or other soft materials may be used to help managing distal contact.

Neither of the following authors nor any immediate family member has received anything of value from or has stock or stock options held in a commercial company or institution related directly or indirectly to the subject of this chapter: Phillip M. Stevens and Mark David Beachler.

This chapter is adapted from Sullivan J: Prosthetic management of osseointegration, in Krajbich JI, Pinzur MS, Potter BK, Stevens PM, eds: *Atlas of Amputations and Limb Deficiencies: Surgical, Prosthetic, and Rehabilitation Principles*, ed 4. American Academy of Orthopaedic Surgeons, 2016, pp 583-595.

Stage 2 Surgery

During stage 2 surgery the muscles are reattached to the periosteum, redundant soft tissues are removed, and a skin flap is attached directly to the distal aspect of the femur, creating an exit site for the abutment. The percutaneous abutment is then fit into the titanium fixture and is held in place by the abutment screw (**Figure 2**). The abutment serves as the attachment point to connect the prosthetic device.[5,6]

Stage 2 surgeries originally occurred approximately 6 months after stage 1.[3] However, efforts have since been made to safely decrease this time. Clinical trials at both Walter Reed National Military Medical Center and University of California, San Francisco, have reduced the time between the stage 1 and stage 2 surgeries to as little as 3 months.[2]

Weight Bearing

After stage 2 surgery, rehabilitation begins with the introduction of standardized weight progression protocols. These can be applied at normal or half speed depending on patient presentation. Normal speed is the standard timeline of progression, whereas half speed is for individuals with less than ideal skeletal conditions. During the normal speed protocol, once cleared by the surgeon, axial weight bearing is initiated on a scale no earlier than 4 weeks after stage 2 using a short training prosthesis (STP)[2] (**Figure 3**). Under the slower speed protocols the progression of rehabilitation is slower, and the weight applied by the patient is decreased.[3]

Short Training Prosthesis

Standard prosthetic componentry can be used to assemble the STP using a four-hole connector with Integrum's custom attachment device. The attachment device secures to the abutment using an Allen key. This STP does not have any features built into it to protect the interosseous fixture against excessive forces like that of a fail-safe device.[5] Therefore, any twisting/torque should be avoided and weight bearing limited to strictly axial loads. The overall length of the STP should approximate the anatomic knee joint center of the contralateral side to allow the patient to kneel to initiate controlled weight bearing.

In the rehabilitation protocols described by Hagberg and Brånemark[3] after fitting with the STP, weight bearing is initiated with 20 kg (approximately 40 lb) of loading, as tolerated, for 30 minutes twice per day. The patient can use a standard home bathroom scale to monitor their progression (**Figure 3**). Weight is increased as tolerated, but no more than 10 kg (20 lb) per week. Pain may be reported during this early stage of rehabilitation and often occurs when offloading the prosthesis. Pain reported at 2 to 3 on a standard 10-point visual analog pain scale is considered safe. Pain ratings above 5 points should be avoided, with the patient returning to lower axial weight loads. This allows the interosseous structures to recover before increasing to the higher loads.

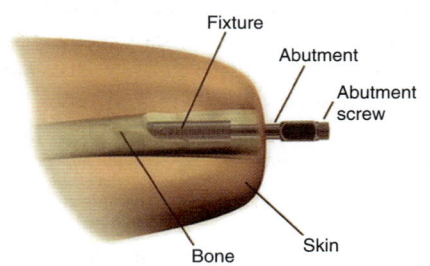

FIGURE 1 Illustration shows the components that make up the OPRA™ Implant System. (Courtesy of Integrum AB, Mölndal, Sweden.)

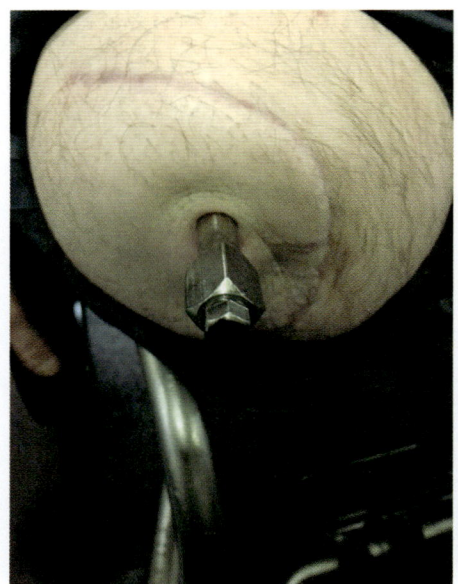

FIGURE 2 Photograph of the percutaneous abutment and retaining bolt after the stage 2 surgery of the Osseointegrated Prosthesis for the Rehabilitation of Amputees (OPRA) osseointegration procedure.

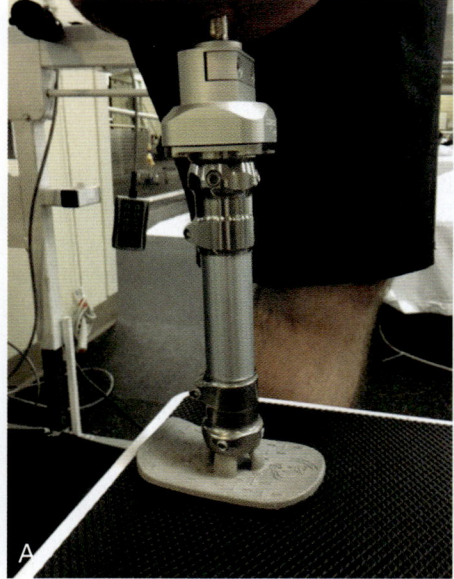 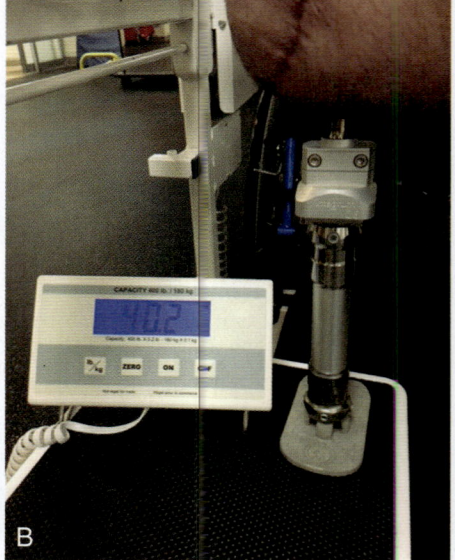

FIGURE 3 Photograph of a short training prosthesis (STP) connected to the percutaneous Osseointegrated Prosthesis for the Rehabilitation of Amputees (OPRA) abutment. **A,** Lateral view demonstrating the height of the STP set to the anatomic knee joint center of the contralateral side. **B,** Anterior view showing the bathroom scale in use to monitor the weight borne through the implant. This is progressively increased until the user can fully bear their weight through the STP.

Chapter 48: Prosthetic Management of Osseointegration

The patient should keep a daily record of pain or discomfort level for each loading session.[3,5]

Full-Length Prosthesis and OPRA Axor II Device

Once the patient has progressed to full weight bearing within acceptable levels of discomfort using the STP, they can progress to a full-length articulating prosthesis. The connection between the full-length prosthesis and the abutment is achieved by using Integrum's OPRA AXOR II device, which attaches to standard prosthetic componentry using a standard four-hole adaptor (**Figure 4**). The AXOR II device is donned and doffed by rotating the outer ring (**Figure 5, A**), which opens up the adjustable jaws of the device allowing for the abutment to seat directly into the AXOR II (**Figure 5, B**). The outer ring, assisted by an internal spring, engages the jaws onto the abutment and then is hand tightened to secure in place[3,5] (**Figure 5, C**).

The AXOR II also serves as a failsafe device. Excessive axial, transverse, or torsional loads or a combination of these loads could cause the bending and/or twisting of either the implant, the abutment, or both during an unexpected fall. The function of the fail-safe device is to protect the intramedullary implant, the abutment, and the retaining screw against these excessive loads. It is designed to release in flexion or rotation either individually or contemporaneously. Flexion release occurs when the prosthetic knee reaches its maximum flexion angle or end point, causing the device to open up (**Figure 6**). Rotational release can occur when an excessive torsional load or torque is placed on the device. This setting comes predetermined by the

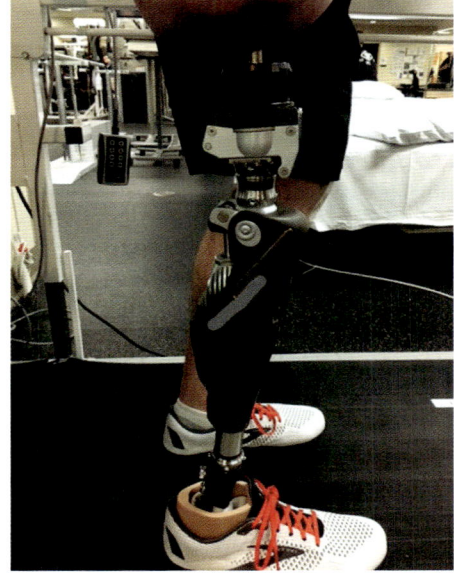

FIGURE 4 Photograph of a full-length definitive prosthesis connected to the user through the AXOR II.

manufacturer. Although a rotational fail-safe mechanism has been engineered into other implant systems, the flexion failsafe mechanism is unique to the AXOR II.

The design of the AXOR II allows the patient to reset the fail-safe mechanism without using any tools or having to replace any parts. Resetting is recommended while sitting down and can be achieved with the prosthesis still attached. If released in rotation the knee can be manually rotated back into place. When resetting the flexion, there can be an abrupt snap back into place. This may cause some discomfort early in the rehabilitation phase. Therefore, taking the prosthesis off the abutment before resetting it manually may be recommended. Once the AXOR II has been reset, the patient can reengage in ambulation. If there is increased pain associated with any fall or excessive load, the medical team should be notified as soon as possible.

Outcomes

A number of publications have presented the clinical outcomes observed in association with the OPRA™ implant system. In a prospective study of 18 patients, Hagberg et al[6] reported improvements in two patient-reported outcomes measures. The widely used Short Form-36 represented a general

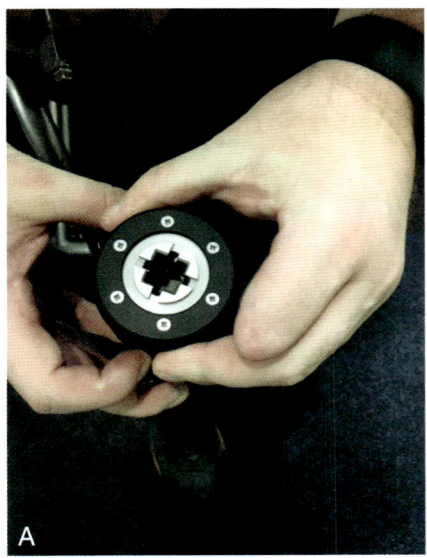
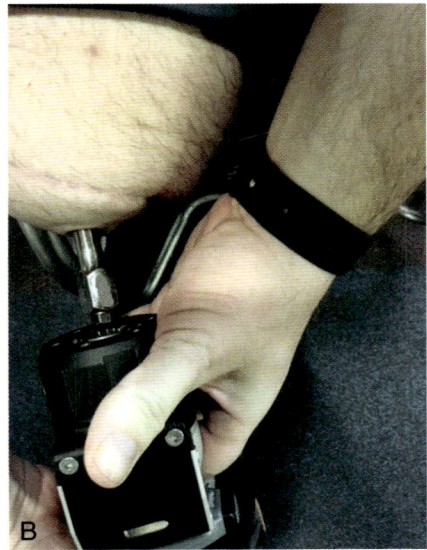
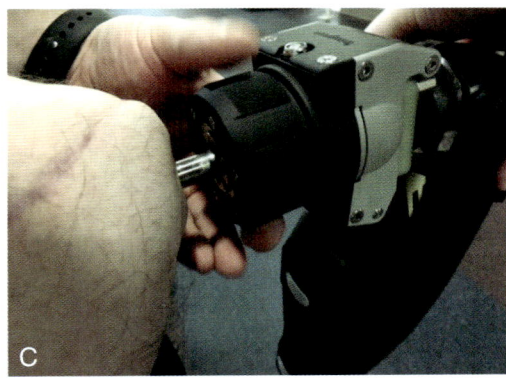

FIGURE 5 Photographs demonstrating the donning of the AXOR II device. **A**, The outer ring is rotated to open the jaws of the mechanism. **B**, The device is positioned over the terminal end of the Osseointegrated Prosthesis for the Rehabilitation of Amputees (OPRA) abutment. **C**, The outer ring is hand tightened, engaging the jaws of the mechanism to secure in place over the abutment.

© 2024 American Academy of Orthopaedic Surgeons — Atlas of Amputations and Limb Deficiencies, Fifth Edition

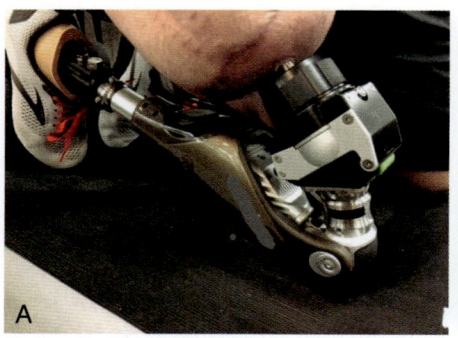 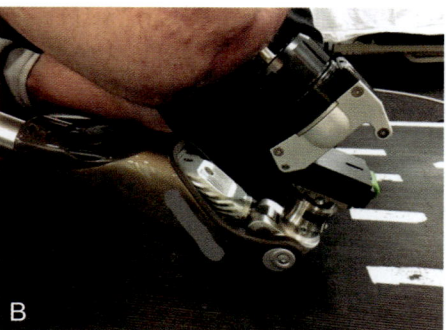

FIGURE 6 **A** and **B**, Photographs of the AXOR II device acting as a fail-safe device against excessive flexion. The device also has a rotational fail-safe mechanism.

measure of quality of life, whereas the cohort-specific Questionnaire for Persons with Transfemoral Amputation (Q-TFA) addressed considerations unique to users of transfemoral prostheses. These same measures have since been used to quantify the improvements experienced and reported by 51 patients at 2 years and 5 years postimplantation.[7,8] These studies have suggested improved health-related quality of life, increased prosthetic use, improved prosthetic mobility, fewer prosthetic problems, and better global health.[6-8]

Press-Fit Implants

Press-fit internal joint replacement implants have been used since the mid 1980s and tend to be favored in younger patients with adequate bone stock and active bone metabolism where biologic fixation through OI into osteoconductive surface can be anticipated. Such implants have been increasingly used and accepted in joint replacement techniques.[9,10]

A number of percutaneous OI implants have been developed with a similar press-fit approach to their bony fixation. These include the Integral Leg Prosthesis (ILP) as a derivative of the original Endo-Exo implant, the Osseointegrated Prosthetic Limb (OPL), the Bone Anchoring Device for Artificial Limbs (BADAL X) implant, and the Percutaneous Osseointegrated Prosthesis (POP).

Endo-Exo-Femur-Prosthesis (Integral Leg Prosthesis)

The ILP implant was first produced in Germany in 1999 and has gone through several design iterations. It is currently manufactured by ESKA Orthopedic in Lubeck, Germany, and it is available in Germany, the Netherlands, and Australia. As with most implant approaches, the implant requires two surgery sessions separated by 6 to 8 weeks.[11,12] In the first stage, the implant stem is press-fit into the medullary canal of the femur. In the second stage, the percutaneous post is attached allowing the attachment of the external limb prosthesis. Partial weight bearing is initiated immediately following the second surgery, with full weight bearing deferred until 4 to 6 weeks postsurgery.[11,12]

One early prospective trial of 22 recipients of the ILP compared a number of outcomes measured with their legacy socket prostheses to those observed 12 months postimplantation and rehabilitation.[13] Compared with the socket prosthesis, all patients significantly improved both prosthesis use and prosthesis-related quality of life as reported by the Q-TFA. The "Global" score of the Q-TFA increased by 68%, whereas weekly prosthesis use increased by 45% from 56 to 101 hours/week. Mean 6-minute walk test values increased significantly from 321 to 423 m (27%), whereas the mean times required to complete the Timed Up and Go test decreased significantly from 15.1 to 8.1 seconds (44%). Oxygen consumption values also demonstrated a significant decrease of 18%.[13]

Although many clinical trials of OI have compared their associated outcomes against those obtained from dissatisfied users of traditional socket users, outcomes associated with the ILP have recently been compared against outcomes collected from highly functional, highly satisfied users of traditional socket prostheses. When matched according to etiology, age, body mass index, limb length, time since amputation, prosthetic component types, and K-level, users of the ILP reported significantly fewer "Problem" scores on the Q-TFA, and significantly higher "Global" scores using the same measure. "Mobility" scores were also higher for those using the ILP, but this difference came just shy of statistical significance.[14]

Osseointegrated Prosthetic Limb

The OPL was developed in Australia in 2013. It is similar in its press-fit design to the ILP. Among the differences between the ILP and the OPL is a material change to titanium. In its first iteration, the implant was provided through a two-stage procedure separated by 4 to 8 weeks.[15] Much like the ILP, in the first stage the intramedullary component is press fit into a reamed femoral medullary canal to allow OI against the porous metals of the implant. In the second stage, a guidewire is used to localize the center of the osseointegrated intramedullary implant. A circular coring device is passed over the guidewire to perforate the skin and permit the insertion of the transcutaneous dual cone component, which is then secured to the intramedullary component.[15]

A defined schedule of progressive weight-bearing increases has been described in the literature, beginning on day 3 following the second stage procedure. At approximately 14 days after stage 2 procedure, patients are fit with their definitive prosthesis. A period of bilateral crutch use is followed by progression to a single crutch in the contralateral extremity, followed by unaided weight bearing.[15]

Muderis et al[15] reported on 53 patients with unilateral transfemoral amputation who underwent their two-stage procedure, of whom 36 had preoperative use of traditional socket prostheses. Compared with their preoperative state, the mean "Global" score of the Q-TFA increased by 75%, whereas the mean physical component summary of the Short Form-36 increased by 27% to 47.29 where it approximated index values of able-bodied patients. Where possible, outcomes measured with legacy socket prostheses were compared against those observed an average of 21.5 months after the stage 1 procedure. Mean 6-minute walk test values increased significantly from 281 to 419 m (49%), whereas the mean times required to complete the Timed Up and Go test decreased significantly from 14.6 to 5.9 seconds (61%).

The two-stage protocols have since been supplemented by the development of a single-state approach to press-fit OI.[16] This approach, reported as routine practice since 2014, reduces the overall time required for definitive osseointegrated reconstruction and rehabilitation to 3 to 6 weeks. In this approach, the components of the stage 1 and stage 2 procedures are combined into a single surgical event with a similar course of progressive weight bearing and ambulation.[16]

Haque et al have also described their protocols for the OI of transtibial limbs.[17] Foundational to this transition is a recognition of the comparative challenges in successfully implanting the cancellous bone of transtibial limbs compared with the more established implanting into the cortical bone of transfemoral limbs.[17] Within their protocols, two different implant styles are described in accordance with the length of the residual limb. For longer residuums with sufficient cortical bone, a more traditional press-fit implant is anticipated. For shorter residuums, a custom-made short-stem implant with coarser surface structure is anticipated.[17] A percutaneous dual cone adapter, similar to those used in their transfemoral applications, will be used to bridge the connection from the implant to the external prosthesis.[17] The rehabilitation pathway for transtibial prosthesis users will largely mimic the pathway previously described for transfemoral prosthesis users, with a similar suit of functional outcomes currently being collected.[17]

BADAL X

A third variant of the press-fit implant with similarities to the ILP and OPL is the BADAL X, manufactured by the Dutch-based OTN Implants. Like its predecessors, the implant is typically placed via two-stage surgery separated by 6 to 8 weeks, though single-stage placement has been reported.[18] Its use has been described in a prospective 1-year follow-up cohort study reporting on 69 transfemoral and 21 transtibial implant recipients.[18] Rehabilitation begins 1 week after the second OI surgery, or 3 weeks after a single-stage OI placement. Load bearing through a full-length prosthesis is modulated according to reported pain values and progressively increased to full body weight.[18] This process occurs over 11 weeks for transfemoral implants and 4 weeks for transtibial implants.

The primary endpoints reported with the OTN implants were the Q-TFA prosthetic use and global scores. Q-TFA prosthetic use, a measure of the amount of normal prosthetic wear per week, increased from 52 ± 39 to 88 ± 18. Calculated as the number of days per week multiplied by the number of hours per day, this suggests that average daily wearing times increased from 7.4 to 12.6 hours. The mean value of the Q-TFA global score, a measure of the users perceived global health and functionality, increased from 40 ± 19 to 71 ± 15. Among their patients, those with short transfemoral residual limbs, half of whom were unable to use a traditional socket prosthesis before OI rehabilitation, experienced the greatest functional improvements. For this cohort, the number of patients describing their current situation as an amputee as "good" or "very good" increased from 38% to 94%.[18]

Prosthetic Attachment of Press-Fit Implants

Connection of commercially available prostheses to the press-fit implants described earlier can be facilitated through a number of prosthetic coupling mechanisms. The connection to the bony implants themselves is accomplished through a percutaneous dual cone adaptor that inserts into the distal aspect of the implant and is held in place by an internal locking screw (**Figure 7**).

One of several taper sleeves is then positioned over the distal cone and secured with a distal screw. In several systems, taper sleeves feature a distal fail-safe ring mechanism designed to shear against excessive rotational forces. Failure at the taper sleeve allows the prosthesis to rotate freely at the fail-safe connection so that rotary forces are not translated proximally to the femoral implant itself.

Taper sleeves feature a distinct outer geometry to facilitate the connection to specific prosthetic connectors (**Figures 8 and 9**). A range of prosthetic connectors have been developed and feature some degree of commercial availability. These engage the taper sleeve proximally and standard endoskeletal prosthetic componentry distally, either via the standard four-hole pattern or a female pyramid adaptor (**Figures 8 through 10**).

The connection between the prosthetic connector and the taper sleeve, which is cycled at least daily by the patient, can be facilitated by several different mechanisms. Common among these are variations of quick-release clamp connectors and connectors with clamp screws that must be secured and

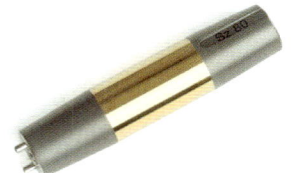 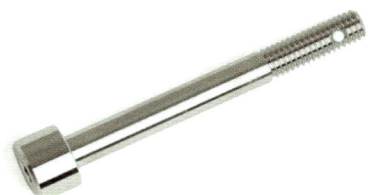

FIGURE 7 Photograph of a percutaneous dual cone adaptor and an internal locking screw. This transition mechanism between the implant and a range of prosthetic connectors is common to all current press-fit implants. (Reproduced from Atallah R, van de Meent H, Verhamme L, Frölke JP, Leijendekkers RA: Safety, prosthesis wearing time and health-related quality of life of lower extremity bone-anchored prostheses using a press-fit titanium osseointegration implant: A prospective one-year follow-up cohort study. *PLoS One* 2020;15[3]:e0230027.)

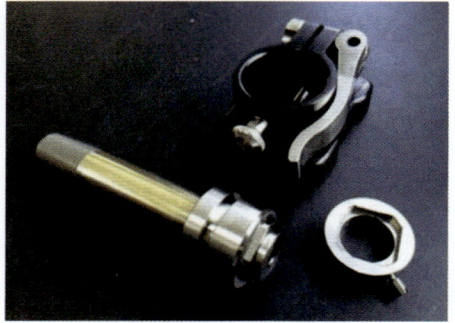

FIGURE 8 Quick-release clamp connector shown with the distal taper sleeve positioned on the dual cone adaptor, distal fail-safe safety ring, and safety pin. The distal aspect of the quick-release prosthetic connector matches the standard four-hole pattern of standard endoskeletal components. (Courtesy of Fred Hernandez.)

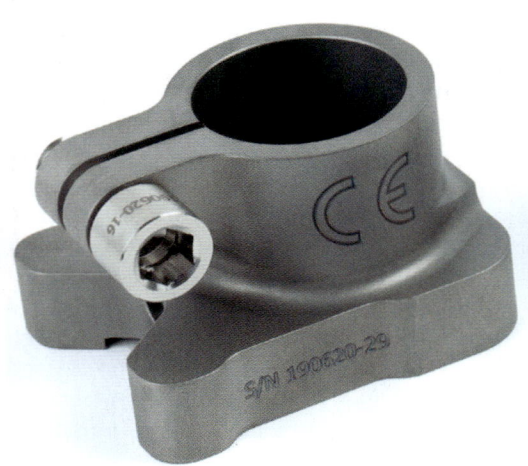
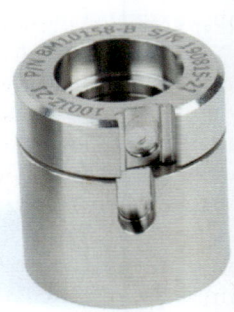

FIGURE 9 Allen key clamp connector shown with its associated distal taper sleeve and failsafe bushing. Once the taper sleeve and fail-safe bushing are affixed to the dual cone adaptor, the connecter is positioned over the taper sleeve and secured into place with an Allen key. A second Allen head screw or grub screw (not shown) on the anterior inferior aspect of the connector engages the distal safety ring of the taper sleeve. The distal aspect of the connector matches the standard four-hole pattern of standard endoskeletal adaptors. (Reproduced with permission from Atallah R, van de Meent H, Verhamme L, Frölke JP, Leijendekkers RA: Safety, prosthesis wearing time and health-related quality of life of lower extremity bone-anchored prostheses using a press-fit titanium osseointegration implant: A prospective one-year follow-up cohort study. PLoS One 2020;15[3]:e0230027.)

released through the use of an Allen wrench (**Figures 8** through **10**). Note that the clamp screw, generally positioned superior and posterior on the connector, should not be confused with the grub screw, generally positioned inferior and anterior on the connector. The latter engages the distal safety ring of certain taper sleeves and is part of the rotary fail-safe mechanism.

Percutaneous Osseointegrated Prosthesis

An additional press-fit implant with a novel distal attachment mechanism is found in the POP. This was the first OI implant to navigate an FDA feasibility trial.[19] Similar to the ILP and OPL in many regards, the POP is differentiated by its narrowed region of porous coating and end-bearing osteotomy collar. As with other press-fit approaches, the POP is installed in a two-stage procedure with a stage 1 implantation of the intramedullary segment to allow OI into the porous coating. Approximately 6 weeks later the stage 2 procedures consist of a coring of the distal residual limb to allow the attachment of the percutaneous post to the intramedullary segment of the implant.[19]

The percutaneous post of the POP system terminates in the geometry of a male Ferrier adaptor, allowing the direct attachment of the external prosthesis through a standard female Ferrier coupler (**Figure 11**). From the distal four-hole pattern of the female Ferrier assembly, traditional prosthetic alignment techniques can be performed, including the addition of requisite spacer plates, double ended female adaptors and offset plates proximal to the knee (**Figure 12**).

The POP feasibility trial reports on the first 10 patients treated with this implant. All proceeded to loading their definitive prosthesis on the day following their stage 2 procedures and to ambulation with an assistive device within 14 days. At 5 weeks, eight patients progressed to independent

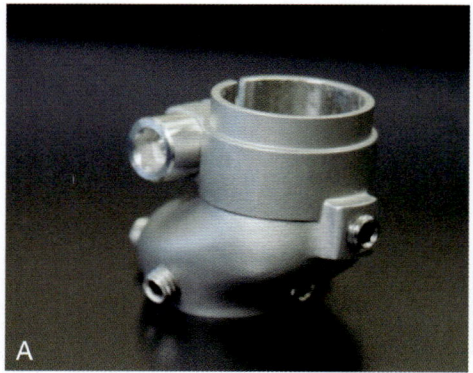
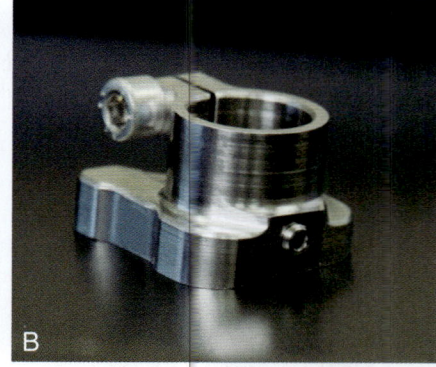

FIGURE 10 Allen key prosthetic connectors with posterior offsets with (**A**) distal standard female pyramid receiver and (**B**) distal standard four-hole pattern. Anterior grub screws engage the distal ring of the taper sleeve's fail-safe mechanism. (Courtesy of Lorin Merkley.)

ambulation with no assistance. A ninth patient was independently ambulating by 12 weeks.[19]

Mean baseline 6-minute walk scores increased significantly from 481 to 585 m at 1-year follow-up. "Global" scores on the Q-TFA increased significantly from 62.5 at baseline to 90.5 at 1 year. The mean "Problem" scores on the same measure decreased significantly from 24.6 to 3.4 over the same interval. The mean "Prosthetic Mobility Score" increased significantly from 64.3 to 90.3 in the first 6 months postimplantation.[19]

Compress

The Compress approach to OI represents a third mechanism of bony attachment.[20] Although new implantations with this approach are not currently occurring, a number of patients have been fitted using this approach, warranting inclusion in this chapter. The Compress was developed by the Biomet Corporation (now Zimmer Biomet) in the 1990s and ultimately received FDA approval for applications in endoprostheses. The Compress is designed to take advantage of the principle that bone

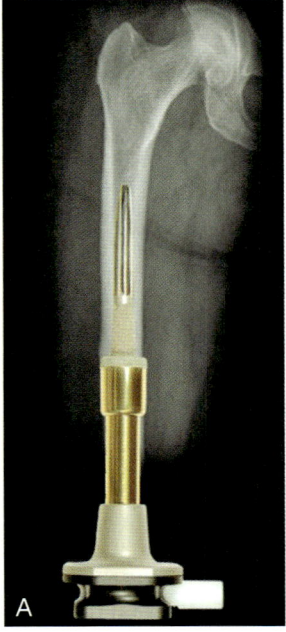 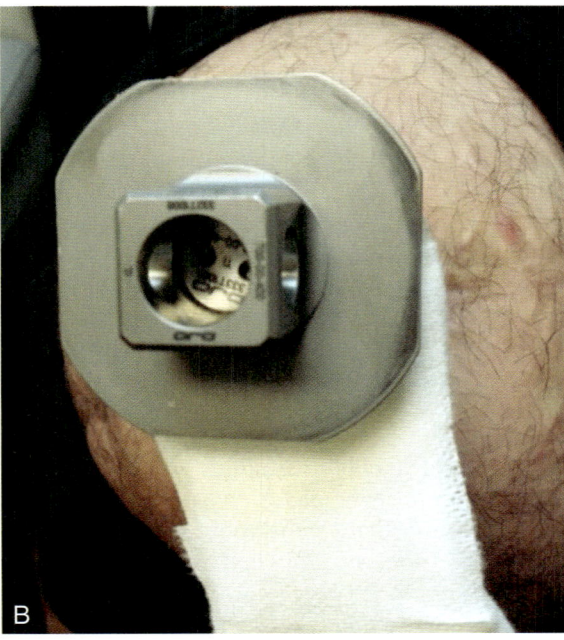 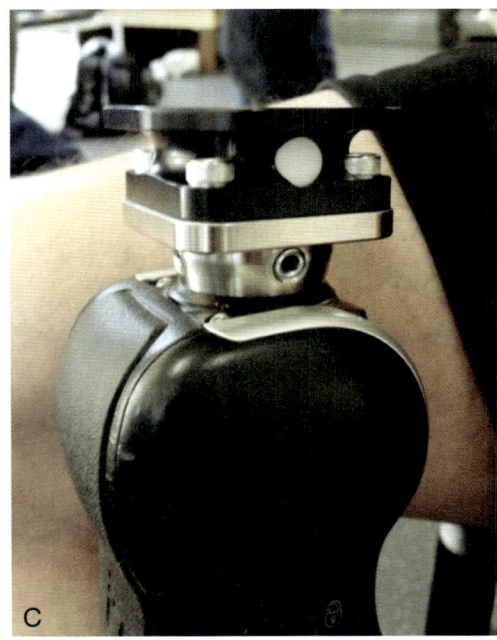

FIGURE 11 Photographs of the Percutaneous Osseointegrated Prosthesis (POP) press-fit implant. **A**, In place of the more common cylindrical taper sleeve, a Ferrier adaptor is fitted over the distal cone, mimicking the geometry of a commercially available male Ferrier coupler. **B**, Distal view of the internal locking screw, locking the Ferrier adaptor in place on the dual cone adaptor. **C**, A commercially available female Ferrier coupler is used at the proximal aspect of the prosthetic knee mechanism. The POP Ferrier adaptor fits within the female Ferrier coupler where it is secured with a standard Delrin pin.

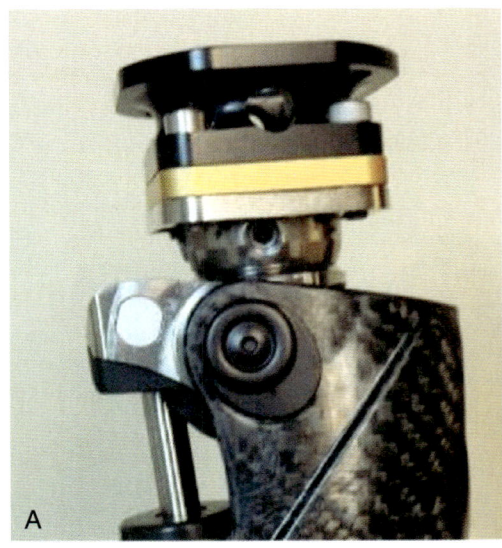 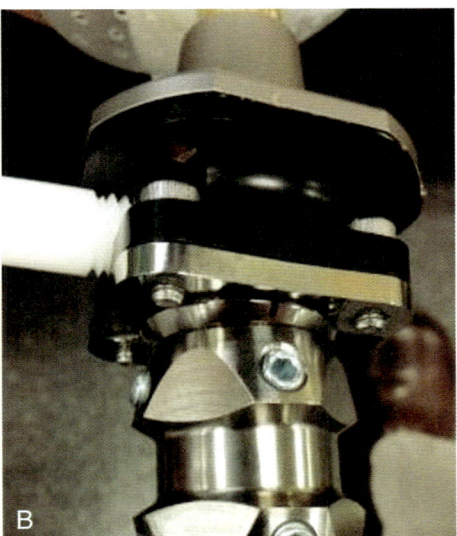 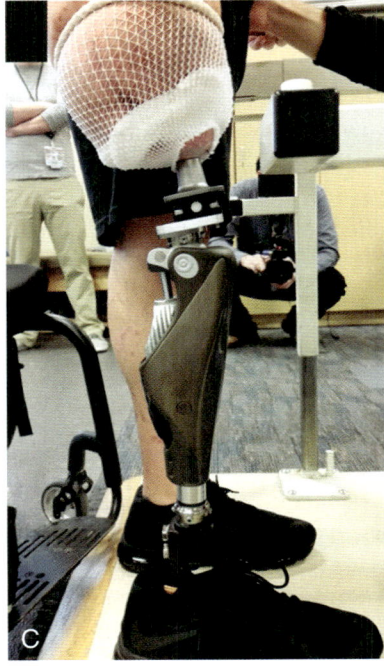

FIGURE 12 Photographs of the prosthetic connections to the Percutaneous Osseointegrated Prosthesis (POP) implant through a standard female Ferrier coupler. Variations include the use of standard spacer plates (**A**), standard alignable endoskeletal components (**B**), and posterior offset plates (**C**).

grows in response to stress. The spindle of the implant is inserted into the medullary canal of the bone until its transected distal edge is set against a firm collar. A series of transosseous pins pass through the bone and the tunneled anchor plug of the implant to anchor the unit at midshaft of the bone. Belleville washers integrated between the transosseous pins and the distal collar are preloaded for 400, 600, or 800 lb of pressure. With the pins in place, these washers are deployed to apply the desired load at the distal end of the bone against the collar to stimulate bone growth.[20]

In 2017, a cohort of authors reported pilot data from 13 patients who had received the Compress transfemoral OI implant under the FDA's custom device regulations.[20] These patients had undergone either two-stage or single-stage implantation. Because of the multicenter nature of these pilot fittings, aggregated outcomes data were not reported.

Prosthetic Alignment Considerations

The alignment of the external prosthesis beneath the percutaneous post and implant-specific adaptors largely follows standard prosthetic principles. Individual implants may be associated with specific offset limits, and this constraint should be considered on an implant-specific basis. Where FDA labels have established clear instructions for use with regard to component selection and alignment constraints, these should be followed. In the absence of such guidelines, implant manufacturers should be consulted.

Following OI, most users of transfemoral prostheses prefer the inherent stability of microprocessor knees. Such knees are associated with reduced risks for stumbles and falls,[21,22] and they may protect the user from fall-related injury to the implant, overlying femur or percutaneous post. In the absence of socket-related suspension limitations, many users are eager to return to activities associated with water exposure, such as taking a standing shower with their prosthesis or wading in bodies of water. Accordingly, water resistance is often an important consideration for this cohort. Where indicated, some users prefer activity-specific prostheses and alignment on a task-specific basis, such as a knee with minimal swing phase resistance aligned in internal rotation to accommodate cycling.

The direct attachment of the femur to the prosthesis may allow users to more fully engage the benefits of stance phase knee flexion resistance. Therefore, prosthetic alignment should facilitate this design feature. Because of the phenomenon of osseoperception, users may more directly feel the forces acting on the prosthetic knee. During early rehabilitation, augmented swing-phase extension dampening may be beneficial in reducing the suddenness of terminal impact in swing phase.

Given the immediate translation of ground reaction forces to the implant–femur interface, some mechanism of force absorption should be considered in the axial, coronal, sagittal, and transverse planes. This often occurs through the choice of prosthetic foot. Feet with vertical shock absorption and multiaxial function, along with endoskeletal axial torque absorbers, are often anecdotally preferred by prosthesis users, with subjective reports of increased comfort at the femoral interface with the use of compliant feet.

In the absence of femoral soft tissues mitigating the forces between the prosthesis and the residual femur, users of osseointegrated prostheses are able to provide an augmented level of feedback to their treating clinicians to pursue a more refined level of dynamic alignment. Alignments may require more clinical attention than those encountered with traditional socket interfaces. However, the consistency of donning an osseointegrated prostheses ensures that prosthetic alignment is more consistent than that observed with traditional socket interfaces.

Sagittal alignment considerations are largely consistent with standard prosthetic principles. Hip flexion contractures can be managed through a flexed alignment proximal to the knee unit with posterior offset plates to align the prosthetic knee beneath the anatomic hip joint. Notably, in contrast to traditional interfaces between the residual femur and the socket, the direct attachment of the prosthesis to the femur is such that hip flexion contractures have been observed to decrease rather quickly through day-to-day use. Thus, any alignment accommodations to a hip flexion contracture should be monitored and reduced as hip extension range of motion is regained.

Some have observed that the anatomic bow of the femur is such that when treating patients with short to midlength residual femurs, some degree of posterior offset may be needed to position the knee beneath the hip joint without undue strain on the low back. Some implant-specific components are designed to provide this posterior offset.

Coronal alignment considerations are largely consistent with standard prosthetic principles. Although the residual femur has been observed in relative abduction despite aggressive socket adduction values,[23] the direct attachment of the femur to the prosthesis allows hip and knee alignment to mimic the Q angle of the sound side limb. Aggressive adduction alignment is often observed with longer residual femurs and in some instances and lateral offset may be indicated. Adduction angles may be more modest with shorter residual femur lengths.

SUMMARY

Although not without their own risks, several approaches to OI have been pursued in recent years in an attempt to eliminate the discomfort and inconvenience of traditional socket prostheses. Common surgical approaches include threaded implants screwed into the medullary canal and press-fit implants inserted into the medullary canal until the transected bone rests on the distal collar of the implant. Implantation protocols can be either single stage or two stage. Each implant is associated with its own rehabilitation pathway with respect to the rate of progression toward full weight bearing. Each implant is associated with a designated means of passing through the skin and connecting to standard prosthetic components. Prosthetists need to understand all constraints related to prosthetic connectors, alignment, and components specific to a given implant. Clinical outcomes with existing implants have been encouraging with increases in prosthetic use and mobility as well as quality of life.

References

1. Hoellwarth JS, Tetsworth K, Rozbruch SR, Handal MB, Coughlan A, Al Muderis M: Osseointegration for amputees: Current implants, techniques, and future directions. *JBJS Rev* 2020;8(3):e0043.

2. Zaid MB, O'Donnell RJ, Potter BK, Forsberg JA: Orthopaedic osseointegration: State of the art. *J Am Acad Orthop Surg* 2019;27(22):e977-e985.

3. Hagberg K, Brånemark R: One hundred patients treated with osseointegrated transfemoral amputation prostheses – Rehabilitation perspective. *J Rehabil Res Dev* 2009;46(3):331-344.

4. Forsberg J, Branemark R: Osseointegration: Surgical management, in Krajbich JI, Pinzur MS, Potter BK, Stevens PM, eds: *Atlas of Amputations and Limb Deficiencies: Surgical, Prosthetic, and Rehabilitation Principles*, ed 4. Amercian Academy of Orthopaedic Surgeons, 2016, pp 575-582.

5. Sullivan J: Prosthetic management of osseointegration, in Krajbich JI, Pinzur MS, Potter BK, Stevens PM, eds: *Atlas of Amputations and Limb Deficiencies: Surgical, Prosthetic, and Rehabilitation Principles*, ed 4. Amercian Academy of Orthopaedic Surgeons, 2016, pp 583-595.

6. Hagberg K, Brånemark R, Gunterberg B, Rydevik B: Osseointegrated transfemoral amputation prostheses: Prospective results of general and condition-specific quality of life in 18 patients at 2-year follow-up. *Prosthet Orthot Int* 2008;32:29-41.

7. Brånemark R, Berlin O, Hagberg K, Bergh P, Gunterberg B, Rydevik B: A novel osseointegrated percutaneous prosthetic system for the treatment of patients with transfemoral amputation: A prospective study of 51 patients. *Bone Joint J* 2014;96-B:106-113.

8. Brånemark R, Hagberg K, Kulbacka-Ortiz K, Berlin Ö, Rydevik B: Osseointegrated percutaneous prosthetic system for the treatment of patients with transfemoral amputation: A prospective five-year follow-up of patient-reported outcomes and complications. *J Am Acad Orthop Surg* 2019;27(16):e743-e751.

9. Aprato A, Risitano S, Sabatini L, Giachino M, Agati G, Massè A: Cementless total knee arthroplasty. *Ann Transl Med* 2016;4(7):129.

10. Asokan A, Plastow R, Kayani B, Radhakrishnan GT, Magan AA, Haddad FS: Cementless knee arthroplasty: A review of recent performance. *Bone Jt Open* 2021;2(1):48-57.

11. Aschoff HH, Kennon RE, Keggi JM, Rubin LE: Transcutaneous, distal femoral, intramedullary attachment for above-the-knee prostheses: An endo-exo device. *J Bone Joint Surg Am* 2010;92(suppl 2): 180-186.

12. Juhnke DL, Beck JP, Jeyapalina S, Aschoff HH: Fifteen years of experience with integral-leg-prosthesis: Cohort study of artificial limb attachment system. *J Rehabil Res Dev* 2015;52(4):407-420.

13. van de Meent H, Hopman MT, Frolke JP: Walking ability and quality of life in subjects with transfemoral amputation: A comparison of osseointegration with socket prostheses. *Arch Phys Med Rehabil* 2013;94(11):2174-2178.

14. Pospiech PT, Wendlandt R, Aschoff HH, Ziegert S, Schulz AP: Quality of life of persons with transfemoral amputation: Comparison of socket prostheses and Osseointegrated prostheses. *Prosthet Orthot Int* 2020;25:309364620948649.

15. Muderis MA, Tetsworth K, Khemka A, et al: The Osseointegration Group of Australia Accelerated Protocol (OGAAP-1) for two-stage osseointegrated reconstruction of amputated limbs. *Bone Joint J* 2016;98-B(7):952-960.

16. Al Muderis M, Lu W, Tetsworth K, Bosley B, Li JJ: Single-stage osseointegrated reconstruction and rehabilitation of lower limb amputees: The Osseointegration Group of Australia Accelerated Protocol-2 (OGAAP-2) for a prospective cohort study. *BMJ Open* 2017;7(3):e013508.

17. Haque R, Al-Jawazneh S, Hoellwarth J, et al: Osseointegrated reconstruction and rehabilitation of transtibial amputees: The Osseointegration Group of Australia surgical technique and protocol for a prospective cohort study. *BMJ Open* 2020;10(10):e038346.

18. Atallah R, van de Meent H, Verhamme L, Frölke JP, Leijendekkers RA: Safety, prosthesis wearing time and health-related quality of life of lower extremity bone-anchored prostheses using a press-fit titanium osseointegration implant: A prospective one-year follow-up cohort study. *PLoS One* 2020;15(3):e0230027.

19. Sinclair S, Beck JP, Webster J, et al: The first FDA approved early feasibility study of a novel percutaneous bone anchored prosthesis for transfemoral amputees: A prospective one-year follow-up cohort study. *Arch Phys Med Rehabil* 2022; 103(11):2092-2104.

20. McGough RL, Goodman MA, Randall RL, Forsberg JA, Potter BK, Lindsey B: The Compress® transcutaneous implant for rehabilitation following limb amputation. *Unfallchirurg* 2017;120(4): 300-305.

21. Stevens PM, Wurdeman SR: Prosthetic knee selection for individuals with unilateral transfemoral amputation: A clinical practice guideline. *J Prosthet Orthot* 2019;31(1):2-8.

22. Sawers AB, Hafner BJ: Outcomes associated with the use of microprocessor-controlled prosthetic knees among individuals with unilateral transfemoral limb loss: A systematic review. *J Rehabil Res Dev* 2013;50(3):273-314.

23. Gottschalk FA, Kourosh S, Stills M, McClellan B, Roberts J: Does socket configuration influence the position of the femur in above-knee amputation? *J Prosthet Orthot* 1989;2(1):94.

Physical Therapy Management of Adult Lower Limb Amputees

Robert S. Gailey, PhD, PT, FAPTA • Anat Kristal, PhD, MScPT •
Ignacio Gaunaurd, PT, PhD, MSPT

CHAPTER 49

ABSTRACT

The physical therapy management of an individual with lower limb amputation is a critical component of the continuum of care. The physical therapist is often introduced to a patient preoperatively in preparation for amputation surgery and is one of the first members of the rehabilitation team to begin treatment postoperatively. From the preprosthetic phase through prosthetic gait training and community reentry, physical therapy interventions can have a profound effect on the outcomes of people with limb loss.

Keywords: amputee; amputation; evidence-based; physical therapy; prosthetics; rehabilitation

Introduction

As members of the rehabilitation team, the prosthetist and the physical therapist often develop a close relationship when working together with individuals with lower limb amputations. The prosthetist is responsible for fabricating a prosthesis that will best suit the lifestyle of the individual patient. The physical therapist has a multifaceted role that includes postoperative care, mobility, and residual limb care. Before the patient can be properly fitted with a prosthesis, the physical therapist helps the amputee become physically prepared for prosthetic training. After the prosthesis is received, the patient must learn how to use and care for it. Prosthetic gait training can be the most frustrating yet rewarding phase of rehabilitation for all involved. The patient must be reeducated in the biomechanics of gait while learning how to use a prosthesis. After success is achieved, the patient may look forward to resuming a productive life. The physical therapist should introduce the patient to higher levels of activities other than just learning to walk. The patient may not be ready to participate in recreational activities immediately; however, providing the names of support and recreational organizations serving the disabled population will enable the individual to seek involvement at the appropriate time.

Preoperative Care

When preoperative care is possible, the physical therapist should begin to establish rapport with the patient during the initial appointment. It is important to earn the patient's trust and confidence. After introductions, the physical therapist should explain the expected timing of events during the rehabilitation process. The unknown can be extremely frightening to many patients. Fears can be addressed by explaining what the future holds and what will be expected of the patient throughout the process. Having another amputee visit and talk with the patient can often assist in this process. The amputee peer visitor should be carefully screened by appropriate personnel and should have a suitable personality for this task. Many hospitals have affiliations with local amputee support groups with members who are certified peer visitors (CPVs) who have received formal training from the Amputee Coalition.[1] Amputees who have successfully completed the CPV training program have been instructed in communication skills, have a basic knowledge of limb loss statistics, have provided references, and should have experience working with healthcare facilities and professionals who serve amputees. When pairing a CPV with a new amputee, consideration should be given to similarities between level of amputation, age, sex, and outside interests.[2] The Amputee Coalition in association with John Hopkins Hospital developed a program called Promoting

---

Dr. Gailey or an immediate family member is a member of a speakers' bureau or has made paid presentations on behalf of Össur and serves as a paid consultant to or is an employee of Össur. Dr. Kristal or an immediate family member serves as a paid consultant to or is an employee of Össur. Neither Dr. Gaunaurd nor any immediate family member has received anything of value from or has stock or stock options held in a commercial company or institution related directly or indirectly to the subject of this chapter.
This chapter is copyrighted by Advanced Rehabilitation Therapy, Inc. Miami FL, 2024.

This chapter is adapted from Gailey RS, Gaunaurd IA, Laferrier JZ. Physical therapy management of adult lower-limb amputees. In: Krajbich JI, Pinzur MS, Potter BK, Stevens PM, eds. *Atlas of Amputations and Limb Deficiencies: Surgical, Prosthetic, and Rehabilitation Principles*. 4th ed. American Academy of Orthopaedic Surgeons, 2016, pp 597-620.

Amputee Life Skills (PALS).[3] This program aims to reduce long-term secondary health effects, such as depression and pain, by improving self-efficacy and quality of life through the implementation of 10 weeks of education specifically designed for those with limb loss. Wegener et al[4] found that the PALS program in conjunction with a peer support group was more effective in decreasing depression, managing pain, and improving function, self-efficacy, and quality of life than standard support group activities. Information on various prostheses, demonstrations of prosthetic capabilities, or videos showing recreational activities may be useful to the patient. The therapist must consider the amount of information the patient is psychologically prepared to absorb. The physical therapist may advise the patient preoperatively on the possibilities of phantom limb sensation and phantom limb pain, and the prevention of joint contracture and loss of mobility, and the benefits of general conditioning.

Acute Postoperative Evaluation

The acute postoperative evaluation consists of several important components. Baseline information is necessary to establish the goals of rehabilitation and formulate an individualized treatment plan. Viewing amputation surgery as a constructive procedure, not a destructive one, is important for all rehabilitation team members. Because preamputation functional capability is a strong predictor for postamputation mobility,[5-12] rehabilitation goals should focus on restoring the amputee to a premorbid lifestyle and preventing further adversity.

A complete medical history should be obtained from the patient or from the medical records to supply information that may be pertinent to the rehabilitation program. During the initial chart review, the physical therapist should note any history of coronary artery disease, congestive heart failure, peripheral vascular disease, hypertension, angina, arrhythmias, dyspnea, angioplasty, myocardial infarction, arterial bypass surgery, diabetes, and renal disease. Any medications that may influence physical exertion or mental status should be recorded. In addition, the cause of the amputation can influence the concomitant medical concerns for the amputee. For example, patients with diabetes should monitor blood glucose levels before, during, and after the exercise to avoid hypoglycemic-related events. Patients with traumatic amputations may present with undetected soft-tissue injuries, nerve damage, fractures, heterotrophic bone formation, or traumatic brain injuries that will need to be addressed if present.[13]

Cardiopulmonary Status

The heart rate and blood pressure of every patient should be closely monitored during initial training and thereafter as the intensity of training increases. If the patient experiences persistent symptoms such as shortness of breath, pallor, diaphoresis, chest pain, headache, or peripheral edema, further medical evaluation is strongly recommended. If the patient's cardiopulmonary status is a concern, relatively inexpensive and simple tools such as the pulse-oximeter, the Dyspnea Index,[2] and the Borg Perceived Exertion Scale[6] may be used to help monitor exertion or to assist the patient by providing guidelines for effort during ambulation. The cause of amputation (dysvascular or traumatic), amputation level, and number of lower limbs lost have a substantial effect on energy expenditure during ambulation.[14] In addition, it is helpful to assess preamputation mobility using self-report measures to assist with predicting postamputation success.

Mental Status

An accurate assessment of the patient's mental status can provide insight about the factors likely to affect future prosthetic care. The physical therapist should assess the patient's cognitive potential to perform activities such as donning and doffing the prosthesis, residual limb prosthetic sock regulation, bed positioning, skin care, and safe ambulation. If the patient does not possess the necessary level of cognition, family members and/or friends should be encouraged to become involved in the rehabilitation process for a successful outcome.

Range of Motion

The range of motion (ROM) of both the upper and lower limbs should be assessed. A measurement of the ROM of the residual limb should be recorded for future reference. Joint contractures can hinder the patient's ability to ambulate with a prosthesis and have been associated with postural imbalances that can contribute to other physical ailments such as low back pain. Every effort should be made by the physical therapist and patient to avoid any loss of ROM. Hip flexion, external rotation, and abduction are the most common contractures in an individual with a transfemoral amputation. Knee flexion is the most frequently observed contracture in a transtibial amputee. During the ROM assessment, the therapist should determine whether the patient has a fixed contracture, or muscle tightness from immobility that may be corrected within a short period of time with ROM therapy.

Strength

The strength of the major muscle groups is typically assessed by manual muscle testing of all limbs including the residual limb and the trunk, to determine the patient's potential skill level to perform activities such as transfers, wheelchair mobility, and ambulation with and without a prosthesis. Hip abductor and extensor strength strongly influence how well a patient will ambulate with a prosthesis, regardless of the level of amputation.[15,16] A formal strengthening program for the residual and contralateral limb will enable the patient to more effectively negotiate stairs and different terrains and participate in sports.[17-19]

Sensation

An evaluation of sensation is useful to the patient and the therapist. Insensitivity of the residual limb and/or intact limb will affect proprioceptive feedback for balance and single limb stance, which in turn can lead to gait difficulties. The patient must be made aware that decreased sensation to pain, temperature, and light touch sensation can increase the risk for injury to the skin and soft-tissue breakdown. Use of a monofilament is a simple, reliable method to assess sensory impairment of the skin over the intact foot or residual limb and determine patients at risk for potential injury or risk for ulceration.[20]

Bed Mobility

The importance of good bed mobility extends beyond simple positional adjustments for comfort or getting in and out of bed. Skills are necessary to maintain correct bed positioning to prevent contractures and to avoid excessive friction of the bedsheets against the suture line or frail skin. If the patient is unable to perform the skills necessary to maintain proper positioning, assistance must be provided. As with most patients, adequate bed mobility is a prerequisite skill for higher level skills such as bed-to-wheelchair transfers.

Balance/Coordination

Balance while sitting and standing is a major concern when assessing the patient's ability to maintain the center of mass over the base of support. Coordination assists with ease of movement and the refinement of motor skills. Introducing balance and coordination exercises early in the rehabilitation program can help improve weight bearing and proprioceptive control on the amputated side and promote symmetric ambulation when undergoing gait training in the later phases of rehabilitation.[21-23] Both balance and coordination are required for weight shifting from one limb to another, thus improving the potential for an optimal gait. After evaluating mental status, ROM, strength, sensation, balance, and coordination, the therapist will have a good indication of what would be the most appropriate initial choice of an assistive device.

Transfers

Early assessment of an amputee's ability to accomplish transfer skills is essential, especially when the rehabilitation team is planning discharge from the acute care setting. Many amputees can be discharged to home if they are able to complete transfers either independently or with limited help. When bed mobility is mastered, the amputee must learn to transfer from the bed to a chair or a wheelchair and then progress to more advanced skills such as transferring to a toilet, a tub, and a car. If moderate to maximal assistance for transfers is necessary, it is not uncommon for the amputee to be referred to an institutional living facility that provides skilled assistance until the amputee becomes more independent.

Potential Ambulation With Assistive Devices

A comprehensive evaluation of the patient's potential for ambulation includes the strength of the intact lower limb and both upper limbs, single limb standing balance, coordination, and mental status. Performance-based outcome measures such as the Amputee Mobility Predictor (AMP) without a prosthesis can be used as a measure of functional capacity before prosthesis fitting, help predict mobility with a prosthesis, and assist with prosthetic prescription and assistive device selection.[24] The selection of an assistive device should match the patient's level of skill, keeping in mind that the required assistive device may change over time. For example, a patient may initially require a walker; however, after proper training, forearm crutches may prove more beneficial as a long-term assistive device. Some patients who have difficulty ambulating on one limb because of obesity, blindness, or generalized weakness can achieve successful ambulation with the additional support provided by a prosthesis.

Setting Goals

The rehabilitation team should establish realistic goals that are consistent with the patient's desired outcomes for employment, social interactions, and recreational endeavors. Regardless of the level of amputation or age, most patients have the ability to return to the lifestyle that they enjoyed before amputation with only minor accommodations.[25-27] Discussing the patient's premorbid lifestyle and goals early in the rehabilitation process can provide the rehabilitation team with valuable information that will enable a personalized treatment plan that is appropriate and motivating.

Immediate Postoperative Treatment

General Management Principles

Generally, the goals of postoperative management for the new amputee are to reduce edema, promote healing, prevent loss of motion, increase cardiovascular endurance, and improve strength. Functional skills must be introduced as early as possible to promote independence in bed mobility, transfers, and ambulation techniques. Patient education concerning the self-care of the residual limb and intact limb can prevent adverse effects such as skin abrasions, excessive edema, delayed healing, loss of ROM, and trauma to the intact limb from overuse. In addition, each member of the rehabilitation team should be aware of the need to assist the patient with the psychological adjustment to limb loss.

Postoperative Dressing

The selection of postoperative dressing varies according to the level of amputation, surgical technique, healing requirements, patient compliance, and preference of the physician. The five major types are soft dressings, nonremovable rigid dressings, immediate postoperative prostheses (IPOPs), removable rigid dressings, and prefabricated postoperative devices. Soft dressings are most often used for patients with vascular dysfunction because regular dressing changes may be needed, and alternative wound environments may be used. The disadvantage to soft dressings is that patients frequently decrease their bed mobility, because they are more hesitant to move the operated limb.[9] Rigid dressings, in addition to controlling edema and providing protection and support, assist in preventing knee flexion contractures in patients with transtibial amputations and provide greater confidence with bed mobility.

The IPOP offers the benefits of rigid dressings and allows ambulation with weight bearing and an assistive device. The IPOP also affords the patient the physiological and psychological advantage of early walking with a prosthetic limb. To date, IPOPs have not been associated with an increased number of falls or injury to the healing residual limb. In amputees with a neuropathic intact limb, providing additional support to the residual limb can potentially reduce foot pressures, improve balance, and reduce the effort of ambulation with an assistive device.

Removable rigid dressings originally were fabricated from plaster and suspended with a variety of supracondylar cuff systems. Currently, it is more common for surgeons to use a commercially available prefabricated copolymer plastic shell with a soft lining and, in some instances, the ability to attach a pylon and foot to create an IPOP. A removable rigid dressing provides the protection and other benefits of the classic rigid dressing with the flexibility of removal for wound inspection or bathing. In addition, socks may be added, or the system tightened for progressive shrinkage of the residual limb. These techniques have been shown to shorten the time to ambulatory discharge from hospital for patients with a temporary prosthesis.

Positioning

When supine, the patient with a transfemoral amputation should place a pillow laterally along the residual limb to maintain neutral rotation with no abduction. If the prone position is tolerable, a pillow should be placed under the residual limb to maintain hip extension. Patients with a transtibial amputation should avoid knee flexion for prolonged periods. A leg rest to elevate the residual limb will help maintain knee extension when using a wheelchair (**Figure 1**). All amputees must be made aware that continual sitting in a wheelchair without any effort to promote hip extension may lead to limited motion during prosthetic ambulation.

Transfers

After bed mobility is mastered, the patient must first learn to transfer from the bed to a chair or a wheelchair and then progress to more advanced transfer skills. In patients who use an IPOP or temporary prosthesis, weight bearing through the prosthesis can assist the patient in transferring and provide additional safety. For patients with transtibial amputation who are not candidates for ambulation, a lightweight transfer prosthesis may allow more independent transfers. A transfer prosthesis is typically fit when the residual limb is healed, and the patient is ready for training. Bilateral amputees who are not fitted with an initial prosthesis will transfer in a "head on" manner in which the patient slides forward from the wheelchair onto the desired surface by lifting the body and pushing forward with both hands.

Wheelchair Propulsion

A wheelchair will be the primary means of mobility for most dysvascular amputees, either temporarily or permanently. The combination of wheelchair and prosthetic use can enhance overall mobility.[28] The amount of energy conserved with wheelchair use compared with prosthetic ambulation is considerable with some levels of amputation.[29] Therefore, amputees should be taught wheelchair skills as a part of their rehabilitation program. Bilateral amputees and older amputees with more severe medical conditions may require greater use of a wheelchair, whereas unilateral and younger amputees with fewer comorbidities will be more likely to use other assistive devices when not ambulating with a prosthesis.[30] Because of the loss of body weight anteriorly, patients are prone to tipping backward while in the standard wheelchair. Adapters can set the wheels back approximately 2 inches (5 cm), thus moving the center of mass away from the axis of rotation to prevent tipping. This is especially helpful when ascending ramps or curbs. An alternative method is the addition of antitipping in place of or in addition to wheel adapters.

Patients who will be long-term wheelchair users for mobility within the community should be fit for a fully adjustable ultralight manual wheelchair. For example, while moving the rear wheels backward would increase chair stability, it would compromise overall maneuverability and place the amputee at increased risk for repetitive strain injuries to the upper limbs during active self-propulsion.[31] Adjustable axle plates can allow the wheels to be set back early in rehabilitation for stability and moved forward to afford the amputee accessibility to the push-rims in a biomechanically safe and efficient position as they become more skilled. Adjustable backrests set at less than 90° can assist the amputee in keeping the center of mass in a forward position when the prosthesis is not worn and recline to greater than 90° to accommodate prosthetic wear. Transtibial amputees also require an elevating leg rest or residual limb support designed to maintain the knee in extension, thus preventing prolonged knee flexion and reducing the dependent position of the limb to control edema. It is also recommended that the wheelchair be fitted with removable armrests to enable ease of transfer to or from either side of the chair.

Ambulation With Assistive Devices

All amputees will need an assistive device for times when they choose not to wear their prosthesis, or on occasions when they are unable to wear their prosthesis secondary to edema, skin irritation, or a poor fit. Some amputees require an assistive device while ambulating with the prosthesis. Although safety is the primary factor when selecting the appropriate assistive device, mobility is an important secondary consideration. The criteria for selection should include the following factors: (1) the ability for unsupported standing balance, (2) the amount of upper limb strength, (3) coordination and skill with the assistive device, and (4) cognition. A walker is chosen when an amputee has fair to poor balance, strength, and coordination. If balance

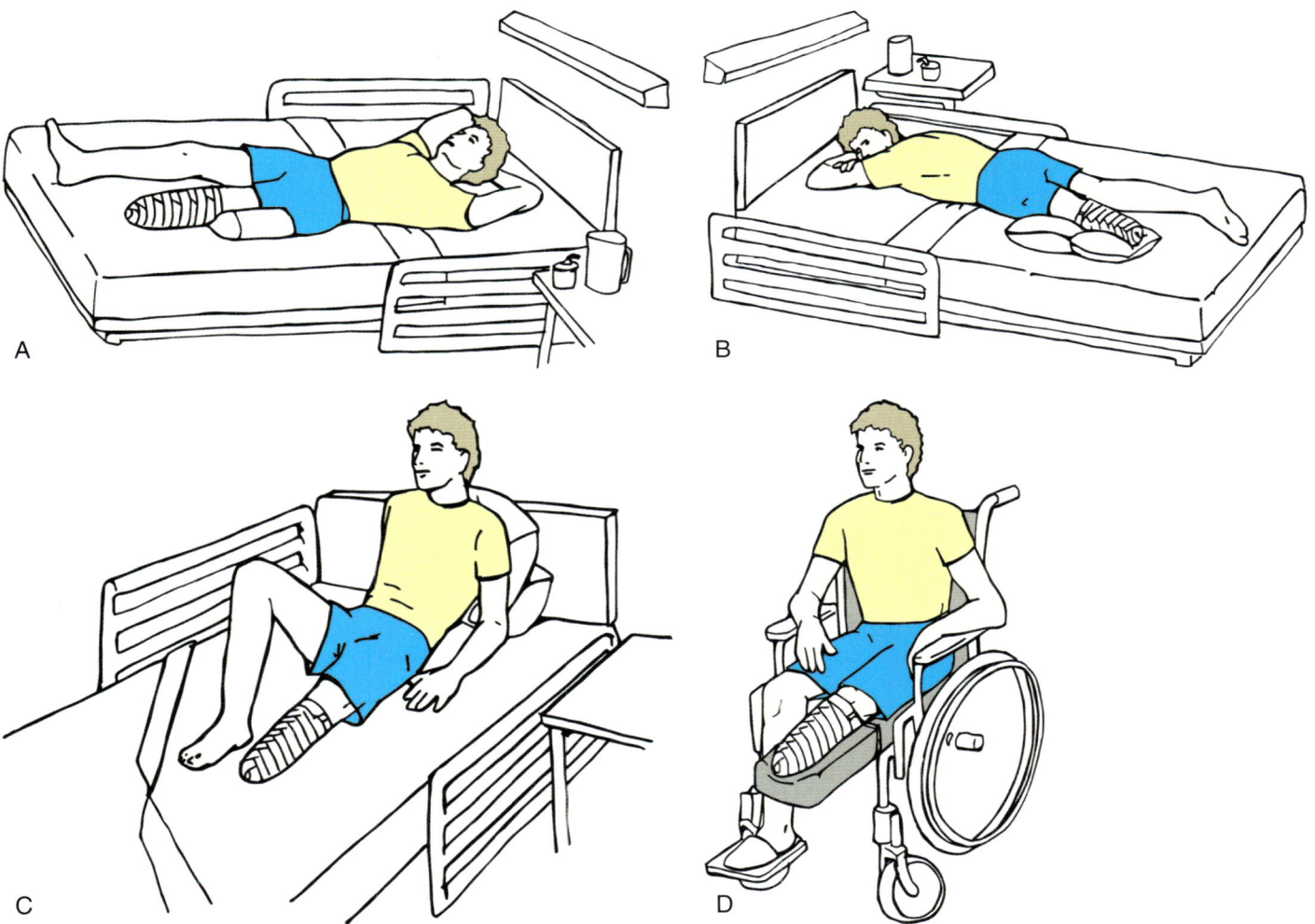

FIGURE 1 Illustrations showing proper positioning of the residual limb. **A**, Neutral hip rotation with no abduction. **B**, Hip and knee extension when prone. **C**, Knee extension when in bed. **D**, Knee extension when sitting. (Copyright Advanced Rehabilitation Therapy, Inc, Miami, FL, 1990. Illustrator, Frank Angulo.)

and strength are good to normal, forearm crutches may be used for ambulation with or without a prosthesis. A quad cane or straight cane may be selected to ensure safety when balance is questionable while ambulating with a prosthesis.

Patient Education

Skin Care

Patients must be instructed about caring for the residual and intact limbs. The care of skin and scar tissue is extremely important to prevent skin breakdown during prosthetic gait training which would delay rehabilitation and lead to further deconditioning. Appropriate skin care is especially important for patients with diabetes mellitus and/or vascular dysfunction because these patients often require additional healing time. Patients must also be taught the difference between weight-bearing and pressure-sensitive areas in relation to the design and fit of the prosthetic socket. They should be instructed to visually inspect their residual limb on a daily basis or after any strenuous activity for evidence of any abnormal pressures from the socket, such as areas of persistent redness.

Inspection of the intact limb after amputation is important because the foot is subject to additional axial and shear force to compensate for prosthetic weight bearing. A hand mirror may be used to view the posterior residual limb and plantar aspect of the foot. Areas of redness should be monitored very closely as potential sites for abrasion or ulcer. Amputees with visual impairment should seek the assistance of a family member for daily inspections.

If a skin abrasion or ulcer develops, the amputee must understand that, in most cases, the prosthesis should not be worn until healing occurs. In some instances, a protective barrier may be used to avert further insult to the integrity of the tissue while permitting continued use of the prosthesis. Without exception, any lesion to the skin should be reported and followed clinically to avoid further complications.

Desensitization

Many amputees experience postoperative skin hypersensitivity as a result of the disruption of the neuromuscular system and associated edema. Progressive desensitization of the residual limb is often necessary for restoring normal sensation, while using wound compression techniques to reduce the edema. Desensitization involves gradually introducing stimuli to reduce the hyperirritability of the limb. For example, a soft material such as cotton cloth or lamb's wool is rubbed around the residual limb, followed by gradually coarser materials such as corduroy. The amputee should progress as quickly as possible to tapping massage with the hand. Eventually, when the suture line has healed, pressure can be applied to the residual limb during transfers, mobility skills, and exercise. These measures will help expedite the ability of the residual limb to wear the prosthesis.

Care of the Prosthesis

The socket should be cleaned daily to promote good hygiene and prevent deterioration of prosthetic materials. The patient should be informed of the best cleansing agent for their socket and liner. In general, laminate plastic, copolymer plastic and silicone materials are cleaned with a damp cloth and mild soap. Foam materials are cleaned with rubbing alcohol. Because some liner materials interact adversely with alcohol, manufacturers' recommendations should be followed. After using the cleansing agent, a clean damp cloth should be used to wipe away any residue. To ensure maximum life and safety of the prosthesis, patients should be reminded that routine maintenance of the prosthesis should be performed by the prosthetist.

Sock Regulation

Prosthetic sock regulation is important to prevent both extreme loading on the distal aspect of the limb and excessive vertical motion or pistoning between the residual limb and the socket. The amputee should always carry extra socks to be added if pistoning or extreme perspiration occurs. Prosthetic socks are available in several thicknesses or plies, permitting the amputee to obtain the desired fit within the socket. The regular interactions between the physical therapist and the newer amputee provide numerous opportunities to reinforce the importance and technique of using prosthetic socks to manage changing limb volume. Socks should be applied wrinkle free with the seam horizontal and on the outside to prevent irritation or abrasion to the skin. Because most prosthetic socks today are seamless this problem has been greatly reduced.

Suspension sleeves and liners are fabricated from a variety of materials such as silicone, urethane, and gel composites. Some of the benefits of these materials include reduced pistoning, better management of unstable limb volume, improved cosmesis, and for some amputees with impaired hand function, easier donning of the prosthesis. Liners not only reduce shear forces over scar tissue and bony prominences, but also act as suspension devices.

Suspension sleeves and liners are widely accepted, but some amputees have problems with skin reactions from the materials used. Fortunately, a wide variety of materials are available with many alternative solutions should this problem become evident.

Donning and Doffing of the Prosthesis

A wide variety of suspension systems are available for all levels of amputation. The methods of donning a prosthesis are too numerous to describe in this chapter; however, it is important that the prosthetist instruct both the amputee and the physical therapist in the proper method of donning and doffing the particular prosthesis. The physical therapist can help patients develop proactive individualized donning strategies during the early phases of prosthetic rehabilitation.

Residual Limb Compression Dressing

Early rigid or semirigid dressings, compression wrapping, or shrinker socks for the residual limb decrease edema, increase circulation, assist in shaping, provide skin protection, reduce redundant tissue problems, reduce phantom limb pain and/or sensation, and desensitize the residual limb. The use of traditional compression wrapping versus the use of residual limb shrinker socks is controversial. Some institutions prefer commercial shrinker socks because they are easy to don. Advocates of compression wrapping suggest that they may provide more control over pressure gradients and tissue shaping.[32]

Many programs prefer to wait until after the sutures or staples have been removed before using a shrinker sock. For amputees with diabetes mellitus, this period is often as long as 21 days. However, compression therapy can begin with wraps or rigid dressings and progress to shrinker socks after the suture line has healed. Compression therapy is a controversial topic, and each rehabilitation team should determine the best course of treatment for their patients. All compression techniques must be performed correctly and consistently to prevent constriction, decreased circulation, poor shaping, and edema. Patient compliance also is an intricate part of the compression program. All wrappings or shrinker socks should be routinely checked and/or reapplied several times per day. The application of a nylon sheath over the residual limb before wrapping or donning the shrinker sock may reduce shearing forces to skin and thus provide additional comfort and safety.

Issues Pertaining to the Intact Limb

The loss of a limb and its substitution by a prosthesis can clearly affect gait biomechanics in most amputees. Therefore, when planning treatment of these patients, management of the intact limb is critical. Preservation of the intact limb may permit continued bipedal ambulation and delay medical complications that can reduce quality of life. One reason for this concern is that the intact limb routinely compensates for the amputee's inability to maintain equal weight distribution between limbs resulting in altered gait mechanics. Two known effects on the intact limb are the altered forces being placed on the weight-bearing surfaces of the foot and the second is the increase in ground reaction forces throughout the skeletal structures of the limb.[33-35]

Amputees with diabetes mellitus may have deviations from normal gait kinematics that increase vertical and shear forces in addition to preexisting abnormal sensation, devascularization, scar tissue, and any foot and/or ankle deformity. Patients with diabetes mellitus have a 50% increased incidence of amputation in the same or contralateral limb within 4 years after the primary amputation.[20] Accordingly, expert care of the intact foot becomes even more critical after amputation for amputees with diabetes mellitus, because their chances of achieving functional ambulation as a bilateral amputee will decline.[36]

Amputations performed because of trauma, congenital causes, or tumor result in a progressively increased risk of musculoskeletal imbalances or pathologies that often lead to secondary physical conditions that affect the patient's mobility and quality of life. Because amputees tend to favor their intact lower limb, it is often stressed in performing daily activities. It has been found that osteoarthritis is more prevalent in the contralateral limb than the residual limb of amputees of those with lower limb amputation.[37,38] The prevalence of osteoarthritis has become an increasing concern, especially with individuals who have lived with an amputation for long periods of time.[39] Over time, the altered forces placed on the skeletal and soft tissues of the intact limb can lead to degenerative conditions.[23] Proper prosthetic fit and physical therapy training increase the probability of having equal force distribution across the intact and prosthetic limbs during ambulation and may decrease the risk of the development of osteoarthritis.[40] The patient should be advised about risks to the intact limb early in the rehabilitation process.

Strategies to Enhance Patient Education

Educating the amputee about self-care and a home exercise program are critical to the ultimate outcome of the rehabilitation process. The most difficult task is ensuring the patient retains the information and complies with instructions. A self-care checklist that the patient can take home may assist in achieving a positive outcome and provides the clinician with a format for ensuring that important points of care are explained.

Preprosthetic Exercises

General Conditioning

Decreased general conditioning and endurance often contribute to the difficulties in learning functional activities, including prosthetic gait. Regardless of age or current physical condition, amputees should begin a progressive general exercise program immediately after surgery, through the preprosthetic period and eventually as part of a daily routine.

There are many possible general strengthening and endurance exercise activities. Examples include using cuff weights in bed, wheelchair propulsion for a predetermined distance, dynamic exercises for the residual limb, ambulation with an assistive device before the prosthesis is fit, lower and/or upper limb ergometer, wheelchair aerobics, swimming, aquatic therapy, lower and upper body strengthening at the local fitness center, and any sport or recreational activity of interest. One or more of these activities should be selected and performed to tolerance initially, progressing to 1 hour or more each day. The advantages of activity extend beyond improving the chances of good ambulation with a prosthesis. Amputees have the opportunity to experience and enjoy activities they may have not thought possible. While still in the hospital or rehabilitation center, they may have access to a physical therapist or fellow amputee who has mastered a particular activity and is available to provide instruction.

Cardiopulmonary Endurance

Because the average physical and cardiac condition of amputees with dysvascular disease is poor, cardiopulmonary endurance training can directly affect functional walking capabilities, particularly distance and the type of assistive device required for walking.[41,42] Aerobic training improves overall ambulation capabilities regardless of the level of amputation.[43]

Aerobic training typically begins immediately after surgery as the patient increases their sitting tolerance and early walking distance. Improving aerobic fitness should be incorporated into the rehabilitation program and remain as a part of the amputee's general fitness after discharge. Initially, most amputees can perform upper limb ergometry safely.[44,45] After balance and strength return, lower limb ergometry may be performed, beginning with the intact limb and progressing to use of the prosthetic limb, when appropriate. As the amputee's level of fitness improves other equipment such as treadmills, stair climbing, and rowing machines may be used. Because amputees enjoy the same activities as nonamputees, swimming and walking may be the exercises of choice for general fitness regardless of age or athletic ability.[46]

Strengthening

Dynamic exercise of the residual limb require little in the way of equipment, just a towel roll and a step stool.[47-49] In addition to increasing strength, these exercises offer benefits such as desensitization, improving bed mobility, and maintaining joint ROM. While lying on an exercise mat, the patient depresses their residual limb into the towel roll and raises their pelvis off the surface for a count of 10 seconds. The four postural positions that strengthen the hip musculature include supine for the hip extensors, side-lying on the sound side for hip abductors, side-lying intact side for adductors, and prone for hip flexor muscles. A transtibial amputee can perform two additional exercises. To strengthen the knee flexors, the patient curls their residual limb over the towel roll or end of the plinth. To strengthen the knee extensors, the patient is prone with a pillow under their thigh, depressing their residual limb into the towel roll. The basic dynamic strength training program[49] for transfemoral and transtibial amputees is shown in **Figure 2**.

As soon as bed or mat exercises can be tolerated, patients should be introduced to the basics of core stabilization,

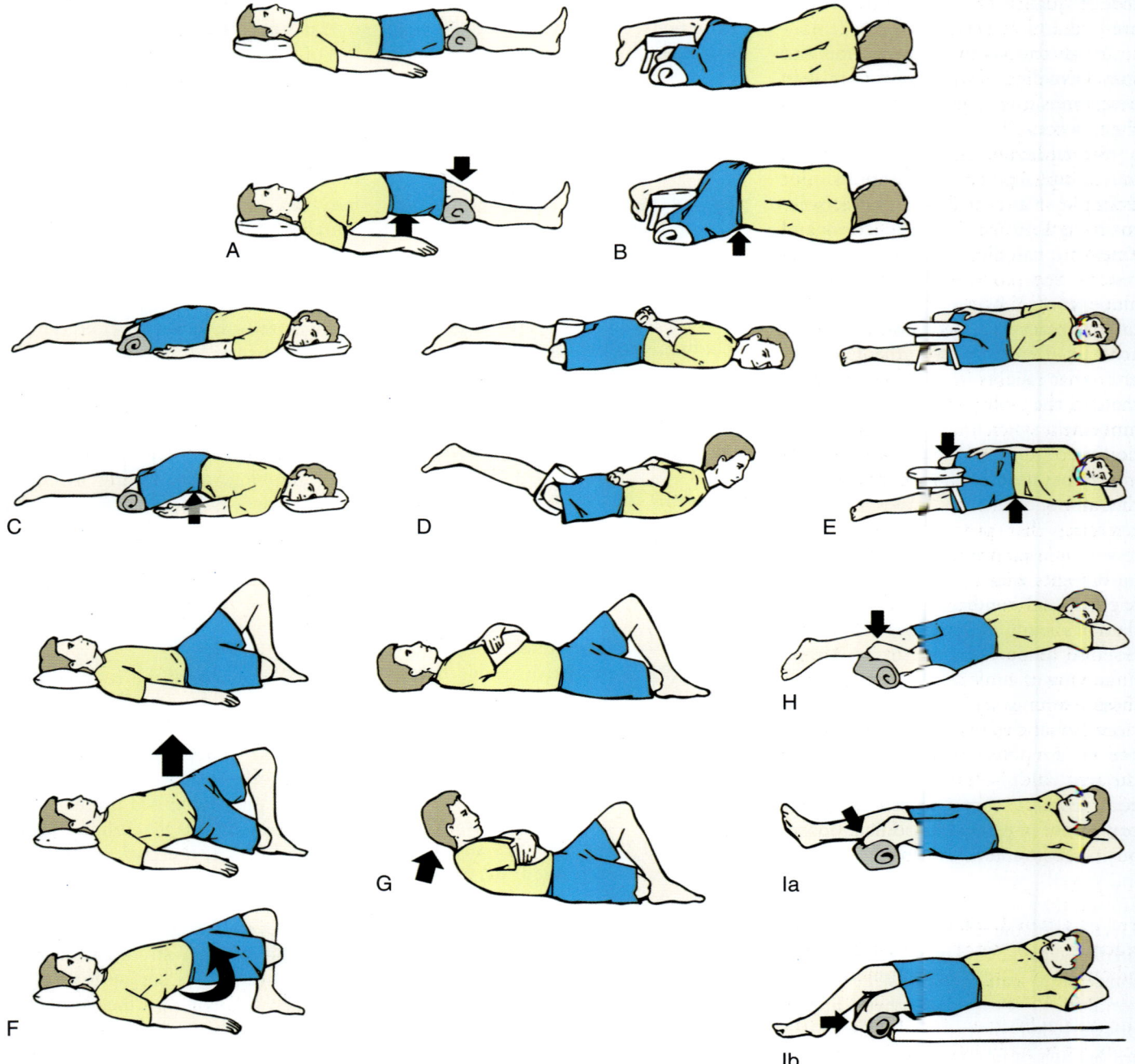

FIGURE 2 Illustrations of strengthening exercises for the residual limb. **A**, Hip extension. **B**, Hip abduction. **C**, Hip flexion. **D**, Back extension. **E**, Hip adduction. **F**, Bridging. **G**, Sit-ups. **H**, Knee extension. **I**, Knee flexion, on table (top), and knee flexion, leg over table (bottom). (Copyright Advanced Rehabilitation Therapy, Inc, Miami, FL, 1989. Illustrator, Frank Angulo.)

which focuses on intervertebral control, lumbopelvic orientation, and whole-body equilibrium, through strengthening of the transversus abdominis and multifidus muscles.[50] Strengthening the core musculature may minimize or prevent some negative effects, including low back pain, gait dysfunction, and functional impairments after lower limb amputation.[51] Core stabilization strengthening can enhance transfer activities, balance, and ambulation by facilitating neuromuscular pathways, increasing strength, and improving balance through the coordination of the synergistic muscles of the trunk. The purpose of core stabilization is to control, prevent, or eliminate low back pain; increase patient education and kinesthetic awareness; increase strength, flexibility, coordination, balance, and endurance; and develop strong trunk musculature to enhance upper and/or lower limb functional activities. Low back pain is a frequent and debilitating impairment in amputees, and it can often limit physical performance and reduce quality of life.⁵²,⁵³ Lower limb amputees have been found to demonstrate alterations in trunk motion and spinal loading during gait that may contribute to a high risk for injury to the low back.⁵⁴

Strengthening should be performed in multiple planes of motions. For example, if a transtibial amputee were to strengthen just the knee flexors and extensor muscles, which primarily control the movement in the sagittal plane, control of the knee in the frontal and transverse plane would not be achieved. With a strengthening program that focuses on all three planes of motion, the ability to control excessive movement when walking in any direction or on uneven terrain will provide improved stability and confidence in the ability to control the prosthesis. Exercises that promote strengthening in multiple planes incorporating rapid movements with concentric and eccentric contractions can assist with prosthetic control and help the amputee respond to the demands of walking.³⁴ Following the receipt of a prosthesis these exercises can be performed in a closed kinetic change posture (**Figures 3** and **4**). Amputees who have access to isotonic and isokinetic strengthening equipment can benefit from using this equipment with few modifications in positioning on the machines.

Range of Motion

Prevention of decreased ROM and contractures is a major concern in the rehabilitation of amputees. Limited ROM can often result in difficulties with prosthetic fit, gait deviations, or the inability to ambulate with a prosthesis. The best way for an amputee to prevent loss of ROM is to remain active. Unfortunately, not all amputees have this option; therefore, proper limb positioning must be maintained long after amputation, especially in sedentary amputees. If ROM has already been lost, the amputee may benefit from many traditional therapy procedures such as passive ROM, contract–relax stretching, soft-tissue mobilization, myofascial techniques, joint mobilization, and other methods that promote increased ROM.

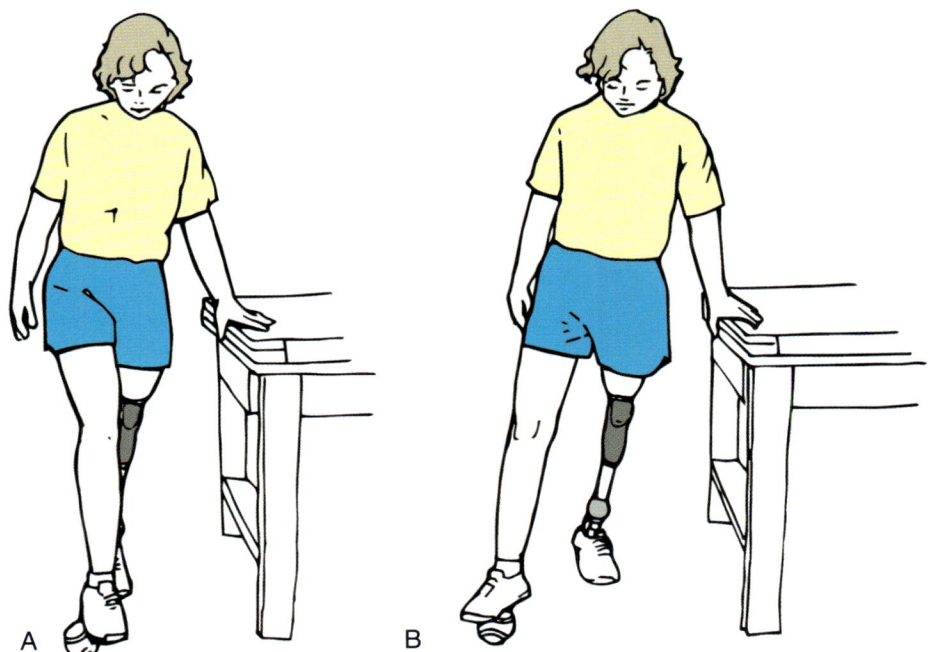

FIGURE 3 Illustrations of the ball roll exercise. **A**, The exercise is performed standing, with a tennis ball placed under the sound limb and the patient holding onto an immovable object. **B**, The ball is rolled quickly 10 to 15 times forward and backward and then side-to-side, followed by clockwise and counterclockwise movements. (Copyright Advanced Rehabilitation Therapy, Inc, Miami, FL, 1994. Illustrator, Frank Angulo.)

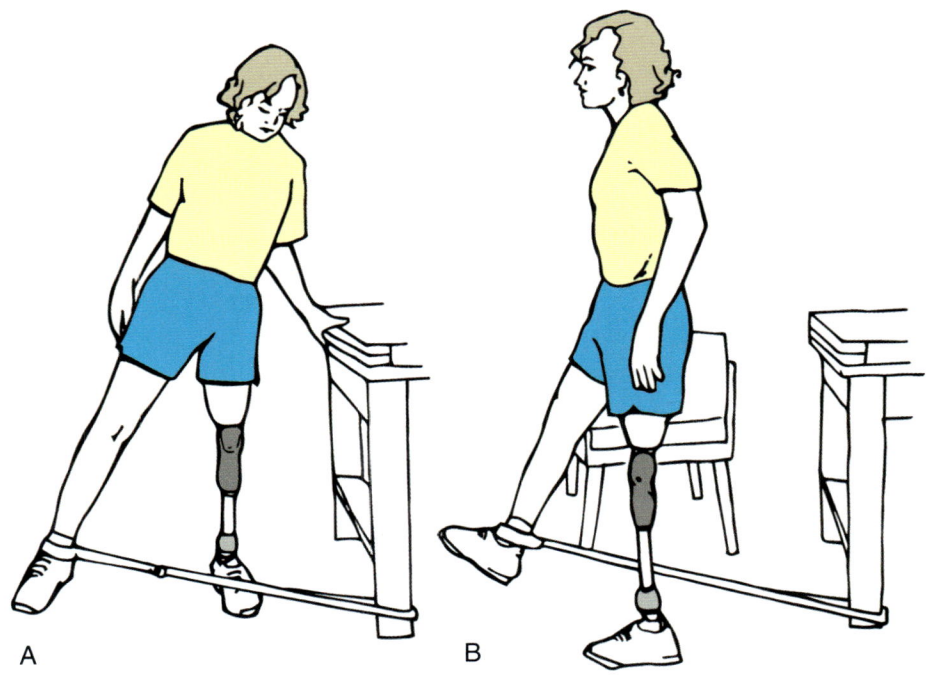

FIGURE 4 Illustrations of resisted elastic kicks. One end of rubber tubing is secured to a sturdy table leg and the other end is placed around the sound ankle. With the patient holding onto a chair, the leg is moved far enough away from the table that the rubber tubing is slightly stretched. The amputee then (1) kicks away from the prosthetic limb while standing sideways to the table (**A**); (2) then, turning 180°, kicks across the prosthetic limb; (3) with their back to the table, kicks forward (**B**); and then, while facing the table, kicks the leg back. (Copyright Advanced Rehabilitation Therapy, Inc, Miami, FL, 1994. Illustrator, Frank Angulo.)

Functional Activities

Encouraging activity as soon as possible after amputation surgery helps speed recovery in several ways. First, it offsets the negative effects of immobility by promoting joint movement, muscle activity, and increased circulation. Second, it helps amputees to reestablish their independence, which may be perceived as threatened because of the loss of a limb. Third, the psychological advantages of activity and independence affect the patient's motivation throughout rehabilitation.

Unsupported Standing Balance

In preparation for ambulation without a prosthesis, all amputees must learn to compensate for the loss of weight of the amputated limb by balancing their center of mass over the intact limb. Although this habit must be broken when learning prosthetic ambulation, balance on a single limb must be learned initially to provide confidence during stand pivot transfers, ambulation with assistive devices, and hopping, depending on the skill level of the patient. An amputee should be able to balance for at least 0.5 seconds to allow for the smooth and safe forward progression of an assistive device during ambulation.

One method of progression begins with the amputee standing in the parallel bars while using both hands for support.[49] After the patient is able to stand in the parallel bars using both arms for support, the hand on the side of the amputation should be removed from the bars. Independent balance is achieved when both hands can be removed from the bars. To improve balance and righting skills, the amputee is challenged by gently perturbing the shoulders in multiple directions or tossing a weighted ball back and forth.[49] Enough time is allowed between perturbations or throws for the patient to regain a comfortable standing posture. Once confidence is gained within the parallel bars, the patient is permitted to practice these skills outside of the parallel bars.

Pregait Training

Balance and Coordination

After the loss of a limb, the decrease in body weight will alter the amputee's center of mass. To maintain the single-limb balance necessary during stance without a prosthesis or ambulate with an assistive device, the amputee must shift the center of mass over the base of support, which is the foot of the intact limb. As the amputee becomes more secure in their single-limb support, reorientation to maintaining the center of mass over both the intact and prosthetic limbs becomes more difficult. Ultimately, the amputee must learn to maintain their center of mass and entire body weight over the prosthesis. Once comfortable with bearing weight equally on both limbs, the amputee can begin to develop confidence with independent standing, and eventually with ambulation.

Orientation

Orientation of the center of mass over the base of support is necessary to maintain balance; thus, the amputee must become familiar with these terms and their relationship. The center of mass is 2 inches (5 cm) anterior to the second sacral vertebra. Although the average person stands with their feet 2 to 4 inches (5 to 10 cm) apart, both the center of mass and base of support vary according to body height.[55] Various methods of proprioceptive and visual feedback may be used to help the amputee to maximize the displacement of the center of mass over the base of support. The amputee must learn to displace the center of mass from side to side, as well as forward and backward[49] (**Figures 5 and 6**). These exercises vary little from the traditional exercises for shifting weight, with the exception that the emphasis is placed on the movement of the center of mass over the base of support, rather than weight bearing into the prosthesis. Increased weight bearing will be a direct result of improved center of mass displacement and will establish a firm foundation for actual weight shifting during ambulation.

Standing on a Single Limb

Bearing weight on the prosthesis is one of the most difficult challenges facing the physical therapist and amputee alike. Without the ability to maintain full single-limb weight bearing and balance for an adequate amount of time (0.5 second minimum), the amputee will exhibit a number of gait deviations including (1) decreased stance time on the prosthetic side, (2) a shortened stride length on the intact side, or (3) lateral trunk bending over the prosthetic limb. Strength, balance, and coordination are

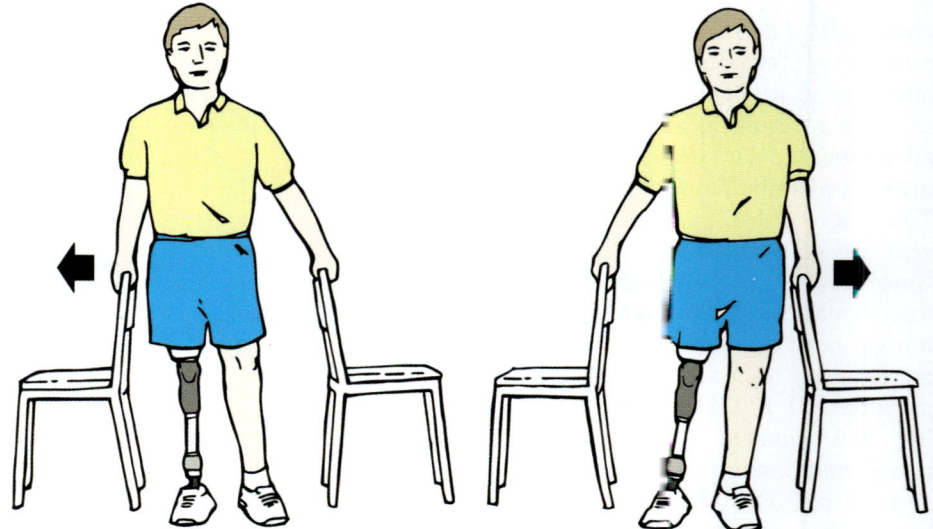

FIGURE 5 Illustration of a method to help the amputee maximize displacement of the center of mass over the base of support using lateral shifting of weight and balance orientation. (Copyright Advanced Rehabilitation Therapy, Inc, Miami, FL, 1989. Illustrator, Frank Angulo.)

Chapter 49: Physical Therapy Management of Adult Lower Limb Amputees

the primary physical factors influencing single-limb stance on a prosthesis. Fear, pain, and lack of confidence in the prosthesis must be considered when an amputee appears reluctant to bear weight on the prosthesis. Adequate weight bearing and balance on the prosthesis before and during ambulation should be emphasized.

Balance on the prosthetic limb while advancing the intact limb should be practiced in a controlled manner so that when it is required in a dynamic situation (such as walking), it can be accomplished with relatively little difficulty. The stool stepping exercise is an excellent method for learning this skill. The amputee stands between the parallel bars, or between two chairs when training at home, with the intact limb in front of a 4- to 8-inches (10- to 20-cm) stool (or block); the height depends on level of ability. The amputee is then asked to step slowly onto the stool with the intact limb while using bilateral upper limb support on the parallel bars. To increase these weight-bearing skills, the amputee is asked to remove the hand on the intact side from the parallel bars. Initially, the speed of the intact leg will increase when upper limb support is removed. With practice, the movement will become slower and more controlled, thus promoting increased weight bearing on the prosthesis (**Figure 7**).

Walking speed and the ability to control intact limb advancement are directly related to the ability to control prosthetic limb stance.[56,57] The following three factors may help the amputee achieve adequate balance over the prosthetic limb: (1) control of the musculature of the amputated side, (2) use of the available sensation at the residual limb–socket interface; and (3) visualization of the prosthetic foot and its relationship to the ground. New amputees will have difficulty understanding these concepts but will attain a greater appreciation of them with time.

Gait Training Skills

Intact and Prosthetic Limb Training

Another factor in adjusting to lower limb amputation is restoration of the

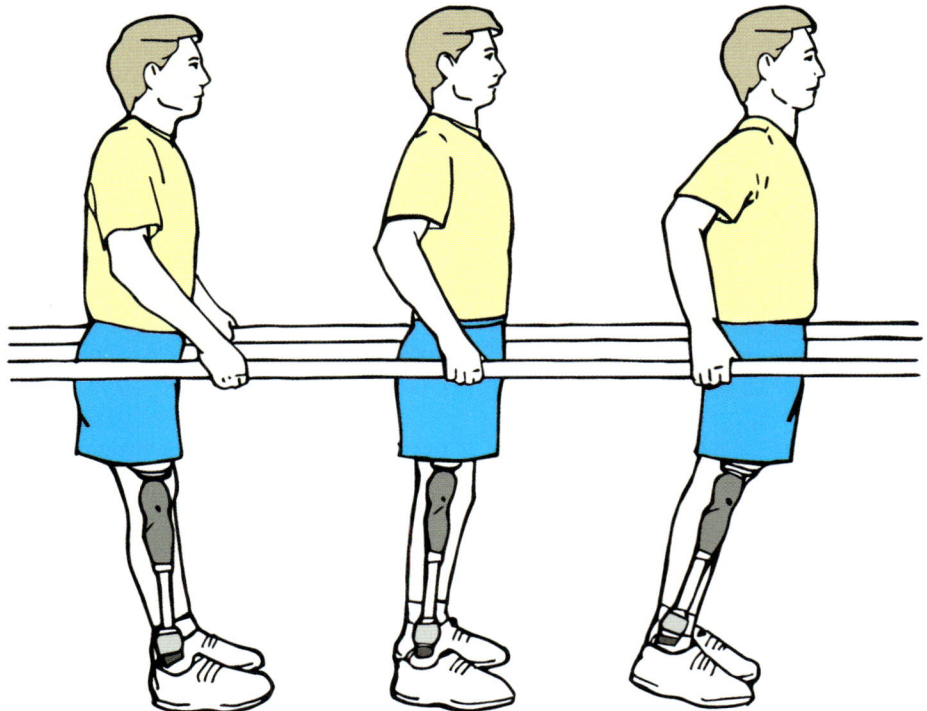

FIGURE 6 Illustration of a method to help the amputee maximize displacement of the center of mass over the base of support using forward and backward shifting of weight and balance orientation. (Copyright Advanced Rehabilitation Therapy, Inc, Miami, FL, 1989. Illustrator, Frank Angulo.)

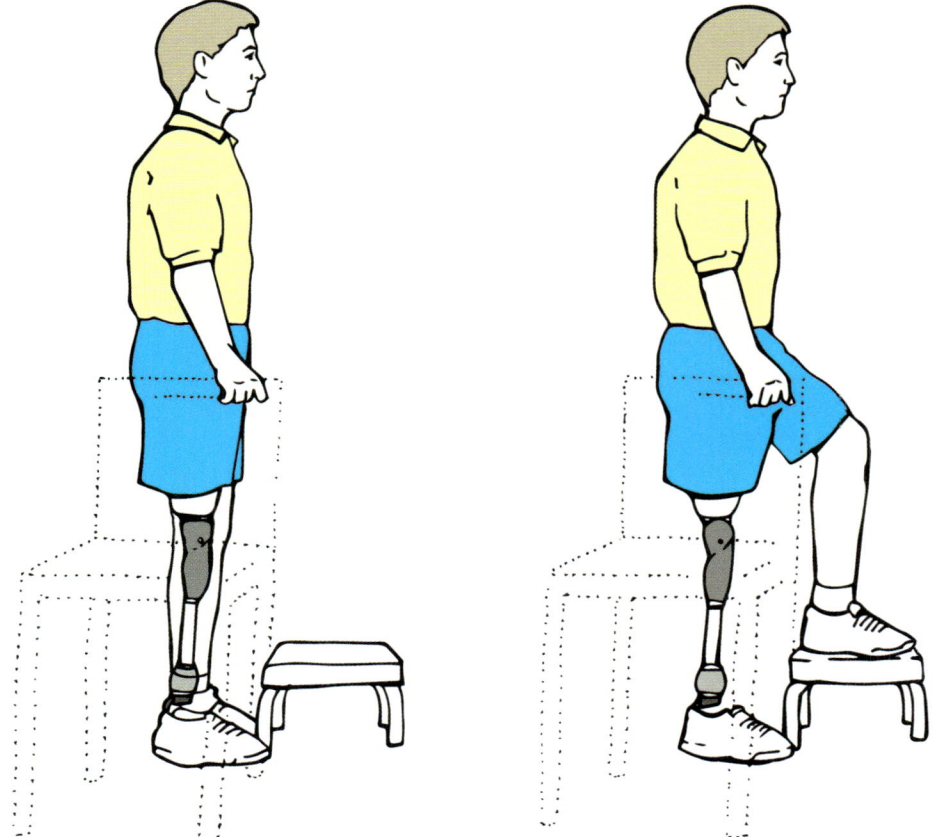

FIGURE 7 Illustrations of the stool-stepping exercise. (Copyright Advanced Rehabilitation Therapy, Inc, Miami, FL, 1989. Illustrator, Frank Angulo.)

gait biomechanics that were unique to the patient before amputation. In other words, not everyone has the same gait pattern. The restoration of function to the remaining joints of the amputated limb should be the goal of gait training. Prosthetic gait training should not alter gait mechanics to suit the prosthesis; rather, the prosthesis should be designed to suit the gait of the amputee. Developments in prosthetics have provided limbs that closely replicate the mechanics of the human leg.

Pelvic Motions

The pelvis moves as a unit with the body's center of mass in four directions: (1) vertical displacement, (2) lateral displacement, (3) horizontal tilt, and (4) transverse rotation. Each motion can directly affect the amputee's gait, resulting in gait deviations and movement asymmetries, with a concomitant increase in energy consumption during ambulation. If restoration of function to the remaining joints of the amputated limb is a goal of gait training, then the pelvic motions play a decisive role in determining the final outcome of the amputee's gait pattern.

Vertical displacement is simply the rhythmical upward and downward motion of the body's center of mass. To replicate able-bodied ambulation, the knee must flex 10° to 15° during loading response, and be fully extended during midstance.[58,59] The transtibial amputee has the ability to flex and extend the knee during the stance phase of gait. Many newer prosthetic knee designs allow limited stance flexion; however, the transfemoral amputee must receive training and have confidence in the knee mechanisms when it flexes slightly during early stance. Frequently, the amputee will exert excessive hip extension throughout the entire stance phase because of the fear the knee might collapse (buckle). Evidence suggests that the contribution of stance phase knee flexion does not appreciably alter the amount of vertical movement during normal walking.[60,61]

Lateral displacement occurs when the pelvis shifts from side to side approximately 2 inches (5 cm). The amount of lateral displacement is determined by the width of the base of support, which is 2 to 4 inches (5 to 10 cm) and the height of the individual. Amputees have to spend an inordinate amount of time on the intact limb, such as when they are on crutches, or during relaxed standing. Therefore, they are adept at maintaining their center of mass over the intact limb and have a habit of crossing midline with the intact foot. Thus, adequate space for the prosthetic limb to follow a natural line of progression is not available. The result is altered forces across the knee joint of the intact limb and an increased dependence on the intact limb during walking. Many transfemoral amputees will abduct the prosthetic limb, potentially increasing the base of support with greater lateral displacement of the pelvis toward the prosthetic side. Although it is frequently observed in transfemoral amputees, an altered base of support may also be seen with transtibial amputees.

Horizontal tilt of the pelvis is normal up to 5°, and any tilt greater than 5° is considered excessive. Excessive horizontal tilt of the pelvis is thought to be related to weak hip abductor musculature, specifically the gluteus medius. Maintenance of the residual femur in adduction by means of the socket theoretically places the gluteus medius at the optimal length-to-tension ratio. If the limb is abducted, however, the muscle shortens in that position and is unable to function properly. The result is a Trendelenburg limp, or the compensatory gluteus medius gait, in which the trunk leans laterally over the prosthetic limb in an attempt to maintain the pelvis in a horizontal position. In addition to hip abductor weakness and altered positioning of the femur and muscles, other biomechanical factors reduce the transfemoral amputee's ability to generate sufficient power at the hip to maintain the pelvis in a horizontal position. These factors include the following: (1) decreased muscle tissue, although the gluteus medius is intact with all transfemoral amputations, the tensor fasciae latae muscle is cut reducing the synergistic capacity of the hip abductor muscles; (2) decreased bone length, the femur bone length is shortened depending on the level of amputation, thus reducing the leverage of the hip in a closed kinetic chain to act on the pelvis; and (3) decrease of speed of contraction—the loss of proprioceptive input from the foot and ankle requires that the hip musculature respond more rapidly with less somatosensory input to postural changes when standing on the prosthetic limb. Even with training, the hip musculature will have difficulty responding rapidly enough to postural changes during walking.

Transverse rotation of the pelvis occurs around the longitudinal axis approximately 5° to 10° forward and backward. The transverse rotation of the pelvis shifts the body's center of mass from one limb to the other and helps to initiate the 30° to 40° of knee flexion during preswing, which is necessary to achieve 60° of knee flexion during the initial swing phase. Knee flexion during preswing is also produced by flexion of the foot and ankle. During preswing, the restoration of transverse rotation of the pelvis becomes of great importance to obtain sufficient knee flexion because most commercially available prosthetic feet do not permit plantar-flexion. A systematic method can be used to teach an amputee about normalization of trunk, pelvic, and limb biomechanics. First, independent movements of the various joint and muscle groups are developed. Second, the independent movements are incorporated into functional movement patterns of the gait cycle. Finally, all component movement patterns are integrated to produce a smooth, normalized gait.

Prosthetic Training Program

In 1989, Gailey and Gailey[48] introduced a functional prosthetic training program that offers a systematic way to establish static and dynamic stability and promote single-limb standing balance over the prosthetic limb. After the amputee has attained a basic level of strength and balance, resistive gait training techniques are implemented to reeducate the amputee in normal gait movements necessary to maximize prosthetic performance and promote economy of gait. Advanced gait training exercises are offered to help the amputee, regardless of level of amputation, to negotiate a variety of environmental conditions that require multidirectional movements and superior dynamic balance. With some minor adaptations, this program also applies for people with bilateral amputations. The time required to progress through the sequence and overall outcomes varies, based on the amputee's physical ability, diagnosis, and motivation. The following sequence of steps is adapted from the Prosthetic Gait Training Program.[48]

1. Dynamic residual limb exercises are used to strengthen muscles (see the section on Preprosthetic Exercise).
2. Proprioceptive neuromuscular facilitation, Feldenkrais techniques, or any other movement awareness techniques may be performed for trunk, pelvic, and limb re-education patterns. These exercises encourage rotational motions, and promote independent movements of the trunk, pelvic girdle and limbs.
3. Pregait training exercises (see the section on Pregait Training).
4. Intact limb stepping within the parallel bars is initiated (**Figure 8**). The amputee steps forward and backward, preswings to initial contact, with both hands on the parallel bars. The purpose of this activity is to familiarize the amputee and physical therapist with the gait mechanics of the intact limb without having to be concerned about weight bearing and balance on the prosthetic limb. This activity also affords the physical therapist an opportunity to palpate the anterior superior iliac spines to gain a feeling for the amputee's pelvic motion, which in most cases is close to normal for the amputee.
5. Prosthetic limb stepping within the parallel bars is similar to intact limb stepping, except the prosthetic limb is used. As the physical therapist palpates the anterior superior iliac spines, a posterior rotation of the pelvis may be observed in some patients. This posterior rotation is often a result of the amputee's attempt to kick the prosthesis forward with the residual limb, in a manner similar to kicking a football. The amputee should feel the difference between the pelvic motion on the prosthetic side and the intact side.
6. To restore the correct pelvic motion, the amputee places the prosthetic limb behind the intact limb while holding on to the parallel bars with both hands. The physical therapist then blocks the prosthetic foot to prevent forward movement of the prosthesis. Rhythmic initiation is used, giving the amputee the feeling of rotating the pelvis forward as passive flexion of the prosthetic knee occurs (**Figure 9**). As the amputee becomes comfortable with the motion, they can begin to move the pelvis actively and progress to resistive movements when deemed appropriate by the physical therapist.
7. After the amputee and physical therapist are satisfied with the passive pelvic motions, the swing phase of gait can be taught with resistive gait training. The amputee steps forward and backward with the prosthetic limb as the physical therapist applies the appropriate resistance to the pelvis to facilitate transverse rotation. The pelvic motions should be facilitated so that the line of progression of the prosthesis remains constant without circumduction and the heel contact occurs within boundaries of the base of support (**Figure 10**). As the amputee improves, the intact side and eventually both hands are released from the parallel bars. There should be little if any loss of efficiency with the motion; however, if there is loss of efficiency, the physical therapist may revert to the previous prerequisite skill to reinforce the proper movement patterns.

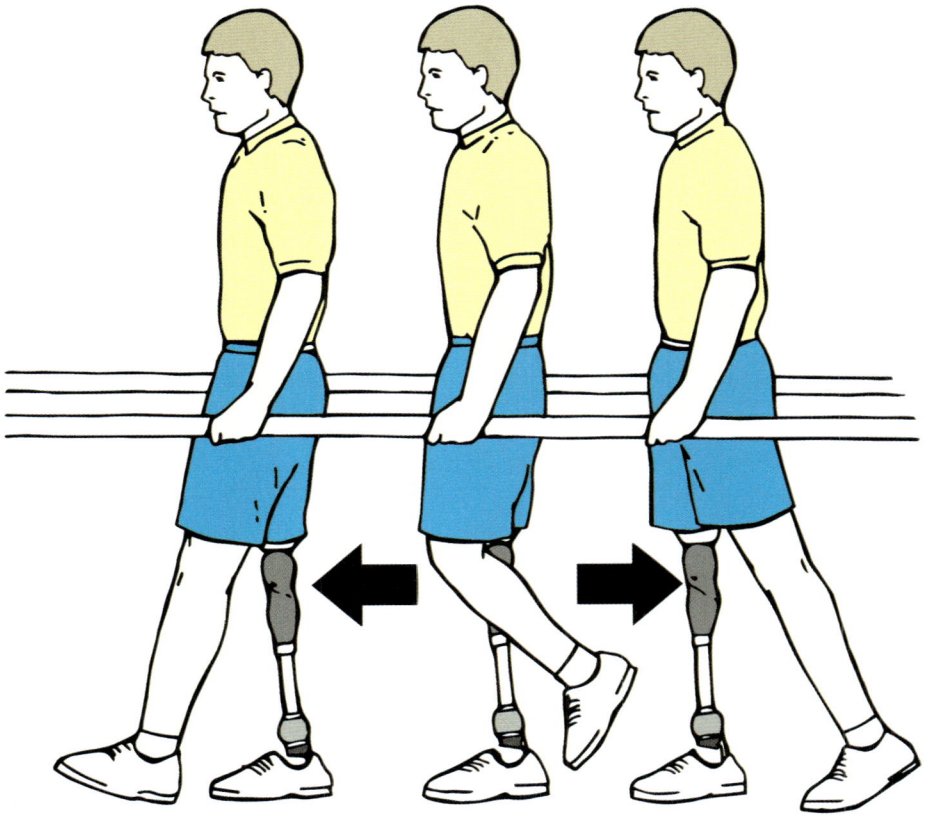

FIGURE 8 Illustration of sound leg-stepping, which is designed to orient the amputee to gait biomechanics. (Copyright Advanced Rehabilitation Therapy, Inc, Miami, FL, 1989. Illustrator, Frank Angulo.)

8. The next step is a return to intact limb stepping with both hands on the parallel bars. The physical therapist will determine if the mechanics are correct and that the intact foot is not crossing midline during initial contact or heel strike. When ready, the amputee will remove the hand on the intact side from the parallel bars. At this time, there may be an increase in the speed of the step, a decrease in step length, and/or lateral leaning of the trunk. These changes may occur as a direct result of the inability to bear weight or balance over the prosthesis. The amputee is verbally cued to remember the skills learned while performing the stool-to-stepping exercise (see the section on Pregait Training). After this skill is adequately perfected, intact limb stepping without any hand support may be practiced until single limb balance over the prosthetic leg is sufficiently mastered.

9. When each of these activities has been performed to an acceptable level of competency, the amputee is ready to combine them and begin walking with the prosthesis. Initially, the amputee will walk within the parallel bars facing the physical therapist. The physical therapist's hands are placed on the amputee's anterior superior iliac spine, with the amputee holding onto the parallel bars. As the amputee ambulates within the parallel bars, the physical therapist applies slight resistance through the hips, providing proprioceptive feedback to the pelvis and involved musculature of the lower limb.

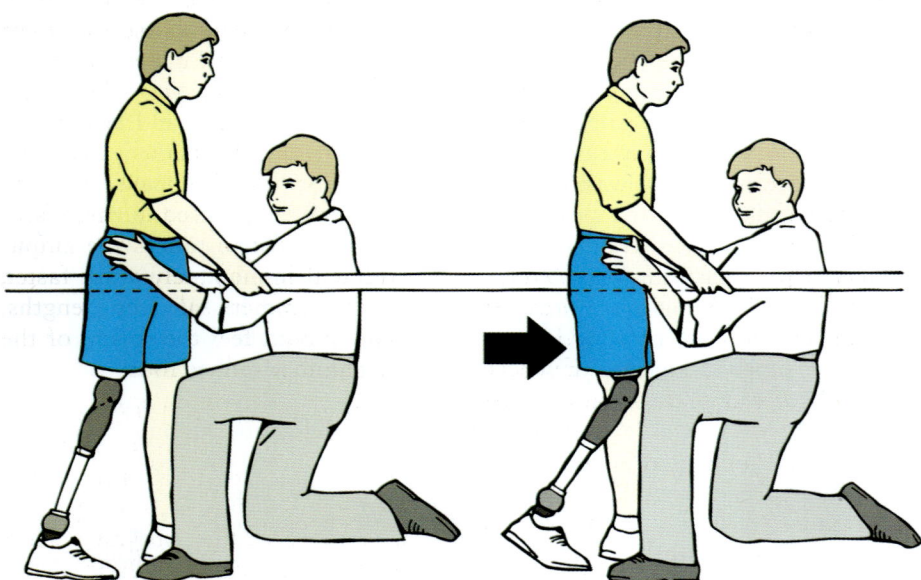

FIGURE 9 Illustration of rhythmic initiation designed to promote transverse rotation of the pelvis. (Copyright Advanced Rehabilitation Therapy, Inc, Miami, FL, 1989. Illustrator, Frank Angulo.)

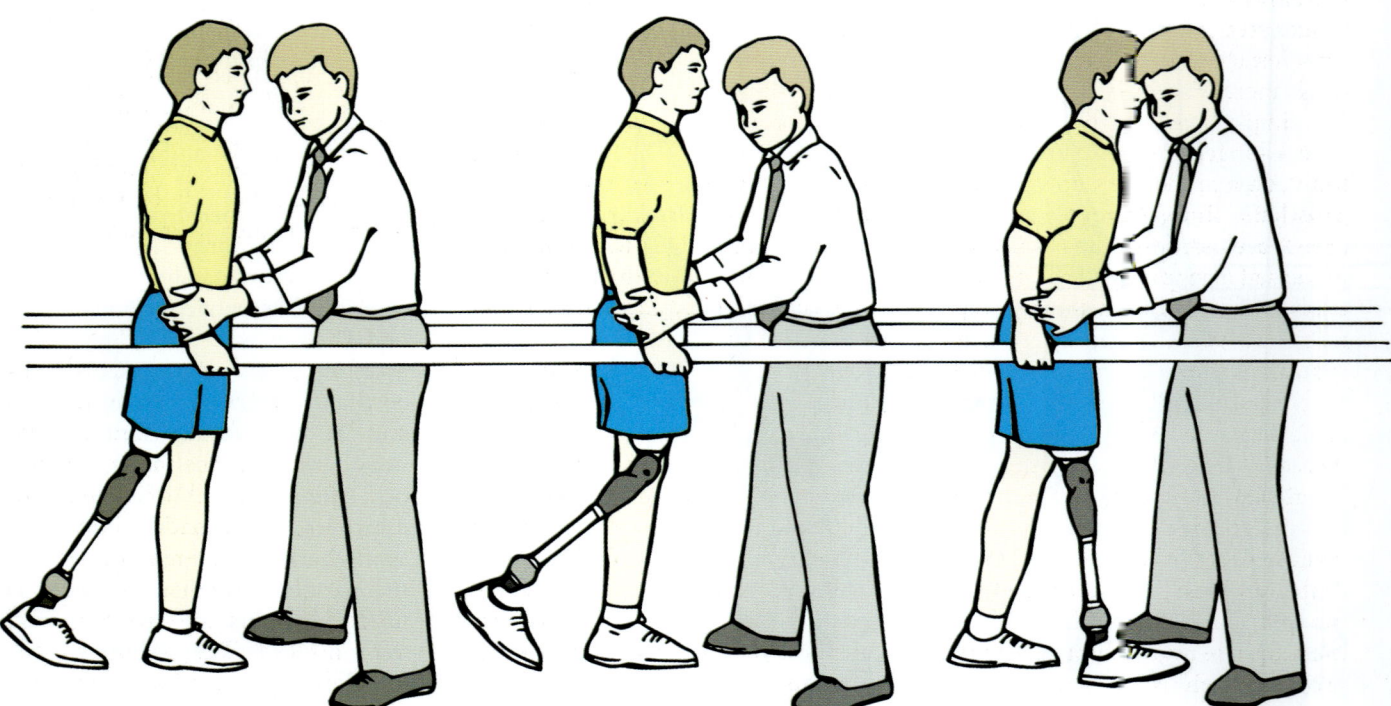

FIGURE 10 Illustration of resistive gait training to facilitate proper pelvic rotation, prosthetic knee flexion, and balance. (Copyright Advanced Rehabilitation Therapy, Inc, Miami, FL, 1989. Illustrator, Frank Angulo.)

10. When both the physical therapist and the amputee are comfortable with the gait demonstrated in the parallel bars, the amputee begins practicing outside of the parallel bars, initially using the physical therapist's shoulders as support and progressing to both hands free when appropriate. The physical therapist may or may not continue to provide proprioceptive input to the pelvis. As the amputee begins to ambulate independently, verbal cueing may be necessary as a reminder to keep the intact foot away from midline to maintain the proper base of support. Maintenance of equal stride length may not be immediately forthcoming because many amputees have a tendency to take a longer step with the prosthetic limb than the intact limb. When adequate weight bearing through the prosthetic limb has been achieved, the amputee should begin to take longer steps with the intact limb and slightly shorter steps with the prosthetic limb. This principle also applies when increasing the cadence. When an amputee increases the speed of walking, a longer step is often taken with the prosthetic limb in compensation, thus increasing the asymmetry. By simply having the amputee take a longer step with the intact limb and a moderate step with the prosthetic limb, increases in gait speed are accomplished without increased asymmetry. If the amputee is observed with a shorter step on the prosthetic side, the cause is typically related to the reluctance to properly roll-over the intact foot. The double support time is increased when the prosthetic limb is entering the stance phase while the intact foot remains in midstance, decreasing the prosthetic limb step length. Confidence that the prosthetic limb will support the amputee allows him or her to progress their body weight over the intact foot without hesitation; this is required for symmetrical step lengths.

11. Trunk rotation and arm swing are important components of restoring the biomechanics of gait. During locomotion, the trunk and upper limb rotate opposite to the pelvic girdle and lower limbs. Trunk rotation is necessary for balance, momentum, and symmetry of gait. Many amputees have decreased trunk rotation and arm swing, especially on the prosthetic side, which may be the result of fear of displacing their center of mass too far forward or backward over the prosthesis. Normal cadence is considered to be 90 to 120 steps per minute, or 67 to 82 meters per minute (2.5 to 3.0 miles per hour).[55] Arm swing provides balance, momentum, and symmetry of gait, and is influenced by the speed of ambulation.[62] As the walking speed accelerates, arm swing increases to permit a more efficient gait. Therefore, amputees who walk at slower speeds will demonstrate a diminished arm swing. Restoring trunk rotation and arm swing is easily accomplished by using rhythmic initiation or passively cueing the trunk as the amputee walks. The physical therapist stands behind the amputee with one hand on either shoulder. As the amputee walks the physical therapist gently rotates the trunk. When the left leg moves forward, the right shoulder is rotated forward and vice versa (**Figure 11**). After amputees feel comfortable with the motion, they can actively incorporate this movement into their gait.

12. Toe load, or the ability to balance full body weight over the prosthetic forefoot during terminal stance, can be difficult but is required to achieve maximum deflection of the footplate of the dynamic energy-storing foot. The ability to balance over the forefoot of the prosthetic foot is best introduced after the amputee has restored their walking biomechanics and demonstrates good walking balance. To facilitate balance over the prosthetic forefoot, the physical therapist walks behind the amputee holding onto a gait belt around their pelvis and resists slightly when the amputee's body weight is over the prosthetic forefoot and the intact limb advances. The focus should be on assisting the amputee to balance over the forefoot with minimum resistance, so that their body weight will deflect the prosthetic footplate. After the physical therapist believes the amputee has achieved balance over the forefoot, the hold on the gait belt can be released during walking. In most instances the amputee will immediately walk faster, with symmetrical step lengths, and should feel the spring of the dynamic response foot.

Amputees who will be independent ambulators and those who will continue to require an assistive device can derive some benefit from this systematic rehabilitation program. Most patients can progress to the point of ambulating outside of the parallel bars. At that time, the amputee must use an assistive device to practice ambulating. Maintaining pelvic rotation, an adequate base of support, equal stance time, and equal stride length all have a direct influence on the energy cost of walking. Trunk rotation will be absent in amputees using a walker as an assistive device. Those ambulating with a cane should be able to incorporate trunk rotation into their gait.

Variations for Disarticulation and Bilaterally Affected Patients

The duration and degree of prosthetic training are unique to each amputee. Many factors influence training, such as age, general health, motivation, and cause and level of amputation. Patients who have had a Syme ankle disarticulation have a major advantage over transtibial amputees because the former group are able to bear some weight distally. The ability to bear weight distally provides better kinesthetic feedback for placement of the prosthetic foot. Because of this capability and the length of the lever arm,

Section 3: Lower Limb

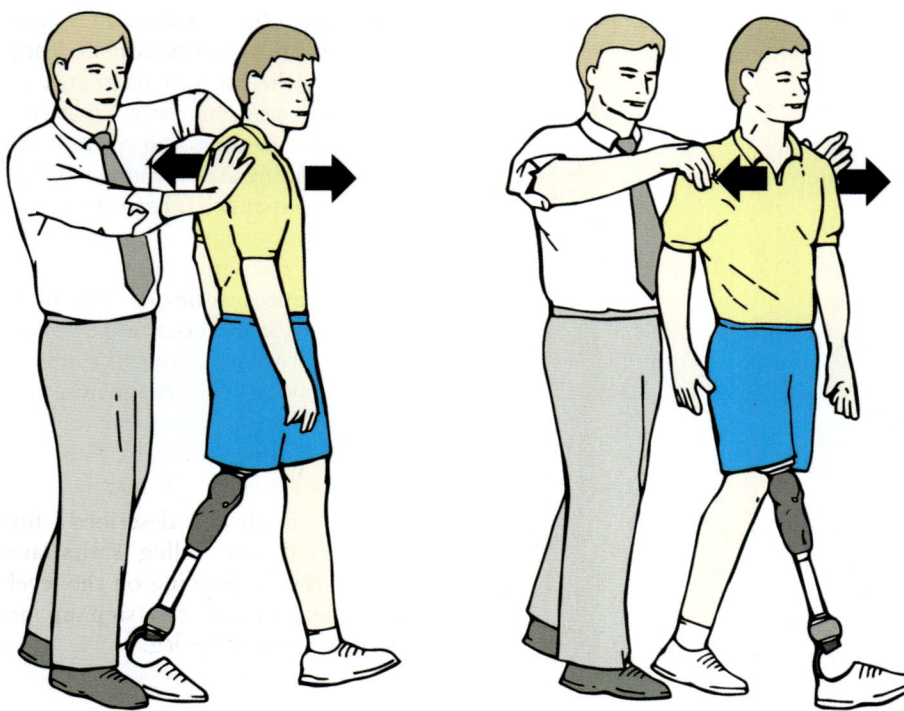

FIGURE 11 Illustration of passive trunk rotation to assist in restoring arm swing for improved balance, symmetry of gait, and momentum. (Copyright Advanced Rehabilitation Therapy, Inc, Miami, FL, 1989. Illustrator, Frank Angulo.)

those with a Syme ankle disarticulation amputation require minimal prosthetic gait training and can progress rapidly with weight shifting and other gait skills; however, they may require practice to achieve equal stride length and stance time.

Patients treated with a knee disarticulation amputation have several advantages over transfemoral amputees, including a longer lever arm, enhanced muscular control, improved kinesthetic feedback and greater distal end weight bearing. Although these advantages may decrease the rehabilitation time, the amputee with a knee disarticulation must learn the same skills as a transfemoral amputee.

Patients who have undergone hip disarticulation and transpelvic amputation also need to master control of the mechanical hip joint as well as the knee joint and foot and ankle assemblies. The gait training procedures are essentially the same as for the transfemoral amputee; however, in some patients the limitations of the mechanical hip joint may require a slight intact limb vaulting action for the foot to clear the ground.

Patients with bilateral lower limb amputation have unique challenges but can become successful ambulators with or without an assistive device. Many bilateral lower limb amputees progress from low-profile prostheses without knee joints (stubbies) to normal-height prostheses with articulating knee joints. The preprosthetic gait training has a greater emphasis on hip strength and core stabilization. The gait training sequence uses the same progression, with the stronger residual limb receiving the initial treatment similar to the intact limb in the unilateral transfemoral amputees. Time and commitment are important for prosthetic success and not all bilateral amputees will be independent prosthetic ambulators. Often, older age is associated with inadequate neurophysiologic integrity and an inability to generate the hip strength and speed of contraction needed to achieve successful use of prosthetic devices. For these reasons, wheelchair mobility training is just as important as prosthetic training. The use of a wheelchair must not be perceived as failure, but rather an alternative mode of mobility.

Advanced Gait-Training Activities

Stairs

Ascending and descending stairs is most safely and comfortably performed one step at a time (step-by-step). Using a purely mechanical prostheses, only a few transfemoral amputees with exceptional ability can descend stairs step-over-step, or by the "jack-knifing" method. Similarly, only a few strong amputees can ascend stairs step-over-step. Most transtibial amputees have the option of either method. Individuals with transpelvic amputations or those who have a hip disarticulation are limited to the step-by-step method.

Most microprocessor and some hydraulic knee devices have made this process easier with "yield rate control" or a mechanical braking system that permits the knee to bend slowly under the amputee's body weight as the intact limb descends to a lower stair. Newer powered prosthetic knee systems have a motor that can help raise the amputee when they ascend the stairs on the prosthetic side as well as control knee flexion when descending the stairs. Regardless of the type of prosthesis, ascending and descending stairs step-over-step requires practice and confidence to perform safely.

Step-By-Step Method

This step-by-step method is essentially the same for amputees at all levels of lower limb amputation. When ascending stairs, the body weight is shifted to the prosthetic limb as the foot of the intact limb is elevated and firmly placed on the stair tread of the next step. The trunk is slightly flexed over the intact limb as the knee extends, raising the body and the prosthetic limb to the same step. The process is repeated for each step with the intact side always leading. When descending stairs, the body weight is shifted to the intact limb as the prosthetic limb is lowered to the step below by eccentrically flexing the knee of the intact limb. After the prosthetic limb is securely in place, the body weight is transferred to the prosthetic limb and the intact limb is lowered to the same step. The process is repeated

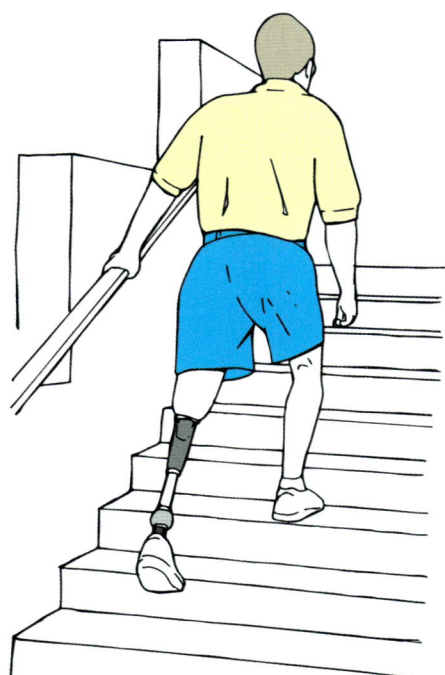

FIGURE 12 Illustration of transfemoral stair ascent by skipping a step for the purpose of increasing speed. (Copyright Advanced Rehabilitation Therapy, Inc, Miami, FL, 1989. Illustrator, Frank Angulo.)

for each step with the prosthetic side always leading the descent.

One of the primary goals for ascending stairs step-over-step is to increase the speed of ascent, but this comes at the cost of increased effort and decreased safety. A variation on the step-by-step method is to simply skip a step. This technique, however, is usually reserved for the most physically fit amputees (**Figure 12**).

Transtibial Amputees
Step-Over-Step Technique

When ascending stairs, the transtibial amputee who cannot dorsiflex their foot and ankle assembly must generate a stronger concentric contraction of the knee and hip extensors to successfully transfer body weight over the prosthetic limb. Descending stairs is very similar to normal descent except that only the prosthetic foot heel is place on the step. This compensates for the lack of dorsiflexion within the foot and ankle assembly. Recent prosthetic ankle designs with active dorsiflexion enable the amputee to place the prosthetic foot flat on the step surface for a more stable base of support.

Transfemoral Amputees
Step-Over-Step Stair Technique

Timing and coordination become critical in step-over-step stair climbing. As the transfemoral amputee approaches the stairs, the prosthetic limb is the first to ascend the stairs by rapid acceleration of hip flexion with slight abduction to achieve sufficient knee flexion to clear the step. Some transfemoral amputees will actually hit the approaching step riser with the toe of the prosthetic foot to passively achieve adequate knee flexion. With the prosthetic foot firmly on the step, usually the toe is against the riser of the step, the residual limb must exert enough force to fully extend the hip so that the intact foot may advance to the step above. With the intact side foot on the higher step, the intact side hip extends, and the hip on the prosthetic side must flex at an accelerated speed to achieve sufficient knee flexion to place the prosthetic foot on the next step above. The strength and coordination required to perform this technique are challenging to accomplish; therefore, very few transfemoral amputees are able or desirous to use the technique.

Descending stairs is achieved by placing only the heel of the prosthetic foot on the stair below, then shifting the body weight over the prosthetic limb. In the absence of a knee with yield rate control, this results in a passive flexion of jackknifing motion of the knee. The intact limb must quickly reach the step below in time to catch the body weight. The process is repeated at a rapid rate until a rhythm is achieved. Most transfemoral amputees who have mastered this skill descend stairs at an extremely fast pace, much faster than would be considered safe for the average amputee.

When the knee of the prosthesis features yield rate control, one-third to one-half of the prosthetic foot should be placed forward to the edge of the stair while the amputee gently contracts the hip extensors against the posterior socket wall, slowing reducing the contractile effort as the stance control mechanism of the prosthetic knee slowly lowers the body to the next step. Considerable practice, strength, and confidence are required to master the skill of descending stairs in a controlled step-over-step manner (**Figure 13**).

Stairs With Crutches

When ascending and descending stairs with crutches, both crutches may be held in the hand opposite the handrail or they can be used in the traditional manner.

Curbs

The same methods described for ascending and descending stairs are used for curbs. Depending on the level of skill, the amputee can step up or down curbs with either leg.

Uneven Surfaces

Unrestricted home and community ambulation requires that the amputee walk over a variety of surfaces such as concrete, grass, gravel, uneven terrain and varied carpet heights. Initially, the new amputee will have difficulty in recognizing the different surfaces secondary to the loss of proprioception. To promote an increased visual and proprioceptive awareness of these differences, time should be spent practicing on various surfaces. In addition, the amputee must realize that in many circumstances, it is important to observe the terrain ahead to avoid hazards such as slippery surfaces or holes that might cause a fall.

Ramps and Hills

Ascending and descending inclines presents a problem for all lower limb amputees because of the lack of dorsiflexion and plantar flexion present in foot and ankle assemblies of most prosthetic feet. Descending is the more difficult task for transtibial amputees and transfemoral amputees with prosthetic knee joints because of the added dilemma of the weight line falling posterior to the knee joint which results in a flexion moment.

When ascending an incline, the body weight should be slightly more

Section 3: Lower Limb

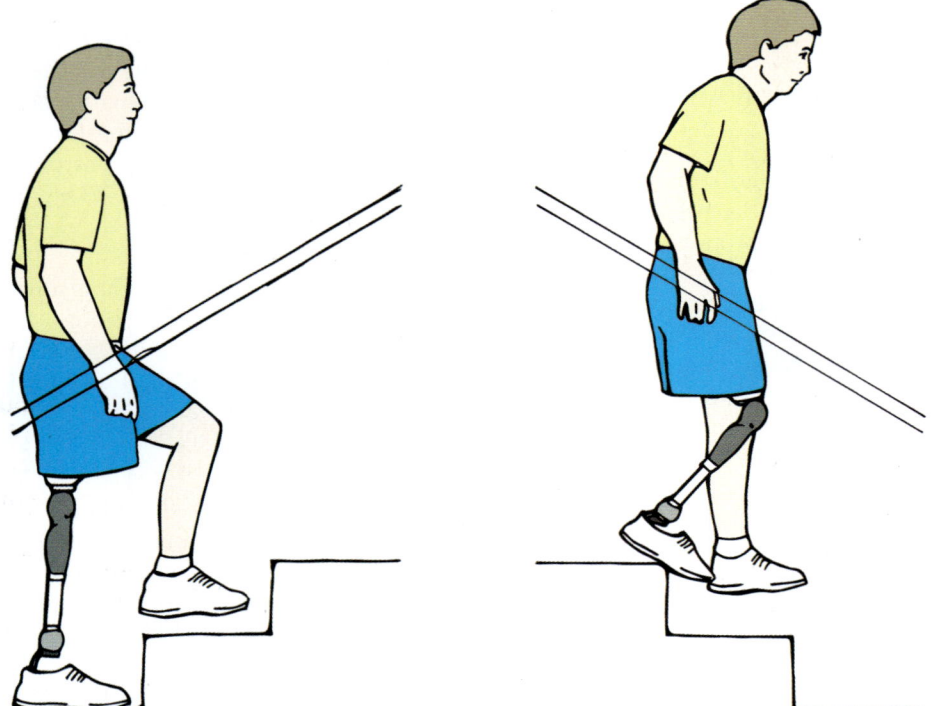

FIGURE 13 Illustration of a transfemoral amputee using a prosthetic knee with controlled stair descent capabilities. When ascending stairs (left), the sound foot is placed on the upper stair. As the knee and hip extend, the body rises and the prosthetic limb is placed on the same stair, enabling the amputee to safely ascend the stairs in a step-by-step manner. When descending stairs (right) one-third to one-half of the prosthetic foot should be placed forward to the edge of the stair lip. The amputee contracts the hip extensors against the posterior socket wall, slowly reducing the effort as the stance control mechanism of the prosthetic knee slowly lowers the body to the next step. (Copyright Advanced Rehabilitation Therapy, Inc, Miami, FL, 1990. Illustrator, Frank Angulo.)

forward than normal to obtain maximal dorsiflexion with articulating foot and ankle assemblies and to keep the knee in extension. Depending on the grade of the incline, pelvic rotation with additional acceleration may be required to achieve maximal knee flexion during swing. Descent of an incline usually occurs at a more rapid pace than normal because of the lack of dorsiflexion and plantar flexion, resulting in decreased stance time on the prosthetic limb. Amputees with prosthetic knees must exert a greater than normal force on the posterior wall of the socket to maintain knee extension. Microprocessor-controlled knee systems can automatically compensate for the increased knee flexion moment by increasing the knee flexion resistance, making descent safer and allowing the amputee to take equal steps with great confidence.

Lower limb amputees can adopt several strategies to aid in ascending and descending inclines. On modest inclines, they may simply adopt shorter equal strides. This method is often preferred because it simulates a more normal appearance as opposed to the sidestepping or zigzag method. However, when ascending and descending steep hills, the amputee will find sidestepping to be the most efficient technique. During ascent, the intact limb should lead, providing the power to lift the body to the next level, while the prosthetic limb remains slightly posterior to act as a firm base by keeping the weight line anterior to the knee. During descent, the prosthetic limb leads but remains slightly posterior to the intact limb. The prosthetic knee remains in extension, again acting as a form of support so that the intact limb may lower the body.

For individuals with transpelvic amputation or a hip disarticulation, sidestepping is the most common alternative regardless of the grade of the incline. Although newer hip joints combined with microprocessor-controlled or powered knee and foot systems have enabled many amputees with this level of amputation to negotiate inclines and declines without sidestepping, the mastery of this skill requires time and practice.

When possible, the most accepted method for navigating a variety of inclines and conditions such as wet surfaces and ice, is placing one hand on another person's shoulder. For example, while walking down an incline, the amputee will walk one step behind an assistant with one hand on the assistant's shoulder. As the two walk slowly down the incline, the speed of descent is controllable, giving the amputee more confidence.

Falling

Controlled falling and lowering to the floor are important skills not only for safety but also as a means to perform activities on the floor. During falling, the amputee must first discard any assistive device to avoid injury and ensure they land on their hands with the elbows slightly flexed to reduce the force and decrease the possibility of injury. As the elbows flex, the amputee should roll to one side to further decrease the impact of the fall. Lowering the body to the floor in a controlled manner is initiated by squatting with the intact limb followed by gently leaning forward onto the slightly flexed upper limbs. From this position, the amputee remains in a quadruped position or assumes a sitting position.

Floor to Standing

Many techniques teach the amputee how to rise from the floor to a standing position and vary with the type of amputation and the skill level of the amputee. The amputee and physical therapist must work closely together to determine the most efficient and safe manner to successfully master this task. The fundamental principle is to have the amputee use the assistive device for balance and the intact limb for power as the body begins to rise.

Exercises for Maximizing Stability Within the Socket

Sidestepping

Sidestepping, or walking sideways, can be introduced to the amputee at various times throughout the rehabilitation program. The patient can begin with simple weight shifting in the parallel bars. With practice, more complex activities can be performed such as unassisted sidestepping around tables or a small obstacle course that requires many small turns. During early rehabilitation, sidestepping provides the amputee with a functional exercise for strengthening the hip abductors; later in the rehabilitation process, it provides an opportunity to progress into multidirectional movements.

Walking Backward

Walking backward is not difficult for transtibial amputees but poses a problem for amputees requiring a prosthetic knee because there is no means of actively flexing the knee for adequate ground clearance. In addition, the posterior forces tend to cause the weight line to fall posterior to the knee, causing a flexion moment, and possible buckling of the knee. There are a few exceptions such as a newer microprocessor and power knees that do actively flex when walking backwards; however these knees require specific movements to activate prosthetic knee flexion. The most comfortable method of backward walking for transfemoral amputees is to vault upward (plantarflex) on the intact foot to obtain sufficient height for the prosthetic limb to clear the ground as it is moving posteriorly. In this maneuver, the prosthetic foot is placed well behind the intact limb with most of the body's weight being borne on the prosthetic toe, which keeps the weight line anterior to the knee. The intact limb is then brought back, usually at a slightly faster speed for a somewhat shorter distance. The trunk is also maintained in some flexion to maintain the weight forward on the prosthetic toe. With a little practice, most amputees become quite proficient in walking backward.

Multidirectional Turns

Changing direction during walking or maneuvering within confined areas is difficult. Situations such as crowded restaurants, elevators, or just simply turning around, are often overcome by "hip hiking" the prosthesis and pivoting around the intact limb. This method is effective but hardly the most aesthetic means of changing direction. When turning to the intact side, two key factors for a smooth transition include maintaining transverse pelvic rotation and performing the turn in two steps. The prosthetic limb is crossed 45° over the intact limb, the intact limb is rotated 180°, and the turn is completed by stepping in the desired direction with the prosthetic limb, leading with the pelvis to ensure adequate knee flexion.

Turning to the prosthetic side is performed in almost exactly the same way, except that slightly more body weight is maintained on the prosthetic toe to keep the weight line anterior to the knee, thus preventing knee flexion. The intact limb is crossed 45° over the prosthetic limb, automatically throwing the weight line forward. The prosthetic limb is as close to 180° as possible without losing balance (135° is usually comfortable), and the turn is completed by stepping in the desired direction with the intact limb. If necessary, the transfemoral amputee may need to be reminded to maintain knee extension by applying a force with the residual limb against the posterior wall of the socket.

Exercise that will reinforce turning skills is follow-the-leader and figure-of-8 drills, in which the amputee follows the physical therapist in making a series of turns in all directions with varying speeds and degrees of difficulty. The level of skill in turning will vary among amputees. All functional ambulators should be taught to turn in both directions regardless of the prosthetic side. Lower limb amputees with poor balance may be limited to unidirectional turns, requiring a series of small steps to complete the turn.

Tandem Walking

Walking with a normal base of support is of prime importance; however, tandem walking can assist with balance and coordination and can improve awareness of the prosthesis. After placing a 2- to 4-inches (5 to 10-cm) wide strip of tape on the floor, the amputee is asked to walk in three ways. The amputee first walks with one foot to either side of the line, then along the line, heel to toe, with one foot in front of the other. Finally, the amputee walks with one foot crossing over in front of the other so that neither foot touches the line, with the left foot always on the right side and vice versa.

Lateral Agility Drills

Lateral agility drills are one of the strategies necessary for moving in different directions. The amputee simply moves sideways for a predetermined distance, starting with slow steps and picking up speed as the movement becomes easier. Amputees who participate in recreational activities that require lateral movements, such as tennis, basketball, and softball, should practice at speeds consistent with their sport. After speed and balance have been established, the drills can include the use of a racquet or ball, adding more complex skills such as swinging the racquet or passing the ball during each repetition.

Braiding

Braiding (cariocas or grapevine step) may be taught either within the parallel bars or in an open area, depending upon the amputee's ability (**Figure 14**). Braiding consists of crossing one leg in front of the other. Care must be given not to bump the prosthetic knee with the intact limb, which will cause it to collapse. Rapidly creating a backward force within the socket with hip musculature will help to maintain stability. As the skill level improves, the amputee will develop the speed of residual limb movement and stability necessary to move confidently in any direction. To improve dynamic balance, the amputee should perform braiding in which the trunk moves in opposition to the pelvic motion. As agility improves, the amputee can vary the speed during the lateral agility drills to further improve prosthetic control in multiple directions.

Section 3: Lower Limb

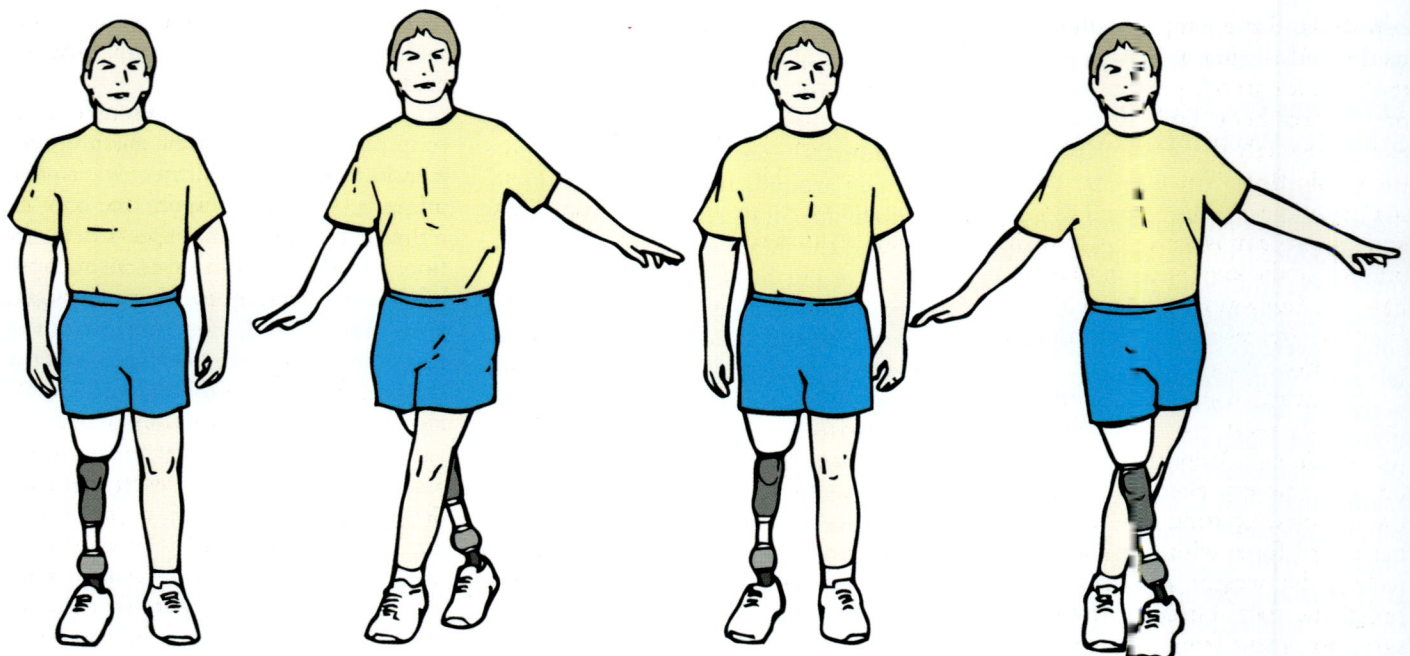

FIGURE 14 Illustration of the braiding exercise that is designed to improve prosthetic control, balance, and coordination by crossing one leg in front of or behind the other in a continuous manner. (Copyright Advanced Rehabilitation Therapy, Inc, Miami, FL. 1989. Illustrator, Frank Angulo.)

Cup Walking Drills

Cup walking is a challenging, low-impact exercise that has been shown to be extremely beneficial in helping amputees to learn to control their prosthesis. Five to 10 disposable cups are placed approximately 12 to 18 inches apart. Paper cups are a good choice because they crush more easily than plastic if stepped on (**Figure 15**). Starting at one end of the row of cups, the amputee slowly raises one leg while stepping forward so that the knee is waist high, or so that a 90° angle is formed at the hip, and then slowly returns the foot to the floor while stepping over the next cup.

When balancing over the prosthetic limb as the intact limb advances, the amputee should focus on three key elements: (1) The buttocks and, for transtibial amputees, the thigh muscles on the prosthetic side are contracted. (2) A downward force through the socket is exerted that creates maximal weight-bearing within the socket. (3) The weight of the body must pass over the prosthetic foot to maintain weight over the great toe of the prosthetic foot.

There are several exercise variations that can be introduced with the

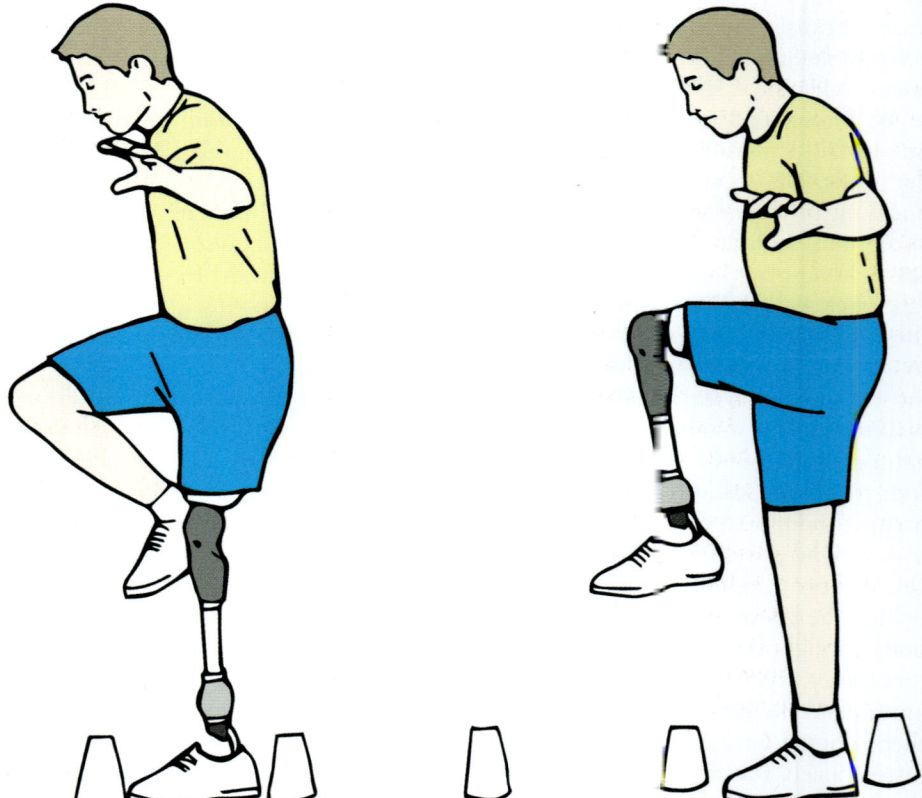

FIGURE 15 Illustration of the cup-walking drill. (Copyright Advanced Rehabilitation Therapy, Inc, Miami, FL, 1990. Illustrator, Frank Angulo.)

cup drills. For example, walking on a compliant or foam surface increases the need for stability within the socket of the prosthetic limb to execute the exercise exactly the way it is performed on a solid floor. The amputee needs to maintain knee stability in all directions and therefore must react faster with the muscles of the knee and hip to maintain balance. Sideways walking will further challenge the residual limb musculature and improve balance.

Backward walking is another skill that will assist in developing prosthetic control. Amputees should focus on the same key elements, contracting the muscles, exerting a downward and backward force within the socket, and feeling the weight progress over the prosthetic foot. Limiting any unnecessary movement from the trunk will be helpful.

Exercises for Maximizing Prosthetic Ankle and Foot Performance

Toe-Box Jumps

For toe-box jumps, four pieces of tape are placed 2 feet apart to form a square. The amputee stands with both feet together, then jumps diagonally to the opposite mark, landing on the toe of the prosthetic foot, using the intact limb for balance. The body weight loads the prosthetic foot; then, as the prosthetic foot plate releases its stored energy, the amputee quickly pushes off using the quadriceps muscles to extend the knee, jumping to the next mark on the lateral side. Again landing on the toe of the prosthetic limb and balancing with the intact limb, the amputee jumps diagonally to the last remaining mark. Initially, a spotter should be present for safety. Timing of the prosthetic foot plate release and the knee extension is the focus of the exercise, as well as learning how to take advantage of the prosthetic foot's energy return.

Lateral Speed Weave

A set of four to five cones are placed in a straight line approximately every 4 feet, with another alternating set of cones placed halfway between and 2 to 3 feet across. The lateral speed weave is designed to promote speed, power, and agility in all directions by having the amputee run forward, to the side, backward, to the side, and forward again. Because of the differences in knee control, transtibial amputees and transfemoral amputees perform this exercise in a slightly different manner.

Agility Drills

To perform agility drills, several cones or cups are placed in two rows (four to six on either side) approximately 6 feet apart. The amputee quickly moves from one cone to another, squatting down to touch each cone as they zig-zag from one cone to another. The key to this exercise is maintaining speed by staying on the toe of the prosthetic foot and using the quadriceps and hip extensor muscles to rapidly extend the prosthetic limb as the amputee turns or rises from the squatting position.

Evidence-Based Amputee Rehabilitation

Evidence-based rehabilitation is defined as "the conscientious and judicious use of current best evidence from clinical care research in the management of individual patients."[63] The practice of evidence-based rehabilitation refers to the integration of current best research evidence and clinical expertise to design a plan of care.[64] Current best research specifically refers to patient-centered studies that provide evidence of efficacy and safety of both assessments and interventions. Clinical expertise refers to the competency clinicians develop through their clinical practice and experience. Clinicians who use current best research evidence are avoiding the risk of implementing dated or inappropriate plans of care.

In rehabilitative medicine, a patient's status is often assessed through the use of outcome measures, either self-report or performance-based. Self-report outcome measures are questionnaires designed to capture patients' perceptions of constructs, such as health, satisfaction, pain, mobility, and balance confidence. Performance-based outcome measures are administered by clinicians and include specific tasks patients need to complete to determine their level of function, mobility, or balance.

The clinical value of outcome measures can vary; however, most instruments have the ability to provide information with respect to one or more of the following aspects of function: (1) determine the current capabilities, (2) determine the functional level of a patient as described by a predefined scale, (3) predict the functional capabilities or mobility of a patient, (4) determine the contribution of specific variables to a measure of function, (5) assist with treatment prescription, (6) detect change over time, and (7) documentation of services.[65] However, the usefulness of outcome measures is far greater than a single score or comparison and should extend to treatment prescription.

Performance-based outcome measures can quantify or categorize the capabilities of a patient as defined by a predetermined value, scale, or description. When a patient completes a performance-based outcome measure, the physical therapist should review the test tasks that were less than satisfactory, identify the impaired body function segment, set appropriate treatment goals, and prescribe the appropriate exercises. After receiving treatment for a period of time, follow-up assessment(s) should be performed to evaluate the change over time. When comparing outcome measure scores there are generally three results that, combined with the knowledge of other patient-related factors, can assist clinicians to determine the effectiveness of current treatments and plan future interventions: (1) Improved test scores suggest the treatment is effective and should continue until the patient's goals are met. (2) No change in test scores can indicate (a) the treatment may be less effective than anticipated and an alternate treatment should be considered, (b) the treatment is effective in maintaining the current level of function and to avoid a decline treatment should continue, and (c) the patient has maximized their functional potential and a maintenance program may be appropriate. (3) A decline in test scores suggests the treatment is ineffective or that the patient's health status is deteriorating as a result of secondary conditions or aging. The value of outcome measures is quantifying the effectiveness of treatment based on the patient's response with repeated testing. For amputee rehabilitation the application of using outcome measures to identify functional limitations for the prescription of targeted exercises is referred to as Evidence-Based Amputee Rehabilitation (EBAR).[66] The following section describes examples of using EBAR for specific tasks included in the Amputee Mobility Predictor (AMP).

Amputee Mobility Predictor

The AMP is a performance-based outcome measure for patients with lower limb loss that is used to determine functional capabilities and mobility. The AMP is used with (AMP Pro) or without (AMP noPro) a prosthesis.[66] The AMP includes 21 tasks that progress in difficulty, starting with sitting balance, transfers from chair to chair, standing, single-limb balance, and a reach test. Next, the AMP progresses to more dynamic tasks that assess elements of locomotion such as step length, step continuity, and the ability to vary cadence, finishing with ascending and descending stairs. The AMP was designed to assess the segments of body function, including strength, endurance, coordination, balance, postural control, power, speed, agility, and the gait of people with lower limb loss. The score assignment is relatively straightforward. A score of "2" is assigned when performed independently and safely, a "1" is scored when performed independently but the patient must use an assistive device for balance or to complete the task, and a "0" is assigned when they are unable to perform the task or they are unsafe. Some tasks have only 0 to 1 grades, but the scoring principles are the same.

Four examples of AMP tasks that assess various levels of mobility and that can be treated with an evidence-based treatment approach are (1) rise from a chair, (2) single-limb standing balance, (3) turning, and (4) stairs. These tasks assess the patient's ability to safely control movement, often related to their center of mass displacement over the base of support while standing or changing postural position, when standing on a narrow base (one limb), changing direction, and negotiating obstacles such as stairs. Patients who can control their center of mass displacement over the base of support are more likely to perform these tasks independently, efficiently, and safely. Therefore, these patients will receive the highest score of "2" for these four selected tasks and would not require treatment for these skills. Conversely, patients who receive a score of either 0 (ie, unsteady or unable) or 1 (ie, require the support of an assistive device or additional steps to complete the turn) would be prescribed target exercises to address their inability to control the center of mass displacement or postural control. Postural control will be the primary skill used as an example for the following treatment descriptions, keeping in mind that other limitations such as strength, coordination, etc. may need to be addressed as well and will be briefly described.

Arise from a Chair

The task of arising from a chair examines a patient's ability to control the center of mass during upward and forward displacements.[67] A score of 2 is given to amputees that are able to rise without using their arms for assistance. Conversely, when amputees use their arms for assistance, the physical therapist must determine which body function segment causes this activity limitation. Arising from a chair involves several body function segments, which include but are not limited to (1) organizational skills, (2) momentum strategies, and (3) dynamic postural stability.[66]

Organizational skills refer to a set of movements performed by patients in preparation to perform a task. Preparatory movements include but are not limited to forward rotation of the trunk and pelvis and knee flexion to reposition the feet closer underneath the pelvis.[68] This set of preparatory movements reduces the distance between the center of mass and base of support and provides greater stability during the transition from sit to stand.[69] If the amputee is not performing these sets of movements, the recommended intervention should include a review of and exercising the order of these movements.

Momentum strategies are used when patients perform a rapid forward motion of the trunk coupled with the contraction of hip and knee extensors to complete the arise from a chair task.[68,69] The generated momentum must be large enough to propel the center of mass from a sitting position to a standing position. In addition, because of the large, generated momentum, this strategy requires fine dynamic postural stability to prevent loss of balance.[68,69] Therefore, the ability to perform arise from a chair independently, efficiently, and safely using momentum strategies requires sufficient trunk and lower limb strength as well as adequate dynamic postural stability.[66]

When amputees use momentum strategies in conjunction with their arms for support, the physical therapist must perform secondary assessments to determine the cause of the activity limitation. A manual muscle test will determine if the amputee has impaired lower limb extensor and/or trunk muscle strength. Amputees with impaired muscle strength are prescribed strengthening exercises based on the specific muscle group at fault. For example, a patient with low hip extensor strength will perform the bridge exercise as presented in **Figure 2, F**; and a patient with moderate muscle strength will perform the partial wall squats exercise.[66] The partial wall squats exercise is performed by having the amputees stand with their back against the wall, place their feet shoulder-width apart, and about 2 feet out from the wall. The exercise begins with amputees sliding their back down the wall while keeping their core muscles engaged and bending their knees until they reach about a 135° angle. The knees should be directly above the ankles. The exercise ends with amputees coming back to a standing position. During descent, the lower limb muscles work eccentrically and, conversely, work concentrically during ascent.[70] The amputees should focus on shifting their center of mass toward the prosthetic limb when performing the exercise with the goal of equal weight-bearing between both lower limbs. Note: A small ball may be placed between the knees to facilitate the equal use of both lower limbs. Also, a small towel can be placed under the prosthetic foot heel to assist with the ankle range of motion.

Single-Limb Standing Balance

The task of single-limb standing balance examines the ability of patients to shift their center of mass over to one foot and maintain balance for 30 seconds. First, the patient is asked to perform the task on the intact limb and then on the prosthetic limb. Single-limb balance involves two main body function segments: (1) lower limb muscle strength and (2) single-limb postural stability.[66] When a patient receives a score lower than "2," the physical therapists should further assess the two key body functions. If the amputee's residual limb muscle strength is impaired, the recommended exercise is stool-stepping[48,66,71] (**Figure 7**). The stool-stepping exercise facilitates amputees to (1) become familiar with the residual limb socket interface during increased weight bearing on the prosthesis and (2) rapidly contract the hip and knee musculature to gain control of the center of mass displacement. Patients with low muscle strength will perform the exercise while holding the parallel bars. As their strength improves, they will perform the task with only one hand for support and then without any support.

If the amputee's single-limb postural stability is impaired, the recommended exercise is ball rolls[48,66] (**Figure 3**). Placing one foot on a tennis ball and moving it in all directions creates disturbances in postural stability. To maintain single-limb postural stability, the hip and knee musculature must perform rapid co-contractions over an extended period of time. Similar to the stool-stepping exercise, a patient may begin performing the exercise while using both arms for support, and as muscle strength improves, less support should be used.

Turning

In the turning task, patients are asked to complete a 180° turn in at maximum three steps.[24,48] The task of turning assesses the patient's ability to control the center of mass displacement from one limb to another while walking on a curved path. Performing a turn involves two main body function segments: (1) dynamic single-limb postural stability and (2) prosthetic control.[66]

Dynamic single-limb postural stability and prosthetic control would need to be evaluated in amputees that receive either a score of "0" (ie, unable to turn without intervention) or "1" (ie, requires more than three steps to complete the task). An additional assessment of dynamic single-limb postural stability would include AMP task #15 that assesses step length. For example, a patient that does not advance the intact limb to a minimum of 12 inches (ie, observed from the toes of the trailing prosthetic limb to the heel of the leading intact limb) will likely have impaired dynamic prosthetic single-limb postural stability. Exercises to improve dynamic prosthetic single-limb postural stability can begin with the previously described stool-stepping exercise. The exercise progression for dynamic single-limb balance and postural stability would include the aforementioned exercises: multidirectional turns, tandem walking, lateral drills, braiding, and cup walking drills (**Figures 14** and **15**). The figure-of-8 drill is especially relevant because the amputee continually alternates the turn direction, which requires continual adjustment in weight shifting and dynamic single-limb postural stability to control the movement.[72] During any turn exercise, the amputee wearing a prosthesis should focus on maintaining normal pelvic forward transverse rotation while rolling over the foot to promote prosthetic knee flexion to advance the prosthetic limb while changing directions. Both forward transverse pelvic rotation and knee flexion are essential motions that enable the amputee to clear the foot off the ground during the swing period and advance the limb forward, completing a normal step length.[73] The goal for the figure-of-8 drill is to complete a 180° turn in three to four steps. As performance of the figure-of-8 improves, the length of the course can shorten to increase the challenge by creating a more acute angle during each directional change.

Stairs

In the stairs task, the amputees are asked to walk up and down a minimum of two stairs, with the maximum of "2" scored for those who can perform the task of stairs, step overstep, without holding onto a railing or an assistive device.[24] The task examines an amputee's ability to control the center of mass upward and forward displacements while maintaining single-limb balance. Performing stair ascent involves three main body function segments: (1) lower limb concentric muscle strength, (2) dynamic single-limb postural stability, and (3) prosthetic control.[66] Stair decent is similar but involves lower limb eccentric strength to control the lowering of the body to the step below. **Figure 13** describes stair ascent and decent in further detail.

When the amputee uses a railing to ascend stairs, the physical therapist should assess all three function segments. As previously described, a manual muscle test will assess the strength of specific muscle groups, single-limb postural stability can be assessed from AMP tasks #8 single-limb standing balance and #15 step length. The targeted exercises can begin with the single-limb bridge exercise (**Figure 2**) alternating stool-stepping exercise (**Figure 7**), and progress to cup-walking drills (**Figure 15**).

When amputees ascend stairs one step at a time (ie, a score of 1 on the AMP), often they will perform the task with the leading intact limb pushing and the trailing prosthetic limb being pulled. Exercises to improve prosthetic control can begin with chair squats, wherein amputees stand with the feet shoulder-width apart and slowly descend to a chair by bending their knees keeping their body weight over their heels. The buttocks touch the chair, and the amputee should push down through their forefoot as they rise to a standing position. If possible, amputees should direct their focus on equal use of both lower limbs to perform this exercise. When amputees are able to perform the chair squats independently and safely using both lower limbs, they should advance to perform the lunge exercise.[66]

The lunge exercise starts with amputees standing in a split stance position, with the prosthetic foot forward and the intact foot about two to three feet back. Next, the amputee is asked to bend the knees and lower the body down until the back knee is a few inches off the ground and then push back up to standing, keeping the weight on the prosthetic foot. For those finding the split stance position difficult to perform, the exercise can begin using parallel bars for support.

The AMP includes multiple tasks that are used to measure the complex phenomena of basic mobility, which have numerous facets. The four AMP tasks discussed above were used to demonstrate how physical therapists can use EBAR to guide interventions. Knowing the body function segments involved in each task performance and how those are assessed enables physical therapists to identify causes for activity limitations. In addition, prescribing targeted exercises for each identified body function impairment can improve the performance of the specific task as well as the total score of the AMP. The application of an EBAR permits clinicians to systematically prescribe treatment, monitor a patient's progress, compare outcome measure results to determine if change over time in functional capabilities and to demonstrate the effectiveness of specific interventions related to the care of people with lower limb loss.

SUMMARY

The physical therapist must work closely with the rehabilitation team to provide comprehensive care for the amputee. An individualized program must be constructed according to the abilities of each patient. The primary skills of preprosthetic training help build the foundation for successful prosthetic ambulation. The degree of success with ambulation may directly influence how much amputees will use their prostheses and may be predictive of their overall level of activity. The primary goal of the rehabilitation team, therefore, should be to make this transitional period as smooth and successful as possible.

References

1. Become a CPV: Amputt coalition website Accessed August 18, 2015. www.amputee-coalition.org/support-groups–peer-support/certified-peer-visitor-program/become-a-cpv/
2. Pasquina PF, Tsao JW, Collins DM, et al: Quality of medical care provided to service members with combat–related limb amputations: Report of patient satisfaction. *J Rehabil Res Dev* 2008;45(7):953-960.
3. PALS: Promoting Amputee Life Skills. Available at: http://www.amputeelifeskills.org/. Accessed August 18, 2015.
4. Wegener ST, Mackenzie EJ, Ephraim P, Ehde D, Williams R: Self-management improves outcomes in persons with limb loss. *Arch Phys Med Rehabil* 2009;90(3):373-380.
5. Czerniecki JM, Turner AP, Williams RM, Hakimi KN, Norvell DC: Mobility changes in individuals with dysvascular amputation from the pre-surgical period to 12 months postamputation. *Arch Phys Med Rehabil* 2012;93(10):1766-1773.
6. Johannesson A, Larsson G, Ramstrand N, Lauge-Pederen H, Wagner P, Atroshi I: Outcomes of a standardized surgical and rehabilitation program in transtibial amputation for peripheral vascular disease: A pro-spective cohort study. *Am J Phys Med Rehabil* 2010;84(4):293-303.
7. Wan-Nar Wong M: Changing dynamics in lower-extremity amputation in China. *Arch Phys Med Rehabil* 2005;86(9):1778-1781.
8. Toursarkissian B, Shireman PK, Harrison A, D'Ayala M, Schoolfield J, Sykes MT: Major lower-extremity amputation: Contemporary experience in a single Veterans Affairs institution. *Am Surg* 2002;68(7):606-610.
9. Taylor SM, Kalbaugh CA, Cass AL, et al: "Successful outcome" after below-knee amputation: An objective definition and influence of clinical variables. *Am Surg* 2008;74(7):607-612.
10. Taylor SM, Kalbaugh CA, Blackhurst DW, et al: Preoperative clinical factors predict postoperative functional outcomes after major lower limb amputation: An analysis of 553 consecutive patients. *J Vasc Surg* 2005;42(2):227-235.
11. Mayfield JA, Reiber GE, Maynard C, Czerniecki JM, Caps MT, Sangeorzan BJ: Survival following lower-limb amputation in a veteran population. *J Rehabil Res Dev* 2001;38(3):341-345.
12. Munin MC, Espejo-De Guzman MC, Boninger ML, Fitzgerald SG, Penrod LE, Singh J: Predictive factors for successful early prosthetic ambulation among lower-limb amputees. *J Rehabil Res Dev* 2001;38(4):379-384.
13. Pasquina PF, Gambel J, Foster LS, Kim A, Doukas WC: Process of care for battle casualties at the Walter Reed Army Medical Center: Part III. Physical medicine and rehabilitation service. *Mil Med* 2006;171(3):206-208.
14. Gailey RS, Wenger MA, Raya M, et al: Energy expenditure of trans-tibial amputees during ambulation at self–selected pace. *Prosthet Orthot Int* 1994;18(2):84-91.
15. Raya MA, Gailey RS, Fiebert IM, Roach KE: Impairment variables predicting activity limitation in individuals with lower limb amputation. *Prosthet Orthot Int* 2010;34(1):73-84.
16. Silverman AK, Fey NP, Portillo A, Walden JG, Bosker G, Neptune RR: Compensatory mechanisms in below-knee amputee gait in response to increasing steady-state walking speeds. *Gait Posture* 2008;28(4):602-609.
17. Vanicek N, Strike SC, Polman R: Kinematic differences exist between transtibial amputee fallers and non–fallers during downwards step transitioning. *Prosthet Orthot Int* 2015;39(4):322-332.
18. Langlois K, Villa C, Bonnet X, et al: Influence of physical capacities of males with transtibial amputation on gait adjustments on sloped surfaces. *J Rehabil Res Dev* 2014;51(2):193-200.
19. Nolan L: A training programme to improve hip strength in persons with lower limb amputation. *J Rehabil Med* 2012;44(3):241-248.
20. Pandian G, Huang ME, Duffy DA: Acquired limb deficiencies. 2. Perioperative management. *Arch Phys Med Rehabil* 2001;82(3 suppl 1):S9-S16.
21. Robbins CB, Vreeman DJ, Sothmann MS, Wilson SL, Oldridge NB: A review of the long-term health outcomes associated with war-related amputation. *Mil Med* 2009;174(6):588-592.

22. Gailey R, McFarland LV, Cooper RA, et al: Unilateral lower-limb loss: Prosthetic device use and functional outcomes in servicemembers from Vietnam war and OIF/OEF conflicts. *J Rehabil Res Dev* 2010;47(4):317-331.
23. Nolan L, Wit A, Dudzinski K, Lees A, Lake M, Wychowanski M: Adjustments in gait symmetry with walking speed in trans-femoral and trans-tibial amputees. *Gait Posture* 2003;17(2):142-151.
24. Gailey R, Roach K, Applegate B, et al: The amputee mobility predictor: An instrument to assess determinants of the lower limb amputee's ability to ambulate. *Arch Phys Med Rehabil* 2002;83:613-627.
25. Brodzka WK, Thornhill HL, Zarapkar SE, Mallory JA, Weiss L: Long-term function of persons with atherosclerotic bilateral below-knee amputation living in the inner city. *Arch Phys Med Rehabil* 1990;71(11):895-900.
26. Medhat A, Huber PM, Medhat MA: Factors that influence the level of activities in persons with lower extremity amputation. *Rehabil Nurs* 1990;13:13-18.
27. Pinzur MS, Gottschalk F, Smith D, et al: Functional outcome of below-knee amputation in peripheral vascular insufficiency. A multi-center review. *Clin Orthop Relat Res* 1993;286:247-249.
28. Laferrier JZ, McFarland LV, Boninger ML, Cooper RA, Reiber GE: Wheeled mobility: Factors influencing mobility and assistive technology in veterans and servicemembers with major traumatic limb loss from Vietnam war and OIF/OEF conflicts. *J Rehabil Res Dev* 2010;47(4):349-360.
29. DuBow LL, Witt PL, Kadaba MP, Reyes R, Cochran V: Oxygen consumption of elderly persons with bilateral transtibial amputations: Ambulation vs wheelchair propulsion. *Arch Phys Med Rehabil* 1983;64(6):255-259.
30. Karmarkar AM, Collins DM, Wichman T, et al: Prosthesis and wheelchair use in veterans with lower-limb amputation. *J Rehabil Res Dev* 2009;46(5):567-576.
31. Fieldler G, Akins J, Cooper R, Munoz S, Cooper R: Rehabilitation of people with lower limb amputation. *Curr Phys Med Rehabil Rep* 2014;2:263-272.
32. May BJ: Stump bandaging of the lower-extremity amputee. *Phys Ther* 1964;44:808-814.
33. Zhu HS, Wertsch JJ, Harris GF, Loftsgaarden JD, Price MB: Foot pressure distribution during walking and shuffling. *Arch Phys Med Rehabil* 1991;72(6):390-397.
34. Mueller MJ, Sinacore DR, Hoogstrate S, Daly L: Hip and ankle walking strategies: Effect on peak plantar pressures and implications for neuropathic ulceration. *Arch Phys Med Rehabil* 1994;75:1196-2000.
35. Katoulis EC, Ebdon-Parry H, Vileikyte L, Kulkarni J, Boulton AJM: Gait abnormalities in diabetic neuropathy. *Diabetes Care* 1997;20(12):1904-1907.
36. Isakov E, Budoragin N, Shenhav S, Mendelevich I, Korzets A, Susak Z: Anatomic sites of foot lesions resulting in amputation among diabetics and non-diabetics. *Am J Phys Med Rehabil* 1995;74(2):130-133.
37. Norvell DC, Czerniecki JM, Reiber GE, Maynard C, Pecoraro JA, Weiss NS: The prevalence of knee pain and symptomatic knee osteoarthritis among veteran traumatic amputees and nonamputees. *Arch Phys Med Rehabil* 2005;86(3):487-493.
38. Kulkarni J, Adams J, Thomas E, Silman A: Association between amputation, arthritis and osteopenia in British male war veterans with major lower limb amputations. *Clin Rehabil* 1998;12(4):348-353.
39. Gailey R, Allen K, Castles J, Kucharik J, Roeder M: Review of secondary physical conditions associated with lower-limb amputation and long-term prosthesis use. *J Rehabil Res Dev* 2008;45(1):15-29.
40. Morgenroth DC, Gellhorn AC, Suri P: Osteoarthritis in the disabled population: A mechanical perspective. *PM R* 2012;4(5 suppl):S20-S27.
41. Perry J, Shanfield S: Efficiency of dynamic elastic response prosthetic feet. *J Rehabil Res Dev* 1993;30(1):137-143.
42. Ward KH, Meyers MC: Exercise performance of lower-extremity amputees. *Sports Med* 1995;20(4):207-214.
43. Kurdibaylo SF: Cardiorespiratory status and movement capabilities in adults with limb amputation. *J Rehabil Res Dev* 1994;31(3):222-235.
44. Davidoff GN, Lampman RM, Westbury L, Deron J: Exercise testing and training of persons with dysvascular amputation: Safety and efficacy of arm ergometry. *Arch Phys Med Rehabil* 1992;73:334-338.
45. Finestone HM, Lampman RM, Davidoff GN, Westbury L: Arm ergometry exercise testing in patients with dysvascular amputations. *Arch Phys Med Rehabil* 1991;72:15-19.
46. Gailey RS: Recreational pursuits of elders with amputation. *Top Geriatr Rehabil* 1992;8(1):39-58.
47. Eisert O, Tester OW: Dynamic stump for lower limb amputees. *Arch Phys Med Rehabil* 1954;33:695-704.
48. Gailey RS, Gailey AM: *Prosthetic Gait Training for Lower Limb Amputees.* Advanced Rehabilitation Therapy Inc., 1989.
49. Gailey RS, Gailey AM: *Strengthening and Stretching for Lower Extremity Amputees.* Advanced Rehabilitation Therapy Inc., 1994.
50. Hodges PW, Julls GA: Motor relearning strategies for the rehabilitation of intervertebral control of the spine, in Liebenson C, ed: *Rehabilitation of the Spine: A Practitioner's Manual*, ed 2. Lippincott Williams & Wilkins, 2003.
51. Kulkarni J, Gaine WJ, Buckley JG, Rankine JJ, Adams J: Chronic low back pain in traumatic lower limb amputees. *Clin Rehabil* 2005;19(1):81-86.
52. Ehde DM, Smith DG, Czerniecki JM, Campbell KM, Malchow DM, Robinson LR: Back pain as a secondary disability in persons with lower limb amputations. *Arch Phys Med Rehabil* 2001;82(6):731-734.
53. Taghipour H, Moharamzad Y, Mafi AR, et al: Quality of life among veterans with war-related unilateral lower extremity amputation: A long-term survey in a prosthesis center in Iran. *J Orthop Trauma* 2009;23(7):525-530.
54. Hendershot BD, Wolf EJ: Three-dimensional joint reaction forces and moments at the low back during over-ground walking in persons with unilateral lower-extremity amputation. *Clin Biomech (Bristol, Avon)* 2014;29(3):235-242.
55. Murray MP: Gait as a total pattern of movement. *Am J Phys Med Rehabil* 1967;16:390-393.
56. Jones ME, Bashford GM, Mann JM: Weight-bearing and velocity in trans-tibial and transfemoral amputees. *Prosthet Orthot Int* 1997;21(3):183-186.
57. Jones ME, Bashford GM, Biokas VV: Weight-bearing pain and walking velocity during primary transtibial amputee rehabilitation. *Clin Rehabil* 2001;15:172-176.
58. Inman VT, Ralson RJ, Todd F: *Human Walking.* Williams & Wilkins, 1981.
59. Saunders JB, Inman VT, Eberhart HD: The major determinants in normal and pathological gait. *J Bone Joint Surg Am* 1953;35(3):543-558.

60. Gard SA, Childress DS: The effect of pelvic list on the vertical displacement of the trunk during walking. *Gait Posture* 1997;5:233-238.
61. Duncan P, Weiner D, Chandler J, Studenski S: Functional reach: A new clinical measure of balance. *J Gerontol* 1990;45:192-197.
62. Murray MP, Drought AB, Kory RC: Walking patterns of normal men. *J Bone Joint Surg Am* 1964;46:335-360.
63. Haynes RB, Sackett DL, Gray JMA, Cook DF, Guyatt GH: Transferring evidence from research into practice: The role of clinical care research evidence in clinical decisions. *ACP J Club* 1996;125(3):A14-A16.
64. Sackett DL, Rosenberg WMC, Gray JAM, Haynes RB, Richardson WS: Evidence-based medicine: What it is and what it isn't. *Br Med J* 1996;312:71-72.
65. Gaunaurd IA, Gailey RS, Pasquina PF: More than the final score: Development, application, and future research of comprehensive high-level activity mobility predictor. *J Rehabil Res Dev* 2013;50(7):vii-xiii.
66. Gailey R, Gaunaurd I, Raya M, Kirk-Sanchez N, Prieto-Sanchez LM, Roach K: Effectiveness of an evidence-based amputee rehabilitation program: A pilot randomized controlled trial. *Phys Ther* 2020;100(5):773-787.
67. Roebroeck ME, Doorenbosch CA, Harlaar J, Jacobs R, Lankhorst GJ: Biomechanics and muscular activity during sit-to-stand transfer. *Clin Biomech (Bristol, Avon)* 1994;9(4):235-244.
68. Schenkman M, Berger RA, Riley PO, Mann RW, Hodge WA: Whole-body movements during rising to standing from sitting. *Phys Ther* 1990;70(10):638-648.
69. Hughes MA, Weiner DK, Schenkman ML, Long RM, Studenski SA: Chair rise strategies in the elderly. *Clin Biomech (Bristol, Avon)* 1994;9(3):187-192.
70. Biscarini A, Contemori S, Dieni CV, Panichi R: Joint torques and tibiofemoral joint reaction force in the bodyweight "Wall Squat" therapeutic exercise. *Appl Sci* 2020;10(9):3019.
71. Yiğiter K, Şener G, Erbahceci F, Bayar K, Ülger ÖG, Akdoğan S: A comparison of traditional prosthetic training versus proprioceptive neuromuscular facilitation resistive gait training with trans-femoral amputees. *Prosthet Orthot Int* 2002;26(3):213-217.
72. Hess RJ, Brach JS, Piva SR, et al: Walking skill can be assessed in older adults: Validity of the figure-of-8 walk test. *Phys Ther* 2010;90(1):89-99.
73. Perry J, Burnfield JM: *Gait Analysis: Normal and Pathological Function.* SLACK, 2010.

Adaptive Lower Limb Prostheses for Sports and Recreation

CHAPTER 50

Francois J. Van Der Watt, CPO, LPO

ABSTRACT

Participation in sports and recreational activities by individuals with lower limb amputation can improve physical and mental health status. Prostheses specifically designed for sports participation can assist lower limb amputees in achieving optimal performance but are not needed to engage in all sports activities. Prosthesis use in sporting and recreational activities is best determined after consultation with a prosthetist, physiotherapist, and other members of the rehabilitation and sports team.

Keywords: adaptive athlete; lower limb amputee; recreational sports; sport prosthetic

Introduction

There are no written records of individuals with amputations or other physical disabilities participating in major organized sporting events from before the beginning of the 20th century. The first record of an amputee participating in a major event is that of George Eyser, who competed in the 1904 Summer Olympic Games.[1] Eyser, who lost his lower left leg in a train accident and used a wooden prosthetic leg, successfully competed against able-bodied athletes and won six Olympic medals (including three gold medals).[1] Taking into account the major differences in physical functioning between able-bodied individuals and those with amputations, his performance represents an outstanding achievement.[2,3]

The first sporting event dedicated to individuals with physical disabilities took place in 1948 at the Stoke Mandeville Hospital, under the initiative of Sir Ludwig Guttmann, a British neurologist of German descent.[4] The first Paralympic Games took place in Rome, Italy, in 1960 and these have since become a regular event held once every 4 years.[5] The number of participants and sports participation has increased in every subsequent Paralympic Games. In the 2016 summer Paralympic Games held in Rio de Janeiro, 4,328 athletes competed from 159 countries.[6,7] Because of the global COVID-19 pandemic in 2019, the 2020 Paralympic Games in Tokyo, Japan, was postponed until 2021. A total of 4,403 athletes from 162 nations competed in 22 sports.[8] Participants were organized into six disability groups to "ensure competition is fair and equal, and that winning is determined by skill, fitness, power, endurance, tactical ability and mental focus, the same factors that account for success in sports for able-bodied athletes."[9]

Approximately 30% of individuals with a lower limb amputation participate in sports, with cycling, fitness, swimming, golf, and walking being some of the favored activities.[10] Generally, an individual who was actively participating in sports before their amputation is more likely to participate in sports after an amputation. Other factors that may have a positive influence on the participation in sports are a younger age, a more distal level of amputation, and a nonvascular amputation.

To better understand participation in recreational and competitive sports by individuals with limb absence or loss, the effects of factors such as physical health, psychological determinants, and technical aids (such as prostheses) must be considered.

Physical Health

Although amputees generally have better physical health than individuals with other physical disabilities such as cerebral palsy or spinal cord injury,[11,12] they still have substantial limitations in physical functioning compared with able-bodied individuals.[13] The rehabilitation period can provide the ideal place, time, and professional care to recover from the amputation and explore the possibility for sports participation for those demonstrating the will and capability to become recreational or competitive athletes. The physical therapist and prosthetist may

---

Neither Francois J. Van Der Watt nor any immediate family member has received anything of value from or has stock or stock options held in a commercial company or institution related directly or indirectly to the subject of this chapter.

This chapter is adapted from Bragaru M, Van Der Watt F: Adaptive lower limb prostheses for sports and recreation, in Krajbich JI, Pinzur MS, Potter BK, Stevens PM, eds: *Atlas of Amputations and Limb Deficiencies: Surgical, Prosthetic, and Rehabilitation Principles*, ed 4. American Academy of Orthopaedic Surgeons, 2016, pp 621-629.

be a source for advice and guidance on the training required and the sport that best suits the individual's skills and capabilities.

Psychological Determinants

The trauma associated with limb amputation is not confined to physical trauma. Psychological trauma is also experienced by many lower limb amputees, who are prone to depression in the first 2 years after an amputation.[14,15] Regular participation in a sport is one method for dealing with depression, and it has proved both physically and psychosocially beneficial for those who have undergone a lower limb amputation.[10,13,16-22] When questioned about the advantages of sports participation, one amputee mentioned the improvement in well-being, the chance to feel useful, and the opportunity to get out of the house and on a path to regaining a social life.[23]

Factors that may promote or deter an individual's participation in sports include past experiences, personal desires and aims, stigma management, coping skills, self-efficacy, disability acceptance, general health, physical capacity, functional outcome, and regional opportunities for participation.[24] Support from family and peers may encourage sports participation.

Technical Aids and Prostheses

The idea of amputees participating in sports is not new, but the understanding of sport prostheses and the role they play in performance is still a developing science. Although some sports can be performed with conventional prostheses not specifically adapted for a particular sport, other sports require a specially designed prostheses. In recent years, there has been an increase in the rate of development of specialized prostheses and prosthetic components used for sports.[25] In 1996, the first Flex-Foot Cheetah (Össur) became available; advancements in sports prosthetic technology have continued since that time. Although the study and understanding of the biomechanics and functioning of prosthetic devices for sports have continued to improve over the past decade, much of the science concerning sport-specific prostheses and their performance is still unknown.[26] Sport-specific components are only one part of the athlete's total package that enables them to participate and achieve advanced performance in sports activities. The limb–socket interface, the method of suspension, and the alignment of prosthetic components are also important factors that continue to develop. A pilot study by Hefner et al suggested that in the development and use of crossover feet, the participants exhibited increased mobility (ie, Timed Up and Go [TUG][27] at comfortable and fast speeds), endurance (ie, distance walked in 6 minutes), and walking performance (ie, walking speed, cadence, sound step length) compared with their energy-storing foot, Similarly. participants reported decreased exertion (ie, lower Borg rating of perceived exertion [RPE][28]) in crossover feet.[29]

Prosthetic Sockets

A prosthetic socket should be custom made to fit the characteristics of the athlete's residual limb. The socket should provide the required support and comfort to allow the athlete to voluntarily move and control the prosthesis during the sports activity. The socket trim lines should be optimized to allow joint mobility without compromising limb support. Muscle atrophy in the residual limbs of amputee athletes is common and requires socket adjustments to accommodate changes in limb shape and volume. It is fairly common to see an increase of up to 17% in the volume of the residual limb during competition or training.[30] Therefore, an adjustable socket may be useful for an athlete with a transfemoral or transtibial amputation. One option for resolving the issue of varying limb volume is an adjustable socket achieved by cutting out targeted socket walls and fitting them with adjustable flaps (**Figure 1**). This approach can use an adjustable cable system to alter the position of the socket walls to increase or decrease the volume of the socket as changes occur in the volume of the residual limb during an activity.

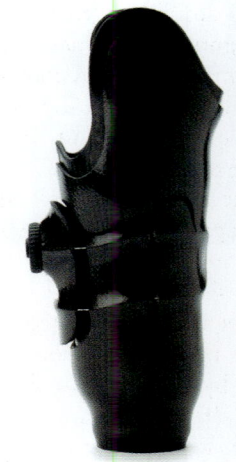

FIGURE 1 Photograph of the RevoFit® (Click Medical), with an adjustable socket for volume fluctuations. (Courtesy of Click Medical LLC.)

At the transfemoral amputation level, subischial or brimless socket designs, which allow increased range of motion and muscle movement, can be considered. These types of sockets are designed for use with a liner to provide skin protection and relief from shear forces applied to the skin of the residual limb by the increased load experienced during sports activities.

Suspension System

The primary function of the socket suspension system is to secure the prosthesis to the athlete's residual limb. The suspension method can also play a critical role in reducing mental fatigue by decreasing the fear of losing the prosthesis during sports participation. The suspension method should be functional and should not limit the joint range of motion. A variety of options is available, and individual needs will determine the most appropriate suspension method. These can include mechanical connections, suction suspension, vacuum suspension, or a combination incorporating two or more suspension methods. The use of an interface liner is most common across all suspension techniques.

Prosthetic Component Choice and Alignment

The prosthetist can choose from a large variety of components that will enable a patient to achieve their best performance in the desired sport. During the dynamic alignment of these components, the manufacturer's recommendations can be helpful because individual component properties and functions differ among manufacturers.

When the need for shock absorption is anticipated and the associated components are incorporated into the prosthetic design, the overall height of the prosthesis must be adjusted accordingly. During running, the compression experienced by shock-absorbing components can affect the timing of ground contact and stride length, and both elements can affect running or agility speed. The selection of the appropriate stiffness for a prosthetic foot can be challenging because the level of amputation, limb length, strength, body weight, and the force production capabilities will vary based on the characteristics of the individual athlete. Secondary, comorbid impairments are also common in traumatic or congenital amputees and should be considered when optimizing the prosthetic setup and alignment for the athlete.

Sport-Specific Prostheses

Distance Running

Recreational running can be one of the simplest forms of exercise for an individual with a lower limb amputation. However, it can be challenging for the novice athlete to learn proper running techniques while using a sport-specific prosthesis. Although jogging with a conventional prosthesis may be more intuitive to a beginning runner, transitioning to a prosthesis specifically designed for running will ultimately be more energy efficient and will help reduce interlimb asymmetries. Because most high-performance, sport-specific feet for running do not have a traditional heel component (**Figure 2**), athletes with a transtibial amputation must adopt new techniques to control and maintain proper knee position during running. Special attention should be paid to prosthetic alignment to help prevent knee hyperextension during initial ground contact when using a sport-specific running prosthesis.

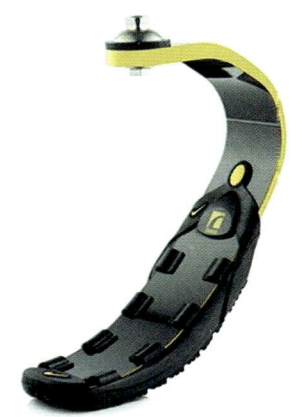

FIGURE 2 Photograph of the Flex-Run foot (Össur), a high performance, sport-specific foot for running. (Courtesy of Össur.)

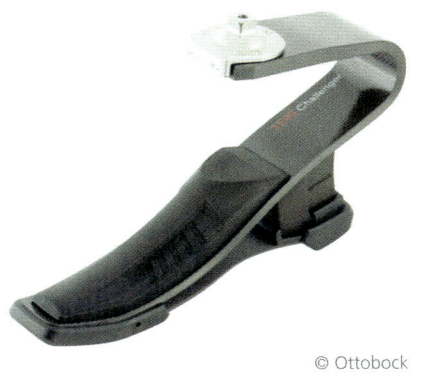

FIGURE 3 Photograph of the Ottobock Challenger foot. This foot is recommended for K3-K4 users. It provides greater energy return and faster cadence speeds than a conventional prosthetic foot. (Courtesy of Ottobock.)

Alternately, the field has seen the emergence of newly engineered crossover feet designed to accommodate a range of activities beyond simple locomotion.[29] Like predecessor high-performance, sport-specific feet, crossover feet incorporate an extended keel that permits users to engage in high-level activities. However, crossover feet also includes elements of more traditional energy storing feet (ie, heel and foot shell) that are not historically present in sport-specific feet. This unique combination of features allows crossover feet to be used both as a daily and sports-specific prosthesis.[29,31] Pilot study data suggest that users experienced significant improvements in most community-based health outcomes in using the crossover feet versus the energy-storing foot. Specifically, participants reported better mobility, balance confidence, and functional satisfaction and less fatigue and activity restrictions.[31] Improvements in performance-based mobility outcome measures across low-level and high-level activities in using crossover feet compared with use of the clinical standard energy-storing foot suggest and indicate that the use of crossover feet may extend the range of activities in which individuals with lower limb amputations can participate using a single prosthesis.[32] This novel foot type improves both low and high mobility outcomes relative to more traditional energy-storing feet[32] (**Figures 3 and 4**).

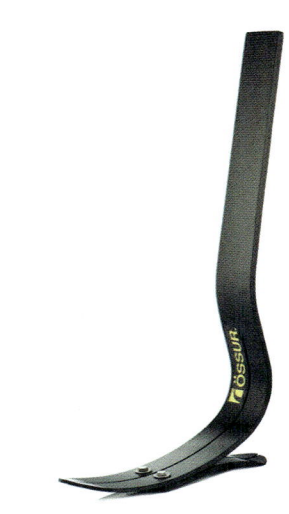

FIGURE 4 Photograph of the Cheetah Xplore foot from Össur. This foot combines energy return properties with flexion, rotation, and good shock absorption. (Courtesy of Össur.)

Running is more challenging for individuals with a transfemoral amputation than those with a transtibial amputation because of the increased interlimb asymmetries experienced at the transfemoral level.[10] The prosthetist attending to a novice transfemoral amputee who wants to participate in distance recreational running should initially consider connecting the

Section 3: Lower Limb

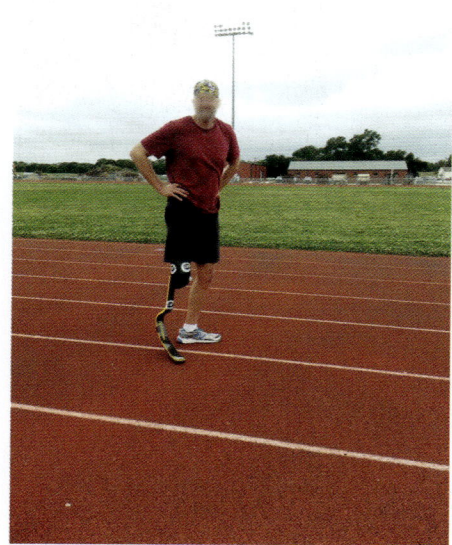

FIGURE 5 Photograph of an athlete with a right above-knee amputation wearing a nonarticulating transfemoral running prosthesis for enhanced knee stability. (Courtesy of Aaron Smith, Gainesville, TX.)

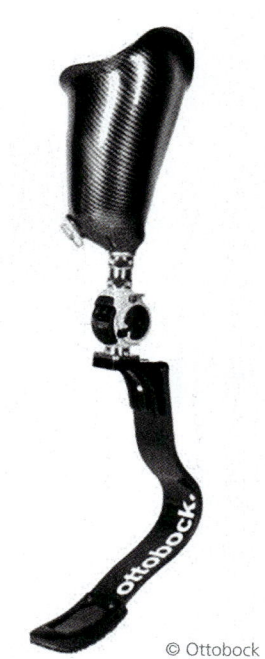

FIGURE 6 Photograph of the 3S80 Fitness Prosthetic Leg (Ottobock). This running prosthesis hydraulically regulates knee motion. (Courtesy of Ottobock.)

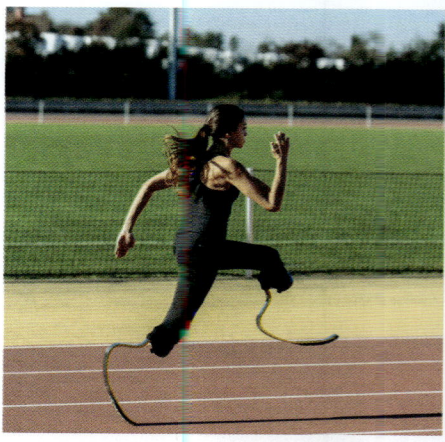

FIGURE 7 Photograph of Abassia Rahmani sprinting with the Cheetah Xtreme foot. (Photographed by Urs Sigg; courtesy of Össur.)

running foot to the socket using a traditional pylon without a prosthetic knee component (**Figure 5**). This approach will assist the amputee in making the transition from a walking gait to a running gait because knee stability during midstance is ensured and will also allow the athlete to become accustomed to using a sport-specific foot for running. For some users, this simple, reliable design may remain their preferred approach for recreational running.

Residual limb length, strength, condition, running experience, and physical and mental ability should be considered when introducing a mechanical knee component for an athlete with a transfemoral amputation. In addition, the athlete's ability to coordinate and control the placement of the prosthetic foot and ensure prosthetic knee stability during the midstance phase of the running gait cycle is important to assess. The use of a running prosthesis with hydraulic regulation of knee motion (**Figure 6**) allows the prosthetist to adjust the rate of flexion and extension during the swing phase and optimize the timing and placement of the prosthetic foot during the initial stance phase of the running gait. Several such knee mechanisms also have a mechanical locking mechanism to assist the athlete when moving around and not running.

When the extension delay of the prosthetic knee during the swing phase cannot be adequately reduced through hydraulic regulation, this delay can be mechanically reduced by lowering the prosthetic knee's horizontal axis and shortening the length of the lower shaft of the prosthesis.[33]

The distance the athlete plans to run also should be considered. The longer the distance, the higher the cost of mental fatigue because the athlete must continually concentrate on maintaining knee stability during the stance phase and optimal prosthetic knee and foot advancement through the swing phase. The prosthetist should align and adjust the components to optimize performance and minimize the physical and mental energy expenditure in the athlete with a transfemoral amputation.

Sprinting

The sport-specific running prosthesis for a transtibial amputee consists of a residual limb socket and a sprinting-specific foot chosen from a line of prosthetic feet made by various manufacturers, including Ottobock, Össur (**Figure 7**), and Fillauer. The method of suspension is determined by the individual athlete's limb configuration and can include any of the suspension approaches discussed. A prosthetic foot for sprinting is generally made of a layered, carbon fiber composite material. Because of the high impact levels encountered, the intense forces applied, and the athlete's training volume, the durability of the foot is limited, and it should be replaced on an annual or biannual basis because the energy-storing properties of carbon fiber feet diminish over time.

A sprinter with a transfemoral amputation can use the same foot components as a sprinter with a transtibial amputation but can choose whether to use a knee component, as the same knee component recommended for distance running can be used for sprinting with some additional knee setting adjustments for sprinting. The athlete's personal preference as well as their running ability and comfort will play a major role in this decision. The coach, the prosthetist, and the rehabilitation professional should be involved in the decision regarding the use of a knee component or not.

Chapter 50: Adaptive Lower Limb Prostheses for Sports and Recreation

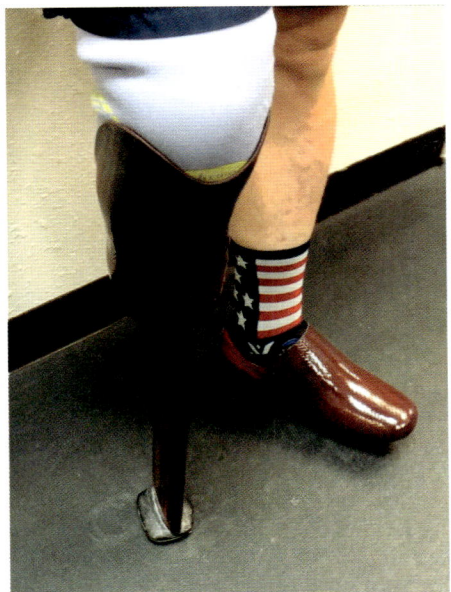

FIGURE 8 Photograph of a cyclist wearing a special cycling prosthesis with a cleat connected directly to the socket. (Courtesy of Francois Van Der Watt, CPO/LPO, Greenwood, AR.)

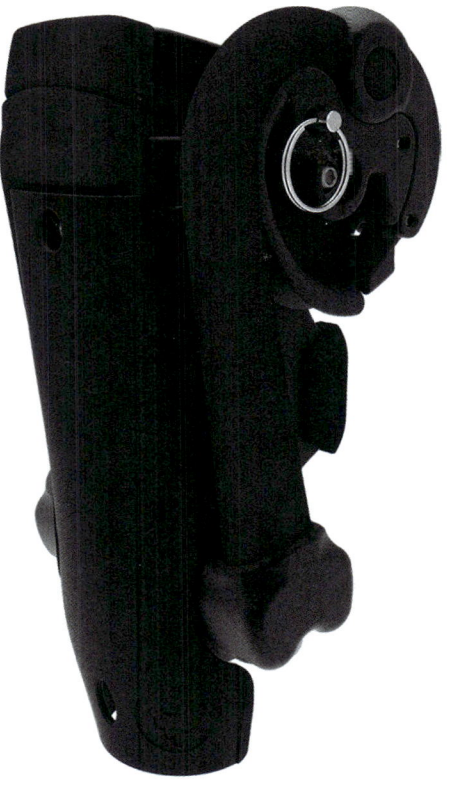

FIGURE 9 Photograph of the Crossover 3G Infinity knee. This knee mimics natural muscle function during cycling in a standing position. (Courtesy of Leftside Industries, Seattle, WA.)

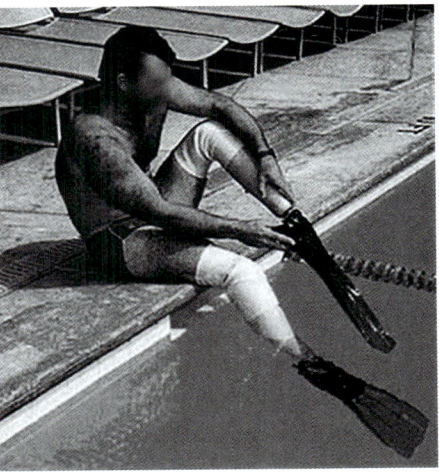

FIGURE 10 Photograph of a swimmer with a bilateral transtibial amputation wearing the Swimankle. (Courtesy of Rampro, Oceanside, CA.)

Cycling

Advancements in technology have allowed amputees to enjoy a wide variety of cycling activities from recreational cycling with family and friends to competitive road racing and mountain biking. The use of a specially designed cycling prosthesis can make cycling easier, however a conventional prosthesis can still be used for everyday cycling activities.

Special attention is needed in selecting the optimal suspension method because a transtibial amputee needs a full range of knee motion and proper alignment to generate power in the downward stroke when cycling. A high-stiffness prosthetic foot without a foot cover or a straight pylon design with the prosthetic foot removed can be used to connect directly to the bike pedal with a shoe cleat. For competitive cycling, the prosthesis can be designed and manufactured with a cleat connected directly to a lightweight exoskeletal socket design (**Figure 8**).

Specialized knee components are available for the cyclist with a transfemoral amputation. These components are designed to allow the user to get into a standing cycling position, which is challenging to achieve and maintain with a conventional mechanical knee component. The Crossover G3 Infinity Knee (**Figure 9**) uses a single-axis pneumatic/hydraulic shock, variable extension dampening bumpers, removeable urethane tendons, and preflexion foam wedges. This allows the cyclist to get in the standing position for the downward power stroke and assists in optimizing foot position during the cycling upstroke.

Swimming

The use of a prosthesis for swimming events is not allowed for Paralympic competitions, although a prosthesis can be used to get to and from the pool or in the swim area. However, an amputee who is a recreational swimmer has a wide variety of prosthetic choices. The method of securing the socket to the residual limb depends on the preference of the user and prosthetist. Currently, the most used method is a sleeve suction suspension system over a cushion liner. Locking liners are also a suspension option. The socket can be designed with or without a foot component; a swimming fin can be attached directly to the prosthetic socket (**Figure 10**). The suspension system should provide a secure and comfortable fit to allow kicking with the prosthesis, without excessive residual limb movement within the socket. The preferred prosthetic design for a swimming prosthesis for a transtibial amputee is a hollow exoskeletal prosthesis, with a hole drilled into the distal shin to allow the water to enter and exit, thus eliminating positive buoyancy. The hole also allows water to drain when the prosthesis is out of the water. The transtibial amputee can use an ankle component like the Freestyle Swim ankle (**Figure 11**). The ankle unit allows the user to adjust and lock the prosthetic foot in up to 70° of plantar flexion for use with swimming fins. The ankles also can lock in a 90° fixed ankle for walking to and from the water.

Care should be taken in component selection because rust and corrosion can damage and limit the function of metal prosthetic components when exposed to salt water and other wet environments.

The type of swimming prosthesis selected for a user with a transfemoral

Section 3: Lower Limb

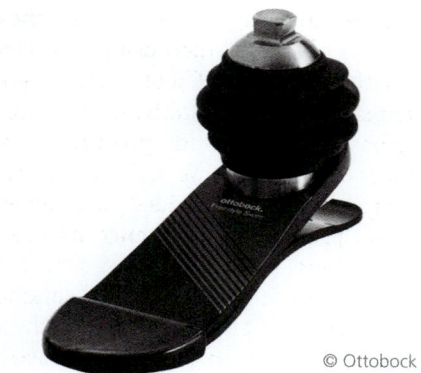

FIGURE 11 Photograph of the Freestyle Swim ankle. This ankle allows an easy transition between swimming and walking. It allows an amputee to walk to the edge of the swimming pool. (Courtesy of Ottobock.)

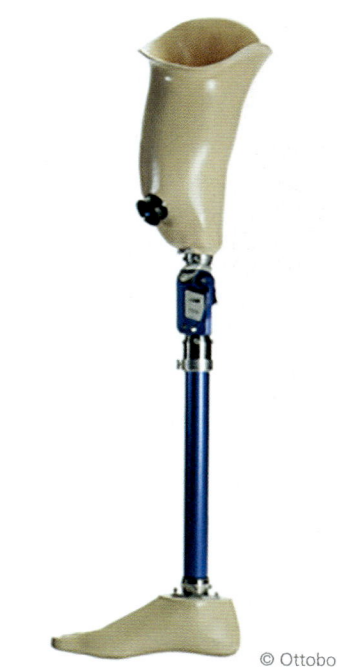

FIGURE 12 Photograph of the Aqualine (Ottobock) waterproof prosthetic system. This prosthesis has a water-resistant coating and a specially designed prosthetic foot that is slip-resistant on wet surfaces. (Courtesy of Ottobock.)

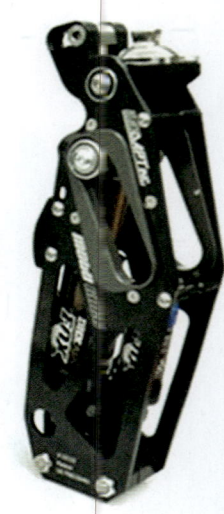

FIGURE 13 Photograph of the Moto Knee 2 (BioDapt). This knee is intended for use during participation in high-impact sports like motocross, snowmobile riding, or various watersport activities. (Courtesy of BioDapt, St. Cloud, MN.)

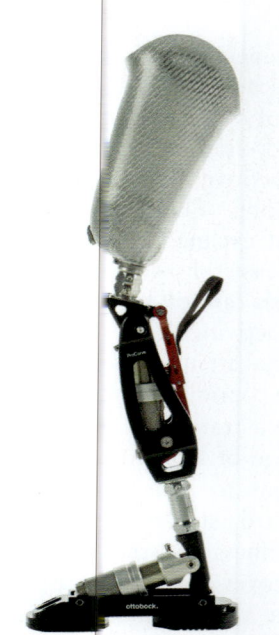

FIGURE 14 Photograph of the ProCarve snow and water sports-specific prosthetic foot and knee system. (Courtesy of Ottobock.)

amputation is an individual and situation-specific decision. Most transfemoral amputees do not elect the use of a swimming prosthesis because of the challenge of suspension and the lack of prosthetic control in the water. The water drag created by a transfemoral prosthetic device can demand substantial energy expenditure, making it more challenging to swim with a device than without one. However, transfemoral prostheses for water-specific sports, which are described in the next section, can be designed for swimming if the transfemoral amputee elects that choice.

Water Sports

The current advancements and developments in sport-specific and activity-specific technologies allow athletes with lower limb amputations to participate in a wide variety of water sports, including surfing, waterskiing, wakeboarding, kiteboarding, fishing, rowing, canoeing, scuba diving, paddleboarding, and water aerobics. The prosthetic parameters to consider are suspension methods, waterproofing and protecting components, and component selection. Conventional prostheses can be protected from water damage and corrosion by using waterproof-specific componentry available from various manufacturers.

The Ottobock Aqualine (**Figure 12**) is an example of a waterproof prosthetic system and is an alternative option for the transfemoral amputee. The components of this prosthesis have a water-resistant coating that provides resistance to corrosion, and the specially designed prosthetic foot, worn without a shoe, is slip-resistant on wet surfaces. The Biodapt Moto Knee 2 (**Figure 13**) or Ottobock ProCarve (**Figure 14**) can be used for water sports like skiing and wakeboarding. This device allows shock-resistant prosthetic knee flexion.

Winter Sports

An athlete with a lower limb amputation who participates in competitive winter sports such as downhill skiing can elect not to use an activity-specific prosthesis but can ski with their sound-side leg using ski poles with outriggers (**Figure 15**). Alternatively, they can ski in a sitting position with a sport-specific mono-ski such as the Shadow Mono-Ski Sports Wheelchair (Sunrise Medical) with outriggers (**Figure 16**).

Alternatively, systems like the Moto Knee 2 (**Figure 11**), the BioDapt Versa Foot 2 (**Figure 17**), and the Crossover G3 Infinity knee (**Figure 9**) allow transfemoral amputees to have resisted knee flexion beyond 60° when in a skiing position. This additional dampening

Chapter 50: Adaptive Lower Limb Prostheses for Sports and Recreation

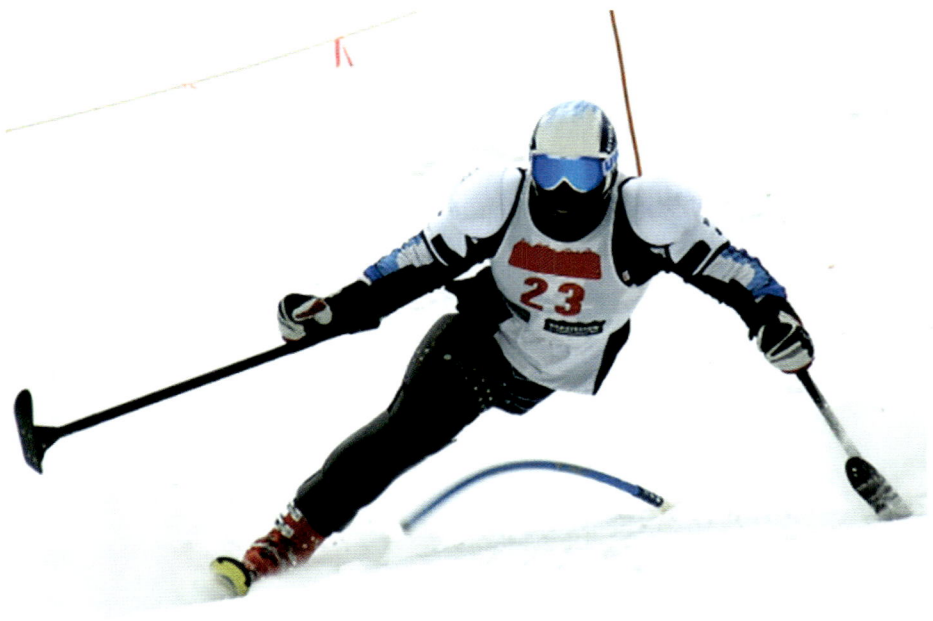

FIGURE 15 Photograph of an amputee participating in downhill skiing without the use of a prosthetic limb. The skier uses his sound-side leg and ski poles with outriggers. (Courtesy of MikeDotta/Shutterstock.com.)

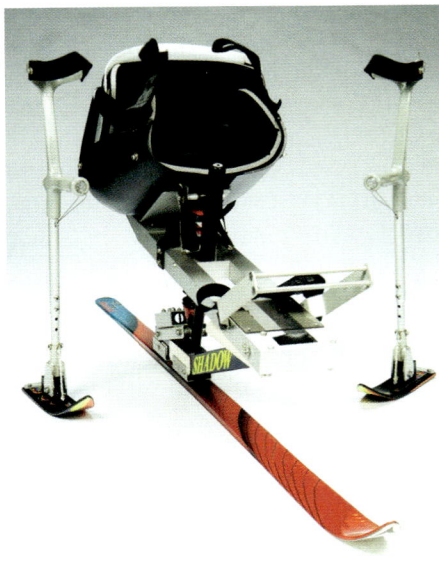

FIGURE 16 Photograph of the Shadow Mono-Ski Sports Wheelchair (Sunrise Medical) with handheld guide skis. (© Science Museum Group. https://collection.sciencemuseumgroup.org.uk/objects/co410448/shadow-mono-ski-sports-wheelchair-england-1993-1995-wheelchair. Accessed June 26, 2022.)

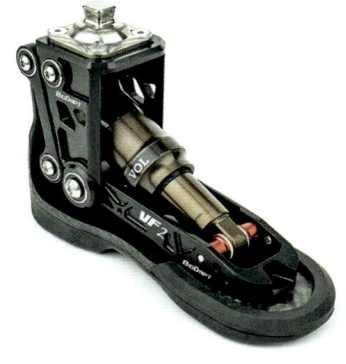

FIGURE 17 Photograph of the Versa Foot 2 (BioDapt). This foot has a shock absorber that controls toe pressure and ankle resistance. (Courtesy of BioDapt, St. Cloud, MN.)

within the knee component allows impact and shock absorption during jumping or high-speed skiing over rough terrain. A ski-specific prosthetic foot has been developed that attaches directly to the ski, thus making a ski boot unnecessary, like the Ottobock ProCarve system (**Figure 14**).

Hybrid Recreational Prostheses

In sporting events, such as Paralympic-level soccer and swimming, prosthesis use is not allowed and soccer players use forearm crutches (**Figure 18**). Some sport activities for amputee athletes do not require a sport-specific prosthesis and may be performed using a conventional prosthesis. These include golf, tennis, baseball, basketball, and soccer. Although specialized prostheses are not required for these activities, certain components can be added to a conventional prosthesis to enhance its use in recreational pursuits. When fitting an athlete with a hybrid or dual-function prosthesis, the treating prosthetist should consider vertical shock absorption properties, linear rotation, and multiaxial movements of the components in relationship to the chosen sport.

Alternatively, a combination shock damper and rotation adaptor can be used to reduce both the torque and the shear forces that act on a residual limb like the Fillauer Durashock (**Figure 19**). This type of device allows the prosthetist to customize the components to the needs of the individual athlete based on their functional impact level and weight.

Various suspension options are available to achieve maximum joint range of motion without compromising suspension when hybrid prostheses are used. A secondary suspension method can be used for athletic pursuits. For example, a seal-in suspension method can be used for daily activities and a secondary locking suspension (**Figure 20**) can be added for sports participation. Because many insurance companies and healthcare organizations do not cover the cost of activity-specific prostheses for sports, a hybrid prosthesis may be a viable option for an active amputee who wants to participate in sports.

Athletic Assessment and Training

Advancements in prosthetic technology should be concomitant with improvements in the athletic performance of an athlete with a lower limb amputation. Sport performance will be heavily influenced by the athlete's skills and abilities, including strength, coordination, flexibility, speed, and endurance. To achieve optimal performance, special training and conditioning are required.

Section 3: Lower Limb

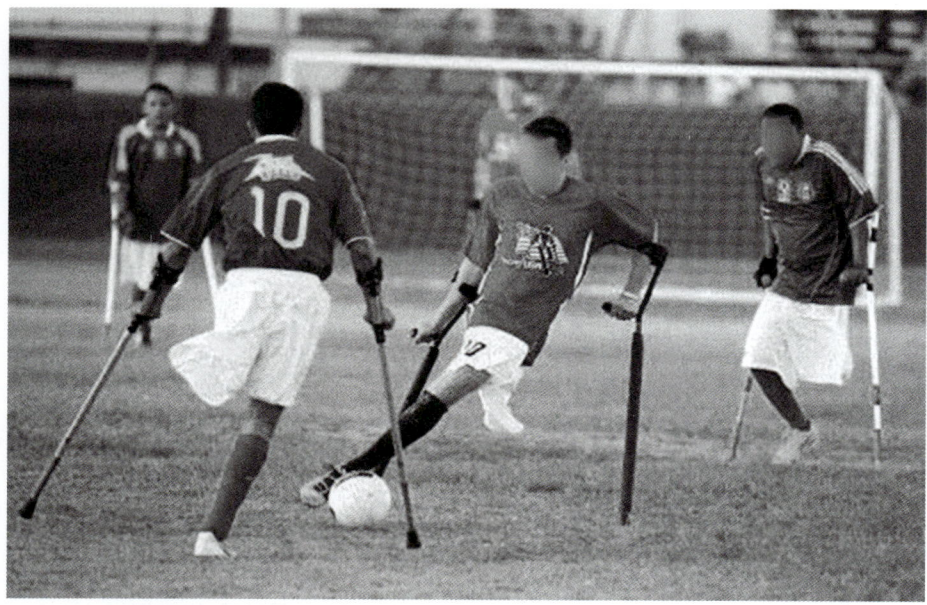

FIGURE 18 Photograph of athletes with lower limb amputations playing soccer. In some sporting events, prosthesis use is not allowed, and players use forearm crutches for mobility assistance. (Courtesy of Burcu Ergin/Shutterstock.)

Using such outcome measurements, a physical training program to improve physical fitness should be developed and incorporated during the rehabilitation process. Such a program should be standardized but flexible enough to adapt to the individual physical characteristics and wishes of the amputee athlete. Exercises to improve cardiopulmonary function, muscle strength, core stability, balance, coordination, and flexibility should be included in the program. The activities of interest and the training intensity should be tailored to the personal characteristics and abilities of the individual, with consideration of the amputation level and the length of the residual limb. It is preferable to present the amputee with a variety of sports opportunities early in the rehabilitation process to enhance rehabilitation and recovery time.

To assess the physical ability of an athlete with a lower limb amputation and create a record to track improvements and progression, the following outcome measures are recommended to be used as described in the CHAMP[34] outcomes tool. The Single-Limb Stance Test to measure balance, the Edgren Side Step Test to measure lateral speed and agility, the t-Test to measure four-directional agility, and the Illinois Agility Test to measure multidirectional running speed and agility.

SUMMARY

Lower limb amputees who actively participate in sports more than an average of two sessions per week may experience an increase in their overall health status as well as a decrease in the psychological burden associated with limb loss. Participation in any sport should be discussed with the rehabilitation team or at least with the treating prosthetist and physiotherapist.

The use of a prosthesis is not compulsory for participating in sports. Activities such as swimming or several wheelchair sports can be fully enjoyed without the use of a prosthesis. If a special sport's prosthesis is needed, the prosthetist is the best source of information and advice. Direct cooperation among all members of the rehabilitation team will ensure that an individual with a lower limb amputation achieves maximal benefits from sports participation.

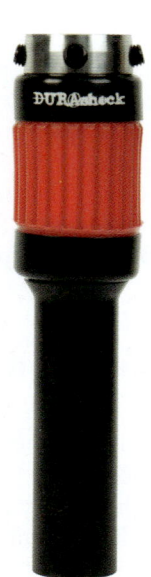

FIGURE 19 Photograph of the Durashock from Fillauer. This device combines a shock damper and rotation adaptor to reduce torque and shear forces that act on a residual limb. (Courtesy of Fillauer, Chattanooga, TN.)

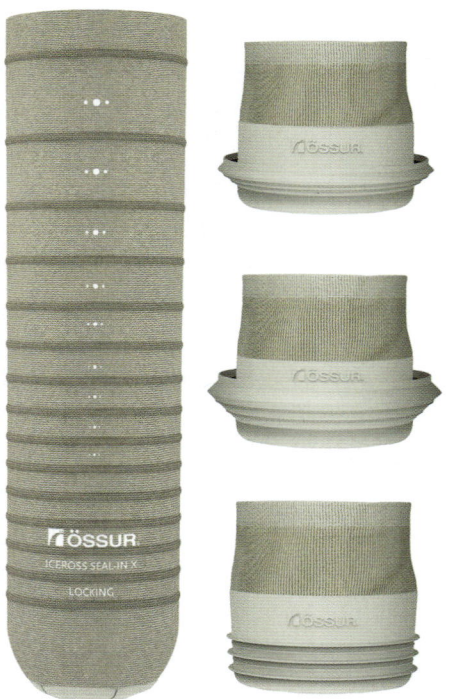

FIGURE 20 Photograph of the Iceross Seal-in X Locking liner system from Össur. This system combines seal-in suction and locking liner suspension. (Courtesy of Össur.)

References

1. George Eyser: Biography: SR/Olympic Sports. Available at: http://www.sports-reference.com/olympics/athletes/ey/george-eyser-1.html. Accessed April 13, 2015.
2. Waters RL, Mulroy S: The energy expenditure of normal and pathologic gait. *Gait Posture* 1999;9(3):207-231.

3. Waters RL, Perry J, Antonelli D, Hislop H: Energy cost of walking of amputees: The influence of level of amputation. *J Bone Joint Surg Am* 1976;58(1):42-46.
4. Sir Ludwig Guttmann: Biography. Available at: http://www.academic-refugees.org/downloads/Guttmann%20Bio.pdf. Accessed April 13, 2015.
5. Paralympic Games. Available at: http://en.wikipedia.org/wiki/Paralympic_Games#Categories. Accessed April 13, 2015.
6. Official Website of the Paralympic Movement. Italy 18-25 September 1960. Available at: http://www.paralympic.org/rome-1960. Accessed April 13, 2015.
7. Official Website of the Paralympic Movement. Rio 2016 Paralympic Games 7-18 September. Available at: https://www.paralympic.org/rio-2016. Accessed July 6, 2021.
8. Wikipedia Contributors: 2020 Summer Paralympics, in *Wikipedia, The Free Encyclopedia*. 2021. https://en.wikipedia.org/w/index.php?title=2020_Summer_Paralympics&oldid=1050650004. Accessed October 22, 2021.
9. Official Website of the Paralympic Movement. Introduction to IPC classifications. Available at: http://www.paralympic.org/classification. Accessed April 13, 2015.
10. Bragaru M, Dekker R, Geertzen JH, Dijkstra PU: Amputees and sports: A systematic review. *Sports Med* 2011;41(9):721-740.
11. Huonker M, Schmid A, Schmidt-Trucksass A, Grathwohl D, Keul J: Size and blood flow of central and peripheral arteries in highly trained able-bodied and disabled athletes. *J Appl Physiol* 2003;95(2):685-691.
12. Mastro JV, Burton AW, Rosendahl M: Attitudes of elite athletes with impairments toward one another: A hierarchy of preference. *Adapt Phys Activ Q* 1996;2(13):197-210.
13. Chin T, Sawamura S, Fujita H, et al: Physical fitness of lower limb amputees. *Am J Phys Med Rehabil* 2002;81(5):321-325.
14. Horgan O, MacLachlan M: Psychosocial adjustment to lower-limb amputation: A review. *Disabil Rehabil* 2004;26(14-15):837-850.
15. Kashani JH, Frank RG, Kashani SR, Wonderlich SA, Reid JC: Depression among amputees. *J Clin Psychiatry* 1983;44(7):256-258.
16. Pitetti KH, Snell PG, Stray-Gundersen J, Gottschalk FA: Aerobic training exercises for individuals who had amputation of the lower limb. *J Bone Joint Surg Am* 1987;69(6):914-921.
17. Chin T, Sawamura S, Fujita H, et al: Effect of endurance training program based on anaerobic threshold (AT) for lower limb amputees. *J Rehabil Res Dev* 2001;38(1):7-11.
18. Valliant PM, Bezzubyk I, Daley L, Asu ME: Psychological impact of sport on disabled athletes. *Psychol Rep* 1985;56(3):923-929.
19. Wetterhahn KA, Hanson C, Levy CE: Effect of participation in physical activity on body image of amputees. *Am J Phys Med Rehabil* 2002;81(3):194-201.
20. Tatar Y: Body image and its relationship with exercise and sports in Turkish lower-limb amputees who use prosthesis. *Sci Sports* 2010;25(6):312-317.
21. Sporner ML, Fitzgerald SG, Dicianno BE, et al: Psychosocial impact of participation in the national veterans wheelchair games and winter sports clinic. *Disabil Rehabil* 2009;31(5):410-418.
22. Rau B, Bonvin F, de Bie R: Short-term effect of physiotherapy rehabilitation on functional performance of lower limb amputees. *Prosthet Orthot Int* 2007;31(3):258-270.
23. Bragaru M, van Wilgen CP, Geertzen JH, Ruijs SG, Dijkstra PU, Dekker R: Barriers and facilitators of participation in sports: A qualitative study on Dutch individuals with lower limb amputation. *PLoS One* 2013;8(3):e59881.
24. Bragaru M: *Sports and Amputation*. GVO drukkers & vormgevers, 2013.
25. Nolan L: Carbon fibre prostheses and running in amputees: A review. *Foot Ankle Surg* 2008;14(3):125-129.
26. Bragaru M, Dekker R, Geertzen JH: Sport prostheses and prosthetic adaptations for the upper and lower limb amputees: An overview of peer reviewed literature. *Prosthet Orthot Int* 2012;36(3):290-296.
27. Podsiadlo D, Richardson S: The timed "Up & Go": A test of basic functional mobility for frail elderly persons. *J Am Geriatr Soc* 1991;39(2):142-148.
28. Borg G: Perceived exertion as an indicator of somatic stress. *Scand J Rehabil Med* 1970;2(2):92-98.
29. Hafner BJ, Halsne EG, Morgan SJ, et al: Functional outcomes in people with transtibial amputation using crossover and energy-storing prosthetic feet: A pilot study. *J Prosthet Orthot* 2018;30(2):90-100.
30. Tingleff H, Jensen L: A newly developed socket design for a knee disarticulation amputee who is an active athlete. *Prosthet Orthot Int* 2002;26(1):72-75.
31. Morgan SJ, McDonald CL, Halsne EG, et al: Laboratory and community-based health outcomes in people with transtibial amputation using crossover and energy-storing prosthetic feet: A randomized crossover trial. *PLoS One* 2018;13(2):e0189652.
32. Halsne EG, McDonald CL, Morgan SJ, Cheever SM, Hafner BJ: Assessment of low-and high-level task performance in people with transtibial amputation using crossover and energy-storing prosthetic feet: A pilot study. *Prosthet Orthot Int* 2018;42(6):583-591.
33. Burkett B, Smeathers J, Barker T: Optimising the trans-femoral prosthetic alignment for running, by lowering the knee joint. *Prosthet Orthot Int* 2001;25(3):210-219.
34. Gailey RS, Gaunaurd IA, Raya MA, et al: Development and reliability testing of the Comprehensive High-Level Activity Mobility Predictor (CHAMP) in male servicemembers with traumatic lower-limb loss. *J Rehabil Res Dev* 2013;50(7):905-918.

Outcome Measures in Lower Limb Prosthetics

CHAPTER 51

Brian Kaluf, CP, FAAOP • Sara J. Morgan, CPO, PhD

ABSTRACT

The administration, interpretation, and communication of clinical outcome measures have emerged as vital competencies for prosthetists and other healthcare clinicians. Several patient-reported and performance-based outcome measures have been designed for or tested with people who have lower limb loss and are deemed well-suited for clinical applications. It is helpful to consider the benefits of outcome measurement and to have useful tips for incorporating these measures into routine clinical practice.

Keywords: amputee; lower limb prosthetics; outcome measures; patient-reported outcome measure; performance-based outcome measure; psychometric property

Introduction

The use of standardized outcome measures has become increasingly important in the provision and management of prosthetic care. When used regularly, outcome measures can improve quality of care and help maximize the overall value of prosthetic rehabilitation. Consistent use of relevant outcome measures can help clinicians predict patient benefit from a prosthetic intervention, document patient improvement, and inform clinical decision-making.[1] Proper selection of high-quality outcome measures, appropriate training in their use, familiarity with their measurement properties, and development of strategies to standardize assessments are equally necessary steps if a practitioner aims to realize the benefits of a measurement program.[2] These steps ensure that routine administration of outcome measures is accompanied by correct interpretation of scores, meaningful discussions about outcomes with patients, family members, and healthcare clinicians, and documentation of clinical changes over time.[3]

It is important to define measurement terms and properties, describe examples of outcome measures that are well-suited to assessment of mobility, pain, and health-related quality of life in people with lower limb loss, and to discuss strategies for incorporating routine outcome measurement into a clinical setting. It is also important to focus on the clinical use of outcome measures, but this information may also be useful for the incorporation of standardized outcome measures in research settings.

Measurement Terms and Properties

Measurement Terms

Clinical measurement is defined as assigning numerals to variables to better understand, evaluate, or compare patients on a specific attribute.[4] Clinicians often measure variables that can be directly observed and are based on physical or physiological properties (eg, height, weight, or temperature). However, many important clinical variables are abstract and require shared definitions and indirect forms of measurement to understand a patient's current state and change over time.[4] These abstract variables (eg, mobility, pain, quality of life) are called constructs, and make up many of the clinical outcomes that are important to patients with limb loss and their practitioners.

Outcome measures are standardized instruments that are developed to quantify constructs of interest. Outcome measures are usually developed for the purposes of discrimination, evaluation, or prediction[4] and can be categorized as patient-reported outcome measures or performance-based

---

Brian Kaluf or an immediate family member serves as a paid consultant to or is an employee of Ability Prosthetics and Orthotics; has stock or stock options held in Ability Prosthetics and Orthotics; has received research or institutional support from Ottobock and Parker Hannifin; and serves as a board member, owner, officer, or committee member of American Academy of Orthotists and Prosthetists. Dr. Morgan or an immediate family member serves as a board member, owner, officer, or committee member of American Academy of Orthotists and Prosthetists.

This chapter is adapted from Stevens PM: Outcome measures in lower limb prosthetics, in Krajbich JI, Pinzur MS, Potter BK, Stevens PM, eds: *Atlas of Amputations and Limb Deficiencies: Surgical, Prosthetic, and Rehabilitation Principles,* ed 4. American Academy of Orthopaedic Surgeons, 2016, pp 645-662.

outcome measures. Patient-reported outcome measures are questionnaires completed by a patient or their caregiver (proxy-reported outcome measures). Patient-reported outcome measures assess a patient's perspective or experience outside the controlled clinical environment. Performance-based outcome measures are assessed by a clinical professional based on observations of patients completing a task or activity, and the scores are not influenced by patient perspectives.[5,6] Performance-based outcome measures are typically administered in a clinical environment, which may not reflect the variety of settings encountered in a patient's daily life. Patient-reported and performance-based outcome measures provide unique and complementary information about a patient's health outcomes, and thus both are recommended for clinical use.

Measurement Properties

An understanding of psychometric properties, such as validity, reliability, and responsiveness to change, is useful to guide the selection of outcome measures.[7] Evidence of a measure's psychometric properties can help clinicians distinguish between measures that are more or less suitable for assessment of a specific patient cohort, treatment, or clinical circumstance.[1,8,9] Validity, reliability, and responsiveness are frequently reported in outcome measurement research and can be examined with statistical methods.[9]

Validity is the extent to which a measure assesses the construct of interest.[4,7,9] A measure's validity can be described as evidence of content validity, criterion validity, and construct validity.[9] Evidence of content validity demonstrates that items within a measure adequately assess all aspects of the construct of interest, and is often based on expert opinion, earlier literature, and other research activities that guided the development of the measure. Evidence of criterion validity demonstrates a relationship between a measure's score and scores on a benchmark measure.[4,9] Similarly, evidence of construct validity demonstrates that a measure's scores correlate with those of another measure of the same construct (convergent validity) and are unrelated to scores from a measure of a different construct (discriminant validity). Evidence of construct validity can also be demonstrated with differences in scores across diverse patient groups (known groups validity).[9] Evidence of validity is often reported in terms of strength of association using correlation coefficients (eg, Pearson product-moment coefficient [r], Spearman rho [ρ]), and with statistical comparison tests for known groups validity.[4] There are no statistical indexes for content validity.[4]

Reliability is the extent to which scores from an outcome measure are consistent and free from error.[4] When a measure is sufficiently reliable, differences between scores can be attributed to real differences in the construct rather than measurement error or noise.[7,9] A measure's reliability can be described as test–retest reliability, rater reliability, and internal consistency.[9] Test–retest reliability is the consistency of scores across timepoints, and rater reliability is consistency of scores across (interrater) or within (intrarater) observers. Intraclass correlation coefficients or kappa statistics are calculated to assess evidence of test–retest and rater reliability, depending on the type of data.[3,4,9] Clinical measures are often considered sufficiently reliable if reliability coefficients are 0.8 or higher,[4] though some suggest that reliability coefficients of 0.9 or higher are needed for the assessment of individual patients over time.[9] Internal consistency is the extent to which items within a measure are related. Cronbach's alpha (α) is used to evaluate internal consistency, and values of 0.7 to 0.9 are considered to be strong.[4]

Responsiveness is the extent to which a measure can detect a change that is clinically important.[7,9] Minimal detectable change (MDC) and minimal clinically important difference (MCID) are estimated values in the units of a particular measure that help clinicians interpret changes in an individual's scores over time. MDC represents the smallest change that exceeds measurement error and can be attributed to a real change in the construct of interest.[4] MDC is related to the reliability of the outcome measure; measures with high reliability have small estimates of MDC. MDC estimates are commonly reported at 90% or 95% confidence intervals (MDC90 and MDC95, respectively).[4,10] MCID represents the minimal change in scores that represents a true and meaningful improvement or worsening in the construct of interest.[4] Estimates of MDC and MCID aid in interpretation of change over time, and facilitate clinical decision-making based on changes in scores.

Ceiling and floor effects are an important consideration when choosing an outcome measure. Measures with ceiling effects are unable to detect meaningful changes in the construct at the highest extremes of the score, and conversely, measures with floor effects are unable to detect changes at the lowest extremes.[3,9,11] These effects are examined by plotting the frequency of scores and examining the shape of the distribution.[10,12] If 15% or more of the scores are at one extreme of the scale, the measure is likely exhibiting a ceiling or floor effect.[13]

Another important concept in measurement is the availability of normative or reference data and criterion scores. Scores on an outcome measure may be challenging to interpret without information about scores that are typical for the general population, or for people who have similar clinical characteristics to the patient being measured. Normative or reference data are data collected from a large sample that provide typical scores as well as information about the spread of data. Normative scores can help clinicians and patients understand what a score means, and how a patient's score is related to scores within a general or representative group. Criterion scores identify a level of the construct that is clinically meaningful and might indicate that the patient is at higher or lower risk for a clinical event (eg, falls).[4]

An outcome measure can never be assumed to be free from error or perfectly accurate, but evidence of acceptable reliability, validity, and responsiveness can increase a clinician's confidence that the measure will provide stable scores and meaningful information throughout a patient's course of care.[3,4,9] It is important to note that the measurement properties of existing outcome measures are often continually researched and refined, and thus there may be a range of values available for each measure under consideration.[3] Comparisons of relative measurement properties between measures can inform selection of outcome measures best-suited for evaluating and guiding clinical decisions for individuals and small patient populations.[3,10]

Mobility, Physical Function, and Balance Measures

Amputee Mobility Predictor (AMP)

The Amputee Mobility Predictor AMP is a performance-based outcome measure developed specifically for individuals with lower limb loss to assess functional capabilities and mobility.[14] It rates performance in 21 tasks involving sitting balance, transfers, standing balance, gait, stair ascent and descent, and use of an assistive device. The AMP can be administered without a prosthesis (AMPnoPRO) or with a prosthesis (AMPPRO). Examples of these tasks are depicted in **Figure 1**. Scores on the AMPnoPRO range from 0 to 43 points, and scores on the AMPPRO range from 0 to 47 points. The AMP has demonstrated excellent interrater and intrarater reliability[14] and a reported MDC90 of 3.4 points.[10] Concurrent validity was assessed by comparing AMPPRO and AMPnoPRO scores with the Amputee Activity Scale and the Six-Minute Walk Test (6mWT).[14] A known groups method was used to establish evidence of construct validity, with AMP scores distinguishing between Medicare Functional Classification Level (MFCL) groups.[14] The MFCL (ie, K-levels) provides guidelines for clinicians to categorize patients into functional levels ranging from K0 through K4 based on rehabilitation potential and ambulatory ability.[15] A recent study found evidence of predictive validity of the AMPnoPRO before initial fitting with future performance on the Two Minute Walk Test (2mWT), the Timed Up and Go (TUG), and MFCL assignment at the end of prosthetic rehabilitation.[16] Reference data are included in the initial article that described the development of the measure,[14] as well as other studies.[17,18]

The AMP was developed to help predict and discriminate between MFCL.[14] The relationship of the AMP score with the MFCL and the 6mWT is strong,[14] and knowledge of AMP score in combination with other patient-related factors (ie, age, amputation level, comorbidities, ability to balance on one leg, and manual muscle testing) can predict the MFCL and potential to ambulate with a prosthesis. However, the AMP developers have cautioned that no clear cut-off scores exist, and AMP scores were overlapping when subjects were grouped based on professional-rated MFCL.[14] Other authors have cautioned against applying AMP cut-off scores for assigning MFCL without assessing other factors.[16,19] Because the initial study evaluated only current prosthesis users, it may not be generalizable to persons with lower limb loss who are still recovering and undergoing rehabilitation following surgery.[11]

Timed Walk Tests (TWTs)

TWTs encompass a variety of performance-based outcome measures that assess readiness to ambulate and the capacity for exercise.[14,20] Initially introduced as the Twelve-Minute Walk Test, more frequently reported TWTs for individuals with lower limb loss are shorter in duration (ie, 2mWT and 6mWT). Required equipment includes a stopwatch and a measuring tape or distance measuring wheel. A TWT should be administered in a quiet area such as a hallway, the walking speed is stipulated by the rater with standardized verbal instructions, the rater should walk behind the patient, and rest should be permitted during the test, if needed[11,21,22] (**Figure 2**). When the test is administered in a hallway, setting up cones 30 m apart and measuring the distance (to the nearest 0.10 m) from the last cone to where the patient stops

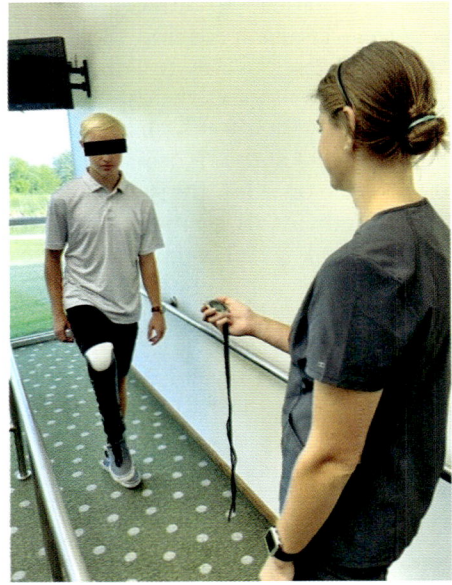

FIGURE 1 Clinical photograph of Amputee Mobility Predictor (AMP) item # 8 single limb standing balance for 30 seconds. (Reproduced with permission from Umbrell C: *Meaningful Measures*. O&P Almanac. 2021, vol 70, No. 7, p 22. https://issuu.com/americanoandp/docs/august_2021_issue/s/13248391.)

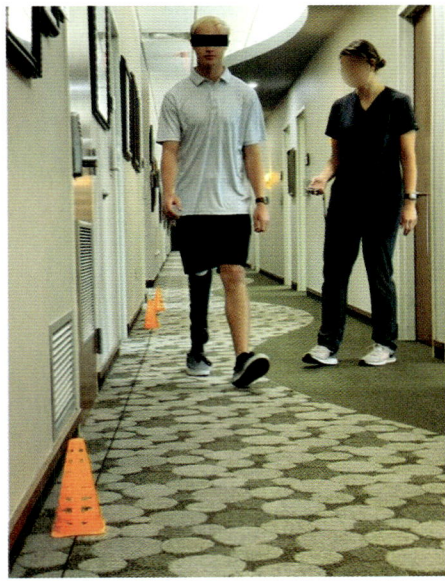

FIGURE 2 Clinical photograph of 10-Meter Walk Test (10mWT) setup with cones for acceleration and deceleration zones. (Reproduced with permission from Umbrell C: *Meaningful Measures*. O&P Almanac. 2021, vol 70, No. 7, p 22. https://issuu.com/americanoandp/docs/august_2021_issue/s/13248391.)

can facilitate scoring of the measure.[22] Shorter standardized walking courses are permitted, but they negatively influence distance travelled and reference values are no longer applicable. The score is reported as distance traveled (m), or average walking speed (m/s) can be calculated.[21]

Six-Minute Walk Test (6mWT)
Typically viewed as a benchmark for assessing walking ability, the 6mWT instructs patients to walk as far as possible in 6 minutes. The 6mWT scores have been shown to differentiate amputation levels[23] as well as MFCL groups (K0–K4).[14] Strong evidence of convergent validity with the Timed Up and Go (TUG) test also has been demonstrated.[24] Evidence of the excellent reliability of the 6mWT has been established in persons with lower limb loss,[23,24] with a reported MDC90 of 45 m.[10] Reference average scores for the different MFCL groups have been reported.[14] In individuals with lower limb loss, a large amount of the variance found in the 6mWT was predicted by age, muscle strength, balance, time since amputation, cause of amputation, and level of amputation.[25] A walking distance of 191 m at the time of discharge from rehabilitation was found to be predictive of sustained prosthesis use 12 months after discharge.[26] While not established separately for persons with lower limb loss, the cut-off for community ambulation is reported as 0.8 m/s[27] or 300 m on the 6mWT,[28,29] and an accepted threshold for a substantial change in walking speed is 0.1 m/s or 50 m on the 6mWT.[30]

Two-Minute Walk Test (2mWT)
A 2mWT has been recommended because some patients with lower limb loss have difficulty walking for 6 minutes, and shorter tests have less administrator burden.[14,20,21] However, if it is important to assess energy cost, heart rate, and oxygen consumption, the 6mWT is preferable to allow individuals with a lower limb loss to reestablish homeostasis while walking.[23] The 2mWT has demonstrated excellent interrater and intrarater reliability with a reported MDC90 of 34.3 m.[10,20]

It was found to have adequate convergent validity with the Houghton Scale and the physical functional scale of the Medical Outcomes Study 36-Item Short Form.[21] The 2mWT has been found to be responsive, with individuals showing an increase in walking distance after rehabilitation.[21] It has also been found to be a significant predictor of ability to walk with a prosthesis, along with the Functional Reach Test.[12] Relevant 2mWT reference values for various subgroups of persons with lower limb loss have been reported.[31]

Ten-Meter Walk Test (10mWT)
The 10mWT measures the time it takes to ambulate over a fixed 10-m walkway, with space to speed up and slow down within the 10 m. The convergent validity of the 10mWT is supported through evidence of correlation with the Barthel Index, Frenchay Activities Index, and Volpicelli Mobility Scale.[32] The distance of 10 m corresponds to the average length of a street crosswalk and represents a real-world environmental situation. In clinical practice, the 10mWT can be administered by asking a patient to walk at a self-selected walking speed and then again at their fastest possible walking speed. This method assesses the capability of individuals with lower limb loss to vary their walking speed. Normative walking speeds on the 10mWT for able-bodied individuals grouped by decade of life offer a useful comparison.[33]

Prosthetic Limb User Survey of Mobility (PLUS-M)
The PLUS-M is a patient-reported outcome measure that assesses a user's perceived degree of difficulty to carry out common mobility-related activities. The PLUS-M is an item bank developed with Item Response Theory, and thus can be administered using fixed-length short forms (12-item short form, 7-item short form) or by Computer Adaptive Testing[34] (**Figure 3**). PLUS-M instruments are scored using a T-score, with a mean of 50 representing the average population score and an SD of 10 points above and below that mean;

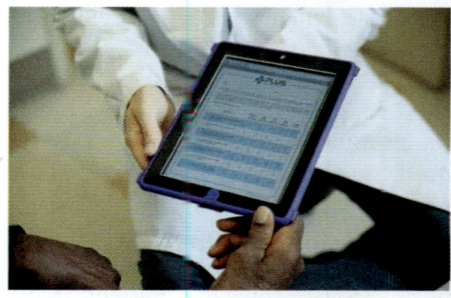

FIGURE 3 Photograph of Prosthetic Limb User Survey of Mobility (PLUS-M™) administration via tablet (iPad). (Courtesy of Brian Hafner, PhD.)

PLUS-M T-scores range from 17.5 to 76.6 points.[34]

The PLUS-M has evidence of good content validity[35,36] and evidence of convergent validity with the AMP, TUG, Prosthesis Evaluation Questionnaire Mobility Subscale (PEQ-MS), Activities-specific Balance Confidence Scale (ABC), and the Patient-Reported Outcomes Measurement Information System Physical Function (PROMIS-PF).[17] Evidence of known groups validity was demonstrated with statistically different scores between MFCL levels.[17] All PLUS-M instruments have demonstrated excellent test–retest reliability, suggesting suitability for use in individual-level comparisons with a reported MDC90 for the 12-item short form of 4.5 points.[37] The PLUS-M instrument user guide provides reference data for patients with lower limb loss with different amputation levels, etiologies, and ages to inform interpretation of scores.[34] This original reference data have since been expanded upon, with a recent publication identifying reference scores across more discrete subgroups of seven age ranges and four amputation etiologies.[38]

Timed Up and Go (TUG)
The TUG test is a performance-based outcome measure designed to assess basic functional mobility in elderly individuals,[39] but has subsequently been tested with people who have lower limb loss.[40] The TUG test takes 3 minutes to administer and requires a stopwatch and a standard chair (seat

height, 46 cm; arm height, 67 cm). The rater starts the stopwatch when they say "go." The patient rises from the chair, then walks 3 m, turns around, returns to the chair, and sits down.[40] The timing ends when the patient is seated. Minor variations in set up, including use of a mark on the ground or a cone as well as the verbal instructions provided to the patient, have been shown to affect TUG times.[41]

The TUG test is said to represent daily function better than other walking tests because it includes common mobility tasks (ie, standing up, walking short distances, turning, and sitting down).[42] The TUG test has demonstrated excellent interrater and intrarater reliability, with a reported MDC90 of 3.6 s.[10,40] Criterion validity has not been assessed because there is no established benchmark for functional mobility;[40] however, the TUG has been used frequently as the benchmark to establish the validity of other outcome measures. Evidence of adequate concurrent validity was established by examining relationships with the Groningen Activity Restriction Scale and the physical and mental subscales of the Sickness Impact Profile and the 68-item Sickness Impact Profile.[40]

The Component TUG is a variation on the TUG that records the time required to complete discrete sections of the TUG.[43] The known groups method has been used to provide evidence that the Component TUG discriminates scores between persons with transtibial and transfemoral limb loss.[43]

The TUG test has been recommended for routine clinical use and research.[8,11,44] Average TUG test times in persons with lower limb loss have been studied to differentiate multiple-time fallers (those reporting two or more falls in the past 6 months)[45] and examine physical, mental, and social factors that affect functional mobility.[46] A fall-risk cut-off score for identifying patients at risk of multiple falls was found to be 19 s.[45] Patient age and ability to balance on one leg were found to predict TUG test scores in 42% of people with lower limb loss.[46]

Activities-Specific Balance Confidence (ABC)

The ABC scale measures a patient's self-rated confidence that they will not fall in 16 situation-specific activities.[47] It was originally developed to assess fall risk in elderly individuals, and it has been evaluated for use with persons with lower limb loss.[48] The original ABC scores were averaged across items and ranged from 0 to 100, with 0 representing no confidence and 100 representing complete confidence. A revised ABC scale with five response options has been developed with Rasch analysis and has demonstrated better measurement properties.[49] Scores on the revised ABC scale range from 0 to 4. Construct validity for the ABC was demonstrated during its development by a panel of experts and patients.[47] The ABC has evidence of concurrent validity with the 2mWT and the TUG test,[48] and evidence of construct validity was evidenced through statistical differences between known groups separated by amputation cause, mobility device use (cane, crutches, or walker), and reported walking ability.[48] The ABC scale has demonstrated excellent intrarater reliability, internal consistency, and test–retest reliability with persons with lower limb loss[37,48] with an MDC90 of 0.49 points for the revised five-level response version.[37] Reference data for the original ABC scale are available for various groups based on the cause of the amputation, the assistive device used, and the ability to perform automatic stepping. Reference data from the revised five-level response version have also been presented.[50] Cut-off scores for the original ABC scale are reported for elderly able-bodied adults with low and moderate mobility and those who are physically active, as well as for fall risk in elderly individuals (ABC fall-risk cut-off = 67).[51,52]

Other Measures

Other relevant outcome measures that address mobility, physical function, or balance, include Amputee Single Item Mobility Measure (AMPSIMM),[53] Berg Balance Scale (BSS),[54] Comprehensive High-level Activity Mobility Predictor (CHAMP),[55] Four Square Step Test (FSST),[56] Houghton Scale,[57] L-test,[22] Narrowing Beam Walking Test (NBWT),[58] and Five Times Sit-to-Stand (5× STS).[59]

Pain and Comfort Measures

Socket Comfort Score (SCS)

The SCS is a patient-reported outcome measure of current perceived comfort in a prosthetic socket.[60] The SCS was introduced as a single-item 11-point scale, with 0 representing the most uncomfortable socket fit imaginable and 10 representing the most comfortable socket fit imaginable.[60] Evidence was found of interrater reliability between prosthetists and physicians, criterion-related validity, and sensitivity to change with socket modification.[60] The minimal detectable change has been measured as an MDC90 of 2.7 points.[37]

An Expanded Socket Comfort Score has been introduced that includes items that ask patients to rate their current, best, worst, and average socket comfort over a 7-day period.[61] The Expanded Socket Comfort Score may provide additional useful information about the variability of socket comfort ratings within or between days. This instrument requires little administrative burden but provides high clinical utility, given the substantial amount of time spent achieving and maintaining an acceptable prosthetic socket interface fit on the residual limb.

Numerical Pain Rating Scale (NRS-11)

The NRS-11 asks patients to rate the intensity of their pain, with 0 representing no pain and 10 representing the worst pain imaginable.[62] Psychometric properties of the NRS-11 have not been directly assessed in persons with lower limb loss. However, NRS-11 is considered appropriate for use in clinical practice because of evidence of validity and reliability across a variety of clinical populations.[63]

Comprehensive Lower-Limb Amputee Socket Survey CLASS

The CLASS is a patient-reported outcome measure that measures prosthetic socket interfaces based on stability, suspension, comfort, and appearance.[64] Each of these determinants of socket fit is rated for the activities of sitting, standing, walking, and ascending/descending stairs. Evidence of internal consistency and content validity have been described.[64]

HRQOL and Multidomain Measures

PROMIS-29

The Patient-Reported Outcomes Measurement Information System (PROMIS) is a collection of patient-reported outcome measures for assessment of a wide variety of health-related constructs that are designed for use across clinical cohorts. PROMIS instruments can be administered as short forms of various lengths or with Computer Adaptive Testing administration. PROMIS-29 is a 29-item short-form that includes brief assessments for eight PROMIS health-related quality of life domains: physical function, fatigue, pain interference, pain intensity, depressive symptoms, anxiety, ability to participate in social roles and activities, and sleep disturbance.[65] Reliability in patients with lower limb loss has been evaluated.[17,37] Reference data for PROMIS-29 have been published for persons with lower limb loss, and have been compared with normative scores from the general population.[66]

Orthotics Prosthetics User Survey (OPUS)

The OPUS was developed to assess functional status, quality of life, and satisfaction with orthotic and prosthetic devices.[67] It consists of the following five indexes (modules) to be administered together or separately: the lower extremity functional scale, the upper extremity functional scale, client satisfaction with device, client satisfaction with service, and health-related quality of life. The OPUS possesses face validity and the developers suggest that construct validity is indicated by OPUS items ranging from easy to difficult to accomplish.[67,68] Evidence of the reliability of the OPUS was demonstrated with internal consistency and test–retest reliability.[10,67] A recent research study demonstrated the challenges and benefits of integrating the OPUS as a clinical management tool in clinical practices.[69] By analyzing the OPUS results, the authors were able to recommend improvements to the overall quality of care by focusing on patient comfort and skin care.

Prosthesis Evaluation Questionnaire (PEQ)

The PEQ is a patient-reported outcome measure designed to evaluate the prosthesis and the prosthesis-related quality of life.[70] The original subscales covered function (usefulness, residual limb health, appearance, and sounds), mobility (ambulation and transfers), psychosocial factors (perceived responses, frustration, and social burden), and a well-being scale.[70]

The PEQ was found to have evidence of construct validity and concurrent validity with SF-36[70] and high internal consistency and test–retest reliability.[10,70] Although it was comprehensive and informative, the entire PEQ consisted of 82 items and the visual analog scale was burdensome to administer. Shorter subscales of the PEQ were designed, with conversion of the visual analog scale to a five-level ordered response (eg, PEQ–mobility subscale [PEQ–MS12/5] for assessing a perceived potential for mobility).[71]

EuroQol 5 Dimension 5 Level (EQ5D5L)

The EQ5D5L is a patient-reported outcome measure that assesses HRQoL on five domains: mobility, self-care, usual activities, pain/discomfort, and anxiety/depression.[72] Additionally, it includes a single-item global health visual analog scale rating. The psychometric properties of this instrument have not yet been examined for persons with lower limb loss, but the EQ5D5L has been used in healthcare economic research into prosthetic interventions and to calculate the Quality-Adjusted Life Years.[73]

Other relevant outcome measures that address HRQOL include the Medical Outcomes Short Form 36 (SF-36)[10,74] and Q-TFA.[75]

Integration of Outcome Measures in Clinical Practice

Routine collection of outcome measures can offer multiple benefits in clinical practice. For the individual practitioner, regular use of outcome measures reinforces ethical practice, increases professional accountability, and facilitates informed clinical decision-making based on standardized assessments of a patient's current condition and changes over time.[8,11,42] At the level of the individual patient, outcome measures have been suggested for use in improving evaluation, measuring treatment effects, estimating prognosis, targeting functional needs, and selecting appropriate prosthetic components.[5,42] If outcome measures are integrated into clinical practice and consistently documented across large patient populations, the aggregated data will be valuable for benchmarking, continuous quality improvement, improving clinical processes, and furthering our knowledge about the real-world effectiveness of prosthetic interventions.

Despite these benefits, integration of routine outcome measurement into prosthetics practice is difficult for many practitioners. Guidance on which outcome measures to use, when to administer outcome measures, and how to increase the efficiency of outcomes measurement can be useful when initiating a measurement plan within a clinical practice.

Choosing an Outcome Measure

Many performance-based and patient-reported outcome measures are well-suited for clinical assessment of people who use prosthetic limbs. Because there is no single outcome measure that is best for all patients or all clinical contexts, it can be useful to select a few measures that provide complementary information about a patient's health status.[2] First, identify health-related constructs that are meaningful to your clinical practice. Consider constructs that are directly affected by prosthetic or rehabilitation interventions that you provide, as well as holistic constructs that might be important to your patients (eg, patient-centric and health-related quality of life). Next, identify outcome measures that assess the constructs of interest, and assess their relative measurement properties (eg, validity, reliability). Desirable outcome measures have acceptable measurement properties, have been evaluated in research samples that are similar to your clinical cohort, and have reference data available to facilitate interpretation. Consider a combination of performance-based and patient-reported outcome measures when possible to evaluate constructs like mobility or balance based on clinical observation and patient perception.

Timing of Outcome Measure Administration

The choice of when to administer outcome measures requires thought and consideration of the purpose for each outcome measure used. Some outcome measures are used to assess the effect of clinical interventions (eg, prosthetic limbs or components). These outcome measures should be administered before the intervention and within a reasonable window following the intervention. Other outcome measures are meant to assess a patient's current status, track their status over time, and compare to reference data. These outcome measures can be assessed at regular intervals (eg, biannually or annually). Some outcome measures are used to assess a construct that might be continually changing from day-to-day (eg, socket comfort). If brief, these outcome measures can be assessed at each appointment to ensure that potential problems are being identified and addressed in a timely manner. A sample measurement plan is provided in **Table 1**.

TABLE 1 Sample Measurement Plan for Patients Who Use Lower Limb Prostheses

Measure	Construct	Timepoint for Measurement			
		All Appointments	Before Delivery	Following Delivery	Biannually
Socket Comfort Score	Socket comfort	X	—	—	—
Amputee Mobility Predictor (AMP)	Mobility (performance)	—	X	X	—
Prosthetic Limb User's Survey of Mobility (PLUS-M)	Mobility (patient-reported)	—	X	X	X
PROMIS-29	Health-related quality of life	—	—	—	X

Promoting Efficiency in Clinical Outcome Measurement

The integration of outcome measurement into a clinical appointment can be challenging given the limited amount of time available. Strategies to improve the efficiency of clinical outcome measurement are thus a key component in routine outcomes measurement. For example, patients may be able to complete patient-reported outcome measures before the clinical appointment, either in the waiting room or online. Performance-based outcome measures often require some set-up before administration. To reduce the time burden on the practitioner, a station or multiple stations can be set up in advance with equipment stored nearby to minimize or eliminate the time required for set-up. Measurement forms for outcome measures used routinely can be printed in advance or set up for collection via electronic tablet to further facilitate measurement. And finally, practicing in advance to ensure proficiency and consistency in data collection, scoring, and interpretation can improve efficiency in outcomes measurement.

SUMMARY

Many of the patient-reported and performance-based outcome measures reviewed have ample evidence of psychometric properties and are recommended for assessing patients with lower limb loss. The information on psychometric properties and the guidance for evaluating, selecting, and adopting outcome measures can facilitate integration into clinical care. The current healthcare environment demands—and useful outcome measures—allow healthcare professionals to measure important aspects of prosthetic rehabilitation and provide results to guide clinical decision-making. Routine use of outcome measures can raise the level of clinical outcome data collected for improved clinical decisions and advancing research evidence.

References

1. Roach KE: Measurement of health outcomes: Reliability, validity and responsiveness. *J Prosthet Orthot* 2006;18:P8-P12.
2. Finch E, Brooks D, Stratford PW, Mayo NE: Physical rehabilitation outcome measures: A guide to enhanced clinical decision making. *Physiotherapy Canada* 2003;55:53-54.
3. Jerosch-Herold C: An evidence-based approach to choosing outcome measures: A checklist for the critical appraisal of validity, reliability and responsiveness studies. *Br J Occup Ther* 2005;68:347-353.
4. Portney LG: *Foundations of Clinical Research: Applications to Evidence-Based Practice*. FA Davis, 2020.
5. Robinson C, Fatone S: You've heard about outcome measures, so how do you use them? Integrating clinically relevant outcome measures in orthotic management of stroke. *Prosthet Orthot Int* 2013;37:30-42.

6. Gailey RS: Predictive outcome measures versus functional outcome measures in the lower limb amputee. *J Prosthet Orthot* 2006;18:P51-P60.
7. Miller LA, McCay JA: Summary and conclusions from the academy's sixth state-of-the-science conference on lower limb prosthetic outcome measures. *J Prosthet Orthot* 2006;18:P2-P7.
8. Condie E, Scott H, Treweek S: Lower limb prosthetic outcome measures: A review of the literature 1995 to 2005. *J Prosthet Orthot* 2006;18:P13-P45.
9. Fitzpatrick R, Davey C, Buxton MJ, Jones DR: Evaluating patient-based outcome measures for use in clinical trials. *Health Technol Assess* 1998;2(14):i-iv, 1-74.
10. Resnik L, Borgia M: Reliability of outcome measures for people with lower-limb amputations: Distinguishing true change from statistical error. *Phys Ther* 2011;91:555-565.
11. Deathe AB, Wolfe DL, Devlin M, Hebert JS, Miller WC, Pallaveshi L: Selection of outcome measures in lower extremity amputation rehabilitation: ICF activities. *Disabil Rehabil* 2009;31:1455-1473.
12. Gremeaux V, Damak S, Troisgros O, et al: Selecting a test for the clinical assessment of balance and walking capacity at the definitive fitting state after unilateral amputation: A comparative study. *Prosthet Orthot Int* 2012;36:415-422.
13. Terwee CB, Bot SD, de Boer MR, et al: Quality criteria were proposed for measurement properties of health status questionnaires. *J Clin Epidemiol* 2007;60:34-42.
14. Gailey RS, Roach KE, Applegate EB, et al: The amputee mobility predictor: An instrument to assess determinants of the lower-limb amputee's ability to ambulate. *Arch Phys Med Rehabil* 2002;83:613-627.
15. Lower limb prostheses. 2021. Available at: https://www.cms.gov/medicare-coverage-database/view/lcd.aspx?LCDId=33787&ContrID=140. Accessed December 9, 2021.
16. Spaan MH, Vrieling AH, van de Berg P, Dijkstra PU, van Keeken HG: Predicting mobility outcome in lower limb amputees with motor ability tests used in early rehabilitation. *Prosthet Orthot Int* 2017;41:171-177.
17. Hafner BJ, Gaunaurd IA, Morgan SJ, Amtmann D, Salem R, Gailey RS: Construct validity of the Prosthetic Limb Users Survey of Mobility (PLUS-M) in adults with lower limb amputation. *Arch Phys Med Rehabil* 2017;98:277-285.
18. Kaluf B: Evaluation of mobility in persons with limb loss using the amputee mobility predictor and the prosthesis evaluation questionnaire–mobility subscale: A six-month retrospective chart review. *Prosthet Orthot* 2014;26:70-76.
19. Dillon MP, Major MJ, Kaluf B, Balasanov Y, Fatone S: Predict the Medicare functional classification level (K-level) using the Amputee Mobility Predictor in people with unilateral transfemoral and transtibial amputation: A pilot study. *Prosthet Orthot Int* 2018;42:191-197.
20. Brooks D, Hunter JP, Parsons J, Livsey E, Quirt J, Devlin M: Reliability of the two-minute walk test in individuals with transtibial amputation. *Arch Phys Med Rehabil* 2002;83:1562-1565.
21. Brooks D, Parsons J, Hunter JP, Devlin M, Walker J: The 2-minute walk test as a measure of functional improvement in persons with lower limb amputation. *Arch Phys Med Rehabil* 2001;82:1478-1483.
22. Deathe AB, Miller WC: The L test of functional mobility: Measurement properties of a modified version of the timed "up & go" test designed for people with lower-limb amputations. *Phys Ther* 2005;85:626-635.
23. Kark L, McIntosh AS, Simmons A: The use of the 6-min walk test as a proxy for the assessment of energy expenditure during gait in individuals with lower-limb amputation. *Int J Rehabil Res* 2011;34:227-234.
24. Lin S-J, Bose NH: Six-minute walk test in persons with transtibial amputation. *Arch Phys Med Rehabil* 2008;89:2354-2359.
25. Raya MA, Gailey RS, Fiebert IM, Roach KE: Impairment variables predicting activity limitation in individuals with lower limb amputation. *Prosthet Orthot Int* 2010;34:73-84.
26. Roffman CE, Buchanan J, Allison GT: Locomotor performance during rehabilitation of people with lower limb amputation and prosthetic nonuse 12 months after discharge. *Phys Ther* 2016;96:985-994.
27. Bowden MG, Balasubramanian CK, Behrman AL, Kautz SA: Validation of a speed-based classification system using quantitative measures of walking performance poststroke. *Neurorehabil Neural Repair* 2008;22:672-675
28. Lerner-Frankel MB: Functional community ambulation: What are your criteria? *Clin Manage* 1990;6:12-15.
29. Lord SE, Weatherall M, Rochester L: Community ambulation in older adults: Which internal characteristics are important? *Arch Phys Med Rehabil* 2010;91:378-383.
30. Perera S, Mody SH, Woodman RC, Studenski SA: Meaningful change and responsiveness in common physical performance measures in older adults. *J Am Geriatr Soc* 2006;54:743-749.
31. Gaunaurd I, Kristal A, Horn A et al: The utility of the 2-minute walk test as a measure of mobility in people with lower limb amputation. *Arch Phys Med Rehabil* 2020;101:1183-1189.
32. Datta D, Ariyaratnam R, Hilton S: Timed walking test – An all-embracing outcome measure for lower-limb amputees? *Clin Rehabil* 1996;10:227-232.
33. Bohannon RW: Reference values for extremity muscle strength obtained by hand-held dynamometry from adults aged 20 to 79 years. *Arch Phys Med Rehabil* 1997;78:26-32.
34. Prosthetic Limb Users Survey of Mobility (PLUS-M™) Version 1.2 Short Forms Users Guide. Available at: http://www.plus-m.org. Accessed December 9, 2021.
35. Morgan SJ, Amtmann D, Abrahamson DC, Kajlich AJ, Hafner BJ: Use of cognitive interviews in the development of the PLUS-M item bank. *Qual Life Res* 2014;23:1767-1775.
36. Hafner BJ, Morgan SJ, Abrahamson DC, Amtmann D: Characterizing mobility from the prosthetic limb user's perspective: Use of focus groups to guide development of the Prosthetic Limb Users Survey of Mobility. *Prosthet Orthot Int* 2016;40:582-590.
37. Hafner BJ, Morgan SJ, Askew RL, Salem R: Psychometric evaluation of self-report outcome measures for prosthetic applications. *J Rehabil Res Dev* 2016;53:797.
38. England DL, Miller TA, Stevens PM, Campbell JH, Wurdeman SR: Normative mobility values for lower limb prosthesis users of varying age, etiology, and amputation level. *Am J Phys Med Rehabil* 2021; December 3 [Epub ahead of print]
39. Podsiadlo D, Richardson S: The Timed "Up & Go": A test of basic functional

mobility for frail elderly persons. *J Am Geriatr Soc* 1991;39:142-148.
40. Schoppen T, Boonstra A, Groothoff JW, de Vries J, Göeken LN, Eisma WH: The Timed "up and go" test: Reliability and validity in persons with unilateral lower limb amputation. *Arch Phys Med Rehabil* 1999;80:825-828.
41. Bergmann JH, Alexiou C, Smith IC: Procedural differences directly affect timed up and go times. *J Am Geriatr Soc* 2009;57:2168-2169.
42. Sansam K, O'Connor RJ, Neumann V, Bhakta B: Can simple clinical tests predict walking ability after prosthetic rehabilitation? *J Rehabil Med* 2012;44:968-974.
43. Clemens SM, Gailey RS, Bennett CL, Pasquina PF, Kirk-Sanchez NJ, Gaunaurd IA: The Component Timed-Up-and-Go test: The utility and psychometric properties of using a mobile application to determine prosthetic mobility in people with lower limb amputations. *Clin Rehabil* 2018;32:388-397.
44. Heinemann AW, Connelly L, Ehrlich-Jones L, Fatone S: Outcome instruments for prosthetics: clinical applications. *Phys Med Rehabil Clin N Am* 2014;25:179-198.
45. Dite W, Connor HJ, Curtis HC: Clinical identification of multiple fall risk early after unilateral transtibial amputation. *Arch Phys Med Rehabil* 2007;88:109-114.
46. Schoppen T, Boonstra A, Groothoff JW, de Vries J, Göeken LN, Eisma WH: Physical, mental, and social predictors of functional outcome in unilateral lower-limb amputees. *Arch Phys Med Rehabil* 2003;84:803-811.
47. Powell LE, Myers AM: The activities-specific balance confidence (ABC) scale. *J Gerontol A Biol Sci Med Sci* 1995;50:M28-M34.
48. Miller WC, Deathe AB, Speechley M: Psychometric properties of the Activities-specific Balance Confidence Scale among individuals with a lower-limb amputation. *Arch Phys Med Rehabil* 2003;84:656-661.
49. Sakakibara BM, Miller WC, Backman CL: Rasch analyses of the Activities-specific Balance Confidence Scale with individuals 50 years and older with lower-limb amputations. *Arch Phys Med Rehabil* 2011;92:1257-1263.
50. Hafner BJ, Amtmann D, Abrahamson DC, Morgan SJ, Kajlich AJ, Salem R: Normative PEQ-MS and ABC scores among persons with lower limb loss, in *Academy Annual Meeting and Scientific Symposium*. Orlando, FL, 2013. Journal of the Proceedings of the 39th Academy Annual Meeting and Scientific Symposium.
51. Myers AM, Fletcher PC, Myers AH, Sherk W: Discriminative and evaluative properties of the activities-specific balance confidence (ABC) scale. *J Gerontol A Biol Sci Med Sci* 1998;53:M287-M294.
52. Lajoie Y, Gallagher S: Predicting falls within the elderly community: Comparison of postural sway, reaction time, the Berg balance scale and the Activities-specific Balance Confidence (ABC) scale for comparing fallers and non-fallers. *Arch Gerontol Geriatr* 2004;38:11-26.
53. Norvell DC, Williams RM, Turner AP, Czerniecki JM: The development and validation of a novel outcome measure to quantify mobility in the dysvascular lower extremity amputee: The amputee single item mobility measure. *Clin Rehabil* 2016;30:878-889.
54. Major MJ, Fatone S, Roth EJ: Validity and reliability of the Berg Balance Scale for community-dwelling persons with lower-limb amputation. *Arch Phys Med Rehabil* 2013;94:2194-2202.
55. Gailey RS, Gaunaurd IA, Raya MA, et al: Development and reliability testing of the Comprehensive High-Level Activity Mobility Predictor (CHAMP) in male servicemembers with traumatic lower-limb loss. *J Rehabil Res Dev* 2013;50:905-918.
56. Dite W, Temple VA: A clinical test of stepping and change of direction to identify multiple falling older adults. *Arch Phys Med Rehabil* 2002;83:1566-1571.
57. Devlin M, Pauley T, Head K, Garfinkel S: Houghton scale of prosthetic use in people with lower-extremity amputations: Reliability, validity, and responsiveness to change. *Arch Phys Med Rehabil* 2004;85:1339-1344.
58. Sawers A, Hafner BJ: Narrowing beam-walking is a clinically feasible approach for assessing balance ability in lower-limb prosthesis users. *J Rehabil Med* 2018;50:457-464.
59. Wilken JM, Darter BJ, Goffar SL, et al: Physical performance assessment in military service members. *J Am Acad Orthop Surg* 2012;20:S42-S47.
60. Hanspal R, Fisher K, Nieveen R: Prosthetic socket fit comfort score. *Disabil Rehabil* 2003;25:1278-1280.
61. Morgan SJ, Askew RL, Hafner BJ: Measurements of best, worst, and average socket comfort are more reliable than current socket comfort in established lower limb prosthesis users. *Arch Phys Med Rehabil* 2021;103(6):1201-1204.
62. McCaffery M: *Pain: Clinical Manual for Nursing Practice*. The C.V. Mosby Company; 1994.
63. Williamson A, Hoggart B: Pain: A review of three commonly used pain rating scales. *J Clin Nurs* 2005;14:798-804.
64. Gailey R, Kristal A, Lucarevic J, Harris S, Applegate B, Gaunaurd I: The development and internal consistency of the comprehensive lower limb amputee socket survey in active lower limb amputees. *Prosthet Orthot Int* 2019;43:80-87.
65. Hays RD, Spritzer KL, Schalet BD, Cella D: PROMIS®-29 v2. 0 profile physical and mental health summary scores. *Qual Life Res* 2018;27:1885-1891.
66. Amtmann D, Morgan SJ, Kim J, Hafner BJ: Health-related profiles of people with lower limb loss. *Arch Phys Med Rehabil* 2015;96:1474-1483.
67. Heinemann AW, Bode R, O'reilly C: Development and measurement properties of the Orthotics and Prosthetics Users' Survey (OPUS): A comprehensive set of clinical outcome instruments. *Prosthet Orthot Int* 2003;27:191-206.
68. Jarl GM, Heinemann AW, Norling Hermansson LM: Validity evidence for a modified version of the Orthotics and Prosthetics Users' Survey. *Disabil Rehabil Assist Technol* 2012;7:469-478.
69. Halsne B, Peaco A: Clinical administration of a standardized patient satisfaction measure, in *Academy Annual Meeting and Scientific Symposium*. Atlanta, GA, 2012. Journal of the Proceedings of the 38th Academy Annual Meeting and Scientific Symposium.
70. Legro MW, Reiber GD, Smith DG, del Aguila M, Larsen J, Boone D: Prosthesis evaluation questionnaire for persons with lower limb amputations: assessing prosthesis-related quality of life. *Arch Phys Med Rehabil* 1998;79:931-938.
71. Franchignoni F, Giordano A, Ferriero G, Orlandini D, Amoresano A, Perucca L: Measuring mobility in people with lower limb amputation: Rasch analysis of the mobility section of the prosthesis evaluation questionnaire. *J Rehabil Med* 2007;39:138-144.

72. EuroQoL. EQ-5D-5L about. 2021. Available at: https://euroqol.org/eq-5d-instruments/eq-5d-5L-about/. Accessed December 9, 2021.
73. Cutti AG, Lettieri E, Del Maestro M, et al: Stratified cost-utility analysis of C-leg versus mechanical knees: findings from an Italian sample of transfemoral amputees. *Prosthet Orthot Int* 2017;41:227-236.
74. Bak P, Müller W-D, Bocker B, Smolenski U: Responsiveness of the SF-36 and FIM in lower extremity amputees undergoing a multidisciplinary inpatient rehabilitation. *Phys Med* 2006;16:280-288.
75. Hagberg K, Brånemark R, Hägg O: Questionnaire for Persons with a Transfemoral Amputation (Q-TFA): Initial validity and reliability of a new outcome measure. *J Rehabil Res Dev* 2004;41(5):695-706.

SECTION 4

Management Issues

Skin Pathologies Associated With Amputation

CHAPTER 52

James T. Highsmith, MD, MS • M. Jason Highsmith, PhD, PT, DPT, CP, FAAOP

ABSTRACT

Skin pathologies are common in association with amputation and, particularly socket-based, prosthesis use. Therefore, it is important for all members of the healthcare team to be familiar with the most common dermatologic maladies observed in the amputee cohort. The most common skin issues and their underlying causes and treatment and management considerations for the multidisciplinary amputation clinic team should be discussed.

Keywords: amputation; blister; dermatitis; rash; ulcer

Introduction

Persons with an amputation or amputations who use artificial limbs require ongoing care of qualified prosthetists to fabricate, fit, align, and maintain their prostheses to maximize function and quality of life. In addition, various healthcare professionals will be involved throughout the amputee's lifespan for a host of additional prosthetic and nonprosthetic issues. Interfacing an artificial limb to human anatomy introduces stress into and upon the body beyond that experienced by nonamputees. These added stressors create health complications to body systems that, at times, require evaluation by other members of the healthcare team.

One such affected body system is the integumentary system. Human skin is composed of cells that communicate with and rely on each other to form tissues, which in turn function together to form an organ. The human body's largest organ is the skin, or integumentary system, which is often taken for granted yet is integral to health and well-being. Skin is vital to maintaining temperature regulation through glandular secretions, vascular constriction or dilation, and contracting the erector pili muscles within the dermis so that hairs on the skin stand up to decrease conduction and convection heat loss. Gross protection of deeper structures is apparent, but the integument is also vital in fluid homeostasis, insulation, sensation, absorption with selective resistance, production of natural moisturizing factors, sun protection, immunologic surveillance, appearance, and more. Many of these functions become impaired because of the artificial prosthesis-to-skin interface and when combined with the complexity of prosthetic provision and maintenance, collaboration between the prosthetist and dermatologist becomes imperative at times to optimize patient outcomes.

Gross anatomic loss after amputation requires altered loading and adapted movement patterns, generally with a prosthesis. With prosthetic use, a socket typically connects the residual limb to artificial joints, limb segments, and ultimately to a terminal device, such as a hand or foot, for environmental interaction. Physiologic changes continue to occur after anatomic loss, for example in the neuromusculoskeletal and vascular systems altering volume and inherent skin function. These changes predispose the limb and body to a multitude of additional signs and symptoms such as pain, motor and sensory dysfunction, thermoregulation, hygiene, infectious as well as cosmetic issues, and scarring.

The prosthetic socket must have an intimate and appropriate fit to the residual limb or many dermatosies may occur. Even an excellent prosthetic fit introduces challenges for the skin. For instance, both air circulation and heat transfer are impeded. Perspiration is likely increased with little to no means of removal. Prosthetic use then exposes moist skin to new materials, chemicals, and considerable mechanical forces. This accumulates increased exposure to injury and irritation and provides little opportunity for healing. Often, this situation is confounded by the fact that many amputees are burdened with a number of other health comorbidities such as vascular disease, diabetes mellitus, obesity, multiple limb loss, pain issues, polytrauma including brain injury, and posttraumatic stress.[1,2] Thus, skin problems in amputees are not solely prosthetic but functionally, economically, medically, socially, and cognitively complex.

It is important to describe the prevalence of dermatologic diagnoses in persons with an amputation or

Neither of the following authors nor any immediate family member has received anything of value from or has stock or stock options held in a commercial company or institution related directly or indirectly to the subject of this chapter: Dr. James T. Highsmith and Dr. M. Jason Highsmith.

amputations; discuss factors, including hygiene, contributing to dermatoses in persons with an amputation or amputations; describe the prevention, presentation, etiology, and management of dermatologic conditions in persons with an amputation or amputations; and describe possible classification systems for dermatologic conditions in persons with amputation.

Epidemiology

Dermatologic issues represent from 12% to as much as 23% of ambulatory visits to primary care, though recent reports show this rate rising in certain populations.[3-5] A recent review of the prevalence of skin problems among amputees reported 15% to 41% of amputees have a dermatologic issue. This is up to a threefold increase in skin problems compared with the general population of nonamputees. The wide range of prevalence was reportedly because of nonstandardized methods of skin assessment based on who was evaluating (ie, patient, clinician, specialist), diagnostic method (ie, patch test, swab test), lack of uniformity in descriptions of problems, and the study setting (ie, country, clinic setting, etiology).[6] Nevertheless, it is clear that persons with limb loss who use prostheses can expect to have increased problems with their skin at rates compared with nonamputees.

In terms of the type and frequency of specific dermatoses in persons with amputation, there is currently no consensus. The study setting has a great deal to do with the rate of certain skin problems, as do comorbidities and numerous confounding variables.[7,8] To give some idea of the rank order of dermatoses, in a study of 745 prosthesis users the most commonly experienced dermatologic conditions were ulcers (27%), followed by irritation (18%), cysts (15%), and calluses (11%) (**Table 1**).[9]

The prosthetist should be familiar with common skin conditions and be prepared to manage them. Additionally, knowledge of less common skin issues is helpful in facilitating a prompt referral to the dermatologist when problems are beyond the scope of routine

TABLE 1 Rank Order of Dermatoses

Rank	Dermatoses	Percentage (%)
1	Ulcers	27
2	Irritation	18
3	Inclusion cyst	15
4	Callus	11
5	Verrucous hyperplasia	9
6	Blister	7
7	Fungal infection	5
8	Cellulitis	2
9	"Other" dermatoses	7

prosthetic care. Hygiene, cutaneous problems, and the classification of cutaneous problems are to be discussed.

Hygiene

Limb amputation inherently brings adaptation, not only in muscular recruitment affecting strength, balance, and higher energy demands but also psychologically, socially, anatomically, and relative to residual limb skin function. The environment within the skin–prosthetic interface is occlusive and includes areas of high stress and friction. For many, the complexities of this environment are compounded by the presence of suction or negative pressure. This atypical (ie, human to device) interface predisposes the residual limb to a multitude of novel, unnatural factors that increase the importance of quality skin hygiene, observation, and management.

If a patient did not experience skin problems before their amputation, it may be reasonable to assume that their preamputation skin care regimen will remain sufficient with the introduction of a prosthesis. However when skin problems arise, it is prudent to initiate prescriptive changes because many amputees have varied and unusual skin hygiene practices.[10] Lack of knowledge and training, cognitive impairment, and other health comorbidities common to patients with amputations could contribute to suboptimal skin care. In many of these patients, poor hygiene contributes to many skin conditions including odor, intertrigo, various infections, eczema, autoeczematization, cysts, and other neoplasms. Therefore, a review of proper instructions for good hygiene practice is not only prudent, but crucial.

Washing practices of the body, residual limb, and prosthetic interface components should generally be a daily routine.[11] Equally important is that prosthetic components be dried or permitted to dry as appropriate, and that they be inspected before use (**Figure 1**). Bathing in the evening is recommended to minimize moisture on the limb as this has been cited as initiating adherence and friction.[12] This was a sound recommendation in early prosthetic literature and is still recommended. Gel liners are currently the most prevalent form of prosthetic suspension[13] and perspiration is known to be problematic with their use. Moisture (ie, perspiration) in gel-lined interfaces can impair suspension but to some extent is unavoidable. Thus, periodic doffing and drying of the interface and residual limb throughout the day should be considered part of routine hygiene practice with the gel-lined suspension systems in current use.

Because the skin is acidic in nature, with a typical pH value near 5, neutral or near-neutral pH cleansers should be used.[12,14] This includes washing with gentle soaps (ie, Dove, Unilever Corporation) and synthetic detergents, or "syndets" (ie, Cetaphil, Galderma Laboratories), using warm water and ensuring all of the cleanser is washed away. Leaving any residual soap or cleanser is a common cause of dry skin and irritant contact dermatitis (ICD). Patients should be instructed to limit the skin-cleansing duration to less than 15 minutes and then blot their skin dry with a towel using a soft touch, pushing motion as opposed to frictional rubbing. This entire process could be both preventive and restorative for many eczematous conditions, xerosis, facilitating normal cutaneous microbial flora, and may be useful to decrease pathogenic bacterial colonization (ie, *Propionibacterium acnes*), which is more commonly seen in most soaps, as nearly all traditional soaps have an alkaline pH.[15] Commonly seen

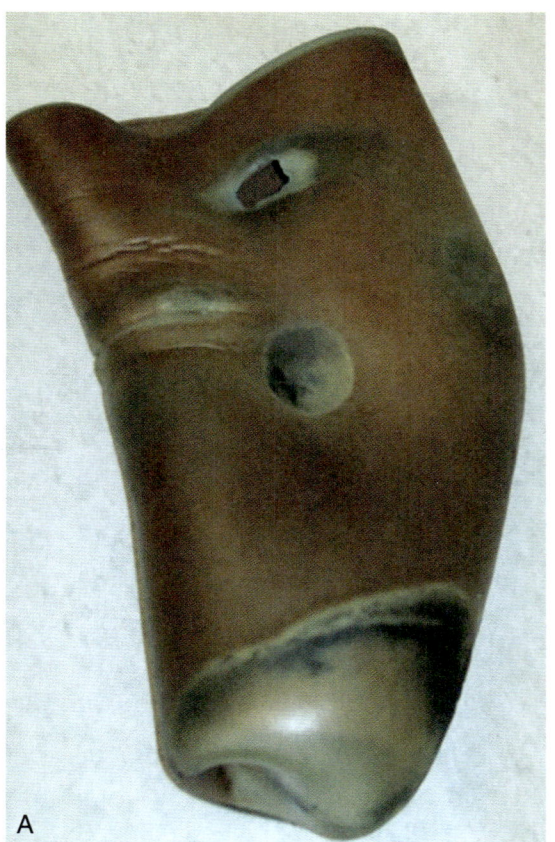
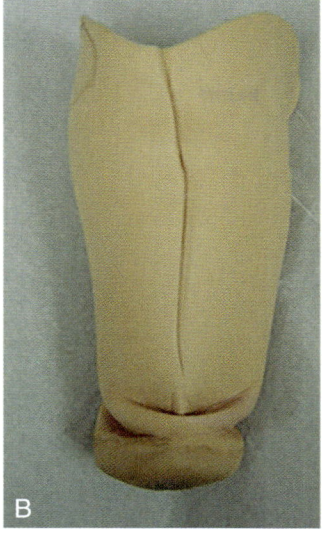
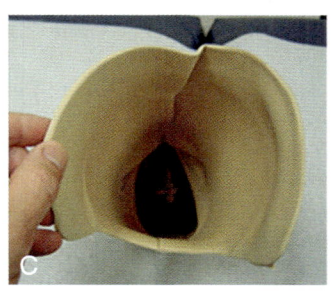
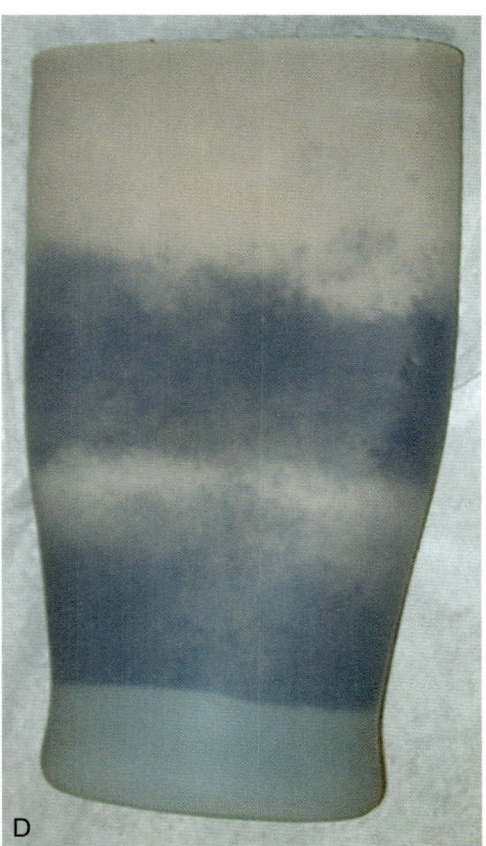

FIGURE 1 Photographs of liners that will contribute to dermatoses because of mechanical failure or the presence of irritants. **A**, Gel liner beyond its useful service life. Note the worn spots where trimlines have worn through the gel proximal to the knee joint and the excess pressure anterior to the knee, at the fibular head, in the popliteal space and distal end. These are all places associated with dermatoses. **B**, Pelite liner in which the patient is proximally constricted leaving a distal air space. Such gaps lead to verrucous hyperplasia. **C**, Pelite liner with contaminants accumulated distally. **D**, Gel liner with mold between the gel and cloth cover.

problems with basic skin care include using hot water, cleansing duration exceeding 15 minutes, using high-alkaline cleansers, not removing all of the cleanser, and rubbing the towel back and forth vigorously across the skin to dry. Each of these factors contributes to more inflammation, contact dermatitis, superficial infections, and generalized dry skin.[16]

Dermatitis

Dermatitis, or eczema, is inflammation of the skin. Inflamed skin may be pruritic (itchy), erythematous, weeping, crusting, vesicular, bullous, or have numerous other irritated presentations. There are multiple causes and types of dermatitis. Selected types of dermatologic conditions and associated etiologies relevant to the care of patients with amputations are discussed here.

Contact Dermatitis

Contact dermatitis occurs when a material or chemical contacts skin and results in signs or symptoms that are typically inflammatory. There are two main forms of contact dermatitis, irritant and allergic. ICD is a nonimmunologically mediated process that occurs when a physical agent is applied long enough or in a high enough concentration to damage cells and disrupt skin integrity and function. ICD is the most common type of contact dermatitis and results from exposure that could cause a reaction in all human skin equally, for example, a strong acid.

A key feature of ICD is that the inflammatory response is limited to the contact site, which often itches or burns, depending on the nature of the contactant. The most common etiologies for ICD include excessive chronic washing with soap and water which can dry and irritate the skin. Chronic excoriation and rubbing further exacerbate the problem. Other predisposing factors include age (worse in the very young and very old), occlusion, and mechanical irritation. Management primarily includes avoiding contact with the offending agent. Other therapeutic modalities include using a physical barrier (ie, Liner-Liner prosthetic sock, Knit-Rite, Inc.) and topical barrier (eg, Desitin paste, Johnson & Johnson Consumer Co, Inc. and A&D ointment, Merck & Co., Inc.), emollients (ie, Aquaphor, Beiersdorf AG), and possibly corticosteroids (eg, hydrocortisone). Frictional ICD (**Figure 2**) is a distinct subtype that results from recurrent low-grade friction and results in hyperkeratosis and lichenification.[14]

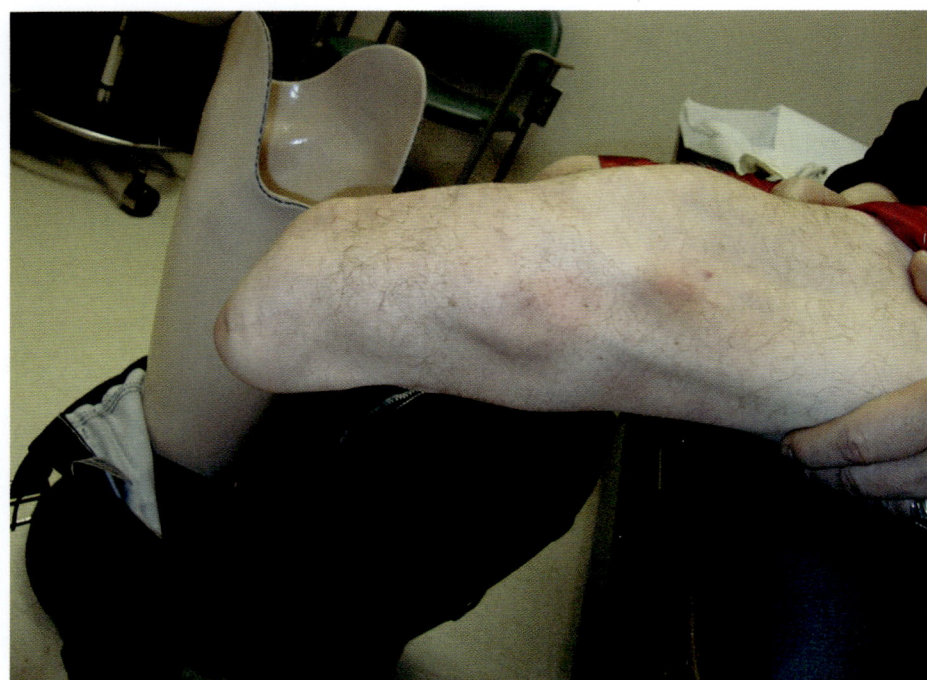

FIGURE 2 Clinical photograph of irritant contact dermatitis (frictional ICD). Note the erythematous areas near the fibular head and anterior and posterior aspects of the lateral femoral condyle. Frictional ICD may present in these areas in association with valgus force coupling during stance phase. Alternatively, the socket may be poorly fit or if the patient is not properly monitoring and adjusting sock-ply during volume change. If the skin fails to blanch with palpation, then a stage I pressure sore has developed which has begun here only at the most proximal erythematous patch near the anterolateral femoral condyle.

However, most friction-related dermatoses are classified later in this chapter; they are typically of higher grade and more directly explain the underlying etiology.

In contrast to ICD, agents triggering an allergic response set off an immunologic hypersensitivity cascade in select persons, generally following repeated allergen exposure. This is referred to as allergic contact dermatitis (ACD) (**Figure 3**). More specifically, ACD is a delayed hypersensitivity reaction to an allergen developing upon reexposure. Lesions from ACD are acutely well-defined involving erythema, edema, and occasionally, vesicles or exudate. Key distinguishing features of ACD include visible reaction upon second but not first exposure. Further, not all persons will react to the offending agent of an ACD, in contrast to irritants that trigger ICD in anyone. Chemicals and materials used in prosthetic fabrication, maintenance, and repair are commonly suspect in contact dermatitis reactions.[17] Varnishes, lacquers, plastics, epoxies, resins, cements, leathers, and others are suspect. Patients with ACD are more likely to have an atopic background (ie, family history of atopic dermatitis, asthma, allergic rhinitis, etc.) in addition to the predisposing factors previously listed for ICD.

Conducting a careful and thorough history is extremely important and necessary to determine if a new exposure outside of the prosthesis (eg, a skin care product) is the offending agent as opposed to a prosthetic component. It may not be possible to differentiate ACD and ICD, especially in the chronic phase, as the signs and symptoms begin to overlap. Patch testing is the benchmark for determining or excluding an immunologic allergen[8,14] (**Figure 4**). One complication with patch testing before completing a thorough history could be that, following the test, the patient's immune system initiates a new response to a material that was historically used without problem in the patient's prosthesis. This would introduce a new problem and could represent a new allergic reaction unrelated to the patient's rash, thus creating a false-positive reaction. In addition, patch testing is not perfect and could fail to detect a true allergy, referred to as a false-negative reaction. False-negative reactions have been estimated to occur in as many as 30% of patients tested.[18] However, if done correctly, discordant reactions are typically observed in less than 5% of tested cases.[19,20] If history and patch testing are successful, removal of the inciting antigen is routinely curative for the dermatitis. If not, then symptom relief becomes the primary goal, at least temporarily. Conservative topical treatment options for symptomatic relief beyond avoidance include antipruritics (eg, Sarna Lotion, Stiefel Co., Research Triangle Park), topical corticosteroids (eg, hydrocortisone), and cool compresses.[10,21,22] In more aggressive cases or if symptoms are refractory to topical therapy, systemic corticosteroid administration may be necessary but should be used with caution.

Nonspecific Eczematization

Although the dermatitis discussed thus far results in inflammation locally at the contact site, there is a possibility of inflammation at a distant site far from the source. A classic example occurs with a dermatophyte fungal infection on a distal extremity that then results in an eczematous patch on the trunk. This has been termed a "dermatophytid," or more simply, an "id" reaction. Other terms such as autoeczematization, autosensitization, angry skin syndrome, and disseminated eczema have all been used to describe this poorly understood process that does not have to be related to an infection. Although unclear, systemic dissemination of an irritant, allergen, or immune cells (ie, activated memory T lymphocytes) likely plays a key role in inflammation at a site distant from the primary inflammatory source and has been speculated to be one source of false-positive reactions in patch testing. Management of id reactions is centered on recognizing and providing

Chapter 52: Skin Pathologies Associated with Amputation

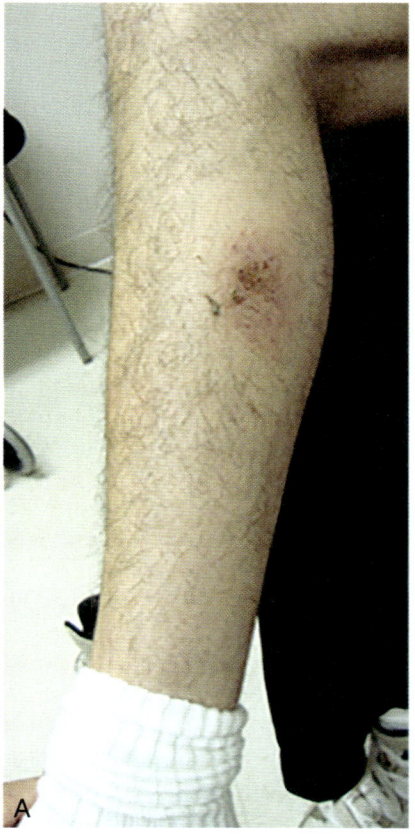

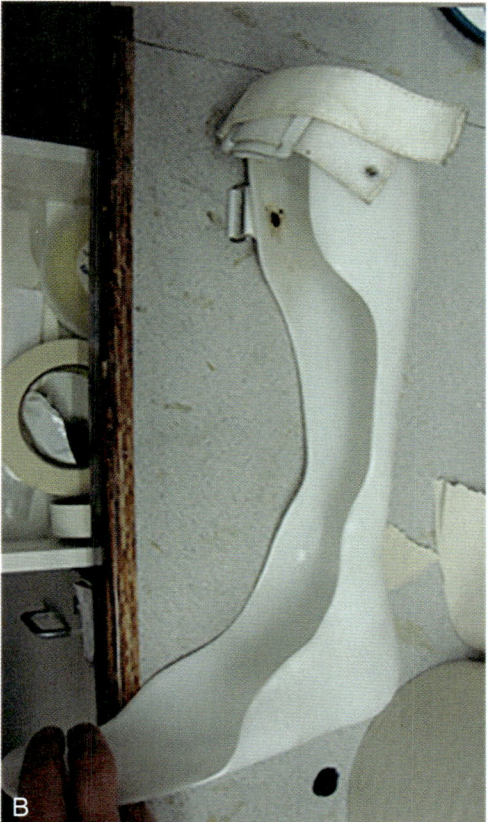

FIGURE 3 Clinical photographs of allergic contact dermatitis (ACD) (Nickel). Suspected ACD in a patient using an ankle-foot orthosis (AFO) in which the cover has come off of the strap rivets, thereby permitting metal to directly contact the skin. **A**, ACD Lesion on skin of lateral leg from contact with the uncovered Nickel AFO strap rivet. **B**, AFO with strap rivets uncovered allowing direct skin contact.

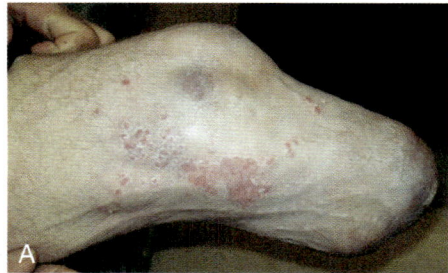

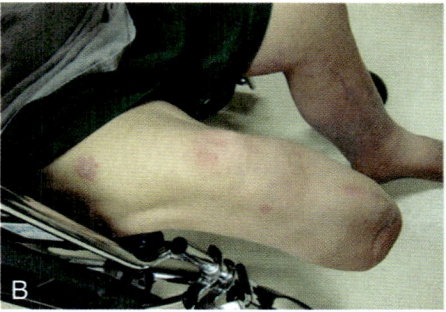

FIGURE 5 Psoriatic plaques presenting on patients' residual limbs are shown. **A**, Note the well-demarcated, pruritic, scaling plaques. **B**, Note the psoriatic plaque on the lateral, proximal right thigh. Psoriasis can result in plaques anywhere upon the body but may be additionally burdensome within the socket region for amputees. Note the stasis dermatitis (**B**) on the patient's left (nonamputated intact) limb as a result of venous insufficiency.

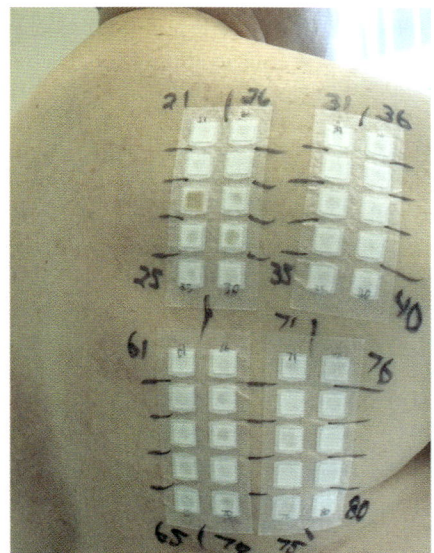

FIGURE 4 Clinical photograph of a patient undergoing patch testing for possible allergens causing allergic contact dermatitis (ACD). The back is used because of the broad surface area and to be able to compare site reactions. Patch testing is the gold standard to diagnose ACD but should be supplemented and corroborated with a thorough patient history.

treatment at the primary source. Emollients and corticosteroids often are the most beneficial in treatment of just the distant eczematous patch(es).

Psoriasis

Psoriasis is a common, chronic immune-mediated systemic inflammatory condition that is characterized by a well-demarcated erythematous patch or plaque with white-colored to silver-colored scales (**Figure 5**). Many patients are genetically predisposed, and an external trigger is possible (eg, infection, hypocalcemia, or medications such as beta blockers). Lesions classically occur on extensor surfaces and are known to occur in areas of friction. In fact, injury may lead to a plaque of psoriasis directly in the traumatized skin that is often linear, as in a scraped knee, known as the Koebner phenomenon (**Figure 6**). For this reason, it is quite possible for psoriasis of the residual limb to develop in an amputee, and it

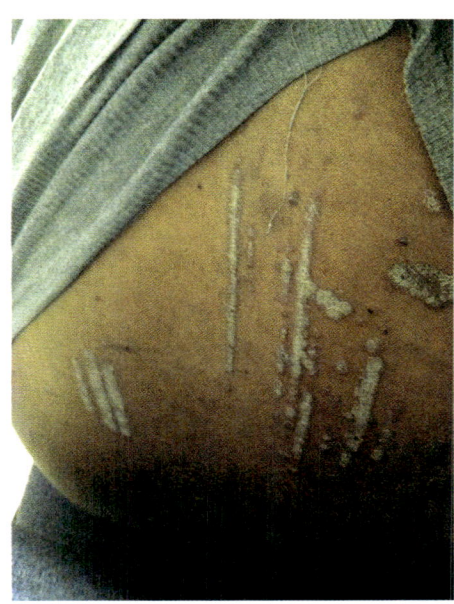

FIGURE 6 Koebner phenomenon. Note the excoriations presenting as linear psoriatic plaques.

would be beneficial to check the elbows, knees, groin, digits, and scalp as well. It is of great service to the patient if the prosthetist can recognize this condition and refer them to their primary care physician or dermatologist. In addition to the skin involvement, approximately one-third of patients have an associated psoriatic arthritis as well as an increased risk of diabetes and cardiovascular complications. Most patients are treated with prescription medications. Topical therapeutic options include corticosteroids, vitamin D creams, retinoids, tar, salicylic acid, and calcineurin inhibitors (eg, tacrolimus).[23] The application of topical therapies is most beneficial if applied when the prosthesis is not on the body, such as during sleeping hours. Collaboration between the prosthetist and dermatologist will ensure prosthetic use is not undermining dermatologic treatment and vice versa in conditions such as psoriasis. Extensive skin involvement, severe symptoms, or arthritis should be managed with systemic therapies such as ultraviolet phototherapy, biologic agents, chemotherapeutic agents, or systemic retinoids.[24]

Intertrigo

Intertrigo is a dermal inflammatory response caused by friction between two skin surfaces that are in constant opposition with each other (**Figure 7**). Areas commonly involved in the nonamputee include the axilla, the submammary areas, and intergluteal cleft. In persons with obesity, intertrigo can develop between tissue folds of the abdomen or thigh and is common on the residual limbs in amputees, particularly where scars are involved. Here, two skin surfaces on either side of an invaginated scar are in constant direct contact while squeezed together inside an artificial interface, often a gel liner.[25] Heat, perspiration, and maceration are present in the semiocclusive environment on the residual limb, coupled with elevated mechanical forces associated with movement that begin breaking down protective keratin and result in inflammation. The compromised tissue is subject to further mechanical irritation and secondary infection. Fissures,

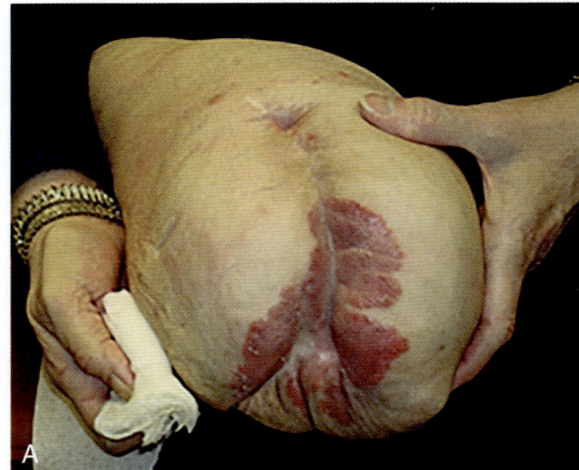 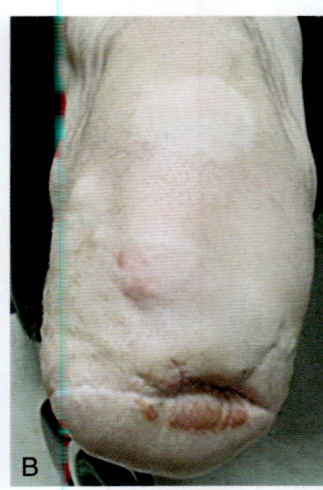

FIGURE 7 Clinical photographs of lesions within opposing skin surfaces of invaginated scars, which are unfortunately common in amputees' residual limbs. These lesions would commonly be referred to as intertrigo. Intertrigo is a nonspecific diagnosis and, when suspected infections or other diagnoses are present, further testing may be indicated. For instance, the left lesion (**A**) is well demarcated and beefy red, so a competing differential diagnosis may be inverse psoriasis and this patient was referred for biopsy as compared to the mild inflammation seen in typical intertrigo (**B**).

eczema, pigment alteration, ulceration, or lichenification can result in chronic cases. Intertrigo is the nonspecific label given to dermatitis in contacting surfaces when no other pathology is present. However, steps should be taken to identify an active comorbid infection or specific underlying pathology. For example, inverse psoriasis may affect just the skin folds as an unusual manifestation of psoriasis and be misdiagnosed as intertrigo. Similarly, many cutaneous infections mimic intertrigo as well, such as erythrasma or fungi. A skin biopsy or microbial culture may be necessary to correctly diagnose underlying pathology in a persistent intertriginous lesion. It is therefore prudent to refer the patient with intertrigo who is unresponsive to conservative treatment beyond a 2-week time period.

General management recommendations include good hygiene practices as previously mentioned, which can be modified as needed along with the application of a topical barrier, emollient, corticosteroid, or some combination thereof, depending on the clinical presentation. Furthermore, appropriately selected, fitted, and aligned prosthetic componentry are vital in minimizing undue stress in the invaginated region. It could be that components are worn beyond their service life, ill-fitting/malfunctioning, or that they are contaminated. Once prosthetic components are functioning optimally, care, maintenance, and cleaning are reviewed with the patient to ensure maximal residual limb protection. Finally, if an underlying cause or secondary infection is isolated, it should be treated as indicated.

Heat Rash

Obstruction of eccrine sweat ducts or malfunction of their integrity is known as miliaria, or more commonly, heat rash (**Figure 8**). Miliaria has been categorized by the depth of pathology and ranges from superficial to deep. Miliaria crystallina is characterized by small subcorneal epidermal clear vesicles that are easily ruptured. Miliaria rubra, or prickly heat, is characterized by occluded sweat that leaks into the lower epidermis or superficial dermis and elicits an inflammatory response with erythematous macules, patches, and papules. These first two types are often described in infants who have been swaddled snugly, creating an excessively warm environment. Miliaria pustulosa may be at the same level as rubra and often occurs after a bout of prickly heat rash. The third

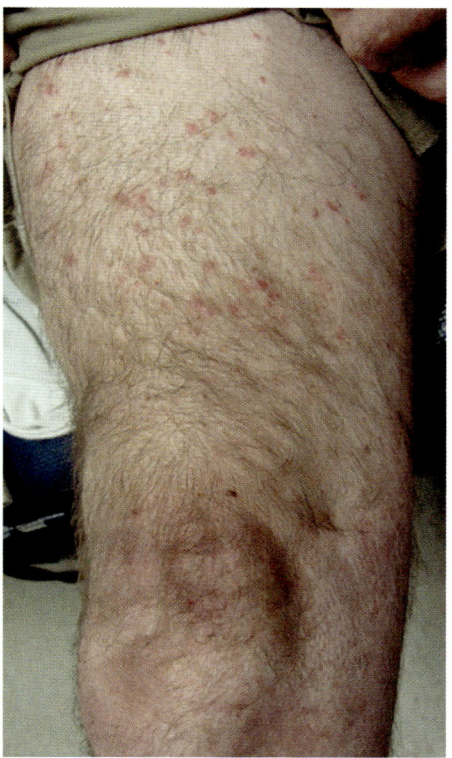

FIGURE 8 Clinical photograph showing miliaria rubra (prickly heat rash) of the distal thigh where skin contacts gel from the patient's suspension system.

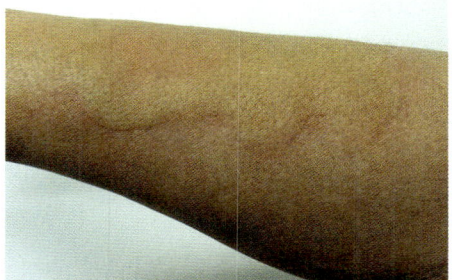

FIGURE 9 Clinical photograph showing urticaria (hives). Note the elevated lesion with a central, pale dermal area.

type, miliaria profunda, results from sweat leaking into the deeper dermis. Among patients with an amputation, prickly heat rash is likely the subtype that will be seen under the prosthetic device because of the artificial interface with sustained exposure to friction and elevated temperatures. Typically, resolution will occur rapidly if the device is not worn for a day or two, usually requiring no further treatment. However, it should be noted that anhidrosis, or a lack of sweating, commonly follows a true heat rash for almost 2 weeks as the ducts need time to repair and restore physiologic function. Because eccrine sweat glands discharge their contents directly onto the skin surface, they are independent of the hair follicle, unlike apocrine and sebaceous glands. Therefore, they are unrelated to epidermal inclusion cyst formation, which is discussed later.

Urticaria

Urticaria is a type of dermatitis commonly referred to as hives (**Figure 9**). Urticaria is characterized by transient pruritic raised wheals formed from central pale dermal edema and surrounded by erythema that blanches with pressure. Individual wheals can resolve as rapidly as within an hour, or persist for an entire day. Wheals that stay in the same location longer than 1 day should be biopsied to rule out an underlying process, such as urticarial vasculitis or systemic lupus erythematosus. However, acute urticaria is defined as lesions that continue to come and go within a 6-week period and chronic urticaria occurs beyond 6 weeks. Physical urticarias are caused by a direct physical agent such as water (aquagenic), brisk stroking of the skin (dermatographism), sweat (cholinergic), cold, heat, solar, pressure, or vibration. Physical urticaria is recognized as a distinct subtype of urticaria but since most cases persist longer than 6 weeks it is generally a chronic urticaria.[26] Although not commonly documented in the prosthetic literature, it is possible to see many of the physical urticarias because of the pressure, heat, and perspiration present in the artificial interface and they should be considered in the differential diagnosis. A careful history should help elucidate if the patient indeed has hives or physical urticaria. Testing physical urticarias should not be done unless the practitioner is trained and equipped to provide treatment for a possible anaphylactic reaction. Treatment of physical urticarias often includes oral antihistamines but topical corticosteroids provide some benefit.[26]

Infection

Skin is equipped with a host of defenses to prevent infection. Defenses have been divided into the innate and adaptive immune systems. The innate system is nonspecific and is known as the first line of defense, composed of components such as the intact skin barrier, antimicrobial peptides (eg, beta defensins, cathelicidins), neutrophils, macrophages, and eosinophils. The adaptive immune system is known as having a delayed but pathogen-specific response with memory, involving Langerhans cells, T cell lymphocytes, B cell lymphocytes, and plasma cells, which produce antibodies. Other barriers to infection include competing normal flora of microbes and the complementary system of proteins, which play a role in both the innate and adaptive immune systems. Trauma, repetitive friction, altered pH, dry skin, and occlusion of the artificial prosthetic interface predispose the host tissue to elevated temperatures, moisture, and maceration that potentially compromises many of these defenses. As a result, microbes may invade the skin resulting in an infection. In persons with an amputation, common skin infections include fungi and bacteria. The classic infectious presentation is localized. Though rare, systemic infections are possible and should be recognized early by constitutional symptoms as seen with an elevated core temperature, accompanied by fever or chills, to avoid serious and even life-threatening complications.[25]

Folliculitis

Folliculitis is defined as hair follicle inflammation (**Figure 10**). It is a common problem related to microbial infection in patients with an amputation. Lesions are characterized by a small pustule centered about a hair follicle. It is more prevalent in individuals with hyperhidrosis, increased hair, or oily skin. Other predisposing factors include obesity, shaving, and friction as seen under a prosthetic device or with tight clothing. Mechanical stress escalates symptoms, particularly in summer months, with higher ambient temperatures, increased perspiration,

Section 4: Management Issues

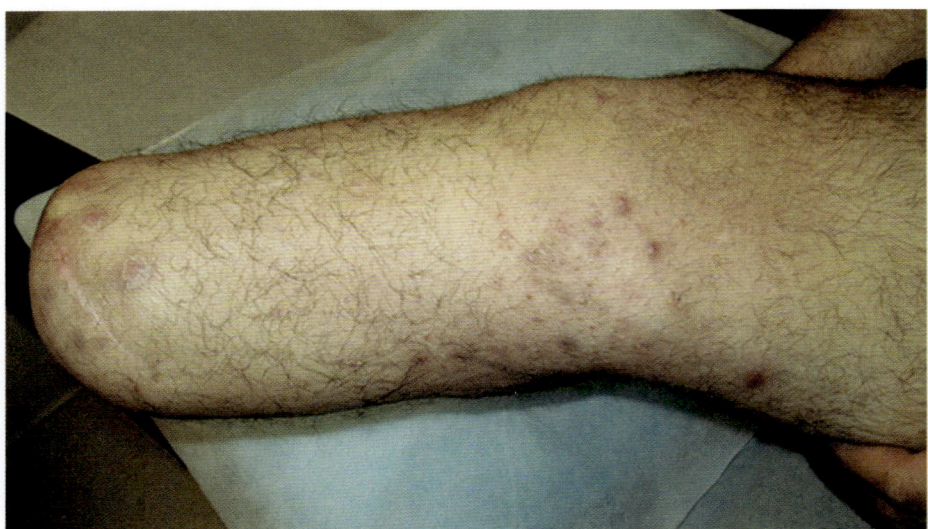

FIGURE 10 Clinical photograph showing folliculitis on a patient's residual limb. A key feature of folliculitis is inflammation, often one or more pustules, centered about a hair follicle.

and exacerbated by the lack of evaporative cooling under the prosthesis.[12,27] These infections are typically caused by the bacteria *Staphylococcus aureus* but other bacteria and even fungi, such as *Malassezia* are also common. It is paramount to recommend against shaving and to emphasize keeping the area cool and as friction-free as possible. Other therapies generally include over-the-counter (OTC) topical antimicrobials (eg, benzoyl peroxide 2% to 5%), prescription topical antimicrobial agents (eg, clindamycin solution, ketoconazole shampoo), and even systemic antibiotics (eg, doxycycline) depending on the severity and microbes involved. For recurrent lesions, permanent laser epilation can also be considered.

Furuncle

A dermal infection deeper than folliculitis is termed a furuncle, or more commonly, a boil.[28,29] A pustule is not visualized in these lesions. Instead, furuncles present as an indurated erythematous nodule, often with tenderness or irritation. Furuncles are generally found on areas of mechanical friction and increased sweating.[10,29] Commonly affected areas include the neck, axilla, and groin, so it is not surprising to see them on the residual limb of a patient with an amputation. Associated systemic disorders include diabetes, immunosuppression, alcoholism, and malnutrition. If more than one follicle is involved the lesion is termed a carbuncle.

Boils are typically caused by *S aureus* and may spontaneously resolve. Furuncles are often managed in a manner similar to that of folliculitis. Recurrent folliculitis or furunculosis may also require antimicrobial soaps or cleansers (eg, chlorhexidine) several times per week, and can be purchased OTC without a prescription, though a discussion with a dermatologist is advisable depending on the previous rate of skin problems and hygiene regimen success among other factors. If the infection involves more surrounding and deeper tissues, it may result in a fluctuant and very painful abscess. An abscess could result in systemic symptoms and a wound culture should be obtained to determine the microbial etiology and susceptibility to antibiotics. Treatment must include incision and drainage of these purulent lesions. Although systemic antibiotics are commonly used, they are generally not necessary as long as the lesion is drained appropriately.

Superficial Fungal Infections

Superficial fungal infections (eg, jock itch, athlete's foot) are also common in the artificial interface.[9] These dermatophytes produce an erythematous annular patch that is a ring of redness (ie, ringworm) along with central clearing or normal-looking skin inside the ring (**Figure 11**). The leading advancing border is typically scaly and flakes when rubbed. Topical antifungal agents are the mainstay of treatment and are available in both off-the-shelf options (eg, terbinafine or clotrimazole) or as a prescription (eg, ciclopirox). Yeast could also affect the skin and would be a distinct fungal infection from the dermatophytes previously discussed. A yeast infection is identified classically as having a beefy red appearance with satellite lesions beyond the primary area of inflammation. *Candida albicans* is the typical yeast involved and is best managed with prescription topical treatment, such as topical nystatin or ciclopirox.

Infection Treatment and Prevention

Improving hygiene practices is the cornerstone for preventing all of the infections discussed.[1] This is important as the skin overlying the residual limb may have altered microbial flora compared with sound limbs in the same person. Levy[10] reported that sound hygiene adherence may be curative in patients with recurrent folliculitis. Other generalized treatment options may include some amount of prosthetic discontinuance[25] and referral to the patient's primary care physician or dermatologist. If the body is being treated for an abscess, the prosthesis and all interfacing soft goods also should be evaluated and cleaned. In chronic, recurrent, or severe infections replacement of soft goods such as socks and gel liners is advised to avoid repeated infections or contamination.[25] For example, soft goods should likely be discarded if an abscess develops in the residual limb or infections involving methicillin-resistant *S aureus* occur.

Volume Change

Limb amputation routinely results in residual limb edema for several weeks postoperatively. Conservative volume management with elevation and a compression garment (ie, shrinker or ACE wrap) is beneficial in controlling and

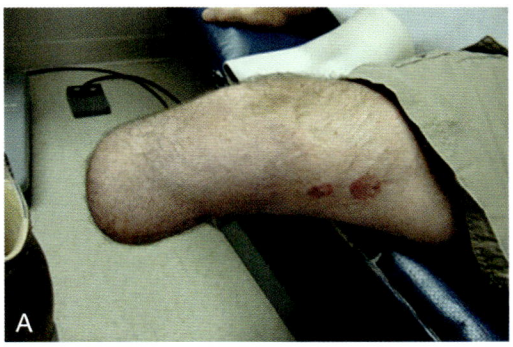 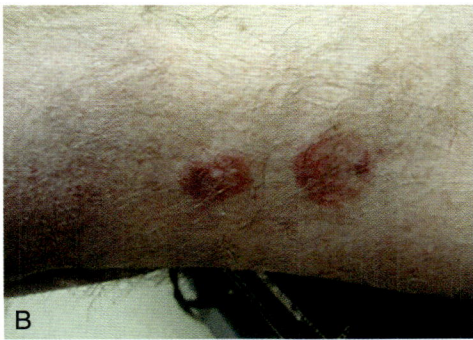 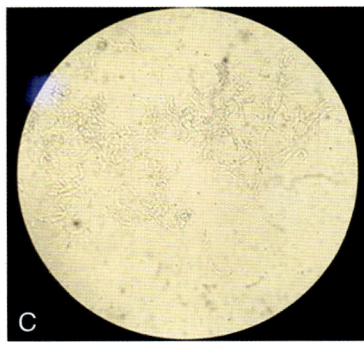

FIGURE 11 **A**, Clinical photograph from a patient presenting with two lesions on the distal medial thigh, beneath the liner of the transtibial prosthesis. **B**, Close-up image from the same patient showing well-demarcated borders with central clearing characteristic of fungal infection. **C**, Potassium hydroxide (KOH) wet mount microscopic view confirming dermatophyte fungal infection. Note the long, slender hyphae characteristic of dermatophytes fungal infections.

reducing the postoperative edema to prepare the limb for prosthetic fitting.[30] Immediate postoperative prostheses, some incorporating negative pressure, are being introduced to facilitate more rapid volume control in addition to early weight bearing.[31,32] Once the preparatory prosthesis is fit, the volume will progressively begin to reduce until the residual limb develops a mature shape. The rapid volume loss experienced in the first year is largely postoperative edema but likely includes additional volume loss from muscular atrophy. Although acute volume reduction will slow approximately 1 year postamputation, the limb will often continue to reduce volume for the remainder of the amputee's life because of many factors, including muscular atrophy and bone demineralization. This volume change process is common but varies between patients. Nevertheless, volume change and the subsequent volume mismatching between the residual limb and prosthetic interface are among the most common and significant sources of dermatologic conditions and impaired function for the prosthesis user. Several specific forms of volume change and their specific medical diagnoses are discussed here.

Prosthesis use results in abnormal mechanical stress being placed on the residual limb. To illustrate this example, note that a typical nonamputee generally experiences 15° to 25° sagittal knee flexion during the loading response for shock absorption purposes. When this happens in transtibial gait, the amputee attempts to regulate the external knee flexion moment by extending the knee. This causes force coupling as pressures increase at the distal anterior tibia and proximal posterior aspect of the socket near the distal hamstring tendon region. As a second example, during mid-stance weight bearing, axial loads in the nonamputee are dispersed through the calcaneal fat pad as well as the arched structure of the foot, with the latter composed of intrinsic and extrinsic muscles and a complex ligamentous array around multiple joints' articular surfaces. When a lower limb is amputated, many of the aforementioned structures are eliminated, requiring structures not designed for load bearing to manage these loads. Specifically, the distal transected ends of the tibia, fibula, and muscle bellies now bear axial loads. It is easy to imagine how this can contribute to abnormal forces and ulceration upon the amputated residuum.

Negative-Pressure Hyperemia

Currently, viable prosthetic suspension options include suction and vacuum (ie, negative pressure). In negative-pressure systems, the prosthesis is held onto the residual limb during unweighting periods (ie, swing phase of gait) via a suction or vacuum.[33] In order for residual limb tissues to be unaffected or minimally affected by the negative pressure, total contact is required. Any loss of contact between the residual limb and interface in the presence of negative pressure will result in a void with lowered resistance to circulation. Fluid is then drawn toward the region of the residual limb closest to the void. The negative pressure pulls lymphatic and circulating blood into the region, creating congestion. If the loss of contact persists, the site will become clearly demarcated, edematous, erythematous, and exquisitely painful (**Figure 12**). The area could begin to weep serosanguinous fluid.[25]

Weight gain is a likely contributor, but any volume change preventing full and total contact could result in this problem. A period of prosthetic disuse may be recommended simply because of the pain that the suction will cause during unweighting. Total contact must be restored in the interface or the problem will persist. Analgesic medication and prosthetic disuse for a short period of time are indicated for pain management from acute symptoms. It is noteworthy, however, that prosthetic discontinuance should be minimized active patients. Temporary padding to restore contact will likely facilitate recovery. However, because the volume change was sufficient to cause this problem in the first place, a cure will likely depend on the fabrication of a new, better-fitting socket.

Friction (Lichenification, Blister, Callus)

Multiple types of forces are being applied to the amputated residual limb during prosthetic use. A very common suspension type in contemporary prostheses includes the gel liner with pin suspension.[11,25,34] When a gel liner is suspending a prostheses via pin lock, the distal end is firmly attached to the bottom of the socket. During movements requiring high degrees of knee flexion, a great amount of friction and stress will be applied to the anterior region of the knee. Patients using pin systems will often complain of knee discomfort if sitting for long periods, as occurs with driving or watching a movie. This friction will result in changes within the skin whereby tissues are attempting to protect themselves from further damage. Initially, blister formation is common, but with time hardening of the skin occurs, leading to hyperkeratosis and acanthosis, termed lichenification (**Figure 13**). Clinically, lichenification can be easily identified with exaggerated skin lines secondary to thickening of cutaneous tissue in the affected area. An isolated affected area is referred to as lichen simplex chronicus when it is caused by chronic manipulation or scratching.[35] Improving prosthetic fit and teaching pressure-relief strategies are recommended as first-line treatment (ie, release the pin lock during prolonged sitting or doff the prosthesis). If indicated, secondary lichenification can be managed with corticosteroids.

Similarly, excess end-bearing as opposed to proportionally distributed loading through total surface bearing could result in distal callusing of the residual limb.[36] Calluses are the skin's protective response to friction and pressure and are generally not problematic. Calluses are caused by an accumulation of terminally differentiated keratinocytes strongly connected by cross-linked proteins in the epidermis.[37] On occasion, excess loads are applied at a pace exceeding the body's ability to form a protective callus and an abrasion or blister could form. Additionally, calluses can lead to skin ulcers or infection. The dermatologist can remove problematic calluses and can culture tissue for infection and treat accordingly. If a blister forms, which are commonly filled with leached plasma from cells exposed to shearing near the stratum spinosum, continued prosthetic use commonly ruptures them. Blisters

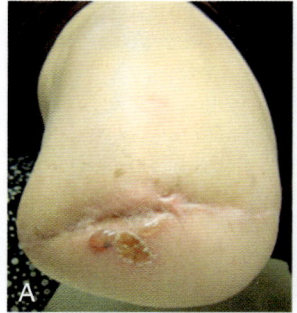 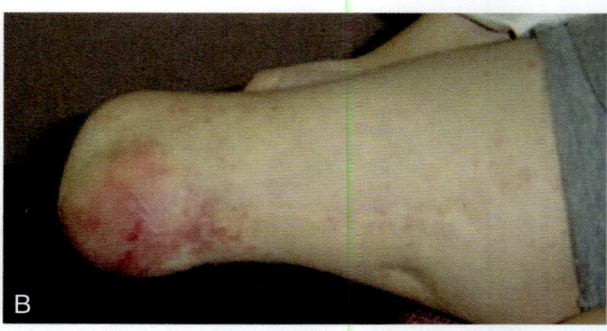

FIGURE 12 **A**, Residual limb presenting with a blister and distal irritation in conjunction with use of a negative-pressure suspension system that resulted in a focal area of suction without total contact. **B**, Classic negative-pressure hyperemia associated with use of a suction suspension prosthesis. Weight gain and an increase in the diameter of the proximal thigh prevents achieving distal contact. Thus, in swing phase there is a constant drawing of fluid to the area of the residuum with the least resistance to fluid flow. Fluid congestion, erythema, and pain result.

can be filled with blood, but can also be infected. Thus, if the fluid is suspect then patients should be referred to their physician. However, blisters are initially sterile and should not be lanced or drained. If blisters rupture, skin should not be removed because it forms a biologic dressing to protect the underlying tissues.

Volume-Related Ulceration

Residual limb ulcers can result from bacterial infections, vascular disease resulting in poor cutaneous nutrition, or focused mechanical pressure from the prosthesis.[25,34,36,38] Concerted efforts to resolve ulcers should be made as long-standing chronic ulcers can become scarred and adherent to deeper tissues, which can complicate healing and future prosthetic use. Chronic ulcers can also develop malignant tissue changes, necessitating referral for biopsy. In the latter cases, additional surgeries expose patients to the risk of systemic anesthesia with further delays in mobility and prosthetic use. No matter the etiology, residual limb ulcerations often result in prosthetic discontinuation until further evaluation.

Decubitus ulcers, or bedsores, are commonly seen on the heels and sacrum of supine-positioned, bed-bound patients. Decubiti can develop on any skin where mechanical pressure is applied focally over a bony

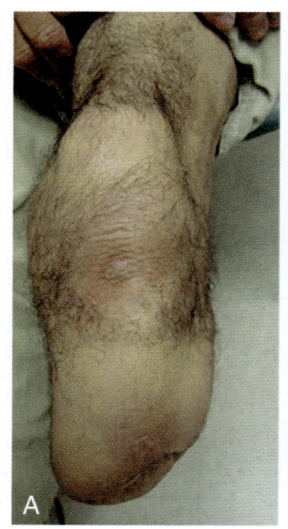 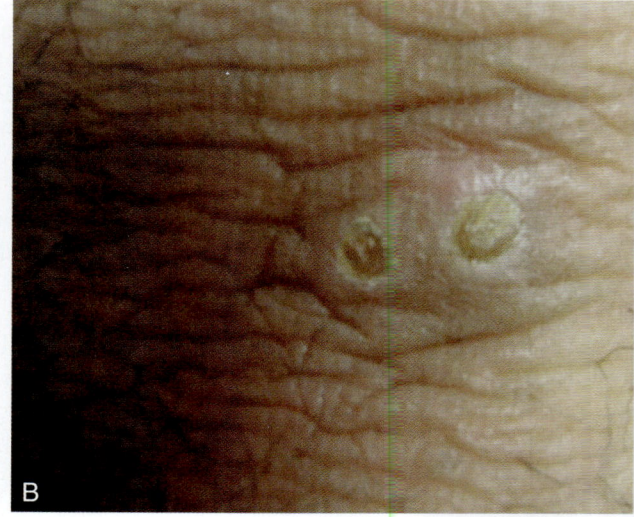

FIGURE 13 **A**, Transtibial residual limb presenting with visible lines characteristic of lichenification. Also present are calluses. **B**, Both the lichenification and calluses are the result of skin attempting to protect itself from high stress, in this case because of patellar bar pressure

prominence. With lower limb prostheses, a poorly fit or aligned socket creates focal pressure and shearing forces over bony prominences (ie, tibial tubercle, femoral condyles) that have been referred to as hot spots (**Figure 14, A**). Unaddressed, the progressive stages of ulceration in this cohort can proceed as follows: irritation and inflammation are introduced to superficial skin layers (stage I). Continued loading further degrades skin integrity allowing the ulcer to erode deeper into the epidermis or dermis (stage II), then into the subcutaneous fascial layers (stage III), and eventually to muscle or bone (stage IV). Sensory deficits compound this problem and are more commonly seen in patients with diabetes and vascular disease. When protective pain sensation is absent, ambulation may likely continue despite the underlying tissue damage, and the pressure sore is further aggravated (**Figure 14, B** through **D**).

Verrucous Hyperplasia

Verrucous hyperplasia (VH), or lymphostasis papillomatosis, is a warty-appearing growth at the distal end of the amputated limb[12,39] (**Figure 15**). Human papillomavirus (HPV), which causes cutaneous warts including genital and common warts, as well as lymphatic stasis, has been proposed as a potential precursor to VH. However, many studies have failed to isolate any viral particles and the condition is almost exclusively a problem in the distal skin of the amputated residual limb, which seems to be the result of a proximal constriction and lack of contact or appropriate contact pressures distally.[12,39,40] The proximal constriction seems to reduce the amount of cutaneous venous, lymphatic, and interstitial fluid return to the proximal circulation. The lack of distal contact and additional fluid presence permits distal congestion, contributing to the warty appearance. The differential diagnosis could include HPV infection, squamous cell carcinoma, or lymphangiosarcoma, which will be discussed later. Nonetheless, the aformentioned mechanism and treatment of VH are generally agreed on by using compression, restoring distal prosthetic contact with the residual limb, and generally optimizing the fit of the prosthetic device.

Topical preparations, radiotherapies, antibiotics, and evaluations by multiple specialists have failed to result in adequate resolution.[12] It has been reported that when total surface-bearing and hydrostatic design sockets were emerging and specific weight-bearing socket designs present at that time minimized distal contact and preferentially loaded proximal tissues, fluid exchange was constricted while creating a space of low resistance in the distal end of the residuum.[10,12,41] These were the standard-of-care socket technologies at that time and, as a result, VH was probably far more common, but unfortunately there are no epidemiologic data to corroborate socket type to this pathology. Nonetheless, successful management has been seen with compression and optimizing socket fit.

Contemporary attempts to more uniformly load the residuum seem to minimize this condition. However, a poorly fit socket or rapid weight gain could create the proximal restriction and distal low-pressure scenario necessary to create VH so the condition still occurs. However, it is probably less common currently than in previous years when total surface-bearing sockets were still novel and not widely used. If an acute situation arises that creates a proximal socket constriction and decreased distal contact pressure, action should be taken immediately to prevent the development of VH. Residual limb compression when out of the socket (ie, ACE wrapping, residual limb shrinker) and distal socket padding during prosthetic use, are a few recommendations to consider while the bodily situation and new socket are being managed. Chronic cases or those with abnormal presentation should be cultured for infection and biopsied. It should be noted that these lesions could be associated with malignancy. For instance, a chronic verrucous hyperplasia situation complicated by extensive ulceration and infection has been reported, and a squamous cell carcinoma developed in the residual limb skin that extended into the bone.[10,42]

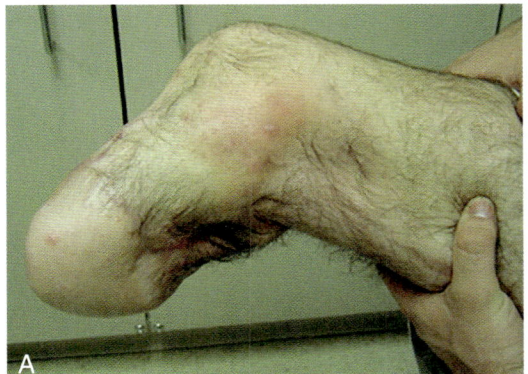 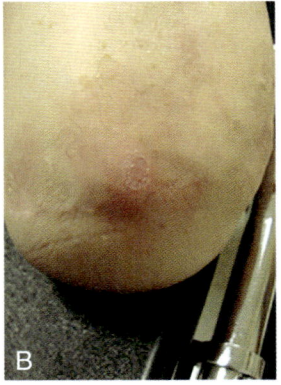 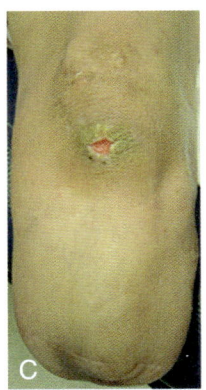 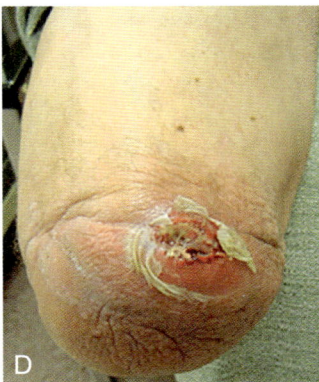

FIGURE 14 **A**, Classic hot spot (decubitus ulcer, stage I) over the medial femoral condyle. **B**, Stage II decubitus characterized by breach of the epidermis. **C**, Stage III decubitus ulcer characterized by penetration into the subcutaneous tissue layers. **D**, Stage IV decubitus with purulent discharge has eroded into muscle tissue.

Section 4: Management Issues

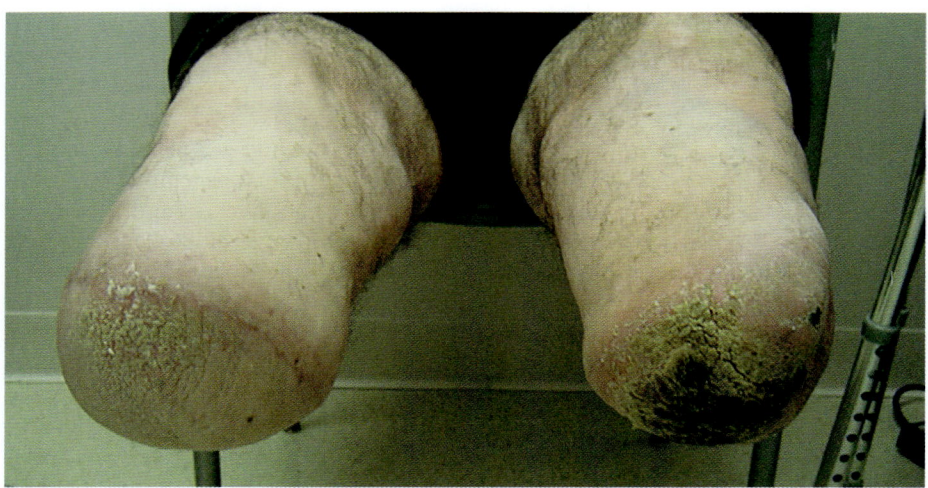

FIGURE 15 Clinical photograph from a patient with bilateral amputation presenting with verrucous hyperplasia secondary to proximal constriction from the prostheses and failure to achieve total contact distally. Medical evaluation to rule out malignancy is indicated in cases this severe. Prosthetic management includes compression when not wearing prostheses and refitting prostheses to ensure total contact without proximal constriction.

Tumor

Tumor is a Latin-derived term (meaning 'to swell') and is often used interchangeably with neoplasia but is not synonymous with cancer. Cancer implies a malignant growth into surrounding or distant tissues (metastasis) that can alter the function of those structures. Tumors are an abnormal proliferation of cellular growth theoretically initiated from an individual cell and may not necessarily invade surrounding structures nor alter their function. Benign tumors do not infiltrate into surrounding organs or typically alter function, as opposed to malignant tumors that lead to cancer.

Normally, each cell has a strictly governed growth cycle with a series of suppressive checks and balances. When a cell begins to express dysplastic or metaplastic changes, these protective processes attempt to halt cellular growth to initiate repair. In the event of numerous errors or an inability to repair the damage, the cell has a final last chance way to prevent cancer formation through preprogrammed cellular death, termed apoptosis. Apoptosis destroys the abnormal cell for the greater good of the host. However, if the cell evades these cell cycle checks-and-balances, as well as apoptosis, then it can replicate and produce many clones that could harbor the same mutations as the parent cell or form many more mutations leading to tumor growth. A complete discussion of carcinogenesis along with all tumors that can affect the skin is beyond the scope of this text. However, a few selected tumors that are very common, or more prevalent in a patient with an amputation, are discussed next.

Benign Growths

Seborrheic Keratoses

Seborrheic keratoses (SKs) are an extremely common, almost universal growth that is seen on the skin of mature adults. SKs are equally prevalent in men and women and have a higher incidence in Caucasian patients. SKs begin to appear after the fourth decade of life and increase in frequency with age thereafter, but occur at a younger age with excessive ultraviolet radiation exposure. A benign clonal proliferation of keratinocytes is the most likely underlying etiology.[43] These common lesions are clinically recognized as a hyperpigmented waxy growth with a "stuck-on" appearance that are generally several millimeters in size but can be several centimeters (**Figure 16**). Although they may have a warty appearance, HPV, which is the virus that causes warts, has very rarely been identified. Simple reassurance without further intervention is recommended for most lesions, but removal with curettage or cryosurgery is reasonable if the lesion is irritated or inflamed. Differentiating these benign growths from true warts or even malignant melanoma may be difficult, so evaluation by a dermatologist is recommended. Similarly, a sudden eruption of dozens of SKs or rapid increases in their size has been noted as a sign of internal malignancy (sign of Leser–Trélat) and should be referred to the patient's primary care physician or dermatologist if noted.

Skin Flaps

Another benign growth that has been described in patients with an amputation is fibroepithelial polyps, also called acrochordons and skin tags. Acrochordons are small, 1 to 3 mm skin-colored to hyperpigmented pedunculated growths that tend to occur on sights of friction and favor the eyelids, axilla, neck, and groin. Friction and weight gain are associated as these lesions may occur within invaginated residual limb scars or a poorly fit prosthesis. Skin tags have also been labeled as a marker for diabetes mellitus.[44] Treatment is not necessary because skin tags are only of cosmetic significance, although snip removal can be done if they become irritated or inflamed.

Neuromas

After amputation of the distal extremity, a potentially painful nerve growth from the distal end of a severed major nerve could develop, termed a neuroma. Neuromas do not appear immediately postoperatively. Most patients use their prosthesis for approximately 9 months before the induction of pain that would suggest a neuroma has formed. Although this delay represents the time needed for the neuroma to grow, it also suggests that more irritation and inflammation from prosthetic use could be required to initiate symptoms or at least be a significant contributing factor. Conservative management should be attempted to improve fit and offload the tender area. However, it is recognized that many of these patients will likely require an additional surgery to remove the tumor at some point.

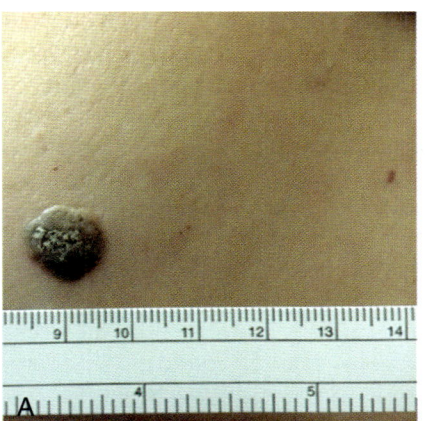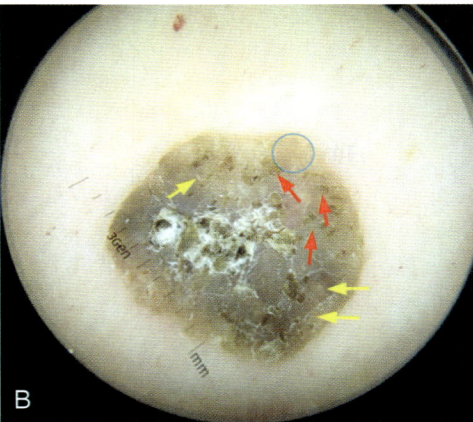

FIGURE 16 A, Presentation of seborrheic keratoses. These benign growths are identified as a hyperpigmented waxy growth of several millimeters with a "stuck-on" appearance. **B**, Dermatoscopic image of the same seborrheic keratosis demonstrating classic findings of comedo-like crypts (red arrows), fingerprint-like structure (blue circle), and white milia-like cysts (yellow arrows).

Following excision of a painful neuroma, most patients had resumed use of their prosthesis by 3 months and all patients studied in a large series were satisfied with the surgery and ultimately were pain free.[45,46]

Cyst

A true cyst is defined as having an epithelial lining, with epidermoid cysts being the most common type of cutaneous cyst. Patients often present for treatment when the lesions are large, irritated, infected, or purely for cosmetic removal. They range in size from a few millimeters, called milia, to several centimeters. Epidermal cysts are typically asymptomatic and usually have a large, dilated keratin-filled pore above them. However, if the keratinous debris within the cyst ruptures into the surrounding dermis, then an intense inflammatory reaction ensues and produces a foul odor if it drains onto the skin surface. Pathogenesis from keratin plugs within the hair follicles of the residual limb is cited as a cause of epidermoid cyst formation as well as when epidermal cells are implanted into the dermis as seen with trauma via the hair follicle. Either way, the infundibular portion of the hair follicle is the suspected site of origin or proliferation. There are multiple interchangeable labels given to epidermoid cysts including: epidermal cyst, epidermal inclusion cyst, infundibular cyst, and keratin cyst.

In nonamputees, these cysts tend to occur on the trunk but could appear in any location and often go completely unnoticed. In prosthesis users, these cysts have most commonly been reported at locations where trimlines terminate and are thought to be caused by trauma with frictional forces. Commonly affected areas in patients with transfemoral amputation are the proximal adductor region, the inguinal crease, and the ischial region. In the patient with transtibial amputation, skin over the pretibial muscle group has been implicated, possibly associated with contraction of these muscles causing stress between pretibial skin and the socket wall during gait. Forces generated from prosthetic use are thought to create an epidermal tissue plug comprised predominantly of keratin. Continued prosthetic use generates forces that drive the keratin plug deeper into a hair follicle. The keratin plug may act as a foreign body to initiate an inflammatory response with infundibular proliferation and thus a cyst develops. The larger the cyst and with repeated rubbing of the prosthetic interface, the more painful and eventually debilitating it will become. These can persist and result in infection, abscess formation, ulceration, and scarring that may complicate prosthetic use, function, and ambulation.[10]

The preferred intervention is surgical removal (ie, excision).[12,28] Infections should be managed as previously described. Restoring appropriate interface pressure is necessary to facilitate breaking a chronic repetitive cycle of cyst formations from the aforementioned process. Pressures can be minimized, or more optimally distributed with appropriately selected interface materials, proper fit and alignment, and good hygiene practices. Other considerations for management include removal of the prosthesis on occasion during prolonged periods of use and ensuring good hygiene practices to remove keratin and debris from skin that could potentially occlude follicles.

Malignant Tumors

Squamous Cell Carcinoma

Although rare, squamous cell carcinoma (SCC) is the most commonly documented malignant tumor to affect the residual limb of amputees[47] and is the second most common malignant cancer of the skin overall. The relatively flat squamous keratinocytes of the epidermis are the cells of origin. In nonamputee patients, the most common source of cellular mutations results from chronic ultraviolet exposure and they are responsible annually for approximately 700,000 cases and 2,500 deaths. SCC is almost three times more prevalent in males than females and is more common in people with fair skin who are older than 50 years. In immunosuppressed patients, there is at least a 65-fold increased risk for the development of SCC.[48] Other risk factors include smoking, HPV infection, earlier skin cancers, radiation, arsenic, lymphedema, chronic sores, chronic inflammation, chronic ulceration, and scarring.[49-51]

A distinct subset of SCC forms a verrucous appearance, termed verrucous carcinoma, and has been documented in the residual limb of amputee patients. These lesions are clinically similar to verrucous hyperplasia or viral HPV infections so a biopsy and possibly a skin culture should be done on chronic warty lesions to exclude malignant potential. HPV has been isolated in verrucous carcinoma and is a predisposing factor. Excision of the affected tissue is the treatment of choice but a residual limb revision leading to a more proximal amputation could be required.

Scar Formation

Scar formation is expected in patients with surgical amputations, but chronic inflammation and chronic ulcerations increase cellular mutations, leading to tumorigenesis, termed a Marjolin ulcer. Marjolin ulcers were initially described in burn scars leading to SCC, but other less common malignancies have been described as occurring in the aforementioned environment and have included basal cell carcinoma, malignant melanoma, and sarcoma.[49,52]

Stewart–Treves Syndrome

Stewart–Treves syndrome is a rare and deadly lymphangiosarcoma that derives from chronic lymphedema and was initially described after radical mastectomies on breast cancer patients.[53,54] Stewart–Treves syndrome has since been used more broadly to describe lymphangiosarcomas that originate in any lymphedematous region, whether congenital or acquired. Technically, lymphangiosarcoma is a poorly chosen term as the cancerous cells appear to originate from blood vessels, not lymphatic vessels. Therefore, a more accurate term, hemangiosarcoma, has been recommended for this condition.[55] Therefore, patients with nonhealing lesions on the residual limb, especially in the presence of edema, must be referred for evaluation by a physician.

Additional Considerations and Presentations

Having a basic understanding of the most common dermatoses that amputees will face is crucial for treatment of a cohort of amputees. On occasion, however, a patient will present with skin signs or symptoms outside of normal. If unsure of the presentation, referral to a dermatologist is always recommended. An eczematous presentation on the chest and leg is fairly common and routine in the practice of a dermatologist and, to a nonamputee, they are not as problematic because they tend not to impair function and mobility. In the amputee, however, misdiagnosing a systemic condition because of localized complications could needlessly impair component selection, access to appropriate treatment, prosthetic use, function, and mobility.

Levy described most amputee skin conditions as "environmental," with a hygiene element thus necessitating changes to the prosthetic environment and hygienic practices to reach resolution.[10,12] Although some componentry and socket theories have evolved and changed, these principles remain unchanged. The occlusive artificial environment and fit within a prosthetic socket are still major factors in setting up dermatologic maladies and quality hygiene practices remain the cornerstone of management. Mechanical stress (ie, friction, pressure) is a major contributor to dermatoses in persons using a prosthesis today and gel liners are introducing a new array of skin challenges.

Pruritus

Pruritus is the cutaneous sensation that leads to the desire to itch or scratch and is the most common symptom affecting the skin.[16] The neurological pathways that transmit itch also transmit pain so itch could be simply a misinterpretation of mild pain. Pruritus may present without any visible lesions. Typically, there is an associated primary cutaneous condition although systemic conditions involving the kidneys, liver, nervous system, and blood cancers (ie, leukemia) are possible. The myriad of reasons that cause itching are beyond the scope of this text. Itching often leads to secondary skin lesions such as excoriations and lichenification. Excoriations can result in pain, cutaneous infections, scars, and a host of additional problems from a compromised skin barrier. Lichenification was previously discussed above with friction but other selected pruritic etiologies, common to persons with limb loss, include xerosis and scar formation (discussed in further detail below). It is imperative to search for and treat the underlying cause of pruritus as first-line management. If the patient fails to improve within 2 weeks of conservative treatment, the severity of symptoms awakens the patient from sleep, or if systemic symptoms are present, then a referral to a physician for systemic evaluation is indicated. It is reasonable to recommend a trial of common antipruritic therapies such as a cold compress for 10 to 15 minutes several times per day (note that ice should not come in direct contact with the skin as this could lead to necrosis), emollients, camphor-menthol (eg, Sarna lotion, Stiefel Co., Research Triangle Park), Pramoxine Hydrochloride (eg, Sarna Sensitive lotion, Stiefel Co., Research Triangle Park), or systemic antihistamines as directed by the package insert, over the counter.

Dry Skin

Xerosis is an extremely common condition and is associated with pruritus. In the elderly, xerosis affects approximately three out of four people over the age of 64.[16,56,57] Xerosis was the most common skin condition observed in a report of 261 outpatient lower limb prosthetic visits but was rarely the primary reason for scheduling a visit with the prosthetist or other clinician.[25] Xerosis is identified by dry, scaly, rough, and possibly itchy skin. Xerosis affects the limbs more than the trunk and is more prevalent in the winter. Xerosis is routinely managed with good hygiene practices and skin moisturizers, such as emollients (eg, Aquaphor, Vaseline, Unilever) or humectants (eg, LacHydrin, urea). A common inciting example would be a prolonged hot bath including excessive washing with soap and concluding with brisk toweling and drying by pulling the towel back and forth along the skin. Long hot tub baths provide short-term symptom relief but heat exacerbates itch and actually pulls further moisture from the skin and increases desquamation.[16] Drag drying also removes potentially protective, superficial epidermal cells and increases friction and dermatitis.

Moisturizers are available OTC and should be applied as instructed on the product label as most help to retard transepidermal water loss. Specifically, a technique referred to as the "soak and smear" method is recommended for dry and scaling skin.[58] With dry skin, a slightly longer duration (20 minutes) lukewarm bath, using a fragrance-free soap or syndet as discussed previously, followed by patting dry with a towel and intentionally leaving a slight amount of moisture that is locked in with the moisturizer at bedtime, preferably in an ointment base such as petrolatum (eg, Aquaphor, Vaseline). Showers of similar length and temperature, or shorter baths have not shown the same benefit. Additionally, chlorinated water soaks as in sitting in a pool or hot tub leads to increased irritation.[58] Unless otherwise instructed, a moisturizing lotion should not be applied to open lesions. In prosthetic management, applying a moisturizer on the residuum immediately before donning a gel liner is not recommended. In such cases, liners with integrated emollients or moisturizers would be preferable but could become a potential chemical irritant. Introduction of new components (ie, changing liner brands) or chemicals (ie, changing moisturizer brands) require skin monitoring for reaction. Another helpful management strategy is to use an air humidifier in bedrooms. Management of xerosis commonly has a seasonal element and is generally a matter of modification of hygiene practices. Patients should be reminded to seek medical advice if symptoms fail to improve or become worse.

Scar

Scars can be a common source of symptoms affecting the residual limb and are an inherent complication of surgery (**Figure 17**). After the initial amputation, the inflammatory stage of wound healing ensues almost immediately. Platelets are the primary player initially and are responsible for platelet-derived growth factor, transforming growth factor (TGF), fibronectin to serve as a provisionary matrix, and other chemoattractants to aid vascular permeability which allows white blood cells, such as neutrophils and macrophages, to clean the wound and reduce infection risk. After about 5 days, the proliferative or granulation stage of healing begins and the focus switches to keratinocytes as the primary cell of significance. These cells of the epidermis begin to leapfrog one another to fill in the wound laterally as well as from deeper hair follicles, if present. Fibroblasts begin producing type III collagen and myofibroblasts act

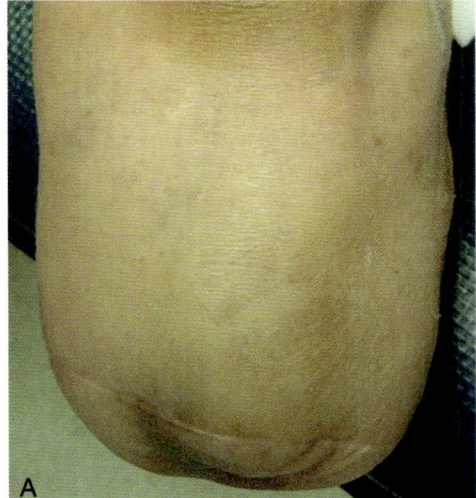
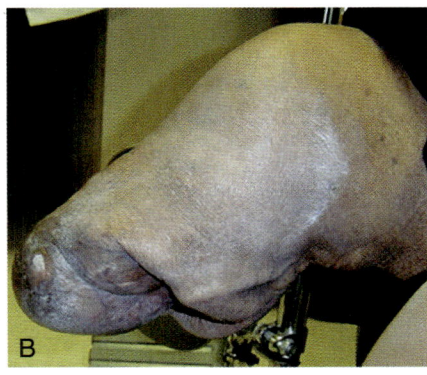
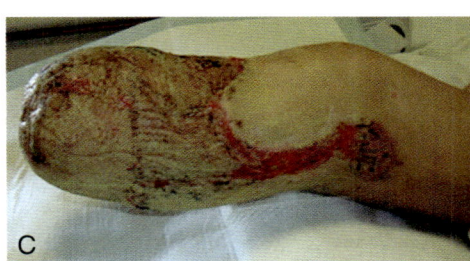
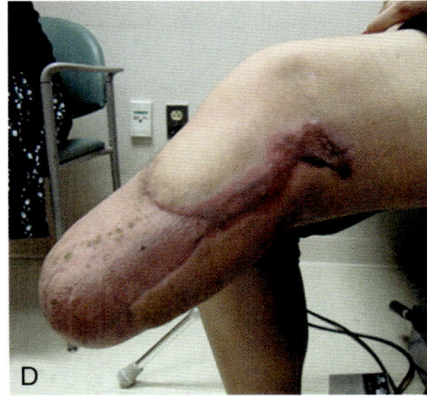

FIGURE 17 **A**, Well-healed, minimally noticeable scar. It is positioned anterior-distal on this transtibial residual limb, characteristic of a typical transtibial amputation with long-posterior flap closure. **B**, Residual limb with mottled, dry distal tissue and excess skin flaps with invaginated scarring (beneath). This limb will be prone to intertriginous lesions in the posterior skin folds and scar area. **C**, Acute, postoperative skin graft covering a residual limb. **D**, The same residual limb presenting subacute scarring.

on the wound to decrease its area with maximal contraction occurring around day 15. Revascularization and angiogenesis occur during this time as well. After nearly 3 weeks, the wound begins maturation and the focus switches to fibroblasts to produce ground substance and more collagen. As time progresses, mature type I collagen replaces type III, and the strength of the scar improves. After 1 year, the scar is fully mature with a peak strength that is about 75% of the prewound strength but it will never attain the strength of normal skin.[59]

Following primary healing, consultation with a physical therapist for scar desensitization and myofascial manipulation may be of benefit to optimize scar strength and healing.[60] Itching, irritation, and pain are common complaints related to scar tissue even when the scar is ideal in appearance. If possible, it is recommended to plan a surgical scar within Langer's cleavage lines as underlying muscles generally run perpendicular and collagen orientation is primarily parallel to these natural skin creases. These tension lines are more apparent with age, smoking, and sun exposure. Cutting parallel to these lines generally results in a more aesthetically appealing fine scar. By contrast, scars widen when these lines are violated. However, removing tension is the most significant factor as high-stressed areas can impede blood flow, scar maturation, and overall healing. Thus, crossing cleavage lines may be necessary at times to relieve tension and optimize healing.[61] It is also important to note that many surgical procedures are done urgently or even emergently to prevent mortality. Underlying comorbidities, smoking, nutritional status, suture selection, undermining, and many other technical aspects of closure have all been known to affect the final outcome of healing and scar formation.

Healing will ideally end with a normal, flat, asymptomatic scar. However, the result may ultimately be an atrophic scar, hypertrophic scar, or keloid. Scars can also break down, ulcerate, or harbor chronic inflammation and even tumor formation (discussed previously). Thin or atrophic scars generally have a white or nearly transparent look with a flat epidermis and very thin dermis to the point where visualization of underlying blood vessels could be possible. Hypertrophic scars are typically elevated above the skin but not beyond the borders of the inciting trauma, whereas keloids have abnormally enlarged collagen bundles and extend beyond the initial site of injury. Hypertrophic scars and keloids are responsible for most mature scar-related symptoms, and treatment is often disappointing. OTC silicone has shown benefit in several studies but intralesional corticosteroids have proven to be most effective in the authors' experience. Laser treatments are effective in some scars. For example, erythematous scars, which are typically younger, improve with laser treatments using wavelengths near 585 nm. Scar revisions are beyond the scope of this text but serve as another management option. However, improvement would not be expected if there was not a significant improvement in the underlying or associated comorbidities previously described. Scar-free healing in humans occurs naturally in utero but does not normally occur otherwise. Nevertheless, this exciting possibility is the focus of intense study and several researchers have documented scar-free healing by altering the chemical wound environment in murine models by decreasing platelet-derived growth factor, neutralizing TGF-β1 or TGF-β2, adding exogenous TGF-β3, or using mesenchymal stem cells.[62,63]

Sweating

Heat loss in normally intact skin occurs by radiation, conduction, convection, and evaporation. Radiation is the transfer of heat from one object to another without contact. At room temperature with normal humidity, 60% to 65% of heat removed from the body is removed via radiation. However, ambient temperature is a major factor in influencing vasomotor responses influencing radiation, whereby colder temperatures cause vasoconstriction and heat is conserved. Contact with a prosthesis impairs radiation heat loss. Similarly, convection requires moving air to remove heat and thus prosthesis to skin contact prohibits air movement and convection. The process of conduction exchanges heat between two contacting surfaces.[12] This is clearly functioning in prosthesis users as interface materials warm up to body temperature, and likely maintain it along with any additional temperature elevations resulting from added forces associated with movement. Evaporation of perspiration from skin is another heat transfer pathway that is impaired during prosthetic use.

Reflex sweating is total body sweating that occurs when any single body part is exposed to the threshold temperature that triggers sweat production. It is a condition associated more commonly with spinal cord injury but has been discussed in association with amputation.[12,64] Reflex sweating induces perspiration in other places of the body even if all other body parts are below the threshold for sweat production. For instance, because of conduction and impairment of all other heat exchange pathways, residual limb skin temperatures may indicate that perspiration is necessary even when the amputee's sound limb, hands, and head are at a comfortable subsweat production temperature. This may lead to perspiration despite otherwise comfortable body temperatures.[12] Simply donning a prosthesis at rest could increase residuum skin temperature by a perceptible 0.5° to 1.0°C.[27] Walking can therefore easily increase residual limb skin temperatures into the perspiration range. Following walking, a 2.0°C reduction or more in temperature is required for amputees to begin to perceive cooling, although they could detect a mere 0.5°C temperature increase as previously mentioned. In summary, amputees who use prostheses are likely to feel warmer and experience total-body, reflex sweating at rates higher than nonamputees.

Hyperhidrosis

Hyperhidrosis is a condition characterized by an abnormal increase in perspiration beyond the typical quantity required for thermoregulation. It can be associated with burden to quality of life from multiple perspectives including in the psychoemotional, aesthetic, and social domains.[65] Sweat glands tend to be highly concentrated in the areas of the hands, feet, axilla, and groin. These locations are where most people tend to have most of their perspiration take place. Primary (or focal) hyperhidrosis occurs with localized sweating, for instance from the scalp, the hands, or the feet. This tends to begin in adolescence and has a familial or genetic component. Alternatively, secondary (or generalized) hyperhidrosis occurs with total body involvement. Secondary hyperhidrosis can start at any point in life, is less likely to be strongly inherited, and could be the consequence of another systemic condition (eg, diabetes, thyroid disorders, menopause). The cause of hyperhidrosis may remain elusive but sympathetic overactivity is involved, and the condition is generally worse in persons who tend to be anxious. Nutrition and food supplements have been found to play a role (ie, stimulants) as can other sensory stimuli (ie, noises, smells).[12,66]

First-line treatment involves using OTC topical antiperspirants, not deodorants, containing aluminum ions (eg, aluminum zirconium, aluminum chloride, aluminum hydroxybromide) which have proved satisfactory in most patients by temporarily occluding sweat gland pores. This is generally initiated with once-daily application at night because of the relative inactivity of sweat glands at this time. After approximately 2 weeks, the patient slowly increases the number of nights between applications to maintain symptom control, ideally once per week.[66] Mild associated irritation or dermatitis is treated with sporadic use of OTC hydrocortisone as needed. The skin should be dry before application because moisture could lead to the formation of irritating hydrochloric acid, therefore, washing just before application should be avoided.

Prescription-strength aluminum chloride may be necessary, or switching to other topical preparations such as anticholinergic agents, boric acid, 2% to 5% tannic acid solutions, resorcinol, or potassium permanganate, but each substance has its own drawbacks. In some patients, systemic anticholinergics (eg, glycopyrrolate) are effective but associated with more adverse events, including blurry vision, dry mouth, difficulty with micturition, and constipation. Although potentially costly and painful because of the necessity of multiple injection sites, some patients have been treated with neuromodulating toxins such as botulinum toxin,[67-70] though minor muscle weakness secondary to diffusion can occur.[71] Furthermore, laser epilation has been recently used as a successful treatment option in axillary hyperhidrosis. Therefore, it is reasonable to presume that improvement would also be seen on the residual limb, so it may also be reasonable to treat the area under the artificial interface with a 1,064 to 1,320 nanometer Nd:YAG laser.[72-74]

Odor

Apocrine sweat is an odorless and sterile substance. Nonetheless, certain bacteria (eg, *Micrococcus* spp. and *Corynebacterium* spp.) modify the secretion into an unpleasant sweaty smell. Rarely, the odor is rancid and patients will present for assistance in management of the foul smell, termed bromhidrosis.[14] Eccrine secretions are also odorless but can soften the skin, allowing bacteria to breakdown keratin also leading to an unpleasant odor. Eccrine bromhidrosis has also been described secondary to ingestion of medications (eg, bromides), foods (eg, garlic), or other metabolic abnormalities. When assisting the patient with an amputation in assessing and managing complaints of odor, the most important aspect is to ensure high-quality hygiene as described previously. A thorough diet and medication history is also encouraged to minimize ingestion of known provocative substances. Topical antimicrobial cleansers (eg, Dial antimicrobial soap, chlorhexidine), prescription antibiotics (eg, clindamycin solution) or a novel glycine-soja stereocomplex agent which has demonstrated promising results, can be attempted for clinical improvement.[75] Finally, odor could emanate from places in the prosthesis not subject to daily hygiene. In cases where odor is a persistent problem, elements of the prosthesis not included in daily cleansing should be investigated by the prosthetist. Such places include between the flexible interface and rigid frame and between the foot shell and foot structure, for example.

Classification Systems

Classification of skin problems is important for multiple reasons. To classify, proper recognition and identification are first necessary. These are early steps in proper management of skin problems. Beyond this, classification is also necessary to facilitate interprofessional dialogue and research. A lack of uniform classification of skin problems is cited as a reason why aggregating epidemiologic data from multiple studies is difficult.[6] This is a valid point. Some studies refer to skin problems by either their diagnosis[8] or by some description of the presenting problem or a combination of both.[36] A classification system has been proposed to either use the morphology or etiology of the amputees' presenting skin problem(s).[6] Both have merit and either may have application depending upon the specific clinical or research question to be answered. However, the etiology of problems may be difficult or, at times, impossible to determine. Therefore, the authors currently consider the morphologic approach to be superior and more useful to both clinical and research teams. The morphologic classification previously recommended is reasonable; however, it may cause some confusion. For instance, infections are listed as both a morphological type as well as in the larger problem list. As difficult a task as it is to create a classification schema, it is necessary. The authors propose a descriptive classification be considered for future interprofessional dialogue and research (**Table 2**).

TABLE 2 Diagnostic Summary of Dermatoses in Amputees

Primary Concern	Specific Diagnosis	Association or Subtype
Dermatitis	a. Atopic dermatitis	—
	b. Contact dermatitis	i. Irritant ii. Allergic
	c. Psoriasis	i. Koebnerization
	d. Lichen planus	—
	e. Intertrigo	—
	f. Urticaria	i. Physical urticaria (pressure)
Infection	a. Bacterial	—
	b. Fungal (nonspecific eczematization)	
	c. Viral	
Volume changes	a. Negative-pressure hyperemia	—
	b. Friction	i. Bullae (blister) ii. Callus iii. Lichenification
	c. Ulceration	i. Pressure sores (decubiti)
	d. Verrucous hyperplasia	—
Tumor	a. Benign	i. Epidermoid (inclusion) cyst ii. Bursa
	b. Malignant	—
Specific concerns	a. Pruritus[a]	—
	b. Xerosis	—
	c. Scarring	i. Atrophic ii. Keloid iii. Hypertrophic
	d. Hyperhidrosis	—
	e. Bromhidrosis	—

[a]In addition to dermatoses previously listed.

Section 4: Management Issues

Summary

Dermatoses are prevalent in persons with amputation compared with the general population, as well as the most prevalent skin conditions reported. Prosthetic use is clearly associated with increased skin issues. Because prosthetic use increases skin problems, prosthetists and other rehabilitation practitioners must first be able to help patients prevent them to the extent possible. When not possible, they must be able to recognize and manage skin problems that occur frequently in this unique cohort. Finally, when skin problems are refractory to routine management or are clearly beyond the experience of the prosthetist, a referral to the primary care physician or dermatologist must be made. When a referral is made for assistance with skin problems, it is vital to include as much history information as possible. This information should include exposures to prosthetic materials and cleaners as well as interventions that have been tried, any changes that have been made, and how long the problem has persisted. At times, prosthetic disuse may be part of the management plan. Interdisciplinary communication and collaboration will ultimately optimize care in such cases.

Commonly occurring dermatoses along with their etiology, morphology, and management have been discussed to facilitate improvements in care and referrals. Finally, classification systems have been considered and introduced. Until tissue and limb regeneration is a reality, exoprostheses will continue as the standard of care. As long as exoprosthetic sockets interface with skin, there will be problems with the skin. Clinicians providing care for persons with limb loss who use prostheses need a fundamental knowledge of how to care for all facets of these unique patients' lives including their skin, the largest and most visible organ system.

References

1. Ziegler-Graham K, MacKenzie EJ, Ephraim PL, Travison TG, Brookmeyer R: Estimating the prevalence of limb loss in the United States: 2005 to 2050. *Arch Phys Med Rehabil* 2008;89(3):422-429.
2. Curran T, Zhang JQ, Lo RC, et al: Risk factors and indications for readmission after lower extremity amputation in the American College of Surgeons National Surgical Quality Improvement Program. *J Vasc Surg* 2014;60(5):1315-1324.
3. Stern RS, Nelson C: The diminishing role of the dermatologist in the office-based care of cutaneous diseases. *J Am Acad Dermatol* 1993;29(5 pt 1):773-777.
4. Bickers DR, Lim HW, Margolis D, et al: The burden of skin diseases: 2004 a joint project of the American Academy of Dermatology Association and the Society for Investigative Dermatology. *J Am Acad Dermatol* 2006;55(3):490-500.
5. Verhoeven EW, Kraaimaat FW, van Weel C, et al: Skin diseases in family medicine: Prevalence and health care use. *Ann Fam Med* 2008;6(4):349-354.
6. Bui KM, Raugi GJ, Nguyen VQ, Reiber GE: Skin problems in individuals with lower-limb loss: Literature review and proposed classification system. *J Rehabil Res Dev* 2009;46(9):1085-1090.
7. Yang NB, Garza LA, Foote CE, Kang S, Meyerle JH: High prevalence of stump dermatoses 38 years or more after amputation. *Arch Dermatol* 2012;148(11):1283-1286.
8. Lyon CC, Kulkarni J, Zimerson E, Van Ross E, Beck MH: Skin disorders in amputees. *J Am Acad Dermatol* 2000;42(3):501-507.
9. Dudek NL, Marks MB, Marshall SC, Chardon JP: Dermatologic conditions associated with use of a lower-extremity prosthesis. *Arch Phys Med Rehabil* 2005;86(4):659-663.
10. Levy SW: Skin problems of the leg amputee. *Prosthet Orthot Int* 1980;4(1):37-44.
11. Hachisuka K, Nakamura T, Ohmine S, Shitama H, Shinkoda K: Hygiene problems of residual limb and silicone liners in transtibial amputees wearing the total surface bearing socket. *Arch Phys Med Rehabil* 2001;82(9):1286-1290.
12. Levy SW, ed: *Skin Problems of the Amputee*. Warren H. Green, Inc., 1983.
13. American Board for Certification in Orthotics, Prosthetics & Pedorthics, Inc: Practice analysis of certified practitioners in the disciplines of orthotics and prosthetics 2014. Available at: https://www.abcop.org/publication/practitioner-practice-analysis. Accessed October 12, 2021.
14. Bolognia JL, Jorizzo JL, Schaffer JV, eds: *Dermatology*, ed 3. Elsevier, Saunders, 2012, No. 1.
15. Tyebkhan G: A study on the pH of commonly used soaps/cleansers available in the Indian market. *Indian J Dermatol Venereol Leprol* 2001;67(6):290-291.
16. Norman RA: Xerosis and pruritus in the elderly: Recognition and management. *Dermatol Ther* 2003;16(3):254-259.
17. Munoz CA, Gaspari A, Goldner R: Contact dermatitis from a prosthesis. *Dermatitis* 2008;19(2):109-111.
18. Nethercott JR, Holness DL: Disease outcome in workers with occupational skin disease. *J Am Acad Dermatol* 1994;30(4):569-574.
19. Ale SI, Maibach HI: Irritant contact dermatitis versus allergic contact dermatitis (Ch 13), in Zhai H, Maback HI, eds: *Dermatoxicology*, ed 6. CRC Press, 2004.
20. Lachappelle J, Maibach HI: *Patch Testing and Prick Testing: A Practical Guide. Official Publication of the ICDRG*. Springer, 2009.
21. Hoare C, Li Wan Po A, Williams H: Systematic review of treatments for atopic eczema. *Health Technol Assess* 2000;4(37):1-191.
22. Green C, Colquitt JL, Kirby J, Davidson P, Payne E: Clinical and cost-effectiveness of once-daily versus more frequent use of same potency topical corticosteroids for atopic eczema: A systematic review and economic evaluation. *Health Technol Assess* 2004;8(47):iii, iv, 1-120.
23. James WD, Berger TG, Elston DM, eds: *Andrews' Diseases of the Skin. Clinical Dermatology*, ed 11. Saunders, Elsevier, 2011.
24. Parisi R, Symmons DP, Griffiths CE, Ashcroft DM: Global epidemiology of psoriasis: A systematic review of incidence and prevalence. *J Invest Dermatol* 2013;133(2):377-385.
25. Highsmith JT, Highsmith MJ: Common skin pathology in LE prosthesis users. *JAAPA* 2007;20(11):33-36, 47.

26. Lang DM, Hsieh FH, Bernstein JA: Contemporary approaches to the diagnosis and management of physical urticaria. *Ann Allergy Asthma Immunol* 2013;111(4):235-241.
27. Peery JT, Ledoux WR, Klute GK: Residual-limb skin temperature in transtibial sockets. *J Rehabil Res Dev* 2005;42(2):147-154.
28. Atanaskova N, Tomecki KJ: Innovative management of recurrent furunculosis. *Dermatol Clin* 2010;28(3):479-487.
29. Highsmith MJ, Cummings S, Highsmith JT: Furunculosis in a transtibial amputee. *Phys Med Rehabil Int* 2014;1(3):4.
30. Smith DG, McFarland LV, Sangeorzan BJ, Reiber GE, Czerniecki JM: Postoperative dressing and management strategies for transtibial amputations: A critical review. *J Rehabil Res Dev* 2003;40(3):213-224.
31. Nawijn SE, van der Linde H, Emmelot CH, Hofstad CJ: Stump management after trans-tibial amputation: A systematic review. *Prosthet Orthot Int* 2005;29(1):13-26.
32. Johannesson A, Larsson GU, Oberg T, Atroshi I: Comparison of vacuum-formed removable rigid dressing with conventional rigid dressing after transtibial amputation: Similar outcome in a randomized controlled trial involving 27 patients. *Acta Orthop* 2008;79(3):361-369.
33. Kahle JT, Highsmith MJ: Transfemoral interfaces with vacuum assisted suspension comparison of gait, balance, and subjective analysis: Ischial containment versus brimless. *Gait Posture* 2014;40(2):315-320.
34. Bruno TR, Kirby RL: Improper use of a transtibial prosthesis silicone liner causing pressure ulceration. *Am J Phys Med Rehabil* 2009;88(4):264-266.
35. Jones RO: Lichen simplex chronicus. *Clin Podiatr Med Surg* 1996;13(1):47-54.
36. Dudek NL, Marks MB, Marshall SC: Skin problems in an amputee clinic. *Am J Phys Med Rehabil* 2006;85(5):424-429.
37. Freeman DB: Corns and calluses resulting from mechanical hyperkeratosis. *Am Fam Physician* 2002;65(11):2277-2280.
38. Salawu A, Middleton C, Gilbertson A, Kodavali K, Neumann V: Stump ulcers and continued prosthetic limb use. *Prosthet Orthot Int* 2006;30(3):279-285.
39. Scheinfeld N, Yu T, Lee J: Verrucous hyperplasia of the great toe: A case and a review of the literature. *Dermatol Surg* 2004;30(2 pt 1):215-217.
40. Kelishadi SS, Wirth GA, Evans GR: Recalcitrant verrucous lesion: Verrucous hyperplasia or epithelioma cuniculatum (verrucous carcinoma). *J Am Podiatr Med Assoc* 2006;96(2):148-153.
41. Levy SW, Allende MF, Barnes GH: Skin problems of the leg amputee. *Arch Dermatol* 1962;85:65-81.
42. Lillis PJ, Zuehlke RL: Cutaneous metastatic carcinoma and elephantiasis symptomatica. *Arch Dermatol* 1979;115(1):83-84.
43. Nakamura H, Hirota S, Adachi S, Ozaki K, Asada H, Kitamura Y: Clonal nature of seborrheic keratosis demonstrated by using the polymorphism of the human androgen receptor locus as a marker. *J Invest Dermatol* 2001;116(4):506-510.
44. Kahana M, Grossman E, Feinstein A, Ronnen M, Cohen M, Millet MS: Skin tags: A cutaneous marker for diabetes mellitus. *Acta Derm Venereol* 1987;67(2):175-177.
45. Paysant J, Andre JM, Martinet N, et al: Transcranial magnetic stimulation for diagnosis of residual limb neuromas. *Arch Phys Med Rehabil* 2004;85(5):737-742.
46. Sehirlioglu A, Ozturk C, Yazicioglu K, Tugcu I, Yilmaz B, Goktepe AS: Painful neuroma requiring surgical excision after lower limb amputation caused by landmine explosions. *Int Orthop* 2009;33(2):533-536.
47. Sarma D, Hansen T, Adickes E: Carcinoma arising in the leg amputation stump. *Internet J Dermatol* 2005;4(1).
48. Jensen P, Hansen S, Moller B, et al: Skin cancer in kidney and heart transplant recipients and different long-term immunosuppressive therapy regimens. *J Am Acad Dermatol* 1999;40 (2 pt 1):177-186.
49. Furukawa H, Yamamoto Y, Minakawa H, Sugihara T: Squamous cell carcinoma in chronic lymphedema: Case report and review of the literature. *Dermatol Surg* 2002;28(10):951-953.
50. American Cancer Society: What are the risk factors for basal and squamous cell skin cancers? https://www.cancer.org/cancer/basal-and-squamous-cell-skin-cancer/causes-risks-prevention/risk-factors.html. Accessed April 21, 2023.
51. Skin Cancer Foundation: Squamous cell carcinoma - Causes and risk factors https://www.skincancer.org/skin-cancer-information/squamous-cell-carcinoma/scc-causes-and-risk-factors/. Accessed April 21, 2023.
52. Kowal-Vern A, Criswell BK: Burn scar neoplasms: A literature review and statistical analysis. *Burns* 2005;31(4):403-413.
53. Gonne E, Collignon J, Kurth W, et al: Angiosarcoma in chronic lymphoedema: A case of Stewart-Treves syndrome. *Rev Med Liege* 2009;64(7-8):409-413.
54. Sharma A, Schwartz RA: Stewart-Treves syndrome: Pathogenesis and management. *J Am Acad Dermatol* 2012;67(6):1342-1348.
55. Schwartz RA, James WD: Stewart-Treves syndrome. Accessed August 1, 2014.
56. Freedberg IM, Eisen AZ, Wolff K, eds: *Fitzpatrick's Dermatology in General Medicine*, ed 5. McGraw-Hill, Inc., 1999, No. 1.
57. Mekic S, Jacobs LC, Gunn DA, et al: Prevalence and determinants for xerosis cutis in the middle-aged and elderly population: A cross-sectional study. *J Am Acad Dermatol* 2019;81(4):963-969.e2.
58. Gutman AB, Kligman AM, Sciacca J, James WD: Soak and smear: A standard technique revisited. *Arch Dermatol* 2005;141(12):1556-1559.
59. Cantu RI, Grodin AJ: *Myofascial Manipulation: Theory and Clinical Application*, ed 2. Aspen Publishers, Inc., 2001.
60. Mensch G, Ellis PM: *Physical Therapy Management of Lower Extremity Amputations*. Aspen Publishing, Inc., 1986.
61. Chaudhry HR, Bukiet B, Siegel M, Findley T, Ritter AB, Guzelsu N: Optimal patterns for suturing wounds. *J Biomech* 1998;31(7):653-662.
62. Ferguson MW, O'Kane S: Scar-free healing: From embryonic mechanisms to adult therapeutic intervention. *Philos Trans R Soc Lond B Biol Sci* 2004;359(1445):839-850.
63. Sabapathy V, Sundaram B, V MS, Mankuzhy P, Kumar S: Human Wharton's Jelly Mesenchymal Stem Cells plasticity augments scar-free skin wound healing with hair growth. *PLoS One* 2014;9(4):e93726.
64. Fast A: Reflex sweating in patients with spinal cord injury: A review. *Arch Phys Med Rehabil* 1977;58(10):435-437.

65. Kang CW, Choi SY, Moon SW, et al: Short-term and intermediate-term results after unclipping: What happened to primary hyperhidrosis and truncal reflex sweating after unclipping in patients who underwent endoscopic thoracic sympathetic clamping? *Surg Laparosc Endosc Percutan Tech* 2008;18(5):469-473.
66. Vorkamp T, Foo FJ, Khan S, Schmitto JD, Wilson P: Hyperhidrosis: Evolving concepts and a comprehensive review. *Surgeon* 2010;8(5):287-292.
67. Kern U, Martin C, Scheicher S, Muller H: Does botulinum toxin A make prosthesis use easier for amputees? *J Rehabil Med* 2004;36(5):238-239.
68. Garcia-Morales I, Perez-Bernal A, Camacho F: Letter: Stump hyperhidrosis in a leg amputee treatment with botulinum toxin A. *Dermatol Surg* 2007;33(11):1401-1402.
69. Charrow A, DiFazio M, Foster L, Pasquina PF, Tsao JW: Intradermal botulinum toxin type A injection effectively reduces residual limb hyperhidrosis in amputees: A case series. *Arch Phys Med Rehabil* 2008;89(7):1407-1409.
70. Kern U, Kohl M, Seifert U, Schlereth T: Botulinum toxin type B in the treatment of residual limb hyperhidrosis for lower limb amputees: A pilot study. *Am J Phys Med Rehabil* 2011;90(4):321-329.
71. Schnider P, Binder M, Auff E, Kittler H, Berger T, Wolff K: Double-blind trial of botulinum A toxin for the treatment of focal hyperhidrosis of the palms. *Br J Dermatol* 1997;136(4):548-552.
72. Goldman A, Wollina U: Subdermal Nd-YAG laser for axillary hyperhidrosis. *Dermatol Surg* 2008;34(6):756-762.
73. Kotlus BS: Treatment of refractory axillary hyperhidrosis with a 1320-nm Nd:YAG laser. *J Cosmet Laser Ther* 2011;13(4):193-195.
74. Letada PR, Landers JT, Uebelhoer NS, Shumaker PR: Treatment of focal axillary hyperhidrosis using a long-pulsed Nd:YAG 1064 nm laser at hair reduction settings. *J Drugs Dermatol* 2012;11(1):59-63.
75. Gregoriou S, Rigopoulos D, Chiolou Z, Papafragkaki D, Makris M, Kontochristopoulos G: Treatment of bromhidrosis with a glycine-soja sterocomplex topical product. *J Cosmet Dermatol* 2011;10(1):74-77.

Chronic Pain After Amputation

LTC Matthew E. Miller, MD • Paul F. Pasquina, MD • LTC David E. Reece, DO

ABSTRACT

Chronic pain after amputation continues to be a substantial problem for both patients and clinicians. Because of the heterogeneous nature of pain and various sources of nociception, proper management often is challenging. Clinicians must place high priority on identifying and aggressively treating pain to not only improve patient comfort but also to allow active participation in rehabilitation. Although a multitude of pharmacologic and nonpharmacologic treatments exist, evidence supporting their clinical effectiveness is limited. Therefore, clinicians should have an understanding of the pathophysiology of pain to best target interventional strategies. Although the goal in managing chronic pain is to reduce pain intensity and frequency, clinicians also must be aware of the functional effect that pain may have on an individual's societal participation and quality of life.

Keywords: amputation; interventional pain and treatment; phantom limb pain; rehabilitation; residual limb pain

Introduction

Managing pain after amputation often is challenging. Aggressive pain control starts in the perisurgical phase and remains a vital part of treatment throughout all phases of recovery after limb loss. The two most recognized categories of pain after amputation are residual limb pain and phantom limb pain. Although these pain syndromes often coexist, they likely have very different pathophysiologies and therefore warrant different treatment strategies. Further complicating pain management strategies are the various phenotypes of pain that exist. Ideally, pain treatment algorithms should be tailored for each individual patient. Often, the pain from the amputation can limit or slow rehabilitation more than the disability from the amputation itself. Although the exact pathophysiology of pain has not been fully discerned, three theories or models (the gate control theory of pain, the neuromatrix theory of pain, and the biopsychosocial model of chronic pain) provide some insight on how the nervous system and environmental factors modulate the experience of pain.[1,2]

This chapter discusses several aspects of postamputation pain, including definitions, basic epidemiology, pathophysiology, and the various treatment options, including both pharmacologic and nonpharmacologic strategies. The available literature on current treatments is reviewed, and strategies are proposed for optimizing effective long-term pain management.

Definitions

The International Association for the Study of Pain defines chronic pain as pain persisting for more than 3 months, but it can also be thought of as maladaptive pain that persists beyond the expected period for the disease state.[3] Postamputation pain can be broadly categorized into two categories: residual limb pain and phantom limb pain. Most individuals experience pain in their residual limb after limb loss. Pain, particularly postsurgical pain, primarily arises from the inflammatory process that occurs after surgical or traumatic tissue damage. The onset of postsurgical residual limb pain is typically immediate and often described as a sharp, pressure-like sensation that is well localized to the distal portion of the residual limb.[4]

Immediately after a limb loss, an individual often continues to feel persistent sensation of a lost body part in the form of touch, pressure, tingling, cold sensation, itching, and motion. This phenomenon is known as phantom sensation. When this abnormal

---

Dr. Miller or an immediate family member has stock or stock options held in Abbvie, Amgen Co, and Pfizer. Dr. Reece or an immediate family member is a member of a speakers' bureau or has made paid presentations on behalf of Abbott, NEVRO, Relievant, and SPR Therapeutics. Neither Dr. Pasquina nor any immediate family member has received anything of value from or has stock or stock options held in a commercial company or institution related directly or indirectly to the subject of this chapter.

This chapter is adapted from Chang MH, Tsao JW: Chronic pain after amputation, in Krajbich JI, Pinzur MS, Potter BK, Stevens PM, eds: *Atlas of Amputations and Limb Deficiencies: Surgical, Prosthetic, and Rehabilitation Principles*, ed 4. American Academy of Orthopaedic Surgeons, 2016, pp 665-676.

sensation becomes unpleasant, it can lead to phantom limb pain, a term first well described during the US Civil War.[5] Some of the more common descriptions of phantom limb pain are as follows: burning, squeezing, knife pressing, and electric shock-like sensations. The frequency and the intensity of phantom limb pain often varies and tends to occur spontaneously. Most phantom limb pain occurs within 8 days after a limb loss, but it may manifest many years after an amputation. Although phantom limb pain typically dissipates in the long term, for some patients the symptoms can be long-standing and have negative consequences on social participation and quality of life. Another term often used when describing phantom limb sensation and pain is telescoping, which refers to a patient's sensation that their missing limb is moving either more proximal or distal than its preamputation anatomic location. It also is common for the location of phantom limb pain to change from affecting an entire limb to just the distal representation of the missing limb.[4]

Epidemiology

In the United States, more than 1.7 million individuals were estimated to be living with limb loss in 2010. This number is projected to increase to 3.6 million by the year 2050. Peripheral vascular disease and diabetes (55%) are the most common causes of amputation, followed by trauma (45%), cancer (<1%), and congenital anomalies (<1%). In the United States, approximately 150,000 surgical amputations are performed annually, mostly for dysvascular indications.[6]

Although previous reports indicate a relatively low prevalence of postamputation pain (in the range of 5% to 10%), more recent surveys indicate that the problem may be much greater. At least one report indicates that of the people with amputations who were surveyed, the prevalence of phantom limb pain ranges from 43% to 80%, and residual limb pain ranges from 43% to 68%.[7] Surveys also indicate that for more than 50% of patients who experience phantom limb pain, their frequency of painful attacks decreases within the first 6 months after amputation. In addition to being discomforting and distressing, phantom limb pain also has a negative effect on quality of life. More than 25% of those with postamputation pain who were surveyed reported that their pain was extremely bothersome, and 85% of these individuals indicated consequential social isolation and an inability to seek and maintain employment.[8,9]

Preexisting pain and poor coping skills may be risk factors for the development of phantom limb pain, particularly for patients with lower limb loss associated with peripheral vascular disease.[10] In some studies, more than 50% of individuals with limb loss express symptoms of depression, which likely has a high correlation with pain intensity.[11] The presence of pain for more than 1 month before amputation has been reported to be associated with an increased incidence of postamputation pain.[12] Hence, it is important to recognize and aggressively treat the patient with preemptive analgesia as well as address signs and symptoms of comorbid depression and anxiety.

Mechanism of Pain

Two broad categories of pain often used to describe postamputation pain are nociceptive and neuropathic. The nociceptive pathway often is thought to mediate residual limb pain, whereas a neuropathic phenomenon is thought to more likely mediate phantom limb pain. Understanding the differences between each pain pathway can be helpful in targeting treatment.

Nociceptive pain is thought to initiate peripherally, typically at the site of tissue or organ damage. Most theories implicate an initial inflammatory cascade, where various sensitizing chemicals—such as bradykinin, serotonin, nitric oxide, and cytokines—are released locally and activate peripheral pain receptors (nociceptors). Once these nociceptors are activated either mechanically or chemically, they generate an electric potential at the distal nerve terminal. If this electric potential exceeds the axon's threshold potential (which often is sensitized or lowered after injury), a resulting action potential then propagates afferently to the dorsal root ganglion and the central nervous system (CNS). After reaching the brain, activation of the somatosensory and limbic systems creates a summative response, causing the patient to experience pain. These basic sequences of pain transmission are referred to as transduction, conduction, transmission, and perception.[13]

In addition to the local inflammatory effect of tissue damage after amputation, the distal ends of transected nerves begin sprouting in a disorganized pattern, forming neuromas, which also may be painful. Neuromas can generate afferent nociceptive action potentials either ectopically or when mechanically irritated. Common sources of mechanical irritation include soft-tissue scarring, inflammation, heterotopic bone formation, or direct pressure from prosthetic sockets. Chronic peripheral nerve firing from neuromas, tissue damage, or inflammation may cause upregulation and sensitization of CNS neurons, contributing to enhanced nociceptive signal transmissions in the spinal cord and the brain. In the face of sustained chronic pain, a persistent, abnormal, unpleasant sensory stimulus leads to peripheral and central sensitization.[14] The term allodynia describes the phenomenon when nonpainful peripheral limb stimulation leads to perceived pain and is frequently associated with neuropathic pain. Other features of neuropathic pain may be paresthesias (ectopic sensations in the limb, typically described as pins and needles) or dysesthesias (ectopic painful sensations in the limb, such as burning and lancinating, knife-like, stabbing pain). Neuropathic pain often is challenging to treat.

Historically, phantom limb pain was considered a psychologic disorder; however, current theories classify the phenomenon as a neuropathic process, with likely involvement at the peripheral, spinal, and supraspinal levels. Some of the proposed theories of phantom limb pain provide potential targets for management (**Figure 1**).

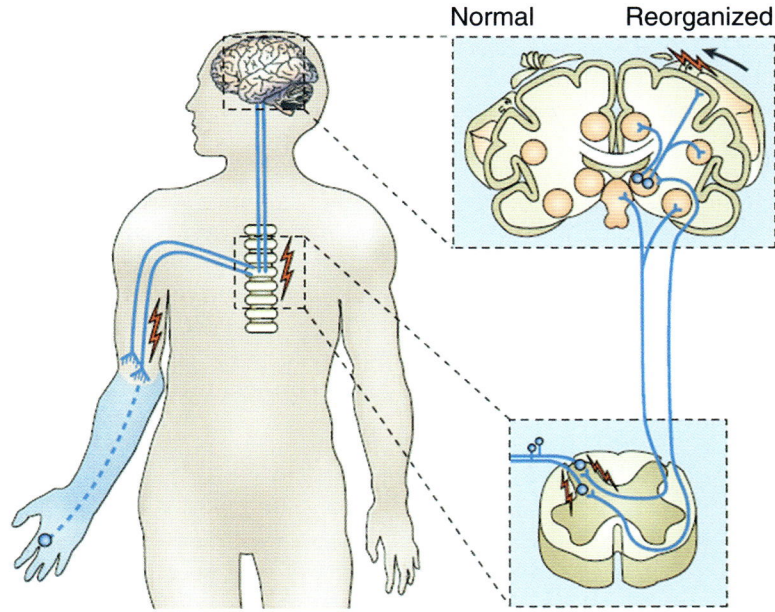

FIGURE 1 Schematic diagram of the areas involved in the generation of phantom limb pain and the primary peripheral and central mechanisms. The peripheral areas include the residual limb and the dorsal root ganglion, and the central areas include the spinal cord and supraspinal centers, such as the brain stem, the thalamus, the cortex, and the limbic system. The proposed mechanisms associated with phantom pain are listed for the peripheral and central nervous systems.

After an injury, the peripheral nervous system, the dorsal root ganglion, and the sympathetic nervous system undergo changes at the cellular level. An increase in the number of transmitters and receptors results in increased sensitivity to pain. These changes affect both ascending and descending pathways within the spinal cord, where the decreased firing of inhibitory interneurons leads to hyperexcitability of painful signals. In addition, downregulation of opioid receptors causes even further excitability of nociceptive signals. Facilitation of N-methyl-D-aspartate (NMDA) receptors at the dorsal horn leads to a wind-up phenomenon and reinforces ectopic activity by A delta and C fibers, which usually carry nociceptive signals, as well as A beta fibers, although these fibers typically are not involved in nociception.[14]

Changes at the cellular level eventually lead to cortical reorganization. Based on the understanding of cortical homunculus and its disproportionate representation of body regions, Ramachandran et al[15] demonstrated that referred sensation of phantom limb pain could be induced when stimuli were applied to the lower part of the face of a person with an upper limb amputation. This phenomenon is likely explained by maladaptive CNS plasticity, where the part of the sensory cortex that was previously mapped to the now amputated limb begins receiving input from other adjacent cortical areas, thereby expanding the receptive field of a missing body part. Reorganization takes place in multiple aspects of the CNS, including the brain stem, the thalamus, the prefrontal cortex, the primary sensory cortex, the motor cortex, the insula, the anterior cingulate cortex, and the parietal cortex. Even in the absence of a limb after amputation, the proprioceptive system still remembers the limb position and creates a proprioceptive memory bank. The resulting disconnect between previous proprioceptive memory and current visual sense makes the patient feel the continued existence of a missing limb.[16] Therefore, the various areas of the brain that are involved in the development of phantom limb pain suggest a complex interplay of visual, sensory, motor, and affective feedback. Further evidence of these pathophysiologic changes is supported through functional MRI studies, which demonstrate reorganization, expansion, and, in certain parts of the brain, even shrinkage in the setting of chronic pain.[17] Fortunately, evidence exists to suggest that these CNS changes are not necessarily permanent. In certain chronic pain conditions such as fibromyalgia, adequate pain control can reverse the CNS changes seen on functional MRI.[18]

Assessment

When assessing individuals with postamputation pain, obtaining a complete history and a thorough physical examination continue to be fundamental in establishing an accurate diagnosis and treatment strategy. Special attention should be focused on assessing a patient's functional status and prosthetic use. A careful examination of the residual limb may reveal common problems, such as skin irritation or breakdown, cyst formation, bursitis, neuromas, heterotopic bone, or myodesis failure. Assessing both prosthetic socket fit and alignment may reveal potential sources of abnormal gait and posture that are causing secondary musculoskeletal pain.[19] Underlying joint pathology should be assessed within the residual limb. Furthermore, clinicians should be reminded that pain from proximal joints or even root injuries may be referred into the distal residual limb. Imaging studies of the residual limb or the spine may help further refine diagnoses. Similarly, laboratory testing should be considered to screen for underlying infection or inflammatory processes.

Screening questionnaires and pain scales, such as the Oswestry Low Back Pain Disability Questionnaire, the McGill Pain Questionnaire, and the Brief Pain Inventory, can help better categorize the quality of pain and functional level. Relying on standard numeric scale assessments of pain, such as the visual analog scale, may have limited clinical value; thus, it also is important to incorporate function-related questions. Some of these questionnaires can be time consuming and may not be practical for use in a busy clinical environment. A recently validated scale, the Defense and Veterans Pain Rating Scale, has a single numeric pain intensity scale plus four supplemental questions to assess sleep, mood, stress, and activity. The main goal of the scale is to provide a simple and quick data-gathering tool to assess how pain affects a patient's function and quality of life[20] (**Figure 2**).

Treatment

Although multiple treatment strategies exist to target the various mechanisms of pain, no single modality is sufficient to treat the heterogeneity and individualized expressions of pain. Strategies to manage postamputation pain include a variety of pharmacologic, nonpharmacologic, and interventional techniques (**Figure 3**).

Adequate pain management begins with preemptive analgesia. Whenever possible, optimal management of postamputation pain should start even before the planned surgery. Existing limb pain before amputation substantially increases the incidence of both residual and phantom limb pain, which emphasizes the importance of aggressive preemptive analgesia.[21] The most commonly used and studied method of preemptive analgesia uses various regional anesthetic techniques. Peripheral nerve and epidural catheters have been used for optimal anesthesia and postsurgical pain management and have been proven to be effective even with devastating and complex traumatic injuries, such as those sustained by wounded service members.

Although regional anesthesia offers greater cardiopulmonary hemodynamic stability compared with general anesthesia, risks include local anesthetic toxicity and the potential for peripheral or central nerve injury.[22] These risks may be decreased by improved techniques, such as real-time ultrasound-guided placement of nerve catheters and readily available intralipid (a reversal agent for local anesthetic toxicity).[23] Therefore, when considering the risk-benefit ratio during the crucial moments after an injury, especially for patients with complex trauma and multiple medical comorbidities, the favorable profile of regional anesthetic should not be ignored. A recent pilot study demonstrated feasibility of peripheral nerve stimulation for postamputation pain in this acute and subacute period, and additional investigations are ongoing.[24]

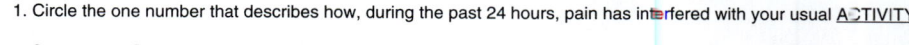
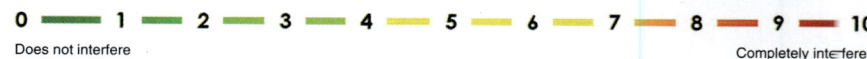
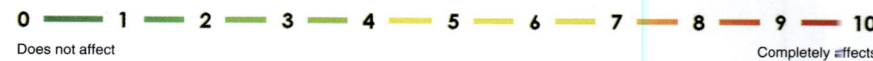
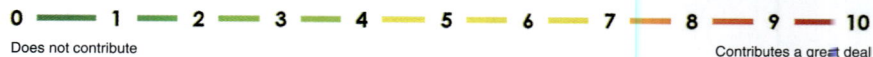

FIGURE 2 Illustration of the supplemental questions for the Defense and Veterans Pain Rating Scale. (Courtesy of the Defense and Veterans Center for Integrative Pain Management, Rockville, MD.)

The use of local anesthesia by means of either a single injection or continuous infusion during the perisurgical period may potentially block the onset of central sensitization and thereby prevent cortical reorganization and the subsequent conversion of pain from acute to chronic. Several review articles, including a Cochrane systematic review, have looked at the evidence for using preemptive analgesia to prevent phantom limb pain. Although numerous studies have been performed, a quality randomized controlled trial (RCT) does not yet exist.[25-28] Among the studies that have demonstrated the effectiveness of regional anesthesia, the incidence of phantom limb pain at 12 months ranged from zero to 8% after the patient received perisurgical epidural analgesia; in comparison, the incidence of development of phantom limb pain in the control group ranged from 27% to 73%.[29] Similar study outcomes in favor of using peripheral nerve catheters with continuous infusion during the postsurgical period exist.[30,31] Although these findings are impressive, several other studies have conflicting results, reporting no benefit in using epidural or peripheral nerve analgesia to prevent postamputation pain.[32-34]

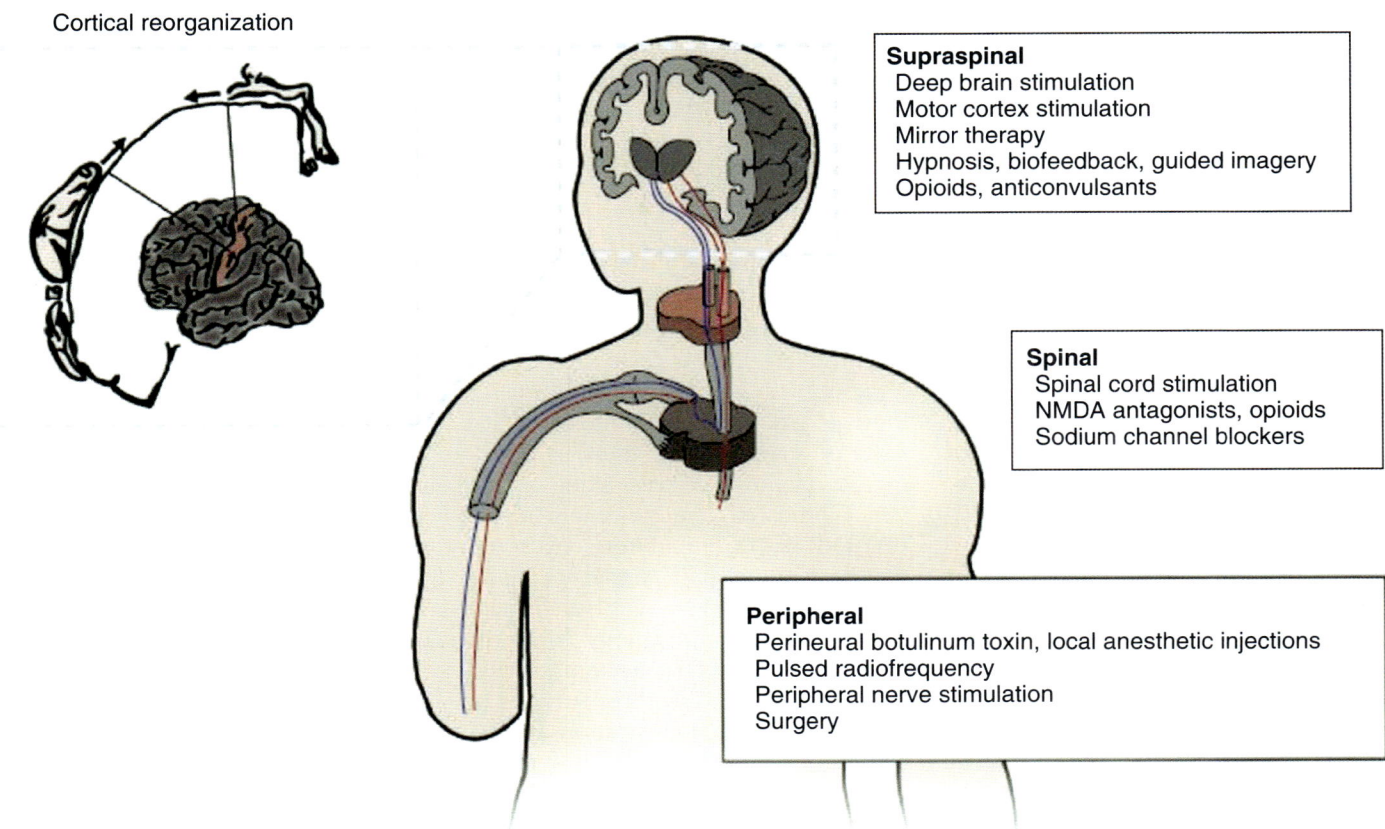

FIGURE 3 Illustration of the treatment modalities for postamputation pain. NMDA = *N*-methyl-D-aspartate

Other pharmacologic agents, such as ketamine, calcitonin, and gabapentin, and nonpharmacologic methods, such as transcutaneous electrical nerve stimulation, show mixed effectiveness as preemptive analgesia. Therefore, more comprehensive RCTs are needed to support their clinical use.[25,35,36]

Pharmacologic Therapies

The most commonly used medications to treat residual and phantom limb pain include opioids, NSAIDs, antidepressants, and anticonvulsants. Although understanding of the mechanism of analgesia and the pathophysiology of nociception has substantially improved, there has not been a corresponding increase in novel drugs introduced in the market.[37] In fact, during the past half century, the number of novel medication classes that have been translated into clinical use beyond the traditional classes has been sparse. Two examples of novel medications include NMDA receptor antagonists and transient receptor potential cation channel subfamily V member 1 receptor blocker, otherwise known as capsaicin.

A Cochrane database review on pharmacologic interventions for phantom limb pain reported that only 13 of 583 existing studies were of good quality.[38] In that report, most of the studied medications fell within the following medication classes: NMDA receptor antagonists, opioids, anticonvulsants, antidepressants, calcitonin, and local anesthetics. Various other reviews also support the use of these medication classes.[25,27,39]

NMDA Receptor Antagonists

Among classifications of medications to manage phantom limb pain, NMDA receptor antagonists have been the most widely studied. NMDA receptor antagonists work by blocking the wind-up phenomenon within the dorsal horn, preventing ectopic discharges and central sensitization. A study using 120 to 180 mg/d of dextromethorphan showed a 50% reduction in chronic phantom limb pain compared with a placebo group.[40] An intravenous dose of 0.4 to 0.5 mg/kg ketamine over a period of 45 minutes to 1 hour also has been shown to be effective in reducing phantom limb pain.[34,41] However, multiple studies looking at the use of up to 30 mg/d of memantine did not yield any benefits.[42,43] The adverse side effects of ketamine include visual hallucinations, and its long-term use can induce liver injury.[44]

Anticonvulsants

Anticonvulsants are commonly used to manage a variety of neuropathic pain conditions and therefore are frequently used for both phantom limb pain and neuropathic residual limb pain. Studies reveal that gabapentin and its cousin pregabalin bind to the α2δ-1 subunit of a voltage-gated calcium channel. A recent study sheds some light on the role of the α2δ-1 receptor.[45] By binding to the α2δ-1 receptor, gabapentin prevents the binding of thrombospondin, a key ingredient in the formation of nerve synapses. This loss of binding of thrombospondin to the α2δ-1 receptor leads to a reduction in CNS synaptogenesis and may partly explain how the gabapentinoid class works in treating pain. Two RCTs looking at the effect of taking gabapentin (up to 2,400 to 3,200 mg/d for 6 weeks) show conflicting results. However, when the results are pooled in a systematic review, the combined results favor the role of gabapentin in reducing phantom limb pain. The adverse effects of gabapentin include sedation, edema, and weight gain.[46,47] Other anticonvulsants, such as topiramate (up to 800 mg/d) have been shown to substantially reduce phantom limb pain in a small number of case series.[48]

Antidepressants

Among various antidepressant medications, amitriptyline is the best studied. Amitriptyline is thought to inhibit serotonin and norepinephrine reuptake and lead to enhancement of descending inhibitory pathways. An RCT by Robinson et al[49] showed that a 6-week trial of amitriptyline titrated up to 125 mg/d did not result in a significant reduction of phantom limb pain compared with a placebo. In contrast, a second RCT by Wilder-Smith et al,[50] using an average dose of 56 mg/d of amitriptyline for 1 month, showed a significant reduction in both residual and phantom limb pain compared with a placebo. The anticholinergic property of this medication causes three common adverse side effects: dry mouth, urinary retention, and sedation. In addition, weight gain is a common report.

Calcitonin

Arendt-Nielsen et al[51] found calcitonin to be useful as an adjunct therapy for various conditions, including phantom limb pain. Although the exact mechanism of its analgesic action is not clear, calcitonin is hypothesized to exert an effect on descending inhibitory pathways within the CNS. Mixed results supporting the use of calcitonin for phantom limb pain have been demonstrated in RCTs. A study by Eichenberger et al[41] involved patients with a median duration of phantom limb pain of approximately 11 years. The treatment group noted no improvement in phantom limb pain after an infusion of calcitonin. Jaeger and Maier[52] studied patients in whom phantom limb pain developed within the first week after an amputation. A single infusion of 200 IU of calcitonin was given to the study group. In more than half of the patients, a reduction in phantom limb pain occurred and was sustained at the 1-year mark. The common adverse side effects of using calcitonin included nausea and flushing.

Opioids

Opioids are clearly the most studied form of analgesia. Morphine is a prototypical opioid derived from opium, which binds to a micro-opioid receptor and has an inhibitory effect on the descending pain signal pathway. Several RCTs have shown benefit with both oral and intravenous forms of morphine in reducing postamputation pain.[53-55] In one RCT, three sessions of daily morphine administration at 0.05 mg/kg bolus followed by 0.2 mg/kg intravenous infusion in a 40-minute period resulted in substantial short-term reductions in both chronic residual and phantom limb pain.[53] The control group receiving intravenous lidocaine at 1 mg/kg bolus followed by 4 mg/kg infusion in a 40-minute period saw a reduction in only residual limb pain. In another study, individuals who used oral morphine (average dose of 112 mg/d) showed a marked reduction in pain (>50%) during an 8-week trial period. The control group, receiving oral mexiletine, showed no improvement in residual and phantom limb pain.[54] A major limitation of both studies was the brief duration of follow-up.

Another RCT looked at the effectiveness of a long-acting morphine. Doses between 70 and 300 mg/d were used with reduction in pain, and the effect remained at 6- and 12-month follow-ups.[55] Tramadol is a unique medication; it acts as a weak opioid and also inhibits the reuptake of both serotonin and norepinephrine. Until recently (2014), tramadol was not categorized as a controlled substance, which led to widespread use. A study by Wilder-Smith et al[50] showed that therapy with a mean tramadol dose of 448 mg/d for 1 month resulted in relief of both residual and phantom limb pain.

When prescribing opioids, it is important to keep in mind the complications that may arise from prolonged use. The long-term use of opioids can lead to osteoporosis, the suppression of endocrine function, the development of opioid-induced hyperalgesia, constipation, and sleep disturbance.[56] In addition, a physical or psychologic dependence on opioids may develop. A physical addiction is characterized by the presence of withdrawal symptoms when abruptly stopping a medication. Therefore, opioid doses should be gradually lowered before discontinuation. A psychologic addiction is characterized by a patient taking an opioid for something other than pain relief. The misuse of opioids may involve taking more than the prescribed dose or diverting (sharing or selling) medications to others. The use of a risk evaluation, such as the opioid risk tool, and mitigation strategies such as patient education can help ameliorate these problems. Such programs involve using questionnaires to assess patterns of use, periodically updating opioid informed consents, counting pills, performing urine drug screens, and being aware of state drug databases.

Polypharmacy

When prescribing several different medications, it is important to be aware of the effects of polypharmacy. It is common to use multiple medications when trying to treat patients with chronic pain. Life-threatening complications, such as serotonin syndrome and Q-T prolongation, can occur with the use of certain antidepressants and opioids.[56] The involvement of a clinical pharmacologist to help treat patients with chronic pain can be a great asset because they can assist with counseling patients and monitoring the proper use of medications.

It is important to remember that the lack of quality evidence does not necessarily preclude the use of certain classes of medications. Nevertheless, studies with more robust evidence will help better guide clinical decision-making processes. In clinical practice, many of the medications listed previously and those in similar classes will continue to be used to manage chronic amputation pain.

Complementary and Integrative Medicine Therapies

Considering the number of adverse reactions associated with many pharmacologic treatments of postamputation pain, it is not surprising that many patients and clinicians explore the use of nonpharmacologic interventions. The advantage of using a variety of complementary and integrative medicine therapies to treat pain is that they tend to be relatively simple, with minimal risk involved, compared with pharmacologic or invasive procedures. Many case reports and uncontrolled studies suggest the beneficial effects of modalities such as acupuncture, biofeedback, guided imagery, yoga, tai chi, relaxation therapy, and transcranial magnetic stimulation. Unfortunately, the quality of evidence that favors the use of these strategies is still lacking.[7,57,58] The transcutaneous electrical nerve stimulation technique is widely used to manage a variety of musculoskeletal conditions and has been studied in patients with postamputation pain as well. A Cochrane review on transcutaneous electrical nerve stimulation use with residual and phantom limb pain shows that although there are no RCTs available, studies suggest a positive trend toward a reduction of postamputation pain.[59]

Among the various controlled ankle motion therapies, mirror therapy has probably gained the most attention. In their 1992 study, Ramachandran et al[15] first introduced the idea of using mirror therapy to treat phantom limb pain. Mirror therapy involves placing a mirror next to the intact limb to create a visual mimic of a limb where the amputated limb would have been (**Figure 4**). Exercise programs involving the movement of the intact limb and visualizing this in the mirror are theorized to reverse a disconnect between visual and proprioceptive feedback of an amputated limb. A functional MRI study by Foell et al[60] showed that mirror therapy could reverse the maladaptive cortical organization within the primary somatosensory cortex and decrease the level of activity within the inferior parietal cortex. The study

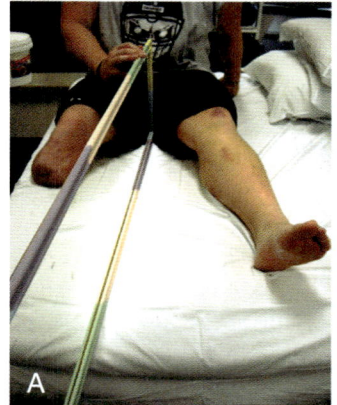 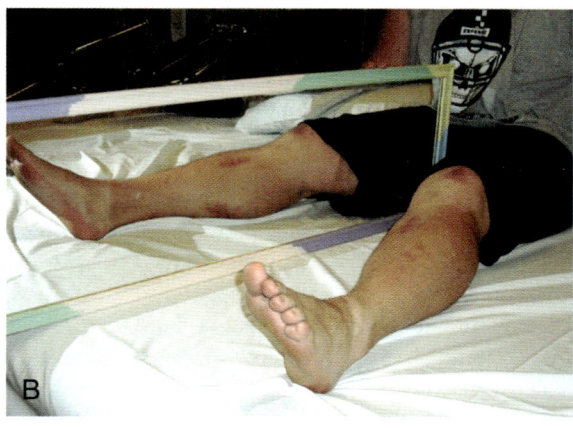

FIGURE 4 **A**, Clinical photograph of a patient with a right transtibial amputation participating in mirror therapy. **B**, Clinical photograph of the same patient showing the effect of mirror therapy for the treatment of phantom limb pain. (Reproduced from Malchow R, King K, Chan B, Weeks S, Tsao J: Pain management among soldiers with amputations, in Walter Reed Army Medical Center Borden Institute, Pasquina PF, Cooper RA, eds: *Care of the Combat Amputee (Textbooks of Military Medicine)*. Department of the Army, 2009, pp 249-250.)

by Foell et al[60] also showed that those patients with less telescoping of the phantom limb were predicted to benefit more from mirror therapy. An RCT by Chan et al[61] showed that after 4 weeks of mirror therapy, all the patients in the mirror therapy group reported a reduction in pain, with a mean decrease of 24 mm on the visual analog scale, whereas the control group failed to show any improvement. A subsequent crossover of the patients showed that a similar level of benefit with mirror therapy was maintained. The results from a small case series suggest that mirror therapy also may play a role in the preemptive treatment of phantom limb pain.[35]

An RCT that looked at cognitive behavioral therapy plus mirror therapy in 59 patients showed that there was no difference in the reduction of anxiety or pain in the cognitive behavioral therapy plus mirror therapy group compared with the group that received only supportive psychotherapy.[62] However, another RCT that looked at the effectiveness of three hypnosis sessions showed a marked decreased in the McGill Pain Questionnaire score compared with the control group after 4 weeks of therapy, showing that hypnosis is effective in treating residual and phantom limb pain.[63]

An obvious need exists for well-designed studies that look at various controlled ankle motion therapies. However, considering the favorable risk-versus-benefit ratio, the use of controlled ankle motion therapies should play an important role in a multimodal treatment strategy to manage chronic postamputation pain.

Peripheral Interventional Techniques

The peripheral nerve is an accessible target for treating patients with chronic postamputation pain. A variety of agents, such as botulinum toxin, corticosteroid, local anesthetic, neurolytic agents (eg, alcohol, phenol), and biologics (eg, tumor necrosis factor) have been injected in and around neuromas to manage postamputation pain. Botulinum toxin may have a role in reducing ectopic discharge in neuromas and depleting substance P (a neurotransmitter) at the dorsal root ganglion. Corticosteroid and tumor necrosis factor are thought to work by means of their anti-inflammatory effects. An RCT that looked at a botulinum toxin injection versus a methylprednisolone acetate–lidocaine injection along a neuroma showed that immediate and sustained relief of residual limb pain occurred in both groups at 6 months but that they had no effect on phantom limb pain.[64] Although many of the available treatment modalities show promise in the treatment of postamputation pain, the lack of high-quality evidence to support these interventions remains a major weakness.[27,65-67]

The local denervation of peripheral nerves by means of radiofrequency (RF) ablation is widely used to treat patients with axial spine pain. The process involves placing a probe on or near the peripheral nerve and heating the probe to 80°C. For postamputation pain, small case reports show that pulsed RF ablation targeting a neuroma can be effective. A notable advantage of pulsed RF over conventional RF ablation is that pulsed RF does not cause permanent damage to surrounding structures because the temperature of the RF probe does not exceed 42°C. To date, no complications associated with pulsed RF have been reported, and this technique may be safer than thermal ablation or cryoablation.[68] The mechanism of analgesia of pulsed RF is not fully understood; however, several studies report that pulsed RF exerts an electric field along the nerve, resulting in prolonged pain signal disruption.

Surgical Treatments

The surgical management of postamputation pain should be reserved for situations in which conservative treatments have failed. Surgical interventions may include, for example, the excision of heterotopic bone, the resection of a neuroma, or the implantation of electrodes in the peripheral nerve, the spinal cord, or the deep brain.

Heterotopic ossification (HO) is the formation of mature lamellar bone outside osseous tissue. These bony projections can lead to residual limb pain and the decreased use of a prosthesis. HO formation is especially common after blast injuries. In a cohort of 213 patients with combat-related injuries, the prevalence of HO was estimated to be approximately 63%.[69,70] Although the incidence of HO in this cohort is high, fewer than 10% of the affected patients require surgical excision. Rates of successful resection have been reported in up to 83% of patients, with most being able to either stop or markedly reduce their use of opioid and/or neuropathic pain medication after 1 year.[69]

As described previously, neuroma formation is expected after peripheral nerve transection; however, not all neuromas are symptomatic. Several studies estimate that symptomatic neuromas occur in approximately 13% to 32% of individuals with acquired amputation.[71] The surgical resection of neuromas is sometimes needed when other conservative methods are unsuccessful. The most common method, historically, of neuroma resection involves transecting the nerve proximal to the neuroma and then burying the end of the nerve within the proximal muscle to protect it from mechanical irritation. Although selected patients who have undergone neuroma resection report excellent relief of residual limb pain, recurrence is common, even after several years.[72,73] Some studies advocate the placement of a silicone cap at the end of a neuroma,[73] although this practice is not widely observed. The use of ultrasonography and magnetic resonance neurography may be helpful in presurgical planning to help better localize symptomatic neuromas.

Recent surgical innovations involve the use of targeted muscle reinnervation (TMR) to treat patients with postamputation neuroma pain. TMR involves reconnecting transected peripheral nerves into the motor end plates of remaining residual limb muscles. Although the technique was originally designed to add myoelectric sites of control for more intuitive prosthetic use, a retrospective study of 15 patients with postamputation neuroma pain who underwent TMR discovered that 14 patients experienced a complete resolution of their pain. TMR is believed to help reduce pain because reinnervation of the residual nerve to a recipient motor nerve branch encourages organized nerve regeneration, thus preventing neuroma recurrence.[74] Pet et al[75] studied the effect of targeted nerve implantation in preventing neuroma-induced pain in two groups by implanting a distal nerve to a partially artificially denervated portion of a motor point within a nearby muscle. In this study, the first group received targeted nerve implantation to prevent occurrence of a neuroma during acute amputation, whereas the second group underwent targeted nerve implantation during neuroma excision. At mean follow-up of 22 months 11 of 12 patients in the first group and 23 of 29 patients in the second group were free of neuroma.[75]

There is some evidence suggesting that reconstructive peripheral nerve surgery also may help reduce phantom limb pain.[76] Reconstructive peripheral nerve surgery is hypothesized to interrupt noxious afferent input from the periphery and prevent central sensitization.[76] Prantl et al[76] examined patients with transtibial amputation who had phantom limb pain. In this study, the sciatic nerve was divided in half in a lengthwise direction proximal to the popliteus fossa. The nerve endings were then reconnected in an end-to-end sling fashion. A substantial reduction in phantom limb pain as well as a decrease in the frequency of occurrences was experienced by 14 of the 15 patients, both of which were sustained after 1 year.

Neuromodulation

The implantation of nerve stimulators is common for treating patients with failed back syndrome and complex regional pain syndrome. Multiple studies also have described the use of a spinal cord stimulator (SCS), a peripheral nerve stimulator, and deep brain stimulation for postamputation pain. Neuromodulation techniques such as SCS or peripheral nerve stimulator should be considered early and can be used in conjunction with the other outlined treatment approaches as opposed to a last-line or salvage procedure. These interventions have been shown to curtain analgesic requirements, thus avoiding side effects and long-term complications such as opioid addiction. Stimulation signals are thought to act by inhibiting the transmission of pain signals via stimulation of the dorsal columns, although mechanisms extend well beyond the gate control theory. For instance, an SCS has been found to improve the hyperexcitability of the wide-dynamic range neurons in the dorsal horn of the spinal cord.

Recently, targeted dorsal root ganglion stimulation has shown promise in managing phantom limb pain, and technology continues to rapidly evolve.[77] Although most reports in the literature are from small case series or retrospective reviews, the success rates of an SCS and deep brain stimulation range from 14% to 83% and 20% to 97%, respectively, with the effects usually lasting several years.[27]

Peripheral nerve stimulation also may be helpful for postamputation pain. Recent advances offer a less invasive technique by using ultrasound guidance to place a percutaneous lead along the distal nerve bundle. In a study by Rauck et al,[78] 16 lower limb amputees with residual and/or phantom limb pain underwent a 2-week home trial of percutaneous peripheral nerve stimulation. Using a novel, single-contact design that selectively stimulated target sensory fibers at 0.5 to 3 cm off the target nerve resulted in comfortable paresthesia without unwanted muscle stimulation. Nine of the 16 patients who tolerated the stimulation reported more than a 50% reduction in pain as well as a corresponding reduction in the Pain Disability Index and sustained improvement at 4 weeks after the end of stimulation.[78]

Future Directions

Continued research is needed to better elucidate the pathophysiologic changes that occur within the nervous system after amputation. In addition, comparative effectiveness studies are lacking to help guide optimal pharmacologic and nonpharmacologic interventional strategies. Outcome measures for such studies should expand beyond pain intensity and include measures of function, quality of life, and behavior. In the future, biomarkers for pain, genome sequencing, the testing of individual neurons, and neuroimaging may help to more accurately define the different phenotypes of pain and better target individualized treatments and minimize adverse effects.[79,80] Targeting specific mechanism-based pathways of pain may prove to be the best therapeutic approach.[81]

SUMMARY

Given the projected increase in the global prevalence of major limb loss, effective pain management in the acute, subacute, and chronic phases of care of individuals with amputation is of critical importance. If untreated, pathophysiologic changes occurring in the peripheral nervous system and the CNS may convert acute pain to chronic pain. Chronic pain should be considered as not only a series of symptoms but also a disease state within itself. Although the proper assessment and management of patients affected by chronic postamputation pain remains challenging, a more thorough understanding of the various pain generators and the physiology of nociception can help better guide clinical practice.

Although beyond the scope of this chapter, the management of complex chronic pain syndromes after amputation often requires the involvement of multiple different specialties and areas of expertise. An ideal pain management team should include a physician with expertise in pain management, a psychiatrist or psychologist, a physiatrist, a physical and occupational therapist, and a clinician skilled and knowledgeable in integrative medicine. Team members should be consistent in their counseling of patients to set realistic expectations that incorporate functionally based goals, rather than solely focusing on reducing pain intensity. By using this approach along with a combination of pharmacologic and nonpharmacologic strategies, it is reasonable to expect that patients will be better able to cope with their pain, improve their functional independence, and pursue more active participation with their families and in their communities.

References

1. Flor H: Phantom-limb pain: Characteristics, causes, and treatment. *Lancet Neurol* 2002;1(3):182-189.
2. Melzack R, Wall PD: Pain mechanisms: A new theory. *Science* 1965;150(3699):971-979.
3. Merskey H, Bogduk N: *Classification of Chronic Pain: Descriptions of Chronic Pain Syndromes and Definitions of Pain Terms*, ed 2. IASP Press, 1994.
4. Jensen TS, Krebs B, Nielsen J, Rasmussen P: Phantom limb, phantom pain and stump pain in amputees during the first 6 months following limb amputation. *Pain* 1983;17(3):243-256.
5. Mitchell SW, Morehouse GR, Keen WW: *Gunshot Wounds and Other Injuries of Nerves*. JB Lippincott, 1864.
6. Ziegler-Graham K, MacKenzie EJ, Ephraim PL, Travison TG, Brookmeyer R: Estimating the prevalence of limb loss in the United States: 2005 to 2050. *Arch Phys Med Rehabil* 2008;89(3):422-429.
7. Moura VL, Faurot KR, Gaylord SA, et al: Mind-body interventions for treatment of phantom limb pain in persons with amputation. *Am J Phys Med Rehabil* 2012;91(8):701-714.
8. Sherman RA, Sherman CJ, Parker L: Chronic phantom and stump pain among American veterans: Results of a survey. *Pain* 1984;18(1):83-95.
9. Sherman RA, Sherman CJ: Prevalence and characteristics of chronic phantom limb pain among American veterans: Results of a trial survey. *Am J Phys Med* 1983;62(5):227-238.
10. Richardson C, Glenn S, Horgan M, Nurmikko T: A prospective study of factors associated with the presence of phantom limb pain six months after major lower limb amputation in patients with peripheral vascular disease. *J Pain* 2007;8(10):793-801.
11. Ephraim PL, Wegener ST, MacKenzie EJ, Dillingham TR, Pezzin LE: Phantom pain, residual limb pain, and back pain in amputees: Results of a national survey. *Arch Phys Med Rehabil* 2005;86(10):1910-1919.
12. Desmond DM, MacLachlan M: Prevalence and characteristics of phantom limb pain and residual limb pain in the long term after upper limb amputation. *Int J Rehabil Res* 2010;33(3):279-282.
13. Raja SN, Dougherty PM, Benzon R: Anatomy and physiology of somatosensory and pain processing, in Benzon HT, Raja SN, Liu SS, Fishman SM, Cohen SP, eds: *Essentials of Pain Medicine*, ed 3. Saunders, 2011, pp 1-7.
14. Flor H, Nikolajsen L, Staehelin Jensen T: Phantom limb pain: A case of maladaptive CNS plasticity? *Nat Rev Neurosci* 2006;7(11):873-881.
15. Ramachandran VS, Stewart M, Rogers-Ramachandran DC: Perceptual correlates of massive cortical reorganization. *Neuroreport* 1992;3(7):583-586.

16. Anderson-Barnes VC, McAuliffe C, Swanberg KM, Tsao JW: Phantom limb pain: A phenomenon of proprioceptive memory? *Med Hypotheses* 2009;73(4):555-558.
17. Kuchinad A, Schweinhardt P, Seminowicz DA, Wood PB, Chizh BA, Bushnell MC: Accelerated brain gray matter loss in fibromyalgia patients: Premature aging of the brain? *J Neurosci* 2007;27(15):4004-4007.
18. Seminowicz DA, Wideman TH, Naso L, et al: Effective treatment of chronic low back pain in humans reverses abnormal brain anatomy and function. *J Neurosci* 2011;31(20):7540-7550.
19. Ehde DM, Czerniecki JM, Smith DG, et al: Chronic phantom sensations, phantom pain, residual limb pain, and other regional pain after lower limb amputation. *Arch Phys Med Rehabil* 2000;81(8):1039-1044.
20. Buckenmaier CC III, Galloway KT, Polomano RC, McDuffie M, Kwon N, Gallagher RM: Preliminary validation of the Defense and Veterans Pain Rating Scale (DVPRS) in a military population. *Pain Med* 2013;14(1):110-123.
21. Nikolajsen L, Ilkjaer S, Krøner K, Christensen JH, Jensen TS: The influence of preamputation pain on postamputation stump and phantom pain. *Pain* 1997;72(3):393-405.
22. Malchow R, King K, Chan B, Weeks S, Tsao J: Pain management among soldiers with amputations, in Walter Reed Army Medical Center Borden Institute, Lenhart MK, Pasquina PF, Cooper RA, eds: *Care of the Combat Amputee (Textbooks of Military Medicine)*. Department of the Army, 2009, pp 234-238.
23. Buckenmaier CI, Blekner L: *The Military Advanced Regional Anesthesia and Analgesia Handbook*. Borden Institute, 2008, pp 6-8.
24. Albright-Trainer B, Phan T, Trainer RJ, et al: Peripheral nerve stimulation for the management of acute and subacute post-amputation pain: A randomized, controlled feasibility trial. *Pain Manag* 2021;12(3):357-369.
25. McCormick Z, Chang-Chien G, Marshall B, Huang M, Harden RN: Phantom limb pain: A systematic neuroanatomical-based review of pharmacologic treatment. *Pain Med* 2014;15(2):292-305.
26. Halbert J, Crotty M, Cameron ID: Evidence for the optimal management of acute and chronic phantom pain: A systematic review. *Clin J Pain* 2002;18(2):84-92.
27. Hsu E, Cohen SP: Postamputation pain: Epidemiology, mechanisms, and treatment. *J Pain Res* 2013;6:121-136.
28. Andreae MH, Andreae DA: Local anaesthetics and regional anaesthesia for preventing chronic pain after surgery. *Cochrane Database Syst Rev* 2012;10:CD007105.
29. Bach S, Noreng MF, Tjéllden NU: Phantom limb pain in amputees during the first 12 months following limb amputation, after preoperative lumbar epidural blockade. *Pain* 1988;33(3):297-301.
30. Madabhushi L, Reuben SS, Steinberg RB, Adesioye J: The efficacy of postoperative perineural infusion of bupivacaine and clonidine after lower extremity amputation in preventing phantom limb and stump pain. *J Clin Anesth* 2007;19(3):226-229.
31. Borghi B, D'Addabbo M, White PF, et al: The use of prolonged peripheral neural blockade after lower extremity amputation: The effect on symptoms associated with phantom limb syndrome. *Anesth Analg* 2010;111(5):1308-1315.
32. Lambert AW, Dashfield AK, Cosgrove C, Wilkins DC, Walker AJ, Ashley S: Randomized prospective study comparing preoperative epidural and intraoperative perineural analgesia for the prevention of postoperative stump and phantom limb pain following major amputation. *Reg Anesth Pain Med* 2001;26(4):316-321.
33. Sahin SH, Colak A, Arar C, et al: A retrospective trial comparing the effects of different anesthetic techniques on phantom pain after lower limb amputation. *Curr Ther Res Clin Exp* 2011;72(3):127-137.
34. Nikolajsen L, Ilkjaer S, Christensen JH, Krøner K, Jensen TS: Randomised trial of epidural bupivacaine and morphine in prevention of stump and phantom pain in lower-limb amputation. *Lancet* 1997;350(9088):1353-1357.
35. Hanling SR, Wallace SC, Hollenbeck KJ, Belnap BD, Tulis MR: Preamputation mirror therapy may prevent development of phantom limb pain: A case series. *Anesth Analg* 2010;110(2):611-614.
36. Karanikolas M, Aretha D, Tsolakis I, et al: Optimized perioperative analgesia reduces chronic phantom limb pain intensity, prevalence, and frequency: A prospective, randomized, clinical trial. *Anesthesiology* 2011;114(5):1144-1154.
37. Kissin I: The development of new analgesics over the past 50 years: A lack of real breakthrough drugs. *Anesth Analg* 2010;110(3):780-789.
38. Alviar MJ, Hale T, Dungca M: Pharmacologic interventions for treating phantom limb pain. *Cochrane Database Syst Rev* 2011;12:CD006380.
39. Griffin SC, Tsao JW: A mechanism-based classification of phantom limb pain. *Pain* 2014;155(11):2236-2242.
40. Ben Abraham R, Marouani N, Weinbroum AA: Dextromethorphan mitigates phantom pain in cancer amputees. *Ann Surg Oncol* 2003;10(3):268-274.
41. Eichenberger U, Neff F, Sveticic G, et al: Chronic phantom limb pain: The effects of calcitonin, ketamine, and their combination on pain and sensory thresholds. *Anesth Analg* 2008;106(4):1265-1273.
42. Maier C, Dertwinkel R, Mansourian N, et al: Efficacy of the NMDA-receptor antagonist memantine in patients with chronic phantom limb pain: Results of a randomized double-blinded, placebo-controlled trial. *Pain* 2003;103(3):277-283.
43. Wiech K, Kiefer RT, Töpfner S, et al: A placebo-controlled randomized crossover trial of the N-methyl-D-aspartic acid receptor antagonist, memantine, in patients with chronic phantom limb pain. *Anesth Analg* 2004;98(2):408-413.
44. Noppers IM, Niesters M, Aarts LP, et al: Drug-induced liver injury following a repeated course of ketamine treatment for chronic pain in CRPS type 1 patients: A report of 3 cases. *Pain* 2011;152(9):2173-2178.
45. Eroglu C, Allen NJ, Susman MW, et al: Gabapentin receptor alpha2delta-1 is a neuronal thrombospondin receptor responsible for excitatory CNS synaptogenesis. *Cell* 2009;139(2):380-392.
46. Bone M, Critchley P, Buggy DJ: Gabapentin in postamputation phantom limb pain: A randomized, double-blind, placebo-controlled, cross-over study. *Reg Anesth Pain Med* 2002;27(5):481-486.
47. Smith DG, Ehde DM, Hanley MA, et al: Efficacy of gabapentin in treating chronic phantom limb and residual limb pain. *J Rehabil Res Dev* 2005;42(5):645-654.
48. Harden RN, Houle TT, Remble TA, Lin W, Wang K, Saltz S: Topiramate for phantom limb pain: A time-series analysis. *Pain Med* 2005;6(5):375-378.
49. Robinson LR, Czerniecki JM, Ehde DM, et al: Trial of amitriptyline for relief of pain in amputees: Results of a

randomized controlled study. *Arch Phys Med Rehabil* 2004;85(1):1-6.
50. Wilder-Smith CH, Hill LT, Laurent S: Postamputation pain and sensory changes in treatment-naive patients: Characteristics and responses to treatment with tramadol, amitriptyline, and placebo. *Anesthesiology* 2005;103(3): 619-628.
51. Arendt-Nielsen L, Hoeck H, Karsdal M, Christiansen C: Role of calcitonin in management of musculoskeletal pain. *Rheumatol Rep* 2009;1(e12):39-42.
52. Jaeger H, Maier C: Calcitonin in phantom limb pain: A double-blind study. *Pain* 1992;48(1):21-27.
53. Wu CL, Tella P, Staats PS, et al: Analgesic effects of intravenous lidocaine and morphine on postamputation pain: A randomized double-blind, active placebo-controlled, crossover trial. *Anesthesiology* 2002;96(4):841-848.
54. Wu CL, Agarwal S, Tella PK, et al: Morphine versus mexiletine for treatment of postamputation pain: A randomized, placebo- controlled, crossover trial. *Anesthesiology* 2008;109(2):289-296.
55. Huse E, Larbig W, Flor H, Birbaumer N: The effect of opioids on phantom limb pain and cortical reorganization. *Pain* 2001;90(1-2):47-55.
56. Benyamin R, Trescot AM, Datta S, et al: Opioid complications and side effects. *Pain Physician* 2008;11(2 suppl):S105-S120.
57. Bolognini N, Spandri V, Olgiati E, Fregni F, Ferraro F, Maravita A: Long-term analgesic effects of transcranial direct current stimulation of the motor cortex on phantom limb and stump pain: A case report. *J Pain Symptom Manage* 2013;46(4):e1-e4.
58. Bradbrook D: Acupuncture treatment of phantom limb pain and phantom limb sensation in amputees. *Acupunct Med* 2004;22(2):93-97.
59. Mulvey MR, Radford HE, Fawkner HJ, Hirst L, Neumann V, Johnson MI: Transcutaneous electrical nerve stimulation for phantom pain and stump pain in adult amputees. *Pain Pract* 2013;13(4):289-296.

60. Foell J, Bekrater-Bodmann R, Diers M, Flor H: Mirror therapy for phantom limb pain: Brain changes and the role of body representation. *Eur J Pain* 2014;18(5):729-739.
61. Chan BL, Witt R, Charrow AP, et al: Mirror therapy for phantom limb pain. *N Engl J Med* 2007;357(21):2206-2207.
62. McQuaid J, Peterzell D, Rutledge T, et al: Integrated cognitive behavioral therapy (CBT) and mirror visual feedback (MVF) for phantom limb pain: A randomized clinical trial. *J Pain* 2014;15(4):S108.
63. Rickard J: *Effects of Hypnosis in the Treatment of Residual Stump and Phantom Limb Pain*. Dissertation. Washington State University, 2004.
64. Wu H, Sultana R, Taylor KB, Szabo A: A prospective randomized double-blinded pilot study to examine the effect of botulinum toxin type A injection versus Lidocaine/Depomedrol injection on residual and phantom limb pain: Initial report. *Clin J Pain* 2012;28(2):108-112.
65. Wolff A, Vanduynhoven E, van Kleef M, Huygen F, Pope JE, Mekhail N: 21. Phantom pain. *Pain Pract* 2011;11(4): 403-413.
66. Dahl E, Cohen SP: Perineural injection of etanercept as a treatment for postamputation pain. *Clin J Pain* 2008;24(2): 172-175.
67. Kern U, Martin C, Scheicher S, Müller H: Treatment of phantom pain with botulinum-toxin A: A pilot study [German]. *Schmerz* 2003;17(2):117-124.
68. West M, Wu H: Pulsed radiofrequency ablation for residual and phantom limb pain: A case series. *Pain Pract* 2010;10(5): 485-491.
69. Potter BK, Burns TC, Lacap AP, Granville RR, Gajewski DA: Heterotopic ossification following traumatic and combat-related amputations: Prevalence, risk factors, and preliminary results of excision. *J Bone Joint Surg Am* 2007;89(3): 476-486.
70. Potter BK, Forsberg JA, Davis TA, et al: Heterotopic ossification following combat-related trauma. *J Bone Joint Surg Am* 2010;92(suppl 2):74-89.

71. Schroeder S: How to address stump neuromas. *Podiatry Today* 2009;22(11). https://www.hmpgloballearningnetwork.com/site/podiatry/how-to-address-stump-neuromas. Accessed January 24, 2023.
72. Sehirlioglu A, Ozturk C, Yazicioglu K, Tugcu I, Yilmaz B, Goktepe AS: Painful neuroma requiring surgical excision after lower limb amputation caused by landmine explosions. *Int Orthop* 2009;33(2):533-536.
73. Ducic I, Mesbahi AN, Attinger CE, Graw K: The role of peripheral nerve surgery in the treatment of chronic pain associated with amputation stumps. *Plast Reconstr Surg* 2008;121(3):908-914.
74. Souza JM, Cheesborough JE, Ko JH, Cho MS, Kuiken TA, Dumanian GA: Targeted muscle reinnervation: A novel approach to postamputation neuroma pain. *Clin Orthop Relat Res* 2014;472(10):2984-2990.
75. Pet MA, Ko JH, Friedly JL, Mourad PD, Smith DG: Does targeted nerve implantation reduce neuroma pain in amputees? *Clin Orthop Relat Res* 2014;472(10):2991-3001.
76. Prantl L, Schreml S, Heine N, Eisenmann-Klein M, Angele P: Surgical treatment of chronic phantom limb sensation and limb pain after lower limb amputation. *Plast Reconstr Surg* 2006;118(7):1562-1572.
77. Eldabe S, Burger K, Moser H, et al: Dorsal root ganglion (DRG) stimulation in the treatment of phantom limb pain (PLP). *Neuromodulation* 2015;18(7):610-616.
78. Rauck RL, Cohen SP, Gilmore CA, et al: Treatment of post-amputation pain with peripheral nerve stimulation. *Neuromodulation* 2014;17(2):188-197.
79. Woolf CJ: Overcoming obstacles to developing new analgesics. *Nat Med* 2010;16(11):1241-1247.
80. Wager TD, Atlas LY, Lindquist MA, Roy M, Woo CW, Kross E: An fMRI-based neurologic signature of physical pain. *N Engl J Med* 2013;368(15):1388-1397.
81. Woolf CJ, Max MB: Mechanism-based pain diagnosis: Issues for analgesic drug development. *Anesthesiology* 2001;95(1):241-249.

Secondary Health Effects of Amputation

CHAPTER 54

Paul F. Pasquina, MD • Brad D. Hendershot, PhD • Brad M. Isaacson, PhD, MBA, MSF, PMP

ABSTRACT

Restoring independence and mobility after amputation remain a primary focus of rehabilitation. However, clinicians who care for individuals with major limb loss should be aware of the long-term health consequences of living with amputation. Evidence indicates that aging with limb loss leads to increased morbidity and mortality from both medical and musculoskeletal complications. It is therefore critical to consider the long-term health risks associated with major limb amputation, as well as understand the pathophysiologic, biomechanical, and psychosocial bases for these increased risks. Familiarity with these secondary effects may help guide optimal management in the acute, subacute, and chronic phases of caring for individuals with amputation, including reducing potential modifiable risk factors, educating patients and families, promoting proper body biomechanics, and optimizing the prescriptions of advanced technologies to help mitigate long-term risks.

Keywords: arthritis; cardiovascular disease; joint degeneration; low back pain; overuse injuries

Introduction

Most healthcare clinicians recognize the immediate challenges for individuals with major limb loss. Restoring mobility and promoting independence with activities of daily living are often the primary focus for both surgical and rehabilitation teams caring for individuals with upper and/or lower limb loss. However, the long-term health consequences associated with limb amputation are frequently underestimated. Issues such as phantom limb pain, prosthetic comfort, and residual limb health may receive more focus than other general health conditions, including diet, exercise, obesity, tobacco use, hypertension, hypercholesterolemia, diabetes, and cardiac disease. In addition, many patients only seek medical attention for problems related to their amputation and may not undergo regular health examinations. Therefore, it is important for all practitioners who interact with individuals with limb loss to be aware of the long-term health risks associated with amputation and to reinforce the importance of healthy life decisions.

Risks for the development of numerous medical and musculoskeletal complications are increased in individuals with major limb loss.[1] Hrubec and Ryder[2] conducted a study commissioned by the US Congress after World War II and reported that the relative risk for death by cardiac disease was 1.6 times greater for veterans with unilateral transfemoral amputation and 3.5 times greater for those with bilateral transfemoral amputation, when compared with age-matched controls with other injuries. Similar findings have been observed for other medical conditions, including long-term musculoskeletal and skin problems. This chapter briefly discusses several complications to highlight their importance in the overall care and well-being of individuals with major limb loss, particularly for optimal long-term outcomes.

Cardiovascular Complications

The prevalence of concomitant cardiovascular disease among patients with acquired lower limb amputation as the result of peripheral vascular disease (PVD) has been estimated to be as high as 75%.[3] In particular, the presence of coronary artery disease, myocardial infarction, congestive heart failure, arrhythmias, abnormal electrocardiographic results, and previous stroke have been associated with perioperative and postoperative mortality.[4] Kannel et al[5] suggested that the loss of a limb because of impaired circulation is a lesser concern for individuals with severe PVD than the morbidity and mortality associated with congestive heart failure, coronary artery disease, and stroke. Huang et al[6] observed 82 patients with symptomatic peripheral artery disease (mean age ± SD, 61.0 ± 12.4 years) and reported that within 21 ± 11 months, 29 patients (35%) underwent amputation and 24 patients (29%) died. Every effort should be made to maximize cardiac function

---

None of the following authors or any immediate family member has received anything of value from or has stock or stock options held in a commercial company or institution related directly or indirectly to the subject of this chapter: Dr. Pasquina, Dr. Hendershot, and Dr. Isaacson.

before amputation surgery, whether using pharmacologic- or revascularization-based therapies.

The rehabilitation of patients who undergo dysvascular-related amputation is particularly challenging because of the high prevalence of associated cardiovascular disease. Preoperative impaired mobility is common among patients with vascular disease, particularly those with associated skin ulceration or symptoms of claudication. Perioperative bed rest, especially in the setting of surgical complications such as wound dehiscence, infection, or venous thrombosis, further contributes to both cardiovascular and musculoskeletal deconditioning. The physiologic effects of deconditioning coupled with the increased metabolic demands required to walk with a transtibial prosthesis (9% to 33% greater demands)[7] or a transfemoral prosthesis (27% to 89% less efficient)[8] also complicate the patient's likelihood of achieving higher levels of ambulation. Davies and Datta[9] reported that only 66% of individuals with dysvascular-related transtibial amputation achieved independent household-level ambulation and only 54% achieved community-level independence; for those with transfemoral amputation, 50% and 29% achieved household and community ambulation, respectively. Even with these challenges, rehabilitation strategies that incorporate specific programs to treat the unique medical issues of each patient can often be effective, especially those that incorporate cardiovascular reconditioning with the traditional approaches of prosthetic fitting and training.[10] Effective rehabilitation strategies also should include adherence to appropriate cardiac precautions such as target levels for heart rate and blood pressure, along with oxygenation monitoring. Although evidence regarding the optimal prosthetic selection is lacking,[11] new advancements in prosthetic components and materials may contribute to enhanced mobility, independence, and quality of life.

It is generally accepted that individuals with acquired amputations as a result of PVD also have a high incidence of comorbid cardiovascular disease; however, there is a greater lifetime risk of cardiovascular disease developing in individuals with trauma-related amputation when compared with their age-matched peers.[2,12] Hrubec and Ryder[2] reported a substantially higher incidence of cardiovascular disease in World War II veterans with traumatic lower limb amputations. In addition, an analysis of Israeli veterans found similar results, reporting a twofold increase in the cardiovascular disease mortality rate in individuals with amputation when compared with a control group matched for age and ethnicity (8.9% versus 3.8%).[12] Although the increased risk of cardiovascular disease may be secondary to factors such as hyperglycemia, hypertension, abdominal obesity, hypercholesterolemia, and hyperlipidemia because of lifestyle and activity restrictions,[13] other physiologic and psychologic factors also can play an important role. Naschitz and Lenger[14] conducted a literature review on possible contributing factors for the development of cardiovascular disease in individuals with traumatic leg amputation. These factors can be behavioral (tobacco and alcohol use); psychologic, especially related to posttraumatic stress (elevated stress hormones and proinflammatory cytokines); social and environmental barriers (resulting in isolation, decreased physical activity, and obesity); dysregulation factors (insulin resistance, sympathetic hyperactivity); and hemodynamic (perturbed arterial flow proximal to the amputation site resulting in intimal wall damage and secondary atherosclerosis). Given the profound influences of cardiovascular disease on overall morbidity and mortality rates, every effort should be made to mitigate modifying risk factors when caring for individuals with limb loss.

Individuals with lower limb amputation also have a higher incidence of abdominal aortic aneurysm. Vollmar et al[15] prospectively evaluated 1,031 male World War II veterans (329 with transfemoral amputation and 702 without amputation). Both groups had comparable arteriosclerotic risk factors, but 5.8% of those with amputation had an abdominal aortic aneurysm, compared with only 1.1% of those without amputation (as confirmed by duplex scanning or arteriography). The increased risk of abdominal aortic aneurysm was attributed to the abnormal hydraulic forces created within the infrarenal aorta as a result of the asymmetric arterial blood flow to the lower limbs after amputation. Therefore, it has been suggested that individuals with lower limb amputation, particularly at a transfemoral or more proximal level, should undergo regular follow-up evaluations to assess the presence of abdominal aortic aneurysm.[16]

Diabetes

Diabetes is the leading cause of nontraumatic lower limb amputation. Although the incidence of amputation in patients with diabetes varies widely across different industrialized and nonindustrialized nations, studies estimate the presence of diabetes increases the relative risk of amputation by a factor of 15 to 20.[17,1] This risk also varies across ethnic and socioeconomically diverse groups.[1] A study by Resnick et al[20] reported that the 8-year cumulative incidence of lower limb amputation for Native American with diabetes was 4.4% and that increased risk was associated with male sex, renal dysfunction, increased ankle–brachial index, and poor glycemic control.

In 2005, the World Health Organization estimated that with appropriate basic management and care of diabetes, up to 80% of all diabetic foot amputations performed were preventable.[21] Aggressive, comprehensive diabetes management, in addition to appropriate screening and treatment of PVD, can prevent many cases of lower limb amputation. Although it is generally understood that diabetes increases the risk of amputation, especially with secondary microvascular disease, the opposite relationship is less well known. As with cardiovascular disease, diabetes is more likely to develop in individuals with traumatic amputation as they age.[22] Individuals with amputation have higher resting insulin levels compared with healthy control patients, which likely reflects a greater insulin resistance. Moreover, this appears to be independent of body mass index, blood pressure, and plasma lipid levels.[23]

Obesity

Weight gain after limb loss can have substantial detrimental effects on overall health, mobility, and quality of life. Kurdibaylo[24] reported that weight gain is greatest during the first year after amputation; the likelihood of obesity increases with more proximal lower limb amputation (37.9%, transtibial; 48.0%, transfemoral) and with bilateral amputation (64.2%). In addition to the overall health risks associated with obesity, excessive weight gain also can contribute to additional challenges to mobility, proper socket fitting (especially with weight fluctuations), and excessive stress on remaining musculoskeletal structures. Within the first 3 months after amputation, tobacco and alcohol use are prevalent (at 55.7% and 72.0%, respectively); of note, despite a mean bodyweight increase of 23 lb during that time, only tobacco use and alcohol consumption were related to development of secondary overuse musculoskeletal conditions.[25] Although individuals with upper limb amputation have been reported to have a higher incidence of overuse injuries to the shoulders, elbows, and wrists,[26] those with lower limb amputation and associated obesity are also more likely to sustain upper limb injuries, particularly when relying on their upper limbs for transferring, wheelchair propulsion, or assisted ambulation. Attention to caloric intake, maintaining a healthy diet, and regular exercise should be incorporated into the early treatment of individuals with both upper and lower limb loss.

Skin Problems

Although upper and lower limb prostheses improve functionality for patients with amputation, the socket interfaces for these devices have been reported to be problematic, especially when fitting individuals with short residual limbs, or those with substantial weight fluctuations, muscular atrophy, or pressure ulcerations.[27-30] Unlike the palms and soles, which are specifically equipped for bearing high loads, residual limb skin is considerably thinner, resulting in the high frequency of skin-related complications associated with prosthesis use.[31] The challenges of socket fitting extend beyond issues of physical comfort and include heat dissipation, excessive sweating,[32,33] skin irritation,[34,35] and, for those with lower limb loss, the inability to walk on challenging terrain.[33] One study investigated skin breakdown in individuals with transfemoral amputation and reported that 30% of patients (26 of 86) had unhealed wounds or damaged skin.[36] Dudek et al[37] retrospectively examined the charts of 745 patients with 828 lower limb amputations. More than 40% reported at least one skin problem, but the cause of amputation (trauma versus PVD) or the presence of comorbid PVD did not correlate with an increased risk of skin problems. The factors associated with an increased incidence of skin problems were amputation level (four times more common with transtibial than transfemoral amputation), being employed or unemployed compared with the retired study cohort, and using either a single cane or no gait aid. Common skin complications included ulceration, epidermoid cysts, follicular hyperkeratosis, calluses, verrucous hyperplasia, atopic eczema, bacterial folliculitis (caused by *Staphylococcus aureus*), tinea infection (caused by *Trichophyton rubrum*), dermatitis, friction erythema, and other rashes.[38] Osseointegration, direct skeletal attachment of an external prosthesis, is becoming a more established treatment option for individuals with lower (and upper) limb amputation; substantially improving upon traditional socket-based prostheses, certainly mitigating skin-related complications but also with potential to provide substantial benefits in functional outcomes and overall quality of life.[39,40]

Musculoskeletal Complications

Degenerative joint disease and other musculoskeletal overuse injuries also have been reported as a long-term consequence of major limb loss. Even with advances in rehabilitation care and prosthetic technology, individuals with major limb loss report a considerably higher prevalence of musculoskeletal conditions, with associated interference in daily activities and reduction in quality of life.[41] For example, among service members with lower limb amputation, the 1-year incidence of developing at least one overuse condition ranges from 59% to 68%;[42] the corresponding incidence for those with upper limb amputation ranges from 60% to 65%.[43] The risks of these complications tend to differ by etiology (traumatic versus vascular), location (upper versus lower limb), and severity (transfemoral versus transtibial amputation). The risk can be further influenced by the duration of time post-injury, because most active ambulators are exposed to continued abnormal body mechanics associated with long-term prosthesis use. Early recognition of these conditions and a more thorough understanding of the mechanisms that contribute to these problems can help guide both rehabilitation and prevention strategies.

Low Back Pain

The frequency and severity of low back pain among individuals with lower limb loss have been well documented, with estimated prevalence ranging from 52% to 89% (substantially higher than the general cohort, 12% to 45%).[44-47] Moreover, a considerable number of individuals with lower limb amputation reported that their back pain was more bothersome than their phantom or residual limb pain and more negatively affected their quality of life.[48] Low back pain is a multifactorial disorder, emphasizing the need for the application of a comprehensive, biopsychosocial model to better understand its development following amputation.[49]

Physical (biomechanical) risk factors likely play a strong contributing role in low back pain development and/or recurrence among individuals with lower limb loss.[50] Focus group interviews have indicated that individuals with lower limb loss perceive uneven postures and compensatory movements of the back as major contributing factors to their pain.[51] Biomechanical studies report larger, more asymmetric trunk movements as common gait features secondary to lower limb loss, including larger forward trunk flexion and sagittal range of motion, as well as lateral trunk flexion (largest in prosthetic stance).[52,53] Repeated exposure to such abnormal trunk motion can predispose individuals with lower limb loss to low back pain through stimulation of embedded nociceptors and/or increasing spinal loads.[54-56] With increasing spinal loads, increased and asymmetric trunk postures and motion impose higher demands on trunk tissues to offset the gravitational and inertial demands of the trunk. Trunk muscle responses are particularly important in responding to spinal loads because of their relatively small moment arms in relation to external forces and/or moments.[57] Among individuals with lower limb loss versus without lower limb loss, measurements of electromyographic activities of the thoracic and lumbar erector spinae identified earlier and more prolonged activations during walking.[58] Because of the cyclic nature of gait, even small increases in load, particularly resulting from muscle forces, could accelerate degenerative joint changes over time.[59] In addition, the presence of pain is likely to further influence these responses, resulting in the recurrence and eventual chronicity of low back pain. Specifically, individuals with transfemoral limb loss, with versus without low back pain, tend to walk with more sustained lumbar rotation toward the prosthetic limb, perhaps because of fear of pain with trunk lateral flexion, which was associated with greater pelvic elevation/hip hiking.[60] Other studies have illustrated either greater axial rotational excursion with low back pain,[61] or oppositional motion patterns in the sagittal and transverse planes.[62] These individuals also have altered coordination and movement variability between the trunk and the pelvis in the frontal and sagittal planes,[63] which are consistent with uninjured individuals with low back pain.

Low back pain is not unique to those with lower limb loss. In a survey of 104 individuals with upper limb loss, 52% reported back pain that was mild ($n = 35$), moderate ($n = 7$), or severe ($n = 12$).[64] These individuals also reported neck pain (45%), as well as pain in the residual (74%) and nonamputated (24%) limbs. However, information for understanding the specific (biomechanical) mechanisms of back pain in populations with upper limb loss is relatively lacking compared with lower limb loss. During bipedal gait, the arms are thought to play a role in regulating angular momentum between the upper and lower body and may contribute to gait stability.[65,66] Biomechanical studies have shown that walking with a restricted or out-of-phase arm swing increases metabolic cost, alters the coordination of movements between the trunk and the pelvis, affects trunk muscle responses, and increases loading in the lower back.[67,68] Investigations of unilateral load carriage (carrying a load in one hand) have demonstrated asymmetric trunk motion, muscle activation, and peak joint loads.[69,70] Upper limb loss may play a similar biomechanical role, particularly regarding postural and muscular asymmetries, whereas habitual use of the nonamputated limb during activities of daily living might support the reported high prevalence of overuse-type injuries and pain in the nonamputated limb.

Psychosocial factors also play an important role in the development and recurrence of low back pain, especially following amputation. Among service members with traumatic amputation, anxiety, fear of movement (ie, kinesiophobia, and employment status are all moderately associated with low back pain-related disability.[71] Greater severity of posttraumatic stress disorder symptoms and more severe depression symptoms are also associated with recurrent low back pain, contributing to a lower quality of life.[72] There is also evidence of somatization among individuals with traumatic amputation;[73] among individuals with low back pain, higher somatization scores have been linked to greater intensity of pain and disability, and lessened likelihood of occupational reintegration.[74] It should be noted that marital status has been associated with a higher risk for low back pain compared with those who are divorced or single, though results from one study do not support such an association with intensity or bothersomeness of low back pain among individuals with lower limb amputation.[45]

Arthritis

Osteoarthritis of the knee and hip joints commonly occurs in older individuals; however, individuals with lower limb loss are at an increased risk for the development of degenerative disease and associated pain at a much younger age, particularly in the knee and hip joints contralateral to amputation. Compared with individuals without amputation, the age-adjusted and body mass–adjusted prevalence ratios for intact-limb knee pain or symptomatic arthritis are 1.3 with transtibial amputation and 3.3 with transfemoral amputation.[75] Similarly, individuals with amputation reported a higher prevalence of hip pain than the general population (15.3% versus 1.1%).[76] These self-reports of pain are supported by radiographic evidence demonstrating joint degeneration.[77-79]

The development of osteoarthritis has been related, in part, to abnormal and repetitive mechanical loading of the affected joints.[80] Individuals with unilateral lower limb loss use compensational walking strategies which transmit larger, more prolonged forces through the contralateral (intact) limb. Limb-loading measurements obtained using formal gait analyses indicated larger peaks, rates, and durations of the vertical ground reaction forces on intact versus prosthetic limbs and relative to uninjured populations.[81,82] Knee adduction moments are another biomechanical measure reflective of medial knee joint loading, although perhaps better associated with the presence and severity of disease than its initiation.[83] Nevertheless, previous investigations have reported greater peak knee adduction moments in intact versus prosthetic limbs[84] and an association with the presence of knee pain,[75] suggesting a potentially greater risk for disease development and progression over time.[85] Muscle and joint contact forces derived from musculoskeletal models identify larger peak loading within the intact limb among high-functioning individuals with unilateral transtibial amputation relative to uninjured controls.[86] It is of note that prosthetic feet that perform more positive ankle work at push-off are associated with reductions in knee adduction moments,[87] although active (versus passive) ankle-foot devices have been shown to provide little benefit regarding biomechanical risk factors for arthritis among young males with transtibial amputation at early points in rehabilitation.[88] The loss of muscular attachments after transfemoral amputation can decrease the mean forces across the ipsilateral (intact side) hip, and this, along with immobilization, can contribute to osteopenia in the nonamputated limb.[78] This reduction in loading has been related to a five-fold decrease in the likelihood of reported pain in the remaining joints of the amputated limb.[75]

The potential occurrence of pathologic joint disorders such as osteoarthritis has been reported to be based on residual limb length; high proximal amputations can create pelvic instability,[89] and transferring loads to a socket-type prosthesis can be more difficult.[90] Joint disorders also can be pronounced in patients with high body mass and lower limb amputations; a 1-lb increase in weight can result in a fourfold increase in compression force on the knee.[91] Kulkarni et al[78] corroborated these biologic principles and noted a threefold increase in the risk of osteoarthritis in the unaffected limb for those with transfemoral compared with transtibial amputations. Therefore, prosthesis users may develop asymmetric gait patterns to alleviate discomfort, with a longer stance occurring on the unaffected limb and a longer swing on the amputated limb during ambulation.[53] Lifestyle and overall activity level modulate risk for joint degeneration and pain.[92]

Osteopenia and Osteoporosis

Bone remodeling is tightly regulated by cells, hormones, and enzymes.[93-95] Although all individuals have cortical and cancellous bone, the quality and mineralization of these osseous tissues vary based on age, activity level, and mechanical loading.[96-99] Physical forces and a minimal effective strain are required to maintain proper bone architecture,[98] and underloading can result in osteopenia and osteoporosis. Both of these skeletal disorders are marked by decreased bone mineral density (BMD) and changes in conformation.[100] Osteopenia and osteoporosis are traditionally measured using dual-energy radiograph absorptiometry and scored based on the number of standard deviations below the mean for young, healthy adults (osteopenia is measured as a T-score between −1.0 and −2.5; osteoporosis is measured as a T-score of −2.5 or less).[101]

Although osteopenia and osteoporosis most frequently occur in elderly postmenopausal women, limb disuse is a primary cause of bone loss and secondary osteoporosis.[26] Nonphysiologic loading and stress shielding can dramatically affect bone health, with cortical erosion noted as early as 6 days after amputation.[102] In 1929, Barber[103] published one of the earliest cases of delayed healing in amputated limbs and reported that osteoporosis occurred in the diaphysis of long bones and appeared to have a "moth-eaten texture." Other studies have corroborated osteoporosis after amputation, and results indicated a reduction in total bone width, an increase in medullary canal width, and a decrease in BMD.[104,105] Most importantly, these factors directly correlated with the time since amputation, often not regained by 12 months of becoming ambulatory,[106] and with the most pronounced effects occurring after protracted periods of unloading.[104]

The main factor resulting in osteopenia and osteoporosis after amputation is believed to be the prosthetic suspension system. Although socket-type prostheses are necessary to restore ambulation, they can exacerbate muscle and skeletal atrophy after amputation because the forces exerted on these tissues do not approach the minimal effective strain threshold.[98,107] MRI studies of high transfemoral amputations have demonstrated pronounced muscle atrophy within the amputated limb for both the cleaved (atrophy range, 40% to 60%) and intact (atrophy range, 0% to 30%) muscles.[53]

In the case of unilateral lower limb loss, the nonamputated limb has an increased likelihood for the development of osteoarthritis, whereas osteopenia or osteoporosis is most likely to develop in the affected limb.[77] Sherk et al[108] evaluated transtibial and transfemoral limb loss with age-matched controls and demonstrated substantial decreases in BMD at the hip and at the distal end of the residual limb. This was most pronounced in individuals with transfemoral amputation. In a study of 75 World War II veterans, Kulkarni et al[78] reported a significant decrease in femoral neck BMD in the amputated limb and significantly lower BMD with transfemoral amputation than transtibial amputation compared with a normal age-matched and sex-matched cohort. Both studies demonstrated that without further medical and rehabilitation interventions, individuals with limb loss may be at an increased risk for osteoporosis and hip fractures. Physical exercise and appropriate prosthetic components are critical for maintaining bone mass and strength.[100]

Economic Effects

In addition to the numerous physical complications that can occur after amputation, there are also economic effects. According to the Amputee Coalition, a standard transtibial prosthesis that allows the user to stand and walk on level ground costs approximately $5,000 to $7,000, and a device that allows the user to become a community walker capable of ascending and descending stairs and traversing uneven terrain costs approximately $10,000.[109] However, these cost estimates may be underreported because several socket changes may be necessary within the first 2 years to accommodate the rapid changes in residual limb volume after amputation.[110]

Smith et al[111] studied individuals with traumatic transtibial amputation and reported that a mean of 1.5 years of continuous prosthetic use were required before an individual was comfortable using a socket, and most patients required four to five prosthetic devices by 5 years after amputation. Another study noted that only 10% of individuals with amputation could traverse a crosswalk in the allotted time, and most individuals were unable to walk continuously for 600 m, the distance required to be an independent community ambulator.[112] These findings increase concern regarding the functionality of current prosthetic devices and the rising healthcare cost for patients. Data from these studies indicate that the cost for individuals who have sustained one major limb loss can exceed $510,000.[113] The economic burden of both limb loss and its associated medical complications can result in healthcare discrepancies and can substantially burden both individuals and the entire healthcare system.[114]

SUMMARY

Major limb amputation is associated with myriad secondary health risks, which individually or collectively can have a substantial negative influence on mobility, morbidity, mortality, and quality of life. Early rehabilitation after amputation, whether because of trauma or disease, should emphasize the promotion of musculoskeletal range of motion, techniques for prosthesis donning and doffing, proper prosthetic fitting and training, restoration of full range of motion and strength, cardiovascular conditioning, and learning proper body biomechanics to mitigate short-term and long-term overuse injuries and secondary musculoskeletal complications. Further understanding of these related risks and developing effective strategies for mitigation is paramount to the successful care of individuals with limb loss to maximize long-term outcomes.

References

1. Robbins CB, Vreeman DJ, Sothmann MS, Wilson SL, Oldridge NB: A review of the long-term health outcomes associated with war-related amputation. *Mil Med* 2009;174(6):588-592.
2. Hrubec Z, Ryder RA: Traumatic limb amputations and subsequent mortality from cardiovascular disease and other causes. *J Chronic Dis* 1980;33(4):239-250.
3. Roth EJ, Park KL, Sullivan WJ: Cardiovascular disease in patients with dysvascular amputation. *Arch Phys Med Rehabil* 1998;79(2):205-215.
4. Hertzer NR: Fatal myocardial infarction following lower extremity revascularization: Two hundred seventy-three patients followed six to eleven postoperative years. *Ann Surg* 1981;193(4):492-498.
5. Kannel WB, Skinner JJ Jr, Schwartz MJ, Shurtleff D: Intermittent claudication: Incidence in the Framingham Study. *Circulation* 1970;41(5):875-883.
6. Huang CL, Wu IH, Wu YW, et al: Association of lower extremity arterial calcification with amputation and mortality in patients with symptomatic peripheral artery disease. *PLoS One* 2014;9(2):e90201.
7. Esposito ER, Rodriguez KM, Ràbago CA, Wilken JM: Does unilateral transtibial amputation lead to greater metabolic demand during walking? *J Rehabil Res Dev* 2014;51(8):1287-1296.
8. Sawers AB, Hafner BJ: Outcomes associated with the use of microprocessor-controlled prosthetic knees among individuals with unilateral transfemoral limb loss: A systematic review. *J Rehabil Res Dev* 2013;50(3):273-314.
9. Davies B, Datta D: Mobility outcome following unilateral lower limb amputation. *Prosthet Orthot Int* 2003;27(3):186-190.
10. Marzolini S, Leung YM, Alter DA, Wu G, Grace SL: Outcomes associated with cardiac rehabilitation participation in patients with musculoskeletal comorbidities. *Eur J Phys Rehabil Med* 2013;49(6):775-783.
11. Cumming J, Barr S, Howe TE: Prosthetic rehabilitation for older dysvascular people following a unilateral transfemoral amputation. *Cochrane Database Syst Rev* 2015;1:CD005260.
12. Modan M, Peles E, Halkin H, et al: Increased cardiovascular disease mortality rates in traumatic lower limb amputees. *Am J Cardiol* 1998;82(10):1242-1247.
13. Shahriar SH, Masumi M, Edjtehadi F, Soroush MR, Soveid M, Mousavi B: Cardiovascular risk factors among males with war-related bilateral lower limb amputation. *Mil Med* 2009;174(10):1108-1112.
14. Naschitz JE, Lenger R: Why traumatic leg amputees are at increased risk for cardiovascular diseases. *QJM* 2008;101(4):251-259.
15. Vollmar JF, Paes E, Pauschinger P, Henze E, Friesch A: Aortic aneurysms as late sequelae of above-knee amputation. *Lancet* 1989;2(8667):834-835.
16. Paes EH, Vollmar JF, Pauschinger P, Mutschler W, Henze E, Friesch A: Late vascular damage after unilateral leg amputation [German]. *Z Unfallchir Versicherungsmed* 1990;83(4):227-236.
17. Carmona GA, Lacraz A, Hoffmeyer P, Assal M: Incidence of major lower limb amputation in Geneva: Twenty-one years of observation [French]. *Rev Med Suisse* 2014;10(447):1997-1998, 2000-2001.
18. Bild DE, Selby JV, Sinnock P, Browner WS, Braveman P, Showstack JA: Lower-extremity amputation in people with diabetes: Epidemiology and prevention. *Diabetes Care* 1989;12(1):24-31.
19. Mier N, Ory M, Zhan D, Villarreal E, Alen M, Tolin J: Ethnic and health correlates of diabetes-related amputations at the Texas-Mexico border. *Rev Panam Salud Publica* 2010;28(3):214-220.
20. Resnick HE, Carter EA, Sosenko JM, et al: Strong Heart Study: Incidence of lower-extremity amputation in American Indians. The Strong Heart Study. *Diabetes Care* 2004;27(8):1885-1891.
21. World Health Organization, International Diabetes Foundation: World Diabetes Day: Too many people are losing lower limbs unnecessarily to diabetes. World Health Organization. News release. 2005. Available at: http://www.who.int/chp/media/news_archive/en/. Accessed February 7, 2015.
22. Yekutiel M, Brooks ME, Ohry A, Yarom J, Carel R: The prevalence of hypertension, ischaemic heart disease and diabetes in traumatic spinal cord injured patients and amputees. *Paraplegia* 1989;27(1):58-62.
23. Peles E, Akselrod S, Goldstein DS, et al: Insulin resistance and autonomic function in traumatic lower limb amputees. *Clin Auton Res* 1995;5(5):279-288.
24. Kurdibaylo SF: Obesity and metabolic disorders in adults with lower limb amputation. *J Rehabil Res Dev* 1996;33(4):387-394.
25. Yepson H, Mazzone B, Eskridge S, Shannon K, Awodele E, Farrokhi S: The influence of tobacco use, alcohol consumption, and weight gain on development of secondary musculoskeletal injury after lower limb amputation. *Arch Phys Med Rehabil* 2020;101(10):1704-1710.

26. Ostlie K, Franklin RJ, Skjeldal OH, Skrondal A, Magnus P: Musculoskeletal pain and overuse syndromes in adult acquired major upper-limb amputees. *Arch Phys Med Rehabil* 2011;92(12):1967-1973.e1.
27. Dillingham TR, Pezzin LE, MacKenzie EJ, Burgess AR: Use and satisfaction with prosthetic devices among persons with trauma-related amputations: A long-term outcome study. *Am J Phys Med Rehabil* 2001;80(8):563-571.
28. Levy SW: Skin problems in the amputee, in Smith DG, Michael JW, Bowker JH, eds: *Atlas of Amputations and Limb Deficiencies: Surgical, Prosthetic, and Rehabilitation Principles*, ed 3. American Academy of Orthopaedic Surgeons, 2004, pp 701-710.
29. Pasquina PF, Bryant PR, Huang ME, Roberts TL, Nelson VS, Flood KM: Advances in amputee care. *Arch Phys Med Rehabil* 2006;87(3, suppl 1):S34-S43.
30. Sullivan J, Uden M, Robinson KP, Sooriakumaran S: Rehabilitation of the trans-femoral amputee with an osseointegrated prosthesis: The United Kingdom experience. *Prosthet Orthot Int* 2003;27(2):114-120.
31. Tortora GJ, Nielsen MT: Structure of the skin, in Roesch B, Trost K, Wojcik L, Muriello L, Raccuia L, eds: *Principles of Human Anatomy*, ed 11. John Wiley & Sons, 2009, p 117.
32. Meulenbelt HE, Geertzen JH, Jonkman MF, Dijkstra PU: Determinants of skin problems of the stump in lower-limb amputees. *Arch Phys Med Rehabil* 2009;90(1):74-81.
33. Hagberg K, Brånemark R: Consequences of non-vascular trans-femoral amputation: A survey of quality of life, prosthetic use and problems. *Prosthet Orthot Int* 2001;25(3):186-194.
34. Salawu A, Middleton C, Gilbertson A, Kodavali K, Neumann V: Stump ulcers and continued prosthetic limb use. *Prosthet Orthot Int* 2006;30(3):279-285.
35. Pierce RO Jr, Kernek CB, Ambrose TA II: The plight of the traumatic amputee. *Orthopedics* 1993;16(7):793-797.
36. Persson BM, Liedberg E: A clinical standard of stump measurement and classification in lower limb amputees. *Prosthet Orthot Int* 1983;7(1):17-24.
37. Dudek NL, Marks MB, Marshall SC, Chardon JP: Dermatologic conditions associated with use of a lower-extremity prosthesis. *Arch Phys Med Rehabil* 2005;86(4):659-663.
38. Lyon CC, Kulkarni J, Zimerson E, Van Ross E, Beck MH: Skin disorders in amputees. *J Am Acad Dermatol* 2000;42(3):501-507.
39. Hebert JS, Rehani M, Stiegelmar R: Osseointegration for lower-limb amputation: A systematic review of clinical outcomes. *JBJS Rev* 2017;5(10):e10.
40. Gerzina C, Potter E, Haleem AM, Dabash S: The future of the amputees with osseointegration: A systematic review of literature. *J Clin Orthop Trauma* 2020;11:S142-S148.
41. Gailey R, Allen K, Castles J, Kucharik J, Roeder M: Review of secondary physical conditions associated with lower-limb amputation and long-term prosthesis use. *J Rehabil Res Dev* 2008;45(1):15-29.
42. Farrokhi S, Mazzone B, Eskridge S, Shannon K, Hill OT: Incidence of overuse musculoskeletal injuries in military service members with traumatic lower limb amputation. *Arch Phys Med Rehabil* 2018;99(2):348-354.
43. Cancio JM, Eskridge S, Shannon K, Orr A, Mazzone B, Farrokhi S: Development of overuse musculoskeletal conditions after combat-related upper limb amputation: A Retrospective Cohort Study. *J Hand Ther* 2021;S0894-1130(21):00075-2.
44. Ehde DM, Smith DG, Czerniecki JM, Campbell KM, Malchow DM, Robinson LR: Back pain as a secondary disability in persons with lower limb amputations. *Arch Phys Med Rehabil* 2001;82(6):731-734.
45. Ephraim PL, Wegener ST, MacKenzie EJ, Dillingham TR, Pezzin LE: Phantom pain, residual limb pain, and back pain in amputees: Results of a national survey. *Arch Phys Med Rehabil* 2005;86(10):1910-1919.
46. Smith DG, Ehde DM, Legro MW, Reiber GE, del Aguila M, Boone DA: Phantom limb, residual limb, and back pain after lower extremity amputations. *Clin Orthop Relat Res* 1999;361:29-38.
47. Devan H, Hendrick P, Hale L, Carman A, Dillon MP, Ribeiro DC: Exploring factors influencing low back pain in people with nondysvascular lower limb amputation: a national survey. *PM R* 2017;9(10):949-959.
48. Taghipour H, Moharamzad Y, Mafi AR, et al: Quality of life among veterans with war-related unilateral lower extremity amputation: A long-term survey in a prosthesis center in Iran. *J Orthop Trauma* 2009;23(7):525-530.
49. Farrokhi S, Mazzone B, Schneider M, et al: Biopsychosocial risk factors associated with chronic low back pain after lower limb amputation. *Med Hypotheses* 2017;108:1-9.
50. Sivapuratharasu B, Bull AM, McGregor AH: Understanding low back pain in traumatic lower limb amputees: A systematic review. *Arch Rehabil Res Clin Transl* 2019;1(1-2):100007.
51. Devan H, Carman AB, Hendrick PA, Ribeiro DC, Hale LA: Perceptions of low back pain in people with lower limb amputation: A focus group study. *Disabil Rehabil* 2015;37(10):873-883.
52. Goujon-Pillet H, Sapin E, Fodé P, Lavaste F: Three-dimensional motions of trunk and pelvis during transfemoral amputee gait. *Arch Phys Med Rehabil* 2008;89(1):87-94.
53. Jaegers SM, Arendzen JH, de Jongh HJ: Prosthetic gait of unilateral transfemoral amputees: A kinematic study. *Arch Phys Med Rehabil* 1995;76(8):736-743.
54. Hendershot BD, Wolf EJ: Three-dimensional joint reaction forces and moments at the low back during overground walking in persons with unilateral lower-extremity amputation. *Clin Biomech* 2014;29(3):235-242.
55. Hendershot BD, Shojaei I, Acasio JC, Dearth CL, Bazrgari B: Walking speed differentially alters spinal loads in persons with traumatic lower limb amputation. *J Biomech* 2018;70:249-254.
56. Yoder AJ, Petrella AJ, Silverman AK: Trunk – Pelvis motion, joint loads, and muscle forces during walking with a transtibial amputation. *Gait Posture* 2015;41(3):757-762.
57. Granata KP, Marras WS: The influence of trunk muscle coactivity on dynamic spinal loads. *Spine* 1995;20(8):913-919.
58. Butowicz CM, Acasio JC, Dearth CL, Hendershot BD: Trunk muscle activation patterns during walking among persons with lower limb loss: Influences of walking speed. *J Electromyogr Kinesiol* 2018;40:48-55.
59. Kumar S: Theories of musculoskeletal injury causation. *Ergonomics* 2001;44(1):17-47.
60. Devan H, Dillon MP, Carman AB, et al: Spinal and pelvic kinematics during gait in people with lower-limb amputation, with and without low back pain: An exploratory study. *J Prosthet Orthot* 2017;29(3):121-129.
61. Morgenroth DC, Orendurff MS, Shakir A, Segal A, Shofer J, Czerniecki JM: The relationship between lumbar spine

kinematics during gait and low-back pain in transfemoral amputees. *Am J Phys Med Rehabil* 2010;89(8):635-643.

62. Fatone S, Stine R, Gottipati P, Dillon M: Pelvic and spinal motion during walking in persons with transfemoral amputation with and without low back pain. *Am J Phys Med Rehabil* 2016;95(6):438-447.

63. Russell Esposito E, Wilken JM: The relationship between pelvis-trunk coordination and low back pain in individuals with transfemoral amputations. *Gait Posture* 2014;40(4):640-646.

64. Hanley MA, Ehde DM, Jensen M, Czerniecki J, Smith DG, Robinson LR: Chronic pain associated with upper-limb loss. *Am J Phys Med Rehabil* 2009;88(9):742-751.

65. Bruijn SM, Meyns P, Jonkers I, Kaat D, Duysens J: Control of angular momentum during walking in children with cerebral palsy. *Res Dev Disabil* 2011;32(6):2860-2866.

66. Ortega JD, Fehlman LA, Farley CT: Effects of aging and arm swing on the metabolic cost of stability in human walking. *J Biomech* 2008;41(16):3303-3308.

67. Collins SH, Adamczyk PG, Kuo AD: Dynamic arm swinging in human walking. *Proc Biol Sci* 2009;276(1673):3679-3688.

68. Callaghan JP, Patla AE, McGill SM: Low back three-dimensional joint forces, kinematics, and kinetics during walking. *Clin Biomech* 1999;14(3):203-216.

69. Corrigan LP, Li JX: The effect of unilateral hockey bag carriage on the muscle activities of the trunk and lower limb of young healthy males during gait. *Res Sports Med* 2014;22(1):23-35.

70. Zhang XA, Ye M, Wang CT: Effect of unilateral load carriage on postures and gait symmetry in ground reaction force during walking. *Comput Methods Biomech Biomed Engin* 2010;13(3):339-344.

71. Butowicz CM, Silfies SP, Vendemia J, Farrokhi S, Hendershot BD: Characterizing and understanding the low back pain experience among persons with lower limb loss. *Pain Med* 2020;21(5):1068-1077.

72. Mazzone B, Farrokhi S, Hendershot BD, McCabe CT, Watrous JR: Prevalence of low back pain and relationship to mental health symptoms and quality of life after a deployment-related lower limb amputation. *Spine (Phila Pa 1976)* 2020;45(19):1368-1375.

73. Durmus D, Safaz I, Adıgüzel E, et al: Psychiatric symptoms in male traumatic lower limb amputees: Associations with neuropathic pain, locomotor capabilities, and perception of body image. *J Mood Disord* 2015;5:164-172.

74. Licciardone JC, Gatchel RJ, Kearns CM, Minotti DE: Depression, somatization, and somatic dysfunction in patients with nonspecific chronic low back pain: Results from the OSTEOPATHIC Trial. *J Am Osteopath Assoc* 2012;112:783-791.

75. Norvell DC, Czerniecki JM, Reiber GE, Maynard C, Pecoraro JA, Weiss NS: The prevalence of knee pain and symptomatic knee osteoarthritis among veteran traumatic amputees and nonamputees. *Arch Phys Med Rehabil* 2005;86(3):487-493.

76. Struyf PA, van Heugten CM, Hitters MW, Smeets RJ: The prevalence of osteoarthritis of the intact hip and knee among traumatic leg amputees. *Arch Phys Med Rehabil* 2009;90(3):440-446.

77. Burke MJ, Roman V, Wright V: Bone and joint changes in lower limb amputees. *Ann Rheum Dis* 1978;37(3):252-254.

78. Kulkarni J, Adams J, Thomas E, Silman A: Association between amputation, arthritis and osteopenia in British male war veterans with major lower limb amputations. *Clin Rehabil* 1998;12(4):348-353.

79. Melzer I, Yekutiel M, Sukenik S: Comparative study of osteoarthritis of the contralateral knee joint of male amputees who do and do not play volleyball. *J Rheumatol* 2001;28(1):169-172.

80. Maly MR: Abnormal and cumulative loading in knee osteoarthritis. *Curr Opin Rheumatol* 2008;20(5):547-552.

81. Pruziner AL, Werner KM, Copple TJ, Hendershot BD, Wolf EJ: Does intact limb loading differ in servicemembers with traumatic lower limb loss?. *Clin Orthop Relat Res* 2014;472(10):3068-3075.

82. Sagawa Y Jr, Turcot K, Armand S, Thevenon A, Vuillerme N, Watelain E: Biomechanics and physiological parameters during gait in lower-limb amputees: A systematic review. *Gait Posture* 2011;33(4):511-526.

83. Mündermann A, Dyrby CO, Andriacchi TP: Secondary gait changes in patients with medial compartment knee osteoarthritis: Increased load at the ankle, knee, and hip during walking. *Arthritis Rheum* 2005;52(9):2835-2844.

84. Lloyd CH, Stanhope SJ, Davis IS, Royer TD: Strength asymmetry and osteoarthritis risk factors in unilateral trans-tibial amputee gait. *Gait Posture* 2010;32(3):296-300.

85. Miyazaki T, Wada M, Kawahara H, Sato M, Baba H, Shimada S: Dynamic load at baseline can predict radiographic disease progression in medial compartment knee osteoarthritis. *Ann Rheum Dis* 2002;61(7):617-622.

86. Ding Z, Jarvis HL, Bennett AN, Baker R, Bull AM: Higher knee contact forces might underlie increased osteoarthritis rates in high functioning amputees: A pilot study. *J Orthop Res* 2021;39(4):850-860.

87. Morgenroth DC, Segal AD, Zelik KE, et al: The effect of prosthetic foot push-off on mechanical loading associated with knee osteoarthritis in lower extremity amputees. *Gait Posture* 2011;34(4):502-507.

88. Esposito ER, Wilken JM: Biomechanical risk factors for knee osteoarthritis when using passive and powered ankle-foot prostheses. *Clin Biomech* 2014;29(10):1186-1192.

89. James U, Oberg K: Prosthetic gait pattern in unilateral above-knee amputees. *Scand J Rehabil Med* 1973;5(1):35-50.

90. Jaegers SM, Arendzen JH, de Jongh HJ: Changes in hip muscles after above-knee amputation. *Clin Orthop Relat Res* 1995;319:276-284.

91. Messier SP, Gutekunst DJ, Davis C, DeVita P: Weight loss reduces knee-joint loads in overweight and obese older adults with knee osteoarthritis. *Arthritis Rheum* 2005;52(7):2026-2032.

92. Welke B, Jakubowitz E, Seehaus F, et al: The prevalence of osteoarthritis: Higher risk after transfemoral amputation? – A database analysis with 1,569 amputees and matched controls. *PLoS One* 2019;14(1):e0210868.

93. Behari J: Elements of bone biophysics, in Behari J, ed: *Biophysical Bone Behaviour: Principles and Applications*. John Wiley & Sons, 2009, pp 1-52.

94. Ross FP, Cristiano AM: Nothing but skin and bone. *J Clin Invest* 2006;116(5):1140-1149.

95. Sela J, Gros UM, Kohavi D, et al: Primary mineralization at the surfaces of implants. *Crit Rev Oral Biol Med* 2000;11(4):423-436.

96. Currey JD: Changes in the impact energy absorption of bone with age. *J Biomech* 1979;12(6):459-469.

97. Rosenbaum TG, Bloebaum RD, Ashrafi S, Lester DL: Ambulatory activities maintain cortical bone after total hip arthroplasty. *Clin Orthop Relat Res* 2006;450(450):129-137.

98. Frost HM: Mechanical determinants of bone modeling. Metab Bone Dis Relat Res 1982;4(4):217-229.

99. Lane JM, Vigorita VJ: Osteoporosis. J Bone Joint Surg Am 1983;65(2):274-278.

100. Giannotti S, Bottai V, Dell'osso G, et al: Disuse osteoporosis of the upper limb: Assessment of thirty patients. *Clin Cases Miner Bone Metab* 2013;10(2):129-132.

101. Cranney A, Jamal SA, Tsang JF, Josse RG, Leslie WD: Low bone mineral density and fracture burden in postmenopausal women. *CMAJ* 2007;177(6):575-580.

102. Barber CG: The detailed changes characteristic of healing bone in amputation stumps. *J Bone Joint Surg* 1930;12:353-359.

103. Barber CG: Immediate and eventual features of healing in amputated bones. *Ann Surg* 1929;90(6):985-992.

104. Cundy T, Grey A: Mechanisms of cortical bone loss from the metacarpal following digital amputation. *Calcif Tissue Int* 1994;55(3):164-168.

105. Schäfer ML, Pfeil A, Renz DM, et al: Effects of long-term immobilisation on cortical bone mass after traumatic amputation of the phalanges estimated by digital X-ray radiogrammetry. *Osteoporos Int* 2008;19(9):1291-1299.

106. Bemben DA, Sherk VD, Ertl WJJ, Bemben MG: Acute bone changes after lower limb amputation resulting from traumatic injury. *Osteoporos Int* 2017;28(7):2177-2186.

107. Todd TW, Barber CG: The extent of skeletal change after amputation. *J Bone Joint Surg Am* 1934;16:53-64.

108. Sherk VD, Bemben MG, Bemben DA: BMD and bone geometry in transtibial and transfemoral amputees. *J Bone Miner Res* 2008;23(9):1449-1457.

109. Mitka M: Advocates seek better insurance coverage for amputees needing limb prostheses. *J Am Med Assoc* 2008;299(18):2138-2140.

110. Sanders J: Pressure ulcer research: Current and future perspectives, in Bader DL, Bouten CH, Colin D, Oomens CW, eds: *Stump-Socket Interface Conditions*. Springer-Verlag, 2005, pp 129-147.

111. Smith DG, Horn P, Malchow D, Boone DA, Reiber GE, Hansen ST Jr: Prosthetic history, prosthetic charges, and functional outcome of the isolated, traumatic below-knee amputee. *J Trauma* 1995;38(1):44-47.

112. Lerner-Frankiel MB, Vargas S, Brown M, Krusell L, Schoneberger W: Functional community ambulation: What are your criteria? *Clin Manag* 1986;6:12-15.

113. MacKenzie EJ, Jones AS, Bosse MJ, et al: Health-care costs associated with amputation or reconstruction of a limb-threatening injury. *J Bone Joint Surg Am* 2007;89(8):1685-1692.

114. Sheehan TP, Gondo GC: Impact of limb loss in the United States. *Phys Med Rehabil Clin N Am* 2014;25(1):9-28.

Surgical Management of Residual Limb Complications

CHAPTER 55

COL Benjamin Kyle Potter, MD, FAAOS, FACS

ABSTRACT

Major limb amputations, regardless of the indication, are fraught with possible, and unfortunately often frequent, complications. For patients with severe medical comorbidities and limited functional potential, complications may devastate an already limited quality of life or represent preterminal events. Conversely, many patients with excellent functional potential cannot achieve their goals because of persistently symptomatic residual limbs that preclude high-level prosthesis use and function. Many of the most frequent complications may be prevented with appropriate patient and amputation-level selections, excellent surgical technique, sound fitting of the prosthesis, and supervised, graduated rehabilitation. Other than overt deep infection or frank wound dehiscence, most complications should be initially managed with a trial of nonsurgical therapies and serial prosthetic socket modifications. However, for patients with persistently symptomatic residual limbs refractory to nonsurgical management and an identifiable cause(s) for symptoms, limited or complete revision surgery may dramatically improve residual limb health, prosthesis use, patient satisfaction, and quality of life.

Keywords: bursitis; heterotopic ossification (HO); infection; neuroma; ulceration

Introduction

Major limb amputations are often a devastating event for patients and their families. Patients with severe medical comorbidities and limited functional reserve often become nonambulatory as a result of amputation, and removal or loss of an injured or diseased limb from younger, healthier patients with superb functional potential nonetheless may severely affect their quality of life. The removal of a diseased or injured limb is ostensibly a simple surgical procedure, but the amputation often results in frequent early and late complications and, unfortunately, countless potential technical errors. Although often maligned as simple, ablative endeavors, amputations should be viewed, approached, and performed as complex reconstructive procedures that, when necessary, offer a patient the best opportunity for maximal functional recovery.

The historical dogma that most individuals with an amputation heal, obtain a prosthesis, and resume normal or somewhat activity-limited lives is unsupported by the available literature. Rather, ample evidence indicates that complications and revision procedures remain frequent after amputation because of a variety of complications.[1-4] Both surgical and functional outcomes after major limb amputations are often poor. However, compelling evidence exists that—particularly when an organic complication or a cause of symptoms is identified in patients with persistently symptomatic residual limbs—appropriate complication management or residual limb revision may relieve symptoms and improve patient function.[3,4] Moreover, it is noteworthy that many of the risk factors for early complications (such as diabetes, anticoagulant use, transfer from another facility, prior revascularization, and renal failure) are not modifiable.[5,6] Expeditious, focused, and competent complication management does not necessarily represent a setback or treatment failure; rather, it presents another opportunity to optimize patient outcomes and improve quality of life.

Early Complications

Delayed Wound Healing, Marginal Necrosis, and Wound Dehiscence

Delayed healing, marginal necrosis of the incision, and frank wound dehiscence represent the most frequent early complications of amputations, with approximately 60% of early residuum complications requiring surgery and up to 42% of all patients requiring revision surgery.[7,8] Likewise, some form of delayed wound healing may affect up to 40% of patients with transtibial amputation.[9,10] The reasons for delayed wound healing are numerous. In patients with dysvascular disease or diabetes, decreased tissue perfusion is frequently responsible. Selection of the appropriate amputation level and healing potential may be determined with

Dr. Potter or an immediate family member serves as an unpaid consultant to Biomet and serves as a board member, owner, officer, or committee member of the Society of Military Orthopaedic Surgeons.

transcutaneous partial pressure of oxygen measurements (values greater than 20 to 30 mm Hg are ideal), an ankle-brachial index (a value greater than 0.5 is ideal), and a clinical evaluation.[11] It should be noted that ankle-brachial index values may be falsely elevated in some patients with dysvascular disease and noncompressible, calcified vessels. Diligent attention to appropriate presurgical perfusion restoration and optimization, even when amputation is required or inevitable, as well as meticulous level selection, perisurgical multidisciplinary care, and surgical technique may dramatically reduce wound healing complications rates.[12] In patients with traumatic injuries, infection, or cancer, it is critical to ensure that only overtly viable tissue flaps are retained and to avoid unnecessary fasciocutaneous flap dissection and stripping. When in doubt, flap viability should be assessed by gross appearance and visible capillary bleeding with the tourniquet deflated and/or demonstrated by means of staged débridement or revision and closure procedures. Fasciocutaneous or myofasciocutaneous flaps also may be assessed intrasurgically with fluorescent, near-infrared, laser-assisted indocyanine green angiography.[13] Although so-called flaps of opportunity (rather than the generally named and described flaps referenced throughout most of this text) may be used by necessity in these patient populations, well-vascularized, described flaps are advocated whenever practicable without substantively affecting residual limb length or amputation level. Incisional negative pressure wound therapy has been demonstrated in a randomized trial to improve the outcomes of orthopaedic fracture wounds at risk and represents a useful adjunct measure after amputation closure.[14]

Current nutritional status and, when practicable, presurgical optimization of such status may be critical in improving healing rates and preventing early complications. Serum albumin levels greater than 3.5 g/dL as well as total lymphocyte counts greater than 1,500 mm³ have been correlated with improved lower limb amputation healing potential.[15,16] For more detailed nutritional assessment, prealbumin levels greater than 20 g/dL serve as a general marker of adequate protein intake.

Delayed healing, in the absence of wound necrosis or overt dehiscence, should be managed with prolonged suture retention, compressive dressing and edema control (ideally an elastic shrinker stocking), close monitoring, and nutritional optimization. Margin necrosis may result from suboptimal surgical technique and may (sometimes) be avoided by using careful tissue handling and tension-free, layered closure with diligent skin edge eversion. Minor edge necrosis or focal wound dehiscence often is managed nonsurgically, with diligent local wound care and close monitoring. Although complete healing and epithelialization is not an absolute prerequisite for initial prosthetic fitting and early wear, adequate time for myodesis and deep tissue healing, as well as documented serial improvement of wounds both before and after fitting, are required. For more extensive edge necrosis, a decision must be made regarding the probable depth of necrosis and the nutritional status and healing potential of the patient, as well as the mobility of adjacent tissues to determine the feasibility of wound excision and delayed primary closure. McCullough[17] recommended excision of the necrotic areas if they extended more than 12 mm from the incision line. Often, this is achievable with concurrent revision closure under minimal tension, without substantive flap elevation and dissection creating risk of additional necrosis, if adequate time has elapsed since the index procedure such that postsurgical edema has largely resolved.

When simple excision and closure are not feasible, simple débridement and healing by secondary intention may be pursued for patients with superficial necrosis and adequate bone coverage. Patients with overt acute or progressive wound dehiscence, particularly caused by trauma (eg, falls onto the residual limb), should be managed with thorough débridement and revision closure if no evidence of deep infection or necrosis exists. More extensive, full-thickness necrosis, with or without dehiscence, frequently requires proximal revision of the amputation (**Figure 1**). In patients without vascular pathology (those with trauma or tumor) for whom such a revision would require extensive residual limb shortening or loss of a joint level, candidacy for free tissue transfer should be assessed by consulting with a microsurgical specialist.

Infection

Wound infections remain common after major limb amputation and are a concern after amputations for diabetes-related and dysvascular foot and limb infections. Infection rates ranging from 13% to 34% also have been reported in several recent studies of trauma-related amputations.[2-4] Infection management starts with prevention. Infection risk may ostensibly be minimized by débriding all nonviable tissue, meticulous flap

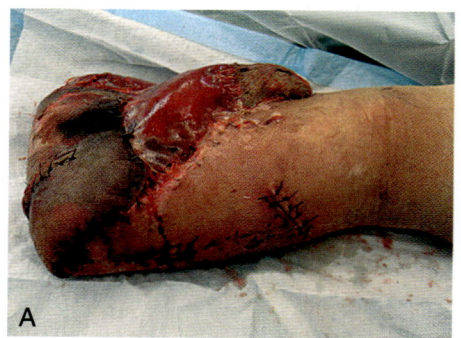 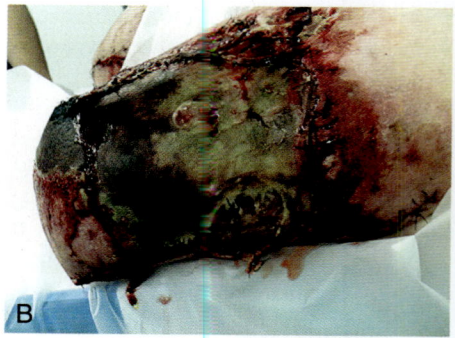

FIGURE 1 **A**, Intrasurgical photograph of a left transtibial amputation complicated by a proximal tibial fracture after medial gastrocnemius flap and dermal substitute placement. Marginal necrosis of the lateral skin incision and epidermolysis and partial necrosis of the posterior myofasciocutaneous flap are seen. **B**, Intrasurgical photograph of a right transfemoral amputation closed with a long posterior flap complicated by catastrophic skin necrosis and resulting infection.

handling, appropriate amputation-level selection, sound sterile technique, staged closures when indicated, perisurgical antibiotic administration, smoking cessation, and nutritional optimization, in addition to tight glucose management for patients with diabetes. For patients undergoing chemotherapy or those with HIV infection, an absolute neutrophil count greater than 1,000 cells/mL and rising (ie, the absence of neutropenia) should be achieved presurgically whenever possible.

Postsurgical fluid collections are common after amputations but are not necessarily an indication for either drainage or débridement. In a series of generally older patients, Singh et al[18] found a 27% rate of early residual limb fluid collections, with most resolving within 30 days. In a separate study of combat-related trauma amputations, Polfer et al[19] reported a 55% rate of early fluid collections; after 3 months, the rate of early fluid collections decreased to 11%. In the absence of clinical indicators of infection, such as erythema, fever, and wound drainage, fluid collections within residual limbs were neither indicative nor predictive of infection.[19]

Established infections within residual limbs are initially managed similar to any other musculoskeletal infection. Superficial infections (such as cellulitis without copious or purulent wound drainage) should be managed with antibiotics and close observation. As a rule, deep infections require formal surgical débridement. In the absence of physiologic instability or sepsis in a patient, broad-spectrum antibiotics should not be used presurgically; they should be administered only after deep tissue cultures are obtained in an otherwise sterile environment. Wound swabs or bedside cultures have no proven utility and frequently demonstrate polymicrobial growth and skin flora contamination. Antibiotic coverage is subsequently narrowed postsurgically based on culture speciation and sensitivities, often in consultation with an infectious disease specialist.

Most patients with deep infections should be treated in a staged fashion. At least one second-look procedure should be performed 24 to 72 hours after the initial thorough surgical débridement to ensure that all residual tissue remains viable and all gross evidence of infection has been eradicated. Despite the absence of controlled studies, antibiotic-impregnated polymethyl methacrylate beads and negative pressure wound therapy with reticulated open-cell foam are useful adjuncts to wound management and infection control between débridement procedures.[20] Provisional anchorage of soft tissues (fascia, myodesis) over antibiotic beads or negative pressure wound therapy sponges with colored monofilament suture between procedures may prevent soft-tissue retraction and facilitate residual limb length and level retention when revision closure is eventually attempted. After all gross infection has been controlled and residual limb wound stability demonstrated, amputation revision and closure over drains is performed, with a period of continued postsurgical antibiotic administration. One study demonstrated that topical antibiotic powder application at the time of wound closure may be effective to prevent and/or treat infections for both primary closure and revision procedures.[21] Residual limb shortening is sometimes required to achieve robust, tension-free closure after a deep infection, but this is generally modest and may be minimized or avoided entirely by adhering to the recommendations previously described. In patients with severe necrotizing soft-tissue infections or massive tissue necrosis, proximal amputation revision may be required.

Joint Contractures

Joint contractures can substantially affect and limit prosthetic fit, use, and function. Contractures that are present presurgically should be assessed and accounted for during surgical decision making, amputation-level selection, and presurgical patient and family counseling. Mild contractures are generally well tolerated and, in some patients, may be improved with focused therapy and nonsurgical management if they do not worsen postsurgically. In select patients, moderate trauma-related contractures may be addressed and improved surgically by lysing adhesions with or without adjacent muscleplasty (eg, quadricepsplasty) and manipulation under anesthesia. Such cases are best addressed in a staged fashion, before (in the elective setting) or after amputation, because the additive pain of concurrent procedures and the inability to tolerate socket use to facilitate joint rehabilitation postsurgically often precludes concurrent residual limb and joint rehabilitation. Severe contractures or overt joint ankylosis should prompt a reevaluation of the planned amputation levels. For example, a patient who is older than 70 years and has severe knee flexion or extension contractures will not optimally benefit from transtibial amputation, and knee disarticulation or transfemoral amputation should be strongly considered.

In patients with normal or nearly normal presurgical range of motion of the proximal joints, contractures are best managed with diligent prevention. Partial foot amputations require careful, balanced tendon reconstructions and should frequently include Achilles tendon lengthening or release intraoperatively. Virtually all other amputation levels simply require dedicated daily therapy for all proximal joints, most notably the knee and elbow. Range of motion and stretching exercise programs are started immediately after the procedure, and patients are encouraged to perform maximal range of motion exercises on their own several times per day between therapy sessions. Both formal and independent therapy are facilitated by good postsurgical pain control and the liberal use of peripheral nerve and epidural catheters. To avoid resting hip and knee flexion, pillows should not be used under a transfemoral residual limb or behind the knee of a patient with a transtibial amputation, even though many patients find resting hip and knee flexion most comfortable for these respective levels. For transfemoral amputations, mandatory flat supine and prone lying for a few hours a day is useful.

Some centers use bracing treatment, splinting, or casting postsurgically, particularly for transtibial amputations. Despite good intentions, however, such interventions create the risk of additional potential complications because decubitus ulcers or eschars may form, even with diligent attention to padding, cutouts, and other precautions (**Figure 2**). In the absence of immediate postsurgical prosthetic placement at an experienced center, splint or cast placement is typically not necessary in a compliant, motivated patient.

Myodesis Failure

The advantages of formal myodesis creation include restoration of physiologic resting muscle tension and greater residual limb control, improved soft-tissue anchorage, and preventing instability, prosthesis shifting, deep bursa formation, and superficial ulceration. Although adductor magnus myodesis, as popularized by Gottschalk,[22] is perhaps most critical for patient function, the author of this chapter advocates myodesis or tenodesis for all transosseous amputation levels and many disarticulations.

Myodesis failure rarely occurs in an attritional, chronic fashion. Most cases are acute or related to trauma or prosthesis use and are noted by the patient (**Figure 3**). Partial tears of a myodesis—without muscle detachment and retraction or soft-tissue instability—verified by both the physical examination and advanced imaging (ultrasonography or MRI), often are managed nonsurgically with a period of rest from prosthesis use and subsequent resumption and rehabilitation. Complete failures in high-functioning patients are best managed with early surgery, before muscle retraction, tendon atrophy, and scarring preclude anatomic myodesis repair.[4]

Late Complications and Residual Limb Pain

Evaluation

Late residual limb complications are common, and revision rates range from 21% to almost 50% in trauma-related amputations.[1-4] Patients who have late residual limb complaints require a thorough evaluation. Although the obvious inclination and clinician bias is to focus almost solely on the residual limb, completing a full, detailed history is critical. Key clinical data include the original injury or disease, evaluation of the amputation level(s) and surgical technique as well as any infections or revision procedures, and patient demographics and medical comorbidities. Recent trauma and change in function or symptoms, age and adjustment frequency of the prosthesis, current and past prosthesis usage, functional goals, and any psychosocial barriers to achieving those goals all require assessment. Next, a thorough skin and residual limb examination is performed, including assessment of myodesis and myoplasty stability and function, palpation for symptomatic neuromas, and assessment of proximate joint range of motion and strength. The prosthesis should be examined for fit and wear. Orthogonal radiographs of the residual limb are then obtained, including weight-bearing radiographs in the prosthesis for lower limb amputations.

A clear tendency in many practices is to avoid revision surgery on any apparently well-healed residual limb and simply refer the patient to the prosthetist, physiatrist, and/or primary care physician. Although the initial management of many late residual limb problems is and should be nonsurgical, many such patients are very uncomfortable, and when this approach is mentioned, it often is rejected. In patients for whom an organic cause of residual limb symptoms is identified and not corrected by a concerted trial of nonsurgical measures, focal or complete revision may dramatically improve patient function, acceptance of the prosthesis, and quality of life.[1,3,4] Exploratory surgery, however, is generally not advocated.

Neuromata and Neurogenic Pain

All transected nerves form neuromas as normal anatomic sequelae. Myriad techniques have been proposed for neuroma and symptom prevention in the acute setting, but no conventional

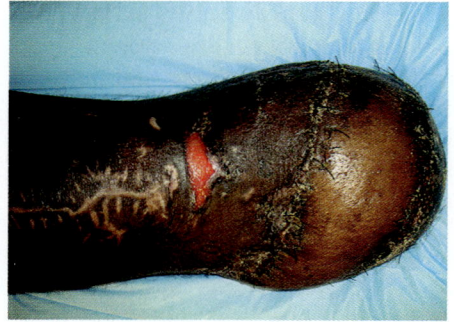

FIGURE 2 Clinical photograph of a left transtibial amputation closed with a distal medial latissimus dorsi free tissue transfer complicated by pressure ulceration over the tibial tuberosity because a postsurgical splint was used.

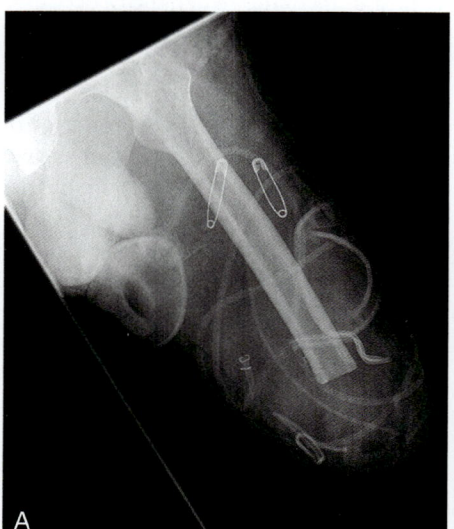
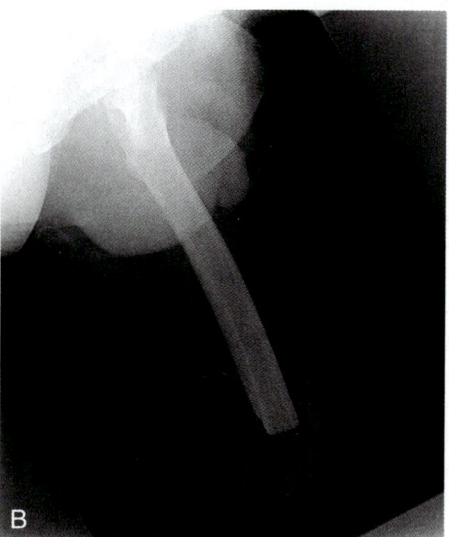

FIGURE 3 **A**, Postsurgical AP radiograph of a left transfemoral amputation closed with two vascular clips on the adductor tendon (intact myodesis) near the distal medial femur. **B**, Lateral radiograph of the same transfemoral amputation 5 months later demonstrating proximal migration of the vascular clips consistent with myodesis failure after the patient felt a pop and noted increased pain and decreased residual limb control.

procedure has proven superior to a simple traction neurectomy (placing the resulting neuroma well proximal to the terminal residuum, ideally in a well-padded location remote and protected from pressure and mechanical stimulation) until recently.

Even if nerves are appropriately managed initially (**Figure 4**), some residual limb neuromas will become symptomatic because of subcutaneous locations, prosthesis use, and long-term atrophy of the soft-tissue envelope. The examination should focus on palpating for neuromas and determining if the symptoms can be reproduced with direct pressure or percussion testing (the Tinel sign). Neuroma-related pain typically manifests as a shock-like stimulus that progresses proximally along the parent nerve and/or distally into the residual phantom limb. The diagnosis of deep neuromas may be confirmed with MRI or ultrasonography localization.[23,24] Suspected distal neuromas also can be confirmed with a diagnostic injection around the proximal nerve and the reassessment of patient symptoms. From a diagnostic perspective, proximal injection is preferred to injection around the neuroma itself because other local sources of pain may be masked by the local anesthetic.

Nonsurgical management is indicated initially for most patients, particularly if the symptoms are intermittent in nature or of recent onset. Prosthetic socket fit can be optimized by avoiding pressure on symptomatic areas. A therapeutic injection of corticosteroid around the neuroma, often under ultrasound guidance, may decrease adjacent inflammation and neuroma irritation. Although the effect is temporary, some patients report lasting relief with such measures. Other less invasive options include percutaneous radiofrequency ablation of the neuroma or the proximal nerve, attempting to deaden the nerve, or inducing a proximal neuroma in continuity, effectively moving the neuroma to a proximal site, hopefully in a more protected and less symptom-prone location.

Because of recent advances and evolving but growing evidence of efficacy for targeted muscle reinnervation and peripheral nerve interface regenerative to prevent or treat symptomatic neuromata and/or phantom pain,[25-27] including for dysvascular patients,[28] this chapter's author no longer advocates simple revision traction neurectomy or most patients requiring surgery for either or both of these indications. Advanced nerve management techniques, including targeted muscle reinnervation and peripheral nerve interface, for neuroma and phantom pain prevention and management (as well as for terminal device control) are discussed in detail elsewhere in this text. Care should be taken with regard to the deinnervation of distal muscle groups useful for current or future myoelectric prosthesis control or needed for distal padding during any revision nerve procedures.

When evaluating patients for possible elective amputation in the setting of preexisting neurogenic pain, such as complex regional pain syndrome (previously known as reflex sympathetic dystrophy), a degree of caution should be exercised. The study by Dielissen et al[29] has disproportionately influenced the literature on this topic, but their series reported 100% recurrence of symptoms in the residual limb after amputation. Generally much better results have been reported by other authors, including the author of this chapter;[30] however, re-amputation for recurrent neuropathic pain does not appear to be effective.[31] At a minimum, therefore, patients seeking elective amputation for pain should be carefully screened by not only the surgeon but also a psychiatrist and a pain management specialist experienced in this area. If the decision to proceed with elective amputation is ultimately made, the amputation must be performed proximal to the level of the associated nerve injury and/or associated pain with strong consideration for concurrent targeted muscle reinnervation and/or regenerative peripheral nerve interface, as discussed elsewhere.

Bursitis

Adventitious bursae represent normal anatomic structures that form in response to repetitive friction. They frequently develop on the terminal residual limbs of active patients with amputations, although palpable bursae develop more commonly in patients with poor soft-tissue coverage over osseous prominences, because of ill-fitting prosthetic sockets, or both. Small, asymptomatic bursae are physiologic and of no consequence if irritation is minimized with intimate prosthetic socket fit.[32] The term bursitis refers to bursae that become inflamed and enlarged because of chronic irritation. Such bursae are generally well circumscribed, transilluminant, somewhat fluctuant, and variably tender masses. Initial treatment is nonsurgical and includes ice, rest, compression, anti-inflammatory medications, and prosthetic modifications.

Aspiration of a bursa should be performed only in patients with suspected septic bursitis, which is manifested by erythema, pain, and/or fever, to avoid seeding an aseptic bursa or inadvertently creating a bursal fistula. Septic bursae require drainage or formal excisional débridement and antibiotic therapy. Conversely, aseptic bursae should not be excised unless the underlying anatomy is concurrently altered to mitigate the risk of bursal recurrence by removing the irritating retained suture or implants, prominent bone contouring, and/or improving stable local soft-tissue coverage via myodesis revision.[33]

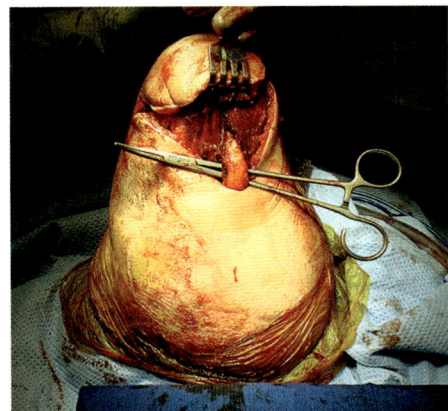

FIGURE 4 Intrasurgical photograph of the posterior aspect of a right transfemoral amputation during revision surgery for a symptomatic sciatic neuroma, demonstrating that the sciatic nerve has been myodesed with the hamstrings into the posterior aspect of the distal femur.

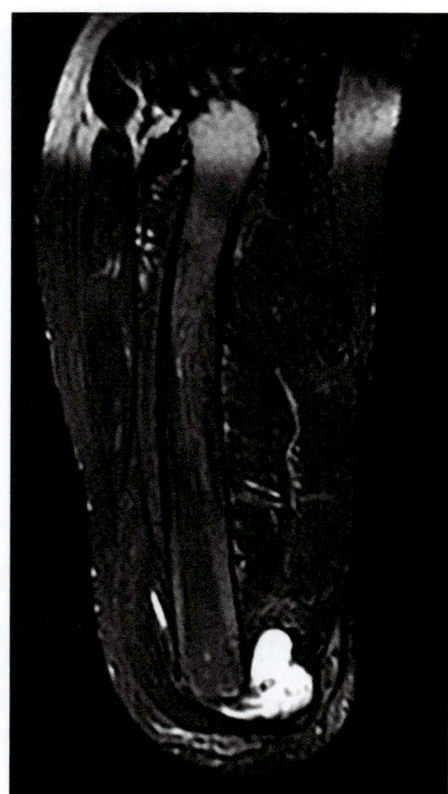

FIGURE 5 Sagittal T2-weighted MRI of a left transfemoral amputation with a symptomatic deep bursa caused by detachment of the hamstring myodesis and demonstrating fluid collection near the distal femur and adjacent detached muscle.

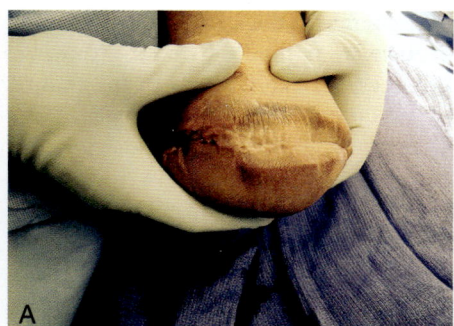 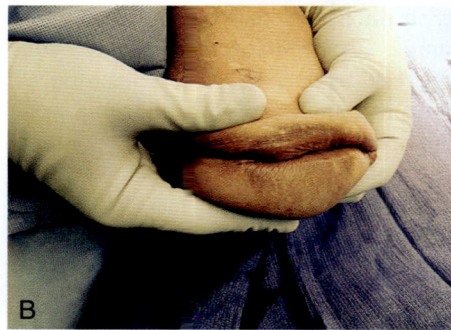

FIGURE 6 **A**, Clinical photograph of a right transtibial amputation with an invaginated scar line adherent to the distal tibia and myodesis. **B**, Clinical photograph demonstrating the resulting hypermobility of adjacent distal soft tissue, causing ulceration of the prominent, mobile skin.

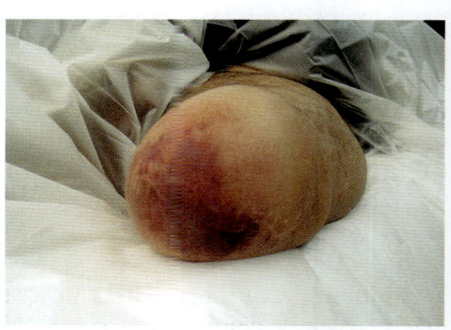

FIGURE 7 Clinical photograph of a left transfemoral amputation with symptomatic, redundant hypermobile soft tissue and reflecting acroangiodermatitis resulting from chronic irritation in the prosthetic socket and the vacuum suspension system.

Deep bursae also may develop over bone, particularly the distal femur in transfemoral amputations if only a quadriceps-hamstring myoplasty has been performed or myodesis failure of these same muscle groups occurs (**Figure 5**). Painful crepitus and palpable grinding with axial loading and shear force may develop. For some patients, prosthetic and liner modifications are successful in stabilizing the distal muscle mass. In those who require surgery, complete bursal excision should be performed concurrent with a stabilizing myodesis of the hamstrings or quadriceps muscles, in addition to retention or restoration of the adductor myodesis. This myodesis is followed by myoplasty of the secondary muscle group, thus creating a myodesis-by-proxy of both residual muscle groups and maximizing residual soft-tissue stability to prevent recurrence. Deep bursal tissue should be sent for culture, but infection is rarely involved in the absence of other clinical indicators. Synovial bodies and particulate debris within bursa are common and are not, in and of themselves, unusual or indicative of infection.

Hypermobile Myoplasty and Redundant Soft Tissues

On some occasions, attempts to construct a viable, robust soft-tissue envelope are overzealous, or soft tissues become lax across time as the residual limb approaches terminal atrophy. More commonly, open amputations are swollen at the time of definitive revision and closure because of distal infection, associated trauma, or reactive hyperemia from tourniquet use. As swelling decreases during the postamputation period, residual limbs that were barely closable intrasurgically may develop abundant and redundant skin and adipose tissue. This problem is then further exacerbated with cutaneous stress relaxation and underlying muscle atrophy. Regardless of the inciting circumstances, the occasional result is a soft-tissue envelope that is both redundant and hypermobile; this is inconsequential for the patient who is asymptomatic and has no skin or instability problems in a well-fitting socket. However, because of skin hypermobility and adjacent scar adherence, recurrent ulceration develops in some patients (**Figure 6**), or they experience uncomfortable and functionally limiting socket instability because of hyperdynamic skin and adipofascial tissue (**Figure 7**). In such instances, scar revision with excision of the redundant fasciocutaneous tissue may provide sound relief and facilitate durable, comfortable socket fitting. For patients with a large amount of loose adipofascial tissue, a longitudinal, generally medial extension of the distal incision for a normal concurrent thighplasty or repair of the residual limb can be advantageous and improve socket fit and comfort. Patients should be counseled that, despite the excision of skin and tightening of the soft-tissue envelope, some subsequent relaxation is to be expected, and symptoms may recur. However, such occurrences are rare in the experience of this chapter's author. Obvious attention is warranted toward not closing the incisions under substantial tension to minimize the risk of postsurgical dehiscence. In the absence of other underlying problems such as bursa, the deep tissues (bone and myodesis) are deliberately not disturbed during these procedures, and patients may resume prosthetic use as soon as their incisions are adequately healed, which is typically within 3 to 4 weeks for healthy patients without comorbid conditions that limit wound healing.

Based on military experience during the Second World War, Dederich[34] first advocated the quadriceps to hamstrings myoplasty for transfemoral amputations. Although this surgical technique was a substantive leap forward for transfemoral amputation management, similar problems may develop when superficial myoplasties are not anchored in sequential layers to the underlying bone or myodesis. In addition to potential symptomatic deep bursa formation, symptomatic shifting of their myoplasties within their prostheses may develop in these patients, causing a sensation of instability and precluding stable socket fitting (**Figure 8**). Some such patients may be treated with socket modifications, and ringlock and multiple ring-lock liners have been found useful for stabilizing the terminal soft tissue in some instances. For patients with persistent instability, limited amputation revision through a lateral approach (leaving the adductor myodesis undisturbed) to convert the myoplasty to a myodesis by anchoring the hamstrings and quadriceps to the terminal femur can be performed, and good results can be anticipated. Near-complete amputation revision is required only if a large bursa is encountered because this may prevent healing of the new myodesis to the femur and adjacent soft tissues.

Inadequate Soft-Tissue Coverage and Skin Problems

Skin problems are common in residual limbs, and a few problems may require surgical management.

The goal of amputation surgery is to construct a viable, robust residual limb to serve as a platform for weight bearing and a stable interface for the prosthetic socket. Skin that is insensate and/or adherent to bone is particularly prone to breakdown and ulceration, and this circumstance should be avoided whenever possible. Nonetheless, up to 57% of individuals with limb loss experience distal ulceration at some point, with 16% to 63% reporting other skin problems.[35]

If scar adherence or invagination is an early problem and sufficient subcutaneous tissue exists to facilitate normal pliability, early scar treatments and mechanical stimulation (scar massage) may be effective in improving or restoring subcutaneous mobility. Mature scar or adherent skin may be managed only with prosthetic modifications to offload and protect affected areas or focal surgical revision with the mobilization of healthy, adjacent full-thickness tissue. De-epithelialization of one side of the incision while advancing the other, generally distal, limb and then tacking the layers sequentially to the deep fascia or periosteum and subsequently to one another in a shingled and overlapping fashion can improve overall coverage durability and thickness. If ulceration develops in an area of otherwise adequate and viable local tissue, meticulous wound care and socket modifications should be immediately initiated. Although activity modification may be required, complete prosthetic rest is not required for most patients. One study found that nearly two-thirds of ulcerations healed within 6 weeks with continued use of the prosthesis, and only 9% of ulcerations worsened.[36] Vacuum-assisted socket systems may be helpful and were found to be safe in a small prospective study of patients with dysvascular disease who had distal ulceration.[37]

Chronic ulcerations should be evaluated for sinus tract formation with sterile probing and/or a sinography. These patients may have an underlying smoldering osteomyelitis that should be evaluated on radiographs and advanced imaging studies, as indicated. Sinus tracts generally will not heal with wound care, may undergo malignant transformation,[38] and should be excised in their entirety at an opportune time, ideally when they are relatively less active and inflamed. Underlying osteomyelitis, if present, should be managed appropriately.

Historical dogma suggests that split-thickness skin grafts (STSGs) perform poorly on residual limbs, particularly in adults.[39] This chapter's author agrees that STSGs should be avoided whenever practicable, particularly on terminal residual limbs or over bone or periosteum. Skin grafts are thinner and less robust than native skin and are, by definition, insensate. Nonetheless, grafts may function reasonably well over robust, healthy muscle. The experiences of this chapter's author with skin grafts in younger, combat-injured patients with amputations has demonstrated an increased surgical revision rate for

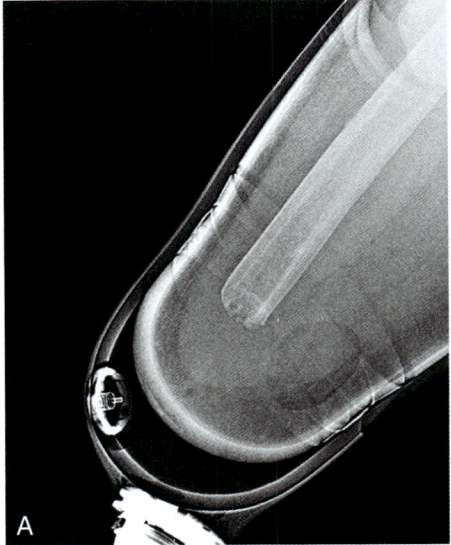 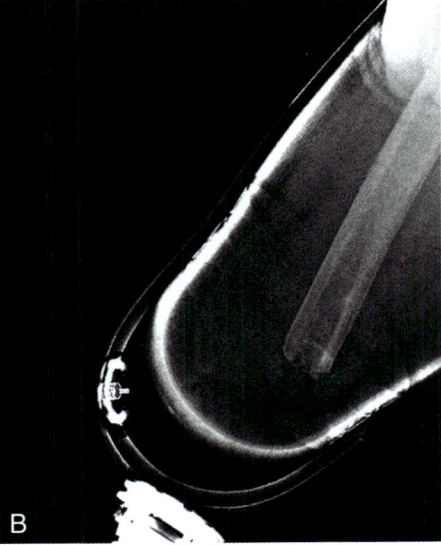

FIGURE 8 AP radiographs of a right transfemoral amputation with a symptomatic, unstable myoplasty in a prosthetic socket demonstrating the femur centered within the socket and the myoplasty reduced (**A**), and the femur medially translated and the quadriceps-hamstring myoplasty subluxated laterally (**B**).

skin graft excision with or without concurrent heterotopic ossification (HO) excision in these patients. Importantly, however, STSGs may serve as a bridge to delayed skin graft excision and local tissue advancement after swelling subsides and pliability returns to the adjacent native skin, successfully facilitating the salvage of important additional residual limb length in the process.[40] When STSGs are necessary, placing synthetic dermal substitutes (eg, Integra [Integra LifeSciences]) before grafting may be helpful for three reasons: (1) The period (typically 10 to 21 days) required for the product to mature provides a litmus test of wound stability and suitability for grafting; (2) the resulting skin graft is supported by a more robust neodermis that may improve tolerance to weight bearing and shear forces, thus resisting ulceration; and (3) if revision surgery becomes necessary and full STSG excision is not feasible, the resulting neodermis may assist in revision wound closure versus sewing directly to unaugmented STSG, which holds suture poorly.

Epidermoid cysts and inflamed sweat glands have a predilection to develop in intertriginous areas subject to chronic irritation from the prosthetic socket edge, such as the popliteus fossa or the inguinal crease. The axillary and antecubital areas also may be affected, albeit much less commonly. When acutely inflamed, these areas may respond to adjustments to prosthetic fit in coordination with meticulous skin care, warm soaks, and antibiotics. Recurrence and chronicity are unfortunately common. After chronic inflammation develops, thick, septated cyst walls often form, and excision of the resulting abscess is sometimes necessary. The excision is easier to perform if the area is relatively quiescent, so a presurgical period of antibiotics and relative prosthetic rest is helpful. Postsurgically, meticulous skin care and prosthetic fit must be implemented to avoid the inevitability of serial recurrence.

Heterotopic Ossification and Bone Spurs

Bone spurs and prominences are common after amputation, but they may be prevented with careful beveling and contouring of the terminal bone, avoidance of excessive periosteal stripping, and adequate padding of the terminal residual limb. Spurs and corners that prove symptomatic and refractory to prosthesis adjustments may be managed with simple excision or shaving, with an effort toward maximizing soft-tissue coverage over and adherence to the affected area.

The complication of HO is problematic for many patients. At least 64% of combat-related amputations and severe limb injuries are affected by HO,[41,42] and rates may exceed 90% for amputations associated with dismounted complex blast injuries.[43] An explosive blast as the mechanism of injury, a final amputation level within the zone of injury, an elevated Injury Severity Score, and traumatic brain injury all are demonstrated risk factors for HO. Fortunately, not all patients are symptomatic, and prosthetic socket modification to offload symptomatic areas is effective for many patients who are symptomatic. Nonetheless, HO excision rates range from 20% to 40%, with a greater likelihood of excision for lower limb amputations and HO that develops beneath STSGs[3,4] (**Figures 9** and **10**). Excision of HO and amputation revision for patients who are persistently symptomatic may be undertaken, with low rates of radiographic (3%) and symptomatic (2%) recurrence, by performing a complete (versus partial) excision at least 6 months after injury.[44] Relatively high perisurgical complication rates occur, but, ultimately, successful relief of symptoms and residual limb length retention are achieved for most patients. Preexisting incisions should be used and any overlying concurrent STSG excised, whenever possible, with an emphasis on longitudinal, soft tissue–sparing dissection as much as practicable.

Although HO in residual limbs has sometimes been considered a problem for patients in the military, a recent study has demonstrated a surprising frequency of HO in civilians who have limb loss. Matsumoto et al[45] reported that HO developed in 36 of 158 civilians (23%) who had undergone amputation. The incidence of HO did not appear to be affected by the indication for amputation, and surgical excision was required in 11% of the affected patients.

Fractures

Fractures are common after amputation. Pierce et al[1] reported a 10% fracture rate in their study of trauma-related amputation outcomes and complications. The risk for proximal fractures appears to be a combination of frequent falls,

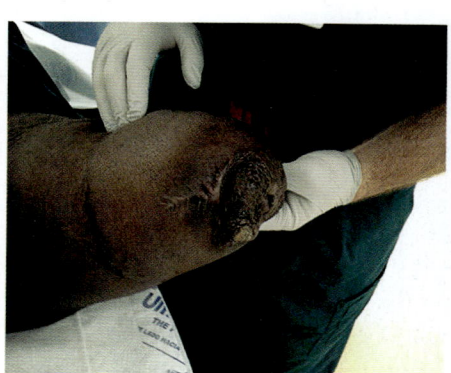

FIGURE 9 Clinical photograph of a left transfemoral amputation with symptomatic distal split-thickness skin graft and underlying heterotopic ossification demonstrating adjacent verrucous skin changes.

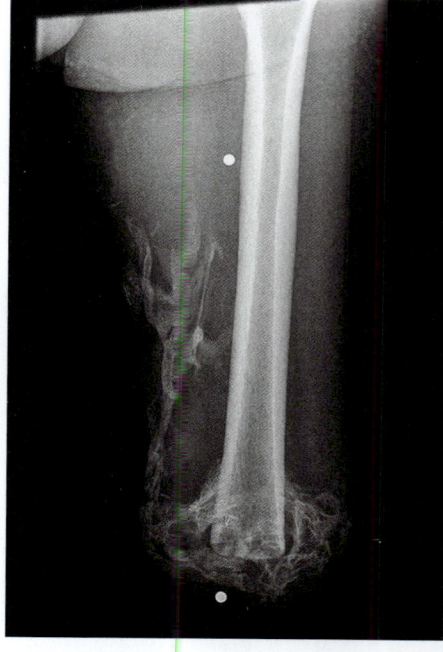

FIGURE 10 AP radiograph of a left transfemoral amputation reflecting heterotopic ossification of the terminal residual limb and tracking along the medial thigh below the split-thickness skin graft.

vulnerable patient populations (such as patients who are elderly or have dysvascular disease), and bone mineral density loss after amputation causing relative or overt osteopenia. Loss of bone mineral density has been demonstrated to affect even individuals younger than 40 years who have trauma-related amputations. Disuse osteopenia and prolonged limited weight bearing are thought to be responsible, which may predispose affected patients to fragility or stress fractures[46] (**Figure 11**).

Bowker et al[47] reported the results of 90 fractures in 85 patients after amputation. Many fractures, excluding those of the hip, were managed nonsurgically, and 97% and 82% of the patients with transtibial and transfemoral amputations, respectively, were able to resume prosthesis wear after healing. They found essentially no indications for re-amputation through the fracture site in this setting. These results mirror the recommendations of Gordon et al[48] for the treatment of acute fractures proximal to trauma-related amputations. They reported a high complication rate but global success in achieving fracture healing and concurrent amputation level and/or residual limb-length salvage.

Tibiofibular Instability and Radioulnar Convergence

Symptomatic tibiofibular instability may develop after transtibial amputation. It affects an unknown proportion of transtibial amputations without a bridge synostosis. Many patients who are symptomatic have associated symptomatic neuromata or osseous prominences that become irritated or compressed by fibular motion within the prosthetic socket. The evaluating physician should test for this clinically by attempting to replicate the patient's symptoms by applying mediolateral tibiofibular compression and gross manipulation of the fibula to assess for a hyperdynamic state. These findings are largely subjective; examiner experience is an asset because some degree of fibular motion is normal, and asymptomatic motion is of no consequence. Some patients may respond to a snugger socket that holds the fibula in a stable position. Patients who are persistently symptomatic may be treated with revision distal synostosis creation (the Ertl procedure), proximal tibiofibular stabilization,[49] or residual fibula excision. Residual fibula excision is generally indicated only for patients with very short fibulae, and the lateral collateral ligament and biceps tendon should be reconstructed by attachment to the proximal tibia with bone anchors to prevent posterolateral knee instability and/or hamstring weakness. Patients with acute tibiofibular instability noted at the time of amputation (**Figure 12**) should likewise be treated with one of these three techniques.

Radioulnar convergence and impingement may similarly affect patients with transradial amputations. Deliberate synostosis creation is not advocated for these patients because all residual pronation/supination would be lost. In fact, the convergence/impingement phenomenon itself is associated with terminal bone spurs or near-synostosis. Patients whose symptoms are refractory to nonsurgical management may undergo limited revision with excision of associated bone spurs or HO and stable interposition grafting with local tendon in an effort to prevent bone-on-bone contact.

SUMMARY

Amputation surgery is fraught with complications because of a combination of complex medical, anatomic, and functional factors. Early complications should be dealt with expeditiously to prevent progression, minimize patient deconditioning, and expedite rehabilitation. Most late or chronic complications should be managed with a diligent trial of nonsurgical management, and, for many patients, such management is sufficient to mitigate the problem or problems. However, for patients with refractory problems and persistently symptomatic residual limbs attributed to an identifiable cause, revision surgery may dramatically improve function, relieve pain, and increase satisfaction and quality of life.

References

1. Pierce RO Jr, Kernek CB, Ambrose TA II: The plight of the traumatic amputee. *Orthopedics* 1993;16(7):793-797.
2. Harris AM, Althausen PL, Kellam J, Bosse MJ, Castillo R: Lower Extremity Assessment Project (LEAP) Study Group: Complications following limb-threatening lower extremity trauma. *J Orthop Trauma* 2009;23(1):1-6.
3. Tintle SM, Baechler MF, Nanos GP, Forsberg JA, Potter BK: Reoperations following combat-related upper-extremity amputations. *J Bone Joint Surg Am* 2012;94(16):e1191-e1196.
4. Tintle SM, Shawen SB, Forsberg JA, et al: Reoperation after combat-related

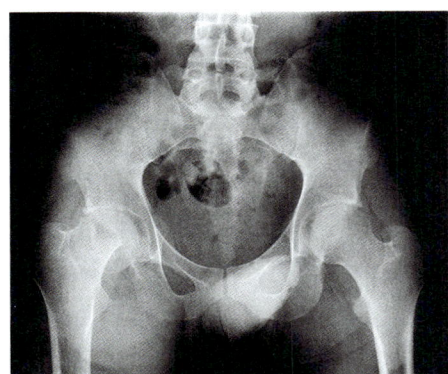

FIGURE 11 AP radiograph of the pelvis of a 26-year-old patient with a right transfemoral amputation (and also a left knee disarticulation) demonstrating a right subcapital femoral neck fragility fracture caused by a fall from standing height resulting from posttraumatic, disuse osteopenia.

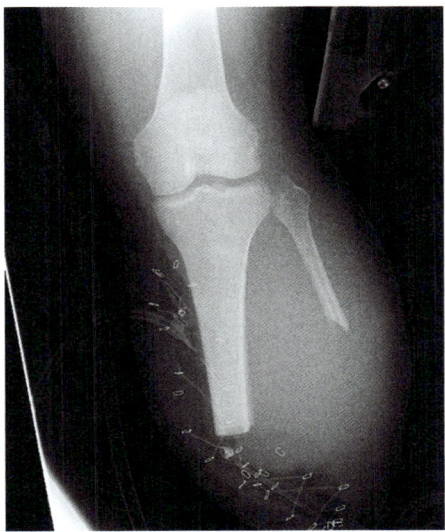

FIGURE 12 Postinjury AP radiograph of a left transtibial amputation demonstrating proximal tibiofibular dissociation and instability with overt dislocation of the proximal tibiofibular joint and valgus angulation of the residual fibula.

major lower extremity amputations. *J Orthop Trauma* 2014;28(4):232-237.
5. Czerniecki JM, Thompson ML, Littman AJ, et al: Predicting reampuation risk in patients undergoing lower extremity amputation due to the complications of peripheral artery disease and/or diabetes. *Br J Surg* 2019;106:1026-1034.
6. Ciufo DJ, Thirukumaran CP, Marchese R, Oh I: Risk factors for reoperation, readmission, and early complications after below knee amputation. *Injury* 2019;50:462-466.
7. Phair J, DeCarlo C, Scher L, et al: Risk factors for unplanned readmission and stump complications after major lower extremity amputation. *J Vasc Surg* 2017;67:848-855.
8. Low EE, Inkellis E, Morshed S: Complications and revision amputation following trauma-related lower limb loss. *Injury* 2017;48:364-370.
9. Jensen JS, Mandrup-Poulsen T, Krasnik M: Wound healing complications following major amputations of the lower limb. *Prosthet Orthot Int* 1982;6(2):105-107.
10. Lexier RR, Harrington IJ, Woods JM: Lower extremity amputations: A 5-year review and comparative study. *Can J Surg* 1987;30(5):374-376.
11. White RA, Nolan L, Harley D, et al: Noninvasive evaluation of peripheral vascular disease using transcutaneous oxygen tension. *Am J Surg* 1982;144(1):68-75.
12. Kelly DA, Pedersen S, Tosenovsky P, Sieunarine K: Major lower limb amputation: Outcomes are improving. *Ann Vasc Surg* 2017;45:29-34.
13. Howard RT, Valerio IL, Basile PL, Nesti L: The use of intraoperative fluorescent angiography to maximize fasciocutaneous flap coverage of battle field extremity injuries. *Plast Recon Surg* 2011;128(4 suppl):79-80.
14. Stannard JP, Volgas DA, McGwin GIII, et al: Incisional negative pressure wound therapy after high-risk lower extremity fractures. *J Orthop Trauma* 2012;26(1):37-42.
15. Dickhaut SC, DeLee JC, Page CP: Nutritional status: Importance in predicting wound-healing after amputation. *J Bone Joint Surg Am* 1984;66(1):71-75.
16. Pinzur MS, Morrison C, Sage R, Stuck R, Osterman H, Vrbos L: Syme's two-stage amputation in insulin-requiring diabetics with gangrene of the forefoot. *Foot Ankle* 1991;11(6):394-396.
17. McCollough NC III: Complications of amputation surgery, in Epps CH, ed: *Complications in Orthopaedic Surgery*, ed 2. JB Lippincott, 1986, vol 2, pp 1335-1367.
18. Singh R, Hunter J, Philip A: Fluid collections in amputee stumps: A common phenomenon. *Arch Phys Med Rehabil* 2007;88(5):661-663.
19. Polfer EM, Hoyt BW, Senchak LT, Murphey MD, Forsberg JA, Potter BK: Fluid collections in amputations are not indicative or predictive of infection. *Clin Orthop Relat Res* 2014;472(10):2978-2983.
20. Barth RE, Vogely HC, Hoepelman AI, Peters EJ: "To bead or not to bead?" Treatment of osteomyelitis and prosthetic joint-associated infections with gentamicin bead chains. *Int J Antimicrob Agents* 2011;38(5):371-375.
21. Pavey GJ, Formby PM, Hoyt BW, Wagner SC, Forsberg JA, Potter BK: Intrawound antibiotic powder decreases frequency of deep infection and severity of heterotopic ossification in combat lower extremity amputations. *Clin Orthop Relat Res* 2019;477:802-810.
22. Gottschalk F: Transfemoral amputation: Biomechanics and surgery. *Clin Orthop Relat Res* 1999;361:15-22.
23. O'Reilly MA, O'Reilly PM, O'Reilly HM, Sullivan J, Sheahan J: High-resolution ultrasound findings in the symptomatic residual limbs of amputees. *Mil Med* 2013;178(12):1291-1297.
24. Henrot P, Stines J, Walter F, Martinet N, Paysant J, Blum A: Imaging of the painful lower limb stump. *Radiographics* 2000;20(Spec No):S219-S235.
25. Dumanian GA, Potter BK, Mioton LM, et al: Targeted muscle reinnervation treats neuroma pain and phantoms in major limb amputees: A randomized clinical trial. *Ann Surg* 2019;270(2):238-246.
26. Valerio IL, Dumanian GA, Jordan SW, et al: Preemptive treatment of phantom and residual limb pain with targeted muscle reinnervation at the time of major limb amputation. *J Am Coll Surg* 2019;228(3):217-226.
27. Kubiak CA, Kemp SWP, Cederna PS: Regenerative peripheral nerve interface for management of postamputation neuroma. *JAMA Surgery* 2018;153(7):681-682.
28. Chang BL, Mondshine J, Attinger CE, Kleiber GM: Targeted muscle reinnervation improves pain and ambulation outcomes in highly comorbid amputees. *Plast Recon Surg* 2021;148(2):376-386.
29. Dielissen PW, Claassen AT, Veldman PH, Goris RJ: Amputation for reflex sympathetic dystrophy. *J Bone Joint Surg Br* 1995;77(2):270-273.
30. Bodde MI, Dijkstra PU, den Dunnen WF, Geertzen JH: Therapy-resistant complex regional pain syndrome type I: To amputate or not? *J Bone Joint Surg Am* 2011;93(19):1799-1805.
31. Hunter GA: Limb amputation and re-amputation in association with chronic pain syndrome. *Prosthet Orthot Int* 1985;9(2):92-94.
32. Ahmed A, Bayol MG, Ha SB: Adventitious bursae in below knee amputees: Case reports and a review of the literature. *Am J Phys Med Rehabil* 1994;73(2):124-129.
33. Stell IM: Management of acute bursitis: Outcome study of a structured approach. *J R Soc Med* 1999;92(10):516-521.
34. Dederich R: Technique of myoplastic amputations. *Ann R Coll Surg Engl* 1967;40(4):222-226.
35. Meulenbelt HE, Geertzen JH, Jonkman MF, Dijkstra PU: Determinants of skin problems of the stump in lower-limb amputees. *Arch Phys Med Rehabil* 2009;90(1):74-81.
36. Salawu A, Middleton C, Gilbertson A, Kodavali K, Neumann V: Stump ulcers and continued prosthetic limb use. *Prosthet Orthot Int* 2006;30(3):279-285.
37. Traballesi M, Delussu AS, Fusco A, et al: Residual limb wounds or ulcers heal in transtibial amputees using an active suction socket system: A randomized controlled study. *Eur J Phys Rehabil Med* 2012;48(4):613-623.
38. Mahaisavariya B, Mahaisavariya P: Marjolin's ulcer complicating a poorly fabricated prosthesis. *Injury* 1991;22(5):423-424.
39. Wood MR, Hunter GA, Millstein SG: The value of stump split skin grafting following amputation for trauma in adult upper and lower limb amputees. *Prosthet Orthot Int* 1987;11(2):71-74.
40. Polfer EM, Tintle SM, Forsberg JA, Potter BK: Skin grafts for residual limb coverage and preservation of amputation length. *Plast Reconstr Surg* 2015;136(2):603-609.
41. Potter BK, Burns TC, Lacap AP, Granville RR, Gajewski DA: Heterotopic ossification following traumatic and combat-related amputations: Prevalence, risk factors, and preliminary result of excision. *J Bone Joint Surg Am* 2007;89(3):476-486.
42. Forsberg JA, Pepek JM, Wagner S, et al: Heterotopic ossification in high-energy wartime extremity injuries: Prevalence and risk factors. *J Bone Joint Surg Am* 2009;91(5):1084-1091.

43. Daniels CM, Pavey GJ, Arthur J, Noller M, Forsberg JA, Potter BK: Has the proportion of combat-related amputations that develop heterotopic ossification increased? *J Orthop Trauma* 2018;32:283-287.

44. Pavey GJ, Polfer EM, Nappo KE, Tintle SM, Forsberg JA, Potter BK: What risk factors predict recurrence of heterotopic ossification following excision in combat-related amputations? *Clin Orthop Relat Res* 2015;473(9):2814-2824.

45. Matsumoto ME, Khan M, Jayabalan P, Ziebarth J, Munin MC: Heterotopic ossification in civilians with lower limb amputations. *Arch Phys Med Rehabil* 2014;95(9):1710-1713.

46. Flint JH, Wade AM, Stocker DJ, Pasquina PF, Howard RS, Potter BK: Bone mineral density loss after combat-related lower extremity amputation. *J Orthop Trauma* 2014;28(4):238-244.

47. Bowker JH, Rills BM, Ledbetter CA, Hunter GA, Holliday P: Fractures in lower limbs with prior amputation: A study of ninety cases. *J Bone Joint Surg Am* 1981;63(6):915-920.

48. Gordon WT, O'Brien FP, Strauss JE, Andersen RC, Potter BK: Outcomes associated with the internal fixation of long-bone fractures proximal to traumatic amputations. *J Bone Joint Surg Am* 2010;92(13):2312-2318.

49. Lewandowski LR, Tintle SM, D'Alleyrand JC, Potter BK: The utilization of a suture bridge construct for tibiofibular instability during transtibial amputation without distal bridge synostosis creation. *J Orthop Trauma* 2013;27(10):e239-e242.

Psychological Adaptation to Limb Amputation

CHAPTER 56

Lakeya S. McGill, MA, PhD • Ellen J. MacKenzie, MSc, PhD • Stephen T. Wegener, MA, PhD

ABSTRACT

How individuals adapt psychologically to the challenges of limb loss varies and depends on several interrelated factors associated with the individual and their environment. Although many individuals adapt successfully, others struggle with symptoms of anxiety, posttraumatic stress, and depression. Early management of these symptoms using a patient-centered, collaborative care approach to care is critical for successful, long-term outcomes. Two approaches are particularly helpful in promoting patient activation: (1) cognitive, behavioral-based self-management programs and (2) peer support and visitation programs. It is helpful for the surgeon and the treatment team to be aware of recommended strategies for promoting an integrated model of care delivery that addresses both physical and psychological symptoms associated with amputation.

Keywords: amputation; anxiety; depression; psychological adaptation

Introduction

The amputation of a limb, whether caused by a traumatic event or chronic local or systemic disease, is a life-altering event. Limb loss invariably affects function and everyday activities. How individuals adapt psychologically to the challenges of limb loss varies and depends on several interrelated factors associated with personal and family resources, coping styles, self-efficacy, resiliency, as well as barriers and facilitators present in social, economic, and physical environments. Most individuals adapt effectively as symptoms of emotional distress, negative body image, and social stigma dissipate across time and functional accommodations occur. However, adaptation is more challenging for some individuals; symptoms linger, impeding recovery and successful reintegration into everyday life. For some, more severe psychological disorders, including anxiety, posttraumatic stress disorder (PTSD), and major depressive disorder, emerge in the months or years after amputation.

The behavioral health consequences of limb loss often are underappreciated when caring for individuals with limb loss.[a] Attention often is focused on surgical management, prosthetic fitting, and physical rehabilitation, without acknowledging and treating the psychological and social needs of the patient and their family. Increasingly, surgical specialties are acknowledging that the traditional biomedical model of disease and disease management is inadequate and must be replaced with a biopsychosocial model, wherein psychological and social factors are addressed together with medical factors to improve patient outcomes and quality of life.[1] It also is becoming increasingly clear that a team approach for caring for individuals with limb loss is critical, and both the patient and the family must be integral members of the team.[2,3]

It is important to review current understanding of the emotional reactions experienced following amputation and the extent to which these reactions evolve into psychological conditions that impede long-term recovery. The benefits of a patient-centered, collaborative care approach to the early treatment of patients undergoing amputation are discussed, and recommendations are provided regarding the role of the surgeon and the treatment team in addressing these adaptation issues.

Common Reactions and Adaptations to Amputation

Data have not supported the assumption that individuals have universal responses to health crises, such as amputation. Stage theory, which exemplifies this concept, predicts that individuals will respond to a crisis or

---

None of the following authors or any immediate family member has received anything of value from or has stock or stock options held in a commercial company or institution related directly or indirectly to the subject of this chapter: Dr. McGill, Dr. MacKenzie, and Dr. Wegener.

[a]Person-first language (eg, individuals with limb loss or amputation) rather than identity-first language (eg, amputees) was used in this chapter; however, both uses are appropriate, with individuals having various preferences for language use. When working with individuals directly, use the language they use to describe themselves.

a loss in specific and predictable ways across time and eventually accept or resolve the emotional crisis.[4] Earlier models of bereavement described successive stages of denial, anger, bargaining, depression, and eventual acceptance. However, more contemporary models of bereavement, such as the Dual Process Model of Coping with Bereavement, hypothesize that grief is a nonlinear, active process unique to each individual and influenced by external factors, such as ongoing stressors and level of support.[5] Similarly, Belon and Vigoda[6] suggested that adaptation after limb loss may involve a more dynamic process, with emotional and coping responses evolving as the individual moves through the process. In addition, traditional models of adaptation do not accommodate the fact that individuals may identify benefits and experience positive growth after physical trauma.[7] Recent literature emphasizes models that conceptualize coping as a transactional process in which the individual's cognitive and behavioral responses interact with social and environmental factors.

From a clinical perspective, it is useful to think of adaptation to an amputation as a process occurring during four phases of care: the preoperative phase (most relevant to those who are losing a limb because of systemic disease), the immediate postoperative phase, the early rehabilitation phase (both inpatient and outpatient), and the longer term adaptation and reintegration phase.[8] Viewing adaptation as a process that occurs across these four phases highlights some of the more critical issues that arise at each point in time and how the health care team may respond to promote effective adaptation. **Table 1** describes these treatment phases and lists the emotional and coping responses a patient may experience. It also provides suggestions on which steps clinicians may take to address potential concerns. Notably, a paucity of data exists to document specific reactions during each treatment phase, and reactions vary tremendously among individuals, with adaptation varying and occurring across the treatment continuum.

It is most important to recognize that if negative emotions and maladaptive responses are not recognized and managed appropriately early in the process, clinical symptoms of anxiety, posttraumatic stress, and depression may result, potentially having a significant effect on long-term outcomes and quality of life.

Prevalence of Anxiety, PTSD, and Depression

The literature on the prevalence of anxiety, PTSD, and depression specifically associated with limb loss is limited, and direct comparison across studies is difficult because of variation in the instruments and methods used, the composition of the study population (eg, differences in demographics, whether the amputation was related to a traumatic event or systemic disease, the circumstances of the trauma, the type and level of amputation, whether the population consists of civilians, veterans, or active-duty service members), and the timing of the assessment after amputation. In addition, most studies are cross-sectional, making it difficult to assess changes in prevalence during the life course of an individual with limb loss and evaluate long-term trajectories of recovery or deterioration. Nevertheless, the preponderance of evidence indicates that rates of psychological distress among individuals with limb loss are higher than those in the general population, calling for a coordinated approach to address the multifactorial needs of patients and their families early in the recovery process. Anxiety, PTSD, and depression are discussed individually, but these symptoms often co-occur among individuals with limb loss.

Anxiety

Generalized anxiety symptoms are common after trauma-related amputations and limb loss resulting from systemic disease. In a systematic review of studies of anxiety and depression following trauma-related limb amputation, Mckechnie and John[9] found rates of generalized anxiety ranging from 25% to 57% across six studies. While an earlier review based primarily on cross-sectional studies of lower limb amputations concluded that elevated symptoms of anxiety often subside after the first year, with levels falling to those found in the general population,[8] a subsequent longitudinal study of all-cause lower limb amputations[10] refuted these conclusions. Singh et al[11] found that although symptoms of anxiety were generally resolved during inpatient rehabilitation, the prevalence of anxiety remained elevated 2 to 3 years after the amputation and was more similar to levels found at the time of admission to rehabilitation (18% at 2 to 3 years compared with 24% at admission). McCarthy et al[10] found similar results in a study of outcomes after 569 lower limb injuries (27% of which eventually underwent amputation); the percentage of those with moderate to severe symptoms of anxiety remained elevated throughout a 2-year follow-up (35%, 30%, 27%, and 29% at 3, 6, 12, and 24 months, respectively). In a more recent study, Melcer et al[12] conducted a retrospective analysis of military and Veterans Administration health data for 440 patients with combat-related lower limb injuries. These included unilateral amputations within 90 days postinjury (early amputation), unilateral amputations more than 90 days postinjury (late amputation), and leg-threatening injuries without amputation (limb salvage). Over the 4 year post-injury observation period, 40% of those with early amputation, 54% of those with late amputation, and 40% of those with limb salvage had been diagnosed with an anxiety disorder based on the International Classification of Diseases, Ninth Revision, Clinical Modification (ICD-9-CM). Individuals with limb salvage had a higher 4-year prevalence of anxiety compared with those with early amputation; however, the prevalence significantly decreased after 1 year for all three groups. Similarly, Mercer et al[13] found that the prevalence of anxiety (based on ICD-9-CM criteria) significantly decreased 5 years postinjury in 318 patients with combat-related upper limb injuries and amputations.

TABLE 1 Common Reactions and Responses to Limb Amputations

Phase	Common Reactions	Role of Surgeon and Treatment Team
Preoperative	A sense of relief that a solution exists for the problem (especially among patients who are dysvascular) Anxiety about effects on function, loss of independence, and change in appearance Early stages of anticipatory grief	Involve surgeon in preparing the patient and family for surgery; a clear explanation of the reason for the amputation and a discussion of alternatives is important Present amputation as a desirable option, not as a last resort Involve patient and family in treatment decision wherever possible Provide access to reliable sources of information about the procedure and the rehabilitation process Link patient and family to resources for individuals with limb loss (eg, the Amputee Coalition of America) Arrange for consultation with behavioral health clinicians, prosthetists, and rehabilitation team members
Immediate postoperative	A range of reactions is expected, from emotional numbness and denial of emotions to feelings of loss and acute distress to optimism and hopefulness about the future A sense of relief caused by surviving a traumatic event or decreased pain	Proactively provide opportunity for the discussion of psychosocial issues Acknowledge that a wide range of emotional reactions is appropriate Support the decision that led to amputation Treat pain early after the surgery Provide a realistic timetable for recovery Involve the patient and the family in discussions about the next steps in the process of recovery Provide referral to a peer visitor program while in the hospital Support follow-through on patient and family connection to resources for individuals with limb loss (eg, the Amputee Coalition of America)
Early rehabilitation	Emotional reactions evolve as the individual confronts functional limitations A wide range of reactions is possible: grief, anxiety regarding future, loss, depression, denial and minimization of change New doubts about the future emerge Maladaptive coping responses (eg, avoidance of social interaction, catastrophic thinking)	Employ early fitting of a prosthesis and mobilization as appropriate Use a support team approach with prosthetists, physical therapists or occupational therapists, social workers, vocational counselors, and psychologists Screen for early signs of depression, anxiety, and PTSD and refer to behavioral health services as needed Engage in self-management training to decrease catastrophic thinking and improve self-efficacy and coping strategies
Long-term adaptation and reintegration into society	Continued adaptation with most returning to baseline emotional health and some experiencing posttraumatic growth Continued elevated risk for depression and anxiety disorders Recognition that adaptation to a new normal will be challenging Concerns regarding employment, social acceptance, and sexual function Financial concerns	Provide ongoing group support for the patient and family members Support connection to the limb loss community (eg, the Amputee Coalition of America) Continue to monitor for maladaptive coping responses and mood disorders Refer to behavioral health services for psychotherapy and pharmacotherapy as needed

PTSD = posttraumatic stress disorder

The literature is mixed regarding the prevalence and trajectory for anxiety symptoms, with some studies reporting rates similar to those of the general population 1 year postinjury and other studies reporting elevated rates 2 to 3 years postinjury. More recent studies suggest that early amputation may contribute to better recovery than limb salvage, as individuals with limb salvage have higher rates of anxiety up to 4 and 5 years postinjury compared with those with early amputation. However, rates of anxiety significantly decreased after 1 year, which is consistent with some previous studies. Additional research is needed to better understand anxiety in this population. Nevertheless, findings consistently show anxiety is a common issue that should be addressed to promote optimal recovery and functional outcomes.

Posttraumatic Stress Disorder

Acute stress reaction often is—although not always—associated with the subsequent development of PTSD, with one study reporting that 78% of individuals with acute stress disorder after a motor vehicle crash subsequently met criteria for PTSD within 6 months.[14] PTSD is a debilitating disorder characterized by re-experiencing the original trauma (eg, flashbacks, intrusive memories); the avoidance of thoughts, activities, and people associated with the trauma (eg, feeling emotionally numb about the traumatic event); negative alterations in cognitions and mood (eg, exaggerated self-blame about the cause of the traumatic event); and hyperarousal (eg, irritability, difficulty concentrating, insomnia). A diagnosis of PTSD can only be made if these symptoms persist for more than 1 month. The adverse

Section 4: Management Issues

consequences of PTSD include high rates of suicide, substance abuse, violence, an inability to maintain intimate and parental relationships, physical illness, and premature mortality.[15] PTSD is commonly present (83% to 90% of the time) with other psychological disorders, including substance use, depression, and panic disorder.[16]

The rates of PTSD after amputation caused by systemic disease appear to be low, most likely because these individuals are more prepared for the surgery and its consequences.[17] However, high rates of PTSD after physical trauma (both civilian and combat related) are well documented in the literature.[18-20] Relatively few studies have focused specifically on the prevalence of PTSD associated with musculoskeletal trauma,[21,22] with even fewer on the prevalence of PTSD after limb amputation.[23-25]

Studies by Melcer et al[24] and Doukas et al[25] are useful in this regard. Both groups of researchers examined the rates of PTSD among service members who sustained major lower limb trauma in Operation Iraqi Freedom, Operation Enduring Freedom, or Operation New Dawn. Both studies reported high overall rates of PTSD. Doukas et al[25] retrospectively examined outcomes in a cohort of 324 service members deployed to Afghanistan or Iraq who sustained a traumatic amputation or limb salvage. At an average of 38 months after injury, 18% screened positive for PTSD using the military version of the Posttraumatic Stress Disorder Checklist (PCL-M)[26] and the scoring criteria proposed by Hoge et al.[27] Interestingly, participants with an amputation had a significantly lower likelihood of PTSD compared with those whose limbs were salvaged (12% among patients with amputation versus 25% among patients with limb salvage). Melcer et al[24] retrospectively examined the military health records of patients who sustained lower extremity injuries: 587 underwent early amputation during the first 90 days after injury, 84 patients had a late amputation more than 90 days after injury, and 117 patients were treated for leg-threatening injuries without amputation. The results of Melcer et al[24] were similar to those of Doukas et al.[25] The 2-year prevalence of a PTSD diagnosis (recorded in the medical record and coded based on the ICD-9-CM criteria) was 19% for early amputations and 30% for limb salvage. Melcer et al[24] also found that patients with late amputations had significantly higher rates of PTSD (33%) compared with those treated with either early amputations or limb salvage. In a follow-up study, the 4-year prevalence of a PTSD diagnosis (based on ICD-9-CM criteria) was 49% for early amputation, 58% for late amputation, and 51% for limb salvage.[12] Although there were no differences between groups, PTSD rates significantly increased over time, particularly during the second year after injury.

Most research has focused on lower extremity injuries, with few studies examining PTSD specifically for upper extremity injuries and amputations. In a follow-up to the study by Doukas et al, Mitchell et al[28] compared outcomes for 155 service members who sustained an upper extremity amputation or limb salvage. Similar to results for lower limb injuries, 19% screened positive for PTSD (based on the PCL-M) at an average of 40 months postinjury; however, PTSD rates were similar across groups, with 19.2%, 21.2%, and 16.7% screening positive for PTSD for patients with unilateral salvage, unilateral amputation, and bilateral amputation, respectively. Melcer et al[13] examined military and Veterans Administration health data for 318 service members with above-elbow amputation, below-elbow amputation, or arm injury without amputation. The 5-year prevalence for a PTSD diagnosis (based on the ICD-9-CM) was high, ranging from 52% to 58%, with no significant differences between the groups. PTSD also significantly increased across years, as the prevalence was 20% at 1 year after injury and 36% at 3 years after injury.

Earlier studies suggested that military patients who had early amputation may have had better outcomes compared with those with limb salvage or especially late amputation. More recent studies demonstrated no differences among these three groups for both upper and lower limb injuries among military patients; however, the rate of PTSD increases over time. In civilians, there is a dearth of high-quality longitudinal studies examining the rates of PTSD following amputation. More research is needed to understand how trends may be similar or different from the military population. Overall, PTSD is a significant issue for individuals with trauma-related injuries and amputations, with rates possibly increasing over time.

Depression

The American Psychiatric Association[29] defines depression as depressed mood or markedly diminished interest or pleasure in activities accompanied by substantial weight change, insomnia or hypersomnia, psychomotor agitation or retardation, loss of energy, feelings of worthlessness, diminished ability to concentrate or recurrent thoughts of death that last for at least 2 weeks that interfere with the activities of daily living. Symptoms of depression are common immediately after limb amputation, with rates ranging from 29% to 41% for patients in rehabilitation.[30-32] In a prospective cohort study of 141 veterans and civilians, Roepke et al[33] found that 40% of patients who underwent dysvascular amputation had at least moderate depressive symptoms before surgery. At 6 weeks after surgery, the cohort had substantial improvement in depressive symptoms, especially among those with greater symptoms at baseline. Depressive symptoms were also generally stable at 4 and 12 months after surgery.

The literature is mixed in its findings about the longer term prevalence of depression and the development of a major depressive disorder among those living with limb loss.[8] In one of the very few community surveys of individuals with limb loss, Darnall et al[34] found that the prevalence of significant depressive symptoms was 29%, a rate that is two to four times greater than that for the general population but similar to rates found for outpatients seeking care for chronic conditions. They found no association between prevalence and recency of amputation. In their study, individuals with trauma-related amputations reported the highest levels of depressive symptomatology (46%) when compared with individuals with limb loss caused by dysvascular disease (38%) or cancer (16%).

In the aforementioned study by Melcer et al,[12] 39% of those with early amputation, 55% of those with late amputation, and 36% of those with limb salvage had been diagnosed with a mood disorder based on the ICD-9-CM over 4 years after injury. Mood disorders include a major depressive disorder and other psychologic conditions, such as persistent depressive disorder (formerly known as dysthymia) and bipolar disorder. Individuals with late amputation had a higher 4-year prevalence of mood disorder compared with those with early amputation and limb salvage; however, the prevalence significantly decreased after 1 year for all three groups. In another study examining outcomes in 318 patients with combat-related upper limb injuries and amputations (above and below elbow), Melcer et al[13] found that the prevalence of mood disorder did not change significantly across postinjury years. There was also no difference in prevalence among individuals with amputation and limb salvage. Mitchell et al[28] compared outcomes for 155 service members who sustained an upper extremity amputation or limb salvage. Forty percent of the sample endorsed having depressive symptoms, and 12% screened positive for possible or probable depression at an average of 40 months after injury. There was no significant difference in rates of depression symptoms or possible diagnosis for patients with amputation and limb salvage.

In reviews of the literature on depression after trauma-related amputations, rates range from 20% to more than 50%, with variation in prevalence again related to the choice of instrument used to assess depression, the timing of the assessment, and the composition of the population surveyed.[9,23] To better understand depression in this population, there is a need for more high-quality studies, particularly examining the longer term prevalence, including greater than 4 to 5 years postamputation. Nevertheless, depression symptoms are prevalent and should be addressed as a part of comprehensive patient care. Studies suggest that depression associated with non–trauma-related amputations may be more related to the underlying chronic condition and overall deterioration in health and function rather than the limb loss itself.[35] This finding suggests that individuals undergoing amputation related to diabetes or other chronic diseases may have very different support and counseling needs than those undergoing amputation because of trauma.[36]

Factors Related to Anxiety, PTSD, and Depression

Multiple factors have been shown to influence the prevalence of anxiety, PTSD, and depression associated with disability and limb loss. Briefly mentioned here are the important roles that pain, negative body image, and social stigma play.

Pain

Several studies have suggested a strong relationship between pain (both residual limb pain and phantom pain) in the early stages of recovery and subsequent psychological distress, including depression and PTSD.[37-41] The lower extremity assessment project (LEAP) study demonstrated that symptoms of negative mood and anxiety present in the early phases of recovery are highly correlated with the long-term persistence of pain.[42] Wegener et al[43] further suggested that the effect of pain on functional outcome is primarily related to its influence on depression and anxiety, providing further support for an integrated approach that adequately addresses the symptoms of emotional distress together with the medical management of physical impairment and pain.

Body Image

The individual's reaction to change in body image may be closely related to the presence of the affective issues described earlier. Individuals with depression or anxiety may be more likely to have a negative body image, and those with a distorted self-image may be more likely to be depressed or anxious.[44] In addition, body image has been shown to predict depression and adaptation to amputation.[45] Changes in the physical body and functional abilities may lead to a negative self-image in some individuals with limb loss. In some individuals, a negative body image may develop because of social discomfort or internalization of stigma expressed by society.[45,46] The individual with a negative self-image may demonstrate distorted views of their body and may be reluctant to participate in social activities, leading to poor participation.

Social Stigma

Social stigma results when individuals with disabilities are viewed differently from those without disabilities; negative assumptions are made about functioning and personality based on physical appearance. In the case of individuals with limb loss, visible impairment exists, which may increase the amount of associated stigma. Perceptions of social stigma are related to depression and adjustment to amputation, such that increased levels of stigma have a negative effect on individuals targeted by the stigma.[45] However, it is unclear whether individuals who report a high level of perceived social stigma are accurate in their perceptions or are distorting their own negative thoughts as coming from others.[44]

Social and Environmental Context Influences Outcomes

Of the limited research examining social determinants of health or disparities in limb amputation, most of the literature focuses on differences in the risk of an amputation. Regarding differences in outcomes, several studies have found a significant association between higher education level and better patient outcomes,[47-51] including mental health.[52,53] Although some studies have found no significant association between education and outcomes, most have found a positive association, and none has found a negative association in which individuals with lower education level have better outcomes. Considering this research, the recently developed American Academy of Orthopaedic Surgeons (AAOS) Clinical Practice Guidelines for the evaluation of psychological factors influencing recovery from adult orthopaedic trauma recommend that clinicians evaluate patients' education level.[54] The AAOS guidelines also mention age, race, sex, income, and employment status as factors that may be associated with greater risk of poor outcomes, including psychosocial functioning. However, there is less research in these areas.

Another important contextual factor to consider is whether an individual is a civilian, veteran, or active-duty service member. Military patients may have better access to state-of-the-art prosthetic devices and prosthetic care compared with civilian patients. Insurance coverage often limits the type and number of prostheses that civilian patients may receive. Compared with civilian patients who have sustained limb loss, military patients with limb loss may benefit from more intensive and specialized rehabilitation (both physical and psychological) early in their recovery.

Clinical and rehabilitation pathways for the treatment of individuals with limb loss have been well established through military amputation care programs.[55] Military personnel often spend more than 1 year in rehabilitation, have ready access to prosthetists, and benefit from targeted reintegration programs. In contrast, very few civilian patients (18% in the LEAP study) receive inpatient rehabilitation,[56] and these programs rarely have the degree of specialized care available in military programs. Furthermore, many civilians have limited or no access to outpatient rehabilitation. Military patients also may benefit from greater access to peer support early in their recovery, which can substantively affect recovery. Peer visitation is an integral part of the military amputee care program and is highly valued among service members with combat-related amputations.[57]

There may be some differences in outcomes based on factors such as level of education, employment status, and military status. These factors may serve as risk or protective factors for individuals with limb loss. Unfortunately, there is limited research in this area. Substantially more research is needed examining the role of personal, environmental, and sociocultural factors in adaptation to limb loss.

Coping Mechanisms Influence Outcomes

How the individual copes with amputation and the subsequent rehabilitation process likely mediates the outcome. Clinically and in research, psychologists and psychiatrists primarily focus on how maladaptive responses, such as catastrophic thinking, influence poor outcomes. Catastrophic thinking is a cognitive coping response to an event that is marked by exaggerated negative expectations and negative appraisals. The literature on pain and disability has pointed to the important role that catastrophic thinking plays in the process of recovery and adaptation to a physical impairment, including limb loss.[37,58,59] Higher levels of catastrophic thinking predict increased pain interference and depressive symptoms in individuals with phantom limb pain.[58] Catastrophic thinking is known to predict pain intensity, disability, and psychological distress independent of the level of physical impairment for individuals with limb loss with phantom limb pain.[60,61] The consistent relationship between catastrophic thinking and the fact that it can be modified through cognitive-behavioral interventions has led to ongoing attention to this coping response in limb loss adaptation.

Less attention has been focused on the positive role that resilience plays in recovery. Resilience refers to patterns of positive adaptation in the face of substantial adversity or risk. In one study, Miller et al[62] evaluated the psychometric properties of the Connor-Davidson Resilience Scale in adults with lower limb amputation. Greater resiliency was significantly associated with higher levels of perceived functional capacity and self-efficacy and lower levels of disability, anxiety, depression, and falls efficacy (ie, concern or fear of falling during a variety of tasks). In adults with upper limb loss, the relationship between resiliency and depression and anxiety has been found to be mediated by activity restriction and positive emotions.[63] Although limited data exist on factors associated with positive adaptation after limb loss, considerable data exist in the broader disability literature that informs the understanding of how individuals with limb loss may successfully adapt after amputation. Both individual and environmental factors have been associated with positive adaptation. Enduring personality characteristics of the individual, such as hopefulness, lower levels of neuroticism, higher levels of agreeableness, and internal locus of control, are associated with better psychosocial adaptation.[64-66] Positive adaptation appears related to specific cognitive styles and coping strategies. Individuals who engage in active coping find meaning and positive aspects of the experience and seek growth.[67-70]

Of particular importance is the concept of self-efficacy and social support as facilitators of a positive coping response. Self-efficacy is the belief that one can perform specific tasks or activities. Individuals with higher self-efficacy are less likely to disengage from the coping process because success is expected. In patients with chronic pain, self-efficacy has been found to mediate the relationship between pain intensity and disability, as well as pain intensity and depression.[71,72] In the LEAP study, low self-efficacy was one of the most important determinants of poor functional outcomes after amputation.[50] Self-efficacy can be both taught and improved.[73] Increased physical and social accessibility, higher levels of social support and family problem solving are all associated with better adaptation and overall well-being.[74,75]

Recognizing the role that catastrophic thinking, self-efficacy, and social support play in adaptation and recovery from limb loss have helped identify effective strategies for managing the psychological consequences.

Managing the Psychosocial Consequences

By adopting certain guiding principles, the health care team can be more attentive to the psychosocial aspects of limb loss and, ultimately, more successful in improving patient outcomes. First, it is critical that the surgeon's care is guided by a biopsychosocial model.[1] Second, the care should comprise a patient-centered approach that widens the focus from the patient's medical needs to the patient's needs as a whole.[76] Finally, working with an established multidisciplinary team allows the surgeon to meet the multifactorial needs of individuals with limb loss in an evolving and demanding health care environment.[2]

The orthopaedic team plays an important role in the early phases of recovery by (1) routinely screening for individuals at risk of psychologic distress, (2) referring patients who meet the clinical criteria for a diagnosable condition to an appropriate mental health clinician, and (3) providing a patient-centered and family-centered environment that promotes peer support and self-management and empowers patients to take charge of their own recovery.[77]

Early Screening and Referral

The early identification of symptoms within a patient-centered and family-centered environment may help prevent the development of more severe conditions and improve overall outcomes. Given the high prevalence of rates of emotional distress in individuals with limb loss, screening—using established instruments that can be completed by patients with basic reading skills—should be conducted as part of routine postoperative follow-up visits. The recommended screening domains and sample instruments are shown in **Table 2**.

With the growing awareness of the multiple factors affecting outcomes after traumatic injury and the onset of chronic disabling conditions, the American Trauma Society in conjunction with two of this chapter's authors and their colleagues developed the Trauma Survivors Network.[78] As part of the services offered by the Trauma Survivors Network, an online recovery assessment tool can be self-administered by patients with either a computer or a mobile device.[79] It assesses risk factors (pain, anxiety, PTSD, depression, and alcohol and/or tobacco use) and protective factors (resilience, social support, self-efficacy for return to work, and managing the financial burden of trauma). The recovery assessment tool provides standardized feedback and recommendations for the patient and the clinician. The surgeon should review the feedback and make recommendations with the patient to establish the basis for follow-up planning and referral. The online version is a convenient alternative to paper-and-pencil screening.

Making an effective referral for in-depth evaluation and treatment by another team member or outside clinician is appropriate when problems are causing significant distress or interfering with an individual's functioning. Early detection of potential problems is one of the most important components of making a good referral. Evidence shows that early intervention for psychological issues enhances outcomes.[80] Having an established team and a network of referral sources facilitates coordinated care for the patient. An effective referral is characterized by the following: a clear question or request, relevant clinical information about the patient, a level of urgency, results from a screening assessment, and willingness to continue to participate in patient care. The referring surgeon should expect the following: (1) a timely response based on the urgency of the situation; (2) an assessment that addresses mental status, affect, mood, life stressors, substance use, and threat of harm to self or others as well as information about the patient's understanding of their medical condition and concerns regarding the current situation, coping style, pain issues, expectations for recovery, and goals for rehabilitation; (3) diagnostic formulation; and (4) recommendations and a treatment plan.[81]

When screening indicates a positive result for a mood disorder, referral to an appropriate mental health specialist is indicated. Surgical endorsement of effective management alternatives for these conditions may promote patient follow-through and provide hope. Several randomized controlled trials have shown that major depression may be effectively managed by medication,[82] psychotherapy,[83] and electroconvulsive therapy.[84] Current treatments of PTSD include pharmacotherapy, such as selective serotonin reuptake inhibitors, and psychotherapies, including cognitive and exposure modalities.[85,86] Although certain psychotherapies and selective serotonin reuptake inhibitors have proved moderately successful for PTSD, both modalities require weeks to months to achieve good results; improvement has not been as significant compared with managing other disorders, such as depression and anxiety. Furthermore, long treatment cycles combined with the stigma associated with the condition are often barriers to seeking and complying with treatment, especially among wounded warriors and veterans.[27]

TABLE 2 Examples of Instruments Used for Screening

Domain	Instrument	Administration Time (minutes)
Depression	Patient health questionnaire	2-3
PTSD	PTSD checklist	5-10
	Five-item screen of the PTSD checklist	1-2
Generalized anxiety disorder	General Anxiety Disorder-7	2-3
Pain	Chronic Pain Grade Scale	2-3
	0-10 numerical rating scale within the Chronic Pain Grade Scale	1

PTSD = posttraumatic stress disorder

Section 4: Management Issues

Psychological Considerations in Osseointegration

Osseointegration that allows for the direct attachment of an external prosthesis to the skeleton in patients with amputation is an elective procedure that is becoming more frequent.[87] This increased frequency is part of a growing effort to incorporate osseointegration, biomimetic control, and sensory/proprioceptive feedback in prosthetic devices. As surgeons and other medical clinicians seek to integrate these technologies into clinical care, patient factors that affect the successful use of the technology should be fully considered.

The patient must understand the procedure, perform postoperative care, and engage in rehabilitation to achieve optimal outcomes. For example, the main complications of osseointegration are infections and skin issues. The patient's ability to recognize and manage these problems is critical and is affected by several factors that can be accurately measured.

There is an established evidence base on the role of psychosocial factors in elective surgeries such as spinal surgery and implantation of nerve stimulators for pain management. Assessment of these patient factors is part of the preoperative process. Indeed, most payors require a psychological evaluation before authorizing nerve stimulator placement. Currently, there are no established protocols for psychological evaluations as part of the osseointegration process. However, guided by established elective surgery evaluation formats for other surgical interventions, appropriate areas for assessment can serve as a starting point and be refined as the data evolve.[88]

Areas for assessment include (1) cognitive factors such as the ability to understand the procedure and guide self-care and catastrophizing; (2) behavioral factors such as substance use, smoking, and exercise; (3) contextual factors such as social support and litigation; and (4) emotional factors such as anxiety, depression, and psychosis.[89] The involvement of the psychologist and the preoperative psychosocial evaluation should be considered part of the process that also includes providing specialized preoperative psychoeducation, evaluating and shaping appropriate management expectations, overseeing mood management, and encouraging preoperative and postoperative monitoring of outcome measures. As with trauma care, surgeons engaged in limb loss care in general and osseointegration in particular should have a psychologist as part of the extended team to meet these assessment and intervention needs.

Promoting Peer Support and Self-management

Most patients undergoing amputation will not meet the criteria for clinical depression, generalized anxiety disorder, or PTSD. However, even those who have subclinical symptoms of distress and anxiety may benefit from services that address maladaptive coping responses and enhance resilience and positive coping mechanisms. These services have the potential to buffer amputation-related stressors, prevent the development of serious mental health problems, and assist in overall recovery. When provided early in the recovery process within a collaborative, patient-centered approach to care, the development of anxiety, PTSD, and depression often can be avoided, and long-term quality-of-life outcomes are improved.

Collaborative, patient-centered models of care emphasize the need for patients and their families to assume greater responsibility for their care and call for clinicians to support patients and families in these activities.[90,91] Empowering patients to take charge of their recovery through increasing self-efficacy and activation is a central component of these models. An increasing body of literature suggests that two approaches are particularly helpful in promoting patient activation: cognitive, behavioral-based self-management programs and peer support and visitation programs.

Self-management

Self-management interventions delivered within an overall context of a collaborative care delivery model have gained widespread application in the management of diabetes, arthritis, and other chronic conditions associated with pain, distress, and functional impairments such as limb loss.[3,72] Many individuals interpret the associated consequences of their conditions as uncontrollable. This decreased self-efficacy and perceived lack of control increase pain and negative emotional responses and lead to further physical and psychosocial disability. Self-management strategies incorporate the principles of cognitive-behavioral theory, which helps patients appreciate the relationship between their thoughts and feelings and behaviors, identify self-defeating patterns of thought, and replace such patterns with adaptive thoughts and behaviors to achieve better outcomes. Cognitive, behavioral-based interventions use active structured techniques to focus on skill acquisition and encourage adaptive coping. Self-management interventions achieve long-term reductions in pain and disability primarily by increasing self-efficacy and decreasing catastrophic thinking rather than instituting specific changes in behavior.

The Promoting Amputee Life Skills (PALS) program is a self-management program designed specifically for individuals with limb loss.[92] This eight-session program is designed to develop skills to improve the quality of life for those who have lost a limb. PALS is designed to be delivered in person in a community setting by trained, volunteer group leaders. Groups generally meet on a weekly basis and are organized according to five topics: (1) an introduction to self-management and key skills (eg, reviews of how limb loss may affect one's life, communication, relaxation, and problem-solving skills); (2) health and activity (focuses on things one can do to make mind and body healthy, including how to manage one's skin and residual limb, be more active, maintain good sleep habits, and make healthy choices related to smoking and alcohol use); (3) managing emotions (explores ways to manage emotional ups and downs, builds positive moods and resilience after limb loss, and identifies strategies for protecting oneself against distress); (4) family and friends (focuses on how amputation affects relationships with family, friends, and social roles and teaches effective strategies for communication in difficult situations); and (5) looking ahead to the future (helps participants identify goals for participating in meaningful activities and maintaining health, identifies the warning signs of setbacks, and teaches skills to help overcome these setbacks).

PALS was compared with support group participation in a randomized controlled trial of 522 individuals with limb loss.[92] Compared with the control group, PALS participants were 2.5 times less likely to report symptoms of depression, reported better function, were less bothered about limitations of everyday function, reported higher levels of general self-efficacy, and reported more positive moods. The effect of the PALS intervention is comparable to those found in other evaluations of self-management courses designed for chronic diseases.[93] The effects were greatest for participants who completed the program, patients younger than 65 years, and those who were less than 3 years postamputation, suggesting that early intervention may be more effective. More information about the original PALS program can be found at the following website: https://www.palsamputeelifeskills.org/.

The VETPALS program was adapted from the original PALS. The modified program consists of a 4-hour workshop plus four 2-hour sessions, and the content is tailored to be appropriate for veterans and military culture. In a randomized controlled trial, Turner et al[94] compared VETPALS to an education control in 147 veterans with chronic limb-threatening ischemia. Relative to the control group (*n* = 76), individuals who participated in VETPALS (*n* = 71) had a greater reduction in depression symptoms and improved satisfaction with their health at 6-month follow-up. The authors also examined the feasibility and acceptability of delivering VETPALS within the Veterans Administration system of care. Results revealed low treatment initiation, as only 56% of participants randomized to VETPALS began the program. However, retention was high for those who began the program, with 93% attending four of five classes and 100% reporting overall satisfaction.

Additional self-management programs may be helpful for patients whose amputation is related to other chronic health conditions, such as diabetes. These programs are available nationwide. For individuals who experience amputation as a result of trauma, the NextSteps self-management program[95] is available in person at trauma centers that participate in the Trauma Survivors Network and online. The online version provides a cost-effective strategy for connecting trauma survivors throughout the United States and teaching them the essential self-management skills. Participants join the online NextSteps program in groups of 8 to 12 individuals and spend 6 weeks working through online lessons (at their own speed) and participating in facilitated online chats.

The self-management literature indicates that programs incorporating social support and peer interaction have the greatest effects in changing behavior and maintaining these gains. Thus, delivering the self-management program in the context of social interaction and support may enhance an individual's perceived ability to carry out the self-care regimen necessary to achieve positive outcomes.

Peer Support

Peer support effectively decreases feelings of isolation, increases optimism for the future, and improves coping abilities and self-efficacy. Peer visits can begin as early as preoperatively in elective procedures or postoperatively during acute hospitalization and continue in the recovery period. An appropriately trained peer visitor can offer support and encouragement that only someone who has successfully gone through a similar experience can provide. Peer visitors also offer practical suggestions for living with an amputation. Peer visitation is an integral part of the United States Armed Forces Amputee Patient Program[55] and is highly valued among service members with combat-related amputations.[57]

The Amputee Coalition has now trained and certified a network of more than 1,000 peer visitors (including patients with amputations and their families) throughout the United States, most of whom are affiliated with one or more health care facilities.[96] A peer visit may be requested from the organization.[97] Both the American Trauma Society and the Amputee Coalition provide resources for establishing hospital-based peer visitation programs. The Amputee Coalition also recently developed a new cell phone application to help amputees connect with a Certified Peer Visitor.

After patients are discharged from rehabilitation, group peer support programs provide ongoing support and the opportunity to connect with the increasing number of individuals who are facing similar challenges in living with limb loss.[98-101] The Amputee Coalition of America has developed a well-established network of more than 300 peer support programs nationwide. The groups are typically based at health care facilities and are registered with the Amputee Coalition.

SUMMARY

Secondary conditions of depression, PTSD, body image, social stigma, and pain are substantial problems for community-dwelling individuals with limb loss. These secondary conditions often are associated with activity limitations, restrictions in participation, and reduced quality of life. Programs and services that empower patients to become active participants in their lifelong care are needed to meet the increasing demands placed on them by an evolving healthcare system that holds consumers and their clinicians accountable for successful outcomes.

Several lines of research suggest various approaches that may enhance outcomes and expand the continuum of care. Brief established and/or validated assessment tools are available to provide early screening. Effective treatments are available to manage depression, anxiety, and PTSD. Recognition is growing that peer mentors and support groups may assist individuals with new impairments with successful adaptation. Self-management training may assist patients in managing subclinical levels of distress and prevent more severe mental health symptoms. Finally, it is well recognized that computer-based health information and support systems disseminate information; link people to needed resources; connect people online who are facing similar challenges; and develop communities of individuals with common interests, aspirations, and needs. Although only recently developed, these programs and services have the potential to be successfully used by individuals with limb loss.

Attention to the psychosocial needs of patients and their families is part of comprehensive care. Effective clinicians are guided by the biopsychosocial model, follow patient-centered care principles, and use a team approach. Integrated models of care delivery that tend to both physical and psychological symptoms associated with an amputation are essential for improving outcomes that matter most to patients.

References

1. Borrell-Carrio F, Suchman AL, Epstein RM: The biopsychosocial model 25 years later: Principles, practice, and scientific inquiry. *Ann Fam Med* 2004;2(6):576-582.
2. Strasser DC, Uomoto JM, Smits SJ: The interdisciplinary team and polytrauma rehabilitation: Prescription for partnership. *Arch Phys Med Rehabil* 2008;89(1):179-181.
3. Wegener ST, Hofkamp SE, Ehde DM: Interventions for psychological issues in amputation: A team approach, in Gallagher P, Desmond D, MacLachlan M, eds: *Psychoprosthetics*. Springer, 2008, pp 91-105.
4. Wortman CB, Silver RC: The myths of coping with loss. *J Consult Clin Psychol* 1989;57(3):349.
5. Fiore J: A systematic review of the dual process model of coping with bereavement (1999-2016). *Omega (Westport)* 2021;84(2):414-458.
6. Belon HP, Vigoda DF: Emotional adaptation to limb loss. *Phys Med Rehabil Clin N Am* 2014;25(1):53-74.
7. Elliott TR, Kurylo M, Rivera P: Positive growth following acquired physical disability, in *Handbook of Positive Psychology*. Oxford University Press, 2002, pp 687-698.
8. Horgan O, MacLachlan M: Psychosocial adjustment to lower-limb amputation: A review. *Disabil Rehabil* 2004;26(14-15):837-850.
9. McKechnie PS, John A: Anxiety and depression following traumatic limb amputation: A systematic review. *Injury* 2014;45(12):1859-1866.
10. McCarthy ML, MacKenzie EJ, Edwin D, et al: Psychological distress associated with severe lower-limb injury. *J Bone Joint Surg Am* 2003;85(9):1689-1697.
11. Singh R, Ripley D, Pentland B, et al: Depression and anxiety symptoms after lower limb amputation: The rise and fall. *Clin Rehabil* 2009;23(3):281-286.
12. Melcer T, Walker J, Bhatnagar V, Richard E, Sechriest VF II, Galarneau M: A comparison of four-year health outcomes following combat amputation and limb salvage. *PLoS One* 2017;12(1):e0170569.
13. Melcer T, Walker J, Sechriest VF II, et al: A retrospective comparison of five-year health outcomes following upper limb amputation and serious upper limb injury in the Iraq and Afghanistan conflicts. *PM R* 2019;11(6):577-589.
14. Harvey AG, Bryant RA: The relationship between acute stress disorder and posttraumatic stress disorder: A prospective evaluation of motor vehicle accident survivors. *J Consult Clin Psychol* 1998;66(3):507-512.
15. Qureshi SU, Pyne JM, Magruder KM, Schulz PE, Kunik ME: The link between post-traumatic stress disorder and physical comorbidities: A systematic review. *Psychiatr Q* 2009;80(2):87-97.
16. Brady KT, Killeen TK, Brewerton T, Lucerini S: Comorbidity of psychiatric disorders and posttraumatic stress disorder. *J Clin Psychiatry* 2000;61(suppl 7):22-32.
17. Cavanagh SR, Shin LM, Karamouz N, Rauch SL: Psychiatric and emotional sequelae of surgical amputation. *Psychosomatics* 2006;47(6):459-464.
18. Grieger TA, Cozza SJ, Ursano RJ, et al: Posttraumatic stress disorder and depression in battle-injured soldiers. *Am J Psychiatry* 2006;163(10):1777-1783.
19. Heron-Delaney M, Kenardy J, Charlton E, Matsuoka Y: A systematic review of predictors of posttraumatic stress disorder (PTSD) for adult road traffic crash survivors. *Injury* 2013;44(11):1413-1422.
20. Zatzick D, Jurkovich GJ, Rivara FP, et al: A national US study of posttraumatic stress disorder, depression, and work and functional outcomes after hospitalization for traumatic injury. *Ann Surg* 2008;248(3):429-437.
21. Aaron DL, Fadale PD, Harrington CJ, Born CT: Posttraumatic stress disorders in civilian orthopaedics. *J Am Acad Orthop Surg* 2011;19(5):245-250.
22. Vincent HK, Horodyski M, Vincent KR, Brisbane ST, Sadasivan KK: Psychological distress after orthopedic trauma: Prevalence in patients and implications for rehabilitation. *PM R* 2015;7(9):978-989.
23. Stevelink SA, Malcolm EM, Mason C, Jenkins S, Sundin J, Fear NT: The prevalence of mental health disorders in (ex-)military personnel with a physical impairment: A systematic review. *Occup Environ Med* 2015;72(4):243-251.
24. Melcer T, Sechriest VF, Walker J, Galarneau M: A comparison of health outcomes for combat amputee and limb salvage patients injured in Iraq and Afghanistan wars. *J Trauma Acute Care Surg* 2013;75(2 suppl 2):S247-S254.
25. Doukas WC, Hayda RA, Frisch HM, et al: The Military Extremity Trauma Amputation/Limb Salvage (METALS) study: Outcomes of amputation versus limb salvage following major lower-extremity trauma. *J Bone Joint Surg Am* 2013;95(2):138-145.
26. Forbes D, Creamer M, Biddle D: The validity of the PTSD checklist as a measure of symptomatic change in combat-related PTSD. *Behav Res Ther* 2001;39(8):977-986.
27. Hoge CW, Castro CA, Messer SC, McGurk D, Cotting DI, Koffman RL: Combat duty in Iraq and Afghanistan, mental health problems, and barriers to care. *N Engl J Med* 2004;351(1):13-22.
28. Mitchell SL, Hayda R, Chen AT, Carlini AR, Ficke JR, MacKenzie EJ: The Military Extremity Trauma Amputation/Limb Salvage (METALS) study: Outcomes of amputation compared with limb salvage following major upper-extremity trauma. *J Bone Joint Surg Am* 2019;101(16):1470-1478.
29. American Psychiatric Association: *Diagnostic and Statistical Manual of Mental Disorders*, ed 5. American Psychiatric Association, 2013.
30. Kashani JH, Frank RG, Kashani SR, Wonderlich SA, Reid JC: Depression among amputees. *J Clin Psychiatry* 1983;44(7):256-258.

31. Cansever A, Uzun O, Yildiz C, Ates A, Atesalp AS: Depression in men with traumatic lower part amputation: A comparison to men with surgical lower part amputation. *Mil Med* 2003;168(2):106-109.
32. Langer KG: Depression in disabling illness: Severity and patterns of self-reported symptoms in three groups. *J Geriatr Psychiatry Neurol* 1994;7(2):121-128.
33. Roepke AM, Turner AP, Henderson AW, et al: A prospective longitudinal study of trajectories of depressive symptoms after dysvascular amputation. *Arch Phys Med Rehabil* 2019;100(8):1426-1433.e1.
34. Darnall BD, Ephraim P, Wegener ST, et al: Depressive symptoms and mental health service utilization among persons with limb loss: Results of a national survey. *Arch Phys Med Rehabil* 2005;86(4):650-658.
35. McDonald S, Sharpe L, Blaszczynski A: The psychosocial impact associated with diabetes-related amputation. *Diabet Med* 2014;31(11):1424-1430.
36. Washington ED, Williams AE: An exploratory phenomenological study exploring the experiences of people with systemic disease who have undergone lower limb amputation and its impact on their psychological well-being. *Prosthet Orthot Int* 2016;40(1):44-50.
37. Hanley MA, Jensen MP, Ehde DM, Hoffman AJ, Patterson DR, Robinson LR: Psychosocial predictors of long-term adjustment to lower-limb amputation and phantom limb pain. *Disabil Rehabil* 2004;26(14-15):882-893.
38. Whyte AS, Niven CA: Psychological distress in amputees with phantom limb pain. *J Pain Symptom Manage* 2001;22(5):938-946.
39. Lew HL, Otis JD, Tun C, Kerns RD, Clark ME, Cifu DX: Prevalence of chronic pain, posttraumatic stress disorder, and persistent postconcussive symptoms in OIF/OEF veterans: Polytrauma clinical triad. *J Rehabil Res Dev* 2009;46(6):697-702.
40. Norman SB, Stein MB, Dimsdale JE, Hoyt DB: Pain in the aftermath of trauma is a risk factor for posttraumatic stress disorder. *Psychol Med* 2008;38(4):533-542.
41. Von Korff M, Simon G: The relationship between pain and depression. *Br J Psychiatry Suppl* 1996;168(30):101-108.
42. Castillo RC, Carlini AR, Doukas WC, et al: Pain, depression, and posttraumatic stress disorder following major extremity trauma among united states military serving in Iraq and Afghanistan: Results from the military extremity trauma and amputation/limb salvage study. *J Orthop Trauma* 2021;35(3):e96-e102.
43. Wegener ST, Castillo RC, Haythornthwaite J, MacKenzie EJ, Bosse MJ, Group LS: Psychological distress mediates the effect of pain on function. *Pain* 2011;152(6):1349-1357.
44. Rybarczyk BD, Nyenhuis DL, Nicholas JJ, Schulz R, Alioto RJ, Blair C: Social discomfort and depression in a sample of adults with leg amputations. *Arch Phys Med Rehabil* 1992;73(12):1169-1173.
45. Rybarczyk B, Nyenhuis DL, Nicholas JJ, Cash SM, Kaiser J: Body image, perceived social stigma, and the prediction of psychosocial adjustment to leg amputation. *Rehabil Psychol* 1995;40(2):95-110.
46. McGill G, Wilson G, Caddick N, Forster N, Kiernan MD: Rehabilitation and transition in military veterans after limb-loss. *Disabil Rehabil* 2021;43(23):3315-3322.
47. Hou WH, Sheu CF, Liang HW, et al: Trajectories and predictors of return to work after traumatic limb injury – A 2-year follow-up study. *Scand J Work Environ Health* 2012;38(5):456-466.
48. Kugelman DN, Haglin JM, Carlock KD, Konda SR, Egol KA: The association between patient education level and economic status on outcomes following surgical management of (fracture) non-union. *Injury* 2019;50(2):344-350.
49. MacDermid JC, Donner A, Richards RS, Roth JH: Patient versus injury factors as predictors of pain and disability six months after a distal radius fracture. *J Clin Epidemiol* 2002;55(9):849-854.
50. MacKenzie EJ, Bosse MJ, Castillo RC, et al: Functional outcomes following trauma-related lower-extremity amputation. *J Bone Joint Surg Am* 2004;86(8):1636-1645.
51. MacKenzie EJ, Bosse MJ, Kellam JF, et al: Early predictors of long-term work disability after major limb trauma. *J Trauma* 2006;61(3):688-694.
52. Bosma H, Sanderman R, Scaf-Klomp W, Van Eijk JTM, Ormel J, Kempen GIJM: Demographic, health-related and psychosocial predictors of changes in depressive symptoms and anxiety in late middle-aged and older persons with fall-related injuries. *Psychol Health* 2004;19(1):103-115.
53. Holtslag HR, van Beeck EF, Lindeman E, Leenen LP: Determinants of long-term functional consequences after major trauma. *J Trauma* 2007;62(4):919-927.
54. American Academy of Orthopaedic Surgeons: Evaluation of Psychosocial Factors Influencing Recovery from Adult Orthopaedic Trauma: Evidence-Based Clinical Practice Guideline. 2019. https://www.aaos.org/globalassets/quality-and-practice-resources/dod/prf-cpg-final-draft-12-3-19.pdf. Accessed September 14, 2021.
55. Gajewski D, Granville R: The United States armed forces amputee patient care program. *J Am Acad Orthop Surg* 2006;14(10 Spec No.):S183-S187.
56. MacKenzie EJ, Jones AS, Bosse MJ, et al: Health-care costs associated with amputation or reconstruction of a limb-threatening injury. *J Bone Joint Surg Am* 2007;89(8):1685-1692.
57. Pasquina PF, Tsao JW, Collins DM, et al: Quality of medical care provided to service members with combat-related limb amputations: Report of patient satisfaction. *J Rehabil Res Dev* 2008;45(7):953-960.
58. Jensen MP, Ehde DM, Hoffman AJ, Patterson DR, Czerniecki JM, Robinson LR: Cognitions, coping and social environment predict adjustment to phantom limb pain. *Pain* 2002;95(1-2):133-142.
59. Hill A, Niven CA, Knussen C: The role of coping in adjustment to phantom limb pain. *Pain* 1995;62(1):79-86.
60. Hill A: The use of pain coping strategies by patients with phantom limb pain. *Pain* 1993;55(3):347-353.
61. Jensen MP, Smith DG, Ehde DM, Robinsin LR: Pain site and the effects of amputation pain: Further clarification of the meaning of mild, moderate, and severe pain. *Pain* 2001;91(3):317-322.
62. Miller MJ, Mealer ML, Cook PF, Kittelson AJ, Christiansen CL: Psychometric assessment of the connor-davidson resilience scale for people with lower-limb amputation. *Phys Ther* 2021;101(4):pzab002.
63. Walsh MV, Armstrong TW, Poritz J, Elliott TR, Jackson WT, Ryan T: Resilience, pain interference, and upper limb loss: Testing the mediating effects of positive emotion and activity restriction on distress. *Arch Phys Med Rehabil* 2016;97(5):781-787.

64. Krause JS, Rohe DE: Personality and life adjustment after spinal cord injury: An exploratory study. *Rehabil Psychol* 1998;43(2):118-130.
65. Elliott TR, Witty TE, Herrick S, Hoffman JT: Negotiating reality after physical loss: Hope, depression, and disability. *J Pers Soc Psychol* 1991;61(4):608-613.
66. Elliott AM, Smith BH, Hannaford PC, Smith WC, Chambers WA: The course of chronic pain in the community: Results of a 4-year follow-up study. *Pain* 2002;99(1-2):299-307.
67. Dunn DS: Well-being following amputation: Salutary effects of positive meaning, optimism, and control. *Rehabil Psychol* 1996;41(4):285-302.
68. Tennen H, Affleck G: Benefit-finding and benefit-reminding, in Snyder CR, Lopez JH, eds: *Handbook of Positive Psychology*. Oxford University Press, 2002, pp 584-597.
69. Kennedy P, Marsh N, Lowe R, Grey N, Short E, Rogers B: A longitudinal analysis of psychological impact and coping strategies following spinal cord injury. *Br J Health Psychol* 2000;5 (pt 2):157-172.
70. Stutts L, Stanaland A: Posttraumatic growth in individuals with amputations. *Disabil Health J* 2016;9(1):167-171.
71. Arnstein P, Caudill M, Mandle CL, Norris A, Beasley R: Self efficacy as a mediator of the relationship between pain intensity, disability and depression in chronic pain patients. *Pain* 1999;80(3):483-491.
72. Lorig K, Holman H: Arthritis self-management studies: A twelve-year review. *Health Educ Q* 1993;20(1):17-28.
73. Bandura A: *Social Foundations of Thought and Action: A Social Cognitive Theory*. Prentice-Hall, Inc., 1986, xiii, 617 pp.
74. Fuhrer MJ, Rintala DH, Hart KA, Clearman R, Young ME: Relationship of life satisfaction to impairment, disability, and handicap among persons with spinal cord injury living in the community. *Arch Phys Med Rehabil* 1992;73(6):552-557.
75. Elliott TR, Shewchuk RM, Richards JS: Caregiver social problem-solving abilities and family member adjustment to recent-onset physical disability. *Rehabil Psychol* 1999;44(1):104-123.
76. Farley FA, Weinstein SL: The case for patient-centered care in orthopaedics. *J Am Acad Orthop Surg* 2006;14(8):447-451.
77. Levin PE, MacKenzie EJ, Roy MJ, Bosse MJ, Ling GS: Psychological, social, and functional manifestations of orthopaedic trauma and traumatic brain injury, in Browner BD, Jupiter JB, Krettek C, Anderson PA, eds: *Skeletal Trauma*. 1, ed 5. Elsevier Saunders, 2015, pp 745-759.
78. Bradford AN, Castillo RC, Carlini AR, Wegener ST, Teter H Jr, Mackenzie EJ: The trauma survivors network: Survive. Connect. Rebuild. *J Trauma* 2011;70(6):1557-1560.
79. Recovery assessment. Available at: http://www.traumasurvivorsnetwork.org/recovery_assessments. Accessed September 13, 2021.
80. Keefe FJ, Rumble ME, Scipio CD, Giordano LA, Perri LM: Psychological aspects of persistent pain: Current state of the science. *J Pain* 2004;5(4):195-211.
81. Wegener ST, Bechtold K, Hill-Briggs F, Johnson-Greene D, Palmer S, Salorio C: Rehabilitation psychology assessment and intervention, in Braddom R, ed: *Physical Medicine and Rehabilitation*, ed 3. Elsevier, 2006, pp 63-93.
82. Entsuah R, Gao B: Global benefit-risk evaluation of antidepressant action: Comparison of pooled data for venlafaxine, SSRIs, and placebo. *CNS Spectr* 2002;7(12):882-888.
83. Roshanaei-Moghaddam B, Pauly MC, Atkins DC, Baldwin SA, Stein MB, Roy-Byrne P: Relative effects of CBT and pharmacotherapy in depression versus anxiety: Is medication somewhat better for depression, and CBT somewhat better for anxiety? *Depress Anxiety* 2011;28(7):560-567.
84. Lisanby SH: Electroconvulsive therapy for depression. *N Engl J Med* 2007;357(19):1939-1945.
85. Jonas DE, Cusack K, Forneris CA, et al: *Psychological and pharmacological treatments for adults with Posttraumatic Stress Disorder (PTSD). AHRQ Comparative Effectiveness Reviews*. Agency for Healthcare Research and Quality (US), 2013.
86. VA/DoD: Clinical practice guidelines for management of posttraumatic stress disorder and acute stress. Available at: https://www.healthquality.va.gov/guidelines/MH/ptsd/VADoDPTSDCPG-Final012418.pdf. Accessed September 14, 2021.
87. Zaid MB, O'Donnell RJ, Potter BK, Forsberg JA: Orthopaedic osseointegration: State of the art. *J Am Acad Orthop Surg* 2019;27(22):e977-e985.
88. Block AR, Marek RJ: Presurgical psychological evaluation: Risk factor identification and mitigation. *J Clin Psychol Med Settings* 2020;27(2):396-405.
89. Block AR, Ohnmeiss DD, Guyer RD, Rashbaum RF, Hochschuler SH: The use of presurgical psychological screening to predict the outcome of spine surgery. *Spine J* 2001;1(4):274-282.
90. Institute of Medicine Committee on Quality of Health Care in A: *Committee on quality of health care in America. Crossing the quality chasm: A new health system for the 21st century* 2001. National Academies Press (US). Copyright 2001 by the National Academy of Sciences. All rights reserved.
91. Bodenheimer T, Wagner EH, Grumbach K: Improving primary care for patients with chronic illness: The chronic care model, Part 2. *J Am Med Assoc* 2002;288(15):1909-1914.
92. Wegener ST, Mackenzie EJ, Ephraim P, Ehde D, Williams R: Self-management improves outcomes in persons with limb loss. *Arch Phys Med Rehabil* 2009;90(3):373-380.
93. Chodosh J, Morton SC, Mojica W, et al: Meta-analysis: Chronic disease self-management programs for older adults. *Ann Intern Med* 2005;143(6):427-438.
94. Turner AP, Wegener ST, Williams RM, et al: Self-management to improve function after amputation: A randomized controlled trial of the VETPALS intervention. *Arch Phys Med Rehabil* 2021;102(7):1274-1282.
95. NextSteps. Welcome to nextsteps. Available at: http://nextstepsonline.org/. Accessed September 13, 2021.
96. Butcher L: Amputee network provides peer support. *Bull Am Coll Surg* 2009;94(9):20-23.
97. Amputee Coalition. Support groups and peer support. Available at: http://www.amputee-coalition.org/support-groups--peer-support/how-to-find-support/. Accessed September 13, 2021.
98. Davison KP, Pennebaker JW, Dickerson SS: Who talks? The social psychology of illness support groups. *Am Psychol* 2000;55(2):205-217.

99. Wells L, Schachter B, Little S, Whylie B, Balogh PA: Enhancing rehabilitation through mutual aid: Outreach to people with recent amputations. *Health Soc Work* 1993;18(3):221-229.

100. Williams RM, Ehde DM, Smith DG, Czerniecki JM, Hoffman AJ, Robinson LR: A two-year longitudinal study of social support following amputation. *Disabil Rehabil* 2004;26(14-15):862-874.

101. Ziegler-Graham K, MacKenzie EJ, Ephraim PL, Travison TG, Brookmeyer R: Estimating the prevalence of limb loss in the United States: 2005 to 2050. *Arch Phys Med Rehabil* 2008;89(3):422-429.

Vocational and Recreational Considerations After Amputation

CHAPTER 57

Helena Burger, MD, PhD • Harvey Naranjo, COTA/L

ABSTRACT

Amputation has a profound influence on an individual's ability to return to work, sport, and some other leisure activities. The goal of postamputation rehabilitation is to allow individuals to integrate back into their communities as independent, productive members, suggesting a return to meaningful employment, recreation, and leisure activities. To better understand the challenges of returning to work and recreation, it is helpful to separately examine the effects of upper and lower limb amputation using the perspectives of the International Classification of Functioning, Disability and Health.

Keywords: adaptive sport; lower limb amputation; recreation; return to work; upper limb amputation; vocational rehabilitation

Introduction

Amputation represents a change in body structure. It has a substantial influence on an individual's quality of life and societal participation (including their ability to work and pursue leisure activities including sport and recreation) and quality of life. To improve quality of life following both lower and upper limb amputation, it is important to enable them to return to work, to recreation, and other leisure activities that they enjoy. These elements should be considered integral to comprehensive rehabilitation programs.

Return to Work

Amputation represents a change in body structure. It has a substantial influence on an individual's ability to perform many activities, on their societal participation (including the ability to work as well as leisure activities such as sport and recreation), and on their quality of life.[1-8] The first article about reemployment and vocational problems after amputation was published in 1955.[9] Interest has since increased in this topic, with more studies conducted on return to work rates and vocational challenges.[3] The number of studies related to return to work among military personnel and veterans has also increased. Such studies have been performed in different countries on five continents, with most originating in North America and several European countries, mainly the Netherlands and the United Kingdom.[3]

The ultimate objective of postamputation rehabilitation is to allow individuals to integrate back into their communities as independent, productive members, suggesting a return to meaningful employment. Although a change in employment may be required, rehabilitation outcomes are generally successful when a person achieves independence in activities of daily living and returns to active employment.[10]

Several factors influence return to work. According to the International Classification of Functioning, Disability and Health,[11] the factors can be divided into the topics of health conditions, body functions and structures, activities, and environmental and personal factors. The factors presented in this chapter follow this classification, with separate considerations for individuals after both lower and upper limb amputations for both war veterans and civilians. Individuals affected by lower limb amputation have different activity limitations and participation restrictions than those affected by upper limb amputation. Although both populations have problems with driving and carrying objects, individuals with lower limb amputation also have problems standing, walking, running, kicking, turning, and stamping. In contrast, individuals with upper limb amputation have problems grasping, lifting, pushing, pulling, writing, typing, and pounding.[12]

Lower Limb Amputation: Return to Work Considerations

The rates of successful return to work differ among studies and are difficult to compare because the inclusion criteria vary considerably.[13,14] The rate of employment is largely dependent upon the definition used and varied in one study between 71.5% and 88.4%.[14] Reported return to work rates range from 43.5%[4] to almost 100%.[1] Most reported rates are between approximately 50% and 66% after a unilateral

---

Neither of the following authors nor any immediate family member has received anything of value from or has stock or stock options held in a commercial company or institution related directly or indirectly to the subject of this chapter: Dr. Burger and Harvey Naranjo.

lower limb amputation and much lower (approximately 16%) after a bilateral lower limb amputation.[13,15-17] Long-term survivors of high-grade osteosarcoma appear to be unique in that this cohort, experiencing no major problems in their employment, with a return to work rate greater than 95%.[18]

Only one study compared the return to work rate of individuals after amputation with the employment rate in the general cohort.[19] The authors found a larger proportion of retired and unemployed individuals among men after amputation and a smaller proportion of students than in the general cohort of Asturias, Spain.[19] Men who had undergone an amputation also attained lower educational levels than the general cohort, whereas no such differences were found in women.

The reemployment rate alone does not provide sufficient information. After lower limb amputation, many patients work only part time or change their job (described in Environmental Factors section). An estimated 15.6% to 50.0% of patients work part time after amputation.[6,13,15] The median return to work was 12 months in most studies, ranging from 1.5 months to 21 years.[6,13,17,20]

Health Status
Negative predictors of return to work include comorbidities,[21,22] level of disability,[23] work-related amputation etiology,[6,21] comorbid major injuries during the event that caused the amputation, problems with residual and contralateral limbs, and phantom and residual limb pain.[4,21,24] Only Ide et al[15] found that both residual limb pain and phantom pain did not influence return to work, but among their patients, those with more severe pain were less satisfied with their work. Ide et al[15] and Fisher et al[16] also reported that the etiology of the amputation did not correlate with satisfaction with working life or return to work.[15,16,25] After amputation, secondary impairments may develop, including hip and knee osteoarthrosis, low back pain, and osteoporosis.[26] These impairments may also influence the ability to work, but research is needed to confirm this relationship.

Body Functions and Structure
Although some studies demonstrate that lower limb amputation decreases muscle strength, causes balance problems, and may decrease range of motion,[27,28] no studies exist on whether these considerations of body functions create problems at work or adversely affect return to work. A relationship seems likely because these factors influence some activities such as walking on level ground, walking on varied terrain, the ability to carry objects, and climbing stairs.[27,28]

Level and Type of Amputation
Between 3.5%[1] and 50.0%[17] of individuals who have undergone lower limb amputation are unable to work.[13,14,21] Approximately 15% of patients (range, 14.0% to 17.6%) retire because of amputation,[16] and 55% stop working within the first 2 years after amputation.[13] After amputation, approximately 25% of employed persons experience periods of unemployment lasting longer than 6 months.[14]

More proximal levels of amputation may decrease return to work rates. Persons with transfemoral amputations have lower return to work rates than those with a transtibial amputation.[6,22,25] Livingston et al[6] reported that no individuals within their cohort returned to work after transfemoral amputation. In contrast, Fisher et al[16] reported no correlation between the level of amputation and scores on an employment questionnaire. Return to work has been reported as lower with multiple amputations.[14] In addition, individuals with transtibial amputation are more willing or able to work than those with successful limb salvage.

Skin
Up to 41% of patients who have undergone lower limb amputation can have different types of skin problems, including wounds.[29] More active individuals have an increased risk for the development of skin problems. Those who are employed, walking without ambulatory aids, and walking in the community have more skin problems than unemployed and retired individuals, than those using two canes, crutches, or a walker, or those walking at home only.[29]

Activities and Participation
Journey et al[2] found that the reintegration into Normal Living Index is a predictor of return to work. However, several studies reporting on return to work after amputation have described the problems individuals reported in their work environments, including walking, climbing stairs, driving, and using public transportation.[1,6,12]

The immediate influence of considerations of activities and participation on return to work has not been directly studied. However, walking distance and restrictions in mobility have a substantial, clinically relevant influence on the individual's ability to return to work.[21] Better physical functioning 3 months after amputation and a lower disability level are positive predictors for return to work.[23,24] Basic physical activities are important considerations in going to and from work and also for some working tasks[12] and can therefore reduce productivity when impeded.[16]

Environmental Factors
Prosthesis
After amputation, a prosthesis is needed that enables the patient to perform their work and is suitable for physical and environmental requirements. Most patients require a prosthesis that decreases the frequency of stumbles and falls, enables good mobility, and allows the individual to perform activities that require divided attention.[30] Some individuals require specific adaptations of the prosthesis. Both the use and wearing comfort of a prosthesis influence return to work in a substantial, clinically relevant manner.[21] Problems with the prosthesis are among the major reasons for reduced productivity.[16]

Climate
Climate is one of the most common environmental barriers for individuals after amputation (in 55.4% of cases).[31] A hot climate can increase sweating and skin problems; a cold climate can influence battery working time for those with a battery-powered prosthesis. However, no studies exist on the

influence of climate on return to work rates or problems at work.

Geography

Physical environment is the second most common environmental barrier (in 54.7% of cases), especially for individuals after lower limb amputation.[31] Walking up and down hills and on uneven terrain is more difficult than walking on smooth, even ground. However, as with climate, no studies exist on the influence of geography on either return to work rates or problems at work.

Type of Work

Although Fisher et al[16] found no difference in employment rate associated with the type of previous work (skilled versus unskilled), 4% to 60% of patients have to change to a different job after lower limb amputation. In most studies, the reported proportion is approximately one-third.[13,22] A general shift from manual to nonmanual employment has occurred, trending toward more administrative and/or scientific/technical work.[4,13] Most individuals move between one and three grades below their preamputation employment classification (ie, from skilled to semiskilled or unskilled occupations).[4] The demands of the job before and after amputation, assessed on a scale ranging from 0 to 16, decreased from a mean of 12.1 to 8.3, respectively.[3] Working before an amputation, increased job involvement before amputation, and decreased workload after amputation are all associated with increased success in return to work.[16,22,24]

Between 28% and 43% of those who undergo lower limb amputation require job adaptations;[7,13] almost one-third remain partially dependent on colleagues.[13] Adaptations needed for each amputation level are well described by Girdhar et al.[12] Two-thirds of patients feel that their productivity is as good as before amputation,[14] and one-fourth work overtime hours.[30] The main reasons for decreased productivity are problems with the prosthesis (48%), transportation difficulties (28%), and other physical problems (20%).[14]

Approximately 57% of the patients were dissatisfied with work reintegration after amputation, citing fewer possibilities for promotion.[13] Livingston et al[6] reported that most patients who returned to work did so at a lower salary, but Wan Hazmy et al[17] found that 40% held the same income. A lower status position and lower income can result in loss of self-esteem and feelings of inadequacy.[32] Individuals with higher income before amputation are more likely to return to work.[6,22] Low income is one of the most common environmental barriers following both upper and lower limb amputation.[31]

Support

Family support, volunteers in the patient's community, survivor groups, health professionals, the possibility of vocational rehabilitation, and the support of colleagues and supervisors have been observed as important factors in successful return to work.[13,16,22]

Transportation Services

After lower limb amputation, many individuals experience problems driving and using public transportation.[1,6,16] Difficulty with transportation is one of the main reasons for decreased productivity;[16] hence, accessible transportation may decrease these problems.

Legal and Social Security Services

Social security systems and services differ greatly among countries; therefore, the results are difficult to compare, and results from one country may not apply to another. When disability benefits exceed work income, individuals may have no interest in returning to work, especially those who are not satisfied with their work. The Dutch system, in which it is possible to combine disability and other benefits proportionally with income from work,[13] seems conducive to stimulating return to work. Importantly, those who return to employment may consume substantially fewer services than unemployed individuals.[4]

Health Services, Systems, and Policies

Effective acute care and comprehensive interdisciplinary rehabilitation that includes vocational rehabilitation is needed after amputation. Vocational rehabilitation intervention increases return to work rates.[14,21-23,32] Authors have found that one-third[33] to one-half[22] of patients need vocational rehabilitation. In addition, many individuals can benefit from workplace assessments.[22] Shorter periods of acute care and less time from injury to amputation surgery are positive predictors of return to work.[22] A prerequisite to such services is health insurance, which is difficult for many amputees to obtain.[18]

Personal Factors

Sex

Millstein et al[14] and Whyte and Carroll[4] reported higher unemployment rates among women than among men, whereas Schoppen et al[13] found this to be reversed among older adults. Wan Hazmy et al[17] reported that more women than men retained their jobs without affecting income (50% versus 31%).

Age

Younger age is a positive predictor for return to work.[14,21,22,24] The unemployment rate was 22% for patients younger than 45 years compared with 48% for those older than 45 years.[14] In the cited study, only one of five individuals who lost their job after amputation was younger than 45 years. Similarly, those who were older at the time of amputation were more dissatisfied with reintegration into work activity.

Education

Having attained a higher educational level is a positive, clinically relevant predictor of return to work.[6,21,24] However, certain pediatric amputations have been associated with reduced rates of graduation from high school and college.[18]

Other Factors

Other factors associated with increased return to work rates include greater motivation, a positive attitude about return to work, being white, being a nonsmoker, possessing higher self-efficacy, and an absence of associated litigation.[23,24] Higher unemployment in the general cohort adversely affects return to work rates.[23]

Upper Limb Amputation: Return to Work Considerations

The employment rates of individuals with upper limb amputation are lower than employment rates for the general community.[33] In Denmark, the unemployment rate of patients with upper limb amputation is twice that of the total cohort.[2] The employment rate may further decrease as time from amputation increases.[33]

Tremendous variability exists in the percentages of patients who successfully return to work after upper limb amputation. As with lower limb amputation, return to work after upper limb amputation depends on the definitions selected.[14] Nevertheless, one study has suggested that more than 90% of individuals reported problems with employment or job seeking after upper limb amputation.[31]

No data exist on whether individuals reemployed after upper limb amputation were working full or part time. The time required to return to work ranges from 5 days to 24 months;[6,34] this time may be shorter for certain populations. Reed[34] reported that farmers return to work 5 days to 6 months after a major upper limb amputation.

Health Status

Individuals with upper limb amputation have higher frequencies of depression and posttraumatic stress disorder symptoms than those with lower limb amputation.[35] Depression has been associated with lower employment rates.[34] Other health concerns that may correlate with lower employment rates include both phantom limb pain[4,14] and residual limb pain.[14,36] Several years after upper limb amputation, overuse syndromes and secondary impairments (such as neck, shoulder, and elbow pain, and carpal tunnel syndrome)[37] can develop and may pose additional problems at work.[37]

Body Functions and Structure
Level and Type of Amputation

Most authors have observed that the level of upper limb amputation affects return to work. Individuals with transradial amputation have a lower unemployment rate (range, 10% to 40%) than those with transhumeral amputation (range, 22% to 57%).[14,38] The return to work rate is even lower for patients after bilateral upper limb amputation.[33,36] Reemployment rates for individuals with finger or partial hand amputation range from 64%[20] to 72%.[5] Individuals with amputation of three or more fingers seldom keep the same job after amputation.[5]

The cause of the amputation also can influence return to work. Very few individuals who sustained work-related amputation returned to the same type of work afterward.[6] The length of time before return to work is increased for individuals with finger amputation because of work-related causes (mean, 7.5 months) compared with those who underwent amputation because of a non–work-related injury (mean, 1.7 months).[8] More individuals with congenital upper limb deficiency are manual workers than are those who have undergone traumatic upper limb amputation. Amputation of the dominant upper limb compared with the nondominant limb does not appear to influence return to work rates or the type of work individuals return to,[5,14,38] even when returning to preamputation vocations.[36]

Skin

With burn-related amputations, the residual limb is often characterized by areas of impaired sensation caused by scarring or skin transplants. This can make fitting an upper limb prosthesis difficult and may present a problem for those who would use their prostheses for work.[39] Individuals who choose not to use a prosthesis when working may be at risk for the development of wounds.

Environmental Factors
Prosthesis

After upper limb amputation, an individual may work with or without the assistance of a prosthesis,[33,40-42] depending on the type of work and the type of prosthesis. Approximately 16% of patients with upper limb amputation indicate the prosthesis is the main factor preventing return to work.[36] However, other sources suggest that using a prosthesis is not a prerequisite for employment. Employed patients who do not use a prosthesis are mainly unskilled workers, which suggests that many prosthetic components are not appropriate for heavy manual work.

Although studies have reported on using a prosthesis for work, not all investigated whether the type of prosthesis affects this decision. Silcox et al[41] reported that the highest percentage of employed individuals with upper limb amputation used a body-powered prosthesis for work (35%), followed by myoelectric prostheses (27%). Approximately 50% of those surveyed indicated that they never used their myoelectric or passive prosthesis for work. In contrast, Pylatiuk et al[40] reported that more than 80% of individuals used their myoelectric prosthesis for work. Myoelectric prostheses are used mainly for occupations that require sitting at a desk or supervising others,[41] handicrafts, or operation of electronic and domestic devices.[40] Similarly, Østlie et al[42] reported that when rated on a scale of 1 to 5, the most useful terminal device for work and/or school appears to be myoelectric hands (mean score, 4.8), followed by body-powered terminal devices (mean, 4.3), myoelectric hooks (mean, 4.1), and cosmetic prostheses (mean, 3.5). Silicone finger prostheses are also used more frequently by individuals who have an occupation that requires sitting at the desk than those who perform manual labor.[5] It is important that all individuals who use their prosthesis for work have a readily available backup prosthesis to avoid interruption of work and activities when the prosthesis needs repair or replacement.

Despite recent advances in upper limb prosthetic technology, the upper limb prosthesis still does not adequately replace the fine dexterous movement and sensation of a human hand. Nevertheless, the use of new components may make the observations of previous studies on return to work obsolete and reduce problems experienced at work.

Climate

As with lower limb amputation, climate has been identified as a potentially important barrier to return to work after upper limb amputation.[31]

Type of Work

Whether an individual will be able to perform the same work as before undergoing upper limb amputation depends on both the type of work and the amputation level. The percentage of individuals who change the type of work they do after a major upper limb amputation varies from 20% to 100%.[6,38] Some authors have suggested that all patients undergoing upper limb amputation have to change the type of work they do.[36]

Studies reported that up to 47% of patients who underwent partial hand amputation had to change the type of work they do.[5,8] Musicians playing string instruments, keyboards, or woodwinds may have to change careers even if they have undergone amputation of a nail and nail bed only.[43] The Hand Injury Severity Score (HISS) can help predict the ability of patients undergoing partial hand amputation to return to their original jobs.[44] HISS assesses injuries to the integument (skin), skeleton (bone), tendon, and nerves of each finger. Most patients with a HISS score of less than 50 are able to return to their original jobs, whereas those with a HISS score of more than 150 are unable to return to their original jobs.[44]

Most patients who must change the type of work they do after amputation previously performed unskilled manual work, such as driving a truck, assisting in a shop, or working in a mine.[4,5,8,14,33,38] Most of these workers changed to clerical work and jobs in the service industries or went back to school.[14,33] Fernández et al[38] reported that the lowest percentage of workers returned to the agriculture sector, whereas Reed[34] reported that all the farmers in his study returned to work very soon after a major upper limb amputation. Improved knowledge of social- and work-related policies within different countries is required to explain those differences.

Modifying a workstation and/or redesigning tasks may make certain job tasks easier or even possible to perform after upper limb amputation.[7,12] The changes needed depend on the task, the level of amputation, and the type of prosthesis.[12]

As with lower limb amputation, individuals have fewer possibilities for job promotions and reduced potential for salary increases after upper limb amputation.[14] Some researchers found that the size of a company did not influence the return to work rate, whereas others concluded that it is a fundamental factor.[38] In France, companies with 5,000 employees or more guarantee return to work (in the same or a different job), whereas in small companies, the amputee's return depends on the company's structure, on the competence and initiative of the individual, and on their ability to perform another job.[38]

Legal and Social Security Services

Although Fernández et al[38] found that social security is not a determining factor regarding return to work, Gallagher et al[31] observed (albeit in a small sample) that more than 50% of amputees perceived laws, regulations, and entitlements as a barrier. Return to work may be facilitated by enlightened employers. Jang et al[36] found that 12% of patients reported lack of social awareness about individuals with disabilities as a barrier for return to work after upper limb amputation.

Health Services, Systems, and Policies

If interdisciplinary rehabilitation programs do not include activities that are important for return to work, the program may not be helpful and may even prevent patients from performing their jobs.[34,44] The time from amputation to the first fitting of a prosthesis must be limited. Resnik et al[45] observed that if this period extends beyond 30 days or 12 weeks, respectively, then patients are less likely to work again.

Vocational rehabilitation and training may help individuals return to their former jobs or reeducate them for new jobs after upper limb amputation, especially for those employed in farming or manual labor before amputation.[7,36] Individuals who are capable of on-the-job training have a higher return to work rate than those who need more extensive vocational preparation.[14]

Personal Factors

Sex

Sex can also affect return to work rates, although observations have been inconsistent. Some researchers found that women have a higher unemployment rate than men after amputation;[4,14] however, Fernández et al[38] found the rate for retired and unemployed men was higher. Burger et al[5] reported that more women than men were able to return to the same job after partial hand amputation.

Age

Individuals younger than 50 years are more likely to return to work than their older counterparts. Similarly, older patient age at the time of amputation results in a reduced rate of return to work, and more older amputees retire.[5,14]

Education

An individual's level of education does not appear to have a substantial influence on remaining employed after amputation, although those with lower educational levels often have to change their job.[5,6,38] Lower educational levels also make vocational rehabilitation more difficult.[33]

Other Factors

Another factor is the year in which the amputation occurred. Patients who underwent amputation during the 1960s and 1970s returned to work more frequently than those who underwent amputation in later years.[38] This is most likely related to environmental factors such as general job market conditions during the different eras and the evolution of social security services.

War Veterans

The results of studies on war veterans are difficult to compare because some report on return to work for military personnel in general, whereas others report on the return to active duty, and some report on military personnel injured by land mines.

The percentage of military personnel with an amputation who returned to work differs greatly, both among countries and also in separate studies within a country. The return to work rate for Iranian soldiers varied from 48% to 61%;[46] the rate for US military personnel injured in Vietnam varied between 70% and 98%.[47] The percentage decreases with a higher level of amputation.[47] Comorbidities also can affect return to work. Several years after the amputation, veterans may be affected by secondary conditions such as back pain (44%) and contralateral knee pain (33%).[46] In addition, approximately 75% of war veterans have psychological problems.[47] The only return to work rate reported for veterans after upper limb amputation was 60%.[46] However, the type of work was not reported in the study.

During the past 15 years, the percentage of military personnel who returned to active duty increased from 2% to 16% in the United States and 85% in the United Kingdom.[48,49] Those who returned to active duty had mainly sustained a partial hand or foot amputation or transtibial amputation. Those with multiple limb amputations have the lowest return-to-duty rate (3%).[48] Military personnel who return to active duty are a mean of more than 4 years older than those who do not,[48] which may relate to the observation that officers and senior enlisted personnel returned to duty at a higher rate than younger personnel (35% versus 7%).[47] Most veterans changed occupation after amputation, with an observable shift toward the civilian sector.[48,49] In the United Kingdom, the mean time to return to work after amputation was 9.9 months (range, 4.5 to 24.3 months).[49] Vocational functional outcomes were worse in those who sustained more severe injuries, although the difference was not significant.[49]

A 1999 study reported that among those injured by landmines, approximately 33% returned to their previous occupation; others had to change employment. Among soldiers surviving a land mine explosion, 10% returned to duty after amputation. The return to work for this group depends on several factors, including ethnicity, the type of prosthesis, and the amount of disability pension.[50]

Adaptive Sport and Recreation

Adaptive sports and recreation has served as a valued rehabilitative resource for individuals living with a limb deficiency or amputation. Encouraging routine participation with adaptive sports and community-based recreation can contribute to the enhancement of an amputee's physical, psychological, and the social aspects of their lives. Early promotion for increased function and socialization through participation in sports and recreation will allow for an amputee to acquire the skills and confidence to physically adapt to the demands of everyday activities; master the use of prosthesis or adaptive equipment; and assist in identifying community resources that will contribute in promoting ongoing independence. Recognizing sports and recreation as an effective strategy for achieving positive rehabilitative physical and emotional outcomes will help pave the way for the maintenance of a safe, active, and inclusive lifestyle for individuals living with amputations or a limb deficiency.

Historically, the utilization of adaptive sports and participation in community recreation was born as a result of the marginalization of people with disabilities by able-bodied people. Participation in sports and recreation provided a venue for the disabled cohort to include amputees to demonstrate their ability, gain recognition, and establish their independence. One of the first records of amputees participating in sports was at Greenwich Hospital during the Napoleonic wars (1799 to 1815) when a team of one-armed patients played a team of one-legged patients in cricket. Another describes a sports festival at Newmarket Heath where two people with leg amputations were each provided with wooden legs to compete in a walking race.[51] Today, adaptive sports and recreation continues to serve as motivation for amputees to remain active and push past perceived societal and physical boundaries presented as a result of living with an amputation or limb deficiency.

According to an article published in the Institute for Health Metrics and Evaluations, it is estimated that in 2017 there were over 57 million people worldwide living with an amputation.[52] The recent conflicts around the world have contributed to the number of amputees and the growing demand for advancements in prosthetic technology, physical environments to be accessible, and for community support to be in place for amputees to thrive. The response to meet this demand has prompted government and private organizations to increase support and funding for the ongoing development of adaptive resources. This event contributed to an improved availability of adaptive sports and recreation programs benefiting amputees of all levels and ages.[53] There are currently many sports and recreation opportunities available for the amputee cohort to participate in with or without a prosthesis or the need for activity-specific adaptive equipment.

Considerations

There are important considerations amputees should take in preparation for participation with adaptive sports or community recreation programs. Once an amputee has identified an adaptive sports program or recreational activity of interest, they should next meet with the program provider to discuss expectations for participation and to obtain the necessary adaptive equipment required to ensure a positive experience.

Early considerations in preparation for participation with sports or recreational activity should include the following:

1. Medical assessment: Is it medically appropriate for the individual to participate in the activity?
2. Activity analysis: What are the required demands of the activity, and can the participant mitigate the demands through grading, modification, or use of adaptive equipment?[54]

3. Equipment: Does the individual have access to the required prosthetic or adaptive equipment?
4. Risks: Determine the level of risk involved with that activity: low, moderate, or high.
5. Expertise: What is the level of experience or certification of the instructor, coach, or event facilitator?
6. Accessibility: Is the individual able to access the location, facility, or terrain where the activity is taking place?
7. Limb care: Limb care/hygiene should be promoted during the activity.
8. Independence: Continued compliance should be encouraged to promote proficiency with the activity.

Opportunities

There are various ways for amputees to participate with sports and recreation. The subsequent list identifies common adaptive sports and recreation resources that may be available locally for amputees for engagement from beginner to advanced levels of participation with or without the use of prosthesis.

Adaptive Sports

Circuit Training/Functional Fitness

Amputees can participate individually or in a group setting. Circuit training or functional fitness is a system of exercises and dynamic movements designed to improve strength, endurance, and physical function (**Figures 1** and **2**). Exercises can be performed with or without the use of a prosthesis. Amputees can participate one handed or from a sitting or standing position. Individuals can perform exercise programs with the use of their own body weight, resistance bands, stationary cardiovascular equipment, or the use of common household items. Exercise programs can be graded or modified to meet personal ability and the individual's level of fitness. Regular training can be performed in a community gym or dedicated exercise space in their home environment. Several adaptive circuit training resources can be found online and in text material. Circuit training promotes increased fitness, a

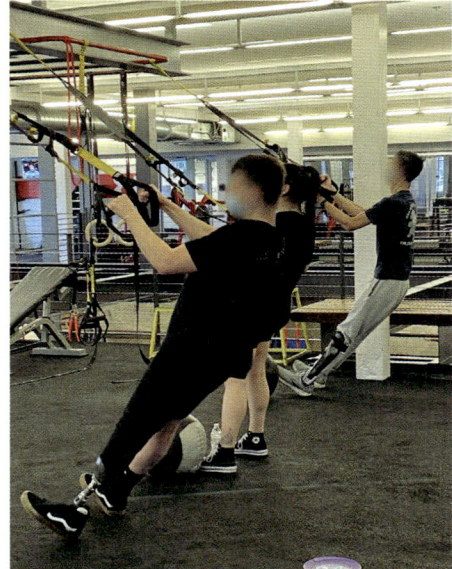

FIGURE 1 Photograph showing community gym group fitness. (Courtesy of Harvey Naranjo, Baltimore, MD, 2021.)

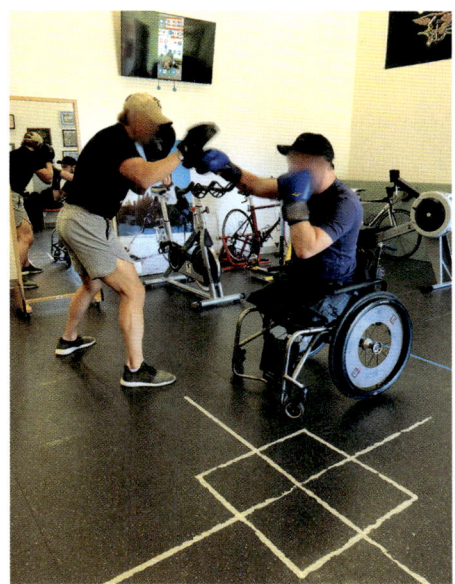

FIGURE 2 Photograph showing community boxing group fitness. (Courtesy of Harvey Naranjo, Bethesda, MD, 2021.)

positive body image, and a reduction in health complications. Current fitness trends also encourage group participation, which facilities socialization and inclusivity.

Adaptive Cycling

Amputees can participate with cycling with the use of cycling-specific (**Figure 3**) adaptive equipment, with or without a prosthesis or with the use of an adaptive bicycle. The type of adaptive bicycle an amputee may use will be dependent on the level of limb loss, cycling experience, and their access to adaptive cycling resources. Amputees can participate on standard bicycles, tandem cycles, handcycles, or recumbent cycles.

Individuals with upper extremity amputations or limb deficiencies may choose to participate one handed or with a prosthesis. Modifications to the gears and brakes will be required to allow access for one-handed control. There are also adaptive options for bilateral upper extremity amputees to cycle. The amputee will require individual training for proficiency and will need to use cycling-specific prosthetics and/or have access to electronic cycling technology. This option and many of the options listed subsequently are

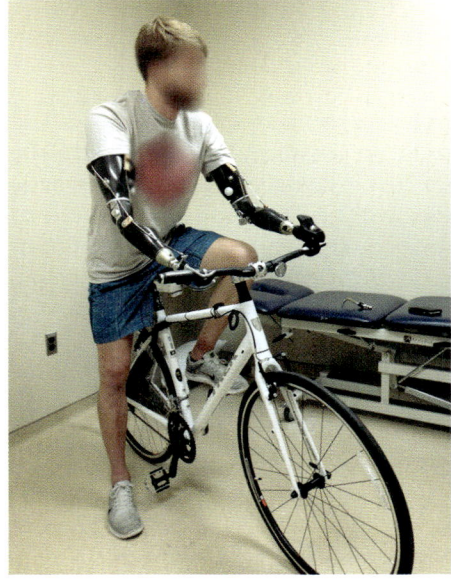

FIGURE 3 Photograph showing a custom adaptive bike fitting. (Courtesy of Harvey Naranjo, Bethesda, MD, 2016.)

only recommended for cycling in a low pedestrian and vehicle traffic area, for example, a dedicated cycling lane or bike trail.

Lower extremity amputees may choose to participate with a prosthesis or with one leg (**Figure 4**). Slight modifications to the bike pedals may be required. If cycling with a prosthetic leg, the amputee will benefit

Section 4: Management Issues

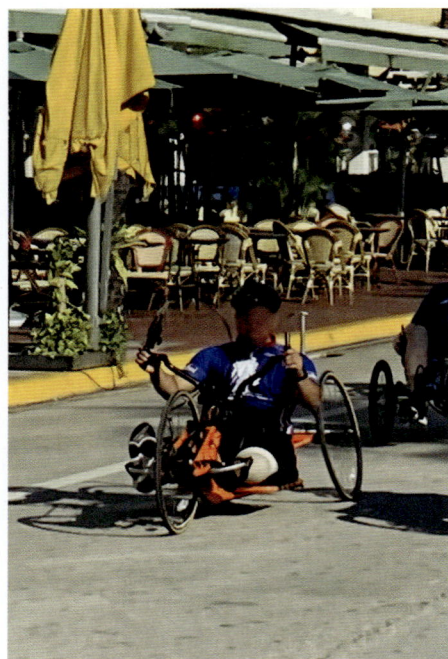

FIGURE 4 Photograph showing a hand cyclist soldier ride. (Courtesy of Wounded Warrior Project, Florida, 2021.)

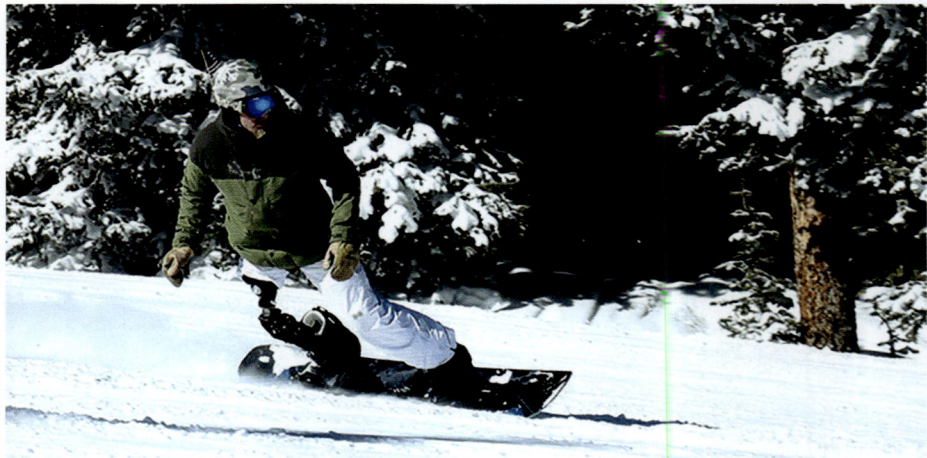

FIGURE 5 Photograph shows an adaptive ski and snowboard clinic. (Courtesy of Vail Veterans Program, Vail, CO, 2018.)

from a cycling-specific prosthesis. The pedal on prosthetic side may need to be shorten or lengthened, and a prosthetic foot will be required to be secured to the bike pedal to allow for the continued connection with the bicycle pedal. A similar prosthetic setup would be the recommendation for each pedal for bilateral lower extremity amputees who want to cycle on a standard bicycle. This option is only recommended for bilateral lower extremity amputees who have demonstrated cycling proficiency and are able to efficiently disengage at least one foot from the bike pedal.

The option for one-legged cycling is also available. With this approach, no special modifications to the bicycle would be necessary, but the amputee will require additional individual training for one-legged cycling proficiency. Using a caged pedal system is recommended. This setup will allow for the sound leg to maintain a connection with the bicycle pedal and allow for a quick release. This option is only recommended for cycling in a low pedestrian and vehicle traffic areas such as a dedicated cycling lane or bike trail.

Handcycling is another alternative for lower extremity amputees of all levels and ages. It enables the amputee to pedal a cycle exclusively using their upper body. Bicycle adaptations for hand propulsion are available for tandem cycles and wheelchairs. There are also some handcycles specifically designed for children. Handcycling is a Paralympic sport, which made its debut in Athens Greece in 2004.[55] Adaptive cycling assists amputees with improving balance, community mobility, and cardiovascular endurance.

Adaptive Skiing and Snowboarding

Adaptive skiing and snowboarding (**Figure 5**) are popular and inclusive sports for people with limb deficiencies or amputations. These sports offer a large variety of adaptive equipment and special techniques to allow the amputee cohort to experience the benefits of skiing and snowboarding. Many resorts have adaptive programs with handicap access offered throughout the resort to include the ski lift, gondolas, and mountains. The method used for the amputee's participation would be dependent on their level of amputation or limb deficiency and their access to a ski-specific or snowboard-specific prosthesis.

Stand-up skiing includes two-track, three-track, four-track, and snowboarding.[56] Stand-up skiing will require the use of ski poles with outriggers to assist with balance, turns, speed control, and stopping. Stand up is the suitable method of participation for upper and lower extremity amputees. Special terminal devices are available to allow for the use of ski poles. Prosthetic feet attachments are also available for direct connection to skis or snowboard. Depending on the method of choice, the amputees could participate with or without use of prostheses. When appropriate the use of a sports socket is recommended when skiing without a prosthesis to protect the residual limb from impact and the environment

Sit-down skiing includes bi-ski, dual-ski, mono-ski, and ski-bike Sit-down skiing (**Figure 6**) is the recommended method for lower extremity amputees who have limited mobility in their legs or choose to participate without the use of prosthesis. When appropriate the use of a sports socket is recommended when sit-skiing without a prosthesis to protect the residual limb from impact or the environment. Sit-skiing requires a seat to be fitted on top of one or two skis and the use of tethers if the amputee requires additional physical assistance. The number of skis used allows for increased or decrease maneuverability and control. The use of ski outriggers is required to assist with balance, turns, speed control, and stopping.

Ski-biking, or snow-biking, is a winter sport that consists of a bicycle-type frame mounted on ski blades. Foot skis are used for balance, turns, speed control, and stopping. This sport

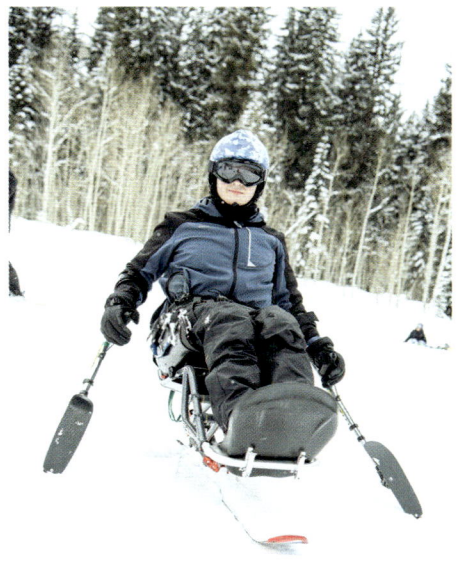

FIGURE 6 Photograph shows an adaptive ski and snowboard clinic. (Courtesy of Vail Veterans Program, Vail, CO, 2022.)

is suitable for both upper and lower extremity amputees with training for proficiency and the appropriate prosthetics or adaptive equipment.

Both adaptive skiing and snowboarding provide competitive or recreational opportunities for the amputee cohort. Athletes can participate in downhill racing, terrain park, and cross country. Skiing and snowboarding help amputees to improve their balance, fitness, confidence, and self-esteem.

Recreation

The Arts

"The Arts are practices that promote healing, wellness, coping and personal change. Traditional healing arts include music art, dance/movement, poetry/writing, and drama therapy."[57] Other practices include laughter and humor, animal-assisted therapy, and cooking or gardening. Amputees can participate with or without a prosthesis or need for specialized adaptive equipment. Key benefits for the amputee or person with a limb deficiency are that it assists with physical function, helps decrease pain, reduces stress, and provides opportunities for inclusivity and self-expression. There are many articles that discuss the positive health benefits of participation in the arts for our disabled cohort.[58]

Leisure Exploration

Leisure exploration is participating in the community and nature when time is free from the demands of work or duty. Leisure exploration is a means for amputees or people with limb deficiencies to be active and be recognized members of their communities. Leisure activities consist of travel, hiking, and fishing or going to the beach or lake. They also include social activities such as attending concerts, bars, and restaurants. Leisure activities are appropriate for amputees and individuals with a limb deficiency of all levels and ages, with or without a prosthesis. Regular participation in leisure activities can promote mental health, environmental accessibility, inclusivity, and community reintegration.

Recreation Technology

Recent advancement in technology has created increased opportunities for the amputee or person with a limb deficiency to socialize or participate in recreation. It provides platforms for amputees to discover other recreation resources, share experiences, and socialize. Social media applications provide a venue for dating, self-expression, and education. Video games and virtual experience platforms provide opportunities for the amputees to reach recreational resources never thought possible.[59] Exploring recreational opportunities through technology would be an alternative where recreation opportunities are limited. Recreation though technology is suitable for amputees and people with a limb deficiency of all levels and ages, with and without a prosthesis. Benefits can include increased participation, function, self-esteem, and socialization.

Resources

- **The Paralympic Games or Paralympics** have been described as "a periodic series of international multi-sport events involving athletes with a range of disabilities. There are winter and summer Paralympic Games, which are held almost immediately following the respective Olympic Games. All Paralympic Games are governed by the International Paralympic Committee (IPC). Given the wide variety of disabilities that Para athletes have, there are several categories in which the athletes compete in based on their disability classification. In Para sports, athletes are grouped by the degree of activity limitation resulting from the impairment."[60]
- **Achilles International** represents "a global organization operating in 25 countries including the United States, (which) transforms the lives of people with disabilities through athletic programs and social connection. Since their founding in 1983, they have empowered over 150,000 athletes of all ages and ability levels to participate in endurance events around the globe."[61]
- **Move United** describes itself as an organization that has been "redefining disability by providing year-round sports and recreation opportunities to people with a wide range of disabilities offering more than 70 different adaptive sports. Through their national network of more than 200 Community Member Organizations, Move United serves over 100,000 individuals with disabilities of all ages each year."[62]
- **National Sports Center for The Disabled** is described as "a world leader in creating and providing adaptive outdoor recreation experiences. As one of the largest and most comprehensive providers of adaptive experiences, they use the power of innovation, recreation and Colorado's great outdoors to improve access, opportunities and possibilities for people living with disabilities."[63]
- **American for the Arts** has asserted, "Our mission is to build recognition and support for the extraordinary and dynamic value of the arts and to lead, serve, and advance the diverse networks of organizations and individuals who cultivate the arts in America. Connecting your best ideas and leaders from the arts, communities, and business, together we can

work to ensure that every American has access to the transformative power of the arts."[64]
- **The Able Gamers Charity** describes its mission as "Creating opportunities that enable play in order to combat social isolation, foster inclusive communities and improve the quality of life for people with disabilities."[65]

Challenges

There are various challenges an amputee or individual with a limb deficiency may encounter as they start to explore participation with adaptive sports or recreation in their communities. Many have had little or no exposure to adaptive sports or recreation programs and may have not received the appropriate training on how to safely adapt to an activity, which can lead to injury or a lack of participation. Others did not receive any education on the numerous sports prostheses and adaptive equipment that are currently available for amputees. Amputees also have encountered challenges with the lack of access to adaptive sports and recreation opportunities in their communities. Many will have to travel outside of their community to access programs. This problem is very challenging when trying to build proficiency with an activity or a sport, especially if the activity or sport requires regular training or team practices.

Another enormous challenge amputees or individuals with limb deficiencies will encounter when trying to access sports and recreation is cost. The price of a sports prosthesis, sports chairs, or adaptive recreation equipment can be very expensive. In addition, travel-related expenses to participate in sports clinics, amputee events, and competitions may be difficult to afford. Most medical insurances only cover basic prosthetic needs and will not cover the cost associated with participation in adaptive sports and recreation. Unfortunately, the resultant lack of participation in peer-supported and motivating activities could lead to exacerbate other underlying medical conditions for amputees, to include their mental health. It is important that people with amputations and limb deficiencies are at least made aware of funding resources for participation through grants, scholarships, and non-profit organizations. They should also be made familiar with using current virtual tools and have increased access to technology to further acquire information and platforms that will provide continued access to adaptive sports and recreation opportunities.

SUMMARY

After lower or upper limb amputation, individuals can experience problems in returning to work and/or adapting to their work environment. Several related factors influence return to work after amputation. Because different inclusion criteria and definitions of return to work are used in studies, and because of the differences in health and social security services and policies in different countries, reaching any strong conclusions is difficult. However, the return to work rate may increase, and problems at work may decrease if patients are included in comprehensive interdisciplinary rehabilitation that includes vocational counseling.

Living with an amputation or limb deficiency does not mean participation with sports or recreation is not an essential need. Many patients with limb loss will gain a greater desire for living a full, active, and healthy lifestyle. Adaptive sports and recreation affords amputees and individuals with limb deficiencies the opportunity to be immersed in meaningful, functional, and purposeful activity. Inspiring continued participation in sport or recreation at any level can provide the important tools necessary to promote increased confidence, self-esteem, and independence to help amputees and people with limb deficiency sustain an enhanced quality of life.

References

1. Narang IC, Mathur BP, Singh P, Jape VS: Functional capabilities of lower limb amputees. *Prosthet Orthot Int* 1984;8(1):43-51.
2. Kejlaa GH: The social and economic outcome after upper limb amputation. *Prosthet Orthot Int* 1992;16(1):25-31.
3. Burger H, Marinček Č: Return to work after lower limb amputation. *Disabil Rehabil* 2007;29(17):1323-1329.
4. Whyte AS, Carroll LJ: A preliminary examination of the relationship between employment, pain and disability in an amputee population. *Disabil Rehabil* 2002;24(9):462-470.
5. Burger H, Maver T, Marinček Č: Partial hand amputation and work. *Disabil Rehabil* 2007;29(17):1317-1321.
6. Livingston DH, Keenan D, Kim D, Elcavage J, Malangoni MA: Extent of disability following traumatic extremity amputation. *J Trauma* 1994;37(3):495-499.
7. van der Sluis CK, Hartman PP, Schoppen T, Dijkstra PU: Job adjustments, job satisfaction and health experience in upper and lower limb amputees. *Prosthet Orthot Int* 2009;33(1):41-51.
8. Sagiv P, Shabat S, Mann M, Ashur H, Nyska M: Rehabilitation process and functional results of patients with amputated fingers. *Plast Reconstr Surg* 2002;110(2):497-503.
9. Boynton BL: The rehabilitation and the re-employment potential of the amputee. *Am J Surg* 1955;89(4):924-931.
10. Nimhurchadha S, Gallagher P, Maclachlan M, Wegener ST: Identifying successful outcomes and important factors to consider in upper limb amputation rehabilitation: An international web-based Delphi survey. *Disabil Rehabil* 2013;35(20):1726-1733.
11. World Health Organization: *The International Classification of Functioning, Disability and Health (ICF)*. World Health Organization, 2001.
12. Girdhar A, Mital A, Kephart A, Young A: Design guidelines for accommodating amputees in the workplace. *J Occup Rehabil* 2001;11(2):99-118.
13. Schoppen T, Boonstra A, Groothoff JW, de Vries J, Göeken LN, Eisma WH: Employment status, job characteristics, and work-related health experience of people with a lower limb amputation in The Netherlands. *Arch Phys Med Rehabil* 2001;82(2):239-245.
14. Millstein S, Bain D, Hunter GA: A review of employment patterns of industrial amputees: Factors influencing rehabilitation. *Prosthet Orthot Int* 1985;9(2):69-78.
15. Ide M, Obayashi T, Toyonaga T: Association of pain with employment status and satisfaction among amputees in Japan. *Arch Phys Med Rehabil* 2002;83(10):1394-1398.

16. Fisher K, Hanspal RS, Marks L: Return to work after lower limb amputation. *Int J Rehabil Res* 2003;26(1):51-56.
17. Wan Hazmy CH, Chia WY, Fong TS, Ganendra P: Functional outcome after major lower extremity amputation: A survey on lower extremity amputees. *Med J Malaysia* 2006;61(suppl A):3-9.
18. Nagarajan R, Neglia JP, Clohisy DR, et al: Education, employment, insurance, and marital status among 694 survivors of pediatric lower extremity bone tumors: A report from the childhood cancer survivor study. *Cancer* 2003;97(10):2554-2564.
19. Fernández A, Revilla C, Su IT, García M: Social integration of juvenile amputees: Comparison with a general population. *Prosthet Orthot Int* 2003;27(1):11-16.
20. Carrougher GJ, Bamer AM, Mandell SP, et al: Factors affecting employment after burn injury in the United States: A burn model system national database investigation. *Arch Phys Med Rehabil* 2020;101(1 suppl):S71-S85.
21. Schoppen T, Boonstra A, Groothoff JW, van Sonderen E, Göeken LN, Eisma WH: Factors related to successful job reintegration of people with a lower limb amputation. *Arch Phys Med Rehabil* 2001;82(10):1425-1431.
22. Hebert JS, Ashworth NL: Predictors of return to work following traumatic work-related lower extremity amputation. *Disabil Rehabil* 2006;28(10):613-618.
23. Sheikh K: Return to work following limb injuries. *J Soc Occup Med* 1985;35(4):114-117.
24. MacKenzie EJ, Bosse MJ, Kellam JF, et al: Early predictors of long-term work disability after major limb trauma. *J Trauma* 2006;61(3):688-694.
25. Journeay WS, Pauley T, Kowgier M, Devlin M: Return to work after occupational and non-occupational lower extremity amputation. *Occup Med (Lond)* 2018;68(7):438-443.
26. Gailey R, Allen K, Castles J, Kucharik J, Roeder M: Review of secondary physical conditions associated with lower-limb amputation and long-term prosthesis use. *J Rehabil Res Dev* 2008;45(1):15-29.
27. van Velzen JM, van Bennekom CA, Polomski W, Slootman JR, van der Woude LH, Houdijk H: Physical capacity and walking ability after lower limb amputation: A systematic review. *Clin Rehabil* 2006;20(11):999-1016.
28. Sansam K, Neumann V, O'Connor R, Bhakta B: Predicting walking ability following lower limb amputation: A systematic review of the literature. *J Rehabil Med* 2009;41(8):593-603.
29. Dudek NL, Marks MB, Marshall SC, Chardon JP: Dermatologic conditions associated with use of a lower-extremity prosthesis. *Arch Phys Med Rehabil* 2005;86(4):659-663.
30. Dasgupta AK, McCluskie PJ, Patel VS, Robins L: The performance of the ICEROSS prostheses amongst transtibial amputees with a special reference to the workplace: A preliminary study. Icelandic Roll on Silicone Socket. *Occup Med (Lond)* 1997;47(4):228-236.
31. Gallagher P, O'Donovan MA, Doyle A, Desmond D: Environmental barriers, activity limitations and participation restrictions experienced by people with major limb amputation. *Prosthet Orthot Int* 2011;35(3):278-284.
32. Schoppen T, Boonstra A, Groothoff JW, De Vries J, Göeken LN, Eisma WH: Job satisfaction and health experience of people with a lower-limb amputation in comparison with healthy colleagues. *Arch Phys Med Rehabil* 2002;83(5):628-634.
33. Davidson J: A survey of the satisfaction of upper limb amputees with their prostheses, their lifestyles, and their abilities. *J Hand Ther* 2002;15(1):62-70.
34. Reed D: Understanding and meeting the needs of farmers with amputations. *Orthop Nurs* 2004;23(6):397-402, 404-405.
35. Cheung E, Alvaro R, Colotla VA: Psychological distress in workers with traumatic upper or lower limb amputations following industrial injuries. *Rehabil Psychol* 2003;48(2):109-112.
36. Jang CH, Yang HS, Yang HE, et al: A survey on activities of daily living and occupations of upper extremity amputees. *Ann Rehabil Med* 2011;35(6):907-921.
37. Burger H, Vidmar G: A survey of overuse problems in patients with acquired or congenital upper limb deficiency. *Prosthet Orthot Int* 2016;40(4):497-502.
38. Fernández A, Isusi I, Gómez M: Factors conditioning the return to work of upper limb amputees in Asturias, Spain. *Prosthet Orthot Int* 2000;24(2):143-147.
39. Kennedy PJ, Young WM, Deva AK, Haertsch PA: Burns and amputations: A 24-year experience. *J Burn Care Res* 2006;27(2):183-188.
40. Pylatiuk C, Schulz S, Döderlein L: Results of an internet survey of myoelectric prosthetic hand users. *Prosthet Orthot Int* 2007;31(4):362-370.
41. Silcox DH III, Rooks MD, Vogel RR, Fleming LL: Myoelectric prostheses: A long-term follow-up and a study of the use of alternate prostheses. *J Bone Joint Surg Am* 1993;75(12):1781-1789.
42. Østlie K, Lesjø IM, Franklin RJ, Garfelt B, Skjeldal OH, Magnus P: Prosthesis use in adult acquired major upper-limb amputees: Patterns of wear, prosthetic skills and the actual use of prostheses in activities of daily life. *Disabil Rehabil Assist Technol* 2012;7(6):479-493.
43. Dumontier C: Distal replantation, nail bed, and nail problems in musicians. *Hand Clin* 2003;19(2):259-272, vi.
44. Matsuzaki H, Narisawa H, Miwa H, Toishi S: Predicting functional recovery and return to work after mutilating hand injuries: Usefulness of campbell's hand injury severity score. *J Hand Surg Am* 2009;34(5):880-885.
45. Resnik L, Meucci MR, Lieberman-Klinger S, et al: Advanced upper limb prosthetic devices: Implications for upper limb prosthetic rehabilitation. *Arch Phys Med Rehabil* 2012;93(4):710-717.
46. Ebrahimzadeh MH, Rajabi MT: Long-term outcomes of patients undergoing war-related amputations of the foot and ankle. *J Foot Ankle Surg* 2007;46(6):429-433.
47. Dougherty PJ: Transtibial amputees from the Vietnam War: Twenty-eight-year follow-up. *J Bone Joint Surg Am* 2001;83(3):383-389.
48. Stinner DJ, Burns TC, Kirk KL, Ficke JR: Return to duty rate of amputee soldiers in the current conflicts in Afghanistan and Iraq. *J Trauma* 2010;68(6):1476-1479.
49. Dharm-Datta S, Etherington J, Mistlin A, Rees J, Clasper J: The outcome of British combat amputees in relation to military service. *Injury* 2011;42(11):1362-1367.
50. Burger H, Marinček C, Jaeger RJ: Prosthetic device provision to landmine survivors in Bosnia and Herzegovina: Outcomes in 3 ethnic groups. *Arch Phys Med Rehabil* 2004;85(1):19-28.
51. Silver JR: The origins of sport for disabled people. *J R Coll Physicians Edinb* 2018;48(2):175-180.
52. McDonald CL, Westcott-McCoy S, Weaver MR, Haagsma J, Kartin D: Global prevalence of traumatic non-fatal limb amputation. *Prosthet Orthot Int* 2021;45(2):105-114.

53. Radocy R: Upper limb prosthetics for sports and recreation, in Pasquina PF, Cooper RA, eds: *Care of the Combat Amputee*. Amazon Fulfillment, 2014, pp 641-668:chap 24.
54. Thomas H: *Occupation-Based Activity Analysis*. SLACK Inc., 2015.
55. Krieger A, Brasile F, McCann C: Sports and recreational opportunities, in Pasquina PF, Cooper RA, eds: *Care of the Combat Amputee*. Amazon Fulfillment, 2014, p 673:chap 25.
56. What is adaptive skiing? 2016. Available at: https://skifederation.org/what-is-adaptive-skiing/. Accessed September 19, 2021.
57. What are the HEALING ARTS? n.d. Available at: https://www.montefiore.org/healingarts-what-are-the-healing-arts. Accessed September 19, 2021.
58. NOAH publications: 2021. Available at: https://thenoah.net/noah-publications/. Accessed September 19, 2021.
59. Miller H: 'It'S my escape.' how video games help people cope with disabilities 2019. Available at: https://www.washingtonpost.com/video-games/2019/10/14/its-my-escape-how-video-games-help-people-cope-with-disabilities/. Accessed September 19, 2021.
60. Paralympic games 2021. Available at: https://en.wikipedia.org/wiki/Paralympic_Games. Accessed September 19, 2021.
61. Our mission n.d. Available at: https://www.achillesinternational.org/who-we-are. Accessed September 19, 2021.
62. Our mission & impact 2021. Available at: https://www.moveunitedsport.org/about-us/our-mission-impact/. Accessed September 19, 2021.
63. Adaptive sports and recreation for people with disabilities 2021. Available at: https://nscd.org/about-nscd-adaptive-sports/. Accessed September 19, 2021.
64. About Americans for the arts 2019. Available at: https://www.americansforthearts.org/about-americans-for-the-arts. Accessed September 19, 2021.
65. The Ablegamers Foundation Inc: Home 2021. Available at: https://ablegamers.org/. Accessed September 19, 2021.

SECTION 5

Pediatrics

The Child With a Limb Deficiency: Classification and Etiology

CHAPTER 58

Chinmay S. Paranjape, MD, MHSc • Anna D. Vergun, MD, FAAOS

ABSTRACT

Pediatric limb deficiencies primarily result from disruptions in formation in utero or as acquired causes from trauma, burns, neoplasm, or infection after birth. Understanding the etiology of limb deficiency in children requires consideration of embryologic limb development in utero and the multiple ways in which those processes can be interrupted. Having a consistent, clear way of classifying these deficiencies enables better communications among members of multidisciplinary teams.

Keywords: amelia; congenital amputation; hemimelia; limb deficiency; longitudinal deficiency; transverse deficiency

Introduction

Relative to adults with limb deficiencies, children with limb deficiencies present with unique challenges. The differences in management between adults and children are driven by differences in etiologies of the deficiency, residual skeletal growth, physiology, psychology, and lifestyle. In a typical center that treats children with limb deficiency, approximately 60% of patients will have a congenital etiology versus 40% who present with an acquired form.[1] Congenital etiologies are often more complex than the usual transverse amputations seen in adults. Therefore, a basic understanding of limb development underscores the root causes of these deficiencies and lays the foundation of the various classifications clinicians use to communicate about pediatric limb deficiencies.

Brief Outline of Embryology

The embryology of limb development will be further detailed elsewhere in this text, but a basic outline is provided here as a foundation for the classification systems and to discuss etiologies.

The appendicular system is composed of the limbs and includes the shoulder and pelvic girdles. Limb buds arise as outpockets from the ventrolateral body wall at 4 weeks' gestation with the upper limbs appearing 1 to 2 days before the lower limbs. Development occurs in three planes with different zones of cells controlling the requisite order of events, resulting in shape.

First, a mesenchymal core from the lateral plate mesoderm forms bones and connective tissues and is covered by a layer of cuboidal ectoderm. Distally, this ectoderm thickens and forms the apical ectodermal ridge (AER). The AER influences the adjacent mesenchyme and causes it to remain undifferentiated. As the limb grows, cells farther and more proximal to the AER begin to differentiate into cartilage and muscle, resulting in proximal-to-distal limb development.

By 6 weeks' gestation, the hand and foot plates form from flattened terminal portions of the limb bud. Programmed cell death within the AER results in creation of fingers and toes, with further growth requiring five intact segments of the AER. The zone of polarizing activity governs radial-to-ulnar limb axis development. Cells in the zone of polarizing activity cluster along the posterior border of the limb and produce vitamin A, which induces Sonic Hedgehog factor. This zone remains in close proximity to the posterior border of the AER to allow proper orientation. Finally, the dorsal ectoderm controls the dorsoventral axis. As the external shape is established, the mesenchyme within the buds condenses and differentiates into chondrocytes. Joint cavities are similarly formed by programmed cell death.

Limb rotation occurs during the seventh week. The upper limb rotates 90° laterally with the extensor muscles adopting a lateral and posterior position and the thumbs laterally. The lower limb instead rotates 90° medially with the extensors anteriorly and the hallux medially.

As a general principle, disruptions to the processes of any of the three zones (AER, zone of polarizing activity, or dorsal ectoderm) will result in limb

---

Dr. Paranjape or an immediate family member has stock or stock options held in Alphatec Spine, OrthoPediatrics and Stryker. Dr. Vergun or an immediate family member serves as a board member, owner, officer, or committee member of Association of Children's Prosthetic and Orthotic Clinics.

This chapter is adapted from Harder JA, Krajbich JI: Limb-deficient child: classification and etiology, in Krajbich JI, Pinzur MS, Potter BK, Stevens PM, eds: *Atlas of Amputations and Limb Deficiencies: Surgical, Prosthetic, and Rehabilitation Principles*, ed 4. American Academy of Orthopaedic Surgeons, 2016, pp 751-758.

absence or malformation. The earlier the insult in the developmental process, the more dramatic the effect.[2]

Etiology

Most pediatric limb deficiencies are congenital, with a smaller portion resulting from traumatic, neoplastic, or infectious etiologies. This stands in contradistinction to that in adults in whom all new amputations are acquired and most commonly secondary to trauma or vascular complications. Furthermore, many congenital limb deficiencies result in multimembral deficiencies that involve other organ systems. Pediatric-specific considerations in treatment are discussed in greater detail in a separate chapter. Accordingly, classification systems and terminology that describe these are more nuanced than those used in the context of transverse, acquired adult deficiencies.

Congenital

Congenital limb deficiencies affect approximately 5 to 10 per 10,000 live births and affect the upper limb at a ratio of 2:1 relative to the lower limb.[1] For most congenital deficiencies, no exact causative factor can be identified. However, with an understanding of embryology, one can gain insight into the intrauterine timing of the causative insult. Most insults occur within the first trimester. Several known factors can influence early skeletal development. These include drugs (eg, thalidomide), toxins (eg, mercury), ionizing radiation, genetics, trauma, and poor intrauterine environments (eg, maternal diabetes). There are evolving data to suggest various modes of inheritance for different congenital deficiencies.[3-5]

Maternal nutritional deficiencies such as folic acid deficiency have been linked to neural tube defects (such as myelomeningocele and spina bifida) but have not been definitively linked to congenital limb deficiency. All the same, nutritional supplements should be part of the antenatal diet because most major organ development occurs before the mother realizes she is pregnant. This highlights the importance of proper diet/nutrition for all women of childbearing age, particularly the ones planning on pregnancy. Later in pregnancy, mechanical and fetal development factors can lead to limb deficiency. A classic example is Streeter dysplasia (or intrauterine constriction band syndrome, amniotic band), which can lead to multimembral amputations with deep constriction bands on the limbs and tissue defects in the trunk and face.

Medical conditions can be associated with congenital limb deficiency and ought to be recognized early because further medical intervention can be lifesaving. In the autosomal recessive condition thrombocytopenia with absent radius syndrome, patients may have severe thrombocytopenia associated with the multimembral limb deficiency. A platelet count is mandatory, and treatment may be necessary to mitigate potential neurologic damage from intracranial hemorrhage. Platelet counts typically improve as the child ages. Likewise, in Fanconi pancytopenia syndrome, another autosomal recessive condition, patients can present with bleeding, pallor, recurrent infections, and reduction limb deformities (absence or deformity of a limb) or dislocated hips. Holt-Oram (hand-heart) syndrome, an autosomal dominant variable penetrance condition, is associated with upper limb reduction deformities and heart defects. Genetic counseling for these patients and their families is critical.

Acquired

As in adults, acquired limb deficiencies in children can follow trauma, burns, infection, and neoplasm. In the Western world, lawnmower injuries, pedestrian-motor vehicle collisions, and thermal or electric burns remain the most common causes of acquired limb loss in children.[6,7] In areas of geopolitical conflict, injuries from ballistic and ordnance explosions remain an unfortunately common etiology of limb loss in children.[8] In colder climates, frostbite remains a rare but potential cause of limb loss in children.

Neoplastic disease of the limbs, namely osteosarcoma and Ewing sarcoma, has largely been historically managed with amputation. As detection abilities improved, neoadjuvant therapies became more common, and limb-salvage options such as reconstructive implants became more durable, so limb salvage has become feasible. Amputation, however, remains an option when a functional and oncologically disease-free extremity cannot be achieved with salvage.[9] For massive benign lesions such as in Klippel-Trenaunay syndrome, Proteus syndrome, or neurofibromatosis 1, limb amputation may result in more functional or even lifesaving outcomes.

Septicemia associated with purpura fulminans remains a common infectious etiology of acquired limb deficiency in infants and children.[10] Purpura fulminans is most commonly associated with meningococcemia. Although the incidence of meningococcus is declining secondary to vaccination efforts,[11] other bacterial strains such as pneumococcus and streptococcus may also result in limb gangrene and subsequent loss. Also, pressor-induced distal limb necrosis may develop in infants on pressors.

Vascular injuries may also result in critical limb ischemia necessitating amputation. These injuries may result from blunt or penetrating trauma and may occasionally be iatrogenic from attempts to obtain peripheral access in the neonatal intensive care unit.[12]

Classification

Classifying congenital limb deficiencies remains paramount in enabling consistent communication among parents and clinicians and in enabling future study of congenital limb deficiencies. Several anatomic classification systems have been described (O'Rahilly,[13] Frantz and O'Rahilly,[14] Swanson,[15] and Gold et al[16]). These systems have defined deficiencies by their relationship to the central axis of the arm and leg. Beginning with the work of Frantz and O'Rahilly, Greek and Latin terminology has been in consistent use to describe congenital deficiencies. These terms are often poorly descriptive but are defined subsequently given the frequency with which they are still encountered in informal communication.

In the 1970s under the guidance of Hector W. Kay, the International Society of Prosthetics and Orthotics (ISPO) designed a more rational classification system to simply and precisely describe deficiencies based on their anatomic and radiographic features.[17] However, this classification does not attempt to address the etiology nor angular or rotational aspects of deformity.

Deficiencies are described as transverse or longitudinal, as detailed in **Table 1**. Individual bones are described based on either total or partial absence. These can be further subdescribed based on the anatomic location within a bone (eg, the proximal one-third), the individual bones (eg, partial or total loss of carpals, metatarsals), or the parts of the bones that are missing. Schemas for describing upper and lower limb deficiencies by the ISPO classification system are provided in **Figures 1** and **2**.

Longitudinal deficiencies may be partial or total and may have normal elements distally with an intercalary defect, as described in **Table 1**. H. J. B. Day, a member of the Kay committee, developed a stylized illustrative system of describing these deficiencies by shading the deficient parts of the limb. Although these are not formally part of the ISPO classification system, they are a useful way of communicating and describing limb deficiencies. An example of tibial deficiency is demonstrated in a Day illustration in **Figure 3**.

Further work is currently underway on refining terminology and classifications of congenital limb deficiency. Gold et al[16] have built on the preexisting ISPO architecture to include etiology as part of the classification. Enabling consistent communication among clinicians and patients remains paramount in providing appropriate care for patients with congenital limb deficiencies and to enable rigorous study of these deficiencies.

For proximal femoral focal deficiency, many use the classification originally described by Aitken.[18] Aitken proposed four groups, A through D. A and B have a present femoral head, whereas C and D have an absent head. A through D are further stratified based on the dysplastic nature of the acetabulum. These are detailed further in **Figure 4**.

TABLE 1	Longitudinal Deficiencies
Term	**Definition**
Amelia	Complete absence of a free limb (excluding the girdle)
Meromelia	Partial absence of a free limb (excluding the girdle)
Terminal deficiency	Absence of all skeletal elements distal to the proximal limit of the deficiency along the designated axis (longitudinal or transverse)
Intercalary deficiency	Absence of the middle tissues between intact proximal and distal elements of a limb
Transverse	Extending across the width of the limb
Longitudinal	Absence extending parallel with the long axis of the limb
Preaxial	Absence along the thumb or great toe side of the limb (radial or tibial)
Postaxial	Absence along the small finger or small toe side of the limb (ulnar or fibular)

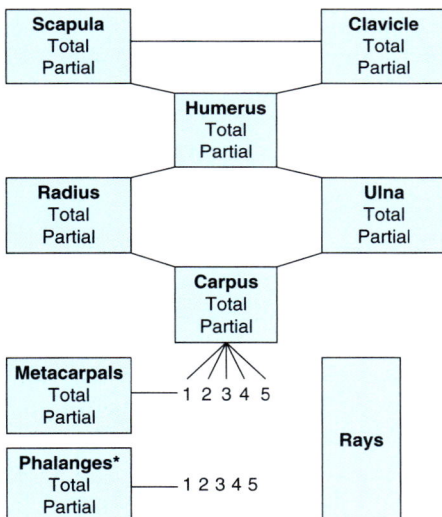

FIGURE 1 Illustration describes longitudinal deficiencies of the upper limb using the International Organization for Standardization classification system. The asterisk indicates that the digits of the hand are sometimes referred to by name: 1 = thumb; 2 = index; 3 = long; 4 = ring; 5 = little (or small). For the purpose of this classification, such naming is depreciated because it is not equally applicable to the foot. (Adapted with permission from Day HJ: The ISO/ISPO classification of congenital limb deficiency. *Prosthet Orthot Int* 1991;15[2]:67-69.)

FIGURE 2 Illustration describes longitudinal deficiencies of the lower limb using the International Organization for Standardization system. The asterisk indicates the great toe, or hallux. (Adapted with permission from Day HJ: The ISO/ISPO classification of congenital limb deficiency. *Prosthet Orthot Int* 1991;15[2]:67-69.)

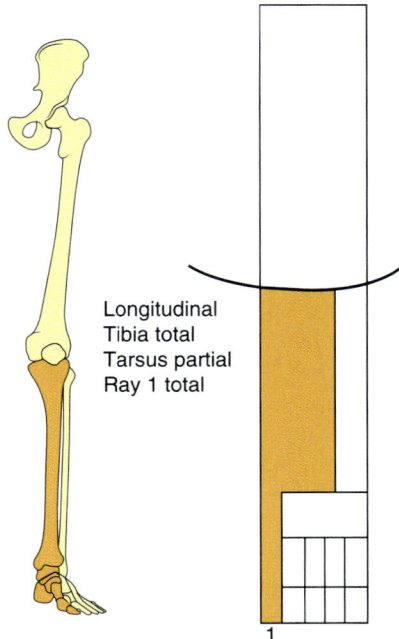

FIGURE 3 Illustration of a longitudinal deficiency shown on the skeleton (left) and in Day's stylized representation (right), which shows the original deficiency and treatment by knee disarticulation. (Adapted with permission from Day HJ: The ISO/ISPO classification of congenital limb deficiency. *Prosthet Orthot Int* 1991;15[2]:67-69.)

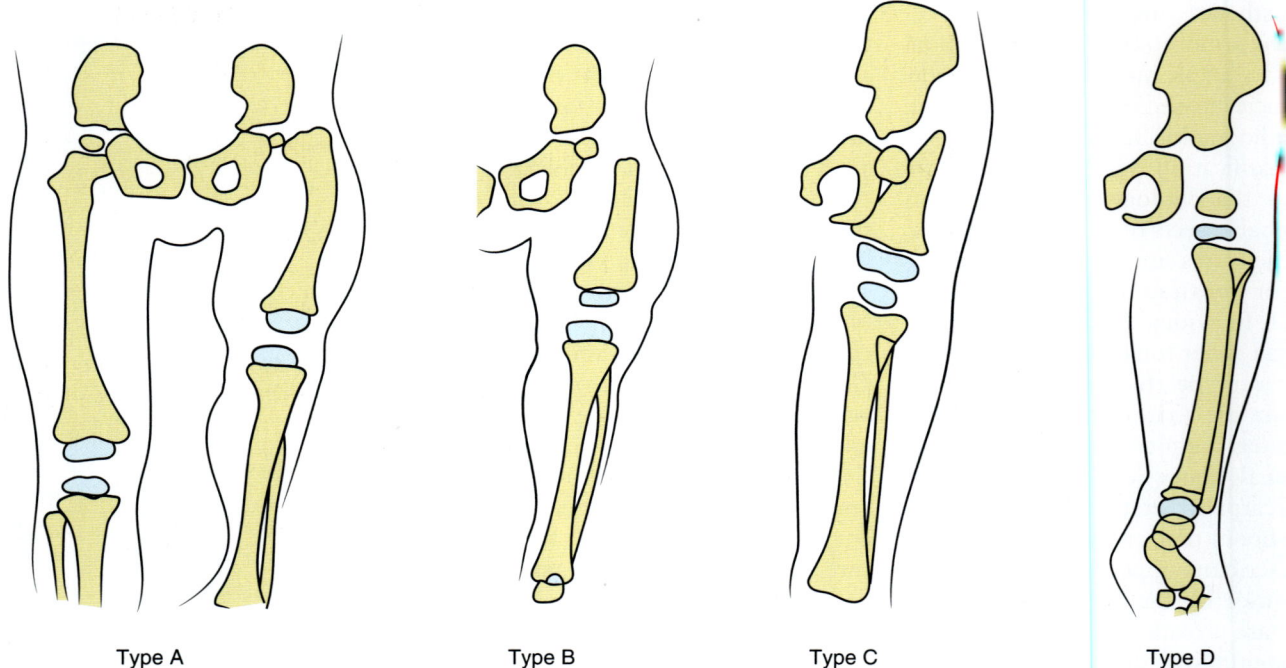

FIGURE 4 Illustration depicting the Aitken classification of proximal femoral focal deficiency. Originally described in 1969, it stratifies patients based on the quality of the acetabulum, femoral head, and proximal femoral shaft.

For tibial deficiencies, the Jones classification is commonly used.[19] It is based on radiographic appearance and also has four types. In type I, the tibia is completely absent radiographically. It is further subclassified into types Ia and Ib based on the status of the distal femoral epiphysis, which is a proxy for the presence of an unossified proximal tibial anlage. In type Ia, the distal femoral epiphysis is hypoplastic, whereas in type Ib it is normal. When the distal femoral epiphysis is normal, the tibial cartilage anlage will ossify with growth, sometimes taking several years to appear radiographically, and the child will typically have an intact knee extensor mechanism. In type II, the proximal tibia is preserved, whereas the distal tibia is absent. In type III, the distal tibia is present with a short segment of tibia, and the proximal tibia is absent. This is the least common and has been postulated to be type Ib that will reveal itself with time and growth.[20] Type IV patients have diastasis of the ankle with a longer fibula displaced proximally at the knee. This classification is delineated in **Figure 5**.

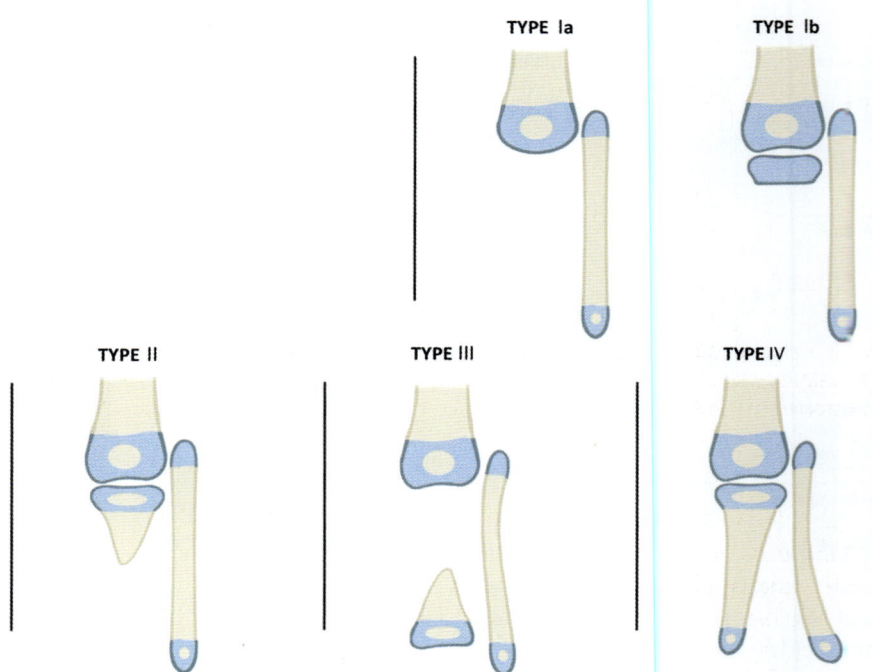

FIGURE 5 Illustration of Jones classification of tibial hemimelia. Jones Ia: tibia is completely absent. Jones Ib: tibia initially absent but has a cartilaginous upper end that may ossify with growth. Jones II: tibia present at upper end but absent at lower end. Jones III: tibia present at lower end but absent at upper end (very rare). Jones IV: tibia and fibula present but diverge at ankle (congenital diastasis of ankle). (Reproduced with permission from the Paley Foundation.)

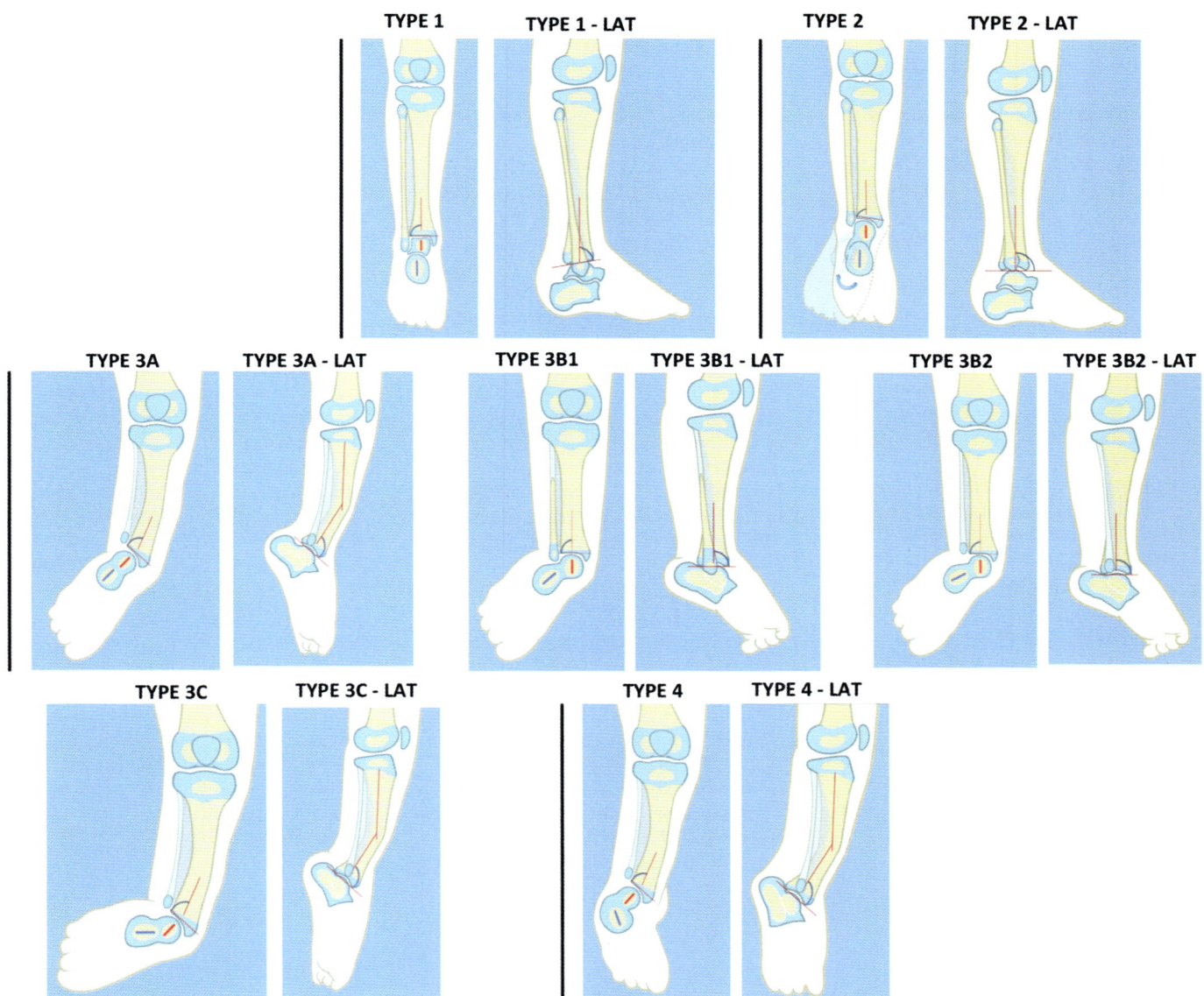

FIGURE 6 Illustrations depicting the Paley classification of fibular hemimelia. Type 1, stable ankle. Type 2, dynamic valgus ankle. Type 3, fixed equinovalgus ankle; 3A, ankle type; 3B, subtalar type; 3C, combined ankle/subtalar type. Type 4, fixed equinovarus ankle. (Reproduced with permission from the Paley Foundation.)

Many classification systems for fibular hemimelia have been proposed, notably by Achterman and Kalamchi,[21] Birch et al,[22] and Paley.[23] Both Birch et al's and Paley's systems account for the significance of the reconstructability of the foot. Where Birch et al's classification relies on radiographs for stratification, Paley's is based solely on the clinical position and stability of the ankle. An example is shown in **Figure 6**.

SUMMARY

Although classifications are useful both in communication and in research, the reader needs to be aware of the limitations of all classifications, particularly with congenital differences. For instance, both tibial and fibular deficiencies can rarely be associated with a bifid femur, where both distal femurs on that side may have variable longitudinal deficiencies of the tibia or fibula. Currently, there are no classifications described for this anomaly. Also, classifications have historically focused on the radiographic features, and they ignore the soft tissues that may also have significant anomalies. The soft tissues are often equally important in determining joint stability and therefore critical for determining treatment and prognosis.

References

1. Ephraim PL, Dillingham TR, Sector M, Pezzin LE, MacKenzie EJ: Epidemiology of limb loss and congenital limb deficiency: A review of the literature. *Arch Phys Med Rehabil* 2003;84:747-761.
2. Sadler T: *Medical Embryology*. Lippincott, Williams and Wilkins, 2012.
3. Ghanem I: Epidemiology, etiology, and genetic aspects of reduction deficiencies of the lower limb. *J Child Orthop* 2008;2:329-332.
4. Norbnop P, Srichomthong C, Suphapeetiporn K, Shotelersuk V: ZRS 406A>G mutation in patients with tibial hypoplasia, polydactyly and triphalangeal first fingers. *J Hum Genet* 2014;59:467-470.
5. Deimling S, Sotiropoulos C, Lau K, et al: Tibial hemimelia associated with GLI3 truncation. *J Hum Genet* 2016;61:443-446.
6. Loder RT, Brown KL, Zaleske DJ, Jones ET: Extremity Lawn-Mower injuries in children: Report by the research Committee of the Pediatric Orthopaedic Society of North America. *J Pediatr Orthop* 1997;17:360-371.
7. Garay M, Hennrikus WL, Hess J, Lehman EB, Armstrong DG: Lawnmowers versus children: The devastation continues. *Clin Orthop Relat Res* 2017;475:950-956.
8. Villamaria CY, Morrison JJ, Fitzpatrick CM, Cannon JW, Rasmussen TE: Wartime vascular injuries in the pediatric population of Iraq and Afghanistan: 2002-2011. *J Pediatr Surg* 2014;49:428-432.
9. Biermann JS, Siegel G: *Orthopaedic Knowledge Update: Musculoskeletal Tumors 4*. Wolters Kluwer, 2020.
10. Morris ME, Maijub JG, Walker SK, Gardner GP, Jones RG: Meningococcal sepsis and purpura fulminans: The surgical perspective. *Postgrad Med J* 2013;89:340-345.
11. Borrow R, Alarcón P, Carlos J, et al: The Global Meningococcal initiative: Global epidemiology, the impact of vaccines on meningococcal disease and the importance of herd protection. *Expert Rev Vaccines* 2017;16:313-328.
12. Markovic MD, Cvetkovic SD, Koncar IB, et al: Treatment of pediatric vascular injuries: The experience of a single non-pediatric referral center. *Int Angiol* 2019;38(3):250-255.
13. O'Rahilly R: Morphological patterns in limb deficiencies and duplications. *Am J Anat* 1951;89:135-193.
14. Frantz CH, O'Rahilly R: Congenital skeletal limb deficiencies. *J Bone Joint Surg* 1961;43(8):1202-1224.
15. Swanson AB: A classification for congenital limb malformations. *J Hand Surg Am* 1976;1:8-22.
16. Gold NB, Westgate MN, Holmes LB: Anatomic and etiological classification of congenital limb deficiencies. *Am J Med Genet A* 2011;155-A(6):1225-1235.
17. Kay HW, Day HJB, Henkel HL: A proposed international terminology for the classification of congenital limb deficiencies. *Orthot Prosthet* 1974;28:33-48.
18. Aitken GT: *Proximal Femoral Focal Deficiency: A Congenital Anomaly*. National Academy of Sciences, 1969.
19. Jones D, Barnes J, Lloyd-Roberts GC: Congenital aplasia and dysplasia of the tibia with intact fibula. Classification and management. *J Bone Joint Surg Br* 1978;60:31-39.
20. Clinton R, Birch JG: Congenital tibial deficiency: A 37-year experience at 1 institution. *J Pediatr Orthop* 2015;35:385-390.
21. Achterman C, Kalamchi A: Congenital deficiency of the fibula. *J Bone Joint Surg Br* 1979;61-B(2):133-137.
22. Birch JG, Lincoln TL, Mack PW, Birch CM: Congenital fibular deficiency: A review of thirty years' experience at one institution and a proposed classification system based on clinical deformity. *J Bone Joint Surg Am* 2011;93(12):1144-1151.
23. Paley D: Surgical reconstruction for fibular hemimelia. *J Child Orthop* 2016;10(6):557-583.

Congenital Limb Deficiencies: Embryology, Genetics, and Associated Syndromes

Ellen M. Raney, MD, FAAOS

ABSTRACT

Management of congenital limb deficiency should begin with an overview of the embryology along with the common or medically concerning associations and the known genetic causes. Cellular proliferation and differentiation occur in response to genetic communication from the apical epidermal ridge and the zone of polarization. Mesenchyme proliferation is stimulated by fibroblast growth factors 2, 4, and 8. The protein Wnt7a along with genes LMX1 and radical fringe are associated with the development of dorsal structures. The gene Engrailed-1 is associated with the development of ventral structures. A Sonic hedgehog gradient influences anterior-posterior development. The process may be disturbed by disruption in the communication mechanisms resulting in limb deficiency. Children with radial longitudinal deficiency always need to be evaluated for nonmusculoskeletal abnormalities including VACTERL syndrome (Vertebral defects, Anal atresia, Cardiac anomalies, Tracheoesophageal fistulas with Esophageal atresia, Renal, and Limb [radial]), thrombocytopenia absent radius, and Fanconi anemia. Longitudinal deficiency of the lower extremity, especially postaxial, is more common and is complicated from a musculoskeletal standpoint but is less likely to be associated with nonmusculoskeletal abnormalities. Inheritance patterns vary for each of the conditions discussed. Genetic consultation is strongly recommended.

Keywords: limb bud; longitudinal; preaxial; postaxial; transverse

Introduction

An inauspicious outpouching on the wall of an embryo undergoes a vastly complicated process to become a functional limb. While elongating, the limb bud develops along axes of proximal to distal, anterior to posterior, and ventral to dorsal in specific temporal sequences. Throughout the development process, cells are proliferating, migrating, and differentiating. Apoptosis cleaves paddles into digits and creates joints. The intricacies of this process involve a network of cues. Rapid advances in biomolecular research continually change the understanding of the control mechanisms. Visceral organs develop simultaneously with the musculoskeletal system. Causative factors of limb deficiency may relate spatially, temporally, or on a molecular basis to simultaneous organ development. Basic understanding of these complex interrelationships helps create more awareness of potentially associated syndromes and inheritance patterns.

Dr. Raney or an immediate family member serves as a board member, owner, officer, or committee member of the American Academy of Pediatrics and the Pediatric Orthopaedic Society of North America.

Limb Bud Development: Structural Aspects

The upper limb bud begins as an outpouching of the lateral plate of the embryo, known as the Wolff crest, at 4 weeks of embryonic growth. Formation progresses from cranial and proximal to caudal and distal. The lower limb bud develops 1 day later than the upper limb. Limb buds develop from the lateral plate mesoderm encased in thickened ectoderm. The inner layer of the thickened ectoderm at the apex of the limb bud is referred to as the apical ectodermal ridge (AER). The AER forms at the border of the future ventral and dorsal ectoderm. The AER influences the proximal to distal outgrowth and differentiation of the mesoderm of the limb bud. The longitudinal growth of the limb bud stems from proliferation of undifferentiated mesoderm immediately under the AER in the progress zone. A small area of mesoderm at the posterior portion of the limb bud, known as the zone of polarizing activity (ZPA), directs the anterior posterior/radioulnar or tibiofibular development including digit type and number (**Figure 1**). The limbs begin as continuous pentagonal paddles, which undergo fissuring through apoptosis. Initially fissures develop to separate the central rays and then the border digits.[1]

Under the influence of the AER, the limb bud mesenchyme forms prechondrogenic condensations, the cells of which will undergo chondrogenic differentiation giving rise to cartilage anlage. The condensations form in a proximal to distal sequence. The cartilage anlage is the precursor to endochondral ossification. Capillary invasion from the trunk into the limb bud accompanies development.

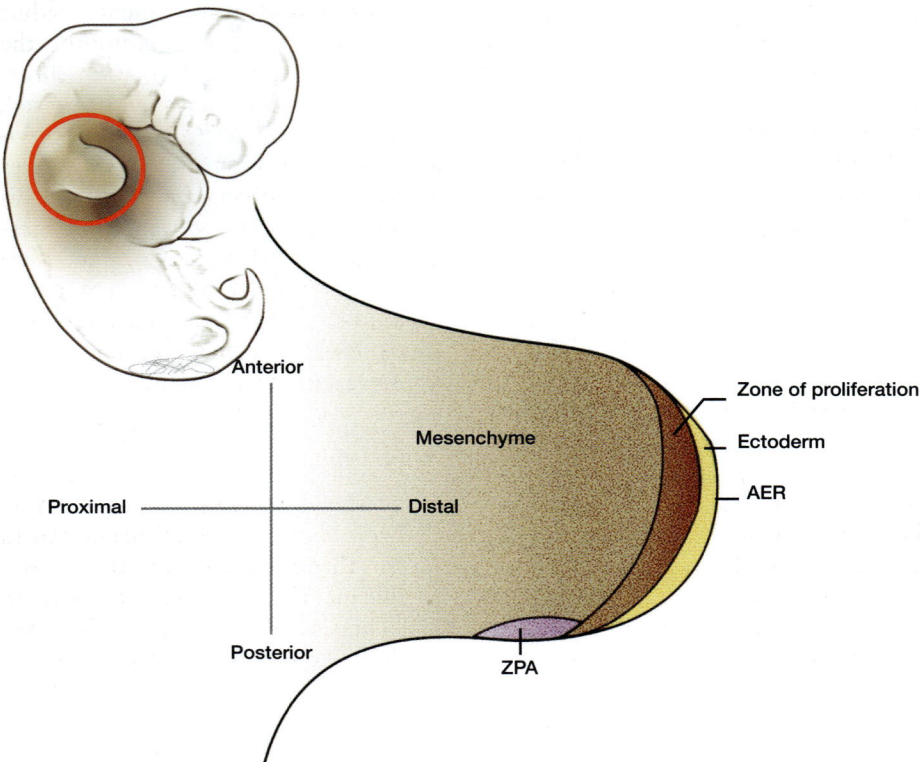

FIGURE 1 Illustration showing the structure of the developing limb bud. AER = apical ectodermal ridge, ZPA = zone of polarizing activity

However, the areas of mesenchymal condensation of the future cartilage anlage remain avascular. As the embryonic period proceeds to the fetal period, chondrocyte proliferation, maturation, and then hypertrophy stimulate vascular invasion and formation of primary centers of ossification. The elements of the physis are visible at this stage. The physis flattens into a platelike shape with the development of the secondary ossification center.

A single end artery is responsible for blood supply to the nascent limb prior to 10 weeks of gestation. The adult pattern of arterial arches forms by 11.5 weeks. The formation of arterial anastomosis provides an element of protection against vascular disruption.[2]

Limb Development Control: Genetic-Molecular Influences

A host of interactive mechanisms creates the cascade of skeletal outgrowth, differentiation, and polarity. The signaling may occur via gradients, cell-to-cell communication, and matrix-to-cell communication.

Fibroblast growth factor (FGF) 8 expressed in the precursors to the ectodermal cells of the AER plays a role in the induction of this structure.[3] Just under the AER lie the mesodermal cells of the progress zone. The continued outgrowth by these undifferentiated mesodermal cells is influenced by FGF 2, 4, and 8 from the AER. Control of the outgrowth requires a balance of FGF 2 upregulation offset by bone morphogenetic protein 2 downregulation.[4]

Factors found in the embryo prior to the formation of the AER determine the dorsoventral patterning. The AER formation occurs along this dorsoventral border. *Wnt7a* in the dorsal ectoderm induces formation of *LMX1* in the mesoderm. The cells in the area of mesoderm with LMX1 undergo dorsalization.[5] The dorsal ectoderm of the limb bud also expresses the gene *radical fringe (r-fng)*, whereas the ventral ectoderm expresses *Engrailed-1*. *Engrailed-1* represses the *r-fng* produced in the dorsal ectoderm, thus creating a border between cells with *r-fng* and those without.[6]

Anterior posterior development is directed by a gradient in Sonic hedgehog (SHH) and retinoic acid. SHH is a secreted protein that is predominant in the ZPA.[7] Skeletal abnormalities may be associated with abnormalities in SHH or disruptions in the gradient that are stabilized by genes that enhance or suppress SHH. The ZPA regulatory sequence functions posteriorly to enhance SHH, whereas GLI3 repressor (GLI3R) functions anteriorly to suppress SHH.[8]

Mesenchymal cell prechondrogenic condensation is associated with cell-to-cell communication. The adhesion molecules N-cadherin and N-cell adhesion molecule are expressed in these areas during condensation and cell recruitment.[9] Cell-to-cell communication is also responsible for differentiation into chondrocytes. Enhanced N-cadherin expression is noted in mesenchymal cell lines treated with transforming growth factor beta 1 or bone morphogenetic protein 2.[10]

Mesenchymal cells also communicate via the production of matrix molecules. Condensing mesenchyme expresses fibronectin, which may function to mediate pattern-specific condensation.[11] Type I collagen is a marker for mesenchymal cells. Chondrocyte progenitor cells begin producing cartilage matrix molecules including type II collagen and the cartilage-specific sulfated proteoglycan, aggrecan. Type II collagen undergoes splicing. Collagen type IIA is noted in the progenitor cells of chondrocytes versus type IIB in the differentiated cells. Type X is most prominent in the maturing hypertrophic chondrocytes. Mature hypertrophic chondrocytes stimulate vascular invasion by releasing an angiogenic factor.[12]

Genetics and Associated Syndromes

Initial evaluation of a child with a congenital limb deficiency always necessitates careful consideration of associated syndromes and abnormalities outside of the musculoskeletal system. These can range from major cardiac and life-threatening hematopoietic conditions to clinically minor alterations in the renal system. The associations correlate with the temporal or molecular insult.

Cardiac, craniofacial, and renal development occur simultaneously with limb development accounting for several of the common associations.

The terminology for limb deficiency generally stems from the area of most severe or most obvious involvement. The treatment team needs to keep in mind that the obvious deficiencies rarely occur in isolation. Potentially subtle proximal abnormalities often drive treatment plans, such as the presence or absence of functioning musculature, joint stability, and joint contractures. For instance, in deciding the best management strategy in children with longitudinal deficiency of the lower limb, not only the presence or absence of a foot but also the intrinsic stability and muscles controlling the knee need to be considered. Similarly, elbow motion and control dictate management of hand anomalies.

Longitudinal Deficiencies of the Upper Limb

Preaxial deficiency of the upper extremity, also known as radial longitudinal deficiency and radial clubhand, may be seen with some of the severe comorbidities including life-threatening cardiac and hematopoietic deficiencies. Distal structures tend to be more involved than proximal structures.[13]

VACTERL and VACTERL-H Association

Radial longitudinal deficiency occurs with multiple organ systems in patients with the VACTERL association (Vertebral defects, Anal atresia, Cardiac anomalies, Tracheoesophageal fistulas with Esophageal atresia, Renal, and Limb [radial]). Most children will have two to three of these conditions. Involvement rarely includes all five organ systems.

The inheritance pattern is unclear for most VACTERL cases. VACTERL association may be associated with hydrocephalus, known as VACTERL-H association. An X-linked specific form has been described.[14]

The SHH pathway is important in the development of each of the organ systems involved in this condition. The SHH pathway, also prominent in the ZPA in limb development, has been implicated in VACTERL association. Mutant mice deficient in the downstream SHH transcription factor known as GLI display deficiencies very similar to VACTERL association.[15] This specific type of GLI mutation has not been noted in humans. Complete loss of the function of SHH interferes with midline developments, causing holoprosencephaly.

Fanconi Anemia

Children with limb deficiencies described earlier in the VACTERL or VACTERL-H constellation should also be evaluated for Fanconi anemia. This syndrome of genomic instability predisposes children to congenital abnormalities, bone marrow failure, and cancer. There is a heterogeneous presentation. In addition to the orthopaedic abnormalities in the VACTERL-H association, another set of recently described conditions includes skin pigmentation, small head, small eyes, central nervous system, otology, short stature (PHENOS).[16] The combination of radial longitudinal deficiency, café au lait spots, and short stature, all common, can be an early warning to the orthopaedic surgeon. Hematologic abnormalities including aplastic anemia, myelodysplastic syndrome, and leukemia may present around school age. The conditions tend to continue to manifest as a person ages. There is a high risk of the development of malignancies.

The inheritance is an X-linked recessive or a heterogenic autosomal pattern. Multiple subtypes exist specific to gene mutations along a common pathway. The 22 gene-encoded proteins involved have been termed the Fanconi anemia pathway or the Fanconi anemia/breast cancer (BRCA) pathway for their association with BRCA susceptibility genes. These genes identified with pathologic variants code for proteins involved in the repair of damaged DNA. The mutations produce increased instability in this repair process. The similarities throughout the subtypes of germline mutations and cellular and organic changes suggest that signal transduction in this pathway regulates organ development.[16,17]

Thrombocytopenia-Absent Radius Syndrome

Radial longitudinal deficiency occurs with life-threatening thrombocytopenia in thrombocytopenia-absent radius syndrome. In this condition, the humerus and ulna are frequently shortened as well. The thumbs are spared, creating a very short, radially deviated extremity with five digits. Lower extremity involvement often manifests as severe genu varum with intra-articular knee deformity, severe knee ligamental deficiency, and femur and tibia malrotation.[18] Additional lower extremity issues can include hip dysplasia, valgus of the ankle and foot, talipes equinovarus, synostoses of the metatarsals, and syndactyly[19] (**Figure 2**). Cardiac and urogenital defects may be seen. Megakaryocytes are precursors to thrombocytes. The deficiency causes severe thrombocytopenia that poses significant risk of bleeding early in life. The risk of perioperative bleeding needs to be considered even after the first year of life, as the thrombocytopenia may persist.

Klopocki et al[20] noted a consistent microdeletion in a segment of the long arm of chromosome 1, specifically 1q21.1, with 25% of cases being a de novo development. The autosomal recessive nature of this rare condition necessitates the presence of healthy carriers, indicating that the 1q21.1 haplotype does not produce an abnormal phenotype.[20] Thrombocytopenia-absent radius syndrome arises when this microdeletion in 1q21.1 is compounded by a mutation in the gene *RBM8A*, the transcription factor of which is ubiquitous in hematopoietic cell lines. The combination of these abnormalities leads to a decrease in coding for Y24 protein, which interferes with cell line development for megakaryocytes and osteoblasts. The association of disruption of the entire cell line of megakaryocytes yet disruption of only a portion of the limb development suggests that this abnormality occurs in a tissue-specific and developmental stage–specific manner.[21]

Holt-Oram Syndrome

Holt-Oram syndrome denotes radial longitudinal deficiency combined with cardiac septal defect. The transmission is autosomal dominant. The phenotypic

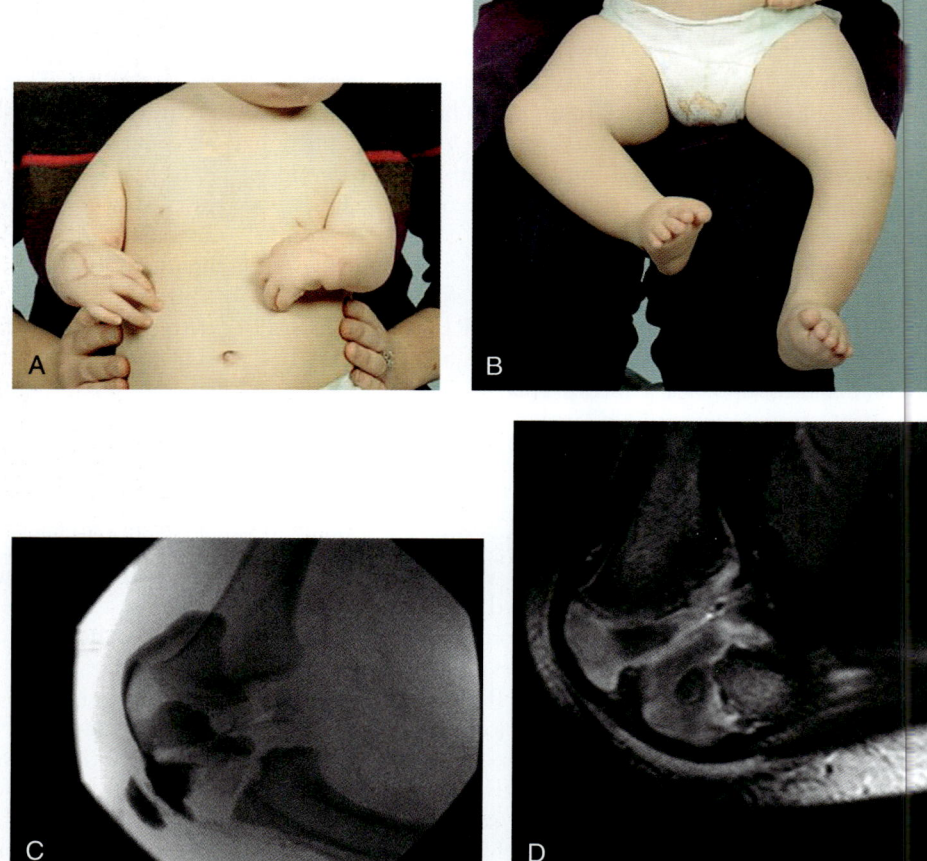

FIGURE 2 **A** through **D**, Images showing a child with thrombocytopenia absent radii. **A**, Clinical photograph showing upper extremity involvement. **B**, Clinical photograph showing lower extremity involvement with varus, knee flexion contractures, and severe external femoral and internal tibial malrotation. **C**, Lateral arthrogram and (**D**) sagittal T2-weighted magnetic resonance image of the left knee demonstrating severe intra-articular deformities including misshapen and flattened femoral condyles and tibial plateau.

variation is wide, from minor cardiac and extremity involvement to severe involvement or either or both.

There is an inconsistent linkage to a gene locus at 12q24.1 producing a transcription factor TBX5, which is key in the development of the limbs and the heart. Multiple mutations in this transcription factor have been described.[22]

Longitudinal Deficiencies of the Lower Extremity

Postaxial Longitudinal Deficiency: Femur and Fibula

Longitudinal deficiencies of the proximal femur and the fibula are often discussed separately based on the most obviously involved segment. However, the wide clinical spectrums of these conditions overlap. Bilateral lower limbs often have asymmetric involvement. Proximal femoral deficiency is commonly associated with distal concerns ranging from tarsal coalition to absence of part or all of the shank and foot. Importantly, the presence or absence of the muscles to control the elements that are present must be considered. Fibular aplasia or hypoplasia is nearly ubiquitously seen with subtle distal femoral valgus from deficiency of the lateral condyle (**Figure 3**). Alternatively, the femur may be short with coxa vara. No consistent pattern of nonskeletal concerns has been defined. The cases are usually sporadic without clear causation. Familial cases have been reported with autosomal dominant inheritance.[23]

Fibular and postaxial limb abnormalities more commonly accompany proximal femoral and acetabular deficiencies, whereas deficiencies of the tibia, with preaxial limb anomalies, are more commonly associated with distal femoral abnormalities, giving support to the theory of defects occurring in tibial versus fibular developmental fields.[23] Upper extremity developmental fields of the radius or ulna also follow along these lines. Ulnar involvement along with proximal femoral and fibular deficiencies has been described in families as the femur-fibula-ulna complex.[24]

Preaxial Longitudinal Deficiency: Tibia

Tibial longitudinal deficiency is quite rare. A large single-institution study of 95 individuals noted bilaterality in 32% of the individuals and that this deficiency has affected first-degree relatives in 3%. The associated anomalies, reported relative to the 125 total involved extremities,

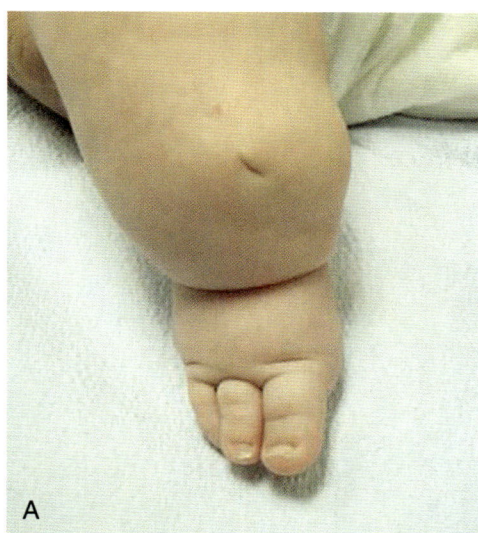
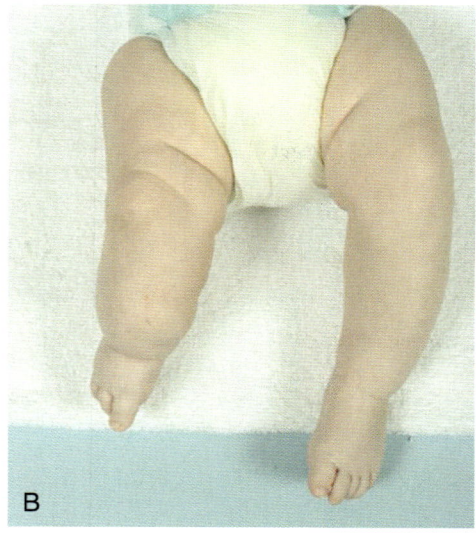
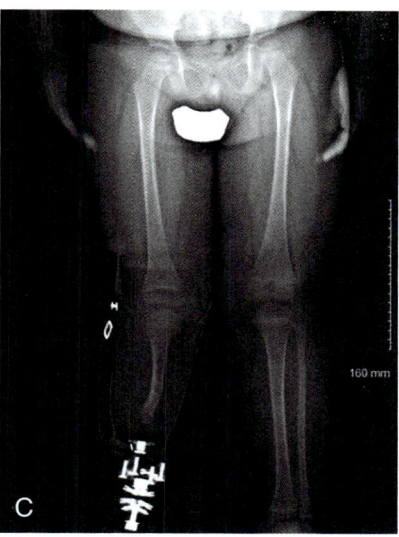

FIGURE 3 **A** and **B**, Clinical photographs of lower extremities including right shank and foot of an infant with fibular longitudinal deficiency, demonstrating severe shortening, tibial flexion deformity with anterior dimple and a three-rayed foot. **C**, Upright anterior posterior radiograph of both lower extremities of the same child at age 5 years after Symes amputation in the first year of life. The child's right femur is now 1 cm shorter than the left. Subtle hypoplasia of the right lateral femoral condyle is able to be seen.

were upper extremity 30%, spine 14%, and visceral 26%.[25] Longitudinal deficiency of the tibia occurring bilaterally in a complex pattern associated with severe foot deformity, preaxial polydactyly of the toes, and triphalangeal thumb has been reported. Older literature uses the term five-fingered hand to refer to the presence of a triphalangeal thumb. Three generations in one family demonstrated autosomal dominant inheritance. Three of seven affected individuals in this family had radial deficiency as well.[26] Similar familial associations have been seen with mutations in the regulatory sequence gene associated with SHH expression in the ZPA. This gene, known as the ZPA regulatory sequence is important in maintaining the SHH gradient that directs tibial to fibular differentiation of the limb bud.[7,8]

GLI3 protein typically possesses a binding domain that binds to SHH and blocks its ectopic expression in the anterior limb bud. When this binding domain is truncated in a GLI3 mutation, tibial hemimelia may be seen.[27]

Transverse Terminal Deficiencies

Transverse terminal deficiencies represent a nonhomogeneous group of failures of formation. The deficiency is characterized by an absence of the primary structural components at a specific level, but commonly small nubbins of digits or skin tags are present at the distal portion of the limb (**Figure 4**). Transverse deficiencies tend to present unilaterally. Associated syndromes and other organ anomalies are not common in this condition. An occurrence with oral microglossia and micrognathia, when present, is termed oromandibular limb hypogenesis. An obvious cause is typically not identified. A vascular insult is hypothesized to represent the final common pathway. Animal models of vascular insult produce similar defects. Maternal thrombophilia presents a higher risk.[28] Multiple limb involvement would increase concerns for teratogenic etiology such as was seen with thalidomide exposure. The deficiencies may be seen with exposure to substances that cause vasoactive events, such as tobacco, cocaine, alcohol, or antihypertensive agents.

Amniotic band syndrome is typically included with the discussion of transverse terminal deficiencies. A recent review from the National Birth Defects Prevention Study distinguished terminal transverse deficiencies from amniotic band syndrome based on the presence of visualized fibrous strands originating from the amniotic lining.[29] This review proposed that amniotic band syndrome is a phenotype distinct

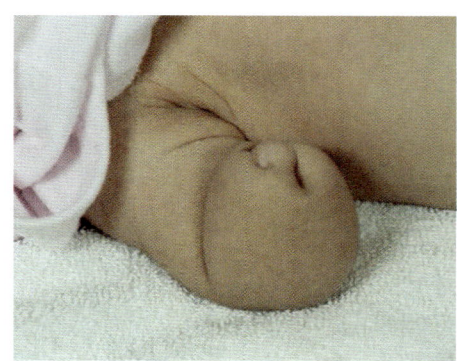

FIGURE 4 Photograph of right upper extremity in a child with terminal deficiency shortly below the elbow with distal soft tissue nubbins.

from transverse terminal deficiency. The deformities produced distal to amniotic bands are often complex. Each involved limb or digit requires separate evaluation. Rigid dysplastic deformities such as talipes equinovarus may also be present (**Figure 5**). Amniotic band syndrome is associated with combined exposure to substances leading to vasodilation such as alcohol and bronchodilators, versus transverse terminal deficiency being associated with the exposure to vasoconstrictive substances such as tobacco and decongestants.[30]

Increasing trends in attention deficit hyperactivity disorder (ADHD) medication use in children over recent

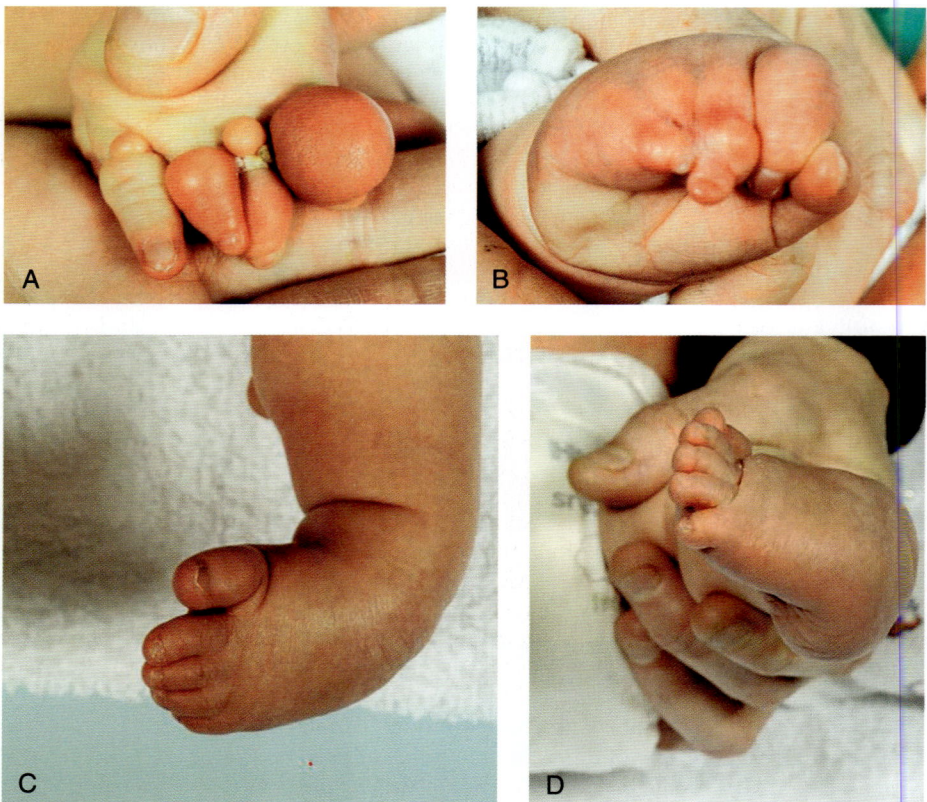

FIGURE 5 **A**, Clinical photographs of right hand (**A**) and left hand (**B**) in a representative child with amniotic band syndrome. Note asymmetry and irregular involvement with soft tissue nubbins distally. **C** and **D**, Clinical photographs of the same child with a dysplastic left talipes equinovarus associated with a deceptively innocuous–looking constriction band on the distal calf. Underlying muscles and tendons may be tethered to the bone at the level of a constriction band.

decades is now evolving into increasing ADHD medication use in women of childbearing years. Recent reports indicate an increased odds ratio (3.3) of transverse limb deficiency in children exposed to stimulant medications for ADHD during pregnancy.[29] Combination medications amphetamine/dextroamphetamine or methylphenidate were most common. This finding was despite the declining use of ADHD medications after the first trimester. Exposure occurred early in pregnancy during the period of limb development. The use of ADHD medication significantly decreased by the second and third month similar to the timing of pregnancy recognition. The occurrence was more common in women pregnant for the first time.

Reports of terminal deficiencies following chorionic villus sampling provide additional insight into the timing of disruption of the limb development process.[2] The risk of this association decreased significantly with chorionic villus sampling performed after 11 weeks as opposed to earlier than 9 weeks. Overlapping theories of proposed mechanisms include hemodynamic disturbance causing vascular disruption, amniotic puncture with mechanical compression and entanglement, and immunologic mechanism stimulating apoptotic cell death.

Disruption of the AER in animal experiments reproduces these deficiencies. As noted previously, the AER secretes FGFs guiding the mesodermal growth and differentiation. Notably, if such FGFs are applied to a limb bud following removal of the AER, the limb growth continues.

SUMMARY

The development of a functional three-dimensional limb requires the coordination of multiple mechanisms of induction and differentiation, much like the care of the child with the congenital limb deficiency requires the coordination of multiple team members. The care of the entire child includes a working knowledge of the potential for musculoskeletal and non-musculoskeletal findings associated with a given deficiency. Knowledge of the basic inheritance pattern can equip the care team to provide the family with counseling regarding the risk of recurrence in siblings and subsequent generations.

References

1. Beatty E: Upper limb tissue differentiation in the human embryo. *Hand Clin* 1985;1:391-403.
2. Firth H: Chorion villus sampling and limb deficiency – cause or coincidence? *Prenat Diagn* 1997;17(13):1313-1330.
3. Fernandez-Teran M, Ros MA: The apical ectodermal ridge: Morphologic aspects and signaling pathways. *Int J Dev Biol* 2008;52:851-871.

4. Niswander L, Martin GR: FGF–R and BMP-2 have opposite effects on limb growth. *Nature* 1993;361:68-71.
5. Riddle RD, Ensini E, Nelson C, Tsuchida T: Induction of the LIM homeobox gene Lmx1 by WNT7a establishes dorsoventral pattern in the vertebrate limb. *Cell* 1995;83:631-640.
6. Rodriguez-Esteban C, Schwabe JWR, De La Pena J, Foys B, Eshelman B, Izpisua Belmonte JC: *Radical fringe* positions the apical ectodermal ridge at the dorsoventral boundary of the vertebrate limb. *Nature* 1997;386:360-386.
7. Riddle RD, Johnson RL, Laufer E, Tabin C: *Sonic hedgehog* mediates the polarizing activity of the ZPA. *Cell* 1993;75:1401-1416.
8. Wieczorek D, Pawlik B, Li Y, et al: A specific mutation in the distant Sonic hedgehog cis-regulator (ZRS) causes Werner mesomelic syndrome while complete the ZRS duplications underlie Haas type polysyndactyly and preaxial syndactyly with or without triphalangeal thumb. *Hum Mutat* 2010;31:81-89.
9. Oberlender SA, Tuan RS: Expression and functional involvement of N-cadherin in embryonic limb chondrogenesis. *Development* 1994;120:177-187.
10. Haas AR, Tuan RS: Abstract: Bone morphogenic protein-2 stimulation of chondrogenesis in multipotential cells – modulation of N-cadherin expression and function. *Mol Biol Cell* 1996;7:424A.
11. Newman SA, Frenz DA, Hasegawa E, Akiyama SK: Matrix driven translocation: Dependence on interaction of amino-terminal domain of fibronectin with heparin like surface components of cells or particles. *Proc Natl Acad Sci USA* 1987;84:4791-4795.
12. Sandell LJ, Sugai JY, Trippel SB: Expression of collagens I, II, X and XI and aggregan mRNA's by bovine growth plate chondrocytes in situ. *J Orthop Res.* 1994;12:1-14.
13. James MA, Green HD, McCarroll R Jr, Manske PR: The association of radial deficiency with thumb hypoplasia. *J Bone Joint Surg* 2004;86-A(10):2196-2205.
14. 314390 VACTERL association with hydrocephalus, X-linked, in *Online Mendelian Inheritance in Man, OMIM (TM).* Johns Hopkins University. Available at: https://www.omim.org/entry/314390?search=vacterl%20association%20with%20hydrocephalus&highlight=%28hydrocephalic%7Chydrocephalus%7Chydrocephaly%29%20association%20vacterl%20with. Accessed December 23, 2021.
15. Kim JH, Kim PCW, Hui CC: The VACTERL association: Lessons from the Sonic hedgehog pathway. *Clin Genet* 2001;59:306-315.
16. Fiesco-Roa MO, Giri N, McReynolds LJ, Best AF, Alter BP: Genotype–phenotype associations in Fanconi anemia: The literature review. *Blood Rev* 2019;37:100589.
17. Che R, Zhang J, Nepal M, Han B, Fei P: Multifaceted Fanconi anemia signaling. *Trends Genet* 2018;34(3):171-183.
18. Schoenecker PL, Cohn AK, Sedgwick WG, Manske PR, Salafsky I, Millar EA: Dysplasia of the knee associated with the syndrome of thrombocytopenia and absent radius. *J Bone Joint Surg Am* 1984;66(3):421-427.
19. Christensen CP, Ferguson RL: Lower extremity deformity associated with thrombocytopenia and absent radius syndrome. *Clin Orthop Relat Res* 2000;375:202-206.
20. Klopocki E, Schulze H, Strauss G, et al: Complex inheritance pattern resembling autosomal recessive inheritance involving a microdeletion in thrombocytopenia-absent radius syndrome. *Am J Hum Genet* 2007;80(2):232-240.
21. Albers CA, Paul DS, Schulze H, et al: Complex inheritance of a low frequency regulatory SNP and a rare null mutation in exon-junction complex subunit RBM8A causes TAR syndrome. *Nat Genet* 2012;44(4):435-441.
22. De Graff E, Kozin SH: Genetics of radial deficiencies. *J Bone Joint Surg Am* 2009;91 suppl 4:81-86.
23. Lewin SO, Opitz JM: Fibular a/hypoplasia: Reviewing documentation of the fibular development field. *Am J Hum Genet* 1996;2:215-238.
24. Lenz W, Zygulska M, Horst J: FFU complex: And analysis of 491 cases. *Genetics* 1993;91:347-356.
25. Clinton R, Birch JG: Congenital tibial deficiency: A 35-year experience at one institution. *J Pediatr Orthop* 2015;35:385-390.
26. Agarwal RP, Jain D, Ramesh Babu CS, Garg RK: A heritable combination of congenital anomalies. *J Bone Joint Surg Br* 1996;78-B:492-494.
27. Deimling S, Sotiropoulos C, Lau K, et al: Tibial hemimelia associated with GLI 3 truncation. *J Hum Genet* 2016;61:443-446.
28. Ordal L, Keunen J, Martin N, et al: 2016 congenital limb deficiencies with vascular etiology: Possible association with maternal thrombophilia. *Am J Med Genet A* 2016;170-A:3083-3089.
29. Anderson KN, Dutton AC, Broussard CS, et al: ADHD medication use during pregnancy and risk for selected birth defects: National birth defects prevention study, 1998-2011. *J Atten Disord* 2020;24(3):479-489.
30. Adrien N, Peterson JM, Parker SE, Werler MM: Vasoactive exposures and risk of amniotic band syndrome and terminal transverse limb deficiencies. *Birth Defects Res* 2020;112:1074-1084.

Development of Locomotor Systems

Phoebe Scott-Wyard, DO, FAAP, FAAPMR

CHAPTER 60

ABSTRACT

Childhood motor development has a considerable effect on the success or failure of prosthetic fitting. Aspects of motor and psychological development can influence prosthetic fitting in children with limb deficiencies; therefore, familiarity of the interplay is imperative for the pediatric practitioner.

Keywords: developmental milestones; embryology; limb deficiency

Introduction

The development of the limbs and motor systems is a complex and orchestrated process, the interruption or disturbance of which can result in limb deficiency or deformity and subsequent disability. Following birth, the developmental processes of the growing child are integral to motor capabilities and should be considered when fitting prosthetic devices. This chapter will review the childhood stages of motor development.

Embryologic Limb Development and Limb Deficiency

Limb development occurs via multiple signaling pathways, each responsible for its own differentiation, yet working in concert with complex interactions, including signaling, regulation, feedback loops, and maintaining the additional axes of development.[1,2] The limbs start to appear at the end of the fourth week and continue to develop through the eighth week after fertilization.

The most critical period of limb development is 24 to 36 days after fertilization (during weeks 4 to 6), when the embryo undergoes rapid tissue proliferation.[3] Often, the mother is not aware of her pregnancy; therefore, exposure to teratogenic agents is difficult to prevent. Inhibition of limb bud development in the fourth week can result in complete absence of the limb, whereas interruption of the growth or development in the fifth week can result in partial absence.

Teratogenic factors affecting limb development include drug use during pregnancy, infections, chorionic villus sampling, or exposure to toxins.[4] Some medications affect limb development, including thalidomide, retinoic acid, and misoprostol. The most famous of these is thalidomide, which was marketed in the 1950s to mothers for management of nausea and vomiting during pregnancy. Thalidomide was available in most European countries and Canada, and it could be obtained without a prescription in Germany. In 1961, Widukind Lenz, a German pediatric geneticist, began investigating an increasing number of children born with severe limb anomalies; his findings resulted in a withdrawal of thalidomide from the market.[5] Thousands of exposed children exhibited phocomelic limb anomalies, facial malformations, and often, internal organ involvement.

Teratogenic causes are often difficult to study, particularly because prenatal history can be complicated by maternal recall bias.[6] Limb deficiencies also can be caused by vascular disruption (eg, amniotic band syndrome, in which fibrous bands constrict the vascular supply to the limbs), vascular malformations (such as Poland syndrome [subclavian artery disruption sequence]), or genetic factors (often a spontaneous point mutation in an otherwise normal family). Of the more than 120 clinically defined congenital limb deficiencies, less than 40% have a known molecular origin.[7] Many limb deficiencies are likely the result of an interaction of genetic and environmental factors (multifactorial inheritance). No racial predilection has been observed. In addition to disruptions in the uterine environment as noted previously, risk factors for congenital limb deficiency include maternal cigarette smoking (longitudinal deficiencies),[8] poorly controlled maternal diabetes (association with longitudinal deficiencies and sacral agenesis with hypoplastic lower extremities),[9] and maternal thrombophilia.[10]

Amniotic band syndrome (also known by more than 30 other names, including congenital constriction band syndrome, amniotic constriction band, and amnion rupture sequence) is a very heterogenous group of clinical anomalies, which can include congenital limb deformities, cleft lip and palate, constriction rings, and talipes equinovarus. There is no unanimously accepted etiology for this constellation of findings.[2] Animal studies have suggested that the

---

Dr. Scott-Wyard or an immediate family member serves as a paid consultant to or is an employee of Hanger Clinics and serves as a board member, owner, officer, or committee member of Association of Children's Prosthetic and Orthotic Clinics.

incidents leading to limb deficiency in amniotic band syndrome may be caused by a cascade of hypoxia, cell damage, hemorrhage, tissue loss, and reperfusion.[4]

Childhood Development

In childhood, development occurs in discontinuous bursts, with complex skills building on simpler skills. A proper understanding of developmental motor milestones (**Table 1**) is important when considering prosthetic prescription in the child with a limb deficiency. Prosthetic fitting should reflect the child's functional needs, not the rather arbitrary chronologic age.[5] Most children with a limb deficiency experience normal development. Those with bilateral upper limb deficiencies can experience a delay in reaching some milestones or miss them completely because of mechanical problems. Parents should be encouraged to treat a child with a limb deficiency in the same manner as they would treat any child, allowing them to explore their environment and develop new skills by experimentation.

Early Development

By 2 months of age, a child may be able to hold their head steady when placed in sitting, allowing for more visual interaction. However, object permanence is still lacking: if an object is removed from sight, the child will continue to stare at the same spot. The child will also smile in response to a face or voice, resulting in more functional social participation.[11]

At 3 to 4 months, a child will be able to bring their hands together in midline, grasping objects and allowing for self-discovery and visual-motor coordination. Palmar and asymmetric tonic neck reflexes are extinguished by this age. The child will stare at their own hand, beginning to understand cause and effect.

When the child is approximately 6 months old, they can sit without support and roll from supine to prone, allowing increased exploration of the environment. The child can transfer objects from hand to hand and begins learning to compare objects. Monosyllabic babbling is also noted at this age. A child this age with an upper limb deficiency could be fitted with a passive prosthesis to free the contralateral limb for manual activities when sitting. However, substantial controversy exists regarding the timing of prosthetic fitting for children with a unilateral upper limb deficiency. Recommendations vary from early fitting to fitting only at the age and time that the child demonstrates a functional or an emotional need for a prosthesis. Some practitioners prefer prosthetic fitting closer to 3 months of age, before the infant develops visually guided reaching.[3] The first prosthesis equalizes the lengths of the upper limbs, provides support when leaned on and during crawling, establishes an early wearing pattern, reduces sensory dependence on the residual limb, and helps in holding large objects.[5,12] A parent can position the prosthesis for optimal use and place objects in the terminal device to help the child become aware of how it can be used. The child does not yet have adequate skills or musculoskeletal excursion to control an activated prosthesis.

By 7 to 8 months of age, the child will begin to exhibit a thumb-finger (pincer) grasp and respond to nonverbal communication (one-step commands with gestures). Cognitively, they will start to have object permanence (eg, finding a hidden toy after seeing it hidden) and will actively compare objects (such as banging two cubes together).

At 10 to 12 months of age, the child will crawl, begin to pull themselves to a standing position, cruise along furniture, and, ultimately, walk independently, allowing for exploration and control of proximity to their parents. The child can follow one-step commands without need for gestures, showing development of verbal receptive language skills. The child with a unilateral lower limb deficiency is ready for prosthetic fitting at this age, with the goals of promoting two-legged standing, reciprocating gait development, and achieving a normal appearance. The prosthesis should be aligned for maximum stability, mimicking the toddler's wide base of support (socket flexion, abduction, and external rotation). For a child with a above-knee limb deficiency, the first prosthesis may not include a mechanical knee unit because of the need for increased function and stability. The practitioner should be aware that the child with a lower limb deficiency may still be transitioning from crawling to walking; therefore, the first prosthetic suspension should be substantial enough to prevent loss or falling off while crawling. Children often do not require any formal gait training or assistive devices. They often can transition to independent walking as do able-bodied children of the same age, using push-toys or hand-held assistance from parents.[13] Children with unilateral congenital transverse upper limb deficiency may never crawl, or may bear weight on the distal end of their limb, causing callousing. They may also use other body parts, such as the elbow, chin, or knee, to assist with bimanual activities.

The child should start to run at approximately 15 to 17 months of age. They can use objects in combination (such as building a tower of three cubes), begin acquisition of object and personal names, and can link actions to solve problems. If considered appropriate by the family and the practitioner, this is the approximate age when the

TABLE 1 Stages of Gross Motor Development

Average Age of Achievement	Developmental Milestone
2 mo	Able to control head in prone position
4 mo	Brings hands to midline, rolls prone to supine
6-8 mo	Sits independently, transfers objects hand to hand
10 mo	Crawls, stands with support
12 mo	Walks independently
2 yr	Jumps
3 yr	Climbs stairs by alternating feet, stands on one foot
4 yr	Hops on one foot, throws ball overhand
5 yr	Skips, dresses independently

child with an upper limb deficiency is ready for fitting with a myoelectric, single-site, voluntary-opening, automatic closing prosthesis, also known as the "cookie cruncher".[3]

By age 2 years, the child should be able to run well, walk up and down stairs (nonreciprocating), and jump. They can build a tower of seven cubes, perform circular scribbling, help in undressing, and speak in three-word sentences. At this time, the child with a unilateral upper limb deficiency may be ready for activation of a terminal device for a body-powered prosthesis. The skills needed are the ability to follow two-step commands, interest in two-handed activities, awareness of the holding functionality of a terminal device, ability to tolerate hand-over-hand therapy, and an attention span of at least 5 minutes. However, this is also the age at which behavior may impede prosthetic training, so individual differences are important to consider before cable activation.

Reciprocating stair climbing usually is attained by 2.5 years of age. Hopping on one foot and climbing occurs closer to 4 years of age. For the child with a limb deficiency above the elbow or with a shoulder disarticulation, a dual-control cable system and elbow lock can be introduced at this age. At 5 years of age, a child is able to skip, copy a triangle, name four colors, dress, and undress. Typically, a child with a unilateral transfemoral limb deficiency is fit with a prosthetic knee joint between ages 3 and 5 years. By age 5 to 6 years, the prosthetic alignment more closely reflects that of an adult. Because this is the age of school initiation, a child's awareness of their limb difference can become acutely apparent, and parents should be encouraged to work closely with the child's school for a smooth transition and introduction of the child to prevent teasing or bullying. Questions about the limb difference are to be expected, and children should be encouraged to provide honest, direct answers.

Development in Middle Childhood and Adolescence

Fine motor abilities continue to progress during middle childhood and adolescence, and psychosocial issues (such as separation from parents) and self-esteem challenges (relationships with peers) become more important. It has been said that a teenager is part child and part adult.[5] Teenagers with a lower limb deficiency may prefer to be fit with cosmetic endoskeletal prostheses so that their peers are less aware of their prosthetic use. Concern about perception of a prosthetic hook or terminal device can compel a teenager with an upper limb deficiency to request changing to a cosmetic or mechanical hand. It is important to provide education regarding function of a cosmetic or mechanical hand. The addition of a cosmetic glove over a mechanical hand reduces efficacy by up to 40%.[13] In addition, it is common for the teenager who does not wear an upper limb prosthesis to request one at this age. Often, the teenager is looking for a replacement for their missing limb and may have unrealistic expectations of the function a prosthetic limb can provide. Psychological support through formal counseling or peer and family support systems can benefit the teenager before initiating prosthetic fitting. This is also the time when adolescents obtain a driver's license, and practitioners should consider referral to an adaptive driving clinic for necessary adaptive equipment and training.

Task-specific prostheses may be beneficial at any age to aid in peer group activity involvement, depending on the child's interest and participation level. Examples include prostheses that aid in playing an instrument (eg, a bow-holding violin terminal device or a guitar pick holder) and sports participation (eg, an upper limb mitt terminal device for catching, a carbon-fiber running leg with a dynamic energy-storing foot, or a handlebar terminal device for cycling).

Psychosocial Development and Special Implications

A review of childhood development would be remiss to not include the psychosocial domain. The first 18 months of life entail rapid expansion of the social and emotional parts of the brain. Initially, the lower limbic system directs reflexive emotional responses in the newborn. Later, frontal lobe activity increases, building emotional regulation and self-control with the help of healthy caregiver attachment. Typically, between 6 and 12 months of age, attachment relationships are developed with responsive caregivers. After 18 months, autonomy begins to emerge in children who have confidence in the child-parent relationship. Around 30 to 54 months, issues with impulse control, gender roles, and peer relationships start to be witnessed. At this time, core values and self-control are learned from caregivers. As the child ages, peers begin to take on more important roles than family, and there is a growing necessity for independence. This can include engaging in risky behavior to impress peers and make sense of novel emotions. Throughout this process, healthy adult caregiver relationships are inherent in the child's ability to develop strong coping strategies and resilience.[14]

Children with lower limb deficiency have greater problems in the arenas of behavioral, emotional, psychological, and social adjustment; however, this has been shown to be ameliorated by a strong social support network.[15] Conversely, higher parental marital discord, paternal anxiety and depression were previously shown to have a negative effect on the mental health of children with lower limb deformities. It is important that the team evaluate the entire family paradigm to appropriately address and circumvent these negative effects on the psychosocial well-being of children with limb deficiencies.[16]

Children who undergo prolonged limb reconstruction with lengthening often experience increased psychological stress, secondary to the long duration, impact on schooling and the potentially high rate of complications of this treatment. Another population that deserves consideration are those undergoing lower extremity rotationplasty, resulting in a posteriorly rotated foot that functions as a knee. Although the cosmesis of the "backwards foot" has been queried in multiple studies, the long-term outcomes in the psychosocial domain have been comparable to those who underwent limb reconstruction or amputation. However, some reported a negative impact on initiating social or intimate relationships. Given the fact that many undergo this operation as children, these are important themes to consider when educating families.[17]

In one study, young adults with unilateral transverse upper limb deficiency reported difficulty with job and education placement, and despite feeling convinced they were suitable for almost any study or job, the perception of others was often more limiting. However, they did not express significant problems with leisure activities, intimate relationships, housekeeping, or transportation.[18]

The most important concerns identified by children with a limb deficiency in one international qualitative study were cosmetic appearance, physical health, body image (particularly if the limb deficiency was due to an acquired amputation), school and sport participation, future job prospects, and social isolation.[19]

Split-hand/split-foot malformation, Cornelia de Lange syndrome, Moebius syndrome, Roberts-SC phocomelia syndrome, and Edwards syndrome are some examples of occurrences of congenital limb deficiency that can coexist with developmental or intellectual delay, which could have a negative impact on physical function and prosthetic management. These children can benefit from involvement of an entire therapeutic team, including physical, occupational, and speech therapists.

SUMMARY

Children are not simply small adults. With the proper understanding of their growth and development along with timely application of prosthetic principles, children with limb deficiencies can be encouraged and supported to achieve a healthy and fulfilling childhood and successful adulthood.

References

1. Moore KL, Persaud TV: *The Developing Human: Clinically Oriented Embryology*, ed 6. WB Saunders, 1998.
2. Dy CJ, Swarup I, Daluiski A: Embryology, diagnosis, and evaluation of congenital hand anomalies. *Curr Rev Musculoskelet Med* 2014;7(1):60-67.
3. Herring JA, Birch JG: *The Child With a Limb Deficiency*. American Academy of Orthopaedic Surgeons, 1998.
4. McGuirk CK, Westgate MN, Holmes LB: Limb deficiencies in newborn infants. *Pediatrics* 2001;108(4):E64.
5. Setoguchi Y, Rosenfelder R: *The Limb Deficient Child*. Charles C. Thomas Publisher, 1982.
6. Werler MM, Pober BR, Nelson K, Holmes LB: Reporting accuracy among mothers of malformed and nonmalformed infants. *Am J Epidemiol* 1989;129(2):415-421.
7. Wilcox WR, Coulter CP, Schmitz ML: Congenital limb deficiency disorders. *Clin Perinatol* 2015;42(2):281-300.
8. Caspers KM, Romitti PA, Lin S, et al: Maternal periconceptional exposure to cigarette smoking and congenital limb deficiencies. *Paediatr Perinat Epidemiol* 2013;27(6):509-520.
9. Garne E, Loane M, Dolk H, et al: Spectrum of congenital anomalies in pregnancies with pregestational diabetes. *Birth Defect Res A Clin Mol Teratol* 2013;94(3):134-140.
10. Ordal L, Keunen J, Martin N, et al: Congenital limb deficiencies with vascular etiology: Possible association with maternal thrombophilia. *Am J Med Genet* 2016;170(12):3083-3089.
11. Behrman RE, Kliegman RM, Jenson HB: *Nelson Textbook of Pediatrics*, ed 17. WB Saunders, 2004.
12. Crandall RC, Tomhave W: Pediatric unilateral below-elbow amputees: Retrospective analysis of 34 patients given multiple prosthetic options. *J Pediatr Orthop* 2002;22(3):380-383.
13. Scott-Wyard P, Yip V, Rotter DB: Limb deficiencies, in Murphy KP, McMahon MA, Houtrow AJ, eds: *Pediatric Rehabilitation: Principles and Practice*, ed 6. Springer, 2020, pp 410-432.
14. Malik F, Marwaha R: *Developmental stages of social emotional development in children*, in StatPearls [Internet]. StatPearls Publishing, 2022.
15. Varni JW, Setoguchi Y: Correlates of perceived physical appearance in children with congenital/acquired limb deficiencies. *J Dev Behav Pediatr* 1991;12(3):171-176.
16. Varni JW, Rubenfeld LA, Talbot D, Setoguchi Y: Determinants of self-esteem in children with congenital/acquired limb deficiencies. *J Dev Behav Pediatr* 1989;10(1):13-16.
17. Bernthal NM, Monument MJ, Randall RL, Jones KB: Rotationplasty: Beauty is in the eye of the beholder. *Oper Tech Orthop* 2014;24(2):103-110.
18. Lankhorst NE, Baars ECT, Wijk IV, Janssen WGM, Poelma MJ, van der Sluis CK: Living with transversal upper limb reduction deficiency: Limitations experienced by young adults during their transition to adulthood. *Disabil Rehabil* 2017;39(16):1623-1630.
19. Chhina H, Klassen AF, Kopec JA, et al: What matters to children with lower limb deformities: An international qualitative study guiding the development of a new patient-reported outcome measure. *J Patient Rep Outcomes* 2021;5(1):30.

Scientific, Technologic, Surgical, and Prosthetic Advances in Pediatric Limb Deficiency

CHAPTER 61

Michael Schmitz, MD, FAAOS • Rebecca Hernandez, CPO, LPO

ABSTRACT

Limb deficiency in children often requires lifelong adaptive measures to improve function, decrease morbidity, and allow for proper development. Targeted muscle reinnervation and regenerative peripheral nerve interfaces are techniques designed to redirect efferent neural impulses to improve both biologic and prosthetic function and decrease residual limb pain. Osseointegration is a technique that links a prosthetic device directly to the appendicular skeleton. Allotransplantation of limbs shows benefit in the upper extremity, however at a cost of the need for lifetime immunosuppression. Refinements in indications, implants, and techniques may lead to use in younger patients. Technologic advancements in fabrication, component modularity and miniaturization, and microprocessor control have improved prosthetic function and durability.

Keywords: 3D scanner printing; allotransplantation; osseointegration; targeted muscle reinnervation

Introduction

Treatment options for pediatric limb deficiency would ideally offer biologic replacement or animated mechanical prostheses that could mimic muscular, neurologic, and skeletally supportive biologic function. Currently, no options can do so without attendant morbidity or functional compromise. However, advances in transplantation science, surgical tissue transfer, mechanical design, fabrication, miniaturization, and microprocessors have led to improvements in both biologic and mechanical function.

Scientific, Technologic, and Surgical Advances

Limb deficiency in children often requires lifelong adaptive measures to improve function, decrease morbidity, and allow for proper development.[1] The goal of limb deficiency treatment is to create a limb facsimile that can functionally replace the deficiency. The ideal replacement would provide afferent tactile, vibratory, and positional sense to the wearer; be able to interpret efferent motor control; translate the efferent motor impulses into physical action; provide structural support; remain pain free; and promote normal function with a low biologic complication rate and high durability. Current prosthetic devices and limb salvage procedures are limited by the bioprosthetic interface, lack of afferent sensation, limited motor control, and componentry unable to replicate biologic function. Surgical techniques create residual limbs with altered anatomy and severed nerves that can become painful neuromas. Developmental advancement, longitudinal limb growth, and elevated activity levels are three factors that make treatment of pediatric patients with limb deficiency more challenging. Refinements in surgical techniques, prosthetic design and fabrication, and rehabilitation can lead to less morbidity and greater function.

Targeted muscle reinnervation (TMR) and regenerative peripheral nerve interfaces (RPNIs) are techniques designed to redirect efferent neural impulses.[2,3] TMR transplants functioning nerves to denervated tissue, whereas RPNI transfers denervated free muscle patch grafts to transected nerves. Both techniques were originally designed to create bioamplifiers of efferent nerve impulses to improve control of myoelectric prostheses and incidentally were found to decrease both phantom limb pain and residual limb pain.[4-8]

Phantom limb pain should be distinguished from residual limb pain in that phantom limb pain refers to central sensation for a body part not present and residual limb pain to pain in the residual limb.[9] Phantom limb pain has a reported prevalence of 7% to 100% and can occur regardless of the etiology of limb loss and persist for an extended period of time.[10-12] Amputation etiology varies the prevalence, with malignancy the highest

---

Dr. Schmitz or an immediate family member serves as a paid consultant to or is an employee of Orthofix, Inc., Orthopediatrics, and Stryker and serves as a board member, owner, officer, or committee member of Pediatric Orthopaedic Society of North America and Scoliosis Research Society. Neither Rebecca Hernandez nor any immediate family member has received anything of value from or has stock or stock options held in a commercial company or institution related directly or indirectly to the subject of this chapter.

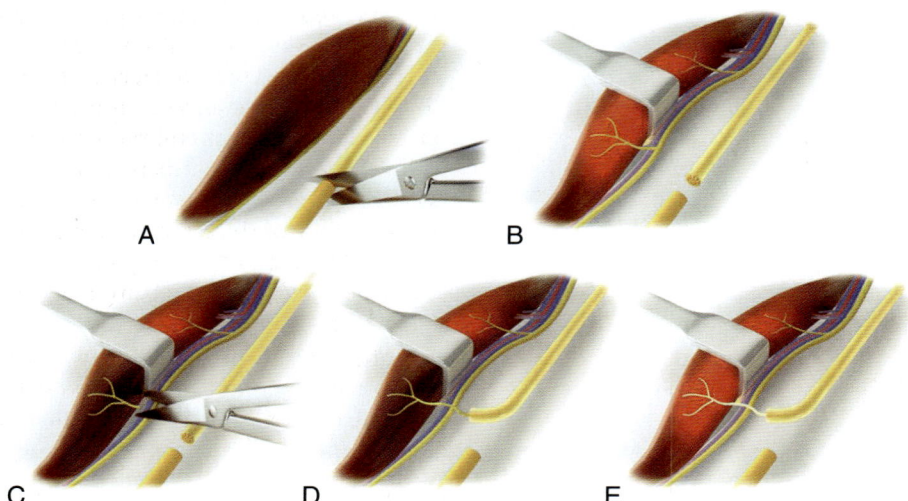

FIGURE 1 Schematic illustration shows targeted muscle reinnervation. **A**, Transection of primary nerve. **B**, Isolation of neurovascular supply to neighboring muscle. **C**, Transection of one discrete motor supplying neighboring muscle, leading to selective muscle deinnervation. **D**, Primary nerve to muscle motor nerve coaptation. **E**, Eventual reinnervation of neighboring muscle with fascicles from primary nerve. (Reproduced with permission from Herr HM, Clites TR, Srinivasan S, et al: Reinventing extremity amputation in the era of functional limb restoration. *Ann Surg* 2021;273[2]:269-279.)

(48% to 90%), trauma highly variable (12% to 83%), and congenital limb loss the lowest (4% to 20%).[10]

Pain in the residual limb or phantom limb pain can significantly alter functional outcomes.[13]

TMR (**Figure 1**) transfers information from larger diameter proximal nerves severed from their muscle effectors to new muscle effectors that can serve as effective electromyographic (EMG) signal generators for receptors in myoelectric prostheses.[14] The large-diameter peripheral nerves can be coapted to smaller nerves close to the entry into vascularized native muscle either primarily or after neuroma excision.[15] The coaptation coordinates the otherwise neuroma-generating regenerative nerve fibers and decreases the incidence of both phantom and residual limb pain.[7,16,17]

RPNIs (**Figure 2**) are nonvascularized free muscle grafts coapted to a distal nerve ending, creating an EMG-generating end plate for the neurosignal.[18] RPNI offers the ability to create multiple EMG generators for prosthetic control after reinnervation without sacrificing native vascularized muscles. RPNI inhibits neuroma formation by providing a denervated biologic target for both sensory and motor nerve ingrowth.[19] Reinnervation of the new target is effective in both preventing and managing neuroma-mediated pain.[8]

The traditional method used to attach both an upper and lower limb prosthesis to a limb requires a bioprosthetic interface of a custom-designed socket. An excellent fit is required to transmit skeletal forces to the end component of the prosthesis. Fit is compromised by volume changes in the limb, dynamic soft tissue, and diaphoresis, which can lead to shear on the skin, pain, and skin breakdown, decreasing quality of life and function.[20]

Osseointegration is a term coined by Brånemark after he found that bone integrated into titanium matrices, during a study of bone flow in rabbit models.[21] Osseointegration refers to direct structural connection between bone and a metallic implant. It has been used successfully in dental implants, maxillofacial reconstruction, and total joint arthroplasties with great success. In some parts of the world, it is an established treatment option for select patients intolerant of traditional sockets.[22]

Current contraindications include skeletal immaturity, peripheral vascular disease, ongoing chemotherapy, immunosuppression, irradiated limbs, and inability to comply with physical therapy and activity restrictions.[23] The most common complication remains infection, but most are superficial and can be managed with oral antibiotics. Shorter term follow-up has shown a 5% to 8% incidence of deep infection requiring additional surgical procedures.[24] Longer term follow-up of a different patient population demonstrated a 10-year cumulative risk of deep infection requiring implant removal at 9%.[25]

Despite these limitations, a meta-analysis of outcomes demonstrated uniform improved function and quality of life with osseointegration compared with traditional socket fittings in transfemoral amputees.[22] In addition, osseointegration offers the potential for osseoperception—the mechanoreceptor-mediated central nervous system (CNS) awareness of prosthetic position and function.[23] A new implant system, the enhanced OPRA (which stands for Osseoanchored Prostheses for the Rehabilitation of Amputees), combines prosthetic skeletal fixation, with connection to implanted neuromuscular interfaces allowing more direct neurocommunication between the user and the prosthetic device.[26]

Proprioception is the sense of body and limb position, movement, and force generation mediated by mechanoreceptors in muscles, tendons, and joint capsules.[27] Afferent impulses from the mechanoreceptors are required to replicate prosthetic proprioception. TMR and RPNI are surgical techniques that can decrease phantom limb pain, decrease neuroma formation, and increase the number of effective EMG signal generators; they do not effectively add afferent neurosignaling.

Agonist-antagonist myoneural interface is a biologic-prosthetic construct that can animate a prosthetic limb to perform more synchronized movements as a limb as opposed to a prosthesis.[28] Two muscles—an agonist and antagonist—are surgically linked in such a manner that contraction of one stretches mechanoreceptors in the other. The link allows afferent communication with the CNS.[29] EMG sensors can trigger myoelectric componentry,

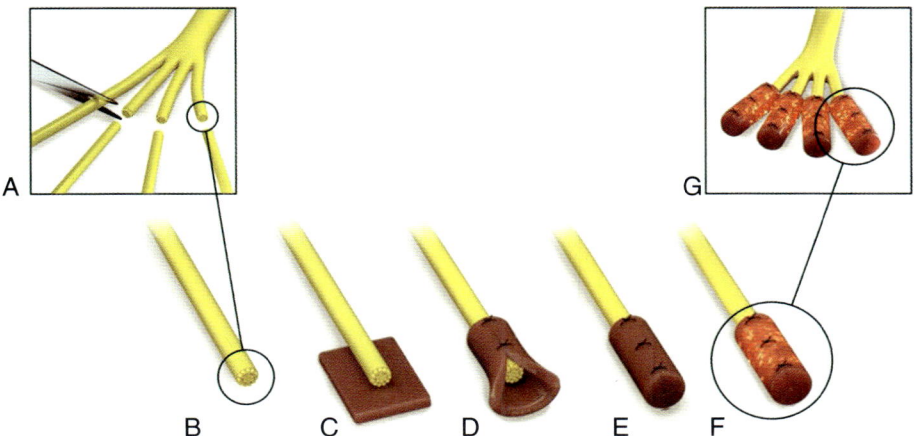

FIGURE 2 Schematic illustration shows regenerative peripheral nerve interface (RPNI) construction. **A,** Transection of primary nerve and intrafascicular split to facilitate reinnervation. **B,** Magnified view of individual nerve fascicle. **C,** Fascicle terminus is placed into deinnervated, nonvascularized free muscle graft procured from remote site. **D,** Suture closure of graft around distal nerve ending. **E,** Completed RPNI construction. **F,** Eventual reinnervation of free muscle graft by terminal nerve fascicle. **G,** Collective view of primary nerve following completion of multiple RPNI construction. (Reproduced with permission from Herr HM, Clites TR, Srinivasan S, et al: Reinventing extremity amputation in the era of functional limb restoration. *Ann Surg* 2021;273[2]:269-279.)

and torque sensors in the prosthesis can provide feedback to the agonist-antagonist muscle loop via functional electrical stimulation. Tuning controller gains can align prosthetic movement and force with CNS perception. The bidirectional signaling between prosthesis and biologic limb is an important step in creating a true bionic limb.[30]

Vascularized composite tissue allotransplantation (VCA) of hands and lower extremities can ideally provide full motor and sensory function with a functional range of motion and strength and restoration of body image.[31] A number of studies have shown that physical functioning, pain, general health, and social functioning of hand transplantation equal that of prosthesis use. Literature suggests improvement in both physical and psychosocial parameters in hand transplantation patients.[32] Lower extremity transplantation has not yet demonstrated equivalent functional results likely because lower extremity prostheses better replicate biologic function.[33]

Similar to solid organ transplants, all VCAs require lifelong immunosuppression to prevent acute and chronic allograft rejection. The immunosuppression protocol is similar to that for kidney transplants including adverse effects as significant as hypertension; diabetes; susceptibility to viral, bacterial, and fungal infections; increased risk of dermatologic, hematologic, oral, and esophageal malignancies; and end organ failure, most commonly renal.[34]

Unlike solid organ failure, limb deficiency is not life-threatening. VCA restores limb function but requires the recipient to accept a chronic treatment that can be life-threatening (immunosuppression). Patient selection should be limited to those with significant functional limitations, sound psychological profile, ability to tolerate a prolonged surgical insult, prolonged rehabilitation, and compliance with a strict pharmacologic regimen post-transplantation. Most VCAs are limited to bilateral hand deficiencies and bilateral transfemoral amputations.

Limb generation or regeneration offers potential for limb function in patients with unreconstructable limbs and those unable or unwilling to accept the ongoing need for immunosuppression. Some vertebrates such as frogs and salamanders can regenerate limbs and organs. In mammals, with rare exception—terminal phalanges in rats and distal fingertips in children—limb injury results in scar formation as opposed to regeneration.[35] Regeneration requires appropriate gene expression, an embryonic extracellular matrix, an immature immune system, appropriate stem cells, and maintenance of these regenerative conditions for a duration long enough to complete limb growth.[36] Investigators have been able to replicate some cellular conditions conducive to regeneration but have not been able to stimulate all tissue types or avoid oncogenic growth.

Prosthetic Advances

Along with surgical advances, there have been numerous prosthetic advances over the past 2 decades for pediatric patients with limb deficiencies. Many of these advances have been adapted from developments in adult components, sized down to fit children; however, there is still continued work to be done to meet the demands of children. Children put the highest demand on their devices with high forces and impact activities, from recreational to highly competitive sports; environmental factors such as sand and mud that can wear away at components; and decreased attention to maintenance. Modular components have made it easier for prosthetists to alter and replace broken parts as well as keep up with growth and angular changes needed because of physiologic changes.[37]

Historically, the prosthetist has been challenged with a limited selection of prefabricated prosthetic feet for the child with a lower limb amputation and was often left to fabricate custom feet or use a traditional SACH (solid ankle, cushion heel) foot. Currently, more manufacturers are offering pediatric-size prosthetic feet in both exoskeletal and endoskeletal designs, allowing for growth adjustments and replacement of commonly broken components. Material advancements such as fiberglass composites (**Figure 3**) have allowed for more durable components.

Posterior mount prosthetic feet are now available in pediatric sizes, offering those with long residual limbs the option of an energy-storing prosthetic foot for both walking and sports activities. For young children, there are also more options for mechanical knees available, starting with knees that are suitable for infants and toddlers for use in their first prosthesis.[38,39] There is a need for more durable hydraulic-controlled prosthetic knees for adolescents approximately age 7 to 10 years as these children are running at varying cadences but are too small for adult prosthetic knees. Additionally, at this age, many children are transitioning into adult-sized prosthetic feet but are under the lower weight ranges for these feet, so the children are left using prosthetic feet that are too stiff for them.

For the teenager and young adult with a higher level amputation, some microprocessor-controlled prosthetic knees (**Figure 4**) have been refined to be more responsive, allow for higher impact activities such as jogging, have a longer battery life per charge, and be more water resistant, allowing for greater use among high-functioning users.

However, for those participating in extreme activities such as water sports and competitive sports, a lighter weight, more durable mechanical knee is not yet available.

One of the greatest areas of advancement in recent years has been in upper extremity technology. Multidigit articulating prosthetic hands offer far more grip patterns than the traditional three-jaw chuck grip. These myoelectric microprocessor-controlled prosthetic hands have apps for user interface and offer both options such as a grip for controlling a computer mouse or for typing. This technology can be partnered with myoelectric pattern recognition to allow for more intuitive and precise control. Some of these prosthetic hands are now being offered in a smaller size, which is suitable for a responsible teenager; however, the challenge lies in getting insurance reimbursement for such devices.

Shape acquisition has traditionally been via applying a cast to a limb. For some patients, three-dimensional (3D) scanners can now aid in obtaining models of the residual limb. Although many 3D scanners are not detailed

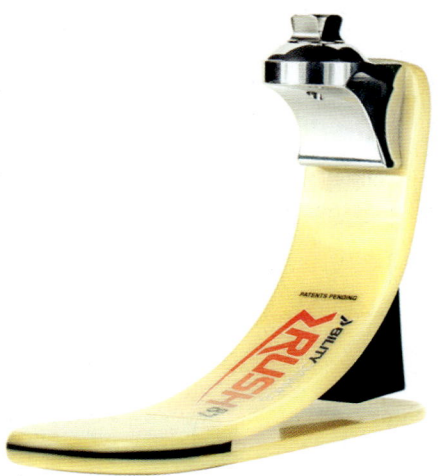

FIGURE 3 Photograph of a fiberglass composite foot. (Reproduced with permission from Rush HiPro [Proteor].)

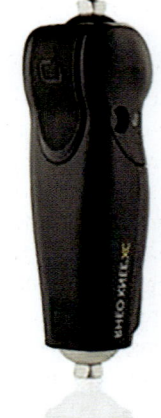

FIGURE 4 Photograph of microprocessor-controlled knees. (Reproduced with permission from Rheo XC [Össur] and Genium [OttoBock].)

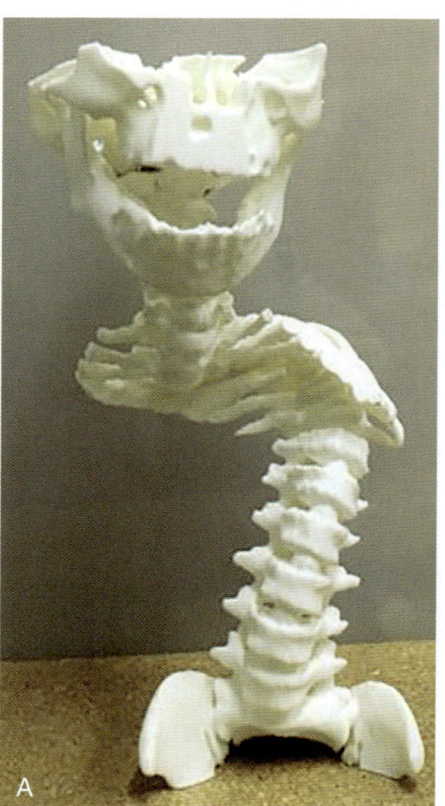
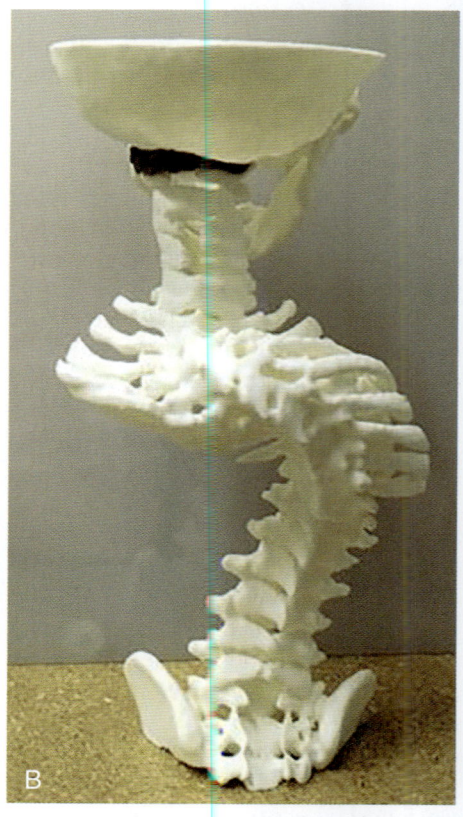

FIGURE 5 **A** and **B**, Photographs of 3D printed spine from preoperative CT for surgical planning.

enough to capture a small residual limb, scanner technology is constantly improving. Computer-aided design/computer-aided manufacturing (CAD/CAM) can be a useful tool in designing sockets or in tooling parts that can aid in the fabrication process of prostheses. Additionally, 3D printed devices can aid in surgical decisions for the orthopaedic surgeon.[40,41] 3D printed preoperative planning models can supplement imaging to provide a greater understanding of complex deformities (**Figure 5**). Customized

3D printed jigs for tumor resection are being used.

Although 3D printed prostheses for upper extremity devices have been glorified in the media as low-cost options compared with a traditional prosthesis, often these are devices that are not durable or well fitting and have not undergone the rigorous testing that mass-produced components have undergone. Some pediatric prosthetists/orthotists are using CAD/CAM and 3D printing to create devices for those previously unaided, such as assistive devices for partial hand amputations, yet this is an area of technology that is still evolving and will likely see great changes in the years to come. For lower extremity components, it is important that they are structurally sound and meet International Organization for Standardization standards to ensure safety and the ability to meet the demands of the very active pediatric patient.

Physically active and highly functioning children will likely carry that lifestyle forward into adulthood. It is important to encourage these children and ensure that they have every opportunity to participate in all mobility activities and sports of their choosing so that they can be highly active and productive adults in their communities.

SUMMARY

A number of advancements in deficiency classification, surgical techniques, prosthetic design, componentry, and CAD/CAM modeling have resulted in expanded reconstructive procedures and prosthetics. Advancements in surgical reconstruction of neural tissue have produced improved postoperative pain scores and prosthetic function and have the potential to offer even greater sensory and motor control of prosthetic limbs. Progress in bidirectional CNS–prosthetic neural feedback creates potential for truly bionic limbs. Vascularized composite allotransplants offer functional limb alternatives but require acceptance of immunotherapy-induced chronic disease. Advancements in materials have yielded more durable prostheses. Miniaturization of adult componentry has advanced pediatric prosthetic capability. CAD/CAM technology offers potential for streamlining prosthetic fabrication and 3D printing can be useful for surgical planning and design but has not been useful in fabrication of durable prosthetics.

References

1. Schoppen T, Boonstra A, Groothoff JW, de Vries J, Göeken LN, Eisma WH: Physical, mental, and social predictors of functional outcome in unilateral lower-limb amputees. *Arch Phys Med Rehabil* 2003;84(6):803-811.
2. Kung TA, Langhals NB, Martin DC, Johnson PJ, Cederna PS, Urbanchek MG: Regenerative peripheral nerve interface viability and signal transduction with an implanted electrode. *Plast Reconstr Surg* 2014;133(6):1380-1394.
3. Cheesborough JE, Smith LH, Kuiken TA, Dumanian GA: Targeted muscle reinnervation and advanced prosthetic arms. *Semin Plast Surg* 2015;29(1):62-72.
4. Bowen JB, Ruter D, Wee C, West J, Valerio IL: Targeted muscel reinnervation technique in below-knee amputation. *Plas Reconstr Surg* 2019;143(1):309-312.
5. Mioton LM, Dumanian GA, Shah N, et al: Targeted muscle reinnervation improves residual limb pain, phantom limb pain, and limb function: A prospective study of 33 major limb amputees. *Clin Orthop Relat Res* 2020;478(9):478-479.
6. McNamara CT, Iorio ML: Targeted muscle reinnervation: Outcomes in treating chronic pain secondary to extremity amputation and phantom limb syndrome. *J Reconstr Microsurg* 2020;36(4):235-240.
7. Dumanian GA, Potter BK, Mioton LM, et al: Targeted muscle reinnervation treats neuroma and phantom pain in major limb amputees: A randomized clinical trial. *Ann Surg* 2019;270(2):238-2426.
8. Hooper RC, Cederna PS, Brown DL, et al: Regenerative peripheral nerve interfaces for the management of symptomatic hand and digital neuromas. *Plast Reconstr Surg Glob Open* 2020;8(6):e2792.
9. Schley MT, Wilms P, Toepfner S, et al: Painful and nonpainful phantom and stump sensations in acute traumatic amputees. *J Trauma* 2008;65(4):858-864.
10. DeMoss P, Ramsey LH, Karlson CW: Phantom limb pain in pediatric oncology. *Front Neurol* 2018;9:219.
11. Krane EJ, Heller LB: The prevalence of phatom sensation and pain in pediatric amputees. *J Pain Symptom Manag* 1995;10(1):21-29.
12. Ephraim PL, Wegener ST, MacKenzie EJ, Dillingham TR, Pezzin LE: Phantom pain, residual limb pain, and back pain in amputees: Results of a national survey. *Arch Phys Med Rehabil* 2005;86(10):1910-1919.
13. Padovani MT, Martins MR, Venâncio A, Forni JE: Anxiety, deression and quality of life in individuals with phantom limb pain. *Acta Ortop Bras* 2015;23(2):107-110.
14. Kuiken TA, Barlow AK, Hargrove L, Dumanian GA: Targeted muscle reinnervation for the upper and lower extremity. *Tech Orthop* 2017;32(2):109-116.
15. Herr HM, Clites TR, Srinivasan S, et al: Reinventing extremity amputation in the era of functional limb restoration. *Ann Surg* 2021;273(2):269-279.
16. Geary M, Gaston RG, Loeffler B: Surgical and technological advances in the management of upper limb amputees. *Bone Joint J* 2021;103-B(3):430-439.
17. Pet MA, Ko JH, Friedly JL, Mourad PD, Smith DG: Does targeted nerve implanation reduce neuroma pain in amputees? *Clin Orthop Relat Res* 2014;472(10):2991-3001.
18. Baldwin J, Moon JD, Cederna PS, Urbanchek MG: Early muscle revascularization and regeneration at the regenerative peripheral nerve interface. *Plast Reconst Surg* 2012;130(1S):73.
19. Woo SL, Kung TA, Brown DL, Leonard JA, Kelly BM, Cederna PS: Regenerative peripheral nerve interfaces for the treatment of postamputation neurom pain: A pilot study. *Plas Reconstr Surg Glob open* 2016;4(12):e1038.
20. Pezzin LE, Dillingham TR, Mackenzie EJ, Ephraim P, Rossbach P: Use and satisfaction with prosthetic limb devices and relaed services. *Arch Phys Med Rehabil* 2004;85(5):723-729.
21. Branemark PI: Vital microscopy of bone marrow in rabbit. *Scan J Clin Lan Invest* 1959;11(38):1-82.
22. Herbert JS, Rehani M, Stiegelmar R: Osseintegreation for lower-limb amputation: A systemic review of clnical outcomes. *JBJS Rev* 2017;5(10):e10.
23. Hoellwarth JS, Tetsworth K, Rozbruch SR, Handal MB, Coughlan A, Al Muderis M: Osseointegration for amputees: Current implants, techniques, and

24. Al-Muderis M, Khemka A, Lord SJ, Van de Meent H, Frölke JP: Safety of osseointegrated implants for transfemoral amputees: A two-center prospective cohort study. *J Bone Joint Surg Am* 2016;98(11):900.

25. Tillander J, Hagberg K, Berlin Ö, Hagberg L, Brånemark R: Osteomyelitis risk in patients with transfemoral amputations treated with osseointegration prostheses. *Clin Orthop Rela Res* 2017;475(12):3100-3108.

26. Zaid MB, O'Donnell RJ, Potter BK, Forsberg JA: Orthopaedic osseointegreation: State of the art. *J Am Acad Orthop Surg* 2019;27(22):e977-e985.

27. Proske U, Gandevia SC: The proprioceptive senses: Their roles in signaling body shape, body position and movement, and muscle force. *Physiol Rev* 2012;92:1651-1697.

28. Clites TR, Carty MJ, Ullauri JB, et al: Proprioception from a neurally controlled lower-extremity prosthesis. *Sci Transl Med* 2018;10(443):eaap8373.

29. Srinivasan SS, Diaz M, Carty M, Herr HM: Towards functional restoration for persons with limb amputation: A dual-stage implementation of regenerative agonist-antagonist myoneural interfaces. *Sci Rep* 2019;9:1981.

30. Bumbasirevic M, Lesic A, Palibrk T, et al: The current state of bionic limbs from the surgeon's viewpoint. *EFORT Open Rev* 2020 5(2):65-72.

31. Reece E, Ackah R: Hand transplantation: The benefits, risks, outcomes, and future. *Tex Heart Inst J* 2019;46(1):63-64.

32. Salminger S, Sturma A, Roche AD, et al: Functional and psychosocial outcomes of hand transplantation compared with prosthetic fitting in below-elbow amputees: A multicenter cohort study. *PLoS One* 2016;11(9):e0162507.

33. Cavadas PC, Thione A, Carballeira A, Blanes M: Bilateral transfemoral lower extremity transplantation: Results at 1 year. *Am J Transplant* 2013;13(5):1343-1349.

34. Bozulic LD, Breidenback WC, lldstad ST: Past, present, and future prospects for inducing donor-specific transplantation tolerance for composite tissue allotransplantation. *Semin Plast Surg* 2007;21(104):213-225.

35. Leppik LP, Froemel D, Slavici A, et al: Effects of electrical stimulation on rat limb regeneration, a new look at an old model. *Sci Rep* 2016;5:18353.

36. Alibardi L: Review limb regeneration in humans: Dream or reality? *Ann Anat* 2018;217:1-6.

37. Hall M, Wustrack R, Cummings D, et al: Innovations in pediatric prosthetics. *JPOSNA* 2021;3(1):221.

38. Geil M, Coulter C: Analysis of locomotor adaptations in young children with limb loss in an early prosthetic knee prescription protocol. *Prosthet Ortho Int* 2014;38(1):54-61.

39. Geil MD, Coulter-O'Berry C, Schmitz M, Heriza C: Crawling kinematics in an early knee protocol for pediatric prosthetic prescription. *J Prosthet Ortho* 2013;25(1):22-29.

40. Shilo D, Emodi O, Blanc O, Noy D, Rachmiel A: Printing the future Updates in 3D printing for surgical application. *Ramban Maomonides Med J* 2018;9(3):e020.

41. Gomez-Palomo JM, Meschian-Coretti S, Esteban-Castillo JL, García-Vera JJ, Montañez-Heredia E: Double lelvel osteotomy assisted by 3D printing technology in a patient with Blount disease. *JBJS Case Connect* 2020;10(2):e0477.

Gait Analysis in the Child With a Limb Deficiency

CHAPTER 62

Michael Aiona, MD, FAAOS

ABSTRACT

Gait analysis is an objective measure to analyze the motion and forces across the joints of the lower extremity. It can define deviations from normal gait and assist in clinical decision making. Gait analysis performed on children with limb deficiency is limited compared with that performed on adults. Energy consumption is greater in children with limb deficiency, with increasing cost as the level of deficiency moves more proximal, similar to adults, although exceptions exist. Children generally place more demands and force across the nonprosthetic side. The biomechanical aspects of the prosthetic foot design can affect the forces across the knee, allowing the clinician and prosthetist to choose which characteristics would be best for the individual patient. However, despite mechanical advantages of certain prosthetic foot designs, patient choice is not always toward the more advanced device. In a specific subpopulation of patients treated with a rotationplasty, controversy still remains regarding the efficacy of a mechanical knee compared with a biologic substitute (ankle) as gait studies differ in their findings. Regardless, the remaining length of the femoral segment and comparative knee axis height are important factors in overall function.

Keywords: gait analysis; limb deficiency; pediatric

Introduction

It is important to know the historical development of motion analysis. The components of a gait analysis, including a description of the three ankle rockers, are key concepts. A literature review will highlight some objective findings relevant to the treatment of the child with a limb deficiency, divided into transfemoral and transtibial levels of deficiency. One specific condition, proximal femoral focal deficiency, is important to discuss with the noted differences in findings, along with gait analysis application and future developments.

History

Upright ambulation is one key evolutionary development that distinguishes humans from other mammals. Whether this occurred to free the upper extremities for more advanced tasks, see over the vegetation, or for more efficient locomotion is still debated. Although Aristotle authored the first known writings on human walking centuries ago, there was limited scientific investigation into this unique human characteristic as observation alone was not sufficiently precise because of perspective and the rapidity of movement. The advent of photography and a wagered bet among some industrialists initiated advancements that led to further insights into ambulation.

Known for his photographic skill documenting the landscapes in the Pacific Northwest for US government, Muybridge developed the technique of sequential serial photographs taken in rapid sequence during the movement of interest, in a quest to determine whether a galloping horse at some point had all four limbs off the ground (because this was not visible to the naked eye). This technique used multiple cameras (24) to take photographs in a timed sequential fashion, requiring the timed sequencing of light exposure and the camera shutter. Indeed, at some point the horse's hoofs were all off the ground during a gallop.[1] He invented the zoopraxiscope, which allowed the pictures to be shown in sequence rapidly, thus the beginning of a motion picture.

This success encouraged Muybridge, while at the University of Pennsylvania, to document many other movements, both in animals and humans. Many photographic sequences of human movement, including ballet, were documented by Muybridge and published in magazines and journals and combined in the book *Animal Locomotion: An Electro-Photographic Investigation of Connective Phases of Animal Movements*. Two more books were published, including *The Human Figure in Motion*, the first extensive book exploring many human movements.[2] Over time, this foundational work was part of the slow but steady scientific investigation into human gait. Others worked on these techniques with a Frenchman, Étienne-Jules Marey, developing a technique called chronophotography, which took 12 pictures per second. Eventually Thomas Edison and

---

Neither Dr. Aiona nor any immediate family member has received anything of value from or has stock or stock options held in a commercial company or institution related directly or indirectly to the subject of this chapter.

colleagues developed the kinetograph, where photographic film was in a long linear loop and was able to be shown through a projector, the Kinetoscope. He has been named the father of motion pictures for this development.

Although descriptions of gait have appeared over the centuries, there are drawbacks to observational gait analysis alone. The single point of observation is unable to incorporate all three dimensions of movement and the rapidity of movement makes precision limited. The addition of video adds more accuracy with its ability to slow down movement, but is not anatomic and lack biomechanical analysis, the ability to measure force.

Combining technical advances and scientific interest, Braune and Fischer[3] incorporated their anatomic measurements to further elucidate the biomechanical functions of the musculoskeletal system, providing the foundation for much of the present-day modeling used in computerized gait analysis. Inman et al[4] at the University of California, San Francisco and Berkeley, with the multidisciplinary team focused research on the biomechanical aspects of gait as it related to prosthetic design, applying their research to the clinical management of WWII veterans with a limb deficiency. Lamoreux[5] developed an exoskeleton to attach to the pelvis and lower extremities with attached potentiometers to more precisely quantify kinematics during walking at various speeds on a treadmill. With the amount of manual work needed to extract and process the data significant and time consuming, it was difficult to move beyond the domain of the research community to the clinical setting.

With computer hardware and software technology advancing, the ability to perform mathematical calculations in a rapid manner held promise for the fledgling field of gait analysis and led to the development of a computerized three-dimensional (3D) gait analysis system. Combining the processing power of computers with the dense amount of data collected, the timely production of the graphs and numerical data became achievable with less human effort. The resultant increase in commercially available 3D gait analysis systems for researchers and clinicians made its clinical application a more widespread reality. Currently, a number of clinical laboratories for both the adult and pediatric population analyze human movement to improve performance and function and manage pathologic conditions.

Gait Analysis

The advantage of instrumented 3D gait analysis is its ability to define lower limb segment motion that is joint centered in three dimensions. It can provide information regarding gait symmetry; parameters such as cadence, step length, and support time; and pathologic motions. Most importantly, it can quantify force, power, and moments across joints that observational analysis is unable to provide.

Evaluation

Each motion analysis center will perform, at minimum, a clinical assessment consisting of a physical examination, 3D joint-centered kinematics, and kinetics. A technical and clinical summary with interpretation of the findings is part of the report. Additional evaluations may include electromyography, foot pressure analysis, foot kinematics, truncal motion, and oxygen consumption, although not all centers have these technical abilities. Because the focus of this chapter is gait analysis in the child with a limb deficiency, the three components of a standard assessment will be presented.

Clinical Assessment

A clinical history is obtained, with a focus on previous treatment and specifically the issue being assessed in that particular subject. A physical examination begins with a static alignment assessment of the trunk and lower extremities in a standing position with spinal alignment. Lower extremity alignment, limb length, and foot alignment with particular attention to any significant deformities or differences are assessed and documented. Dynamic assessment includes range of motion of the hip, knee, and ankle along with strength assessment. Motor control and tone assessment may also be evaluated. These important measures add valuable information in the final clinical interpretation of the gait study along with any treatment recommendations.

Kinematics

Kinematics describe the motion of lower extremity joints and limb segments, including the trunk. A set of retroreflective sphere-shaped markers are attached to anatomic points on the trunk and lower extremities specific to the proprietary motion analysis system used (**Figure 1**). Infrared cameras track the marker movement, with the frequency of data collection dependent on the rapidity of the movement of interest (**Figure 2**). The data are processed through

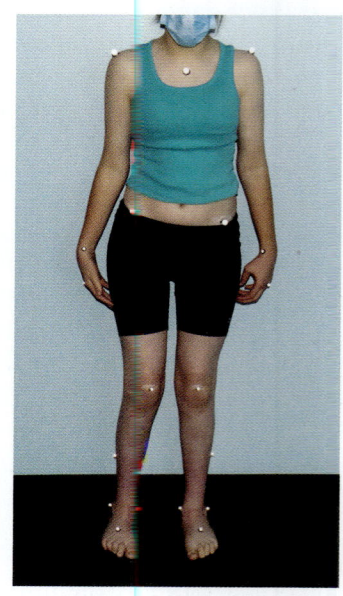

FIGURE 1 Clinical photograph showing typical retroreflective marker set on anatomic positions. (Courtesy of Motion Analysis Center, Shriners Hospital for Children, Portland, Oregon.)

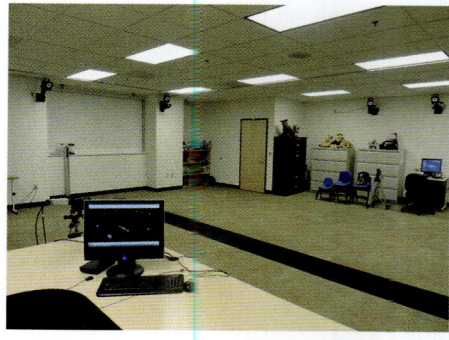

FIGURE 2 Photograph shows typical motion analysis with the walkway and cameras. (Courtesy of Motion Analysis Center, Shriners Hospital for Children, Portland, Oregon.)

proprietary algorithms to generate a graphical representation of the trunk and lower extremity segment movements in three dimensions (**Figure 3**). Most of the clinical laboratories assume the foot is a rigid segment, although some have recently developed segmental foot models.

A complete gait cycle is defined from initial foot contact until it once again contacts the ground. Stance phase, 60% of the gait cycle, is divided into components: loading response, midstance, terminal stance, and preswing. Swing phase (40%) has three components: initial, mid, and terminal swing. Each of these events has defined specific kinematic and timing components.

Walking requires power generation to move the body center of mass forward. The displacement magnitude in all three planes while moving forward determines the amount of energy required, with less excursion translating into less energy consumption. Saunders et al[6] described the major determinants of gait, which focused on movements of the pelvis and lower limb that minimized the displacement of the center of mass in normal gait, which is approximately 5° in all three planes. The greater compensatory motion at each joint to maintain this minimal excursion, the greater the energy cost as well. For example, athletes in the 110-m hurdle sprint are virtually performing leg splits to clear the hurdles

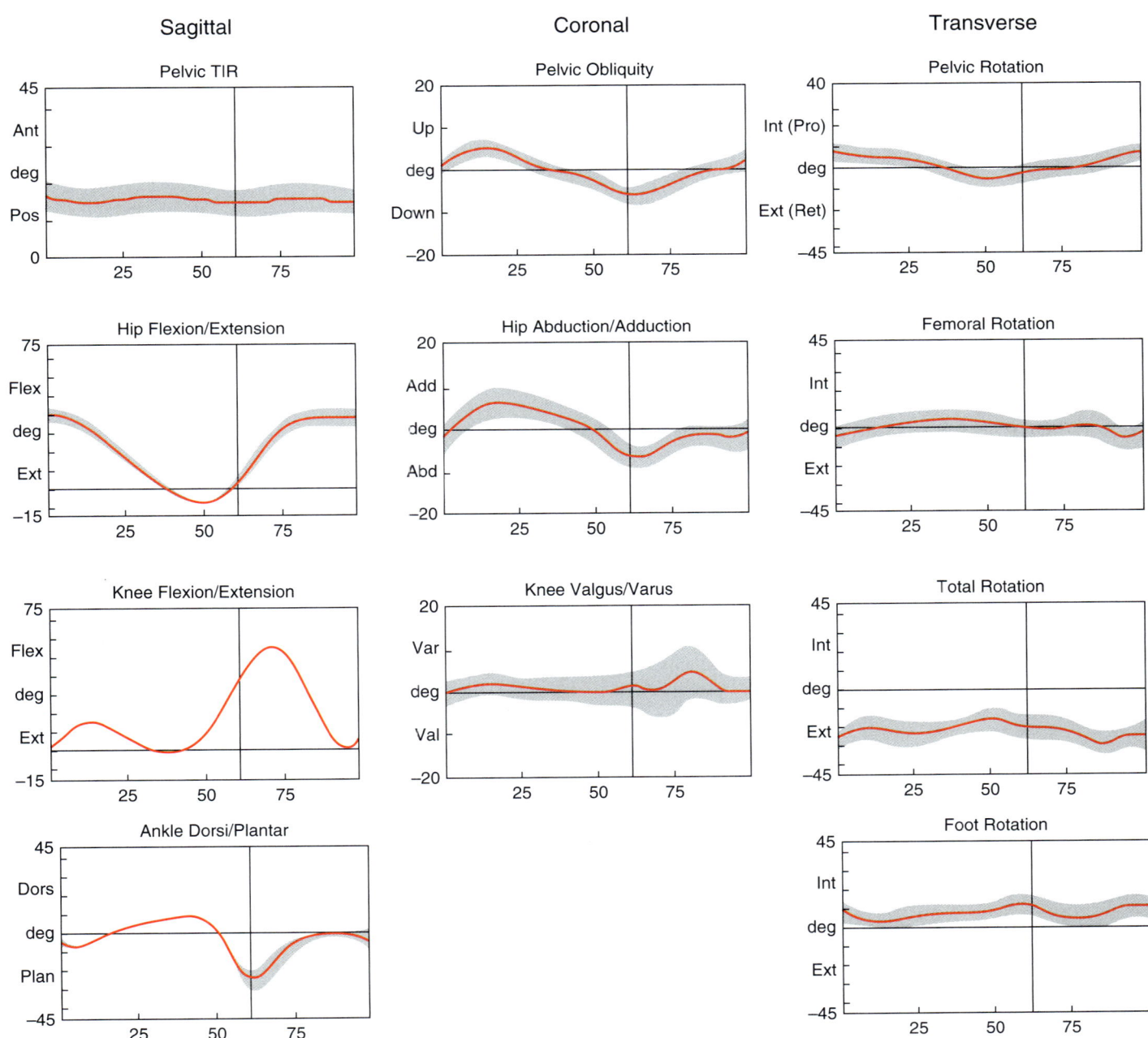

FIGURE 3 Kinematic graphs of the sagittal, coronal, and transverse planes. deg = degree, Ab = abduction, Ad = adduction, Dors = dorsiflexion, Ext = extension, Flex = flexion, Plan = plantar. (Courtesy of Motion Analysis Center, Shriners Hospital for Children, Portland, Oregon.)

rather than jumping over the hurdles to minimize the up-and-down movement of their center of mass.

Kinetics

Kinetics in gait describes the forces affecting the motion of the limbs. Maintaining an upright posture requires controlling the bending moment across each joint. Some joints such as the hip three degrees of freedom, whereas others such as the ankle are much more limited to one plane of motion. When a foot is on the ground, body weight (force) is applying a bending moment across the joints of the lower extremity. The moments at each joint can be calculated using the components of the ground reaction force (GRF), measured by force plates embedded in the walkway, the motion graphs, and anthropomorphic data. The magnitude of this moment (M) is the product of the distance (D) from the joint axis of rotation times body weight ($M = F \times D$) and can be resolved into three planes: sagittal, coronal, transverse (**Figure 4**). It is

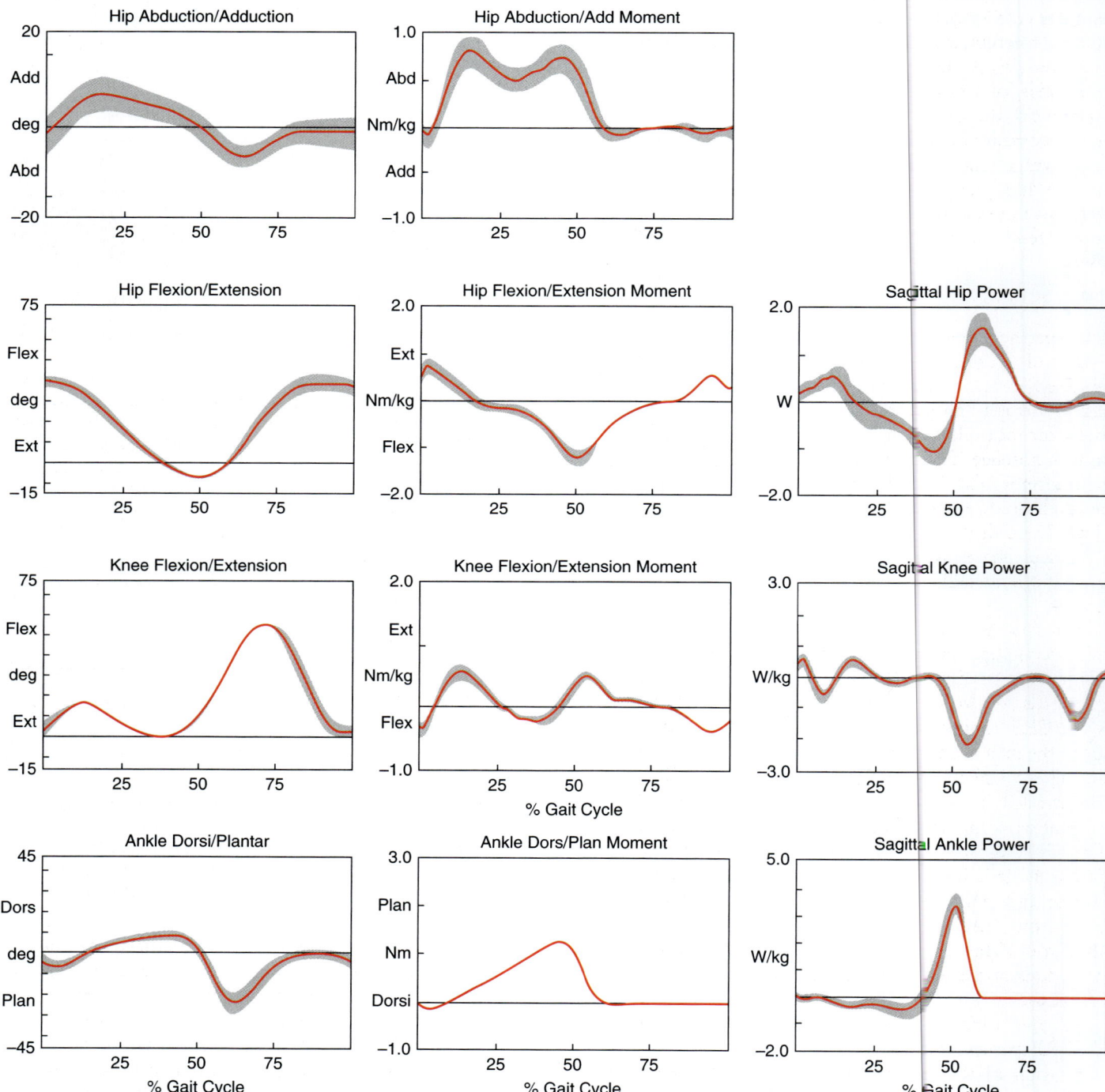

FIGURE 4 Kinetic graphs. Abd = abduction, Add = adduction, Dors = dorsiflexion, Ext = extension, Flex = flexion, Plan = planar. (Courtesy of Motion Analysis Center, Shriners Hospital for Children, Portland, Oregon.)

bending the joint into a specific direction. The body controls this movement tendency by a reactionary force generated through muscle contraction and joint stabilizing soft tissue such as ligaments. Eccentric contraction, the elongation of a muscle while contracting, controls the velocity of joint motion to ensure the coordinated smooth movement of the trunk, pelvis, and joints of the lower extremity. Most of the muscle function is eccentric in normal walking.

Power (W) is joint angular acceleration times joint moment calculated at any point of the gait cycle. Concentric muscle contraction produces most of the power at the ankle, A2 push-off and the hip, H3 pull-off. The knee generates minimal power and is under more eccentric control and absorbing power.

Ankle Rockers

One specific area of focus is the design of various prosthetic foot/ankle replacements. This component is part of virtually all prosthetic devices, except for foot fillers in those with partial foot absence. The prosthetic foot is an important modulator of force across the ankle with extension to proximal joints. Three distinct ankle movements in stance phase were described by Perry and Burnfield[7] as the three ankle rockers.

The first is ankle plantar flexion from initial heel contact to foot flat, comprising the first 15% of the gait cycle. This passive motion is produced by the GRF applied at the heel, posterior to the axis of rotation of the ankle, causing it to plantarflex. This motion is controlled by eccentric contraction of anterior compartment musculature of the tibia, mostly the tibialis anterior (**Figure 5**). It is important to note the GRF at this point is posterior to the axis of the knee, causing it to move into flexion. This must be controlled by eccentric contraction of the quadriceps (**Figure 6**).

As the tibia advances forward, the GRF passes anterior to the axis of rotation of the ankle. This causes the ankle joint to move into dorsiflexion. This second rocker is controlled by the eccentric contraction of

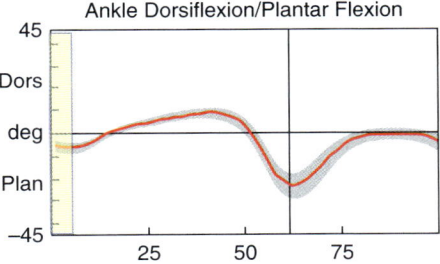

FIGURE 5 Ankle sagittal kinematic graph. The shaded area represents first ankle rocker, controlled plantar flexion of the ankle. (Courtesy of Motion Analysis Center, Shriners Hospital for Children, Portland, Oregon.)

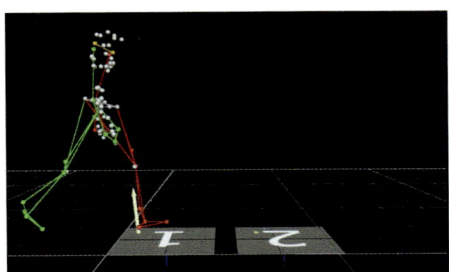

FIGURE 6 Sagittal view-whole body marker set with ground reaction force (GRF). First ankle rocker demonstrating the GRF vector represented by the arrow is posterior to the ankle axis and the knee axis. The ankle is moving into plantar flexion and the knee into flexion. (Courtesy of Motion Analysis Center, Shriners Hospital for Children, Portland, Oregon.)

the posterior calf musculature. This is energy absorbing in nature (**Figure 7**). The GRF moves anterior to the axis of the knee, causing it to move into extension (**Figure 8**). The knee is inherently stable in full extension and is assisted into this position by the movement of the GRF anteriorly, controlled by the ankle foot function.

Later in stance, the ankle now transitions from dorsiflexion to plantar flexion. This active event is push-off and represents the third rocker (**Figure 9**). This power generation by muscle concentric contraction of the gastrocnemius-soleus complex is part of the propulsive force to move the limb and body forward (**Figure 10**).

A significant amount of research is devoted to studying various designs of the prosthetic foot, focusing on replicating the three rocker functions of the ankle to varying degrees. In

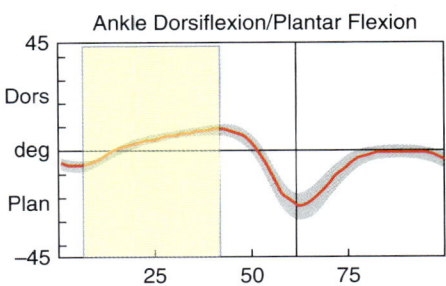

FIGURE 7 Ankle sagittal kinematic graph. The shaded area represents second ankle rocker, controlled ankle dorsiflexion. (Courtesy of Motion Analysis Center, Shriners Hospital for Children, Portland, Oregon.)

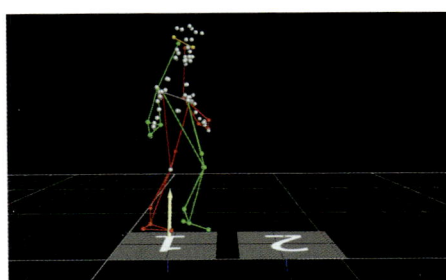

FIGURE 8 Sagittal view-whole body marker set with ground reaction force (GRF). Second ankle rocker. The GRF is anterior to the ankle axis and knee. The ankle is moving into dorsiflexion and the knee into extension. (Courtesy of Motion Analysis Center, Shriners Hospital for Children, Portland, Oregon.)

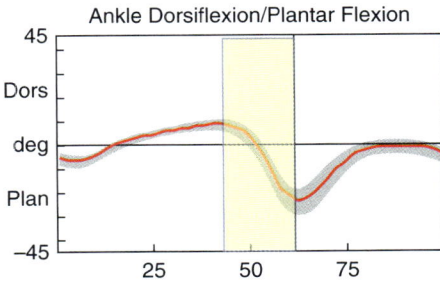

FIGURE 9 Ankle sagittal kinematic graph. The shaded area represents third ankle rocker, active plantar flexion producing power. (Courtesy of Motion Analysis Center, Shriners Hospital for Children, Portland, Oregon.)

each amputee population, the rocker of focus may vary. For example, in the more active adult with a traumatic amputation, power generation may be the focus. In contrast, in the pediatric population, with other congenital deficits, second rocker may take precedence depending on knee function and more proximal involvement as the effect of the GRF on the knee is controlled by the biomechanical characteristics of the prosthetic foot and ankle. If a child has an unstable knee in extension or hyperextends to a significant degree, a foot-ankle design that maintains the GRF posterior to the knee axis may be a consideration. If quadriceps weakness is an issue, then moving the GRF more anterior to the axis of the knee would promote passive extension of the knee and reduce quadriceps demand (**Figure 11**). This can be achieved by prosthetic design and alignment with more functional ankle plantar flexion and biomechanical characteristics of the prosthetic foot and its sagittal plane alignment.

Adult Versus Pediatric Populations With Limb Deficiency

Significantly greater use of gait analysis in the adult amputee compared with children is reflected in the literature. Unfortunately, much of this adult research does not translate to the child. Unlike the adult population where most of the limb deficiency is the result of an insult (trauma) or disease process (tumor, vascular) to an otherwise intact musculoskeletal system, the child with limb deficiency presents a unique challenge. By definition, any child with a limb deficiency has an immature musculoskeletal system, one with remaining skeletal growth and maturing muscle strength and function. As muscles provide the power for walking and physical activity, its development as the child grows will have differing effects depending on the age of the child. Changes do not occur linearly with time, with the onset of puberty a demarcating event for physical change. A 7-year-old child differs from the 14-year-old in terms of skeletal size, alignment, and muscle strength.

Etiology adds another layer of uniqueness. Most commonly congenital in origin, this diagnostic category can present with many associated findings and deficiencies. This can range from missing digits to significant abnormalities involving all three joints of the lower extremity. Secondary muscle deficiencies, as well, will affect the gait efficiency of the child. Just the absence of a foot does not define the extent of involvement of the limb. Although diagnostic categories exist, each child can present a unique clinical picture.

With traumatic causes, this is usually in an otherwise normal developing musculoskeletal system, one with more power to compensate for the loss compared with congenital causes. The trauma amputee generally has an underlying intact musculoskeletal system proximal to the amputation. This simplifies management as gait compensations can be minimized by the prosthetic design. The challenge is the greater activity level and demand of this otherwise healthy young amputee.

Research and Clinical Studies

Research

Outcome measures for optimizing function are numerous. Although described in an adult population, Fey et al[8] articulated a number of them including muscle activation, joint work, limb power, self-selected walking speed, peak moments, range of motion, kinematic symmetry, metabolic cost, and extensive patient-reported surveys in the area of prosthetic design. It is important to interpret research regarding the principal outcome measured and then determine its applicability to each clinical situation. Each measure influences each wearer differently, with some factors in conflict when determining optimal device design and choice.

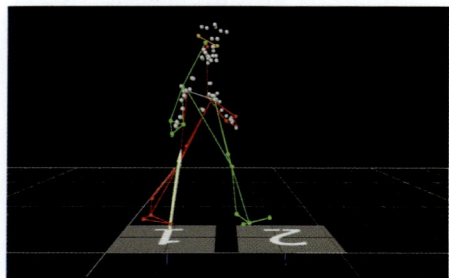

FIGURE 10 Sagittal view-whole body marker set with ground reaction force (GRF). Third ankle rocker. The GRF is on the forefoot and with the ankle motion graph moving into plantar flexion. (Courtesy of Motion Analysis Center, Shriners Hospital for Children, Portland, Oregon.)

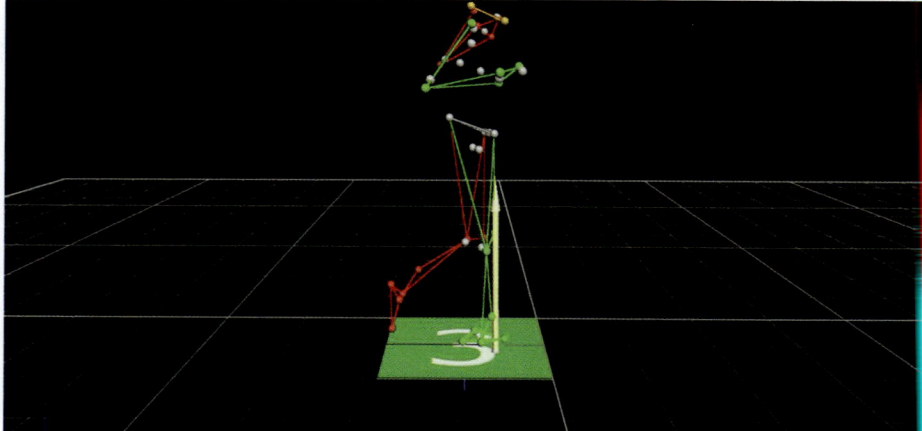

FIGURE 11 Sagittal view-whole body marker set with ground reaction force (GRF). An example of a prosthetic foot of a stiffer configuration causing the GRF to rapidly move anterior the knee axis, driving it into extension. (Courtesy of Motion Analysis Center, Shriners Hospital for Children, Portland, Oregon.)

Impact

Ashley et al[9] described the increased energy consumption and increased work needed in 56 children with amputations. Jeans et al[10] studied a heterogenous group of 73 children with varying levels of limb deficiency. Their findings noted the more proximal the level of amputation, the greater the physiologic cost, with transfemoral and hip levels having VO_2 cost of 151% to 161%. However, unlike the adult population, children with knee disarticulation and transtibial amputation actually functioned with a normal walking speed with no increase in energy cost. This demonstrates the uniqueness of the pediatric population and why translating some findings in the adult population must be done with great care.

Engsberg et al[11] studied children with transtibial amputation, noting they have increased loads on the nonprosthetic limb compared with the prosthetic side. This study contrasted the findings of Lewallen et al[12] who noted no increase in sagittal plane moments comparing intact with the amputated side. These articles point to a deficit in the literature as many studies have small sample sizes (four and six in these two studies), which may be one explanation for the different findings.

Gait symmetry has been investigated by many authors, focusing on the GRF and/or joint motion, especially relevant in the traumatic amputee with an otherwise normal musculoskeletal system. Because children have complex disorders, the goal of minimizing the compensations made both on the ipsilateral limb and the contralateral limb to achieve an efficient gait will take precedence over symmetry. What has generally been shown is the overworking of the noninvolved limb to compensate for the limb-deficient side, performing more work or taking greater impact during gait. The ipsilateral limb compensations are the more proximal joints altering their motion and force for the deficiency present.

In summary, the child with a limb deficiency has increased energy cost, as the deficiency moves anatomically more proximal. However, unlike the adult, children undergoing knee disarticulation have much better function and this should be one goal in management of some cases. The noninvolved limb does take more impact and compensations can be made by both limbs. These can be identified by gait analysis and provide some guidelines for management.

Transtibial Amputation

Research has been focused on the power generation of various prosthetic foot design, using 3D gait analysis as one measurement tool to assess it in a clinical population.

In children, studies have focused mainly on foot design. The varying stiffness and energy effects of each foot design can influence the movement of the more proximal joints. Schneider et al[13] demonstrated differences between the traditional solid ankle, cushioned heel (SACH) foot and Flex-Foot on the kinematics and kinetics in gait in 12 children. The Flex-Foot returned more energy than the SACH foot (66% versus 21%) with greater differences at higher gait speeds (70% versus 19%).

Jeans et al[14] compared gait after Syme and transtibial amputation in children. They noted the transtibial level of amputation allowed a statistical increase in ankle power generation, with varying foot designs simulating differing ankle motion. Yet no demonstrable increased patient satisfaction was noted with the high-performance foot, with many subjects preferring the lower functioning design.

McMulkin et al[15] performed a comparative study of three prosthetic feet in a group of 16 children with a transtibial amputation level. The feet included two multiaxial designs and an energy-storing nonarticulated design. Although the more sophisticated design demonstrated greater ankle peak power generation with increased motion, the subjective preferences were equally distributed with the apparent biomechanical advantage not universally preferred.

Colborne et al[16] studied children with transtibial amputations, comparing the SACH and Seattle foot designs. They found the Seattle foot design had small increases in stride length and velocity, with less resistance to midstance dorsiflexion. Their gait analysis findings demonstrated a persistent knee flexor moment with the SACH foot, whereas the Seattle foot allowed a more normal knee extensor moment.

Zernicke et al[17] noted differences in knee moments dependent on the prosthetic foot with the SACH foot producing a flexor moment at the knee with a CAPP (Child Amputee Prosthetic Project) foot maintaining the center of pressure more on the forefoot that may enhance stability of the knee in five children with a prosthetic knee.

In summary, the prosthetic foot design affects the point of application of the GRF and regulates its position on the proximal joints. All three ankle rockers affect knee function. A stiffer prosthetic foot that limits dorsiflexion function may keep the GRF anterior to the axis of the knee and provide an extending force to the knee. In some children, an anterior cruciate ligament deficiency may require maintaining some knee flexion to maintain stability, whereas in others, weak muscular function may need compensation by maintaining passive knee extension, which may be inherently more stable. Last, the A2 power generation has been the focus of many prosthetic foot designs. However, in children, although some technical advantages are demonstrated, personal preference is not fully influenced by this parameter. Because prosthetic devices have properties based on mechanical design and material characteristics, applying this to a growing immature musculoskeletal system in children with differing physical demands and desires at varying ages presents a unique challenge.

Transfemoral Amputation

Goldberg et al[18] compared the use of cadaver anthropomorphic norms versus actual measurement of the residual limb and prosthesis when performing estimates of moments in the pediatric population. Although differences at the hip and knee in stance phase were not found, the inertial couple in swing demonstrated differences at those joints. Their recommendation was to use direct measurements if swing phase kinetics are relevant. Dumas et al[19] published similar concerns in the adult population with transfemoral amputations. These studies demonstrate the challenges in the pediatric population, with the varying morphology of each child at varying ages.

Bell et al[19] described gait changes in adults with transfemoral amputations. Because of anatomic muscle attachments, the loss of adductor function in more proximal amputations resulted in greater abductor drift and greater difficulty with mechanical and anatomic alignment. They emphasized the need to maintain as much femoral length for function. This needs to be kept in mind when treating the pediatric patient as options for residual segment length are present. Jeans et al[14] noted patients with knee disarticulation have better energy efficiency compared with patients with transfemoral deficiency as residual length is presumably greater.

Geil et al[21,22] challenged the traditional teaching of initial treatment of the child with congenital transfemoral deficiency with a nonarticulated knee prosthesis, transitioning to an articulated one as the child matured. An early knee protocol was initiated, with initial prosthetic fitting having an articulated knee, used as the child crawled and then stood during normal development. Using gait analysis, patients in whom an early knee protocol was used demonstrated greater knee flexion and fewer adaptations than those in the traditional management protocol.

Controlling the mechanical knee is a challenge in prosthetic design. Andrysek et al[23] described their research into designs specifically in the pediatric population and its challenges. No specific device is recommended, just the challenges of creating a variable friction mechanism as the acceleration/deceleration of the knee varies with both speed and phase of gait.

In summary, a knee disarticulation or femoral segment of greatest length provides the greatest function for a child with limb deficiency. The management at an early age should consider the implication of an articulated knee sooner than traditionally, although this requires the coordination with the physical therapy, prosthetist, and orthopaedic surgeon.

Clinical Study

Although proximal femoral focal deficiency is a distinct clinical entity, it manifests with varying degrees of femoral length and associated anomalies. This broad clinical variation influences treatment options, which can vary from amputation to extensive reconstructive procedures. As the adult literature clearly demonstrates the advantages of a biologic knee to a mechanical one, the treatment goal in children is to create some sort of biologic knee when retention of the existing one is not an option. Rotationplasty, a unique surgical procedure, converts the ankle joint into a biologic knee joint with the foot becoming the transtibial lever arm. The outcomes of this procedure have been investigated using gait analysis.

Fowler et al[24] found advantages of rotationplasty over Syme amputation and prosthetic management. They noted significant improved gait kinematics in the nine patients treated with rotationplasty with less stance phase vaulting and more importantly, less abnormal nonprosthetic limb kinetic abnormalities such as excessive hip power absorption/generation and knee power generation at varying speeds. Fuchs et al[25] described the advantages of the biologic knee of the rotationplasty compared with the prosthetic knee with closer-to-normal kinematics and superior knee motion with a resulting more coordinated gait pattern.

Benedetti et al[26] published their review of 16 patients with rotationplasty with noted decreased knee GRF of 6% and an increase of knee range of motion of 25°. They noted the importance of knee height as an average difference of 5.8% resulting in pseudoknee flexion.

In contrast, Floccari et al[27] compared three management groups in this population: an equinus prosthesis alone, rotationplasty, and those with ankle disarticulation and transfemoral prosthesis. All required up to 170% more energy. Many gait deviations were noted with knee motion significantly different and with the prosthetic knee having greater motion. Functional scores, including patient happiness, did not differ among the group. In their conclusions, the authors noted their findings contradict previous studies regarding the advantages of rotationplasty in this diagnostic category.

In summary, these studies compared management differences with outcomes such as gait and satisfaction. In this uncommon condition, the variation in clinical presentation and treatment present challenges in comparative outcomes research. As age adds a significant variable, so does the choice of outcome to be evaluated. It may explain the conflicting results noted with rotationplasty compared with other management schemes including amputation. With technologic advances, the comparisons of a mechanical versus a nonideal biologic knee will become even more challenging. An important finding is the need to make the thigh segment as equal to the contralateral side as possible, seemingly less than approximately a 5% difference. This should be addressed as the child grows, as options are greater than when an adult.

Role of Gait Analysis in Clinical Practice

Gait analysis in the pediatric population is not as extensive as in the adult population because the number of studies is quite small in comparison. However, the information provides a guide for the role of gait analysis in the clinical setting for an individual subject. Gait and function are most affected by limb-length inequality, alignment, joint stability, and power generation (muscle component). The ability to objectively produce kinematic and kinetic parameters will provide additional important information to guide management decisions. It is important to be aware of prosthetic findings, but also the effect on the intact limb. Significant deviations can be identified and recommendations can be made including therapy, prosthetic redesign, or surgical management. The difficulty is deciding what specific outcome is desired and how it applies to actual daily life outside the laboratory.

As gait analysis is equipment intense and not portable, the evaluation occurs in a laboratory setting. It requires space, control of vibration, specialized technically trained personnel, and controlled lighting. It generally can only evaluate walking because only a few laboratories are able to perform running evaluations.

Wearable sensors will provide some of that additional information if they can be validated for use in the pediatric population. Inertial motion units, a combination of accelerometer and gyroscopic devices, are being used as devices that can be worn by the individual and generate data without the need for a camera system. Their continued miniaturization allows attachment to the lower extremity, collecting data such as number of steps, step and stride length, and velocity. Symmetry can be measured as well. These devices are ideal for measuring daily activity and function. Insole pressure-sensitive devices placed into shoes can map foot pressures during walking, but then correlation to joint motion is still being developed. Accurate segment motion and incorporation of force in the actual living environment is still challenging but necessary for translation of prosthetic research to the actual patient. Poitras et al[28] reviewed the literature and presented the challenges on validating inertial motion unit precision in the laboratory and its use in the clinical setting.

SUMMARY

Since ancient times, gait has been observed and analyzed. Advances in technology has taken the observation component to one of greater accuracy. Two specific technologic advances, laboratory-based 3D gait analysis and community-based activity as measured by inertial motion units, complementary in data provision, will advance care for the child with a limb deficiency along with improved mechanical design. Their incorporation into the clinical setting is still a challenge but should be considered an important component that provides objective information that can assist the multidisciplinary team in their treatment of the child with a limb deficiency.

References

1. Muybridge E: *Animal Locomotion*. J.B. Lippincott, 1888.
2. Muybridge E: *The Human Figure in Motion*. Dover Publications, 1955.
3. Braune W, Fischer O: *The Human Gait*. Springer Science and Business Media, 2012.
4. Inman VT, Ralston HJ, Todd F: *Human Walking*. Williams and Wilkins, 1981.
5. Lamoreux LW: Kinematic measurements in the study of human walking. *Bul Prosthet Res* 1971;10(15):3-84.
6. Saunders JB, Inman VT, Eberhart HD: The major determinants in normal and pathological gait. *J Bone Joint Surg Am* 1953;35-A(3):543-558.
7. Perry J, Burnfield J: *Gait Analysis: Normal and Pathologic Function*. Slack Incorporated, 1994.
8. Fey NP, Klute GK, Neptune R: The influence of energy storage and return foot stiffness on walking mechanics and muscle activity in below-knee amputees. *Clin Biomech (Bristol, Avon)* 2011;26(10):1025-1032.
9. Ashley RK, Vallier GT, Skinner SR: Gait analysis in pediatric lower extremity amputees. *Orthop Rev* 1992;21(6):745-749.
10. Jeans KA, Browne RH, Karol L: A effect of amputation level on energy expenditure during overground walking by children with an amputation. *J Bone Joint Surg Am* 2011;93(1):49-56.
11. Engsberg JR, Lee AG, Patterson JL, Harder JA: External loading comparisons between able-bodied and below-knee-amputee children during walking. *Arch Phys Med Rehabil* 1991;72(9):657-661.
12. Lewallen R, Dyck G, Quandury A, Ross K, Letts M: Gait kinematics in below-knee child amputees: A force plate analysis. *J Pediatr Orthop* 1986;6(3):291-298.
13. Schneider K, Hart T, Zernicke RF, Setoguchi Y, Oppenheim W: Dynamics of below-knee child amputee gait: SACH foot versus Flex foot. *J Biomech* 1993;26(10):1191-1204.
14. Jeans KA, Karol LA, Cummings D, Singhal K: The comparison of gait after syme and transtibial amputation in children: Factors that may play a role in function. *J Bone Joint Surg Am* 2014;96(19):1641-1647.
15. McMulkin ML, Osebold WR, Mildes RD, Rosenquist RS: Comparison of three pediatric prosthetic feet during functional activities. *JPO J Prosthetics Orthot* 2004;16(3):78-84.
16. Colborne GR, Naumann S, Longmuir PE, Berbrayer D: Analysis of mechanical and metabolic factors in the gait of congenital below knee amputees. A comparison of the SACH and Seattle feet. *Am J Phys Med Rehabil* 1992;71(5):272-278.
17. Zernicke RF, Hoy MG, Whiting WC: Ground reaction forces and center of pressure patterns in the gait of children with amputation: Preliminary report. *Arch Phys Med Rehabil* 1985;66(11):736-741.
18. Goldberg EJ, Requejo PS, Fowler EG: The effect of direct measurement versus cadaver estimates of anthropometry in the calculation of joint moments during above-knee prosthetic gait in pediatrics. *J Biomech* 2008;41(3):695-700.
19. Dumas R, Brånemark R, Frossard L: Gait analysis of transfemoral amputees: Errors in inverse dynamics are substantial and depend on prosthetic design. *IEEE Trans Neural Syst Rehabil Eng* 2017;25(6):679-685.
20. Bell JC, Wolf EJ, Schnall BL, Tis JE, Tis LL, Benjamin KP: Transfemoral amputations: The effect of residual limb length and orientation on gait analysis outcome measures. *J Bone Joint Surg Am* 2013;95(5):408-414.
21. Geil MD, Safaeepour Z, Giavedoni B, Coulter CP: Walking kinematics in young children with limb loss using early versus traditional prosthetic knee prescription protocols. *PLoS One* 2020;15(4):e0231401.
22. Geil MD, Coulter CP: Analysis of locomotor adaptations in young children with limb loss in an early prosthetic knee prescription protocol. *Prosthet Orthot Int* 2014;38(1):54-61.
23. Andrysek J, García D, Rozbaczylo C, et al: Biomechanical responses of young adults with unilateral transfemoral amputation using two types of mechanical stance control prosthetic knee joints. *Prosthet Orthot Int* 2020;44(5):314-322.
24. Fowler EG, Hester DM, Oppenheim WL, Setoguchi Y, Zernicke RF: Contrasts in gait mechanics of individuals with proximal femoral focal deficiency: Syme amputation versus Van Nes rotational osteotomy. *J Pediatr Orthop* 1999;19(6):720-731.
25. Fuchs B, Kotajarvi BR, Kaufman KR, Sim FH: Functional outcome of patients with rotationplasty about the knee. *Clin Orthop Relat Res* 2003;415:52-58.

26. Benedetti MG, Okita Y, Recubini E, Mariani E, Leardini A, Manfrini M: How much clinical and functional impairment do children treated with knee rotationplasty experience in adulthood? *Clin Orthop Relat Res* 2016;474(4):995-1004.

27. Floccari LV, Jeans KA, Herring JA, Johnston CE, Karol LA: Comparison of outcomes by reconstructive strategy in patients with prostheses for proximal femoral focal deficiency. *J Bone Joint Surg Am* 2021;103(19):1817-1825.

28. Poitras I, Dupuis F, Bielmann M, et al: Validity and reliability of wearable sensors for joint angle estimation: A systematic review. *Sensors (Basel)* 2019;19(7):1555.

Psychological, Social, and Socioeconomic Aspects of Limb Deficiencies

CHAPTER 63

Catherine B. McClellan, PhD

ABSTRACT

It is important to outline the psychological, social, and socioeconomic variables affecting the lives of children with limb deficiencies along with health-related quality of life for youth with limb deficiency and other psychosocial factors, including body image, prosthesis use, and participation in leisure and social activities. The social dynamics and socioeconomic status for the pediatric limb deficiency population play a prominent role. Caregiver/parent support, surgical support, and behavioral interventions for youth with limb deficiency should be considered, along with developmental tasks and caregiver expectations for the pediatric limb deficiency population. Health care clinicians can support children and families by setting developmentally appropriate expectations for parents and youth, connecting families of youth with limb deficiency, and helping to prepare youth for unwanted/unexpected attention and unique social dynamics.

Keywords: health-related quality of life; parent support; pediatric limb differences; psychosocial; socioeconomic

Introduction

Youth with pediatric limb deficiencies represent a heterogeneous population with a broad range of presentations. High levels of resiliency and overwhelmingly positive adjustment unite this population.[1,2] Health care professionals caring for the pediatric limb deficiency population have the privilege and challenge of working with patients and their families during the most dynamic phase of human development. Working with patients with pediatric limb deficiency can be intensely rewarding for those who provide their care. These youth are able to interact meaningfully with their medical care clinicians and can be models of the human ability to adapt and grow to meet challenges.

Pediatric patients with limb deficiency differ considerably from adults with limb deficiency, with the pediatric population demonstrating higher functioning in psychological, social, and other domains. Health care clinicians working with children with limb deficiency benefit from an understanding of the developmental, psychological, social, and socioeconomic influences on the lives of their patients. This knowledge can improve the collaborative efforts of multidisciplinary medical teams, parents, and patients as they plan for future orthopaedic care.

The psychosocial well-being of youth with limb deficiency is imperative and also includes psychological adjustment, including social, emotional, academic, and overall well-being. It is important to review the socioeconomic influences of and developmental considerations for youth with limb deficiency. There are several ways the health care clinicians and parents can promote positive identity, social skills development, and graduated independence in health care behaviors.

Psychological Functioning

Although the phrase "children are not small adults" applies to most medical fields, the phrase "child amputees are not adult amputees" rings especially true. There are considerable differences between the adults and children with limb deficiency, including etiology of the limb difference, global health status, developmental processes, comorbid mental health concerns, and psychosocial functioning.[3,4] Adults have higher rates of acquired amputation secondary to trauma and/or disease processes, with lower limb deficiency typically associated with disease process and upper limb deficiency with traumatic injuries.[3] Adults with upper limb deficiency, especially females and those from certain ethnic groups, experience high rates of mental health concerns, including 50% higher rates of posttraumatic stress disorder and depression symptoms.[4]

Whereas adult limb deficiency is most often associated with acquired amputation secondary to trauma and chronic illness, the pediatric limb deficiency population has a 3:1 ratio of congenital to acquired limb deficiency. Congenital limb differences occur in 1

Neither Dr. McClellan nor any immediate family member has received anything of value from or has stock or stock options held in a commercial company or institution related directly or indirectly to the subject of this chapter.

of every 1,943 births, with higher rates of upper limb deficiency relative to lower limb deficiency.[5] Acquired pediatric amputations occur at an average age of 6 years and are more common in males (3:1 male to female ratio), with finger and toe amputations comprising most (93%) acquired pediatric amputations.[6] Acquired amputations can also occur secondary to surgical conversions of a congenital limb deficiency. From a psychological perspective, higher rates of congenital relative to acquired limb deficiency may translate into lower rates of trauma sequelae and emotional and social adjustment for the pediatric limb deficiency population. However, approximately 75% of acquired pediatric limb deficiencies are secondary to trauma,[5,7] and the experience of having a limb deficiency and a visible body difference, at a minimum, presents unique challenges to patients and their families.

Just as the origin of the limb deficiency (congenital versus acquired) can result in different lived experiences, the location and severity of limb deficiency can also affect the daily lives of children in different ways. Youth with upper limb deficiency may face challenges completing tasks of daily living, differences in nonverbal communication, and in the expression of physical affection. Persons with upper limb deficiency may try to conceal their difference, and the interpersonal effect of their limb deficiency is more likely to occur within their closer and more intimate relationships. In contrast, youth with lower limb deficiency may be less able to keep up with their peers in walking and athletics, potentially limiting their participation in certain social activities. Persons with lower limb deficiency are less able to conceal their difference, resulting in greater public attention; however, lower limb deficiency has less of an effect on closer interpersonal relationships.

As noted previously, the psychological health and peer relationships of youth with limb deficiency are generally comparable with those of the normative population.[8] Importantly, qualitative research evaluating the experiences of youth with limb deficiency across three countries (Canada, Ethiopia, and India) reveals that most youth endorse some feelings of distress surrounding their limb deficiency, with worries about how their limb deficiency may affect their future employment opportunities, feeling different from their peers, and frustrated with feeling left out of social and sports activities. Coping strategies as well as emotional and instrumental support mediated the effect of limb deficiency on youth perceptions of themselves.

Feelings of "being different" for youth with limb deficiency are aggravated by frequent encounters of unwanted attention or focus on their limb deficiency, reportedly one of the more psychologically troublesome experiences of youth with visible physical differences.[9] Importantly, the degree to which a youth is bothered by this unwanted attention appears to moderate the effect of this attention on feelings of well-being.[9] Specifically, youth who are able to tolerate unwanted attention without feeling emotionally activated demonstrate greater resilience and improved well-being relative to those who are very bothered by this unwanted attention. The psychological functioning of youth with limb deficiency is complex and mediated by many variables, including internal resources, modeling of responses by caregivers, access to supportive resources, and limb deficiency–specific features, such as the degree to which their limb deficiency restricts access to typical developmental experiences and rites of passage.

Health-Related Quality of Life

Health-related quality of life (HR-QOL) has emerged as an outcomes tool to assess the effect of a health condition on global and specific (eg, emotional, social, school, physical) aspects of functioning. Self-report is the gold standard of HR-QOL; however, pediatric HR-QOL inventories typically include both self- and parent-reported ratings. HR-QOL in adult amputees is affected by age and degree of functional impairment,[10] adjustment to amputation and use of artificial limb,[11] and level of education, back pain, and phantom limb pain.[12]

As a whole, the HR-QOL of the pediatric limb deficiency population is comparable with that of the general population; however, some differences exist.[13,14] The self- and parent-reported HR-QOL of youth with unilateral upper limb deficiency are comparable with those of the healthy control population;[14] however, youth with lower and/or multiple congenital limb deficiency rated their physical and social HR-QOL lower than those of the general population.[16] Lower HR-QOL scores for youth with lower limb deficiency, relative to upper limb deficiency, may be attributable to the reduced participation in social and athletic activities secondary to accessibility, pain, and mobility. Importantly, when compared with other chronic health conditions, the parent report and self-report for youth with congenital limb deficiency are significantly higher than those of their peers with chronic health conditions (eg, diabetes, asthma, epilepsy), regardless of sex, age, or the type, severity, or site of the limb deficiency.[9]

Sex also appears to play a role in the HR-QOL of the pediatric limb deficiency population. Girls and young women with limb deficiency endorse greater social stigma and social concerns relative to boys and young men.[1] The site of limb deficiency and number of limb deficiencies more often affect the HR-QOL of females relative to males. Specifically, females with bilateral limb deficiency and/or lower limb deficiency experience less social inclusion, lower emotional health, and higher levels of physical impairment relative to males with unilateral or bilateral lower limb deficiency.[9]

In addition to sex and site/number of amputations, there is evidence that parents of youth with limb deficiency view their child's HR-QOL in a more negative light than do the youth themselves. For example, parent ratings of school functioning for all youth with congenital limb deficiency were significantly lower than those of the general population.[16] The discrepancy between parent and patient-reported HR-QOL is not unique to the limb deficiency population. Although parents of physically healthy children typically overestimate their child's HR-QOL, parents of youth with health conditions typically underestimate their child's HR-QOL.[17] The discrepancies between parent-proxy and youth self-report appear to be especially large in domains of emotional well-being.[18]

Lower parent-reported HR-QOL, relative to youth self-report, may reflect underlying parental fears or concerns about their child's ability to perform as well as their same-age peers. In work examining the HR-QOL of youth with congenital lower limb deficiency, an age by reporter difference emerged. Specifically, parent ratings of younger children's (8 to 11 years) HR-QOL in areas of autonomy, mood/emotions, and self-perception were significantly lower than child self-report.[13] In contrast, parent and youth self-report for older children (12 to 18 years) did not reveal significant differences in perceptions of HR-QOL. For many parents, concerns about their child with limb deficiency are not fully assuaged until the child can demonstrate their ability to meet age-expected milestones.

The HR-QOL for youth with limb deficiency is indeed strong, both compared with their physically typical peers and when compared with youth with other chronic medical conditions. Although youth with upper limb amputations, as a whole, are comparable with youth without amputations, there is evidence that girls experience greater social stigma and concerns relative to boys.[1] Youth with lower limb deficiency appear to face greater challenges in areas of social and physical HR-QOL relative to their peers with upper limb deficiency. Of particular note are the discrepancies between self and parent ratings in areas of social, academic, and physical HR-QOL, which suggests that parents may anticipate greater struggles with HR-QOL than the children themselves experience.

Participation

Research investigating the HR-QOL of youth with limb deficiency provides both global and specific information on a variety of functions. Examining participation rates in recreational and leisure activities provides additional insight into possible reasons for lower HR-QOL. According to the World Health Organization (2001), participation in recreation and leisure activities provides another way to capture the general well-being and health status of youth and adults. Participation in structured and unstructured activities contributes to the development of physical and social skills, builds confidence, improves communication, and can serve as a buffer to adverse childhood events.[19,20]

Participation in recreational, social, skill-based, physical, and self-improvement activities does not differ for youth with congenital lower limb deficiency, relative to same-age peers without limb deficiency.[13] However, adolescents with limb deficiency had less diversity in activities and lower frequency of participation in social and skill-based activities. Future work should clarify the factors driving these lower participation rates. Other work has shown that youth with lower or multiple limb deficiency, relative to those with upper unilateral limb deficiency, have higher rates of school absences, lower participation in physical education, and higher rates of pain.[16] Youth with lower limb deficiency face greater functional impairments secondary to difficulties with walking and pain, leaving them less able to participate in physical education.

Prosthesis Use

Prosthesis use and availability directly affect the range and degree of participation in certain activities. Adult amputees who are able to use a prosthesis enjoy positive outcomes, including decreased phantom limb pain and improved mental health, HR-QOL, and employment.[21,22] Prosthesis use for adults is affected by several socioeconomic variables including geography, race/ethnicity, access to inpatient rehabilitation facility, and funding for prostheses with the lifetime-estimated costs of prostheses far exceeding insurance coverage.[23]

In the pediatric population, prosthesis use can offer gains in functionality and social acceptance, and many parents seek out early use of a prosthesis to maximize their child's function.[24] Benefits of prosthesis wear appear to vary depending on the reason or goal of wearing the prosthesis, with youth preferring prostheses designed for specific tasks relative to those for general use, which were noted to be heavy and more of a hindrance than a help.[25] In the United Kingdom, the importance of sports participation in the lives of children resulted in funding for sports prostheses for all youth with acquired or congenital limb deficiency who would benefit from a prosthesis to engage in sport.[26] Prostheses can also be a means of reducing unwanted attention.[24] Work examining prosthesis use for youth with transradial limb deficiency revealed cosmesis to be one of the primary reasons for wearing a prosthesis.[27]

At the same time, the functional abilities of youth with transradial limb deficiency appear to be equivalent for prosthesis wearers relative to nonwearers. These youth also enjoyed similar or higher HR-QOL scores relative to their peers, regardless of their use of a prosthesis.[2] Other work has revealed possible nuanced differences between these two groups, with nonwearers being less likely to desire normal limbs and more likely to face questions from others who are more readily able to notice the limb deficiency.[24]

Body Image and Self-Perception

As noted previously, prosthesis use in youth with limb deficiency can be more about self-perception and body image than functionality, especially for youth with upper limb deficiency. Body image is also linked to the psychological well-being of youth with limb deficiency.[14] The awareness of and focus on body image, which includes a person's attitudes and perception of their own body, peaks in the adolescent phase of development.[28] Body image is an important predictor of psychological functioning in adolescents, especially as it affects peer relationships and dynamics.[29] Regardless of sex, lower levels of body satisfaction correlate with lower HR-QOL in adolescent amputees.[9]

Work evaluating self-reported body image in adolescents with limb deficiency reveals differences in youth with congenital relative to acquired limb deficiency. Body image for youth with congenital limb deficiency was similar to the standardization sample; however, youth with acquired amputation had greater rates of body image dissatisfaction.[14] Similar to other work, body image significantly correlated with psychological adjustment.

Body image reflects specific, as opposed to global, aspects of self-perception. The self-perception of youth with limb deficiency varies both between and within youth with limb deficiency. Youth describe mixed feelings surrounding their limb deficiency, with very few endorsing exclusively positive or negative feelings about their limb deficiency. As children age, they are more accepting and less ashamed of their limb difference, and many youth are proud of their ability to overcome and accept their difference.[24]

Social Dynamics

Social dynamics and perceived social support play an important role in the lives of youth with limb deficiency. Children and adolescents spend most of their days in school, and this is where most of their social dynamics occur. The social environment of the school setting, which includes dynamics with teachers, classmates, and friends, is the strongest predictor of emotional and psychological functioning.[30]

Bullying represents a significant threat to the social environment of youth. Over the past 2 decades, there has been an increased focus on the immediate and longer term effects of bullying on the well-being of youth. Youth with disabilities face a disproportionate degree of bullying relative to their physically able peers.[31] Within the pediatric orthopaedic population, approximately 39% endorse moderate to severe bullying experiences, which is higher than the general population (20% to 35%).[32] Individuals with foot deformity experienced significantly higher rates of moderate to severe bullying (80%) than their peers with other orthopaedic conditions, including youth with multiple orthopaedic diagnosis (55%), chronic pain (39%), fracture/acute injury (37%), and scoliosis (33%).

Romantic Relationships

Romantic relationships and the desire for intimacy are a hallmark of adolescence and an important variable in personal development and global well-being.[33] By the age of 17 years, most adolescents have had at least one romantic relationship, with 70% of youth surveyed reporting having experienced a romantic relationship within the previous 18 months.[34] For persons with limb deficiency, body image concerns, social stigma, and participation in social rituals (such as school dances or sporting events) can complicate romantic relationships. In the adult literature, persons with limb deficiency share the same interest and desire for intimacy as individuals without physical disabilities, yet are often viewed by society as being asexual, or unattractive.[35] Adults with acquired amputations express increases in body image concerns and difficulties reestablishing their sexual identity postamputation.[35] There is a paucity of research examining how pediatric congenital or acquired amputations affect the development of romantic relationships and sexuality of youth with limb deficiency. However, literature exploring adolescent romantic interests and sexual experience indicates that youth with physical disabilities are generally as sexually experienced as their nondisabled peers, with the exception being youth with severe physical disabilities.[36] There is a need for longitudinal research to understand the nuanced ways in which limb deficiency affects adolescent sexual identities, self-perceptions of sexual attractiveness, and satisfaction with their romantic relationships.

Socioeconomic Status

Socioeconomic status (SES) refers to the social standing or class of an individual or group, typically measuring a combination of education, income, and occupation (American Psychological Association). SES is a strong predictor of physical and mental health, with lower SES youth suffering higher levels of mood disorder, substance use, and suicide attempts.

Much of the work investigating the connections between SES and limb deficiency has focused on adults who undergo amputation during their adult years. There are no available studies comparing the SES of large cohorts of adults who experienced pediatric acquired limb deficiency with that of the general population. However, researchers have compared educational and employment outcomes for pediatric cancer survivors treated with amputation with those treated with limb-sparing and nonsurgical intervention.[37] Participants with upper limb deficiency were less likely to graduate college, with a 63% nongraduation rate compared with the 47% nongraduation rate of those with lower limb deficiency, and a 37% rate for the limb-sparing/nonsurgical group. Rates of unemployment mirrored those of educational attainment, with highest unemployment rates for adults with upper limb deficiency (20%), followed by those with lower limb deficiency (approximately 15%) and those who had nonsurgical (10%) or limb-sparing treatment (9%). Low income (<$20,000 per year) was highest in the amputation group (37% to 35%); however rates of low income were also high for the nonsurgical (27%) and limb-sparing (25%) groups. Although this research contributes to the understanding of the adult SES of pediatric cancer survivors, it is important to note that this research only included outcomes for pediatric cancer survivors treated in 1970 to 1986. Given the improvements in pediatric oncology since that time, current-day outcomes may be more positive.

The outcomes for adults with congenital limb deficiency, relative to persons who experienced acquired amputation in childhood, appear to be more positive. Adults with congenital limb deficiency have normative life experiences that are comparable with those adults without limb deficiency, including rates of marriage, becoming a parent, unemployment status, and active participation in healthy adult activities.[38,39] The education levels of persons with congenital limb deficiency were higher than those of the general population, suggesting that persons with congenital limb deficiency may pursue careers that require higher education and that are less dependent on their physical functioning. Although full-time employment was lower than that of the general population, adults with congenital limb deficiency enjoyed higher rates of full-time employment relative to persons with acquired amputations in adulthood. Researchers did find that adults with congenital limb deficiency were more likely to receive disability pension and more likely to retire early, frequently because of chronic pain. Importantly, participants in these studies were from countries that enjoy universal health insurance with fewer financial restrictions on their ability to access prosthetic care, receive inpatient rehabilitation, and multidisciplinary care relative to those without access to these resources. Additionally, persons with unilateral upper limb deficiency were overrepresented in this work, with authors suggesting that these outcomes do not necessarily reflect those of the entire congenital limb deficiency population.

Unlike adults with limb deficiency, youth with limb deficiency are in phases of rapid physical growth, resulting in a greater total number of prostheses across the lifespan. Depending on the age at amputation and the site of amputation, youth who use prostheses average 6 to 22 prosthetic devices before they reach age 18 years.[40] Prosthetic and repair costs from time of injury to age 18 years can range from $66,000 to $216,000 per single lower limb amputation. These costs do not include the indirect cost of care for the patient and family. For example, time away from work and school for medical appointments can be difficult to achieve for families, especially families who live a long distance from where they receive their medical care. Time away from work resulting in decreased income can be especially challenging for lower income families.

Given the considerable financial and time demands that can be part of caring for a youth with limb deficiency, it is not surprising to find that SES affects the experiences of youth with limb deficiency. For example, family income has been shown to play a role in the lives of youth with limb deficiency, such that lower family income and lower body image correlated with lower quality of life.[14] Importantly, there is evidence that lower SES correlated with higher rates of birth defects, including congenital limb deficiency.[41] In the pediatric limb deficiency population, Alaskan Natives/Native Americans, populations that have historically experienced disparities in health care and lower SES, are disproportionately represented for congenital limb deficiency.[42]

Critique of the Literature

Research on the psychosocial functioning of youth with limb deficiency is not without its limitations. The pediatric limb deficiency population is highly diverse and includes a broad range of presentations. For example, sample populations of youth with limb deficiency can include youth with mild limb deficiencies, such as a missing digit, along with youth who have multiple limb deficiencies. However, because limb deficiencies are relatively rare, it can be challenging to obtain large-enough sample sizes to make meaningful comparisons between groups of persons with limb deficiency. The context and supports available for youth with limb deficiency may also affect psychosocial outcomes, limiting the generalization of results. For example, the outcomes of youth living in countries with universal health insurance and ready access to multidisciplinary medical teams may not be generalized to youth living in impoverished countries. Research in the pediatric limb deficiency population would also benefit from greater use of objective rating scales, especially when discrepancies are noted between parent-reported and self-reported outcome, such as HR-QOL. For example, parents of youth with limb deficiency endorse lower academic functioning than do youth themselves; however, without teacher report, specific academic outcomes, and measurement of functional ability, the understanding of this difference is not clear.

Support and Intervention for Youth and Families With Limb Deficiency

Parental/Caregiver Support

Parents and caregivers new to the world of limb deficiencies benefit from support and guidance from their medical team, both for medical and psychosocial adjustment. Parents of youth with prenatal limb deficiency diagnosis report feelings of anger, guilt, and shame in the prenatal and postnatal period.[24] Caregivers of youth with congenital limb deficiency are often in the position of having to make major medical decisions before their child is old enough to fully understand and communicate their assent.[43] Parents need support to manage grief and concerns surrounding their child's future well-being.

Medical teams can support parents by remaining cognizant of parents' emotional responses to their child's health status. This can provide parents an opportunity, without their child present, to process and ask questions about their child's limb deficiency or need for amputation. Similarly, permitting parents to view their child's residual limb following amputation but before anesthesia has been reversed was shown to be a valuable experience for parental coping.[44] Connections with other families experiencing similar limb deficiencies, along with support from family and friends, are helpful to parents.[43] Parents also report feeling reassured as their child develops following the standard milestones and exhibits greater capabilities than they initially expected.[24]

There is extensive support surrounding the role of parent behavior in promoting adaptive responses to medical procedures.[45,46] Specific parent behaviors, including providing reassurance, apologizing, and criticism, have been found to be distress-promoting parent behaviors, whereas using humor, encouraging use of coping skills, and distraction are considered coping-promoting parent behaviors. In general, coaching parents to be open and emotionally regulated about their child's limb deficiency can set a positive tone and can help children feel less shame and vulnerability, as well as the development of adaptive coping behaviors.

Surgical Support

For youth facing amputation, presurgical behavioral health consultation can improve the physical and emotional outcomes in children and adolescents, including reductions in anxiety, less pain medication, and better global coping.[47] The goals of a presurgical consultation are to ensure that the patient and family have a complete understanding of all options available to them, to clarify their reasons for amputation, and to identify psychological factors, such as depression or excessive anxiety, that merit intervention before surgery. Consultation should include a collaborative and personalized plan for ways to maintain the patient's social, academic, and family functioning and realistic expectations for recovery.

Health care clinicians can support families by acknowledging and being sensitive to their feelings of grief and loss. Amputation, as an example, can be an insult to bodily integrity and a unique loss for which there are few social norms and/or community-supported grief processes. Youth and families may express distress surrounding the disposal of the amputated body parts. Part of effective presurgical planning includes educating families about disposal of the amputated body parts. Some families express a desire to memorialize their child's amputation, be it for cultural or emotional reasons. Other families seek alternative disposal options that reflect their personal values, such as donating the amputated body part to medical researchers.[48] Health care clinicians should be able to discuss the options available to families and hospitals and should have established policies that can support the families as they consider amputation disposal. Cremating amputated body parts can require coordination between health care facilities and local funeral homes. Other disposal options can also require advanced planning, such as making a plaster mold or donating the limb to research. Having information available to patients and families during presurgical consultation demonstrates sensitivity to the loss they experience.

Supporting Youth With Limb Deficiency

There exist a variety of interventions/supports for youth with visible physical differences, such as those found in youth with limb differences. Overarching goals of these interventions are to promote positive thinking about appearance, raise self-esteem and confidence, and develop the social skills required to address appearance-based negative responses from others. Residential social camps, social skills training, behavioral therapy, and cognitive behavioral therapy are some of the more common interventions for youth with visible physical differences. In a systematic review of these interventions for youth with visual differences, researchers found little to no support for residential social camps improving the self-esteem, social experiences, and psychological well-being of the campers.[49] Social skills training, cognitive behavioral therapy, and behavioral therapy appear to provide some benefits; however, the lack of appropriate outcome measures and rigorous study design limits interpretation of the literature. Importantly, other qualitative work has shown that youths with limb deficiency do not necessarily think that they need to discuss their limb deficiency with parents or psychologists.[24]

Adolescents in particular benefit from developing a sense of community, especially with same-age peers and young adults who can model adaptive coping with amputation. Judicious use of the internet can provide youth and families with a sense of community and camaraderie with their limb deficiency peers and parents. For the adolescent with limb deficiency, a helpful peer group is one that is accepting of physical differences and that can provide a positive influence and buffer some of the social-emotional effects of feeling different from one's peers. Additionally, although summer camps for youth with limb deficiency have not yet demonstrated measurable change in emotions or behavior, qualitative interviews reveal that opportunities to engage in structured and unstructured activities with similar peers can be an overwhelmingly positive experience resulting in feelings of belonging and validation that are hard to achieve without exposure to other youth with limb deficiency.

Supporting Academics and Activities

With work showing lower rates of participation in physical education and greater absences for youth with late-life depression, it is critical that families work with school teams to develop accommodations that can help youth manage discomfort, participate, and avoid any educational gaps secondary to missed school. Collaboration between educators, medical teams, and families in the development of educational plans, such as a 504 or Individualized Education Plan, can help to reduce the effect of limb deficiency on academics. Similarly, supporting youth as they pursue extracurricular interests is important, as these activities can keep adolescents engaged in prosocial interests, promote positive identity development, and broaden their peer groups.

Developmental Considerations

The developmental needs of youth with limb deficiency are important in guiding parental expectations and behaviors (**Table 1**). In their earliest years, children have the developmental task of establishing a secure attachment to

TABLE 1 Developmental Tasks of Childhood and Promotion of Adaptive Behaviors for Parents of Youth With Limb Deficiencies

Age Range	Developmental Task	Child Consideration	Parent Considerations
0-18 mo	Establishing secure connection with attentive, loving, and validating caregiver Exploring their world	Infants and toddlers closely observe and read parents to guide for their own responses	Treat residual limb with same confidence and affection granted to other limbs. Strive to model calm and adaptive approach during medical visits or possible setbacks/developmental lags in ambulation. Develop adaptive responses to questions and comments from others less familiar with limb deficiency.
18 mo to 3 yr	Identify and express feelings adaptively Gains in independence while still very much seeking/requiring parental attention for comfort and security	High activity level—easy frustration and tantrums Still developing language skills—tantrums can reflect underlying frustration with communication skills Toddlers not necessarily aware of their limb deficiency—preschool peers typically accepting of visible differences at this age	Initiate graduated independence in self-care routines, including aspects of residual limb care and prosthetic care (if appropriate). Continue to set and maintain firm and consistent limits surrounding safety and critical routines; permit flexibility and choice when possible to avoid unproductive power struggles. Encourage feelings identification and be thoughtful about parental expressions of intense/uncomfortable feeling.
4-5 yr	Growing awareness of time and the connection between behaviors and consequences Developing socially appropriate behavior and social engagement	Many questions about their world (Why? How? When?) Enjoyment of participation in multiple activities—increased interested in social activities	Help child start to develop an adaptive narrative/identity surrounding limb deficiencies and simple phrasing to explain their limb difference to peers and others. Children at this stage may show increased curiosity about their limb differences. Answer questions in a candid but simple manner. Bite-sized pieces of information, consider using drawings or manipulatives to provide developmentally appropriate explanations. Correct misinformation. Continue to provide names and ways to express emotions.
School age (6-11 yr)	Accepting, following, and internalizing rules Developing mastery of social skills, reasoning skills, and increasing independence Selecting adult role models (often of same sex)	Enhanced cognitive and social skills development permits greater flexibility Gains in abstract reasoning can increase grief over missing limb as children are more able to grasp the permanent nature and possible future implications of limb deficiency Unexpected attention or bullying can be a significant challenge for youth with limb deficiency	Children may have stronger emotional responses about their limb deficiency than they had at previous ages. Continue to model adaptive coping using neutral and true responses while also validating their feelings. Work with your child to collaboratively problem solve and gradually increase expectations for independence in self-care and higher levels of responsibility. Provide a structure/scaffold with clearly defined expectations to set up the child for success and deliver natural and prompt consequences for meeting or not meeting expectations. Avoid power struggles. Introduce child to a number of role models; identify a few role models with limb differences (online or in person). Increase opportunities for time with friends, ideally with youth who share prosocial interests (eg, athletics, scouting, band).
Adolescence (12-18 yr)	Establishing identity separate from parents—emotional separation from parents Experimentation with differing values and development of own values Development of future adult relationship with parents and family members	Period of increased focus on appearance—puberty can be especially challenging Increased capacity for abstract thought—a period of greater creativity, idealism, and engagement with causes and interests	Monitor for indicators of low mood, social unease, or self-esteem; limb deficiency may increase feelings of difference for some youth. Provide opportunities for healthy peer involvement while maintaining firm rules and limits for safety (curfew, internet use). Permit flexibility for areas (clothing, hairstyle) that allow for safe expression of independence. Gradually transfer self-care responsibilities, including keeping track of appointments, care of medical equipment, and knowledge of their medical history. Have youth take the lead in medical appointments and decision making when possible. Educate teens about their medical team members and how to communicate with medical team when there are concerns.

Modified from Center for Parenting Education. https://centerforparentingeducation.org.

their caregiver and are not necessarily cognizant of or bothered by their difference. At the earlier ages, parents can set healthy routines and model adaptive behavior and responses to the queries of family and others who express curiosity surrounding the child's limb deficiency. As children start school and have stronger reasoning skills, they have questions about their limb deficiency and benefit from exposure to other peers and adults with limb deficiency who serve as positive role models.

During the school-age years, youth understand their limb deficiency more completely, and some experience grief responses surrounding their limb deficiency. Providing youth with social activities and sports can help to ensure that they establish strong peer relationships and have many opportunities to develop social skills. School-age youth are also increasingly independent in aspects of their care, making this a good time to establish expectations and natural consequences to avoid future power struggles. In their adolescent years, youth are more aware of their appearance, which can affect their social confidence and emotional well-being. Adolescent years represent a period of identity development in which many youth experiment with values, appearance, and behaviors to cultivate an identity separate from their parents. All adolescents, regardless of their orthopaedic status, benefit from monitoring of their mood and behavior, especially given the increases in suicidal ideation of young people.

Role of Health Care Clinicians in Psychosocial Adjustment

Parents and youth with limb deficiency need and seek the expert guidance of medical clinicians for critical information about limb deficiency, treatment planning, and ongoing care. By emphasizing ability, instilling pride, and modeling adaptive approaches to uncomfortable situations, persons working with the pediatric limb deficiency population are in a unique position to support families and youth.

Demonstrating sensitivity to family needs is one way that the medical community can support youth with limb deficiency. Effective communication is key in all aspects of medical care. Medical terminology, although critically important for communicating within the medical world, can feel insensitive and harsh to patients and families. Research has demonstrated that use of some specific medical terminology, including the term morbidly obese, negatively affects patient engagement and the quality of the patient-clinician relationship.[50] Patient engagement is critical to the development of trusting and candid relationships with medical clinicians, which in turn can affect medical outcomes. Children and adolescents, who are in the midst of developing their sense of self-worth and identity, may be especially vulnerable to negatively perceived medical terminology.

Health care clinicians can also support families by acknowledging and striving to improve the significant underrepresentation of female and minority orthopaedic clinicians. This underrepresentation has effects on patient comfort level, willingness to obtain care, and adherence to medical clinician treatment recommendations.[51] Being aware of this effect, showing humility, curiosity, and respect for all groups and cultures can reduce the effect of underrepresentation on the patient-clinician dynamic. Striving to connect families, especially those new to pediatric limb deficiency, to others who share their demographics is another way to bridge this gap in the near future.

Emphasizing positively framed language and sensitivity to patient preferences is also critical to the development of a trusting and supportive clinician-patient dynamic. As an example, the term "stump" is neither attractive nor sensitive to the needs of children and adolescents who may be hyperaware of their body appearance, even at a very young age. Using terms such as limb differences and residual limb provides subtle, but important, shifts in language use. Following the patient's lead by asking how they prefer to refer to their residual limb can be empowering and validating to the patient and their family. Some patients prefer not to differentiate their residual limb, and simply refer to their residual limb as their short leg or arm. Other families find it helpful to use more playful terms, including naming their residual limb or using family terms or nicknames that feel both comfortable and empowering.

The unexpected stares and comments of others is a certainty that awaits most youth with visible physical differences. Literature summarized previously reveals that this unexpected attention can invoke feelings of shame and difference from others, and is one of the more troublesome experiences for youth with limb deficiency.[24] Parents and clinicians can support youth by validating the child's discomfort while also normalizing the curiosity of others. Health care clinicians who have worked with many youth with limb deficiency can model or describe adaptive responses to unexpected attention. The simple act of validating frustration can help a youth feel heard and improve the patient-clinician connection.

SUMMARY

Youth with limb deficiency are a resilient group with overwhelmingly positive outcomes. Their psychosocial functioning is strong and similar to their same-age physically typical peers, and higher than that of youth with other major health concerns. Comparisons between youth with upper versus lower or multiple limb deficiencies suggest that youth with congenital and transradial limb deficiency fare especially well in their psychosocial health. Social dynamics and body image, especially the feelings of social isolation experienced by girls and young women, are a source of stress for individuals with limb deficiency. An area of greatest psychosocial need is the effective management of unwanted and unexpected attention from others, which youth with limb deficiency experience at a higher than average rate.

Importantly, youth tend to express mixed feelings surrounding their limb deficiency, with many youth expressing pride in their abilities and greater feelings of self-acceptance as they emerge into adulthood. Future research would benefit from the addition of objective rating scales, for example, teacher-report tools to clarify the discrepancy between parent and youth reports of academic functioning. Small sample sizes and the heterogeneity of this population affect the generalizability of this literature, but recent research efforts to make comparisons across countries of varying SES and resource allocation are a positive indicator.

Parents of youth with limb deficiency seek the guidance of health care clinicians, presenting an opportunity for clinicians to support families in a multitude of ways. Emphasizing the human capacity to adapt, promoting coping and personal achievement, and connecting families within the limb deficiency community are important ways to support youth with limb deficiency. Future goals include developing surgical and nonsurgical protocols that include ways to promote effective coping, encouraging parents to set developmentally appropriate expectations for independence, and screening for psychosocial adjustment concerns.

The review of the psychosocial and socioeconomic functioning of youth with limb deficiency provides a generally optimistic outlook for this population. Although body image and social acceptance are areas of concern for the pediatric limb deficiency population, these concerns tend to improve with age, and many young adults with limb deficiency report particular pride in their physical achievements. Parents tend to express greater concerns for their youth with limb deficiency than the youth themselves; however, these concerns lessen as parents see their child meet goals and expectations over the years. There is reason to have hope for the socioeconomic outcomes for youth with limb deficiency, especially as medical interventions advance, yet ethnic and economic disparities continue to affect those with the fewest resources and least access to quality medical care. Armed with knowledge and skills, health care clinicians working with the pediatric limb deficiency population can set the stage to promote adaptive coping, acceptance of body differences, and support parents/youth as they progress through their developmental milestones.

References

1. Hermansson L, Eliasson AC, Engstrom I: Psychosocial adjustment in Swedish children with upper-limb reduction deficiency and a myoelectric prosthetic hand. *Acta Paediatr* 2005;94(4):479-488.

2. James MA, Bagley AM, Brasington K, Lutz C, McConnell S, Molitor F: Impact of prostheses on function and quality of life for children with unilateral congenital below-the-elbow deficiency. *J Bone Joint Surg Am* 2006;88(11):2356-2365.

3. Ziegler-Graham K, MacKenzie EJ, Ephraim PL, Travison TG, Brookmeyer R: Estimating the prevalence of limb loss in the United States: 2005 to 2050. *Arch Phys Med Rehabil* 2008;89(3):422-429.

4. Armstrong TW, Williamson MLC, Elliott TR, Jackson WT, Kearns NT, Ryan T: Psychological distress among persons with upper extremity limb loss. *Br J Health Psychol* 2019;24(4):746-763.

5. Mai CT, Isenburg JL, Canfield MA, et al: National population-based estimates for major birth defects, 2010-2014. *Birth Defects Res* 2019;111(18):1420-1435.

6. Borne A, Porter A, Recicar J, Maxson T, Montgomery C: Pediatric traumatic amputations in the United States: A 5-year review. *J Pediatr Orthop* 2017;37(2):e104-e107.

7. Bryant PR, Pandian G: Acquired limb deficiencies. 1. Acquired limb deficiencies in children and young adults. *Arch Phys Med Rehabil* 2001;82(3 suppl 1):S3-S8.

8. Bae DS, Canizares MF, Miller PE, Waters PM, Goldfarb CA: Functional impact of congenital hand differences: Early results from the Congenital Upper Limb Differences (CoULD) Registry. *J Hand Surg Am* 2018;43(4):321-330.

9. Ylimäinen K, Nachemson A, Sommerstein K, Stockselius A, Norling Hermansson L: Health-related quality of life in Swedish children and adolescents with limb reduction deficiency. *Acta Paediatr* 2010;99(10):1550-1555.

10. Migaou H, Kalai A, Hassine YH, Jellad A, Boudokhane S, Frih ZBS: Quality of life associated factors in a North African sample of lower limbs amputees. *Ann Rehabil Med* 2019;43(3):321-327.

11. Christensen J, Ipsen T, Doherty P, Langberg J: Physical and social factors determining quality of life for veterans with lower-limb amputation(s): A systematic review. *Disabil Rehabil* 2016;38(24):2345-2353.

12. Michielsen A, van Wijk I, Ketelaar M: Participation and health-related quality of life of Dutch children and adolescents with congenital lower limb deficiencies. *J Rehabil Med* 2011;43(7):584-589.

13. Demirdel S, Ülger Ö: Body image disturbance, psychosocial adjustment and quality of life in adolescents with amputation. *Disabil Health J* 2021;14(3):101068.

14. Johansen H, Dammann B, Andresen IL, Fagerland MW: Health-related quality of life for children with rare diagnoses, their parents' satisfaction with life and the association between the two. *Health Qual Life Outcome* 2013;11:152.

15. Johansen H, Damman B, Andersen LØ, Andresen IL: Children with congenital limb deficiency in Norway: Issues related to school life and health-related quality of life. A cross-sectional study. *Disabil Rehabil* 2016;38(18):1803-1810.

16. Eiser C, Morse R: Quality-of-life measures in chronic diseases of childhood. *Health Technol Assess* 2001;5(4):1-157.

17. Sheffler LC, Hanley C, Bagley A, Molitor F, James MA: Comparison of self-reports and parent proxy-reports of function and quality of life of children with below-the-elbow deficiency. *J Bone Joint Surg Am* 2009;91(12):2852-2859.

18. Easterlin MC, Chung PJ, Leng M, Dudovitz R: Association of team sports participation with long-term mental health outcomes among individuals exposed to adverse childhood experiences. *JAMA Pediatr* 2019;173(7):681-688.

19. Law M: Participation in the occupations of everyday life. *Am J Occup Ther* 2002;56(6):640-649.

20. Akarsu S, Tekin L, Safaz I, Göktepe AS, Yazicioğlu K: Quality of life and functionality after lower limb amputations: Comparison between uni- vs. bilateral amputee patients. *Prosthet Orthot Int* 2013;37(1):9-13.

21. Raichle KA, Hanley MA, Molton I, et al: Prosthesis use in persons with lower- and upper-limb amputation. *J Rehabil Res Dev* 2008;45(7):961-972.

22. Pasquina CP, Carvalho AJ, Sheehan TP: Ethics in rehabilitation: Access to prosthetics and quality care following amputation. *AMA J Ethics* 2015;17(6):535-546.

23. de Jong IGM, Reinders-Messelink HA, Janssen WGM, Poelma MJ, van Wijk I, van der Sluis CK: Mixed feelings of children and adolescents with unilateral congenital below elbow deficiency: An online focus group study. *PLoS One* 2012;7(6):e37099.

24. Sims T, Donovan-Hall M, Metcalf C: Children's and adolescents' views on upper limb prostheses in relation to their daily occupations. *Br J Occup Ther* 2019;83(4):237-245.

25. Department of Health and Social Care: *First Children Receive Sports Limbs on the NHS*. Department of Health and Social Care, 2017.

26. Vasluian E, de Jong IGM, Janssen WGM, et al: Opinions of youngsters with congenital below-elbow deficiency, and those of their parents and professionals concerning prosthetic use and rehabilitation treatment. *PLoS One* 2013;8(6):e67101.

27. Mäkinen M, Marttunen M, Komulainen E, et al: Development of self-image and its components during a one-year follow-up in non-referred adolescents with excess and normal weight. *Child Adolesc Psychiatry Ment Health* 2015;9:5.

28. Davison TE, McCabe MP: Adolescent body image and psychosocial functioning. *J Soc Psychol* 2006;146(1):15-30.

29. Varni JW, Rubenfeld LA, Talbot D, Setoguchi Y: Determinants of self-esteem in children with congenital/acquired limb deficiencies. *J Dev Behav Pediatr* 1989;10(1):13-16.

30. Rose CA, Simpson CG, Moss A: The bullying dynamic: Prevalence of involvement among a large-scale sample of middle and high school youth with and without disabilities. *Psychol Sch* 2015;52(5):515-531.

31. Carrillo LA, Sabatini CS, Brar RK, et al: The prevalence of bullying among pediatric orthopaedic patients. *J Pediatr Orthop* 2021;41(8):463-466.

32. Collins WA, Welsh DP, Furman W: Adolescent romantic relationships. *Annu Rev Psychol* 2009;60:631-652.

33. Carver K, Joyner K, Udry JR: National estimates of adolescent romantic relationships, in Florsheim P, ed: Cambridge University Press, 2003, pp 291-329.

34. Murray C: Gender, sexuality and prosthesis use: Implications for rehabilitation, in Murray C, ed: *Amputation, Prosthesis Use, and Phantom Limb Pain: An Interdisciplinary Perspective*. Springer Science + Business Media, 2010, pp 115-127.

35. Cheng MM, Udry JR: Sexual behaviors of physically disabled adolescents in the United States. *J Adolesc Health* 2002;31(1):48-58.

36. Marina N, Hudson MM, Jones K, et al: Changes in health status among aging survivors of pediatric upper and lower extremity sarcoma: A report from the childhood cancer survivor study. *Arch Phys Med Rehabil* 2013;94(6):1062-1073.

37. Johansen H, Østlie K, Andersen LØ, Rand-Hendriksen S: Adults with congenital limb deficiency in Norway: Demographic and clinical features, pain and the use of health care and welfare services. A cross-sectional study. *Disabil Rehabil* 2015;37(22):2076-2082.

38. Sjoberg L, Nilsagard Y, Fredriksson C: Life situation of adults with congenital limb reduction deficiency in Sweden. *Disabil Rehabil* 2014;36(18):1562-1571.

39. Loder RT, Dikos GD, Taylor DA: Long-term lower extremity prosthetic costs in children with traumatic lawnmower amputations. *Arch Pediatr Adolesc Med* 2004;158(12):1177-1181.

40. Yang J, Carmichael SL, Canfield M, Song J, Shaw GM: National Birth Defects Prevention Study: Socioeconomic status in relation to selected birth defects in a large multi-centered US case-control study. *Am J Epidemiol* 2008;167(2):145-154.

41. Canfield MA, Mai CT, Wang Y, et al: The association between race/ethnicity and major birth defects in the United States, 1999-2007. *Am J Public Health* 2014;104(9):e14-e23.

42. Murray CD, Fox J: Body image and prosthesis satisfaction in the lower limb amputee. *Disabil Rehabil* 2002;24(17):925-931.

43. Jaraway D, Perry S, Phillips M, Ziegler P, Wolgemuth A, Scott SD: Preparing parents to help support their child post-amputation for bone cancer. *ORNAC J* 2013;31(4):13-19, 24-25.

44. Dahlquist LM, Power TG, Carlson L: Physician and parent behavior during invasive pediatric cancer procedures: Relationships to child behavioral distress. *J Pediatr Psychol* 1995;20(4):477-490.

45. McMurtry C, McGrath PJ, Chambers CT: Reassurance can hurt: Parental behavior and painful medical procedures. *J Pediatr* 2006;148(4):560-561.

46. Webb N, ed: *Helping Children and Adolescents With Chronic and Serious Medical Conditions: A Strengths-Based Approach*. John Wiley & Sons, Inc, 2010.

47. Hanna E: "What do you want to do with the leg?" A critical narrative review of the understandings and implications of disposal in the context of limb amputations. *Sage Open* 2019;9(2):1-8.

48. Jenkinson E, Williamson H, Bryon-Daniel J, Moss TP: Systematic review: Psychosocial interventions for children and young people with visible differences resulting from appearance altering conditions, injury, or treatment effects. *J Pediatr Psychol* 2015;40(10):1017-1033.

49. Albury C, Strain WD, Brocq SL, et al: The importance of language in engagement between health-care professionals and people living with obesity: A joint consensus statement. *Lancet Diabetes Endocrinol* 2020;8(5):447-455.

50. Sullivan LW, Mittman IS: Keynote address: The need for greater racial and ethnic diversity in orthopaedic surgery. *Clin Orthop Relat Res* 2011;469(7):1809-1812.

Principles of Amputation in Children

Chinmay S. Paranjape, MD, MHSc • Anna D. Vergun, MD, FAAOS

ABSTRACT

Amputations in children and adults require different considerations. In children, remaining growth, other potential deficiencies, healing and remodeling potential, and familial needs and expectations drive the principles outlined herein. A collaborative, multidisciplinary approach is needed between surgeons, physiatrists, prosthetists, physical and occupational therapists, and families to achieve a good outcome.

Keywords: congenital limb deformity; limb deficiency; pediatric amputation; Van Nes rotationplasty

Introduction

Limb deficiencies in children and adults are different owing to differences in etiology and physiology. In children, limb deficiencies most commonly result from errors in formation rather than from trauma or vascular insufficiency.[1] Remaining growth lends to variability in limb size and motor development and creates a potential for terminal overgrowth. Many physiologic differences exist between children and adults and must be considered by the treating team. Children have improved healing potential and, when associated with congenital limb deficiency, less commonly experience phantom pain, though they may experience phantom sensations.[2,3] Painful sensations may be more prevalent when associated with oncologic or traumatic etiologies of limb loss.[4,5] They are more likely than their adult counterparts to have multiple extremity involvement in addition to cognitive or behavioral challenges because of comorbid conditions.[6,7] Finally, children are more likely to place increased physical demands on their residual limbs and prostheses, requiring replacement every 12 to 24 months compared with every 3 to 5 years.[8] These factors must be considered when planning for amputation or salvage to improve the use of prostheses in children. As a result, pediatric limb deficiencies may be best managed at specialized centers with experience and a multidisciplinary team composed of therapists, prosthetists, physiatrists, and orthopedic surgeons. In this chapter, the authors present several guiding principles for the treating surgeon.

Goals of Care

When addressing pediatric limb deficiency, the treating team should attempt to (1) optimize function during childhood while (2) optimizing future function in adulthood and (3) minimizing the total number of procedures required. Typically, optimal management during growth yields optimal final adult outcome. However, there are situations in which those two goals must be separately considered. In these instances, optimal function in adulthood (most of the individual's life) must be prioritized. All the same, management during growth must be palatable to both the child and the family.

Consider the case of a 3-year-old child with unilateral localized gigantism of a foot undergoing a foot amputation. A foot amputation now would create a residuum that is too long in adulthood to accommodate a foot prosthesis. Addressing that problem with a transtibial amputation in childhood would create a secondary issue with recurrent terminal overgrowth. As a result, a resection of the distal tibia combined with a Boyd amputation addresses both issues. If the length of the tibia is adequate for an adult transtibial residuum at the time of the Boyd amputation in childhood, then a proximal tibial epiphysiodesis can be performed concurrently. Immediately following the surgery, the length of the residuum will still be too long. However, several years later, the growth of the contralateral limb should provide a sufficient difference to accommodate a standard transtibial prosthesis.

Surgical Principles

Several general principles are useful in optimizing eventual function following amputation in children:

1. Maximize length of the residual limb.
   a. Preserve epiphyseal plates when possible and consider limb length inequalities.
   b. Use soft-tissue rearrangements/grafting when needed to increase the available limb length.

Dr. Paranjape or an immediate family member has stock or stock options held in Alphatec Spine, OrthoPediatrics, and Stryker. Dr. Vergun or an immediate family member serves as a board member, owner, officer, or committee member of Association of Children's Prosthetic and Orthotic Clinics.

2. Amputate through joints (disarticulation) rather than through bone (transosseous) when possible.
3. When transosseous amputation is necessary, consider a primary osteochondral capping procedure to prevent terminal bony overgrowth.
4. Preserve joint function (especially in the knee).
5. Address proximal limb abnormalities (ie, stability, morphology) if coincident with distal pathology.
6. Prepare to address other health concerns:
   a. Associated genetic syndromes.
   b. Associated organ/structural abnormalities (cardiac, renal, spine).
   c. Upper extremity and multiple limb deficiencies: consider the goal of function rather than simply normalizing anatomy—children may function better with native sensation and adaptations using residual limbs more efficiently than through limb replacement by means of prostheses. For many children, having more than one prosthesis is cumbersome. Meta-analyses of data available since the 1980s demonstrates a 20% nonwear rate of prosthesis for a variety of reasons.
   d. Consider additional challenges posed by cognitive and/or motor delay.

Principles 1 and 2: Maximizing Limb Length and Considering Growth

The treating surgeon must consider final limb length at skeletal maturity. At the time of initial consultation, the current and projected limb length discrepancies, both with and without treatment, should be mapped out. Several prior publications discuss different methods of accurately predicting limb length discrepancies and are beyond the scope of this chapter.[9-11] However, some heuristics exist to provide rough estimates of limb lengths at maturity as assessed on initial physical examination.

One assumption is that infants with congenital deficiencies will continue to grow proportionally. For example, if the deficient long bone is 60% of the length of the opposite long bone at birth, it will be about 60% of the contralateral unaffected long bone length at skeletal maturity. On examination, with both limbs in full extension, the examiner should see where the distal end of the limb is relative to the longer side. At full maturity, untreated, the deficient limb will end at approximately the same level relative to the other side. With previously described predictions for final limb length, this proportion can be used to provide a rough prediction of final limb length of the deficient limb to enable informed discussion of management options. Conversely, early treatment without consideration of growth can be disastrous. For example, amputation above the level of the distal femoral physis in an infant may initially appear to have an appropriate length. However, because of the missing 70% to 80% of femoral growth from the distal physis, the residuum at maturity will grow only slightly longer, resulting in such a tiny proximal femur that the amputation level will function like an amputee with a hip disarticulation at maturity.[12]

A notable exception to using the aforementioned assumptions is when trauma has caused complete growth arrest in a physis of interest. Instead, the relative contributions of the relevant proximal and distal physes should be referenced and used to provide a prediction. The authors of this chapter reference the proximal femur as contributing to 15%, the distal femur to 35%, proximal tibia 30%, and distal tibia 20% of the final length of the limb. Two additional assumptions are then made: (1) girls stop growing at 14 years of age and boys at 16 years of age, and (2) growth arrest is complete. Next, the average growth in millimeters per year from each contributing femoral or tibial epiphyseal plate can be calculated. Note that infections may cause partial physeal arrest and that this method may not be valid. Instead, the growth inhibition method or Moseley's straight-line method may be used. For a bit more accurate residual limb length determination, skeletal age combined with either Moseley or Paley method can be employed.

Generally, a longer residuum results in improved function.[13-15] This is true for both ambulatory and nonambulatory children. In ambulators, the longer lever arm affords greater power and distributes forces within the socket over a larger area. In nonambulators, longer limbs improve balance when seated and with transitional movements.[16] No ideal length for amputated long bones has been identified. The minimum required length is determined by the length required to keep the prosthesis in place. This is a moving target with advancements in liners and with the advent of transosseous integration. Recent studies of osseointegration in adults have demonstrated increased prosthesis use, walking speed, and decreased energy expenditure. The stoma site between the implant and skin requires careful hygiene to prevent infection, but the technology remains promising.[17-18] The technique and potential complications related to growth have not yet been studied in children. Short residua can be lengthened distal to tendinous insertions to allow for more appropriate prosthesis wear using limb lengthening techniques (Figure 1). The maximum length is based on the desire for equal joint heights (eg, the knee for transfemoral amputees) and the interposed bulk of soft tissue between the residuum and the mechanical joint. Variable knee heights have similar function when walking on level ground, and studies have demonstrated more normal gait parameters with lowered center of mass and hinge with prostheses.[19] In the experience of the authors, minor problems with variable knee heights include difficulty fitting into stadium seating, pain under the longer thigh when sitting because of a short tibial segment, and increased pressure from chairs on the posterior thigh.

Principle 3: Using Soft-Tissue Grafting to Increase the Available Limb Length

Traumatic amputations and postradiation oncologic resections may affect the soft-tissue envelope, with the temptation to allow for primary closure by resecting more bone. The reconstructive surgery ladder progresses from local wound care, primary closure, split-thickness skin grafting, local skin flaps, pedicled flaps, and finally to free flaps. Orthoplastic principles may help achieve longer residuum by allowing staged soft-tissue coverage to allow retention of diaphyseal long bone and native joints.[20] This in turn may maximize functional outcome. Several case examples of these principles were outlined by Fleming et al[21] in an adult military cohort suffering traumatic amputations caused by war. Therapies discussed by his group included rotational flaps, free flaps, split-thickness skin grafts, tissue expanders, and bio-composite dermal substitutes. They noted that preservation of residuum length requires management considerations of both the underlying bony segment and its associated soft-tissue envelope.

When following the reconstructive ladder, Fleming et al recommend:

1. Consideration of split-thickness skin grafting should outweigh conversion to higher functional amputation levels just for skin coverage
2. Consideration of tissue expanders and negative wound therapies to allow for delayed primary closure
3. Consideration of atypical local skin flaps, albeit in the zone of injury
4. Progression through the reconstructive ladder to allow retention of native diaphyseal bone and proximal articulations

In a pediatric traumatic amputation cohort, the benefits of residual length with orthoplastic considerations should be weighed with principles 4 and 5 described next (**Figure 2**).

Principles 4 and 5: Prevention of Terminal Overgrowth by Disarticulation Versus Cartilage Capping

Nearly 50% of transosseous amputations experience terminal bony overgrowth, likely as a result of periosteal reaction with penciling of the terminal bone. This principle was first noted by Ernst Marquardt, who observed that overgrowth never occurred after amputation through joints.[22] Age and location of amputation are the most

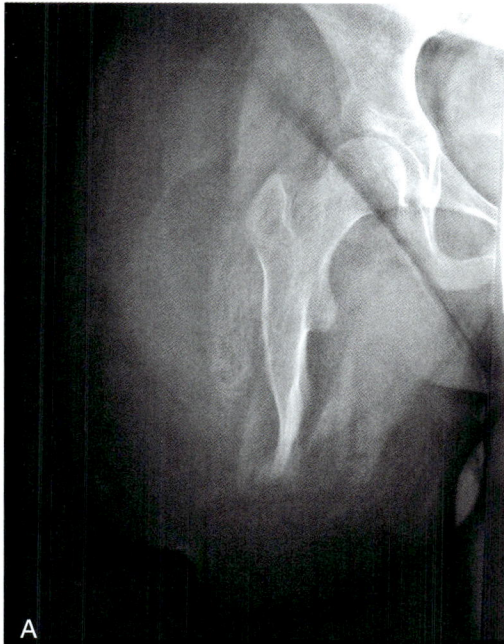 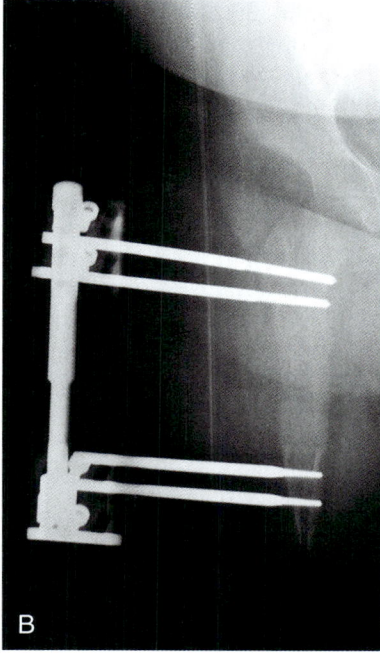

FIGURE 1 AP radiographs of a short femoral residual limb (**A**) that was associated with poor control of the prosthesis. The femur underwent an osteotomy and lengthening of 9 cm (**B**) with an external fixator. The amount of length achieved was limited by pain over the distal tip during the lengthening process, but this pain abated during the consolidation phase. The mild hip flexion contracture present before lengthening resolved once the patient was using their new prosthesis.

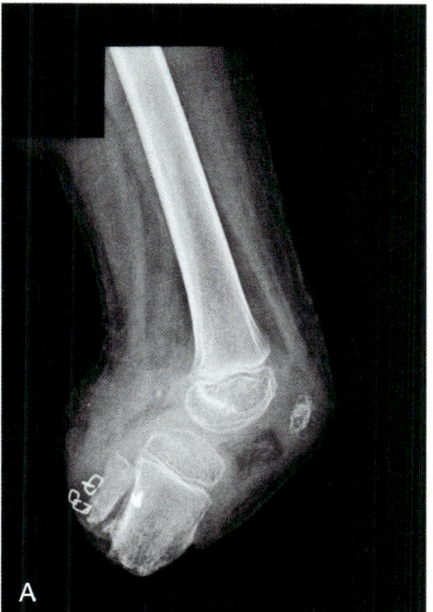 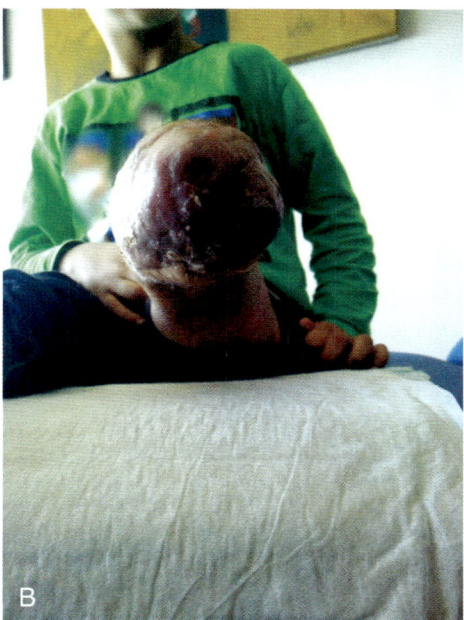

FIGURE 2 Lateral radiograph (**A**) and clinical photograph (**B**) of a 4-year-old boy who was injured by a bomb blast, resulting in a traumatic tibial amputation. The left tibial segment was extremely short with inadequate soft-tissue coverage, but the extensor mechanism remained intact. The full thickness tissue loss over the distal residuum and the tibial periosteum was treated with skin graft. After the grafted tissue hypertrophies and matures, it will function well inside a standard transtibial prostheses. With normal growth, the proximal tibia will increase by an additional 6 to 8 cm at maturity.

influential factors in overgrowth. Overgrowth is not observed in children older than 12 years or in disarticulations.[23] Overgrowth is rare in the forearm but common in the arm and lower extremity amputations.[23]

Overgrowth can result in the need for multiple reoperations.[24] The recurrent overgrowth can persist into the third decade of life. This painful, recurrent problem is best avoided by ensuring that the bone end always has a native or grafted cartilage cap, which can prevent overgrowth in 90% of cases.[25] Several synthetic caps have been tried but suffer from complications as a result of inflammatory foreign body reactions.[26] Autografts from iliac crest can be successful but are complicated by donor site pain and difficulty with fixation between the recipient bone and graft.[27] Fibular head autografts have been used for tibial residuum capping successfully[24] (Figure 3).

Principle 6: Preserve Joint Function (Especially in the Knee)

Evolution and natural selection have optimized normative human anatomy for bipedal gait efficiency. Therefore, metabolic efficiency is improved by preserving native joints[28] and performing as distal an amputation as reasonably allowable.[29-31] Energy costs are substantially increased for above-knee versus below-knee amputations. Compared with unimpaired individuals, unilateral transfemoral amputation led to 49% higher oxygen consumption relative to 9% with transtibial amputation.[13] Jeans et al[30] determined that children with through-knee amputations had similar oxygen consumption and velocity compared with those with transtibial amputations on level ground. On uneven ground, the mechanical knee cannot adapt, causing difficulty with gait. Computer-assisted devices can anticipate movement, and early subjective experiences suggests this may be improved with the advent of osseointegrating prostheses, although these modalities are currently

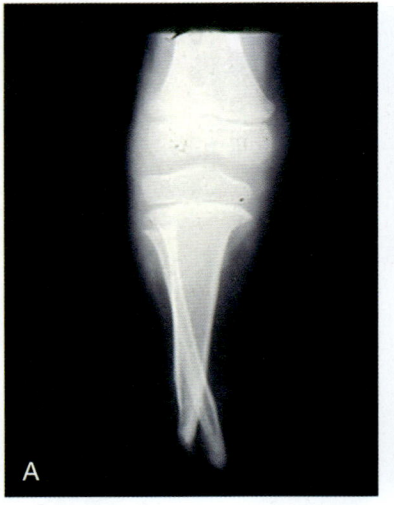
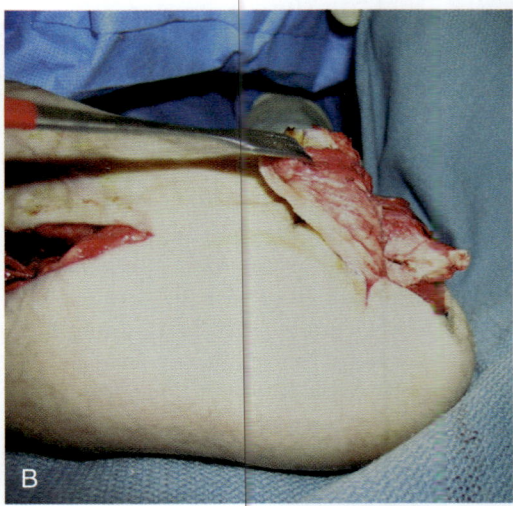
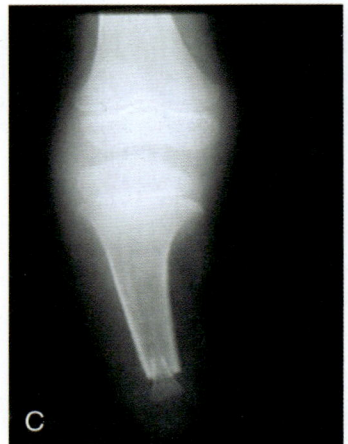
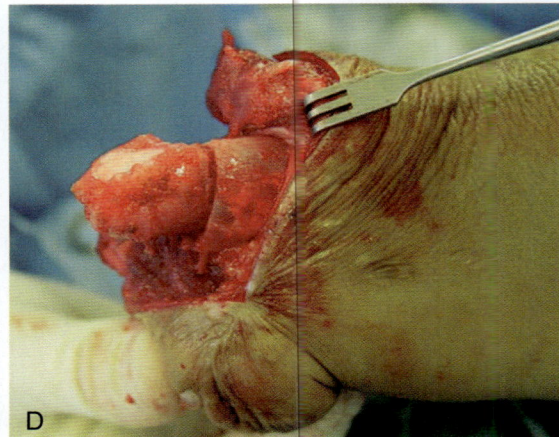

FIGURE 3 AP radiograph (**A**) and intraoperative photograph (**B**) of tibial residual limb overgrowth. AP radiograph (**C**) and intraoperative photograph (**D**) of osteochondral capping using an ipsilateral fibular head autograft (modified Marquardt technique as described by H.G. Watts). In the preoperative radiograph, the fibula appears longer, but the tibia is a subcutaneous bone and is often symptomatic first.

reserved for adults.[32] Rotationplasty, described subsequently, can allow for preservation of knee joint function even in the setting of transfemoral amputation.

Principle 7: Address Ipsilateral Proximal Limb Abnormalities

Limb deficiency syndromes can result in coincident ipsilateral hip and knee instability. In the case of proximal femoral focal deficiency (PFFD), hip instability and/or severe coxa vara, depending on the severity of the PFFD, is present. The majority have associated fibular hemimelia and its manifestations. Flexion knee contractures are also common, as is external rotation deformity. The Aitken classification groups patients based on presence or absence of the femoral head (A/B versus C/D) and severity of dysplasia of the hip acetabulum (normal, A; mildly dysplastic, B; severely dysplastic, C; and absent, D).[33] Knee fusion is a common surgery to address the issues of very short femur and contractures around both the knee and hip. The knee should be fused in full extension at the time of rotationplasty or foot ablation to align the limb in the sagittal plane of the trunk[12] and to increase the lever arm of the thigh bone (fused tibia and femur) to stretch out contractures and improve muscle efficiency.

Principle 8: Preparation to Address Other Health Considerations and Planning

Genetic Concerns

Lack-of-formation deficiencies have been found to have variable inheritance modes. Parents often desire to know this information, especially if the condition is transmissible. Coxa vara and some tibial deficiencies have an autosomal dominant inheritance pattern. Total absence of hands and feet has been reported in multiple members of Brazilian families in an autosomal recessive mode. PFFD has been reported to have multiple inheritance modes in the literature.[34] This is a growing field, and there will likely be more somatic and/or germline variants discovered in the future.

Psychologic Considerations

For elective surgery, families must accept the need for an amputation or a structural change in the residuum with a goal to improve function and/or simplify prosthetic fit. An amputation imparts a sense of finality and is often emotional for the parents who are already experiencing a sense of loss. Drotar et al[6] described five stages of parental reactions following the discovery of a congenital anomaly: shock, denial, sadness and anger, adaptation, and reorganization. Many parents discover the anomaly at birth, although the frequency of antenatal diagnoses is growing because of improvements in ultrasonography. It is reasonable to assume that parents will struggle to make any decision before the adaptation stage, so extensive counseling and multiple medical opinions are requisite. It is the authors' experience that most families with a newborn with a limb loss/difference benefit from medical and surgical counsel every 2 to 3 months during the first 9 to 12 months of life as they have variable ability to grasp information at the different stages of reactions. It is very important to note that the child born with limb loss/difference experiences no sense of loss, but instead experiences their parents' emotional reactions.

Parents often feel pressure to make early decisions about an amputation. Although plausible that amputations are psychologically easier for the child if done before long-term memory is developed, no evidence validates this assumption. Traditionally, this age was thought to be 3 to 4 years. However, evidence suggests that even very early traumatic events can be recalled.[35] Finally, the well-being and self-esteem of the child is most closely tied to social support from classmates, parents, teachers, and friends.[7] Parental depression and anxiety and marital discord in families have also been associated with increased childhood depression and anxiety. Therefore, parental well-being and comfort with the decisions they are making is paramount. A prosthesis or an orthosis can be fashioned to fit the extremity for functional purposes until the family is ready to make a decision about surgery. In these situations, patients and/or families often reach a point where they prefer a more cosmetic prosthesis or orthosis and will reconsider an amputation as a logical progression toward that end.

Surgical Timing

Intervention should not impede but rather assist a child in achieving normal motor milestones. Delaying surgery until the age of 9 to 12 months will help decrease the risks of anesthesia in infants. As an example, a child needing an elective foot amputation for a fibular or tibial deficiency should be delayed until the child is pulling to stand, typically age 10 to 14 months.

Recognizing and addressing concomitant hip dysplasia is another important consideration. Taking advantage of the remodeling potential of the acetabulum is advantageous and requires appropriate timing. Coxa vara may be protective, but severe varus deformity can cause blunting of the lateral acetabular lip or levering of the head out of the socket inferiorly with hip abduction. A proximal femoral valgus producing osteotomy, femoral shortening, and a possible acetabular osteotomy may be protective of hip function in such children.

Perisurgical Pain Control

In light of the increasing recognition of phantom limb pain and sensations in children, there have been several modalities that have demonstrated benefits. Gabapentin, tricyclic antidepressants, opioids, regional neuraxial blockade, mirror therapy, acupuncture, and psychotherapy have all been described in the literature and summarized nicely by DeMoss et al.[4]

Upper Limb Deficiencies

Beyond initial treatment for traumatic injuries, many upper extremity deficiencies do not require surgical intervention. Specifically, for children with congenital amputations, nubbins on the residuum may provide sensation and traction. They are particularly helpful with use of touchscreens. These should not be removed unless there is a specific issue such as with hygiene or repeat trauma.

For unilateral upper limb deficiency, prostheses are controversial. James et al[36] suggested that there were no quality of life or functional differences in individuals with and without prostheses for below-elbow amputations. Interestingly, early exposure to prostheses led to continued use in adulthood. However, individuals tended to choose the simplest prosthesis despite being exposed to increasingly complex devices.[37] Individuals with bilateral upper limb deficiencies can often compensate well using their lower limbs. This should be considered before any planned lower extremity surgery. The Krukenberg procedure should be considered for bilateral hand amputees.[38]

Syme Versus Boyd Amputation

These eponymous amputations are used about the ankle. Both have similar complication rates and results, but they differ in rehabilitation and complication profiles. Syme's amputation involves ankle disarticulation with retention of the heel pad tissue.[39] Boyd's[40] amputation is a transcalcaneal amputation with resection of the talus and tibiocalcaneal arthrodesis.

Although a Syme in adults typically involves resection of the medial malleolus, in children, diminished growth of the malleoli renders this unnecessary. A Syme is typically less technically challenging to perform than a Boyd, has decreased acute postsurgical wound complications, has no need for a postsurgical cast, and has a shorter time to fitting a prosthesis. These come at the cost of posterior heel pad migration and less reliable weight bearing on the distal end of the residuum.[41,42] Birch et al reported that posterior heel pad migration is typically asymptomatic and does not affect function within the prosthesis.

A Boyd amputation in adults results in a longer residual limb with a bulbous end. This is not always the case in children because the residual limb is often hypoplastic. The distal tibia and its physis are often resected, shortening the residual limb and allowing for correct positioning of a subluxated calcaneus beneath the tibia and decreasing soft-tissue tension of the wound clsure. In very young children, it can result in a residual limb ending at the contralateral mid-calf at skeletal maturity. In the authors experience, the resultant bulk from the calcaneus is nicely contoured as part of the calf within the prosthesis and provides a good cosmetic result as well as self-suspension within the prosthesis. Relative to a Syme, a Boyd can be more technically demanding, have increased wound complications with rates as high as 15%, result in nonunion of the tibiocalcaneal arthrodesis, and requires casting and increased rehabilitation time before prosthesis fitting. Most postsurgical wound complications are with soft-tissue healing that can be managed with local wound care.[43]

Congenital Tibial Pseudarthrosis
Congenital tibial pseudarthrosis can be a difficult clinical entity. Especially when multiple attempts for union have failed, special caution is required. Amputation through the nonunion site can be tempting. Unfortunately, overgrowth of the residuum can result in complications, and distal end capping procedures can also result in nonunion. In this case there are two options. (1) A Syme or Boyd amputation is performed to improve the length of the residuum and to decrease the likelihood of overgrowth. This may still result in persistent nonunion, but this is rarely symptomatic in a prosthesis and often does not require treatments.[43-45] (2) The surgeon can perform a transtibial amputation well above the pseudarthrosis site where the bone quality appears normal and plan for a primary residuum capping with an osteochondral autograft. In this case, the first metatarsal from the amputated foot often fits well in the tibial canal.

Van Nes Procedures
Rotationplasty was originally described by Borggreve[46] in Germany for management of tuberculosis of the knee. The procedure substitutes a 180° externally rotated ankle for the knee in patients with a femoral deficiency. Van Nes later modified the procedure to treat congenital femoral focal deficiency.[47] It has since been applied for primary tumor resection about the knee and other needs for knee reconstruction in children.[48,49] Long-term follow-up studies have demonstrated acceptable cosmesis, similar energy-efficient gait parameters and function relative to transfemoral amputation.[28,50,51] In children, the foot and ankle joint will adapt in a way that avoids long-term arthrosis.[52]

Van Nes rotationplasty requires a stable hip joint and ankle mortise. Accordingly, any concomitant hip dysplasia or coxa vara should be treated. The procedure can be employed in Aitken type A, B, C, and D femoral deficiencies. For mild fibular deficiency where the tip of the fibula ends at the mortise, there is still good postsurgical function (unpublished case study from senior author of this chapter, Association of Children's Prosthetic-Orthotic Clinics Annual Meeting, Banff, Canada 2012).

Various surgical techniques have been described to achieve rotationplasty. The knee joint is resected with epiphysiodesis of one or both epiphyseal plates at the knee. The limb is externally rotated 180°, and the tibia is then fused to the remaining femur via various available fixation methods. Details of this procedure are described elsewhere in this book. An example for a patient treated at our institution for a distal femoral osteogenic sarcoma is provided in **Figure 4**, and for a patient with PFFD, Aitken type C is provided **Figure 5**. In the authors' experience, a common pitfall is to leave the neo-femoral segment too long, and the surgeon should err on the side of additional acute shortening or perform a pan genu epiphysiodesis at the index procedure.

Multiple Limb Deficiencies
Global consideration of whole-body function is critical in children with multiple limb deficiency. Task performance hinges on synergistic function of the entire body. Children with multiple limb deficiencies must learn to substitute other parts of their body. Motor milestones are typically not delayed; instead they achieve the milestones with modifications that are appropriate for their individual physical limitations. Surgery is rarely indicated for these children. Amputation or surgical correction of the feet or remnants of the feet should not be done if they substitute for hands, even if surgery would provide better gait or improved prosthesis use. The authors have written another chapter in this book specifically dedicated to this topic.

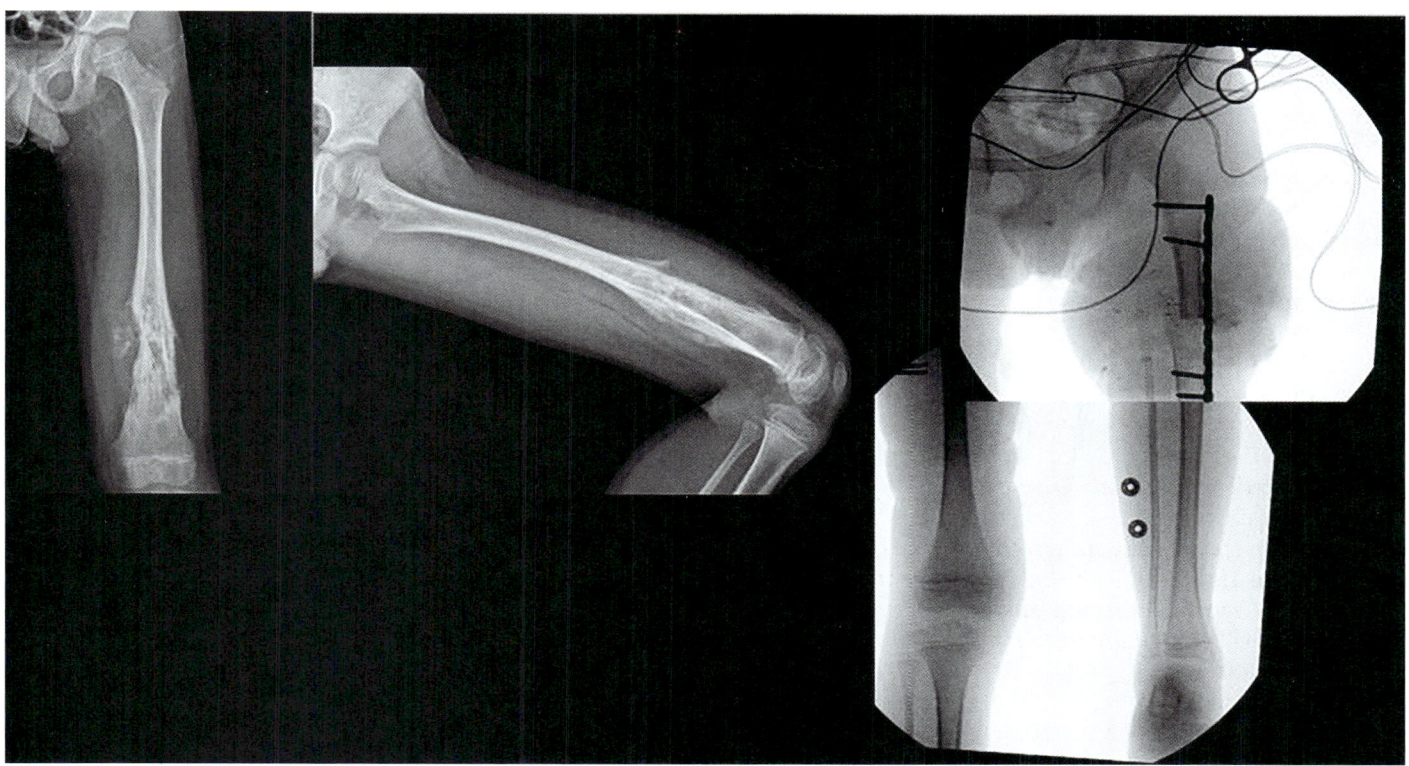

FIGURE 4 Presurgical and postsurgical radiographs of a 6-year-old boy with osteogenic sarcoma of the left distal femur that required neoadjuvant chemotherapy, followed by wide resection and Van Nes rotationplasty of the left tibia. Note the relative heights of the neo-knee relative to the native knee at time of index procedure as well as orientation of the ankle. The overall new thigh segment was left too long and will likely require additional intervention in the future.

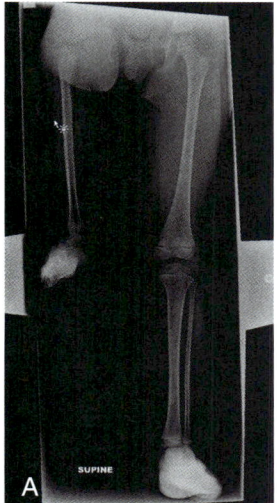 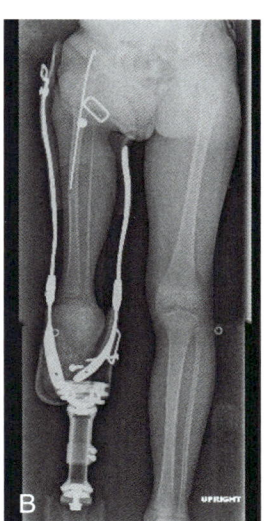 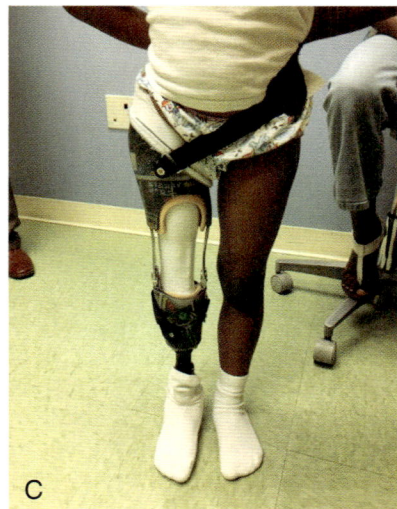 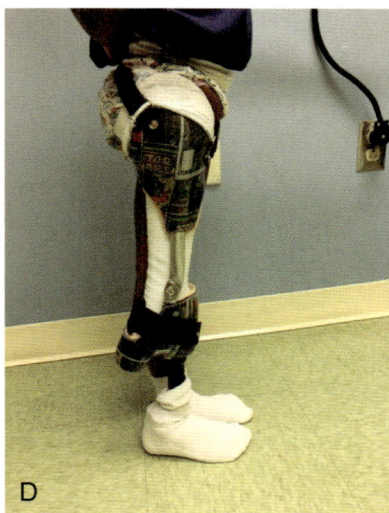

FIGURE 5 Standing hip, knee, ankle radiographs of a child with Aitken type C PFFD before surgery (**A**) and after Van Nes rotationplasty (**B**). Photographs standing with prosthesis from the front (**C**) and side (**D**) after van Nes rotationplasty.

SUMMARY

Adhering to several surgical principles can result in acceptable results in pediatric patients undergoing amputation. These principles are based on the child's growth and its effects on the residuum length and potential for terminal bony overgrowth. Treating children with congenital limb reductions and multiple limb involvement often requires a multidisciplinary approach. Surgical planning requires a thorough evaluation of the child, prediction of limb differences at maturity, and consideration of the family's and patient's needs and expectations in the context of the patient's whole body.

References

1. Borne A, Porter A, Recicar J, Maxson T, Montgomery C: Pediatric traumatic amputations in the United States: A 5-year review. *J Pediatr Orthop* 2017;37(2):e104-e107.
2. Wilkins KL, McGrath PJ, Finley AG, Katz J: Phantom limb sensations and phantom limb pain in child and adolescent amputees. *Pain* 1998;78(1):7-12.
3. Wilkins KL, McGrath PJ, Finley GA, Katz J: Prospective diary study of nonpainful and painful phantom sensations in a preselected sample of child and adolescent amputees reporting phantom limbs. *Clin J Pain* 2004;20(5):293-301.
4. DeMoss P, Ramsey LH, Karlson CW: Phantom limb pain in pediatric oncology. *Front Neurol* 2018;9:219.
5. Poor Zamany Nejatkermany M, Modirian E, Soroush M, Masoumi M, Hosseini M: Phantom Limb Sensation (PLS) and Phantom Limb Pain (PLP) among young landmine amputees. *Iran J Child Neurol* 2016;10:42-47.
6. Drotar D, Baskiewicz A, Irvin N, Kennell J, Klaus M: The adaptation of parents to the birth of an infant with a congenital malformation: A hypothetical model. *Pediatrics* 1975;56(5):710-717.
7. Varni JW, Setoguchi Y: Correlates of perceived physical appearance in children with congenital/acquired limb deficiencies. *J Dev Behav Pediatr* 1991;12(3):171-176.
8. Hall M, Cummings D, Welling R Jr, et al: Essentials of pediatric prosthetics. *J Pediatr Orthop Soc N Am* 2020;2:1-15.
9. Kelly PM, Diméglio A: Lower-limb growth: How predictable are predictions? *J Child Orthop* 2008;2(6):407-415.
10. Paley D, Bhave A, Herzenberg JE, Bowen JR: Multiplier method for predicting limb-length discrepancy. *J Bone Joint Surg Am* 2000;82(10):1432-1446.
11. Sanders JO, Karbach LE, Cai X, Gao S, Liu RW, Cooperman DR: Height and extremity-length prediction for healthy children using age-based versus peak height velocity timing-based multipliers. *J Bone Joint Surg Am* 2021;103:335-342.
12. Louer CR, Scott-Wyard P, Hernandez R, Vergun AD: Principles of amputation surgery, prosthetics, and rehabilitation in children. *J Am Acad Orthop Surg* 2021;29:e702-e713.
13. Huang CT, Jackson JR, Moore NB, et al: Amputation: Energy cost of ambulation. *Arch Phys Med Rehabil* 1979;60:18-24.
14. McQuerry J, Gammon L, Carpiaux A, et al: Effect of amputation level on quality of life and subjective function in children. *J Pediatr Orthop* 2019;39:e524-e530.
15. Feick E, Hamilton PR, Luis M, et al: A pilot study examining measures of balance and mobility in children with unilateral lower-limb amputation. *Prosthet Orthot Int* 2016;40:65-74.
16. Highsmith MJ, Lura DJ, Carey SL, et al: Correlations between residual limb length and joint moments during sitting and standing movements in transfemoral amputees. *Prosthet Orthot Int* 2016;40:522-527.
17. Frölke PM, Leijendekkers RA, van de Meent H: Osseointegrated prosthesis for patients with an amputation. *Unfallchirurg* 2017;120:293-299.
18. Al Muderis M, Lu W, Li JJ: Osseointegrated prosthetic limb for the treatment of lower limb amputations: Experience and outcomes. *Unfallchirurg* 2017;120(4):306-311.
19. Ramakrishnan T, Schlafly M, Reed KB: Effect of asymmetric knee height on gait asymmetry for unilateral transfemoral amputees. *Int J Curr Adv Res* 2017;6:6896-6903.
20. Parry IS, Mooney KN, Chau C, et al: Effects of skin grafting on successful prosthetic use in children with lower extremity amputation. *J Burn Care Res* 2008;29:949-954.
21. Fleming ME, O'Daniel A, Bharmal H, Valerio I: Application of the orthoplastic reconstructive ladder to preserve lower extremity amputation length. *Ann Plast Surg* 2014;73:183-189.
22. Marquardt E, Correll J: Amputations and prostheses for the lower limb. *Int Orthop* 1984;8(2):139-146.
23. Jahmani RA, Paley D: Stump overgrowth after limb amputation in children, in Fujioka M, ed: *Limb Amputation*. Intech Open, 2019.
24. Fedorak GT, Watts HG, Cuomo AV, et al: Osteocartilaginous transfer of the proximal part of the fibula for osseous overgrowth in children with congenital or acquired tibial amputation: Surgical technique and results. *J Bone Joint Surg Am* 2015;97(7):574-581.
25. O'Neal M, Bahner R, Ganey T, Ogden J: Osseous overgrowth after amputation in adolescents and children. *J Pediatr Orthop* 1996;16:78-84.
26. Tenholder M, Davids JR, Gruber HE, Blackhurst DW: Surgical management of juvenile amputation overgrowth with a synthetic cap. *J Pediatr Orthop* 2004;24:218-226.
27. Fedorak GT, Cuomo AV, Watts HG, Scaduto AA: Management of terminal osseous overgrowth of the humerus with simple resection and osteocartilaginous grafts. *J Pediatr Orthop* 2017;37:e215-e221.
28. McClenaghan BA, Krajbich JI, Pirone AM, Koheil R, Longmuir P: Comparative assessment of gait after limb-salvage procedures. *J Bone Joint Surg Am* 1989;71:1178-1182.
29. Mengelkoch LJ, Kahle JT, Highsmith MJ: Energy costs and performance of transfemoral amputees and non-amputees during walking and running: A pilot study. *Prosthet Orthot Int* 2017;41(5):484-491.
30. Jeans KA, Browne RH, Karol LA: Effect of amputation level on energy expenditure during overground walking by children with an amputation. *J Bone Joint Surg Am* 2011;93:49-56.
31. Jeans KA, Karol LA, Cummings D, Singhal K: Comparison of gait after syme and transtibial amputation in children: Factors that may play a role in function. *J Bone Joint Surg Am* 2014;96(19):1641-1647.
32. Kunutsor SK, Gillatt D, Blom AW: Systematic review of the safety and efficacy of osseointegration prosthesis after limb amputation. *Br J Surg* 2018;105(13):1731-1741.
33. Aitken GT: Proximal femoral focal deficiency: A congenital anomaly, in Aitken GT, ed: *National Academy of Sciences*. National Academy of Sciences, 1969.
34. Ghanem I: Epidemiology, etiology, and genetic aspects of reduction deficiencies of the lower limb. *J Child Orthop* 2008;2:329-332.
35. Wang Q, Peterson C: Your earliest memory may be earlier than you think: Prospective studies of children's dating of earliest childhood memories. *Dev Psychol* 2014;50:1680-1686.
36. James MA, Bagley AM, Brasington K, Lutz C, McConnell S, Molitor F: Impact of prostheses on function and quality of life for children with unilateral congenital below-the-elbow deficiency. *J Bone Joint Surg Am* 2006;88:2356-2365.
37. Crandall RC, Tomhave W: Pediatric unilateral below-elbow amputees: Retrospective analysis of 34 patients given multiple prosthetic options. *J Pediatr Orthop* 2002;22:380-383.
38. Swanson AB: The Krukenberg. *J Bone Joint Surg* 1963;46-A:1540-1610.
39. Syme J: On amputation at the ankle joint. *Lond Edinb Mon J Med Sci* 1843;26:93-96.

40. Boyd HB: Amputation of the foot, with calcaneotibial arthrodesis. *J Bone Joint Surg* 1939;21:997-1000.
41. Eilert R, Jayakumar S: Boyd and Syme amputations in children. *J Bone Joint Surg* 1976;58-A:1138-1141.
42. Maffulli N: Longitudinal deficiency of the fibula. Operative treatment. *J Bone Joint Surg Am* 1997;79:794-795.
43. Westberry DE, Davids JR, Pugh LI: The Boyd amputation in children: Indications and outcomes. *J Pediatr Orthop* 2014;34:86-91.
44. Jacobsen ST, Crawford AH, Millar EA, Steel HH: The Syme amputation in patients with congenital pseudarthrosis of the tibia. *J Bone Joint Surg Am* 1983;65:533-537.
45. Guille JT, Kumar SJ, Shah A: Spontaneous union of a congenital pseudarthrosis of the tibia after Syme amputation. *Clin Orthop Relat Res* 1998;351:180-185.
46. Borggreve J: Kniegelenksersatz durch das in der Beinlängsachse um 180 gedrehte Fussgelenk. *Arch Orthop Unfall-Chir* 1930;28:175-178.
47. Van Nes CP: Rotation-plasty for congenital defects of the femur. *J Bone Joint Surg Br* 1950;32:12-16.
48. Krajbich JI, Carroll NC: Van Nes rotationplasty with segmental limb resection. *Clin Orthop Relat Res* 1990;256: 7-13.
49. Kotz R, Salzer M: Rotation-plasty for childhood osteosarcoma of the distal part of the femur. *J Bone Joint Surg Am* 1982;64-A:959-969.
50. Alman BA, Krajbich JI, Hubbard S: Proximal femoral focal deficiency: Results of rotationplasty and Syme amputation. *J Bone Joint Surg Am* 1995;77:1876-1882.
51. Hanlon M, Krajbich JI: Rotationplasty in skeletally immature patients. Long-term followup results. *Clin Orthop Relat Res* 1999;358:75-82.
52. Gebert C, Hardes J, Vieth V, Hillmann A, Winkelmann W, Gosheger G: The effect of rotationplasty on the ankle joint: Long-term results. *Prosthet Orthot Int* 2006;30:316-323.

Role of Limb Lengthening in the Pediatric Amputee

Mark T. Dahl, MD, FAAOS • Stewart G. Morrison, MBBS • Andrew G. Georgiadis, MD, FAAOS

ABSTRACT

Residual limb length should be considered when optimizing gait, function, and satisfaction in the patient living with amputation. When an amputation residual limb is short, functional prosthetic fitting is challenging to achieve and hence a prosthesis may require anchorage more proximally. In the pediatric amputee, additional considerations are present, including the remaining potential growth of both limbs, which in the amputated limb will depend on the physes that are preserved.

Accurate terminology when measuring and comparing residual limb length is important and may be measured in relative (compared with the other limb) or absolute terms. Length modulation may involve epiphysiodesis or distraction osteogenesis, as used in the practice of limb lengthening. Lengthening of amputation residual limbs is a highly specialized application of distraction osteogenesis, and considerations include management of the residual soft-tissue envelope, the length and quality of bone available for fixation, and the effect of lengthening on remaining joints.

When approached diligently, residual limb lengthening can be used and has been described in the arm, forearm, thigh, and leg. The technologic development of internal motorized lengthening nail mitigates some of the complications presented by external fixators.

Keywords: amputation; distraction osteogenesis; external fixation; limb lengthening; motorized internal lengthening nails

Introduction

Congenital and acquired limb loss is a disabling condition that can significantly affect a person's quality of life. There are additional considerations when managing amputation in the pediatric patient that have implications for residual limb length (RLL), including the preference for transarticular rather than transosseous amputation, when possible, due to the problem of bone overgrowth; and the moving target of limb length difference in the growing patient, both pertaining to the amputated extremity as well as the contralateral limb. The presence or absence as well as the function and expected remaining growth of physes in both limbs must be considered. Congenital and developmental etiologies are overrepresented in this population compared with adult amputees, each bringing with it unique bone and soft-tissue difference in the limb that must be considered as a part of surgical and prosthetic intervention, to achieve the best function.

When an amputation residual limb is short, functional prosthetic fitting is challenging to achieve and hence a prosthesis may require anchorage more proximally. This may condemn the limb to function as an amputation of a more proximal level, increasing energy consumption during gait in the lower extremity, and reducing comfort and dexterity in the upper extremity. An overview of considerations and treatment strategies with regard to limb length management in the childhood amputee is presented.

Measuring RLL

RLL can be measured in absolute or proportional terms. Absolute length may be quantified in centimeters or inches as bone length radiographically, or bone length relative to a soft-tissue point (such as a flexion crease), or the RLL difference relative to the other limb (known as clearance from a prosthetic fitting perspective).[1]

Proportional methods may also be used; for example, a residual limb may be 70% the length of the contralateral limb, or described in terms of anatomic landmarks (the residual limb ends at the level of the contralateral distal tibial metaphysis). Additionally, in the patient with bilateral amputation, proportionality may be considered in relation to torso length, arm span, or other anatomic considerations.

When considering pediatric patients or implications for gait, a proportional method may be more informative. The physician should be aware, however, that prosthetic componentry is usually measured in absolute terms.

Dr. Dahl or an immediate family member has received royalties from Stryker and serves as a paid consultant to or is an employee of NuVasive and Stryker. Neither of the following authors nor any immediate family member has received anything of value from or has stock or stock options held in a commercial company or institution related directly or indirectly to the subject of this chapter: Dr. Morrison and Dr. Georgiadis.

Background of Distraction Osteogenesis

Bone lengthening was first described by Codivilla in 1905; however, it was Ilizarov who developed the modern methods of distraction osteogenesis, commonly known as the Ilizarov method.[2]

The factors Ilizarov viewed to be important for osteogenesis at an osteotomy site are:

1. Maximum preservation of extraosseous and endosteal blood supply
2. Stable circular external fixation
3. A delay before distraction begins
4. A lengthening rate of 1 mm per day divided in multiple small increments
5. A period of stable neutral fixation after distraction is complete
6. Functional use of the limb throughout treatment

The techniques of distraction osteogenesis as well as distraction histogenesis are useful not only for limb lengthening but also for the management of nonunions, bone deficits, and angular deformity.[3,4]

Such techniques were traditionally achieved using fine wire fixation, eponymously referred to as an Ilizarov apparatus or ring fixator. The innovation of hexapod style frames, commonly referred to as Taylor spatial frames, was a significant technologic advancement, but retained the disadvantages of earlier fixators of being cumbersome, uncomfortable, difficult to apply, and association with high complication rates.[5]

The introduction of the intramedullary skeletal kinetic distractor (Orthofix) intramedullary lengthening nail hailed the arrival of all-internal solutions for distraction osteogenesis, and these ratchet-based devices were driven by patient movement. The Fitbone (Orthofix) motorized intramedullary nail is activated by external remote control, and this was rapidly followed by the development of a second remote controlled nail, the PRECICE (NuVasive). Both implants are activated by an external signal, radiofrequency and magnetic, respectively.

These devices are useful in the context of residual limb lengthening, and both companies have developed modified devices specifically for short amputation residual limb lengthening (**Figure 1**).

Although motorized internal lengthening nails are less cumbersome and have been demonstrated to have lower rates of certain complications compared with their external fixation predecessors, some difficulties remain, and new problems have been introduced. The same limits of soft-tissue tolerance are present. New problems exist with the size limitations of the devices, particularly when trying to fit them within short residual limbs.

RLL Considerations

A residual limb should be long enough to allow comfortable and functional fitting of a prosthesis that does not impede the function or motion of more proximal joints, and be able to act as a functional lever arm within that prosthesis. A residual limb should not be so long, however, such that there is insufficient longitudinal space for prosthetic componentry to gain maximal achievable function. Preserving length is crucial in pediatric patients; for example, because the distal epiphyseal plate contributes 75% of longitudinal femoral growth, transfemoral amputation results in a very short final residual limb.[6]

Because of the type of amputations often performed in children, excessive length thought initially to be of advantage in retaining as much of the limb as possible may indeed hinder performance. Adolescents with Syme amputations were found to have higher self-reported function and satisfaction when their residual limb ended at the level of their contralateral tibial middiaphysis; a longer residual limb resulted in a limb with insufficient clearance space for the fitting of an energy return prosthesis and more prosthetic complications.[7] In both this setting as well as amputations performed for vascular overgrowth syndromes, well-timed epiphysiodesis or even acute intercalary shortening may be of utility in achieving ideal limb lengths at skeletal maturity.

Additionally, the local soft-tissue envelope (most evident in amputation posttrauma), as well as proximal joint stability and function (most important in congenital and developmental etiologies), needs be considered in a pediatric population.

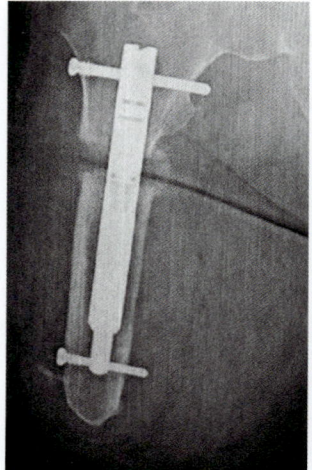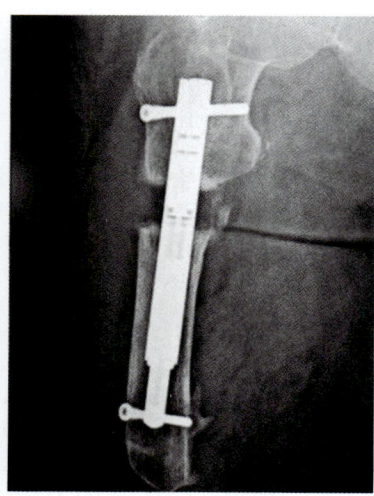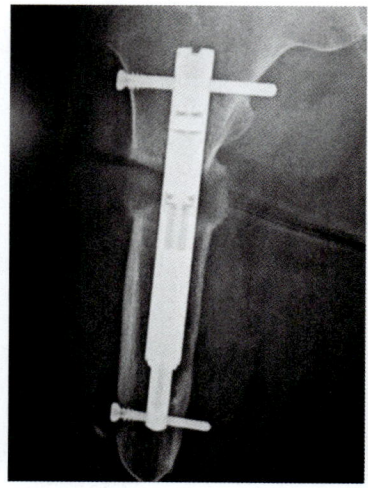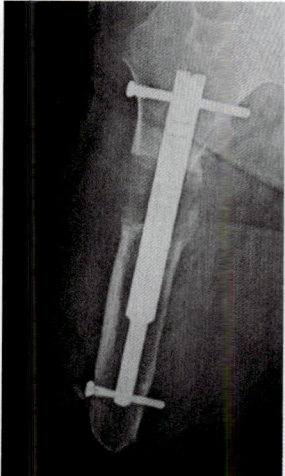

FIGURE 1 AP plain radiographs showing progressive femoral residual limb lengthening using an intramedullary motorized nail. Normotrophic regenerate can be appreciated throughout.

Lengthening

If indeed the residual limb is so short that more proximal prosthetic fitting is required, and the patient possesses a soft-tissue envelope that will tolerate it, residual limb lengthening may be of benefit. It is also unknown how much length will be necessary to benefit an individual patient.

The minimum RLL for adequate prosthetic fitting is highly variable, although studies have suggested bone length for a successful transtibial prosthesis should be 15 cm and for a transfemoral prosthesis 25 cm.[8-10]

The paucity of English language literature on residual limb lengthenings consists of brief case reports and small series.[8,11,12] Limb lengthening via distraction osteogenesis is an involved process even in complete limbs, requiring impeccable surgical technique, regular follow-up, and a nuanced and proactive approach to arising complications. Limb lengthening in the residual amputated limb adds further considerations, and should only be embarked upon by a surgeon and team confident in the technique, and a patient who has provided consent informed by comprehensive discussion.

External Fixation Technical Considerations

External fixation can be used to lengthen very short residual limbs, and although bone size, patient comfort, and wire or pin site complications may present problems, the most important limitation is the soft tissue's ability to stretch with the lengthened bone. Embarking on lengthening with anything less than generous soft-tissue coverage is a recipe for disaster.

Preoperative planning is critical. The patient should be measured so that rings of appropriate diameter are selected. Next, fixation is planned, with a combination of tensioned wires and half-pins. An atlas of cross-sectional anatomy is reviewed and closely correlated with any previous limb surgery, so that wires and pins do not impale or tether neurovascular structures. Ilizarov-specific atlases are available for this purpose.[13] Novel wire and pin placement, such as longitudinal pulling wires and cables,[14,15] can be used to minimize movement (travel) of the pin and wire (**Figure 2**). The cases discussed at the end of this chapter should be reviewed for some site-specific techniques regarding fixation placement.

Corticotomy is the act of cutting the bone via a low-energy technique that maintains maximal local vascularity to produce good regenerate bone. It is difficult in residual limb lengthening because of previous scarring, as well as the often extremely short distances between Ilizarov rings and fixation points. A corticotomy that fractures into a pin or wire site can destabilize the entire construct.

The transfixion wires or pins used in external fixation travel through the soft tissues of a limb by pressure necrosis, whereas the trailing edge of the wire/pin heals by secondary intention, similar to that seen in bone transport. This is much more pronounced than in nonamputation limb lengthening, where presumably the nondisrupted soft-tissue and skin attachments distal to the lengthening site and device allow for more evenly distributed traction by the underlying bony segment being moved. Soft tissues can be pushed ahead of the moving bone segments by a process of compressing the proximal skin and soft tissue with elastic wrapping, thereby recruiting additional tissue for lengthening of the bone. Reoperation to release tethered skin, or add additional fixation or sutures is common. When advancing bone threatens the skin integrity, lengthening must be slowed or stopped.

Motorized Nail Technical Considerations

The development of intramedullary motorized lengthening nails has hailed a paradigm shift in the field of limb lengthening, and the technology has been applied to amputation residual limbs. A major limitation is initial bony segment length and desired magnitude of lengthening. Minimum length for standard devices is approximately 150 mm; lengthening shorter segments therefore requires cutting of the implant, or implanting the device in a way that it extends beyond the length of the bone (perhaps in the trochanteric region). Specially designed residual limb lengthening nails exist. The Freedom Nail from NuVasive uses a double deployment mechanism to allow 100 mm of

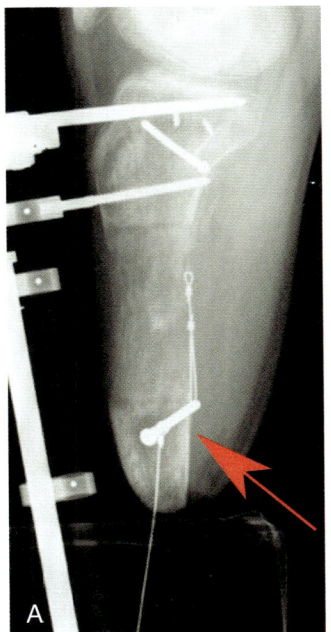
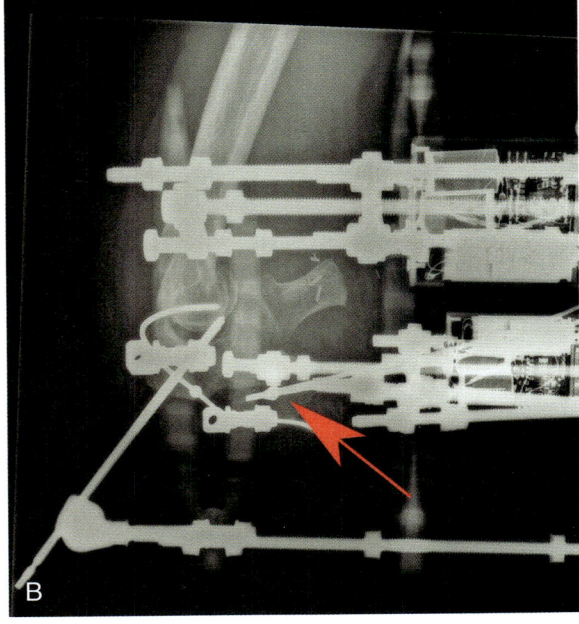

FIGURE 2 **A**, Lateral radiograph of a short proximal tibial residual limb undergoing lengthening by distraction osteogenesis with an external fixator. **B**, Lateral radiograph of a short forearm residual limb undergoing lengthening. Both are examples of pulling cables exiting the skin (red arrows) through the end of a residual limb, to reduce wire travel through skin. (Panel A, Courtesy of Professor Rainer Baumgart.)

lengthening from a nail starting length of only 130 mm, but these may not be available in all jurisdictions.

The use of these devices in children is limited by additional factors, including intermedullary canal size, the presence of actively growing physes (the crossing of which with an intramedullary nail may cause physeal arrest), and in the proximal femur, the blood supply of the femoral head and its anastomosis in the piriformis fossa—therefore, trochanteric-entry nails should be used. Recently developed techniques of extramedullary lengthening with modified or new devices, to overcome these pediatric considerations, have been published, but it is not yet known whether these techniques have been used in a residual limb lengthening situation.[16,17]

Intramedullary systems often allow only one or two interlocking screws per segment, which may be inadequate for the disuse osteopenia encountered in amputation residual limbs. Novel solutions may be required for achieving adequate fixation through which to lengthen.

Specific Applications

The Arm

Upper limb prosthetic technology has advanced significantly in recent years, but RLL remains important for function. The presence and location of the deltoid insertion must be considered when attempting humeral residual limb lengthening. Bernstein et al[1] report on a series that includes 10 humeral residual limb lengthenings, in one case achieving a length increase of a massive 438%, though of course these proportions depend on what is measured. The amputations were of traumatic, congenital, or burn etiologies. The patients in the series had a mean age of 13.7 years. All the skin problems that occurred were in patients who had previously sustained burns or trauma to their limb.

The Forearm

Forearm residual limb lengthening is essentially ulnar lengthening, with the ulna being the forearm bone of the elbow. Ulnar lengthening can be successful even in markedly short amputations. It is important to assess for the presence and function of a flexor mechanism (ie, a functioning biceps brachii or brachialis, inserting into the radial tuberosity and ulna, respectively). **Figure 3** shows the

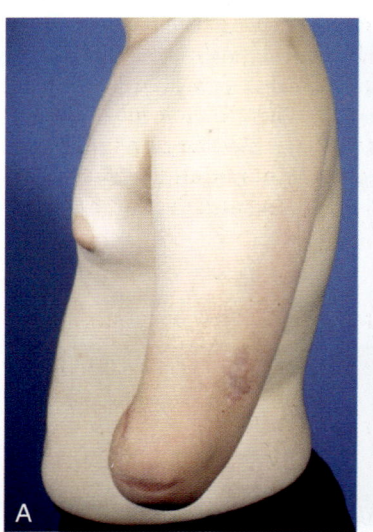
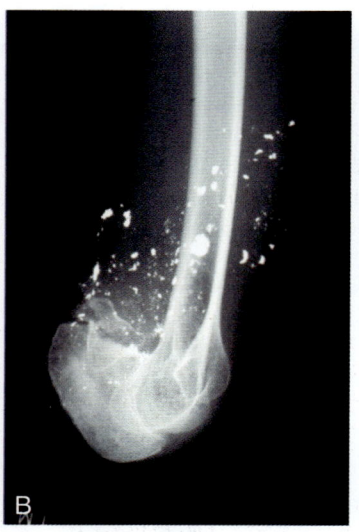
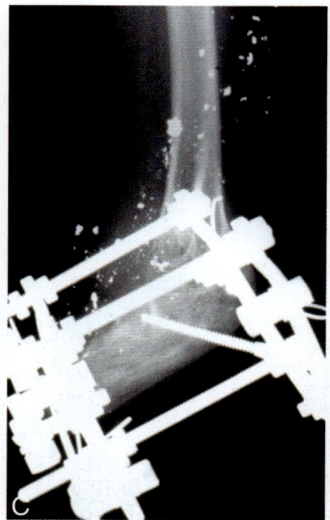
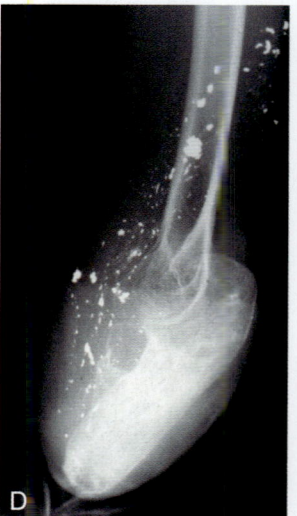
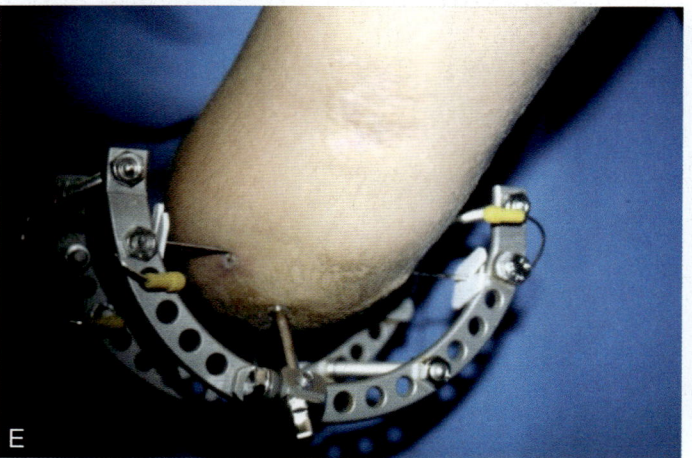
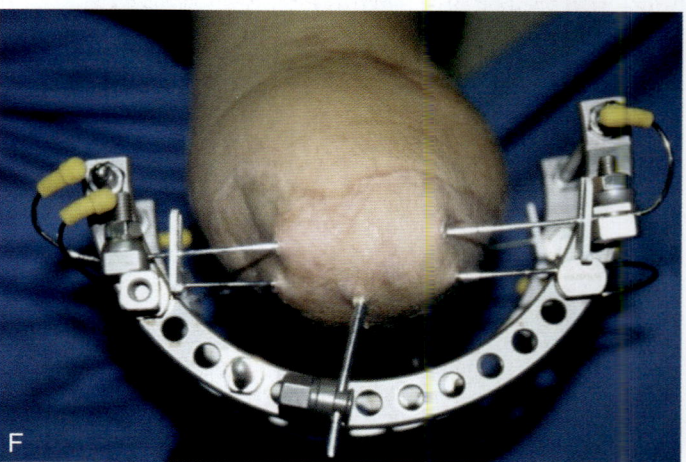

FIGURE 3 Clinical photograph showing a very short below-elbow residual limb with good elbow motion (**A**) undergoing lengthening. Lateral radiographs (**B**) before, (**C**) during, and (**D**) after lengthening. **E** and **F**, Clinical images of the external fixator during lengthening. In the plain radiograph with the fixator in place, appreciate the oblique pin placement.

Chapter 65: Role of Limb Lengthening in the Pediatric Amputee

left arm of a 14-year-old boy who sustained a gunshot wound. A 5-cm residual ulna residual limb had been salvaged along with a portion of the mobile flexor muscles, which provided an adequate soft-tissue envelope.

A modified Ilizarov fixator was preassembled using two half-rings connected together with three threaded rods. The proximal fragment was secured with a transverse, tensioned 1.8-mm wire, as well as a 4-mm half pin, directed obliquely and distally, thereby providing stability adjacent to the lengthening site, but entering skin at a point far remote to it (infection at a lengthening site is a disaster). Distally, two transverse wires are placed after placing the skin on traction distally, to recruit skin and lessen skin issues during the lengthening process. Finally, a distal half pin is placed almost longitudinally, again decreasing the force on skin.

Lengthening was stopped as distal skin became thin, reaching the preoperative goal of 5 cm lengthening, which doubled the RLL.

Figure 4 shows an amputation as a result of an industrial accident of the dominant arm of a skeletally mature male in whom good elbow joint motion was retained, but there is inadequate length for prosthetic fitting. The patient underwent initial lengthening with an external fixator, spanning the elbow to increase stability, with a pulling cable used to minimize skin travel of the wire. Seven centimeters of length was achieved, with progressive distal skin thinning. Following this, a myocutaneous free flap was applied to provide generous distal soft-tissue envelope. A motorized internal lengthening nail then allowed 5 cm of further length to be achieved.

The Femur

Figure 5 shows bilateral femoral amputation after an improvised explosive device injury. The right side required hip disarticulation-type prosthesis, resulting in poor gait. Sequential radiofrequency-activated motorized lengthening nails were used to achieve 8 cm each, allowing for transfemoral-style prosthetic fitting and independent ambulation.

Figure 6 shows traumatic transfemoral amputation in an 8-year-old child after a train accident. The patient underwent 8 cm of lengthening with a circular external fixator, using two convergent half-pins for proximal fixation and two maximally convergent smooth wires for distal fixation.

The Tibia

A case of external fixator (Ilizarov) lengthening of a short tibial residual limb in an 18-year-old patient who had sustained traumatic amputation at the age of 5 years is described by Eldridge et al.[18] They used a two-ring construct, noting that at 5 weeks, as expected the problem of skin thinning distally became apparent. This was managed with two procedures to place wires through the distal skin, transverse to the limb, which were then attached to elastic bands running longitudinally to a third ring on the frame. Although helpful initially, each of these sets of wires eventually cut out and

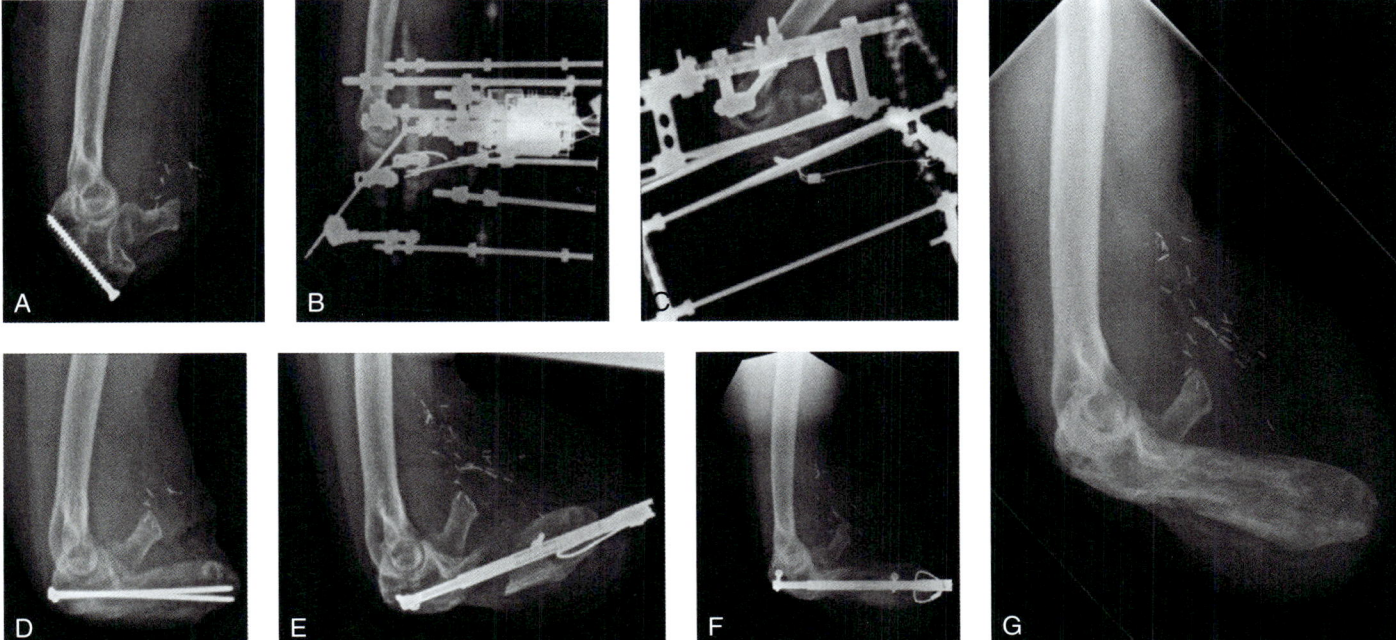

FIGURE 4 Plain lateral radiographs of a forearm lengthening using a series of two circular fixators (**A**, before lengthening; **B** and **C**, two successive external fixation lengthenings). At the end of lengthening, the ulna was provisionally fixed by long intramedullary screws to decrease second fixator time (**D**). Subsequent lengthening was performed with off-label use of an intramedullary motorized nail, which was cut with a diamond-tipped burr to diminish length, capped with the Silastic plug from the packaging to mitigate skin protrusion, and a pulling cable was used for distal fixation (**E**, early in lengthening; **F**, awaiting consolidation; **G**, consolidated lengthening site after implant removal). Total lengthening care ended in quadrupled ulnar length.

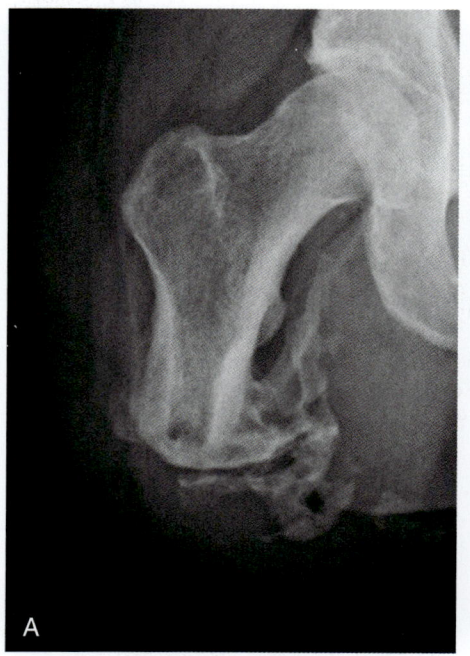
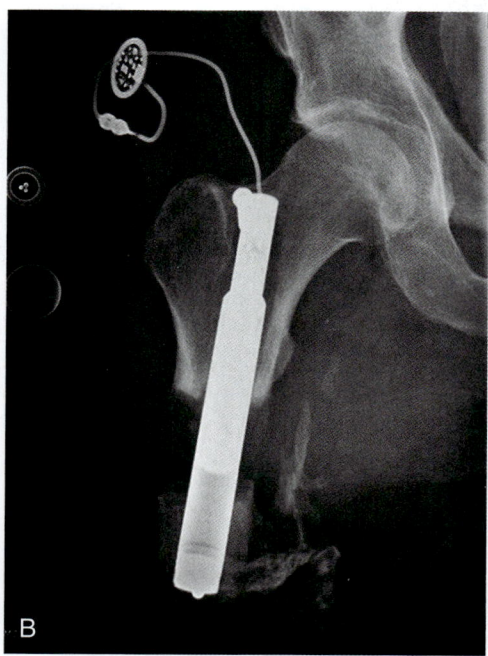
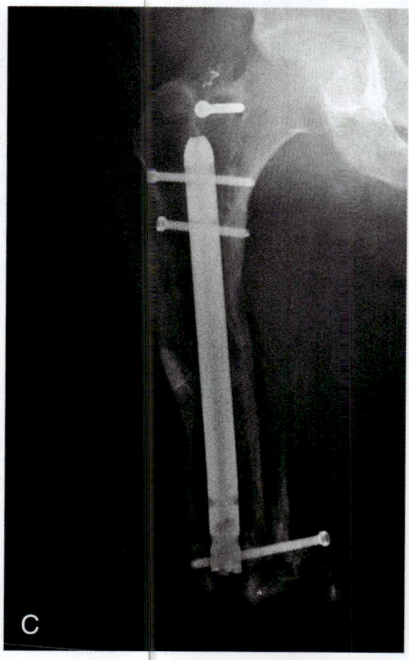
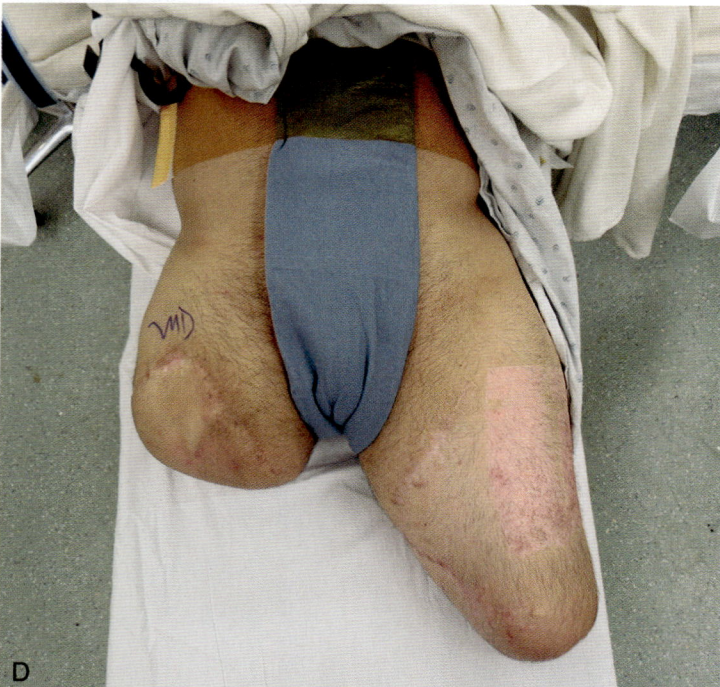
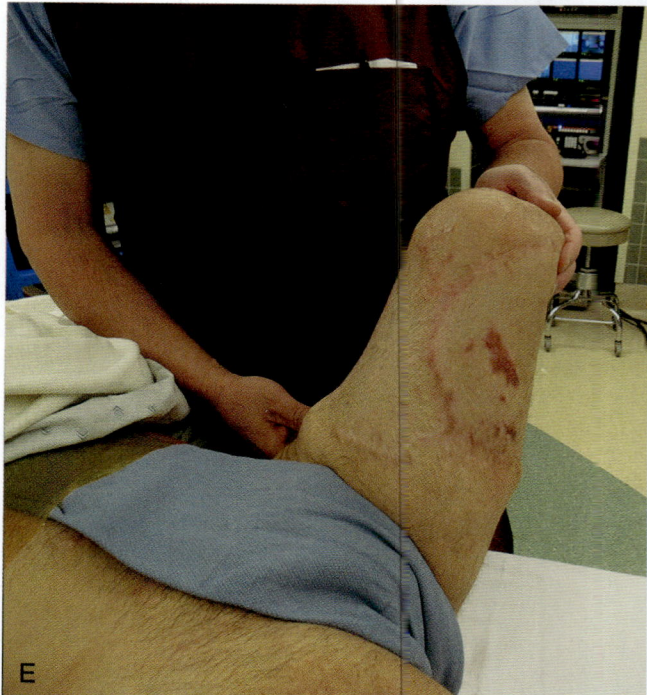

FIGURE 5 Images of the right femur. Plain AP radiographs (**A**) before lengthening, (**B**) during lengthening, and (**C**) after consolidation imaging. **D** and **E**, Clinical images of a double transfemoral amputee after an improvised explosive device injury.

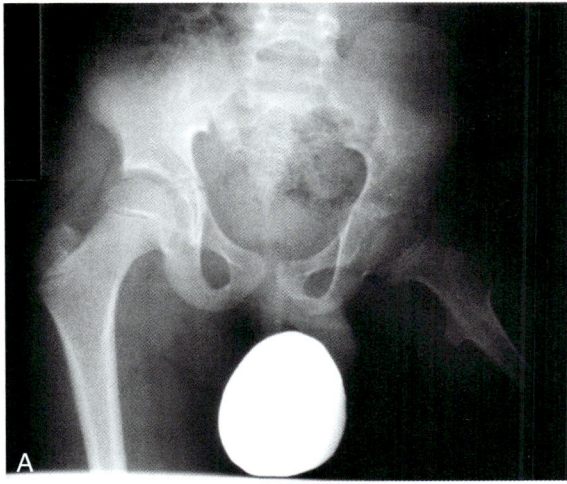 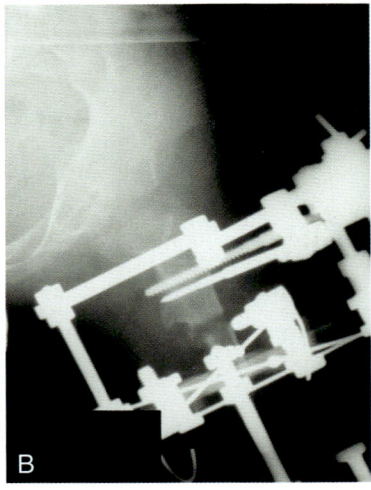 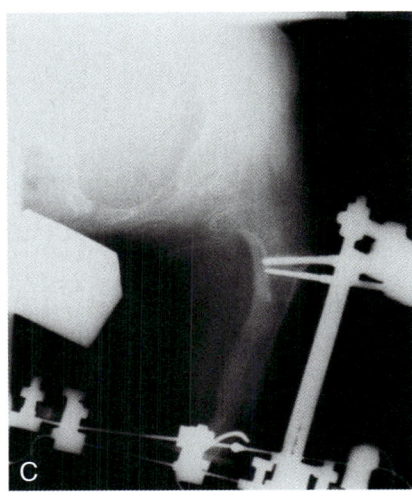

FIGURE 6 Plain AP radiographs demonstrating a short left transfemoral amputation. This patient was an 8-year-old child involved in a remote train accident with 9.5 cm of residual femur (**A**). A circular external fixator was used with maximally divergent convergent half-pins proximally and maximally divergent smooth pins distally (**B**), with successful lengthening of 8 cm (**C**). Total treatment time was 3.5 months.

ultimately skin problems necessitated a free myocutaneous flap. The authors recommend proactive skin coverage before lengthening, rather than as a salvage solution once problems are encountered.

As with any tibial lengthening, posterior bony consolidation occurs quicker than the less well vascularized anterior cortex, hence putting the lengthening site at risk of premature consolidation, as encountered and described by Toon et al.[19] Prevention of premature consolidation requires meticulous corticotomy technique, regular postoperative radiographs, and a method for proportionally faster distraction posteriorly if required. This may be achieved via the use of hexapod type systems or drop hinges, the use of both, however, being limited by the space available within the frame. These are advanced reconstruction techniques that require the oversight of an experienced limb reconstruction surgeon.

Complications

Fixation

Short residual segment length presents a technical challenge for surgical lengthening. All methods of distraction osteogenesis rely on adequate fixation in the distracted segment with pins, screws, wires, etc. Osteopenic bone may not provide sufficient pullout strength for implants and device failure can result (**Figure 7**), so more than one point of fixation is ideal in the distracted segment. Wire loops can be used to achieve purchase if the distal end of an intramedullary device is longer than the bone segment (**Figure 8**). Similarly, proximal segment bone stock can be poor, in which case additional rafting implants can be placed external to a lengthening nail but adjacent to its proximal portion, so as to provide push-off.

Contractures

Joint contractures adjacent to a prosthetic fitting may respond to soft-tissue stretching by serial casting and tendon releases. Metallic wires and pins are well tolerated through even unhealthy skin. Overcorrection of joint contracture is necessary, because of soft-tissue memory, and contractures will otherwise tend to recur. Burn contractures are often resistant to these treatments and can be managed with progressive

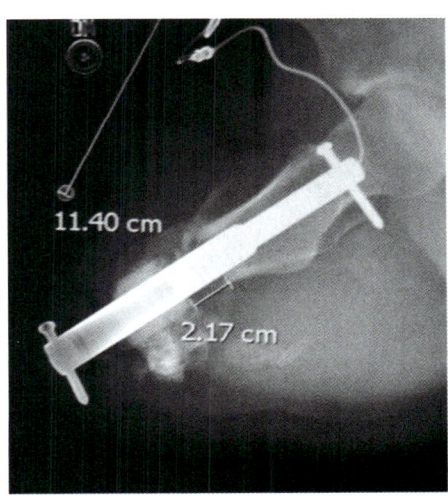

FIGURE 7 Plain lateral radiograph of a femoral residual limb undergoing intramedullary motorized residual limb lengthening. A single point of contact in osteopenic bone may result in loss of fixation. A traumatic femoral residual limb was just long enough for distal screw fixation through heterotopic bone, but implant pullout occurred after 2 cm of lengthening (notice the screw at left is no longer within bone).

stretching using circular external fixation (**Figure 9**). Ilizarov termed this phenomenon distraction histogenesis,[20] using it to great effect in other applications, such as joint contractures adjacent to nonunions.

 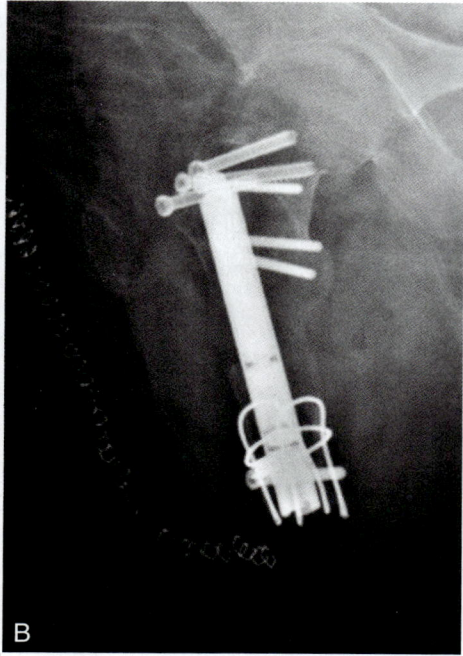 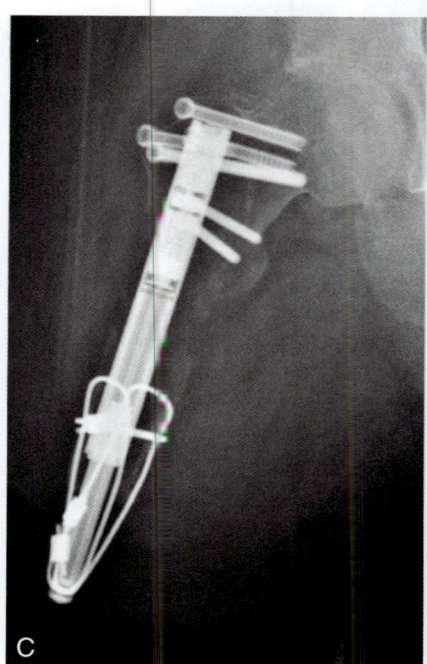

FIGURE 8 Plain AP radiographs of the femur demonstrating a fixation strategy for osteopenic bone (**A**). **B** and **C**, Two screws have been placed above the nail to prevent nail cutout, two screws adjacent to the nail to prevent the side-to-side migration and double cables have been routed through the interlocking screw holes at the end of the rod, and through the bone, as the rod is too long for traditional fixation. (Courtesy of Munjed Al Muderis, FRACS, FRCS (Ortho), MBChB.)

Soft-Tissue Strategies

A principle of traumatic amputation surgery is to preserve as much viable soft tissue as possible.[21] Combining preoperative soft-tissue assessments by a plastic surgeon, lengthening surgeon, prosthetist, and physical therapist, goals can be aligned for an individual patient. The following is a partial list of strategies to provide improved soft-tissue coverage. An orthoplastic reconstructive ladder is also described for conceptualizing the preservation of RLL by various soft-tissue strategies.[22]

Deep stretching can be done as a method to mobilize skin and soft tissue from underlying bone. This is difficult to measure, document, and assess. One of the chapter authors has had success in some patients using techniques to direct soft tissues distally before and during the lengthening process.

Preoperative soft-tissue advancement can be performed when asymmetric distal tissues are present.

Park et al[23] described the preservation of a gastrocnemius and heel flap preserved in a patient with multiple injuries resulting from a motor vehicle accident. A high transtibial amputation 4 weeks post injury was necessary because a deep wound infection developed. A gastrocnemius and a heel pad flap, containing the posterior tibial artery and nerve, was used to cover the end of the bony tibial residual limb, which was 5.5 cm long.

Gallico et al and Shenaq et al describe microvascular free tissue transfer for secondary amputation residual limb salvage and suggest that it is possible after infection has been eradicated.[24,25]

The use of prelengthening tissue expanders has been described,[26] but expanding the skin without the underlying soft tissues of muscle and fat can lead to rapid contraction of the tissue and thin end-bearing surfaces.

There is at least one report of phantom limb pain being exacerbated by Ilizarov residual limb lengthening,[27] but this would not be expected in residual limb lengthening in which phantom limb pain is absent preoperatively.

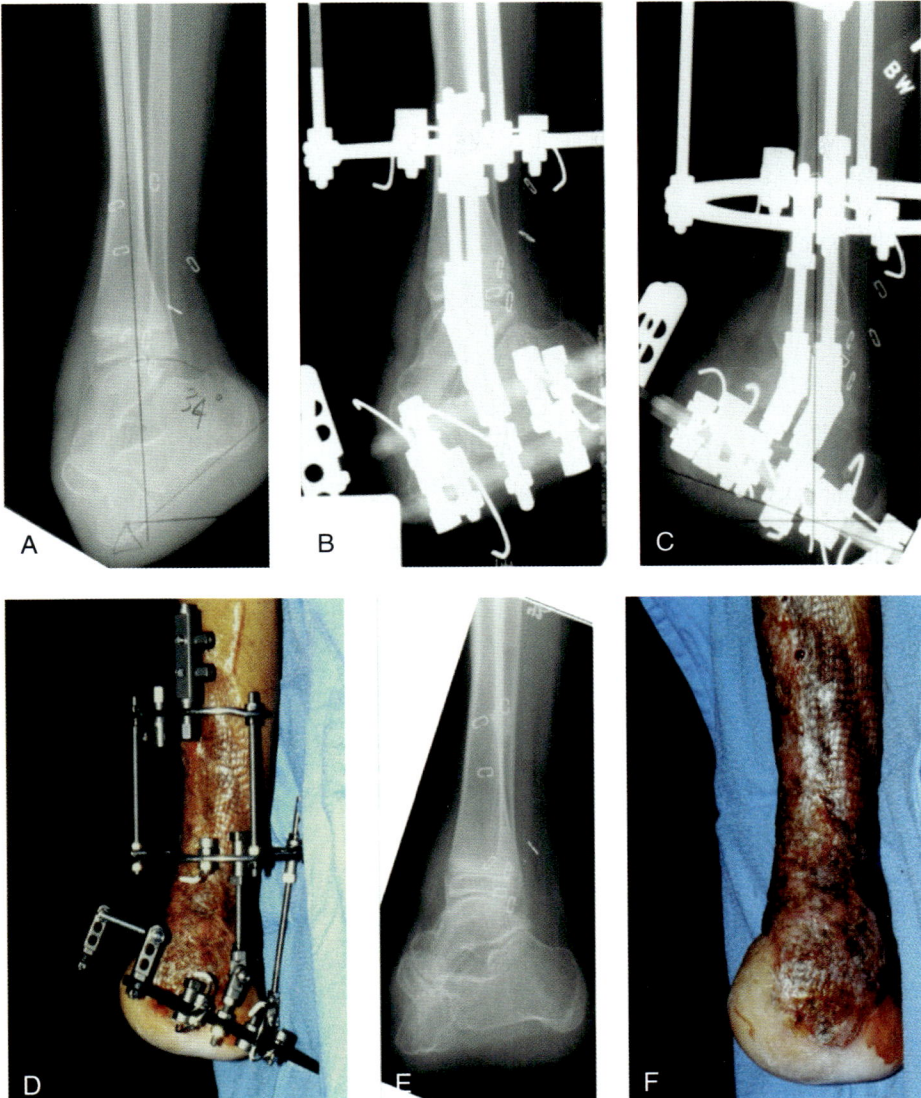

FIGURE 9 Clinical and plain radiographic images from a 12-year-old boy who sustained extensive burns and Chopart level amputation. At this level, the tibialis anterior insertion is absent, equinus contracture developed because of unopposed ankle plantar flexion (**A**). Correction with external fixation was performed (**B**, onset of treatment; **C** and **D**, terminus of treatment). The corrected position was maintained for twice the duration of correction, as soft-tissue rebound is expected to occur. Final result is a braceable Chopart amputation with neutral ankle alignment (**E** and **F**).

SUMMARY

Adequate RLL allows a lower consumption of energy and a more efficient gait using a prosthesis.[28] Amputation in pediatric patients has additional implications for RLL because of remaining growth, and as such, careful planning of ideal RLL is important in maximizing their satisfaction and function as young adults. Bone lengthening by distraction osteogenesis is an option in the appropriately selected patient but is more challenging than lengthening in other settings.

Good soft-tissue cover that is durable is a prerequisite before lengthening, as the need for bone length can result in protrusion of the bone through the skin. Lengthening can be achieved via external fixator, or where possible, intramedullary motorized nails, but should be performed by an expert in the field after close consultation with patient and prosthetist. Plastic surgery to achieve an adequate soft-tissue envelope may be best performed preemptively, rather than after problems arise.

References

1. Bernstein RM, Watts HG, Setoguchi Y: The lengthening of short upper extremity amputation stumps. *J Pediatr Orthop* 2008;28(1):86-90.
2. Birch JG: A brief history of limb lengthening. *J Pediatr Orthop* 2017;37 (suppl 2):S1-S8.
3. Ilizarov GA: The tension-stress effect on the genesis and growth of tissues: Part II. The influence of the rate and frequency of distraction. *Clin Orthop Relat Res* 1989;239:263-285.
4. Ilizarov GA: Clinical application of the tension-stress effect for limb lengthening. *Clin Orthop Relat Res* 1990;250:8-26.
5. Dahl MT, Gulli B, Berg T: Complications of limb lengthening. A learning curve. *Clin Orthop Relat Res* 1994;301:10-18.
6. Griffet J: Amputation and prosthesis fitting in paediatric patients. *Orthop Traumatol Surg Res* 2016;102(1 suppl):S161-S175.
7. Morrison SG, Thomson P, Lenze U, Donnan LT: Syme amputation: function, satisfaction, and prostheses. *J Pediatr Orthop* 2020;40(6):e532-e536.
8. Bowen RE, Struble SG, Setoguchi Y, Watts HG: Outcomes of lengthening short lower-extremity amputation stumps with planar fixators. *J Pediatr Orthop* 2005;25(4):543-547.
9. Volpicelli LJ, Chambers RB, Wagner FW Jr: Ambulation levels of bilateral lower-extremity amputees. Analysis of one hundred and three cases. *J Bone Joint Surg Am* 1983;65(5):599-605.
10. Waters RL, Perry J, Antonelli D, Hislop H: Energy cost of walking of amputees: The influence of level of amputation. *J Bone Joint Surg Am* 1976;58(1):42-46.
11. Latimer HA, Dahners LE, Bynum DK: Lengthening of below-the-knee amputation stumps using the Ilizarov technique. *J Orthop Trauma* 1990;4(4):411-414.
12. Mertens P, Lammens J: Short amputation stump lengthening with the Ilizarov method: Risks versus benefits. *Acta Orthop Belg* 2001;67(3):274-278.
13. Catagni MA: *Atlas for the Insertion of Transosseous Wires and Half-Pins: Ilizarov Method*, ed 2. Medi Surgical Video, 2003.

14. Baumgart R, Hinterwimmer S, Krammer M, Mutschler W: Central cable system--fully automatic, continuous distraction osteogenesis for the lengthening treatment of large bone defects. Article in German. *Biomed Tech (Berl)* 2004;49(7-8):202-207.

15. Quinnan SM, Lawrie C: Optimizing bone defect reconstruction-balanced cable transport with circular external fixation. *J Orthop Trauma* 2017;31(10):e347-e355.

16. Dahl MT, Morrison SG, Laine JC, Novotny SA, Georgiadis AG: Extramedullary motorized lengthening of the femur in young children. *J Pediatr Orthop* 2020;40(10):e978-e983.

17. Shannon C, Paley D: Extramedullary internal limb lengthening. *Tech Orthop* 2020;35(3):6.

18. Eldridge JC, Armstrong PF, Krajbich JI: Amputation stump lengthening with the Ilizarov technique. A case report. *Clin Orthop Relat Res* 1990;256:76-79.

19. Toon DH, Khan SA, Wong KHY: Lengthening of a below knee amputation stump with Ilizarov technique in a patient with a mangled leg. *Chin J Traumatol* 2019;22(6):364-367.

20. Aronson J: Experimental and clinical experience with distraction osteogenesis. *Cleft Palate Craniofac J* 1994;31(6):473-481.

21. Burgess EM, Zettl JH: Amputations below the knee. *Artif Limbs* 1969;13(1):1-12.

22. Fleming ME, O'Daniel A, Bharmal H, Valerio I: Application of the orthoplastic reconstructive ladder to preserve lower extremity amputation length. *Ann Plast Surg* 2014;73(2):183-189.

23. Park HW, Jahng JS, Hahn SB, Shin DE: Lengthening of an amputation stump by the Ilizarov technique. A case report. *Int Orthop* 1997;21(4):274-276.

24. Gallico GG III, Ehrlichman RJ, Jupiter J, May JW Jr: Free flaps to preserve below-knee amputation stumps: Long-term evaluation. *Plast Reconstr Surg* 1987;79(6):871-878.

25. Shenaq SM, Krouskop T, Stal S, Spira M: Salvage of amputation stumps by secondary reconstruction utilizing microsurgical free-tissue transfer. *Plast Reconstr Surg* 1987;79(6):861-870.

26. Persson BM, Broome A: Lengthening a short femoral amputation stump. A case of tissue expander and endoprosthesis. *Acta Orthop Scand* 1994;65(1):99-100.

27. Novikov K, Subramanyam K, SV K, Chegurov O, Kolesnikova E, Mundargi A: Ilizarov stump lenthening can aggravate phantom limb pain – A case report. *Arch Bone Jt Surg* 2018;6(3):240-243.

28. Gailey RS, Wenger MA, Raya M, et al: Energy expenditure of trans-tibial amputees during ambulation at self-selected pace. *Prosthet Orthot Int* 1994;18(2):84-91.

Traumatic Amputations of the Lower Extremity in Children and Adolescents

Robin C. Crandall, MD, FAAOS

ABSTRACT

Major lower extremity amputations from trauma in children and adolescents are not common. These injuries are devastating and are associated with many potential and expected complex complications that are not present in adult age groups. Incorporation of a realistic and compassionate team strategy will maximize best outcomes.

Keywords: angular deformity; bony overgrowth; limb reconstruction; pediatric lower extremity traumatic amputation

Introduction

Injuries in children that are severe enough to result in a major lower extremity amputation are not common. Cumulatively, many of these patients exist despite major advances in limb salvage, revascularization procedures, and limb replantation. Complications are particularly common in the pediatric patient with a traumatic amputation and need to be anticipated early. Not only are the typical complications of infection, delayed healing, compartment syndromes, and chronic pain issues present but also bony overgrowth, progressive angular deformity with or without physeal damage, and poor residual limb durability into adult life. It is of fundamental importance that the surgical team recognize an injury that ultimately is best managed by a level of amputation. If an amputation decision is made, the team then must finally try to create a residual limb that is durable and supports the high level of activity in these young individuals.

First, information on overall etiology and incidence data relevant to the pediatric lower extremity trauma amputee is provided. Next, current decision-planning strategies regarding reconstruction versus amputation in pediatric patients affected by major lower extremity traumas are discussed. Specific levels are then addressed, including ankle-level amputation, transtibial amputation, knee disarticulation, and above-knee amputation. Each level includes specific complicating issues, key aspects of surgical techniques, and current prosthetic strategies. Partial foot amputations, which represent a high percentage of pediatric lower extremity amputations, are outside the scope of this chapter. Before final conclusions, psychological and medical legal issues should be discussed.

Etiology and Incidence

The exact incidence of major (ankle-level and above) pediatric lower extremity traumatic amputations is not known. Most traumatic amputations occurring in the United States in children and adolescents involve fingers and toes. In a study of emergency department visits from 1990 to 2002, with an amputation diagnosis in children, 91% of these were to fingers.[1] Borne et al[2] studied data in children from 2002 to 2011 using the National Trauma Data Bank, noting 54% finger and 20% toe amputations. Major lower extremity amputations in this study showed 5.9% foot and ankle, and 14.8% transtibial amputations and transfemoral amputations of the 2,238 amputations identified. Conner,[3] using the Kids Inpatient Database, also noted that of 956 pediatric traumatic amputations in 1 year (2003) severe enough to require hospitalization, 64% were to fingers and toes, with foot and leg combined at 10%. The Borne study indicates that a per-year incidence of ankle-level and above traumatic amputations would average approximately 93 per year, a number nearly identical in the Conner review.[2,3] National Trauma Data Bank data, however, are not all inclusive because they do not have specific data from private or nontrauma centers. Inclusion of data is highly encouraged from trauma centers but not mandated. A significant additional factor is that in studies on young adults, lower extremity traumatic injuries that ultimately result in amputation are amputated months to years after initial hospitalization and are not part of initial database searches.[4]

The etiology and mechanism of primary injury that results in a lower extremity amputation in children varies with age and which region of the world or portion of the United States the patient lives. In the study by Loder et al[5] of 165 pediatric traumatic amputees treated in the upper Midwest over a 20-year period, the most common mechanism was powered lawn mower (PLM) trauma (69 of 165) followed by farm machinery (57 of 165) and then motor vehicle collision (38 of 165). The Borne et al[2] study of the entire United States

Neither Dr. Crandall nor any immediate family member has received anything of value from or has stock or stock options held in a commercial company or institution related directly or indirectly to the subject of this chapter.

further reflected PLM as the primary mechanism of major lower extremity amputation in young children (age 5 years or younger), but motor vehicle collision was most common in children older than 12 years. This study also indicated farm machinery was the second most common overall mechanism, which caused mostly finger and toe amputations (83%). Intentional and unintentional firearms trauma accounted for 6.1% of all pediatric amputations with 80% in the adolescent age bracket. Firearms trauma in 16- to 17-year-olds resulted in high levels of major lower extremity amputation (48% transfemoral amputations and transtibial amputations) with identified vascular injury from firearms in 64% of transtibial amputations and 75% of transfemoral amputations. Siracuse et al[6] noted higher risk of amputation in firearm trauma compared with nonfirearm penetrating trauma. Other causes of major lower extremity amputations in children include train injuries, thermal injury, and explosion.[2,3,5]

PLM trauma in the United States remains a significant cause of major lower extremity amputation, notably backover trauma in young children. Children with small body size can be hard to see and operators using hearing protection are unable to sense them when in proximity (**Figure 1**). A six times higher likelihood of severe lower extremity amputation in children younger than 5 years has been noted when comparing with those aged 6 years and older.[2] In the 25-year study by Ren et al[7] of PLM injuries in children, an estimated 1,641 backover injuries occurred, 70% in children younger than 5 years. This study also noted a significant decrease in PLM injuries from 1990 to 2014. The decrease in PLM-related injury may be due to increased public awareness in addition to improved safety features. Multiple studies have shown that in evaluating the rate of PLM trauma versus age, a bimodal pattern is clearly present with a peak in ages 1 to 5 years and a second peak in ages 10 to 17 years.[2,3,6] Younger children are generally struck by PLMs; older children are usually injured when operating PLMs. Males

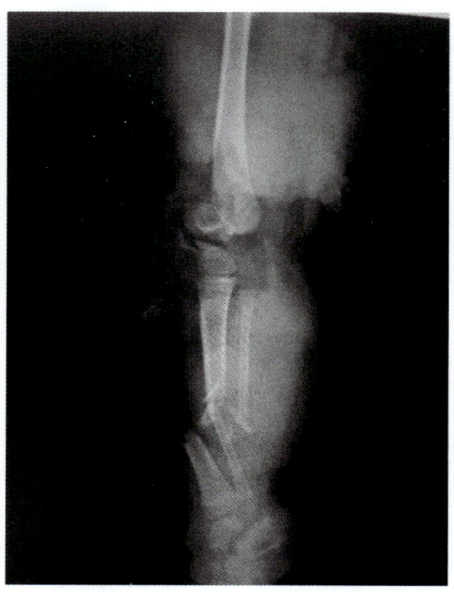

FIGURE 1 Lateral radiograph showing severe mangled extremity in a child from powered lawn mower (PLM) backover trauma. With adequate perfusion, reconstruction should be attempted but possibility of amputation should be discussed early and not framed as failure.

were predominant in all age groups, with higher percentages of males in older age groups.[2,3] Quantification of exact PLM types involved in injury is needed. This is particularly true of zero radius mowers that require backup to fully operate steering. Currently, safety features on non–zero radius mowers include no mow in reverse and have been present on most equipment since 2004 (American National Standards Institute/Outdoor Power Equipment Institute B71.1-2003). Safety features can be bypassed either by override switches provided by the manufacturer or by nonauthorized fixes often presented on social media video.

Worldwide, etiologies that cause major traumatic lower extremity amputations in children are different. Ahmad et al[9] reported a series of traumatic amputations primarily involving the lower extremities in children and adolescents from northern India. These authors indicated road trauma followed by train accidents as the most common mechanisms. Roche and Selvarajah[10] retrospectively reviewed 83 major pediatric lower extremity amputations in the United Kingdom, noting accidents on the road accounting for 63%, nearly a third being pedestrians struck by a bus. Train and farm trauma followed with surprisingly no PLM listed as a mechanism.

Landmine explosion trauma continues to be a significant etiology and unfortunately involves a high percentage of children and adolescents.[11] Soroush et al[12] studied 3,713 landmine victims from Iran during the period 1988 to 2003. These authors identified 1,499 amputations with 41% in patients age 18 years or younger; most of the amputations being transtibial. The primary reason for encountering a landmine was walking with livestock for grazing. The actual number of worldwide traumatic amputations involving children from landmines is unknown. It is established that landmine blast injuries are fatal in 21.1% of these pediatric patients because of their small body mass and proximity of organ systems to the blast, compared with 10.7% in adults.[13]

Decision Making: Reconstruction Versus Amputation

A key factor in managing severe pediatric lower extremity trauma is the surgical team's initial strategy and planning regarding a large array of modern treatment options. With the advent of wound vacs, improved macrovascular and microvascular vessel repair techniques, free flap transfers, and improved antibiotic and medical management strategies, more limbs are being salvaged.[14-18] Surgeon bias and lack of available resources, particularly vascular team availability, can be important factors. In a study of young patients with amputations that occurred during military service, the main reason for an immediate or primary lower extremity amputation following trauma appears to be prolonged loss of circulatory status, especially with crush injuries to popliteal or posterior tibial vessels.[19]

Prolonged or unrecognized compartment syndrome with perfusion loss in comatose or obtunded individuals can necessitate an amputation early in treatment. With reasonable perfusion or the ability and team resources to obtain perfusion, reconstruction or limb salvage should be the initial approach. Careful preoperative and surgical assessment must be carried out. Systematic débridement of open injuries with documentation of tissue viability, nerve loss, and bone loss is needed. Major nerve loss should not be regarded as a reason for amputation.[20] With PLM and farm machinery trauma, multiple surgical débridement procedures and assessments will be needed to eliminate multiple infective organisms.[5,21,22] It is expected that with high-velocity, explosion, or firearms trauma, tissue that initially appeared viable may not be. In children or adolescents, injuries severe enough to consider amputation may also involve damage to neighboring physes, other extremities, or organ systems. Children and adolescents have a more robust ability for wound healing after trauma than adults.[23]

One of the most difficult challenges facing patients, families, and clinician is making the decision that an amputation will be required. The surgical team must understand that long-term outcome should be predicated on long-term function, not a mindset to preserve a limb at all costs. If the surgical team frames an amputation of a severely mangled extremity as an unsuccessful outcome, the family is deprived of crucial information.[24] A painful, insensate lower extremity with poor joint mobility and lacking durable skin coverage will likely be functionally inferior to a converted amputation. However, even though cosmesis is likely severely altered, a sensate or even partially sensate extremity with a plantigrade foot that can support walking and normal shoe wear is the key factor in successful reconstruction outcome. The distinction does blur because major trauma–damaged extremities are not identical (**Figures 2** through **4**).

Studies comparing long-term follow-up of strictly pediatric patients undergoing traumatic major lower extremity amputation versus limb salvage are not available. Adolescent patients treated at pediatric centers are often lost to follow-up upon graduation.

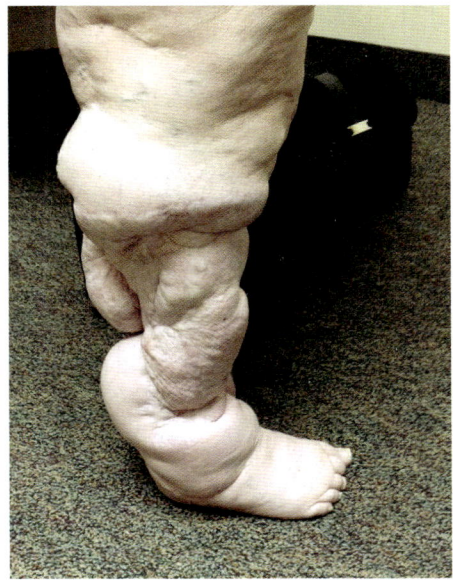

FIGURE 2 Photograph many years after reconstructive limb salvage following a motor vehicle accident; the patient considers herself pain free, although a cane is required full time for ambulation. The foot is plantigrade, but because of extrinsic/intrinsic imbalance custom shoe wear is needed.

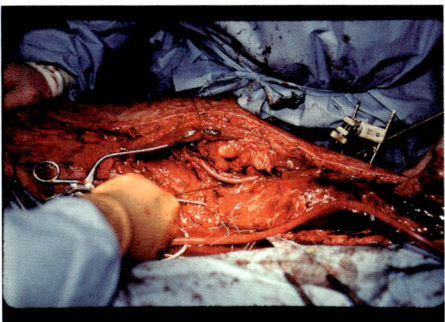

FIGURE 3 Intraoperative photograph from a patient following a fall while water-skiing resulting in severe knee hyperextension and complete popliteus artery disruption. Segmental reconstruction of popliteus artery and fasciotomies were carried out. The limb remains viable but is chronically painful with severe joint stiffness of knee and ankle. The patient and family refused further surgery or consideration of amputation.

Pediatric patients are often blended in studies with adult trauma patients. Overall numbers of major lower extremity amputations in children following trauma are small. In Baldwin et al's[25] multiple-center systematic review of 726 pediatric open fractures of the tibia, only 9 limbs required amputation. In one study comparing 18 patients with amputation versus 21 patients with microvascular reconstruction, reconstruction was thought to be better long term even though initial cost was higher.[26] In contrast, another study comparing 27 patients who underwent limb salvage using free flaps with 18 patients with transtibial amputation noted that significantly more patients who had reconstruction considered themselves disabled[27] ($P < 0.05$). In Busse et al's[14] multicenter comparison of 384 limb salvage cases with 161 primary amputations, both groups were associated with high rates of self-reported disability, 40% to 50% with worsening over time. Functional outcomes from both groups were not significantly different and costs were significantly higher in the reconstructed group. Importantly, most of the patients in whom limb salvage failed would opt for early amputation if they could decide again. Ladlow et al[28] noted in a study of young adult patients injured during military service comparing reconstruction versus amputation that the group with unilateral amputation demonstrated significant functional advantage. It is important to distinguish success as not just tissue viability but patient functionality. This is particularly important in active pediatric patients with many decades of life remaining. Prosthetic advances with respect to materials, componentry, and socket design have also improved function in patients with an amputation, most notably at the transfemoral level.[29]

Replantation of a fully amputated lower extremity in children is controversial. Anecdotal case reports in children with long-term follow-up are documented in the literature.[30,31] In a recent analysis of 50 years of replantation surgeries, fewer attempts and a decreased success rate have been noted in the United States with regard to all types of replantation.[32]

If a decision is made to amputate a lower extremity in a child, regardless of level, Krajbich[33] listed the following important general guidelines:

1. Preserve length
2. Preserve physes
3. Avoid a transosseous amputation
4. Preserve the knee joint

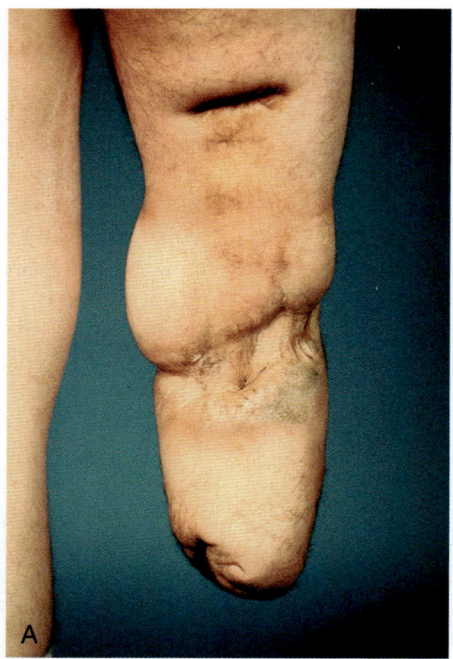
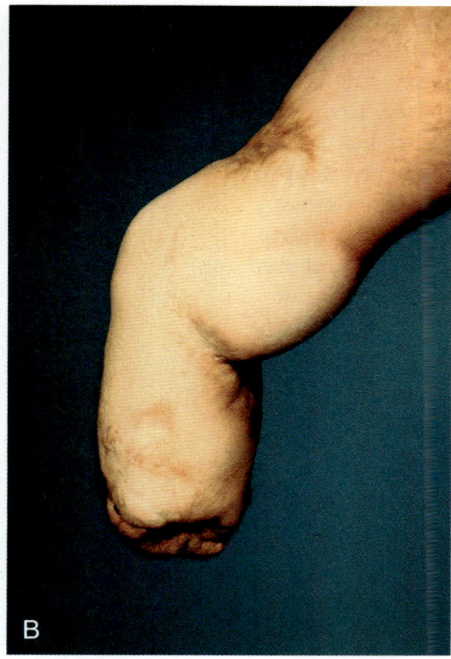

FIGURE 4 Clinical photographs from a pediatric patient with traumatic transtibial amputation who underwent initial reconstruction with failure and eventual amputation. The patient is pain free and capable of distance running with a modern dynamic response prosthesis. Multiple scars and skin-grafted areas have not affected prosthetic wear. **A**, Posterior view showing reconstruction of popliteal space. **B**, Lateral view of residual limb.

It is valuable that the patient and family are educated in rehabilitation strategies and prosthetic choices. Visits from other children who have undergone amputation, psychological consultation, and presentation of the amputation as a good treatment option and not a failure are very helpful. Rehabilitative efforts that improve balance and ambulation need to be incorporated very early.[34]

Traumatic Ankle-Level Amputations

A severely mangled or injured foot may require more than a partial foot amputation. This is particularly true with extreme hindfoot trauma.[35] It is difficult to obtain long-term data of large numbers of pediatric or adolescent patients with a traumatic ankle-level amputation. Many children with traumatic ankle-level amputations are initially treated at community hospitals or trauma centers, not necessarily pediatric centers. In a systematic review by Braaksma et al,[36] of 238 children with Syme amputation 94% were congenital. It is of extreme importance that the surgical team consider Syme or modified ankle-level amputation such as Boyd rather than a transtibial level amputation.[37] Although the usual surgical flap is posterior in a Syme or Boyd amputation, in trauma all possibilities should be considered, including anterior, medial, lateral, or sagittal flaps, to avoid transtibial level amputation. Transtibial amputations in children will generate a vexing array of complications, including diminished residual limb growth, bony overgrowth, and angular deformity, which are discussed in the next section. Ankle-level amputations are well tolerated in children with excellent survivability into adulthood.[38-40]

Usual surgical details of the Syme and Boyd amputation have been described. **Figure 5** shows details of the posterior flap as described by Wagner.[41] In the Syme amputation it is important to keep the talocalcaneal dissection on bone, particularly medially to avoid vascular damage. Removal of the Achilles tendon from the calcaneus should be done carefully to avoid buttonholing through the skin; all parts of the calcaneus should be removed. Leaving residual calcaneal apophysis is common and may lead to a more bulbous residual limb or heel pad

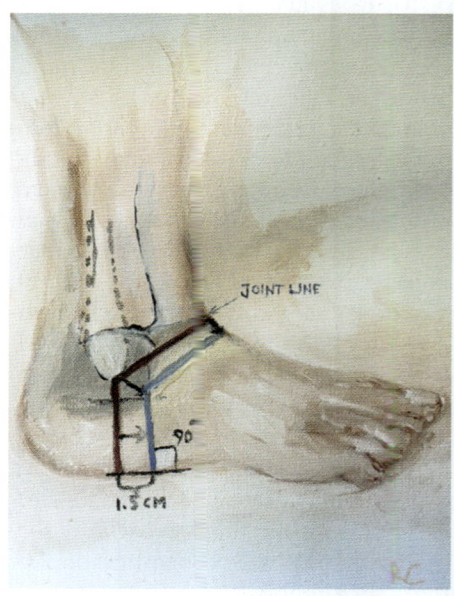

FIGURE 5 Illustration demonstrating traditional Syme incision with apex of incision at malleolar tips following joint line anterior and perpendicular to plantar axis distally (red line). For stage one or trauma with swelling, enlarging 1 to 1.5 cm anterior to joint line and 1 to 1.5 cm distal and anterior to malleoli will allow a closure without sacrificing critical skin (blue line).

migration. In trauma, modifications may often be necessary. Frequently, inadequate skin coverage occurs. Malleolar excision may help in wound closure. In PLM and farm machinery trauma, multiple contaminating organisms may be anticipated[5,21,42,43] and multiple surgical débridements needed. After final wound débridement has been accomplished, the team should not be reluctant to use split-thickness skin graft if needed. It has been shown by Parry et al[44] that the presence of skin grafts on a child's amputated limb does not adversely affect outcome or cause greater prosthetic problems. Full-thickness coverage over weight-bearing areas may be accomplished in later staged procedures; anything that avoids the transtibial level in a child is a major success.

Although ankle-level amputations avoid the complications of transtibial levels, it is crucial to create an ankle-level amputation that is not too long. A pediatric Syme amputation is easier to fit and allows for more generally available prosthetic component options if somewhat shorter than the sound side. Morrison et al[39] recently documented this concept showing improved function in children with shorter residual limb Syme amputation in a study of 47 patients with Syme amputation. Others have published studies on this concept.[45] The Chopart amputation where talus and calcaneus are preserved can be very awkward to manage, as well as Syme or Boyd procedures, if tibial growth is normal on the amputated side. In adult groups, Chopart level ablation has been shown to create much difficulty in successful prosthetic fitting[46] (Figure 6). A shoe lift is often needed on the sound side. Fortunately, in children, length can be manipulated by physeal arrest.

Physeal arrest to improve prosthetic options, cosmesis, and potential function in the child with ankle-level amputation should be carried out at an age that will allow at least 4 to 6 cm of shortening. Green-Anderson-Messner charts[47] are used in this planning and have been shown to be very effective where proximal tibial and fibular physes are ablated.[48] This is often carried out during early adolescence (Figure 7). Drill ablation is the preferred method; however, both drill or screw physeal arrest has shown similar outcomes in nonamputee patient groups.[49] To avoid varus deformity or proximal fibular migration, proximal fibular arrest is also recommended. It has been shown that if less than 2 years of growth remain, proximal fibular arrest may not be needed.[50]

Physeal arrest should be done with caution in young children in light of higher risk of complications, including asymmetric arrest and rare articular deformity possibilities.[51] A criticism of physeal arrest in the patient with Syme amputation is the possibility of decreasing ambulation without a prosthesis. It has been shown that after age 11 years in the child with Syme amputation, there is a general lowering of ability to walk without a prosthesis, also dependent upon walking environment.[52] Physeal arrest can be done distally at the ankle, but care must be taken not to create a distal tibial-fibular synostosis. Following severe trauma, a spontaneous synostosis may also occur at the ankle. In young children, a varus knee deformity can result from the distal tibial-fibular synostosis[53] (Figure 8).

Severe hindfoot and plantar trauma such as shredding or explosion injury can present difficulties as the usual

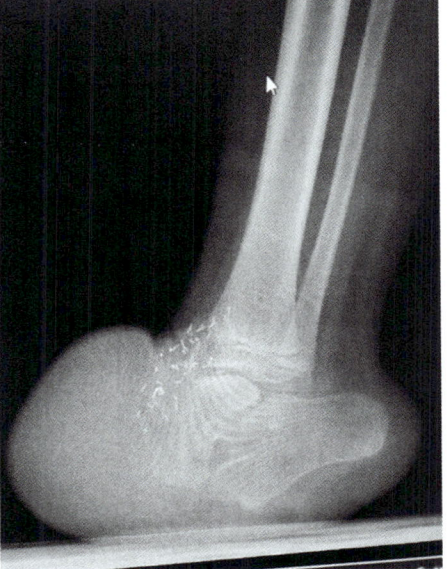

FIGURE 6 Radiograph showing lateral view of traumatic Chopart amputation with plantar-directed calcaneus and bulky soft tissue, which will be extremely difficult to fit with a prosthesis.

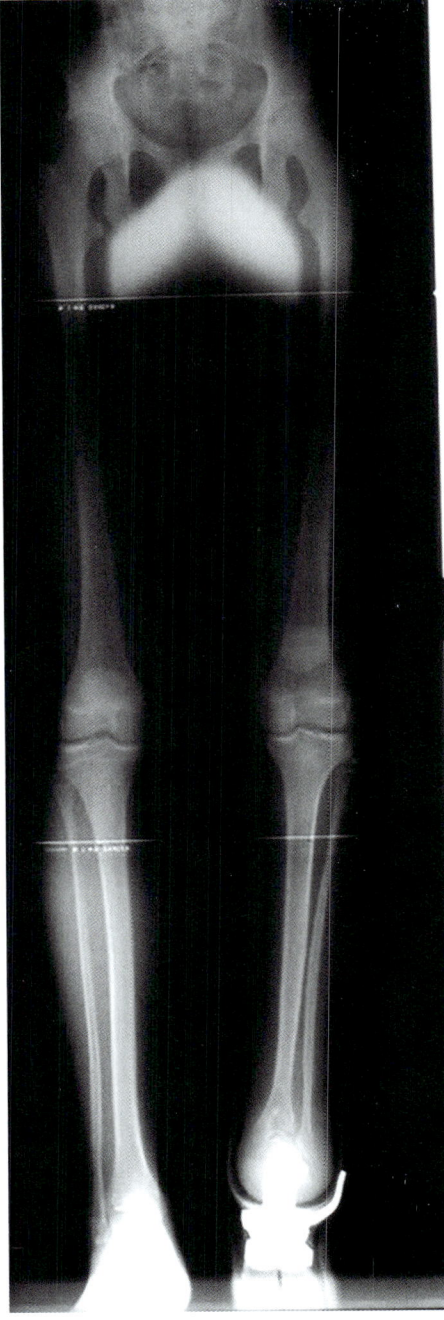

FIGURE 7 Standing AP radiograph with prosthesis on. Proximal tibial and fibular physeal arrest in this patient with a traumatic Syme amputation allows for shortening and ease in fitting foot/ankle prosthetic components and a more cosmetically appealing appearance.

flap for a Syme procedure may not be possible. In such cases, calcanectomy with secondary tissue coverage or primary Syme amputation using anterior flap are options.[54] Atesalp and Yildiz[55] described using the anterior flap Syme procedure successfully in 42 cases of

Section 5: Pediatrics

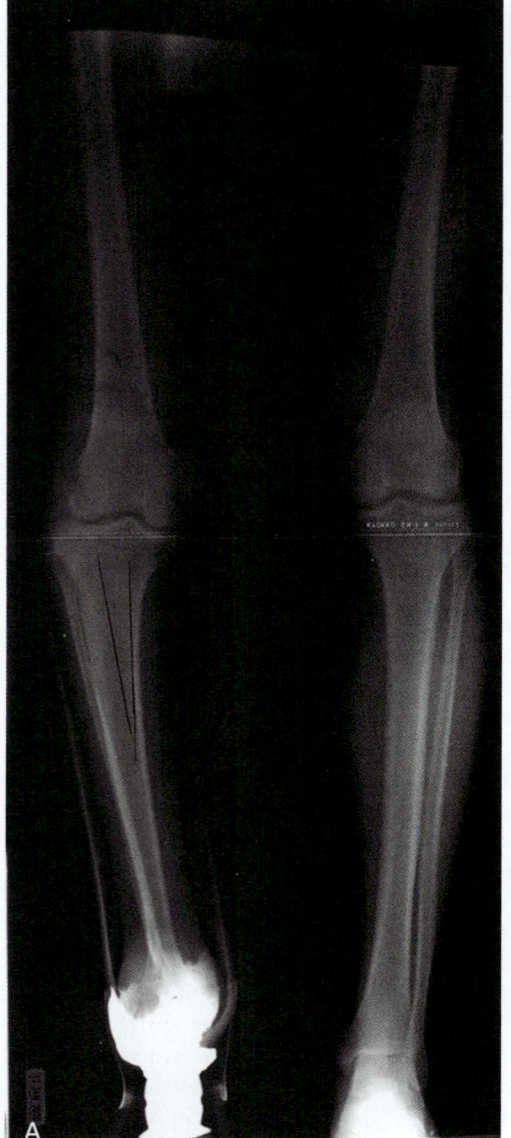

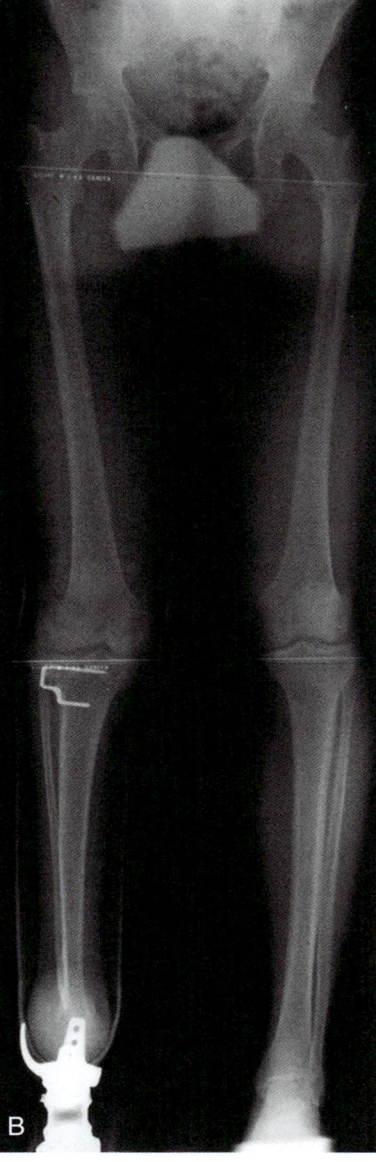

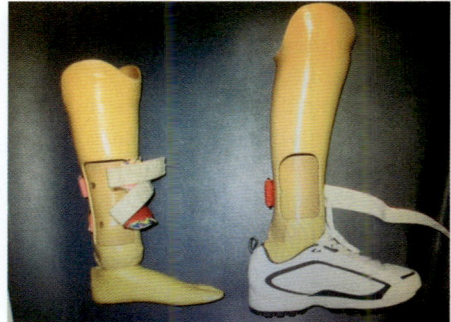

FIGURE 9 Clinical photograph of lightweight Syme prosthesis with a window that allows accommodations for light dressing applications early and cooling distally.

FIGURE 8 Standing AP radiograph with prosthesis on. Distal-tibial-fibular synostosis in a patient with a Syme amputation in whom a varus deformity has developed, requiring proximal tibial osteotomy for correction. Recognition of this deformity earlier would allow correction by guided growth. **A**, Traumatic Syme amputation and development of varus deformity of the right residual limb. **B**, Following correction using proximal tibial osteotomy.

Postoperative care is of major importance in an injury so severe as to create an ankle-level amputation. Most of these wounds are left open initially; however, negative-pressure wound therapy devices have been shown to be useful in the amputated extremity[17,60,61] and can be incorporated into a rigid or semirigid dressing. In children, early dressing changes should be done under anesthesia with appropriate re-débridement and wound assessment as needed. Regional anesthesia applications are particularly important in these children.[62] After the wound is closed and a final rigid or semirigid dressing applied, the wound should not be inspected until follow-up in clinic. Interval semirigid dressings can continue for 4 to 6 weeks followed by residual limb shrinker dressings and a lightweight temporary prosthesis (**Figure 9**).

Final prosthetic choices in patients with an ankle-level amputation are more limited than with transtibial levels because of limited space for the foot and ankle component. In the new amputee, keeping the early prostheses light and easy to don and doff is important for early activity. In the early postoperative interval, a windowed socket may be needed to accommodate swelling and, in some individuals, useful long term. Capability of improved ankle motion with a modular design has been noted in multiple different prosthetic devices.[63] Overall functional differences between children with transtibial dynamic response components versus patients who have undergone Syme amputation with less

landmine trauma after primary radical débridement. In cases so severe that no reasonable attached flap is present, free flap coverage has been successfully incorporated in large heel defects in primarily nonamputee groups.[56-58] Cross leg flap may be considered and has shown success in salvage of a Syme residual limb in a 5-year-old child.[59]

Complications of Syme procedures include posterior heel pad migration, a condition not seen in Boyd procedures.[40] Most of the heel pad migration cases in children often seen in congenital fibular deficiency diagnoses can be accommodated with prosthetic modification. Neuroma formation in a pediatric ankle-level amputation residuum appears to be rare, an advantage of ankle-level ablations. In the systematic literature search by Braaksma et al[36] that included 238 children with Syme amputation, no neuromas were reported.

mobile ankle and foot components are small; both groups fortunately function at high levels. Studies show that the increased ankle motion seen in the high-performance feet does not reflect in peak power advantage or Pediatric Outcomes Data Collection Instrument sports/physical subscale.[64]

Transtibial Amputation Levels

If an injury in a child or adolescent is thought to be serious enough to require a diaphyseal or transtibial amputation, the team providing treatment as well as patient and family need to be prepared for complications that can continue through the entire pediatric lifespan. This section will systematically describe potential complications and appropriate solution options. Transtibial-level amputation in children and adolescents represent a high percentage of patients undergoing major traumatic lower extremity amputation.[2,5] In a blended study of all major lower extremity traumatic amputations carried out in the United States from 2011 to 2012, 48% were transtibial.[15]

Pediatric patients undergoing transtibial procedures function at a level nearly equal to the ankle-level amputee.[64] This reflects the importance of a functional knee joint in both groups. Once the knee is lost, gait velocity has been shown to significantly decrease and metabolic costs increase.[64,65] Preservation of the knee is thus a mantra in the treatment considerations of patients undergoing transtibial-level amputation.

Regardless of mechanism or etiology, many traumatic pediatric transtibial amputations begin as type IIIb lower leg injuries that were not amenable to or failed reconstruction attempts.[66] Although it is generally recommended to obtain early and robust wound coverage to avoid amputation, Clegg et al[67] noted delays of soft-tissue coverage were not predictors of amputation in a study of 140 consecutive blended pediatric and mainly adult patients with type IIIb injuries. These authors noted 20 of these patients (15%) had secondary amputations because of refractory osteomyelitis as cause in 52%.

If a transtibial amputation is decided, there is no specific technique because the variability of soft-tissue damage is nearly infinite. Generally, the principle of using a robust posterior flap applies, but the major decision surgically in trauma is length versus skin coverage.[68,69] A high rate of revision surgery after the initial amputation is expected; this rate was 42% in one study.[14] Gailey et al[70] has noted that the metabolic cost and heart rate are decreased in patients with longer versus short transtibial amputation. Thus, striving for a longer residual limb is of value. This must, however, be balanced with the advantage of robust tissue coverage to prevent deep tissue injury with resultant tissue breakdown in the transtibial amputee.

Much literature exists objectifying deep tissue loads in patients undergoing transtibial amputation and risk factors for residual limb failure. Henrot et al[71] and Portnoy et al[72,73] identified thin muscle flap, minimal adipose tissue, sharp bone edges/osteophytes, and sensory impairment as major nonprosthetic risk factors. Split-thickness skin grafts are necessary adjuncts to wound closure but should be avoided on weight-bearing sites. The presence of skin grafts on the pediatric transtibial residual limb has been shown to not diminish successful outcome.[44]

During the initial amputation, careful attention to dividing nerve tissue is needed to decrease post-operative neuroma complications. MRI is useful in neuroma diagnosis[72] (**Figure 10**). In general, it is recommended gently pulling each amputated nerve and dividing such that they retract. It is preferable to ligate each nerve, in particular large diameter nerves, to avoid hematoma from vasa nervorum. There are no studies of specific neuroma numbers or nerves most commonly involved in traumatic pediatric transtibial-level amputation. If after amputation a neuroma develops that does not respond to nonsurgical management, simple traction neurectomy may be needed, with recurrence in 42%.[74]

Targeted muscle reinnervation (TMR) has been proposed to improve outcome and prosthetic tolerance.[75-77]

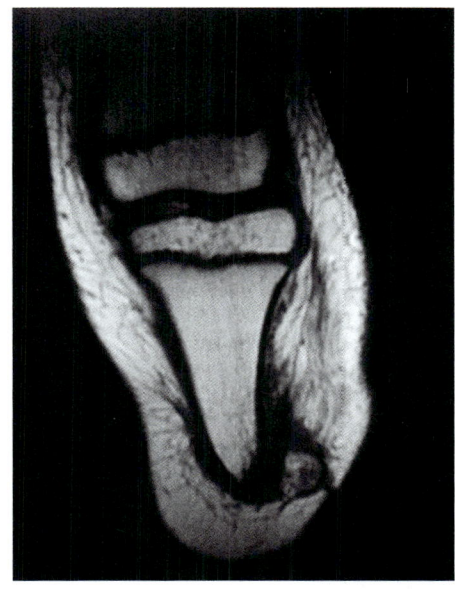

FIGURE 10 Following fibulectomy and end capping of tibia, MRI shows neuroma of the superficial peroneal nerve in a patient with a traumatic transtibial amputation.

In adult literature, Nigam et al[78] noted in transtibial-level amputations neuromas most commonly involved superficial peroneal followed by sural, saphenous, and deep peroneal. The posterior tibial nerve was rarely involved. These authors indicated that in neuroma excision better results were noted in TMR versus simple excision in pain control outcome. Further studies of pediatric traumatic transtibial neuromas and TMR are needed.

Bony overgrowth represents a well-established significant complication of pediatric transtibial amputation, with higher percentages in younger patients[79] (**Figure 11**). Most overgrowth is managed by serial resection of the symptomatic affected bone if not amenable to prosthetic modification. Multiple resections, however, yield a shorter residual limb. To prevent multiple serial overgrowth resection surgical procedures in patients younger than 12 years, end capping procedures have been proposed, usually as secondary procedures months to years after primary amputation.[80-83] There are no specific long-term studies of end capping in immediate primary traumatic pediatric transtibial amputations. If infection possibility has been minimized, using biologic material from the amputated

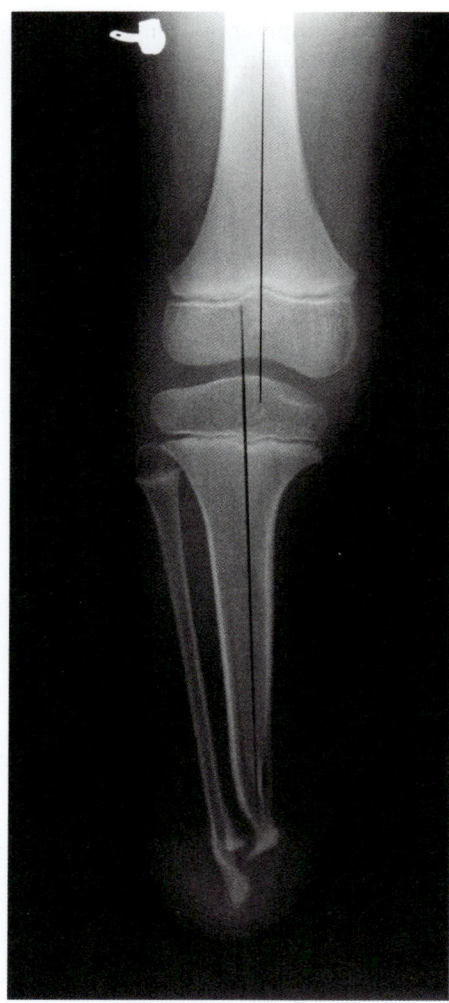

FIGURE 11 AP radiograph showing bony overgrowth following transtibial amputation.

specimen such as distal metatarsal or calcaneal tuberosity may be of value to reduce tibial overgrowth.[83] The study by Benevenia et al[83] showed success in 9 of 10 patients; similarly, the study by Fedorak et al[80] of 50 tibial caps using proximal fibula had 22% complications overall, but in 90% the overgrowth issue was resolved. A study using iliac crest as the biologic cap showed failure in three of four patients.[81]

A transtibial amputation in a very young child will result in a very short residual limb when the child reaches adulthood, a major complication of diaphyseal level selection. This is intuitive in the patient with a transfemoral amputation where distal femoral physis contributes to 70% of femoral growth but also occurs particularly in young patients with a transtibial amputation with proximal tibial physis preservation.[84] Very short residual limbs resulting after traumatic transtibial amputation are generally difficult to fit and may require bulky knee joint, thigh lacer prosthetic devices to help unload the residual limb. Even though a residual limb from transtibial amputation is short, function can be excellent and thus not a reason to revise higher and eliminate the knee. A small cohort of young adults with extremely short residual tibial length with fibular head excision have shown good function regardless of a very short lever arm.[85] Lengthening of the tibia has been successfully used in children with transtibial amputation with short residual limbs to improve function but can be difficult with relatively high complications.[86] In pediatric patients with very short residual limbs following traumatic transtibial amputation, fibular excision can be used to diminish possible overgrowth issues and to facilitate wound closure. The fibula may then be used as a cap on the distal tibia, as described earlier[80] (Figure 12).

Free-flap tissue transfer in children for large soft-tissue defects has been shown to be valuable with high success rates.[87] Free flaps can be of significant help in salvaging a transtibial residual limb from becoming a higher level, or to preserve a longer residuum.[18,58,88-90] Long-term durability of an insensate free flap in the active patient with a transtibial amputation can be an issue, with one study showing four of five patients needing surgical revision for deep tissue ulceration.[88] Numerous flap donor sites have been successful in blended adult and pediatric studies usually including latissimus dorsi, gracilis, parascapular flap, foot fillet, lateral thigh, and groin. Many of the free flaps used in children with traumatic

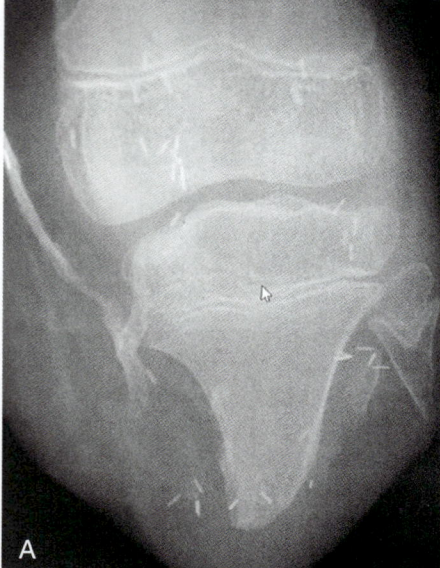
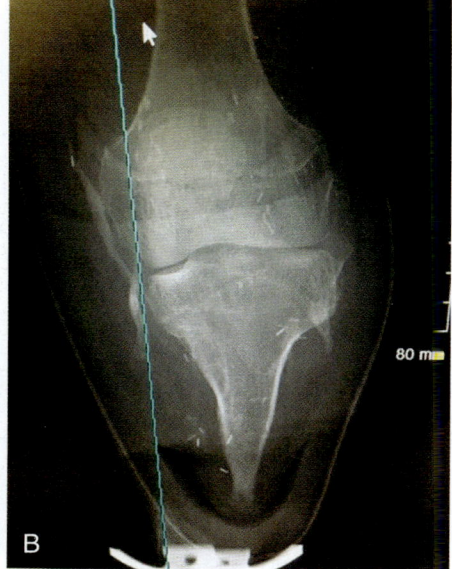

FIGURE 12 **A**, AP radiograph showing prefibulectomy of short transtibial traumatic amputation. **B**, AP radiograph showing postfibulectomy with end capping of the tibia used with success in a patient with a short transtibial amputation.

injuries are for defects around the foot and ankle. Rectus abdominis free flaps have also been used in traumatic injuries in children for tibial coverage as well as heel defects.[56] A free fillet foot flap to salvage a transtibial-level amputation in a 2-year-old child at 17-year follow-up demonstrated excellent results with no breakdown issues.[91] Additional long-term studies of free flaps in trauma-related transtibial amputation in children and adolescents are needed to evaluate durability years after the free flap procedure.

Angular deformity of the knee may develop in children after traumatic transtibial amputation. In one study, a progressive knee varus occurred after spontaneous or surgically created synostosis between tibia and fibula. Surgical correction was needed in 10 of 12 patients[53] (**Figure 13**). Angular deformity can occur without a synostosis and was noted in 38% of pediatric

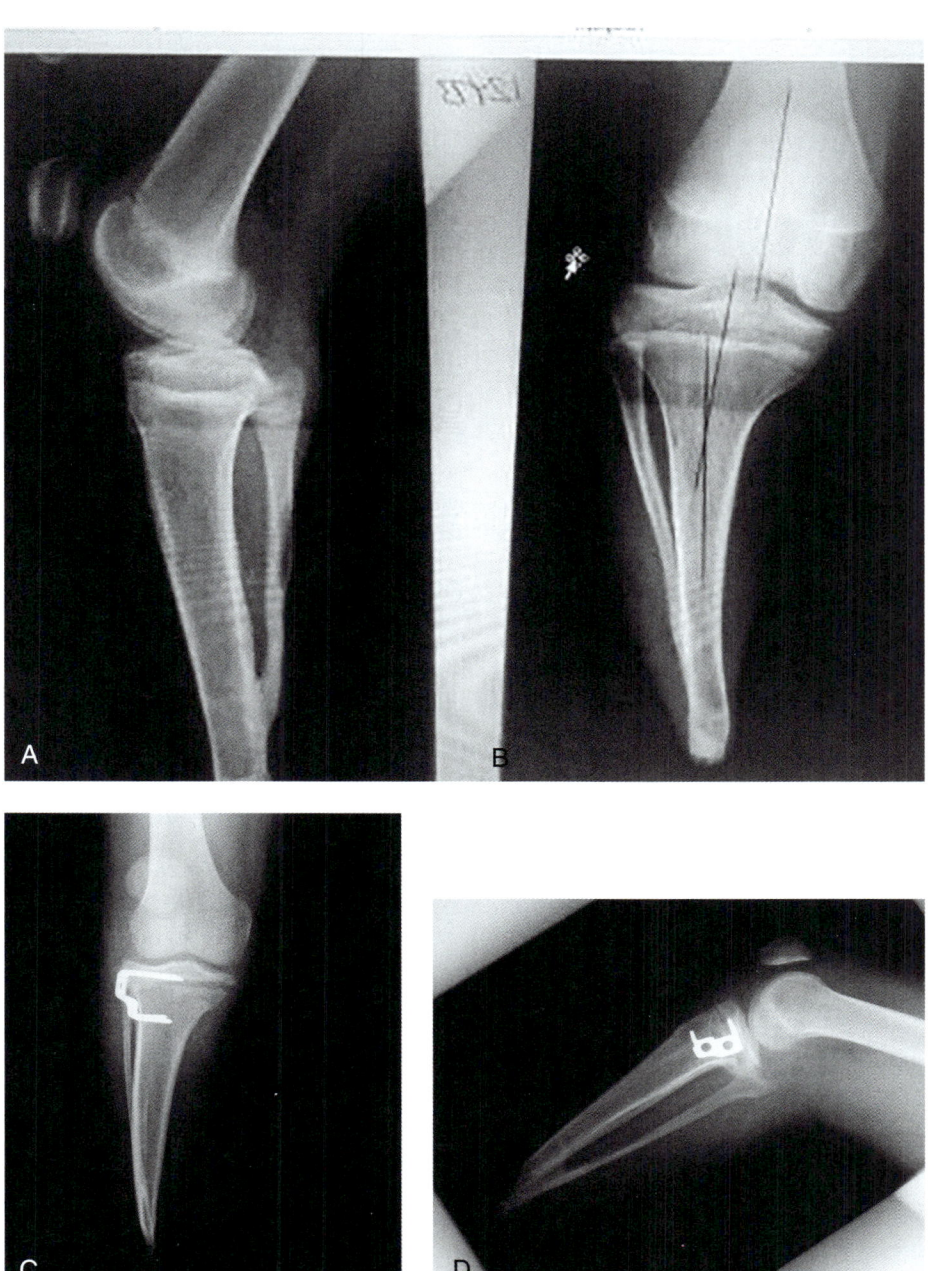

FIGURE 13 Radiographs showing significant varus deformity in an adolescent that occurred following traumatic transtibial amputation after spontaneous synostosis of tibia and fibula. Progressive knee varus occurred after spontaneous (**A** and **B**) or surgically created synostosis between tibia and fibula (**C** and **D**). Recognition of this deformity early will allow for guided growth rather than osteotomies. **A**, AP radiograph showing varus deformity following spontaneous synostosis between the tibia and fibula in a patient with a traumatic transtibial amputation. **B**, Lateral radiograph showing synostosis. **C**, AP radiograph following osteotomy for varus deformity. **D**, Lateral radiograph showing synostosis following osteotomy.

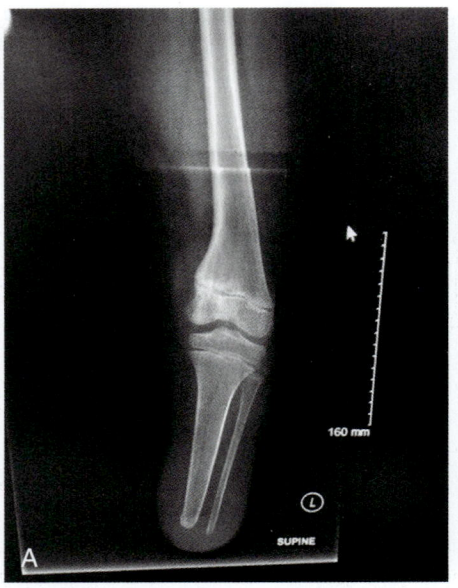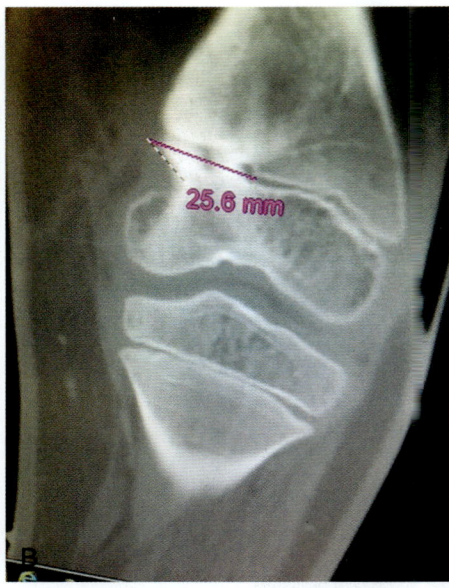

FIGURE 14 Images showing concomitant medial physis injury in a patient with a transtibial amputation that resulted in progressive varus deformation requiring bar excision and guided growth. **A**, AP radiograph showing varus deformity following medial physis injury. **B**, CT showing medial bar formation on distal femur.

patients with transtibial amputation with varus, valgus, and recurvatum issues.[92] Injuries severe enough to create a transtibial amputation may cause damage to a physis near the area of injury. If unrecognized, late deformity may result (**Figure 14**).

Interval standing radiographs with the patient wearing a prosthesis are valuable because deformity can be hidden by the prosthesis (**Figure 15**). Regardless of etiology, if deformity is recognized early, correction with hemiphyseal guided growth should be carried out, avoiding osteotomy needed in older patients.[93]

Fitting a prosthesis on the patient with a traumatic transtibial amputation may begin soon after primary wound healing. An exact timetable on trauma patients is impossible because of possible skin graft maturity and general patient debilitation differences from the original injury. Use of immediate postoperative prosthesis rigid dressings have generally been replaced by rigid removable dressings and have been shown to be of value in adult and pediatric patients.[94-96] At the time of initial fitting, prosthetists need to work closely with parents and physical therapists so that painful areas can be identified and early socket or alignment modification carried out.[29] The first prosthesis should be simple, lightweight, and modular so socket changes can be made easily. Early goals should emphasize donning and doffing, pain control, edema control, walking, and balance control.[34] Patients and family members need to be informed that with major trauma-related injury, residual limb swelling will persist for many months followed by atrophy, necessitating more frequent socket changes for perhaps 1 year after injury. It has been objectively noted that children with acquired amputations require a longer period of rehabilitation than do children with congenital amputations.[97]

Through-Knee Amputation Level

Amputation at the through-knee level should be considered instead of the transfemoral level, if possible, in pediatric patients when transtibial amputation is impossible. This is particularly true in very young children in whom a loss of the distal femoral physis in a 3-year-old may create a residual limb so short as an adult that prosthetic fitting is nearly impossible or hip disarticulation prosthesis is necessary (**Figure 16**). This finding becomes much more of a hard sell in older adolescents where excess length and distal residual limb bulk can significantly decrease prosthetic options, making microprocessor prosthetic knee component nearly impossible to incorporate.

In a study of primarily adult trauma patients, physicians were less satisfied with clinical, cosmetic, and functional recovery in the knee disarticulation group. The knee disarticulation group had slower self-selected walking speeds than either transtibial or transfemoral amputation levels.[98] Another study of military patients who underwent amputation comparing through-knee versus transfemoral amputation levels, however, showed no differences measured by the Prosthesis Evaluation Questionnaire, Low Luminance Questionnaire, 36-Item Short Form Health Survey, and Tegner Activity Scale with follow-up averaging 66 months.[99]

Through-knee amputations performed during childhood are commonly carried out for congenital conditions such as certain types of proximal femoral focal deficiency or tibial longitudinal deficiency, but are uncommon in lower extremity pediatric trauma. Functional long-term studies comparing pediatric trauma–related through-knee versus transfemoral outcomes are needed.

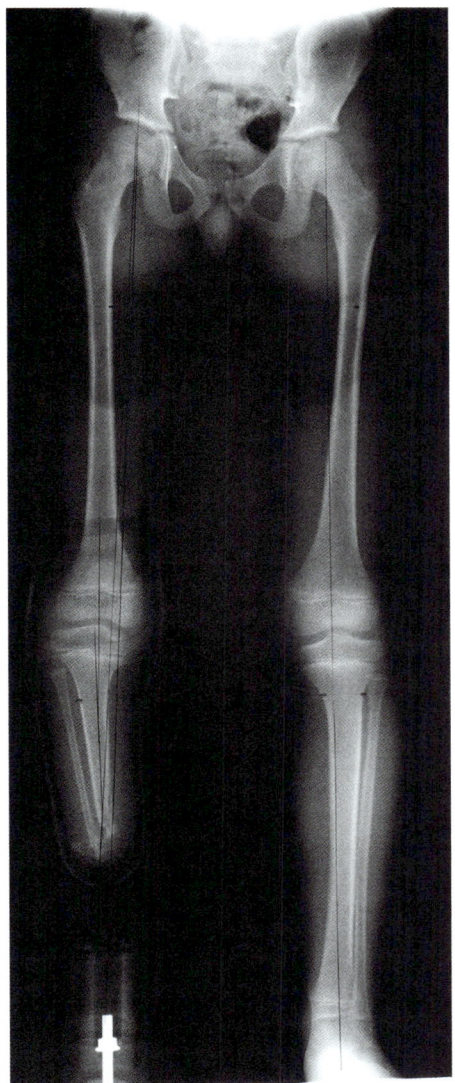

FIGURE 15 Standing AP radiograph from a patient wearing a prosthesis is valuable for detecting early varus deformities, which may be hidden by the prosthetic device.

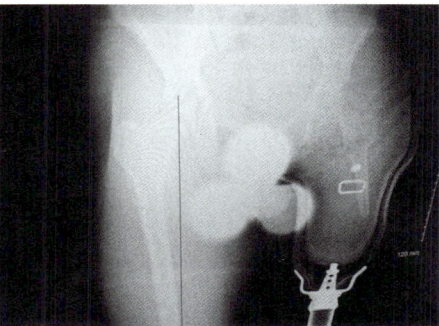

FIGURE 16 AP radiograph of transfemoral amputation in a young child will result in an extremely short residual limb at maturity, making prosthetic fitting difficult and prone to failure.

The advantages of end-bearing, longer lever arm/quadriceps power, minimal use of proximal suspension systems, and elimination of bony overgrowth are major benefits of through-knee–level selection in children. Just as in the ankle-level amputation, length can be adjusted in children by physeal arrest to avoid the residual limb being too long. Arresting the distal femoral physis at an age to allow 8 to 10 cm of shortening will allow multiple easily obtainable prosthetic component choices with improved cosmesis without disruption of knee axis. This implies that generally any adolescent patient with a newly acquired through-knee amputation should undergo distal femoral physeal arrest at the time of amputation (**Figure 17**).

The surgical techniques for trauma-related pediatric through-knee amputations are variable, as in traumatic transtibial-level selection. Depending on where most of the soft-tissue damage is, closure may be with posterior flap, sagittal flaps, or less common, medial, lateral, or anterior. The surgical team should strive to obtain robust tissue, preferably gastrocnemius-soleus as coverage over the femoral condyles. Trauma directed anteriorly will probably configure best for posterior flap coverage with major soft-tissue damage anterior. For sagittal flap coverage, some skin distal to the joint line is needed; however, large soft-tissue loss posteriorly can be tolerated (**Figure 18**). Most through-knee amputations now are carried out for vascular etiologies using a variety of techniques, but predominantly posterior flaps.[100-104] It is important that, because of significant variability in trauma-related amputation, the surgeon is not committed to one specific technique but will strive for reasonable wound closure regardless of flap placement. Distal condylar excision with care to preserve the physis with partial or total patellectomy may facilitate closure and decrease bulk for prosthetic fitting.[102,105] Long-term outcome studies comparing different surgical flaps and techniques of this uncommon level of pediatric traumatic amputation are needed.

The end-bearing advantage of the through-knee level with longer lever arm is advantageous in children because it simplifies suspension compared with transfemoral levels. Formerly, these children, especially young children, were started with simple pylon-type prostheses, with later addition of a mobile prosthetic knee. It has been shown, however, that young children will use the prosthetic knee if provided. In major trauma, a simple lightweight pylon shell may still be useful early if grafted or flap sites have not matured.[106] Early prosthetic fittings may incorporate simple modular knees with axis distal to the joint; however, the long-term goal should be a closer prosthetic knee placement to the sound side. As noted earlier, distal femoral physeal arrest will greatly facilitate that outcome.

Transfemoral Amputation Levels

Pediatric transfemoral traumatic amputations represent a most challenging level for patients and families and all members of the treating team. Rehabilitation is more prolonged and difficult, prosthetic decisions are suddenly more complex, and surgical decisions are no less difficult. The goal of pain-free walking without the need for aids can require a prolonged interval of time. Without the knee, metabolic need based on oxygen consumption rises significantly.[65,107,108] Structural complicating issues such as bony overgrowth, soft-tissue coverage problems, neuroma formation, and short residual limbs all are major challenges covered in this section.

Transfemoral-level traumatic amputations in pediatric patients represent the most severe civilian injuries possible and may often result in death before the patient arrives at a treatment facility. Although exact death rates are not precisely known in pediatric patients with transfemoral injuries, an overall mortality rate of 15% has been proposed for patients with major lower extremity limb loss.[109,110] Handling these patients in the field quickly and appropriately is of significance. Many transfemoral amputation injuries,

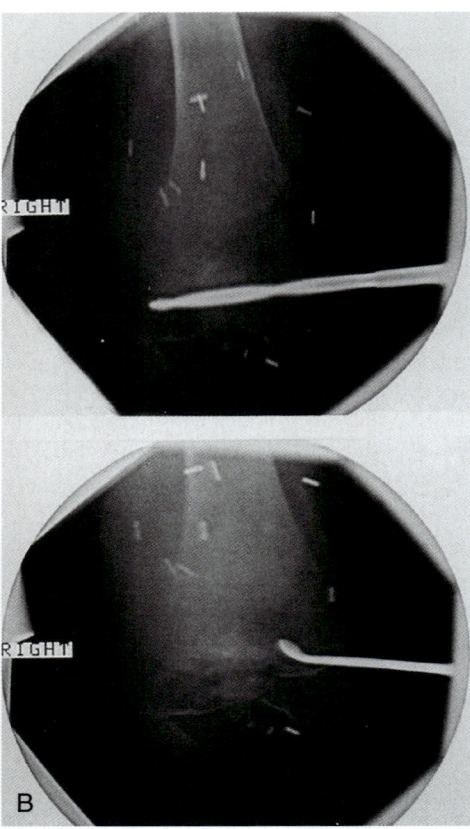

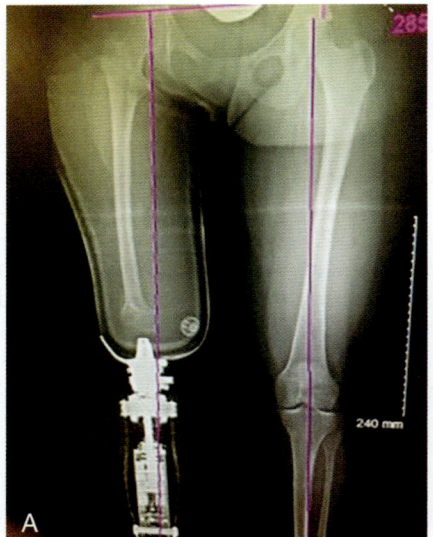

FIGURE 17 **A**, AP radiograph following through-knee amputation showing benefit of physeal arrest, allowing for more prosthetic options and improved cosmetic knee axis at maturity. **B**, AP radiograph of intraoperative physeal arrest done at time of initial surgery in traumatic knee disarticulation.

particularly firearms trauma, involve vascular damage, with critically injured patients requiring stabilization followed by prolonged hospitalization.[2] Proper placement of a tourniquet when shock is absent may save 90% of these lives in an analysis of battle injuries.[111]

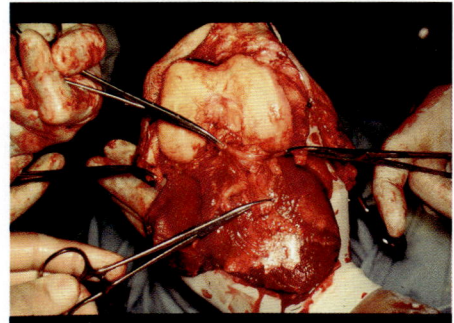

FIGURE 18 Intraoperative photograph shows, regardless of whether posterior flap or sagittal flaps are used, the gastrocnemius should be used to cover the femoral condyle in knee disarticulation.

Loss of the distal femoral physis, especially in young children, will result in an extremely short residual limb as an adult, a significant and expected complication of pediatric transfemoral amputation. Length of the femoral residual limb correlates highly with failure of prosthetic use long term, with one study showing only 50% prosthetic use in adult patients with transfemoral level amputation.[112] It is important, if possible, during the initial surgery to create an adductor myodesis to the distal femur. With loss of distal adductor muscle attachments and preservation of proximal hip flexor and abductor attachment, the short residual femur will become flexed and abducted, creating a very difficult prosthetic fitting challenge.[113,114] Residual femoral length correlates highly with functional outcome as shorter residual femur length results in greater torso and pelvis excursion as well as slower self-selected walking speed.[115] Walker et al[116] reported four cases of femoral lengthening in patients undergoing transfemoral amputation with substantial functional improvement but with significant complications and protracted treatment times. Intramedullary devices have also been used to lengthen transfemoral residual limbs.[117] Because residual femoral length may be the major predictor of long-term prosthetic success, additional studies are needed on pediatric patients undergoing femoral lengthening as a result of transfemoral amputation. Socket design can be nearly impossible to objectify as to what is the best option for patients with a short residual limb following transfemoral amputation, a crucial factor to success being simply overall comfort.[118]

Osseointegration implant systems may represent a future solution option for the patient with a short residual limb following transfemoral amputation in particular. Several implant devices are available, with most being used in individuals who have undergone transfemoral amputation.[119] Approval in the United States is only under FDA Humanitarian Device Exemption.[120] Osseointegration offers the potential for not only lengthening the femoral lever arm but also eliminating the difficult socket/suspension systems. Bony integration of these prosthetic devices may be particularly robust in pediatric patients, an advantage but also a potential disadvantage if implant removal becomes necessary. A recent comprehensive review of this concept by Hoellwarth et al[121] is available.

Bony overgrowth in the pediatric residual limb following traumatic transfemoral amputation is not as common as in the patient group with transtibial amputation but represents as significant a challenge. A penciled, nearly subcutaneous femoral segment may be practically impossible to fit with a prosthesis. Overgrowth of the femur in children is fourth most common following humerus, fibula, and tibia, and its symptoms can be equally severe and create significant prosthetic fitting issues.[122,123] Biologic capping procedures similar to those discussed for transtibial amputation have been used in transfemoral levels to prevent overgrowth. However, no series of capping results for strictly pediatric transfemoral amputation are available.[124]

Symptoms of tenderness over the overgrowth site may be managed initially by socket modification or steroid injection in overlying bursal tissue. Overgrowth requiring surgical revision may be needed in less than 10%.[79] Heterotopic ossification can occur with regularity in young adults with combat-related injury, in particular with blast trauma. However, no specific series of thigh segment heterotopic ossification in children following traumatic amputation is available.[125] If surgical excision becomes necessary for femoral overgrowth, care must be taken to redo the myodesis or assess for myodesis failure. With painful exuberant bone spurring overgrowth not associated with overgrowth penciling, the previous myodesis, if present, will need to be taken down and then re-repaired following bone excision (**Figure 19**).

Neuroma formation in pediatric patients undergoing traumatic transfemoral amputation appears to be less common than in adult patients and may occur more commonly in extreme or blast trauma. In a study of landmine explosion trauma in young male soldiers (average age 26 years), of 527 lower extremity amputations neuromas developed in 75, 31% at the transfemoral level.[126] These patients responded well to simple excision. As mentioned previously, TMR may hold promise in patients with transfemoral amputation as a way to avoid neuromas and help actuate future microprocessor electronic prosthetic components.[127] TMR has also been suggested to be carried out at the time of initial surgery, primarily to improve pain.[128]

Traumatic transfemoral amputation may often create difficulties in skin closure. It is important to remember that ultimate prosthetic functional success or failure is often predicated on femoral length. Drastic early shortening to obtain closure may eliminate walking with a prosthesis, especially in children with transfemoral amputation as they age and the residual limb gets even shorter. Many of these complex thigh wounds require some patience and can be managed with customary débridement, wound vacs, and split-thickness skin graft procedures without excessive femoral shaft shortening. After swelling has been eliminated and postamputation atrophy has occurred, residual limb revision can often be carried out with elimination of less durable grafted skin (**Figure 20**). Vertical rectus abdominis myocutaneous pedicle flaps can be used for large femoral defects and have been shown to be useful in transfemoral amputation.[128] Free flap procedures in patients with transfemoral amputation are much less common

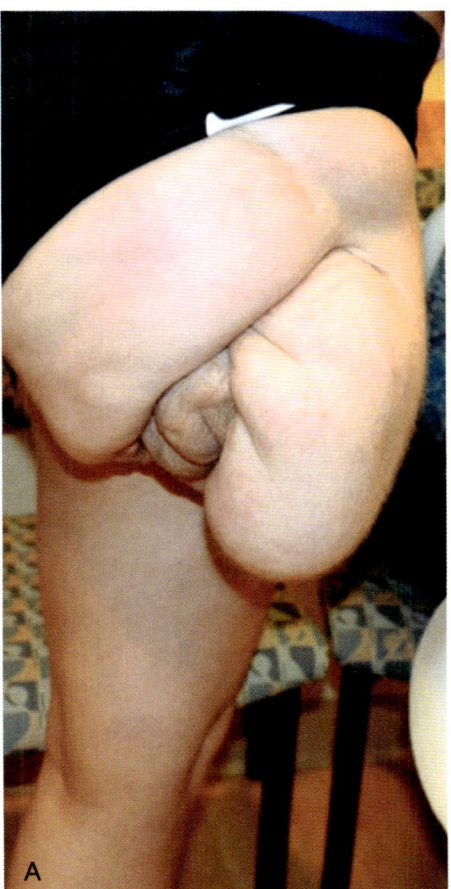

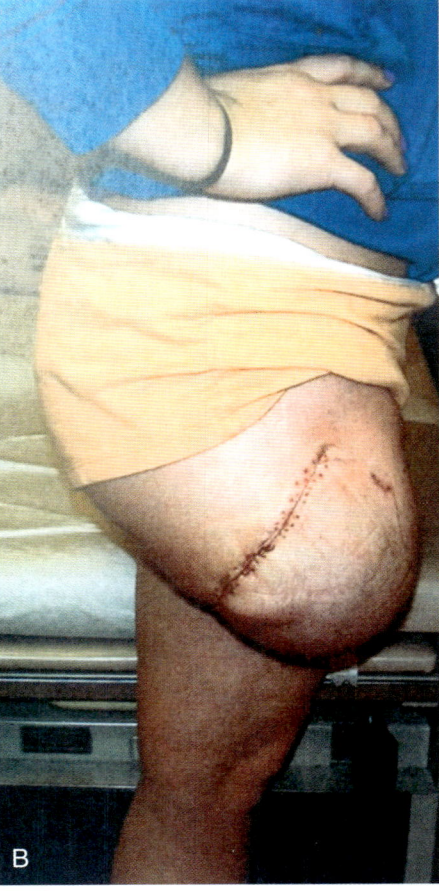

FIGURE 19 Intraoperative photograph of distal femoral spurring in an adolescent with a transfemoral amputation requiring excision. This is not the same as overgrowth penciling noted in younger age groups. Following excision, repair of adductor myodesis is needed.

FIGURE 20 Photograph shows removal of previous split-thickness skin grafts needed at initial injury allows for improved functional result without excessive femoral shortening in later revision. **A**, Lateral view of transfemoral amputation prior to revision. **B**, Lateral view after revision.

than in transtibial amputation groups, but some success has been shown using latissimus dorsi donor tissue.[129]

As soon as pain is under reasonable control and primary healing has occurred, ambulatory rehabilitation with prosthetic fabrication can begin. Recent prosthetic advances have particularly helped the pediatric patient who has undergone a transfemoral amputation. Gone are the days of quadrilateral sockets, parachute cord posterior knee check straps, elastic band extension assist with free hinged knees, and simple prosthetic feet. Unless the residual limb is short, waist strap band suspension is rarely used. The patient with a transfemoral amputation walks smoother, falls less, has narrower stance width, and simply looks less noticeably impaired. Fitting a child who has recently undergone transfemoral amputation with a rigid pylon prosthesis is unnecessary, as young children with an amputation can be successfully fit with a mobile prosthetic knee at first fitting.[106]

As the child with a transfemoral amputation progresses into adolescent age and body weight increases, adult-size components are needed. Programmable microprocessor knee components become available but add additional cost. Studies have shown cost effectiveness as well as improved energy expenditure in these high technology components,[130,131] but this must be balanced with the practicality of breakdown issues and proximity of available team support in highly active pediatric patients; playing a dirty sandlot football game is different from commuting to an office job. Microprocessor knee joints that sense excessive knee motion in stance and swing phase markedly help the patient who has undergone an amputation gain confidence in balance, decrease self-reported falls, and increase gait velocity.[132]

This section is not meant to provide a comprehensive discussion of all transfemoral prosthetic options but to encourage the incorporation of a team approach in discussion of pediatric multiple prosthetic options in patients with varied activity levels.

Pain Issues in the Pediatric Patient With a Traumatic Lower Extremity Amputation

Pain can be a significant problem in all levels of pediatric traumatic lower extremity amputation.[133] Pain in the patient with an amputation is generally divided into nonpainful phantom-like sensations of the missing residual limb segment, phantom painful sensation of the missing segment, and residual limb postoperative pain. In a study of adults who have undergone amputation, which dominate the literature, phantom sensations and phantom limb pain (PLP) were highly prevalent both 8 days and 6 months after surgery (67% to 90%); however, postoperative residual limb pain present in 57% at 8 days decreased to 22% at 6 months.[134] In the Krane and Heller[133] study of pediatric-only patients comparing those with traumatic amputations and those with congenital and neoplastic amputations, 100% had phantom sensations with the most also having PLP; resolution of PLP occurred in only 35%. Studies have shown that the severity of preoperative pain correlated with higher incidence of postoperative PLP.[133,135] Other studies, however, have not shown a correlation of preoperative limb pain with PLP.[136] Wilkens et al[137] noted that patients with an amputation who are younger than 6 years had a 47% incidence of phantom sensation, but 100% of the older patient group had phantom sensation. PLP in this study was noted in 3.7% of those with a congenital amputation and 47% of those with a surgical amputation. Many of the studies in the literature are retrospective and questionnaire-based with variable response rates, making data objectification difficult. In a comprehensive review of PLP in children with cancer who have had an amputation, it has been suggested that controlled prospective trials are needed.[138] This suggestion would also apply to children with traumatic lower extremity amputation.

It is important for the team providing treatment to differentiate PLP, a difficult diagnosis to treat, from postamputation residual limb pain. In a traumatic amputation, residual infection from retained foreign material or deep suture may be present as well as bone spurring, overgrowth, and neuroma formation. Bone scans, C-reactive protein levels, and MRI may be useful in diagnosis of structural treatable pain issues in the residual limb. Consultation with the prosthetist is important. Changing the liner or socket may be a simple solution to residual limb pain.

Other treatments have been proposed for management of PLP. At the time of initial amputation, recent studies have proposed TMR as treatment for alleviating neuroma formation as well as development of PLP.[139] Continuous nerve block for 6 days has been shown to reduce PLP for at least 1 month but no benefit was noted at 12 months.[140] Suggested pharmacologic treatment for the child with PLP includes gabapentin, amytriptyline, and opioids.[141,142] Mirror therapies, which place a mirror juxtaposed to the sound limb side, show promise, but randomized studies are needed in children with traumatic lower extremity amputation.[143] Future studies of all forms of treatment for pediatric lower extremity trauma-related PLP are needed.

Psychological Issues in Children With Trauma-Related Lower Extremity Amputation

Major lower extremity loss in a child or adolescent creates the potential for devastating long-term psychological effects on patients, family members, and extended families. Many traumatic lower extremity amputations are particularly devastating because there is no preoperative preparation as in patients with cancer or congenital etiologies, just a terrible sudden loss. Initial trauma clinicians, such as surgeons or intensivists, are oriented in a pathologic way to save the patient's life or solve the structural problem that exists. Psychological consultation and interaction, which can be immediately helpful, is often delayed. Many affective disorders can occur with a sudden severe traumatic event. Families can get torn apart, severe patient depression is common, and patients may refuse to even consider prosthetic fitting with some refusing to even look at their residual limb for months to years.

Studies of strictly pediatric trauma-related major lower extremity amputation-related psychological problems are needed. In two studies from India of psychiatric comorbidity after traumatic limb amputation that were blended with pediatric and adult patients (71.2% to 81% younger than 30 years), major depressive disorder occurred in 63% to 71.2%, suicidal ideation in 30.5%, and posttraumatic stress disorder in 20.3%.[144,145] In tumor-related pediatric amputation, acceptance of the surgery appears better if pain was present before the amputation.[146] In traumatic amputation, a completely normal nonpainful extremity is lost, a significant difference in comparing oncology literature.

In a blended study of congenital and acquired child amputees, perceived parent, teacher, classmate, and friend social support are noted to be of significant importance in self-esteem development and in overcoming the negative effect and psychological strain of limb loss.[147] Psychometric outcome measurement tools such as the Child Amputee Prosthetics Project Functional Status Inventory for Preschool Children are useful.[148] PedsQL (Pediatric Quality of Life Inventory) is also a proven useful tool for evaluating age groups 2 to 16 years.[149] It is important that the team providing treatment engage in early and follow-up dialogue with patients and families to help identify whether depression is a problem and have effective resources for treatment. The devastation of untreated or poorly treated depression cannot be overemphasized.

Medical-Legal Issues With Children and Adolescents With Traumatic Lower Extremity Amputation

Lawsuits after injuries severe enough to create a major lower extremity amputation in a pediatric patient occur, but few objective data are available documenting percentages of product or personal/family liability versus physician or provider liability. In the study by Galey et al[150] of malpractice in pediatric orthopaedics, the number one lawsuit was fracture diagnosis issues followed by misdiagnosis of developmental dysplasia of the hip. In the study by Matsen et al[151] of overall orthopaedic malpractice claims, one-third involved amputations, brain injury, and nerve injury, with 41% involving failure to protect structures in the surgical field. Settlement compensation formulas for limb loss include past and future medical expenses, past and future loss of wages, past and future pain and suffering, past and future mental anguish, past and future enjoyment of life, disability, and scarring and disfigurement. Other liability issues can involve the trauma surgical team if inappropriate, delayed, unnecessary, or poorly done procedures leading to amputation are carried out.

Inadequate informed consent for surgical interventions can occur.[152] In one study, elective surgery carried more legal risk (61%) than trauma surgery, with informed consent issues representing 5.3% of legal cases.[152] Advances in technology and product safety have likely reduced amputation numbers,[7] but if technology fails, lawsuits can be triggered.[154]

SUMMARY

Major lower extremity amputations in children and adolescents represent many significant orthopaedic challenges. It is of key importance to be aware of potential and expected complications in these young patients. Progressive angular deformity can be skillfully hidden by a good prosthetic team until it is too late for guided growth procedures. It should be recognized that significant complications of diaphyseal amputations exist. Overall, a residual limb that is durable for many decades of life needs to be created. It is important to interact compassionately with patients and families, realizing the devastation of a sudden traumatic limb loss in a child or adolescent.

References

1. Hostetler SG, Schwartz L, Shields BJ, Xiang H, Smith GA: Characteristics of pediatric traumatic amputations treated in hospital emergency departments: United States, 1990-2002. *Pediatrics* 2005;116(5):e667-e674.
2. Borne A, Porter A, Recicar J, Maxson T, Montgomery C: Pediatric traumatic amputations in the United States: A 5-year review. *J Pediatr Orthop* 2017;37(2):e104-e107.
3. Conner KA, McKenzie LB, Xiang H, Smith GA: Pediatric traumatic amputations and hospital resource utilization in the United States, 2003. *J Trauma* 2010;68(1):131-137.
4. Stinner DJ, Burns TC, Kirk KL, et al: Prevalence of late amputations during the current conflicts in Afghanistan and Iraq. *Mil Med* 2010;175(12):1027-1029.
5. Loder RT, Brown KL, Zaleske DJ, Jones ET: Extremity lawn-mower injuries in children: Report by the Research Committee of the Pediatric Orthopaedic Society of North America. *J Pediatr Orthop* 1997;17(3):360-369.
6. Siracuse JJ, Farber A, Cheng TW, Jones DW, Kalesan B: Lower extremity vascular injuries caused by firearms have a higher risk of amputation and death compared with non-firearm penetrating trauma. *J Vasc Surg* 2020;72(4):1298-1304.e1.
7. Ren KS, Chounthirath T, Yang J, Friedenberg L, Smith GA: Children treated for lawn mower-related injuries in US emergency departments, 1990-2014. *Am J Emerg Med* 2017;35(6):893-898.
8. Fletcher AN, Schwend RM, Solano M, Wester C, Jarka DE: Pediatric Lawn-Mower Injuries Presenting at a Level-I Trauma Center, 1995 to 2015: A danger to our youngest children. *J Bone Joint Surg Am* 2018;100(20):1719-1727.
9. Ahmad J, Gupta AK, Sharma VP, Kumar D, Yadav G, Singh S: Traumatic amputations in children and adolescents: a demographic study from a tertiary care center in Northern India. *J Pediatr Rehabil Med* 2016;9(4):265-269.
10. Roche AJ, Selvarajah K: Traumatic amputations in children and adolescents: demographics from a regional limb-fitting centre in the United Kingdom. *J Bone Joint Surg Br* 2011;93(4):507-509.
11. Bilukha OO, Brennan M, Woodruff BA: Death and injury from landmines and unexploded ordnance in Afghanistan. *J Am Med Assoc* 2003;290(5):650-653.
12. Soroush A, Falahati F, Zargar M, Soroush M, Khateri S, Khaji A: Amputations due to landmine and unexploded ordinances in post-war

Iran [published correction appears in *Arch Iran Med*. 2009;12(1):105]. *Arch Iran Med* 2008;11(6):595-597.

13. Surrency AB, Graitcer PL, Henderson AK: Key factors for civilian injuries and deaths from exploding landmines and ordnance. *Inj Prev* 2007;13(3):197-201.

14. Busse JW, Jacobs CL, Swiontkowski MF, Bosse MJ, Bhandari M; Evidence-Based Orthopaedic Trauma Working Group: Complex limb salvage or early amputation for severe lower-limb injury: A meta-analysis of observational studies. *J Orthop Trauma* 2007;21(1):70-76.

15. Low EE, Inkellis E, Morshed S: Complications and revision amputation following trauma-related lower limb loss. *Injury* 2017;48(2):364-370.

16. Kauvar DS, Sarfati MR, Kraiss LW: National trauma databank analysis of mortality and limb loss in isolated lower extremity vascular trauma. *J Vasc Surg* 2011;53(6):1598-1603.

17. Shilt JS, Yoder JS, Manuck TA, Jacks L, Rushing J, Smith BP: Role of vacuum-assisted closure in the treatment of pediatric lawnmower injuries. *J Pediatr Orthop* 2004;24(5):482-487.

18. Organek AJ, Klebuc MJ, Zuker RM: Indications and outcomes of free tissue transfer to the lower extremity in children: Review. *J Reconstr Microsurg* 2006;22(3):173-181.

19. Brown KV, Ramasamy A, McLeod J, Stapley S, Clasper JC: Predicting the need for early amputation in ballistic mangled extremity injuries. *J Trauma* 2009;66(4 suppl):S93-S98.

20. Bosse MJ, McCarthy ML, Jones AL, et al: The insensate foot following severe lower extremity trauma: An indication for amputation? *J Bone Joint Surg Am* 2005;87(12):2601-2608.

21. Lubicky JP, Feinberg JR: Fractures and amputations in children and adolescents requiring hospitalization after farm equipment injuries [published correction appears in *J Pediatr Orthop*. 2010;30(8):944]. *J Pediatr Orthop* 2009;29(5):435-438.

22. Dormans JP, Azzoni M, Davidson RS, Drummond DS: Major lower extremity lawn mower injuries in children. *J Pediatr Orthop* 1995;15(1):78-82.

23. Hollander JE, Singer AJ, Valentine S: Comparison of wound care practices in pediatric and adult lacerations repaired in the emergency department. *Pediatr Emerg Care* 1998;14(1):15-18.

24. Humbyrd CJ, Rieder TN: Ethics and limb salvage: Presenting amputation as a treatment option in lower extremity trauma. *J Bone Joint Surg Am* 2018;100(19):e128.

25. Baldwin KD, Babatunde OM, Russell Huffman G, Hosalkar HS: Open fractures of the tibia in the pediatric population: A systematic review. *J Child Orthop* 2009;3(3):199-208.

26. Hertel R, Strebel N, Ganz R: Amputation versus reconstruction in traumatic defects of the leg: Outcome and costs. *J Orthop Trauma* 1996;10(4):223-229.

27. Georgiadis GM, Behrens FF, Joyce MJ, Earle AS, Simmons AL: Open tibial fractures with severe soft-tissue loss. Limb salvage compared with below-the-knee amputation. *J Bone Joint Surg Am* 1993;75(10):1431-1441.

28. Ladlow P, Phillip R, Coppack R, et al: Influence of immediate and delayed lower-limb amputation compared with lower-limb salvage on functional and mental health outcomes post-rehabilitation in the U.K. Military. *J Bone Joint Surg Am* 2016;98(23):1996-2005.

29. Griffet J: Amputation and prosthesis fitting in paediatric patients. *Orthop Traumatol Surg Res* 2016;102(1 suppl):S161-S175.

30. Hierner R, Berger AK, Frederix PR: Lower leg replantation decision-making, treatment, and long-term results. *Microsurgery* 2007;27(5):398-410.

31. Zubairi AJ, Hashmi PM: Long term follow-up of a successful lower limb replantation in a 3-year-old child. *Case Rep Orthop* 2015;2015:425376.

32. Noh K, Hacquebord JH: 50+ years of replantation surgery experience: Are we progressing or regressing? *Plast Aesthet Res* 2020;7:50.

33. Krajbich JI: Lower-limb deficiencies and amputations in children. *J Am Acad Orthop Surg* 1998;6(6):358-367.

34. Eshraghi A, Safaeepour Z, Geil MD, Andrysek J: Walking and balance in children and adolescents with lower-limb amputation: A review of literature. *Clin Biomech (Bristol, Avon)* 2018;59:181-198.

35. Penn-Barwell JG, Bennett PM, Gray AC: The 'could' and the 'should' of reconstructing severe hind-foot injuries. *Injury* 2018;49(2):147-148.

36. Braaksma R, Dijkstra PU, Geertzen JHB: Syme amputation: A systematic review. *Foot Ankle Int* 2018;39(3):284-291.

37. Westberry DE, Davids JR, Pugh LI: The Boyd amputation in children: Indications and outcomes. *J Pediatr Orthop* 2014;34(1):86-91.

38. Finkler ES, Marchwiany DA, Schiff AP, Pinzur MS: Long-term outcomes following syme's amputation. *Foot Ankle Int* 2017;38(7):732-735.

39. Morrison SG, Georgiadis AG, Dahl MT: Lengthening of the humerus using a motorized lengthening nail: A retrospective comparative series. *J Pediatr Orthop* 2020;40(6):e479-e486.

40. Davidson WH, Bohne WH: The Syme amputation in children. *J Bone Joint Surg Am* 1975;57(7):905-909.

41. Wagner FW: *Atlas of Limb Prosthetics: Surgical, Prosthetic, and Rehabilitation Principles*. O and P virtual library project, Digital Resource Foundation: chap 17A.

42. Vollman D, Smith GA: Epidemiology of lawn-mower-related injuries to children in the United States, 1990-2004. *Pediatrics* 2006;118(2):e273-e278.

43. Harkness B, Andresen D, Kesson A, Isaacs D: Infections following lawnmower and farm machinery-related injuries in children. *J Paediatr Child Health* 2009;45(9):525-528.

44. Parry IS, Mooney KN, Chau C, et al: Effects of skin grafting on successful prosthetic use in children with lower extremity amputation. *J Burn Care Res* 2008;29(6):949-954.

45. Osebold WR, Lester EL, Christenson DM: Problems with excessive residual lower leg length in pediatric amputees. *Iowa Orthop J* 2001;21:58-67.

46. Brodell JD Jr, Ayers BC, Baumhauer JF, et al: Chopart amputation: Questioning the clinical efficacy of a long-standing surgical option for diabetic foot infection. *J Am Acad Orthop Surg* 2020;28(16):684-691.

47. Anderson M, Green WT, Messner MB: Growth and predictions of growth in the lower extremities. *J Bone Joint Surg Am* 1963;45( ):1-4.

48. Burger K, Farr S, Hahne J, Radler C, Ganger R: Long-term results and comparison of the Green-Anderson and multiplier growth prediction methods after permanent epiphysiodesis using Canale's technique. *J Child Orthop* 2019;13(4):423-430.

49. Troy M, Shore B, Miller P, et al: A comparison of screw versus drill and curettage epiphysiodesis to correct leg-length discrepancy. *J Child Orthop* 2018;12(5):509-514.

50. Boyle J, Makarov MR, Podeszwa DA, Rodgers A, Jo CH, Birch JG: Is proximal fibula epiphysiodesis necessary when performing a proximal tibial epiphysiodesis? *J Pediatr Orthop* 2020;40(10):e984-e989.

51. Sinha R, Weigl D, Mercado E, Becker T, Kedem P, Bar-On E: Eight-plate

epiphysiodesis: Are we creating an intra-articular deformity? *Bone Joint J* 2018;100-B(8):1112-1116.

52. Morrison SG, Thomson P, Lenze U, Donnan LT: Syme amputation: function, satisfaction, and prostheses. *J Pediatr Orthop* 2020;40(6):e532-e536.

53. Segal LS, Crandall RC: Tibia vara deformity after below knee amputation and synostosis formation in children. *J Pediatr Orthop* 2009;29(2):120-123.

54. Crandall RC, Wagner FW Jr: Partial and total calcanectomy: A review of thirty-one consecutive cases over a ten-year period. *J Bone Joint Surg Am* 1981;63(1):152-155.

55. Atesalp S, Yildiz C: Disarticulation at the ankle using an anterior flap. *J Bone Joint Surg Br* 2000;82(3):462.

56. Aboelatta YA, Aly HM: Free tissue transfer and replantation in pediatric patients: Technical feasibility and outcome in a series of 28 patients. *J Hand Microsurg* 2013;5(2):74-80.

57. Piper ML, Amara D, Zafar SN, Lee C, Sbitany H, Hansen SL: Free tissue transfer optimizes stump length and functionality following high-energy trauma. *J Reconstr Microsurg Open* 2019;4(2):e96-e101.

58. Lin CH, Mardini S, Wei FC, Lin YT, Chen CT: Free flap reconstruction of foot and ankle defects in pediatric patients: long-term outcome in 91 cases. *Plast Reconstr Surg* 2006;117(7):2478-2487.

59. Mahajan RK, Srinivasan K, Ghildiyal H, et al: Review of cross-leg flaps in reconstruction of posttraumatic lower extremity wounds in a microsurgical unit. *Indian J Plast Surg* 2019;52(1):117-124.

60. Armstrong DG, Lavery LA, Boulton AJ: Negative pressure wound therapy via vacuum-assisted closure following partial foot amputation: What is the role of wound chronicity? *Int Wound J* 2007;4(1):79-86.

61. Sumpio B, Thakor P, Mahler D, Blume P: Negative pressure wound therapy as postoperative dressing in below knee amputation stump closure of patients with chronic venous insufficiency. *Wounds* 2011;23(10):301-308.

62. Shah RD, Suresh S: Applications of regional anaesthesia in paediatrics. *Br J Anaesth* 2013;111(suppl 1):i114-i124.

63. Crandall RC, Anderson TF, Backus B, Frucci T: Clinical evaluation of an articulated, dynamic-response prosthetic foot in teenage transtibial and Syme-level amputees. *J Prosthet Orthot* 1999;11(4):92-97.

64. Jeans KA, Karol LA, Cummings D, Singhal K: Comparison of gait after Syme and transtibial amputation in children: Factors that may play a role in function. *J Bone Joint Surg Am* 2014;96(19):1641-1647.

65. Waters RL, Perry J, Antonelli D, Hislop H: Energy cost of walking of amputees: The influence of level of amputation. *J Bone Joint Surg Am* 1976;58(1):42-46.

66. Jeans KA, Browne RH, Karol LA: Effect of amputation level on energy expenditure during overground walking by children with an amputation. *J Bone Joint Surg Am* 2011;93(1):49-56.

67. Clegg DJ, Rosenbaum PF, Harley BJ: The effects of timing of soft tissue coverage on outcomes after reconstruction of type IIIB open tibia fractures. *Orthopedics* 2019;42(5):260-266.

68. Bowker HK: Atlas of Limb Prosthetics. O and P Library; 1984 :chap 18A.

69. Burgess EM: The below knee amputation *Bull Prosthet Res* 1968;10:9-19.

70. Gailey RS, Wenger MA, Raya M, et al: Energy expenditure of trans--tibial amputees during ambulation at self-selected pace. *Prosthet Orthot Int* 1994;18(2):84-91.

71. Henrot P, Stines J, Walter F, Martinet N, Paysant J, Blum A: Imaging of the painful lower limb stump. *Radiographics* 2000;20 Spec No:S219-S235.

72. Portnoy S, van Haare J, Geers RP, et al: Real-time subject-specific analyses of dynamic internal tissue loads in the residual limb of transtibial amputees. *Med Eng Phys* 2010;32(4):312-323.

73. Portnoy S, Siev-Ner I, Shabshin N, Kristal A, Yizhar Z, Gefen A: Patient-specific analyses of deep tissue loads post transtibial amputation in residual limbs of multiple prosthetic users. *J Biomech* 2009;42(16):2686-2693.

74. Pet MA, Ko JH, Friedly JL, Smith DG: Traction neurectomy for treatment of painful residual limb neuroma in lower extremity amputees. *J Orthop Trauma* 2015;29(9):e321-e325.

75. Souza JM, Cheesborough JE, Ko JH, Cho MS, Kuiken TA, Dumanian GA: Targeted muscle reinnervation: A novel approach to postamputation neuroma pain. *Clin Orthop Relat Res* 2014;472(10):2984-2990.

76. Bowen JB, Wee CE, Kalik J, Valerio IL: Targeted muscle reinnervation to improve pain, prosthetic tolerance, and bioprosthetic outcomes in the amputee. *Adv Wound Care (New Rochelle)* 2017;6(8):261-267.

77. Eberlin KR, Ducic I: Surgical algorithm for neuroma management: A changing treatment paradigm. *Plast Reconstr Surg Glob Open* 2018;6(10):e1952.

78. Nigam M, Webb A, Harbour P, Devulapalli C, Kleiber G: Symptomatic neuromas in lower extremity amputees: implications for pre-emptive–targeted muscle reinnervation. *Plast Reconstr Surg Glob Open* 2019;7(8 suppl):80-81.

79. Abraham E, Pellicore RJ, Hamilton RC, Hallman BW, Ghosh L: Stump overgrowth in juvenile amputees. *J Pediatr Orthop* 1986;6(1):66-71.

80. Fedorak GT, Watts HG, Cuomo AV, et al: Osteocartilaginous transfer of the proximal part of the fibula for osseous overgrowth in children with congenital or acquired tibial amputation: Surgical technique and results. *J Bone Joint Surg Am* 2015;97(7):574-581.

81. Jahmani R, Robbins C, Paley D: Iliac crest apophysis transfer to treat stump overgrowth after limb amputation in children: Case series and literature review. *Int Orthop* 2019;43(11):2601-2605.

82. Davids JR, Meyer LC, Blackhurst DW: Operative treatment of bone overgrowth in children who have an acquired or congenital amputation. *J Bone Joint Surg Am* 1995;77(10):1490-1497.

83. Benevenia J, Makley JT, Leeson MC, Benevenia K: Primary epiphyseal transplants and bone overgrowth in childhood amputations. *J Pediatr Orthop* 1992;12(6):746-750.

84. Christie J, Lamb DW, McDonald JM, Britten S: A study of stump growth in children with below-knee amputations. *J Bone Joint Surg Br* 1979;61-B(4):464-465.

85. Carvalho JA, Mongon MD, Belangero WD, Livani B: A case series featuring extremely short below-knee stumps. *Prosthet Orthot Int* 2012;36(2):236-238.

86. Bowen RE, Struble SG, Setoguchi Y, Watts HG: Outcomes of lengthening short lower-extremity amputation stumps with planar fixators. *J Pediatr Orthop* 2005;25(4):543-547.

87. Parry SW, Toth BA, Elliott LF: Microvascular free-tissue transfer in children. *Plast Reconstr Surg* 1988;81(6):838-840.

88. Gallico GGIII, Ehrlichman RJ, Jupiter J, May JW Jr: Free flaps to preserve below-knee amputation stumps: Long-term evaluation. *Plast Reconstr Surg* 1987;79(6):871-878.

89. Kasabian AK, Colen SR, Shaw WW, Pachter HL: The role of microvascular free flaps in salvaging below-knee amputation stumps: A review of 22 cases. *J Trauma* 1991;31(4):495-501.

90. Kim SW, Jeon SB, Hwang KT, Kim YH: Coverage of amputation stumps using a latissimus dorsi flap with a serratus anterior muscle flap: A comparative study. *Ann Plast Surg* 2016;76(1):88-93.

91. Chen L, Yang F, Zhang ZX, Lu LJ, Hiromichi J, Satoshi T: Free fillet foot flap for salvage of below-knee amputation stump. *Chin J Traumatol* 2008;11(6):380-384.

92. Ranade A, McCarthy JJ, Davidson RS: Angular deformity in pediatric transtibial amputation stumps. *J Pediatr Orthop* 2009;29(7):726-729.

93. Gyr BM, Colmer HGIV, Morel MM, Ferski GJ: Hemiepiphysiodesis for correction of angular deformity in pediatric amputees. *J Pediatr Orthop* 2013;33(7):737-742.

94. Reichmann JP, Stevens PM, Rheinstein J, Kreulen CD: Removable rigid dressings for postoperative management of transtibial amputations: A review of published evidence. *PM R* 2018;10(5):516-523.

95. Gendron B, Andrews KL: The use of rigid removable dressings for juvenile amputees: A case report. *J Assoc Child Prosthetic Orthotic Clin* 1991;26:4.

96. Johannesson A, Larsson GU, Oberg T, Atroshi I: Comparison of vacuum-formed removable rigid dressing with conventional rigid dressing after transtibial amputation: Similar outcome in a randomized controlled trial involving 27 patients. *Acta Orthop* 2008;79(3):361-369.

97. Ülger Ö, Sener G: Functional outcome after prosthetic rehabilitation of children with acquired and congenital lower limb loss. *J Pediatr Orthop B* 2011;20(3):178-183.

98. MacKenzie EJ, Bosse MJ, Castillo RC, et al: Functional outcomes following trauma-related lower-extremity amputation [published correction appears in *J Bone Joint Surg Am*. 2004;86-A(11):2503]. *J Bone Joint Surg Am* 2004;86(8):1636-1645.

99. Polfer EM, Hoyt BW, Bevevino AJ, Forsberg JA, Potter BK: Knee disarticulations versus transfemoral amputations: Functional outcomes. *J Orthop Trauma* 2019;33(6):308-311.

100. Mazet M, Hennessy CA: Knee disarticulation: A new technique and joint mechanism. *J Bone Joint Surg Am* 1966;48(1):126-139.

101. Wagner FW Jr: Management of the diabetic neurotrophic foot. Part II. A classification and treatment program for diabetic, neuropathic, and dysvascular foot problems, in *Instructional Course Lectures, The American Academy of Orthopaedic Surgeons*. Vol 28. CV Mosby, 1979, pp 143-165.

102. Bowker JH, San Giovanni TP, Pinzur MS: North American experience with knee disarticulation with use of a posterior myofasciocutaneous flap. Healing rate and functional results in seventy-seven patients. *J Bone Joint Surg Am* 2000;82(11):1571-1574.

103. Murakami T, Murray K: Outcomes of knee disarticulation and the influence of surgical techniques in dysvascular patients: A systematic review. *Prosthet Orthot Int* 2016;40(4):423-435.

104. Albino FP, Seidel R, Brown BJ, Crone CG, Attinger CE: Through knee amputation: technique modifications and surgical outcomes. *Arch Plast Surg* 2014;41(5):562-570.

105. Burgess EM: Disarticulation of the knee. A modified technique. *Arch Surg* 1977;112(10):1250-1255.

106. Geil MD, Safaeepour Z, Giavedoni B, Coulter CP: Walking kinematics in young children with limb loss using early versus traditional prosthetic knee prescription protocols. *PLoS One* 2020;15(4):e0231401.

107. van Schaik L, Geertzen JHB, Dijkstra PU, Dekker R: Metabolic costs of activities of daily living in persons with a lower limb amputation: A systematic review and meta-analysis. *PLoS One* 2019;14(3):e0213256.

108. Russell Esposito E, Rábago CA, Wilken J: The influence of traumatic transfemoral amputation on metabolic cost across walking speeds. *Prosthet Orthot Int* 2018;42(2):214-222.

109. Delhey P, Huber S, Hanschen M, et al: Significance of traumatic macroamputation in severely injured patients: an analysis of the Traumaregister DGU®. *Shock* 2015;43(3):233-237.

110. Barmparas G, Inaba K, Teixeira PG, et al: Epidemiology of post-traumatic limb amputation: A national trauma databank analysis. *Am Surg* 2010;76(11):1214-1222.

111. Kragh JF Jr, O'Neill ML, Walters TJ, et al: Minor morbidity with emergency tourniquet use to stop bleeding in severe limb trauma: Research, history, and reconciling advocates and abolitionists. *Mil Med* 2011;176(7):817-823.

112. Hagberg E, Berlin OK, Renström P: Function after through-knee compared with below-knee and above-knee amputation. *Prosthet Orthot Int* 1992;16(3):168-173.

113. Gottschalk F: The importance of soft tissue stabilization in transfemoral amputation: English version. *Orthopade* 2016;45 suppl:S1-S4.

114. Gottschalk F: Transfemoral amputation. Biomechanics and surgery. *Clin Orthop Relat Res* 1999;361:15-22.

115. Bell JC, Wolf EJ, Schnall BL, Tis JE, Tis LL, Potter BK: Transfemoral amputations: the effect of residual limb length and orientation on gait analysis outcome measures. *J Bone Joint Surg Am* 2013;95(5):408-414.

116. Walker JL, White H, Jenkins JO, Cottle W, Vander Brink KD: Femoral lengthening after transfemoral amputation. *Orthopedics* 2006;29(1):53-59.

117. Kuiken TA, Butler BA, Sharkey T, Ivy AD, Li D, Peabody TD: Novel intramedullary device for lengthening transfemoral residual limbs. *J Orthop Surg Res* 2017;12(1):53.

118. Kahle J, Miro RM, Ho LT, et al: The effect of the transfemoral prosthetic socket interface designs on skeletal motion and socket comfort: A randomized clinical trial. *Prosthet Orthot Int* 2020;44(3):145-154.

119. Al Muderis M, Khemka A, Lord SJ, Van de Meent H, Frölke JP: Safety of osseointegrated implants for transfemoral amputees: A two-center prospective cohort study. *J Bone Joint Surg Am* 2016;98(11):900-909.

120. *Humanitarian Device Exemption Osseoanchored Prostheses for the Rehabilitation of Transfemoral Amputees (OPRA)*. U.S. Food and Drug Administration, 2019. Accessed June 29, 2021. Available at: https://www.accessdata.fda.gov/scripts/cdrh/cfdocs/cfhde/hde.cfm?id=H050004

121. Hoellwarth JS, Tetsworth K, Rozbruch SR, Handal MB, Coughlan A, Al Muderis M: Osseointegration for amputees: Current implants, techniques, and future directions. *JBJS Rev* 2020;8(3):e0043.

122. Aitken GT: Surgical amputation in children. *J Bone Joint Surg Am* 1963;45:1735-1741.

123. O'Neal ML, Bahner R, Ganey TM, Ogden JA: Osseous overgrowth after amputation in adolescents and children. *J Pediatr Orthop* 1996;16(1):78-84.

124. Pfeil J, Marquardt E, Holtz T, Niethard FU, Schneider E, Carstens C: The stump capping procedure to prevent or treat terminal osseous overgrowth. *Prosthet Orthot Int* 1991;15(2):96-99.

125. Potter BK, Burns TC, Lacap AP, Granville RR, Gajewski DA: Heterotopic ossification following traumatic and combat-related amputations. Prevalence, risk factors, and preliminary results of excision. *J Bone Joint Surg Am* 2007;89(3):476-486.

126. Sehirlioglu A, Ozturk C, Yazicioglu K, Tugcu I, Yilmaz B, Goktepe AS: Painful neuroma requiring surgical excision after lower limb amputation caused by landmine explosions. *Int Orthop* 2009;33(2):533-536.

127. Kuiken TA, Barlow AK, Hargrove L, Dumanian GA: Targeted muscle reinnervation for the upper and lower extremity. *Tech Orthop* 2017;32(2):109-116.

128. Frantz TL, Everhart JS, West JM, Ly TV, Phieffer LS, Valerio IL: Targeted muscle reinnervation at the time of major limb amputation in traumatic amputees: early experience of an effective treatment strategy to improve pain. *JBJS Open Access* 2020;5(2):e0067.

129. Wamalwa AO, Khainga SO: VRAM flap for an above knee amputation stump. *JPRAS Open* 2019;23:11-18.

130. Brodtkorb TH, Henriksson M, Johannesen-Munk K, Thidell F: Cost-effectiveness of C-leg compared with non-microprocessor-controlled knees: a modeling approach. *Arch Phys Med Rehabil* 2008;89(1):24-30.

131. Seymour R, Engbretson B, Kott K, et al: Comparison between the C-leg microprocessor-controlled prosthetic knee and non-microprocessor control prosthetic knees: A preliminary study of energy expenditure, obstacle course performance, and quality of life survey. *Prosthet Orthot Int* 2007;31(1):51-61.

132. Fuenzalida Squella SA, Kannenberg A, Brandão Benetti Â: Enhancement of a prosthetic knee with a microprocessor-controlled gait phase switch reduces falls and improves balance confidence and gait speed in community ambulators with unilateral transfemoral amputation. *Prosthet Orthot Int* 2018;42(2):228-235.

133. Krane EJ, Heller LB: The prevalence of phantom sensation and pain in pediatric amputees. *J Pain Symptom Manage* 1995;10(1):21-29.

134. Jensen TS, Krebs B, Nielsen J, Rasmussen P: Phantom limb, phantom pain and stump pain in amputees during the first 6 months following limb amputation. *Pain* 1983;17(3):243-256.

135. Nikolajsen L: Postamputation pain: studies on mechanisms. *Dan Med J* 2012;59(10):B4527.

136. Burgoyne LL, Billups CA, Jirón JL Jr, et al: Phantom limb pain in young cancer-related amputees: Recent experience at St Jude children's research hospital. *Clin J Pain* 2012;28(3):222-225.

137. Wilkins KL, McGrath PJ, Finley AG, Katz J: Phantom limb sensations and phantom limb pain in child and adolescent amputees. *Pain* 1998;78(1):7-12.

138. DeMoss P, Ramsey LH, Karlson CW: Phantom limb pain in pediatric oncology. *Front Neurol* 2018;9:219.

139. Bogdasarian RN, Cai SB, Tran BNN, Ignatiuk A, Lee ES: Surgical prevention of terminal neuroma and phantom limb pain: A literature review. *Arch Plast Surg* 2021;48(3):310-322.

140. Ilfeld BM, Khatibi B, Maheshwari K, et al: Ambulatory continuous peripheral nerve blocks to treat postamputation phantom limb pain: A multicenter, randomized, quadruple-masked, placebo-controlled clinical trial. *Pain* 2021;162(3):938-955.

141. Rusy LM, Troshynski TJ, Weisman SJ: Gabapentin in phantom limb pain management in children and young adults: report of seven cases. *J Pain Symptom Manage* 2001;21(1):78-82.

142. Thomas CR, Brazeal BA, Rosenberg L, Robert RS, Blakeney PE, Meyer WJ: Phantom limb pain in pediatric burn survivors. *Burns* 2003;29(2):139-142.

143. Barbin J, Seetha V, Casillas JM, Paysant J, Pérennou D: The effects of mirror therapy on pain and motor control of phantom limb in amputees: a systematic review. *Ann Phys Rehabil Med* 2016;59(4):270-275.

144. Sahu A, Gupta R, Sagar S, Kumar M, Sagar R: A study of psychiatric comorbidity after traumatic limb amputation: A neglected entity. *Ind Psychiatry J* 2017;26(2):228-232.

145. Samdani AJ, Azhar A, Shahid SM, et al: Homozygous frame shift mutation in ECM1 gene in two siblings with lipoid proteinosis. *J Dermatol Case Rep* 2010;4(4):66-70.

146. Clerici CA, Ferrari A, Luksch R, et al: Clinical experience with psychological aspects in pediatric patients amputated for malignancies. *Tumori* 2004;90(4):399-404.

147. Varni JW, Setoguchi Y, Rappaport LR, Talbot D: Psychological adjustment and perceived social support in children with congenital/acquired limb deficiencies. *J Behav Med* 1992;15(1):31-44.

148. Pruitt SD, Varni JW, Seid M, Setoguchi Y: Functional status in limb deficiency: Development of an outcome measure for preschool children. *Arch Phys Med Rehabil* 1998;79(4):405-411.

149. Varni JW, Limbers CA, Burwinkle TM: Parent proxy-report of their children's health-related quality of life: An analysis of 13,878 parents' reliability and validity across age subgroups using the PedsQL 4.0 generic core scales. *Health Qual Life Outcomes* 2007;5:2.

150. Galey SA, Margalit A, Ain MC, Brooks JT: Medical malpractice in pediatric orthopaedics: A systematic review of US Case Law. *J Pediatr Orthop* 2019;39(6):e482-e486.

151. Matsen FA III, Stephens L, Jette JL, Warme WJ, Posner KL: Lessons regarding the safety of orthopaedic patient care: an analysis of four hundred and sixty-four closed malpractice claims. *J Bone Joint Surg Am* 2013;95(4):e201-e208.

152. Bhattacharyya T, Yeon H, Harris MB: The medical-legal aspects of informed consent in orthopaedic surgery. *J Bone Joint Surg Am* 2005;87(11):2395-2400.

153. Tarantino U, Giai Via A, Macrì E, Eramo A, Marino V, Marsella LT: Professional liability in orthopaedics and traumatology in Italy. *Clin Orthop Relat Res* 2013;471(10):3349-3357.

154. Gifford DG: Technological triggers to tort revolutions: Steam locomotives, autonomous vehicles, and accident compensation. *J Tort Law* 2018;11(1):71-143.

Congenital Longitudinal Deficiencies of the Upper Limb

Krister Freese, MD, FAAOS • Stephen Butler, MBBS(Hons), FRACS(Orth), FAOrthA, PFET(Hand Surgery)

ABSTRACT

Radial and ulnar longitudinal deficiencies are the two most common congenital longitudinal deficiencies of the upper limbs and are characterized by a partially or completely absent radius or ulna, respectively. Radial longitudinal deficiency often is associated with abnormalities of other organ systems, including cardiac and renal systems, which can be potentially lethal and require a comprehensive medical evaluation. Ulnar longitudinal deficiency tends to be associated with other musculoskeletal abnormalities. Treatment aims to improve function and appearance and is best provided in a well-resourced setting in the context of a long-term relationship between the child, their family, and the hand surgeon.

Keywords: humeral hypoplasia; radial hypoplasia; radial longitudinal deficiency; thumb hypoplasia; ulnar longitudinal deficiency; upper limb hypoplasia

Introduction

Radial longitudinal deficiency (RLD) and ulnar longitudinal deficiency (ULD) are the two most common congenital longitudinal deficiencies of the upper limbs. These conditions historically were described as radial or ulnar clubhand, but this term is no longer commonly used. The deficient bone may be partially or completely absent. In the 2013 classification by Kerby Oberg, Paul Manske, and Michael Tonkin, and approved by the International Federation of Societies for Surgery of the Hand[1], these deficiencies are classified as malformations of the upper limb resulting from a failure of formation of the radial–ulnar (fetal anterior-posterior) axis[1,2] (also known as preaxial [radius] or postaxial [ulna] longitudinal deficiencies).

Radial Longitudinal Deficiency

Clinical Features

RLD is characterized by partial or total absence of the radius and a short, bowed ulna that can result in profound radial and palmar displacement of the hand and the carpus. In severe forms the ulna is approximately two-thirds of its normal length. The humerus is often shorter than normal, and in rare cases may be absent.[3] The elbow may be stiff and the thumb may be absent or hypoplastic. The index and middle fingers also may be stiff; the ring and small fingers are usually flexible.

RLD often is bilateral and asymmetric. Bilateral deficiency is twice as likely in those with syndromic RLD, as is having concurrent thumb hypoplasia.[4] Thumb hypoplasia severity is correlated to RLD severity.[4-6] The wrist is unstable because of a lack of radial carpal support, and grip is weak because this instability is combined with finger stiffness. Children with RLD have difficulty reaching away from the body because of radial deviation of the wrist and bowing of the ulna. Children with manifestations of radial and thumb deficiencies may have difficulty attaining independence with activities of daily living, such as fastening buttons and performing personal hygiene.

Etiology

Two recent Northern European population studies showed that the incidence of RLD is 0.4 to 1.6 per 10,000 live births.[7,8] Recent Congenital Upper Limb Differences (CoULD) data[4] suggest that 32% of children with RLD have an associated syndrome (**Table 1**). Golbfarb et al[9] found that 67% of children with RLD had an associated syndrome or musculoskeletal condition. Scoliosis was the most common associated musculoskeletal condition. Other limb anomalies include humeral hypoplasia, radioulnar synostosis, radial head dislocation, and stiff digits.[10,11] The most common syndromes associated with RLD are VACTERL (vertebral malformations, imperforate anus, cardiac defects, tracheoesophageal fistula, renal abnormalities,

---

Dr. Freese or an immediate family member serves as a board member, owner, officer, or committee member of the Pediatric Orthopaedic Society of North America. Neither Dr. Butler nor any immediate family member has received anything of value from or has stock or stock options held in a commercial company or institution related directly or indirectly to the subject of this chapter.

This chapter is adapted from James MA, Peck KM: Congenital longitudinal deficiencies of the upper limb, in Krajbich JI, Pinzur MS, Potter BK, Stevens PM, eds: *Atlas of Amputations and Limb Deficiencies: Surgical, Prosthetic, and Rehabilitation Principles*, ed 4. American Academy of Orthopaedic Surgeons, 2016, pp 823-830.

and limb defects) and Holt–Oram syndrome; others that are less common but critical to diagnose preoperatively are thrombocytopenia absent radius (TAR) syndrome, Diamond–Blackfan anemia (also known as congenital hypoplastic anemia), and Fanconi syndrome (also known as Fanconi anemia). Patients with TAR syndrome have severe RLD but usually have a hypoplastic thumb present. Those with Holt–Oram syndrome are more likely to have both RLD and radioulnar synostosis.[4] The unclassifiable thumb or five-fingered hand are more common in patients with TAR syndrome or Holt–Oram syndrome and should alert the surgeon to the possible presence of these syndromes.[4,9,12]

VACTERL is a sporadic condition that includes anomalies of multiple different systems: vertebra, anus, cardiac, trachea/esophagus, renal, and limbs (including RLD).[13,14] Holt–Oram syndrome is an autosomal dominant condition that is characterized by cardiac septal defects as well as RLD.[8] Diamond–Blackfan anemia, Fanconi syndrome, and thrombocytopenia absent radius syndrome are bone marrow failure syndromes that may present as RLD. These conditions should be diagnosed preoperatively and treated by a pediatric hematologist because they are treatable and potentially lethal if not diagnosed and treated.[15]

Thalidomide, a teratogenic agent prescribed as a sedative in the late 1950s, resulted in various limb malformations, including RLD.[16] Other teratogens also may cause this malformation, depending on the timing of maternal exposure.

Diagnostic Studies

Children with RLD should undergo a complete physical examination, a thorough family history should be obtained, and a geneticist should be consulted. Radiographs of the entire upper limb (humerus, elbow, forearm, wrist, and hand—both sides) are essential to assess for associated abnormalities and to classify the condition. A spine radiograph should be obtained to evaluate for congenital spine anomalies associated with VACTERL.

A complete blood count (bone marrow failure syndromes), a cardiac echocardiogram (VACTERL and Holt–Oram syndrome), a renal ultrasonography (VACTERL), and a chromosomal breakage test (Fanconi syndrome) also are indicated.

Classification

Bayne and Klug[17] classified RLD into four types based on the extent of radial hypoplasia demonstrated on radiographs. James et al[5] combined Bayne and Klug's classification with the modified Blauth classification for thumb hypoplasia to create a modified version that included children with carpal or thumb deficiencies in the presence of a normal radius.[17] Additionally proximal longitudinal deficiency has also been included in modifications of the classification (**Tables 2 and 3**).

Treatment

The treatment of RLD is based on improving function and appearance. Functional impairments may be caused by thumb hypoplasia or absence, wrist instability with radial deviation and

TABLE 1 Most Common Syndromes Associated With Radial Longitudinal Deficiency

Syndrome	Inheritance Pattern	Associated Anomalies
VACTERL	Sporadic	Vertebral malformations, imperforate anus, cardiac defects, tracheoesophageal fistula, renal abnormalities, and limb defects
Holt–Oram syndrome	Autosomal dominant	Cardiac septal defects and radial dysplasia
Fanconi syndrome	Autosomal recessive	Pancytopenia and radial dysplasia
Thrombocytopenia absent radius syndrome	Autosomal recessive	Thrombocytopenia, absent radii, mildly hypoplastic thumbs present
Diamond–Blackfan anemia	Inherited, but heterogeneous	Anemia and reticulocytopenia; growth retardation; craniofacial, upper limb, heart, and urinary system malformations

TABLE 2 Modified Bayne Classification of Radial Longitudinal Deficiency

Type	Thumb	Carpus	Distal Radius	Proximal Radius	Humerus
N	Hypoplastic or absent	Normal	Normal	Normal	Normal
0	Hypoplastic or absent	Absence, hypoplasia, or coalition	Normal	Normal, radioulnar synostosis, or congenital dislocation of the radial head	Normal
1	Hypoplastic or absent	Absence, hypoplasia, or coalition	>2 mm shorter than the ulna	Normal, radioulnar synostosis, or congenital dislocation of the radial head	Normal
2	Hypoplastic or absent	Absence, hypoplasia, or coalition	Hypoplasia	Hypoplasia	Normal
3	Hypoplastic or absent	Absence, hypoplasia, or coalition	Physis absent	Variable hypoplasia	Normal
4	Hypoplastic or absent	Absence, hypoplasia, or coalition	Absent	Absent	Normal
5	Hypoplastic or absent	Absence, hypoplasia, or coalition	Absent	Absent	Proximal upper extremity hypoplasia including abnormal glenoid and proximal humerus

TABLE 2 Modified Bayne Classification of Radial Longitudinal Deficiency (continued)

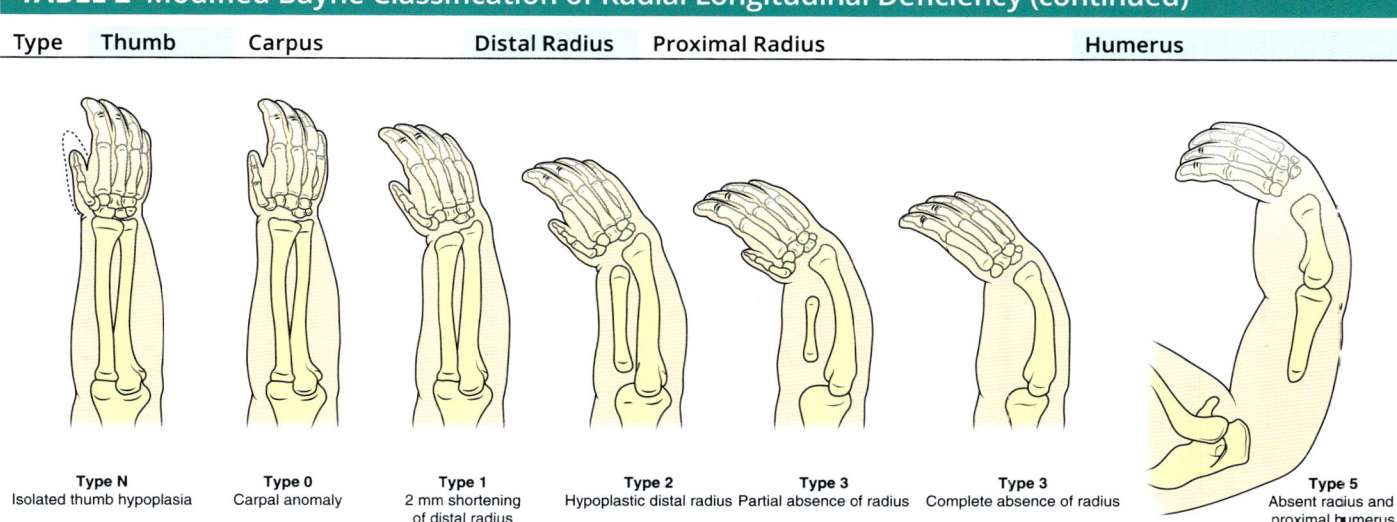

Illustration redrawn from Forman M, Canizares MF, Bohn D, et al: Association of radial longitudinal deficiency and thumb hypoplasia: An update using the CoULD registry. *J Bone Joint Surg Am* 2020;102(20):1815-1822.

TABLE 3 Modified Blauth Classification of Hypoplastic Thumb

Type	Characteristic
I	Mild shortening or narrowing of the thumb
II	Thumb–index web space narrowing, hypoplastic intrinsic thenar muscles, and metacarpophalangeal joint instability
III	Type II hypoplasia plus:
	A: Extrinsic muscle abnormalities, hypoplastic metacarpal, and stable carpometacarpal joint
	B: Extrinsic muscle abnormalities, partial metacarpal aplasia, and unstable carpometacarpal joint
IV	Pouce flottant (floating thumb)
V	Absent thumb

Illustration redrawn from Forman M, Canizares MF, Bohn D, et al: Association of radial longitudinal deficiency and thumb hypoplasia: An update using the CoULD registry. *J Bone Joint Surg Am* 2020;102(20):1815-1822.

palmar flexion of the hand in relation to the forearm, and an overall shortened arm. Controversy still exists concerning the best way to surgically address the radially deviated wrist, although most pediatric hand surgeons agree that children fare better with surgical rather than nonsurgical treatment. Kotwal et al[18] reviewed 446 patients with RLD types 3 or 4 with a minimum follow-up of 5 years. A total of 309 patients were treated surgically, and 137 patients were treated nonsurgically. Despite the high recurrence of deformity after centralization, improvements in the surgically treated group included the appearance and alignment of the wrist and hand, finger

Section 5: Pediatrics

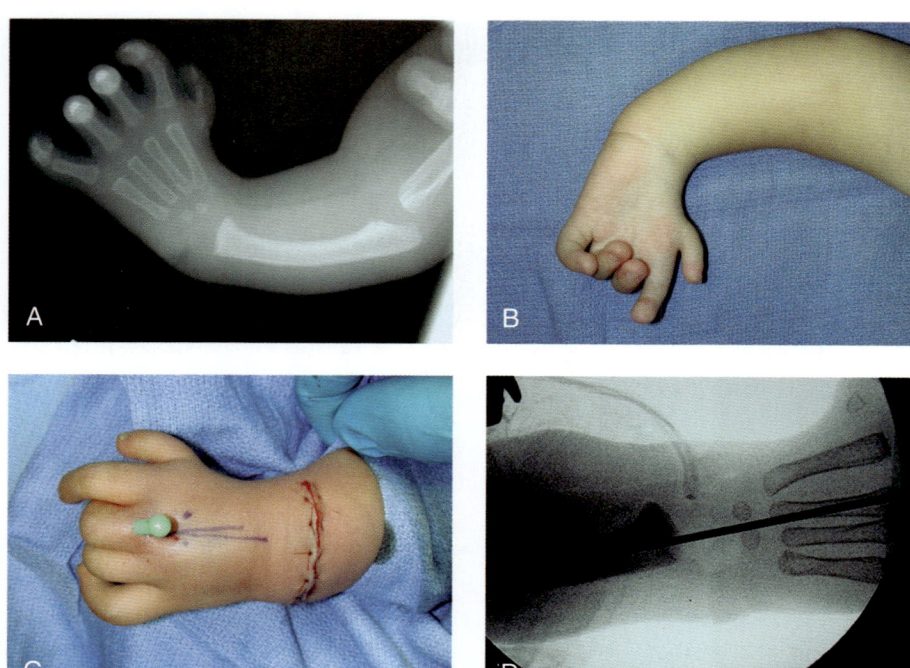

FIGURE 1 Images of a type 4 radial longitudinal deficiency and a type IIIB hypoplastic thumb in a child. **A**, AP radiograph. **B**, Clinical photograph of the limb. **C**, Postoperative photograph after centralization. **D**, AP radiograph after centralization, with intramedullary fixation in place.

and wrist range of motion, and grip strength (**Figure 1**).

Although there have been no studies investigating any change in the natural history of RLD after stretching and splinting, they are still used to lengthen the soft tissues along the radial side of the ulna, place the hand in a more functional position for use, and can aid future realignment procedures. Serial long-arm, flexed-elbow casts can be used to stretch the radial and palmar soft tissue, and splints can be used to maintain correction. Splints can be applied to the radial side of the forearm to push or along the ulnar side to pull the hand ulnarly. In addition to splinting, parents should be taught how to stretch out a hand that exhibits radial deviation—a process that should be done several times per day.

Centralization and radialization are two techniques for repositioning the hand onto the distal end of the ulna. Centralization aligns the long finger metacarpal and the ulna; radialization, as proposed by Buck-Gramcko,[19] placed the hand in ulnar deviation and aligned the index metacarpal with the ulna to diminish the recurrence of radial deviation. Both techniques are complicated by the recurrence of deformity and growth retardation from damage to the distal ulnar physis. Radialization is less widely used,[20] and less well reported compared with centralization; however recent literature also supports its use.[21,22]

If stretching exercises and splinting are insufficient, distraction can stretch the soft tissues to allow centralization. Goldfarb et al[23] described the use of a ring external fixator for soft-tissue distraction before centralization, gaining an average of 16 mm of distraction and enabling centralization without tension, thus minimizing the risk of damage to the ulnar physis. Nanchahal and Tonkin[24] showed that carpal realignment was possible in five of six patients who had soft-tissue distraction with an external fixator system before centralization, but if only centralization was performed, carpal realignment occurred in only one of six patients. However, a recent study reported that despite the ease of centralization after soft-tissue distraction, radial deviation was more likely to recur in those who underwent distraction versus the group who did not have distraction.[25]

After centralization, wrist motion is reduced;[17] thus, centralization is contraindicated when the ipsilateral elbow has an extension contracture because the child may need radial deviation and flexion to reach their mouth.

In addition to a high risk of recurrence of deformity, centralization places the distal ulnar physis at risk for early growth arrest, which is a devastating complication in an already shortened upper limb. More modern centralization techniques that avoid carpal notching seem to be at a lower risk of causing ulnar physeal arrest or slowing.[26] An ulna osteotomy is recommended at the time of centralization procedures if the ulna bow exceeds 30°.[27] However, remodeling of the ulna may occur during distraction before centralization, reducing the ulna bow and potential need for osteotomy. Soft-tissue releases combined with tendon transfers and long-term splinting at night may improve wrist alignment while preserving wrist motion. For types 3 and 4 deficiencies, Wall et al[28] recommended the initiation of splinting and stretching, followed by releasing constricted radial soft tissues at the wrist with a volar bilobed flap for coverage of the radial side for a child aged 1 to 2 years. For a child aged 5 to 6 years, microvascular transplantation of the first metatarsophalangeal joint to the radial side of the wrist is considered, which was originally described by Vilkki;[29] however, most patients do not proceed further with the transfer because they are satisfied with both function and appearance. This approach maintains wrist motion and does not endanger the distal ulnar physis.

For adolescents with recurrent radial deviation, ulnocarpal arthrodesis is a salvage option. Pike et al[30] reported on 12 children with RLD who underwent ulnocarpal arthrodesis (11 patients underwent ulnocarpal epiphyseal arthrodesis, and one patient underwent traditional ulnocarpal arthrodesis). All achieved wrist stability and a decrease of 42° in radial deviation. Patients did, however, undergo a reduction of prehension following the arthrodeses, with a

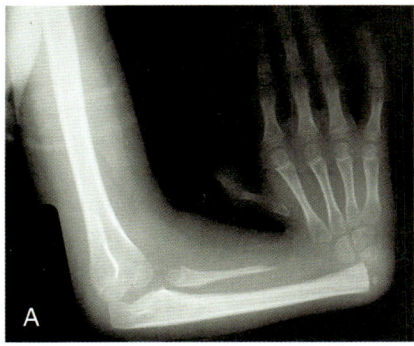 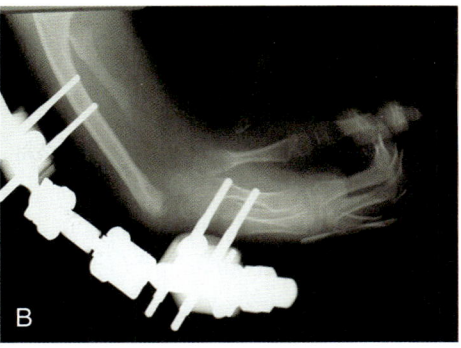 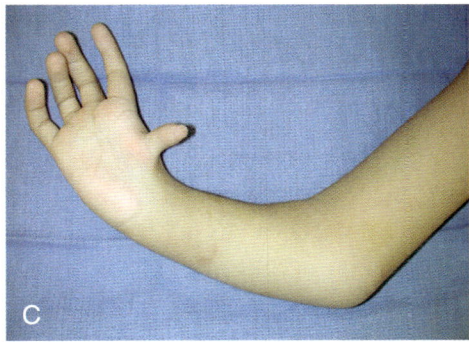

FIGURE 2 **A,** AP radiograph of a child with type 3 radial longitudinal deficiency and a type IIIB hypoplastic thumb. **B,** AP radiograph obtained after applying an external fixator for soft-tissue distraction. **C,** Clinical photograph obtained after soft-tissue distraction and centralization.

reduction in finger total active range of motion of 35° to 39°.

Ulnar lengthening has been used to treat RLD (**Figure 2**). Farr et al[31] reported eight ulnar lengthenings, noting an average increase of 75%, but correction of radial deviation and ulnar bowing was not maintained. Yoshida et al[32] reported on their experience of repeated lengthenings of patients with type 4 RLD. With their initial lengthening, length increased 89% and then regressed to 70%; after the second lengthening, length increased to 102%, with the final length increase averaging 83%. Yoshida et al[32] recommended a second lengthening after skeletal maturity. Peterson et al[33] reported on nine patients who underwent 13 ulnar lengthenings, achieving an average length of 4.4 cm with each lengthening. These authors commented that the process was long and arduous for both families and surgeons, and fraught with complications. They recommended that this procedure be limited to the mature adolescent or teenager who has excellent family support.

Vascularized second metatarsophalangeal joint transfer has been used to stabilize the carpus and allow physeal growth. Vilkki[29] originally described this technique of transferring the second metatarsophalangeal joint along with the second ray to the radial aspect of the distal forearm. This technique provides structural support in addition to allowing growth resulting from the transposed toe phalanx physis. de Jong et al[34] reported an 11-year follow-up, noting an average of 28° of radial deviation, average active wrist motion of 83°, and continued ulnar growth. The surgical procedure is technically demanding, and complications were reported in more than 50% of patients, resulting in subsequent procedures. Recently vascularized proximal fibula has been used in an attempt to improve the physeal growth rate compared with second metatarsophalangeal joint transfer, and avoids the cosmetic disadvantage of sacrificing the second toe. This technique, however, has been reported only on type 3 cases of RLD, and long-term follow-up is lacking.[35]

Another challenge with the surgical correction of RLD is soft-tissue coverage after the deviated wrist is corrected. The radial-side skin often is under substantial tension, and the ulnar-side skin often is redundant. Multiple techniques have been described to treat this, including the bilobed flap described by Evans et al,[36] which addresses the skin coverage issue by rotating the ulnar-side skin to the dorsum and the dorsal-side skin to the radial side. The bilobed flap can potentially lead to tip necrosis and cosmesis issues because of excessive ulnar skin. VanHeest and Grierson[37] and VanHeest[38] used a dorsal rotation flap that rotates the excessive ulnar skin radially. Subjective satisfaction with scar appearance was reported.[37]

Pollicization is generally performed as a staged procedure after centralization for those with hypoplastic thumbs of Blauth IIIB severity or worse, however combining the procedures has been reported.[39] It should be noted that the functional results of pollicization are worse in patients with more severe RLD.[40] In severe RLD the index finger is typically stiff with hypoplastic extrinsic components, and some surgeons will not perform a pollicization, especially in the setting of ulnar prehension.[20] Pollicization in the setting of stiff index fingers, however, has been reported with good functional results.[41]

Ulnar Longitudinal Deficiency
Clinical Features

The most important functional deficiencies in ULD involve the elbow and the forearm.[42] The ulna is partially or totally absent, and a cartilaginous anlage is often present.[43] The radius is typically shortened and bowed. The elbow is abnormal and commonly a radiohumeral synostosis is present. Typically, the entire arm is hypoplastic. The shoulder tends to be internally rotated. The carpus and the hand are almost always involved, with 90% of affected limbs missing digits, 70% demonstrating thumb abnormalities, and 30% demonstrating syndactyly.[43] Unlike RLD, the hand is typically aligned with the wrist but can be in ulnar deviation.

ULD is most commonly unilateral.[44] Children with severe elbow contractures, radiohumeral synostosis, or bilateral ULD have more severe limitations in function. They may have difficulty completing activities of daily living, especially personal hygiene and dressing. Children with radiohumeral synostosis and absent, deformed, or stiff fingers have the most limited function.[45,46] In contrast to radial longitudinal deficiency, lower extremity deficiencies are commonly associated with ULD. A recent study found that 17% of patients with fibular or femoral deficiencies had an associated upper limb congenital anomaly, most commonly ULD.[44] Patients with bilateral lower extremity involvement were more likely to have ULD.

Incidence and Etiology

Two recent epidemiologic studies of Northern European populations showed that the incidence of ULD is 0.2 to 0.4 per 10,000 live births.[7,8] Flatt[47] found that RLD is approximately four times as common as ULD. Unlike RLD, ULD is usually sporadic and not associated with systemic conditions.[43] It may be associated with other musculoskeletal malformations, including coxa vara, proximal femoral focal deficiency, fibular deficiency, phocomelia, scoliosis, absent digits, and radial ray deficiencies. Approximately 40% of children with ULD have associated contralateral upper limb abnormalities.[48] Syndromes associated with ULD include Weyers oligodactyly, Cornelia de Lange syndrome, ulnar mammary syndrome, Langer and Reinhardt-Pfeiffer type mesomelic dysplasias, Pillay syndrome, ulnar fibular dysostosis, and femoral-fibular-ulnar deficiency syndrome.[46,49,50]

Diagnostic Studies

Radiographic imaging is necessary to determine the extent of ULD and classify the condition. Bilateral radiographs of the upper limbs are essential to evaluate for associated musculoskeletal anomalies, such as phocomelia, radiohumeral synostosis, absent digits, thumb hypoplasia, and syndactyly. Radiographs of the spine also should be obtained to evaluate for scoliosis.[51]

Classification

Multiple classification systems have been proposed for ULD, focusing on elbow and forearm anomalies. The classification system by Kummel[52] addressed the elbow joint and whether radiohumeral synostosis or dislocation of the radiocapitellar joint is present. Ogden et al[53] classified ULD based on the length of the ulna. The classification system by Bayne[54] combined ulnar length and elbow morphology[43] (Table 4). Cole and Manske[55] approached classification of ULD differently and based their system on the characteristics of the thumb and the first web (Table 5).

Because the entire upper limb is involved, it is difficult to develop a classification system that addresses all associated anomalies. Therefore, some clinicians combine classification systems to develop a comprehensive plan to treat all the upper limb anomalies associated with ULD.

Treatment

The goals of treatment of children with ULD include improving the position and function of the affected limb. Splinting of the wrist may prevent worsening of the ulnar deviation, but to date this is not supported by published literature. Procedures to address hand anomalies include syndactyly release, first web space deepening, index pollicization (Figure 3), opponensplasty, and thumb metacarpal osteotomy.

Children with substantial internal rotation of the upper limb caused by ULD may have difficulty reaching their face and head with the ipsilateral hand. If they are able to perform activities of daily living, treatment may not be necessary. For persistent limitations, an external rotation osteotomy of the

TABLE 4 Modified Classification of Ulnar Longitudinal Deficiency

Type	Ulna	Radius	Elbow	Wrist/Hand
0	Normal	Normal	Stable	Absent or hypoplastic digits; carpal absence or coalition
1	Hypoplastic; distal and proximal epiphysis present	Mildly bowed	Stable	Mild ulnar wrist deviation; absent or hypoplastic digits
2	Partial aplasia; distal portion absent; ulnar anlage	Bowed	Variable stability; radial head may dislocate posterolaterally	Mild ulnar wrist deviation
3	Absent; no anlage	Straight	Unstable; posterolateral radial head dislocation; may have severe elbow flexion deformity	Less ulnar wrist deviation; severe carpal and digital deficiencies
4	Absent; ulnar anlage	Severely bowed	Radiohumeral synostosis; humeral internal rotation; forearm pronation	Ulnar wrist deviation
5	Absent	Straight	Radiohumeral synostosis; humeral bifurcation or large medial condyle	Less ulnar wrist deviation; severe carpal and digital deficiencies

TABLE 5 Manske and Cole Classification of Thumb and First Web Space Anomalies Associated With Ulnar Longitudinal Deficiency

Type	Characteristic
A	Normal thumb and first web space
B	Mild first web space and thumb deficiency
C	Moderate to severe first web space and thumb deficiency (loss of opposition, malrotation, thumb index syndactyly, no extrinsic tendon function)
D	Absent thumb

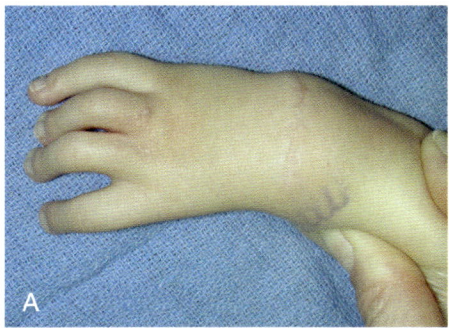 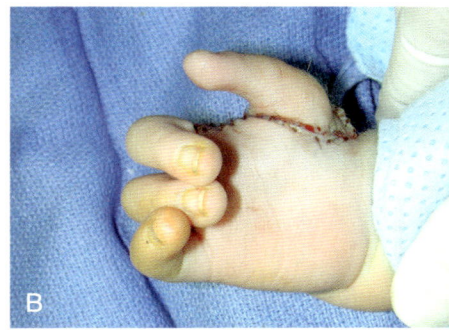

FIGURE 3 **A**, Clinical photograph of the hand of a child with type V absent thumb. **B**, Postoperative photograph of the hand after pollicization.

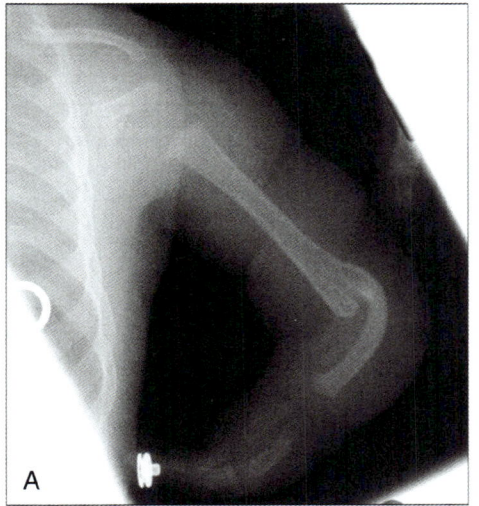 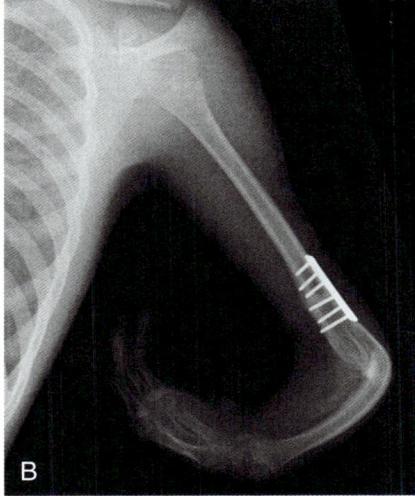

FIGURE 4 **A**, AP radiograph of a child with ulnar longitudinal deficiency. **B**, Postoperative AP radiograph of the same child taken several years later after humeral osteotomy.

humerus places the hand in a more functional position (**Figure 4**).

Surgery for radiohumeral synostosis will not improve motion,[56] but a forearm rotational osteotomy may place the hand in a more functional position.[47] For children with partial ulnar deficiency, painful elbow instability, and limited forearm rotation, a one-bone forearm procedure can confer stability and reduce pain.[57-59]

Excision of the ulnar anlage, a fibrocartilaginous structure, is a controversial procedure for the treatment of ULD. Although some surgeons have hypothesized that the ulnar anlage fails to grow with the radius and acts as a tether, which leads to increased ulnar deviation and progressive wrist deformity,[48] progressive ulnar deviation deformity has not been consistently noted by others. Ulnar anlage resection appears most appropriate when progressive deformity of the wrist or elbow is present or if the bowing of the radius increases.[60]

A recent case report of two patients with Bayne type I ULD reported successfully treating mild but symptomatic shortening of the ulna with a z-shaped ulnar lengthening osteotomy.[31] While long-term results are lacking this may be an option in the symptomatic patient with mild bony deformity.

Transverse Deficiencies

Transverse deficiencies of the upper extremity can be seen in a heterogeneous group of diagnoses including symbrachydactyly, amelia, segmental deficiencies, and amniotic band syndrome. Clinically, the distinction between symbrachydactyly and a segmental transverse deficiency can be made by the presence of ectodermal elements. Patients with a foreshortened limb with nubbins and nail elements are diagnosed with symbrachydactyly. Transverse deficiencies are often unilateral. They are commonly confused with amniotic band syndrome. Frequently, patients will be given a diagnosis of amniotic band syndrome in the perinatal period. Patients with amniotic band syndrome will usually have multiple bands on different limbs and fenestrated acrosyndactyly. An accurate diagnosis is important in counseling families. Patients with amniotic band syndrome and a transverse amputation may develop bony overgrowth at the end of their residuum. When this occurs surgical resection may be necessary in the symptomatic patient. Additionally, overgrowth can recur until skeletal maturity. Patients with other causes of their transverse deficiency are unlikely to experience this phenomenon.

Historically, patients with unilateral congenital amputations were fit with a prosthesis at a young age. However, in a recent comparison of patients who do and do not wear prosthetics in the setting of a unilateral congenital below elbow deficiency, no functional improvement was found in the group of patients wearing prosthetics.[61] This may be a limitation of current prosthetics but also highlights the baseline functional abilities of these patients. Our current practice is to fit patients with a prosthetic aimed at completing a specific task or function (eg, participating in a favorite sport, riding their bicycle). This prosthesis is not usually meant for full-time wear.

SUMMARY

RLD and ULD are failures of formation of the radius and ulna, respectively. Transverse deficiencies can also occur. These conditions may be associated with other musculoskeletal conditions and syndromes. Treatment aims to improve function and appearance and is best provided in a well-resourced setting in the context of a long-term relationship between the child, their family, and the hand surgeon.

References

1. Tonkin MA, Tolerton SK, Quick TJ, et al: Classification of congenital anomalies of the hand and upper limb: Development and assessment of a new system. *J Hand Surg Am* 2013;38(9):1845-1853.
2. Ezaki M, Baek GH, Horii E, Hovius S: IFSSH Scientific Committee on congenital conditions. *J Hand Surg Eur Vol* 2014;39(6):676-678.
3. Goldfarb CA, Manske PR, Busa R, Mills J, Carter P, Ezaki M: Upper-extremity phocomelia reexamined: A longitudinal dysplasia. *J Bone Joint Surg Am* 2005;87(12):2639-2648.
4. Forman M, Canizares MF, Bohn D, et al: Association of radial longitudinal deficiency and thumb hypoplasia: An update using the CoULD registry. *J Bone Joint Surg Am* 2020;102(20):1815-1822.
5. James MA, McCarroll HR Jr, Manske PR: The spectrum of radial longitudinal deficiency: A modified classification. *J Hand Surg Am* 1999;24(6):1145-1155.
6. James MA, Green HD, McCarroll HR Jr, Manske PR: The association of radial deficiency with thumb hypoplasia. *J Bone Joint Surg Am* 2004;86(10):2196-2205.
7. Koskimies E, Lindfors N, Gissler M, Peltonen J, Nietosvaara Y: Congenital upper limb deficiencies and associated malformations in Finland: A population-based study. *J Hand Surg Am* 2011;36(6):1058-1065.
8. Ekblom AG, Laurell T, Arner M: Epidemiology of congenital upper limb anomalies in Stockholm, Sweden, 1997 to 2007: Application of the Oberg, Manske, and Tonkin classification. *J Hand Surg Am* 2014;39(2):237-248.
9. Goldfarb CA, Wall L, Manske PR: Radial longitudinal deficiency: The incidence of associated medical and musculoskeletal conditions. *J Hand Surg Am* 2006;31(7):1176-1182.
10. Bauer AS, Bednar MS, James MA: Disruption of the radial/ulnar axis: Congenital longitudinal deficiencies. *J Hand Surg Am* 2013;38(11):2293-2302.
11. James MA, McCarroll HR Jr, Manske PR: Characteristics of patients with hypoplastic thumbs. *J Hand Surg Am* 1996;21(1):104-113.
12. Wall LB, Piper SL, Habenicht R, Oishi SN, Ezaki M, Goldfarb CA: Defining features of the upper extremity in Holt-Oram syndrome. *J Hand Surg Am* 2015;40(9):1764-1768.
13. Quan L, Smith DW: The VATER association Vertebral defects, anal atresia, T-E fistula with esophageal atresia, radial and renal dysplasia: A spectrum of associated defects. *J Pediatr* 1973;82(1):104-107.
14. Beals RK, Rolfe B: VATER association: A unifying concept of multiple anomalies. *J Bone Joint Surg Am* 1989;71(6):948-950.
15. Chirnomas SD, Kupfer GM: The inherited bone marrow failure syndromes. *Pediatr Clin North Am* 2013;60(6):1291-1310.
16. Lamb DW: Radial club hand: A continuing study of sixty-eight patients with one hundred and seventeen club hands. *J Bone Joint Surg Am* 1977;59(1):1-13.
17. Bayne LG, Klug MS: Long-term review of the surgical treatment of radial deficiencies. *J Hand Surg Am* 1987;12(2):169-179.
18. Kotwal PP, Varshney MK, Soral A: Comparison of surgical treatment and nonoperative management for radial longitudinal deficiency. *J Hand Surg Eur Vol* 2012;37(2):161-169.
19. Buck-Gramcko D: Radialization as a new treatment for radial club hand. *J Hand Surg Am* 1985;10(6 pt 2):964-968.
20. Wall LB, Kim DJ, Cogsil T, Goldfarb CA: Treatment of radial longitudinal deficiency: An international survey. *J Hand Surg Am* 2021;46(3):241.e1-241.e11.
21. Bhat AK, Narayanakurup JK, Acharya AM, Kumar B: Outcomes of radialization for radial longitudinal deficiency: 20 limbs with minimum 5-year follow-up. *J Hand Surg Eur Vol* 2019;44(3):304-309.
22. Mittal S, Garg B, Mehta N, Kumar V, Kotwal P: Randomized trial comparing preliminary results of radialization and centralization procedures in Bayne Types 3 and 4 radial longitudinal deficiency. *J Pediatr Orthop* 2020;40(9):509-514.
23. Goldfarb CA, Murtha YM, Gordon JE, Manske PR: Soft-tissue distraction with a ring external fixator before centralization for radial longitudinal deficiency. *J Hand Surg Am* 2006;31(6):952-959.
24. Nanchahal J, Tonkin MA: Pre-operative distraction lengthening for radial longitudinal deficiency. *J Hand Surg Br* 1996;21(1):103-107.
25. Manske MC, Wall LB, Steffen JA, Goldfarb CA: The effect of soft tissue distraction on deformity recurrence after centralization for radial longitudinal deficiency. *J Hand Surg Am* 2014;39(5):895-901.
26. Vuillermin C, Butler L, Ezaki M, Oishi S: Ulna growth patterns after soft tissue release with bilobed flap in radial longitudinal deficiency. *J Pediatr Orthop* 2018;38(4):244-248.
27. Vuillermin C, Wall L, Mills J, et al: Soft tissue release and bilobed flap for severe radial longitudinal deficiency. *J Hand Surg Am* 2015;40(5):894-899.
28. Wall LB, Ezaki M, Oishi SN: Management of congenital radial longitudinal deficiency: Controversies and current concepts. *Plast Reconstr Surg* 2013;132(1):122-128.
29. Vilkki SK: Vascularized joint transfer for radial club hand. *Tech Hand Up Extrem Surg* 1998;2(2):126-137.
30. Pike JM, Manske PR, Steffen JA, Goldfarb CA: Ulnocarpal epiphyseal arthrodesis for recurrent deformity after centralization for radial longitudinal deficiency. *J Hand Surg Am* 2010;35(11):1755-1761.
31. Farr S, Petje G, Sadoghi P, Ganger R, Grill F, Girsch W: Radiographic early to midterm results of distraction osteogenesis in radial longitudinal deficiency. *J Hand Surg Am* 2012;37(11):2313-2319.
32. Yoshida K, Kawabata H, Wada M: Growth of the ulna after repeated bone lengthening in radial longitudinal deficiency. *J Pediatr Orthop* 2011;31(6):674-678.
33. Peterson BM, McCarroll HR Jr, James MA: Distraction lengthening of the ulna in children with radial longitudinal deficiency. *J Hand Surg Am* 2007;32(9):1402-1407.
34. de Jong JP, Moran SL, Vilkki SK: Changing paradigms in the treatment of radial club hand: Microvascular joint transfer for correction of radial deviation and preservation of long-term growth. *Clin Orthop Surg* 2012;4(1):36-44.
35. Yang J, Qin B, Li P, Fu G, Xiang J, Gu L: Vascularized proximal fibular epiphyseal transfer for bayne and klug type III radial longitudinal deficiency in children. *Plast Reconstr Surg* 2015;135(1):157e-166e.
36. Evans DM, Gateley DR, Lewis JS: The use of a bilobed flap in the correction of radial club hand. *J Hand Surg Br* 1995;20(3):333-337.
37. VanHeest A, Grierson Y: Dorsal rotation flap for centralization in radial longitudinal deficiency. *J Hand Surg Am* 2007;32(6):871-875.

38. VanHeest A: Wrist centralization using the dorsal rotation flap in radial longitudinal deficiency. *Tech Hand Up Extrem Surg* 2010;14(2):94-99.

39. Luangjarmekorn P, Pongernnak N, Yamprasert N, Kitidumrongsook P: Single-stage radialization and pollicization for radial longitudinal deficiency with thumb hypoplasia. *Tech Hand Up Extrem Surg* 2019;24(2):71-78.

40. De Kraker M, Selles RW, Van Vooren J, Stam HJ, Hovius SE: Outcome after pollicization: Comparison of patients with mild and severe lonitudinal radial deficiency. *Plast Reconstr Surg* 2013;131(4):544e-551e.

41. Al-Qattan MM: Pollicization of the index finger requiring secondary fusion of the new metacarpophalangeal joint. *J Hand Surg Eur Vol* 2016;41(3):295-300.

42. Miller JK, Wenner SM, Kruger LM: Ulnar deficiency. *J Hand Surg Am* 1986;11(6):822-829.

43. Bednar MS, James MA, Light TR: Congenital longitudinal deficiency. *J Hand Surg Am* 2009;34(9):1739-1747.

44. Walker JL, White HD, Jacobs CA, Riley SA: Upper extremity anomalies in children with femoral and fibular deficiency. *J Pediatr Orthop B* 2020;29(4):399-402.

45. Blair WF, Shurr DG, Buckwalter JA: Functional status in ulnar deficiency. *J Pediatr Orthop* 1983;3(1):37-40.

46. Johnson J, Omer GE Jr: Congenital ulnar deficiency: Natural history and therapeutic implications. *Hand Clin* 1985;1(3):499-510.

47. Flatt AE, ed: *The Care of Congenital Hand Anomalies*, ed 2. Quality Medical Publishing Inc., 1994, pp 411-424.

48. Schmidt CC, Neufeld SK: Ulnar ray deficiency. *Hand Clin* 1998;14(1):65-76.

49. Ramirez RN, Kozin SH: Ulnar mammary syndrome. *J Hand Surg Am* 2014;39(4):803-805.

50. Al-Qattan MM, Al-Sahabi A, Al-Arfaj N: Ulnar ray deficiency: A review of the classification systems, the clinical features in 72 cases, and related developmental biology. *J Hand Surg Eur Vol* 2010;35(9):699-707.

51. Kozin SH: Upper-extremity congenital anomalies. *J Bone Joint Surg Am* 2003;85(8):1564-1576.

52. Kummel W: Die Missbildungen der Extremitaeten durch Defekt, Verwachsung und Ueberzahl. *Bibliotheca Medica* 1895;3:1-83.

53. Ogden JA, Watson HK, Bohne W: Ulnar dysmelia. *J Bone Joint Surg Am* 1976;58(4):467-475.

54. Bayne LG: Ulnar club hand (ulnar deficiencies), in Green DP, ed: *Operative Hand Surgery*. Churchill Livingstone, 1982, vol 11, pp 245-257.

55. Cole RJ, Manske PR: Classification of ulnar deficiency according to the thumb and first web. *J Hand Surg Am* 1997;22(3):479-488.

56. Jacobsen ST, Crawford AH: Humeroradial synostosis. *J Pediatr Orthop* 1983;3(1):96-98.

57. Gogoi P, Dutta A, Sipani AK, Daolagupu AK: Congenital deficiency of distal ulna and dislocation of the radial head treated by single bone forearm procedure. *Case Rep Orthop* 2014;2014:526719.

58. Kitano K, Tada K: One-bone forearm procedure for partial defect of the ulna. *J Pediatr Orthop* 1985;5(3):290-293.

59. Sénès FM, Catena N: Correction of forearm deformities in congenital ulnar club hand: One-bone forearm. *J Hand Surg Am* 2012;37(1):159-164.

60. Broudy AS, Smith RJ: Deformities of the hand and wrist with ulnar deficiency. *J Hand Surg Am* 1979;4(4):304-315.

61. James MA, Bagley AM, Brasington K, Lutz C, McConnell S, Molitor F: Impact of prostheses on function and quality of life for children with unilateral congenital below-the-elbow deficiency. *J Bone Joint Surg Am* 2006;88(11):2356-2365.

Pediatric Hand Deficiencies

Krister Freese, MD, FAAOS • Rashmi Agarwal, MD

CHAPTER 68

ABSTRACT

Congenital hand deficiencies and abnormalities present unique diagnostic and therapeutic challenges. Each patient requires an individual approach to manage specific priorities including increasing function, pain reduction, and improved aesthetics. Common deficiencies include symbrachydactyly, syndactyly, longitudinal deficiencies, and polydactyly. Improved basic knowledge of pediatric hand deficiencies will aid surgeons and clinicians in choosing the optimal treatment strategy for their patients.

Keywords: congenital hand deficiency; polydactyly; symbrachydactyly; syndactyly

Introduction

The birth of a child with an upper limb deficiency may elicit many confusing parental emotions. Medical professionals should address parental concerns and expectations in a compassionate, honest, and forthright manner. Parents may grieve that their infant is not the perfect child that they had anticipated or voice anger that prenatal evaluations did not detect their child's hand difference. Many parents feel an intense need to do something, either surgical or prosthetic, to make their child normal and whole. Conflicting advice from well-meaning friends and relatives may contribute to parental stress.

Despite frequently voiced parental concerns, a recent self-concept scale study demonstrated that overall, children with congenital anomalies possessed equal self-concept to healthy children.[1] Interestingly, children with more mild anomalies had worse scores than children with more severe anomalies.

As infants begin to explore their environment, they learn to use their unique physical capabilities to their best advantage. Deficits in function will be augmented through the use of the other hand, or if needed feet. The child's growing awareness of their abnormality is usually the result of comments from playmates, siblings, or well-meaning adults. The child usually does not become self-conscious until approximately the age of 6 or 7 years. Peer pressure may cause the child with a unilateral abnormality to conceal the hand in a pocket or to reject an otherwise successful prosthesis.

Other points of psychological stress occur during adolescence when concerns arise over attractiveness. Feelings may be further complicated by impending marriage and the prospect of offspring with similar abnormalities. Access to knowledgeable genetic counseling is essential, particularly at that time. Increased use of patient-reported outcomes measures has allowed for improved evaluation of subjective measures not normally available to clinicians. The PROMIS score especially has demonstrated utility in the congenital hand cohort without evidence of a ceiling effect. Early studies have demonstrated decreased function, however low scores for depression, anxiety, and pain. Qualitative studies looking at the psychosocial effects of congenital hand differences have also become of increasing interest—there is a high stress level in the patient cohort as well as the parents, regarding the functional deficits, hand appearance, social interactions, and emotional reactions.[2]

Upper Limb Kinesiology

The hand allows children to explore their environment and to manipulate objects within that environment. The hand should be able to maneuver in space under volitional control and should be able to reach the body and the area in front of the body. Using both visual and tactile clues, a child must be able to aim the hand so that it can precisely approach an object. The object is then grasped by the closing fingers and adducting the thumb. The hand must also be capable of releasing the object from its grasp.

The two major types of grasp are precision prehension and power prehension.[3] Precision prehension is used

---

Dr. Freese or an immediate family member serves as a board member, owner, officer, or committee member of the Pediatric Orthopaedic Society of North America. Neither Dr. Agarwal nor any immediate family member has received anything of value from or has stock or stock options held in a commercial company or institution related directly or indirectly to the subject of this chapter.

This chapter is adapted from Langer JS: Pediatric hand deficiencies, in Krajbich JI, Pinzur MS, Potter BK, Stevens PM, eds: *Atlas of Amputations and Limb Deficiencies: Surgical, Prosthetic, and Rehabilitation Principles*, ed 4. American Academy of Orthopaedic Surgeons, 2016, pp 843-854.

to hold relatively small objects with modest force, whereas power prehension is used to hold larger objects, often with greater force. In precision prehension, the object is secured between the distal phalanx of the thumb and the index finger or within the thumb, index, and middle fingers. The fingers are usually extended at the interphalangeal joints, and the metacarpophalangeal (MCP) joints are partially flexed. The object itself usually does not contact the palm.

The three most common forms of precision grasp or pinch are palmar pinch, lateral pinch, and tip pinch. With palmar pinch, the flat palmar pads of the thumb and fingers secure opposite sides of the object being grasped. With lateral pinch, the palmar surface of the thumb's distal phalanx is brought against the radial border of the index finger. Because this posture is often used to grasp and twist a key, this pattern is also known as key pinch. Tip pinch provides contact with the distal end of the distal phalanx of the thumb with the distal phalanx of the index or of the index and middle fingers. Tip pinch is used to pick up small objects such as a pin or a dime from a tabletop.

Power prehension involves the ulnar digits (most often the ring and little fingers), whereas the radial digits (the index and middle fingers) are used primarily in precision prehension. The hand also plays an important role in nonprehensile activities. These activities usually involve the transmission of force through the terminal portion of the limb to another object. Nonprehensile activities include keyboarding or button pushing, pushing open a swinging door, or throwing a punch. The hand may also be used to cradle or hold objects against the chest or to support objects such as a tray. Congenitally anomalous hands without prehensile capability are often used with great dexterity to perform these nonprehensile functions.

Prostheses

A purely cosmetic prosthesis to conceal the abnormality may be some parents' first choice but may ultimately prove to be a hindrance. Any decision-making process should include a frank discussion of poor outcomes when a cosmetic prosthesis covers the sensate skin of an anomalous hand should be openly discussed. Although a cosmetic upper limb prosthesis may facilitate rehabilitation after a traumatic amputation, it is usually an impediment to a child with congenital amputation who possesses a mobile hand and wrist, even without fingers. Cosmetic prostheses may become a source of conflict between parent and child if the child regards the prosthesis as an obstacle rather than an aid. The child may feel that the prosthesis functions only to please parents who are embarrassed by their appearance. If a prosthesis is to be successfully integrated into the child's life, it must help the child either accomplish otherwise impossible activities or perform meaningful activities with greater facility.

Prostheses have not yet been designed to replicate sensation, leading to limited utility for children with unilateral conditions. If the affected side is able to function as a helper hand for the unaffected side, especially with wrist motion and/or at least one functional digit, a prosthesis may be more of an obstruction than an aid. Some prosthesis designs may augment the single-digit hand, allowing for a surface to pinch again, such as an opposition paddle or a partial hand prosthesis.

On occasion, the removal of a functionless part may facilitate prosthetic fitting. Approximately 50% of individuals with congenital lower limb amputations require surgical revision before prosthetic fitting, whereas only approximately 10% of congenital anomalous upper limbs fit for prostheses require surgical revision.[4] Consultation between the surgeon and prosthetist helps the surgeon understand which anomalies will obstruct prosthetic donning and wear. Portions of the affected limb that are useful for prehension without a prosthesis should never be amputated.

A recent advancement in prosthetic care is three-dimensional prosthetic printing, which provides a low-cost alternative to traditional cosmetic or functional prosthetic devices.[5,6] This patient driven and family-driven modality gives the child or family the ability to easily customize and alter the prosthesis and may aid in the emotional adjustment to their disability. These prostheses can be lightweight, durable, and easily replaced as a child grows and has different needs. Cooperation between clinicians and engineers has led to multiple designs available online as open-source blueprints, which can be used and modified to fit a specific child's desired function. This area will continue to grow and develop as the technology continues to advance.

Clinical Presentation

Although congenital upper limb abnormalities are increasingly diagnosed by prenatal ultrasonography, they typically are first diagnosed at birth. Identification of congenital limb anomalies on prenatal ultrasonography has been cited as low as 30% and as high as 80%, with significant variation based on the type of malformation.[7-9] Parents often have a deep need to understand the nature of their child's abnormality and the potential treatments available. Early consultation with experienced physicians and therapists is helpful for most families. In some cases, a prenatal consultation with a congenital hand surgeon can provide the family with insight into their child's condition.

Classification

The Oberg, Manske, and Tonkin (OMT) classification of congenital anomalies of the hand and upper limb was proposed in 2010 as a replacement for the Swanson International Federation of Societies for Surgery of the Hand classification system. The OMT system uses increasing knowledge of molecular and developmental pathways, and relates them to clinically relevant anomalies. It separates malformations from deformations and dysplasias. Malformations are subdivided according to the axis of formation and differentiation and involvement of the whole limb or the hand plate alone. It has been updated twice, in 2014 and 2020, with the most recent version shown in **Table 1**.[10] The classification has demonstrated high intraobserver reliability and substantial interobserver agreement.

Conditions in which body parts are absent are referred to as failures of formation. These have been classified by etiology in the modified Swanson/International Federation of Societies for Surgery of the Hand system (**Table 2**). In most patients, the anatomic border between normal tissue and absent elements is indistinct and gradual; a blend of dysplastic and hypoplastic tissue typically forms a transition zone that may extend the entire length of the limb. One exception is amniotic band syndrome, where there is highly localized intrauterine trauma to the growing limb and there may be an abrupt transition from normal tissue to absent elements (**Figure 1**). In these limbs, the anatomy proximal to the area of abnormality is usually normal.

Conditions in which the absence is most intense in the distal portion of the limb are usually referred to as terminal deficiencies (**Figure 2**). The entire limb, including the chest, must be evaluated to fully understand these abnormalities. Distal anomalies involving the hand, such as syndactyly, may be associated with chest abnormalities in children with Poland syndrome.

Symbrachydactyly

The most common forms of terminal limb deficiency are related to the symbrachydactyly sequence of abnormalities.[11-13] The term symbrachydactyly literally refers to a hand with syndactyly of short fingers. Manifestations may be as mild as slightly shortened middle phalanges or as severe as a very short forearm segment with digital nubbins protruding from its distal end. Children with intermediate forms may have only a thumb or only a thumb and little finger with small nubbins representing the undeveloped fingers. Mild hypoplasia of the ipsilateral humerus is common, as is dysplasia or hypoplasia of the forearm. When multiple digits are involved, the central three digits are usually the most profoundly affected. Many patients with symbrachydactyly have primitive digits, often termed nubbins. These bud-like, incompletely formed digits often include small fingernails. In many instances, digital flexor and

TABLE 1 Oberg, Manske, and Tonkin Classification 2020

1. Malformations
   a. Entire upper limb: abnormal axis formation (early limb patterning)
      i. Proximodistal axis
         1. Brachymelia
         2. Symbrachydactyly spectrum (with ectodermal elements)
            a. Poland syndrome
            b. Whole limb excluding Poland syndrome (various levels: humeral to phalangeal)
         3. Transverse deficiency (without ectodermal elements)
            a. Amelia
            b. Segmental (various levels: humeral to phalangeal)
         4. Intersegmental deficiency (phocomelia)
            a. Proximal (humeral: rhizomelic)
            b. Distal (forearm: mesomelic)
            c. Proximal plus distal (hand to thorax)
         5. Whole limb duplication/triplication
      ii. Radioulnar (anterior-posterior) axis
         1. Radial longitudinal deficiency
         2. Ulnar longitudinal deficiency
         3. Ulnar dimelia
         4. Radiohumeral synostosis
         5. Radioulnar synostosis
         6. Congenital dislocation of radial head
         7. Forearm hemiphyseal dysplasia, radial (Madelung deformity), or ulnar
      iii. Dorsoventral axis
         1. Ventral dimelia
         2. Dorsal dimelia
      iv. Unspecified axis
         1. Shoulder
            a. Undescended (Sprengel)
            b. Abnormal shoulder muscles
         2. Upper to lower limb transformation
   b. Hand plate: abnormal axis differentiation (late limb patterning/differentiation)
      i. Proximodistal axis
         1. Brachydactyly
         2. Symbrachydactyly (with ectodermal elements)
         3. Transverse deficiency (without ectodermal elements)
         4. Cleft hand (split hand foot malformation)
      ii. Radioulnar (anterior-posterior) axis
         1. Radial longitudinal deficiency, hypoplastic thumb
         2. Ulnar longitudinal deficiency, hypoplastic ulnar ray
         3. Radial polydactyly
         4. Triphalangeal thumb
            a. Five-finger hand
         5. Ulnar dimelia (mirror hand)
         6. Ulnar polydactyly
      iii. Dorsoventral axis
         1. Dorsal dimelia (palmar nail)
         2. Ventral dimelia (hypoplastic/aplastic nail)
      iv. Unspecified axis
         1. Soft tissue
            a. Cutaneous (simple) syndactyly
         2. Skeletal
            a. Osseous (complex) syndactyly
            b. Clinodactyly
            c. Kirner deformity
            d. Synostosis/symphalangism
         3. Complex
            a. Syndromic syndactyly (eg, Apert hand)
            b. Synpolydactyly
   c. Not otherwise specified
2. Deformations
   a. Constriction ring sequence
   b. Not otherwise specified

(Continued)

TABLE 1 Oberg, Manske, and Tonkin Classification 2020 (Continued)

3. Dysplasias
   a. Variant growth
      i. Diffuse (whole limb)
         1. Hemihypertrophy
         2. Aberrant flexor/extensor/intrinsic muscle
      ii. Isolated
         1. Macrodactyly
         2. Aberrant intrinsic muscles of hand
   b. Tumorous conditions
      i. Vascular
         1. Hemangioma
         2. Malformation
         3. Others
      ii. Neurological
         1. Neurofibromatosis
         2. Others
      iii. Connective tissue
         1. Juvenile aponeurotic fibroma
         2. Infantile digital fibroma
         3. Others
      iv. Skeletal
         1. Osteochondromatosis
         2. Enchondromatosis
         3. Fibrous dysplasia
         4. Epiphyseal abnormalities
         5. Pseudarthrosis
         6. Other
   c. Congenital contracture
      1. Arthrogryposis multiplex congenita
         a. Amyoplasia
         b. Distal arthrogryposis
         c. Other
      2. Isolated
         a. Camptodactyly
         b. Thumb in palm deformity
         c. Other
   d. Syndromes

Reproduced with permission from Goldfarb CA, Ezaki M, Wall LB, Lam WL, Oberg KC: The Oberg-Manske-Tonkin (OMT) classification of congenital upper extremities: Update for 2020. *J Hand Surg Am* 2020;45(6):542-547. © 2020 by the American Society for Surgery of the Hand.

TABLE 2 Modified Swanson/International Federation of Societies for Surgery of the Hand Classification

Type	Description
I	Failure of formation of parts (arrest of development)
II	Failure of differentiation (separation) of parts
III	Duplication
IV	Overgrowth (gigantism)
V	Undergrowth (hypoplasia)
VI	Congenital constriction band syndrome
VII	Generalized skeletal abnormalities

extensor tendons insert into the nubbin, enabling children to move the tip of the digit proximally (**Figure 3**). Some characteristic patterns of digital absence have been noted and are summarized in **Table 3**.

The symbrachydactyly sequence is relatively uncommon, occurring in approximately 0.6 per 10,000 live births. Boys are more frequently affected than girls (73%). Only 7% have been associated with other anomalies and 7% have an associated family history. The left upper limb is involved more often than the right upper limb (67%).[14,15]

When the right side is involved, a diagnosis of Poland syndrome should be considered. Though most cases of

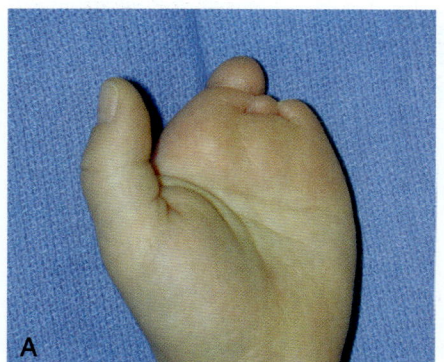 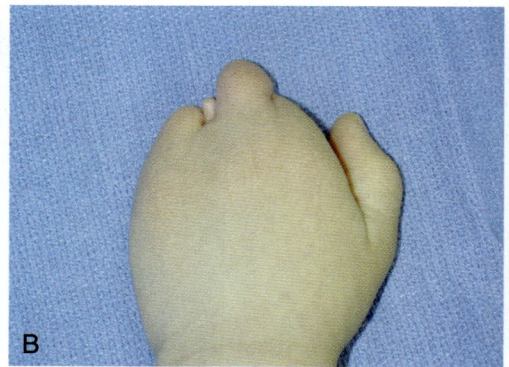 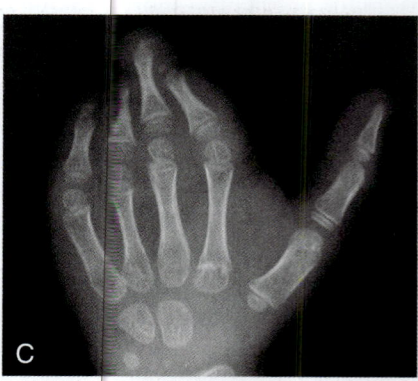

FIGURE 1 Photographs demonstrating early congenital amniotic rupture sequence with amputation and syndactylization of the index, middle, ring, and little fingers. **A**, Palmar view demonstrating interdigital sinuses. **B**, Dorsal view. **C**, AP radiograph showing tapering of the distal end of the proximal phalanx of the ring finger.

isolated symbrachydactyly involve the left side, 61.1% of Poland syndrome patients have symbrachydactyly on the right side. Poland syndrome involves the unilateral absence or hypoplasia of the pectoralis major muscle with associated symbrachydactyly.

Imaging Studies

Radiographs of the entire upper limb should be obtained usually between 1 and 2 years of age. Earlier radiographs are unlikely to change management and should be avoided. The limb will grow in proportion to the contralateral side. Radiographs of young children may underestimate the extent of bone formation, particularly in syndactylized fingers. Portions of the anomalous fingers and carpus often include unossified cartilage.

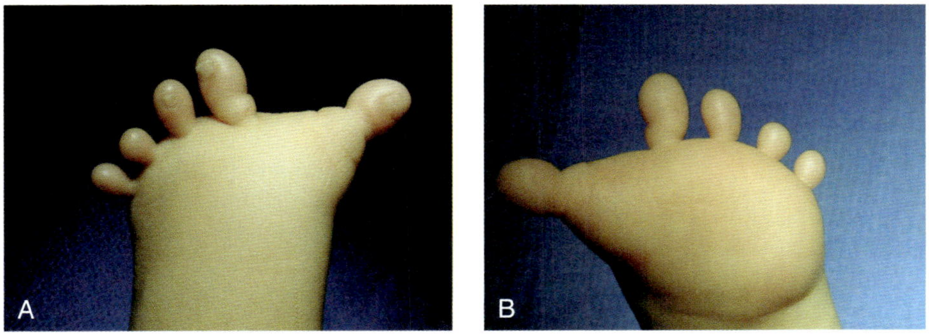

Classification

The original classification groups symbrachydactyly under three categories: I, failure of formation; II, failure of differentiation; and V, undergrowth. This has since been revised in the OMT classification to consider the condition to be a malformation in the failure of axis formation/differentiation of the entire limb and hand plate. The most useful classification is based on the number of functional digits as that may help guide treatment—adactylous, monodactylous, bidactylous versus multidigit.

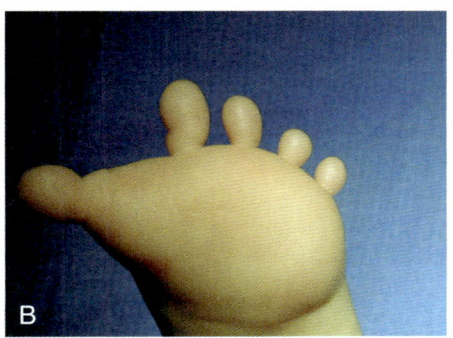

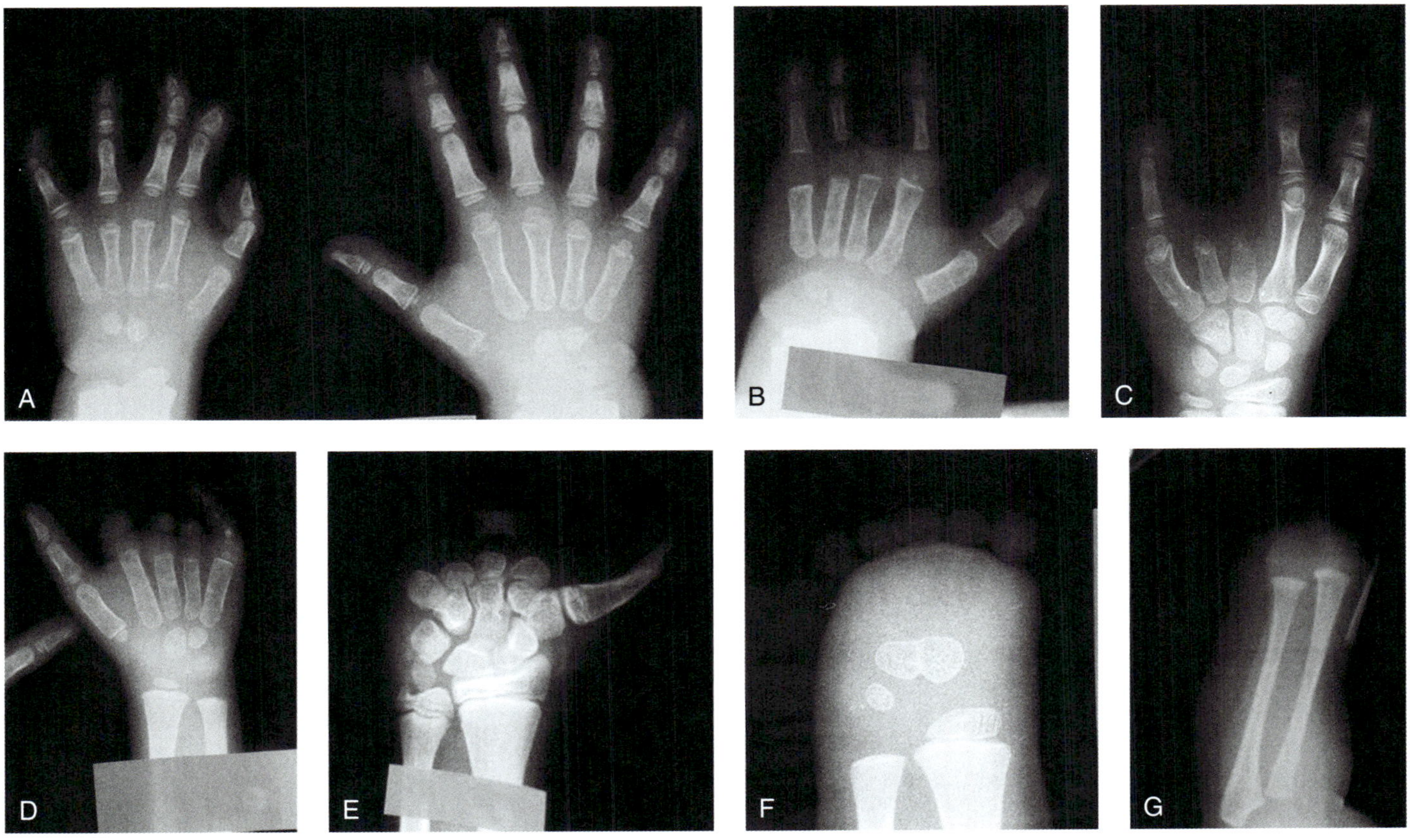

FIGURE 2 Dorsal (**A**) and palmar (**B**) photographs of a terminal transverse deficiency characterized by persistent digital nubbins without bony phalangeal elements.

FIGURE 3 Radiographs demonstrating the variable morphology of unilateral symbrachydactyly. **A**, Five-digit–type hand with biphalangeal thumb and biphalangeal fingers (left) is smaller than the contralateral, normal hand. **B**, Four-digit–type hand with four biphalangeal digits and one digital nubbin. **C**, Three-digit–type hand includes a narrowed syndactylized web between the biphalangeal thumb and biphalangeal ring finger. **D**, Two-digit–type hand shows limited ossification of the distal phalanx within the nubbin index, middle, and ring fingers. **E**, Monodigital-type hand consists of a widely abducted thumb metacarpal. **F**, Carpal-type hand with five soft-tissue nubbins. **G**, Wrist disarticulation-type hand with a single digital nubbin.

TABLE 3 Classification of Common Types of Digital Absence

Type of Hand	Characteristics
Symbrachydactyly	
Five digits with biphalangeal thumb	All fingers triphalangeal
	Incomplete simple syndactyly of the index, middle, and ring fingers
Five digits with biphalangeal thumb	Biphalangeal index, middle, and ring fingers
	Triphalangeal little finger
	Incomplete simple syndactyly of the index, middle, and ring fingers
Five digits with biphalangeal thumb	Monophalangeal index, middle, and ring fingers
Three digits with biphalangeal thumb	Nubbin index and middle fingers
	Monophalangeal ring finger
	Biphalangeal little finger
Two digits with monophalangeal thumb	Nubbin index, middle, and ring fingers
	Monophalangeal little finger
Monodigital with monophalangeal thumb	Nubbin index, middle, ring, and little fingers
Aphalangeal	
Adactylous with five metacarpals	Five nubbins
Adactylous with two metacarpals	Thumb metacarpal
	Little finger metacarpal
	Digital nubbins
Carpal	Digital nubbins
	No metacarpals or phalanges
	Mobile carpus
Wrist disarticulation level	Digital nubbins
	No wrist motion
	No carpal, metacarpal, or phalangeal elements
Short transradial level	Extremely short forearm
	Digital nubbins

Reproduced from Light TR: Hand deficiencies, in Smith DG, Michael JW, Bowker JH, eds: *Atlas of Amputations and Limb Deficiencies: Surgical, Prosthetic, and Rehabilitation Principles,* ed 3. American Academy of Orthopaedic Surgeons, 2004, p 857.

Associated Findings

Poland syndrome is the ipsilateral finding of symbrachydactyly and chest abnormality.[11-13,15-19] Interestingly, the proximal chest abnormality is more common with the milder, more distal forms of symbrachydactyly than with more profound limb abnormalities. The most frequently associated chest abnormality is absence of the sternocostal head of the pectoralis major muscle. More profound chest abnormalities include total absence of the pectoralis major muscle, rib abnormalities, and asymmetric nipple location. As girls mature, ipsilateral breast hypoplasia may become more evident. Poland syndrome may be because of disruption of the subclavian artery during embryonic development leading to limb undergrowth.

Functional Deficits

The function of the hand at baseline should be considered when planning intervention. Individual digital function may be compromised by syndactyly, interphalangeal joint instability, or angulation.

An untreated adactylous hand will be unable to perform prehension tasks but can serve as a helper hand, assisting the contralateral extremity. It may also function to hold objects against the body or a surface. A monodactylous hand usually has only a thumb and may be able to grasp between the thumb and the palmar surface. They also may be able to press and hook using the finger alone. The bidactylous hand may be capable of prehension if the two digits can actively touch one another but will have weaker grip.

Adactylous hands with wrist motion are used to cradle objects against the trunk and to hold objects in place for manipulation by the unaffected hand. The adactylous hand can hold a piece of paper in place while the other hand holds the pen or pencil to draw or write on the paper.

Differential Diagnosis

A hand that possesses only the thumb and little finger has, in the past, been referred to as an atypical cleft hand.[20,21] It is important to recognize, however, that these two-digit hands are unrelated to cleft hand, an autosomal dominant condition often with bilateral hand and foot involvement.

Surgical Treatment

Because symbrachydactyly is usually unilateral, most affected children are remarkably facile at performing activities of daily living.[22] As a result, some parents may choose to wait before surgical intervention until functional deficits become evident. Intervention can range from removal of nubbins if problematic to syndactyly releases and joint-stabilizing procedures.

Nonprehensile activities such as typing may be improved by the stabilization of unstable interphalangeal joints by capsulodesis, chondrodesis, or arthrodesis (**Figure 4**). Angulation of digits, usually the result of a trapezoidal middle phalanx, may be treated by a closing wedge osteotomy. Pinch may be improved by repositioning a digit through a rotational osteotomy or lengthening to allow the fingers to converge.

When a soft-tissue digital sleeve is redundant and devoid of skeletal elements, puckering of the tip will demonstrate the insertion of extrinsic flexor and extensor tendons. In such digits, it is possible to reconstruct a short, mobile digit by a nonvascularized proximal phalanx transfer from the foot to the hand.[23] Complications from this procedure may include joint instability, premature epiphyseal closure, and infection and graft loss with inconsistent functional outcomes. There have been variable reports on the donor site morbidity as well, making the decision to proceed with transfer more equivocal.[24,25] In fact, a recent review of nonvascularized toe phalangeal transfers reported on the potential substantial morbidity of this procedure, including gait abnormality, abnormal appearance, and toe instability.[24]

The monodactylous hand consisting of only a mobile, actively motored thumb is capable of nonprehensile activities such as stabilizing a shoelace, but incapable of either power or precision grasp. Construction of an ulnar-sided buttressing digit by distraction lengthening, toe-phalanx transfer, or free toe transfer may allow the hand to achieve meaningful prehension. A prosthesis that provides a passive ulnar-sided buttress may also make prehension possible (**Figure 5**).

When a hand is devoid of fingers, the microvascular transfer of both second toes has been suggested.[26] This has been described as a two-stage procedure, the first to put a digit in the thumb position then to place a digit positioned for pinch. Though this procedure is technically possible, the results are variable—the most frequent reason for secondary operations being limited digital motion. Indications for the procedure are also changing, as success may depend on the degree of normalcy of the proximal anatomy.[26,27]

Syndactyly

Syndactyly is the physical joining or tethering of fingers or toes. It is the most common congenital hand difference, occurring in two to three in 10,000 live births. It occurs more often in males than females. Approximately 50% of cases occur bilaterally. It can be sporadic or inherited, usually autosomal dominant with variable expressivity and incomplete penetrance.

Clinical Presentation and Classification

Classification is based primarily on the type and extent of tissues involved. When syndactylization extends the entire length of a digit, the condition is termed complete syndactyly. When the web involves only part of the length of the digit, it is termed an incomplete syndactyly. When skeletal and nail elements of the syndactylized

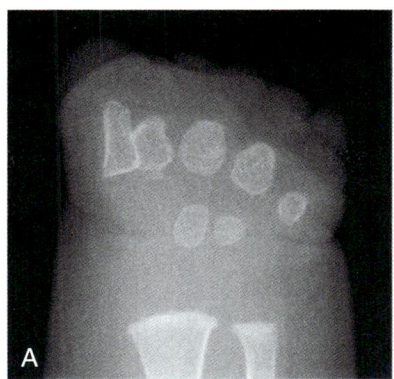
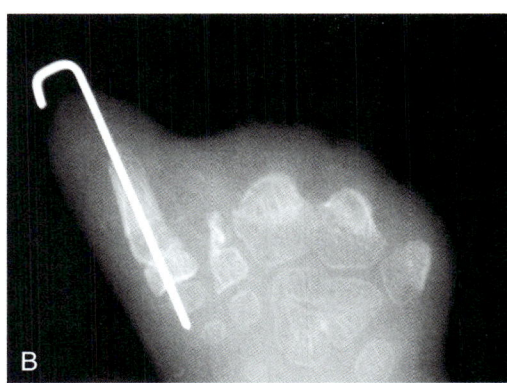
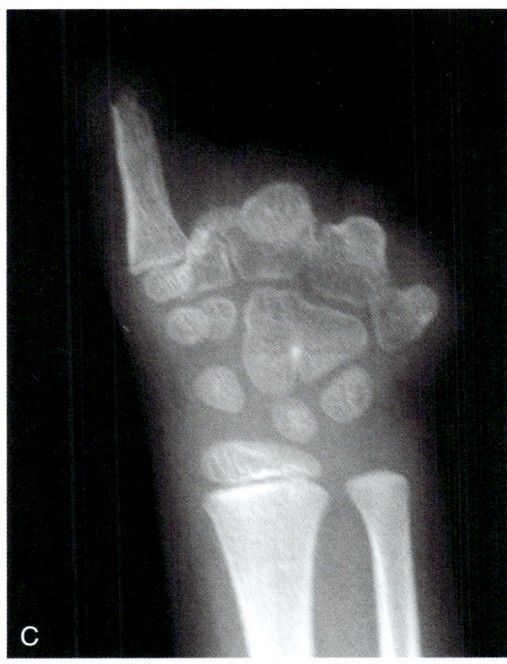

FIGURE 4 Radiographs of an adactylous hand treated with a transverse osteotomy. **A**, Preoperative radiograph showing the five small metacarpal elements, which had limited thumb metacarpal motion. **B**, Transverse osteotomy of the thumb metaphysis allowed insertion of intercalated bone graft from the adjacent index metacarpal. **C**, Additional length allowed improved monodigital function.

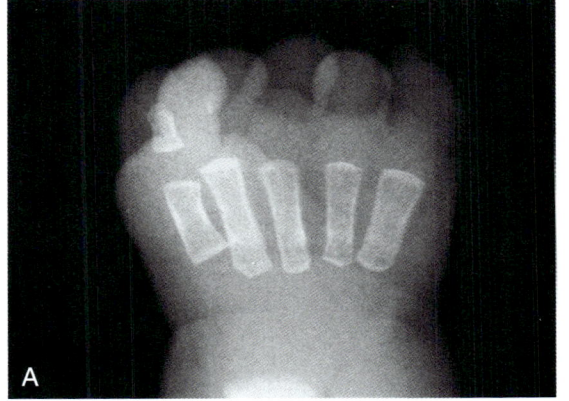
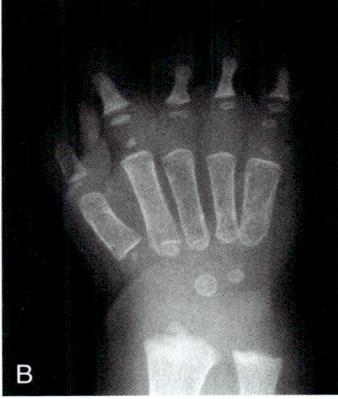

FIGURE 5 Radiographs showing the reconstruction of a monodactylous hand. **A**, Preoperative radiograph of the hand with a monophalangeal thumb and empty finger skin sleeves. **B**, Nonvascularized toe phalangeal grafts from the third and fourth toe proximal phalanges enhance digital stability, length, and dexterity.

digits are separate, the syndactyly is said to be simple. When digital skeletal and/or nail elements are fused, the syndactyly is termed complex (**Figure 6**). Acrosyndactyly refers to syndactyly in which the ends of the fingertips are joined and a proximal fenestration exists. This is the sine qua non of amniotic band syndrome. Syndactyly of the digits containing angulated phalanges is termed complicated syndactyly.[27]

Surgical Treatment

Surgical release of syndactylized digits will enhance digital independence. Even short digits consisting of only a proximal phalanx may benefit from separation. Index finger radial abduction may be increased and pinch improved when a short index finger is released from the middle finger. Syndactyly release must provide skin coverage of the adjacent lateral surfaces of the released digits and create a proper web space commissure. Because the surface area of two syndactylized digits is less than the skin surface area of two separated digits, a full-thickness skin graft is necessary to supplement local flaps. Graft can be obtained from the antecubital fossa or ulnar aspect of the hand. Hair-bearing areas should be avoided as they can become problematic in adolescents.

Many skin flap techniques have been used for the separation of syndactylized digits.[28-32] Successful surgical procedures cover the surface of both digits with durable skin, create an appropriate web space floor, and accommodate growth of the digit without secondary contracture (**Figure 7**). Flap tissue may be derived either from the dorsum of the hand, from the palmar aspect of the hand, or from a combination. Dorsal flaps provide the best skin color match when the web space is viewed from the dorsum but may result in a hypertrophic scar across the interdigital commissure. A palmar flap provides a better commissure contour but results in the shifting of pink palmar skin into the web space. Because the web space is usually viewed from the dorsum, the difference in color is particularly noticeable in dark-skinned individuals.

The web space floor normally begins just distal to the MCP joint and slopes to the edge of the palmar commissure, approximately 40% of the length of the proximal phalangeal segment. The web palmar commissure is supple enough to allow interdigital abduction of up to 45°. Skin incisions on the palmar and dorsal surfaces of the syndactylized digits should be planned to avoid longitudinal scars crossing digital flexion creases because these scars tend to contract with growth. Zigzag incisions may be planned to interdigitate skin flaps to achieve full closure of one digit or partial closure of two adjacent digits. The primarily closed skin flaps should be tension free. Interdigital dressings are maintained until all wounds have healed.[32,33] When multiple digits are

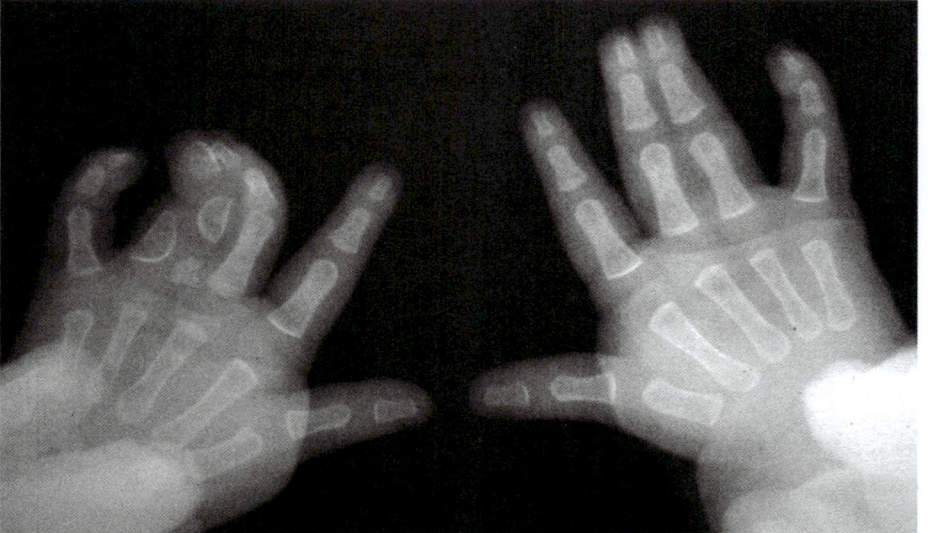

FIGURE 6 Radiograph showing a patient with syndactyly of both hands. The left hand demonstrates a complete, complex central synpolydactyly, whereas the right hand demonstrates a complete simple syndactyly.

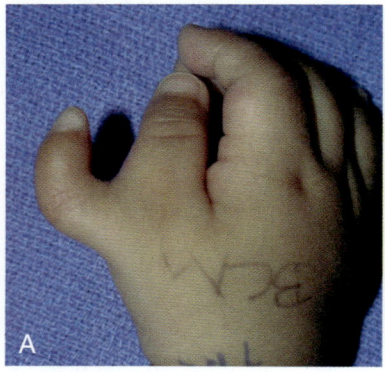 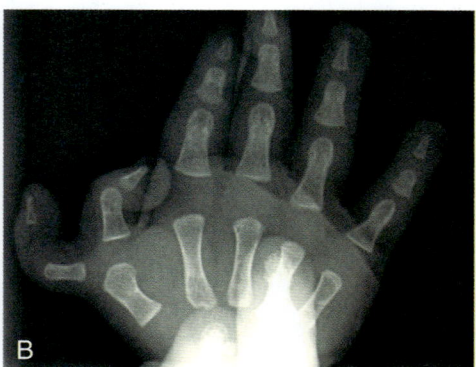 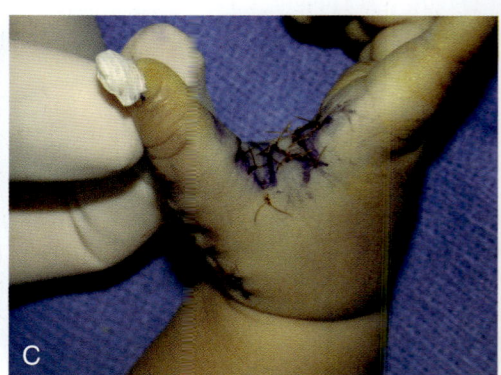

FIGURE 7 Images showing thumb polydactyly, consisting of two biphalangeal digits and a narrow first web space. **A**, Clinical photograph. **B**, Radiograph. **C**, Reconstruction includes removal of the skeletal elements of the radial digit, reconstruction of the collateral ligament of the metacarpophalangeal joint, first web space release, and Z-plasty.

syndactylized, surgeries should be staged to avoid releasing both sides of a digit during a single operation.[34] There have been promising studies looking at synthetic skin graft substitutes—a series by Wall et al[35] demonstrated very little web creep, visual satisfaction, and no complications at 1 year follow-up.

Complication rates are low (0.3%), and included graft loss or neurovascular injury. Surgery is contraindicated in patients with super digits (two metacarpals supporting one digit or one metacarpal supporting two or more digits), complex syndactyly in which the fingers move in unison, hands that lack active muscle control, and adults with functional syndactylized digits.

Early Amniotic Rupture Sequence

The term early amniotic rupture sequence refers to a collection of congenital abnormalities including upper and lower extremity banding, oligodactyly, hemangiomas, acrosyndactyly, talipes equinovarus, and cleft lip and palate.[36,37] There is a lack of consensus on the etiology or defining features of the early amniotic rupture sequence. It is also known as amniotic band syndrome, constriction band syndrome, and annular band syndrome, among others. The overall incidence is approximately 0.98 to 1.16/10,000 live births.

Clinical Presentation

Patients may present with a wide range of involvement from a single band on an extremity to a more global presentation including body wall defects, internal organ abnormalities, and craniofacial abnormalities. Most patients have three extremities involved, with the upper limbs more involved than the lower limbs.

Surgical Treatment

Treatment is focused on improving function and cosmesis. Areas of indentation may be effectively treated by excision of indented skin and constricting underlying fascia. A layered closure combined with local rotation flaps will improve the contour of the limb or digit. When deep bands compress underlying nerves, compromising distal neurovascular function, decompression and nerve grafting may be helpful. Although data are limited, nerve decompression in isolation has failed to demonstrate an improvement in neurologic function, perhaps because the nerve compression is long-standing.[38] Acrosyndactyly may be addressed using traditional syndactyly release techniques. If an interdigital sinus is present, it should be excised at the time of syndactyly release. Partial digital transfer (on-top plasty) and bone-lengthening procedures may be considered to improve function.

Complications

Because the level of amputation through the forearm or phalangeal bones often passes through the bone's diaphysis, bony overgrowth frequently occurs. Diaphyseal bony overgrowth results in tapered ends of fingers. The most distal bone grows faster than the soft-tissue coverage, resulting in tender, poorly padded fingertips or recurrent problems with prosthesis fit. Revision of the ends of these digits or limb ends should be generous to minimize the likelihood of recurrent overgrowth.

Polydactyly

Polydactyly takes many forms. In black children, postaxial (ulnar) polydactyly is the most common form, whereas in white children, preaxial (radial) polydactyly is more frequent. Central polydactyly is less common than either preaxial or postaxial polydactyly.[39] Polydactylous digits are rarely supernumerary, that is, they rarely represent parts additional to a normal hand.[31] Most often, digits with polydactyly are structurally abnormal.[40] The challenge of surgery is not simply to remove sufficient tissue but rather to retain tissue sufficient to optimally reconstruct the retained digits.[41-44]

Classification

Preaxial polydactyly takes many forms. Adrian Flatt classified the six that involve biphalangeal thumbs (**Figure 8**); this was modified by Wassel to include the seventh type, the triphalangeal thumbs.

Central polydactyly often presents in combination with syndactyly.[39] Three types have been described based on the characteristics of the duplicated digit. Type I duplications are not attached to the adjacent finger by osseous or ligamentous attachments. Type II duplications have a normal-appearing digit but share a joint or bifid metacarpal with the adjacent finger—they are further subclassified by the absence (IIa) or presence (type IIb) of syndactyly. Type III have a complete duplicate ray including a full metacarpal.

Postaxial polydactyly may span a spectrum of presentations. All are characterized by supernumerary digits on the ulnar side of the hand, but these may

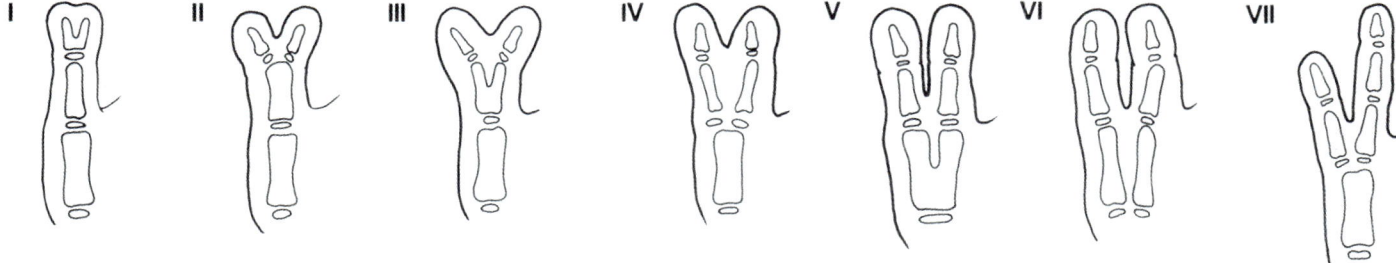

FIGURE 8 Illustration of Wassel's original classification scheme for thumb polydactyly, which has been modified to demonstrate the most common form of thumb polydactyly (type IV), in which two proximal phalanges each possess separate secondary ossification centers.

range from nubbins to well-developed, functional digits. The more commonly used classification is by Temtamy and McKusick—type A are well-formed digits with an osseous connection with the rest of the hand, and type B are incompletely formed with a skin bridge alone.

Ulnar dimelia (mirror hand) is an unusual abnormality characterized by duplication of the postaxial border of the hand with seven or eight fingers.[45] Neither the thumb nor the radius is present. Surgery on the preaxial proximal ulna is useful in expanding the arc of elbow flexion and extension but does not provide forearm rotation. Because there is an overabundance of flexor musculature and relative paucity of extensor musculature, release of the wrist flexion contracture may be necessary. Deletion of two or three digits with pollicization of one of the digits along the preaxial border will improve the cosmetic appearance of the hand and modestly improve function.[46]

Clinical Presentation

Patients often present just after birth when the anomaly is discovered. Parents may require some reassurance regarding development of fine motor skills in the early ages. Some children may have undergone an attempt at suture ligation, which may leave a scar or skin tag that may require revision in the future. Most surgeons defer surgical intervention to at least 1 to 2 years of age when the digits are larger and technically easier to reconstruct.

Type B postaxial polydactyly is common in patients of African descent, at 1/100 to 300 live births, but uncommon in white children at 1/1500 to 3000. The presence of type B postaxial polydactyly in a white child should raise suspicions for a concomitant syndrome and referral to genetics is warranted.

Surgical Treatment

Simply amputating one of the duplicate digits may result in an inadequate residual digit that is smaller than its counterpart on the opposite side. This effect can be decreased by soft-tissue coaptation (**Figure 9**). Incisions are planned to facilitate the coapting of soft tissues from both digits to provide optimal soft-tissue

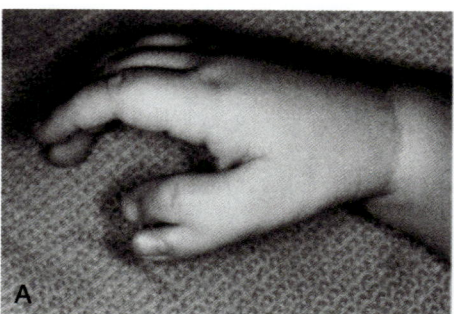 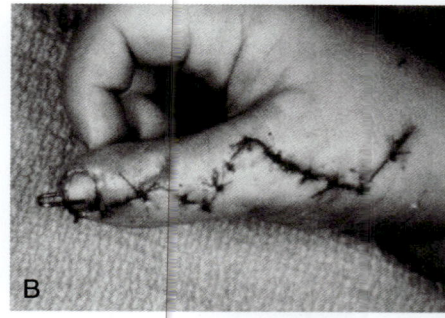

FIGURE 9 Photographs of a Wassel type IV thumb duplication. **A**, Preoperative photographs demonstrate angulation of the larger ulnar thumb metacarpophalangeal (MCP) and the interphalangeal joint levels. **B**, Surgical reconstruction of the thumb included a soft-tissue coaptation flap from the excised radial digit, a closing wedge osteotomy of the thumb metacarpal, and an opening wedge osteotomy of the proximal phalanx to achieve appropriate longitudinal alignment of the digit. The radial collateral ligament of the MCP joint was reconstructed, and the abductor pollicis brevis muscle reinserted in the retained digit.

bulk. Angular deformity in either phalanx or metacarpal should be corrected by osteotomy. Surgical reconstruction aims to achieve a digit in which the carpometacarpal, MCP, and interphalangeal joints are parallel. The longitudinal axis of the metacarpals and phalanges should be perpendicular to the three joints. Correction of angulation is usually achieved by a closing wedge osteotomy and secured with Kirschner wires. An opening wedge osteotomy using a segment of excised bone as intercalated graft is occasionally indicated. Correction of angulation is usually achieved by osteotomy or rebalancing of the flexor pollicis longus tendon.[47] Reconstructed thumbs that demonstrate excessive late angulation yield the worst patient satisfaction scores.[47-49]

Type I deformities may present as simply a wide distal phalanx and nail, in which case no treatment is indicated.[50] If two nails are present, two treatment alternatives may be considered: (1) excision of one nail with the underlying bone or (2) central resection of adjacent nail borders and underlying bone, combined with longitudinal phalangeal osteotomies, to narrow the distal phalanx. The latter technique, known as the Bilhaut-Cloquet procedure, requires care in nail matrix repair, articular surface alignment, and physeal alignment to avoid creating a stiff interphalangeal joint with a longitudinal nail ridge. Osteotomies should be performed distal to the physis to avoid growth disturbance.

Type II duplications consist of two undersized distal phalanges seated atop a somewhat widened proximal phalangeal distal articular surface. The more radial digital element has a collateral ligament along its radial border, whereas the ulnar digit has a collateral ligament along its ulnar border. The two digits abut with adjacent articular facets and are bound by pericapsular tissue. In most instances, it is preferable to excise the more radial digit because it is usually less well developed. The broad distal articular surface of the proximal phalanx may need to be tapered to a size appropriate to the distal phalanx. The collateral ligament that initially secured the radial aspect of the deleted radial digit must be retained to stabilize the radial aspect of the new interphalangeal joint. Retained flexor and extensor tendons must be examined to ensure that the course and insertion of residual tendons are centered.

Type III abnormalities are usually treated by eliminating the radial digit. Type IV abnormalities are the most common and usually require deletion of the radial digit, narrowing of the metacarpal head, and reconstruction of the collateral ligament. The intrinsic muscles that originally inserted into the more radial thumb are reinserted into the hood of the residual ulnar thumb component. Type V abnormalities usually require deletion of the more radial digit and reinsertion of the intrinsic muscle insertion into the residual ulnar digit. Type VI abnormalities may require shifting of the more distal portion of the radial digit onto the more proximal portion of the ulnar digit.

For central polydactyly, surgical planning has to be individualized to provide the best functional and cosmetic outcome and may include attention to skin closure, rebalancing of flexor and extensor tendons, and reconstruction of collaterals to restore joint stability. Revision is often required after surgery and some physicians advocate for ray resection to create a more functional and cosmetic hand compared with a stiff, reconstructed finger.

Postaxial polydactyly of the digit joined only by soft tissue may be treated by simple excision with care to ligate the neurovascular pedicle proximally and avoid a painful neuroma. When the most ulnar digit articulates with the metacarpal head in a fashion similar to that in the Wassel type IV thumb duplication, simple digital excision will result in an inadequate residual digit. It may be necessary to narrow the metacarpal head, but it should be recognized that the metacarpal head of the little finger, unlike that of the thumb, contains a physis. Thus, care must be taken to preserve physeal growth. If the hypothenar musculature inserts into the more ulnar little finger, its insertion must be detached from the skeletal elements being resected and reinserted into the retained radial little finger. Similarly, the ulnar collateral ligament of the deleted digit must be retained and reconstructed to stabilize the ulnar aspect of the residual little finger MCP joint.

Wrist Disarticulation and Short Transradial Amputation

In cases where the degree of deformity of the terminal portion of the limb is severe enough to impede function or cause pain, wrist disarticulation may be necessary. One option in these cases would be the Krukenberg procedure that has been suggested as a reconstructive alternative for children with congenital absence of the hand, particularly in those with profound contralateral abnormalities, associated blindness, or a lack of access to prosthetic care.[51,52] The distal radius and ulna are surgically separated by division of the interosseous membrane and resurfacing the radial aspect of the ulna and the ulnar aspect of the radius. This creates a prehensile limb that will also allow prosthetic fitting. Because the cosmetic disadvantage of this procedure is substantial, its use in patients with unilateral absence is controversial.

Short transradial amputation is a common level of terminal deficiency, which is effectively treated with prosthetic management. Surgical reconstruction is rarely necessary, although Seitz[53] reported distraction lengthening of a very short ulna to facilitate suspension of a conventional myoelectric prosthesis. Initial prosthetic management begins with a passive hand. The sophistication of the prosthesis can be increased as the child matures. However, in a recent comparison of patients who do and do not wear prosthetics in the setting of a unilateral congenital below elbow deficiency no functional improvement was found in the group of patients wearing prosthetics.[54] This may be a limitation of current prosthetics but also highlights the baseline functional abilities of these patients.

Timing of Management

Although surgical reconstruction of an anomalous hand can begin during the first year of life, recent literature supports a delay in surgical intervention until the child is at least 2 years of age. There is concern about the effects of anesthesia on the developing brain. However, in the case of a single short anesthetic exposure, the anesthesia literature is equivocal.[55,56] In many cases, a delay may be advantageous to the surgeon. Delaying the procedure allows for increased size of the extremity to be operated on, making procedures technically easier.

Some procedures, such as nonvascularized toe-phalanx transfer, must be performed early for optimal revascularization and subsequent growth.[12,57] Children undergoing digit-shifting procedures, such as pollicization or cleft hand reconstruction, may benefit from intervention before beginning school. The ideal timing of these procedures has not been defined and the plasticity of children's brains would not necessarily preclude later intervention.

Systemic consideration may cause surgery to be delayed until children are older. For example, children with thrombocytopenia with absent radius syndrome have low platelet counts at birth, but these usually gradually increase with age. Surgical reconstruction usually should be delayed until the child's platelet count is at least $60,000/mm^3$. Centralization of the wrist, which is typically done within the first year of life, may sometimes be delayed in these children until 3 or 4 years of age.

Decisions regarding the reconstruction or deletion of digits are best made when children are young. It is inappropriate to place the burden for deciding whether a digit is to be deleted on an adolescent. Parents should not be encouraged to allow children to decide for themselves when they are older because this serious decision places inappropriate pressure on adolescents and diminishes the responsibility of parents.

SUMMARY

When treating a child with a congenital hand deficiency, the surgeon is tasked with providing an accurate diagnosis, assessing function, offering a prognosis, and counseling the patient and family about potential surgical and nonsurgical treatments. Most children with congenital hand differences and deficiencies will adapt to their environment and situation in creative and efficient ways. The role of surgeons is to identify situations and difficulties that may be improved by either targeted use of prostheses and assistive devices or specific goal-oriented surgical reconstructions to improve aesthetics and function.

References

1. Andersson GB, Gillberg C, Fernell E, Johansson M, Nachemson A: Children with surgically corrected hand deformities and upper limb deficiencies: Self-concept and psychological well-being. *J Hand Surg Eur Vol* 2011;36(9):795-801.

2. Pino PA, Zlotolow DA, Kozin SH: What's new in congenital hand surgery. *J Pediatr Orthop* 2020;40(8):e753-e760.

3. Light TR: Kinesiology of the upper limb, in *Atlas of Orthotics*, ed 2. Mosby-Year Book, 1985, pp 126-138.

4. Aitken GT, Pellicore RJ: Introduction to the child amputee, in *Atlas of Limb Prosthetics: Surgical and Prosthetic Principles*. Mosby Year-Book, 1981, pp 493-500.

5. Gretsch KF, Lather HD, Peddada KV, Deeken CR, Wall LB, Goldfarb CA: Development of novel 3D-printed robotic prosthetic for transradial amputees. *Prosthet Orthot Int* 2015;40(3):400-403.

6. Burn MB, Ta A, Gogola GR: Three-dimensional printing of prosthetic hands for children. *J Hand Surg Am* 2016;41(5):e103-e109.

7. Gray BL, Calfee RP, Dicke JM, Steffen J, Goldfarb CA: The utility of prenatal ultrasound as a screening tool for upper extremity congenital anomalies. *J Hand Surg Am* 2013;38(11):2106-2111.

8. Dicke JM, Piper SL, Goldfarb CA: The utility of ultrasound for the detection of fetal limb abnormalities – A 20-year single-center experience. *Prenat Diagn* 2015;35(4):348-353.

9. Buckwalter V JA, Shah AS: Presentation and treatment of poland anomaly. *Hand (N Y)* 2016;11(4):389-395.

10. Goldfarb CA, Ezaki M, Wall LB, Lam WL, Oberg KC: The Oberg-Manske-Tonkin (OMT) classification of congenital upper extremities: Update for 2020. *J Hand Surg Am* 2020;45(6):542-547.

11. Blauth W, Gekeler J: Symbrachydactylias. *Handchirurgie* 1973;5(3):121-174.

12. Buck-Gramcko D: The role of nonvascularized toe phalanx transplantation. *Hand Clin* 1990;6(4):643-659.

13. De Smet L, Fabry G: Characteristics of patients with symbrachydactyly. *J Pediatr Orthop B* 1998;7(2):158-161.

14. Woodside JC, Light TR: Symbrachydactyly - diagnosis, function, and treatment. *J Hand Surg Am* 2016;41(1):135-143.

15. Beals RK, Crawford S: Congenital absence of the pectoral muscles: A review of twenty-five patients. *Clin Orthop Relat Res* 1976;119:166-171.

16. Goldberg MJ, Mazzei RJ: Poland syndrome: A concept of pathogenesis based on limb bud embryology. *Birth Defects Orig Artic Ser* 1977;13(3D):103-115.

17. Ireland DC, Takayama N, Flatt AE: Poland's syndrome. *J Bone Joint Surg Am* 1976;58(1):52-58.

18. Wilson MR, Louis DS, Stevenson TR: Poland's syndrome: Variable expression and associated anomalies. *J Hand Surg Am* 1988;13(6):880-882.

19. Catena N, Divizia MT, Calevo MG, et al: Hand and upper limb anomalies in Poland syndrome: A new proposal of classification. *J Pediatr Orthop* 2012;32(7):722-726.

20. Barsky AJ: Cleft hand: Classification, incidence and treatment. Review of the literature and report of nineteen cases. *J Bone Joint Surg Am* 1964;46:1707-1720.

21. Miura T, Suzuki M: Clinical differences between typical and atypical cleft hand. *J Hand Surg Br* 1984;9(3):311-315.

22. Goodell PB, Bauer AS, Oishi S, et al: A functional assessment of children and adolescents with symbrachydactyly. *J Bone Joint Surg Am* 2017;99(13):1119-1128.

23. Cavallo AV, Smith PJ, Morley S, Morsi AW: Non-vascularized free toe phalanx transfers in congenital hand deformities--the Great Ormond Street experience. *J Hand Surg Br* 2003;28(6):520-527.

24. Garagnani L, Gibson M, Smith PJ, Smith GD: Long-term donor site morbidity after free nonvascularized toe phalangeal transfer. *J Hand Surg Am* 2012;37(4):764-774.

25. Raizman NM, Reid JA, Meisel AF, Seitz WH Jr: Long-term donor-site morbidity after free, nonvascularized toe phalanx transfer for congenital differences of the hand. *J Hand Surg Am* 2020;45(2):154.e1-154.e7.

26. Kay SP, Wiberg M: Toe to hand transfer in children: Part 1. Technical aspects. *J Hand Surg Br* 1996;21(6):723-734.

27. Kaplan JD, Jones NF: Outcome measures of microsurgical toe transfers for reconstruction of congenital and traumatic hand anomalies. *J Pediatr Orthop* 2014;34(3):362-368.

28. Bauer TB, Tondra JM, Trusler HM: Technical modification in repair of syndactylism. *Plast Reconstr Surg* 1956;17(5):385-392.

29. Eaton CJ, Lister GD: Syndactyly. *Hand Clin* 1990;6(4):555-575.

30. Flatt AE: Treatment of syndactylism. *Plast Reconstr Surg Transplant Bull* 1962;29:336-341.

31. Light TR: Congenital anomalies: Syndactyly, polydactyly and cleft hand, in Peimer CA, ed: *Surgery of the Hand and Upper Extremity*. McGraw-Hill, 1996.

32. Toledo LC, Ger E: Evaluation of the operative treatment of syndactyly. *J Hand Surg Am* 1979;4(6):556-564.

33. Miyamoto J, Nagasao T, Miyamoto S: Biomechanical analysis of surgical correction of syndactyly. *Plast Reconstr Surg* 2010;125(3):963-968.

34. Goldfarb CA, Steffen JA, Stutz CM: Complex syndactyly: Aesthetic and objective outcomes. *J Hand Surg Am* 2012;37(10):2068-2073.

35. Wall LB, Velicki K, Roberts S, Goldfarb CA: Outcomes of pediatric syndactyly repair using synthetic dermal substitute. *J Hand Surg Am* 2020;45(8):773.e1-773.e6.

36. Foukes GD, Reinker K: Congenital constriction band syndrome: A seventy year experience. *J Pediatr Orthop* 1994;19:973-976.

37. Ogino T, Saitou Y: Congenital constriction band syndrome and transverse deficiency. *J Hand Surg Br* 1987;12(3):343-348.

38. Jones NF, Smith AD: Congenital constriction band syndrome causing ulnar nerve palsy: Early diagnosis and surgical release with long-term follow-up. *J Hand Surg Am* 2001;26A:467-473.

39. Tada K, Kurisaki E, Yonenobu K, Tsuyuguchi Y, Kawai H: Central polydactyly: A review of 12 cases and their surgical treatment. *J Hand Surg Am* 1982;7(5):460-465.

40. Marks TW, Bayne LG: Polydactyly of the thumb: Abnormal anatomy and treatment. *J Hand Surg Am* 1978;3(2):107-116.

41. Cheng JC, Chan KM, Ma GF, Leung PC: Polydactyly of the thumb: A surgical plan based on ninety-five cases. *J Hand Surg Am* 1984;9(2):155-164.

42. Ezaki M: Radial polydactyly. *Hand Clin* 1990;6(4):577-588.

43. Miura T: Duplicated thumb. *Plast Reconstr Surg* 1982;69(3):470-481.

44. Tada K, Yonenobu K, Tsuyuguchi Y, Kawai H, Egawa T: Duplication of the thumb: A retrospective review of two hundred and thirty-seven cases. *J Bone Joint Surg Am* 1983;65(5):584-598.

45. Barton NJ, Buck-Gramcko D, Evans DM: Soft-tissue anatomy of mirror hand. *J Hand Surg Br* 1986;11(3):307-319.

46. Barton NJ, Buck-Gramcko D, Evans DM, Kleinert H, Semple C, Ulson H: Mirror hand treated by true pollicization. *J Hand Surg Br* 1986;11(3):320-336.

47. Tonkin MA: Thumb duplication: Concepts and techniques. *Clin Orthop Surg* 2012;4(1):1-17.

48. Xu YL, Shen KY, Chen J, Wang ZG: Flexor pollicis longus rebalancing: A modified technique for Wassel IV-D

thumb duplication. *J Hand Surg Am* 2014;39(1):75-82.e1.

49. Goldfarb CA, Patterson JM, Maender A, Manske PR: Thumb size and appearance following reconstruction of radial polydactyly. *J Hand Surg Am* 2008;33(8):1348-1353.

50. Wassel HD: The results of surgery for polydactyly of the thumb: A review. *Clin Orthop Relat Res* 1969;64(64):175-193.

51. Bora FW Jr, Nicholson JT, Cheema HM: Radial meromelia: The deformity and its treatment. *J Bone Joint Surg Am* 1970;52(5):966-979.

52. Swanson AB: The Krukenberg procedure in the juvenile amputee. *J Bone Joint Surg Am* 1964;46:1540-1548.

53. Seitz WH Jr: Distraction osteogenesis of a congenital amputation at the elbow. *J Hand Surg Am* 1989;14(6):945-948.

54. James MA, Bagley AM, Brasington K, Lutz C, McConnell S, Molitor F: Impact of prostheses on function and quality of life for children with unilateral congenital below-the-elbow deficiency. *J Bone Joint Surg* 2006;88(11):2356-2365.

55. Grabowski J, Goldin A, Arthur LG, et al: The effects of early anesthesia on neurodevelopment: A systematic review. *J Pediatr Surg* 2021;56(5):851-861.

56. Warner DO, Zaccariello MJ, Katusic SK, et al: Neuropsychological and behavioral outcomes after exposure of young children to procedures requiring general anesthesia: The Mayo Anesthesia Safety in Kids (MASK) Study. *Anesthesiology* 2018;129(1):89-105.

57. Goldberg NH, Watson HK: Composite toe (phalanx and epiphysis) transfers in the reconstruction of the aphalangic hand. *J Hand Surg Am* 1982;7(5):454-459.

Upper Limb Prostheses for Children

Robert D. Lipschutz, CPO, BSME

ABSTRACT

Fitting children with upper limb prostheses has many similarities to and many differences from adult prosthetic fittings. The components used in adult and pediatric devices are somewhat analogous in design, shape, and function. However, differences are present in the size of the components, the etiology of the deficiency or amputation, the level of family involvement, and the required accommodations for future growth and component designs. Most adults with upper limb amputations are young men who have sustained traumatic injuries, while congenital limb differences are the most common reason for fitting a child with an upper limb prosthesis. All prosthetic fittings are unique to the situation and the individual. Common factors for choosing the timing, components, and complexity of upper limb prostheses to children are dependent on residual limb length, age at the time of fitting, and current functional needs.

Keywords: acquired limb loss; congenital limb deficiency; longitudinal deficiency; transverse deficiency

Introduction

The decision to fit an individual with a limb prosthesis, regardless of the etiology or cause of the limb difference, seems to be obvious. Strange as it may seem, fitting upper limb prostheses to some children with upper limb differences has been a topic of controversy for many years. Most parents will pursue fitting of prostheses to their child if their child has had a traumatic amputation or one because of disease or illness. However, fitting a child with a congenital limb difference is not an absolute. Many factors weigh into the decision of whether to fit children with prostheses including level of limb difference, prosthesis options, aesthetics of the device, and experiences of the prosthetist and doctor. Compounding this dilemma are the current approaches and design foci of new prosthetic options for children and young adults.[1-7] Several of these fitting approaches, that is, 3-D printed kits and sharing of scanned files, remotely to fabricate a prosthesis for the child, eliminate the prosthetist (and entire healthcare team) from the clinical evaluation and fitting process. This direction is somewhat concerning to clinicians, but the families and healthcare professionals need to be aware of these options to insure appropriate safety and provisions for children/families seeking prosthetic care.

The development of new components for children has been almost nonexistent for the past decade. Manufacturing of mechanical digits and some designs of externally powered hands are being made in smaller sizes. Additionally, newer methods of electromyogram (EMG) acquisition and processing referred to as pattern recognition are being introduced to younger individuals with limb differences and amputations. Currently, because of the size and weight, the hardware for these systems along with the smaller hands are not applicable to younger children, but may be beneficial for some adolescents or young adults.

Although some studies have alluded to the minimal benefits of fitting children with upper limb prostheses, others have demonstrated their usefulness in improving self-esteem, acceptance among peers, and efficiency in manual activities.[8-12] Regardless of these conclusions, each child and family is unique and has its own reasons and desires when considering prosthetic fitting. Success in fitting a child with an upper limb prosthesis is also subject to a multitude of variables, and requires educating the family and providing the appropriate resources from the community and dedicated healthcare team.

General Considerations

When a family is considering fitting their child with a prosthesis, they should have a thorough understanding and acceptance of the influence of amputation/limb difference etiology, component options, functional benefits, cyclic wearing patterns, the child's motivation level, and the challenges

Robert D. Lipschutz or an immediate family member serves as a board member, owner, officer, or committee member of the Association of Children's Prosthetic and the Orthotic Clinics.

associated with prosthetic use. At first, the parents will make the decision for their child; later in life, the child will be encouraged to become involved in the process of selecting a prosthesis that they feel will be most beneficial to them, along with the corresponding components.

The primary etiology for upper limb amputations in children is congenital anomalies. In such patients, it is essential that the parents understand and accept the differences in their child's upper limb. In a child with an acquired amputation caused by trauma, infection, tumor, or other injury, it may be even more difficult for the child and family to accept the amputation, and greater demands may be expected of both the prosthesis and prosthetist.

Education should be provided about the associated benefits and limitations of various prosthetic fittings and components, such as terminal devices, wrists, and elbows. The child and family also need to be able to clearly express their goals and desires for the prosthetic fitting (whether the device will be aesthetic, prehensile, or have some combination of aesthetic and prehensile attributes) and recognize that such preferences may change throughout the child's life. Periodically, through their growing years, children may express a reluctance to wear an upper limb prosthesis. This reluctance will often begin with nonverbal cues when the child is quite young and progress to complete rejection when the child has the ability to verbally communicate. Children and young adults have the ability to change their minds and often go through a cyclic pattern of use and rejection of upper limb prostheses. Throughout childhood and adolescence, children will have the ability to try a variety of styles and components, allowing them to make a more educated decision on the prosthetic design of choice and use as they become adults.

The commitment of the family, the child, and the clinical team to the prosthetic fitting process is paramount in achieving success.[13,14] Over the past few decades, the approaches of clinical teams and families toward the fitting and use of upper limb prostheses have changed[15]—with fewer absolutes and more gray zones. The clinical team should discuss the pros and cons of prosthetic fitting, including voluntary nonuse by the child. If the child is fit with a prosthesis, a thorough effort must be made to train the child to use it and to incorporate the prosthesis into their daily activities. Parents often express that they are too busy, or do not want to spend the few moments that they have together with their child struggling over donning and practicing with the prosthesis. Unfortunately, unless the family is willing to invest adequate time in the training process, it is unlikely that the child will accept the prosthesis without constant assistance in donning the device and reminders of how and when to use their prosthesis.

Along with family and peer support, professional training by a skilled occupational therapist is also beneficial. Although many occupational therapists have limited training in working with upper limb prostheses, there are many centers that specialize in the care of children and have therapists with the required experience. If the therapist does not have the experience working with upper limb prostheses, they should seek the assistance of the prosthetist or an experienced therapist to provide training and support.

The clinical characteristics of children with upper limb deficiencies vary widely. Longitudinal limb deficiencies are less common than transverse deficiencies; therefore, prosthetic fittings are more common in patients with transverse deficiencies.[16,17] A discussion of the principles of prosthetic fitting must begin with the distal-most amputations and deficiencies and progress through more proximal amputation levels. The components appropriate for different levels of limb absence in specific age groups are to be discussed.

Digital Absence

Congenital deficiencies are rarely the cause of isolated absences of a digit or digits. Syndromes such as Streeter dysplasia (often referred to as amniotic band syndrome), Möbius syndrome, or Poland syndrome may infrequently cause digital absence, but these disorders are uncommon, and prosthetic restoration of individual fingers is rare in affected patients. In the pediatric cohort, trauma is more likely the cause of digital amputations. Potential causes include injuries sustained from paper shredders, farming equipment, and fireworks.

Historically, the main prosthetic intervention for digit amputation has been an aesthetic replacement of the finger for functional and psychological reasons. The function of these digits is limited and often interferes with the child's ability to perform manual tasks. Prostheses for this level of amputation that meet the aesthetic needs of the child and family often are very expensive and do not last for long periods of time because of the child's continued growth and active lifestyle. However, this may prove beneficial as an option, especially for older children and those with an acquired digital amputation.

Newly developed designs of mechanical digits may also be of benefit to the adolescent and younger adult. Manufacturers of individual articulated fingers have made options available for the pediatric cohort. These designs can be cable driven via movement of proximal joints such as the wrist, or passively positional using the contralateral hand, leg, or other surface to preposition the digit in the desired amount of proximal-interphalangeal and distal-interphalangeal (DIP) flexion (**Figure 1**). The passively positional designs are quite strong and incorporate ratcheting mechanisms to prevent extension of the digit once the prepositioning force is removed. To extend the finger, it is either fully flexed and released or a trigger on the dorsum of the finger is pressed to release the finger (extension) lock, permitting the finger to spring back into full extension.

Partial Hand With No Digits Remaining and Wrist Disarticulation

Partial hand amputations with no digits remaining (eg, transverse deficiency of the carpals, partial) are much more common in children than adults. When an adult sustains a traumatic partial

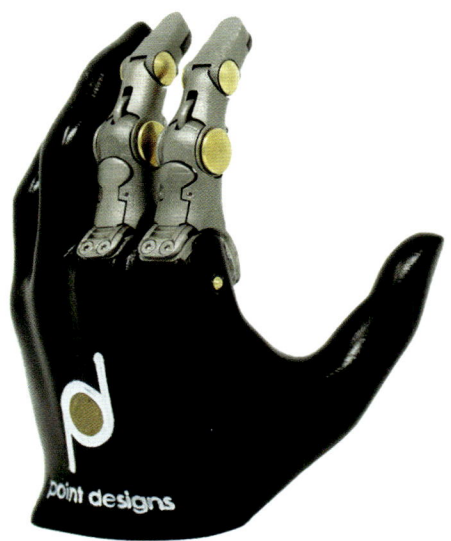

FIGURE 1 Photograph of point digit on a model. (Courtesy of Point Designs, LLC, Lafayette, CO.)

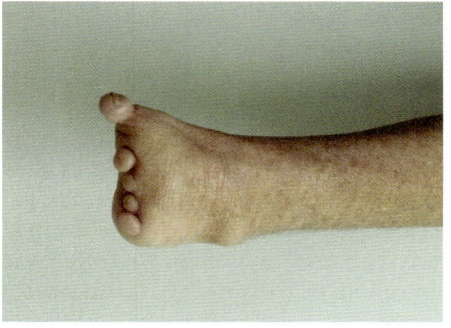

FIGURE 2 Clinical photograph of a transcarpal congenital limb deficiency with nubbins and physiologic wrist motion. (Courtesy of the Shirley Ryan AbilityLab, Chicago, IL.)

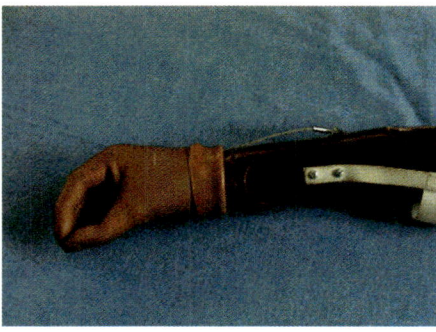

FIGURE 4 Photograph of a forearm prosthesis with a distal opening at the end of the forearm that exposes the distal residual limb to allow tactile feedback. (Courtesy of the Shirley Ryan AbilityLab, Chicago, IL.)

hand amputation, it is rare to have all five rays completely absent, with a single row of carpal bones remaining. In children with these and other congenital limb differences, the limbs often have small finger-like remnants on the distal end of their limb, referred to as nubbins (**Figure 2**). Associated with a row or rows of carpal bones may be the presence of movement (ie, wrist flexion and extension). Despite the differences between such amputations and wrist disarticulations, the prosthetic fitting principles are to be addressed together because of the similar limb lengths and overlapping prosthetic interventions, particularly when residual wrist and hand motion is limited.

A residual limb of this length allows the child to perform many tasks without a prosthesis in a physiologic position that is close to normal. The manipulation of objects and the performance of bimanual tasks are only minimally affected because the end of the affected limb is nearly at the level of the contralateral hand (**Figure 3**).

Prosthetic fitting at this amputation level has both advantages and disadvantages. Encouraging wear of the prosthesis allows the child to become accustomed to its use and emphasizes the benefits of incorporating the prosthesis into daily activities. However, covering the end of the residual limb

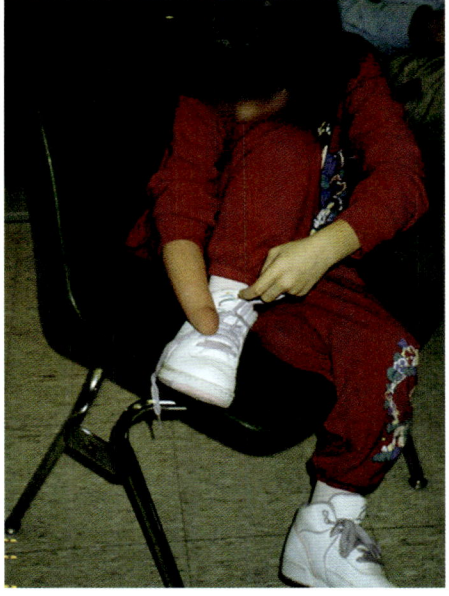

FIGURE 3 Clinical photograph of an approximately 5-year-old girl with a longer residual limb and minimal functional impairment. (Courtesy of the Shirley Ryan AbilityLab, Chicago, IL.)

decreases tactile feedback, which is an important aspect of manual dexterity and development. Some retention of tactile feedback may be accomplished by leaving an opening at the end of the forearm of the prosthesis so that the distal residual limb is exposed (**Figure 4**). However, it is unclear whether this provision benefits long-term prosthetic use and acceptance.

As with any long residual limb, there are challenges of fitting components and maintaining prosthetic limb-length equality with the contralateral side. Epiphysiodeses of the radial and ulnar styloids have been suggested as a potential means of creating space for prosthetic components. However, opponents of this surgical approach cite the disadvantage of the exaggerated limb-length discrepancy if the individual chooses not to wear a prosthesis.

Fitting Infants

The age of a child at the first fitting with an upper limb prosthesis varies from clinic to clinic and according to the level of the limb deficit. At the partial hand and wrist disarticulation levels, it has been widely accepted that infants (younger than 1 year) can be fit with a prosthesis at approximately 6 months of age when they are obtaining sitting balance and are beginning to explore their environment bimanually.[6,14,15,18] The optimal fitting age varies from child to child and may be affected by many variables, including the effect of having infants sleep on their backs to decrease the risk of sudden infant death syndrome. Limited tummy time may delay upper body development and coordination, thus delaying the benefits gained from using an upper limb prosthesis. For very young children, passive prostheses are the most widely accepted options for decreasing the difference in length between the residual limb and contralateral hand, maintaining sitting balance, directing lines of site for spatial relations when manipulating objects and encouraging bimanual activities. It has been suggested that the earlier prosthetic fitting begins, the more likely the child and family will be to accept the device; however, this topic is debatable.

In infants, the passive terminal devices may have the appearance of an open hand, a crawling hand, or a mitt. Standard terminal devices and wrist units are discouraged at these levels of limb absence because they make the prosthesis too long. Instead, proximally hollowed terminal devices and/or gloves filled with a flexible material are generally used. These modifications permit the socket to protrude into the proximal aspect of the terminal device to attain limb-length equality.

At this early age, an infant's limbs have little bony definition and, thus, will not require the prosthetic accommodations for a bulbous distal end. This, however, will become necessary as the child matures. The shape of the socket is very generic, and reliance on sleeves or minimal harnessing for suspension is preferred. Socket construction for an infant's prosthesis often consists of a thin, lightweight lamination with a removable (onion-skin) layer to accommodate growth. A semiflexible thermoplastic material, such as Surlyn (Dupont), is often used for this removable layer (or inner socket) because it provides a hygienic environment with ease of cleaning and allows direct lamination of the rigid socket without a separator. Laminating directly over the semiflexible thermoplastic material permits the two sockets to temporarily bond together until such time that the prosthetist and the family deem it appropriate to remove the inner socket because of growth. This will become evident, as the child's limb no longer fits well into the socket. When this transition occurs, the prosthetist should check the trim lines of the remaining laminated socket because the edges most likely will be sharp and require smoothing.

Additional volume management is often necessary because the child grows rapidly during this stage. Limb volume may be managed by initially oversizing the socket and using fitting socks that can be reduced in thickness and ultimately eliminated as the child grows. However, the thickness of the original sock should be limited because it further increases the size and bulk of the forearm, which is already larger because of the addition of the onion-skin layer. Although the preemptive use of an inner socket layer and additional fitting socks will ultimately prolong the useful life of the prosthesis, too large a forearm will be noticeable and unacceptable to the family.

Fitting Toddlers and Preschoolers

Similar components may be used when fitting a toddler (1 year to younger than 3 years) and a preschooler (aged 3 to 5 years). Although no exact age exists at which the child will be fit with a prosthesis that has grasping capabilities, the introduction of a child's first prehensile terminal device often is accomplished at the toddler stage. The main factors that necessitate the recommendation for most new prosthetic fittings at this developmental stage include anatomic changes to the limb and the child's capacity to use prosthetic designs with expanded capabilities. If designed appropriately with growth accommodations, the child's first prosthesis should last approximately 1 year, at which time the child will be approximately 18 months of age—an appropriate age for fitting a prosthesis with a prehensile terminal device.

At 18 months of age, toddlers with transverse deficiencies of the carpals may or may not have sufficient space for a prehensile terminal device in their prosthesis without having a length discrepancy of their forearm and hand. Congenital anomalies are rarely isolated to one structure, and these deficiencies are generally no exception. A discrepancy in the length of the ipsilateral humerus and/or radius and ulna is frequently associated with a transverse deficiency of the carpals. Shortening of these additional structures may be beneficial as standard prosthetic components may be used without resulting in a longer prosthetic arm compared with the noninvolved arm.

Terminal devices for toddlers may be similar to the passive devices previously mentioned or passive devices with prehensile capabilities (**Figure 5**). They may have flexible, conformable fingers or true articulations with spring-loaded or elastic-loaded closing force. Some may also be designed with the anticipation of adding a cable for body-powered use at a later date. These designs may be of various shapes, including hooks, hands, and the CAPP (Fillauer) terminal device (**Figure 6**). Arguments have been made for the functional abilities of one design compared with another; however, the most important aspect is

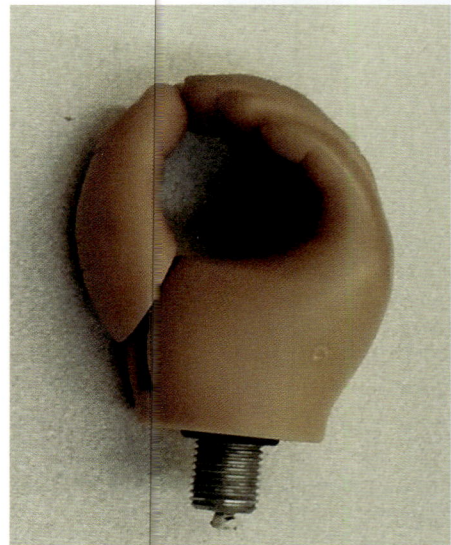

FIGURE 5 Photograph of a passive terminal device with prehensile capabilities. (Courtesy of the Shirley Ryan AbilityLab, Chicago, IL.)

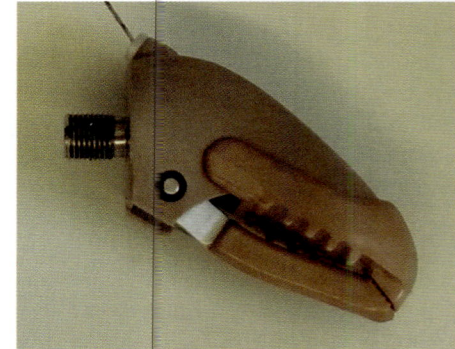

FIGURE 6 Photograph of the child-size CAPP terminal device, which has a wide palmar face and a friction cover for secure prehension. (Courtesy of the Shirley Ryan AbilityLab, Chicago, IL.)

acceptance by the family and actual use of the prescribed prosthesis.

If the child has substantial movement in their residual limb (wrist flexion and extension), opposition posts may be a more beneficial approach over the traditional passive prostheses. Opposition posts are typically frame-type devices that fit over the forearm and have a distal extension that provides a platform to which the motion of the residual limb will oppose during wrist flexion. Adjustability of the platform position is generally provided to allow grasping of objects of varying sizes and shapes. The efficacy of these devices may be more pronounced in individuals with bilateral involvement.[19]

Body-powered terminal devices also may be used, which require a harness to provide cable activation of the prehensor. This transition will likely be new to the child and family and may require greater education and training for donning, use, and adjustments.

Arguments also have been made that toddlers do not have the cognitive ability and coordination for these types of devices, so an externally powered prosthesis is the most appropriate design for this age.[6] Externally powered options consist of electric hand terminal devices with one of two common EMG-based input strategies that are both myoelectrically controlled. Toddlers are commonly fit with a single-site, voluntary-opening, automatic-closing electronic scheme. This type of electronic control is analogous to that of mechanical body-powered voluntary-opening terminal devices. This often is referred to as a cookie crusher or St. Anthony's circuit and was designed by T. Walley Williams III and Tom Haslam in the late 1980s.[20] This input design requires a single electrode, which is typically mounted in the socket over the child's wrist extensors, and requires muscle activation to signal opening of the hand. After the extensor signal falls below the open threshold, the hand is driven closed by means of either electric power or a spring, such as that used in the Scamp Hand (RSLSteeper). The placement of the electrode over the extensors is not only intended for this initial design and function but also in anticipation of future designs in which dual-site myoelectric systems will use wrist extensors for hand opening and wrist flexors for hand closing. If appropriate, this latter strategy may be planned for by incorporating an electrode dummy into the socket with the goal of later converting the current prosthesis into dual-site control without the need to fabricate an entirely new device. For a small percentage of toddlers, dual-site myoelectric prostheses may be used in the initial fitting because children with longer limbs have an innate ability to move the end of their residual limb by means of extensors and flexors, and they may have the cognitive abilities to use this agonist–antagonist muscle strategy for their first prehensile design.

Another method of controlling an externally powered prosthesis may be accomplished by incorporating force-sensing resistors (FSRs) or Flex Strips versus EMG sensing electrodes. These input devices can have force or bending moments applied to them, respectively, to enable a proportional output signal to the motor for either opening or closing of the hand. As in the aforementioned opposition post, the child must have adequate motion distal to the styloids that will enable the end of the limb to flex and extend, thus contacting the FSRs or creating a deflection of the Flex Strips. Because of the complexity of this agonist–antagonist method of control, these strategies may be plausible for the preschoolers or may need to wait until at least adolescence.

Regardless of the strategy for controlling the electric hand, a battery is required. Limbs of this length have adequate mechanical advantage and may well tolerate this added weight. The challenge, however, for these residual limb lengths is where to place the battery without compromising the aesthetics of the prosthesis. The battery must be either incorporated into the forearm, making the forearm more bulky and cylindrical, or tethered on a cable, necessitating a more proximal attachment such as on a triceps cuff (**Figure** 7). Neither option is optimal.

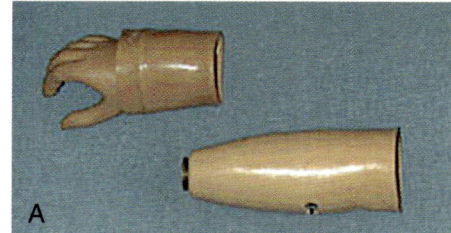

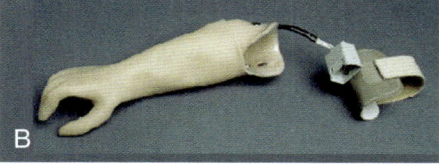

FIGURE 7 **A**, Photograph of a prosthesis with a bulky forearm with an incorporated battery. **B**, Photograph of a battery tethered on the triceps cuff of the prosthesis. (Courtesy of the Shirley Ryan AbilityLab, Chicago, IL.)

Fitting School-Age Children, Adolescents, and Young Adults

After a child reaches school age and beyond, if they have been previously fit with a prosthesis, a wearing pattern has typically been developed. The aforementioned component options (passive, body-powered, and externally powered) are still available and appropriate as the child grows. Depending upon the size of the child/young adult; the smaller multiarticular hands that have been recently introduced to the market are worth exploring. As the category describes, multiarticular hands have the ability to be positioned in several different hand grasp/grip patterns versus the historic palmar prehension or three-point opposition of electronic hands for children. Although with any component having more moving parts/motors, they are more susceptible to breakdown, these children are getting to the age that they may have more of an appreciation of how to use and care for their prostheses.

One difference that may become progressively apparent when examining the residual limb is the anatomic definition that has developed. For transverse deficiencies of the carpals, partial hand amputations, or wrist disarticulations, a bulbous distal end has now developed, which is both a benefit and a detriment. The benefit of these contoured limbs is the ability to provide suspension of the prosthesis by securing adequate purchase of the bulbous distal limb. Drawbacks include the difficulty of designing a prosthesis that permits easy donning. As the child's limb shape begins to develop, it may be necessary to explore different donning and suspension options. With the distal end of the residuum being more bulbous in shape, expandable sockets via cut-out doors/windows, elastic straps, or flexible materials (bladders) may be necessary to facilitate passing this wider distal limb into the socket. Other socket designs may use custom silicone liners with lanyards (straps) for suspension. Custom liners will be fabricated with an increased thickness proximal to the bulbous limb, thus decreasing the amount of circumferential discrepancy on the outer circumference of the liner and permitting easier donning. These lanyard straps are passed through a slot at the distal end of the socket (similar to that of transfemoral prostheses), are reflected back to the proximal aspect of the socket, and may be secured via a chafe with Velcro on either side of the lanyard or a clasp buckle. Self-suspension of any upper limb prosthesis has the benefit of reducing or eliminating harnessing and potentially decreasing the amount of force being transmitted to the contralateral axilla by means of the harness. In these instances, it may also enable the socket trim lines to be lowered, distal to the humeral epicondyles, and thus permitting active pronation and supination of the forearm.

As previously mentioned, an additional benefit of the limb definition may be the option of using alternative means of input to EMG for control of an externally powered prosthesis. In myoelectric prostheses, electrodes must be in contact with muscle bellies. In traditional designs for this amputation level, electrodes are mounted over the wrist flexors and extensors at the proximal aspect of the forearm, requiring a socket that encompasses most of the forearm. For those individuals with available carpal (wrist) motion, control is obtained by bending Flex Strips or initiating contact against opposing FSRs. These designs require that the socket not limit wrist motion within the prosthesis.

Transradial Level

Transradial amputations in adults are usually the result of trauma or tumor. In children, it is more likely because of a congenital transverse deficiency of the forearm (predominantly in the upper one-third of the forearm, leaving a short or very short limb). Children with transverse deficiencies often have residual nubbins, which are usually smaller than those on longer limbs and do not disrupt prosthetic fitting. Although fitting children with this level of limb absence may be somewhat controversial, differing opinions are less directed at the length and use of the prosthetic limb and more at the long-term use of a prosthesis and the improvement in the child's quality of life.[8,9] Despite not having a hand or long residual limb, children with this limb length will often find ways to use the residual limb for tasks, such as opposing the residual limb against the other arm with an object captured between, holding an object in the cubital fold of the residual limb, or trapping an object under their axilla. However, these methods are generally used in positions in which visualization is less directed at the environment and is more within their personal body space. Wearing a prosthesis will afford children the ability to manipulate objects farther away from their body as well as provide prehensile capabilities in the terminal device. These benefits may enhance the task being performed. Contrary to the previously described levels of amputation, these limbs often are quite short and could conceivably benefit from orthopaedic lengthening techniques. However, evidence has shown that this is rarely performed, and when lengthening is performed, complications often arise.[21]

Fitting Infants

In addition to moving bimanual tasks toward more functional lines of sight, additional reasons for fitting a prosthesis to an infant with a transradial-level deficit are analogous to reasons for fittings at longer limb levels and will be pertinent throughout the remainder of this chapter. Early fittings begin at approximately 6 months of age and consist of passive terminal device options. Fabrication often consists of removable inner sockets for growth and lightweight, laminated outer sockets that are pigmented to match the child's skin. The appearance of these prostheses often results in a proximal section that is larger than the forearm or glove that is being applied, thus creating an abrupt transition from the socket to the forearm (**Figure 8**). Because of material limitations associated with vinyl used in many glove types, it is challenging to stretch the prefabricated glove over this socket circumference.

These prostheses are suspended by means of a small sleeve or lightweight figure-of-8 or chest strap harness. Because children have a way of wiggling out of their prostheses (especially when the residual limb is short), it is beneficial to have a harness in place to prevent loss of the device. Applying the prosthesis and the harness to an infant is challenging. Parents, therapists, and prosthetists alike finding it difficult to keep the infant's limb in the socket while simultaneously securing the harness in place. This situation can be a source of frustration for parents and caretakers and an impetus for trying a sleeve for suspension.

A suspension strategy that is gaining more popularity in pediatric fittings is the use of high-density silicone sockets. Some have integrated silicone sleeves, while others are of suction suspension design with very small (peewee) valves. This flexible material may be reflected proximally, donned onto the limb, and rolled back over the child's limb, where it provides compressive forces to suspend the device. In these designs, the entire outer surface, including the socket, is fabricated from silicone and is customarily a one-piece design. Although the appearance is more satisfactory than laminated sockets and vinyl gloves, these designs are not easily modified and can be somewhat restrictive to active elbow flexion and extension.

Chapter 69: Upper Limb Prostheses for Children

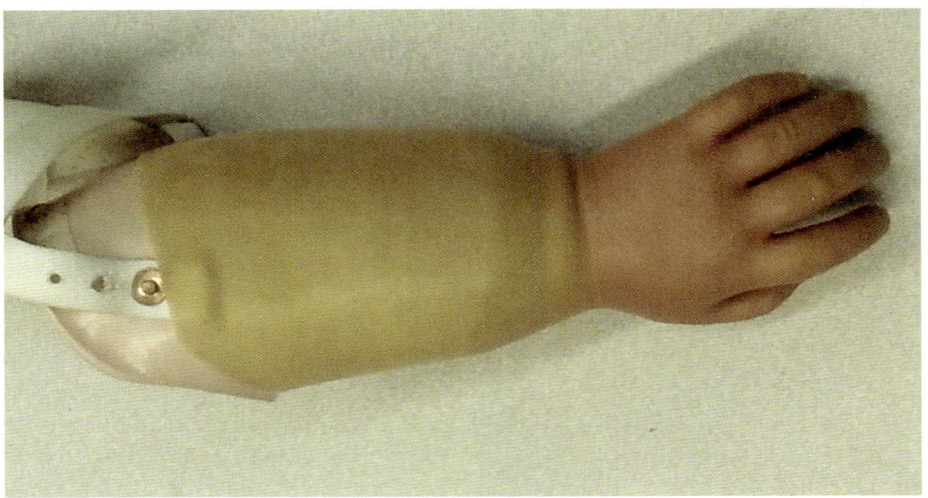

FIGURE 8 Photograph of a passive transradial prosthesis for an infant of approximately 6 months of age. The prosthesis has a removable inner socket for growth and a lightweight, laminated outer socket that is pigmented to match the child's skin. These prostheses often result in a proximal section that is larger than the forearm, thus creating an abrupt transition from the socket to the forearm. (Courtesy of the Shirley Ryan AbilityLab, Chicago, IL.)

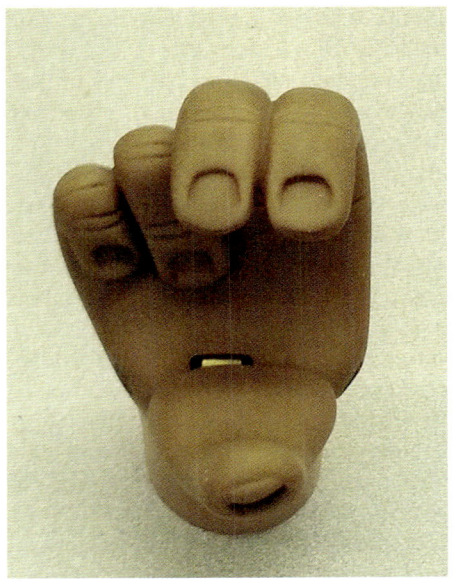

FIGURE 9 Photograph of a voluntary closing terminal device with sculpted fingers for a toddler or preschool-age child. (Courtesy of the Shirley Ryan AbilityLab, Chicago, IL.)

Fitting Toddlers and Preschoolers

The decision to either keep the current design or try an alternative prosthetic approach is generally made when a child achieves the milestone of either outgrowing the current device or beginning to investigate their environment to the degree that the child's family feels a new design is warranted. As with the previously described limb levels, passive, passive with prehensile capabilities, cable-activated, or myoelectric prostheses may be chosen. In contrast, however, adequate room generally exists between the distal end of the residual limb and the final length of the terminal device in all of these prosthetic strategies.

A child's cognitive ability to use a body-powered prostheses may present a challenge, but training by a skilled occupational therapist usually remedies problems.[5,6] The aesthetics of a cable-driven prosthesis tends to be the greater challenge as many parents prefer to have a prosthesis for their child that does not have a harness nor a hook terminal device. Regardless of the degree of function permitted with a given terminal device, if it is not acceptable in application or appearance to the family, they will not be motivated to put it on the child, and the fitting will likely fail.

Voluntary-opening terminal devices are limited to the split-hook design, the CAPP terminal device, or mechanical hands. Voluntary-closing terminal devices for children are available in a variety of shapes and colors, including those with sculpted fingers (**Figure 9**). Because parents often desire a more lifelike prosthesis for their child, they often choose devices with a hand-like appearance. More conventional mechanical hands with voluntary opening or voluntary closing activation patterns are an available option but are much more difficult for the child to operate, largely because of the gloves that cover them. When a glove is applied over a mechanical hand, it dramatically decreases the mechanical efficiency of the system by increasing the forces required for operation.[22] Spring tension in the hands may be reduced for easier opening; however, this also proportionally decreases the grasping force of the hands, especially voluntary-opening hands.

Myoelectric prostheses are another popular option because they provide a hand-like terminal device with a glove. These alternatives also do not require gross body movements for use. The motor, which is housed within the hand, provides the necessary force to open and close the device against the resistance of the glove. However, the weight of the electric hand must be considered because most children with transverse deficiencies of the forearm have transradial limbs in the proximal one-third of their anatomic forearm length, which puts their short residual limbs at a mechanical disadvantage relative to the mass of the hand and the forearm. In addition, as described previously, such systems require a battery, which adds more weight to the prosthesis distal to the residual limb. Although these batteries have become substantially smaller in recent years, they still add weight that must be overcome by flexion of the residual limb.

Cookie-crusher strategies are the most popular for a first electric prosthesis, especially in children younger than 4 years. At this limb level, a single-control (voluntary opening) pattern may be elicited much more easily than a dual-control (voluntary opening and closing) pattern. Training a child with a short transradial deficiency to contract antagonistic muscles is much more difficult than for a child with a longer residual limb because there is less tissue movement at the end of the shorter residual limb. Asking the child to wiggle the end of their arm is a typical training prompt, but it does not always elicit a consistent response in a child younger than 3 years.

Prosthetic sockets are much more invasive for shorter residual limbs than for longer limbs. They often cross the elbow joint proximally to provide stability and obtain purchase on the limb. Proximal extensions of the socket also distribute forces over a larger surface area, thus decreasing pressure. Many prosthetists choose self-suspending sockets when designing prostheses for children of this age. Traditional Münster socket designs are appropriate for this limb length. They incorporate high and tight anterior-posterior trim lines that straddle the biceps tendon and extend above the olecranon, respectively. Because of this design, they require a donning technique in which the soft tissues are drawn into the socket by means of a pull sock, or donning aid, a technique that is often difficult to master for both the parents and the child. Additionally, because of its proximal extension and containment, the Münster socket reduces the range of motion (both flexion and extension) at the elbow when worn. In response to these issues, a hybrid socket design that incorporates principles of moderately tight anterior-posterior and mediolateral trim lines may be used. This design will facilitate easier donning (although a donning aid may still be needed), but it will not limit range of motion of the prosthesis as dramatically, and the aesthetics of the static and dynamic use of the prosthesis will not be affected. Lower trim lines allow greater range of flexion for midline and cephalic activities.

When a child with this limb level flexes their limb completely, the radius and ulna seem to disappear within the soft tissue. This anatomical change makes it difficult to capture and maintain suspension through the full range of flexion without having high, anterior trim lines. The dramatic difference in children's limb shapes when the elbow is extended also makes socket fit more difficult. Many of these children have substantial ligamentous laxity about the elbow and are capable of hyperextending their elbows (**Figure 10**). When doing so, the radial head frequently subluxates anteriorly, causing a bulge

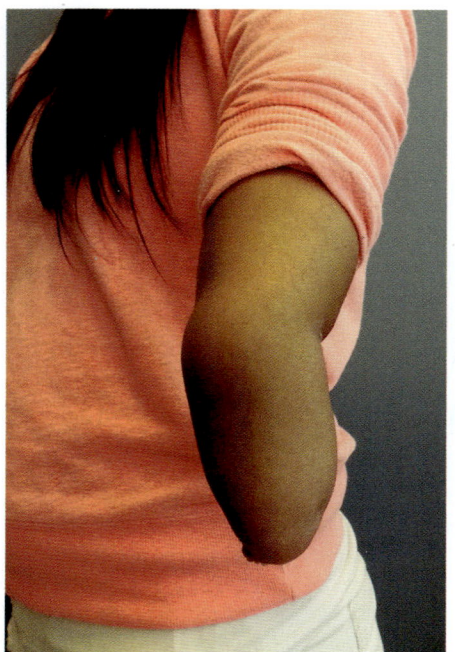

FIGURE 10 Clinical photograph shows hyperextension of a transradial limb. (Courtesy of the Shirley Ryan AbilityLab, Chicago, IL.)

in the anterolateral aspect of their cubital fold. This change in limb shape must be considered to create a comfortably fitting socket.

Fitting School-Age Children, Adolescents, and Young Adults

As mentioned for other amputation levels, if a child has developed a wearing pattern with a particular style of prosthesis, they are likely to continue with that design. However, as children grow older they may want a prosthesis that is more accepted by their peers (hand-like terminal devices). All of the aforementioned prosthetic control options (passive, body-powered, and externally powered) are available for children of school age or older whose residua are at the transradial level. Externally powered hands are a good option for these children because they add aesthetic value, require minimal movement to activate, and maintain prehensile capabilities. At these ages, the child would most likely prefer to have volitional control of both opening and closing; therefore, a cookie-crusher circuit often is replaced with a dual-site control strategy. It may be challenging to educate the child to perform these movements and accurately capture their EMG in a myoelectric control strategy. The residual limb is often quite short, and when the muscles on the medial aspect of the forearm (those assumed to be wrist and finger flexors) are contracted, the residual limb becomes even shorter, resulting in space between the skin and electrode. It is imperative that the medial electrode be well situated on the limb to capture this surface electromyographically. Unfortunately, this electrode begins to encroach on the medial epicondyle because it must be located more proximally to maintain skin contact during muscle contraction.

An additional challenge with electronic hands for school-aged children may be changes in the grasp patterns of the hand. The two main aforementioned hand grasp patterns for children's electronic hands were that of palmar prehension (three-jaw-chuck) and oppositional grasp.[4,23] Several hands, including Variety Ability Systems Inc. (now an Ottobock product) and RSLSteeper, make prosthetic hands with the palmar prehension pattern, and the hands are available in a variety of age-correlated sizes, ranging from 0 to 2 for infants and toddlers through 7 to 11 for adolescents. The Electrohand 2,000 line from Ottobock also is available in a range of similar sizes; however, this design provides a more three-point oppositional-type grasp (**Figure 11**). When transitioning to larger hands, this oppositional grasp pattern is no longer available, so a young adult must adapt to a palmar prehension pattern or use one of the smaller multiarticular hands. In multiarticular hands, prehensile patterns may be selected through various means of mode selection such as co-contraction, double-impulse, triple-impulse, long opening, or pattern recognition control.

Transhumeral Level

Limb lengths at the transhumeral level of amputation or deficiency vary quite dramatically. Children with a very short ulna may be fit prosthetically as

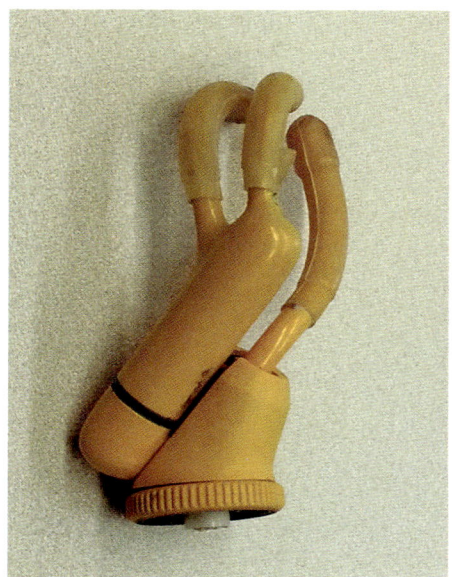

FIGURE 11 Photograph of a pediatric, externally powered hand with oppositional grasp. (Courtesy of the Shirley Ryan AbilityLab, Chicago, IL.)

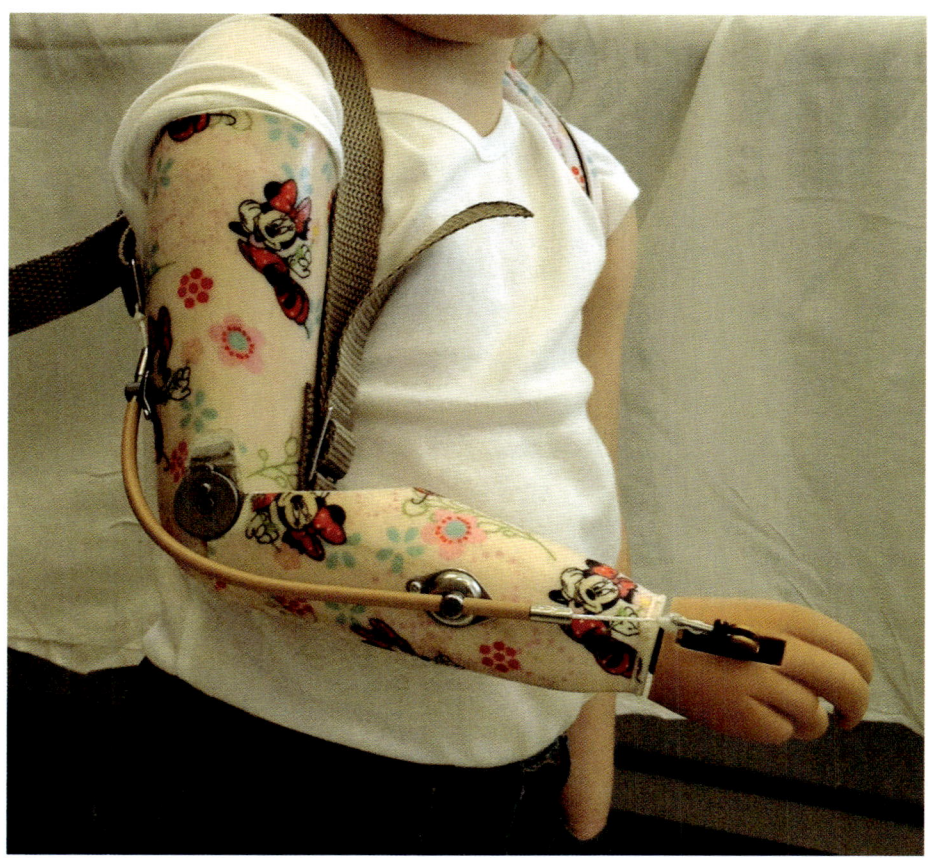

FIGURE 12 Clinical photograph of a prosthesis with outside hinges and a step-lock style mechanism. (Courtesy of the Shirley Ryan AbilityLab, Chicago, IL.)

if they have an elbow disarticulation. Relatively long congenital transhumeral deficiencies also are frequently observed. The most challenging fittings are those with mid-length to short transhumeral limbs because of the fairly substantial mechanical disadvantage along with the frequent need for revisions that further shorten the limb segment. Such revisions often are necessary because of the absence of the distal humeral epiphysis, making the limb prone to bony overgrowth (often referred to as spiking). As this distal bone is removed to relieve spiking and damage to the internal soft tissue, the residual limb becomes shorter, thus losing more leverage for controlling a prosthesis.

Fitting Infants

Children with deficiencies through the humerus may also be fit early. However, a lack of consensus exists as to when to introduce components that are more complex and when to expect the child to gain the ability to control the prosthesis entirely with the involved limb.[1,3,13,18] First fittings for these children include passive prostheses, most of which do not have articulating joints or prehensile terminal devices. Prosthetic elbows are usually omitted because they would require a prohibitively sophisticated feature that could vary the amount of friction between loading and unloading during activities such as crawling. The resistance to elbow movement in the sagittal plane would need to be low when pre-positioning the hand for activity; however, resistance to the weight of the child when leaning on the device would need to be high to prevent inadvertent elbow flexion. In many instances, this first prosthesis will resemble a banana arm—a transhumeral prosthesis with no elbow articulation but with a severe flexion bow that permits the child to easily reach midline with the terminal device. The aforementioned terminal device may be a passive hand or a spring-loaded component that permits objects (eg, bottles and rattles) to be held.

Fitting Toddlers and Preschoolers

Articulating joints often are incorporated into prostheses for children older than 20 months of age. The method of activation, however, will depend on the child's cognitive abilities, the family's willingness to participate in the functional use of the device, and the clinical team's experience in fitting and training the child with these added components. Friction elbows that are passively flexed and extended enable the forearm and terminal device to stay in place for bimanual tasks. However, if substantial force or weight is placed through the terminal device or on the forearm of the prosthesis, the elbow may inadvertently flex or extend. This could be a source of frustration for the young prosthesis user.

Instead of a passive frictional component, a component with a positive locking feature may be used (either outside locking hinges or an internal locking elbow). Outside hinges with a step-lock style mechanism may be used, especially for longer limbs (**Figure 12**). Step-lock mechanisms permit the user to manually flex the elbow to a greater degree of flexion, which then blocks the joints from going into extension. To bring the arm back into extension, the joints must be maximally flexed, which then releases the lock and permits full extension of the elbow. This movement is analogous to that mentioned in the passively positional fingers discussed in the section on Digital Absence.

For those elbows with alternating locking and unlocking, the mechanism should be easily activated by attaching a loop or other form that is readily grasped by the parent or the child's contralateral hand (Figure 13). The aforementioned elbows may be successfully combined with a body-powered terminal device if a Bowden cable system is used.

Active locking and unlocking mechanism with the typical combined motions of glenohumeral extension, glenohumeral abduction, and shoulder depression is a sophisticated task that is reserved for experienced, older children. Most children cannot complete this complex combination of motions until they are at least age 5 years of age.[5,18] Devices that use a fairlead cable and housing approach require that, after the child has the elbow locked in the desired position of flexion, they must have enough remaining body excursion to open the terminal device. Because of the cabling configuration, such a process is challenging for a young child and is proportionately more difficult for those with shorter limbs.

Active control of the prosthetic elbow and the terminal device may be facilitated when an electronic hand is used in combination with a mechanical elbow such as within a hybrid prosthesis. Electronic elbow choices for children of this age are no longer available because the only suitable pediatric electronic elbows have been discontinued by their manufacturers. The use of larger pediatric electronic elbows is reserved for older children, children with bilateral limb loss above the elbow, or those with shoulder disarticulations. If active use of the elbow and the hand is desired in a toddler or a preschool-age child, a hybrid prosthesis consisting of a body-powered elbow combined with an externally powered hand must be chosen.

Fitting School-Age Children, Adolescents, and Young Adults

As the child grows older, they have the cognitive ability to perform some of the more complex body movements required to activate transhumeral body-powered and externally powered prostheses. In school-age children with recently acquired amputations resulting from trauma or tumor, there may be greater motivation to use prostheses with more complex controls compared with their age-matched counterparts with congenital deficiencies. This may arise because those with a recent amputation have been accustomed to living with an active elbow. At this age, the elbow locking/unlocking functions generally may be controlled by means of the previously described ipsilateral shoulder movements. In addition, powered prosthetic components, such as electronic elbows and terminal devices, may be introduced to provide function without the limitations of insufficient body excursion. Based on the research of the author, there are no electronic elbows currently being offered for children. Electronic terminal devices are analogous to those described previously and some may be combined with electronic elbows in an externally powered prosthesis or a hybrid design.

Shoulder Disarticulation Level

Congenital shoulder disarticulation levels for an infant are either true shoulder disarticulations (transverse deficiency of the arm, complete), often referred to as amelia, or a variety of longitudinal deficiencies in which most or all of the humerus is absent, with only a phocomelic hand or digits present. Other anomalies are frequently concomitant with these limb deficiencies and often take precedence in the care and treatment of the very young child. Acquired shoulder disarticulations are uncommon in children, but they can result from tumors, and traumatic events such as automobile, electrical, and farm equipment injuries.[24]

Fitting Infants

Shoulder disarticulation prostheses for infants are cumbersome and ineffective. Because of this, in children with amelia or phocomelia, prosthetic fittings are frequently delayed. Although early fitting contributes to successful prosthesis use, in these patients, prosthetic fittings are impractical because they may inhibit the achievement of infant developmental milestones by preventing rolling and mobility. It may be feasible to begin prosthetic fitting when sitting balance is achieved; however, this milestone may be delayed if the child's body asymmetry makes it difficult for them to balance when sitting.

If a prosthesis is provided for these children, it often will have a passive friction shoulder (or no shoulder joint), a friction elbow, and a passive terminal device. A passive elbow would be used for infants at the shoulder disarticulation level because of the inability of the infant to actively position the prosthetic arm in space. The therapist and parents must show the child how to use the prosthesis. Friction settings on these elbows tend to be set quite high because the infant is not expected to preposition the elbow at such a young age, while the parents and therapists have the strength to do so.

Fitting Toddlers and Preschoolers

If a child with a congenital shoulder disarticulation and their family have successfully adopted the prosthesis at

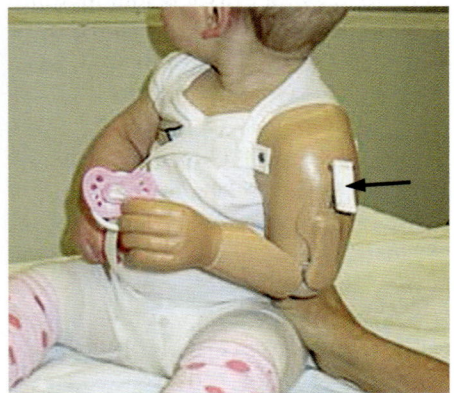

FIGURE 13 Clinical photograph of a prosthesis with an alternating locking mechanism that is manually activated by pulling and releasing the webbing (arrow) attached to the elbow cable lock. (Courtesy of the Shirley Ryan AbilityLab, Chicago, IL.)

the toddler to preschool stage, they will most likely continue with prosthetic fittings. In addition to the components mentioned for the infant user, the toddler may have a prehensile terminal device that is either passively prehensile or activated by cable excursion. Because glenohumeral flexion is not an option for controlling the cable system, excursion is limited to scapular and biscapular protraction. It may be worth considering an externally powered terminal device combined with electrical activation schemes through a harness using scapular protraction or shoulder elevation and a harness pull switch mounted across the child's back or on the waist belt, respectively, or via shoulder elevation to contact an FSR with the socket to control the terminal device. Electronic control of the terminal device decreases the amount of excursion necessary to activate the component as compared with a body-powered component. Such externally powered prostheses may be configured with volitional control of opening with automatic closing or with volitional opening and closing of the terminal device. Although myoelectric control would eliminate the need for significant excursion to activate a component, it is very difficult to teach such control to a child of this age with this proximal a level of limb difference.

Fitting School-Age Children, Adolescents, and Young Adults

In addition to children with congenital shoulder disarticulation limb absence, school-age children, adolescents, or young adults may have sustained a traumatic event that necessitated a shoulder disarticulation. Depending on the size of the child, component selection may vary.

Most prosthetic shoulders include friction-regulated flexion–abduction joints. However, adolescents and young adults may benefit from a shoulder joint that offers both locking and free-swinging positions in the sagittal plane, combined with the friction abduction component. The decision to incorporate such a shoulder joint is highly dependent upon the size of the child. A free-swinging arm feature may improve

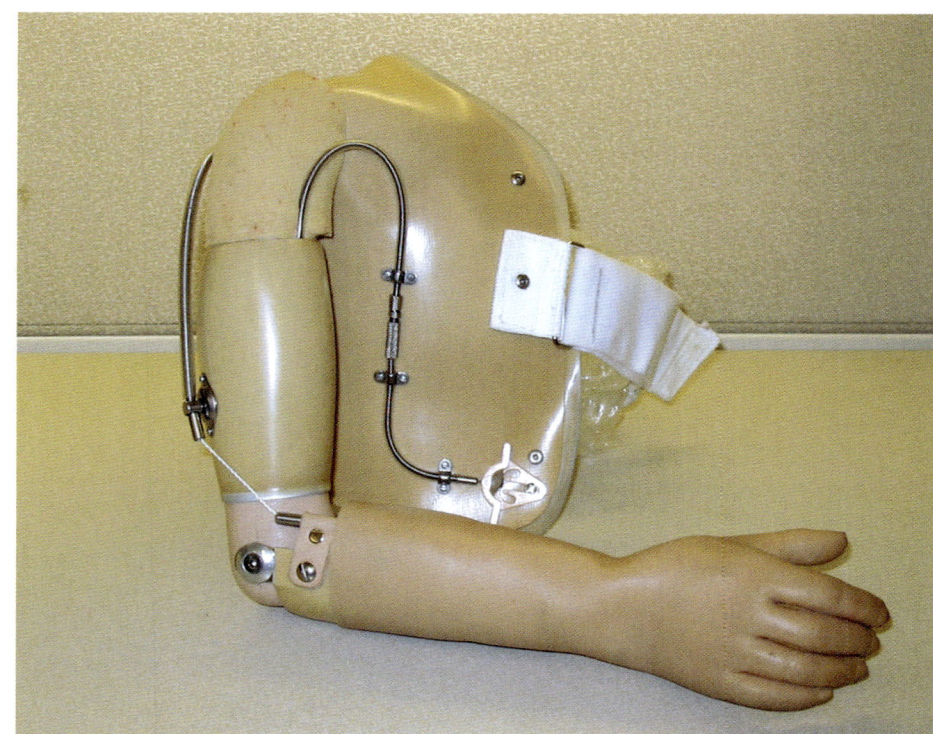

FIGURE 14 Photograph of a shoulder disarticulation prosthesis with hybrid control. (Courtesy of the Shirley Ryan AbilityLab, Chicago, IL.)

comfort while walking and may translate to improved wear and compliance.

The available components distal to the shoulder are the same as those described for the transhumeral amputation level. Because excursion for shoulder disarticulations is even more limited, it is essential to use either a hybrid control (**Figure 14**) or a completely externally powered prosthesis if an active elbow and a terminal device are required. Unfortunately, as previously cited, there are no externally powered elbows available for children. Therefore, the child would be ineligible for a completely powered prosthesis until they reached a size at which they could benefit from an adult, commercially available elbow such as the Espire Elbow (Steeper Group), the Utah Arm (Fillauer/Motion Control), or the Ergo and Dynamic Arm (Ottobock).

Bilateral Shoulder Disarticulation

Complete, bilateral upper limb absence in children is primarily seen in those individuals who have congenital deficiencies, whereas if this were not present at birth, it would most likely have been a result of an electrical injury.[2,18,25] It has been well documented that prosthetic use is quite challenging for these children (and adults). If available, at a young age these children with bilateral shoulder disarticulation should be trained to use other parts of their anatomy (such as feet and legs) for grasping and manipulating objects. Individuals may be quite successful at using their feet like hands and can develop excellent coordination and dexterity. Prostheses fittings in these children may be attempted but are frequently unsuccessful because the benefits often do not outweigh the drawbacks.[26]

SUMMARY

Successful fitting of upper limb prostheses for pediatric patients involves a team effort, with the child and family at the core of this team. All team members need to be educated on the pros and cons of prosthetic fitting, functional benefits and limitations of available devices, and appropriate control schemes and training. Infants will often use their prostheses for very different functions than toddlers, school-age children, and young teens. The level of limb absence or amputation has a great influence on the use of prostheses. As in all prosthetic fittings, the shorter the residual limb and the higher the level of the limb difference or amputation, the more challenging is fitting, achievement of good functional outcomes, and prosthesis acceptance. Additionally, the child may choose to use, or not use the prosthesis throughout their growing years and adulthood. This cyclic prosthesis acceptance and rejection needs to be appreciated and supported, with the child and family provided assurance that they are always welcome to revisit prosthetic fitting at any time.

References

1. Supan T: Prosthetic and orthotic management, in Bowker JH, Michael JW, eds: *Atlas of Limb Prosthetics: Surgical, Prosthetic, and Rehabilitation Principles,* ed 2. Mosby Year Book, 1992, pp 761-766.
2. Clark MW, Atkins DJ, Hubbard SA, Patton JG, Shaperman J: Prosthetic devices for children with bilateral upper limb deficiencies: When and if, pros and cons, in Herring JA, Birch JG, eds: *The Child With a Limb Deficiency.* American Academy of Orthopaedic Surgeons, 1998, pp 397-403.
3. Patton J: Prosthetic components for children and teenagers, in Meier R, Atkins D, eds: *Comprehensive Management of the Upper-Limb Amputee.* Springer-Verlag, 1989, pp 99-120.
4. Sauter W: Electric pediatric and adult prosthetic components, in Meier R, Atkins D, eds: *Comprehensive Management of the Upper-Limb Amputee.* Springer-Verlag, 1989, pp 121-136.
5. Brenner C: Electric limbs for infants and pre-school children. *J Prosthet Orthot* 1992;4:184-190.
6. Schuch CM: Prosthetic principles in fitting myoelectric prostheses in children, in Herring JA, Birch JG, eds: *The Child With a Limb Deficiency.* American Academy of Orthopaedic Surgeons, 1998, pp 405-416.
7. Hubbard SA, Kurtz I, Heim W, Montgomery G: Powered prosthetic intervention in upper extremity deficiency, in Herring JA, Birch JG, eds: *The Child With a Limb Deficiency.* American Academy of Orthopaedic Surgeons, 1998, pp 417-431.
8. James MA, Bagley AM, Brasington K, Lutz C, McConnell S, Molitor F: Impact of prostheses on function and quality of life for children with unilateral congenital below-the-elbow deficiency. *J Bone Joint Surg Am* 2006;88(11):2356-2365.
9. Wagner L, Bagley A, James M: Reasons for prosthetic rejection by children with unilateral congenital forearm total deficiency. *J Prosthet Orthot* 2007;19(2):51-54.
10. Davids JR, Wagner LV, Meyer LC, Blackhurst DW: Prosthetic management of children with unilateral congenital below-elbow deficiency. *J Bone Joint Surg Am* 2006;88(6):1294-1300.
11. Wright FV, Hubbard S, Naumann S, Jutai J: Evaluation of the validity of the prosthetic upper extremity functional index for children. *Arch Phys Med Rehabil* 2003;84(4):518-527.
12. Lerman JA, Sullivan E, Barnes DA, Haynes RJ: The Pediatric Outcomes Data Collection Instrument (PODCI) and functional assessment of patients with unilateral upper extremity deficiencies. *J Pediatr Orthop* 2005;25(3):405-407.
13. Patton J: Training the child with a unilateral upper-extremity prosthesis, in Meier R, Atkins D, eds: *Functional Restoration of Adults and Children With Upper Extremity Amputation.* Demos Medical Publishing, 2004, pp 297-315.
14. Gaebler-Spira D, Lipschutz R: *Pediatric Limb Deficiencies in Pediatric Rehabilitation,* ed 4. Demos Medical Publishing, 2010, pp 334-360.
15. Blakeslee B: *The Limb-Deficient Child.* University of California Press, 1963.
16. Frantz C, O Rahilly R: Congenital skeletal limb deficiencies. *J Bone Joint Surg Am* 1961;43(8):1202-1224.
17. Schuch M, Pritham C: International Standards Organization terminology: Application to prosthetics and orthotics. *J Prosthet Orthot* 1994;4:29-33.
18. Patton J: Developmental approach to pediatric prosthetic evaluation and training, in Meier R, Atkins D, eds: *Comprehensive Management of the Upper-Limb Amputee.* Springer-Verlag, 1989, pp 137-149.
19. Mahoney L, Frankovitch K: Use of opposition posts in children. *J Assoc Child Prosthet Orthot Clin* 1991;26(1):33.
20. Fairley M, Williams TWIII: The O&P EDGE. 2013. Available at: http://www.oandp.com/articles/2013-03_09.asp. Accessed November 5, 2015.
21. Bernstein RM, Watts HG, Setoguchi Y: The lengthening of short upper extremity amputation stumps. *J Pediatr Orthop* 2008;28(1):86-90.
22. Smit G, Bongers RM, Van der Sluis CK, Plettenburg DH: Efficiency of voluntary opening hand and hook prosthetic devices: 24 years of development? *J Rehabil Res Dev* 2012;49(4):523-534.
23. Trost F, Rowe D: Externally powered prostheses, in Bowker JH, Michael JW, eds: *Atlas of Limb Prosthetics: Surgical, Prosthetic, and Rehabilitation Principles,* ed 2. Mosby Year Book, 1992, pp 767-778.
24. McClure SK, Shaughnessy WJ: Farm-related limb amputations in children. *J Pediatr Orthop* 2005;25(2):133-137.
25. Friedman L: Functional skills in multiple limb anomalies, in Meier R, Atkins D, eds: *Comprehensive Management of the Upper-Limb Amputee.* Springer-Verlag, 1989, pp 150-164.
26. Setoguchi Y, Patton J, Shida-Tokeshi J: Pediatric case studies of upper extremity limb deficiencies, in Meier R, Atkins D, eds: *Functional Restoration of Adults and Children With Upper Extremity Amputation.* Demos Medical Publishing, 2004, pp 322-324.

Pediatric Physical Therapy

CHAPTER 70

Colleen P. Coulter, PT, DPT, PhD, PCS • Jill Cannoy, PT, DPT

ABSTRACT

Children with congenital and acquired limb deficiencies receive the best quality care when a multidisciplinary team specializing in pediatrics evaluates the child, provides appropriate interventions, and recognizes the challenges in working with this patient cohort. Using knowledge of growth, sensorimotor and cognitive development, and orthopaedics, pediatric physical therapists play an integral role in the team treating children with limb loss and limb differences. The physical therapist often serves as a liaison between the family and other team members and promotes family-centered care that focuses on the child's function and participation in the home and the community.

Keywords: congenital; limb deficiency; limb loss; pediatric; physical therapy

Introduction

The World Health Organization (WHO) recognizes that children experience rapid growth and substantial changes in physical, social, and psychological development during their first 2 decades of life, and that a child's development depends on and is influenced by factors in the child's environment as well as the wishes, beliefs, and actions of parents and caregivers.[1] In addition, children experience the intensity and effects of disability and health-related conditions differently from adults.[1] The Children and Youth Version of the World Health Organization's International Classification of Functioning, Disability and Health (ICF-CY) uses terminology that classifies these challenges and problems in the following areas: body structures and function, activity limitations, and participation. Healthcare clinicians use the ICF-CY framework and terminology to document and measure health-related issues and design interventions for their young patients that include both the child and their family.

Within the construct of the ICF-CY, surgeons, orthotists, prosthetists, and therapists that treat children are very aware of and confident with identifying, measuring, and treating impairments of body structure and function, such as limb differences, the physiologic effects of trauma and disease, limitations to joint range of motion, vital signs, and pain. Although such limitations of body structures and function need to be addressed, these are best accomplished with goals that consider and optimize a child's developmental age, function, and family's beliefs and wishes, and engage the child within their family, school, and community environments. The ultimate goal of pediatric rehabilitation is for children to participate in activities with their families and within their schools and communities.

Children with limb loss and limb differences have benefited from increased societal awareness and acceptance of individuals with limb loss. Commonly featured in social media and TV advertisements are stories of wounded warriors, Paralympic athletes, and children who wear prostheses. An unfortunate consequence of war has been the increased number of wounded soldiers who are seeking rehabilitation and prostheses that enable them to resume function beyond what was previously imagined. Similarly, children with amputations and limb differences continue to challenge their capabilities by participating in camps, school and community events, and competing in sports with their peers.

Manufacturers have assisted in meeting these demands by developing various pediatric prosthetic components, such as running feet for children[2,3] and adaptive feet for rock wall climbing and cycling.[4] In addition, developments in pediatric suspension systems now allow children to wear prostheses without the need for suspension belts. However, a persistent major gap remains in the development of pediatric prosthetic knee technology that will keep up with the ever-growing demands and wear and tear placed on prosthetic components during a child's everyday activities and play.

Dr. Coulter or an immediate family member serves as a board member, owner, officer, or committee member of Association of Children's Prosthetic and Orthotic Clinics. Neither Dr. Cannoy nor any immediate family member has received anything of value from or has stock or stock options held in a commercial company or institution related directly or indirectly to the subject of this chapter.

By providing surgical options besides amputation, advances in surgical reconstruction and limb salvage techniques continue to influence the decisions of families of children in whom bone tumors are diagnosed.[5,6] Even children diagnosed with congenital longitudinal deficiencies of the femur, tibia, and fibula are benefiting from these surgical innovations.[7,8] Physical therapists and prosthetists should be aware of these advances to fully understand the options available to each family as they make difficult decisions for their patients.

In pediatric patients with acquired limb loss, the physical therapist's role is well defined. The primary goal is to restore both children and adolescents to the function they possessed before the trauma or surgery that precipitated the amputation. This restoration is initially done through wound care, edema control, shaping of the residual limb, preserving range of motion, and strengthening and functional exercises.

For children with congenital limb loss, the physical therapy goals and management strategies are different. These children naturally develop abilities to perform age-appropriate activities by incorporating the impaired limbs into their movement stratgies.[9,10] Because children with congenital limb loss do not know any differently, learning to move with a deficient limb is normal for them as they automatically integrate their affected limbs into their motor, sensory, and cognitive development. Regardless of the type of deficiency, the size, shape, strength, and flexibility of the deficient limb provides both sensory and motor input that guides the child's motor development. Even infants and toddlers with moderate to severe lower limb deformities will attempt to pull to stand and cruise if they have intact neurologic development. Accordingly, the physical therapist needs to be knowledgeable in all areas of gross motor, fine motor, and cognitive development and be able to anticipate the limitations that may be caused by a limb deficiency.[9,10] The physical therapist should also be aware of current pediatric prosthetic technologies and surgical options available for the different classifications of limb deficiencies.

In children with congenital limb deficiencies, the physical therapist often acts as an advocate, teacher, and mentor to the child and their family, anticipating immediate and future functional challenges. In centers specializing in pediatric limb deficiencies, the physical therapist frequently acts as a liaison between the family and other team members, empowering the parents to be the primary providers of care and promoting family-centered care.[9]

Early and ongoing education is imperative to educate and empower the child and family about possible surgical, prosthetic, and therapy options. Regardless of whether the child is born with a limb difference or sustained a limb loss resulting from illness or trauma, education is crucial for understanding of the child's condition and available treatment options. Many factors determine the education provided to child and family that include: the severity of the child's limb deficiency; associated medical and/or neurologic impairments, involvement of multiple limbs; the child's age; and the family's beliefs and wishes. The distance the family lives from the center and their ability to actively participate in their child's care will further influence the amount of clinical interaction.

Home programs are necessary for optimal surgical, prosthetic, and rehabilitation outcomes and to enable the parents and family to assist in the child's care. Videotaping therapy sessions is an excellent teaching tool for both parents and community-based physical therapists involved in the treatment of a child. Digital photography makes it easier to personalize therapy sessions, and document progress. Web-based commercially available exercise programs are also excellent resources for home programs, some of which include specialized sections addressing rehabilitation for individuals with amputations.[11] Exercise manuals can be modified to provide age-appropriate activities for infants and young children with limb loss and limb differences.[12,13]

Postoperative Considerations

Postoperative care for children who have amputations whether to address a congenital limb deficiency, or because of sarcoma, illness, vascular condition, or trauma, is similar to that of adults.[14] When appropriate and depending on the center's protocols, postop care should begin with wound care, swelling/edema control, shaping of the residual limb, bed mobility, transfers, mobility training, range of motion, strengthening, home exercise program, and parent education that addresses the above interventions.[14] Swelling is common with both acquired and elective amputations. Edema control begins with postoperative dressings and continues with elastic bandage wraps and shrinkers after the wound is adequately healed. Properly applied dressings may control postoperative edema and facilitate prosthetic fitting.[9,10,14] The type of postoperative dressing is determined by the surgeon based on surgical procedure, the age and activity level of the child, with additional variables, such as the distance of the child's residence from the treatment center and parental preferences taken into consideration. After the wound is healed, edema control remains important. The principles for compression in infants and children with an amputation are approximately the same as those for adults.[10,14] However, most children are too small for commercially available over-the-counter prosthetic shrinkers, necessitating the use of small elastic bandages and custom shrinker socks sewn with various sizes of soft elastic tubular bandages. Frequently used are strips of tape to secure the shape of the elastic bandage as it is being wrapped and extending the wrap around proximal structures to provide greater stabilization for security because of the child's increased activity during the postoperative period (**Figure 1**). Detailed written instructions and videos of the techniques of applying elastic compression, elastic wrapping or stockings, should be provided to parents and caregivers.

Children who have a rotationplasty require a unique wrapping technique to control edema and shape the limb

Chapter 70: Pediatric Physical Therapy

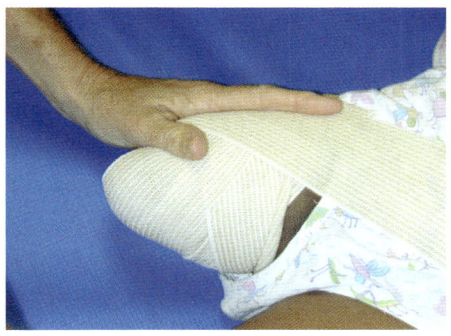

FIGURE 1 Clinical photograph of elastic wrapping of the residual limb of an 8-year-old child with a short transfemoral amputation after revision for femoral overgrowth. The elastic bandage is wrapped around the waist for stabilization and high on the adductor area to control edema proximally.

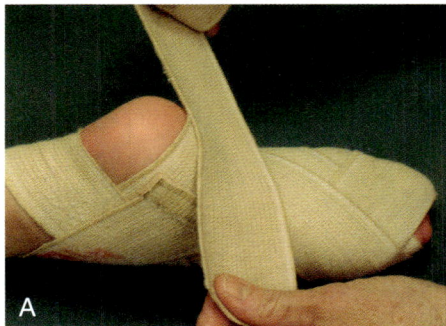 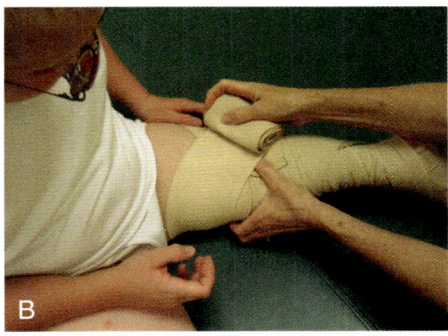

FIGURE 2 Clinical photographs of elastic bandage wrapping techniques for a 12-year-old boy after rotationplasty. **A**, The foot and ankle are wrapped, including the toes. **B**, The elastic bandage extends up the limb in a figure-of-8 pattern and includes the proximal thigh. An additional elastic bandage is necessary to continue around the waist for stabilization of the wrap and for edema control proximally.

proximally (**Figure 2**). Typically, substantial swelling occurs in the foot, ankle, and calf areas as well as above and below the surgical incision. The foot is wrapped, incorporating the toes and ankle separately as is done for an acute ankle sprain.[15] The wrapping continues up the limb in a figure-of-8 configuration, extending beyond the surgical site proximally and, if possible, around the waist to secure the wrapping. Control of proximal swelling that typically occurs after a rotationplasty is managed by using custom-sewn tights from elastic tubular stockings, compression shorts, and, even, support stockings. The amount of compression should allow an adequate degree of wound healing and should take into consideration the child's tolerance to pressure.

Physical Therapy Treatments

Range-of-motion, strengthening, mobility, gait training, and functional activities depend on a child's age, medical and neurologic condition, motivation, and interests, as well as the family's ability to assist in the child's care. The following factors should be considered when developing therapy goals and home programs: (1) every child is unique and develops at their own rate; (2) a child with multiple limb loss has special needs, and treatment interventions must be prioritized; (3) the environment needs to be adapted to the child for maximal function; (4) the child with a limb deficiency may have associated medical, neurologic, or orthopaedic impairments that will influence function and intervention; and (5) surgical amputations and revisions may take place at different developmental ages, so treatment should be centered on age-appropriate functions.[9,10] General expectations and limitations associated with common congenital lower limb deficiencies are listed in **Table 1**.

Early intervention is important to provide optimal outcomes and prevent the development of secondary disabilities. Family-centered services provide for maximal intervention.[9,10] Exercise programs should be created with the parents' input, taking into account their ability to perform the recommended interventions. Goals should be age-appropriate, functionally based, and within the limits of the degree of the limb deficiency or amputation level(s). With positive parental input, the child is likely to develop and grow with their peers and achieve all that they dream possible.

Infants (Birth to <12 Months)

When a child is born with a limb deficiency, where available, a referral should be made to a limb deficiency center that specializes in the management of congenital limb differences.[10,16-18] At the center, the family meets with the physician and other team members to identify the infant's strengths and briefly outline possible future surgical, prosthetic, and therapeutic strategies that address the infant's physical impairments. Intervention should focus on assisting the infant to achieve motor and cognitive milestones in the context of their physical limitations.[9]

Families often come to their first clinic visit with a multitude of questions and fears about their child's future and severity of the limb deficiency. Information is often gathered from many sources, including well-meaning family and friends plus Internet medical web sites and social media, such as Facebook groups, each having varying opinions about the infant's care. The physical therapist can help and, if needed, redirect the family's understanding of their child's condition by using dolls with differing levels of amputations, videos, and photographs of children with similar limb differences, and samples of prostheses appropriate for the child. All are useful teaching tools for parents and can ease their anxiety and fears concerning the surgical, prosthetic, and therapeutic management of their child. The relationships between the specialized medical team including the physical therapist and the family begins at this point.

Introducing the family to other families with children who have similar limb differences is one of the most powerful interventions.[9,10,16] The effects of family networking are lasting and help ease parental fears and concerns for their child's future. However, the therapist should monitor and decipher information given to parents

TABLE 1 Lower Limb Functional Outcomes and Special Considerations in Children With Lower Limb Deficiencies

Deficiency	Outcomes and Considerations
Unilateral Syme disarticulation	No limitations are expected in daily activities. Able to participate in age-appropriate activities and sports, such as bicycling, skiing, dancing, and gymnastics. Assistive devices are not required.
Unilateral transtibial level	No limitations are expected in age-appropriate daily activities. Able to participate in age-appropriate sports and activities, such as bicycling, skiing, dancing, and gymnastics. Assistive devices are not required.
Bilateral transtibial level	Limitations may occur on uneven surfaces, curbs, and stairs. Participates in age-appropriate sports with limitations. May require adaptive physical education or wheelchair for sports. Rides a bicycle with adaptations. Assistive devices are not required for ambulation. Uses a wheelchair as backup.
Unilateral knee disarticulation or transfemoral amputation level	May have limitations in age-appropriate daily activities. Requires adaptation to ride a bicycle; may ride without prosthesis. Able to participate in sports; adaptations may be required. Assistive devices are not required; uses crutches or wheelchair as backup.
Bilateral knee disarticulation or transfemoral level	Limitations expected ascending and descending stairs with possible challenges on uneven surfaces and curbs. Encounters difficulty riding a bicycle; needs adaptations. Adaptive physical education is required. Uses a wheelchair for sports and as backup for mobility. Has limitations in sports and age-appropriate activities. May require assistive devices, although most do not.
Unilateral hip disarticulation	Limitations are expected on uneven surfaces, curbs, and steps. (Children with congenital deficiencies are quite functional; children with acquired loss have more difficulties.) Bicycling is difficult with prosthesis; may ride without prosthesis. Has limitations in running and sports; requires adaptations in sports. Uses a wheelchair for sports and as backup for mobility. May use crutches or cane for moderate to longer distances. May use crutches and no prosthesis.
Bilateral hip disarticulation	Wheelchair is used for primary mobility; power mobility may be necessary if associated upper limb involvement. Prosthesis use is for standing, exercise, and short-distance mobility. Requires assistive devices. Uses a wheelchair for sports.

Multiple limb loss, medical conditions, trauma, and neurologic impairments may influence the functional outcomes.

Adapted with permission from Coulter O'Berry C: Physical therapy management in children with lower extremity limb deficiencies, in Herring JA, Birch JG, eds: *The Child With a Limb Deficiency.* American Academy of Orthopaedic Surgeons, 1998, pp 319-330.

because not every parent is ready for all the information at the first visit. Too much initial information may increase parental anxiety and fosters fears that may focus on disabilities rather than abilities.

An infant with a congenital limb deficiency will benefit greatly from early intervention. According to the American Physical Therapy Association, early intervention is based on six important principles: (1) the rapid growth and development in the first years of life provide the foundation for later development; (2) infants can actively interact, form attachments, and are capable of learning; (3) parents are the main providers of care and early learning experiences; (4) parents of children with special needs may require assistance or instruction in caring for their children; (5) the interaction between the biologic insult and environmental factors influences the developmental outcome; and (6) structured programming may improve the abilities of infants and young children.[19]

Intervention should begin by evaluating the infant's gross and fine motor development to establish baseline records for the range of motion, strength, neurologic function, and movement patterns. In addition, the infant's ongoing motor development should be monitored regularly as he or she grows and learns to roll, sit, pull to stand, and walk.[10] These assessments should include any changes to range of motion, functional strength, weight bearing, and symmetry of both posture and movement.

Among infants with congenital limb deficiencies, asymmetry of movement is common. When asymmetry is present, parents and caregivers can be taught exercises for positioning, handling, and play, so that they foster symmetric movements as the infant develops. Parents are encouraged to move their infants to both sides and not be afraid of increasing the deformity or injury to the involved limb. They are taught to help the infant roll and transition into and out of sitting, kneeling, and standing equally to both sides. Symmetry and balance of movements during early motor activities are precursors to weight shifting in standing, cruising, and walking.[5-10]

In infants with congenital limb deficiencies or acquired limb amputations, range-of-motion exercises are designed to minimize the development of contractures and prepare the limb for future prosthetic fitting and function. With certain levels of limb deficiency, characteristic contractures and deformities are present. For example, longitudinal deficiencies of the tibia and the fibula are commonly associated with anomalies of the foot and ankle. These deficiencies may affect surgical, prosthetic, and orthotic management and hinder gross motor development. For example, a contracture of the foot may impact future options of a rotationplasty or limb lengthening in an infant with a proximal femoral focal deficiency (PFFD) with associated partial longitudinal deficiency of the fibula.

Similarly, hip flexion, abduction, and external rotation contractures are anticipated in infants with PFFD and those with short transfemoral limb loss.[16,20] Instruction should be provided regarding both positioning and range-of-motion exercises. Early prosthetic fittings can be considered if the loss is unilateral. Parents and caregivers can be taught how to maintain mobility at the hips, knees, and ankles during simple caregiving activities such as diapering, picking up the infant, dressing, feeding, and play.[9,10,16] Parents should be instructed in range-of-motion and positioning exercises.[9,10] Hip and knee flexion contractures are common in infants who are born with short residual limb segments of the femur and tibia, respectively, as well as resulting from constrictive amniotic bands or a traumatic amputation.[9,10] Prosthetic fittings have been used to manage knee flexion tightness in an infant as young as 6 months who was born with a very short unilateral transtibial amputation.[9,10]

Prosthetic fitting is recommended after the infant begins to pull to stand, typically at approximately age 8 to 12 months.[16,17,21,22] During this period, infants with longitudinal tibial and fibular deficiencies often have undergone elective amputations and are ready for the initiation of prosthetic fittings. Postoperative wound care, edema control, limb protection, and range-of-motion exercises constitute the important physical therapy interventions at this stage. The benefits of early fittings are threefold: (1) flexion contractures are minimized; (2) symmetric weight bearing may be achieved for early, age-appropriate crawling, kneeling, and standing activities; and (3) the infant receives early sensory and proprioceptive feedback that truly prepares them for more functional prosthetic fittings at later developmental stages. An added benefit is that parents are involved early in the management of their child's care.[9,10,23] To maximize the benefits of a more anatomic prosthesis as the infant grows, it is recommended that the infant who would benefit from early prosthetic fitting have regular physical therapy to work on transitions and activities that are preparatory for crawling, standing, and walking.

Matching an infant's function with available prosthetic components allows the infant to parallel normal development. Infants with knee disarticulation and transfemoral amputation levels have demonstrated the ability to control a prosthetic knee and incorporate knee functions in early developmental activities, such as creeping and crawling, pulling to stand, half kneeling, and tall kneeling play[23-26] (**Figure 3**). Even infants with PFFD have demonstrated the ability to control prosthetic knee function in an unconventional prosthetic fitting with a short prosthetic tibial section using a hinged knee or an internal knee, depending on the length of the limb segments[23-26] (**Figure 4**). Prosthetic alignment should consider the developmental activities of the infant and may need to be modified frequently as the infant develops and motor skills mature. The physical therapist and the prosthetist should work closely together to address alignment issues for the infant.

Infants born with multiple limb deficiencies with or without neurologic and medical involvement will require frequent therapeutic interventions and may take longer to acquire motor skills. Intervention should begin as soon as possible, focusing on all developmental parameters. Where available, referral to early intervention services is important as well as monthly monitoring by the limb deficiency team to update home programs and record changes in development, range of motion, and strength[9,10,16,19,27] (**Figure 5**).

Toddlers (12 to <36 Months)

By the first year, the toddler should be pulling to stand and, if appropriate, wearing a definitive prosthesis. Surgical intervention may be necessary at this age to correct deformities or perform a primary elective amputation. When surgeries are performed, postoperative management remains imperative for optimal prosthetic fit and function. When the toddler is ready for prosthetic fitting, instructions are given for donning and doffing, skin care, and

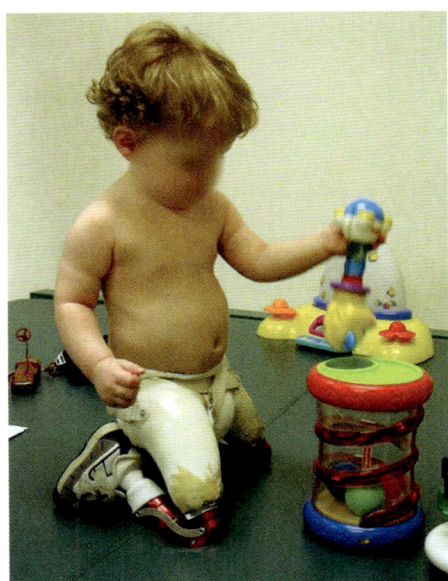

FIGURE 3 Clinical photograph of a 16-month-old child with congenital bilateral longitudinal deficiencies playing in a kneeling position. Knee disarticulations were performed at age 9 months, with prosthetic fitting at age 11 months. This child crawls, pulls to stand, cruises, and pushes a walker. The prostheses are not finished cosmetically because of the need for frequent alignment changes as the child develops.

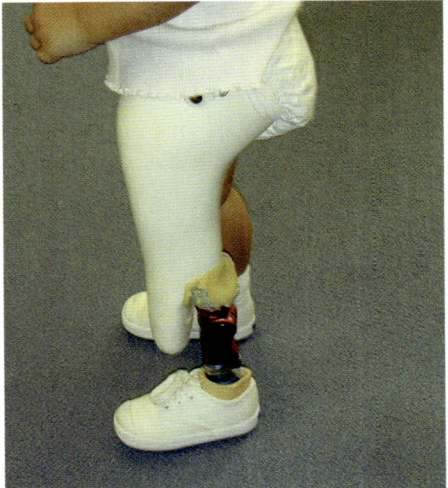

FIGURE 4 Clinical photograph of an 18-month-old child with a proximal femoral focal deficiency (PFFD) fitted in a traditional high proximal socket for containment of the hip because of the PFFD. A knee unit is placed distally. Although there is a short tibial segment, the knee is used appropriately in gait and all functional developmental activities.

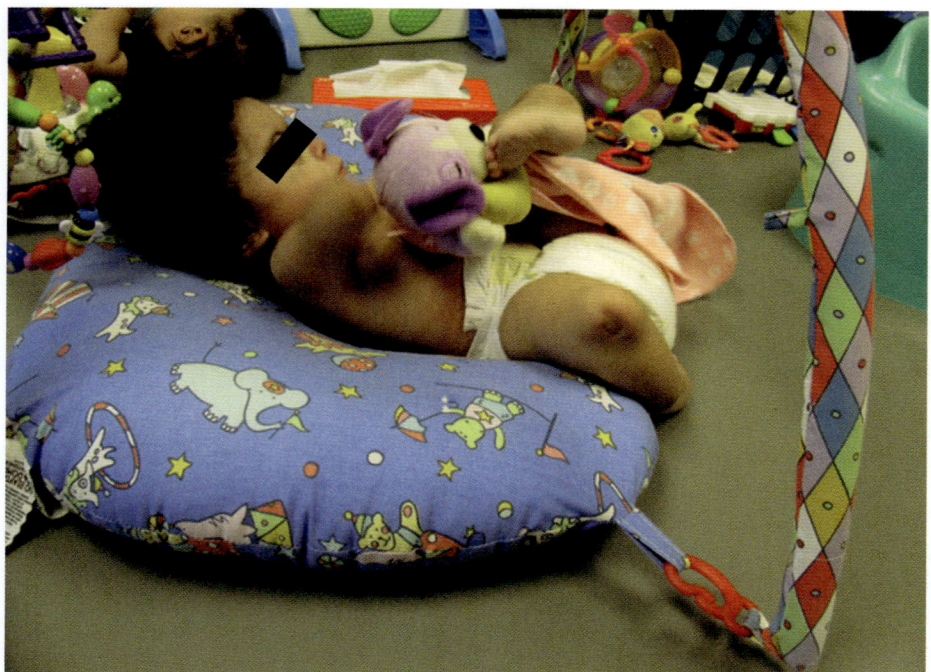

FIGURE 5 Clinical photograph of a 15-month old toddler diagnosed with Cornelia de Lange syndrome. The child has longitudinal deficiencies of the upper and lower extremities as well as visual, cardiac, and gastrointestinal impairments. The physical therapist is working with the mother on positions for ways to adapt placement of toys so the child can reach and explore toys and objects. This child can also use his feet to play when placed in sidelying.

wearing of the prosthesis. It is common for infants and young children with knee disarticulations or higher levels of amputations to reject their prostheses. Initially, the prosthesis interferes with mobility and hinders overall movements, such that toddlers are more mobile in crawling and creeping activities without it. It is not until the toddler spends more time in standing and cruising activities that the prosthesis is readily accepted. The use of articulating knees in infants and toddlers has decreased some of these frustrations, allowing more normal gross motor functions by providing freedom and symmetry in patterns of movement through the actions offered by the prosthetic knee.[28] Studies in which toddlers with at or above the knee levels of limb loss fit with prosthetic knees in their first prosthesis were observed in developmental play activities documented prosthetic knee flexion and extension during climbing up and sliding down a small slide, squatting in play, balancing in half kneel and kneeling, transitioning up to stand, and playing on the floor[23-26] (**Figure 6**). The studies concluded that prosthetic knee functions in these young toddlers precluded knee function in walking but rather aided in the subject's ability to play in sitting and kneeling leading into transitions for standing and walking. In 2020, Geil et al published the results of a multisite study that examined kinematic outcomes during walking in three separate groups of young children. Subjects in group 1 were fit with an early knee (EK) protocol, group 2 had a traditional protocol without a prosthetic knee (TK), and the third group were children without lower limb amputations.[29] Children in the two prosthetic groups had unilateral limb loss and had been treated either at one site with the TK protocol or at another with the EK protocol. Children in the EK group achieved swing phase prosthetic knee flexion averaging 59.8° ± 8.4°. Children wearing prosthetic limbs walked slower than age-matched peers. In most instances, walking speed and step length increased with age in the EK group, similar to the control group. However, this trend was not observed in the TK group. Clearance adaptations were present in both limb loss groups. Observed adaptations were twice as prevalent in the TK group versus the EK group; however, the groups differed in age and etiology. Children with limb loss provided with an articulating knee component in their first prosthesis incorporated knee flexion during swing phase and showed fewer gait adaptations than children in the TK protocol.[29]

A therapy program for a toddler at the prewalking and early walking stages should stress symmetry of posture and movement as well as control of weight shifting over the prosthesis.[9,10] Developmental screening and assessment tools can be used for examples of age-appropriate activities and assist in forming home programs.[9,10,30-32] Exercises should be fun and incorporated into a toddler's everyday play. Push toys and walkers are adjuncts to treatment. Most toddlers with single limb deficiencies do not require special assistive devices, but adaptations may be necessary to assist in ambulation for those with multiple limb loss.

Preschool and Young Childhood Years (36 Months to <6 Years)

As the child begins walking with the prosthesis, treatment again focuses on age-appropriate activities. Activities such as marching to music, climbing on small gym equipment, and riding a tricycle are excellent gross motor activities. Home exercise programs still include range of motion to prevent the progression of contractures.

The frequency of therapy visits at this stage will depend on the child's mastery of walking, the child's age-appropriate function, and the family's ability to follow through with home exercise programs. The physical therapist should monitor the child's development during clinic or prosthetic visits approximately every 4 to 6 months and make recommendations for changes of prosthetic components that parallel the child's motor development.[30-32] The prosthesis should be closely monitored for appropriate fit and function as the child grows. Prosthetic feet with

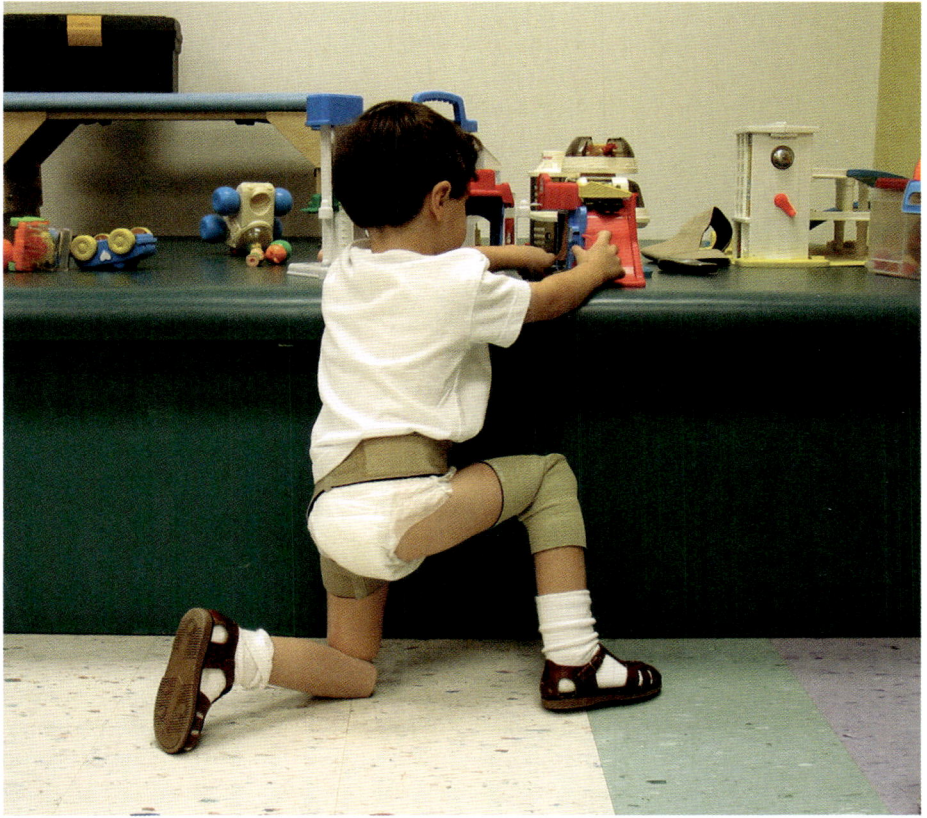

FIGURE 6 Clinical photograph of a 2-year-old child with congenital bilateral tibial deficiencies playing in a half-kneeling position. Note the knee disarticulation level on the left side and the Syme ankle disarticulation level on the right side. This child was fitted with an articulating knee unit at age 11 months. He was walking independently by age 15 months.

dynamic-response keels as well as those that enable adaptability to uneven terrain continue to become available in smaller and smaller sizes and may be indicated at this stage if available.

Physical therapy can take place at the child's preschool or home and can be an effective means of educating the child's teachers, classmates, and other family members. Preschool staff will be less apprehensive about having a child with special needs if they are well informed and taught strategies on managing the prosthesis and adapting the environment as needed. Toilet training is a major obstacle at this age for children with transfemoral or knee disarticulation prostheses. Typically, belts are required for suspension, making it difficult to pull pants up and down. Therapy can address this issue as well as dressing at home and in school.

In addition, certain surgical interventions, such as a Van Nes rotationplasty for the child with PFFD, may be performed this age. After each surgery, wound healing, edema control, pressure wrapping, and range-of-motion and functional strengthening exercises are implemented. The child may require additional physical therapy postoperatively until independent function is restored.

Elementary Years (6 to 12 Years)

Initial amputations secondary to trauma or bone tumors commonly occur from 6 to 12 years of age.[5,6] In addition, children with congenital limb deficiencies may undergo surgical revisions for overgrowth or to correct developing deformities. At this age, if available, children may receive technologically advanced prosthetic components that will require additional gait training and balance exercises.[10,26]

If possible, gait training should begin with the aid of parallel bars, teaching the child how to operate the prosthetic components, such as flexing and extending the prosthetic knee and learning how to sit, stand, and squat. Multidirectional weight shifts and stepping patterns progressing to walking on level surfaces with or without assistive devices should be instructed.

At approximately 7 years of age, the child's gait parallels that of an adult.[33] The child is able to participate actively in an exercise program and is less dependent on their parents. After the child is walking and the prosthesis is fitting well, outpatient physical therapy should change focus to encourage participation in community and school recreational and sports activities. Specialty sports medicine physical therapy may be appropriate. It is important to remember that exercises and activities should be age appropriate and meaningful for the child and family. If possible, the physical therapist from the limb deficiency center should visit the child's school as a way of educating teachers, school therapists, and classmates about the child's limb difference and prosthesis. Again, instruction and exercises should focus on age-appropriate activities, sports, and recreation.

Rotationplasty

Rehabilitation of the child with a rotationplasty is both challenging and rewarding. Children who have a rotationplasty from trauma or bone tumors with no associated hip pathology have gait patterns similar to those with transtibial function.[34] Children who have had rotationplasty as the treatment of PFFD may have challenges relating to hip instability, as well as physiologic derotation that may be addressed either surgically or with prosthetic fitting.[20,35] These conditions can influence the gait pattern of the child. Regardless of the underlying etiology, range-of-motion and strengthening exercises of the hip, ankle, foot, and toes are imperative. Immediate postoperative management typically includes 6 to 8 weeks of restricted weight bearing, with instruction in isometric, active, and active-assisted hip, ankle, and foot range-of-motion exercises. Because the child attends frequent physical therapy for postoperative care, the physical therapist may be asked to monitor and assist the surgeon and family with wound care.[10]

As with the postoperative management of amputations and other reconstructive surgeries, edema control; limb shaping; range-of-motion exercises of the hip, foot, ankle, and toes; and isometric strengthening of the hip and ankle are initiated. The child's orthopaedic surgeon should guide the initiation and progression of active and active-assisted exercises, weight bearing, and overall activity requiring ongoing communication and updating the child's progress. Healing is different in every child, with delays in wound healing commonly observed in children receiving chemotherapy for the treatment of bone cancer. Although both flexibility and strength are imperative for optimal prosthetic knee function, gaining range of motion of the ankle, foot, and toes should precede strengthening. Ankle range of motion powers prosthetic knee function. Restrictions of ankle and foot active and passive range of motion will interfere with proper gait and, in some children, cause pressure marks, skin breakdown, pain, and foot and midfoot breakdown. In extreme situations, rupture of the Achilles tendon has occurred. Similarly, tightness of the plantar fascia will influence toe and foot function. Toes are excellent initiators of prosthetic knee motion and act to stabilize the foot inside the socket. Proper alignment of the anatomic ankle–foot complex and the prosthetic knee joints is necessary to optimize the foot's ability to flex and extend the prosthetic knee.[10]

Ankle dorsiflexion of 0° to 30° is adequate for prosthetic knee function. Optimal plantar flexion beyond 50° to 60° is desired.[9,10,34] The greater the available plantar flexion, the more streamlined is the relationship of the foot with the proximal segment, creating a larger excursion of prosthetic knee motion. Strength of the hip, ankle, foot, and toes leads to optimal prosthetic knee power after adequate range of motion is achieved. Exercises are necessary to facilitate ankle movements at speeds, excursions, and strengths common to knee function, using the foot's anatomy in an opposite orientation (**Figure 7**).

Limb Lengthening

Surgical management to address limb-length discrepancies of the femur, tibia, or fibula is typically initiated during the elementary years. Advances in surgical procedures and devices have provided options to address limb length discrepancies and deformities because of congenital limb differences, trauma, and bone tumors. The goal is to equalize limb lengths and deformity correction.[7,8] Limb reconstruction and lengthening procedures can be done as a single surgical procedure (osteotomy) or as a gradual process allowing the skin, fascia, muscles, and nerves to slowly increase in length together with the bones.[36] Lengthening and angular correction devices include expandable intramedullary nails, growing rods, and external fixators.[8] Angular deformities and limb length differences in either acquired or congenital deficiencies can be addressed through guided growth, complete or partial growth arrest epiphyseal (growth) plates or osteotomies. Limb reconstruction procedures can be staged across several years, requiring extensive physical therapy and guidance for the child and the family. Common goals for therapy include maintaining range of motion of the hip, knee, and ankle, strengthening the limb, weight bearing as prescribed by the surgeon, increasing endurance and overall conditioning, and restoring function and activity level during the lengthening process.[36-41] These children should be kept as active as possible, attending school and participating in recreational activities as permitted.

Adolescence (13 to 17 Years)

Malignant bone tumors are most common in the first and second decades of life.[5,6] Children and their families are faced with surgical options for limb salvage, amputation, or rotationplasty depending on the size, location, and characteristics of the tumor as well as the activity and functional levels of the child, taking into account cultural, psychological, and family issues.[5] Because physical therapists may play a role in educating the child and the family about the functional outcomes of each surgical procedure and the early and late effects of chemotherapy, therapists should be knowledgeable about these challenges.[42]

The child who undergoes a limb salvage procedure encounters numerous physical challenges. Physical therapy goals include regaining mobility and strength, progressive weight bearing, improving cardiovascular endurance, pain management, scar mobility, and independence in transfers.[10] Age-appropriate activities, which include activities of daily living, are incorporated in the exercise program. The therapist must always remember, however, that the primary goal for a child with a bone tumor is to survive the malignancy. The aggressive nature of these tumors and the morbidity associated with their treatment can substantially limit the goals of physical therapy. Each limb salvage procedure is unique, and therapy must be performed under the close direction of the orthopaedic surgeon.[40,42]

For a child who elects or requires an amputation for local control of a tumor, an immediate postoperative prosthesis may be used if appropriate. Postoperative physical therapy treatment includes edema control; wound healing; and range-of-motion, strengthening, and balance exercises necessary to prepare the child for prosthetic fit and function.[10]

Preadolescents and adolescents with congenital limb deficiencies may undergo surgical reconstructions and revisions to correct deformities and overgrowth in limbs that are less functional.[43] This is often the child's choice, based on potential improvements with regard to function and optimal prosthetic fitting. When necessary, the ongoing management of longitudinal deficiencies of the femur, tibia, and fibula may require a continuation of the limb-lengthening processes.

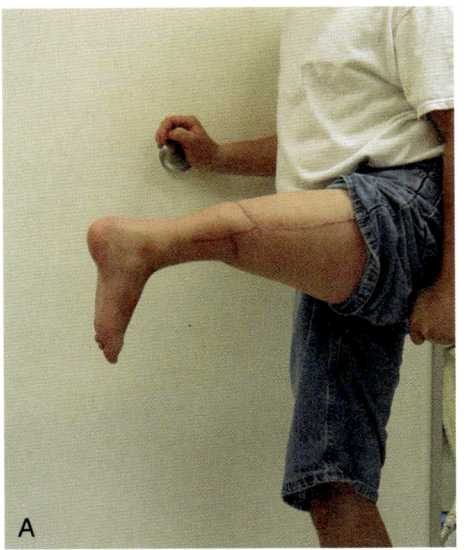 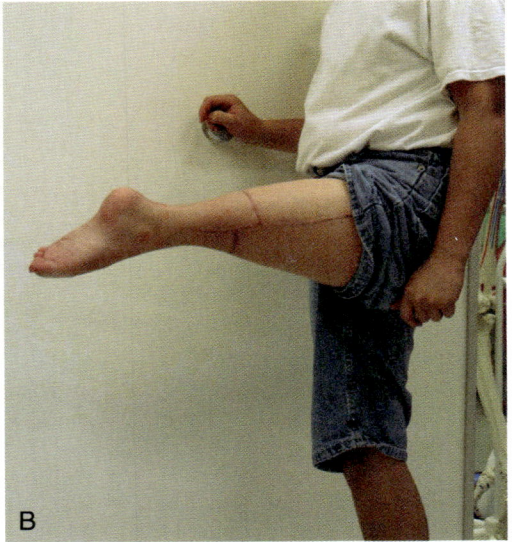 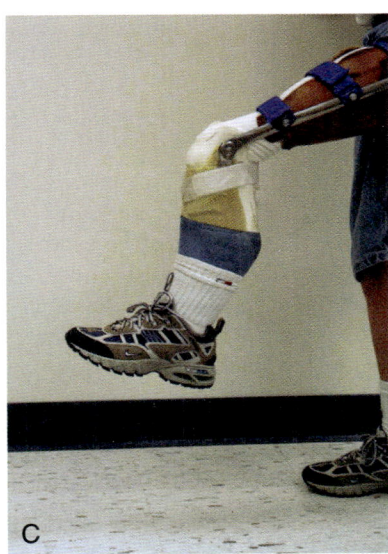

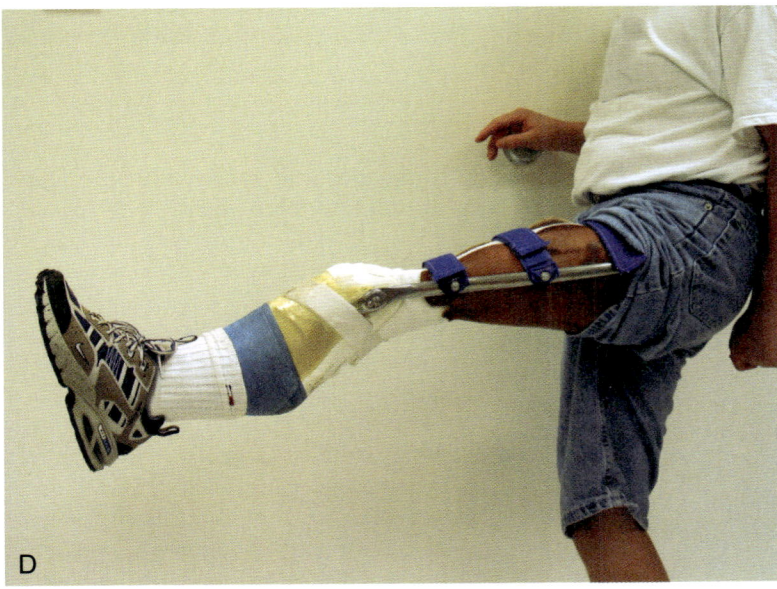

FIGURE 7 Clinical photographs of a 15-year-old boy who underwent a rotationplasty because of osteosarcoma using his foot and ankle to power a prosthetic knee 12 weeks after surgery. **A**, The foot in plantar flexion. **B**, The foot in dorsiflexion. **C** and **D**, The same foot and ankle positions with the boy wearing the prosthesis. The prosthesis is not cosmetically finished because of the need for frequent alignment changes to accommodate gains in plantar flexion and range of motion.

Phantom limb sensation is common in adolescents with acquired amputations resulting from trauma and tumors,[10,44] but is less frequent in those with congenital limb deficiencies after reconstructions or elective ablations. The phantom limb sensations and pain of adolescents can become intense. If left untreated, phantom limb sensations can become debilitating and interfere with prosthetic wear and daily activities. Referral to a pain management team may be beneficial. Physical therapy interventions of phantom limb sensation and pain may include: desensitization of the residual limb through massage, gentle rubbing, and taping, and compression; mirror therapy through the facilitation of an illusion of an unaffected limb;[45] and weight bearing when appropriate.[9] Targeted muscle reinnervation is now being used for pain management in adults and children following acquired amputations. Targeted muscle reinnervation is a surgical technique that reassigns severed motor nerves to proximal motor units of proximal muscles for muscle reinnervation and pain control during or following amputation.[46]

Learning to drive a car is a very age-appropriate activity for adolescents. The physical therapist should know of local resources to assess the adolescent's abilities and the need for adaptations and modifications to the car. Accessibility issues are more apparent as the adolescent prepares for college and independent living away from their family. Universities and colleges typically have a department dedicated to students with special needs and accessibility issues.[47]

Sports and Recreation

Children and adolescents of all ages with limb deficiencies with and without amputations and prostheses should be encouraged to participate in sports and recreational activities with their peers. The psychological effects of sports participation should be recognized.[48,49] Improving self-esteem and confidence; gaining independence; learning to compete, win, and lose; developing decision-making and problem-solving skills; and participating as a team member are a few of the benefits that individuals carry throughout their lives as they participate in recreational and competitive sport programs. Improvement in physical fitness; the development of balance, strength, coordination, and motor skills; increased endurance; and weight control also are benefits of physical activity.[9] Adaptive sports and recreational programs have developed throughout the United States for individuals with all types of physical impairments.

In the United States, laws have been enacted that require children and adolescents to be educated in the least restrictive environment. The Individuals with Disabilities Education Act provides free and appropriate education for children with disabilities.[10,19] Physical therapy and adaptive physical education in schools are included in this legislation. In addition, special adaptations and sports prostheses are available, depending on the degree and level of impairment. Advances in prosthetic technology are assisting people with amputations to compete in major sporting events at national and international levels.[48-50] The Challenged Athletes Foundation is an excellent resource for geographically located programs.[50] The Orthotic and Prosthetic Activities Foundation[51] provides financial and technologic assistance to individuals with physical disabilities who require orthotic and prosthetic services. Exposing children and adolescents to these opportunities and referring them to local sports and recreational programs is one of the most important roles of a therapist (Figure 8).

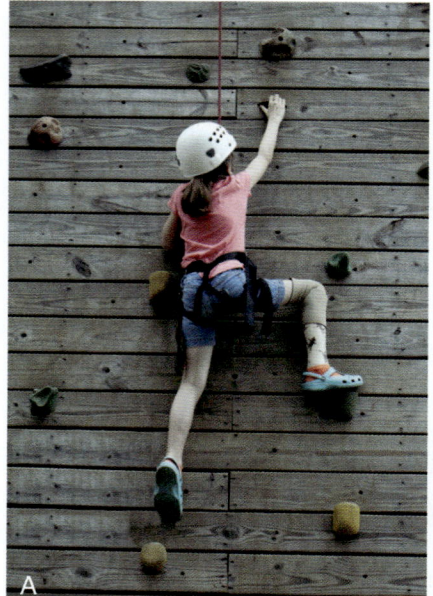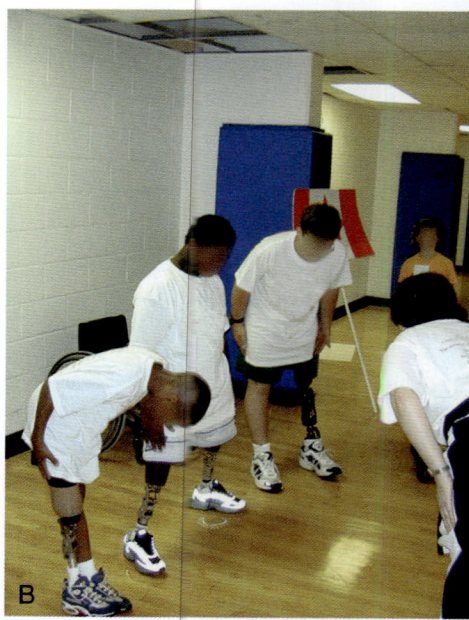

FIGURE 8 **A**, Photograph of an adaptive climbing program for children with physical challenges. **B**, Photograph of a karate class for children with limb deficiencies.

Multiple Limb Loss With and Without Neurologic Impairments

Infants, children, and adolescents with congenital or acquired multiple limb loss have special needs. They require more intensive and regular therapeutic interventions.[9,10,28] Typically, delays in development occur, the severity of which often depends on the degree of limb loss and other associated medical or neurologic impairments. Special mobility aids, wheelchairs, and adaptations to the environment may be necessary. Prioritization of surgical, prosthetic, and therapeutic interventions is required to meet the goals of both the child and the family. It is important not to overburden the child with multiple new prosthetic devices at the same time.[9,10,27]

In infants, children, or adolescents with both neurologic involvement and amputation, the neurologic impairment has a greater influence on functional limitations than the amputation, whether acquired or congenital. Examples of acquired limb loss with neurologic pathology include a traumatic head injury with traumatic amputation, prematurity with intravenous infiltrate causing ischemia leading to amputation, meningococcemia causing brain and musculoskeletal insults, and myelomeningocele (spina bifida) with amputation. Treatment should focus on neurologic function as well as balance and stability associated with the prosthesis. Typically, the prosthetic limb is the sounder and more stable limb. Strong communication and collaboration are necessary between the family, school, community, and limb deficiency team for optimal outcomes.

SUMMARY

Every infant, child, and adolescent is different and has expectations and goals unique to their needs. Many factors influence the goals when treating these patients. Age-appropriate functional activities that meet patient and family goals should guide physical therapy interventions. Treatments should be fun, meaningful, and coordinated with the child's family, schoolteachers, and community physical and occupational therapists. Physical therapists who work with infants, children, and adolescents are teachers, coaches, mentors, and advocates for the child and the family.

References

1. World Health Organization: ICY-CY International Classification of Functioning, Disability and Health: Children and Youth. Available at: http://apps.who.int/iris/bitstream/10665/43737/1/9789241547321_eng.pdf. Accessed September 23, 2021.
2. Össur: Junior solutions. Available at: http://www.ossur.com/prosthetics/juniorsolutions. Accessed September 23, 2021.
3. Fillauer: Pediatric formula foot. Available at: https://www.fillauer.com. Accessed September 23, 2021.
4. Fillauer TRS Inc: El Dorado Z-AXIS climbing foot. Available at: http://www.trsprosthetics.com. Accessed September 23, 2021.
5. Gorlick R, Bielack S, Teot L, et al: Osteosarcoma: Biology, diagnosis, treatment, and remaining challenges, in Pizzo PA, Poplack DG, eds: *Principles and Practice of Pediatric Oncology*. Lippincott Williams & Wilkins, 2011, pp 1015-1044.
6. Hawkins DS, Bolling T, Dubois S, et al: Ewing sarcoma, in Pizzo PA, Poplack DG, eds: *Principles and Practice of Pediatric Oncology*. Lippincott Williams & Wilkins, 2011, pp 987-1014.
7. Fabregas J, Whitesell R: Congenital longitudinal deficiency of the tibia, in Krajibich I, Pinzur M, Potter B, Stevens P, eds: *Atlas of Amputations and Limb Differences*, ed 4. American Academy of Orthopaedic Surgeons, 2016, pp 873-880.
8. Jobst C: Long bone lengthening in children. *Tech Orthop* 2020;35(3):189-194.
9. Coulter C: Pediatric physical therapy, in Krajibich I, Pinzur M, Potter B, Stevens P, eds: *Atlas of Amputations and Limb Differences*, ed 4. American Academy of Orthopaedic Surgeons, 2016, pp 803-814.
10. Stanger M, Coulter C, Giavedoni B: Limb deficiencies and amputations, in Palisano R, Orlin M, Schreiber J, eds: *Campbell's Physical Therapy for Children*, ed 5. Elsevier, 2017, pp 272-293.
11. Medbridge Education: Available at: https://www.medbridgeeducation.com/. Accessed September 26, 2021.
12. Jaeger L, Ascher G, Atlee J, eds: *Home Program Instruction Sheets for Infants and Young Children*, ed 3. Therapy Skill Builders, 1987.
13. Diamant RB, ed: *Positioning for Play: Home Activities for Parents of Young Children*. Therapy Skill Builders, 1992.
14. Webster J, Crunkhorn A, Sall J, Highsmith J, Pruziner A, Randolph B: Clinical practice guidelines for the rehabilitation of lower limb amputation. An update from the department of veterans affairs and department of defense. *Am J Phys Med Rehabil* 2019;98(9):820-829.
15. Borra V, Berry DC, Zideman D, Singletary E, De Buck E: Compression wrapping for acute closed extremity joint injuries: A systematic review. *J Athl Train* 2020;55(8):789-800.
16. Gillespie R: Principles of amputation surgery in children with longitudinal deficiencies of the femur. *Clin Orthop Relat Res* 1990;256:29-38.
17. Fisk JR, Smith DG: The limb deficient child, in Smith DG, Michael JW, Bowker JH, eds: *Atlas of Amputations and Limb Deficiencies: Surgical, Prosthetic and Rehabilitation Principles*, ed 3. American Academy of Orthopaedic Surgeons, 2004, pp 773-777.
18. Krebs DE, Fishman S: Characteristics of the child amputee population. *J Pediatr Orthop* 1984;4(1):89-95.
19. Chiarello L, Catalino T: Infants, toddlers, and their families: Early intervention services under IDEA, in Palisano R, Orlin M, Schreiber J. eds: *Campbell's Physical Therapy for Children*, ed 5. Elsevier, 2017, pp 703-722.
20. Torode I: Congenital deficiencies of the femur, in Krajibich I, Pinzur M, Potter B, Stevens P, eds: *Atlas of Amputations and Limb Differences*, ed 4. American Academy of Orthopaedic Surgeons, 2016, pp 889-900.
21. Tooms RE: The amputee, in Lovell WW, Winter RB, eds: *Pediatric Physical Therapy*, ed 3. Lippincott Williams & Wilkins, 1999, pp 378-428.
22. Kalamchi A, ed: *Congenital Lower Limb Deficiencies*. Springer-Verlag, 1989.
23. Geil MD, O'Berry C: Temporal and spatial parameters of crawling in children with limb loss: Implications on prosthetic knee prescription. *J Prosthet Orthot* 2010;22(1):21-25.
24. Geil MD, Coulter-O'Berry C, Schmitz M, Heriza C: Crawling kinematics in an early knee protocol for pediatric prosthetic prescription. *J Prosthet Orthot* 2013;25(1):22-29.
25. Geil M, Coulter C: Analysis of locomotor adaptations in young children with limb loss in an early prosthetic knee prescription protocol. *Prosthet Orthot Int* 2014;38(1):54-61.
26. Giavedoni BJ: *The Use of Prosthetic Knees in Infants and Toddlers: Alignment*. Canadian Association for Prosthetics and Orthotics, 2000, pp 25-26.
27. Cuomo A, Watts H: The child with multiple limb deficiencies, in Krajibich I, Pinzur M, Potter B, Stevens P, eds: *Atlas of Amputations and Limb Differences*, ed 4. American Academy of Orthopaedic Surgeons, 2016, pp 953-960.
28. Wilk B, Karol L, Halliday S, et al: Transition to an articulating knee prosthesis in pediatric amputees. *J Prosthet Orthot* 1999;11:69-74.
29. Geil MD, Safaeepour Z, Giavedoni B, Coulter CP: Walking kinematics in young children with limb loss using early versus traditional prosthetic knee prescription protocols. *PLoS One* 2020;15(4):e0231401.
30. Dole R, Schreiber J: Measurement, in Palisano R, Orlin M, Schreiber J, eds: *Campbell's Physical Therapy for Children*, ed 5. Elsevier, 2017, pp 15-29.
31. Bayley N, ed: *Bayley Scales of Infant Development*. Psychological Corporation, 1969.
32. Folio MR, Fewell RR, eds: *Peabody Developmental Motor Scales*. George Peabody College for Teachers, 1974.
33. Harborne R, Dusing S: Motor development and control, in Palisano R, Orlin M, Schreiber J, eds: *Campbell's Physical Therapy for Children*, ed 5. Elsevier, 2017, pp 30-77.
34. Gupta SK, Alassaf N, Harrop AR, Kiefer GN: Principles of rotationplasty. *J Am Acad Orthop Surg* 2012;20(10):657-667.
35. Ackman J, Altiok H, Flanagan A, et al: Long-term follow-up of Van Nes rotationplasty in patients with congenital proximal focal femoral deficiency. *Bone Joint J* 2013;95-B(2):192-198.
36. Morrison S, Georgiadis A, Dahl M: What's new in limb lengthening and deformity correction. *J Bone Joint Surg Am* 2020;102(16):1391-1396.
37. Catagni MA, Guerreschi F: Management of fibular hemimelia using the Ilizarov method, in Herring JA, Birch JG, eds: *The Child With a Limb Deficiency*. American Academy of Orthopaedic Surgeons, 1998, pp 179-193.
38. Paley D: Lengthening reconstruction surgery for congenital femoral deficiency, in Herring JA, Birch JG, eds: *The Child With a Limb Deficiency*. American Academy of Orthopaedic Surgeons, 1998, pp 113-132.
39. Coglianese DB, Herzenberg JE, Goulet JA: Physical therapy management of patients undergoing limb lengthening

40. Shehadeh A, El Dahleh M, Salem A, et al: Standardization of rehabilitation after limb salvage surgery for sarcomas improves patients' outcome. *Hematol Oncol Stem Cell Ther* 2013;6(3-4):105-111.

41. American Physical Therapy Association: Guide to physical therapist practice Part 1. A description of patient/client management. Part 2: Preferred practice patterns. *Phys Ther* 1997;77(11):1160-1656.

42. Marcheese V, Thomas K, Morris S: Pediatric oncology, in Palisano R, Orlin M, Schreiber J, eds: *Campbell's Physical Therapy for Children*, ed 5. Elsevier, 2017, pp 381-397.

43. Cuomo A: Principles of amputation surgery in children, in Krajibich I, Pinzur M, Potter B, Stevens P, eds: *Atlas of Amputations and Limb Differences*, ed 4. American Academy of Orthopaedic Surgeons, 2016, pp 765-777.

44. Ness KK, Hudson MM, Ginsberg JP, et al: Physical performance limitations in the childhood cancer survivor study cohort. *J Clin Oncol* 2009;27:2382-2389.

45. Rothgangel A, Braun S, deWitte L, Beurskens A, Smeets R: Development of a clinical framework for mirror therapy in patients with phantom limb pain: An evidence-based practice approach. *Pain Pract* 2015;16:1-13.

46. Kiuken TA, Barlow AK, Hargrove L, Dumanian GA: Targeted muscle reinnervation for the upper and lower extremity. *Tech Orthop* 2017;32(2):109-116.

47. Best US colleges and universities for wheelchair accessibility. Available at: http://www.oocities.org/ketchum4/bestcollegesanduniversitiespg2.htm. Accessed September 27, 2021.

48. Bragaru M, Van Der Watt F: Adaptive lower limb prostheses for sports and recreation, in Krajibich I, Pinzur M, Potter B, Stevens P, eds: *Atlas of Amputations and Limb Differences*, ed 4. American Academy of Orthopaedic Surgeons, 2016, pp 621-630.

49. Radocy R: Upper limb adaptive prostheses for vocation and recreation, in Krajibich I, Pinzur M, Potter B, Stevens P, eds: *Atlas of Amputations and Limb Differences*, ed 4. American Academy of Orthopaedic Surgeons, 2016, pp 379-388.

50. Challenged Athlete's Foundation: Available at http://www.challengedathletes.org. Accessed September 27, 2021.

51. The Orthotic & Prosthetic Activities Foundation (OPAF): http://www.opaf-firstclinics.org. Accessed September 23, 2019.

Occupational Therapy for Children With Upper Limb Deficiencies

Wendy Hill, BScOT • Vivian J. Yip, OTD, MA, OTR/L

ABSTRACT

Comprehensive care of a child with an upper limb difference includes occupational therapy. To provide the best outcomes for this patient cohort, it is helpful to review prosthetic and nonprosthetic care and prosthetic and therapy options, as well as understand the role of the occupational therapist. The importance of family-centered care and the involvement of a comprehensive team should be recognized. Considerations are needed to accommodate the uniqueness of each child, family, and situation.

Keywords: occupational therapy; pediatric; prosthetics; training; upper limb deficiency

Introduction

Children are adaptable. A child born without an arm or a hand, with a limb difference, or who has an acquired upper limb amputation is capable of learning how to complete necessary tasks and participate in desired activities. If children are fitted with a prosthesis at an early age, encouraged to wear it, and taught how to use it, they will learn how to accomplish important activities using the prosthesis. If a child (or their family) chooses not to wear a prosthesis, he or she will learn to do these activities in other ways, often using other parts of the body to compensate for the missing limb or by incorporating adaptive equipment or tools into their daily life.

Unilateral congenital transradial limb deficiency is a common level of limb loss seen in pediatric prosthetic clinics throughout the world.[1-4] The treatment of upper limb deficiency differs slightly from clinic to clinic, but most clinics offer prosthetic fitting as a common treatment option for children. Regardless of the decision to elect or decline a prosthetic fitting, the child should be regularly evaluated by the management team. The team of specialists in an upper limb clinic can assess the child as he or she develops and address concerns or issues that may arise or evolve over time. Experienced clinicians can be identified through the Association of Children's Prosthetic and Orthotic Clinics (ACPOC). This organization promotes multidisciplinary team development and collaboration and supports research and education for professionals involved in caring for children who need orthopaedic interventions.[5] Information on clinical teams who provide care for children with limb differences is available from ACPOC and can serve as an additional resource.

The prosthetic options for children with upper limb loss include passive or cosmetic prostheses, body-powered or cable-activated prostheses, and externally powered prostheses. When children become involved in extracurricular activities and sports, more than one type of prosthesis may be required. Children who are fitted with a prosthesis often have an active-grasping prosthesis for daily use and may also have a passive prosthesis with activity-specific recreational attachments or a passive cosmetic option.

It is important to be aware of the psychological effect experienced by a family or a child with a limb deficiency. The desire to have a prosthesis may be rooted in the child's or the family's desire to appear "normal" to the outside world, possibly to avoid stares and questions from strangers, or to assuage the guilt parents may feel regarding the cause of the limb deficiency. A prosthesis may help the child and/or the family come to terms with the child's condition, and a cosmetic prosthesis may promote comfort in social situations. However, addressing the root of these concerns through a qualified counsellor is important. A prosthesis will not resolve feelings of guilt or social discomfort.

As children develop, they will decide if they need a prosthesis and what type of prosthesis they prefer. Being fit with prostheses during childhood allows the exploration of various options and provides experience on which to base prosthetic decisions later as life activities and/or priorities change.

Neither of the following authors nor any immediate family member has received anything of value from or has stock or stock options held in a commercial company or institution related directly or indirectly to the subject of this chapter: Wendy Hill and Dr. Yip.

The Team and First Assessment

The members of the clinical team will vary depending on the clinic but may consist of a physician (pediatrician or physical medicine specialist), an orthopaedic surgeon, a prosthetist, an occupational therapist (OT), a physical therapist, a social worker, a case manager, a child-life specialist, a nutritionist, a psychologist, and a psychiatrist. The first encounter with the clinical team can be intimidating for families, so it is important not to overwhelm them by introducing too many care clinicians at the initial meeting. One of the main goals of the first meeting is to build rapport with the family and child because the clinic may be providing care for many years. Some clinics treat children until they are 18 years of age, whereas others follow the patient into adulthood. If the family is having difficulty accepting or coping with the limb loss, further psychosocial counselling should be recommended.

Pediatric care involves the entire family unit. The activities or interests that are important to the family will form the basis of the child's treatment by the team. If the family wants the child to be fit with a prosthesis, information and appropriate prosthetic options should be presented by the prosthetist and/or the OT. When funding is secured, the prosthetist will begin building an appropriate prosthesis. The OT typically has a role in evaluating the child as he or she works with a temporary prosthesis and may provide feedback to assist the prosthetist so that the device can be fabricated in the most functional position for this stage of development. The child and the family will then attend prosthetic training sessions with the OT to learn how to use the prosthesis and incorporate it into daily activities.

The role of an OT is to maximize independence in occupations (meaningful and purposeful everyday life activities).[6] These include the activities of daily living (ADLs) and the instrumental activities of daily living (IADLs). ADLs are activities oriented toward taking care of one's own body. For a child, this may include bathing, grooming, hygiene, toileting, dressing, and feeding. IADLs may include play participation, exploration, school activities, and social participation with peers and the community.[6] As children develop, these activities will change and may include participation in hobbies, sports, and work activities. The OT provides skilled services in collaboration with the family and the team to facilitate full engagement in the child's everyday life activities. For a child with upper limb loss, the OT assists the family in solving problems in accomplishing ADLs and/or IADLs with or without a prosthesis. The OT evaluates the development, behavior, and performance skills of the child to establish family-centered goals and interventions and provides information and resources to educate the family so that the child can work toward optimal participation in ADLs and IADLs.

The involvement of other team members can help the family to accept and cope with the limb difference. The OT will follow the child's development, help the parents focus on the child's strengths and abilities, and address concerns about the child's ability to participate in future activities.[7] Many aspects of the child's life, health,[8] and relationships may be included in the team assessment (**Table 1**).

Unilateral Transradial Deficiency

Prosthetic Considerations

When a family decides to pursue prosthetic fitting for their child, the options for appropriate types of prostheses should be presented at the first consultation appointment and at subsequent appointments over the years as new technologies or components become available and the needs of the child or family have changed. The options for a prosthesis are dependent on the age of the child, the level of amputation, and the availability of funding. Practice guidelines vary regarding the age when the first prosthesis is prescribed. A 2006 review of the literature determined that the age of the first fitting varied worldwide, with the age ranging from 2 to 25 months.[9] The aim of the study was to determine if fitting a prosthesis before 2 years of age was related to lower rates of rejection and better functional outcomes at an older age. The authors concluded that the guidelines for prosthetic prescription procedures are based on experience, not on evidence. Currently, the literature shows that most clinics that fit prostheses to children with upper limb differences

TABLE 1 Items That May Be Included in the Team Assessment

Birth history
Medical history
Previous therapy interventions
Health history of parents, siblings, and other extended family members who may have a limb difference
Developmental status
Cognitive function
School-grade level and performance
Socioeconomic status of parents and/or guardians
Family and child's daily routine
History of the patient's use of a prosthesis if one was previously used
Activities of daily living assessment and instrumental activities of daily living assessment—how they are completed (with assistance, using equipment, age appropriateness)
Identification of individuals who provide the most care for the patient
Patient and parent social skills, thoughts about limb difference, coping skills and techniques
Inspection of the residual and sound limbs related to skin integrity, residual limb length, pain, edema, bony prominences, range of motion, and strength
Discussion of interests, goals, and the things the family wants the child to accomplish (with or without a prosthesis) (aesthetics versus function)
Information about prostheses and other adaptive equipment and strategies, as appropriate

agree that there are benefits to fitting a passive prosthesis between the ages of 3 and 9 months.[2,10]

Shaperman[11] conducted a survey of fitting practices for children with transradial limb loss in pediatric prosthetic clinics throughout North America. She concluded that most children with unilateral transradial limb absence have their first fitting when they can sit (approximately at age 6 months) and are later fit with an active-grasping prosthesis when the child demonstrates awareness of cause and effect and attempts to hold objects (between ages 10 and 18 months). A recent survey of clinicians working with children in different parts of the world reported that most clinics fit an active prosthesis, either body-powered or externally powered, between 1 and 3 years of age.[10] Because there is limited evidence-based research on the best age for fitting the first prosthesis, it is important to collaborate with the child's parents to determine what is in the best interest of their child and family.

There are various reasons why children with congenital upper limb differences may be fitted with a prosthesis at different ages or stages of development. The home situation may be overwhelming for some families, and they may be unable to comply with the requirements of prosthetic care when the child is a toddler. A family may want to wait until the child is able to verbalize his or her wants and needs or may not have access to care when the child is young. Regardless of the reason, prosthetic fitting in an older child has its own considerations. The child will likely be able to express his or her opinions, and his or her level of motivation will need to be considered. It is likely that an older child will have adapted to efficiently completing ADLs with compensatory techniques and will not find a prosthesis useful for these tasks. If fitted, the child may only consider a cosmetic option for special occasions or an activity-specific prosthesis to participate in sports or activities such as art or playing musical instruments. If the child decides to incorporate an active prosthetic option into ADLs and IADLs, he or she must be prepared to allot time for training with the prosthesis to achieve proficient use.

The First Passive Prosthesis

The goals of fitting the first passive upper limb prosthesis at an early age are twofold. First and foremost, it allows the family to establish a consistent wearing pattern and become accustomed to incorporating the prosthesis into the family's lifestyle. When a child age 2 or 3 years is fit with a prosthesis for the first time, parents often struggle to keep the prosthesis on the child. This may be because the child is accustomed to using his or her residual limb in daily activities and the added weight, heat, and diminished sensation while wearing the prosthesis forces the child to do tasks in an unfamiliar manner. Second, a prosthesis that is fitted around the time the child is mastering sitting can be incorporated into the acquisition of gross motor skills. It provides length extension and support on the missing side to aid with sitting balance, reaching forward while sitting, prone play, crawling, and pulling to a standing position (**Figure 1**).

When a child wears a prosthesis as a regular part of the daily routine, he or she learns to manipulate toys in the true midline of the body, instead of a skewed midline closer to the missing limb when a prosthesis in not worn. The prosthesis helps establish a more upright posture from a young age and encourages body symmetry. The neuronal group selection theory of brain development described by Meurs et al[9] implies that if a child wears a prosthesis during the early phases of development, a representation of the limb with a prosthesis will be established in the brain. If the prosthesis is used as the child develops motor skills, the child will have motor functioning abilities with and without the prosthesis.[9] The clinical experiences of the authors of this chapter reinforce this theory because children who establish an early wearing pattern tend to incorporate the use of the device into their daily routines and use it to accomplish daily tasks. A study by Hahamy et al looked at cortical reorganization in children born with one hand who

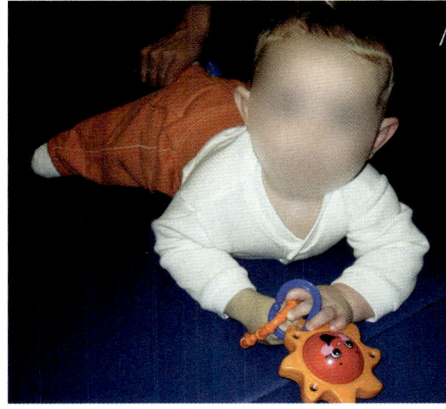

FIGURE 1 Photograph of a child with a passive upper limb prosthesis that provides support in prone play.

do not use a prosthesis. They determined that the residual limb or other body parts that function in place of the hand (lips, feet) are represented in the area of the brain associated with hand function.[12]

The prosthetist and OT provide the parents with a home program when the passive prosthesis is fitted. This program should include instructions for initial wearing time and how to progress to full-time wear. Full-time wear is considered to be all waking hours, with removal of the prosthesis for napping and bathing. The parents should monitor the child for signs (such as localized areas of redness around the brim of the socket or on the distal end of the residual limb) that the prosthesis is becoming too small and in need of adjustment.

The home program should also provide instruction for hygiene and cleaning of the residual limb and the prosthesis. The inner socket should be cleaned daily with a soft, moist cloth (with a mix of soap and water or alcohol and water) or a baby wipe. The outside of the prosthesis should be cleaned as often as the child's hand is cleaned, such as when there is obvious dirt or food on it. Certain types of prosthetic gloves are more prone to staining than others. If there is a polyvinyl chloride glove covering the hand, it will be easily stained by food dyes, ink, clothing dyes, and other agents. Stains should be cleaned promptly with alcohol or they will be very difficult to remove. Many of the newer prosthetic hands and gloves for children are made of silicone and are more easily cleaned.

As part of a home program, it is helpful to include a list of toys or activities that will encourage use of the prosthetic arm in bimanual play. If the child does not pay attention to the side with the prosthesis, interesting toys can be attached over the hand with straps or handles. Toys that can be placed in the mouth or that make noise may be highly interesting to very young children. A fun game can be made by placing toys with large handles on the prosthetic hand and encouraging the child to remove them. The child can be encouraged to hold down a toy with the prosthesis while playing with or manipulating the toy with the other hand. Deep pots or buckets filled with blocks or smaller toys to dump or pick up are fun for some children. Playing with large balls or large stuffed animals encourages bimanual arm use, as does playing pat-a-cake or other rhyming songs with arm gestures.

Regular follow-up with the family is essential to monitor progress with the wearing schedule, comfort, and fit of the prosthesis as well as the child's achievement of developmental milestones. These will be factors in deciding when to fit the next prosthesis. If the prosthesis is too snug before the child is considered developmentally ready, the prosthesis can be lengthened or the socket can be adjusted to allow more time for the development of gross motor skills and improved cognitive readiness.

It is important that the fitting process does not have unnecessary delays that would leave the child without a prosthesis after a wearing schedule has been established. If possible, the fitting for a new prosthesis should be started before the previous device has been completely outgrown. This will ensure any progress made in wearing and using the prosthesis is not lost.

The First Active Prosthesis

The appropriate time to fit a child with the first active prostheses varies among practitioners and in different parts of the world, although most agree that it should occur before age 3 years.[10] Some centers follow a developmental approach to fitting a child with a myoelectric hand, meaning that the child is considered ready if he or she is cognitively ready and is walking and no longer requires arm extension for balance. Other centers fit a body-powered prosthesis when the child meets their readiness criteria; an externally powered prosthesis would be considered if the child proves to be a good user of the body-powered device. In Germany, the family is given the choice of either a myoelectric or body-powered prosthesis when the child is between the ages of 2 and 4 years.[13] In the United Kingdom, prosthetic centers follow guidelines established by the British Society for Rehabilitation Medicine. These guidelines recommend fitting children for a first passive prosthesis between the ages of 4 to 15 months, and then fitting the first active prosthesis, either a body-powered device or a myoelectric device, between the ages of 15 months and 3 years.[14]

When a child has outgrown the passive prosthesis and is considered ready for a prosthesis with active prehension, the team, including the family, must determine what type of prosthesis will best meet the child's needs. To ensure the child's success with an active prehension prosthesis, the family must be committed to attending the training appointments and complying with the requirements of the home program.

Body-Powered Prostheses for Young Children

When the child has outgrown the first passive prosthesis and/or has demonstrated a readiness to use a terminal device for grasping, an active-grasping prosthesis should be considered. The criteria to determine readiness are as follows: (1) the child can follow simple one- or two-step directions; (2) he or she has an attention span of at least 5 to 10 minutes; (3) the child attempts to hold objects with his or her residual limb or the terminal device; and (4) the child tolerates being handled by the OT.[15,16]

During general development, the child may be ready for formal training between 20 and 26 months of age.[15,16] The child's behavior, ability to attend to simple instructions, and motor development will influence the progress during prosthetic training. A home program for the family will guide parents how to assist the child in learning the control motions of opening and closing the terminal device and promote follow-through with using the prosthesis.

Toddlers with a transradial deficiency are typically fit with the elbow preflexed in the socket. This allows the terminal device to be in a midline position without the child exerting much effort, and the prosthesis will be prepositioned adequately for two-handed activities. When the prosthesis is positioned with the elbow in extension, which is more appropriate for adults or older children, toddlers tend to ignore the prosthesis, and more effort is needed for appropriate midline use of the prosthesis.[15,16] A well-balanced harness that is slightly snug and does not have a center ring will help the very young child easily learn the control motion.

Initial prosthetic training should begin at a height-appropriate table for the child to learn the basic control motion. The OT should sit behind the child and use both hands to guide the child. For voluntary opening terminal devices, one hand should be on the shoulder joint for stabilization and one hand on the forearm of the prosthesis to assist with humeral flexion for opening the terminal device[15,16] (**Figure 2**). The therapist should call attention to the open terminal device with verbal cues. The child is encouraged to use the sound hand to place an object in the open terminal device while the OT guides the prosthesis from humeral flexion to humeral extension to close the terminal device securely on the object. It is important to use repetitive bimanual tasks to teach the control motion, including activities such as stringing beads, opening nesting barrels, and opening markers. The child should be encouraged to use the prosthesis for gross motor activities and all daily tasks. For voluntary closing terminal devices, training will be similar, however humeral flexion will close the terminal device and humeral extension will open the device. Clinics' fitting philosophies

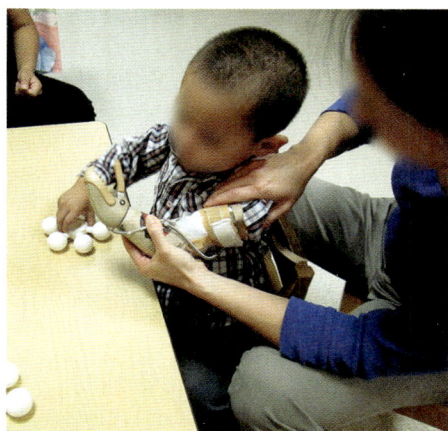

FIGURE 2 Clinical photograph of a therapist positioning a transradial prosthesis to assist with terminal device operation.

of when to fit voluntary opening versus voluntary closing terminal devices may vary and should be individualized to the child's development and the intended tasks for the prosthesis.

As the child progresses and understands the basic control motion, he or she needs to learn various prosthetic skills and refinements. These include prepositioning the terminal device, accurate placement of objects inside the terminal device, opening the terminal device close to the body, keeping the terminal device closed when reaching forward, and refining the basic control motion to include shoulder abduction. All of these skills are learned by the child through practice and performing age-appropriate bimanual activities on a daily basis and during prosthetic training with the OT. Training activities and functional tasks described in the following section on externally powered prostheses also can be used in body-powered prosthesis training.

Externally Powered Prostheses for Young Children

Externally powered prostheses generally refer to those devices operated using myoelectric control. However, activation also can be accomplished with switches, touchpads, or linear transducers. Children with longitudinal deficiencies who have digits at the distal end of the residual limb may prefer to use the movement they have in the distal end to push against or activate a switch or touchpad to control a prosthetic hand.

Egermann et al[13] described the following keys to success in a pediatric upper limb prosthetic rehabilitation program. A myoelectric prosthesis should be fitted at a specialized center, and the child should be managed by a specialized multidisciplinary team. The child should train with an OT and be regularly monitored to assess use of the prosthesis and for changing prosthetic needs. The center should provide timely support for maintenance and repair of the prosthesis.

Myoelectrode Site Selection

When fitting a young child with the first myoelectric prosthesis, a simple one-muscle system is often used to operate the hand. When the muscle is contracted, the hand opens. When the muscle is not contracting, the hand closes and remains closed. This is often referred to as the "cookie crusher" control strategy. Initially, the electrode sensitivity will be set quite high so that any activity of the muscle will cause the hand to open. This is intentional because it draws attention to the hand and reinforces the cause–effect concept. In some fitting centers, children are fitted right away with a two-muscle system where the extensors are used to open the hand and flexors are used to close the hand. Dr. Liselotte Hermansson,[17] an occupational therapist in Sweden, describes a structured training program for young children learning to use a myoelectric prosthesis using two muscles.

When fitting a toddler or very young child with a myoelectric prosthesis, finding appropriate muscle sites to place an electrode is generally not challenging. The muscles can be palpated during the assessment; however, the electrode is generally placed on the forearm extensors close to the lateral epicondyle. The size of the standard electrode will usually encompass much of the extensor muscle belly, producing a strong signal when the muscle is contracted.

During the appointment to select the myoelectrode site, it is a good idea to place an electrode on the forearm in the approximate location on the extensor muscle and secure it with a cuff or strap if the child allows. A single-function toy modified to operate with a standard electrode can be used to establish the cause–effect concept at this early stage. A toy that lights up, makes sounds, or moves is highly reinforcing for young children (**Figure 3**). When the child is asked to wiggle his or her "little arm," the child sees that something happens as a result. This will encourage the child to continue to activate the muscle to see the resulting action of the toy. This technique works well when the child is sitting quietly, either with the parents or with the OT, and is able to attend to the toy. A small room with a limited number of people is recommended for this training. The OT may want to gently hold the child's forearm when he or she is being asked to wiggle it so the child does not wiggle the whole arm instead of the muscles in the forearm. A child's prosthetic hand also can be used in place of the toy for the purpose of site selection and cause–effect training. Some children respond well to a prosthetic hand as opposed to a toy; however, because the hand is not attached to the child's forearm, operating a hand in this way is still an abstract concept and may not generalize into the ability to control the prosthetic hand after the prosthesis is fabricated.

When the child is old enough to have a sustained attention span of at least 10 minutes and the ability to follow simple instructions, the myoelectrode site selection process and socket fitting can take place with the aid of computer software. Several manufacturers have software for evaluating and visualizing muscle signals, but the MyoBoy tester (Ottobock) is most often used for pediatric patients because it is the only software with a virtual child's prosthetic hand.[18] The MyoBoy tester allows muscle signals to be viewed in real time, and the child can see a virtual hand moving in real time as he or she activates the electrode (**Figure 4**). If the child can isolate the muscle on command, the electrode sensitivity can be adjusted to an appropriate level, eliminating guesswork. For young children,

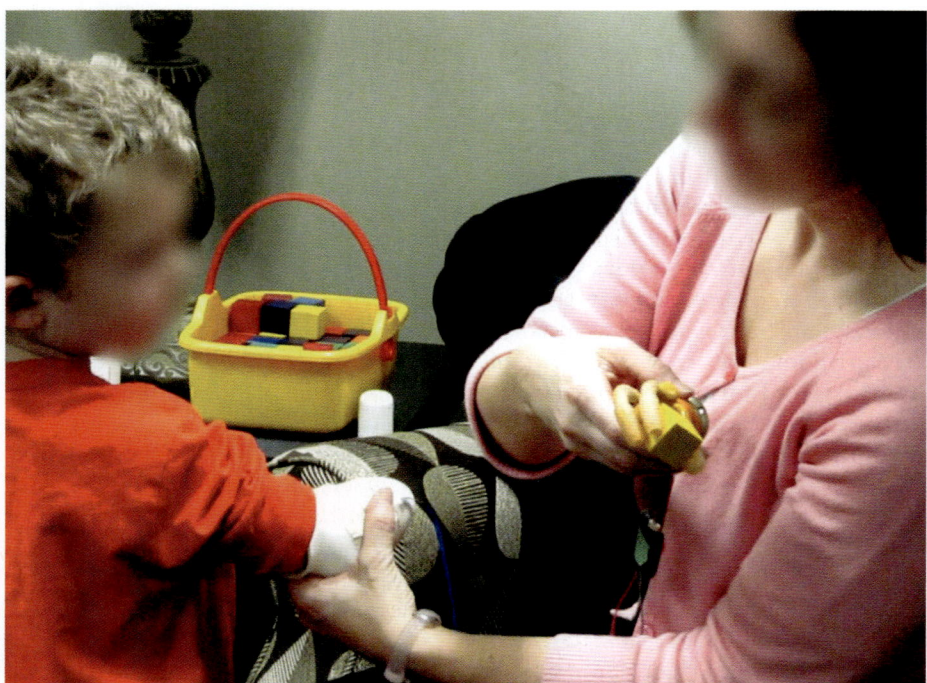

FIGURE 3 Clinical photograph of a therapist using a test socket with a prosthetic hand during myoelectrode site selection.

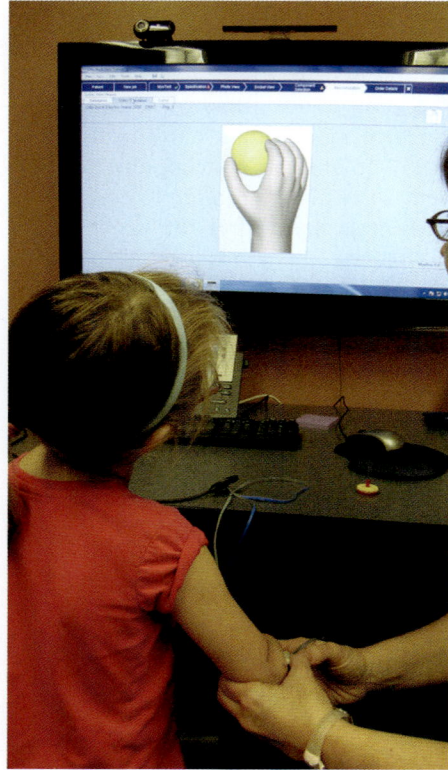

FIGURE 4 Clinical photograph of a therapist working with a child to determine myoelectrode site selection using computer software. The child can see a virtual hand moving in real time as the electrode is activated.

the computer software may not be motivating, so attention will be quickly lost. If this happens, it is more important to know that the child understands the concept of contracting the muscle to cause something to happen than to sit for extended periods of time practicing this control. It may be necessary to distract the child with other toys or games to ensure that he or she keeps the socket on long enough to ensure a good fit and intimate contact with the electrode.

Control Training

When a toddler is fit with the first active-grasping prosthesis, it will likely be used in a passive manner initially. It is important to manage the expectations of the parents so they do not assume that the child will immediately be able to pick up objects with the prosthesis and manipulate them voluntarily. This will occur gradually over time and will require regular prompting and intervention by the parents and/or the OT.

When the prosthesis is completed and the prosthetist is satisfied with the fit and suspension, training can begin. Training should occur in a small but comfortable room with the parents, child, and OT; the number of distracting toys or people should be limited. Toys or objects brought in for training should be kept out of sight until needed by the OT. If the child is shy or anxious, he or she can be seated on a parent's lap. If comfortable with the OT, the child can be seated on the floor facing the OT or at a small child-size table. The OT may at times want to be behind the child to hold the prosthesis or to demonstrate actions.

The child is asked to wiggle the "little arm" within the socket. If the parents use different terminology to refer to the residual limb, the OT should use the familiar term so the child understands the instructions. Sometimes, using a sticker on the outside of the socket close to the distal end of the residual limb on the side where the electrode is located can help the child understand the motion required. The child can be asked to try to "touch" the sticker or move toward it with the little arm. When he or she sees that the hand moves, it will reinforce the muscle movement. The OT should draw attention to the movement of the hand when the child activates the muscle. Repetition is important at this early stage. The OT should continue to ask the child to wiggle or move toward the sticker, and the child should be praised for opening the hand. The child's attention span will dictate how long this training will last.

If the child opens the hand consistently, small toys, such as blocks, play animals, plastic rings, and colorful paper, can be placed in the opened hand to maintain interest. Often the child will want to remove the object from the hand. By extending the arm to pull a toy away, the extensor muscles will contract, causing the hand to open. This also reinforces the control of the hand. If the child enjoys the repetitiveness of dropping toys on the floor, the game of putting objects in the hand and having the child drop them can be a fun training activity.

When the child wants to move around the room, toys with handles, such as ride-on toys (a rocking horse or tricycle) or push-toys (grocery carts, strollers, or toy lawnmowers), should be introduced. These toys encourage bimanual play. It is safer and easier to hold on with both hands while on a ride-on toy. If the child allows, the OT or parent should help position the prosthetic hand on the handle of the toy. It is important to let the child explore using the hand in his or her own way for periods of time and watch closely for opportunities to intervene. When the OT helps to position the hand on objects or handles, it demonstrates to the child how the hand can be useful. This is important even if the child is not at a stage when he or she can consistently open the hand when asked. By pointing out these opportunities to parents during training sessions, the OT can reinforce how the parents can continue training in the home environment.

With very young children, it is important to give frequent breaks during training or to have multiple short training sessions. The OT must recognize signs of resistance and judge when to push the child to attempt to use the hand and when to pull back and allow the child to play independently. If the OT is too demanding, the child may pull the arm away or hide it behind his or her back and use only the sound arm for play. Training progress can be lost if the child resists wearing the arm or bringing it into play because people are paying too much attention to the activation of the hand.

If the child is resistant to training strategies to open the hand, it is best to let the child explore through play and use the prosthesis passively as he or she has done in the past. This will allow the child to become comfortable with the weight and size of the prosthetic arm and the sounds that occur when the hand is opened. If cognitive awareness is present and the OT is confident that the child has made the connection between contracting the muscle and activating the hand, success has been achieved. This may be the only expectation at the first training session. Some children make the connection within the first 10 minutes of training, whereas others may need several sessions to fully understand how to activate the hand.

Over the course of weeks or months through a detailed home program and the support of the OT, the child is expected to progress from using the hand passively to using it actively. The process of learning to use a myoelectric hand can be categorized into the following stages that require specific skills:[17,19] (1) The awareness that moving the muscle causes the prosthetic hand to open and close. (2) The ability to open the hand on command, although the child tends to use it passively for support. (3) The child attempts to place objects in the hand or position the hand but requires assistance or support because of the weight of the prosthesis. Support may be provided by the side of the body (**Figure 5**), a tabletop, the parent, the OT, or someone else. (4) The ability to successfully grasp objects spontaneously, without needing support for the weight of the prosthesis. (5) The ability to hold and carry objects while keeping muscles quiet and releasing objects when desired (**Figure 6**). (6) The ability to grasp objects in various positions around the body and at different heights. (7) The ability to coordinate use of both hands smoothly and spontaneously. (8) The ability to adjust the opening width of the prosthetic hand based on the size and softness of the object being grasped (grasping delicate objects without crushing them). (9) The ability to grasp and/or release objects while the arm is moving or the object is moving (**Figure 7**). (10) The ability to grasp, hold, or release objects when not looking at the hand.

Children progress at different rates, and their individual personalities and age of maturation are factors in how they use their prostheses. Some children learn to activate the hand and will do this when commanded or reminded; however, they tend to use the prosthesis in a passive manner most of the time. Others require very little prompting to use the hand for grasping and will routinely use it to complete bimanual tasks, although they still will require assistance to position the wrist appropriately.

Much of the training and progression of skills occurs at home. The home program should reinforce what has been discussed during training sessions, such as expectations for wearing and using the prosthesis, care and maintenance information, and the implementation of suggested activities that encourage use of the prosthesis. Some activities to encourage bimanual play (**Figure 8**) are described in **Table 2**.

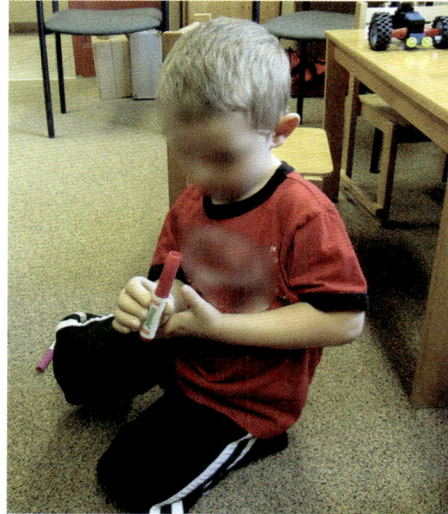

FIGURE 5 Clinical photograph of a boy using body support for the initial control of a terminal device.

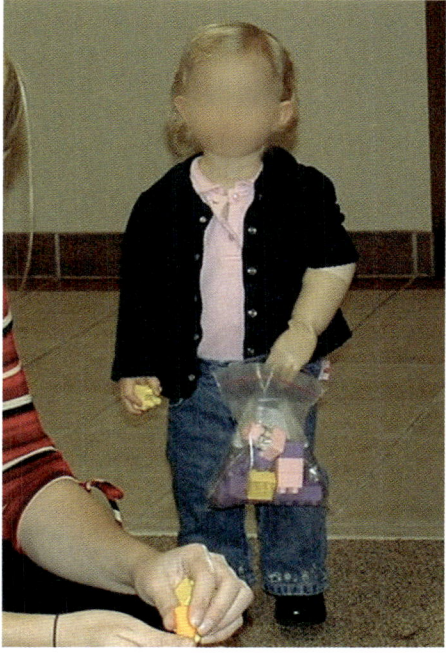

FIGURE 6 Photograph of a child carrying an object with her prosthetic hand. The muscle must be kept quiet to prevent release of the object.

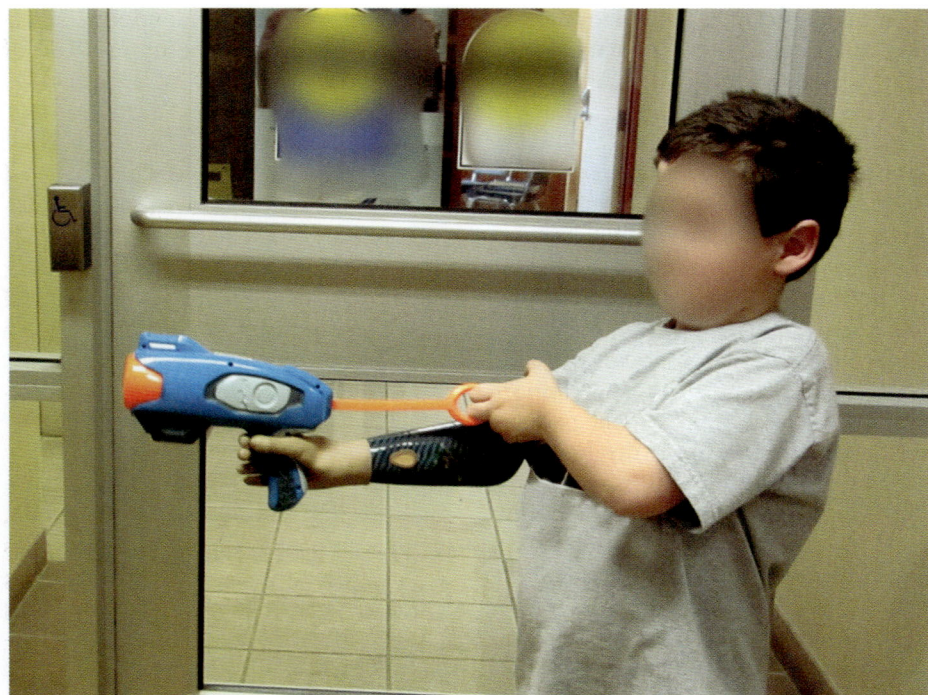

FIGURE 7 Photograph of a child controlling a terminal device while his arm is in motion.

When activities are chosen for training, it is important to note the opening width of the prosthetic hand. All items should easily fit into the prosthetic hand for bimanual play, including handles on toys. Parents should be made aware that the smallest size prosthetic hands have a limited opening width and should take this into account when purchasing toys for the home.

Subsequent Prostheses and Changing Control Strategies

As the child develops and ages, the ability to follow instructions improves and the possibilities for controlling a prosthesis also increase. When the first myoelectric prosthesis is outgrown, a decision must be made about when to introduce a two-muscle control system. Children are usually ready to switch to a two-site control system at 4 years of age or older. At this point, they have better control over movement of the distal end of the residual limb and have generally outgrown the behavioral challenges characteristic of many 2- and 3-year-old children. Their attention spans are longer and they follow instructions well. The age for introducing a two-muscle control system is variable because it depends on how well the child has learned to control the one-muscle system and how well the prosthesis has been integrated into daily use at home. If the child continues to require prompting to use the hand for grasping and struggles with consistent control, it is not appropriate to switch to a more difficult control strategy.

When introducing a two-muscle control system, the forearm extensors and flexors are used if possible. The child must learn to activate and relax each muscle separately for independent control of the opening and closing functions of the hand. Initially, the OT should explain to the child how to move the residual limb to activate the muscles by flexing and extending the wrist or the intact arm. For some children, asking them to close their eyes and move both sides in the same manner will help them to achieve this technique. For some children, holding the residual limb and asking them to (make a muscle) on one side of the arm and then the other will be effective. For others who have soft tissue or nubbins at the end of the residual limb, it is helpful to draw a face on the end of the arm and have them move the tissue in different ways to make changes to the face. This may reinforce the desired muscle action.

When the muscle bellies can be palpated and the child understands the action required to contract both muscles, visual feedback can be very helpful to practice the motions. Computer

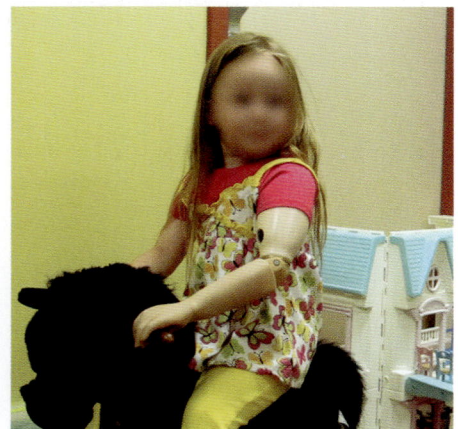

FIGURE 8 Clinical photograph of a child using a rocking horse, a toy that encourages bimanual play.

TABLE 2 Suggested Activities to Encourage Bimanual Play
Holding onto a rolling pin to roll out dough
Pinch dough to make marks
Hold handles on push toys, such as a stroller, a grocery cart, or a lawnmower
Hold onto riding toys, such as bouncers, tricycles, or a play car with a steering wheel
Hold containers, such as a bag of chips, a box of raisins, a bottle of bubbles, a bag of toys, a small pail for sand and water
Hold a pot to stir
Hold a bag or purse to put items in or to empty
Play with two-handed musical instruments, such as a toy drum, maracas, and cymbals

software can be used to show signals or a virtual hand in real time.[18] Initially, it is useful to show the signals and have the child concentrate on making contractions with one muscle and then the other. There are training games within the software that reinforce sustaining signal strength while relaxing the opposing muscle. Frequent breaks may be required during training because of muscle fatigue. If the computer software is confusing or too abstract for the child, a prosthetic hand can be used at this stage of training.

In some children with congenital limb loss, the anatomy of the musculature in the residual limb is not the same as the intact limb and sometimes there are co-contractions of the extensor and flexor muscles. This may delay the change to a two-site control strategy or it may make it impossible to make the change. In these cases, alternative control strategies can be considered, depending on the prosthetic components being used. For example, in a rate-sensitive control system, a big or fast contraction of a muscle opens the hand and a small or slow contraction of the same muscle closes the hand. The Vario (Ottobock) one-muscle control system operates much like a "cookie crusher" system but provides proportional control over the speed of opening the hand by contracting the muscle and proportional control over closing the hand by the rate of muscle relaxation. When the child is able to use these alternative control methods, he or she will have finer control of opening and closing the hand. This allows more confidence when using the hand for everyday activities.

As a child ages into adolescence, if he or she continues to only have one available muscle site, and if funding and space in the prosthesis allow, pattern recognition could be considered as an alternative control option. Pattern recognition uses information from many muscles within the prosthetic socket and maps to individual functions of the prosthetic hand.[20] As long as muscle movements are consistent, co-contraction of muscles does not interfere with control of the hand.

Therefore, the child who cannot use two-site proportional control because of co-contraction can successfully use pattern recognition to control opening and closing of a hand as long as the muscle patterns look different from each other.

Progression of Training

When the basic operation of the hand has been mastered, the use of the hand can be refined. Activities presented in therapy should initially require repetition to ensure that the hand is working properly and that the child is consistently able to open and close the hand. Some ideas for initial skill-building activities include moving or stacking blocks or cones, playing tic-tac-toe with wooden blocks, playing board games that require the movement of objects (**Figure 9**), and removing caps from markers for coloring. During these initial skill-building activities, the arm may require support from the OT or the child to remove the weight factor when activating the hand. These activities encourage the child to use the hand in a dominant manner and provide opportunities to operate the hand. If the activities are motivating and fun, most children will willingly participate. When the fit of the prosthesis and function of the hand are deemed to be satisfactory, training can continue using functional activities to reinforce more natural use of the hand in the home environment.

Functional Activity Training

Training activities should be fun and relevant to the child's age and developmental level. For preschool-age children, imaginative play and gross motor activities are popular. Tabletop and gross motor activities should vary to keep the child's interest and attention. Children at this age enjoy many activities, such as drawing; coloring; building with construction blocks; blowing bubbles; playing simple card games; pretend play in a kitchen, workshop, or grocery store; dressing in costumes or adult clothing; parachute games; playing with dolls or stuffed animals; making objects with dough; and participating in outdoor playground activities. Self-care skills, such as fastening buttons, zippers, or laces, can be practiced by dressing up in oversized clothes or dressing and undressing dolls or stuffed animals. This is easier for the children initially, and they can progress to practicing these skills on themselves.

As children approach school age, attention should be given to skills required in the school setting such as cutting with scissors, tying shoelaces independently, starting zippers on coats, and stabilizing and opening bags with zippers and individually wrapped

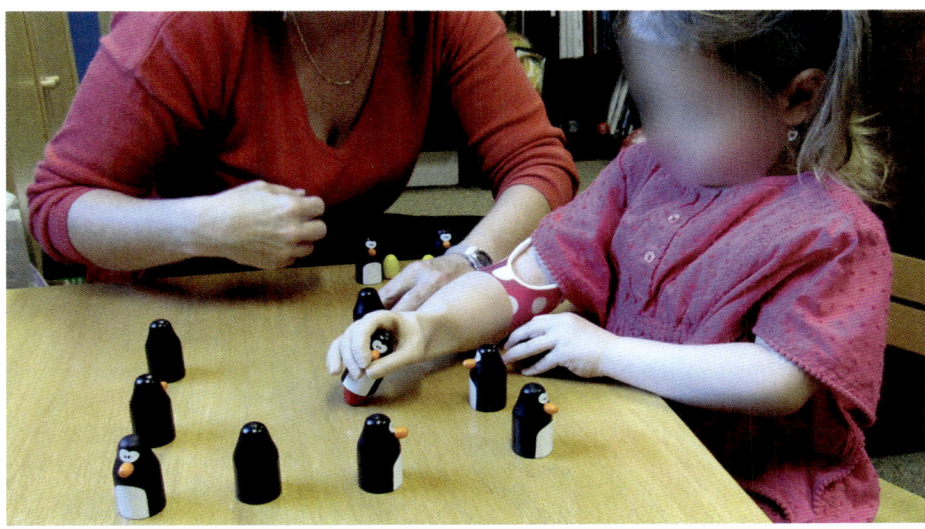

FIGURE 9 Clinical photograph of a child engaging in a skill-building activity to encourage repetitive use of her prosthetic hand.

Section 5: Pediatrics

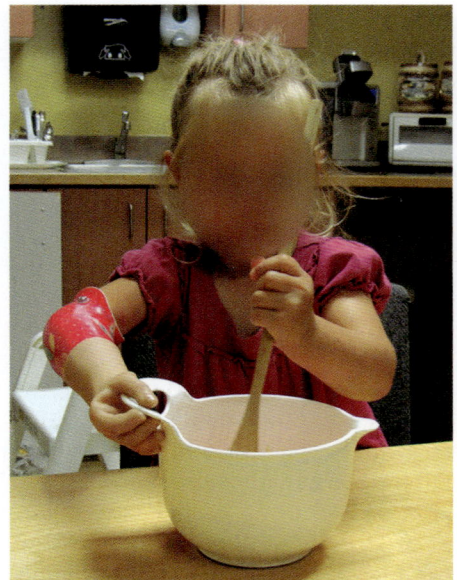

FIGURE 10 Photograph of a child stirring a pot. This task provides bimanual functional activity training.

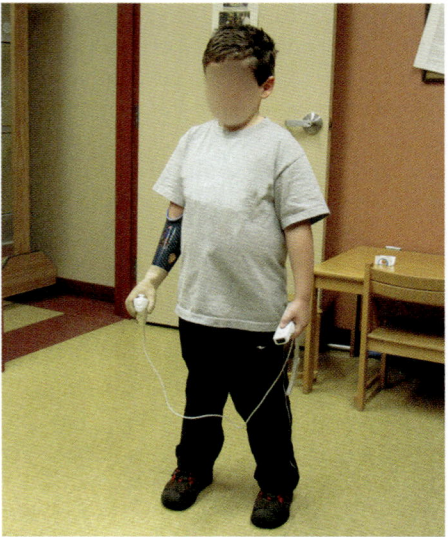

FIGURE 11 Clinical photograph of a child demonstrating that active video games requiring movement in three dimensions can be used to provide function training that encourages movement of both arms.

snack items. Outdoor play and learning to skip rope are important as well.

Children near school age or slightly older may enjoy time spent baking or helping to prepare snacks or food. Younger children may be able to hold a bowl and stir to make pudding (**Figure 10**) or roll out dough to make cookies. Many bimanual tasks can be practiced in the kitchen, such as opening packages, measuring, pouring, cutting food, washing hands and dishes, spreading out a tablecloth, putting on an apron, and wrapping and putting away food.

One of the factors to consider in training is whether the prosthesis will stay on the child and function appropriately when the child is active and sweating. Games or sports involving running and full-body movement can be used to evaluate this concern. Racquet sports such as badminton and tennis or catching and throwing games are a good choice because they require the use of both hands. Swinging, playing on a teeter-totter, and climbing up ladders or rope walls are also good choices. When space is limited or the child prefers video games, active games that require movement in three dimensions can be effective in encouraging children to use both hands to hold remotes while moving in a limited space (**Figure 11**).

Unilateral Transhumeral and Shoulder Disarticulation-Level Deficiencies

First Passive Prosthesis: Fitting and Training

The choice of whether to fit a child with a unilateral transhumeral or shoulder disarticulation congenital deficiency with a prosthesis is the same as for children with a unilateral transradial deficiency. If the family is motivated to pursue prosthetic fitting, committed to attending follow-up appointments for therapy, and amenable to participating in a home program for the child, a passive fitting can be considered at the same developmental timeframe as that previously described for a child with a transradial deficiency. The goal of the first prosthesis is to establish a wearing pattern, accustom the child to the weight of the prosthesis, and include it during play.

A passive prosthesis at this level consists of an intimately fitted socket, a humeral segment, a passive friction elbow, a forearm segment, a wrist, and a terminal device. The terminal device options include a passive hand, a mitt, or a voluntary-opening terminal device (eg, a passive hook or Child Amputee Prosthetics Project terminal device [CAPP TD#1] with an adult to assist with passive grasping ability).

A passive arm with a friction elbow and wrist can provide support and help with balance as a child learns to sit and, eventually, to walk. It should be worn throughout the child's waking hours as long as it does not interfere with gross motor skills. Most children with a residual limb at this level will not crawl on all four limbs. They usually learn to scoot on their bottoms and use other methods to transition to a prone posture or standing. A physical therapist may be consulted if there is a delay in the child achieving gross motor milestones. The parent will need to position the forearm of the prosthesis for various activities. For example, the elbow should be in an extended position to help with balance in sitting or when reaching forward to play. When the child begins walking, the elbow should be positioned in extension to help with balance. When the child is comfortable walking, he or she can be encouraged to bring the terminal device forward to push or carry large items.

The First Active Prosthesis

The readiness criteria used for determining when to transition to an active prosthesis for the child with a transhumeral limb loss is the same as for the transradial level. The prosthesis is intended to be used as an assisting or "helper" hand. This is especially true when referring to higher-level upper limb loss. As the function of more joints needs to be replaced, it becomes more complicated and time consuming to control these motions. For children with a deficiency at the transhumeral level, elbow flexion and extension, wrist rotation, and hand grasp and release need to be considered. When fitting a child, especially with the first active-grasping prosthesis, the hand or terminal device will be the focus of control, with the other joints remaining as passive friction joints that are manually positioned.

Body-Powered Prosthesis: Transhumeral Level

The first transhumeral prosthesis for a young child will operate with a single control cable. It is initially easier for a young child to focus only on operating the terminal device and then learn how to operate the elbow lock at a later stage. The same control motions (shoulder flexion and extension) are used for transradial and transhumeral prostheses. After the child has learned how to consistently open and close the terminal device on objects, prepositioning of the wrist and elbow or forearm is introduced. The length of the residual limb will affect the type of prosthetic elbow used. There are two types of elbow units available for children—an internal elbow with a turntable and an elbow with outside joints. The elbow joint with a turntable is used if an older child is able to tolerate the extra weight and if the residual arm length is short enough to accommodate the size of the component. The overall length of the prosthesis should not compromise the child's comfort and functional position at a table when performing two-handed activities. A young child is usually fit with outside elbow joints with a pull tab to lock and unlock the elbow when the child is not developmentally ready and does not have adequate shoulder depression and extension to activate the elbow lock from the control strap on the harness. The child or an adult caring for the child can activate the pull tab to preposition the elbow for activities.

An older child who is able to use his or her sound hand on the pull tab to activate the elbow lock can use his or her ipsilateral leg or a table to assist with prepositioning the forearm. If an older child has adequate shoulder depression and extension, the elbow lock control strap may be attached to the harness. The child may initially need hands-on assistance to learn the control motions of shoulder depression and extension. The terminal device at the friction wrist will be prepositioned in the same way as for a transradial prosthesis. For example, the terminal device will be rotated upward (supinating the terminal device instead of upward and downward movement) for holding cards or rotating it downward (pronating the terminal device) for holding onto a rolling pin or a bike handle.

The developmental readiness criteria that should be met before adding a dual-control cable system are usually accomplished at age 4 to 5 years and include (1) mastering operation of the terminal device; (2) ability to tolerate one full rubber band on the hook; (3) understanding the control motion for elbow lifting and locking; and (4) attaining adequate strength and range of motion to operate the dual-control cable system.

The child should be taught the control motions of humeral flexion and scapular abduction. The combination of these two motions helps maintain the forearm in a certain position after lifting. When the elbow is locked, humeral flexion will allow the terminal device to open. When the elbow is unlocked, humeral flexion lifts the forearm and scapular abduction keeps the forearm in position before locking the elbow. The elbow-lock cable is separate from the dual-control cable system. The child may need a more hands-on approach to learn shoulder extension and scapular depression to control the elbow lock. The OT can stand in front or at the back of the child and guide the prosthesis through the control motion. Learning this motion takes time and practice. It is important to provide a variety of bimanual activities in standing and sitting positions that require the child to preposition the forearm, such as buttoning a shirt, tying shoelaces, or pushing a cart.

Externally Powered Prostheses: Transhumeral Level

The options for controlling a prosthesis at the transhumeral level depend on the anatomic presentation of the residual limb. If the child has a longitudinal deficiency and there are residual digits present, the considerations will be different. The digits should then be used to activate control of the terminal device within the socket using either force-sensing resistors or switches. If the child has a transverse deficiency, the triceps muscle is usually chosen for myoelectric control of the opening function of the prosthetic hand. Physiologically, this is the muscle most closely associated with opening the hand. Extending the elbow and opening the hand is more natural than flexing the elbow to open the hand. Also, when the triceps is used in a one-site control system, it is easier to learn to quiet this muscle than the biceps to allow the hand to maintain a grasp while carrying objects. When children lift large objects, it often triggers activation of the biceps muscle. Therefore, in the first myoelectric prosthesis, the triceps is the muscle of choice, and when the child is ready to switch to a two-muscle control system, the biceps is a logical choice for activating the closing function of the hand.

When teaching the child to activate the appropriate muscle, the terminology used must be consistent with the terms that the parents use at home to refer to the residual limb or any nubbins that might be present. As with a transradial-level deficiency, the child must learn to move the tissue at the distal end of the residual limb to activate the muscle. If there are nubbins present, it is much easier for the child to understand the instruction of "move your nubbins up like you are trying to hold something" or "move your nubbins down like you are stretching them out." Touching or tickling the area to be activated may help. It may also be helpful to hold the residual limb so the child does not misunderstand and activate shoulder muscles.

When the child seems to understand the action required, an electrode can be placed on the desired muscle belly and held in place with a cuff or strap. It can then be used to activate either a modified toy or prosthetic hand to reinforce the concept of moving the muscle to cause some action and, eventually, to open the hand.

The fitting process for this deficiency level is the same as described in the transradial section. A cast is taken encapsulating the shoulder, a trial socket is fabricated, and the final prosthesis is then fabricated to match as closely as possible the length of the intact arm for the humeral and forearm segments. A chest strap is used to secure the prosthesis and aid with suspension.

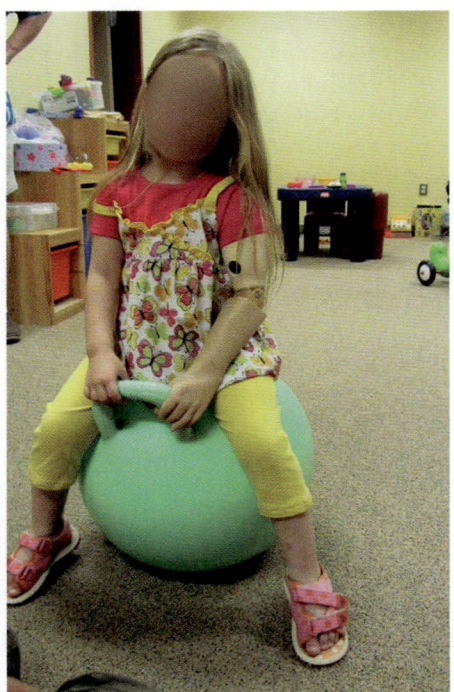

FIGURE 12 Clinical photograph of a child with a transhumeral prosthesis demonstrating the importance of positioning the prosthetic forearm so that the child can focus on functional use of the terminal device.

The strategies for training with an externally powered transhumeral prosthesis are the same as those used with a transradial prosthesis. The focus is on learning to control the hand. Initially the OT or parents will need to position the elbow and wrist in an optimal position for using the hand. Eventually, the child will be able to preposition the hand to function independently (**Figure 12**).

Elbow and wrist units for children will remain as passive or manually locking joints, unless there is a reason to switch to a powered elbow. Powered components such as elbows and wrists add a substantial amount of weight to the prosthesis and are often unnecessary for children who have an intact contralateral hand to use for positioning the prosthetic hand. If an externally powered elbow is considered, control of the elbow should be separate from control of the hand. A simple method is to incorporate a pull switch into the chest strap harness attached to the humeral segment so that when the child abducts the arm, the elbow moves.

Body-Powered Prostheses: Shoulder Disarticulation Level

The readiness criteria used for a young child with a transradial deficiency are similar to activating/fitting a child with a shoulder disarticulation-type prosthesis. As with transradial and transhumeral prostheses, the initial focus is on control of the terminal device. However, in adolescents with a shoulder-level deficiency, positioning of the prosthetic shoulder in flexion/extension and abduction/adduction need to be considered, as well as control of the elbow, wrist, and terminal device. The shoulder may initially be placed in a fixed position of slight flexion and abduction to aid with function and simplify positioning. The young child needs to be able to tolerate some frustration and have a good power source to control the terminal device. A single-control cable with a contralateral thigh strap is recommended for initial active operation of the terminal device. The terminal device will operate with shoulder girdle elevation and trunk rotation, which is a difficult motion for a young child to perform. When teaching the control motion, it is necessary to stabilize the lower trunk and have the child use trunk flexion to open the terminal device. Because the shoulder disarticulation prosthesis has limited function, it will take much effort by the family to encourage the child to wear and use this type of prosthesis. The OT will use the same techniques and provide the child with bimanual activities to encourage use and skill development.

The readiness to learn how to operate the forearm lift and elbow lock operation is the same for a transhumeral prosthesis. The prosthesis will need a dual-control cable rather than a single-control cable, and the elbow lock can be connected to a chin nudge control. The child will use shoulder girdle elevation and trunk rotation on the prosthetic side, while stabilizing the lower trunk to lift the forearm. The elbow lock will be locked and unlocked when the nudge button is pushed by the child's chin. The child should learn the motion as a combined motion of forearm lifting and elbow locking from the beginning. A flexion stop, which limits the full range of motion of the forearm, may initially be used for safety. When the child has established good control of the forearm motion, the flexion stop may be removed.

Externally Powered Prostheses: Shoulder Disarticulation Level

When the shoulder joint is absent, the muscles chosen to operate the terminal device for myoelectric control must be proximal to the shoulder. The orientation of the electrode on the muscle fibers of the chosen muscle will be important to consider. Myoelectric control at this level becomes more complex because the muscles required to operate the functions of the prosthetic hand are not physiologically associated with the intended function and are sometimes confusing for a child to learn.

Other options for control at this level are use of push switches or force-sensing resistors; the latter provide proportional control based on proportional pressure on the surface of the touchpad. Push switches can be used when the child can elevate, depress, protract, and retract his or her shoulder to activate control over various prosthetic components. A single switch can be used with a simple "cookie crusher" control circuit to operate a prosthetic hand. Dual-action switches can be used to operate elbow motion, where a small shoulder motion activates elbow flexion and a larger shoulder motion activates elbow extension.[21] When fitting a child at this level, it is best to begin simply with control of the terminal device as the only powered component.

Transcarpal and Partial Hand Deficiencies

Amputation levels distal to the wrist have many functional advantages over those above the wrist. If the length of the forearm is equal to the contralateral limb and the wrists are equal in length, body posture will be symmetric. The limb can be very useful as a support for holding objects while manipulating objects with the dominant hand. If there are any nubbins present on the residual limb, they may also be used to manipulate objects.

Many children with a deficiency at this level prefer to use their residual limb and do not tolerate full-time wear of a prosthesis. The advantages of kinesthetic feedback and proprioception will usually outweigh the grasping function of a prosthesis. It is important, however, to offer prosthetic options to these children because their needs and desires will change as they age.

The most common choice for an assistive device for these children is an opposition post (**Figure 13**), which is sometimes referred to as a paddle or opposition splint. This is a simple device that attaches to the limb with a distal and proximal bracelet and provides a flat, hard surface to oppose the distal residual limb. The pad of the post can be covered with a friction surface to assist with more adequate grip. The opposition post allows the child to hold objects using the remaining part of the palm by flexing at the wrist. Using utensils, markers, toothbrushes, and toys with handles becomes much easier with the ability to hold with both "hands." The opposition post typically needs to be customized for thin, medium, or thick objects. A child may be fit with multiple posts for different activities. An opposition post for thin objects, such as paper or playing cards, will not be able to hold large objects, such as a baseball bat or bike handle (**Figure 14**).

A push-button multipositional post may be used so that the child can be fit with one post for various activities.

Some parents or children will want to pursue prosthetic fitting despite the fact that the prosthesis will likely be longer than the contralateral limb. Before proceeding with a fitting, it may be helpful to demonstrate the expected overall length to parents using a drawing of the limb with the additional space required for wrist units and a terminal device. The parents can then make an informed choice to continue with the fitting or to explore other options and adaptations.

If a myoelectric prosthesis is chosen, site selection and training will follow the same process as described in the transradial section of this chapter.

Bilateral Upper Limb Deficiency

The team approach is crucial in the care of a child with bilateral or multiple limb loss. The therapist, prosthetist, and team can provide assistance with home activities, instructions, adaptive equipment, and psychosocial support. A child with high-level congenital limb loss may not reach developmental milestones within the typical time frames. He or she may need additional time to acquire gross and fine motor skills and will perform tasks in an adapted manner. The child should be encouraged to move and use all available limbs during play. Parents should be reminded not to overdress the child because there is less skin surface area for heat dissipation. Excessive clothing also restricts the child's movements, making it difficult to achieve motor skills. Ample range of motion and flexibility in the trunk and remaining lower limbs will be helpful in completing tasks and activities.

For a child with high-level bilateral upper limb loss, prostheses may assist with eating, writing, and limited dressing and hygiene; however, prostheses cannot provide complete independence. The child will need to rely on modified body movements, adaptive equipment, mouth use, and foot use for many self-care tasks. The development of foot skills will occur naturally if the child is given the opportunity to use his or her feet. Providing age-appropriate fine motor activities will enhance the dexterity and use of the child's toes. The feet provide sensory feedback and

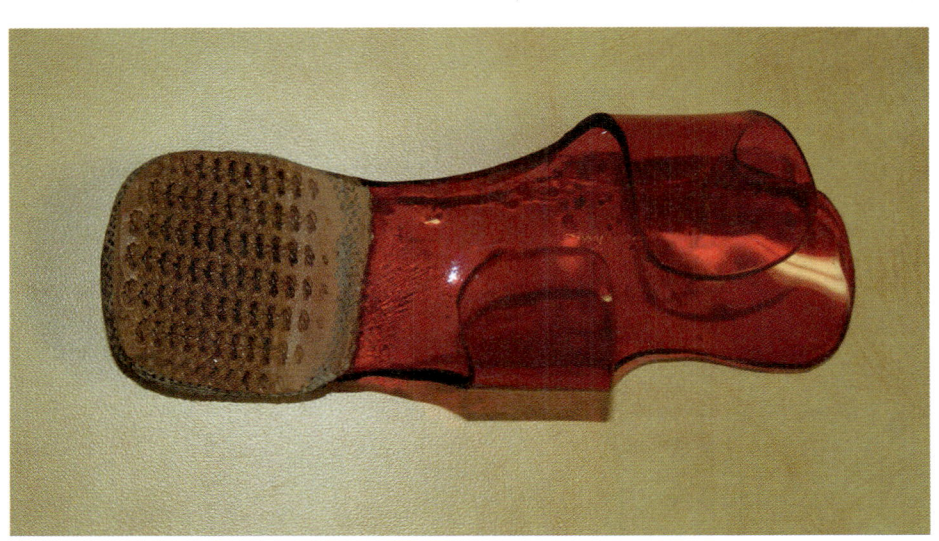

FIGURE 13 Photograph of an opposition post, which is a commonly used prosthetic device for a child with a partial hand deficiency. The device attaches to the limb with a distal and proximal bracelet and provides a flat, hard surface and a post for opposition.

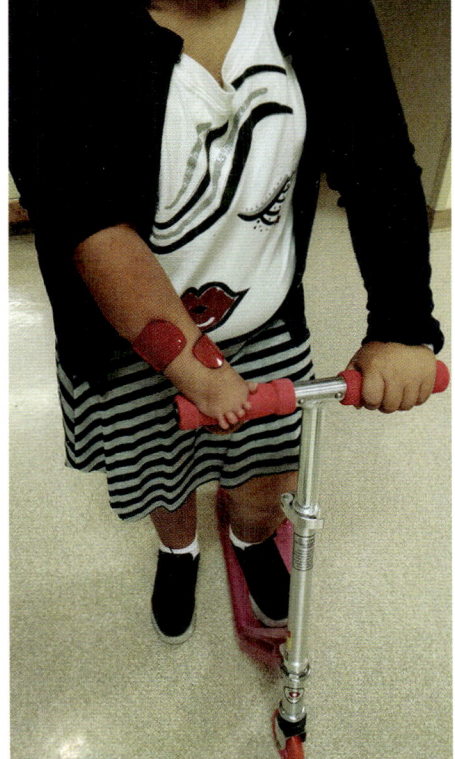

FIGURE 14 Clinical photograph of a child using a larger-sized opposition post that fits the handle of a scooter.

precision that prostheses do not provide. Most children prefer to use foot skills over using their prosthesis/prostheses (**Figures 15** and **16**).

For a child missing both arms with residual arm lengths that can touch each other, the child will likely become accustomed to using a bimanual pattern to perform daily tasks. The child is able to feel the objects in his or her residual arms and can manipulate the objects to incorporate them into activities, including self-feeding with a fork or spoon, teeth brushing, grooming, hygiene, and writing (**Figure 17**). If the child chooses not to use prostheses, he or she will use compensatory techniques and may require adaptive equipment to complete some tasks.

Prosthetic Considerations

If a family decides to pursue fitting for their child with one or two prostheses, early fitting is preferable to establish a consistent wearing pattern. Often, early fitting is not possible because of the child's delays in attaining motor skills and family concerns. For children with bilateral upper limb loss, there is not a formula or standard method of fitting because each case is different and often complex. In some instances, it is beneficial to fit the child with one prosthesis initially to evaluate how he or she adapts before considering fitting both arms. It may be beneficial to fit the nondominant side if there is some functional use of the dominant side (**Figure 18**). Alternatively, it may be beneficial to fit the side with more length and range of motion to better incorporate the prosthesis into specific tasks or activities. Many factors must be taken into consideration by the team during the prosthetic prescription phase. It is extremely important that the prosthesis or prostheses do not interfere with the child's development. The prostheses should be made as lightweight as possible by using endoskeletal prosthetic components. Terminal devices should be carefully chosen because the prosthesis will be used for dominant-hand tasks. It is important to establish a consistent wearing pattern; however, it should be expected that the prosthesis will not be worn full-time.

Passive Prosthetic Fitting

For a child with bilateral transradial limb deficiencies, he or she can be fit with a prosthesis when good sitting balance has been achieved. The team and family can decide if one or two prostheses are beneficial for the child because the child will likely use the prostheses to support body weight and perform simple tasks. For a child with bilateral transhumeral loss or amelia, the child is more likely to be fit when he or she is safely walking. Children with bilateral amelia or those with very short transhumeral limb deficiencies may need to wear a helmet for protection when learning to walk because of the inability to protect themselves from falls.

The child with amelia at the shoulder level can be fit with one prosthesis initially. Typically, the single prosthesis will be fit on the side opposite of the child's dominant foot so that the dominant foot may assist with positioning

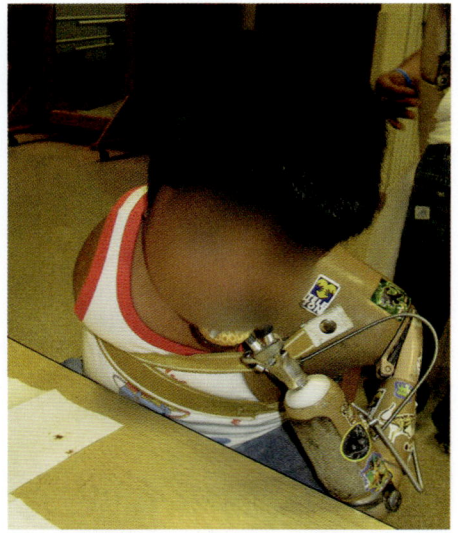

FIGURE 15 Clinical photograph of a child with a bilateral upper limb deficiency using a shoulder disarticulation prosthesis with a hook for self-feeding.

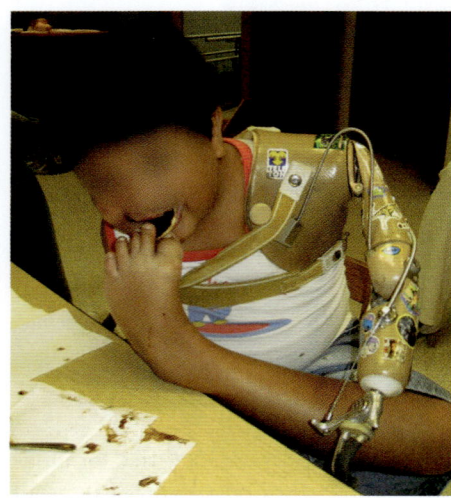

FIGURE 16 Clinical photograph of the child in Figure 15 using his foot for self-feeding.

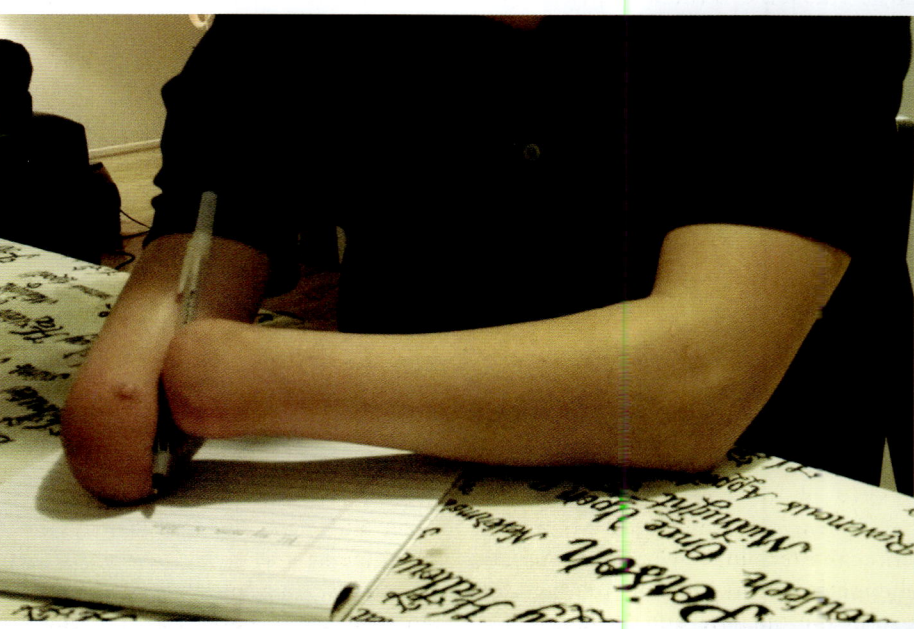

FIGURE 17 Clinical photograph of a child demonstrating bimanual use of residual limbs.

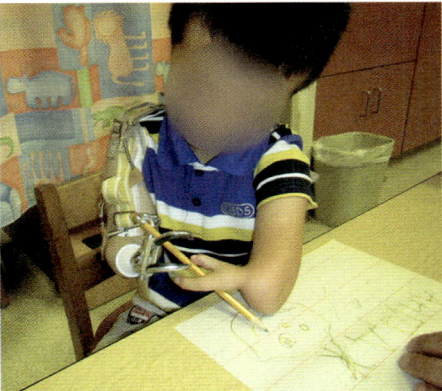

FIGURE 18 Clinical photograph of a child with bilateral limb deficiencies using his dominant limb to position an object in the terminal device of his prosthesis.

of the prosthesis. This prosthesis will not be used to support body weight for activities such as crawling.

Bilateral Transradial Body-Powered Prostheses

The criteria for readiness for fitting with an active prosthesis are the same as the readiness criteria for a unilateral fitting.

Initial control training for bilateral transradial cable-activated prostheses begins with the OT assisting as one prosthesis is moved into humeral flexion to demonstrate how the terminal device opens and then placing an object into the terminal device. This training continues until the child initiates the control motion and the OT assists the child in closing the terminal device. When the child is at a table, he or she can learn to push objects with the opposite limb or with the second prosthesis (if both sides are fit) into the open terminal device. The child needs to learn to time the closure of the terminal device with the grasping of the object. The child will continue to practice until the control motion is refined. He or she is then taught the second control motion, biscapular abduction to open the terminal device near the midline of the body. More advanced skills include learning how to preposition the terminal devices adequately, eliminating cross-control, refining the size of the opening and closing of the terminal device, and repositioning an

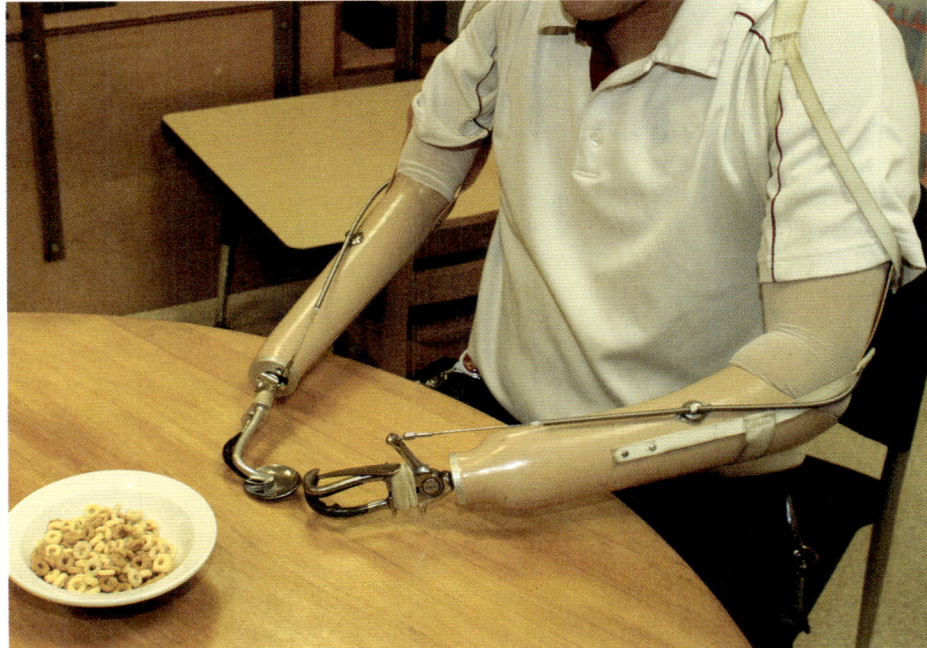

FIGURE 19 Clinical photograph of a bilateral upper limb amputee using one hook to position a utensil in the second hook.

object in the terminal device by using one hook to position the other hook (**Figure 19**).

Bilateral Transhumeral Body-Powered Prostheses

The length of the residual transhumeral limb, shoulder range of motion, and strength all must be adequate for the child to successfully operate transhumeral prostheses. A child with short residual limb length and weakness typically has difficulty lifting the weight of the prostheses to place the terminal device in the best position for function and gains little from the prostheses.

Initial prosthetic control training should begin with a single-control cable system and a pull tab to operate the elbow. The single-control cable system requires less force to open the terminal device when the forearm is at 90° of flexion. Children between the ages of 2 and 3 years typically do not have the range of motion, strength, or understanding to operate a dual-control cable system. The training on how to open and close the terminal device is the same as that given for a transradial prosthesis. An adult assists with prepositioning the forearm with the pull tab to operate the elbow.

When the child has mastered opening and closing the terminal device, he or she will next be taught how to preposition the terminal devices, preposition the turntable on a positive locking elbow (if one is used), eliminate cross-control (if possible), transfer an object from one terminal device to the other, and refine the size of the opening of the terminal device.

Bilateral Amelia at the Shoulder Level

If a child with bilateral amelia at the shoulder level is fitted, the child will likely only be fitted on one side. The child may progress to bilateral fitting; however, this is not recommended because of the excessive weight, discomfort, decreased mobility, and lack of functional use of the prostheses. The child is more likely to be fitted with bilateral cosmetic prostheses rather than bilateral functional prostheses.

The child with bilateral amelia is more likely to be fitted with electric components for an active prosthesis. The push-button switch control will be placed at the top part of the shoulder disarticulation socket. The child will use shoulder elevation to activate the button to open the terminal device.

When the child relaxes the shoulder away from the button, the terminal device will close.

The OT assists the child in learning the control motion and places objects in the terminal device. The OT or other adults may need to assist the child to preposition the shoulder, elbow, and wrist. The child may incorporate the prosthesis into play, learning how to grasp and release objects from a table, carry lightweight objects, scribble, color with markers, or eat with a swivel spoon secured inside the terminal device.

A shoulder disarticulation prosthesis for children is typically limited to use in tabletop activities. The goals of functional prosthetic training should include eating, printing, writing, typing, and carrying objects. These children may need adaptations to the environment and may use adaptive equipment, foot skills, and compensatory techniques to complete most activities of daily living ADLs.[16]

Acquired Upper Limb Deficiency

In children with an acquired amputation, the OT interventions and strategies used will vary based on the child's age and the amputation level. Considerations for acquired amputations will be very similar to amputations in adults. If a nontraumatic amputation is planned in advance, the preoperative phase is a great opportunity to discuss and prepare the child and family for surgery and postoperative care. The limb may have been ill (ie, osteosarcoma or vascular disease) for weeks or months before surgery. This is the ideal time to provide education and review proper body mechanics to incorporate the amputated limb into tasks and activities following surgery. In the preoperative and prehabilitation timeframe, the child and family may benefit from alternative techniques or adaptive equipment to help perform daily activities. After surgery, areas to address include wound management, edema control, desensitization, range-of-motion exercises, and maximizing independence in ADLs. Depending on when the OT becomes involved in the care of the child, some of these areas may have been addressed. The child will likely be seen by therapists in an acute care setting before being referred to a prosthetic center.

When the child is first seen in the prosthetic clinic, the acute care instructions should be reviewed. The OT should review desensitization techniques and procedures for mobilization of scar tissue, address phantom sensation or phantom pain, and review range-of-motion exercises for all of the joints of the upper limb (not just the closest joint to the amputation). For example, in a child with a transradial amputation, shoulder range of motion is as important as elbow range of motion. The limb should be wrapped with a self-adhering elastic bandage until edema is controlled. If the bandage is not being applied evenly or consistently at home, a silicone liner can be used instead. The silicone liner also can be helpful in keeping scar tissue supple and for shaping the limb in preparation for prosthetic fitting.

When the wound has healed and edema is resolved, a prosthesis can be considered. The prosthetic options for a child with an acquired amputation are the same as previously discussed for congenital limb deficiencies. If the child is older, he or she may prefer to have an active-grasping prosthesis as the first primary device because all of the child's experience before the amputation was accomplished with two-handed performance of tasks. Replacing the grasp on the amputated side will be viewed as necessary to continue to do things in the accustomed manner. If the child is younger, the grasping patterns may not have been as well established and the perception of need for a prosthesis may not be the same.

For a child with a very short residual limb or with sensitive areas on the residual limb, an active-grasping prosthesis may not be immediately tolerated. The weight of an externally powered prosthesis may cause too much stress on the short residual limb. Also, the forces transferred to the residual limb when using a body-powered or externally powered prosthesis to lift or carry objects may not be tolerated. For these children, a passive or cosmetic prosthesis may be a better initial option, or they may prefer not to wear a prosthesis.

Time should be allocated to address concerns about performing ADLs. For the older child who was previously independent in self-care activities, adaptations should be considered to allow the child to regain independence, even before a prosthesis has been fabricated. This may mean adding zipper pulls to coats to allow the child to use the residual limb to pull up a zipper, using elastic shoelaces or teaching one-handed methods to tie a shoe, and addressing grooming concerns. For the child who has lost the dominant hand, strategies for changing hand dominance for writing, eating, and other daily tasks should be addressed.

Activity-Specific Prostheses

Some children who wear a prosthesis for daily activities may also require a specialized grip or device for recreational or other activities. Activities such as riding a bicycle, swimming, and playing sports or musical instruments require a custom grip for security and comfort while participating in the activity. In some cases, a child may only want to wear a prosthesis for a specific sport or activity and will not wear a prosthesis for other daily activities. Often in competitive sports a prosthesis is not worn because of comfort, safety, or sports regulations. Bike riding can be a concern because the child must be able to securely grip the handlebars but needs to also be able to safely release in case of a fall. The residual limb should never be fastened to the bike handle, however, a special socket can be made to mount on the bicycle so that the residual limb can fit into the socket to provide better steering control (**Figure 20**).

A passive prosthesis can be used with interchangeable terminal devices in place of a hand when being used for specific activities. In some cases, a body-powered prosthesis can be used with a recreational attachment without the use of the harness. Terminal devices are available for many sports including hockey, basketball, baseball, swimming, gymnastics, golf, archery, martial arts, skiing, etc. Terminal devices are also available for playing musical instruments (drums, violin, guitar), weightlifting, kayaking, riding a bicycle, gardening, meal preparation, eating, and using various woodworking or mechanic's tools. These devices all come with a threaded bolt that can be inserted into a standard wrist unit in a prosthesis and can be easily swapped out by the child or the parent for the activity at hand. If multiple attachments are being provided, a quick-disconnect wrist unit may be incorporated into the prosthesis for efficiency in changing TDs.

The OT should spend time training the child to safely perform the desired activity using the optimal recreational attachment and ensure they can remove and insert the various attachments being provided. Training may involve going to outside facilities or sporting areas to practice using the appropriate device. Adjustments or customizations may be necessary to ensure the child can perform the desired activity. A team approach works best to ensure the child's needs are met.

OT Intervention When a Prosthesis Is Not Worn

There are many reasons why an individual will choose to wear or not to wear a prosthesis, and there are studies demonstrating that children will function well whether they wear a prosthesis or not.[4,22-27] However, it is important to continue to discuss prosthetic options and new technologies and components as they become available so that families can make informed decisions for the best care of their children. Care should always be customized for the lifestyle of each child and their family.

For children who decline wearing a prosthesis, regular monitoring by the team remains necessary because the needs of the child and family may change over time. The factors that affect the decision of whether to try a prosthesis may change. In some instances, family issues or other medical concerns make prosthetic fitting a lesser priority, or the functional benefits are not perceived by parents to be sufficient to warrant fitting at an early age. The personality of the child may be a factor. In a rambunctious toddler who is already having problems with general behavioral management, the parents may find fitting of a prosthesis and training to be an unrealistic expectation.

Although the child may function well in performing daily tasks without a prosthesis, the OT should determine how tasks are accomplished so that bad habits, such as poor posture and overusing other body parts (especially teeth for opening packages), can be addressed early to prevent long-term problems. Modifications may be beneficial to allow the child to be independent in dressing and eating. For example, pulling up pants may be easier to accomplish if a loop is sewn into the pants on the side of the residual arm. Zippers on jackets may be easier to fasten with a zipper pull that fits the residual limb. The child can be taught to tie shoelaces with one hand, or shoes can be adapted with elastic laces or fabric hook-and-loop closures. Handles of utensils can be adapted so the residual limb can be used for eating (**Figure 21**).

The OT can help anticipate functional issues and find solutions for performing daily activities. Because each child has differing needs and abilities based on the level of limb loss/absence and personalities and aptitudes, the solutions available are variable. OTs are trained to assess the needs of the child and family and determine whether a change in technique, use of adaptive equipment, or changes to the environment will result in increased functional independence. When assessing the child who does not wear a prosthesis, the OT will address age-appropriate skills in the areas of self-care, including

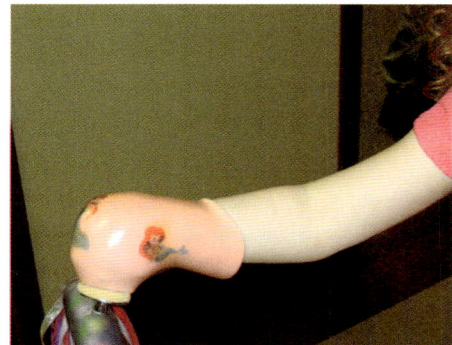

FIGURE 20 Photograph showing an example of adaptive equipment. A special socket is mounted on the handlebar of a bicycle so that the residual limb can fit into the socket to provide better steering control.

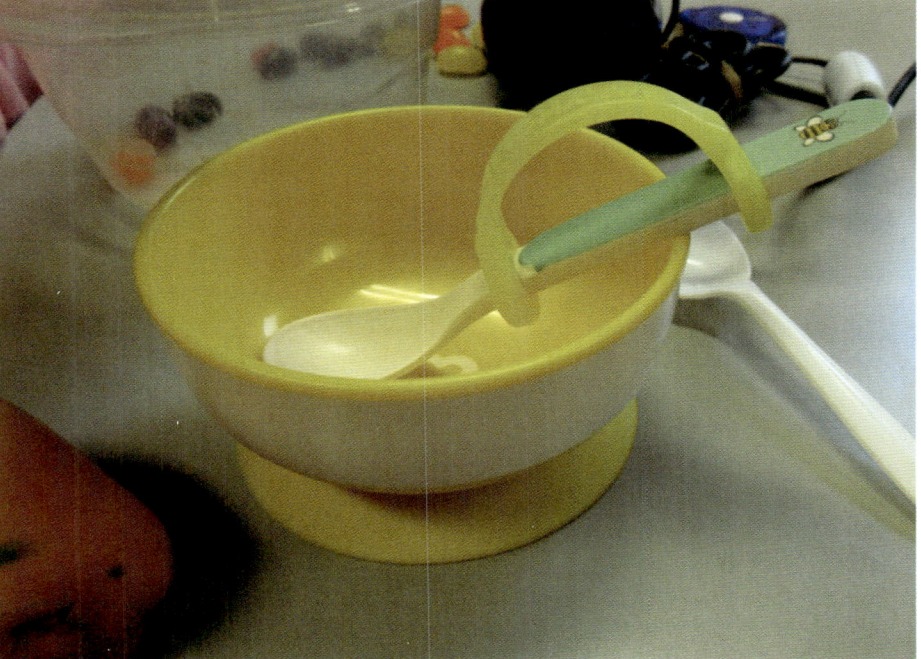

FIGURE 21 Photograph showing an example of adaptive equipment. A special handle is attached to a spoon to allow independent eating using the residual limb.

self-feeding, bathing, toileting and dressing, as well as home activities, school activities, and recreational activities. Home activities may include household chores, and helping with cleaning and making meals.

School activities that may require intervention include desktop activities like holding papers down, opening packages and items for arts and crafts, using playground equipment, and meeting requirements for music or gym classes. It is important for the OT to maintain open communication with the parents and to be available as a resource to the parents and school and/or daycare as functional issues arise. For example, swinging on monkey bars is very difficult when using a prosthesis because maintaining suspension of the prosthesis is usually a concern when it is supporting the child's body weight. If the child wants to play a musical instrument, a strap may be devised to aid in supporting the instrument. Holding a skipping rope may require the rope to be tied around the residual limb, or the handle of the rope can be modified with a fabric hook-and-loop fastener or elastic strap. In some instances, children need to attempt a desired task before they realize they need assistance to find an alternative method to complete it.

SUMMARY

The care of children with upper limb differences has a variety of considerations. The OT and prosthetist provide the family with the education and knowledge to make appropriate prosthetic fitting decisions for their child. There is no single plan of care for every child with an upper limb difference, and there may be trials and errors before the ideal plan is realized. The plan of care is dynamic and should adapt as the child progresses through different stages of development. There may be stages of wearing and not wearing of a prosthesis throughout childhood. The OT should be available to assist with changes in the child's functional ability. The OT will assist with learning to use a prosthesis and incorporating it into ADLs if that is the choice of the child and family. The OT also helps to ensure that the child is able to independently complete ADLs and IADLs that are important to the family, whether the child wears a prosthesis or not.

Because each child is unique, the care for children with upper limb differences is best provided by a unified team of specialists in an upper limb clinic where the needs and goals of the child and the family are the central part of the treatment plan.

References

1. Burger H, Marincek C: Upper limb prosthetic use in Slovenia. *Prosthet Orthot Int* 1994;18(1):25-33.
2. Curran B, Hambrey R: The prosthetic treatment of upper limb deficiency. *Prosthet Orthot Int* 1991;15(2):82-87.
3. Davids JR, Wagner LV, Meyer LC, Blackhurst DW: Prosthetic management of children with unilateral congenital below-elbow deficiency. *J Bone Joint Surg Am* 2006;88(6):1294-1300.
4. Kuyper M-A, Breedijk M, Mulders AH, Post MW, Prevo AJ: Prosthetic management of children in The Netherlands with upper limb deficiencies. *Prosthet Orthot Int* 2001;25(3):228-234.
5. The Association of Children's Prosthetic-Orthotic Clinics: Mission-vision-objectives. Available at: http://www.acpoc.org/mission.asp. Accessed August 25, 2015.
6. American Occupational Therapy Association (AOTA): Occupational therapy practice framework: Domain and process (3rd edition). *Am J Occup Ther* 2014;68(suppl 1):S1-S48.
7. Hubbard S: Powered upper limb prosthetic practice in paediatrics, in Mazumdar A, ed: *Powered Upper Limb Prostheses: Control, Implementation, and Clinical Application*. Springer-Verlag, 2004, pp 85-115.
8. Canavese F, Krajbich JI, LaFleur BJ: Orthopaedic sequelae of childhood meningococcemia: Management considerations and outcome. *J Bone Joint Surg Am* 2010;92(12):2196-2203.
9. Meurs M, Maathuis CG, Lucas C, Hadders-Algra M, van der Sluis CK: Prescription of the first prosthesis and later use in children with congenital unilateral upper limb deficiency: A systematic review. *Prosthet Orthot Int* 2006;30(2):165-173.
10. Hill WL, Hermansson LN: Treatment for children with upper limb difference in various parts of the world: Preliminary findings. *J Prosthet Orthot* 2022; February 4 [Epub ahead of print].
11. Shaperman JL: Early upper limb prosthesis fitting: When and what do we fit. *J Prosthet Orthot* 2003;15(1):11-17.
12. Hahamy A, Sotiropoulos SN, Henderson Slater D, Malach R, Johansen-Berg H, Makin TL: Normalisation of brain connectivity through compensatory behaviour, despite congenital hand absence. *Elife* 2015;4:e04605.
13. Egermann M, Kasten P, Thomsen M: Myoelectric hand prostheses in very young children. *Int Orthop* 2009;33(4):1101-1105.
14. Ibbotson V: Abstract: Congenital upper limb deficient children fitting philosophies in the UK. Instructional Course Abstract: ISPO World Congress, Vancouver, Canada. International Society for Prosthetics and Orthotics, 2007, p 27.
15. Patton J: Occupational therapy, in Smith DG, Michael JW, Bowker JW, eds: *Atlas of Amputations and Limb Deficiencies: Surgical, Prosthetics, and Rehabilitation Principles*, ed 3. American Academy of Orthopedic Surgeons, 2004, pp 813-829.
16. Shaperman J: *Child Amputee Prosthetics Project Manual: Regents of the University of Los Angeles*. Shriners Hospital for Children–Los Angeles Unit, 1997.
17. Hermansson LM: Structured training of children fitted with myoelectric prostheses. *Prosthet Orthot Int* 1991;15(2):88-92.
18. Ottobock website: MyoBoy: Measure-train–simulate–document. Available at: http://professionals.ottobock.ca/cps/rde/xchg/ob_us_en/hs.xsl/6961.html?id=teaser2#teaser2. Accessed September 23, 2015.
19. Hermansson LL: *Assessment of Capacity for Myoelectric Control Manual*. Orebro University Hospital: Liselotte Hermansson, 2011.
20. Johnson SS, Mansfield E: Prosthetic training: Upper limb. *Phys Med Rehabil Clin N Am* 2014;25(1):133-151.
21. Hubbard S: Myoelectric prostheses for the limb-deficient child, in Jaffe K, ed. *Physical Medicine and Rehabilitation Clinics of North America*. WB Saunders, 1991, pp 847-866.
22. Biddiss EA, Chau TT: Upper limb prosthesis use and abandonment: A survey of the last 25 years. *Prosthet Orthot Int* 2007;31(3):236-257.
23. de Jong IG, Reinders-Messelink HA, Janssen WG, Poelma MJ, van Wijk I,

van der Sluis CK: Mixed feelings of children and adolescents with unilateral congenital below elbow deficiency: An online focus group study. *PLoS One* 2012;7(6):e37099.

24. Deans S, Burns D, McGarry A, Murray K, Mutrie N: Motivations and barriers to prosthesis users participation in physical activity, exercise and sport: A review of the literature. *Prosthet Orthot Int* 2012;36(3):260-269.

25. James MA, Bagley AM, Brasington K, Lutz C, McConnell S, Molitor F: Impact of prostheses on function and quality of life for children with unilateral congenital below-the-elbow deficiency. *J Bone Joint Surg Am* 2006;88(11):2356-2365.

26. Routhier F, Vincent C, Morissette MJ, Desaulniers L: Clinical results of an investigation of paediatric upper limb myoelectric prosthesis fitting at the Quebec Rehabilitation Institute. *Prosthet Orthot Int* 2001;25(2):119-131.

27. Vasluian E, de Jong IG, Janssen WG, et al: Opinions of youngsters with congenital below-elbow deficiency, and those of their parents and professionals concerning prosthetic use and rehabilitation treatment. *PLoS One* 2013;8(6):e67101.

General Principles of Limb Salvage Versus Amputations in Children

CHAPTER 72

Federico Canavese, MD, PhD • Joseph Ivan Krajbich, MD, FRCS(C)

ABSTRACT

The major advances in medical technology in the past 20 to 30 years have led to an increasing number of treatment options for patients facing a potential loss of limb. In terms of surgical options, both a variety of limb salvage techniques and more sophisticated, more functional amputation techniques and prosthetic appliances are now available to the treatment team. The rational choice of the procedure is primarily influenced by the age of the patient as well as many other factors such as etiology, comorbidities, functional demand, healing potential, and overall life expectancy. Moreover, the choice of treatment must also consider the socioeconomic reality of the patient.

It is important to describe the main options the patient with a limb-threatening event faces and the factors influencing the decisions.

Keywords: amputation surgery; developing countries; infections; limb salvage; trauma; tumors

Introduction

Very few subspecialties of orthopaedic surgery have experienced as marked an evolution as the field of limb-sparing surgery in the past 30 to 40 years. What used to be a routine amputation treatment for a variety of conditions can currently be, in many instances, treated by a limb-sparing surgery. Even when amputation is necessary, the current techniques frequently allow for the creation of more functional, more distally amputated residual limb. The advances in imaging (MRI, CT), surgical techniques such as microvascular surgery, external fixators' techniques, nerve repair, increased sophistication of internal fixation and vacuum suction dressing for complex wounds, to name just the most important ones, have opened a field for innovative techniques of limb salvage and reconstruction.

In addition, a wide availability of allograft tissue, especially bone, the advent of commercially available biologic modifiers of bone healing such as bone morphogenetic proteins, and advances in the fields of anesthesia and resuscitation have further contributed to the evolution of limb-sparing surgery.

Although it was probably management of malignant tumors of the extremities that led the way in limb-sparing surgery, these techniques are now widely used in any situation where the limb is at risk, such as trauma, infection, vascular abnormalities, and in children with congenital limb deficiencies.

Congenital limb deficiencies in children are more frequent and have less specialized care in developing countries.[1] These inequalities and imbalances are highlighted by epidemiologic data and surveillance records of the various countries, and have been reported and analyzed by the World Health Organization.[2,3] The monumental compendium *Congenital Malformations* by J. Warknay, dealing with the etiology and clinical manifestations of congenital diseases, is considered to be a milestone not only for the field of teratology but for the whole human biology.[4,5] Congenital limb deficiencies comprise most abnormalities requiring specialized care, to which will be added posttraumatic, vascular, and infectious conditions. Therefore, it is important to always refer to the history of teratology and to the current knowledge of embryo teratology and teratogenesis. Knowledge of the anatomy of congenital limb deficiencies, their classification systems,[6-10] and the embryo-teratogenic development[11,12] are important references to guide the choice of treatment and improve care.[13-15]

Despite the aforementioned information, amputation remains the procedure of choice in many instances. Insensate, poorly perfused, functionally useless reconstructed limb is a poor alternative to properly selected and performed amputation and modern prosthetics fitting.

The best procedure for a given problem or situation depends on multiple factors, both objective and subjective. Age and skeletal maturity in children, etiology of the affliction, anatomic involvement, comorbidities, and overall life expectancy of the patient are objective criteria. Functional demands and

---

Dr. Canavese or an immediate family member serves as a board member, owner, officer, or committee member of EPOS. Dr. Krajbich or an immediate family member serves as a board member, owner, officer, or committee member of Scoliosis Research Society.

cultural and psychological acceptance of a given procedure are of a nature that is more subjective. The availability of specialized surgical expertise, modern medical technology, and specialized prosthetic and orthotic services will also play a significant role in a given procedure choice.

Even when amputation, either terminal or intercalary, is required, various limb salvage techniques can be used to make the residual limb more functional. In this sense, the anatomy of congenital limb deficiencies and the study of experimental models of such deficiencies are of fundamental help.[6-10,16-18]

It is imperative to help the reader in the decision making regarding the best approach to a given problem, based on objective principles and published outcome studies.

Differences in Etiology in the Pediatric Age Group Versus Adult Patients

The etiology of amputations is different between adult and pediatric patients (Table 1). In adults, most amputations are performed for complications of peripheral vascular disease, followed by trauma and tumors. The most frequent causes of amputation in children are congenital limb deformities, tumors, trauma, and infections. Other rare conditions are less common. In children as well as in adults, causes of amputations show regional variations and can vary with the type of socioeconomic conditions of each region.[19-33] In this respect, a more up-to-date approach to the most frequent causes of amputation in children as congenital limb deficiencies, tumors, trauma, and infections must also consider the socioeconomic reality of the patient.[1]

Skeletal growth and potential for remodeling have a significant effect on the outcome of both a pediatric amputation and a limb-sparing surgery, particularly in the younger child. For example, a very young child who undergoes an transfemoral amputation will have an extremely short residual limb at skeletal maturity because of the loss of the distal femoral physis, causing a loss of approximately 1.2 cm per year until the end of growth. Similarly, a 10-year-old child who has a successful total femur endoprosthesis will have a lower limb discrepancy at maturity because of the loss of both proximal and distal femoral physis of the affected leg and the continuing growth of the contralateral limb. Remaining growth must be taken into account when limb-sparing surgery or amputations are planned so as to provide the best esthetic and functional outcomes as children have higher functional demand compared with adults (who are more sedentary are often more overweight).

Stunted growth, painful overgrowth, and growth disturbances such as limb shortening and/or limb deviation can develop in children. Moreover, treatment can be lengthy with significant psychological consequences. In some cases, treatment can last several years, thus leading young amputees and their caretakers to face decades of potential pain, psychological consequences, and difficulties with daily life activities such as eating, playing, and doing schoolwork. In some other cases, when neoplasms are the cause of amputations, the emotional aspect is particularly important because of the evolution of the disease and the expectations of surgery.[19-33] The context presented previously, and partly analyzed, is broad and difficult. However, it is an opportunity to consider and take note of the multiplicity and richness of the scientific achievements of recent decades, which have made it possible to face complex situations, solve difficult problems, and find methods and solutions that were judged to be at the limit of the possible, for example, the unthinkable rebirth of many amputees and the success of the Paralympic Games that has made everyone aware of the incredible lives of so many young amputees.

Peripheral Vascular Disease

Vascular amputations are almost exclusively performed in adult patients. In the adult age group, major causes of amputation are diabetes and/or peripheral arterial disease resulting in painful limb, poor limb perfusion, untreatable ulcers, or gangrene (with or without infection). The prevalence of peripheral arterial disease in the general population ranges between 12% and 14%, affecting up to 20% of adults older than 70 years. In this situation, the emphasis is primarily on prevention of ischemia by medical and surgical means. Once a limb becomes nonviable, standard amputations such as transtibial and transfemoral are usually used.

Trauma Amputations

Traumatic amputations are more frequent in adults compared with children.

In children, amputations secondary to trauma represent approximately 5% of all injuries. Every year, approximately one-third of traumatic amputation injuries occur among children younger than 18 years.[34,35] Approximately 80% of all

TABLE 1 Etiology and Frequency of Amputations According to Patients (Pediatric Versus Adult) and Etiology

Etiology	Adults	Children	Sex Ratio	Limb
Peripheral vascular disease	++++	−	M = F	LE
Trauma	+++	+	M > F	LE > UE 8:2 in children 2:1 in adults
Tumors	++	++	M = F	LE > UE
Infections	++	++	M = F	LE > UE
Burns				
Electric injuries	+	+/−	M > F in adults	LE = UE
Chemical burns	++	+/−		
Thermal burns	++	+++	M = F in children	
Cold injuries	++	+/−		

F = female, LE = lower extremity, M = male, UE = upper extremity amputations affect the lower limb with the remainder in the upper limb,[36,37] and most cases of major amputations following trauma in children involve the lower extremity, in particular the tibia. More than 95% of amputations secondary to trauma in children equally affect the foot or toes and the hand or fingers.[38] Hostetler et al found most traumatic amputations involve fingers caught in closing doors in children (predominantly males) younger than 2 years. However, such amputations are often minor and, in most cases, do not compromise upper limb function. Older children, preadolescents, and adolescents experience a higher proportion of more serious amputation injuries, mostly related to high-energy trauma (lawn mower accidents, bike, motorbike, and road traffic accidents). In particular, studies have found that road traffic accidents are responsible for approximately two-thirds of amputations in older children.[36-38] Those percentages are significantly higher in adults. In children, skeletal immaturity predisposes to higher rate of complications such as terminal overgrowth.[39,40] However, such complications are less severe in the pediatric populations compared with adult patients.

Malignant Tumors

Amputation has long been the mainstay of treatment of soft-tissue and bone tumors. During the past 2 to 3 decades, limb-sparing surgery has become increasingly popular. Currently, limb-sparing procedures have become the first choice of treatment (when technically feasible) of bone and soft-tissue sarcomas, whereas amputations are performed in selected cases only.[41-43] Limb-sparing techniques provide slightly better functional outcome compared with amputations. de Bari et al reported that patients undergoing amputation for Ewing sarcoma or osteosarcoma had poorer outcome compared with patients undergoing limb-sparing surgery. In particular, they found increased pain, decreased function, less satisfactory emotional appearance, and poorer gait.[41] However, patients with amputations for bone and soft-tissue sarcomas experience fewer complications from the surgery compared with patients with limb-sparing surgeries, although complications from limb-sparing techniques are usually manageable. Overall, the rate of local recurrence after amputation is similar to limb-sparing procedures, ranging from 5% to 10%. Similarly, long-term survival is the same, ranging from 70% to 80% in the two patient populations.

Burn Injuries

Burn injuries are more frequent in adults compared with children. Burns can be subclassified as thermal (fire, frostbite), electrical, and chemical.[44-49]

Electric Injuries

High-tension electric burns potentially leading to amputations usually involve adult workers or electrical installation vandals[44,50] and are less common in children. The passage of electric current through the human body can produce diverse and serious injuries to the brain, heart, muscles, and skin. This is because the human body conducts electricity very well. High-voltage electric injuries often cause burns and blunt trauma. Direct contact with electric current can be lethal, and the extent of lesions is related to the voltage of current. As a rule of thumb, it must be remembered that burns secondary to electricity are often much worse than they initially appear. Electrical burns have a tendency to affect a relatively small body surface compared with burns because of hot liquids or fire. However, electric burns can cause a deep tissue injury.[44-46,50] Injuries result from both the luminous bridging when current is shorted and the direct conduction of the current through the patient. Fractures resulting from severe muscle contractions or falls (also known as indirect injuries) characterize patients as victims of electric burns. Mortality rate ranges between 3% and 15% and are related to the length of electrical contact.[44,46,47,50]

Chemical Burns

Amputations because of chemical burns are uncommon. Overall, amputations secondary to chemical burns are more frequent in adults compared with children. Chemical burns can result from exposure to acid, alkaline, or petroleum solutions. As a rule of thumb, alkali burns tend to be deeper and more serious than burns secondary to acid products.

Thermal Burns

Cooking-related injuries are a common problem worldwide, resulting in more pediatric burns than any other cause. However, thermal burn injuries resulting in amputations are relatively uncommon. The proportion of thermal injuries leading to amputation is particularly high in countries where the custom is to place the fire at floor level, thus predisposing to burns to children who crawl or play inside or around the home. Also, the habit of leaving young, inexperienced children to prepare meals for themselves and siblings is responsible for such injuries in a high proportion of cases. In a significant amount of those patients, burns can be complicated by infection, leading to amputation to reduce the mortality rate.[45,47-49]

Frostbite and Nonfreezing Cold Injuries

Frostbite and nonfreezing cold injuries have frequently affected fit, adult active people such as climbers, expedition members, skiers, mountaineers, and agriculture workers. Frostbite and nonfreezing cold injuries are rare in children, except in countries at high latitudes. Frostbite and nonfreezing cold injuries can be responsible for amputations; the need for amputation is correlated to the duration of cold exposure rather than the temperature. In particular, frostbite injuries can have significant repercussions on the distal end of the extremities (ie, toes and fingers). The spectrum of injuries is heterogeneous, varying from minimal tissue loss with mild long-term sequelae, to major necrosis of the distal limbs with subsequent major amputations and resultant phantom limb pain. Injury to the epiphyseal plate of phalanges in children living in high northern latitudes is not uncommon.[49]

Infections (Purpura Fulminans)

Purpura fulminans is an infrequent but potentially catastrophic condition that follows a meningococcal infection. In recent years, probably because of prompt diagnosis and effective aggressive resuscitation, most children with fulminant meningococcemia have survived. The development of an effective vaccine has had a major effect on the incidence of this condition, with new cases becoming rarer and almost solely confined to the very young age group. However, survivors are at increased risk for complications because of poor tissue perfusion such as soft-tissue loss, autoamputations, and surgical amputations.[34] Following extremity amputations and soft-tissue healing, major issues with the residual extremities often persist. Residual limb overgrowth, growth disturbances, and scar contractures are common results. Custom prosthetic fitting is often required for this patient population.[34]

Limb Salvage Techniques and Amputations: Principles, Indications, and Contraindications in Trauma, Malignant Tumors, Infections, and Burn Injuries

There are many different types of limb-sparing techniques as well as several types of limb amputations, depending on the nature of the disease. In terms of surgical options both a variety of limb-sparing techniques and more sophisticated, more functional amputation techniques and prosthetic appliances are now available to the treatment team.

In children, skeletal immaturity predisposes to a higher rate of complications as the limb continues to grow, leading to stunted growth, painful overgrowth, and growth disturbances such as limb shortening and/or limb deviation. Transosseous amputations in children are characterized by significant appositional bone growth, not usually seen in adults. In addition, children have higher functional demand compared with more sedentary adults and have lower phantom limb incidence compared with adults.[34,38,51]

Trauma

Severe traumatic injuries of the extremities can be managed with amputations or limb salvage techniques. In terms of surgical options, both a variety of limb salvage techniques and more sophisticated, more functional amputation techniques and prosthetic appliances are available to the treatment team. The rational choice of the procedure is primarily influenced by the severity of the injury, the location of the injury, the time of ischemia, and the presence of neurologic compromise.[35-37]

Even in the acute situation of trauma the main principles of optimizing the functional outcome of the affected limb and limbs should be applied. This is particularly so in children in whom limb(s) need to remain functional for decades. Preserving the length, major epiphyseal plates, and proximal joints and minimizing transosseous amputations is of major importance. Vascular repairs, nerve repairs, use of discarded parts for fashioning end-bearing residual limbs, shortening osteotomies to provide soft-tissue coverage for the articular end of the bone to preserve the distal epiphyseal plate and prevent the overgrowth phenomena all can be used in this situation provided that the treating team is cognizant and well versed in these principles and techniques.

The decision to perform an amputation is usually taken immediately as part of primary treatment (primary amputation) or during hospital stay when the nature of the trauma and associated complications make persistence with an attempt at limb salvage unwise (secondary amputation).

In severe injuries to the extremities, primary amputation is usually necessary as part of lifesaving treatment. Primary amputations should be performed as a damage control procedure, when hemorrhage is incontrollable or when ischemia has lasted for more than 6 hours. The main objective is to stabilize and resuscitate the patient. Primary amputations are also indicated in incomplete traumatic amputations with a distal remnant that is significantly injured (crush injuries).

However, ischemia exceeding 4 hours, segmental muscle loss exceeding two compartments, and bone loss greater than one-third of the length of the bone are not absolute indications for primary amputations, and limb-sparing techniques can be considered. Absent or reduced plantar sensation is not an indication for primary amputation.

In skeletally mature patients (adolescents and adults), in case of amputation, whether primary or secondary, joints and length should be preserved as much as possible and, when needed, transtibial and transfemoral amputations should be preferred to transarticular amputations at the more proximal joint. In every case the functional proximal joint should be salvaged whenever possible (knee, hip). Energy expenditure for a transtibial amputee is approximately twice less compared with transfemoral cases. Bilateral transtibial cases incur an extra energy cost of more than 40%, whereas those with bilateral amputations where one level is transfemoral may have to double their energy costs simply to ambulate.[36-38]

Soft-tissue coverage is often an issue in severely injured patients. Adequate techniques should be used for limb salvage procedure and amputation levels should be optimized.[39,40]

Malignant Tumors

Malignant bone tumors are likely the most important diagnostic category in terms of a limb salvage versus amputation decision. There are several reasons for this.

The first one is the fact that the surgical decision has a major implication in terms of the patient's survival and potential future functionality. Overall, when malignant bone and soft-tissue tumors can be properly excised and adequate resection margins performed, limb salvage surgery, as opposed to amputation, is the standard treatment in patients with sarcomas of the extremities. It is mandatory that the procedure chosen allow for wide resection with clean margins of the tumor unless a palliative procedure is deliberately chosen. Residual, even microscopic, tumor will almost certainly lead to local recurrence, with its effect on patient survival.

Second, the procedure should be carefully weighted in terms of survival, longevity, and long-term complications. This is particularly so in young children with major skeletal growth ahead of them.

Third, with modern sarcoma protocols of neoadjuvant chemotherapy, with a surgical procedure usually planned several weeks, sometimes even months, after the diagnosis and initial staging, there is time to gather all the relevant information about the lesion such as all the modern imaging, accurate diagnosis, accurate staging, and chemotherapy response to select and plan the optimal procedure for the given patient. It also allows for assembly, if needed, of the multisubspecialty team and procurement of the needed surgical equipment and possible implants such as endoprosthesis or allograft bone of the appropriate size.

Last, the procedure chosen under the circumstances must ensure viable limb, which is sensate and functional, because insensate, poorly perfused, painful, poorly functional limb is a poor substitute for a well-fashioned amputation residual limb fitted with a well-crafted modern prosthesis.

The location of the tumor, resection margins, risk of recurrence, potential complications, and limb function must be considered when planning limb-sparing surgery and amputations.

Limb-sparing surgery should be preferred to amputation if the tumor is located in the extremity skeleton (limbs) if adequate wide resection margins can be achieved, if the recurrence risk is no greater and survival is no worse than with amputation, if potential complications do not exceed potential benefits, if the proposed limb-sparing technique is enduring and not associated with a high number of complications, leading to secondary procedures and frequent hospitalizations, and if predicted limb function is equal to or better than that potentially obtained with amputation.

When the patient's life expectancy is reduced (usually because of the presence of metastatic disease) and palliation is the primary goal of the orthopaedic treatment, the procedure selected should be the one that is the least likely to produce significant morbidity, ensures the fastest recovery, and allows for the best pain control and functional outcome. That usually means either endoprosthetic replacement or amputation.

Relative contraindications to performing limb-sparing techniques are pathologic fractures (fracture hematoma extending beyond compartment limits), inappropriately performed biopsy, infection of the surgical site, predicted limb-length discrepancy more than 8 to 10 cm, extensive soft-tissue involvement, poor response to preoperative chemotherapy, and when vascular bypass is not feasible when tumor invades major neurovascular structures.[37,38,50,51]

Outcomes for different surgical procedures are very often comparable (**Table 2**). The choice of one procedure versus another must be based on a discussion with the patient and their family and after assessing the features of the tumor. Treatment must be tailored to each patient.

Infections (Purpura Fulminans)

Patients who have had purpura fulminans are at increased risk for complications because of poor tissue perfusion such as soft-tissue loss, autoamputations, and surgical amputations.

Identification of viable tissues, use of adequate imaging techniques, limb function, and potential complications must be considered when planning amputations in survivors from purpura fulminans.[34]

Before performing a surgical amputation, it is mandatory to wait for clear demarcation between viable and nonviable tissues. In particular, attention should be paid to a delay in surgical amputation until gangrene (necrosis) is clearly established and demarcated, particularly with respect to deep tissues, as it will allow selection of the right level of amputation. There is no need for early amputation as long as no life-threatening wet gangrene is present in the extremities.

Adequate imaging techniques should be used before surgical amputation is performed. In particular, a technetium bone scan will help with determining clear demarcation of the necrotic tissue and aid in selection of the level of amputation.

To preserve limb function, the surgeon should preserve joints (in particular, the knee and ankle) whenever possible, as well as length, to avoid short residual limbs. In particular, transosseous amputations should be avoided whenever possible (metaphyseal-diaphyseal segment resection with shortening but preservation of the distal epiphysis and joint surface if need be), that is, Syme amputation versus transtibial amputation.[40,44,45]

Complications are relatively frequent, even after amputations. It should be kept in mind that epiphyseal plates beneath areas of skin necrosis and limbs free of amputation are also at risk of developing growth arrest.[34]

The treating surgeon must be prepared to use innovative and sometimes unorthodox techniques to address the bone and soft-tissue issues (both early and late) in these patients to achieve optimal functional results.[39]

Burn Injuries

Amputation is sometimes required as part of lifesaving burn care. However, it is required for nonsalvageable limbs.[24-33] Amputations are also performed in cases with extensive tissue necrosis or in cases complicated by infection. In cases of extensive tissue necrosis or in cases complicated by infection, amputation

TABLE 2 Surgical Options: Types of Limb-Sparing Surgeries

Limb-Sparing Techniques
Local tissue flaps, transfers, and excisions
Autologous transfers
Allograft transplants
Endoprosthetics
Composite systems
Intercalary resections
Bone transfers

can reduce the mortality rate. The role of the limb salvage is relatively limited in this group of patients and consists almost solely of securing soft-tissue coverage over the exposed deep tissues. Skin grafts, skin flaps on occasionally bone-shortening osteotomies, can be of benefit. Flaps, skin grafts, and vacuum suction dressings may need to be used to address the remaining wound.[29-33]

Overall, in children, bone overgrowth is known to occur in less than 10% of burn amputations. The type of burn does not influence overgrowth, and lower limb amputations are more likely to show overgrowth than upper limb ones.[26] Moreover, burn-related amputations are often combined with other associated injures (polytrauma) that can make care more challenging.

Techniques Available for Limb Salvage and Optimization of Amputation Levels

There have been developments in multiple areas to improve the outcome of limb-sparing techniques and amputations. Although it was probably management of malignant tumors of the extremities that led the way in limb-sparing surgery, the techniques are now widely used in any situation where the limb is at risk, such as trauma, infection, vascular abnormalities, and in children with congenital limb deficiencies. Even when amputation, either terminal or intercalary, is required, various limb salvage techniques can be used to make the residual limb more functional.

Several techniques are available for limb salvage and optimization of amputation levels. The best procedure for a given problem or situation depends on multiple factors, both objective and subjective. Age and skeletal maturity in children, etiology of the affliction, anatomic involvement, comorbidities, and overall life expectancy of the patient in question are objective criteria. Functional demands, and cultural and psychological acceptance of a given procedure are of a more subjective nature. The availability of specialized surgical expertise, modern medical technology, and specialized prosthetic and orthotic services will also play a significant role in a given procedure choice.[41-49,52-54]

Overall, several categories of limb-sparing procedures can be identified: (1) local tissue flaps, transfers, and excisions; (2) autologous transfers; (3) allograft transplants; (4) endoprosthetics; (5) composite systems; (6) intercalary resections; and (7) bone transfers (Table 2).

Significant bone and soft-tissue losses can be reconstructed with different techniques, the main goals being to provide biologic reconstruction, to restore bone stocks, and to preserve joint kinematics as much as possible. In particular, recent growing devices in children are useful not only to bridge the surgical defect but also to correct a residual limb-length discrepancy.

Amputations

Overall, amputations can be divided into three main groups: (1) transarticular; (2) transosseous; and (3) intercalary (Table 3). Despite technical progress made by limb-sparing procedures, amputation remains a procedure of choice in many instances. Insensate, poorly perfused, functionally useless reconstructed limb is a poor alternative to properly selected and performed amputation and modern prosthetics fitting. In general, there are more potential complications with limb salvage than amputation. However, complications from limb-sparing techniques are usually manageable.[41-49,52-57]

SUMMARY

Thanks to major advances in medical and surgical care, the treatment team usually has several options for treatment of a young patient facing a potential limb loss. The choice between various types of limb-sparing surgery and amputation is based on several factors frequently unique to the individual patient. The patient's age, etiology of the disorder, degree of tissue pathology/damage, available surgical, medical, and prosthetic expertise, potential complications, socioeconomic circumstances, and in some cases cultural and parental preferences all have to be considered in making the decision of which way to proceed.

References

1. Perenchio MT, Ricci F: Cerebral palsy in the developing world, in Canavese F, Deslandes J, eds: *Orthopaedic Management of Children with Cerebral Palsy.* Nova Science Publishers, Inc., 2015, pp 388-392.
2. EUROCAT Guide 1.4: *Instruction for the Registration of Congenital Anomalies.* EUROCAT Central Registry, University of Ulster, 2013.
3. WHO/CDC/ICBDSR: *Birth Defects Surveillance: A Manual for Programme Managers.* World Health Organization, 2014.
4. Warkany J: *Congenital Malformations.* Year Book Medical Publishers, 1971.
5. Wilson JG: Presentation of the Howland Award to Josef Warkany, Children's Hospital Research Foundation. Cincinnati, Ohio, USA. *Pediat Res* 1970;4:427-430.
6. Frantz CH, Rapids G, O'Rahilly R: Congenital skeletal limb deficiencies. *J Bone Joint Surg Am* 1961;43-A(8):116-138.
7. Barrow MV: A brief history of teratology to the early 20th century. *Teratology* 1971;4:109-119.

TABLE 3 Surgical Options: Types of Amputation

Amputations		
Transosseous amputation	Transfemoral or above-knee amputation	
	Transtibial or below-knee amputation	
	Transhumeral amputation	
	Transforearm amputation	
Transarticular amputation	Syme amputation (ankle disarticulation)	
	Boyd amputation	
	Transknee amputation	
Intercalary	Rotationplasty	
	Upside-down tibia technique	

8. Gold NB, Westgate MN, Holmes LB: Anatomic and etiological classification of congenital limb deficiencies. *Am J Med Genet* 2011;155A(6):1225-1235.
9. Oberg KC: Classification of congenital upper limb anomalies: Towards improved communication, diagnosis, and discovery. *J Hand Surg* 2019;44(1):4-14.
10. Wilcox WR, Coulter CP, Schmitz ML: Congenital limb deficiency disorders. *Clin Perinatol* 2015;42(2):281-300.
11. Bamshad M, Watkins W, Dixon M, et al: Reconstructing the history of human limb development: Lessons from birth defects. *Pediatr Res* 1999;45:291-299.
12. Barham G, Clarke NM: Genetic regulation of embryological limb development with relation to congenital limb deformity in humans. *J Child Orthop* 2008;2(1):1-9.
13. Aston SA, James G: *Wilson's Six Principles of Teratology*. Embryo Project Encyclopedia. Available at: http://embryo.asu.edu/handle/10776/7893. Accessed September 2, 2021.
14. Jelínek R: Review: The contribution of new findings and ideas to the old principles of teratology. *Reprod Toxicol* 2005;20:295-300.
15. Finnell RH: Teratology: General considerations and principles. *J Allergy Clin Immunol* 1999;103(2 pt 2):S337-S342.
16. Moon A: Mouse models for investigating the developmental basis of human birth defects. *Pediatr Res* 2006;59:749-755.
17. Demirtaş MS: *The Pathogenesis of Congenital Anomalies: Roles of Teratogens and Infections* [Online First]. IntechOpen. Available at: https://www.intechopen.com/online-first/72507. Accessed September 23, 2021.
18. Liu A, ed: *Animal Models of Human Birth Defects*. Springer, 2020.
19. Hostetler SG, Shwartz L, Shields BJ, Xiang H, Smith GA: Characteristics of pediatric traumatic amputations treated in hospital emergency departments: United States, 1990-2002. *Pediatrics* 2005;116:e667-e674.
20. Goldner RD, Fitch RD, Nunley JA, Aitken MS, Urbaniak JR: Demographics and replantation. *J Hand Surg Am* 1987;12:961-965.
21. Roche AJ, Selvarajah K: Traumatic amputations in children and adolescnets: demographics from a regional limb fitting centre in the United Kingdom. *J Bone Joint Surg Br* 2011;93:507-509.
22. Loder RT: Demographics of traumatic amputations in children. Implications for prevention strategies. *J Bone Joint Surg Am* 2004;86:923-928.
23. Vollman D, Smith GA: Epidemiology of lawn-mower-related injuries to children in the United States, 1990-2004. *Pediatrics* 2006;118:e273-e278.
24. Love SM, Grogan DP, Ogden JA: Lawn-mower injuries in children. *J Orthop Trauma* 1988;2:94-101.
25. Farley FA, Senunas L, Greenfield ML, et al: Lower extremity lawn-mower injuries in children. *J Pediatr Orthop* 1996;16:669-672.
26. Klimish J, Carmichael KD, Muradov P, Evans EB: Prevalence of stump overgrowth in pediatric burn patient amputations. *J Pediatr Orthop* 2011;31:216-219.
27. Rai J, Jeschke MG, Barrow RE, Herndon DN: Electrical injuries: A 30-years review. *J Trauma* 1999;46:933-936.
28. Luz DP, Millan LS, Alessi MS: Electrical burns: A retrospective analysis across a 5-years period. *Burns* 2009;35:1015-1019.
29. Baker MD, Chiaviello C: Hosehold electrical injuries in children. Epidemiology and identification of avoidable hazards. *Am J Dis Child* 1989;143:59-62.
30. Dim EM, Amanari OC, Nottidge TE, Inyang UC, Nwashindi A: Bilateral lower limb amputations in a Nigerian child following high-voltage electrical burns injury: A case report. *Malys Orthop J* 2013;7:45-47.
31. Loro A, Franceschi F: Prevalence and causal conditions for amputation surgery in third world: Ten years experience at Dodoma regional hospital Tanzania. *Prosthet Orthot Int* 1999;23:217-224.
32. Dissanaike S, Boshart K, Coleman S, et al: Cooking-related paediatric burns: Risk factors and the role of differential cooling rate among acommonly implicated substances. *J Burn Care Res* 2009;30:593-598.
33. Kennedy PJ, Young WM, Deva AK, Hertsch PA: Burns and amputations: A 24-years experience. *J Burn Care Res* 2006;27:183-188.
34. Canavese F, Krajbich JI, LaFleur B: Orthopedic sequelae of childhood meningococcemia: Management considerations and outcome. *J Bone Joint Surg Am* 2010;92:2196-2203.
35. Akahane T, Shimizu T, Isobe K, et al: Evaluation of postoperative general quality of life for patients with osteosarcoma around the knee joint. *J Pediatr Orthop B* 2007;16:269-272.
36. Waters RL, Perry J, Antonelli D, Hislop H: Energy cost of walking of amputees: The influence of level of amputation. *J Bone Joint Surg Am* 1976;58:42-46.
37. Mavrogenis AF, Coll-Mesa L, Gonzalez-Gaitano M, et al: Criteria and outcome of limb salvage surgery. *J BUON* 2011;16:617-626.
38. Donati D, Benedetti MG, Catani F, Berti L, Capanna R: Gait analysis after rotationplasty hip surgery for malignant tumor of the proximal femur. *Rev Chir Orthop Reparatrice Appar Mot* 2004;90:561-568.
39. Canavese F, Kuang A, Krajbich JI: Application of the Vacuum Assisted Closure in pediatric patients with orthopedic sequelae of meningococcemia: Report of a case successfully treated. *J Pediatr Orthop B* 2009;18:388-391.
40. McClenaghan BA, Krajbich JI, Pirone AM, Koheil R, Longmuir P: Comparative assessment of gait after limb-salvage procedures. *J Bone Joint Surg Am* 1989;71:1178-1182.
41. de Bari A, Krajbich JI, Langer F, Hamilton EL, Hubbard S: Modified Van Nes rotationplasty for osteosarcoma of the proximal tibia in children. *J Bone Joint Surg Br* 1990;72:1065-1069.
42. Winkelmann WW: Hip rotationplasty for malignant tumors of the proximal part of the femur. *J Bone Joint Surg Am* 1986;68:362-369.
43. Davids JR, Meyer LC, Blackhurst DW: Operative treatment of bony overgrowth in children who have an aquired or congenital amputation. *J Bone Joint Surg Am* 1995;77:1490-1497.
44. Alman BA, Krajbich JI, Hubbard S: Proximal femoral focal deficiency: Results of rotationplasty and Syme amputation. *J Bone Joint Surg Am* 1995;77:1876-1882.
45. Roux N, Pieterrs S: Prosthetic management 56 years after rotationplasty due to proximal femoral focal deficiency (PFFD). *Prosthet Orthot Int* 2007;31:313-320.
46. Ackman J, Altiok H, Flanagan A, et al: Long-term follow-up of Van Nes rotationplasty in patients with congenital proximal focal femoral deficiency. *Bone Joint J* 2013;95-B:192-198.
47. DiCaprio MR, Friedlaender GE: Malignant bone tumors: Limb sparing versus amputation. *J Am Acad Orthop Surg* 2003;11:25-37.
48. Dasmin J, Pous J, Ghanem I: Therapeutic approach to severe congenital limb discrepancies: Surgical treatment versus prosthetic management. *J Pediatr Orthop B* 1995;4:164-170.

49. Van Nes CP: Transplantation of the tibia and fibula to replace the femur following resection; turn-up-plasty of the leg. *J Bone Joint Surg Am* 1948;30:854-858.
50. Torode IP, Gillepsie R: Rotationplasty of the lower limb for congenital defects of the femur. *J Bone Joint Surg Br* 1983;65:569-573.
51. Krajbich JI, Carroll NC: Van Nes rotationplasty with segmental limb resection. *Clin Orthop Rel Res* 1990;256:7-13.
52. Harris RI: Syme's amputation: The technical details essential for success. *J Bone Joint Surg Br* 1956;38:614-621.
53. Boyd RH: Amputation of the foot with calcaneotibial arthrodesis. *J Bone Joint Surg Am* 1939;21:997-1001.
54. Kotz R, Salzer M: Rotationplasty for childhood osteosarcoma of the distal part of the femur. *J Bone Joint Surg Am* 1982;64:959-969.
55. Aksnes LH, Bauer HC, Jebsen NL, et al: Limb-sparing surgery preserves more function than amputation: A Scandinavian sarcoma group study of 118 patients. *J Bone Joint Surg Br* 2008;90:786-794.
56. Pisters PW, O'Sullivajn B, Maki RG: Evidence based recommendations for local therapy for soft tissue sarcomas. *J Clin Oncol* 2007;25:1003-1008.
57. Varan A, Yazici N, Aksoy C, et al: Treatment results of pediatric osteosarcoma: Twenty-years experience. *J Pediatr Orthop* 2007;27:241-246.

Prosthetic Considerations in the Pediatric Lower Limb Amputee

CHAPTER 73

Brian J. Giavedoni, MBA, CP, LP

ABSTRACT

As a well-established subspecialty within the field of orthotics and prosthetics, pediatric prosthetics continues to advance in both treatment protocols and technological innovations. The fitting of a prosthesis on a child with a limb deficiency requires a thorough knowledge of the child's presentation, whether congenital or traumatic. Additional considerations in these children are the initial need for family-centered care and the long-term, developmental timing of care that will be required over the patient's lifetime.

Keywords: amputation; congenital limb difference; lower limb deficiency; pediatrics; prosthetics

Introduction

Congenital limb differences require an understanding of the anatomic anomaly and all of the associated developmental, physical, and physiologic implications. In the management of pediatric limb anomalies, the child is a continuously changing patient in whom body size, limitations, and physical potential mimic the age-appropriate developmental advances expected in able-bodied children. The support and participation of the patient's family, technologic advances, and the practitioner's skill and experience all contribute to the prosthetic fitting outcome. The prosthetic prescription for a child is very different from that for an adult with a similar level of limb loss.

Lifelong and family-centered care are two additional distinctions in the treatment of a child with a limb deficiency. Unlike their adult counterparts, children often have no input in initial surgical planning or prosthetic prescription. All decisions are made by parents in consultation with the treatment team that often includes a physician, a prosthetist, a therapist, and a social worker. Prosthetic issues unique to children with limb differences encompass anticipated physiologic growth, healing potential, and tissue metabolism. In addition, the child who grows into adulthood with a congenital deficiency is often viewed as an adult amputee with minimal attention being paid to the underlying cause of the amputation, such as congenital malformation.

The incidence of congenital limb deficiency is approximately one out of 2,000 live births.[1] Children with upper limb deficiencies outnumber those with lower limb deficiencies by a ratio of 3:1, and they often have multiple limb anomalies and other comorbidities or syndromes[2] (**Figure 1**). A comprehensive examination of a child with a congenital limb difference should include facial, spinal, and pelvic evaluations so that other conditions can be quickly identified. If a syndrome is involved, the limb difference may not be the most pressing medical issue.

Lower Limb Fitting Strategies

The prosthetic socket is the foundation of a well-designed and functional prosthesis and must be intimate, anatomically correct, and comfortable. The socket represents the interface between the patient's body and technology. A poor socket fit will negate the advantages of good technology. Generally, a prosthesis for a child should be designed to last at least 12 months, although its useful duration is heavily dependent on the activity level and play habits of the child. A prosthesis that becomes unusable in less than 1 year may indicate that either the initial socket fit was too aggressive or it did not take into account both longitudinal and circumferential growth.[3] From a global perspective, the ability to grow a prosthesis to coincide with the child's physiologic growth is an important consideration for the prosthetist. Although manufacturers have provided an ever-increasing number of prosthetic components, the most desirable options are those in which parts are modular and can be added or exchanged to increase height or those made of materials that can be adjusted after fabrication.

Lower limb socket designs and components vary with the age, activity level, and functional requirements of the individual child. Most children with a lower limb deficiency will want to walk, run, and play in the same manner as their able-bodied peers. Knowledge gained over the past 10

Neither Brian J. Giavedoni nor any immediate family member has received anything of value from or has stock or stock options held in a commercial company or institution related directly or indirectly to the subject of this chapter.

years has demonstrated that protecting a young child (6 years or younger) from falling by incorporating a locking knee into a transfemoral-level prosthesis is not only unnecessary but may prove counterproductive. Studies have suggested that early knee placement in a prosthesis can reduce the adaptation of clearance options during the development of ambulation.[4-6]

Although many component options are available for pediatric patients, the choice of whether to use a particular option must be based on sound clinical judgment. Manufacturers began producing pediatric component lines in the late 1980s and, over time, have substantially increased the variety of components available for most functional amputation levels. Lower limb milestones are used to help determine the best component match. While focus on gait is paramount, crawling, tall kneeling, and pulling to stand mark the onset of prosthetic intervention and the amputation level determines only a general prescription. The general consensus is that children progress to mature gait patterns between the ages of 2 to 4 years.[7] The role of the prosthetist is to determine the necessary and optimal blend of socket and componentry to best compliment and support the milestone.

Stance control knees, which are frequently selected for adult amputees, are often unnecessary for the child with lower limb loss. For children, a step-over-step strategy for descending stairs is often impossible in a device with activated stance control. Step-over-step running is effortless if a child is exposed early to this activity, and it is hampered by a knee with prosthetic stance control. In the experience of this chapter's author, most children request deactivation of the stance control feature in their knees so that their activity level is not reduced. Similarly, although a locking knee may be appropriate for geriatric patients, it is rarely appropriate in the pediatric cohort. If increased knee stability is required, simple alignment modifications can be made to articulating knees to increase stability.

Although suction sockets provide an intimate, secure solution to both suspension and ease of donning for adults, these sockets are generally ill-suited to the growing child. Relatively small variances in volume can substantially affect both fit and the ability to maintain a vacuum seal. Similarly, although various types of gel liners provide comfort, these liners increase the need for hygienic practices to avoid the commonplace occurrences of yeast and fungal infections. In addition, liners add weight and bulk to an already visually oversized prosthesis. However, if justified clinically, liners can afford both suspension and the ability to increase the lifespan of the prosthesis by allowing changes to the liner thickness to compensate for growth (**Figure 2**).

Experience has demonstrated that most healthy, active pediatric amputees easily achieve a K4 (**Table 1**) activity level through their developing years and into their 20s and 30s. Because of the high activity level of many children, pediatric lower limb components may be subjected to tremendous wear and tear. When catastrophic failure is not the reason for replacement of a prosthesis, physiologic growth is usually the inciting factor. Generally, a child will grow 12 inches (30.38 cm) per year, thus warranting the need to replace a prosthetic foot, and, in most cases, requiring a new socket or an entirely new prosthesis.

In both upper and lower limb prosthetic management, a common dilemma

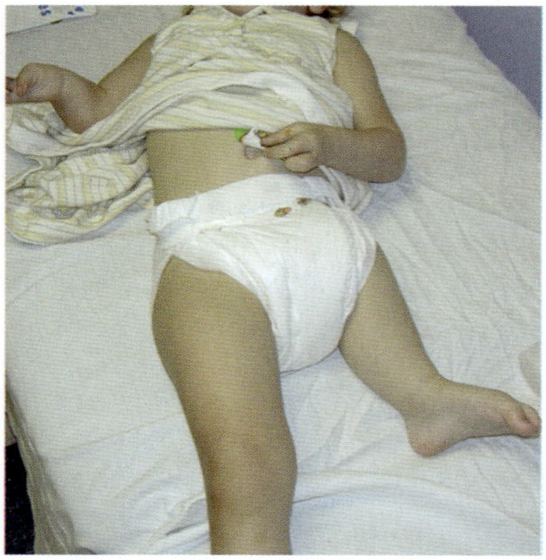

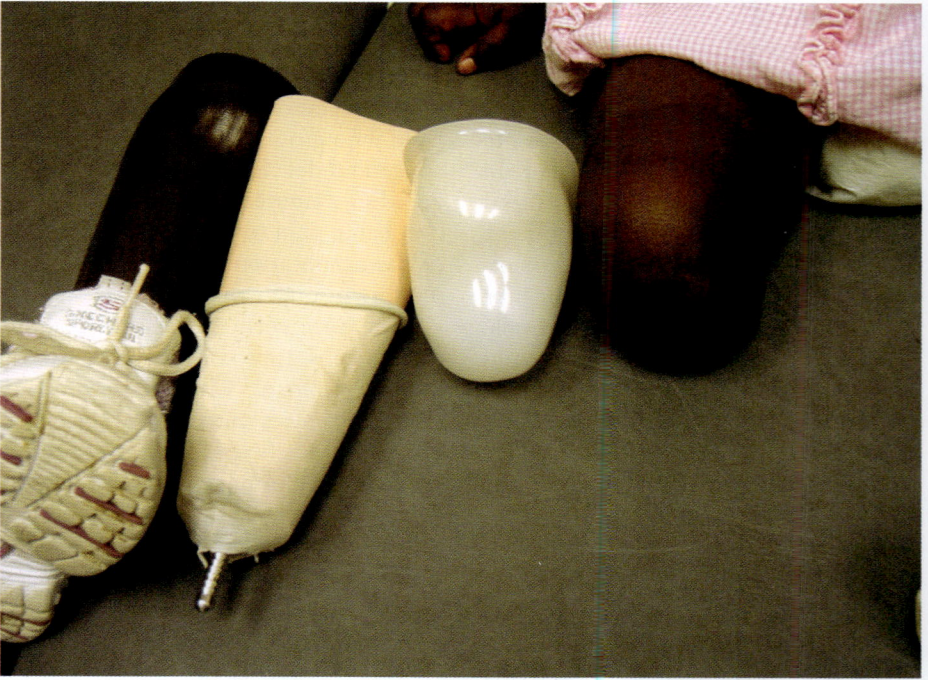

FIGURE 1 Photograph of an infant with multiple congenital limb anomalies, including left proximal focal femoral deficiency and right and left ulnar deficiencies.

FIGURE 2 Photograph of the limb of a child with a very short transtibial amputation. A pin liner (center) can be used for suspension over a thin thermoplastic inner socket (right). The outer prosthesis is shown on the far left.

Chapter 73: Prosthetic Considerations in the Pediatric Lower Limb Amputee

TABLE 1 Local Coverage Determination (LCD): Lower Limb Prostheses (L33787). Centers for Medicare and Medicaid Services

K Levels	K levels indicate a person's potential for prosthetic use, often as required by insurance carriers for coverage of a prosthesis
K-0	Does not have the ability or potential to ambulate or transfer safely with or without assistance and a prosthesis does not enhance their quality of life or mobility.
K-1	Has the ability or potential to use a prosthesis for transfers or ambulation on level surfaces at fixed cadence. Typical of the limited and unlimited household ambulator.
K-2	Has the ability or potential for ambulation with the ability to traverse low-level environmental barriers such as curbs, stairs, or uneven surfaces. Typical of the limited community ambulator.
K-3	Has the ability or potential for ambulation with variable cadence. Typical of the community ambulator who has the ability to traverse most environmental barriers and may have vocational, therapeutic, or exercise activity that demands prosthetic utilization beyond simple locomotion.
K-4	Has the ability or potential for prosthetic ambulation that exceeds basic ambulation skills, exhibiting high impact, stress, or energy levels. Typical of the prosthetic demands of the child, active adult, or athlete.

Reprinted from the US Centers for Medicare and Medicaid Services' Medicare Coverage Database. https://www.cms.gov/medicare-coverage-database/view/lcd.aspx?LCDId=33787

is whether to replace the entire prosthesis or only the failed or outgrown components. As a general rule, the entire device should be replaced if (1) the major components (hand, foot, or knee) have excessive wear; and (2) the socket requires replacement because of growth or surgical revision.

Growth Management in Children

Growth in children is a physiologic reality, and their open epiphyseal plates represent a major difference between children and adults. In adults undergoing amputation, adequate space can be allowed to accommodate both an optimal socket design and a good selection of prosthetic components. This is not the case in pediatric patients in whom transosseous amputations are rare. Rather, an elective amputation in a child with a congenital limb deficiency is usually performed through the most distal joint. Disarticulation preserves the distal epiphyseal plates, prevents residual bone overgrowth, and improves weight-bearing ability and the stability of the prosthetic socket on the residual limb. This approach, however, presents the prosthetist with the unique challenge of providing a prosthetic fitting for a very long upper or lower residual limb; optimal component selection is rarely a reality in this situation.

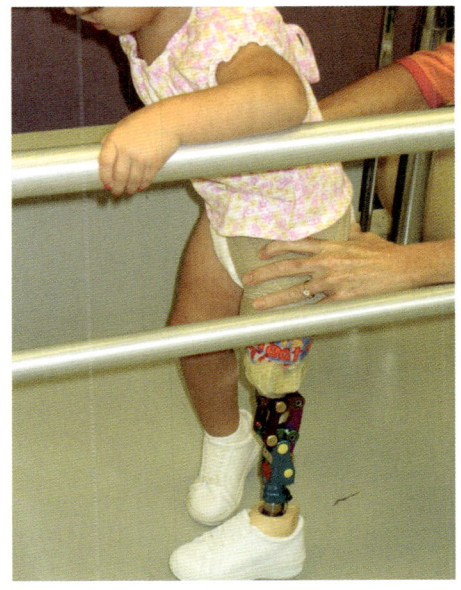

FIGURE 3 Photograph of a child with a lower limb prosthesis in which dynamic alignment has been achieved without the aid of alignment jigs or hardware because of space limitations.

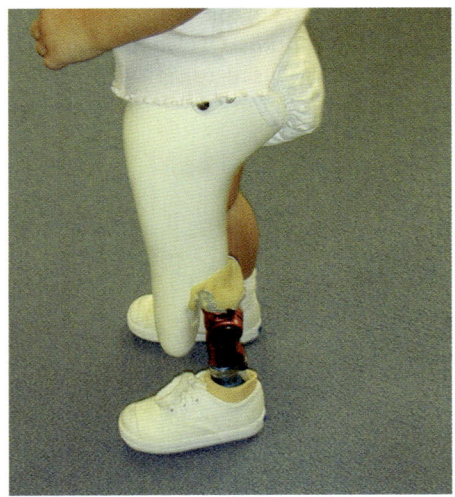

FIGURE 4 Photograph of a child with a proximal focal femoral deficiency fitted with a single-axis knee. The knee center is better approximated by mounting the knee joint posterior to the distal aspect of the limb (on the heel).

In the lower limb, prosthetic components that can be aligned are commonplace for adult amputees but are generally contraindicated in pediatric patients because of spatial limitations. The art of attaching a socket to a lamination plate directly with no built-in alignment capability continues to be standard practice (**Figure 3**). When a knee disarticulation is performed, the lack of additional clearance for the knee results in a lower knee center than on the contralateral side. In some instances, the knee center can be better approximated by mounting the knee joint posterior to the distal aspect of the limb (**Figure 4**). Any level of knee bending allows for shortening of the overall length of the entire limb, which affords ground clearance for the swing-through phase of gait.

An underlying goal for all clinicians involved in the prosthetic care of children is to ensure that surgical management ultimately leads to the best possible prosthetic outcomes in adulthood. When staged or timed appropriately, epiphyseal plate arrests can maintain the functional benefits of distal end bearing while creating increased clearance for prosthetic components over time. Epiphyseal plate arrest may be performed in patients treated with knee or ankle disarticulation. This practice of epiphyseal plate arrest varies depending on the medical center in which the patient is treated, but it can provide the necessary space to allow for superior prosthetic components that would not otherwise be possible because of spatial limitations. The eventual creation of equal knee center heights is often more relevant to the mature amputee because of aesthetic concerns that usually manifest in young adulthood and functional concerns, such as a prosthetic knee that can accommodate the limited legroom on airplanes.

The use of socks to adjust or accommodate changes in limb volume is a common practice in both adult and pediatric patients. Initially, a parent will aid the child in donning and doffing the prosthesis. Proper alignment of the residual limb within the socket is critical for comfort and good function. Socks can range from one ply to five plies in thickness. Thermoplastic socket designs with frame support allow for increased flexibility and volume control by adjusting the socket with heat if necessary, or adding interface padding behind the inner socket to increase support areas.

Bony Overgrowth and Angular Deformities

Most elective amputations in children with congenital limb differences are planned to preserve bone growth by preserving the distal epiphyseal plates. In patients with traumatic or acquired amputations, a transdiaphyseal amputation may be performed, frequently resulting in terminal overgrowth[8] (**Figure 5**). In general, after bony overgrowth begins, prosthetic wearing tolerance quickly decreases and prosthesis nonuse is common. Very few prosthetic interventions are available to reduce the pain associated

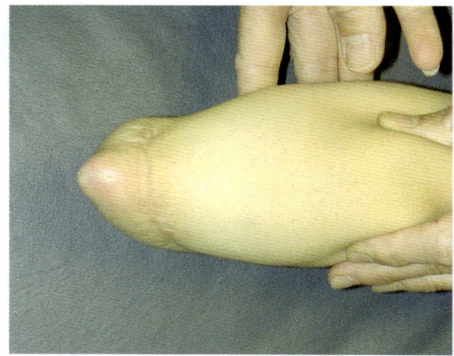

FIGURE 5 Clinical photograph showing terminal bony overgrowth that will require surgical intervention.

with such overgrowth. The presence of a small bursa, detected by palpation, is a classic sign of the onset of overgrowth. These bursae generally require surgical treatment. A number of surgical options are available, and some are more successful than others at preventing recurrences.

Angular deformities are very common in patients with congenital limb deficiencies. In a patient with longitudinal deficiency of the fibula, there is a high incidence of genu valgus, often resulting in angles greater than 35°. However, biomechanical principles dictate that the ground reaction force from a prosthetic foot pass near or through the center of the knee. With an angular deformity at the knee, the foot is outset to accommodate the limb. The resultant medial distal hump can be sizable, and it often poses a challenge in wearing pants (**Figure 6**). Angular deformities can be treated with either guided growth surgery or osteotomy. Consultation between the prosthetist and the pediatric orthopaedic surgeon is necessary to determine the need and timing of surgical interventions.

Bilateral Lower Limb Deficiencies

Prosthetic fitting for patients with bilateral lower limb loss requires clinical experience in recognizing the correct prosthetic pathways to optimize outcomes. In general, fitting of a bilateral transtibial or Syme ankle disarticulation prosthesis is initiated when the

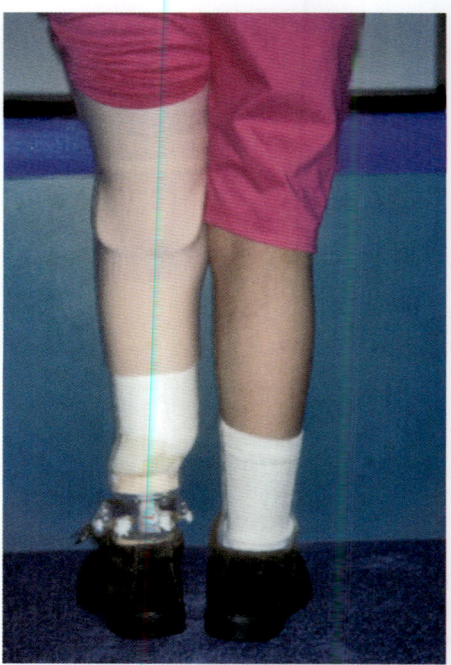

FIGURE 6 Photograph of a child with a prosthesis designed to provide proper alignment for angular issues. The patient had fracture nonunion and transtibial amputation.

child reaches the pull-to-stand stage of development. Bilateral prosthetic fitting is similar to unilateral fitting except in alignment challenges. In a child with a bilateral longitudinal deficiency of the fibula, flexed knees are common and must be considered when aligning the prosthesis. Genu valgus may also be present and will require incorporation into the prosthetic alignment.

Patients with bilateral transfemoral amputations or knee disarticulations begin with short nonarticulated stubby prostheses (stubbies) or may start with knees incorporated into the devices to help achieve clearance and allow for tall kneeling during play. The knees are kept very low to the ground, often attached directly to the surface of the feet. The decision of whether to initially add knees requires expertise and sound clinical judgment. The first prosthesis is usually best designed with stubby feet. This strategy provides the child the opportunity to develop balance and coordination with the prosthesis and frees the child's hands for other tasks. Historically, stubby feet were attached to a saucer. The rocker motion provided balance training and core

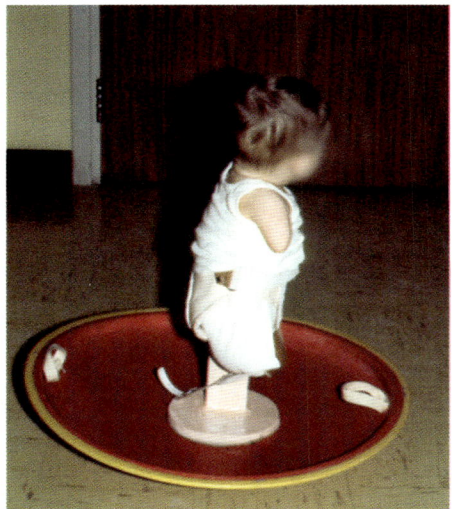

FIGURE 7 Photograph of a child with quadrilateral amputations using a prosthetic socket with a saucer setup for balance training and core trunk strengthening.

strengthening. Although the saucer technique is now rarely used, it remains a sound viable practice for the quadrilateral amputee (**Figure 7**). After standing stability and good core strength are achieved, adding knees to subsequent prostheses has proven to be an effective transitional step as the child reaches developmental milestones.

SUMMARY

The management of children with lower limb deficiencies is challenging and complex. Clinical practice guidelines for the pediatric patient are often anecdotal and based heavily on mentoring experiences. A child with bilateral congenital or acquired amputation warrants special consideration. Understanding the physical and physiological differences of a child with a limb deficiency is necessary to optimize prosthetic fittings and provide quality care over the lifetime of the patient.

References

1. Centers for Disease Control and Prevention: Data and statistics on birth defects. Accessed October 8, 2021. Available at: https://www.cdc.gov/ncbddd/birthdefects/data.html.
2. Wilcox WR, Coulter CP, Schmitz ML: Congenital limb deficiency disorders. *Clin Perinatol* 2015;42(2):281-300, viii.
3. Morrissy RT, Giavedoni B, Coulter-O'Berry C: The limb-deficient child, in Wood W, Winter RB, Morrissy RT, Weinstein SL, eds: *Lovell and Winters Pediatric Orthopaedics*. Lippincott Williams & Wilkins, 2001, pp 1217-1272.
4. Geil M, Coulter C: Analysis of locomotor adaptations in young children with limb loss in an early prosthetic knee prescription protocol. *Prosthet Orthot Int* 2014;38(1):54-61.
5. Geil M, Coulter-O'Berry C: Temporal and spatial parameters of crawling in children with limb loss: Implications on prosthetic knee prescription. *J Prosthet Orthot* 2010;22(1):21-25.
6. Geil MD, Coulter-O'Berry C, Schmitz M, Heriza C: Crawling kinematics in an early knee protocol for pediatric prosthetic prescription. *J Prosthet Orthot* 2013;25(1):22-29.
7. Sutherland DH, Olshen R, Cooper L: The development of mature gait. *J Bone Joint Surg Am* 1980;62(3):336-353.
8. Aitken GT, Pellicore RJ: Introduction to the child amputee, in Bowker, HK, Michael JW, eds: *American Academy of Orthopaedic Surgeons: Atlas of Limb Prosthetics Surgical and Prosthetic Principles*. Mosby-Year Book, 1981, pp 493-500.

Hip Disarticulation and Hemipelvectomy in Children: Surgical and Prosthetic Management

Joseph Ivan Krajbich, MD, FRCS(C) • Todd DeWees, MHA, CPO

ABSTRACT

Hip disarticulation and hemipelvectomy (transpelvic amputation) are uncommon in pediatric patients. However, in acute situations, it is helpful to be familiar with the surgical approaches and prosthetic options for children undergoing high-level lower limb amputations. Classification based on etiology may affect overall patient management. The components available for prosthetic fitting may be limited based on the age of the patient.

Keywords: hemipelvectomy; high-level pediatric amputee; hindquarter amputation; hip disarticulation; prosthetic management; surgical management

Introduction

Pediatric amputees represent between 10.3% and 11.7% of the overall amputee population.[1,2] Patients with hip disarticulations and hemipelvectomies (transpelvic amputations) represent approximately 2% of the amputee population.[1] Therefore, pediatric patients with high-level lower limb amputations represent only 0.2% of the overall amputee population. Because of the very small number of children with hip disarticulation or hemipelvectomy, surgeons and prosthetists often have limited experience in treating these patients, who have special needs and require special considerations. It is likely that only tertiary referral centers for pediatric limb deficiency treat enough of these children to collect adequate objective data to establish both surgical and prosthetic treatment principles. Besides congenital absence of the lower extremity (amelia) or rare instance of other complex congenital abnormality, the traumatic injury, sepsis, malignant neoplasm, and vascular malformation are among the main etiologic causes of these high-level amputations. Consequently, virtually any practicing orthopaedic surgeon can face an acute situation where hip disarticulation or hemipelvectomy is necessary to save the life of a child. It is therefore important to be familiar with the basic management principles that guide treatment and prosthetic fitting to provide these children with optimal care.

Surgical Management: Anatomic Considerations

In most instances of acquired high-level amputation, the surgical treatment is likely to be dictated by the type of injury or the condition leading to the amputation. Therefore, the surgeon should be well versed in the anatomy and the surgical exposures around the hip and pelvis and be able to adapt the approach to the individual circumstances.

Children usually have a healthy proximal blood supply, resilient tissues, and good healing potential. All three main blood supplies to the proximal part of the limb can be used as dictated by the circumstance. A posterior gluteal flap based on gluteal vessels, an anterior flap based on external iliac/femoral vessels, and a medial flap based on the obturator vessels can all be used. It is important to be aware that the bony pelvis and the proximal femur serve as attachments to a host of central skeleton muscles. Their loss or loss of their anchorage can lead to secondary issues related to pelvic floor support, abdominal wall integrity, and spinal balance.

The pelvis is also the site of several internal organs whose preservation or removal will depend on the existing pathology and surgeon's skill. Because a procedure of this magnitude will have a substantial effect on the patient's quality of life and future health, an intimate knowledge of the underlying pathology and pelvic anatomy is imperative. Not infrequently, a multidisciplinary team consisting of an orthopaedic surgeon, pediatric general surgeon, urologist, vascular surgeon, and even a plastic surgeon is called on to maximize safety of the procedure and preservation of organs and tissue. The goal is to optimize recovery potential with the maximum residual function attainable under the circumstances. In rare circumstances when neurovascular supply to the distal part of the extremity is preservable and the distal part of the extremity

---

Dr. Krajbich or an immediate family member serves as a board member, owner, officer, or committee member of Scoliosis Research Society. Neither Todd DeWees nor any immediate family member has received anything of value from or has stock or stock options held in a commercial company or institution related directly or indirectly to the subject of this chapter.

itself is relatively uninvolved by the pathologic process, more complex reconstructive procedures can be attempted (rotationplasty, tibia to pelvis fusion, or articulation).

Terminology and Classification

Hip Disarticulation

In general, in hip disarticulation, it is assumed that there is loss of the bony structures distal to the pelvic side of the hip joint. That is, all of the femur is absent, but the pelvis, including the acetabulum, is intact and present. The integrity of the soft tissues can vary with etiology. A special case is the presence of a very short femoral segment that cannot serve as a functional proximal femur for the purpose of prosthetic fitting. In such instances, the child will likely require a hip disarticulation–like prosthetic fitting. This is a relatively important point. In a very young child facing transfemoral amputation, the loss of the distal femoral epiphyseal plate will lead to insufficient growth in the remaining femur and may preclude a functional transfemoral prosthetic fitting when the child becomes older. Such a child may eventually require a hip disarticulation–like prosthesis (**Figure 1**). In some congenital deficiencies, such as phocomelia, a hip disarticulation–like prosthesis may be required if the vestigial limb cannot provide enough function to support transfemoral amputation–like prosthesis. Despite this, every effort should be made to preserve as much length of the proximal femur as possible. Even a relatively small fragment can potentially be lengthened in the future as long as there is an adequate soft-tissue envelope. Even modest proximal femoral lengthening may lead to a better anchor for a prosthesis.

Hemipelvectomy

Partial or complete hemipelvectomy is also called transpelvic or hindquarter amputation. The limb loss involves not only the whole limb but also a portion of the central skeleton (the pelvis and potentially pelvic organs). Congenital deficiency of this magnitude is not unheard of but clearly very rare (**Figure 2**). Even acquired deficiency is quite uncommon. Malignant tumor, acute trauma, or rarely surgical separation of pygopagus conjoined twins are among the causes of this radical intervention. The complexity of the surgical approach, if needed, and prosthetic fitting depend on the presence and integrity of the remaining bony pelvis, the soft-tissue structures, and the underlying pathologic process. The extent of amputation can vary from a limb removal, including only a portion of the bony pelvis, to complete hemipelvectomy, including part of the sacrum and part or all of several pelvic organs (gastrointestinal tract, lower urinary tract, and reproductive organs) (**Figure 3**). In such a situation, it is mandatory that a well-coordinated team of several surgical subspecialists is assembled to achieve an optimal outcome. When possible, careful planning of the procedure should be undertaken to optimize the achievement of the primary goal of the surgical procedure, which is complete control of the disease process (adequate surgical margins in the case of malignant tumor resection) yet allowing for an optimal anatomic and functional result. Especially in very young children, future additional surgical intervention(s) and potential prosthetic fitting will very much depend on the presence of any preserved skeletal and soft-tissue elements.

Classification According to Etiology

Similar to other limb deficiencies in children, high-level lower limb loss can be either acquired (trauma, neoplasm, or sepsis) or congenital (amelia), phocomelia (intercalary deficiency), or another type of loss (conjoined twins).

Trauma

Trauma likely accounts for most high-level amputations in the lower limbs. Motor vehicle crashes (the child is usually a pedestrian), lawnmower injuries, and injuries sustained in a war zone are high-energy injuries that devastate the proximal soft tissues. Frequently, these injuries are complicated by massive wound contamination and loss of bony integrity. Because these are serious, life-threatening injuries, resuscitation of the child by establishing cardiopulmonary stability is the first priority. Stopping major blood loss is an integral part of this effort. Initially, simple manual pressure and packing is all that can be done. After the patient's condition has stabilized and adequate ventilatory support and fluid resuscitation have been accomplished, careful assessment of the extent of the injuries is necessary for a rational approach.

Surgical control of major bleeding and débridement of contaminated tissue is the next mandatory step. At this point, the treatment

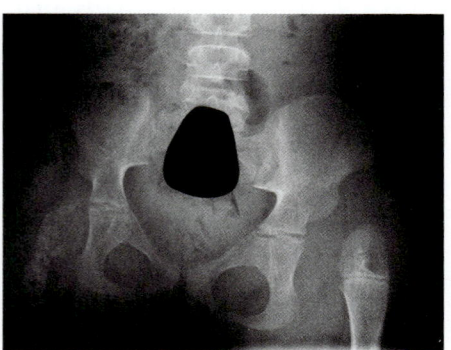

FIGURE 1 AP radiograph of the pelvis of a child with right-sided phocomelia. The patient will be fitted with a functional hip disarticulation prosthesis.

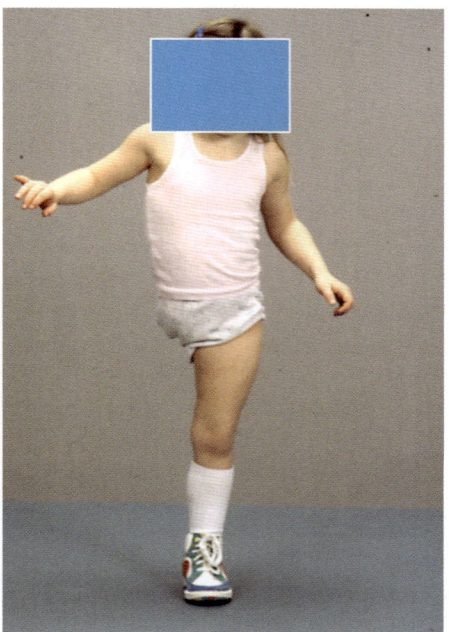

FIGURE 2 Congenital deficiency of the hemipelvis. (Courtesy of Joseph Ivan Krajbich MD, FRCS(C), Portland, Oregon.)

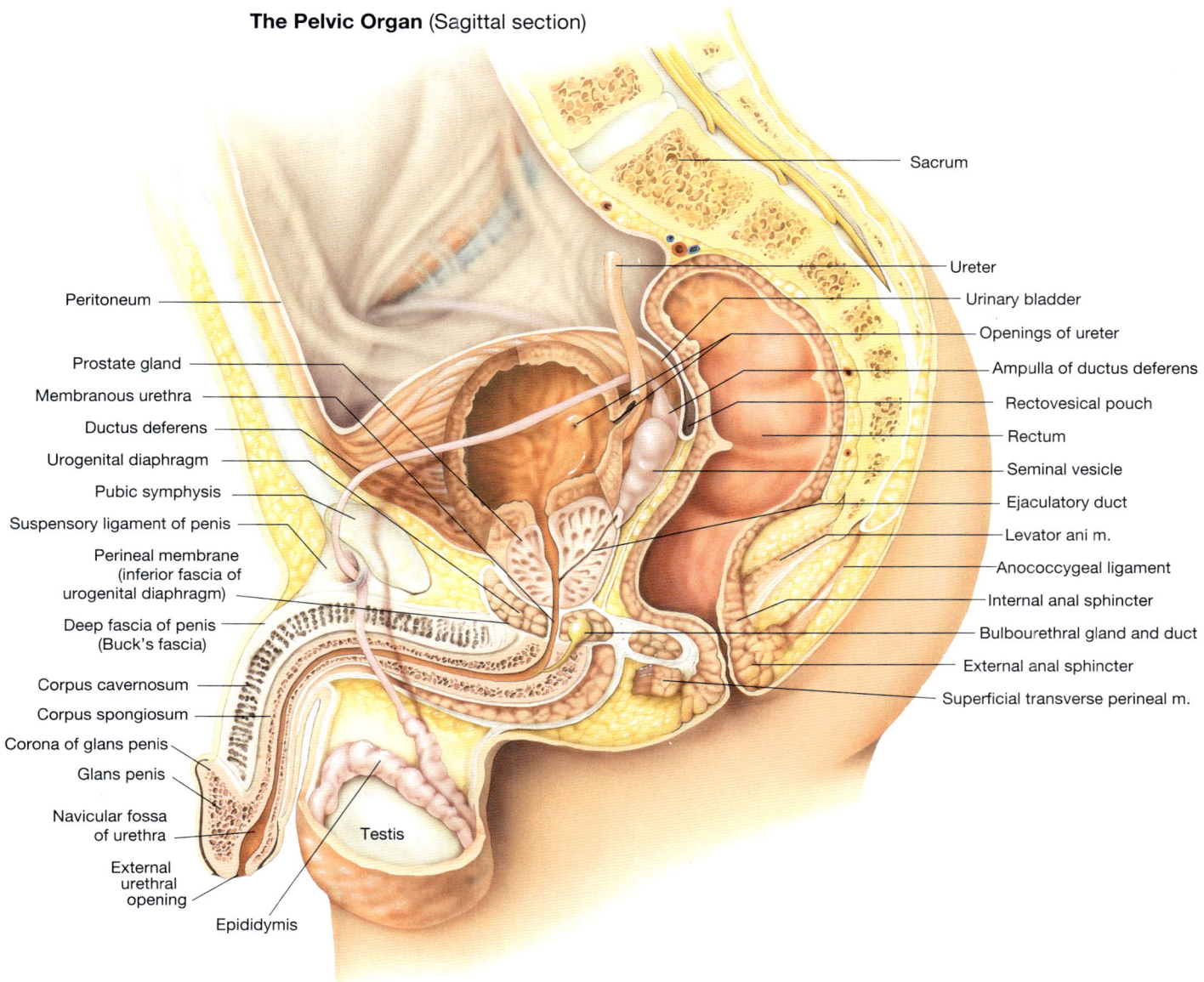

FIGURE 3 Pelvic anatomy. Any of these structures can be involved in as significant pelvic trauma or pelvic neoplasm. (Reproduced with permission from Anatomical Chart Company © Wolters Kluwer. All right reserved.)

team must decide if any emergent limb salvage procedure can be used. Revascularization is an important consideration because a relatively short window of a few hours exists in which an avascular limb can be saved. Attempts should be made to preserve and use any relatively intact and viable tissue to increase the length of the limb and diminish functional loss. As already mentioned, the ability to preserve the distal femoral physis can be of major importance in the functional outcomes of very young children. A major impediment of instituting such reconstructive procedures in the setting of acute trauma is the absence of an onsite specialized surgical team. Transfer of the child to an institution with these capabilities should be considered if feasible.

Additional interventions can be instituted after the patient is stabilized. Treatment by experienced surgeons in an operating room setting may lead to more judicial débridement and may optimize the survival of remaining tissues. A number of débridements with the wound remaining temporarily open or managed with vacuum suction dressing may be necessary before final wound closure. Any needed bone or soft-tissue reconstruction can be part of this process.[3-5]

Additional techniques can be used to obtain optimal functional results for each patient. Bone transport, rotationplasty, free flaps, rotational flaps, and composite vascularized graft all can be used.[6-9]

Neoplasms

In children, Ewing sarcoma is the most common neoplasm found in the proximal femur or pelvis; however, osteogenic sarcoma and some soft-tissue sarcomas also occur at these sites. Among the soft-tissue sarcomas in children with neurofibromatosis type 1 (von Recklinghausen disease), peripheral nerve sheath sarcoma is the most frequently encountered neoplasm.

Because modern management of these tumors has shifted toward chemotherapy and limb salvage, a primary amputation is performed only in a situation in which limb salvage is not possible because of the involvement of vital structures and inability to otherwise obtain clear resection margins.[10-15] Primary amputation is a relatively rare treatment in a modern pediatric oncology surgical practice. In the experience of one of this chapter's authors (JIK), primary amputation is most likely in a patient with pelvic neurofibrosarcoma. This neoplasm is resistant to chemotherapy and radiation therapy and frequently involves several vital structures in the pelvis; a complete hemipelvectomy is often the only chance for a cure. Failure of a primary limb salvage procedure, such as endoprosthetic or allograft replacement in the femur or internal hemipelvectomy on the pelvic side, is another situation where hip disarticulation or formal hemipelvectomy may be required. Substantial postoperative complications are possible.[15-17]

Sepsis

Purpura fulminans septicemia, necrotizing fasciitis, and other causes of infected gangrenous limbs may necessitate proximal limb amputation as a lifesaving measure.[18] The surgical principles used to manage septic shock will apply. Cardiopulmonary resuscitation, fluid resuscitation, the administration of massive doses of antibiotics, and débridement of any obvious necrotic contaminated tissue are also critical to the patient's survival. However, the need for an emergent proximal amputation usually does not apply in patients with purpura fulminans. Associated systemic sepsis generally leads to ischemia of various body parts, which quite commonly includes the limbs. In this situation, limbs or parts of a limb can become ischemic but are not contaminated by infection (dry gangrene). In such a situation, it is necessary to wait until the final demarcation of necrotic and viable tissue occurs before deciding on the level of amputations. This final demarcation may take several days or even weeks and is usually quite distal to what may initially appear. Very proximal amputation is rarely necessary.

In any of these situations, the usual course of treatment involves multiple débridements and delayed wound closure until a healthy, uninfected wound is obtained. Modern, complex wound care techniques, such as vacuum-assisted dressings, flaps, and skin grafts, are usually used to achieve wound closure.[4]

Congenital Defects

Unilateral Congenital Absence of the Whole Limb

Unilateral congenital absence of the whole limb, also known as amelia, is a rare condition (**Figure 2**). The treatment mainstay is prosthetic fitting determined by the extent of the pelvic involvement. Surgical intervention is limited to the treatment of secondary effects of such a limb deficiency.

Phocomelia

Lower limb phocomelia is not technically a hip disarticulation. Quite frequently, however, a small deficient, minimally functional foot contributes little to limb function other than perhaps acting as an improved anchor for a prosthetic socket. Children with lower limb phocomelia frequently require hip disarticulation–like prostheses. Surgical intervention is rarely indicated unless the position or alignment of the affected limb at the pelvis interferes with prosthetic fitting. In such patients, a realignment procedure may be indicated. Many of these children have other limb deficiencies and warrant an individualized approach to maximize their function.

Separated Conjoined Twins

Pygopagus conjoined twins (Siamese twins) may be candidates for a separation procedure. After separation, either one or usually both children will have a hemipelvectomy-like situation. Separation is a very complex surgical procedure performed by a multidisciplinary surgical team, and it usually requires double teams of general pediatric surgeons, pediatric urologists, pediatric orthopaedic surgeons, and pediatric plastic surgeons. The soft-tissue defects can be quite large and may require prolonged treatment before the child is ready for prosthetic fitting.

Hemipelvectomy in Very Young Children

The absence of a hemipelvis has a substantial influence on the development of a child's spine and contralateral hip. The loss of abdominal wall integrity, paraspinal muscle integrity, and iliopsoas integrity all lead to early paralytic-like lumbar scoliosis convex to the side of the absent hemipelvis. The remaining hemipelvis is at the caudal end of the scoliotic curve and tilts into abduction. Consequently, the remaining hip is forced into an adducted position with respect to its acetabulum. This leads to uncovering of the femoral head and, in a young child, the development of further hip dysplasia and eventually hip subluxation. Both surgical and prosthetic techniques are needed to treat these patients (**Figure 4**).

Initially, prosthetic treatment incorporates a spinal brace into the prosthetic design (**Figure 5**). However, a progressive worsening of the deformity may require surgical management. Surgical management of scoliosis and/or osteotomies around the hip, on the femoral as well as the pelvic side, may be required. In some of these children, other organ deficiencies and their management (eg, colostomies and other enterostomies) can make treatment even more challenging. A child with a colostomy or enterostomy on the prosthetic side may be more functional without a prosthesis; a walker or crutches and a swing-through gait may provide more effective locomotion.

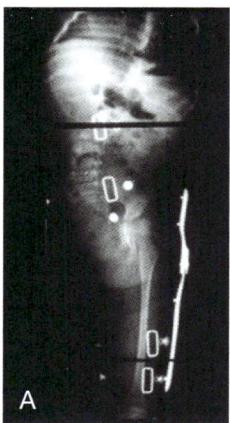 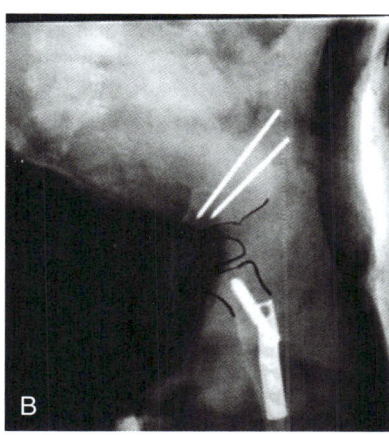 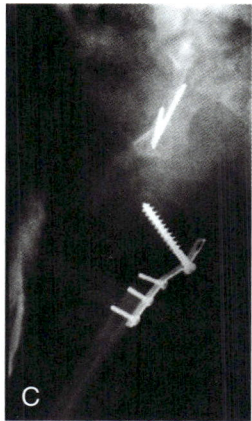

FIGURE 4 **A**, Radiograph demonstrating the pelvic obliquity with acetabular—femoral adduction and hip subluxation in a young child with hemipelvectomy. **B** and **C**, Radiographs of surgical correction using innominate Salter osteotomy and femoral varus osteotomy.

Prosthetic Management

As previously stated, pediatric patients with hip disarticulation or hemipelvectomy are a small and specialized population. Studies of adults with hip disarticulations or transpelvic amputations have traditionally shown high prosthetic rejection rates[19,20] because of the combination of socket discomfort and the high-energy cost of ambulation. Although these factors exist in the pediatric population, prosthesis rejection rates have been found to be as low as 10%.[21]

It should be noted that there are important differences between pediatric patients with high-level lower limb loss and their adult counterparts. The first major physiologic distinction is the rate of energy consumption. For pediatric patients with hip disarticulation and transpelvic amputation, the oxygen consumption cost has been reported at 151% and 161% of normal, respectively.[22] Their adult counterparts have energy consumptions levels reported as high as 200% of normal.[23] A second difference between pediatric and adult amputees is the most common causes of amputation. In adults older than 60 years, the most common causes are vascular disease or trauma. In pediatric patients, the primary causes of amputation are tumor or congenital amputation.[1] In addition, the smaller body mass of a pediatric patient, particularly at younger ages, decreases the force on weight bearing within the socket. This in turn decreases the need for additional padding or thermoplastic material to create a comfortable socket. Lessening the materials required reduces the overall weight of the prosthesis without compromising the structure.

Prosthetic fitting in pediatric patients is complicated by their constantly changing body size, changes in functional levels, the limited availability of appropriately sized prosthetic components, and conflict between the weight of the prosthesis and its durability. These challenges can be mitigated by following the sound prosthetic fitting principles of good communication, regular patient follow-up, appropriate component selection, and flexibility in prosthetic design.

Biomechanics and Prosthetic Alignment

No studies that show differences in the biomechanics of gait between pediatric and adult patients treated with hip disarticulation or transpelvic amputation are available; therefore, the descriptions of the gait biomechanics of hip disarticulation and transpelvic amputation will follow the descriptions of Radcliffe,[24] Raiford and Epps,[25] and Solomonidis et al.[26] At initial contact, the ground reaction line runs posterior to the ankle, anterior to the knee, and anterior to the hip. Solomonidis et al[26] subdivided and described hip disarticulation gait in terms of axial force, anterior-posterior knee moment, anterior-posterior hip moment, medial-lateral hip moment, and torque. The axial force follows a double-bump pattern, which reaches a maximum force at approximately 20% of the gait cycle, maintaining a force approximately equal to body weight to 50% of the gait cycle, and then diminishing to zero at toe-off. The anterior-posterior knee moment begins with a small extension force until 30% of the gait cycle; at that point, it increases to its maximum force, which is maintained to 55% of the gait cycle. At that point, it gradually decrease to zero at toe-off. The anterior-posterior hip moment is described as a flexion moment caused by contact of the hip joint with the flexion limiter. There is a brief reversal of this force between 10% and 20% of the gait cycle and then the force returns to an extension moment, which reaches its maximum just before toe-off. The medial-lateral hip moment follows that of an able-bodied individual, with the moment adducting the hip with a maximum force at 35% of the gait cycle.

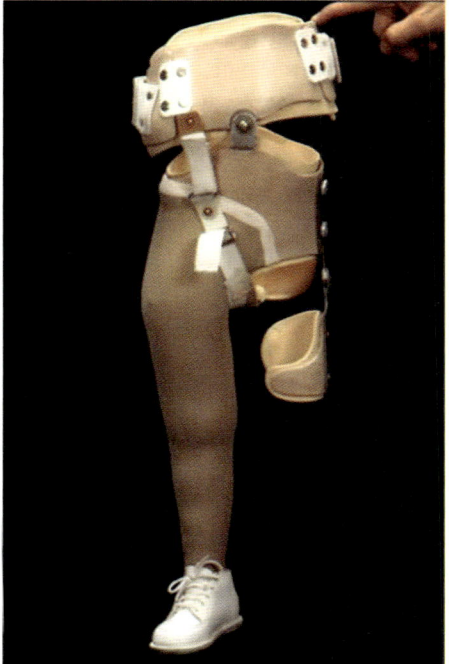

FIGURE 5 Photograph of a hemipelvectomy prosthesis with a thoracic extension to control 2° of scoliosis.

Torque was also shown to be very similar to that of able-bodied individuals, with maximum force occurring at approximately 50% of the gait cycle in the internal direction.[24-26] This brief description of the biomechanics highlights both the similarities and differences between hip disarticulation and normal gait.

Prosthetic alignment in a pediatric patient with a high-level lower limb amputation should follow similar biomechanical principles to that of an adult. The primary goals are to allow maximum stability in stance and necessary mobility in the swing phase of gait. However, the alignment of the prosthesis should not be overly stabilized. The adult standard of placing the weight line 1.0 to 1.5 inches anterior to the knee joint at midstance[27] should be scaled appropriately for the size of the pediatric patient. For example, the aforementioned offset may be appropriate for an adult with a hip-to-floor length of 91 cm, but a pediatric patient with a hip-to-floor length of 45 cm would require a midstance offset of approximately 0.5 to 0.75 inch.

Hip Disarticulation Versus Transpelvic Amputation

The prosthetic care of pediatric patients with hip disarticulation or transpelvic amputation is often similar. It is necessary at this point to delineate important and specific differences in the management of these two high-level amputations. These differences are primarily centered on the pelvic anatomy and socket designs.

For the patient with a hip disarticulation and a fully intact hemipelvis, weight-bearing forces are distributed over both bony and soft-tissue surfaces. This distribution allows the prosthetist to maintain maximum control over the prosthetic device by taking advantage of the ischial tuberosity, high anterior and posterior socket walls, and containment of the iliac crest. It should be noted that patients with very short femurs or those with phocomelia with a deficient foot located at the hip are fitted with a prosthesis as though they had a hip disarticulation. Although they technically do not have a hip disarticulation, these nonfunctional distal elements necessitate prosthetic treatment with a hip disarticulation–style prosthesis.

Conversely, because the patient with a transpelvic amputation may have few, if any, of these bony structures, weight bearing will be necessary through hydrostatic forces applied to the soft tissues of the amputated side. Suspension of the prosthesis for a patient with a transpelvic amputation may be further enhanced by the use of a suction socket to help maintain intimate contact with the soft tissues.[28] Both styles of sockets will likely require iliac crest containment of the contralateral side to improve coronal plane stability, which is typically done through the use of a single-piece socket with a flexible posterior element. The transpelvic socket design often includes the addition of a lumbar or thoracic extension on the amputated side. This extension is integral to the socket and designed to address the likely development of scoliosis, which is almost universal in this patient population (**Figure 5**). This design allows easy donning of the prosthesis while maintaining enhanced rotational control. The transpelvic socket typically has a taller proximal trim line in an attempt to reduce the risk of induced scoliosis. The patient with a hip disarticulation may be able to obtain contralateral iliac crest containment using a two-piece prosthetic design with the segments connected with nylon or polyethylene terephthalate straps. The advantages of this design over a one-piece socket are reduction in overall socket weight and increased comfort.

In the patient with bilateral high-level amputation, the use of prostheses is rare except for therapeutic standing. For this population, the primary purpose of a prosthetic socket is to provide a balanced pelvis for sitting, spinal support, and containing abdominal viscera.

Pediatric Considerations

Pediatric patients tend to be more active and have a higher functional level, decreased oxygen consumption, and more pressure-tolerant soft tissues, and they may be more motivated than adults with the same level of amputation.[29] These advantages, however, are offset by the disadvantages of limited choice in prosthetic components, high prosthetic weight relative to body mass, and the limited experience of clinicians in treating children with high-level lower limb amputation.

Limitations in prosthetic components specifically designed for pediatric patients represent a substantial barrier to producing a prosthesis that is functional, durable, and sufficiently lightweight. Weight is extremely important considering that the typical adult prosthesis for a high-level lower limb amputation weighs between 5.75 and 6.20 kg.[23] This means that for the typical 6-year-old child weighing approximately 21 kg,[30] a prosthesis built with adult components and based on adult principles would represent greater than 25% of the child's body mass.

Current options for pediatric hip joints include the Fearless Hip (DAW Industries), the 7E8 hip joint (Ottobock), and 3K51 Modular Hip Joint (Streifeneder-BroadBay). Knees produced for pediatric amputees provide a larger variety of options, though not as many as available to adult patients. When choosing a knee, mechanical or pneumatic options should be considered because they tend to be lighter in weight than hydraulic options. When the knee is to be used in functional gait, the selection of a polycentric option is encouraged. A polycentric knee will provide an effective shortening of the prosthetic limb in the swing phase of gait. This knee style is the only pediatric prosthetic component that provides this benefit because polycentric hip joints are currently available only in adult sizes. A polycentric hip such as the Helix 3D hip may be appropriate for older teenage amputees. The foot component of the prosthesis provides the greatest variety of pediatric options, nearly equaling those available to the adult amputee. When selecting components for a child's prosthesis, the goals of minimal weight and high durability are often at odds, but both must be a priority to achieve a successful outcome.

The anatomy of a pediatric patient with a high-level lower limb amputation should be taken into special consideration when attempting to produce a good fitting and high-functioning prosthetic device because of a combination of factors, including body size and the cause of amputation. The small body size, particularly of a preteen, often provides only minimal surface area for weight bearing and control of the prosthesis. Structures such as the ischial tuberosity may be too small to provide sufficient surface area for a classic socket design. In some children, the anatomy may also create additional fitting complications, such as a child with a congenital hip disarticulation who has a nonfunctional proximal femoral segment or a child with a congenital transpelvic amputation with a partial but atrophic hemipelvis.

Casting and Modification

Although casting methods for hip disarticulation and transpelvic amputees are substantially different, both procedures start with a thorough physical examination. Whenever possible, this should include the examination of pelvic radiographs to provide a full understanding of the remaining bony structure. An interview with the patient and family is also indispensable in determining functional level and realistic goals, as well as providing appropriate education to patients and their families. Only after establishing this knowledge base should the casting process begin.

Hip Disarticulation

Prosthetic casting for the patient with a hip disarticulation should follow the principles applicable to an anatomic hip disarticulation socket.[31,32] This casting method relies primarily on containment of the hemipelvis, including the ischial tuberosity and pubic ramus. To obtain an intimate socket fit with this design, the patient is placed in snug-fitting casting socks suspended over the shoulders to maintain suspension. Electrical tape is then applied from the sound-side greater trochanter anteriorly around to lay superior to the iliac crest on the amputated side. The tape is then continued across the lumbar region and over the top of the sound-side iliac crest. Finally, the tape is continued across the midline, thus well defining the waistline above the iliac crest (**Figure 6**). This is an excellent method of defining the waist without distorting the shape of the impression through the use of tubing. Following this step, bony landmarks and areas of notable anatomy should be marked on the casting garment with an indelible marker and appropriate measurements taken.

Casting is now ready to begin. A combination of plaster and fiberglass bandage is used during this process. This quick and clean method provides excellent tissue compression while sacrificing very little in shape capture. When applying the casting medium, complete coverage of the amputated side, including the ischial tuberosity and the pubic ramus, is necessary. The cast should be extended completely around the waist to provide two distinct advantages: (1) it suspends and compresses the mold and (2) it will provide a mold for the pelvic support for the sound side. After the casting tape is applied, a casting stand may be used to provide weight bearing and stability while the clinician uses their hands to mold the contours of the socket. At this point in the casting procedure, anterior and posterior casting wedges should be used to achieve a snug anterior-posterior dimension[33] and preshape the socket. For younger children, it may be more practical for a clinician to provide support and stability because the support surface of a casting stand may be too large for a child. The mold should be removed at the anterior midline. After removal, it should be examined to ensure that the appropriate shape has been captured. If the resulting cast does not have easily identifiable relief for all bony structures, recasting is necessary. This may appear to be an unnecessary step; however, when modifying an unfamiliar socket shape it is better to smooth than to sculpt.

Transpelvic Amputation

Casting for the child with a transpelvic amputation should be performed using the suspension casting technique. This method of casting provides an excellent approximation of the hydrostatic pressures that the patient will experience in the prosthetic socket.[34,35] It has the added advantage of freeing the practitioner's hands to mold around any residual pelvic anatomy and provide the cast the desired shape.

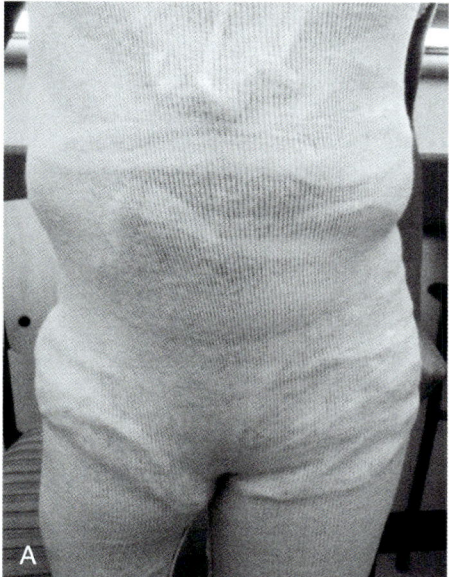 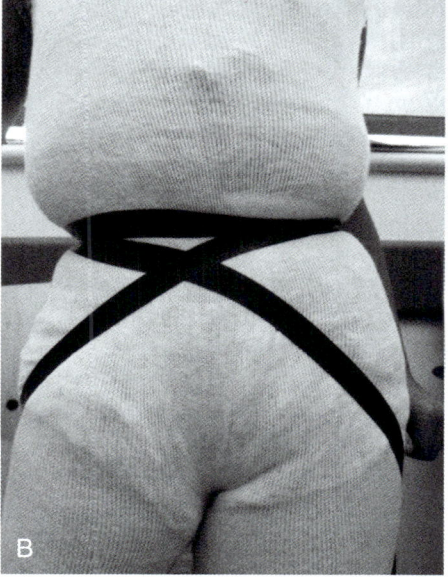

FIGURE 6 Clinical photographs depicting the casting technique for a hip disarticulation prosthesis. **A**, The patient with casting garment applied, providing little definition to the waist groove. **B**, Tape is applied to define and accentuate the waist groove.

The process of preparing a cast for the child with a transpelvic amputation begins with the application of a casting garment of sufficient strength to provide support for at least 50% of the patient's body weight because 50% or more of their weight will be supported by the sound-side lower limb. Any residual pelvic anatomy as well as the sound-side bony structures should then be marked with an indelible pencil. The patient is then wrapped in casting media; fiberglass is recommended rather than plaster because fiberglass provides superior compression of the soft tissues. A combination of plaster and fiberglass may also be used to better delineate any bony anatomy. This mold should wrap around the sound side at the waist groove in the same manner as described for the hip disarticulation casting procedure. The medial border of the cast should extend well past the midline of the body. This is important because the medial trim line of the socket will extend as far across the midline as possible to prevent herniation of the viscera.[36] After the casting material is applied, anterior and posterior casting blocks may be used to provide the socket the appropriate shape. This increases control for the patient and creates the proper anterior shape for placement of the hip joint lamination plate.

Before filling and modification of the model, it should be checked against measurements taken at the time of molding. This is particularly important of the anterior-posterior dimension because this provides the basis for control of the prosthetic limb. If the anterior-posterior dimension of the cast is greater than the measurement, it can be decreased by cutting through the floor of the cast and overlapping the cut. This should allow sufficient adjustment to the anterior-posterior dimension. The cast should be then filled and modified as appropriate for the type of socket being fabricated.

Prosthetic Design

Ages 9 to 18 Months

At the time a child starts to demonstrate the desire to pull to stand, it is appropriate to begin prosthetic treatment of a child with a high-level lower limb amputation. The child with amputation at this level may be delayed in reaching the pull-to-stand milestone, depending on the cause of amputation. For example, the child who has undergone amputation for tumor removal will likely be delayed because of extensive medical interventions and hospitalizations. It is also beneficial to begin educating the child's family as early as possible because this relationship will be extremely important in the ultimate success of prosthetic intervention. A simple lightweight design consisting of a laminated socket, hip joint, pylon, and foot is suggested (**Figure 7**). Examples of appropriate prosthetic hips would include the 7E8 hip joint and 3K51 Modular Hip Joint. Foot options include offerings by various manufacturers, such as Trulife, Kingsley MFG Company, and TRS Incorporated. These prosthetic feet are lightweight, simple, and stable, and they meet the needs of weight-bearing support appropriate for early locomotion. Early gait often requires additional support in the form of furniture cruising, an appropriate push toy, or a walker. Children in this age group also greatly benefit from the intervention of a physical therapist, preferably with pediatric prosthetic experience.

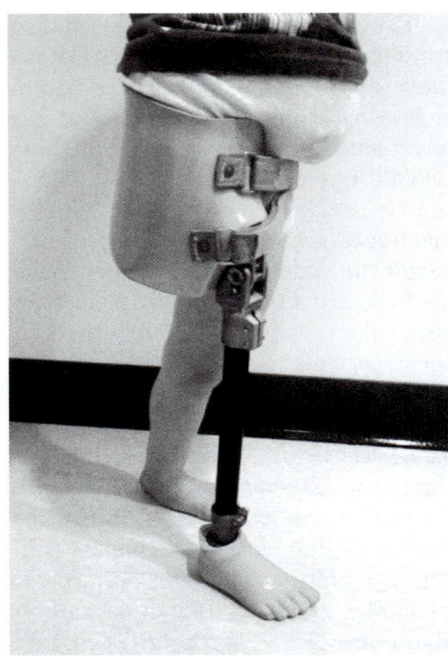

FIGURE 7 Photograph of an initial hip disarticulation prosthesis with a hip joint, no knee, and a basic foot. Note the anterior bulge of an ostomy bag, which further complicated this fitting.

Ages 18 to 48 Months

As the child grows, the first substantial change in prosthetic design is the addition of a monocentric manual locking knee (**Figure 8**), which provides the child with continued stability as well as allows the knee to bend for sitting activities and eliminating the protrusion of the foot while sitting (a substantial drawback in a monolithic pylon system). Examples of this type of knee include the 3K41 knee (Streifeneder) or 3R30 knee (Ottobock). These and similar knees have the additional advantage of being very lightweight, thereby reducing the energy cost of gait. In contrast, patients in this age range with a transfemoral amputation would be fitted with an articulated knee.[37] Patients with transfemoral amputations and knee disarticulations have better control of their prosthetic devices because of the longer lever arm of the prosthesis.

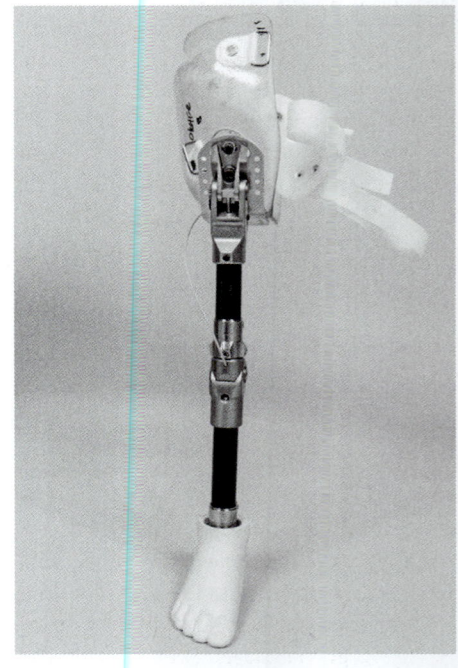

FIGURE 8 Anterior photographic view of a hip disarticulation prosthesis in the dynamic alignment phase. Components include a hip joint, a locking knee, and a basic foot.

Ages 4 to 8 Years

As the child grows and matures, the transition to functional knees and more dynamic feet is the appropriate next step. The transition to a knee that flexes and extends as the prosthesis moves through the swing phase of gait allows a more natural and rapid gait.[38] An additional benefit can be gained by using a polycentric knee, which, when flexed, creates a functional shortening of the distal segment of the prosthesis. This in turn reduces the need for gait compensations such as vaulting, hip hiking, or circumduction. Examples of this type of knee are the Total Knee Junior (Össur) and the PK-400 (TiMed). When selecting a knee for children in this age group, it is important to keep in mind the weight and durability of the component as well as the clearance above the foot because an overly long knee could result in uneven knee centers.

After the required prosthetic foot size exceeds approximately 13 cm, foot options expand. It is important to remember the balance between a dynamic foot and the stability necessary to control the hip and knee in stance. Examples of feet that provide this balance include the TruPer Foot (College Park) and the Child's Play Foot (Trulife). These feet as well as other prosthetic feet provide the function necessary for a stable and efficient gait.

When a patient is transitioning from a locked knee to a functional prosthetic knee, it is highly beneficial for the patient to be treated by a physical therapist with experience in pediatric prosthetic gait training. The therapist can be a valuable resource and will greatly improve the likelihood of a successful prosthetic outcome.[39]

Ages 8 to 12 Years

For a child with a hip disarticulation or transpelvic amputation who is age 8 to 12 years, a full spectrum of pediatric prosthetic components are available because the body size is generally sufficiently large. These options include the pediatric 7E8 hip (Ottobock), which allows for alignment adjustability and a spring extension assist.

For children in this age range, prosthetic knee choices are similar to those available for children of age 4 to 8 years. Exceptions include four-bar pneumatic knees such as the TK-4P0C (DAW Industries). This type of knee is slightly longer than those previously mentioned and requires a greater body height for adequate clearance above the foot. These knees are advantageous because they functionally decrease in length when flexed and pneumatic control allows greater control of the knee motion through the swing phase. The swing-phase control is achieved with a smaller weight penalty compared with hydraulic-controlled knees, which is important in maintaining efficient gait. A few more prosthetic foot options are available, and more dynamic carbon fiber options are appropriate. Children of this age usually have adequate muscular strength and body awareness necessary to control a prosthetic hip and knee over a more dynamic foot (**Figure 9**). When selecting components for a specific patient, it is important to keep in mind not only the patient's needs and desires but also the interplay of the components and their increasing complexity.

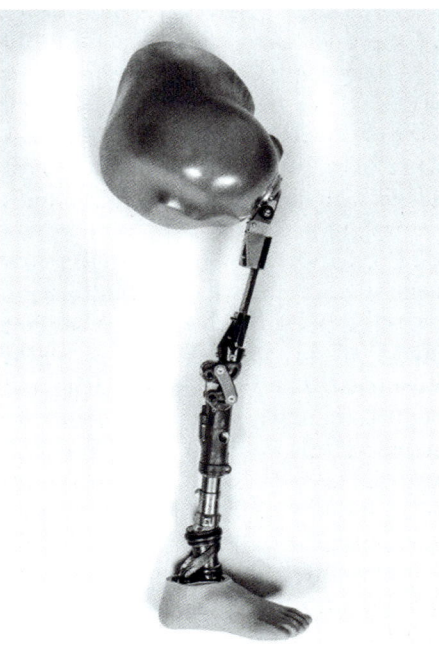

FIGURE 9 Lateral photograph of a hip disarticulation prosthesis with the Littig Hip, a pneumatic knee, and a carbon fiber foot.

Ages 13 to 21 Years

The principles applicable to patients age 13 to 21 years also apply to very active patients of all ages with high-level lower limb amputations. As pediatric patients enter this age group, they approach adult stature, but their body mass is usually less than that of adults. This is especially true for female patients, who physically mature approximately 2 years ahead of males.[40] For a pediatric patient with a nearly adult-sized body, the full spectrum of adult components is available for use in creating the appropriate prosthesis.

The socket can now be altered to include the use of soft thermoplastics or gel to provide increased comfort and improved pressure distribution. In this older pediatric population, the objections to using such materials are negated because the prosthesis represents a smaller percentage of total body mass and therefore has a smaller relative drag on walking efficiency. The use of many types of materials may be appropriate if the goals of comfort and prosthetic control are maintained. Alterations can range from the simple addition of gel in the area of the ischial tuberosity and ramus to a full flexible inner socket with a rigid frame to a complete custom gel interface. The needs of the patient should be paramount in making decisions, keeping in mind that socket discomfort is the primary reason for rejection of hip disarticulation or transpelvic prostheses.[20]

The selection of a hip joint for these patients is limited to the few hip joints on the market, which have changed little from the first hip joints used in the early 1950s. This is true with the notable exceptions of the 7E9 hydraulic hip joint and the Helix 3D hip (Ottobock). The Helix 3D hip is a polycentric joint with hydraulic control of both the swing and stance phases of gait. In addition, this joint is designed to link hip flexion and extension with transverse plane hip rotation.[41] These design advantages allow for the functional shortening of the prosthesis during swing using a polycentric mechanism and a gait pattern that very closely simulates that of able-bodied peers.[26,42]

Drawbacks to the Helix 3D hip include cost and the need to use the C-Leg knee (Ottobock) and a compatible foot (also from Ottobock). Another potential drawback is the incompatibility of a microprocessor-controlled knee with the lifestyle of many pediatric patients, which can potentially expose the device to water, impact, and dirt. The patient must also be responsible enough to routinely charge the device. Although these knees have proven beneficial in some patients, the use of microprocessor components in lower limb prostheses is not recommended until the later teenage years when growth is complete.

Multiaxial knees with either pneumatic or hydraulic control of the swing phase of gait may also be appropriate for patients in this age group. Although hydraulic knees can be an excellent choice, they are slightly heavier than pneumatic knees, which may be a consideration particularly in a patient with a low body mass. Knees in this category include the 1325A knee (ST&G Corporation) and the Total Knee 2000/2100 (Össur). An additional knee choice is a knee similar to the KX06 knee (Endolite), which provides hydraulic control of both the swing and stance phases while maintaining a polycentric design that is important to toe clearance.

Patients in this age group may also benefit from the addition of a rotation adapter such as the 4R57 (Ottobock). This component, which is typically installed directly above the prosthetic knee, allows the patient to rotate the prosthetic leg a full 360° at that point. This allows a patient to more easily enter the front seat of a car or to cross their legs. This device also allows the patient to move the prosthetic foot away from the gas and brake pedals when driving an automobile.

The choice of a prosthetic foot should be dictated by the activity level of the patient and their need for more stability or more mobility. Because it is important to carefully consider how the function of the foot will affect the other components in the prosthesis, the foot should be the last of the major components selected when formulating a prosthetic prescription. For example, the use of a carbon fiber foot with a long spring, such as the Silhouette (Freedom Innovations), may induce a greater knee flexion moment at heel strike while creating enhanced energy return as the patient transitions from terminal stance into swing. This provides a more dynamic but less stable prosthesis, which may be entirely appropriate for a highly active patient. However, the selection of a foot that has greater heel compliance, decreases the knee flexion moment at heel strike, and produces a more biomechanically stable prosthesis may be more appropriate for a patient who requires more stability because of activity level or environment.

SUMMARY

Both the surgical approach and subsequent prosthetic fitting can be quite challenging in a pediatric patient with a hip disarticulation or a transpelvic amputation. These children require an individualized approach depending on the integrity of their remaining tissue. The initial amputation procedure should concentrate on preserving as much bony skeleton as possible and, in young children, preserving the critical epiphyseal plates to enhance functional benefits as the child ages. Most of these children require a multidisciplinary team approach, both in the initial acute phase of treatment and until skeletal maturity and beyond. The successful fitting of hip disarticulation or transpelvic prosthetic devices in pediatric patients is a complex task. Successful prosthesis use can be confounded by limitations in available componentry, extreme levels of activity, and the ever-changing body of the growing child. The constantly changing pediatric patient will require closer follow-up than an adult patient as well as the establishment of a positive, trusting relationship with both the patient and their family. Outcomes are determined by careful attention to the needs of the specific pediatric patient and their family as well as socket fit, component selection, alignment, and the expertise of the members of the medical team.

References

1. Shurr D, Coot T, Buckwalter J, Cooper R: Hip disarticulation: A prosthetic follow-up. *Orthot Prosthet* 1983;37(3):50-57. Available at: http://www.oandplibrary.org/op/1983_03_050.asp. Accessed November 24, 2015.
2. Jeans KA, Browne RH, Karol LA: Effect of amputation level on energy expenditure during overground walking by children with an amputation. *J Bone Joint Surg Am* 2011;93(1):49-56.
3. Bramer JA, Taminiau AH: Reconstruction of the pelvic ring with an autograft after hindquarter amputation: Improvement of sitting stability and prosthesis support. *Acta Orthop* 2005;76(3):453-454.
4. Canavese F, Krajbich JI, LaFleur BJ: Orthopaedic sequelae of childhood meningococcemia: Management considerations and outcome. *J Bone Joint Surg Am* 2010;92(12):2196-2203.
5. Labler L, Trentz O: The use of vacuum assisted closure (VAC) in soft tissue injuries after high energy pelvic trauma. *Langenbeck's Arch Surg* 2007;392(5):601-609.
6. Boehmler JH, Francis SH, Grawe RK, Mayerson JL: Reconstruction of an external hemipelvectomy defect with a two-stage fillet of leg-free flap. *J Reconstr Microsurg* 2010;26(4):271-276.
7. Eldridge JC, Armstrong PF, Krajbich JI: Amputation stump lengthening with the Ilizarov technique: A case report. *Clin Orthop Relat Res* 1990;256:76-79.
8. Park HW, Jahng JS, Hahn SB, Shin DE: Lengthening of an amputation stump by the Ilizarov technique: A case report. *Int Orthop* 1997;21(4):274-276.
9. Sara T, Kour AK, Das De S, Rauff A, Pho RW: Wound cover in a hindquarter amputation with a free flap from the amputated limb: A case report. *Clin Orthop Relat Res* 1994;304:248-251.
10. Carter SR, Eastwood DM, Grimer RJ, Sneath RS: Hindquarter amputation for tumours of the musculoskeletal system. *J Bone Joint Surg Br* 1990;72(3):490-493.
11. Gebert C, Gosheger G, Winkelmann W: Hip transposition as a universal surgical procedure for periacetabular tumors of the pelvis. *J Surg Oncol* 2009;99(3):169-172.
12. Griesser MJ, Gillette B, Crist M, et al: Internal and external hemipelvectomy or flail hip in patients with sarcomas: Quality-of-life and functional

outcomes. *Am J Phys Med Rehabil* 2012;91(1):24-32.
13. Grimer RJ, Chandrasekar CR, Carter SR, Abudu A, Tillman RM, Jeys L: Hindquarter amputation: Is it still needed and what are the outcomes? *Bone Joint J* 2013;95-B(1):127-131.
14. Han I, Lee YM, Cho HS, Oh JH, Lee SH, Kim HS: Outcome after surgical treatment of pelvic sarcomas. *Clin Orthop Surg* 2010;2(3):160-166.
15. Wirbel RJ, Schulte M, Mutschler WE: Surgical treatment of pelvic sarcomas: Oncologic and functional outcome. *Clin Orthop Relat Res* 2001;390:190-205.
16. Apffelstaedt JP, Driscoll DL, Spellman JE, Velez AF, Gibbs JF, Karakousis CP: Complications and outcome of external hemipelvectomy in the management of pelvic tumors. *Ann Surg Oncol* 1996;3(3):304-309.
17. Hillmann A, Hoffmann C, Gosheger G, Rödl R, Winkelmann W, Ozaki T: Tumors of the pelvis: Complications after reconstruction. *Arch Orthop Trauma Surg* 2003;123(7):340-344.
18. Brandt MM, Corpron CA, Wahl WL: Necrotizing soft tissue infections: A surgical disease. *Am Surg* 2000;66(10):967-970.
19. Nowroozi F, Salvanelli ML, Gerber LH: Energy expenditure in hip disarticulation and hemipelvectomy amputees. *Arch Phys Med Rehabil* 1983;64(7):300-303.
20. New York University: *Lower-Extremity Prosthetics*. New York University, 1973.
21. Schnall BL, Baum BS, Andrews AM: Gait characteristics of a soldier with a traumatic hip disarticulation. *Phys Ther* 2008;88(12):1568-1577.
22. Hector WK, Newman JD: Relative incidences of new amputations: Statistical comparisons of 6,000 new amputees. *Orthot Prosthet* 1975;29(2):3-16. Available at: http://www.oandplibrary.org/op/1975_02_003.asp. Accessed November 24, 2015.
23. Glattly HW: A statistical study of 12,000 new amputees. *South Med J* 1964;57(11):1373-1378.
24. Radcliffe CW: The biomechanics of the Canadian-type hip-disarticulation prosthesis. *Artif Limbs* 1957;4(2):29-38.
25. Raiford RL, Epps CH Jr: Experiences with the Canadian hip disarticulation prosthesis in the juvenile. *J Natl Med Assoc* 1974;66(1):71-75.
26. Solomonidis SE, Loughran AJ, Taylor J, Paul JP: Biomechanics of the hip disarticulation prosthesis. *Prosthet Orthot Int* 1977;1(1):13-18.
27. Zaffer SM, Braddom RL, Conti A, Goff J, Bokma D: Total hip disarticulation prosthesis with suction socket: Report of two cases. *Am J Phys Med Rehabil* 1999;78(2):160-162.
28. Sabolich J, Guth T: The CAT-CAM–H.D.(tm): A new design for hip disarticulation patients. *Clin Orthot Prosthet* 1988;12(3):119-122.
29. Littig D, Lundt J: The UCLA anatomical hip disarticulation prosthesis. *Clin Orthot Prosthet* 1988;12(3):114-118.
30. Houdek MT, Kralovec ME, Andrews KL: Hemipelvectomy: High-level amputation surgery and prosthetic rehabilitation. *Am J Phys Med Rehabil* 2014;93(7):600-608.
31. Pasquina P, Cooper R: *Care of the Combat Amputee*. Office of the Surgeon General, 2009.
32. van der Waarde T, Michael JW: Hip disarticulation and transpelvic amputation: Prosthetic management, in Bowker J, Michael J, eds: *Atlas of Limb Prosthetics: Surgical, Prosthetic, and Rehabilitation Principles*, ed 2. Mosby-Year Book, 2002.
33. Stark G: Overview of hip disarticulation prostheses. *J Prosthet Orthot* 2001;13:50-53.
34. Fernández A, Formigo J: Are Canadian prostheses used? A long-term experience. *Prosthet Orthot Int* 2005;29(2):177-181.
35. Wilk B, Karol L, Halliday S, Cummings D, Haideri N, Stephenson J: Transition to an articulating knee prosthesis in pediatric amputees. *J Prosthet Orthot* 1999;11:69-74.
36. Average Weight for Children by Age. Available at: http://www.buzzle.com/articles/average-weight-for-children-by-age.html. Accessed October 7, 2015.
37. Isakov E, Susak Z, Becker E: Energy expenditure and cardiac response in above-knee amputees while using prostheses with open and locked knee mechanisms. *Scand J Rehabil Med Suppl* 1985;12:108-111.
38. Lundt JE, Littig DH, Choi GE: Das ESSA-3D-Hüftexartikulationsgelenk-System und sein Einfluß auf den Energiebedarf bei einseitig Amputierten. *Orthop Technik* 1995;9:773-785.
39. Tanner JM: *Foetus Into Man: Physical Growth From Conception to Maturity*. Castelmead Publications, 1989, pp 6-23.
40. Ludwigs E, Bellmann M, Schmalz T, Blumentritt S: Biomechanical differences between two exoprosthetic hip joint systems during level walking. *Prosthet Orthot Int* 2010;34(4):449-460.
41. Rommers GM, Vos LD, Groothoff JW, Eisma WH: Clinical rehabilitation of the amputee: A retrospective study. *Prosthet Orthot Int* 1996;20(2):72-78.
42. Blumentritt S, Ludwigs E, Bellman M, Boiten H: Das neue Hüftgelenk Helix[3D]. *Orthop-Technik* 2008;5:345-350.

Transfemoral Amputations and Knee Disarticulation: Surgical Principles and Prosthetic Management

CHAPTER 75

Jorge A. Fabregas, MD, FAAOS • David B. Rotter, CPO

ABSTRACT

When considering amputations above the knee in the pediatric cohort, there are two main options: knee disarticulation or a traditional transfemoral amputation. Both amputations have their benefits and disadvantages. Lever arm length, potential limb length, and expected complications should be considered before proceeding with either procedure.

Keywords: knee disarticulation; myodesis; terminal overgrowth; transfemoral amputation

Introduction

Several factors distinguish the care of pediatric limb deficiencies versus adult amputations. Data suggest that 70% of the children seen in pediatric clinics have a congenital limb deficiency, and the remaining 30% have acquired amputations resulting from causes such as trauma and sarcomas.[1] For the child who has a congenital limb deficiency, both advantages and challenges need to be addressed. Children who are born with a limb deficiency are incredibly adaptable because they know no other existence. The use of a prosthesis often becomes second nature if it is incorporated during the child's growth and development. When not wearing their prostheses, children also learn locomotion strategies, such as hopping, scooting, and crawling, which allows for the development of greater balance and strength in their sound limb. Patients with bilateral lower limb deficiency use their upper limbs and torso to propel themselves forward on the ground when not using prostheses, thus affording greater muscle development and dexterity.

Challenges in care relate to the appearance of the affected limb. Congenital limb deficiencies can be associated with other anomalies, such as irregular bone and muscle development, joint instability, and joint malrotation.[2] Data further suggest that 40% of patients have multiple limb involvement, potentially increasing prosthetic fitting challenges.[3] Bony overgrowth is a challenge specific to a transosseous amputation. The terminal bone overgrowth can eventually overtake the soft-tissue envelope, potentially resulting in bone piercing through the skin.[4]

When given the opportunity, it is always preferable for the surgeon to perform a knee disarticulation that preserves the end-bearing surfaces, allows for additional growth through the distal femoral epiphyseal plate, and avoids terminal bony overgrowth. In the pediatric cohort, knee disarticulation is considered preferable to transfemoral amputation for many reasons. The primary concern in a growing child is that the development of the affected limb will keep pace with the sound limb. Knee disarticulation preserves the femoral epiphysis, allowing the growth mechanism in the femur to be unaffected. An end-bearing limb with primarily intact thigh musculature makes a knee disarticulation functionally superior to a transfemoral amputation.[5,6]

Surgical Principles

In the pediatric patient, the indications to perform transfemoral amputation or a knee disarticulation are very broad. They can vary widely from congenital anomalies, as in the case of tibial deficiency, to traumatic lawn mower accidents, to oncologic cases.[7] Data suggest a gradual decline in sport/physical functioning with higher level amputations. However, the literature suggests that amputation level did not affect pain scores, happiness, or basic mobility.[8]

When dealing with any level of amputations in children there two main fundamental principles. The first principle is to preserve as much length as possible. The longer lever arm allows for greater power and ease of prosthetic use.[9] The second principle is to attempt to perform a disarticulation whenever possible; in part for the longer lever arm, but also to avoid the dreaded complication of terminal overgrowth.

In attempting to conserve energy, the child's innate biologic potential allows for the surgeon to use surgical techniques that would have been likely unsuccessful in adults. In an adult there may be a reluctance to attempt wound closures under tension, and also skepticism about using split-thickness skin grafts. A split-thickness skin graft, even over large areas of the residual limb, may be tolerated relatively well by the child, while in an adult it can be fraught with complications.[10]

Dr. Fabregas or an immediate family member serves as a paid consultant to or is an employee of Astura Medical. David B. Rotter or an immediate family member serves as a board member, owner, officer, or committee member of Association of Children's Prosthetic and Orthotic Clinics.

Disarticulations preserve the epiphyseal plate and ensure continued longitudinal growth. This is critical when dealing with transfemoral amputations. In amputations at this level, sacrificing the distal femoral physis, which accounts for 70% of the longitudinal growth of the femur, the residual limb length may provide a challenging prosthetic option if it is too short. What may have appeared to be a long transfemoral amputation in a very young child could potentially be extremely short in an adult.

Disarticulation precludes the development of terminal overgrowth or appositional growth of the transected bone. The prominent condyles usually atrophy, thereby eliminating the cosmetic objection to this type of surgery that is present when performed in adults. It should also be borne in mind that there is also an attempt made to provide enough space on the distal residual limb to accommodate knee components. The desired length of the residual limb, even in a knee disarticulation, must be discussed with the prosthetist to achieve an ideal outcome. It is not uncommon to perform a distal femoral growth arrest to achieve this ideal length. If the patient is skeletally mature and an epiphysiodesis is not an alternative, intercalary resection is also a viable option.

Complications

Terminal overgrowth is the most common complication in through-bone amputations.[11] This particular complication is unique to growing bones.

Initially, preventive management at the time of amputation should be undertaken. Surplus bones may be used to biologically cap the residual limb. The fibular head, metatarsal head, and even the distal tibia, or fibula, can be salvaged. Unfortunately, biologic capping for transfemoral overgrowth, when performed as a revision, leaves limited biologic caps. Tricortical iliac crest autograft, a technique described by Davids in which a tricortical allograft along with an apophyseal plate is used to cap the femur, can be employed.[12,13]

There are several other causes of complications requiring surgical intervention.

Adventitious bursae formation may develop in an area of terminal overgrowth. Conservative treatment, including aspiration or steroid injections, for symptomatic bursae is only a temporary measure. The underlying pathology needs to be addressed to ultimately resolve the problem, whether it is because of poor prosthetic fitting or spur formations. Bone spurs can be differentiated from terminal overgrowth in that they occur in the periphery of the residual limb, as opposed to the terminal portion.

Postoperative and traumatic scarring can also hinder prosthetic fitting.

Neuroma formation can also occur as a result of transecting the nerve at the time of amputation. Revision surgery may occur in up to 4% of these patients;[14] however, most can be managed with socket adjustment.[12,13] Targeted muscle innervation is an option when neuroma formation becomes debilitating and precludes prosthetic wear despite adjustments.

Phantom limb pain also has been described. Fortunately, if it occurs in children younger than 10 years the phantom sensation tends to disappear. Unfortunately, however, there are multiple reports in teenage amputees with varied treatment modalities and inconsistent outcomes.

Postamputation pain is another source of disability in the amputee. This is a complex condition that can be traced to the residual limb, spinal cord, brain, or a combination of these locations. The mainstay of treatment is largely medical, but several other options are being studied.[15]

Surgical Technique: Transfemoral Amputation

Pediatric transfemoral surgical techniques do not differ significantly from those of adults. Transfemoral amputation levels illustrate the importance of muscle reconstruction. The goals of reconstruction after transfemoral amputation are to regain muscle balance and to better position the limb so that it can sustain some weight on the side of the thigh. The transfemoral amputee can support very little weight directly on the end of their residual limb.

To balance the thigh muscles, the surgeon must perform myodesis (attachment of muscle to bone). The surgeon can secure the muscle by drilling holes into the bone and suturing the muscle directly to bone or by securing it onto the periosteum.

Because the adductor and extensor muscles of the hip attach at the lower end of the thigh, their insertion is sacrificed in a transfemoral amputation. The net effect is an unbalanced residual limb. Without a myodesis there is tendency for the limb to stay in a flexed and abducted position. Myodesis will provide a stronger residual limb that is more balanced and centered in the muscle mass. Myodesis can also provide benefits in reducing the adductor roll. The adductor roll is soft-tissue redundancies that can form high on the inner thigh and become bothersome with prosthetic fit. The cause of the adductor roll is believed, in part, to be caused by retraction of the muscles that are no longer held in place by a distal anchor. Myodesis is not a simple task. Muscles do not generally hold sutures well. In that case, the fascia may be the best available anchor point. Meticulous dissection should be performed to enable a good fascial layer to be sutured later.

When performing an amputation on a congenital limb deficiency the possibility of hip instability should always be considered. Hip instability may need to be addressed to provide an adequate fulcrum for a proper lever arm to function.

Indications for a knee disarticulation are congenital deficiency, a nonfunctional knee, and when reconstruction is not an option. Knee disarticulation is the preferred surgical option over a transfemoral amputation on a growing child, so that risks of overgrowth are obviated, length is preserved, and muscle transection is minimized.

Surgical Technique: Knee Disarticulation

This surgery can be performed with the patient in a supine or lateral position. A sterile tourniquet is preferred, and a posterior-based or anterior-based flap can be used. The patella is excised at the time of the original amputation to minimize the risk of future patellofemoral pain. The patellar tendon and hamstrings are sutured to the cruciate residuum or the knee capsule to achieve appropriate myodesis (**Figure 1**).

Prosthetic Management

When to Begin Prosthetic Care

The literature suggests that it is appropriate to begin prosthetic fitting when a child reaches the developmental milestone of independently pulling to a standing position.[7-9] However, varying opinions exist in the literature on when to provide a child with an articulated knee. Earlier studies suggested waiting until age 3 years,[10] but the more contemporary approach suggests that a child should be provided with an articulating knee early during development, in line with the pull-to-stand milestone.[11,16] The benefits of early fitting with an articulating knee include permitting a child to crawl and kneel even before standing is achieved.[17-23]

Early Suspension and Knee Systems

If a summary statement can be made about suspension systems and knee components for the pediatric patient, it is that one can influence the other. This fact is most apparent when a child with a congenital limb deficiency is fitted with their first prosthesis. Component selection often is predicated on space allowance.

Just as liner technology has become ubiquitous for adult suspension systems, liners have steadily become an ideal suspension choice for the pediatric cohort. Liners are easy for parents to put on very young children. In addition, the elastic nature of the material allows for expansion as the child grows. Liners provide secure suspension, generally eliminating the need for a suspension belt. If the residual limb is short and lacks sufficient leverage, a belt can be used to augment suspension and stability. The disadvantage of using liners is that length is added to the end of the residual limb. If a liner system is chosen for suspension, the remaining overall length must be measured, and a decision must be made to determine which knee articulation system can be used.

Examples of some liner and suspension considerations in the first prosthetic fitting for a child are shown in **Figure 2**. It is important that parents be instructed on how to apply the liner and chosen suspension system. The prosthetist may use a temporary socket to determine the overall height of the prosthesis. In fitting the child shown in **Figure 2**, outside hinges were selected because there was insufficient space for an articulating knee below the socket,

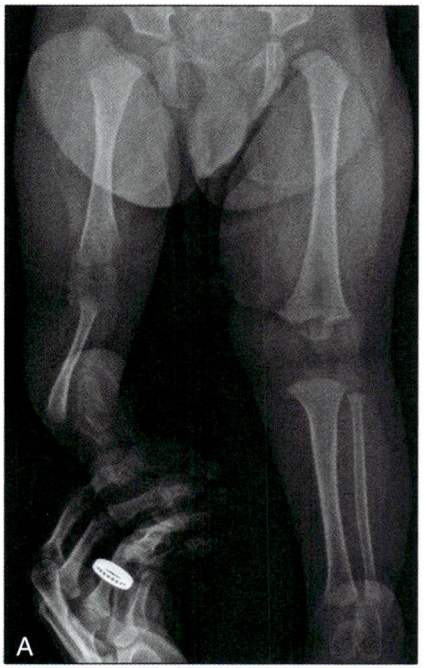 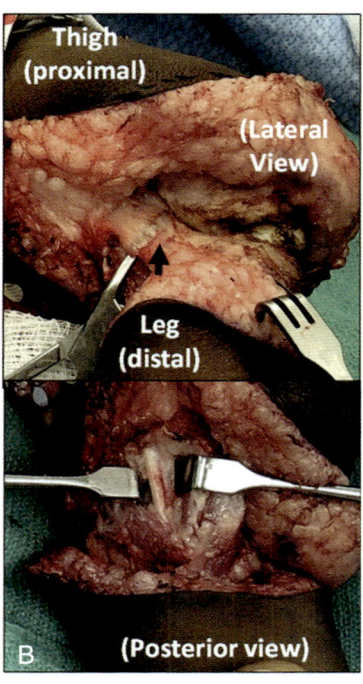 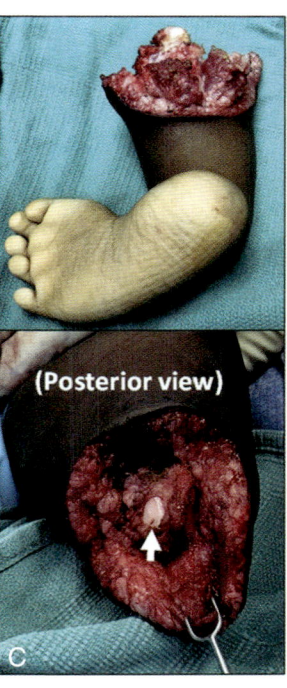 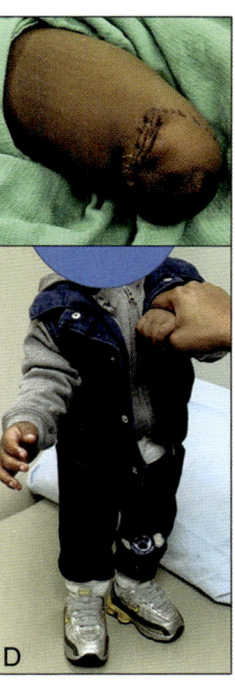

FIGURE 1 Radiograph and clinical photographs showing knee disarticulation. **A**, Radiograph from a 9-month-old male child with Jones type 1a tibial deficiency with the absence of entire tibia and extensor mechanism. It was decided to proceed with amputation before walking age. **B**, The patient was in the lateral position with the apex of the fish-mouth incision at the joint line with a larger anterior flap. After anterior dissection and arthrotomy, dissection was continued medially and laterally. There were no medial hamstring tendons or extensor mechanism encountered anteriorly, although the iliotibial (IT) band required division laterally (black arrowhead). Dissection then continued posteriorly, where the popliteus neurovascular structures were isolated before ligation. In tibial deficiency, the posterior dissection may be hindered by the knee flexion contracture. In these cases, it may be advantageous to primarily strip the gastrocnemius origin to allow extension, then isolate, and ligate the neurovascular bundle. **C**, The amputated part and residual limb (note dysmorphic distal femur with single condyle—white arrowhead—void of notch or cruciate ligaments) are shown. **D**, Final closure with anterior skin flap (posterior flap was trimmed to eliminate redundancy) and clinical photograph showing prosthesis use at 6 weeks after surgery. (Reproduced with permission from Louer CR Jr, Scott-Wyard P, Hernandez R, Vergun AD: Principles of amputation surgery, prosthetics, and rehabilitation in children. *J Am Acad Orthop Surg* 2021;29[14]:e702-e713, Figure 5.)

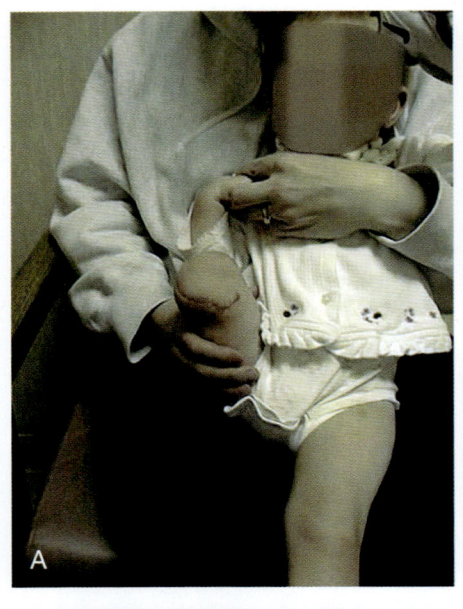
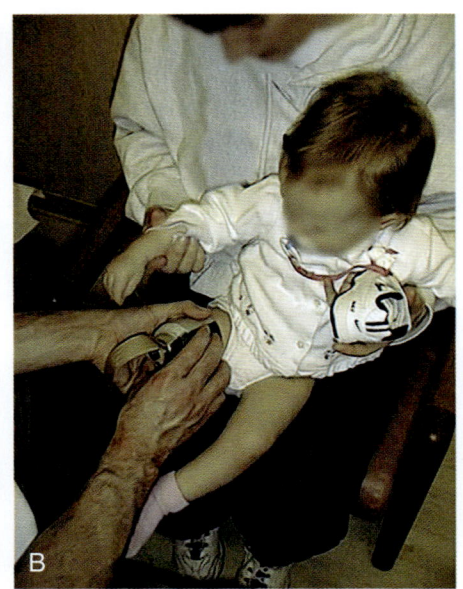
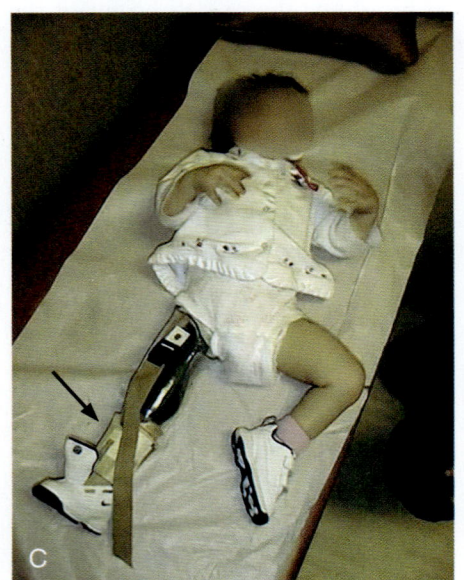
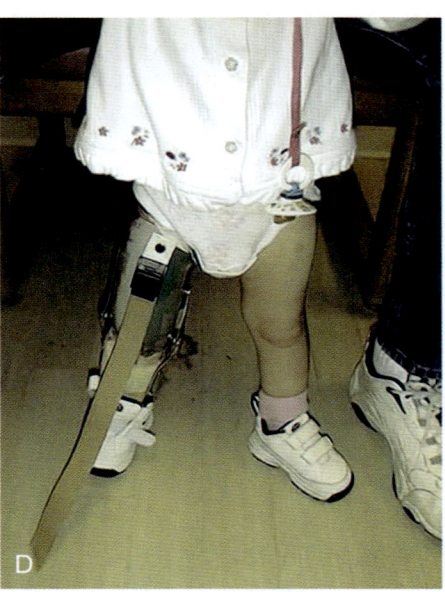

FIGURE 2 Clinical photographs demonstrating some steps and considerations in the first prosthesis fitting of 6-month-old child. **A**, The right limb was revised to a knee disarticulation because the child was born with an absent tibia and a nonfunctioning limb distal to the knee. **B**, The parent is instructed on the application of the gel liner. **C**, The donned liner is shown within the clear socket of the prosthesis. A distal lanyard was fed through the bottom of the socket to create a lanyard-style suspension system that is secured with a plastic clip. Also pictured is an exoskeletal wood block (arrow) attached to the temporary socket that is used to determine the overall height. After the appropriate height is determined, articulation can be added to the knee. **D**, Outside hinges were used because of insufficient space for an articulating knee below the socket. (Courtesy of David B. Rotter, CPO, David Rotter Prosthetics, LTD, Joliet, IL.)

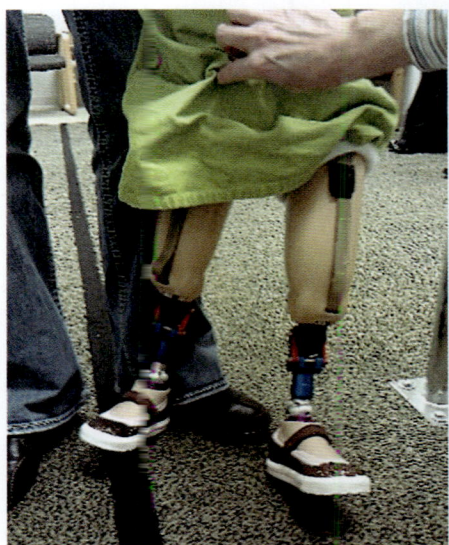

FIGURE 3 Clinical photograph of endoskeletal components being fitted. (Courtesy of David B. Rotter, CPO, David Rotter Prosthetics, LTD, Joliet, IL.)

and the knee center would be impractically low. This would impede the child from crawling. A common strategy used with outside hinges is to couple them with an anterior elastic strap attached proximally to the socket and distally to the shin section. The elastic strap allows the child to crawl with a bent knee and is snug enough to ensure immediate knee extension on standing. This strap can be tightened or loosened depending on the child's ability to control the articulation throughout their maturation and development.

In patients with bilateral transfemoral amputations or knee disarticulations, matching the anatomic knee center is no longer a primary consideration. The prosthetist may choose to use bilateral endoskeletal knee joints (**Figure 3**) Initially, such prostheses may be intentionally shortened to minimize the risk of injury from falls. However, as these children grow and stability increases, length is added to the shin sections to create better overall symmetry.

The Growing Child

The main factor influencing component selection is the space available distal to the socket. As a child grows and the relative distance between the distal end of the socket and the ground increases, a greater range of component choices becomes available. As more distance is gained, suspension options become less of a fitting consideration.

Despite a steady increase in component offerings for the pediatric cohort, selection remains limited, which is especially true for pediatric knee systems. As a child grows and gains sufficient clearance, various four-bar mechanical knee systems can be used (**Figure 4, A**). Polycentric knee mechanisms offer several advantages, specifically for pediatric fittings. The greater range of motion present when kneeling is practical and helpful both for an infant who is crawling and an older child who kneels on the ground during play (**Figure 4, B**).

As greater clearance is achieved with a child's continued growth, the patient can be fitted with a polycentric five-bar mechanism (**Figure 4**). The advantage of this system is the increased stability present with a mechanical locking feature at heel strike or when pressure is exerted on the heel of the foot. This feature allows for greater inherent stability as the child becomes more active and traverses uneven terrain during play and sport activities.

The Active Child

Almost all children will eventually want to use their prostheses to run. This process might start with a double hop on the sound limb to a single hop on the prosthesis and will eventually progress to running leg over leg. Most pediatric knee prostheses have a manual friction setting that is good for level, steady-speed walking but does not provide sufficient resistance to heel rise when running. The child will compensate by using an abducted circumduction motion, swinging through a stiff leg, or having the leg shank fully flexed and rebounding off the posterior aspect of the socket back into extension. Being highly adaptable, children will use their ingenuity to resolve any design shortcomings of the prosthetic knee. As the shank length gets longer, the effective pendulum length of the prosthesis elongates, increasing its swing-phase duration, thus making it increasingly difficult to run with prosthetic knees with only friction resistance.

A few fluid-controlled prosthetic knees have been designed to address this deficit within the pediatric cohort (**Figure 5, A**). At present, further development of fluid-controlled prosthetic knee systems is needed to better accommodate the growing and increasingly more active child.

Polycentric prosthetic knees can be coupled with highly responsive pediatric carbon fiber prosthetic feet (**Figure 5, B**); however, such dynamic prosthetic feet will subject the prosthetic knee mechanism to greater torques in swing as the child goes from walking to running. This further supports the need for mechanisms that will provide greater swing phase control for pediatric patients.

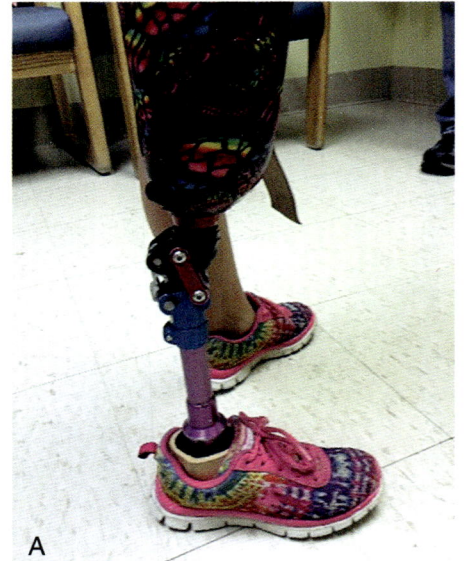
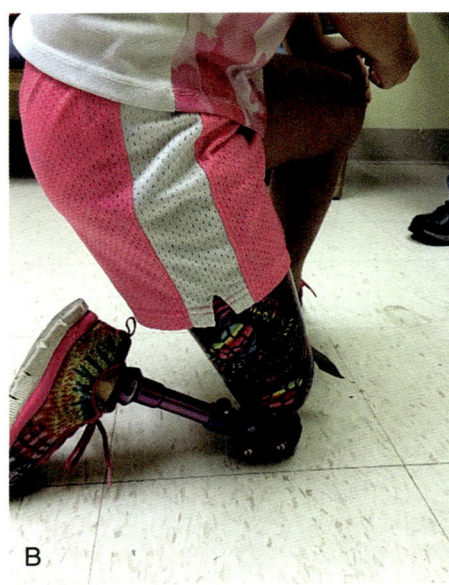

FIGURE 4 **A**, Clinical photograph of a pediatric four-bar prosthetic knee. **B**, Clinical photograph of the advantages of using a four-bar prosthetic knee system, which include greater range of flexion to allow kneeling. (Courtesy of David B. Rotter, CPO, David Rotter Prosthetics, LTD, Joliet, IL.)

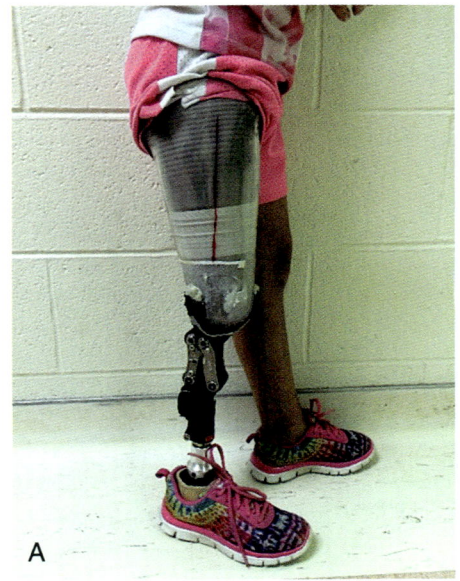
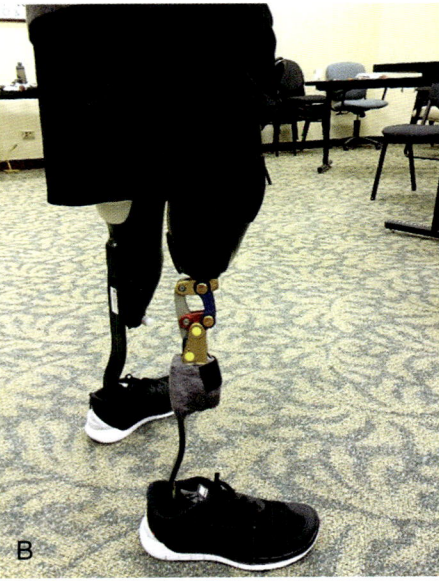

FIGURE 5 **A**, Clinical photograph of a fluid-controlled pediatric prosthetic knee. **B**, Clinical photograph of responsive carbon fiber prosthetic feet. (Courtesy of David B. Rotter, CPO, David Rotter Prosthetics, LTD, Joliet, IL.)

Transitioning to Adult Components

As a child becomes an adolescent, the prosthetist is encouraged to consider adult components as soon as their limb length and body weight allow. Adult prosthetic components offer a far greater array of choices for fluid-controlled prosthetic knees and dynamic prosthetic feet to accommodate the active adolescent. Endoskeletal components can adapt the standard pediatric 22-mm diameter pylon to an adult 30-mm pylon, which allows for mixing and matching of adult and pediatric components.

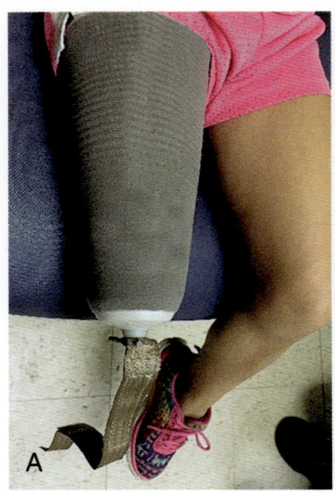 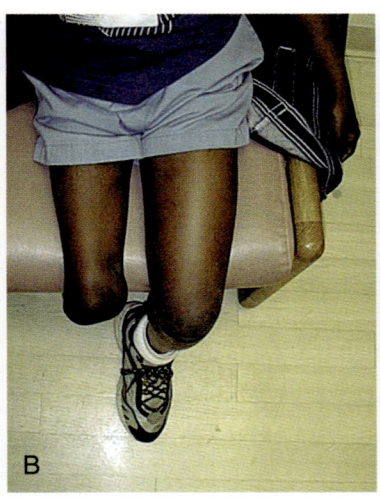 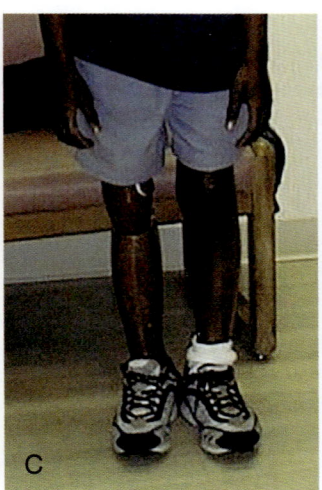 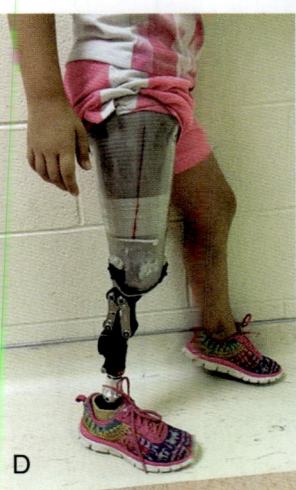

FIGURE 6 Clinical photographs of suspension prostheses. **A**, Locking liner with lanyard strap. **B**, Knee disarticulation with palpable prominent condyles. **C**, Supracondylar medial door suspension. **D**, Seal-in liner. (Courtesy of David B. Rotter, CPO, David Rotter Prosthetics, LTD, Joliet, IL.)

As previously mentioned, liner technology is used extensively in pediatric fittings. When a child is young and the bony anatomy is difficult to palpate, an elastomeric liner will provide good soft-tissue load bearing in addition to a secure form of suspension (**Figure 6, A**). As the child with a knee disarticulation grows older and their anatomy becomes more defined, more traditional means of suspension, such as a suspension system with a supracondylar door, can be used (**Figure 6, B and C**). This type of suspension will reduce the distal build height of the prosthesis and allow a more symmetric knee center.

A modern variant to true suction suspension is a seal-in liner (**Figure 6, D**), which can be used after a child develops sufficient dexterity and strength to don and doff the liner independently. Given the rapid growth considerations that must be accounted for, true suction suspension is challenging in pediatric prosthetic management.[13] The seal-in liner system offers a better alternative because it does not have to fit as snugly as a true suction socket. The initial fit can be intentionally loose, requiring the use of fitting socks. As the limb grows, removal of the interface socks will accommodate growth and maintain a reasonable socket fit. Importantly, a positive suction suspension is preserved throughout the initial socket fitting and subsequent growth accommodations (**Figure 7**).

Congenital Anomalies

Children born with congenital anomalies may have unique fitting challenges. A prosthetist may encounter uniquely formed limbs and must think creatively to accommodate the anatomy into a functional prosthesis. The most commonly seen congenital deformity managed with a transfemoral prosthesis is a proximal femoral focal deficiency, which is also known as partial longitudinal deficiency of the femur. Proximal femoral focal deficiency results in a shortened anatomic femoral length, which raises the ipsilateral ankle and foot closer to the height of the contralateral knee.

Three potential courses of action exist for pediatric patients with congenital anomalies at or distal to the knee. The first option is to fit the limb as is with a modified extension prosthesis (**Figure 8**). The foot is placed in full equinus to accommodate the donning of pants. The articulation is placed as proximally as possible to gain ground clearance during swing and should be as compact as possible to allow comfortable sitting. This option accommodates the anatomy the child was born with and allows the child's input into future decision-making if rotationplasty or ankle disarticulation is considered at a later date.

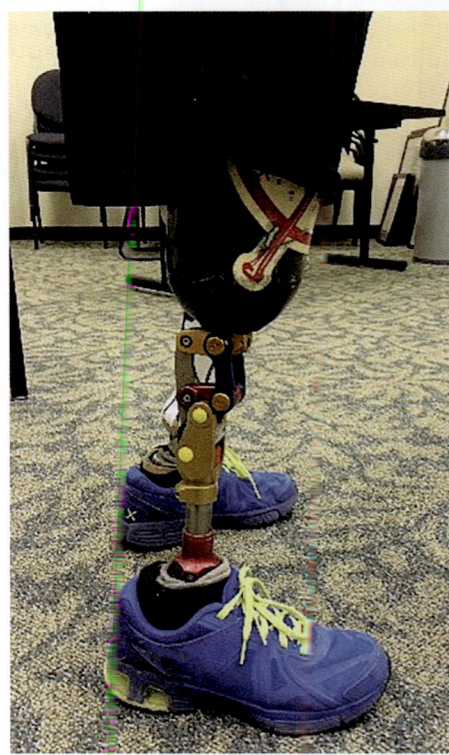

FIGURE 7 Clinical photograph of a pediatric polycentric five-bar prosthetic knee. (Courtesy of David B. Rotter, CPO, David Rotter Prosthetics, LTD, Joliet, IL.)

The second option is for the surgeon to perform rotationplasty of the foot (also known as Van Nes rotationplasty). In this procedure, the surgeon rotates the affected foot 180° to allow the foot to function as a quasi-knee joint (**Figure 9, A and B**). The dorsiflexors act as knee flexors, and the plantar flexors act as knee extensors.[12] Outside hinges should be used on the prosthesis to contour around the malleoli and create a mechanical joint center that is congruent with the anatomic joint center to create a smooth reaction at the joint (**Figure 9, C**). As the child grows older and larger, stronger outside hinges are required to accommodate the forces generated in gait. The foot is positioned in full equinus to generate maximum power for each movement. The shape of the foot in equinus allows for good suspension over the heel as it becomes prominent enough for self-suspension. Suspension can be achieved using an anterior door, a strap over the heel, or a stovepipe-style cushion insert in the distal foot portion.

After rotationplasty, it is common for the foot to start to derotate back to its original position with the passage of time. As this occurs, the prosthetist must creatively fashion the articulations to maintain a semblance of fluid ankle articulation. If the joint incongruity becomes too severe, surgery is required to reset the limb at an appropriate angle.

The third option for patients with congenital anomalies at or distal to the knee is surgical ablation of the foot with a Syme ankle disarticulation. The advantage of this procedure is that it allows the fitting of traditional prosthetic knee components. The disadvantages include the loss of a functional joint under physiologic control. In some instances, the decision to perform a Syme ankle disarticulation can be delayed until the child is old enough to make their own decision regarding the procedure (**Figure 10**).

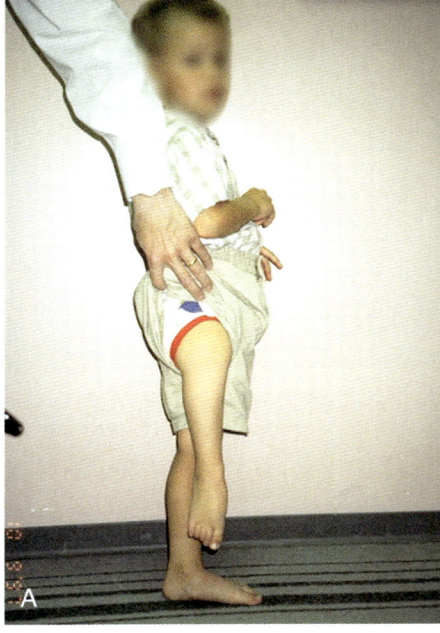
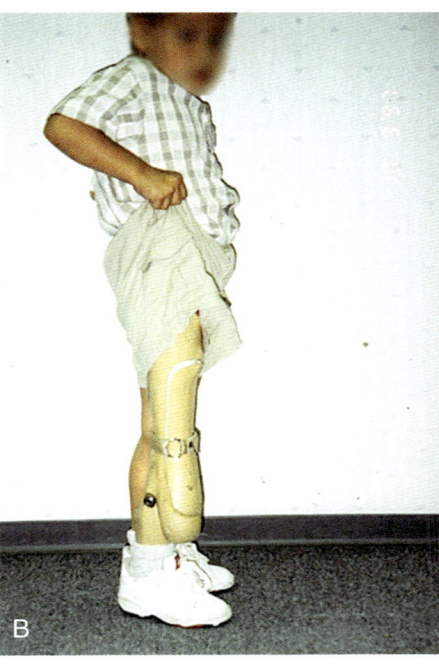

FIGURE 8 Clinical photographs of a child with a proximal femoral focal deficiency. **A**, Untreated. **B**, The child wearing an extension prosthesis. (Courtesy of David B. Rotter, CPO, David Rotter Prosthetics, LTD, Joliet, IL.)

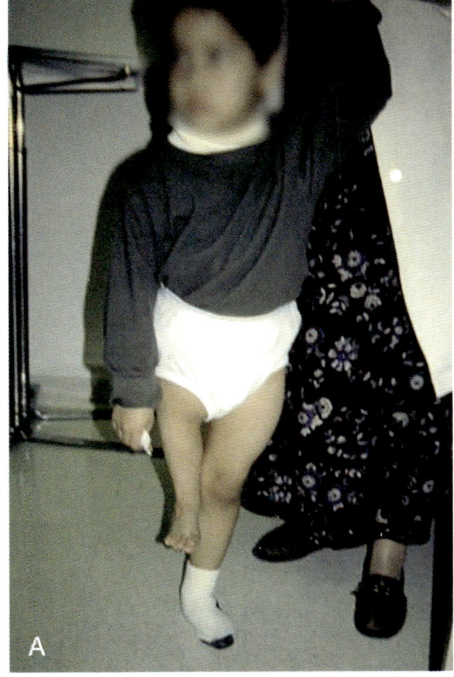
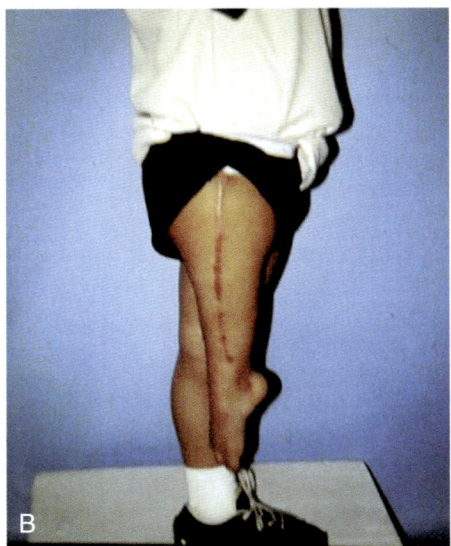
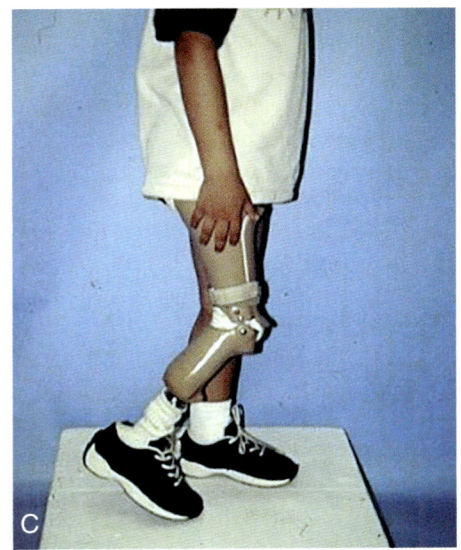

FIGURE 9 Clinical photographs of a child before (**A**) and after (**B**) rotationplasty. **C**, Photograph of a pediatric rotationplasty prosthesis. (Courtesy of David B. Rotter, CPO, David Rotter Prosthetics, LTD, Joliet, IL.)

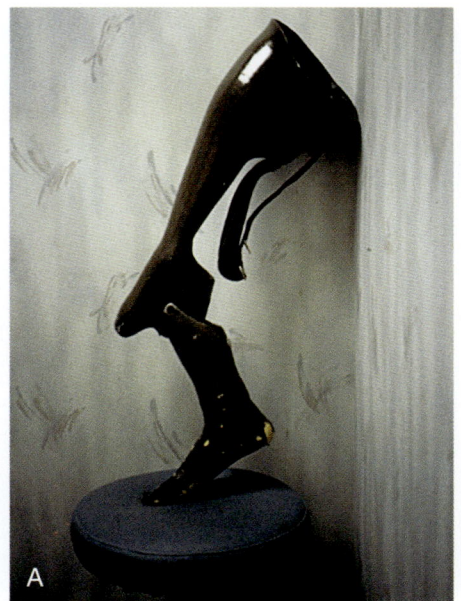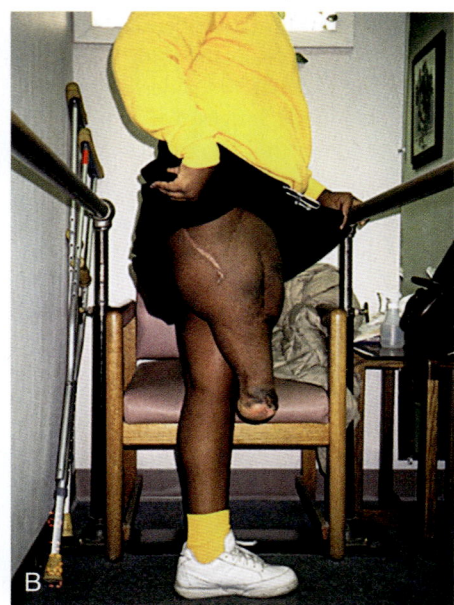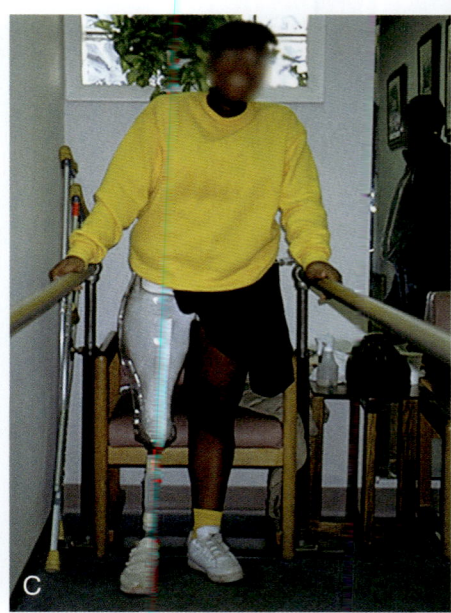

FIGURE 10 **A**, Photograph of a prosthesis worn before elective foot ablation. **B**, Clinical photograph of a limb after foot ablation. **C**, Clinical photograph of the fitting of traditional prosthetic knee components in an adolescent. (Courtesy of David B. Rotter, CPO, David Rotter Prosthetics, LTD, Joliet, IL.)

SUMMARY

If knee disarticulation and transfemoral amputation are compared, several factors must be taken into consideration, including muscle preservation, lever arm, complication potential, shape, and prosthetic suspension. Muscle preservation is achieved in knee disarticulation, but partially on a transfemoral amputation. Myodesis attempts to counteract this difference, but clearly a biologic muscle attachment has its benefits. Terminal overgrowth is impossible in knee disarticulation but possible in transfemoral amputation.

It is important to compare/take into account lever arms when performing an amputation. The knee disarticulated limb will ideally be 10 to 15 cm shorter, to account for the prosthetic knee joint in the future.

Children who require transfemoral prostheses may have a wide range of limb shapes and fitting challenges. Children who have a congenital limb deficiency are likely to have atypical bone shapes, muscle placements, and joint irregularities, and may have multiple limb involvement. When surgery is the appropriate course of action to remove a nonfunctioning residual limb distal to the knee, a disarticulation procedure is preferred. Children with acquired transtibial amputations are more susceptible to bony overgrowth.

The prosthetist must be mindful of the limitations in the available components to construct a prosthesis for the child with a limb deficiency caused by a transfemoral amputation or a knee disarticulation. This is especially true for the youngest patients undergoing first-time fittings. Congenital anomalies such as proximal femoral focal deficiency offer unique challenges and have a separate fitting protocol.

The pediatric patient with a transfemoral amputation, a knee disarticulation, or a lower limb congenital anomaly is faced with unique challenges. Those challenges should be viewed by the prosthetist as unique opportunities to fashion a well-functioning device that will improve the quality of life for the growing child.

References

1. Challenor YB: Limb deficiencies and amputation surgery in children, in Molnary GE, ed: *Pediatric Rehabilitation*. Williams and Wilkins, 1985.
2. Aitken GT, Pellicore RJ: Introduction to the child amputee, in Bowker HK, Michael JW, eds: *Atlas of Limb Prosthetics: Surgical, Prosthetic, and Rehabilitation Principles*. CV Mosby, 1981, pp 493-500.
3. Gibson D: Child and juvenile amputees, in Banjerjee S, Khan N, eds: *Rehabilitation Management of Amputees*. Williams and Wilkins, 1982, pp 394-414.
4. Aitken GT: Overgrowth of the amputation stump. *Interclin Info Bull* 1962;1:1-8.
5. Loder RT, Herring JA: Disarticulation of the knee in children: A functional assessment. *J Bone Joint Surg Am* 1987;69(8):1155-1160.
6. Hughes J: Biomechanics of the through-knee prosthesis. *Prosthet Orthot Int* 1983;7(2):96-99.
7. Aitken GT: Surgical amputation in children. *J Bone Joint Surg* 1963;45:1735-1741.
8. McQuerry J: Effect of amputation level on quality of life and subjective function in children. *J Pediatr Orthop* 2019;39(7):e524-e530.
9. Waters RL, Perry J: Energy cost of walking of amputees: The influence of level of amputation. *J Bone Joint Surg* 1976;58:42-46.
10. Parry IS, Mooney KN, Chau C, et al: Effects of skin grafting on successful prosthetic use in children with lower extremity amputation. *J Burn Care Res* 2008;29(6):949-954.
11. O'Neal ML, Bahner E, Ganey TM, Ogden JA: Osseous overgrowth

11. after amputataion in adolescent and children. *J Pediatr Orthop* 1996;16:78-84.
12. Aitken GT: The child with an acquired amputation. *Inter Clin Bull* 1968;7:1-15.
13. Davids JR, Meyer LC, Backhurst DW: Operative treatment of bone overgrowth in children who have an acquired or congenital amputation. *J Bone Joint Surg Am* 1995;77A:1490-1497.
14. Modest JM, Raducha JE, Testa EJ, Eberson CP: Management of post-amputation pain. *R I Med J* 2020;103:19-22.
15. Morrissy RT, Giavedoni BJ, Coulter-O'Berry C: The limb-deficient child, in Morrissy RT, Weinstein SL, eds: *Lovell and Winter's Pediatric Orthopaedics*, ed 5. Lippincott Williams & Wilkins, 2001, vol 2, pp 1217-1272.
16. Fedorak GT, Watts HG, Cuomo AV, et al: Osteocartilaginous transfer of the proximal part of the fibula for osseous overgrowth in children with congenital or acquired tibial amputations: Surgical technique and results. *J Bone Joint Surg Am* 2015;97:574-581.
17. Coulter-O'Berry C: Physical therapy management in children with lower extremity limb deficiencies, in Herring JA, Birch JS, eds: *The Child With a Limb Deficiency*. American Academy of Orthopaedic Surgeons, 1998, pp 319-330.
18. Krebs DE, Edelstein JE, Thornby MA: Prosthetic management of children with limb deficiencies. *Phys Ther* 1991;71(12):920-934.
19. Stanger M: Limb deficiencies and amputations, in Campbell SK, Palisano RJ, Vander Linden DW, eds: *Physical Therapy for Children*. WB Saunders, 1994, pp 325-351.
20. Wilk B, Karol L, Halliday S: Characterizing gait in young children with a prosthetic knee joint. *Phys Ther Prod* 1999;10:20.
21. Giavedoni BJ, Coulter-O'Berry C, Geil M: Movement masters. *Adv Direct Rehab* 2002;11:43-44.
22. Thompson GH, Leimkuehler JP: Prosthetic management, in Kalamchi A, ed: *Congenital Lower Limb Deficiencies*. Springer-Verlag, 1989, pp 211-235.
23. Van Nes C: Rotation-plasty for congenital defects of the femur: Making use of the ankle of the shortened limb to control the knee joint of a prosthesis. *J Bone Joint Surg Br* 1950;32:12-16.

Congenital Deficiencies of the Femur

Joseph Ivan Krajbich, MD, FRCS(C) • Ian P. Torode, MD, FRACS*

CHAPTER 76

ABSTRACT

To appropriately treat a child with a limb deficiency, it is first necessary to understand the natural history of the condition and the associated functional implications. It is also important to be able to adequately communicate important findings to the child's parents and family members. Some children can be treated with a simple procedure, whereas others will require a number of major reconstructive surgeries to achieve optimal function. Because treatment may extend over many of the childhood years, the support of the family is essential to achieve the best outcome for the child.

Keywords: absence; deficiency; deformity; femur

Introduction

Although the femur is the largest skeletal component in the lower limb, congenital deficiencies of the femur must be considered along with the associated anomalies that frequently coexist in the lower segments of the limb. The degree of femoral involvement/deficiency combined with the deficiency of the skeletal components distal to the knee joint makes each patient's presentation almost a unique one. Therefore, surgeons must deal with a spectrum of disorders whose management depends not only on solely femoral deficiency but involvement of the whole limb. The functional compromise that can arise from a more distal deficiency may play an important role in the plan for managing a femoral deficiency. Other associated deficiencies particularly of the upper extremities influence the overall management of the child. The relationship between these additional deficiencies is briefly discussed in this chapter as they relate to femoral deficiencies. The diagnosis, management, and treatment of femoral deficiencies from the antenatal period to maturity are also addressed. The terms congenital short femur and proximal femoral focal deficiency (PFFD) and some more commonly used classifications are used because they adequately differentiate the extremes of longitudinal deficiencies, particularly regarding management.

Etiology

Congenital deficiencies of the femur differ from other typical skeletal anomalies in the extent of the variations and influence of distal extremity involvement on management. Currently, in most cases, the etiology of the condition is unknown. There are a few exceptions. Bilateral femoral involvement is said to be associated with maternal diabetes and with femoral–facial syndrome as is rare Goltz syndrome, which is associated with a gene mutation on the X chromosome[1,2] (**Figure 1**). Of causative agents, the drug thalidomide is the best known because it caused a number of limb deficiencies in the 1960s when it was briefly used to control early pregnancy nausea in expecting mothers. Thalidomide-induced deficiencies had a more phocomelic-like, intercalary type of involvement. The drug was never approved for use by the FDA in the United States, sparing this country's many young families of the trauma of having a newborn child with significant skeletal abnormalities.

Based on current knowledge of human embryology and intrauterine development, it is clear that most noxious insults must happen very early in fetal life. The lower limb is in place with all the important elements present by 8 weeks of gestation. It is likely that whatever intrauterine insult has taken place, it could very well be before the mother was even aware of being pregnant.

Presentations

Congenital deficiencies of the femur have essentially three modes of presentation for orthopaedic management. These modes are a prenatal presentation, which is detected using

---

Dr. Krajbich or an immediate family member serves as a board member, owner, officer, or committee member of Scoliosis Research Society.

*Deceased.

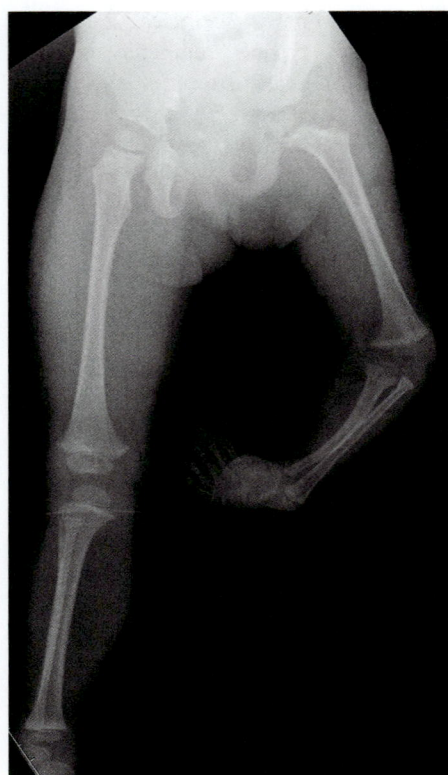

FIGURE 1 Radiograph of the lower limbs of a female infant with Goltz syndrome demonstrates the hypoplastic left lower limb.

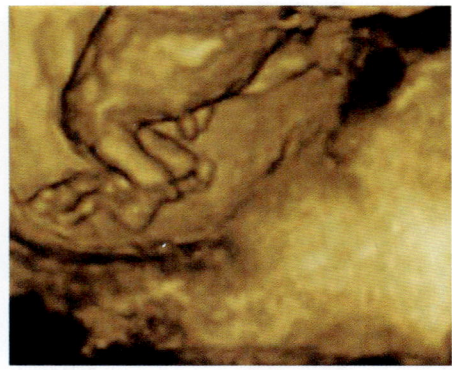

FIGURE 2 Prenatal ultrasonography image shows a bowed and short tibia, a foot in valgus, and a slightly short but intact femur. After birth, the child will be best treated with foot ablation (usually in the second year of life when the child wants to walk) and prosthetic fitting.

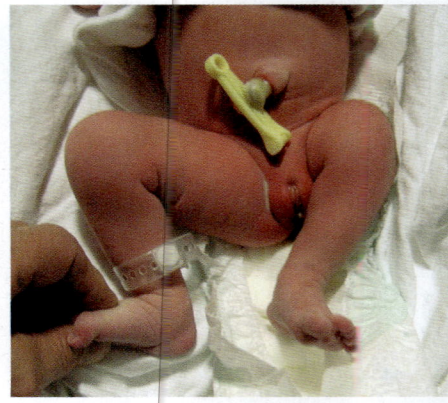

FIGURE 3 Photograph of a newborn female with a very short left femur, with a good foot and normal-appearing leg.

ultrasonography, initial detection at the time of birth, and later referral of an older child who had not been evaluated earlier or only partially because of some extenuating circumstance, such as residence in a remote area without access to a surgeon with expertise in managing limb deficiencies or other socioeconomic or religious factors, or possibly a relatively mild involvement whose significance may not have been initially appreciated.

Prenatal Presentation

In developed countries, many pregnant women have an ultrasonography examination during pregnancy. Because the first ultrasonography examination performed at approximately 12 weeks' gestation may be cursory and done only for pregnancy confirmation, a substantial number of skeletal limb deficiencies may be overlooked. Limb deficiencies may not be detected until the 20-week ultrasonography examination, which may present an issue if pregnancy termination is a consideration.[3] The orthopaedic surgeon may be asked to provide advice on the likely extent and natural history of a detected limb deficiency (**Figure 2**).

The surgeon should be able to reasonably differentiate between a congenitally short femur and a true PFFD. In cases in which the available information does not allow a definite opinion, some reassurance of a favorable outcome may still be possible and will help to decrease the parents' distress and potential feelings of guilt during the remainder of the pregnancy.

Postnatal Presentation

Ideally, the newborn will be treated by the same surgeon who provided prenatal advice. This continuity of care prevents the dissemination of well-intentioned but often erroneous information given by family members and the nursing staff, most of whom are unfamiliar with such an abnormality. If a diagnosis has not been made before birth, the pediatrician will refer the infant to a surgeon for care; the treating surgeon should address any misinformation received by the infant's family and offer reassurance. The family will want to know if the child will walk. Even in infants with a true PFFD, the surgeon can offer reassurance that the child will walk, even if a prosthesis may be needed, as long as the condition is unilateral (**Figure 3**).

Delayed Presentation

In some instances, there may be a delay in the child being seen for treatment. If an older child is referred for treatment, the surgeon may need to allocate considerable time to explain the child's condition and review management options with the parents.

Classification Systems

The numerous classification systems for congenital femoral deficiencies suggest that no single system is satisfactory for all patients. The Hamanish classification system[4] demonstrates that there are many radiologic appearances and degrees of severity in congenital femoral deficiencies (**Figure 4**). Gillespie and Torode[5] categorized congenital longitudinal femoral abnormalities into two major groups. At the moderate end of the severity scale is the congenital short femur, and at the more extreme end is the true PFFD. Later, Gillespie[6] revised the classification system by adding a third group that consisted of children with a very short femoral residual limb, which is often fused to the tibia. In this group, no intervention around the knee is necessary (**Figure 5**) unless a rotationplasty procedure is considered. The revised

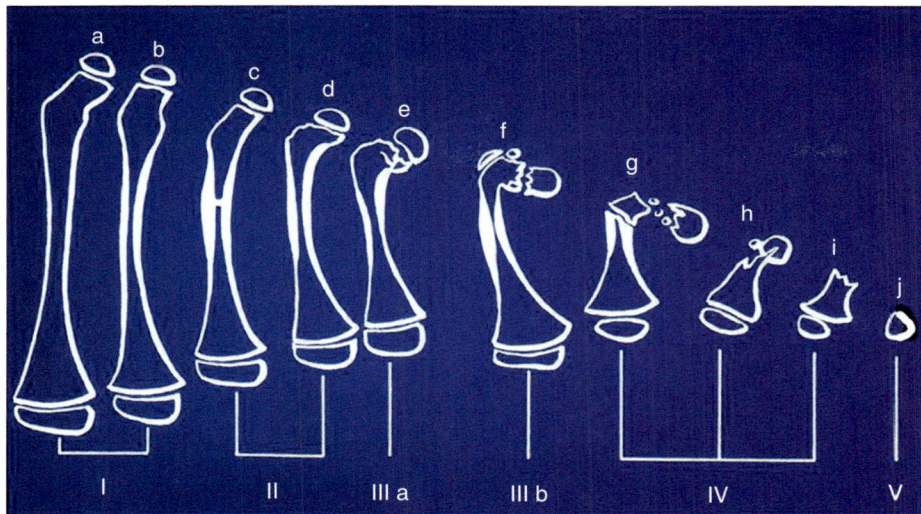

FIGURE 4 Illustration of the Hamanishi classification system for femoral deficiency. This system demonstrates the large number of variations that may be present, ranging from a virtually normal femur (a) to a vestigial bone (j).

Gillespie classification system is useful in formulating a management plan and is readily understood by parents. In most instances, the Gillespie classification system helps the surgeon determine if reconstruction or prosthetic assistance would be the most appropriate course of management.[7] The true PFFD itself has been a subject of a number of classifications by itself. The most widely used is the classification by Aitken[8] (**Figure 6**).

The Aitken classification divides PFFDs into four types. Type A includes children with a radiographically abnormal proximal femur, with a pseudarthrosis that will ossify progressively with time and a varus proximal femoral deformity. These femora can be reconstructed. A type B deficiency is more severe, with a persistent defect between the femoral head in the acetabulum and the femoral shaft. These femora may be reconstructible. In type C and D deficiencies, no femoral head is present, and there is no discernible acetabulum. From embryologic studies, it is known that a hip develops from a single cartilage enlage. The cleft that appears in this cartilage block is the nascent hip joint. So, it can be said if there is no acetabulum, there is no femoral head and vice versa. It follows that attempts to reconstruct a hip joint in this situation will likely not be feasible. In Aitken type C deficiency, the femur is of reasonable size with somewhat bulky proximal end In type D deficiencies, the femur is rudimentary and tapered proximally, and no proximal reconstruction should be attempted[8] (**Figure 7**).

The classification by Paley and Stannard[9] is useful for guiding surgical intervention and reconstruction, particularly in patients with more severe proximal femoral and diaphyseal deficiencies. On one end of the severity spectrum, congenital femoral deficiency management involves treatment of a modest limb-length difference, and at the other end is a gross limb discrepancy and the need for prosthetic assistance (**Figure 8**).

Within this spectrum is a dividing line between patients who can be treated with limb reconstruction and those who are best treated with limb ablation and prosthetic restoration (**Figure 9**). The additional confounding factor is that many of these children have associated involvement of the distal part(s) of the extremity. For the extremity to be rendered functional by either surgical or prosthetic means (or their combination), several parameters have to be considered. Pelvic femoral articulation has to be at least moderately stable with reasonable range of motion. The same goes for the knee joint and ankle joint to allow for relatively normal biomechanical alignment and function and to potentially withstand a lengthening procedure. To address these issues in a simple treatment guiding algorithm,

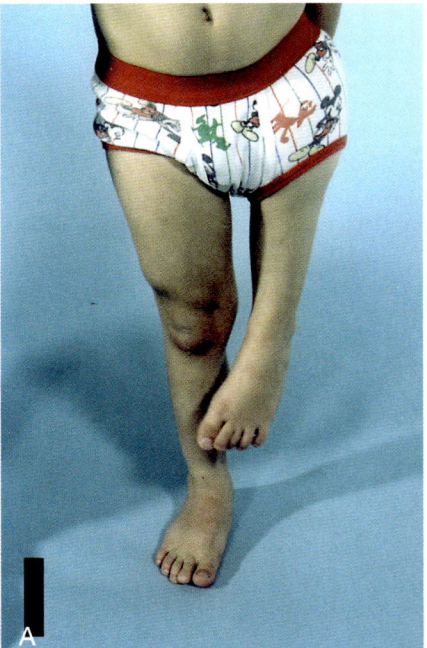
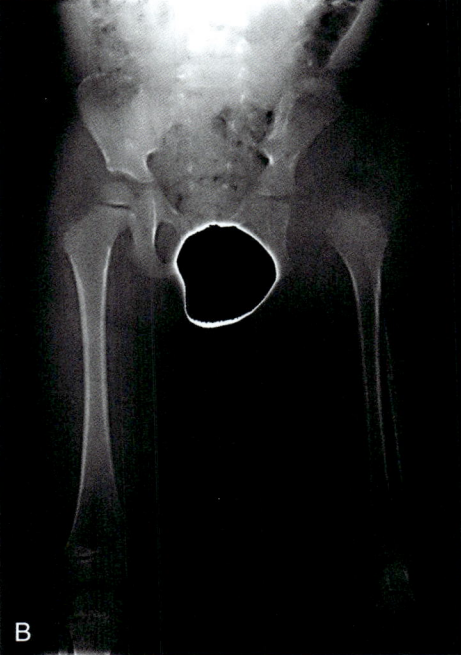

FIGURE 5 Clinical photograph (**A**) and radiograph (**B**) of a child with Gillespie group C proximal femoral focal deficiency.

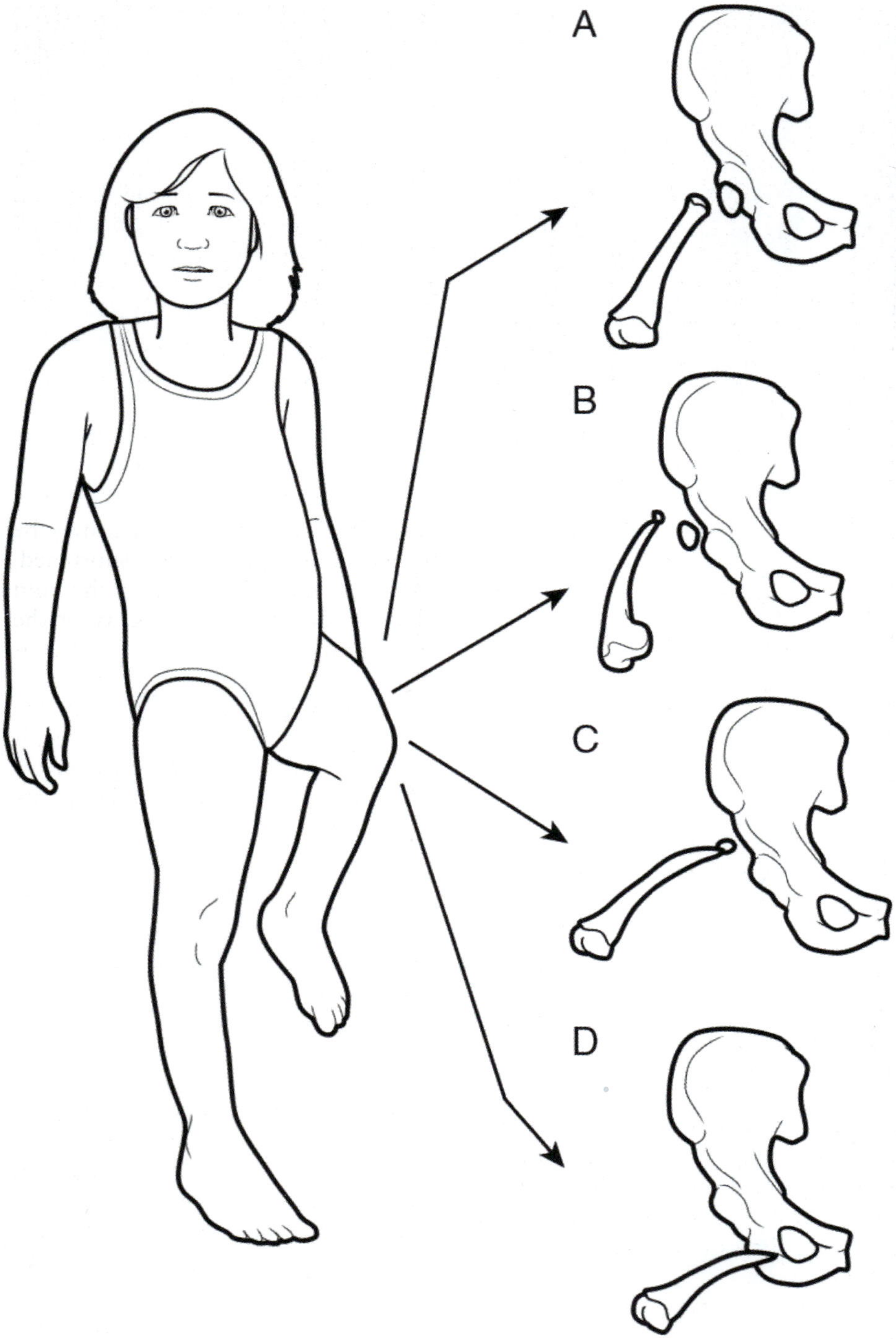

Section 5: Pediatrics

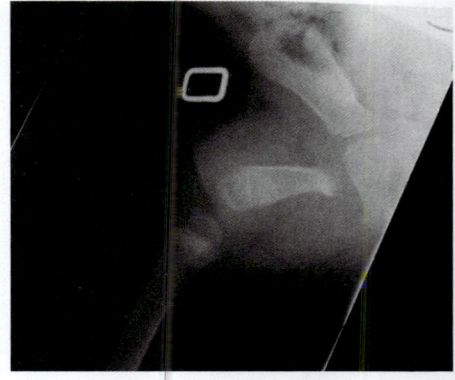

FIGURE 7 Radiograph of a high-grade (Aitken type D) proximal femoral focal deficiency.

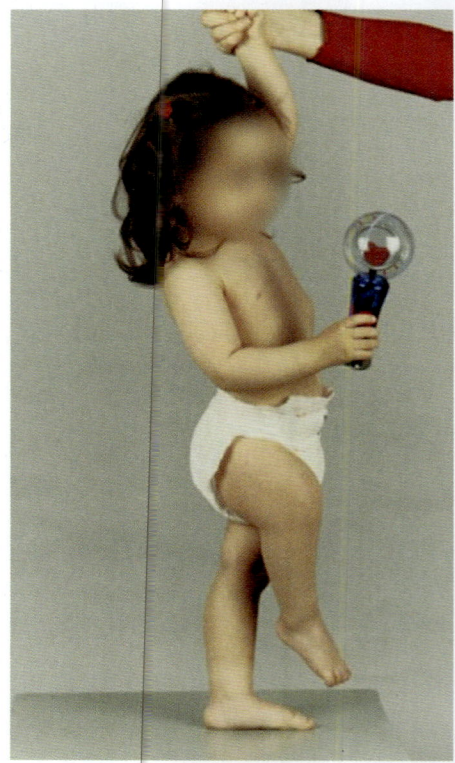

FIGURE 6 Illustration of the Aitken classification of femoral deficiency. **A**, In a type A deficiency, there is stability, with a bulbous proximal femur and a femoral head in the acetabulum. **B**, In a type B deficiency, the femur is more spindle shaped proximally, which implies a lack of connection between the ossified bone in the acetabulum and the femur. The lack of stability is accompanied by failure of ossification and the continued existence of motion between the femur and pelvis. **C**, In a type C deficiency, the femoral head is lacking, and the femur is less well developed. A tuft of ossification is seen at the proximal femur, but there is no articular relationship between the femur and acetabulum. The acetabular development is poor. **D**, In a type D deficiency, the femoral deficiency is severe, and there is no proximal tufting. The acetabular development is poor, the hip is unstable, and there is a marked limb-length discrepancy.

FIGURE 8 Standing lateral photograph of a girl with a congenital short right femur.

Krajbich and Alman proposed a classification based on (1) reconstructability of the hip joint and (2) integrity of the ankle/subtalar joint in patients with PFFD (Tables 1 and 2).

It is also important to recognize that management decisions are influenced by the mores of the society in which the patient resides, the skill and experience of the surgeon, and the wishes of the family.

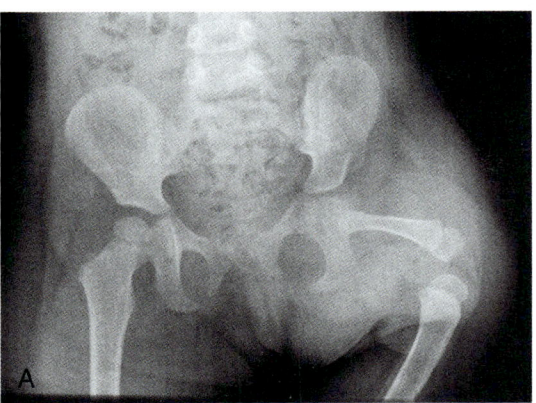 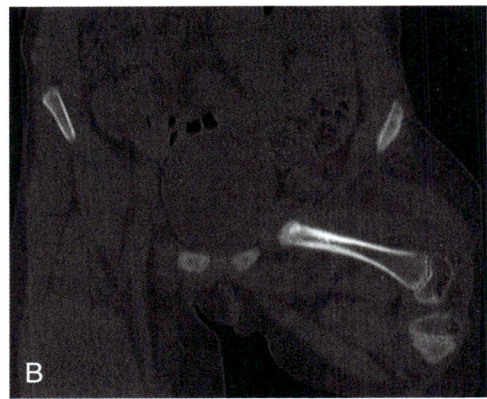 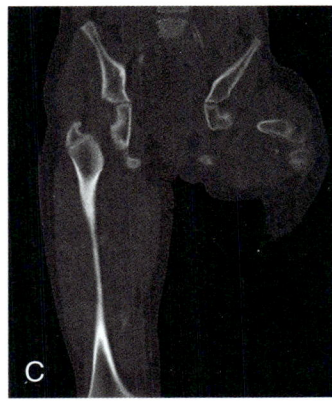

FIGURE 9 A, AP radiograph of the pelvis of a 3-year-old girl with marked femoral deficiency. Note the bulbous proximal femur. CT scans of the pelvis of the child at 8 years old shows the femur lying anterior to the superior pubic ramus, with the proximal end adjacent to the bladder (**B**) and the ossified femoral head fused to the ischium (**C**).

TABLE 1 Classification of Proximal Femoral Focal Deficiency as Proposed by Krajbich and Alman

Type I	The hip can be reconstructed (Aitken type A and most Bs)
Type II	Nonreconstructable hip joint (Aitken C, D, and some Bs)
Subtype A	Functional ankle/subtalar joint complex
Subtype B	Nonfunctional ankle/subtalar joint complex

TABLE 2 Treatment of Proximal Femoral Focal Deficiency as Proposed by Krajbich and Alman

Ia	Hip reconstruction and either limb equalization procedure or knee fusion with rotationplasty
Ib	Hip reconstruction and either Syme's amputation and prosthetic restoration below the knee or knee fusion and prosthetic restoration at the knee level
IIa	Knee fusion and rotationplasty
IIb	Knee fusion and Syme's amputation

Clinical Examination

The patient will typically lie or stand with the affected limb in a position of flexion and external rotation. Examination of the hip may reveal telescoping, which is a sign of a true higher grade PFFD and indicates a likely lack of integrity between the femoral shaft and the head and neck or a complete absence of the hip joint (Aitken type C and D, Krajbich type II). In infants, the hip flexion deformity is often relatively fixed. It becomes less fixed in patients with a congenital short femur, whereas it remains fixed in patients with true PFFD. The affected knee will often demonstrate laxity in the AP plane of the joint. This is particularly true if there is associated fibular hemimelia involving the distal part of the extremity. Paradoxically, the laxity is more obvious in patients with lesser degrees of limb shortening, because the contractures around the knee with the PFFD will often disguise the instability.

Below the knee, it is important to assess the presence and degree of tibial and fibular involvement. True tibial hemimelia associated with PFFD is relatively rare. However, some degree of fibular hemimelia is present in most PFFD patients. The whole spectrum of fibular deficiency can be encountered in these patients. In milder cases, the degree of shortening may be minimal, but in more severe cases, not only the fibula is absent, but the tibia may be bowed and significantly shortened, with a linear dimple over the mid tibia. In the foot, the integrity of the ankle joint, the extent of tarsal coalitions, and the number of rays in the foot must be considered. Although the number of rays is readily apparent, it is often less important than the integrity of the ankle and subtalar joints (**Figure 10**).

Radiographic Features

Plain radiographs will complement and clarify clinical findings. In an infant, a radiograph of the lower half of the patient's body will provide useful information and is mandatory for full assessment. It allows for a useful reference point between a normal and abnormal limb in the unilateral case. Bilateral involvement is not common but not that rare either. In the bilateral involvement the degree of deficiency can be quite asymmetrical with the less involved side sometimes manifesting only as acetabular dysplasia (**Figure 11**).

In a patient with a milder level of congenital short femur, the femur will be short with a degree of midshaft sclerosis and an anterolateral bow. The proximal femur will be ossified, and there may be a varus deformity. The external rotational deformity and valgus of the distal femur will become more obvious over time. In patients with a higher level of congenital short

Section 5: Pediatrics

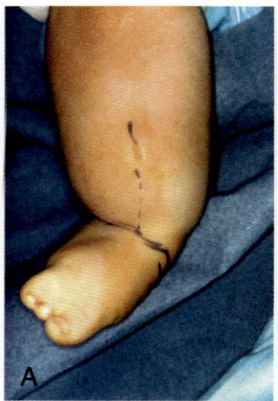 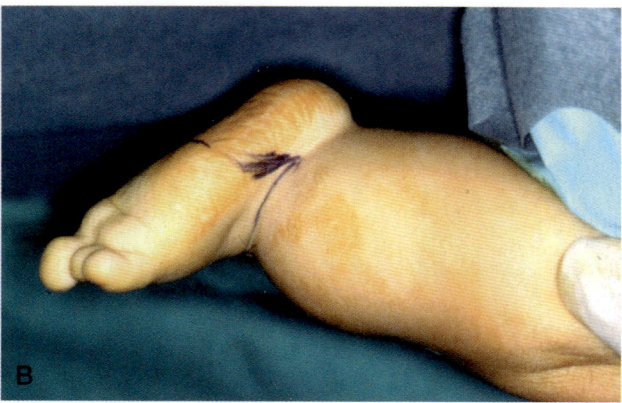

FIGURE 10 **A** and **B**, Clinical photographs of a nonfunctional foot in a child with fibular hemimelia associated with proximal femoral focal deficiency and planned Symes amputation.

femur, the femur will be shorter than in those with a milder deformity, it will lack ossification proximally, and the proximal femur will be bulbous. The presence of a reasonably well-formed acetabulum almost always implies the presence of unossified femoral head. Radiographic findings can be confirmed with ultrasonography, but it is important to note that the varus of the femoral neck will make the unossified greater trochanter proud, and this can be interpreted as a congenital dislocation. The findings can be confirmed with MRI (**Figure 12**). Although sedation may be required in infants, MRI may be performed if there is doubt about the diagnosis or confirmation is needed.

In children with a true PFFD, the femur is very short, the proximal end is poorly developed, and there is substantial involvement of the diaphysis. The acetabulum can be dysplastic or absent, and ossification of the femoral head is delayed or completely absent. The foot lies at the level of the contralateral knee. Below the knee, the tibia and fibula can be variably involved. At the milder end of the severity spectrum, the tibia and fibula may appear equal in length or minimally shorter than the contralateral side, whereas at the more severe end of the spectrum, the fibula is absent and the tibia is short and bowed anteriorly. In these patients, the foot is in equinus, and the talus is subluxated posterolaterally to the tibia.

As time passes, ossification continues, and the outcome for an individual patient becomes clearer. Clinical findings and radiographic features will usually allow the surgeon to develop a working plan for the child, so the family can understand the likely course of the disorder; however, accurate classification of a deficiency is difficult to determine in some children. For example, clinical findings suggested a true PFFD in a 3-year-old girl. Radiographic findings showed a bulbous proximal femur and a femoral head that was present but completely ossified to the ischium. The proximal femur was located anterior to the superior pubic ramus and posterior to the femoral neurovascular bundle.

Abnormality of the hip joint is a hallmark characteristic in these children, but true dislocation of a developed femoral head from the acetabulum is rare. For example, **Figure 13** shows a three-dimensional reconstruction of the hip of a child who appeared to have a dislocated femoral head, but the femoral head and neck were actually markedly underdeveloped. During an attempted open reduction of the femur, a complete lack of development of the pubic segment of the acetabulum was found; the proximal femur was returned to the presurgical articulation.

Treatment Planning

If the infant is examined by the surgeon in the first few weeks after birth, the parents should be reassured that the deficiency is not the mother's fault, there is no specific treatment necessary for the deficiency, no surgery will be necessary in the child's first year of life, and the deficiency will not prevent the child from crawling or pulling to a standing position. No special physiotherapy is required. The family should be reassured that the child will be able to walk. Parents should be informed if their child is a candidate for surgical reconstruction, with the goal of the

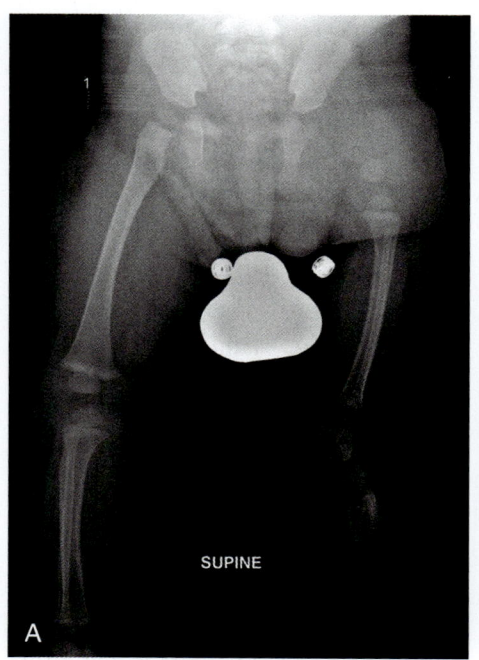 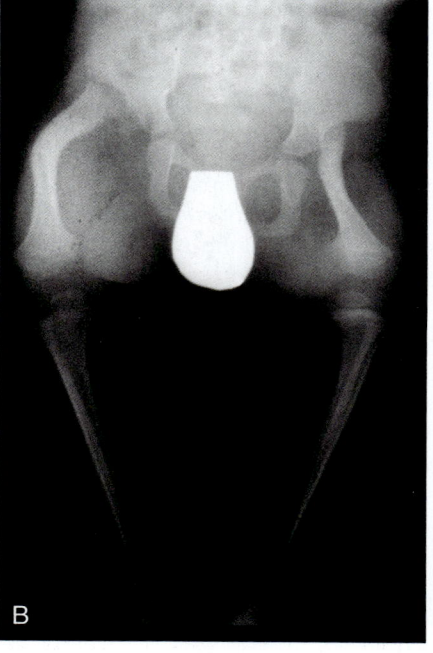

FIGURE 11 Radiographs of (**A**) unilateral and (**B**) bilateral proximal femoral focal deficiency.

Chapter 76: Congenital Deficiencies of the Femur

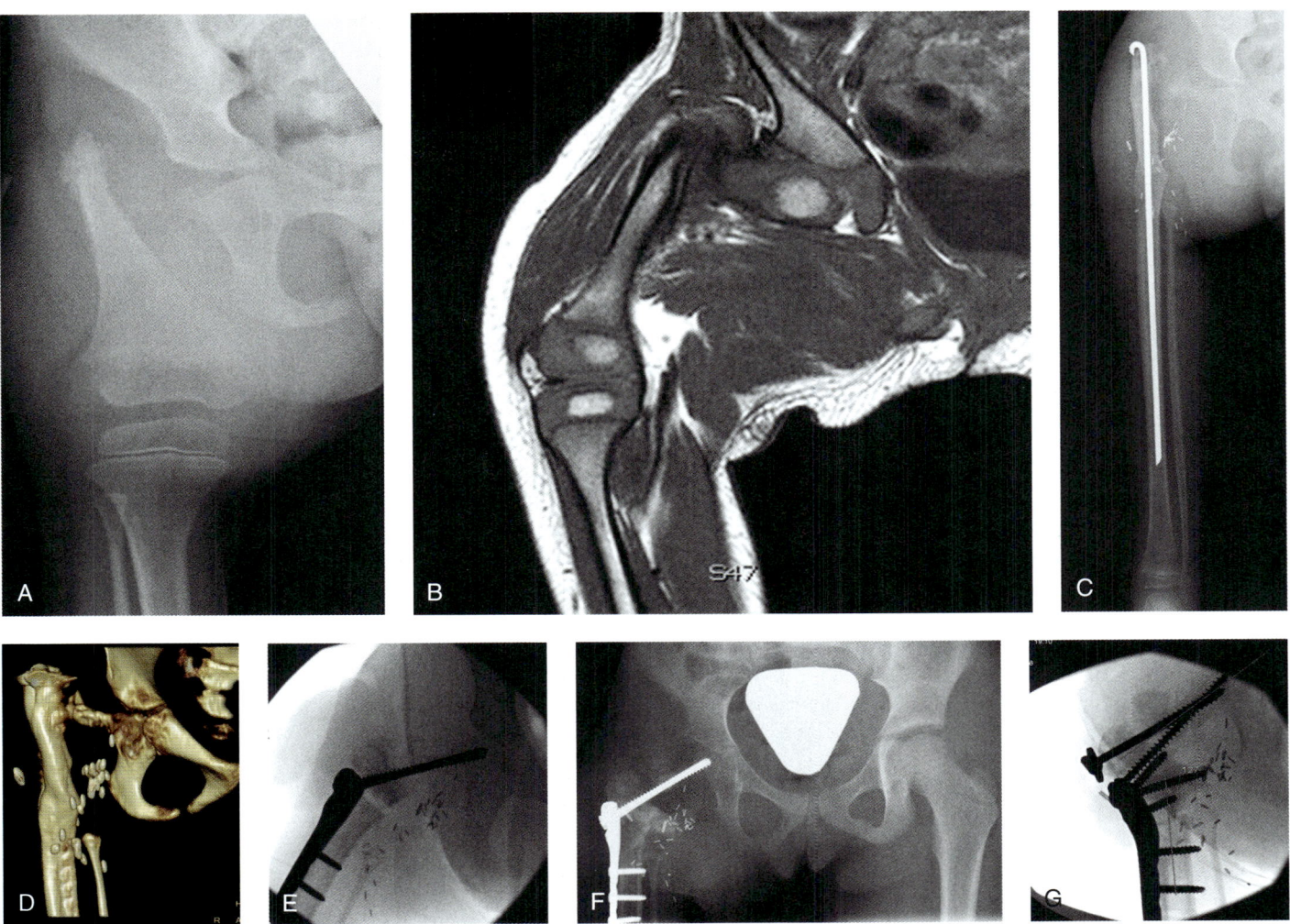

FIGURE 12 Hip reconstruction in type I proximal femoral focal deficiency. **A**, Radiograph of type Ia (Aitken type B) proximal femoral focal deficiency. **B**, MRI demonstrating a femoral head inside the acetabulum. **C**, Radiograph after rotationplasty. **D**, Three-dimensional CT scan before hip reconstruction. **E**, Radiograph of valgus shortening osteotomy. **F**, Radiograph of persistent ossification defect. **G**, Radiograph of bone graft of the defect and revision of internal fixation with compression across the defect.

child be able to walk with their own feet, or whether the femoral or foot and ankle deficiency will necessitate a prosthesis for ambulation. A management plan should be formulated and discussed with the family early in the child's life. It is expected that these children will undergo several surgical procedures over their growing years, which can be a source of anxiety for the family. However, if the family is informed of the treatment plan ahead of time and is aware of the serial steps, they will likely be involved in the process and experience less anxiety.

In patients with lesser degrees of femoral deficiency and a good foot and ankle, judicious use of epiphysiodesis and/or femoral/tibial lengthening should lead to satisfactory outcomes. In a child with a more severe deficiency, such as a typical congenital short femur with the foot at the midshaft level of the contralateral tibia, the expected limb-length discrepancy at maturity requiring accommodation is approximately 20 cm. Resolving such a discrepancy in a series of smaller surgical steps is less daunting and more readily achievable.

In a child with a good foot and ankle and a minor degree of fibular hemimelia, the management plan should include tibial lengthening (expected gain of 4 to 5 cm) in the preschool years, pelvic lengthening and correction of acetabular dysplasia using the Hall modification of the Salter innominate osteotomy technique (expected gain of 2 cm),[10] and correction of the coxa vara (expected gain of 2 cm) as two separate procedures to lessen a change of hip subluxation or even subluxation through a sacroiliac joint. Instead of lengthening the femur with a frame, an alternative plan is to wait and lengthen the femur with intramedullary nails using a pertrochanteric approach when the child is approximately 10 years of age (expected gain of 5 cm), coupled with a judicious contralateral epiphysiodesis (expected gain of approximately 3 cm), followed by a final femoral lengthening using a nail when the patient is a teenager.

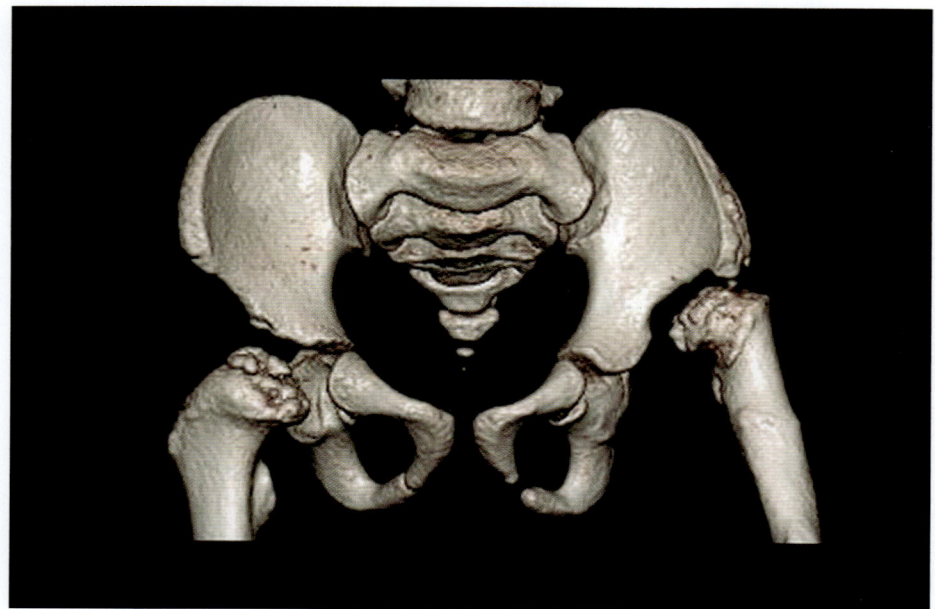

FIGURE 13 Three-dimensional CT scan of the pelvis of a child showing a deficient left femur articulating with a pseudoacetabulum that had been stable for 3 years.

A guided-growth system can be used to correct valgus malalignment of the distal femur, and the rotational malalignment can be addressed at the time of femoral lengthening (**Figure 14**).

If the condition of the foot and ankle is poor and the tibia is bowed, a foot ablation (Syme amputation) and prosthetic fitting are indicated.[11,12] Knee valgus in later childhood can be managed with a temporary hemiepiphysiode.[13] A guided-growth system using a plate can readily correct the valgus. Although children can generally tolerate a difference in knee heights and a prosthesis can readily cope with leg-length issues, a contralateral epiphysiodesis or a femoral lengthening can be considered for some patients (**Figure 15**).

In more severe cases, the femoral deficiency is the most obvious abnormality; however, the integrity of the foot and ankle requires early assessment. Experience has shown that attempts to salvage a marginally functioning foot will compromise long-term function. If the foot is saved, there is often great reluctance to undergo foot amputation until the child reaches the teenage years and becomes aware of the functional limitations of the saved foot (**Figure 16**).

Children with a poor foot and ankle and a femur that is not reconstructable (Krajbich IIb) may be best treated with foot ablation and knee fusion. This surgery can be done as soon as ossification around the knee is adequate. Patients with a tiny femur that is often already fused to the tibia (Gillespie group C) are included in this group. In this group, no knee fusion is usually needed.

Children with a good foot and ankle and a poor femur are candidates for rotationplasty. This procedure is done through the knee and combined with a knee fusion. If the child's parents do not want the child to be treated with a rotationplasty, the child should be treated with methods used for a patient with a poor foot.

In a child with a stable femur (albeit short) and a femoral head in the acetabulum, there is a role for delayed treatment and further investigation before committing the child and family to several surgical procedures, including at least two femoral lengthening procedures. In the child with a poor foot, the need for below-knee reconstruction

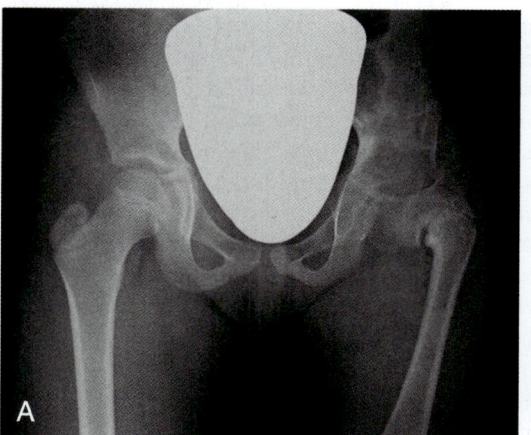
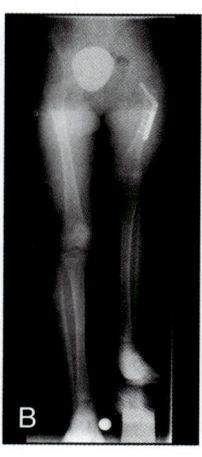
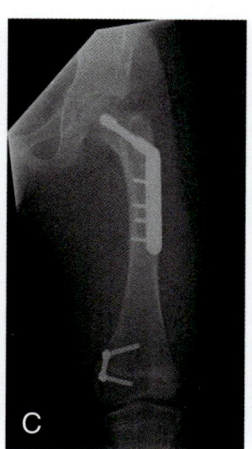
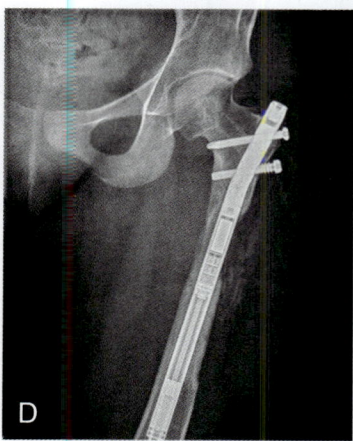

FIGURE 14 Radiographs of the patient shown in Figure 5. **A**, AP radiograph of the pelvis taken when the child was 9 years old. The shadow of the carbon fiber block used to lengthen the left hemipelvis can be seen. The femoral head and neck have ossified in varus. **B**, Standing radiograph of the legs and pelvis after correction of the coxa vara. **C**, Radiograph of the femur after correction of coxa vara. A guided-growth system using a plate is in place to treat the genu valgum. **D**, Radiograph of the left femur after lengthening using a PRECICE nail (Ellipse Technologies).

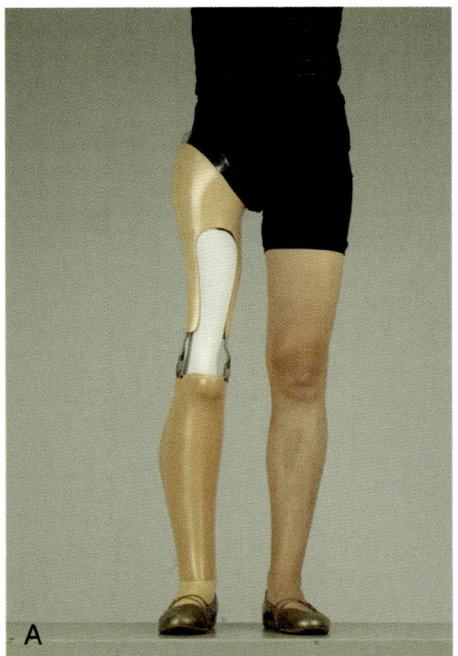
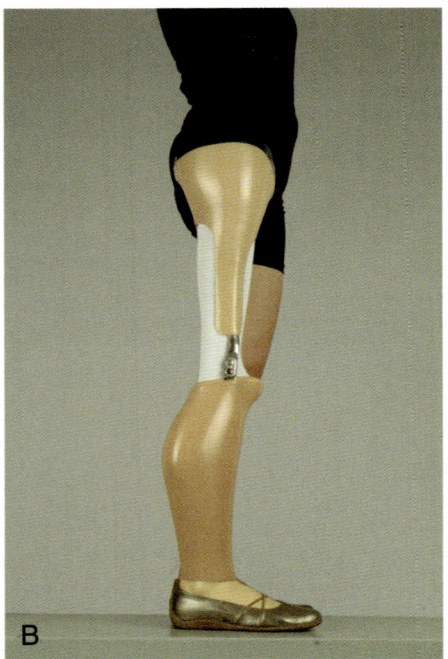
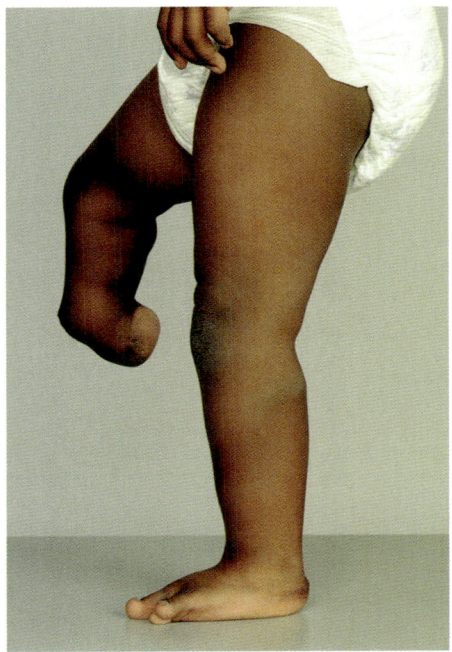

FIGURE 15 AP (**A**) and lateral (**B**) photographic views of a rotationplasty prosthesis.

FIGURE 16 Clinical photograph of the lower limbs of a young boy who was treated with a foot ablation but did not undergo correction of the tibial kyphosis. This deformity substantially compromises prosthetic fit and comfort.

and tibial lengthening can be avoided, and length can be attained by a prosthesis after foot ablation.[9]

Surgical Techniques

Foot Ablation

In patients requiring foot ablation, it is preferable to use a Syme amputation approach or ankle disarticulation. A Boyd amputation can be used, but the talus and os calcis are often fused and difficult to deliver distally. The Boyd procedure provides no functional gain in these patients. A useful adjunct is to divide the Achilles tendon through a small incision at approximately the junction of the middle and distal thirds of the leg. This allows a simpler delivery of the talus and calcaneus for the posterior capsular resection and removal of those bones for either a Syme or Boyd procedure. It should be noted that the tibial kyphosis commonly seen in children with more severe deficiencies should be corrected by a tibial osteotomy with internal fixation at the time of the foot ablation. Failure to do so may compromise long-term prosthetic fitting and comfort (**Figure 17**).

Knee Valgus

Knee valgus in a femoral deficiency is often overlooked. Hypoplastic lateral femoral condyle is a relatively common feature of congenital femoral deficiencies and is always present in lesser or greater degree in instances of associated fibular longitudinal deficiency (fibular hemimelia) (**Figure 18**). Previously, a distal femoral opening osteotomy with a fibular graft was advocated to gain some length and stimulate growth. Although the outcome was usually satisfactory, correction with a hemiephysiodesis is a much simpler procedure and can be done as an outpatient procedure.[13,14] Correction of the genu valgum also needs to be done when a foot ablation has been performed. If correction is not done, the prosthetic leg will often be aligned to the tibia, which will magnify knee valgus, or alternatively, the prosthetic fitting would allow for a bulge in the lateral aspect of the prosthesis so that the prosthetic limb is correctly aligned to the patient. It is also necessary to appreciate that the genu valgum may be disguised by the external rotation deformity of the femur, which may require correction

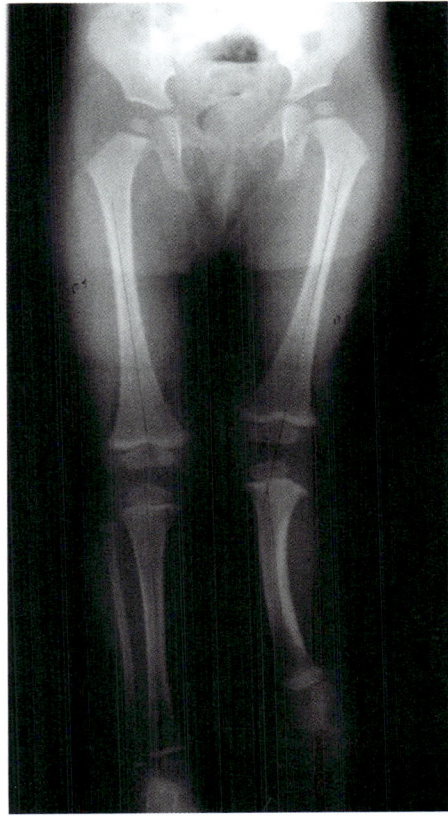

FIGURE 17 Radiograph of knee valgus deformity secondary to lateral femoral condyle hypoplasia as a result of associated fibular hemimelia.

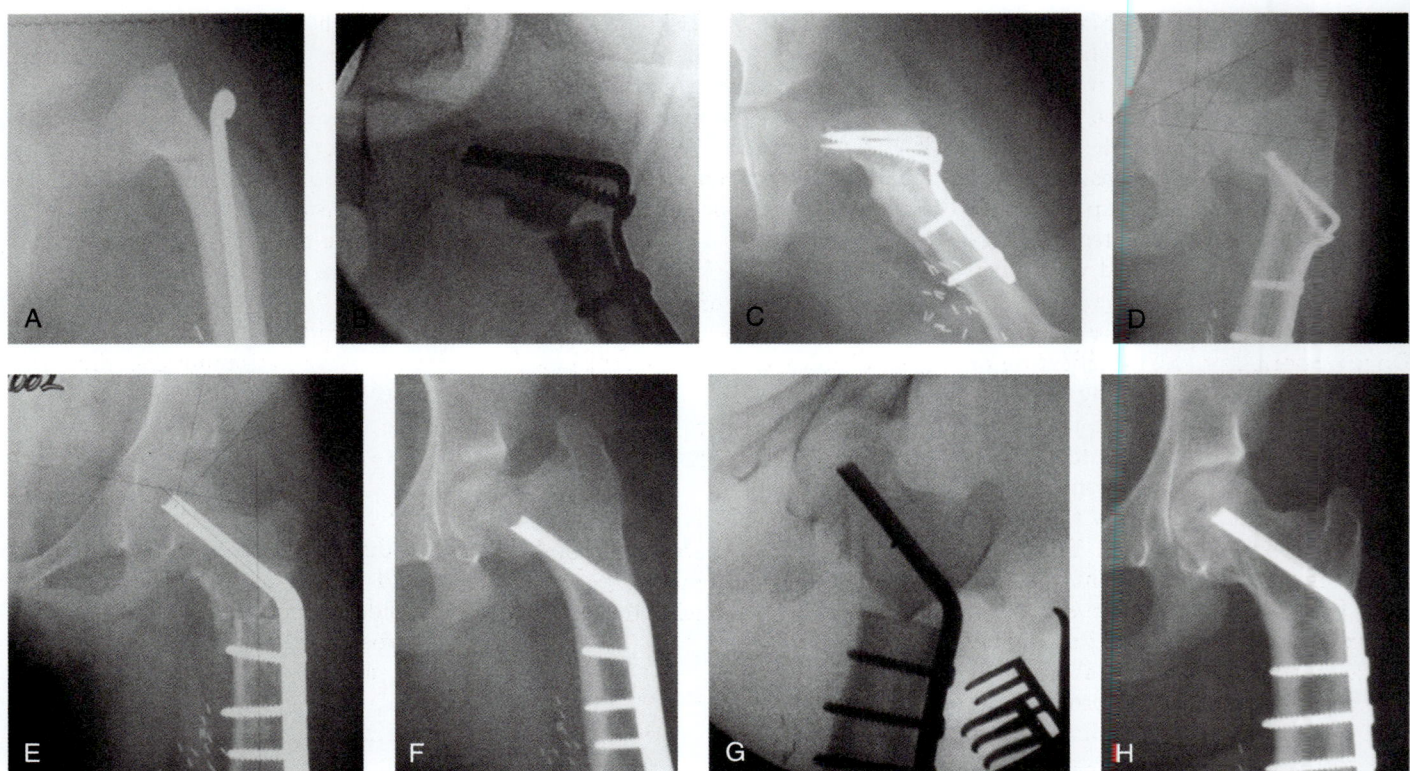

FIGURE 18 **A** through **H**, Radiographs of recurrent varus deformity as the child matures. Two revision osteotomies were required over the years to achieve the final result at skeletal maturity.

in addition of correcting the knee valgus by osteotomy or derotation at the time of femoral lengthening.

Correction of Coxa Vara

In a patient with a completely ossified intact femur, the procedure to correct coxa vara is relatively straightforward. It is, however, important that it is performed at a relatively young age before development and worsening of acetabular and femoral head dysplasia. In more complicated instances, particularly if there is an ossification defect (pseudarthrosis), coxa vara correction is more difficult and requires either a soft-tissue release or femoral shortening. Rather than compromise the soft-tissue integrity of muscle units, the use of femoral shortening is preferred. It is necessary to adequately correct the coxa vara so the healing of the compromised bone of the proximal femur is not impaired because of poor biomechanics. In these patients, the use of bone morphogenetic protein has been advocated to stimulate ossification.[9] To achieve at least 120° of neck shaft angle is recommended. There is a significant tendency for the varus recurrence particularly when the initial procedure needs to be performed at a young age. It can be expected that the correction will need to be repeated, sometimes even several times.

Correction of Acetabular Dysplasia

Acetabular dysplasia is common in children with a congenital deficiency of the femur, but it may be overlooked on radiographic studies because the shorter limb may be abducted. If the hip subluxates during lengthening, it is very difficult to resolve the problem. It is better to overtreat children with acetabular dysplasia. A modification of the Hall modification of the Salter innominate osteotomy has been used with consistent results.[10] This modified procedure uses iliac crest bone grafts and a carbon fiber insert to provide immediate stability because these grafts tend to collapse when used alone in small children with dysplasia and require protection in the spica cast. In unpublished studies, none of the children treated with this modified procedure had hip subluxation during subsequent femoral lengthening procedures.

Hip Reconstruction in the Absence of Proximal Femur

In the more severe degree of PFFD (Aitken type C and D, Krajbich II), true hip joint reconstruction is not possible. There is no true acetabulum and no femoral head. The distal femoral fragment articulates with soft tissues on side of the pelvis. This leaves femoral pelvic articulation relatively unstable with compromised abductor and extensor strength. This compromises the child's gait. Significant Trendelenburg lurch is always present, and in the case of prosthetic use, an ischial bearing socket is recommended. The surgical intervention has not been widely used in this situation. However, there are possible alternatives. Steele originally described femoral iliac fusion where the knee functions as a hip (personal communication). Knee extension substitutes for hip flexion and vice versa. This original version of the procedure is rarely used currently. Most recently Dungl reported on the modification of this procedure by performing fusion of the residual distal femur to the pelvis using modified Chiari osteotomy with femur in a horizontal position with the knee somewhat anterior to the pelvis (personal communication). The knee again functions as a hip joint with the knee flexion simulating hip extension and vice versa. The femoral fragment is left relatively long, and no ablation of the epiphyseal plate is performed. This is to give better biomechanical advantage to the knee extensors and flexors (quadriceps and hamstrings). Good long-term results have been reported (**Figures 19** and **20**).

Brown[19] modified the procedure even further by fusing the femoral segment to the pelvis in a 180°-rotated position to allow for knee flexion to provide hip flexion and knee extension hip extension. Further studies are needed to determine if it is better to preserve motion at the expense of energy and joints or provide stability by fusing the femur to the pelvis.

Tibial Lengthening

A minor degree of tibial shortening is often present in children with femoral deficiency. Tibial lengthening of approximately 4 to 5 cm is readily achievable in these children during the preschool years. If there is any doubt about the stability of the foot and ankle, a calcaneal wire should be used. If a knee flexion contracture develops, a simple orthotic extension from the frame will suffice during the lengthening phase.

Knee Fusion

Knee fusion is one of the mainstays procedures in treatment of a true PFFD where femoral reconstructive procedure is not feasible (most of Aitken type B, C, and D). It was King[16] who originally described the procedure in this situation. Procedure allows for a single thigh bone while getting rid of the flexion contracture and guiding gradual correction of the hip flexion and abduction contracture by providing sufficient lever arm to allow for stretching of contracted soft tissues. A knee fusion can be performed as soon as the ossification centers around the knee are present. The need to retain or remove the epiphyseal plates around the knee will depend on the degree of deficiency of the femur and tibia and the expected desired length at maturity. Usually both can be safely removed. Not too infrequently the thigh is left too long, negatively influencing prosthetic fitting, function, and cosmesis. The distal aspect of the new thigh should be shorter than the contralateral side at maturity to accommodate the prosthetic knee. If the fusion is held by a smooth pin or nail, growth will continue if a epiphyseal plate has been retained for that purpose if needed (**Figure 21**).

Femoral Lengthening

Many femora have been lengthened using a frame; however, the advent of lengthening nails has provided a

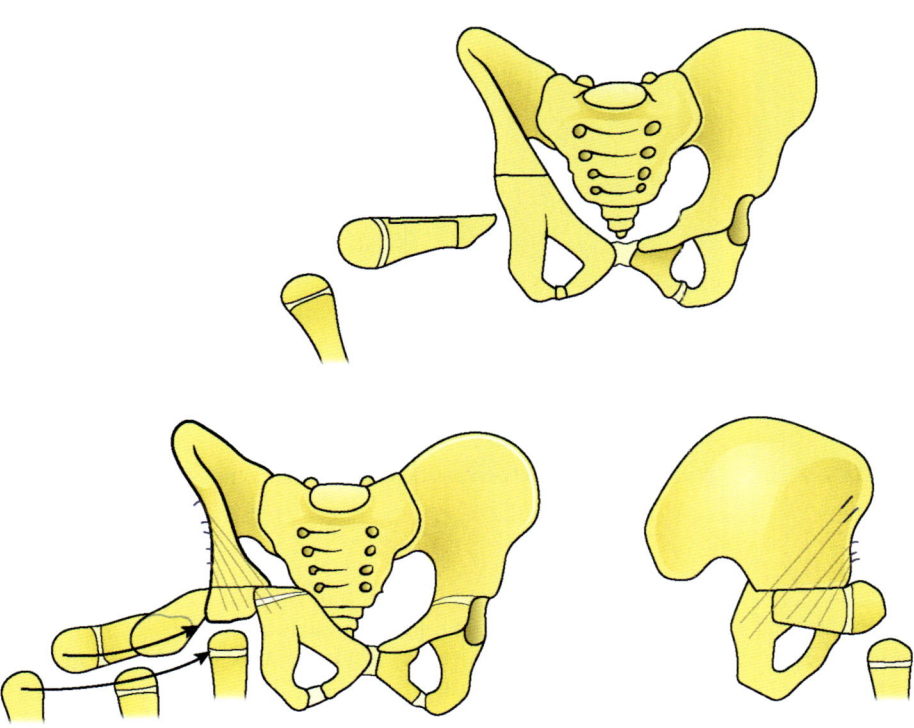

FIGURE 19 Illustration depicting the Dungl operation. (Courtesy of Professor Pavel Dungl, Prague, Czech Republic.)

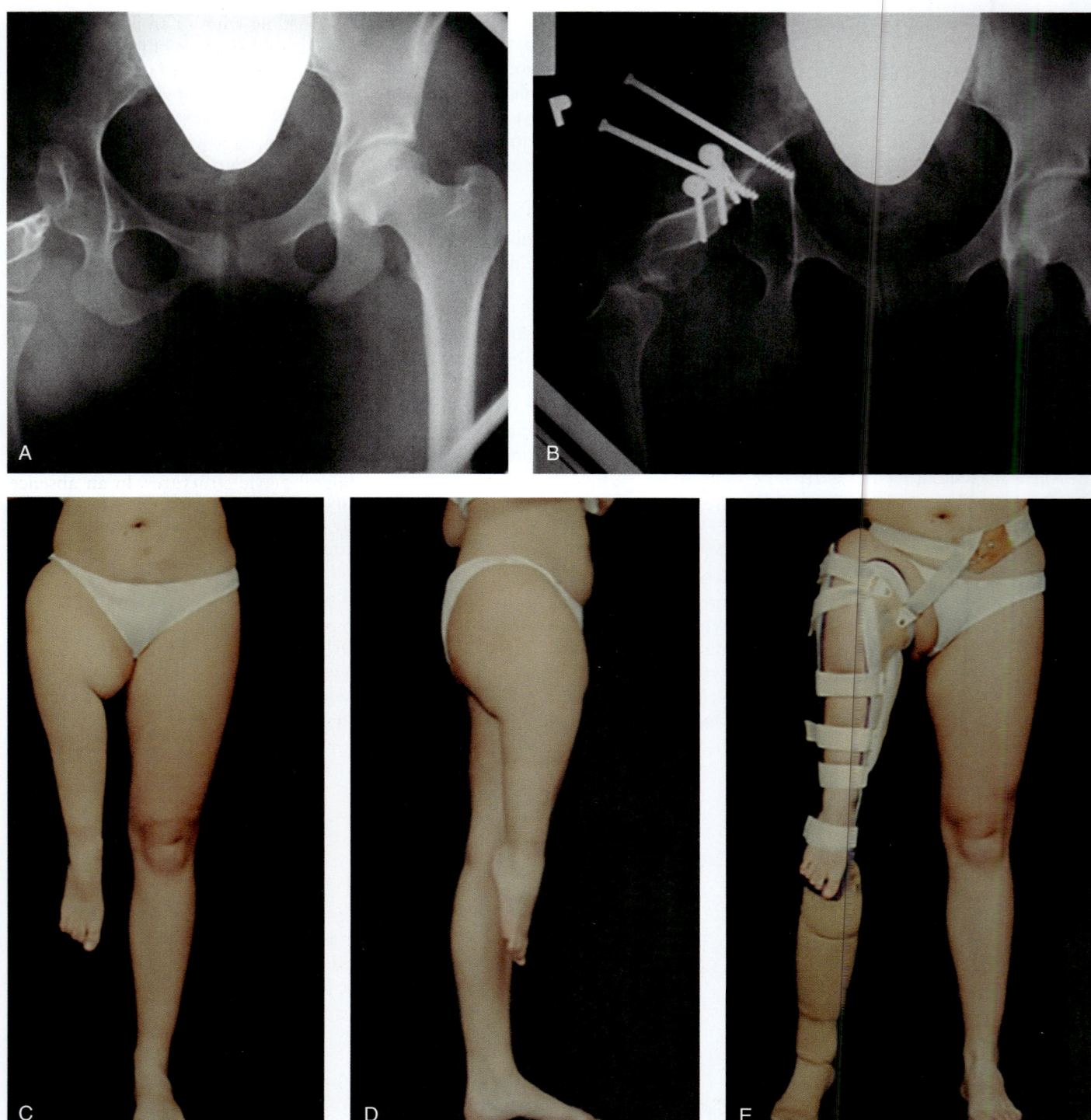

FIGURE 20 **A** and **B**, Radiographs and **C** through **E**, clinical photographs showing the clinical outcome of the Dungl operation. (Courtesy of Professor Pavel Dungl, Prague, Czech Republic.)

method that is more acceptable because it avoids the considerable scarring and muscle entrapment that accompanies the use of a frame. Excellent results have been obtained with various nails, which are produced by various manufacturers and are usually the individual surgeon's choice. The femur must be large enough to accommodate the nail. In addition, although a lateral bow can be accommodated with an osteotomy, an anterior bow is often more distal, and a second osteotomy or a shorter nail may be required. These issues should be addressed when planning the procedure. For a teenager, a two-stage correction using a corrective osteotomy and nail followed by

Chapter 76: Congenital Deficiencies of the Femur

lengthening with a nail is preferable to the use of a frame around the thigh for an extended period of time.

Rotationplasty

The major advance in rotationplasty was changing the site of rotation from the tibia[15,16] to the knee, as described by Torode and Gillespie.[17] With experience, the safety net provided by using a tibial osteotomy can be avoided to completely rotate the leg through the knee.[18] It is much easier to adjust limb length through the knee. Children treated with rotationplasty generally achieve excellent mobility; however, a degree of Trendelenburg lurch is present with the severity depending on the status of the hip joint and supporting lateral pelvic structures. In an absence of the hip joint, an alternative approach is stabilization of the limb by fusing the distal femur to the pelvis.[19] The knee is retained in a rotated position to provide flexion and extension close to the hip. The distal femoral epiphyseal plate should be ablated to prevent excessive growth.

It is important to consider the future growth of the retained epiphyseal plates and the need for additional procedures to prevent compromise of future function that could result from leaving the limb too long.

Rotationplasty Prosthesis

The rotationplasty prosthesis consists of three components: proximal thigh component, external knee supporting hinges, and foot socket. The proximal component can be either ischial bearing in the case of absent hip joint, or thigh suspending in the case of a patient with a stable hip joint (**Figure 16**). Care should be taken to place the hinges at the axis of rotation of the ankle/subtalar joint complex in cases of associated higher grade of fibular hemimelia with equinovalgus deformity at the ankle. Radiographic determination of optimal positioning of the hinges will be aided by placing markers on the skin. As children grow and make use of their new knee, the range of plantar flexion may increase. However, the temptation

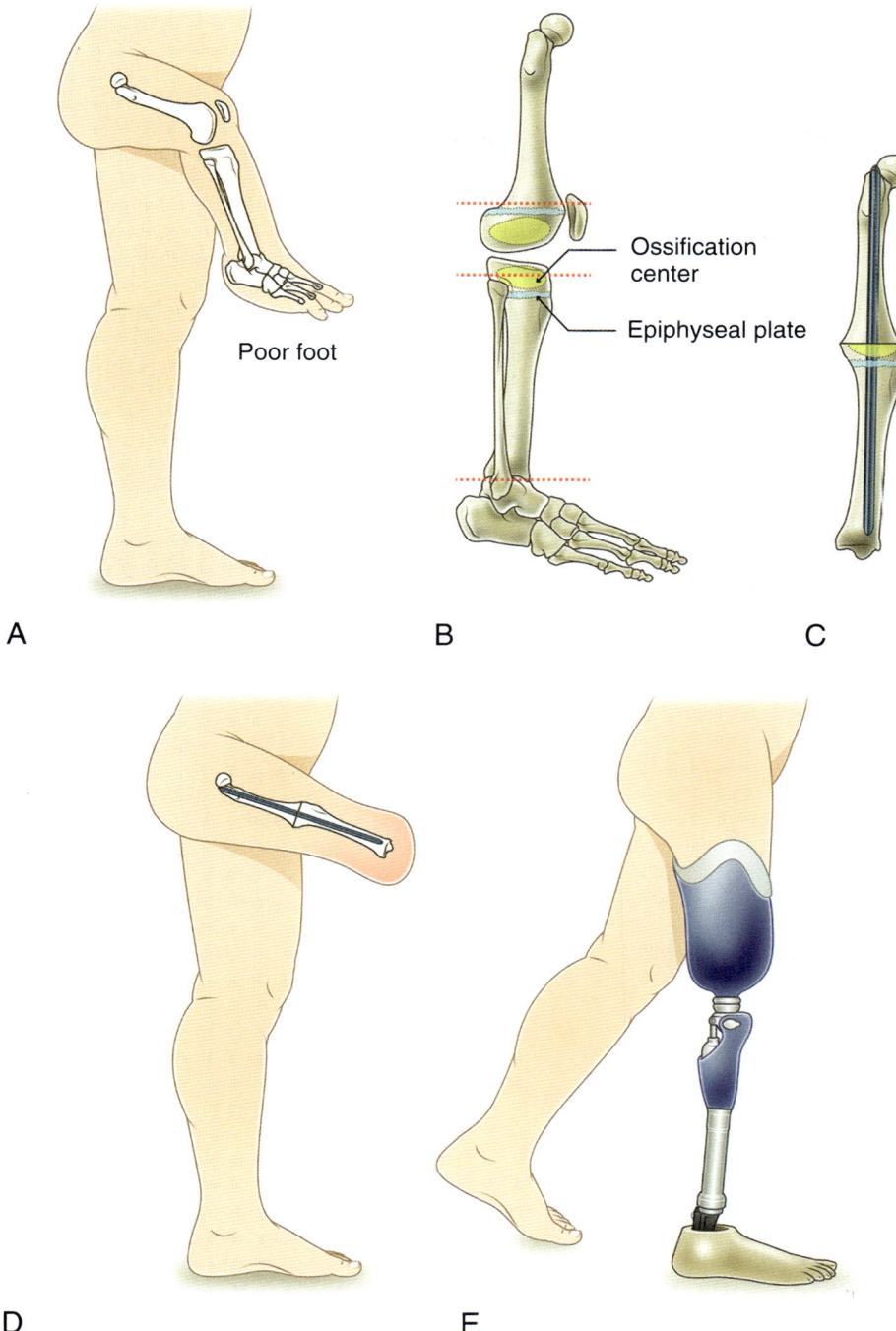

FIGURE 21 Diagrammatic representation of the procedure to fuse the knee and ablate the foot. **A**, The deficient limb is not suitable for a rotationplasty; a foot ablation and knee fusion is planned. **B**, The skeleton of the limb is shown, with possible resection levels at the knee marked by the dotted lines. In this example, the proximal tibial epiphyseal plate is retained, and the distal femoral epiphyseal plate is removed. The decision regarding these levels depends on the desired overall limb length at maturity as indicated by the distal dotted line incorporating the combination of existing segmental lengths and the available growth potential. **C**, The final position of the femur and tibia, with fixation using an intramedullary nail. Rotational control is superfluous because the foot has been amputated. **D**, The limb after foot ablation and knee fusion. **E**, The patient fitted with a prosthesis.

to make the prosthesis as cosmetically pleasing as possible by casting the foot in maximal plantar flexion should be avoided because the joint will become inflamed as it operates at its limit, reducing the load-bearing capacity of the calcaneus and allowing for more pistoning in the prosthesis so that the joints are no longer optimally aligned.

Distal Femoral Focal Deficiency

Distal femoral focal deficiency is discussed as a separate entity for several reasons. First, in terms of occurrence, it is quite rare. There are isolated case reports in the English language literature but no patient studies.[20-23] Second, the ossification of the proximal femur is intact, and the function of the hip joint itself appears normal, although Taylor et al[22] reported a case of distal deficiency associated with a hip dislocation.

The clinical appearance of a distal femoral focal deficiency is similar to that of a severe PFFD, with the foot of the affected limb at the level of the contralateral knee. However, instability occurs through the diaphyseal defect of the distal femur. The knee joint may be nonexistent because the distal femoral condylar component may be fused to the proximal tibia.

In this setting, the child will require a prosthesis for ambulation. Alignment of the limb through fusion of the proximal femoral segment to the tibia will restore stability to the limb and allow better prosthetic function. Rotationplasty is another option to improve stability and function. This procedure should achieve a better gait than seen in patients after rotationplasty for PFFD because of relatively normal hip joint.

SUMMARY

Although congenital deficiencies of the femur are uncommon, the diagnosis can be demystified by knowledge of the natural history of the condition and an understanding of the expected development of the limb. At the milder end of the severity spectrum, management is essentially the same as that provided for a limb-length discrepancy, unless the distal segments of the limb are substantially involved. At the severe end of the spectrum, most children will be best managed by prosthetic fitting. Within these extremes, there will be children in whom the potential exists for essentially normal function; reconstructive procedures and femoral lengthening are justified in these patients. In some instances, the desire for reconstruction and normalization needs to be tempered by an appreciation of the number of surgical procedures and years of a child's life that will be involved in the attempt to achieve those goals. A close collaboration between the treating surgeon and the prosthetic team is essential for optimal care of children with a congenital deficiency of the femur.

References

1. Jones KL: Femoral hypoplasia: Unusual facies syndrome, in Jones KL, ed: *Smith's Recognizable Patterns of Human Malformations*, ed 4. WB Saunders, 1988, pp 268-269.
2. Goltz RW, Peterson WC, Gorlin RJ, Ravits HG: Focal dermal hypoplasia. *Arch Dermatol* 1962;86:708-717.
3. Filly AL, Robnet-Filly B, Filly RA: Syndromes with focal femoral deficiency. *J Ultrasound Med* 2004;23(11):1511-1516.
4. Hamanishi C: Congenital short femur: Clinical, genetic and epidemiological comparison of the naturally occurring condition with that caused by thalidomide. *J Bone Joint Surg Br* 1980;62(3):307-320.
5. Gillespie R, Torode IP: Classification and management of congenital abnormalities of the femur. *J Bone Joint Surg Br* 1983;65(5):557-568.
6. Gillespie R: Classification of congenital abnormalities of the femur, in Herring JA, Birch JB, eds: *The Child With a Limb Deficiency*. American Academy of Orthopaedic Surgeons, 1998, pp 63-72.
7. Fixsen JA, Lloyd-Roberts GC: The natural history and early treatment of proximal femoral dysplasia. *J Bone Joint Surg Br* 1974;56(1):86-95.
8. Aitken GT: Proximal femoral focal deficiency: Definition, classification and management, in Aitken GT, ed: *Proximal Femoral Focal Deficiency: A Congenital Anomaly*. National Academy of Sciences, 1968, pp 1-22.
9. Paley D, Guardo F: Lengthening reconstruction surgery for congenital femoral deficiency. https://paley-institute.org/wp-content/uploads/Lengthening-Reconstruction-Surgery-for-Congenital-Femoral-Deficiency.pdf. Accessed April 21, 2023.
10. Millis MB, Hall JE: Transiliac lengthening of the lower extremity: A modified innominate osteotomy for the treatment of postural imbalance. *J Bone Joint Surg Am* 1979;61(8):1182-1194.
11. Syme J: Amputation at the ankle joint. *Lond Edinb Mon J Med Sci* 1843;3:93.
12. Birch JG, Walsh SJ, Small JM, et al: Syme amputation for the treatment of fibular deficiency: An evaluation of long-term physical and psychological functional status. *J Bone Joint Surg Am* 1999;81(11):1511-1518.
13. Métaizeau JP, Wong-Chung J, Bertrand H, Pasquie P: Percutaneous epiphysiodesis using transphyseal screws (PETS). *J Pediatr Orthop* 1998;18(3):363-369.
14. Blount WP, Clarke GR: Control of bone growth by epiphyseal stapling: A preliminary report. *J Bone Joint Surg Am* 1949;31(3):464-478.
15. Kritter AE: Tibial rotation-plasty for proximal femoral focal deficiency. *J Bone Joint Surg Am* 1977;59(7):927-934.
16. King R: Providing a single lever in proximal femoral focal deficiency: A preliminary report. *J Assoc Child Prosthet Orthot Clin* 1966;6:23.
17. Torode IP, Gillespie R: Rotationplasty of the lower limb for congenital defects of the femur. *J Bone Joint Surg Br* 1983;65(5):569-573.
18. Krajbich I: Proximal femoral focal deficiency, in Kalamchi A, ed: *Congenital Lower Limb Deficiencies*. Springer-Verlag, 1989, pp 108-127.
19. Brown KL: Resection, rotationplasty, and femoropelvic arthrodesis in severe congenital femoral deficiency: A report of the surgical technique and three cases. *J Bone Joint Surg Am* 2001;83(1):78-85.
20. Tsou PM: Congenital distal femoral focal deficiency: Report of a unique case. *Clin Orthop Relat Res* 1982;162:99-102.
21. Gilsanz V: Distal focal femoral deficiency. *Radiology* 1983;147(1):105-107.
22. Taylor BC, Kean J, Paloski M: Distal focal femoral deficiency. *J Pediatr Orthop* 2009;29(6):576-580.
23. Joseph B: Distal focal femoral deficiency, in Loder RT, Torode I, Joseph B, Nayagam S, eds: *Paediatric Orthopaedics: A System of Decision-Making*. Hodder Arnold, 2009, pp 269-271.

Rotationplasty: Surgical Techniques and Prosthetic Considerations

CHAPTER 77

Joseph Ivan Krajbich, MD, FRCS(C) • Sabrina Jakobson Huston, CPO

ABSTRACT

Rotationplasty is a surgical technique that maximizes the functional potential of children and young adults who are faced with potentially high-level terminal amputation of the lower extremity or were born with a significant intercalary lower limb deficiency, such as proximal femoral focal deficiency. It is helpful to be familiar with the surgical techniques for acquired and congenital deficiencies and prosthetic management of the residual limb.

Keywords: Aitken types A through D; limb salvage; osteosarcoma; proximal femoral focal deficiency; rotationplasty

Introduction

Rotationplasty, which is also referred to in the literature as a Borggreve procedure, a Van Nes rotationplasty, or a tibial or femoral turnaround procedure, has undergone several modifications since its original description. The principle of rotationplasty, however, remains the same: a healthy, functional joint (usually the ankle) is used as a substitute for the loss of a more proximal joint (usually the knee). For the ankle to function as a biologic knee substitute, it must be brought up to the level of the contralateral knee and turned 180° to function in the plane and range of a normal knee (**Figure 1**). The foot distal to the ankle joint is then a below-knee component of the limb and is fitted with a transtibial-like prosthesis (**Figure 2**). Ideally, the child's function then resembles that of a patient who has undergone a transtibial amputation.

Borggreve[1] first described the procedure in 1930 for a patient with tuberculosis of the knee. In the 1950s, Van Nes[2] published a variation of the procedure, which was used for congenital limb deficiency. Rotationplasty and its subsequent modification gained some popularity for the management of congenital femoral deficiencies,[3-5] most frequently proximal femoral focal deficiency (PFFD), and it has been used in several pediatric orthopaedic surgery centers, primarily in North America and Europe. In the late 1970s in Vienna, Austria, Salzer et al[6] modified the procedure for limb salvage in patients with osteosarcoma of the distal femur. The procedure was further adapted for use in salvage of limbs with tumor in the proximal tibia and also for lesions involving the proximal femur, where the rotated knee can be used as a substitute for a hip joint. Since then, rotationplasty has been applied in a variety of conditions where the distal part of the limb with the functional distal joint can be salvaged, but a proximal joint cannot be salvaged. The greatest barrier to the wider acceptance of this technique appears to be unfamiliarity with the procedure.[7-9]

In addition to a cooperative patient and their family, an optimal functional outcome in these procedures requires a successful surgical outcome, a diligent rehabilitation regimen, and expert prosthetic fitting. The rotationplasty prosthesis, albeit relatively inexpensive in terms of the prosthetic components, requires significant expertise on the part of the prosthetist to achieve a functionally optimal outcome.

Surgical Considerations

Indications

The primary reason for rotationplasty, compared with a terminal transfemoral amputation, is to provide a patient with a biologic knee substitute that would improve gait efficiency, energy consumption of ambulation, and the ability to walk on uneven surfaces. Ideally, the resulting function is very similar to that of a transtibial amputation.

The indications for rotationplasty or its various modifications can be classified into two main categories: (1) congenital lower limb deficiency (usually but not always PFFD) and (2) acquired deficiency with rotationplasty as a form of limb salvage. The underlying condition is most frequently a

---

Dr. Krajbich or an immediate family member serves as a board member, owner, officer, or committee member of Scoliosis Research Society. Neither Sabrina Jakobson Huston nor any immediate family member has received anything of value from or has stock or stock options held in a commercial company or institution related directly or indirectly to the subject of this chapter.

Section 5: Pediatrics

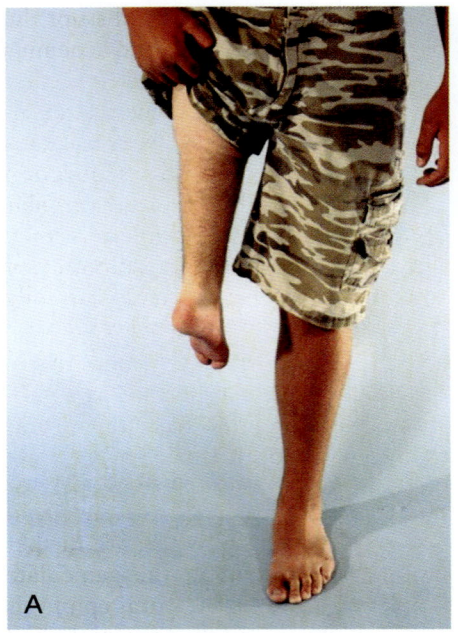
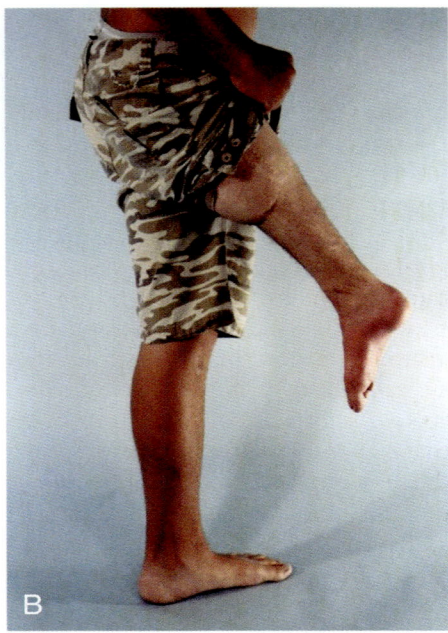

FIGURE 1 AP (**A**) and lateral (**B**) clinical photographs of a male patient treated with rotationplasty.

malignant tumor in a child or a young adult, but it is also used in other etiologies, such as trauma, infection, and the failure of previous limb salvage or other reconstruction procedures.

The surgical technique differs for each category, so each has a separate description in this chapter. However, some general principles apply to both categories.

Prerequisites

The joint to be transferred or rotated must have functional range of motion, and its nerve supply must be intact. Vascular supply to the distal part of the limb must be preservable or reconstructible. Motor supply to the newly reconstructed joint must be present and functional.

Absolute Contraindications

The absolute contraindications are a failure to satisfy the prerequisites. A poorly perfused or insensate foot with restricted range of motion is a poor substitute for other reconstructive methods or transfemoral amputation and restoration with modern transfemoral amputation prosthesis. The procedure is contraindicated in patients with malignant tumors where adequate oncologic resection margins do not allow for major nerve preservation.

Relative Contraindications

The relative contraindications are primarily subjective. In the opinion of one this chapter's authors (J.I.K.), the primary reason that this procedure is not more widely performed, particularly in patients with PFFD and young (first and second decade) patients with cancer, is the treating surgeon's unfamiliarity with the procedure. The somewhat odd appearance of the reconstructed limb can occasionally be a deterrent. Functional expectations, particularly in patients with a tumor, also play an important role.[10] An active lifestyle versus a relatively sedentary lifestyle but better cosmesis with potential multiple reoperations in the future may weigh on the child and any parental decision regarding the procedure chosen. The patient and the family must be comfortable with the decision to proceed with the proposed surgical approach. A lack of appropriate prosthetic services can also be a relative contraindication; however, this criterion should be limited only to very underserved areas or countries. The prosthetic componentry is relatively simple, and the skill for making the prosthesis is acquirable and learnable. Having a well-functioning rotationplasty limb and prosthesis allows excellent function resembling that of a transtibial amputation. Having a

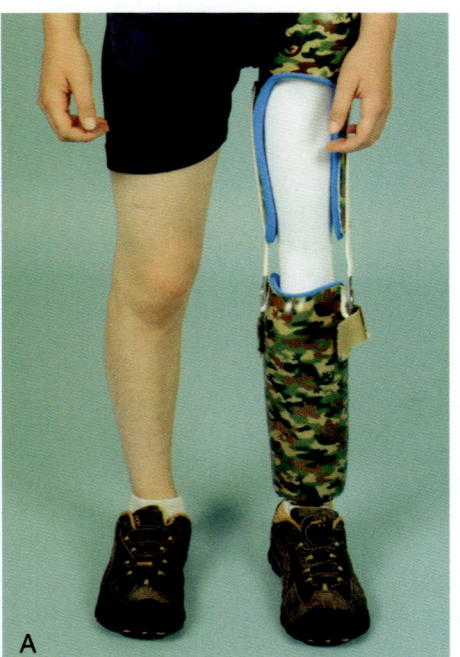
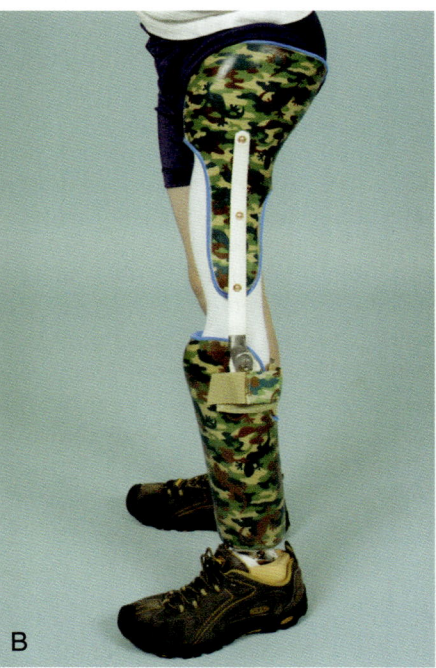

FIGURE 2 Clinical photographs of front (**A**) and side (**B**) views of a child with a rotationplasty prosthesis.

functioning biologic knee-like joint provides for improved energy consumption in gait and improved agility and ability to walk on uneven surfaces.[11-15]

Rotationplasty for Children With PFFD

PFFD is a congenital abnormality of the femur that varies in severity from a deficit primarily in the subtrochanteric region of the femur to virtual complete absence of the femur[16-20] (**Figure 3**). For the purpose of this discussion, only true PFFD versus congenital short femur as described by Gillespie and Torode[21] will be considered. The most frequently used PFFD classification was developed by Aitken,[22] and all four types (A through D) are potentially suitable for rotationplasty if the child has a relatively normal foot and ankle complex. The presence or absence (or various degrees of dysplasia) of the hip is not a contraindication to the procedure. In patients with a reconstructible hip (Aitken types A and B) and who are deemed not be candidates for femoral reconstruction and limb equalization procedures, hip reconstruction is usually performed as a second procedure 1 or 2 years after rotationplasty. In addition, in normalizing the hip joint, the procedure allows for fine-tuning of the rotationplasty as to the length and rotation of the new thigh.[23]

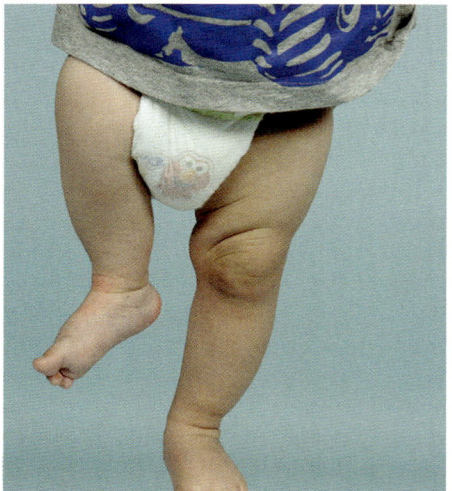

FIGURE 3 Clinical photograph of the lower extremities of a young child with proximal femoral focal deficiency before rotationplasty.

The rotationplasty procedure has been modified several times since first being introduced by Van Nes.[2] Initially, the rotation was performed through the diaphysis of the tibia and the fibula, either alone or combined with knee fusion.[4,5,24] The addition of knee fusion has been a major contribution to the surgical treatment of PFFD, with or without rotationplasty. It was first described by King and Marks[25] and has become a standard part of PFFD treatment.[25-27] A single-bone thigh is aligned under the hip joint, thus allowing for restoration of the biomechanical axis of the limb in the sagittal plane.[25-27] Taking advantage of knee fusion, Gillespie[28] and Torode and Gillespie[29] incorporated a substantial portion of the rotation through the knee fusion and the remainder through the tibial diaphysis.[30] Still, the relatively common phenomena of derotation led one of this chapter's authors (J.I.K.) to modify the procedure even further. In most patients, the entire rotation is carried through the knee fusion, which necessitates detachment of all muscle and tendon structures crossing the knee joint and careful mobilization of the neurovascular bundles to ensure a viable functional limb.[23] Muscles and tendons are then reattached so they line up in the plane of the adjacent joint motion, thus less likely contributing to derotation.

Surgical Technique

The child is placed on a radiolucent table in a supine position, with the affected limb draped free. The posterior tibial and anterior tibial arterial pulses are marked on the skin for easy location and later monitoring. A lazy S incision is made over the knee area starting proximally and laterally, crossing the knee anteriorly at the level of the joint and curving medially and distally. The practice of one of this chapter's authors (J.I.K.) is to first identify and dissect free the peroneal nerve on the lateral side. The biceps femoris and pes anserinus muscles and tendons are divided at the level of the knee joint. The two heads of the gastrocnemius muscles are detached as close to their origin on the femoral condyles as possible.

Care must be taken not to disrupt the nerve supply to the gastrocnemius muscle because this muscle, together with the soleus, will become the reconstructed knee's primary extensor. This process allows for good visualization of the popliteal fossa neurovascular bundle. The patellar tendon is then divided, and complete capsulotomy of the knee joint is performed, carefully protecting the posterior neurovascular structures. The collateral and cruciate ligaments, if present, also are divided. The remaining muscular structures (semimembranosus and popliteal) are then identified and divided, which allows for good exposure of the popliteal artery and vein, which are further mobilized by dividing the geniculate branches. The distal femoral epiphysis and metaphysis and the proximal tibial epiphysis and portions of the metaphysis are thus exposed. The distal femoral epiphysis together with its physis and a portion of metaphysis are excised. The extent of proximal tibial excision depends on length of the remaining femur. If the femur is very short, only a portion of the epiphysis preserving the epiphyseal plate is excised. If the femur is of a reasonable length, the whole epiphysis is removed together with the physis and a small portion of the metaphysis (approximately 5 mm). The extent of the metaphyseal excision of the femur is to some degree guided by the ease of rotation of the distal part of the extremity. Complete 180° rotation must be achievable without vascular compromise. The previously marked peripheral pulses are carefully monitored with a sterile Doppler probe. Any compromise in circulation must be addressed by additional dissection and mobilization of the vessels and/or additional shortening of the femoral metaphysis.

The procedure is then completed by arthrodesis of the tibia, which is rotated 180° to the femur using intramedullary fixation of a Rush rod and securing the rotation alignment with either a cross pin or a small plate (**Figure 4**). Maintaining good vascular perfusion as monitored by Doppler is critical at this stage. Any compromise must be

Section 5: Pediatrics

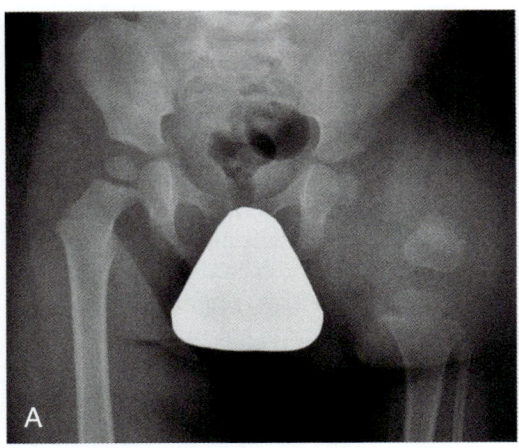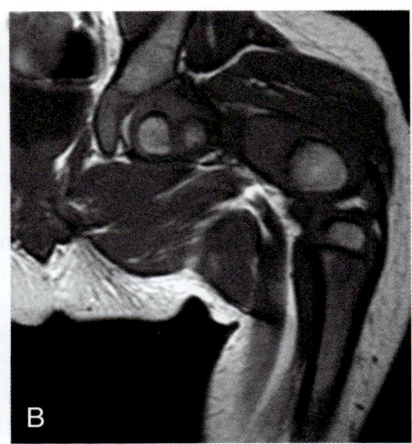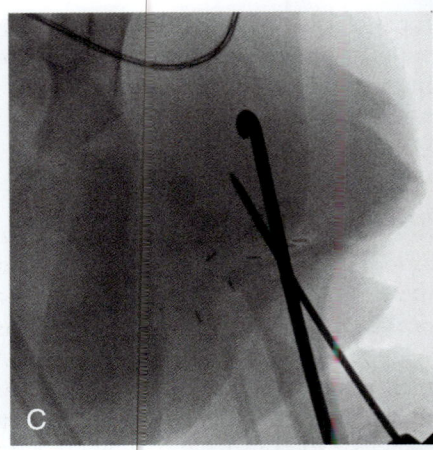

FIGURE 4 AP radiograph (**A**) and MRI (**B**) from a child with left-sided proximal femoral focal deficiency (Aitken type B). **C**, Intraoperative radiograph from the same child with a completed rotationplasty. A Rush rod and cross pin were used to control the rotation.

addressed immediately by further vessel decompression and mobilization. In very rare instances, the rotation can be controlled by cast immobilization without an internal cross pin, allowing less-than-perfect rotation but obviating the need for implants. The final desired rotation can be achieved in 1 or 2 weeks during a cast change under anesthesia.

Before skin closure, the distal portion of the quadriceps is attached to the gastrocnemius to maximize knee extension power. Skin closure is sometimes facilitated with the trimming of excess skin.

Postsurgical Care

Initially (first 24 hours) the peripheral circulation of the surgically treated extremity is very carefully monitored. Any perceived compromise of the circulation has to be aggressively investigated and managed. The child's limb is immobilized in a hip spica-like dressing or a cast for 6 weeks, after which intensive rehabilitation with physical therapy is started (**Figure 5**). After both the arthrodesis and soft tissue have healed, the child is fitted with a rotationplasty prosthesis and begins physical therapy–guided gait training.

Alternative Technique

Brown[31] described a modification of the rotationplasty technique for patients with Aitken types C and D longitudinal deficiencies of the femur in an attempt to provide such patients with a stable hip. Arthrodesis of the distal femur to the side of the pelvis is performed with the leg rotated 180°, similar to the procedure described by Winkelmann[32] for tumors of the proximal femur and the hip (as described later in this chapter). Frequently, a very short femoral segment and an abnormal knee in these

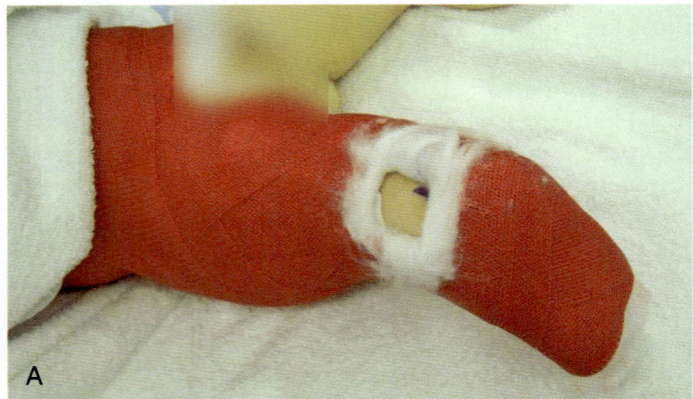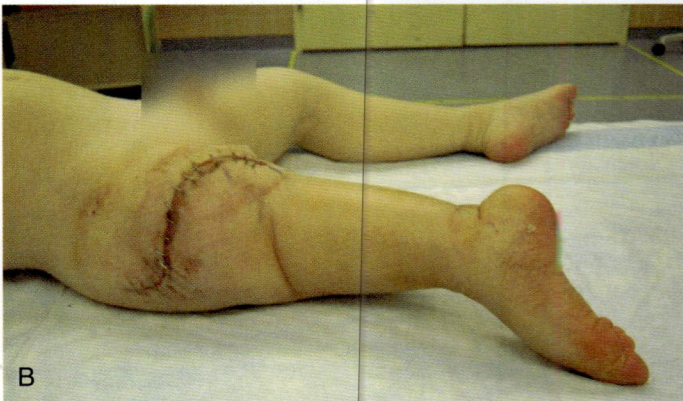

FIGURE 5 **A**, Clinical photograph of postoperative hip spica cast immobilization. **B**, Clinical photograph of early healing with postoperative appearance.

higher grade PFFDs limits the number of patients suitable for this procedural variant.[31,33]

Rotationplasty as a Limb Salvage Procedure

Rotationplasty has been used in limb salvage surgery for malignant tumors of the lower limb.[34] The procedure allows for wide margins in tumor resection similar to that accomplished by high transfemoral amputation if the sciatic nerve can be preserved without compromising tumor-free margins. The blood supply to the distal part of the limb can be spared by dissecting the femoral artery free (if tumor-free margins can be attained) or resecting the vessel together with the tumor and restoring circulation by anastomosing the proximal femoral artery and vein to the popliteal artery and vein.[6,34,35]

Surgical Technique

As with most tumor resection procedures, careful procedural planning is just as important as the actual surgical execution. Careful staging of the lesion with detailed MRI showing the tumor extension, particularly near the neurovascular structure, is critical in determining which vessels to preserve or resect. One of this chapter's authors (J.I.K.) routinely obtains full-length radiographs of both lower limbs to plan the level of bone osteotomies in the proximal tibia and femur. The goal of the procedure is to have the thighs of equal (or very near equal) length at the end of the procedure.[36] The new rotationplasty thigh consists of the hip joint, the proximal femoral fragment, the tibia minus the proximal epiphysis, and small portions of the proximal metaphysis. The 180°-rotated ankle joint then substitutes for the knee. A relatively common mistake is to make the new thigh too long (not enough resection), which detracts from both cosmetic appearance and the functional result of the limb. To prevent these problems, the femur should be transected just below the lesser trochanter and the attachment of gluteus maximus muscles, and several centimeters of the proximal tibial metaphysis are also resected.

In the operating room, the patient is placed on the operating table in the supine position, and the surgical limb is draped free from the toes to almost the umbilicus to ensure easy access to the proximal femoral and external iliac arteries.

Skin incisions are marked on the thigh, planning cylindroid resection of the skin of the mid and distal thigh (**Figure 6**). More obliquely oriented incisions are required distally to account for the relative diameter mismatch of the distal limb and proximal part of the limb. Incisions are extended vertically, proximally, and distally. Proximally, the extension is placed anterolaterally, allowing access to both the anterior vessels and lateral part of the proximal femur. Distally, the extension is medial, allowing for access to the medial part of the proximal tibia for ease of reconstruction. Additional skin incisions are made in the cylindroid portion (which will be resected) to gain easy access to the structure or structures to be preserved (the sciatic nerve and the femoral popliteal artery and veins), still carefully preserving adequate margins around the tumor.

The saphenous vein is frequently dissected and preserved to obtain additional venous drainage of the limb. All the muscles of the thigh are transected at the level of the planned proximal femoral osteotomy. The fascia lata can be transected somewhat further distally so that it can be used for lateral thigh soft tissue toward the end of the procedure. Distally, the pes anserinus tendons are transected at the level of the tibial osteotomy, and the biceps femoris is detached from the fibular head. Care must be taken to protect and carefully mobilize the peroneal nerve at its entry

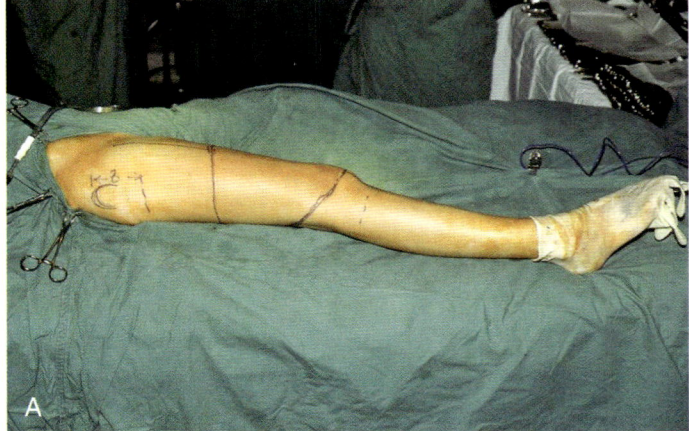
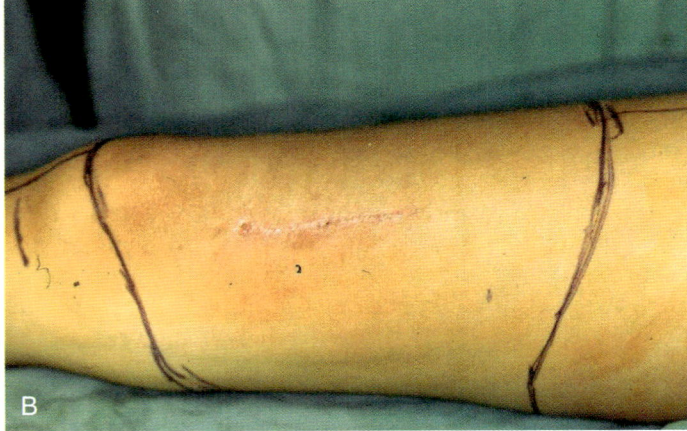

FIGURE 6 **A**, Intraoperative photograph of planned incision for rotationplasty in a patient with a lower limb tumor. **B**, Intraoperative photograph of the biopsy track, which is easily removed with the resected tumor.

into the anterior compartment of the leg. The heads of the gastrocnemius are transected near their origin on the femoral condyles. Maintaining appropriate tumor resection margins is critical at this stage and dictates the proximal extent of transection. Every care must be taken not to violate the tumor margin and to preserve the nerve supply of the gastrocnemius as it exits the posterior tibial nerve. The patellar tendon is detached distally without entering the knee joint proper. The sciatic nerve is dissected free posteriorly along its entire exposed length. The femoral popliteal artery and vein are dissected free if the tumor margins allow; if not, the vessels are isolated proximally and distally, and after the femoral and tibial osteotomies are completed, the vessels are divided to be reanastomosed. A portion of the thigh and the knee containing the tumor is removed after final transection of the soft tissue (popliteal muscle and periosteum at the tibial osteotomy site), while carefully protecting the trifurcation branches of the popliteal vessels.

The thigh is then reconstructed by bringing the leg portion proximally, externally rotating it 180°, and internally fixing the proximal femoral fragment to the proximal tibia (**Figure 7**). If the vessels were resected, vascular anastomosis is now performed to reestablish circulation to the limb. Relatively little is needed in terms of remaining muscle and soft-tissue reconstruction. The vessels, if preserved, and the sciatic nerve are gently coiled around the muscles, avoiding sharp kinks. The iliotibial band is anchored to the tibia to stabilize the lateral side, and the gastrocnemius heads are attached to the remaining proximal portion of the quadriceps. Skin flaps are trimmed for easy closure and closed in layers over a drain; a hip spica-like dressing is applied.[37]

For lesions arising in the proximal tibia, the procedure has been modified to allow for resection of most of the tibia, leaving only the distal metaphysis/epiphysis and the ankle joint (**Figure 8**). Proximally, the osteotomy is

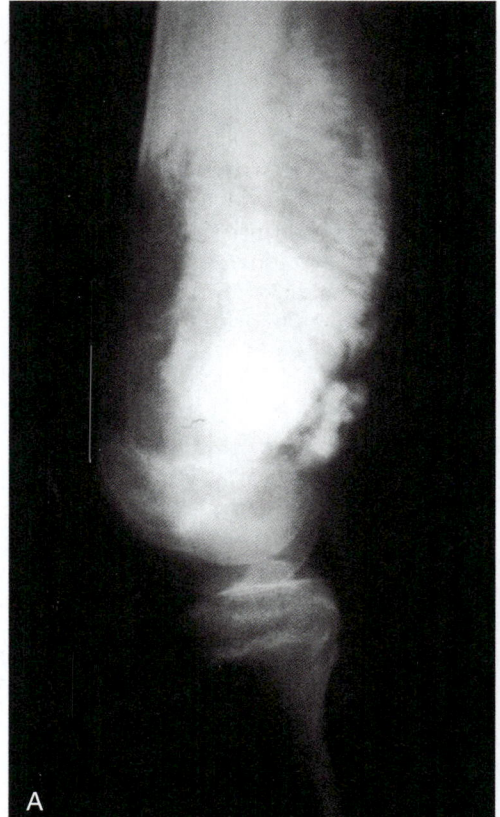
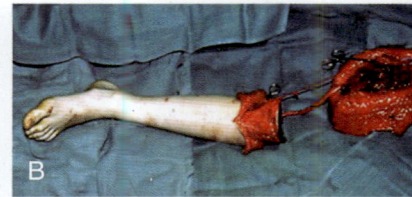
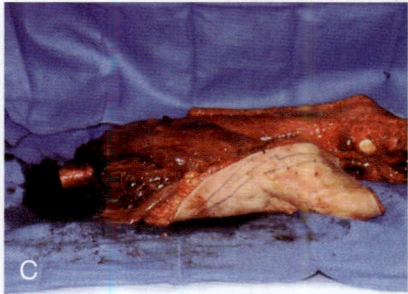
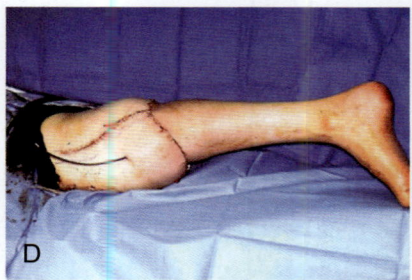

FIGURE 7 Preoperative and intraoperative images from a child with a diagnosis of osteosarcoma. **A**, Preoperative lateral radiograph shows distal femoral osteosarcoma. **B**, Intraoperative photograph of the distal part of the limb connected only by the sciatic nerve. The femoral artery and vein were resected with the tumor part, and the child will have vascular reanastomosis. **C**, Intraoperative photograph of the resected portion of the thigh, including the tumor. **D**, Intraoperative photograph of extremity appearance at the conclusion of the surgical procedure. Normal neurovascular function of the distal limb is checked before leaving the operating room.

through the distal femoral metaphysis. The reconstruction is somewhat more complex because the new ankle/knee is powered by the thigh musculature. Good balance between the dorsiflexors (knee flexors) and the plantar flexors (quadriceps) must be achieved[38,39] (**Figure 9**). As a rule, patients with this reconstruction require a longer period of rehabilitation to maximize their new knee/ankle function compared with more commonly performed rotationplasty for distal femoral lesions. However, in the experience of one of the authors of this chapter (J.I.K.), their eventual function is superior because the powerful thigh muscles (quadriceps and hamstrings) power the new knee. Their gait in the prosthesis is indistinguishable from those who have a transtibial amputation.

Rotationplasty also has been adopted for reconstruction after tumor resection of lesions of the proximal femur involving the hip joint. In this situation, nearly the whole femur, including the femoral head and possibly the acetabulum, is resected together with the thigh soft tissues. The distal femoral metaphysis is then attached (via arthrodesis) to the pelvis after being rotated 180°. This allows the original knee to function as a uniplanar hip joint (flexion/extension),

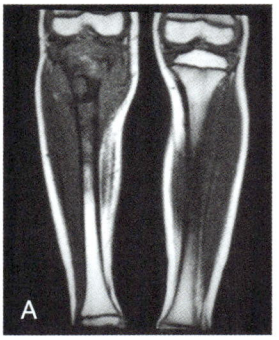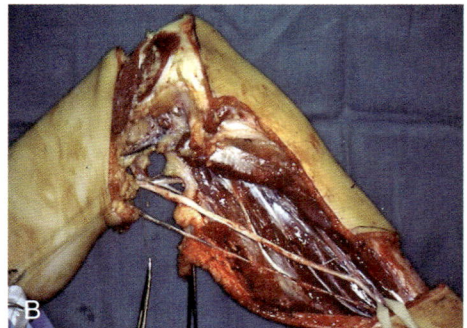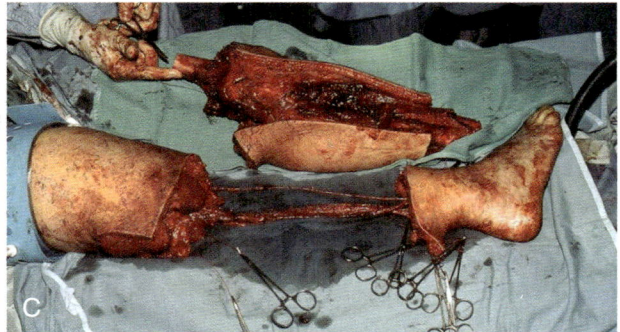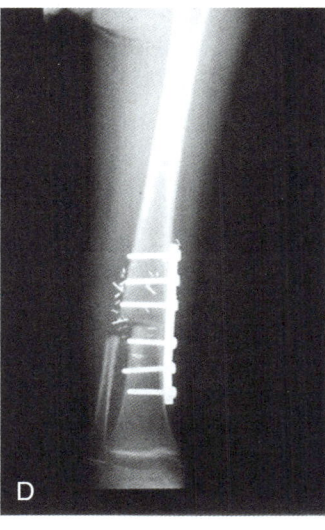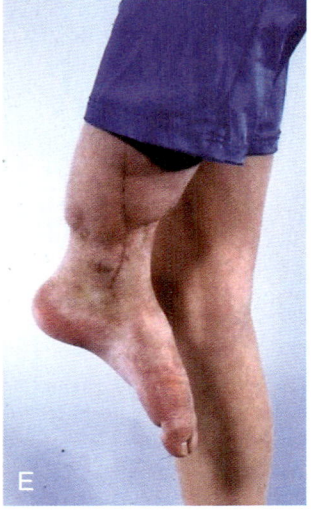

FIGURE 8 Images from a patient with osteosarcoma involving the proximal half of the tibia and the knee. **A**, Coronal cut MRI shows a large osteosarcoma with bone destruction and soft-tissue extension in the right proximal tibia. **B**, Intraoperative photograph of dissection that is isolating the neurovascular structures to be preserved. **C**, Intraoperative photograph of removal of the tumor. A wide margin is obtained throughout. **D**, AP radiograph at completion of the rotationplasty. **E**, Clinical photograph of the healed limb.

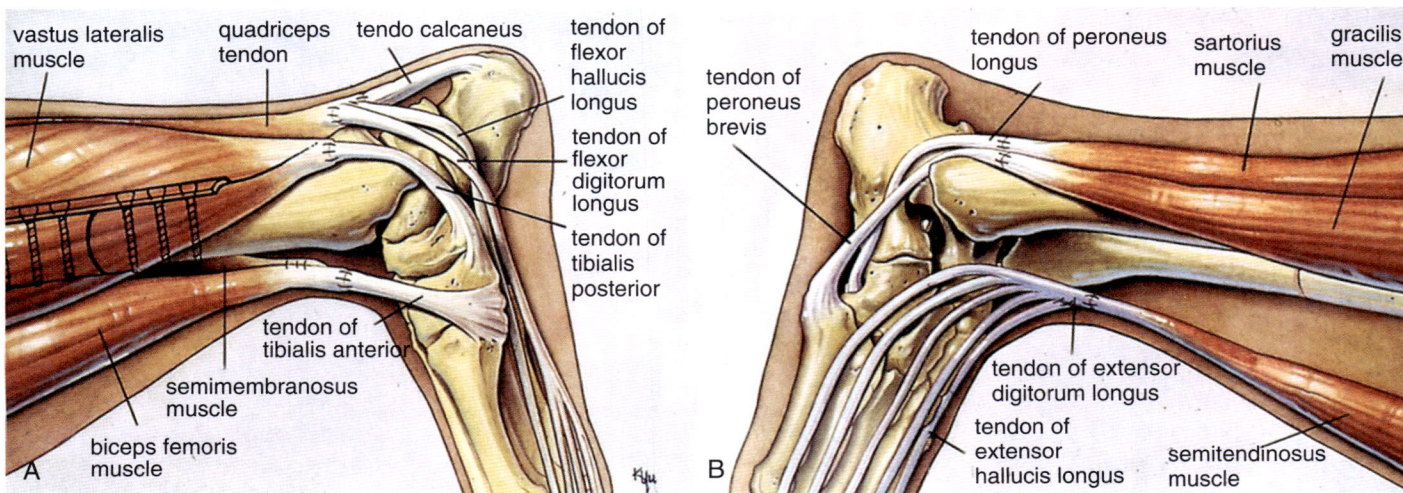

FIGURE 9 Illustrations of individual tendon-muscle reattachments in the case of rotationplasty performed for a tumor in the proximal tibia. **A**, Lateral view. **B**, Medial view.

and the ankle again functions as a new knee joint (**Figure 10**). The gluteus maximus is reattached to the quadriceps tendon to provide hip extension, and the iliopsoas, the tensor fascia lata, and the sartorius are used for the new hip flexion.[32,40,41]

Most of these procedures are performed for malignant tumors requiring major resection to maximize a child's chances for survival. However, other etiologies, such as early or late failure of other limb-sparing reconstructions, including infection, tumor recurrence, the failure of endoprosthetic replacement, or a massive allograft replacement, can be salvaged with rotationplasty (**Figures 11** and **12**). Likewise, massive tissue loss of the proximal part of the limb because of trauma or infection can be salvaged by rotationplasty if the alternative is a high-level amputation.

Rehabilitation

As would be expected, regardless of etiology, these procedures require a substantial period of recovery and rehabilitation. Gradual progression from gentle range of motion exercises,

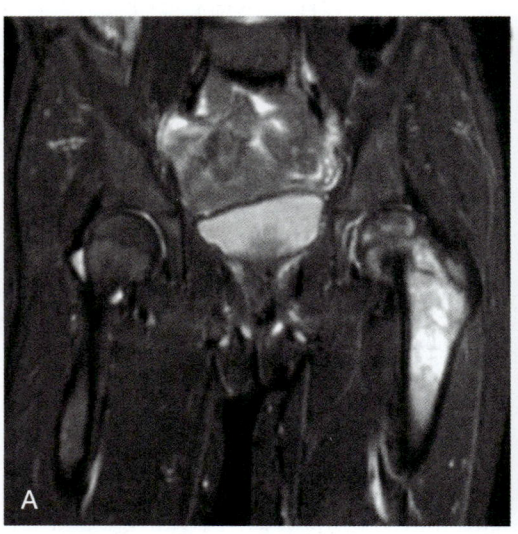 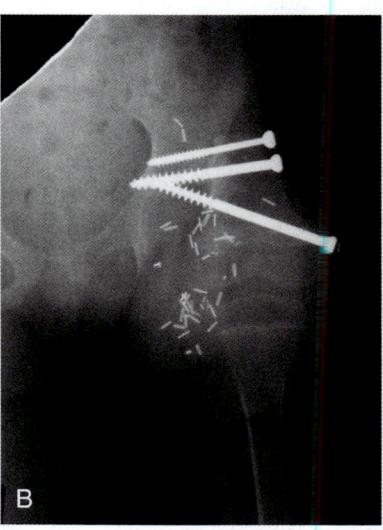

FIGURE 10 **A**, MRI from a child with Ewing sarcoma of the proximal femur. **B**, AP radiograph from a patient after rotationplasty. The patient had a distal femoral epiphysiodesis as a second procedure after chemotherapy was completed.

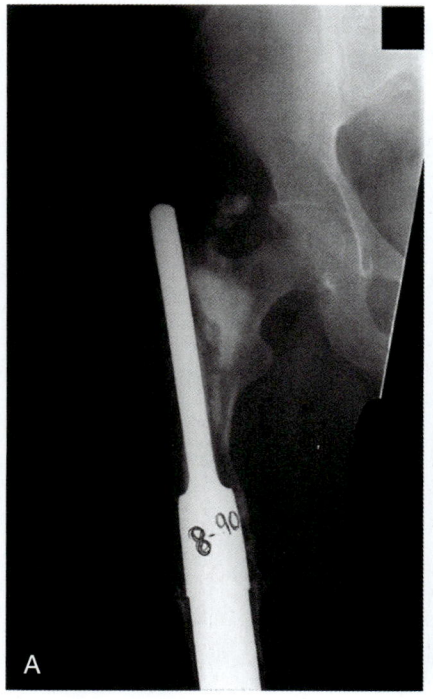 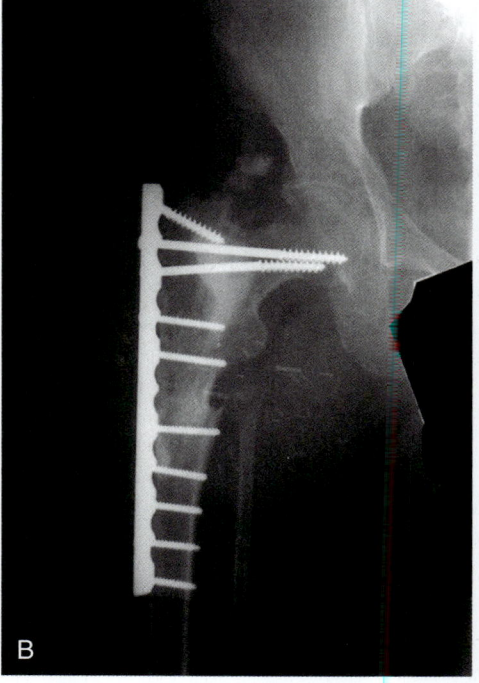

FIGURE 11 **A**, AP radiograph of a failed endoprosthesis in a patient with osteosarcoma. **B**, AP radiograph of the limb after being salvaged with rotationplasty.

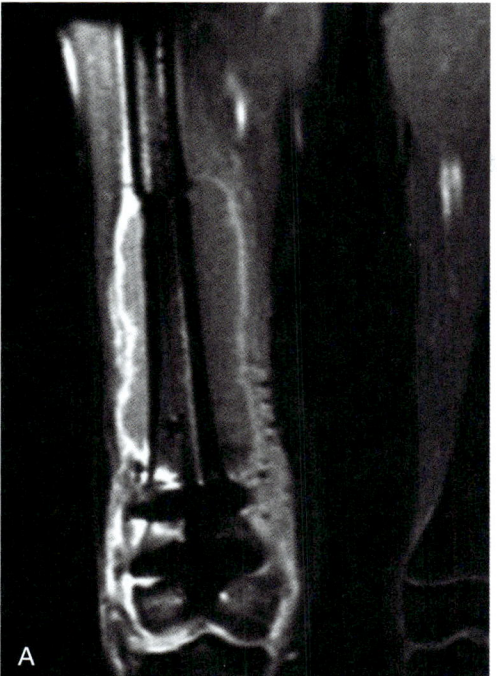 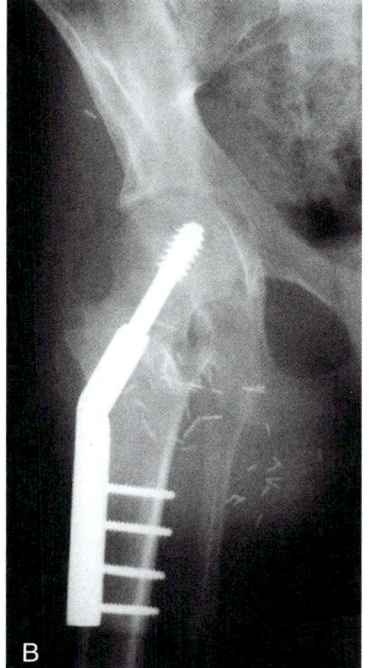 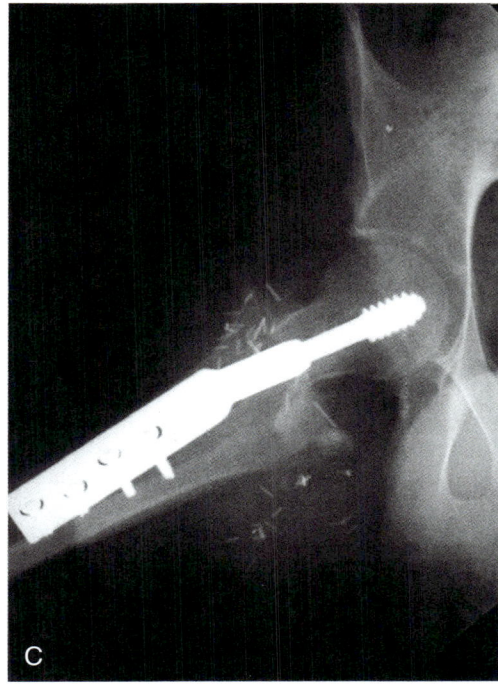

FIGURE 12 Imaging studies demonstrating failed primary treatment and reconstruction for sarcoma. **A**, MRI of a large tumor recurrence. AP (**B**) and frog-lateral (**C**) radiographs of a modified rotationplasty performed as a salvage procedure.

gradual strengthening, and, finally, gait training with the new rotationplasty prosthesis require substantial time and care from the physiotherapy and prosthetic teams.

Prosthetic Considerations

Advancements in limb salvage surgery have given the patient with a lower limb tumor more treatment options. In the past, children with a diagnosis of malignant tumors of the lower limbs usually faced amputation of the affected limb. Transfemoral amputation, hip disarticulation, or transpelvic amputation were the typical outcomes.[42]

Being a rare congenital deformity, PFFD is characterized by an incomplete or absent femur. It can be unilateral or bilateral. Fibular hemimelia is often associated with the condition, occurring in 70% to 80% of the PFFD population.[37] Surgery and prosthetic intervention are necessary for bipedal ambulation for a child with unilateral PFFD.[37]

Rotationplasty is an option for children with tumors of the distal or proximal third of the femur and the proximal tibia[42] and congenital PFFD. Clinically, the patient has a foot rotated 180° and an ankle that functions as a knee (**Figure 1**). The advantage of rotationplasty versus a Syme disarticulation in the child with PFFD—or proximal leg amputations for children with lower limb tumors—is the elimination of a mechanical prosthetic knee. Studies have reported more efficient energy-efficient ambulation after rotationplasty than with a mechanical knee.[7,11,12]

For children who have undergone rotationplasty because of tumor resection or PFFD, the prostheses are similar, but the design and the fit may differ. Because the population of patients with a rotationplasty is relatively small, only a limited number of prosthetists have experience in fitting rotationplasty prostheses. The collaboration of an experienced multidisciplinary team is paramount for a positive prosthetic outcome.

Prosthesis Molding

In preparation for molding the prosthesis, a pantaloon-style garment should be tailored to aid in the molding process and for the patient's modesty. With the patient standing, the residual limb is molded in a vertically extended position, with the foot in maximum hyperplantar flexion and the hips square to the body. If the patient is unable to stand, they should lie on their sound side, with the hips stacked, the limb in line with the torso, and the foot in maximum plantar flexion. On the pantaloon-style garment, the sulcus, the medial and lateral malleoli, the calcaneal tuberosity, the navicular, and the sustentaculum tali should be referenced. If a cut strip is used to remove the mold, it should be placed in a posterior position to avoid distorting bony prominences.

For the patient with PFFD, the shape of the thigh should be captured by wrapping one turn around the waist and then continuing to wrap the residual limb proximally to distally. Stability and flexibility of the hip are critical in the patient with Aitken types C and D deficiency.[18] The socket will resemble a ship's funnel shape,[42] having a high lateral wall to contain the residual tissue. The patient with a lower limb tumor may not require a thigh section as high as the ischial level. The wrap should be started above the level of the surgical site. While the molding material is still soft, the prosthetist places the web of their hand on the distal plantar calcaneus and their thumb in the sustentaculum tali.

The standing patient is then asked to bear weight moderately. If the patient is lying down, the prosthetist should apply pressure with the web of their hand to the distal plantar calcaneus, with their thumb in the sustentaculum tali. With the opposite hand, the sulcus is defined to create a weight-bearing shelf distal to the calcaneus. The sustentaculum tali groove will control mediolateral motion of the foot and provide navicular relief in the socket; the sulcus will aid in suspension. The mold is then removed.

Model Modification

Modifications to the positive model on the foot section will include the malleoli, navicular buildup, sulcus relief, sustentaculum tali groove relief, and extension of the distal toes by 0.50 to 0.75 inch. Reduction of the thigh section will depend on the amount of residual tissue.

Diagnostic Socket

A clear diagnostic socket is fabricated to determine fit, suspension, and joint placement. A mold of clear thermoplastic is draped over the modified mold. A vertical line is marked on the lateral and anterior foot and thigh sections to reference the relationship of the foot and thigh before removing the plastic from the model. These sections are fit separately.[43] The foot section is checked for ease of donning, relief of bony prominences, and for adequate clearance over the malleoli with the ankle flexed and extended. Patients with PFFD and fibular hemimelia may use a combination of the subtalar joint for dorsiflexion and the talocrural joint for plantar flexion; this causes the calcaneus to be in hypereversion in dorsiflexion, thus affecting the placement of the mechanical knee joint.

The foot should slip easily through the ischial level thigh section. The residual thigh tissue and surgical site should be contained in the proximal socket or a thigh lacer. For the patient with PFFD, an intimate fit of the thigh section and a high lateral wall will control rotatory issues proximally and distally in the prosthesis.

The lateral malleolus is then marked on the diagnostic socket. Initial joint placement is at the apex of the lateral malleolus (anatomic medial malleolus) and slightly distal to the ankle with 5° of external rotation.[3] A squaring jig is used to attach the medial joint to the foot section. The relationship of the foot socket to the thigh section is determined by using the vertical reference lines marked on the lateral side. The thigh section is attached perpendicular to the floor. The anatomic foot may not be perpendicular to the floor because of a lack of range of motion in plantar flexion.

With the patient bearing weight in the diagnostic socket, there should be sufficient clearance distally for the toes.[43] If adequate space distally is not available, ingrown toenails may develop. Appropriate suspension in the foot socket comes from the posterior dorsal strap, the heel shelf, and the sulcus depression.[44] Aitken types C and D deficiencies may require a hip joint and a pelvic band to prevent the thigh from sliding out of the proximal socket.[20] Trim lines are established with the patient both sitting and standing. A second check socket may be necessary to correct the fit of the socket.

The floor-to-socket height of the prosthesis is determined. The ankle will not be at the same height as the contralateral knee in the child who is skeletally immature.[42] The patient with Aitken type C or D PFFD may require the prosthetic side to be higher to compensate for the pelvis dropping at midstance during the gait cycle because of a dysplastic acetabulum or absence of the acetabulum and the bulk of the thigh tissue. A dynamic alignment jig is attached to the socket using transfemoral bench alignment.

Dynamic Alignment

Extensive physical therapy is critical for an acceptable prosthetic outcome for the patient with a newly acquired rotationplasty. The best outcome is achieved by dynamically aligning the prosthesis in a diagnostic socket. To accommodate socket and alignment changes as the patient progresses, physical therapy should occur with the patient using an unfinished, temporary prosthesis. The temporary prosthesis may be used for an undetermined amount of time, depending on the patient's status. A patient with a lower limb tumor who is simultaneously undergoing cancer treatment, physical therapy, and prosthetic fitting will need more time before being fit with a definitive prosthesis.

Dynamic alignment is similar to the thigh lacer and joint procedure.[1] Relative motion will exist in the socket because of the many axes of the ankle joint and the relationship of the single axis of the mechanical joint, but the relative motion should be minimal. Improper proximal or distal joint placement may cause pistoning in the socket. Joint placement for a patient with PFFD may not be in the line of progression because of derotation or subtalar/ankle motion.

During the gait cycle, a loading response may be absent after initial contact because of a decrease in knee extension in the swing phase.[7] Sliding the foot forward will aid knee extension at the loading response. Medial and lateral deviations can be corrected with foot placement beneath the socket or repositioning the joint placement in the transverse plane. During the prosthetic swing phase, vaulting on the sound side may be caused by insufficient knee flexion resulting from a lack of range of motion in the new anatomic knee. The cause of insufficient knee flexion may be a posterior strap that is too proximal, a long prosthesis, or a lack of proper suspension. At initial contact, the knee joints should be fully extended, and the patient will be able to feel the stop of the joints.

Weak adductors produce a Trendelenburg gait in the patient with PFFD. It may be reduced but not eliminated with an intimate fitting socket and a high lateral wall. Therapy will minimize or eliminate

Trendelenburg gait in the patient with a lower limb tumor.

Components

The selection of pediatric-specific components is limited. The available space beneath the prosthesis for components will not only limit the prosthetist's selection but also affect durability and cosmesis for the prosthesis. As the child grows, a wider range of components becomes available. Distal component selection follows the traditional transtibial protocol. The child and their parents can choose between an endoskeletal prosthesis and an exoskeletal prosthesis.

The ankle has more planes of motion than the knee; therefore, the rotationplasty prosthesis needs mechanical joints to control medial and lateral motion of the foot and ankle.[44] It is critical that knee joints have extension stops and can withstand the activity level of the child. Stainless steel prosthetic joints are durable and preferred for the active child. Polycentric joints will replicate anatomic knee joint mechanics as the knee flexes and extends. Unfortunately, these joints are bulkier and not available in pediatric sizes. Adjustable extension stop joints may be needed if the child does not have full range of motion at the knee.

Finished Prosthesis

The definitive prosthesis should have a soft lining in the laminated foot section, which not only provides comfort but also aids in suspension. The distal and proximal sections are connected with medial and lateral knee joints. The proximal section of the prosthesis will differ in the patient with PFFD, in that it will have a laminated shell that extends to the ischial level to contain the proximal tissue and have a high lateral trim line. It will resemble a ship's funnel.

The patient with a lower limb tumor may need only a leather corset, but it should contain and be above the surgical site. If the contours of the thigh are unusual, the leather will have to be molded to the plaster model. A soft thermoplastic thigh section also is an option.

Special Considerations

Rotationplasty prostheses for the pediatric population have unique requirements and challenges. The patient must be frequently evaluated by the prosthetist for prosthetic changes, which will include growth adjustments, socket changes, and maintenance. The prosthetist must inform the multidisciplinary team of any pertinent changes. Loss of range of motion, strength, or derotation[31] will require reevaluation by other specialists on the team.

The ankle of the child who is skeletally immature will not be even with the contralateral side. For an integral part of a rotationplasty procedure, the surgeon will plan the length of the thigh so that the ankle is at the level of the contralateral knee when the patient is skeletally mature.[42]

Cosmesis can be compromised because of limited clearance between the floor and the socket, resulting in a bulky appearance to the lower section of the prosthesis. Limited plantar flexion range of motion places the foot under the anatomic heel, with the anatomic toes facing posteriorly instead of downward. Donning pants may be difficult, and they may have a bulky appearance in the sagittal plane.

SUMMARY

Rotationplasty in all its variations allows for biologic reconstruction of the proximal joint (usually a knee) by a more distal joint (usually an ankle) in a variety of pathoetiologic situations. Fitting a prosthesis for a child who has undergone rotationplasty is challenging and requires considerable time. The availability of pediatric components and space confinements can limit prosthetic component selection. The patient's changing health and rehabilitation status may prolong the time before the fitting of a definitive prosthesis. A multidisciplinary team is required for positive surgical and prosthetic outcomes. With careful selection of patients, attention to surgical details, and a dedicated rehabilitation and prosthetic team, excellent functional results with minimal long-term complications can be expected.

References

1. Borggreve J: Kniegelenksersatz durch das in der Beinlangaschse 180-Grad-gedrehte Fussgelenk. *Arch Orthop Unfall-Chir* 1930;28:175.
2. Van Nes CP: Rotationplasty for congenital defects of the femur: Making use of the ankle of the shortened limb to control the knee joint of a prosthesis. *J Bone Joint Surg* 1950;32:12.
3. Hall JE, Bochmann D: The surgical and prosthetic management of proximal femoral focal deficiency, in *A Symposium Proximal Femoral Focal Deficiency: A Congenital Anomaly*. National Academy of Sciences, 1969, pp 77-81.
4. Hall JE: Rotation of congenitally hypoplastic lower limbs to use the ankle joint as a knee. *Inter Clin Inform Bull* 1966;6(2):3.
5. Kostuik JP, Gillespie R, Hall JE, Hubbard S: Van Nes rotational osteotomy for treatment of proximal femoral focal deficiency and congenital short femur. *J Bone Joint Surg Am* 1975;57(8):1039-1046.
6. Salzer M, Knahr K, Kotz R, Kristen H: Treatment of osteosarcomata of the distal femur by rotation-plasty. *Arch Orthop Trauma Surg* 1981;99(2):131-136.
7. Ackman J, Altiok H, Flanagan A, et al: Long-term follow-up of Van Nes rotationplasty in patients with congenital proximal focal femoral deficiency. *Bone Joint J* 2013;95-B(2):192-198.
8. Hanlon M, Krajbich JI: Rotationplasty in skeletally immature patients: Long-term followup results. *Clin Orthop Relat Res* 1999;358:75-82.
9. Knahr K, Kotz R, Kristen H, et al: Clinical evaluation of patients with rotationplasty, in Enneking WE, ed: *Limb Salvage in Musculoskeletal Oncology*. Churchill Livingstone, 1987, pp 429-434.
10. Varni JW, Setoguchi Y: Correlates of perceived physical appearance in children with congenital/acquired limb deficiencies. *J Dev Behav Pediatr* 1991;12(3):171-176.
11. Alman BA, Krajbich JI, Hubbard S: Proximal femoral focal deficiency: Results of rotationplasty and Syme amputation. *J Bone Joint Surg Am* 1995;77(12):1876-1882.
12. Fatone S: Gait biomechanics and prosthetic management for children with PFFD. *ACPOC News* 2003;9(1):5-13.
13. Knahr K, Kristen H, Ritschl P, Sekera J, Salzer M: Prosthetic management and functional evaluation of patients with

13. resection of the distal femur and rotationplasty. *Orthopedics* 1987;10(9):1241-1248.
14. McClenaghan BA, Krajbich JI, Pirone AM, Koheil R, Longmuir P: Comparative assessment of gait after limb-salvage procedures. *J Bone Joint Surg Am* 1989;71(8):1178-1182.
15. Murray MP, Jacobs PA, Gore DR, Gardner GM, Mollinger LA: Functional performance after tibial rotationplasty. *J Bone Joint Surg Am* 1985;67(3):392-399.
16. Aitken GT: Proximal femoral deficiency, in Swinyard CA, ed: *Limb Development and Deformity: Problems of Evaluation and Rehabilitation*. C. C. Thomas, 1969.
17. Amstutz HC: The morphology, natural history, and treatment of proximal femoral focal deficiency, in *A Symposium on Proximal Femoral Focal Deficiency: A Congenital Anomaly*. National Academy of Sciences, 1969, pp 50-76.
18. Crandal RC: Proximal femoral focal deficiency. *ACPOC News* 2007;13(1):5-25.
19. Fixsen JA, Lloyd-Roberts GC: The natural history and early treatment of proximal femoral dysplasia. *J Bone Joint Surg Br* 1974;56(1):86-95.
20. Krajbich JI: Proximal femoral focal deficiency, in Kalamchi A, ed: *Congenital Lower Limb Deficiencies*. Springer-Verlag, 1989, pp 108-127.
21. Gillespie R, Torode IP: Classification and management of congenital abnormalities of the femur. *J Bone Joint Surg Br* 1983;65(5):557-568.
22. Aitken GT: Proximal femoral deficiency: Definition, classification and management, in *A Symposium on Proximal Femoral Focal Deficiency: A Congenital Anomaly*. National Academy of Sciences, 1969.
23. Krajbich JI: Lower-limb deficiencies and amputations in children. *J Am Acad Orthop Surg* 1998;6(6):358-367.
24. Kritter AE: Tibial rotation-plasty for proximal femoral focal deficiency. *J Bone Joint Surg Am* 1977;59(7):927-934.
25. King RE, Marks TW: Follow-up findings on the skeletal lever in the surgical management of proximal femoral focal deficiency. *Inter Clin Inform Bull* 1971;11(3):1.
26. King RE: Providing a single skeletal lever in proximal femoral focal deficiency: A preliminary case report. *Inter Clin Inform Bull* 1966;6(2):23.
27. King RE: Some concepts of proximal femoral focal deficiency, in *A Symposium Proximal Femoral Focal Deficiency: A Congenital Anomaly*. National Academy of Sciences, 1969.
28. Gillespie R: Principles of amputation surgery in children with longitudinal deficiencies of the femur. *Clin Orthop Relat Res* 1990;256:29-38.
29. Torode IP, Gillespie R: Rotationplasty of the lower limb for congenital defects of the femur. *J Bone Joint Surg Br* 1983;65(5):569-573.
30. Friscia DA, Moseley CF, Oppenheim WL: Rotational osteotomy for proximal femoral focal deficiency. *J Bone Joint Surg Am* 1989;71(9):1386-1392.
31. Brown KL: Resection, rotationplasty, and femoropelvic arthrodesis in severe congenital femoral deficiency: A report of the surgical technique and three cases. *J Bone Joint Surg Am* 2001;83(1):78-85.
32. Winkelmann WW: Type-B-IIIa hip rotationplasty: An alternative operation for the treatment of malignant tumors of the femur in early childhood. *J Bone Joint Surg Am* 2000;82(6):814-828.
33. Steel HH, Lin PS, Betz RR, Kalamchi A, Clancy M: Iliofemoral fusion for proximal femoral focal deficiency. *J Bone Joint Surg Am* 1987;69(6):837-843.
34. Kotz R, Salzer M: Rotation-plasty for childhood osteosarcoma of the distal part of the femur. *J Bone Joint Surg Am* 1982;64(7):959-969.
35. Jacobs PA: Limb salvage and rotationplasty for osteosarcoma in children. *Clin Orthop Relat Res* 1984;188:217-222.
36. Krajbich JI: The method of predicting the level of the knee in the modified Van Nes rotationplasty, in *Program Book: Pediatric Orthopaedic Society of North America Annual Meeting, Toronto, Canada*. Pediatric Orthopaedic Society of North America, 1987.
37. Krajbich J, Bochmann D: Van Nes rotationplasty in tumor surgery, in Bowker JH, Michael JW, eds: *Atlas of Limb Prosthetics: Surgical, Prosthetic, and Rehabilitation Principles*, ed 2. Mosby-Year Book, 1992, pp 885-899.
38. de Bari A, Krajbich JI, Langer F, Hamilton EL, Hubbard S: Modified Van Nes rotationplasty for osteosarcoma of the proximal tibia in children. *J Bone Joint Surg Br* 1990;72(6):1065-1069.
39. Hillmann A, Hoffmann C, Gosheger G, Krakau H, Winkelmann W: Malignant tumor of the distal part of the femur or the proximal part of the tibia: Endoprosthetic replacement or rotationplasty Functional outcome and quality-of-life measurements. *J Bone Joint Surg Am* 1999;81(4):462-468.
40. Hillmann A, Rosenbaum D, Gosheger G, Hoffmann C, Rödl R, Winkelmann W: Rotationplasty type B IIIa according to Winkelmann: Electromyography and gait analysis. *Clin Orthop Relat Res* 2001;384:224-231.
41. Shih C, Carroll NC: Modified Van Nes rotationplasty for the treatment of proximal femoral osteosarcoma in children. *J Bone Joint Surg Br* 1985;1:81-86.
42. Alexander I: *The Foot: Examination and Diagnosis*, ed 2. Churchill Livingstone, 1990, pp 29-40.
43. Banziger E: Rotation plasty prostheses: A prosthetist's perspective. *ACPOC News* 2001;7(1):1-16.
44. Sinclair W, Maale G: Springfield D: Distal femur rotation-plasty prosthesis. *Orthot Prosthet* 1985;39(2):48-51.

Congenital Longitudinal Deficiencies of the Fibula

CHAPTER 78

Michael Schmitz, MD, FAAOS • Rebecca Hernandez, CPO, LPO

ABSTRACT

Congenital longitudinal deficiency of the fibula is an abnormality affecting the lateral aspect of the lower extremity (postaxial deficiency) in a wide spectrum of severity and involvement. The degree of involvement of various parts of the extremity will dictate the treatment decisions and ultimate function. Successful limb salvage requires a stable, plantigrade painless foot, a stable ankle, and equalized limb lengths at skeletal maturity. Foot and ankle function are predictive of limb salvage success. Foot ablation and prosthetic treatment offers excellent functional outcomes in patients not amenable to limb salvage.

Keywords: fibular hemimelia; longitudinal deficiency of the fibula; SHordt; SUPERankle

Introduction

Congenital longitudinal deficiency of the fibula or fibular hemimelia, as the condition is frequently called, is also described as postaxial deficiency of the lower limb. The latter term most accurately describes the actual condition because the entire lateral (postaxial) aspect of the limb is affected to various degrees (**Figures 1** and **2**). It is a spectrum of disease where, at a minimum, the limb manifests a mild degree of fibular dysplasia, a ball-and-socket ankle joint, a lax (dysplastic) anterior cruciate ligament, and a mildly hypoplastic lateral femoral condyle. At the other end of the spectrum, fibular deficiency can include femoral shortening, knee valgus from a significantly dysplastic lateral femoral condyle, complete absence of the cruciate ligaments, complete absence of the fibula, a shortened bowed tibia, stiff equinovalgus deformity of the ankle, and a dysplastic foot with hindfoot coalitions and absent lateral rays. It is important to focus on the various presentations of congenital fibular deficiencies; classification systems; factors that influence the choice and types of treatment; and prosthetic consideration for patients treated with foot ablation.

Incidence

Fibular deficiency is the most common hemimelia[1] with an incidence of 5.7 to 20 cases per million births[2] as well as the most common congenital long bone deficiency occurring in 1 to 2/100,000 births.[3] The deficiency is twice as common in males as in females, and can be unilateral (usually right) or bilateral.[4]

Etiology

Various mechanisms including absence of the anterior tibial artery,[5] defects in muscle development,[1] disruption of the apical ectodermal ridge expression,[6] and developmental field defects[7] have been proposed as etiologic factors. However, at present, the etiology remains unknown. Most cases are sporadic, while some are associated with a syndrome and other abnormalities.[3] Teratologic insults including radiation, busulfan, and retinoic acid have been identified.

Associated Abnormalities

The spectrum of fibular deficiency includes varying degrees of deformities of the limb including the pelvis, femur, knee, tibia, ankle, and the foot.[8] It is important for the clinician to identify associated abnormalities as they will often significantly impact treatment decisions.[9-12] The most common abnormalities in the femur are proximal femoral focal deficiency, congenital short femur, and coxa vara.[10,11] Distal femoral valgus can lead to genu valgum which

---

Dr. Schmitz or an immediate family member serves as a paid consultant to or is an employee of Orthofix, Inc., Orthopediatrics, and Stryker and serves as a board member, owner, officer, or committee member of Pediatric Orthopaedic Society of North America and Scoliosis Research Society. Neither Rebecca Hernandez nor any immediate family member has received anything of value from or has stock or stock options held in a commercial company or institution related directly or indirectly to the subject of this chapter.

This chapter is adapted from Giavedoni BJ: Congenital longitudinal deficiencies of the fibula, in Krajbich JI, Pinzur MS, Potter BK, Stevens PM, eds: *Atlas of Amputations and Limb Deficiencies: Surgical, Prosthetic, and Rehabilitation Principles*, ed 4. American Academy of Orthopaedic Surgeons, 2016, pp 865-872.

Section 5: Pediatrics

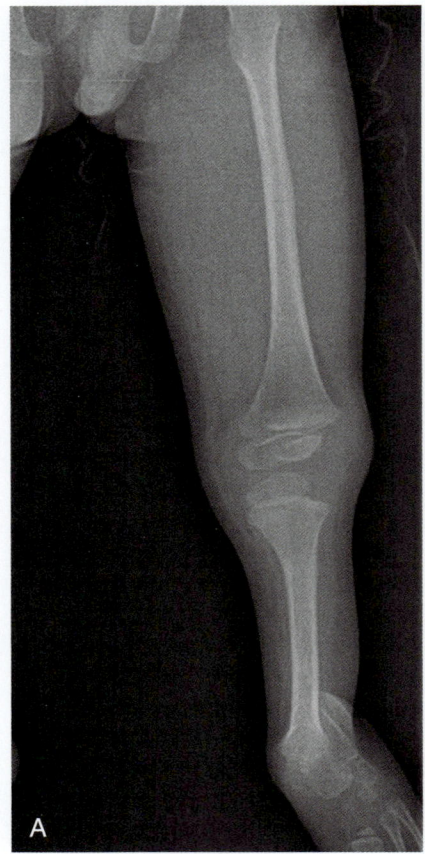 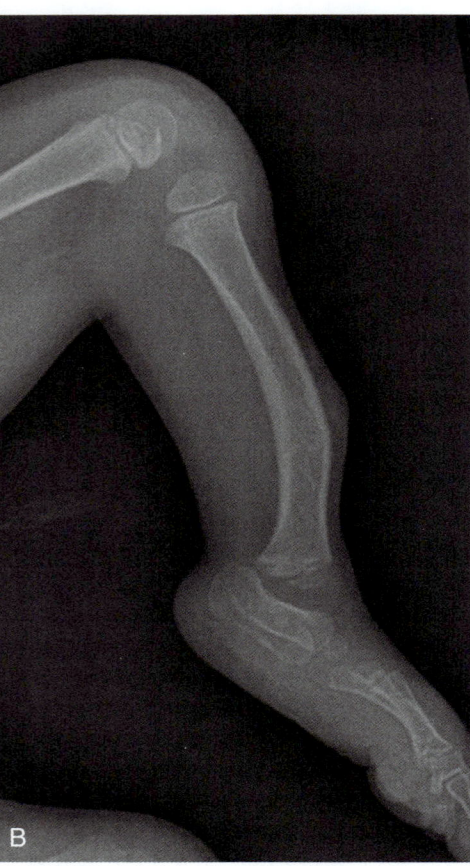

FIGURE 1 AP (**A**) and lateral (**B**) projections of longitudinal deficiency of the fibula. Note the length deficiency, ankle abnormality, foot deficiency, and anterior tibial bow. Note complete tarsal coalition on the lateral view. Radiographic and clinical appearance of fibular deficiency demonstrating anterior dimple foot deficiency, length deficiency, ankle abnormality, and tibial bow.

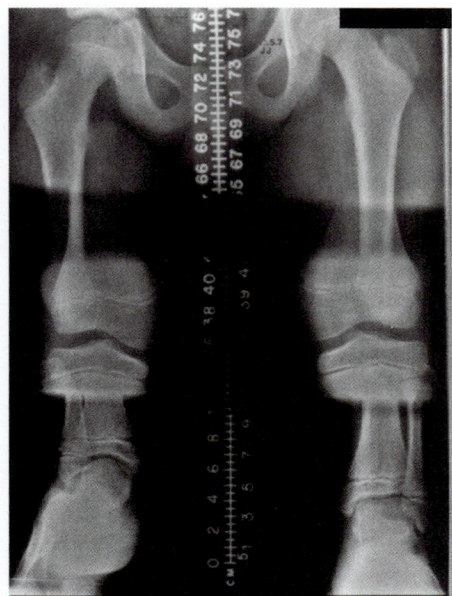

FIGURE 2 A scanogram demonstrates mild limb length discrepancy and ball and socket ankle typical of mild fibular deficiency.

can be associated with patellar instability.[11] The cruciates are often absent, with clinical laxity but rarely functional instability.[11] Foot abnormalities include ball and socket ankle,[13] tarsal coalitions,[14] and absent lateral rays. The tibia can be dysplastic or bowed, possible secondary to a residual fibrotic remnant of the fibula restricting normal growth.[1]

In addition, the upper extremity may be involved and range from syndactyly to a hypoplastic or aplastic ulna.[9,15,16] While upper extremity abnormalities do not affect ambulation they can limit donning and doffing capability. In cases of bilateral upper extremity abnormalities, the feet may be required for prehension.

Classification

A classification system should aid the clinician in choosing the most effective interventions for a given problem, provide information useful for counseling the patient and parents regarding diagnosis, and serve as a basis for future studies of the patient cohort. Ideally, the classification system should further define the deficiency with variables that are known to affect the outcome and that help to identify effective interventions. The identification of these determinant variables must be reproducible to allow researchers to appropriately define populations for study.

The variables that have the greatest effect on outcome in fibular deficiency are limb length discrepancy, ankle function, foot function, and the presence and extent of upper extremity abnormalities.

Coventry et al[17] published a classification system based on radiographic appearance of the fibula and the presence of associated abnormalities. The system did not address function. Type I involves a unilateral deficiency with a hypoplastic fibula, no foot involvement, and a substantial limb-length discrepancy. Type II is a unilateral abnormality, with nearly complete or complete absence of the fibula. Type III is a bilateral abnormality with complete absence of the fibula and a proximal femoral focal deficiency or upper limb involvement or involvement of the contralateral foot or tibia.[17]

Achterman and Kalamchi[18] presented a simplified classification system based only on the radiographic appearance of the fibula. It is most applicable for retrospective evaluation when only radiographs are available for review. In type IA abnormalities, the entire fibula is present but dysplastic, and in type 1B there is a partial absence of the proximal fibula and the distal fibula does not support the ankle. A type II abnormality is characterized by complete absence of the fibula. The authors recommended limb length equalization for near normal fibulas (type IA) and early amputation for absence or deficiency associated with an unstable ankle (IB and II).

Birch et al[19] reported on a retrospective review of 104 patients with fibular deficiencies treated at one institution between 1971 and 2005. They noted that both the Achterman and Kalamchi and Coventry and Johnson classification scheme's treatment-predictive value was poor. In addition, they found that femoral shortening was of a magnitude that it impacted the overall treatment plan in greater than 80% of the patients. They proposed a simplified classification system based on the clinical status of the foot and the overall limb length discrepancy expressed as a percentage. This allowed the classification system to be applied at birth and was found to more accurately predict management at their institution.

Type I

Foot with three or more rays capable of providing a stable weight-bearing base with or without reconstructive procedures.

IA—Limb length inequality 0% to <6%
IB—Limb length inequality 6% to 10%
IC—Limb length inequality 11% to 30%
ID—Limb length inequality >30%

Type II

Foot unsalvageable.

IIA—Intact upper extremities
IIB—Bilateral lower extremity involvement and upper extremity dysfunction that may require foot substitution for function

Paley developed a classification scheme describing the foot, ankle, and tibial deformities associated with fibular hemimelia. Each type is prescriptive for specific reconstructive procedures and limb lengthening (**Figure 3**).

All Paley types have fibular shortening with Type I characterized by a stable ankle and foot. Type II is a stable ankle with dynamic valgus but stable foot. Type III is characterized by a fixed equinovalgus ankle with Type IIIa characterized by ankle valgus, Type IIIb by subtalar valgus, and Type IIIc by both ankle and subtalar valgus. Type IV describes a fibular deficiency associated with a fixed equinovarus ankle.

Each type is associated with a procedure or combination of procedures designed to combine foot and ankle realignment into a plantigrade position and lengthen the limb.

Type 1—Lengthening
Type 2—Shortening osteotomy realignment distal tibia and soft-tissue release to align foot and ankle and relatively lengthen the fibula followed by tibial lengthening
Types 3 and 4—Shortening osteotomy realignment distal tibia and soft-tissue release with subtalar osteotomy as needed followed by lengthening.

Clinical Findings

The deficiency is usually apparent at birth, manifested as variable shortening of the fibula and an equinovalgus foot with a stiff hindfoot. There may be associated shortening and distal valgus of the femur and the tibia with apex anterior angulation and an anterior skin dimple over the apex. Frequently, lateral rays of the foot are missing and there is syndactylization of the toes (**Figure 4**). Knee cruciate deficiency and lateral femoral condyle hypoplasia can produce clinical knee laxity and genu valgum. The patient should be fully examined to assess upper extremity abnormalities as well as contralateral deficiencies. Radiographs of bilateral lower extremities with a ruler are obtained to assess total limb length inequality as a percentage and assess angular deformities.

Treatment

Treatment of the fibular deficiency is directed toward functional optimization of the affected limb to allow the child's development to parallel that of an unaffected child as closely as possible. An accurate assessment of the extent of determinate variables of total limb length discrepancy, ankle function, foot function, bilaterality, and upper extremity function will allow the clinician to develop a treatment plan that minimizes complications and maximizes functional outcomes. Treatment options include no treatment or only a shoe lift or foot orthosis in very mild cases, contralateral shortening with epiphysiodesis to equalize limb lengths, surgical restoration of the affected limb via stabilization and alignment of the foot and ankle combined with limb equalization techniques, and restoring use of the limb with the aid of a prosthesis, usually after foot ablation. It is important to present a realistic assessment of complications and consequences of lengthening included native or lengthening-induced hip and knee instability when deciding to pursue a course of limb reconstruction or ablation.

The options, indications, risks, and benefits should be discussed early with the parents as some decisions are best made before the child is able to participate in the decision-making process.[20]

Factors in Decision-Making

Historically, treatment decisions were based upon the radiographic appearance of the fibula and the presence of associated abnormalities.[17,18,21] Relative preservation of the fibula was seen as an indication for lengthening and reconstruction, with fibular absence an indication for foot ablation and prosthetic fitting. Bilateral involvement often did not require length equalization but may require treatment to create a functional foot (**Figure 5**). Foot substitution for absent hand prehension was seen as a relative contraindication for foot ablation.

In a 2011 review of experience, Birch et al demonstrated that radiographic appearance of the fibula is was not predictive for the patients treated at his institution. A preservable foot, defined as a painless, plantigrade foot able to support weight bearing with or without reconstructive procedures, and total limb length discrepancy were much more appropriate factors to consider in the choice of amputation or limb salvage treatment for children in congenital fibular deficiency.[19] Subsequent retrospective reports have shown that foot and ankle deformity are the most predictive factors of overall success in limb reconstruction procedures.

Section 5: Pediatrics

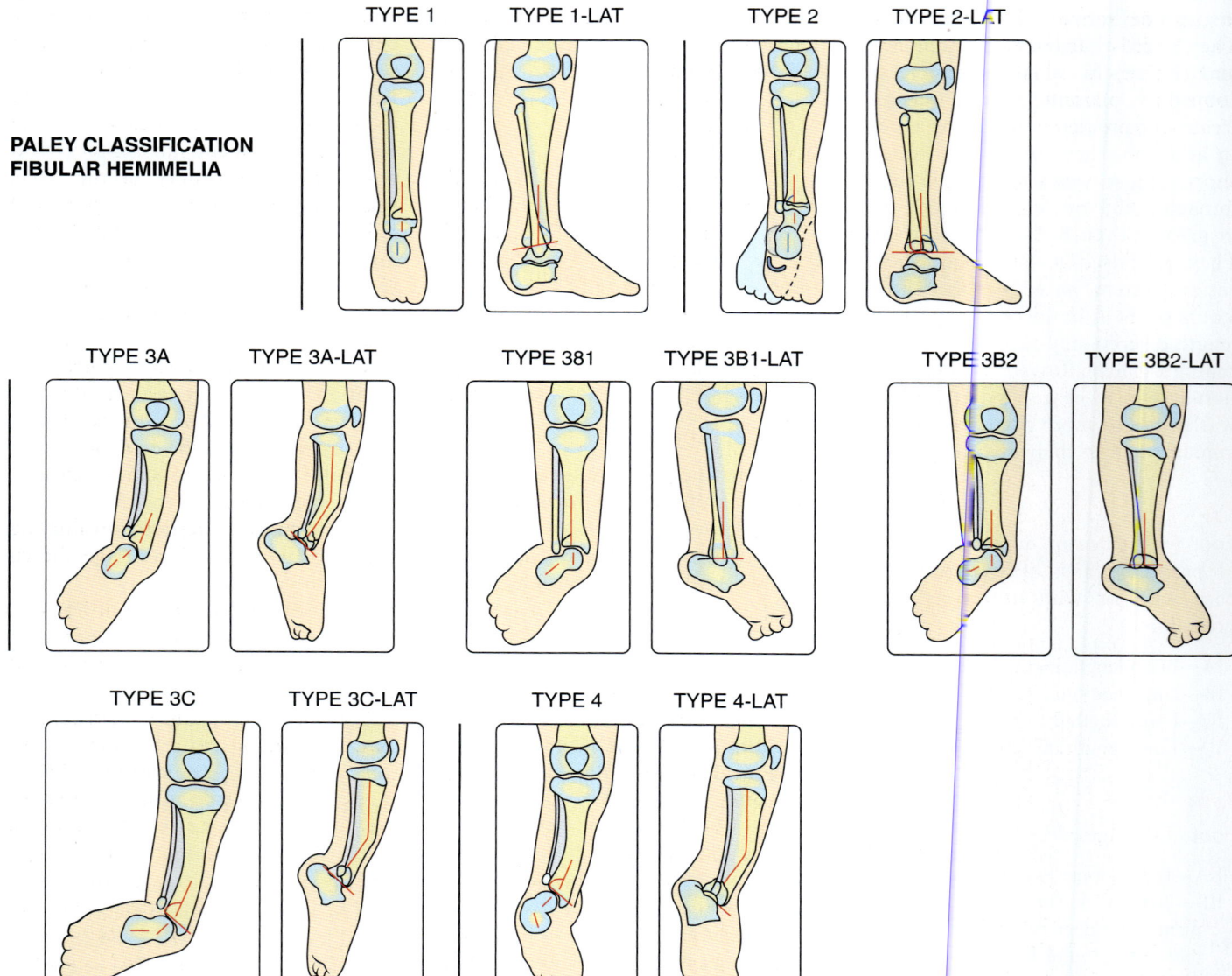

FIGURE 3 Schematic illustration shows the Paley classification based upon deficiencies/deformities requiring reconstruction to create stable plantigrade foot and equal limb lengths. (Reproduced with permission by the Paley Foundation.)

Advancements in limb lengthening and reconstruction offered viable limb salvage opportunities for congenital fibular deficiencies.[20-25] A plantigrade, painless foot that can function as a support, a limb length that can be equalized, and a stable hip and knee are requirements for consideration for limb salvage. If limb reconstruction is not possible, foot ablation and subsequent prosthetic fitting allow one operation and one hospital stay to correct the foot, ankle, and length deformity via prosthetic substitution for the deficiency. Comparisons of reconstruction and amputation patients achieve nearly equivalent functional results but lengthening patients require more surgery, more hospitalization, greater surgical and hospital costs, and have more complications.[23,26] Randomized group comparisons have not been reported and matched group comparisons are confounded by heterogeneity in both deficiency and surgical reconstruction procedures. A matched group comparisons between amputation and staged reconstruction for patients with severe fibular deficiency demonstrated no significant differences in self-reported quality of life, treatment satisfaction, and function. However, at the time of the evaluation, all of the reconstruction patients had future planned surgical procedures.

Limb salvage requires procedures to create a plantigrade, painless foot, equalized limb lengths at skeletal maturity, and correction of angular deformities. This may include an Achilles lengthening, peroneal lengthening, a tibial osteotomy to neutralize plafond malalignment, a hindfoot osteotomy to neutralize the hindfoot, and metatarsal osteotomies to allow for shoe wear. Lengthening can be accomplished through the tibia, femur, or both, and can be performed concurrently with angular correction of both the tibia and femur.

The Birch classification is specific in lengthening recommendations.[19] Limb length discrepancy less than 6% can be treated with a lift or epiphysiodesis. Six to 10% should require an epiphysiodesis or single-stage lengthening. Discrepancies of 11% to 30% require at least one lengthening and may require either two or a bifocal lengthening. Patients with more than 30% limb length discrepancy require extensive lengthening and may be best treated with amputation and prosthetic fitting.[10,12,19,20,22]

Paley has developed a comprehensive treatment algorithm based upon his classification scheme describing the ankle and foot abnormalities. His recognition that many reconstruction failures were because of residual or recurrent foot and ankle deformity led him to develop the SHordt and SUPERankle procedures, described elsewhere, that combine foot and tibial osteotomies with extensive soft-tissue releases to neutralize coronal and sagittal plane angular deformities before limb lengthening.

A retrospective review of fibular deficient patients, including those with foot and ankle pathology classified and treated with the Paley algorithm, demonstrated 47% with excellent results. Complications included pin tract infections (25%), recurrent foot deformities (31%), rocker bottom foot (26%), knee subluxation, and fixed flexion deformity of the knee, suggesting that extensive foot and ankle reconstruction combined with limb lengthening is not problem-free. The authors did note a significantly decreased chance of foot deformity recurrence if the initial foot and neo-ankle reconstruction were performed before age 5. Long-term evaluation of fibular hemimelia patients treated with Syme amputation and prosthetic demonstrates function similar to age-matched controls.

Retrospective reports evaluating reconstructive procedures have shown varied outcomes.

Indications and contraindications for reconstruction and amputation remain relative. Longer length and a functional foot suggest reconstruction. An unreconstructable foot regardless of limb length is an indication for amputation.[19,22,26] A meta-analysis evaluating cumulative results of 169 cases in seven studies concluded that patients who underwent amputation had greater satisfaction and fewer procedures and complications than limb reconstruction patients. If the patient has associated upper extremity functional deficits requiring foot substitution for prehensile function early amputation should be avoided.

Foot ablation can be accomplished with either a Syme or Boyd amputation.[12,23,26] Tibial angular deformity can be addressed at the time of amputation with an osteotomy and fixation with a removable pin (**Figure 6**). A Syme amputation can be associated with posterior migration of the heel pad and growth of an inadvertently retained calcaneal apophysis that requires subsequent resection.[12] Because the Syme procedure is a true disarticulation, the whole calcaneus, including the apophysis, must be removed and the Achilles sectioned to avoid heel pad migration. Matched comparisons of patients with Syme or Boyd amputations show

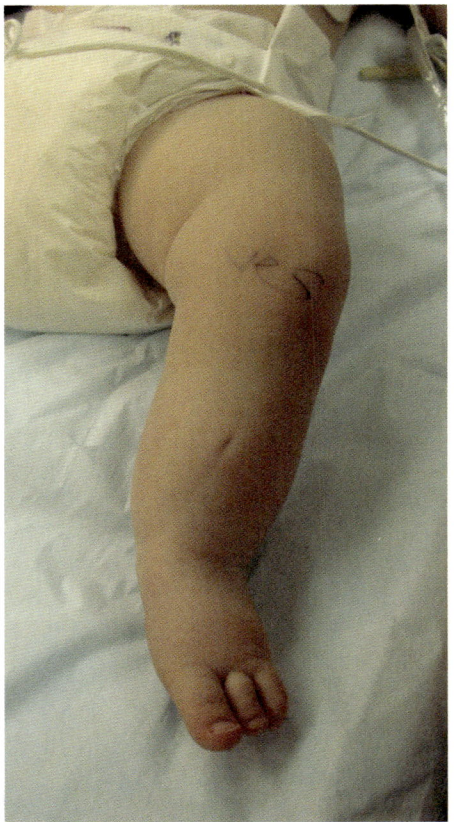

FIGURE 4 In this clinical photograph, note dimpling of skin over the apex of the anterior tibial bow, equinovalgus foot, and absent lateral rays.

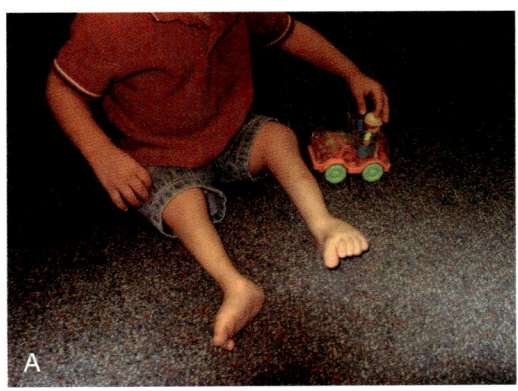
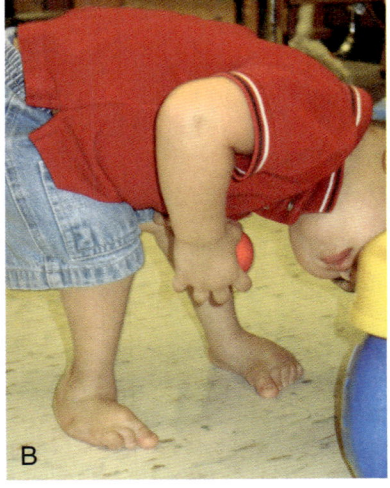

FIGURE 5 Photographs (**A** and **B**) showing bilateral fibular deficiencies with functional, braceable plantigrade feet after Achilles lengthenings.

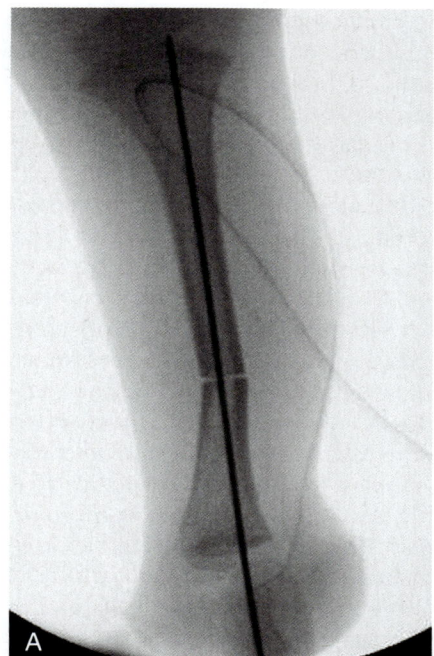
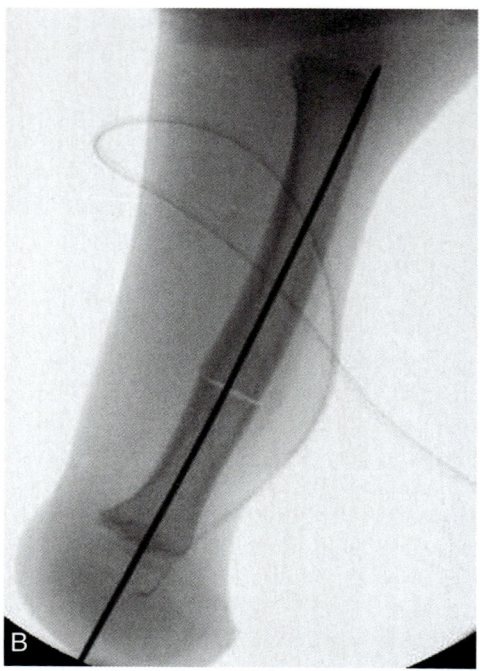

FIGURE 6 AP (**A**) and lateral (**B**) projections of complete fibular deficiency treated with Syme amputation and tibial osteotomy secured with a percutaneous Kirschner wire that will be removed in the office once the osteotomy has healed.

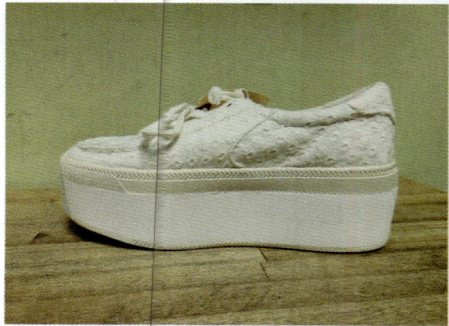

FIGURE 7 Photograph showing a shoe lift that may be used before or during the lengthening process, typically used with an ankle foot orthosis to provide ankle stability.

fewer complications with the Boyd procedure.[12] The Boyd procedure is more successful in aligning the heel pad in a plantigrade position but can be technically more difficult to perform, especially if there is significant equinus. Subsequent angular deformities of the tibia or femur at the knee should be anticipated and may require later treatment with hemiepiphyseal stapling or osteotomy.[11,12,19]

Orthotic Considerations

If a child with fibular deficiency will be undergoing limb reconstruction and lengthening, they may need orthotic devices before, during, or immediately after their surgical treatment. This typically consists of shoe lifts and/or ankle foot orthoses (AFOs) before or between lengthenings. A shoe lift is used to approximately equalize leg lengths, with the affected side slightly shorter to allow for clearance of the limb during swing phase (**Figure 7**). The AFOs are used for positioning and correction of deformity as well as normalizing biomechanical forces across the plantar surface of the foot and at the ankle, and to protect and stabilize the leg while healing after reconstruction. If a shoe lift is less than 2 inches and the foot is in a plantigrade position, an AFO may not be necessary. Generally, a lift greater than 2 inches will require support and stability at the ankle provided by an AFO.

Prosthetic Considerations

If the child is not a lengthening candidate, or the family opts for an ablation of the foot, a prosthesis is used to restore function. The common adage of "children are not small adults" needs to be reinforced whenever the design of a prosthesis is considered. Function and ability to undergo change to accommodate growth are the two most important outcomes the prosthetist is tasked to provide when dealing with the pediatric amputee and overall prosthesis design.

There are several socket designs that can be used for a child with a Syme level or Boyd amputation, depending on the bony anatomy. Shaving or remodeling of the malleoli is strongly discouraged so that socket design can take advantage of the difference between the widest aspect of the malleoli and the area just proximal to it for self-suspension. The circumferential difference between these two landmarks dictates the design of the socket. The lesser the difference of these two dimensions, the more likely that the prosthesis will require secondary suspension. The greater the difference between these two areas the more likely that the design moves in the direction of an anatomically self-suspending socket with the extreme being an obturator, opening, or door that will allow passage of the residual limb.

A removable or segmented liner socket incorporates a full foam liner that has been built up to the same circumference as the distal bulbous heel and a laminated shell is then formed over this insert (**Figure 8, A**). The patient dons the liner first then slips this into the laminated outer socket. An atrophied residual limb with a small heel pad is best suited for this design and the degree of cosmetic restoration will be very good. The silicone or bladder prosthesis uses an inner elastic area that stretches to permit passage of the bulbous end. This design is favored for those with upper extremity involvement as it eliminates the use of liners and sleeves (**Figure 8, B**).

The obturator or medial opening design is used infrequently in children and only when the distal end of the residuum is large and the medial malleolus is prominent; because of

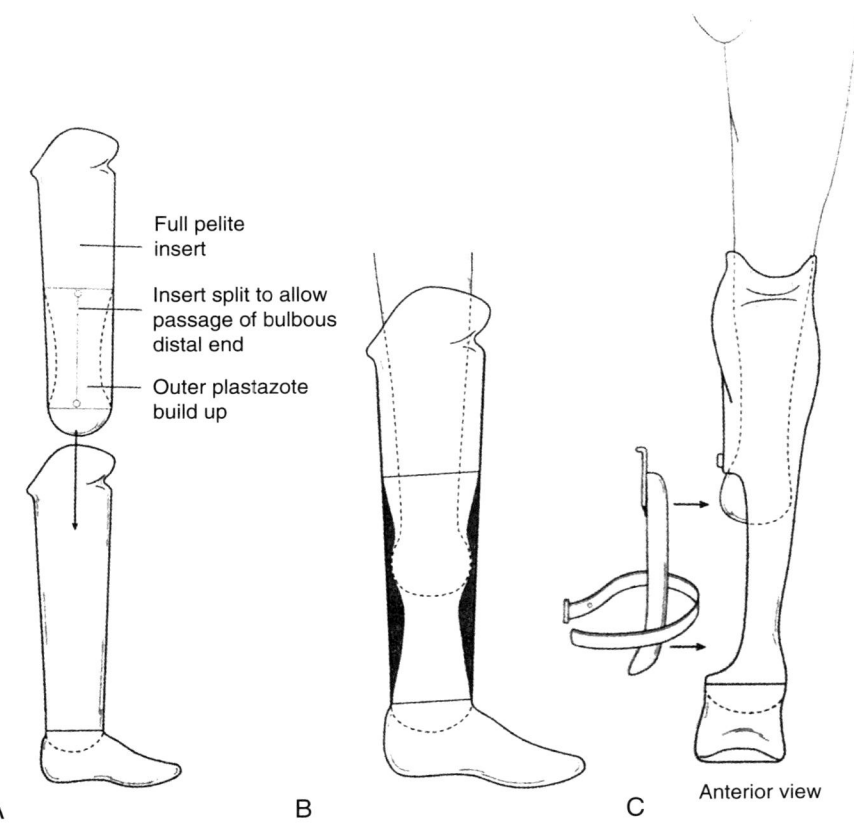

FIGURE 8 Illustrations of different types of Syme-level prostheses. **A**, Prothesis with segmented Pelite liner that allows donning of the liner over the bulbous end, which is then inserted into the outer socket to lock the residual limb into the prosthesis. **B**, Prosthesis with bladder design that allows insertion of the bulbous end into the prosthesis, with the silicone bladder expanding into a hollow air chamber and then constricting back onto the residual limb. **C**, Prosthesis with lateral obturator (door) that is removed to allow passage of the bulbous end and then is locked back into place to secure the limb. (Reprinted from Bowen RE, Otsuka NE, Doty SA: The child with a limb deficiency, in Weinstein S, Flynn JM, Crawford HA, eds: *Lovell and Winter's Pediatric Orthopaedics*, ed 8. Wolters Kluwer, 2021, pp 1466-1536.)

inherent weaknesses in the design, catastrophic failure along the distal aspect of the opening is a common occurrence (**Figure 8, C**). As the child continues to grow longitudinally, the limb generally tends to slim out. It is therefore important to remember that the design of the socket for the pediatric patient changes when followed through their physiological growth.[27] The socket brim takes on a supracondylar appearance to better encapsulate the knee and afford added protection. In most cases, a well-designed prosthesis can remain functional from 12 to 14 months, depending on the child's rate of growth. Component failure caused by normal wear and tear is more common in pediatric prostheses than in comparable adult devices.

Accommodation of the anterior tibial bowing found in the longitudinal deficiency of the fibula is usually accommodative since most children or adults have a relatively low pain threshold to pressure placed on the tibial crest. In many cases, a mild bowing can be accommodated within the prosthesis. In cases where the bowing is more severe, straightening should be considered. This author has been fortunate to work alongside physicians who perform the tibial osteotomy to straighten the bone during the foot ablation procedure at the "pull to stand" stage of development in the child. The challenge of dealing with a severe bowing is the prosthetic foot placement. As the tibia grows, the aspect distal to the apex of the bow continues to grow or migrate posterior, making correct foot placement more complicated.

Pediatric prosthetic foot options present a big challenge for children with a Syme level or Boyd amputation because of limited clearance for components as most basic prosthetic feet require at least 6 cm of clearance. The greater the technology and function, the more space that is required. In the Boyd amputation, the calcaneus remains intact and is fused to the tibia, resulting in an amputation longer than the Syme and it is far more challenging to accommodate a prosthetic foot because of near zero clearance.

In the younger child, a custom-made foot may be required using a carbon or fiberglass footplate, foam for shaping, and a leather covering. Newer options for off-the-shelf feet include a TRS Syme Little foot (**Figure 9**). Recently, posterior mounted carbon composite feet have become available in pediatric sizes, allowing for greater function for those with long residual limbs (**Figure 10**). Previously, many children with long residua have been unable to use the energy-storing properties of carbon feet because of clearance restraints. These posterior carbon pylons can be easily adjusted for growth. If the child has had an epiphysiodesis, other options for distal components are possible because of the great leg length discrepancy between the sound limb and the residual limb (**Figure 10**). Components are chosen carefully to allow a reasonable amount of vertical growth to maintain a level pelvis through routine height adjustments.

The two most common comorbidities with longitudinal fibular deficiency and a foot ablation circle back to the knee, genu valgum and knee laxity, pose a considerable challenge to fitting (**Figure 11**). As is the case with most angular issues, alignment must not deviate from biomechanical principles and optimized functional outcomes. As mentioned above, increasing the height of the medial and lateral socket

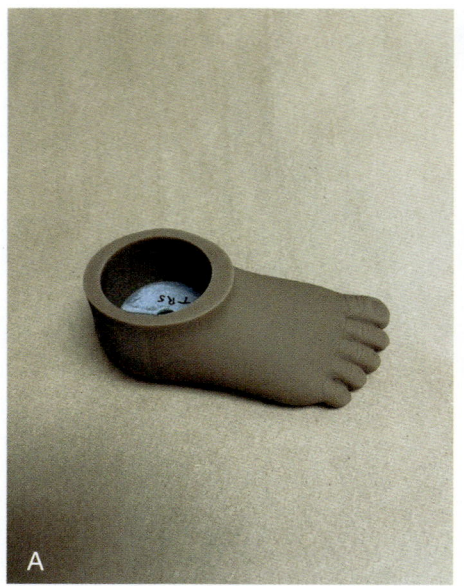
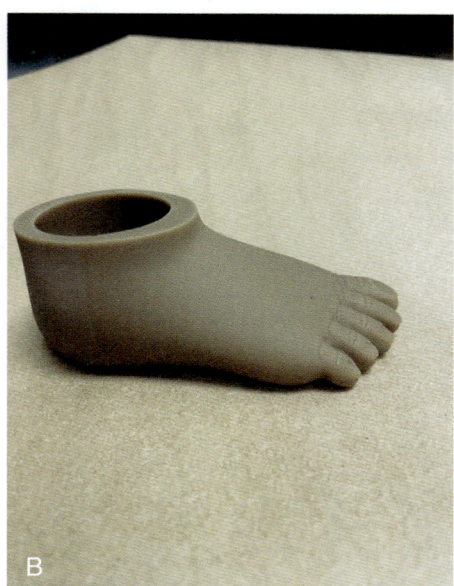

FIGURE 9 Superior (**A**) and lateral (**B**) photographs of a TRS Little Foot (Fillauer) which is an off-the-shelf foot demonstrating minimal clearance requirements for a child with a Syme or Boyd amputation.

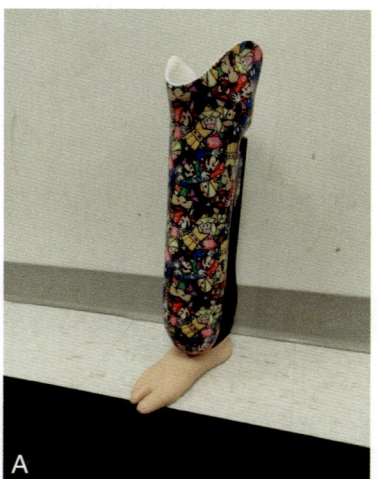
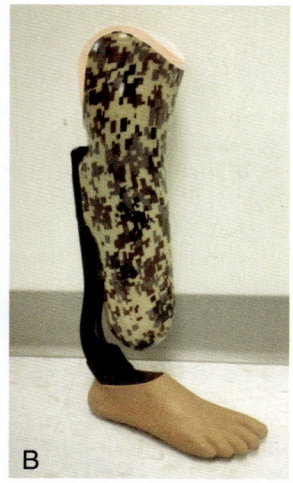
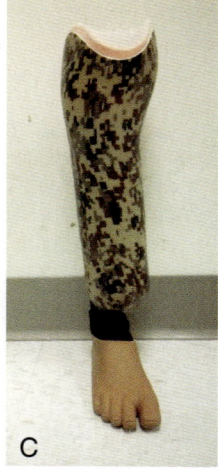

FIGURE 10 Oblique (**A**), lateral (**B**), and anterior (**C**) clinical photographs of a Syme prostheses with posterior mounted feet that allow children with long residual limbs and limited clearance to take advantage of the energy-storing properties of carbon fiber prosthetic feet.

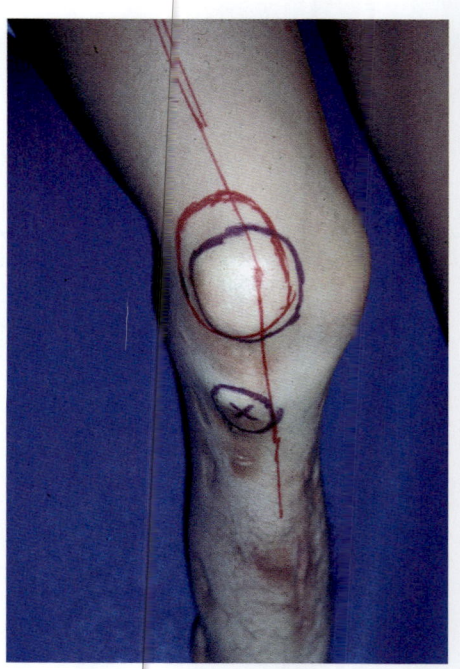

FIGURE 11 Photograph showing clearly marked patella alta with lateral patellar subluxation and severe genu valgus that pose increased challenges to socket design.

walls affords control and protection to the knee. Foot placement (**Figure 9**) is routinely inset so that the ground reaction force falls through the center of the knee and reduces any additional stresses that would be otherwise present.[28]

By understanding the anatomical differences of the congenital longitudinal fibular deficiency contrasted to the traumatic Syme amputation, the prosthetist can better fit and adjust alignment expectations for optimal outcomes. Prosthetic fit should be comfortable while maintaining a balance between intimate fit and reasonable growth potential before the child or teen requires a new prosthesis. Above all, anticipating future needs and maximizing outcomes before skeletal maturity is an ongoing challenge with the pediatric patient.

SUMMARY

Congenital longitudinal fibular deficiency is a postaxial deficiency of the lower limb variably affecting femoral length and lateral condyle, cruciate ligaments, fibular length, ankle and foot anatomy. The deficiency is clinically manifested as limb shortening, variable knee and ankle instability, and deficiencies in foot function. Treatment is directed at correcting anatomic and functional deviations through limb sparing reconstruction or limb ablation combined with prosthetic fitting. Native foot and ankle deformity/function are predictive factors for success in limb reconstruction procedures.

References

1. Fordham LA, Applegate KE, Wilkes DC, Chung CJ: Fibular hemimelia: More than just an absent bone. *Semin Musculoskelet Radiol* 1999;3(3):227-237.
2. Froster U, Baird P: Congenital defects of the lower limbs and associated malformations: A population based study. *Am J Med Genet* 1993;45(1):60-64.

3. Ghanem I: Epidemiology, etiology, and genetic aspects of reduction deficiencies of the lower limb. *J Child Orthop* 2008;2(5):329-332.
4. Reed MH, ed: *Normal and Abnormal Development in Pediatric Skeletal Radiology*. Williams and Wilkins, 1992, pp 349-392.
5. Levinsohn E, Hootnick D, Packard DS Jr: Consistent arterial abnormalities associated with a vareity of congenital malformations of the human lower limb. *Invest Radiol* 1991;26(4):364-373.
6. Baek GH, Kim JK, Chung MS, Lee SK: Terminal hemimelia of the lower extremity: Absent lateral ray and a normal fibula. *Int Orthop* 2008;32(2):263-267.
7. Lewin S, Opitz J, Reynolds J: Fibular A/hypoplasia: Review and documentation of the fibular developmental field. *Am J Med Genet* 1986;25(2):215-238.
8. Pavone L, Viljoen D, Ardito S, et al: Two rare developmental defects of the lower limbs with confirmation of the lewin and opitz hypothesis on the fibular and tibial development field defects. *Am J Med Genet* 1989;33(2):161-164.
9. Birch J, Lincoln T, Mack P: Functional classification of fibular deficiency, in Herring JA, Birch JG, eds: *The Child with Limb Deficiency*. American Acadamy of Orthopaedic Surgeons, 1998, pp 161-170.
10. Miller L, Bell D: Management of congenital fibular deficiency by Ilizarov Technique. *J Pediatr Orthop* 1992;12(5):651-657.
11. Stevens P, Arms D: Postaxial hypoplasia of the lower extremity. *J Pediatr Orthop* 2000;20(2):166-172.
12. Fulp T, Davids JR, Meyer LC, Blackhurst DW: Longitudinal deficiency of the fibula. Operative treatment. *J Bone Joint Surg Am* 1996;78(5):674-682.
13. Takahura Y, Tamia S, Masuhara K: Genesis of the ball-and-socket ankle. *J Bone Joint Surg Br* 1986;68(5):834-837.
14. Grogan D, Holt G, Ogden J: Talocalcaneal coalition in patients who have fibular hemimelia or proximal femoral focal deficiency. A comparison of the radiographic and pathological findings. *J Bone Joint Surg Am* 1994;76(9):1363-1370.
15. Holmes L: *Common Malformations*, 1 ed. Oxford University Press, 2011.
16. Bohne W, Root L: Hypoplasia of the fibula. *Clin Orthop Relat Res* 1977;125:107-112.
17. Coventry M, Einer W, Johnson J: Congenital absence of the fibula. *J Bone Joint Surg Am* 1952;34(4):941-955.
18. Achterman C, Kalamchi A: Congenital deficiency of the fibula. *J Bone Joint Surg Br* 1979;61(2):133-137.
19. Birch JG, Lincoln TL, Mack PW, Birch CM: Congenital fibular deficiency: A review of thirty years' experience at one institution and a proposed classification system based on clinical deformity. *J Bone Joint Surg Am* 2011;93(12):1144-1151.
20. Patel M, Paley D, Herzenberg J: Limb-lengthening vs amputation for fibular hemimelia. *J Bone Joint Surg Am* 2002;84(2):317-319.
21. Epps C, Schneider P: Treatment of hemimelias of the lower extremity. Long-term results. *J Bone Joint Surg Am* 1989;71(2):273-277.
22. Naudie D, Hamdy RC, Fassier F, Morin B, Duhaime M: Management of fibular hemimelia: Amputation or limb lengthening. *J Bone Joint Surg Br* 1997;79-B(1):58-65.
23. McCarthy JJ, Glancy GL, Chnag FM, Eilert RE: Fibular hemimelia: Comparison of outcome measurements after amputation and lengthening. *J Bone Joint Surg Am* 2000;82(12):1732-1735.
24. Choi I, Kumar S, Bowen J: Amputation or limb-lengthening for partial or total absence of the fibula. *J Bone Joint Surg Am* 1990;72(9):1391-1399.
25. Herring J: Symes amputation for fibular hemimelia: A second look in the Ilizarov era. *Instr Course Lect* 1992;41:435-436.
26. Walker JL, Knapp D, Minter C, et al: Adult outcomes following amputation of lengthening for fibular deficiency. *J Bone Joint Surg Am* 2009;91-A(4):797-804.
27. Cummins D, Kapp S: Lower limb pediartic prosthetics: General considerations and philosophy. *J Prosthet Orthot* 1992;4:203.
28. Gibson D: Child and Juvenile amputee, in Banjerjee S, Khan N, eds: *Rehabilitation Management of Amputees*. William and Wilkins, 1982, pp 394-414.

Congenital Longitudinal Deficiency of the Tibia

CHAPTER 79

Jorge A. Fabregas, MD, FAAOS • Rebecca C. Whitesell, MD, MPH, FAAOS

ABSTRACT

Congenital deficiency of the tibia or tibial hemimelia is characterized by partial or complete absence of the tibia. Many of these patients have other associated anomalies. Although the true incidence of this condition is unknown, it has a bilateral presentation in approximately 30% of patients. Treatment varies depending on the amount of tibia that is absent and the presence or absence of the extensor mechanism.

Keywords: Brown procedure; congenital limb deficiency; congenital longitudinal deficiency; Syme ankle disarticulation; tibial deficiency; tibial hemimelia

Introduction

Congenital longitudinal deficiency of the tibia is the term used to describe a longitudinal deficiency of the tibial (medial) side of the lower limb. The tibia and the medial aspect of the foot are involved to various degrees. This condition has been known by many names in the literature, including tibial hemimelia, tibial meromelia, tibial anomaly, congenital tibial absence, congenital aplasia/dysplasia of the tibia, and congenital preaxial deficiency of the lower extremity.[1-3] The two most frequently used terms in modern literature and practice are congenital longitudinal deficiency of the tibia and tibial hemimelia.

Congenital longitudinal deficiency of the tibia is defined as partial or complete absence of the tibia, with a relatively unaffected fibula. Associated limb anomalies that occur in conjunction with the tibial deficiency include varying degrees of limb shortening, an equinovarus foot, knee joint abnormalities, and longitudinal deficiencies of the foot.[4-7] Frequently, there is bilateral involvement (up to 30% in some case series), and patients may have other limb anomalies such as proximal femoral focal deficiency (PFFD), a lobster claw hand deformity, or radial longitudinal deficiency of the upper limbs. The incidence of longitudinal congenital deficiency of the tibia has historically been estimated as one in one million live births in the United States,[8] but the true current incidence of the disease has not been reported. The database of the National Center on Birth Defects and Developmental Disabilities of The Centers for Disease Control and Prevention groups all limb deficiencies into either upper or lower limb deficiencies. The annual incidence of reduction deformity in the lower limbs is approximately two in 12,000 births; however, further data identifying only tibial deficiencies are unavailable.[9]

Clinical Presentation

In some instances, congenital longitudinal deficiency of the tibia can be difficult to distinguish from the much more common fibular deficiency, especially because it is difficult to precisely palpate and differentiate the soft, cartilaginous tibia and fibula in a small infant. The best clinical clue is that patients with a fibular deficiency always have an equinovalgus foot deformity, whereas patients with tibial deficiency almost always have an equinovarus foot deformity[6,10] (**Figure 1**). If there are associated ray abnormalities in the foot, patients with fibular deficiencies will have lateral ray deformities or deficiencies, and patients with tibial deficiencies will have medial ray deformities or deficiencies. The knee should be evaluated for the presence of a palpable patella, quadriceps, and a patella tendon. It should also be determined if there is active extension of the knee (functional quadriceps) because this will guide surgical decision-making.

History

Otto is widely accepted as the first person to report on a patient with tibial hemimelia in the English literature in 1841.[1] In 1877, Albert described the transference of the fibula to the distal aspect of the femur to create a fibulofemoral arthrodesis. In the early 1900s, Myers[1] described fibular transfer to recreate a knee joint. Helferich, Patrona, Motta, Busachi, and Joachimstal all individually reported single procedures in which they made slight modifications to Albert's described procedure to achieve a fibulofemoral arthrodesis.[1]

Dr. Fabregas or an immediate family member serves as a paid consultant to or is an employee of Astura Medical. Neither Dr. Whitesell nor any immediate family member has received anything of value from or has stock or stock options held in a commercial company or institution related directly or indirectly to the subject of this chapter.

Brown[11] was the first to report on a series of three patients in which he performed a fibulofemoral transfer to recreate the knee joint.

In 1961, Frantz and O'Rahilly[12] were the first to attempt to define a unified language to describe all limb deficiencies. Jones et al[13] were the first to create a classification system designed specifically to distinguish types of tibial deficiencies (known as the Jones classification). In an effort to create a classification system that would help dictate potential surgical interventions, Kalamchi and Dawe[7] modified the Jones classification scheme.

After Brown[11] first described his fibular transfer technique in 1965, a substantial number of articles regarding tibial hemimelia were published until the early 1980s. By the early 1980s, some authors estimated there were up to 300 reported cases of the deficiency.[3] Since the 1980s, there have been relatively few articles published regarding this deficiency, and most of the current literature focuses on the genetic aspects of the disorder. Tibial hemimelia is unique among congenital limb deficiencies because it is genetically transmitted in a substantial number of patients.[3] For example, bilateral tibial deficiency associated with central cleft defect is inherited as an autosomal dominant condition.

Classification

The ideal classification system for congenital longitudinal deficiency of the tibia would incorporate treatment guidelines, help determine a prognosis, and aid in future research. The classification system would categorize the deficiency by the variables known to affect the patient's outcome and help identify potential interventions.

In tibial deficiencies, quadriceps function and strength, the length of the tibial remnant, the degree of ankle joint and foot involvement, and any associated musculoskeletal anomalies help determine potential interventions and can affect the patient's overall outcome.[6,14] The Jones classification system, which was published in 1978, remains the most widely used system to describe tibial deficiencies.[13] This system, however, is based on radiographic appearance and does not incorporate any of the variables known to influence patient outcomes. The classification system developed by Kalamchi and Dawe[7] attempts to incorporate some clinical factors in the classification scheme, but this system is less widely used by clinicians. Most recently, Weber[15] developed a classification and scoring system, but it is a rather detailed system and has not achieved wide popularity among clinicians.

Jones System

In the Jones classification system, groups are separated by radiographic appearance.[13] In type 1 deficiencies, the tibia is not visible on radiographs. In type 1a deficiencies, the proximal tibia is completely absent, and the distal femoral epiphysis is hypoplastic. In type 1b deficiencies, the proximal tibia is absent on radiographs, but unossified small tibial cartilaginous anlage can be viewed by ultrasonography, arthrogram, and MRI, or can be appreciated on surgical dissection. The most distinguishing radiographic characteristic between type 1a and type 1b deficiencies is the normal distal femoral epiphysis in a type 1b deficiency. Williams et al[4] performed surgical dissections on several patients classified as having a type 1b deficiency and found no tibial anlage despite that finding in the patient cohort used to create the Jones classification in which all type 1b patients had a tibial anlage on surgical exploration.[13] An additional distinguishing feature between Jones type 1a and type 1b deficiencies is a lack of quadriceps function (absent active knee extension) in the type 1a group.

In type 2 deficiencies, the proximal tibia is visible on radiographs, but the tibia is substantially shortened, with the distal part at least partially absent or substantially hypoplastic. In type 3 deficiencies, the distal tibial epiphysis is visible as either a fully ossified entity or as localized calcification with the proximal tibia poorly defined. Type 3 deficiencies are very rare. In type 4 deficiencies, the tibia is shortened, and there is tibiofibular diastasis. The Jones classification is very useful for defining various tibial deficiencies based on radiographic appearance, but outcome-based factors, such as quadriceps strength, foot anomalies, and overall limb length are not used as a basis for classification.[13]

Kalamchi and Dawe System

The Kalamchi and Dawe[7] classification system is based on the type and degree of deformity, which the authors proposed would lead to defined treatments. Three groups are described based on clinical and radiographic findings. Type I is characterized by total absence of the tibia, proximal fibular migration, and distal femoral epiphysis hypoplasia on radiographs. Clinically, patients with type I deficiency have knee flexion contractures greater than 45°, no quadriceps function, marked equinovarus foot deformity, and, occasionally, medial ray deficiencies. Type II deficiency is defined as distal tibial aplasia. On radiographs, the proximal fibular migration is not as severe as in type I, and the distal femoral metaphyseal width and epiphyseal ossification are normal. Clinically, patients with

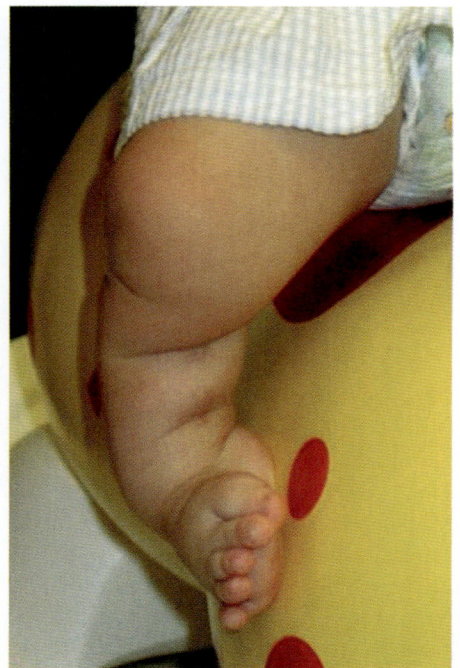

FIGURE 1 Clinical photograph of a 3-month-old infant with an absent tibia showing the typical equinovarus position of the foot. Note the dimpling along the medial border of the missing tibia.

type II deficiency have milder knee flexion contractures (25° to 45°), positive quadriceps function, and a relatively normal knee joint articulation. Type III deficiency is defined as dysplasia of the distal tibia, with diastasis of the tibiofibular syndesmosis. Radiographically, the distal tibia shows varying degrees of hypoplasia and shortening, the amount of syndesmotic diastasis can vary, the foot is in varus, and the talus may have a nearly vertical orientation. Clinically, patients with type III deficiency have normal knee joints and well-developed quadriceps function.

Weber System

In 2008, Weber[15] proposed a new classification and scoring system for tibial deformities. The classification system was developed to create a more modern system that incorporates correct anatomic terms, all types of deficiencies, and the inclusion of a scoring system to weight various associated anomalies in accordance with their effects on clinical decisions. The classification system identifies seven types of tibial deficiencies (I through VII), and five of the types have subgroups, depending on whether a cartilaginous tibial anlage is present or absent. The higher the number assigned to the classification, the more severe the tibial deficiency.

The scoring system assigns points for the presence or absence of a patella and the state of the hip, the femur, the fibula, the foot, and associated muscle function. The scoring system has a minimum score of 0 and maximum assigned value of 39; the higher the score, the less severe the impairment.

Type I is tibial hypoplasia, and type II is tibial fibular diastasis; these types have no subgroups. Type III is distal aplasia, type IV is proximal aplasia, type V is biterminal aplasia, type VI is agenesis with double fibulae, and type VII is tibial agenesis with a single fibula. Types III through VII each include two subgroups: in subgroup a, cartilaginous anlage is present; in subgroup b, cartilaginous anlage is absent.

Paley Classification

In 2003, and later modified in 2015, Paley proposed a new classification system to ensure it as an accurate descriptor of the level of tibial deficiency. It attempts to create a direct relationship between classification type, treatment, and prognosis. There are five main types, but as many as 11 subtypes (**Figure 2**).

Paley type I has hypoplastic nondeficient tibia: genu valgum with relative overgrowth of proximal fibula, plafond present and normal. Paley type II has proximal and distal tibial epiphysis present, but with a dysplastic ankle. They are further subdivided into A, B, and C. Paley type III is characterized by the presence of proximal tibia and knee joint, medial malleolus present, and tibio-fibular diastasis present. Further subdivision into A and B takes place. Paley type IV, with two subtypes, describes distal tibial aplasia; and type V, which has three subtypes, has complete tibial aplasia. There are modifiers to describe the presence or absence of associated deficiencies and duplications.

Comparisons

Despite the efforts of Kalamchi and Dawe[7] and, most recently, Weber,[15] the classification system most widely accepted and used by surgeons remains the Jones system.[13] Although the Kalamchi and Dawe[7] system more clearly defined the clinical correlates of each type of deformity, it did not add any new information regarding patient treatment. Weber's classification is more thorough, includes all variants (no matter how rare they may be), and attempts to provide a scoring system to indicate outcomes; however, it is rather difficult to understand, is cumbersome to use, and its reproducibility is questionable. All three classification systems (**Figure 3**) fail to incorporate the importance of associated foot anomalies in the decision-making process for amputation versus limb salvage.

On the other hand, the Paley classification does not fit the mold of the other classifications. Even though it does incorporate foot anomalies into its description, it mainly is a classification system designed to guide different limb reconstruction options. Amputations as an option are not described in this classification system and, as we have discussed, limb reconstruction may not be viable option for all patients.

Foot Abnormalities

Although Kalamchi and Dawe[7] addressed the knee and tibial deformity in their classification system, there is no scheme that has incorporated the degree of foot deformity. Radiographic and clinical examination may show duplication or absence of the medial rays (**Figure 4**). The degree of tibial deficiency does not correlate with the degree of foot abnormality.[5] Dissection studies[4,5,16] have further defined the various anomalies. The investigators found that nearly all of the patients had subtalar coalitions, as well as various other midfoot and hindfoot coalitions. The cuboid was larger than normal. The talus was elongated, and its joint surfaces were in abnormal sagittal alignment. These dissection studies found abnormal muscle and tendon development. Vascular anomalies are common, and they have been defined as being similar to the embryonic vascular structure of the distal limb with a prominent two-vessel system.[17]

Although foot anomalies are not incorporated into the classification schemes for tibial deformities, they are important in clinical practice for prognosis and determination of appropriate surgery. The more deformed the foot, the more likely amputation is the appropriate surgical option. Nearly normal or normal feet is an indication for reconstruction surgery. Knowledge of abnormal vasculature may be beneficial in determining surgical flap or reconstruction options. Miller and Armstrong[16] advocate the use of arteriography to help in this process.

Other Associated Anomalies

In addition to foot abnormalities, tibial deficiencies are frequently associated with other skeletal anomalies. A review of several of the largest patient studies found that hip and hand abnormalities are the most common associated anomalies.[6,10,13,18] The most common hip abnormalities include developmental hip dysplasia, PFFD,

Section 5: Pediatrics

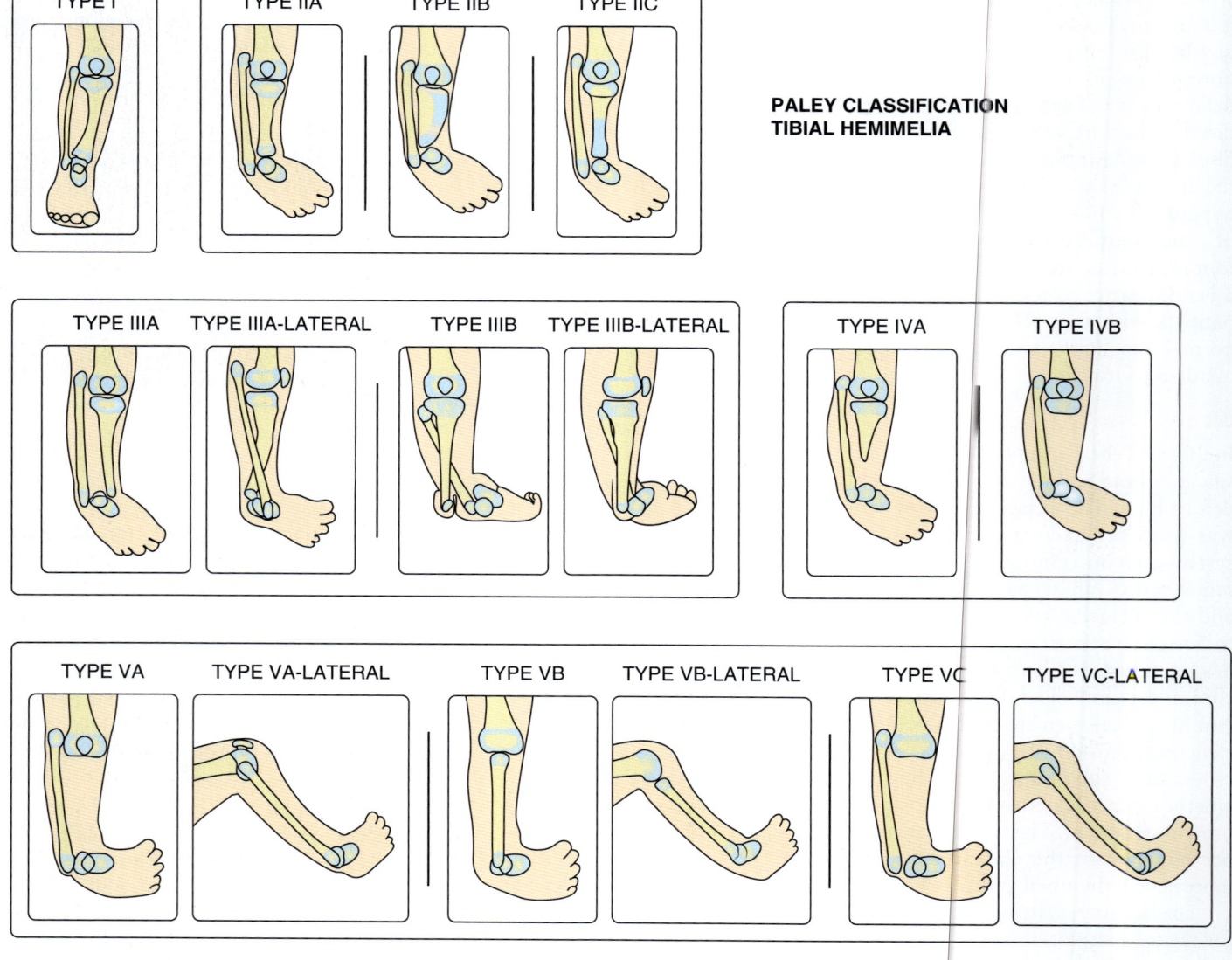

PATHOANATOMICAL VARIANTS

- Metatarsals	+ Metatarsals	+ Fibula	+/- Femur
- Tarsals	+ Tarsals	+ Femoral condyle	+ Distal tibia remnant

FIGURE 2 Illustration of the Paley classification of tibial hemimelia. (Reproduced with permission by the Paley Foundation.)

coxa valga, and a congenitally shortened femur.[19,20] The most common hand anomalies include a lobster claw hand and thumb abnormalities.[7,21] Schoenecker et al[10] described a 21% incidence of spine abnormalities, including hypoplastic vertebra and hemivertebra, in their patient cohort. Visceral anomalies, including hypospadias, imperforate anus, cardiac abnormalities, hernia, cryptorchidism, and learning disabilities, also have been documented.[7,13]

There are two defined conditions involving tibial deficiency. Warner syndrome involves tibial dysplasia, triphalangeal thumbs, and prehallucal polydactyly. The second group of disorders involves tibial deficiency, split-hand deformity, and femoral bifurcation or ulnar defects (also known as split hand/foot malformation with failure of long deficiency). Tibial deficiency has been identified as a rare component (not present in all patients) of various other syndromes, including Gollop-Wolfgang complex and Langer-Giedion syndrome.[22,23]

Etiology

The etiology of most tibial deficiencies is unknown, but several theories have been proposed in the literature. Given the skeletal and vascular anomalies found on dissection, some authors have suggested an embryologic incident in approximately the fifth gestational week.[2,12,17] In the early 20th century, tibial deficiency occurred in several

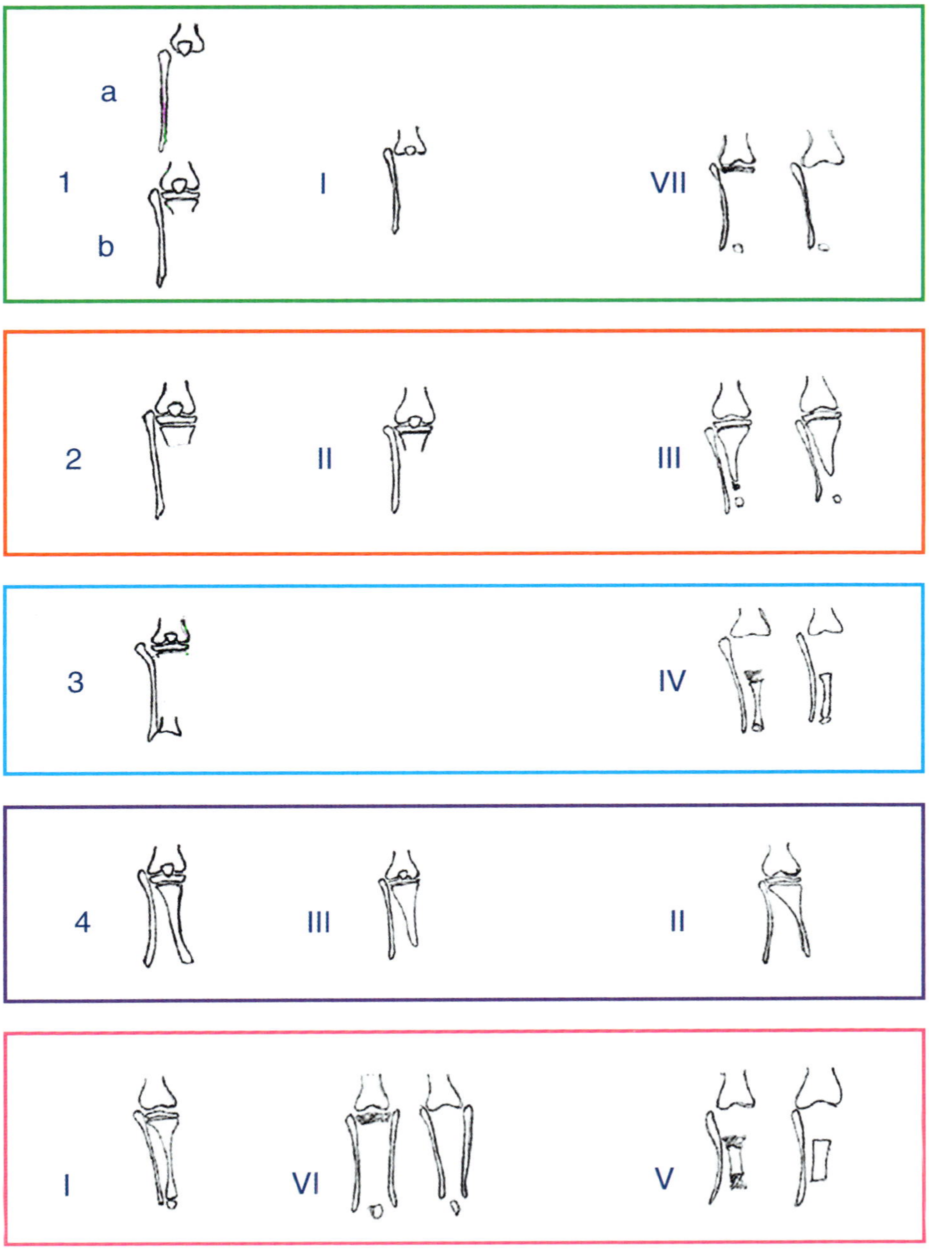

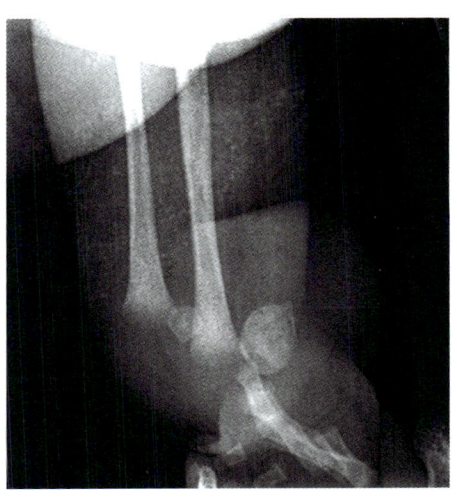

FIGURE 4 AP radiographs showing a tibial deficiency with an abnormal distal tibia and medial rays.

FIGURE 3 Illustration comparing the common characteristics of three classification systems (Jones, Kalamchi and Dawe, and Weber) for congenital longitudinal deficiencies of the tibia. Jones types 1a and 1b, Kalamchi and Dawe type I, and Weber type VII all demonstrate absence of the tibia (green box). Jones type 2, Kalamchi and Dawe type II, and Weber type III all demonstrate the presence of the proximal tibia with absence distally (red box). Jones type 3 and Weber type IV demonstrate the absence of the proximal tibia, with the distal tibia present (blue box). Jones type 4, Kalamchi and Dawe type III, and Weber type II demonstrate diastasis of the distal tibiofibular joint (purple box). Weber types I, VI, and V do not have any corresponding types in the other classification systems (pink box).

patients who had been exposed to thalidomide in utero.[6]

Because of several case reports of similar congenital abnormalities in family members, some authors have suggested genetic transmission.[6,21,24,25] Clark[21] documented an autosomal dominant inheritance pattern with variable penetrance. Pashayan et al[25] documented a review of several reports of family inheritance in a father and daughter, a father and son, and a father and daughter/daughter and daughter. McKay et al[24] documented an autosomal recessive inheritance pattern.

A single genetic mutation that leads specifically to tibial deficiency has yet to be identified. A *PITX1* gene mutation was implicated as being associated with various malformations of the lower limbs, including clubfoot, polydactyly, and tibial deficiency.[26] A genetic mutation at chromosome 17p13.3 has been implicated in split-hand/split-foot syndrome in patients with long bone deficiency syndrome. Cho et al[27] identified a 404 G > A mutation in the sonic hedgehog *cis*-regulator in patients with tibial hemimelia–polydactyly–triphalangeal thumb syndrome.

Surgical Planning

The goal of any surgical intervention for tibial deficiency is to obtain nearly normal knee function with as normal a gait as possible. Before proceeding with any surgical intervention, the patient must be thoroughly evaluated. The association of tibial deficiency with multiple syndromes has been well documented, and the involvement of any syndrome should be considered when planning surgery. Other limb anomalies, such as bilaterality, may play a role in the overall functional outcome of the patient. Tibial hemimelia can sometimes be associated with PFFD. In these patients, the treatment of PFFD takes precedence. In a patient who has a very short limb with no extensor mechanism associated with PFFD, consideration should be given to arthrodesis of the fibula to the femur in combination with a Syme ankle disarticulation to increase the lever arm of the femoral segment.

The foot must be considered in surgical planning. Anatomic variations in the foot may preclude limb salvage. Congenital anomalies, such as coalitions, instability, and missing rays, must all be considered. Universal recurrence of a deformed, rigid plantigrade foot and a substantial limb-length discrepancy at maturity can be problematic. Amputation and prosthetic fitting are usually the preferred treatment for substantial foot deformity.

The next management decision concerns the functionality of the knee. The most important deciding factor in the treatment of tibial deficiency is the presence of active knee extension,[5] which implies an adequate active quadriceps muscle. Quadriceps function is a prerequisite for a successful Brown procedure or any procedure other than a knee disarticulation. It may be possible to identify the extensor mechanism clinically, which is the preferred method. Other techniques, such as arthrography, direct surgical exploration, ultrasonography, CT, or MRI (**Figure 5**), can be used but are rarely needed. The extensor mechanism should be considered inadequate or absent if a trained physical therapist and/or physician is unable to identify active knee extension after a careful examination.

Treatment Options

The classification system described by Jones et al[13] is used in the following discussion of treatment options for tibial deficiencies.

Jones Type 1a Deficiency

In a type 1a tibial deficiency, there is complete absence of the tibia seen on the radiograph taken at birth. In a type 1a deficiency, the infant's contracted limb is positioned proximal and lateral to the femoral condyles, with an absent patella but normally functioning hamstrings. The foot is in extreme varus and is nonfunctional. There is no extensor mechanism, which precludes the possibility for reconstruction.

Knee Disarticulation

Most patients with complete tibial hemimelia will require knee disarticulation. Loder and Herring[5] reported on functional outcomes in children treated with knee disarticulation and prosthetic fitting. Gait analysis showed nearly normal gait velocity (81%) and energy expenditure within normal range. Although their speed for a 50-yard dash was below the fifth percentile, an appropriate prosthesis allowed for both a stable knee and return to recreational sports.[5] In one study, approximately 17% of the patients returned to recreational skiing after a knee disarticulation.[14]

Knee disarticulation is usually indicated when the child begins to pull to stand. In some patients, surgery may be delayed past this milestone up to 1 year of age. This allows additional time for the parents to be convinced of the nonfunctionality of the limb and the need for amputation.

A knee disarticulation is performed using a long curved transverse incision, with the anterior flap larger than the posterior flap. The dressing, with or without a plaster shell, must be secured with suspension above the pelvis.

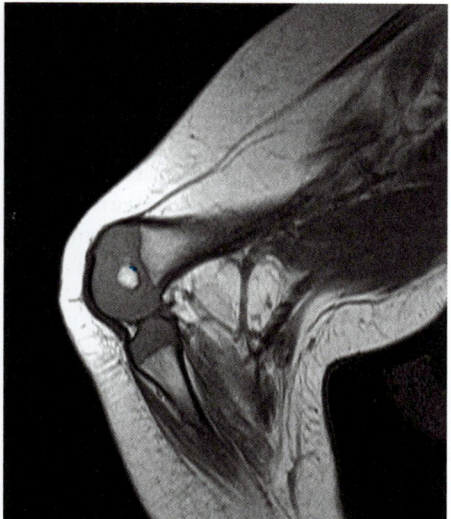

FIGURE 5 Sagittal MRI of the lower limb of a child with tibial deficiency showing absence of an extensor mechanism.

Compression garments can be used to control swelling for 2 to 3 weeks postoperatively, followed by prosthetic fitting. Some patients may require epiphysiodesis later in life to accommodate prosthetic componentry and achieve symmetric knee levels.

Brown Procedure

Centralization of the fibula (Brown procedure) combined with a Syme ankle disarticulation has been mentioned often in reference to type 1 tibial deficiencies. This procedure is likely successful only in patients with a type 1b deficiency because the complete lack of an extensor mechanism (as in a type 1a deficiency) is said to be a contraindication. This procedure is distinct from synostosis of the fibula to the tibia. Apparently, although not observed by Brown and Pohnert,[28] there are tibial deficiencies in which the extensor mechanism occasionally will insert into the fibula. This would make the Brown procedure a more viable option.

A lack of the proximal portion of the tibia is associated with a lack of an extension mechanism across the knee. Failure of the Brown procedure has resulted from the unopposed action of the hamstrings across the knee joint, which leads to flexion contracture and difficult (if not impossible) prosthetic fitting. In most patients, the Brown procedure results in less functionality because of recurrent knee flexion contractures.

The family of the patient should be fully counseled before a Brown procedure is performed because of the high failure rates and probability of an eventual knee disarticulation. Although early studies reported successful outcomes, many surgeons have been unable to reproduce those outcomes.

The Brown[11] procedure attempts to produce a limb with a useful knee segment. The procedure entails transposing the fibula into the intercondylar notch. This allows the fibula to undergo hypertrophy and become a tibia-like structure, resulting in adequate knee function. A successful procedure can produce a proprioceptive knee with active knee extension and flexion. Although the procedure was described by Myers[1] and by Sulamaa and Ryoeppy,[29] it was popularized by Brown[11] after he published a case series of three patients with tibial deficiencies.

Key points in performing a Brown procedure include shortening the femur, remodeling the upper fibula, and creating a long posterior flap for the Syme ankle disarticulation to avoid wound closure problems if no attempt is made to preserve the foot. A longitudinal incision is made along the lateral border of the quadriceps. The absence of the tibial remnant, which should have been determined preoperatively with MRI, should be confirmed. If a tibial remnant is present, transfer should be delayed until the segment is ossified. If the tibial remnant is absent, the surgeon can proceed with the fibular transfer. The epiphysis is dissected and half of its attachment to the soft tissue is maintained to preserve the epiphyseal blood supply. The proximal fibula is cut with a knife to fit into the condylar notch area of the femur. Muscle balance is established and immobilization is provided in a reduced and extended position.

Based on outcomes, it is unclear if results of the Brown procedure justify its use. Loder and Herring[5] reported poor results in 53 of 55 patients who were treated with fibular transfer for congenital absence of the tibia. Although the Brown procedure invariably results in varus and valgus instability, this does not usually pose a substantial problem because it can easily be corrected with a prosthesis. However, the progressive development of flexion contractures is a complication that cannot be accommodated with a prosthesis. Flexion contractures are unremitting because of the unopposed hamstrings, and they frequently lead to the need for knee disarticulation. Attempted preservation of the foot also is controversial. An unstable ankle results in the permanent use of a brace, unless an arthrodesis is performed. Despite the aforementioned controversies, Simmons et al[30] reported that patients were satisfied with the results of their Brown procedure based on the patients' own objective assessment of their daily functioning. In 2016, Birch reported on his 37-year experience and reached the conclusion that the Brown procedure universally failed at his institution.[1]

Jones Types 1b and 2 Deficiencies

In patients with type 1b and 2 tibial deficiencies, the proximal tibia is present, but the distal portion is absent. Importantly, the hamstrings and quadriceps are both present and function normally. Unlike patients with a type 1a deficiency, these patients typically have instability and problems occur distally. The foot is in varus and is displaced medially. In infants, the proximal tibia may not be initially apparent at birth and may be cartilaginous.

Although fusion of the fibula to the tibia may result in excellent outcomes, if the proximal tibial segment has not ossified (is still cartilaginous), surgery should be delayed until ossification occurs. This will facilitate fusion between the fibula and the tibia. After fibular tibial synostosis is performed, a Syme ankle disarticulation can be done at 1 year of age, followed by prosthetic fitting (**Figure 6**). This primary

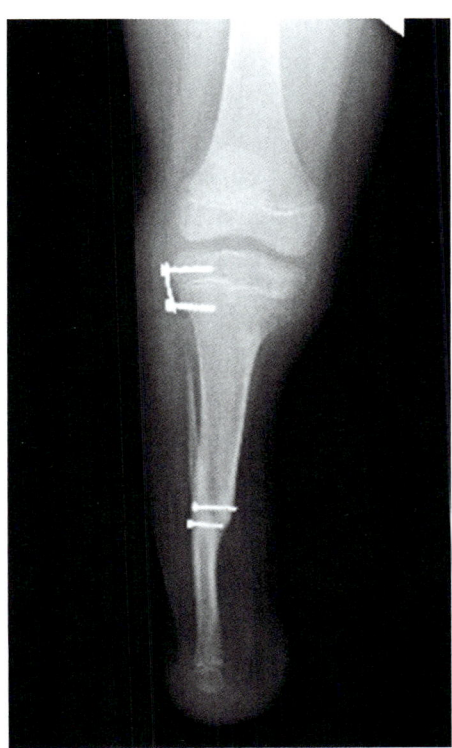

FIGURE 6 AP radiograph of child with a Jones type 2 tibial deficiency who was treated with synostosis of the fibula to the tibial remnant and a Syme ankle disarticulation.

reconstruction of the proximal tibial remnant via fusion to the fibula by translation to the more medial position is the favored procedure of the authors of this chapter. A Syme ankle disarticulation is typically needed because of ankle instability. Salvage of the deformed foot will lead to a rigid nonfunctional foot, whereas ankle disarticulation will allow a prosthesis to be fitted so that patients can participate in normal activities.

The fibular centralization procedure can be performed by end-on-end fusion of the tibia to the fibula, followed by fixation with a medullary rod or by side-to-side fusion with screw fixation and cast immobilization to maintain alignment. In both techniques, removal of the proximal fibula should be considered to avoid prosthetic fitting difficulties and allow more mobility of the fibula. This will lead to more appropriate mechanical alignment under the tibial remnant.

Jones Type 3 Deficiency

In patients with a type 3 tibial deficiency, the knee is unstable, and the tibial remnant is present distally. The patient typically has good quadriceps function and a very small proximal tibial remnant. A unique amorphous osseous structure develops characteristics of the distal tibial shaft. Distinction must be made between patients with a type 3 tibial deficiency and those with a short tibia and a varus foot.[17] In patients with a short tibia, the full tibia is present and clearly seen on radiographs. Depending on the anatomy of the ankle, some patients may be considered candidates for tibial lengthening. With tibial lengthening, however, there tends to be severe varus deformity of the limb. Type 3 tibial deficiency is rare, and few studies have been published. Based on the limited available data, patients achieve good function after a modified Syme ankle disarticulation or a Copart amputation.[31]

Jones Type 4 Deficiency

In a type 4 tibial deficiency, diastasis of the distal tibia and fibula causes a severe rigid varus foot positioned between the fibula and tibia. Moderate limb shortening is present, and there is no articular surface of the tibiotalar joint. Care must be taken to differentiate this condition from clubfoot. The correct diagnosis of a type 4 deficiency may not be apparent until resistance to clubfoot correction is encountered. These patients are candidates for a Syme ankle disarticulation.

A functional articulation of the foot at the ankle joint is possible, but it is extremely rare. In some instances, an attempt to retain the foot is reasonable if the condition is less severe or if a contralateral deficiency is present. In either case, surgery should be delayed until the child has reached walking age. Some techniques of tibial lengthening and foot repositioning may permit a plantigrade foot to be retained;[32] however, this may be difficult because of talocalcaneal coalitions, deformities, and other congenital foot anomalies.

Reconstruction of the ankle may result in a limb-length discrepancy of greater than 8 cm. In a study of patients who had a type IV deficiency, nine of 10 patients were treated with ankle reconstruction, and the foot was retained.[10] However, five of those nine patients eventually elected conversion to a Syme ankle disarticulation because of concerns regarding the resultant limb-length discrepancy and the magnitude of the lengthening required.

In some of these patients, the ankle joint may appear normal on the initial examination and the only apparent abnormality is a severe clubfoot. On close examination mild hypoplasia of the first ray (big toe) is usually present. Robert Gillespie referred to this condition as forme fruste of tibial hemimelia. In many of these patients the usual treatment of the clubfoot leads to multiple recurrences with Syme's amputation, not a rare final treatment for these patients (personal communication).

SUMMARY

Congenital longitudinal deficiencies of the tibia can have various clinical and radiographic presentations. Regardless of the type of tibial deficiency, the characteristics of the patient, the psychological and financial effects on the patient and family, the need for multiple surgeries, and the possibility of eventual knee disarticulation should all be considered in the decision-making process before treatment begins. It is imperative that the family be fully informed about treatment options and expected outcomes.

References

1. Myers H: Congenital absence of the tibia: Transplantation of the head of the fibula. Arthrodesis at the ankle joint. *Am J Orthop Surg* 1905;23(1):72-85.
2. Epps CH Jr, Tooms RE, Edholm CD, Kruger LM, Bryant DD III: Failure of centralization of the fibula for congenital longitudinal deficiency of the tibia. *J Bone Joint Surg Am* 1991;73(6):858-867.
3. Wehbé MA, Weinstein SL, Ponseti IV: Tibial agenesis. *J Pediatr Orthop* 1981;1(4):395-399.
4. Williams L, Wientroub S, Getty CJ, Pincott JR, Gordon I, Fixsen JA: Tibial dysplasia: A study of the anatomy. *J Bone Joint Surg Br* 1983;65(2):157-159.
5. Loder RT, Herring JA: Fibular transfer for congenital absence of the tibia: A reassessment. *J Pediatr Orthop* 1987;7(1):8-13.
6. Epps CH Jr, Schneider PL: Treatment of hemimelias of the lower extremity: Long-term results. *J Bone Joint Surg Am* 1989;71(2):273-277.
7. Kalamchi A, Dawe RV: Congenital deficiency of the tibia. *J Bone Joint Surg Br* 1985;67(4):581-584.
8. Brown FW: The Brown operation for total tibial hemimelia, in Aitken GT, ed: *Selected Lower-Limb Anomalies: Surgical and Prosthetics Management.* National Academy of Sciences, 1971, p 20.
9. Centers for Disease Control and Prevention: Birth defects: Data and statistics. Available at: http://www.cdc.gov/ncbddd/birthdefects/data.html. Accessed September 1, 2015.
10. Schoenecker PL, Capelli AM, Millar EA, et al: Congenital longitudinal deficiency of the tibia. *J Bone Joint Surg Am* 1989;71(2):278-287.
11. Brown FW: Construction of a knee joint in congenital total absence of the tibia (paraxial hemimelia tibia): A preliminary report. *J Bone Joint Surg Am* 1965;47(4):695-704.
12. Frantz CH, O'Rahilly R: Congenital skeletal limb deficiencies. *J Bone Joint Surg Am* 1961;43(8):1202-1224.
13. Jones D, Barnes J, Lloyd-Roberts GC: Congenital aplasia and dysplasia of the tibia with intact fibula: Classification and management. *J Bone Joint Surg Br* 1978;60(1):31-39.
14. Christini D, Levy EJ, Facanha FA, Kumar SJ: Fibular transfer for congenital absence of the tibia. *J Pediatr Orthop* 1993;13(3):378-381.
15. Weber M: New classification and score for tibial hemimelia. *J Child Orthop* 2008;2(3):169-175.
16. Miller LS, Armstrong PF: The morbid anatomy of congenital deficiency of the tibia and its relevance to treatment. *Foot Ankle* 1992;13(7):396-399.
17. Hootnick DR, Levinsohn EM, Randall PA, Packard DS Jr: Vascular dysgenesis associated with skeletal dysplasia of the lower limb. *J Bone Joint Surg Am* 1980;62(7):1123-1129.
18. Aitken GT: Amputation as a treatment for certain lower-extremity congenital abnormalities. *J Bone Joint Surg Am* 1959;41(7):1267-1285.
19. Sedgwick WG, Schoenecker PL: Congenital diastasis of the ankle joint: Case report of a patient treated and followed to maturity. *J Bone Joint Surg Am* 1982;64(3):450-453.
20. Wolfgang GL: Complex congenital anomalies of the lower extremities: Femoral bifurcation, tibial hemimelia, and diastasis of the ankle. Case report and review of the literature. *J Bone Joint Surg Am* 1984;66(3):453-458.
21. Clark MW: Autosomal dominant inheritance of tibial meromelia: Report of a kindred. *J Bone Joint Surg Am* 1975;57(2):262-264.
22. van de Kamp JM, van der Smagt JJ, Bos CF, van Haeringen A, Hogendoorn PC, Breuning MH: Bifurcation of the femur with tibial agenesis and additional anomalies. *Am J Med Genet* 2005;138(1):45-50.
23. Stevens CA, Moore CA: Tibial hemimelia in Langer-Giedion syndrome: Possible gene location for tibial hemimelia at 8q. *Am J Med Genet* 1999;85(4):409-412.
24. McKay M, Clarren SK, Zorn R: Isolated tibial hemimelia in sibs: An autosomal-recessive disorder? *Am J Med Genet* 1984;17(3):603-607.
25. Pashayan H, Fraser FC, McIntyre JM, Dunbar JS: Bilateral aplasia of the tibia, polydactyly and absent thumb in father and daughter. *J Bone Joint Surg Br* 1971;53(3):495-499.
26. Klopocki E, Kähler C, Foulds N, et al: Deletions in PITX1 cause a spectrum

of lower-limb malformations including mirror-image polydactyly. *Eur J Hum Genet* 2012;20(6):705-708.

27. Cho TJ, Baek GH, Lee HR, Moon HJ, Yoo WJ, Choi IH: Tibial hemimelia-polydactyly-five-fingered hand syndrome associated with a 404 G>A mutation in a distant sonic hedgehog cis-regulator (ZRS): A case report. *J Pediatr Orthop B* 2013;22(3):219-221.

28. Brown FW, Pohnert WH: Construction of a knee joint in meromelia tibia (congenital absence of the tibia): A fifteen-year follow-up study. *J Bone Joint Surg Am* 1972;54(6):1333.

29. Sulamaa M, Ryoeppy S: Congenital absence of tibia. *Acta Orthop Scand* 1963;33(1-4):262-270.

30. Simmons ED Jr, Ginsburg GM, Hall JE: Brown's procedure for congenital absence of the tibia revisited. *J Pediatr Orthop* 1996;16(1):85-89.

31. Fernandez-Palazzi F, Bendahan J, Rivas S: Congenital deficiency of the tibia: A report on 22 cases. *J Pediatr Orthop B* 1998;7(4):298-302.

32. Blauth W, Hippe P: The surgical treatment of partial tibial deficiency and ankle diastasis. *Prosthet Orthot Int* 1991;15(2):127-130.

Syme, Boyd, and Transtibial Amputation in Children: Surgical and Prosthetic Management

Heather Kong, MD, FAAOS • Rebecca Hernandez, CPO, LPO

ABSTRACT

Special considerations must be taken when managing lower limb amputations in pediatric patients. Treatment decisions in both acquired and congenital deficiencies are affected by the underlying etiology or disease process. Surgical and technical pearls may also help to minimize both short-term and long-term complications from amputation, such as bony overgrowth, soft-tissue migration, and residual limb-length discrepancy. Pediatric patients also have unique activity and prosthetic requirements compared with adult patients.

Keywords: ankle; Boyd; lower limb deficiency; pediatric; Syme; tibial

Introduction

Pediatric patients with congenital or acquired lower limb amputations require special considerations to maximize their function and minimize complications. Clinician should become familiar with a wide range of etiologies for lower limb amputation and their treatment implications. The growing skeleton introduces some unique challenges to the management of amputations, but also provides opportunities for growth modulation and deformity correction. Prosthetic management for pediatric patients varies depending on their anatomy, size, and functional needs.

General Considerations

Pediatric lower limb deficiencies or differences can be broadly categorized as either congenital or acquired.[1] Congenital conditions include transverse, both terminal and intercalary (ie, terminal aplasia, phocomelia), or longitudinal deficiencies (ie, tibial hemimelia, fibular hemimelia). Acquired etiologies for amputation include traumatic, infectious, oncologic, dysvascular, and neurogenic causes. Amputations through the tibial diaphysis or ankle joint are commonly used when the foot or ankle joint are not viable or functional.

The treatment of pediatric patients requiring lower limb amputation may differ from that for adult patients in several ways. In cases of elective amputation, the timing of amputation should correlate with the patient's developmental milestones. It is generally recommended that lower extremity amputation be performed at 6 to 10 months of age, when children are pulling to stand and starting to walk.[2] Their gait pattern and velocity will continue to mature until age 3 to 4 years, at which time they may be candidates for more dynamic prostheses or activity-specific prostheses.[2,3] During childhood, patients typically require a new prosthesis every 12 to 24 months, compared with every 3 to 5 years for adults. This is due to both the continued growth of the limb as well as the increased activity level and demands of pediatric patients.

Pediatric patients with both congenital and acquired amputations must be monitored until skeletal maturity for any associated bony deformity or joint instability. This may include hip dysplasia or instability, angular deformity around the knee joint, or growth disturbance from trauma or infection.[4] The residual limb length may also need to be optimized for an ideal prosthetic fit. Surgical options can include hemiepiphysiodesis for angular deformity, epiphysiodesis for a long residual limb, or gradual lengthening of a short tibial segment. Transtibial amputations are also prone to bony overgrowth in skeletally immature patients, who require close monitoring and often additional surgical management.[5-8]

Many studies in adult patients have shown differences in energy expenditure, function, and patient satisfaction based on the level of amputation. This is especially evident when comparing transfemoral versus transtibial amputations.[9-11] However, studies have shown that pediatric patients with amputation through the knee or distal have the same walking speed and oxygen consumption as children of the same age without amputation.[10,12] A comparative gait study between pediatric patients with Syme and transtibial amputation showed small differences in the prosthetic ankle range of motion, but comparable Pediatric Outcomes Data Collection Instrument scores.[13]

Neither of the following authors nor any immediate family member has received anything of value from or has stock or stock options held in a commercial company or institution related directly or indirectly to the subject of this chapter: Dr. Kong and Rebecca Hernandez.

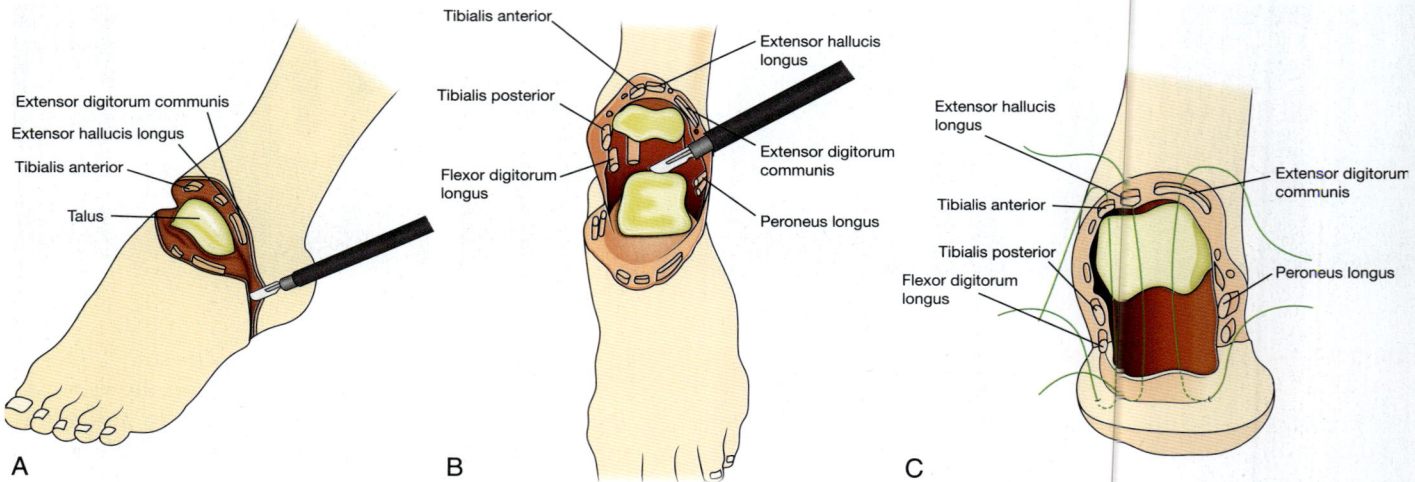

FIGURE 1 Illustration of surgical technique for Syme amputation. **A**, The conventional Syme skin incision is modified when the fibula is absent. **B**, With maximum plantar flexion of the talus, the subperiosteal dissection of the talus and calcaneus is carried out. **C**, The extensor tendons are attached to the anterior heel pad. (Reprinted with permission from Davidson WH, Bohne WH: The Syme amputation in children. *J Bone Joint Surg Am* 1975;57[7]:905-909.)

McQuerry et al[14] reported that Pediatric Outcomes Data Collection Instrument scores were similar between pediatric patients of various amputation levels in the subcategories of pain, happiness, transfers, and basic mobility. There was a trend toward poorer sports and physical function in patients with transtibial amputation compared with transfemoral amputation.

Both elective and unexpected amputations can create significant stress and anxiety for patients and their families. Pediatric patients who have undergone amputation and their families significantly benefit from a multidisciplinary treatment team, including orthopaedic surgeons, prosthetists, physical and occupational therapists, psychologists or behavioral health specialists, and social workers. There are many additional community resources and support networks for families, both locally and nationally.[15,16]

Syme Amputation

The Syme amputation is a true disarticulation of the ankle joint with maintenance of the heel pad for end weight bearing[17-19] (**Figure 1**). The malleoli are left intact. Its advantages include relative technical ease, decreased wound complications, and quick time to prosthetic fitting. The residual limb length and distal soft-tissue envelope allow patients to bear weight reasonably well without donning a prosthesis. In pediatric patients, amputation through the tibiotalar joint also avoids the potential for bony overgrowth seen with transosseous amputations.

The potential disadvantage of a Syme amputation is migration of the heel pad over time (8% to 45%).[20-22] A systematic review of pediatric Syme amputations reported a 28% incidence of heel pad migration (49 of 176 children).[23] Posterior heel pad migration is most common (**Figure 2**), although varus or valgus migration has also been reported. Heel pad migration can often be managed with prosthetic adjustments and may not require revision surgery.[24] Several technical modifications have been described to decrease the risk of heel pad migration. The anterior edge of the heel pad can either be sutured to the anterior ankle joint capsule or extensor tendons.[18] Tenodesis of the Achilles tendon or peroneal tendons have also been described in an attempt to balance the residual forces on the heel pad.[25,26]

The surgical technique for the Syme amputation most often describes extraperiosteal excision of the calcaneus, carefully preserving heel fat pad with its fibrous septae. The technique of subperiosteal excision of calcaneus has also been described and once secured to the distal tibia, it can potentially decrease the risk of heel pad migration

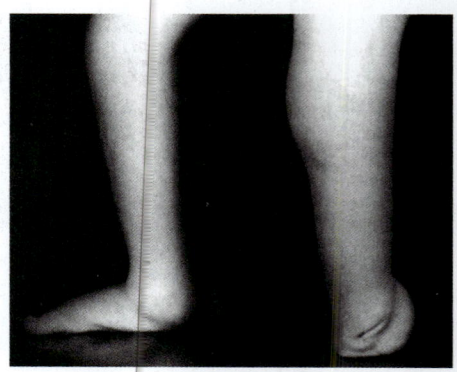

FIGURE 2 Clinical photograph demonstrating posterior migration of the heel pad after Syme amputation. (Reprinted with permission from Davidson WH, Bohne WH: The Syme amputation in children. *J Bone Joint Surg Am* 1975;57[7]:905-909.)

and maintain the hydraulic function of the heel pad.[15,22] Some authors have noted that the calcaneal periosteum (with or without the calcaneal apophysis) can later ossify and essentially create a Boyd-type amputation[21] (**Figure 3**). Other authors have noted that the ossified remnants of the periosteum or calcaneus can cause painful weight bearing or prosthetic fit, and therefore they advocate for extraperiosteal excision of the calcaneus.[19,20] Typically, the malleoli do not need to be resected in pediatric patients.

Although the residual limb length after a Syme amputation can allow end-bearing without a prosthesis and

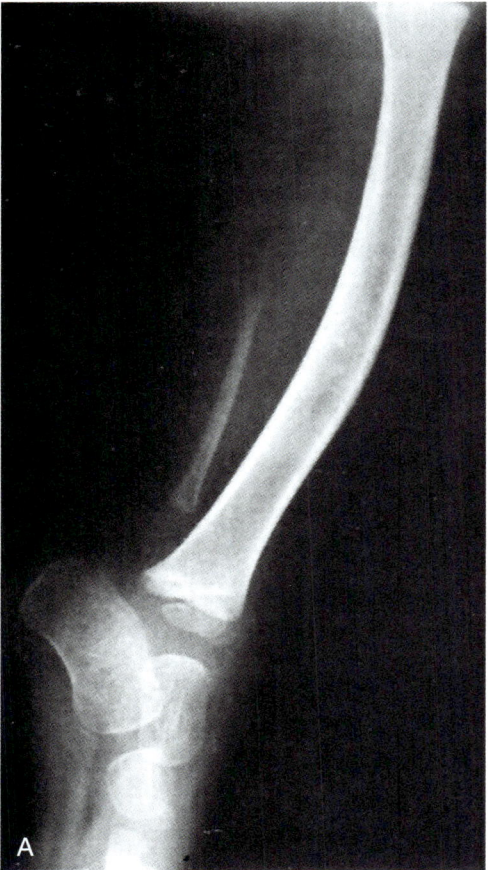 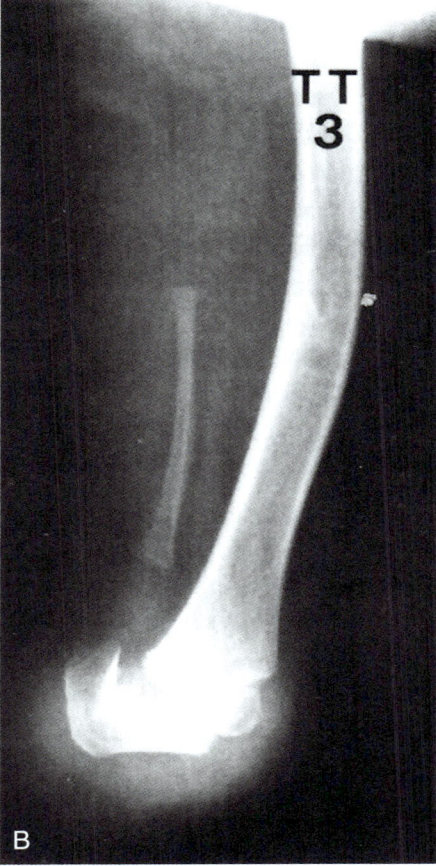 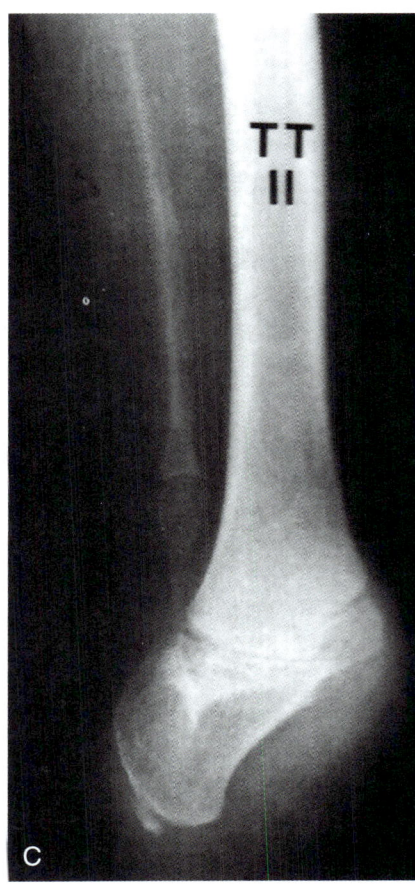

FIGURE 3 Serial radiographs showing calcaneal overgrowth after Syme amputation. **A**, Preoperative radiograph from a patient with partial absence of the fibula and proximal focal femoral deficiency. The calcaneus was removed subperiosteally and a Syme amputation was performed when the child was age 2 years, 6 months. **B**, At the age of 3 years 6 months after the Syme amputation, there is ossification in the cartilaginous calcaneal epiphysis. **C**, At the age of 11 years, the calcaneus has almost completely reformed from the periosteum and cartilage cells that were left at the time of amputation. (Reprinted with permission from Eilert RE, Jayakumar SS: Boyd and Syme ankle amputations in children. *J Bone Joint Surg Am* 1976;58[8]:1138-1141.)

potentially improve energy expenditure, a residual limb that is too long can limit prosthetic options. This is less likely to be an issue in patients with congenital deficiencies, because the involved limb is usually already shorter. At the time of skeletal maturity, a limb-length difference of 8 to 18 cm will provide enough clearance for a more dynamic or advanced prosthesis.[2,27] Morrison et al suggested that the optimal residual limb length be tailored to the patient's level of function and activity, as well as preferred prosthetic option, rather than maximizing length in all patients[28] (**Figure 4**). If additional shortening is needed, surgical options include epiphysiodesis in a skeletally immature patient or acute shortening osteotomy of either the femur or tibia in skeletally mature patients.

Boyd Amputation

The Boyd amputation is also performed at the level of the ankle, but involves removal of the talus and arthrodesis of the calcaneus to the distal tibia[29,30] (**Figure 5**). Preservation of the calcaneus and heel pad for weight bearing most closely replicates the native foot and can maximize end-bearing potential without a prosthesis. It prevents the heel pad migration seen often with the Syme amputation. The disadvantages include the necessity for bony fixation and healing, leading to a longer time to achieve weight bearing and prosthetic fit.

The incision and most of the dissection for the Boyd amputation is identical to that for the Syme amputation. Once the talus is removed, a saw is used to create parallel cuts in the distal tibia and superior articular surface of the calcaneus. The calcaneal cut should also be parallel to the plantar aspect of the heel pad. The anterior process of the calcaneus is then removed with the rest of the foot. The calcaneus and heel pad are then fixed to the distal tibia with a single or multiple Kirschner wires (**Figure 6**). The residual limb is typically placed in a cast and the patient must not bear weight until bony fusion is achieved and the Kirschner wires are removed, usually approximately 6 weeks postoperatively. Complications can include nonunion (5%) and wound healing complications (6%).[21,31] Skin necrosis or wound dehiscence can occur because of excessive length and tension on the closure. Significant flap necrosis can occur if the posterior tibial vasculature is disrupted.

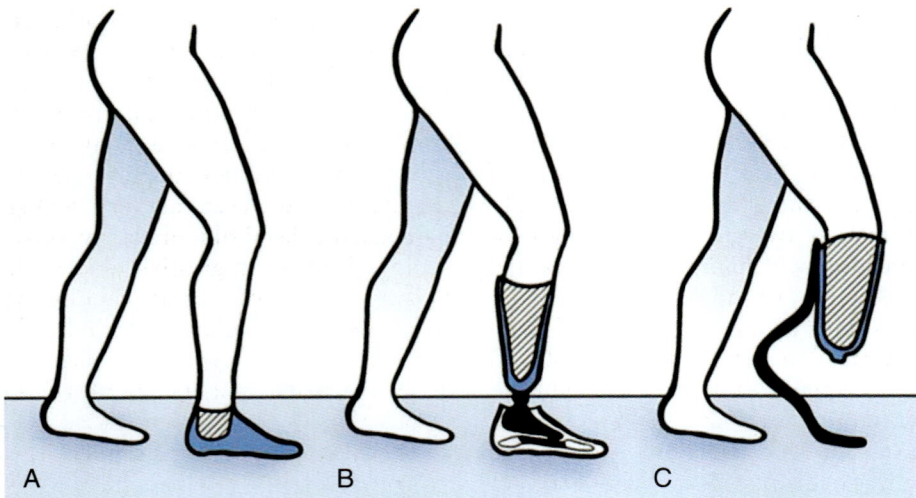

FIGURE 4 Illustration of prosthesis types and the necessary clearance of the limb. **A**, Rigid single-axis type prosthesis with little capacity for energy return or shock absorption. **B**, Prosthesis with heel/forefoot spring capacity. **C**, Spring foot for running, mounted to socket posteriorly. (Reprinted with permission from Morrison SG, Thomson P, Lenze U, Donnan LT: Syme amputation: Function, satisfaction, and prostheses. *J Pediatr Orthop* 2020;40[6]: e532-e536.)

the calcaneus. The Achilles tendon may be significantly contracted with notable equinus position of the calcaneus. More extensive dissection and soft-tissue release may be required to bring the calcaneus into appropriate position beneath the tibial plafond to avoid fusing the calcaneus in an equinus position. If this is not possible, a Syme amputation may be more appropriate. Subtalar coalitions and other abnormalities may be seen in the shape or alignment of the talus and calcaneus. This requires careful planning to ensure the appropriate plane of osteotomy as well as optimal position of the calcaneus for weight bearing.[15,19] The distal fibula may also need to be resected depending on the level of distal tibial osteotomy and whether the distal tibial physis is removed. In some situations, it may even be possible to incorporate the distal fibular anlage into the calcaneotibial fusion.[31]

The additional length provided by a Boyd amputation can be advantageous in situations where the residual tibial segment is quite short. This can improve energy expenditure and allow easier end-bearing without a prosthesis. However, similar to the

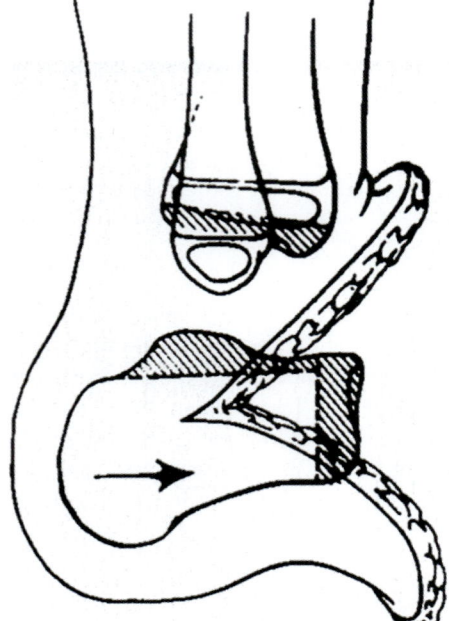

FIGURE 5 Illustration of surgical technique for Boyd amputation. The shaded areas are to be resected in fashioning the fusion site. It is important to shift the calcaneus anteriorly so that it will sit squarely under the distal tibia. When there is fixed ankle equinus, the Achilles tendon may require sectioning. (Reprinted with permission from Blum CE, Kalamchi A: Boyd amputations in children. *Clin Orthop Relat Res* 1982;165:138-143.)

In patients with congenital deformities involving the ankle joint, most commonly in fibular longitudinal deficiencies, special care must be taken during the resection and positioning of

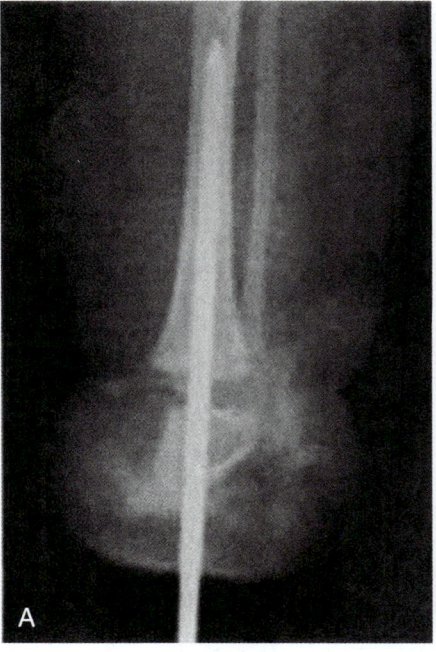
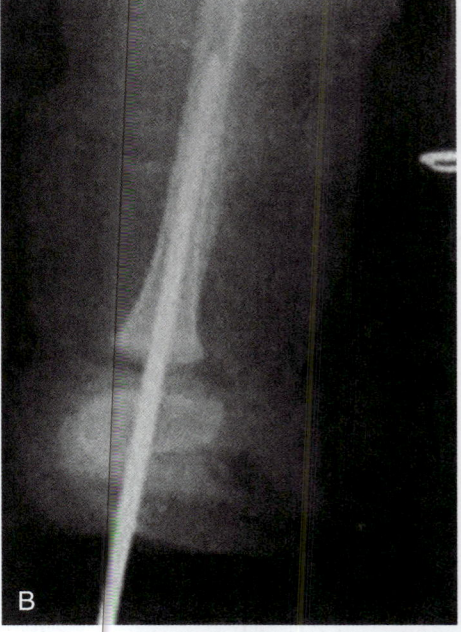

FIGURE 6 Intraoperative AP (**A**) and lateral (**B**) radiographs showing alignment of the fusion site and intramedullary threaded pin fixation after Boyd amputation. (Reprinted with permission from Blum CE, Kalamchi A: Boyd amputations in children. *Clin Orthop Relat Res* 1982;165: 138-143.)

Syme amputation, excessive length of the residual limb can limit prosthetic options. The simplest prosthetics require at least 2 to 3 cm of clearance, whereas more dynamic prosthetics require 8 to 18 cm of residual limb-length difference.[2,27] If further shortening of the residual limb is anticipated, the distal tibial physis can be resected at the time of amputation. Proximal tibial epiphysiodesis can also be performed at the appropriate time during skeletal growth/maturity.[31] It should also be noted that overgrowth of the residual calcaneus can also increase the residual limb length or lead to challenges with prosthetic fit.[21] The bulkiness of the terminal aspect in Boyd amputation can also affect the prosthetic fitting. The trap door opening in the prosthesis may be required for donning of the prosthesis. The cosmesis of the prosthesis can also be an issue in many of these patients.

Transtibial Amputation

Transtibial amputations are rarely electively performed in skeletally immature patients because of the risk of bony overgrowth (4% to 50%).[5-8] However, both congenital and acquired conditions such as traumatic injury or malignancy may result in a tibial diaphyseal or metaphyseal amputation. A transtibial amputation also has less end-bearing potential and less robust soft-tissue coverage compared with a transarticular amputation.

Studies have shown that children younger than 12 years at the time of acquired amputation have the highest rates of overgrowth requiring revision surgery.[5] Children with congenital amputations or who are older than 12 years have a lower incidence of overgrowth.[5,8] Younger age is associated with more repeat revisions.[5] Metaphyseal and diaphyseal amputations appear to have similar rates of overgrowth.[8] The bony overgrowth may also be accompanied by bursa or neuroma formation, skin ulceration, or infection (**Figure 7**).

An attempt should first be made to manage the bony overgrowth with prosthetic adjustments. If unsuccessful, several surgical techniques have been described to manage this issue. Simple resection alone often leads to recurrent overgrowth and loss of length. Various autogenous osteochondral grafts can be used to cap the end of the bone, including the iliac crest, proximal or distal fibula, and metatarsal heads[32-34] (**Figure 8**). Use of a synthetic cap has also been described, which can potentially decrease donor site morbidity.[32,35,36] Resection alone can lead to recurrent overgrowth in as high as 85% of cases, synthetic caps in 30% to 77% of cases, and biologic caps in 10% to 29% of cases.[7,33,34] The Ertl procedure has also been described to potentially improve end-bearing and decrease bony overgrowth in transtibial amputations[37-40] (**Figure 9**). However, in very young patients, the distal tibiofibular synostosis may lead to progressive tibia vara, perhaps because of the unequal rates of the growth of the tibia and fibula.[41,42] Furthermore, the synostosis did not appear to change quality of life or outcome scores in adult patients.[43-45]

Angular deformity or a significantly shortened tibial residual limb may arise either iatrogenically or from the underlying disease process. This can affect prosthetic fit, comfort, and biomechanics. The tibial segment should be at least 10 to 12 cm in length, and ideally between 12 and 17 cm, to allow for appropriate prosthetic fit. Several reports in the literature have described the use of a multiplanar external fixator to gradually correct angular deformity

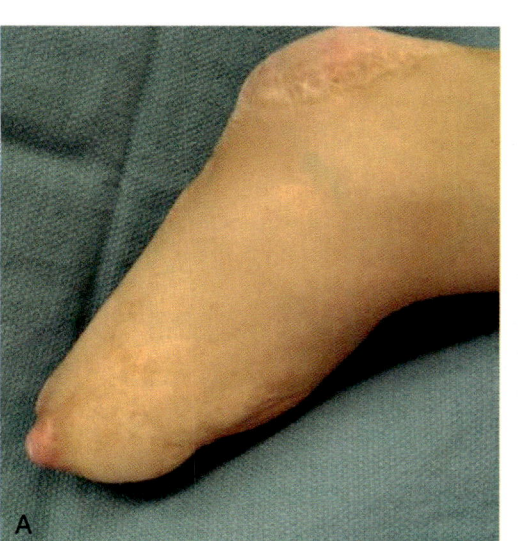
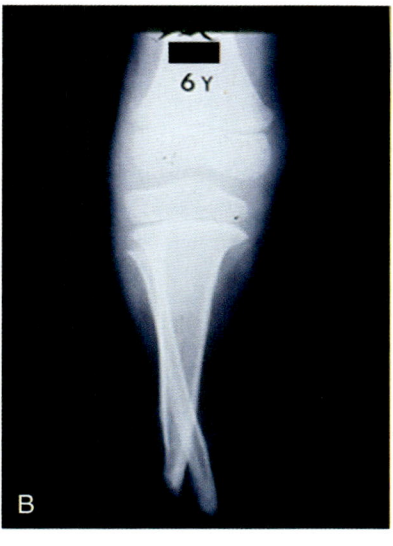

FIGURE 7 **A**, Preoperative clinical photograph of tibial residual limb. **B**, AP radiograph of tibial residual limb overgrowth. (Reprinted with permission from Fedorak GT, Watts HG, Cuomo AV, et al: Osteocartilaginous transfer of the proximal part of the fibula for osseous overgrowth in children with congenital or acquired tibial amputation: Surgical technique and results. *J Bone Joint Surg Am* 2015;97[7]:574-581.)

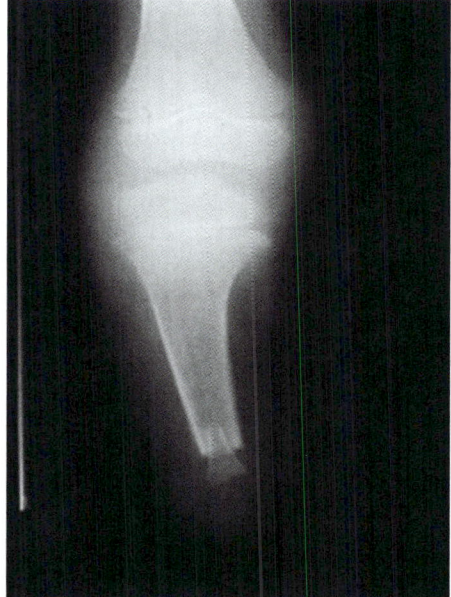

FIGURE 8 Postoperative AP radiograph of osteocartilaginous transfer of the proximal fibula for tibial residual limb overgrowth. (Reprinted with permission from Fedorak GT, Watts HG, Cuomo AV, et al: Osteocartilaginous transfer of the proximal part of the fibula for osseous overgrowth in children with congenital or acquired tibial amputation: Surgical technique and results. *J Bone Joint Surg Am* 2015;97[7]:574-581.)

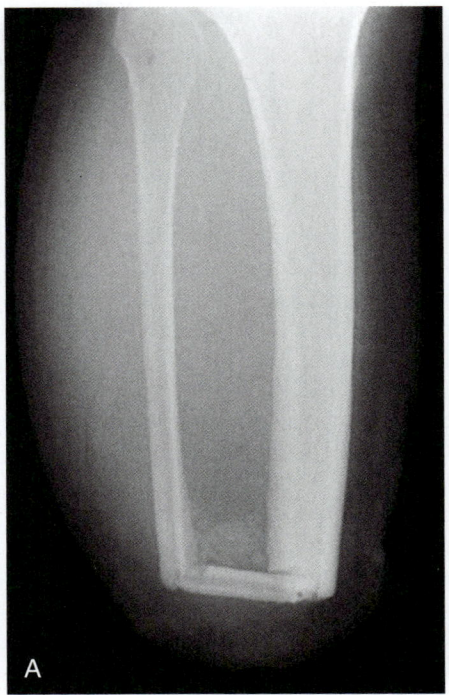 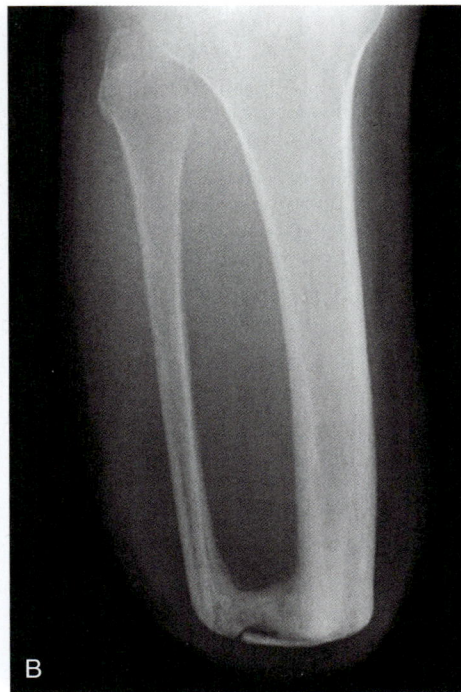 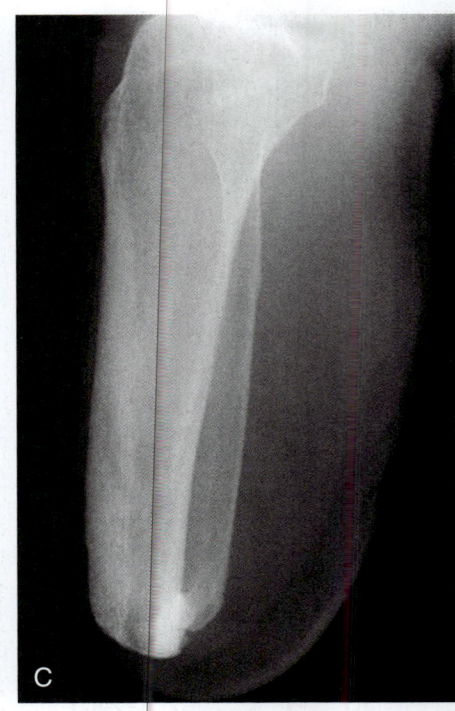

FIGURE 9 Radiographic example of the Ertl procedure. **A**, AP radiograph of the lower extremity obtained immediately postoperatively demonstrating an osteomyoplastic transtibial amputation. Note the placement of an autogenous fibular strut across the distal aspect of the amputated tibia and fibula. AP (**B**) and lateral (**C**) radiographs of the extremity obtained 36 months postoperatively. (Reprinted with permission from Taylor BC, Poka A: Osteomyoplastic transtibial amputation: The Ertl technique. *J Am Acad Orthop Surg* 2016;24[4]:259-265. © 2016 by American Academy of Orthopaedic Surgeons.)

or increase the length of the tibial segment.[4,46,47] Growth modulation may also be an option depending on the patient's age and degree of deformity. If performing lengthening or deformity correction of the residual tibial segment, careful preoperative planning is essential to minimize complications such as joint stiffness or contractures, joint instability, or distal soft-tissue breakdown.

Prosthetic Management

Many factors make fitting a prosthesis on a child different from on an adult. Rapid skeletal growth, angular deformities requiring unique prosthetic alignment, limited clearance for distal components, and increased functional demand on the prosthesis are a few challenges presented to the prosthetist when treating a pediatric patient.

A prosthesis for a young child should be designed to allow some growth to prolong the life span of the prosthesis. The socket design must account for longitudinal and circumferential growth, which can be accomplished by using a greater number of socks or a thicker liner at the time of initial fit, gradually decreasing sock ply or liner thickness at the child grows.[2] The addition of removable, multidurometer distal end pads and higher trim lines can accommodate longitudinal bony growth. Using modular components that can be lengthened or replaced as the child grows when possible is advantageous. In general, by the time the child has outgrown the socket, the components have failed or begun to fail because of wear and tear.

Although expanding, the variety of components available to the pediatric population does not yet compare with the wide variety available for the adolescent or adult population. Because of the high demands with significant and repeated forces, often resulting in failures and requiring small and lightweight designs, development of pediatric componentry specific to pediatrics seems to pose a challenge to the prosthetic manufacturing industry. Advancing materials and manufacturing processes in recent years have provided lighter, more durable and responsive components for children. Exoskeletal designs continue to be more appropriate for younger children because of increased durability. The introduction of endoskeletal designs permit increased modularity of components allowing for ease of adjustments, repairs, and replacement of components.

Prosthetic treatment should coincide with normal development and activity. For infants and toddlers, the prosthesis should have simple components and design, possibly a foam or rubber foot that would allow for easy transitions from sitting to crawling, tall kneeling to stand, cruising, and finally independent ambulation (**Figure 10**). Early walkers have a flat-footed wide base of support with hip and knee flexion. This should be accounted for in the alignment by having more dorsiflexion relative to the typical adult bench alignment.

Prosthetic foot requirements change as the child reaches preschool age and a gait pattern develops with a heel strike at loading response and heel rise at terminal stance through toe-off. At

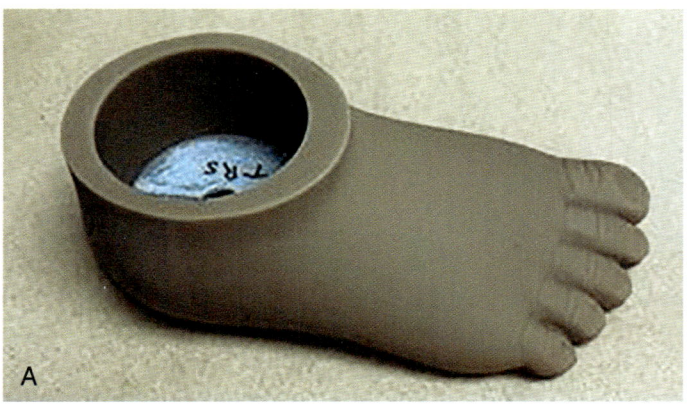 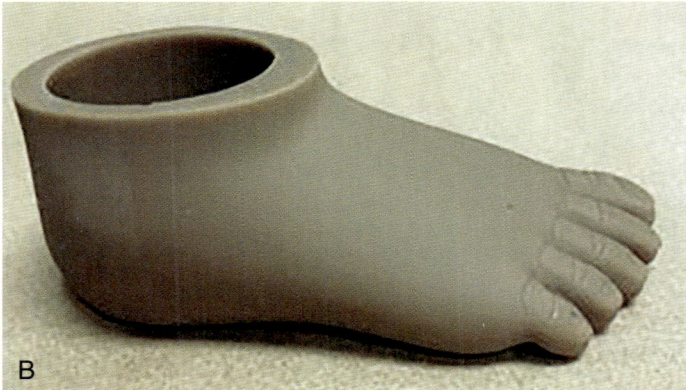

FIGURE 10 Superior (**A**) and lateral (**B**) photograph of a TRS Lil' Foot (Fillauer), which is an off-the-shelf foot prosthesis demonstrating minimal clearance requirements for a child with a Syme or Boyd amputation.

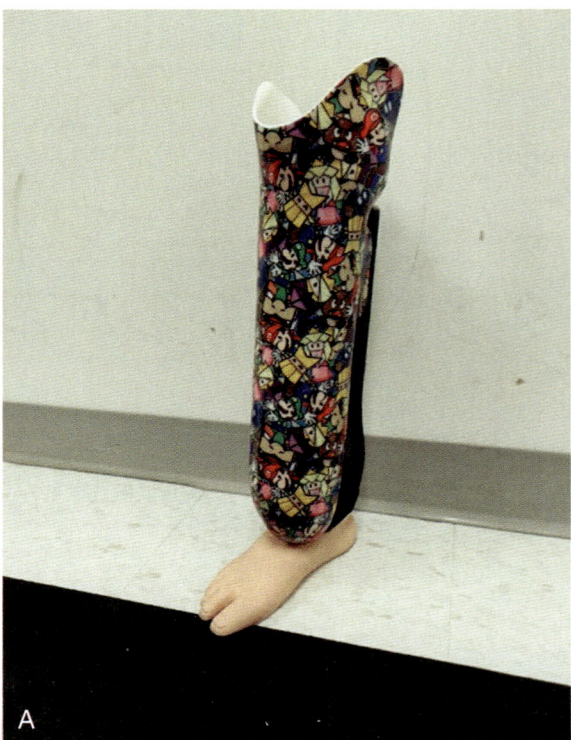 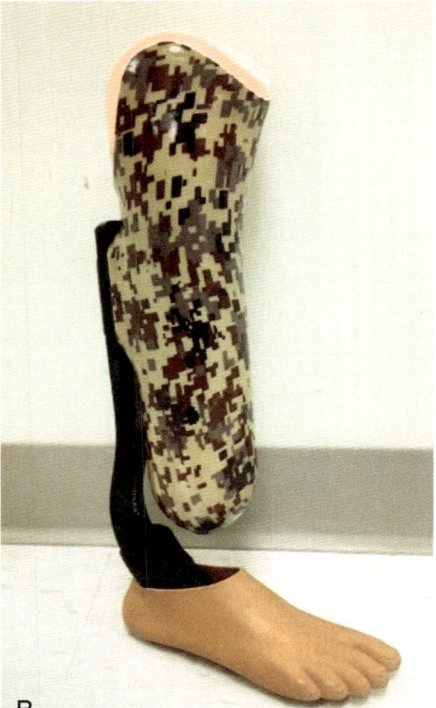 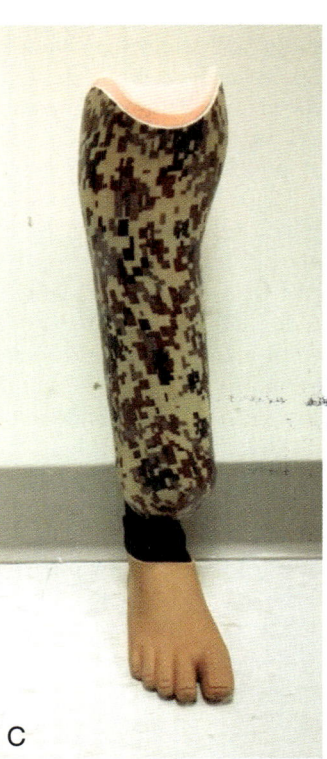

FIGURE 11 Anterior (**A**), lateral (**B**), and anterior (**C**) clinical photographs of a Syme prosthesis, in which posterior-mounted prosthetic feet allow children with long residual limbs and limited clearance to take advantage of the energy-storing properties of carbon fiber prosthetic feet.

this age, prosthetic feet typically have a heel rise to accommodate a standard children's athletic shoe. The heel still provides compression at heel strike but provides a greater lever arm for toe-off at terminal stance.

As children continue to reach developmental milestones, such as running, jumping, and playing sports, more high-performing, dynamic response and energy-storing prosthetic feet become appropriate. These typically become available at 15 to 16 cm in length. Recently, posterior-mounted prosthetic feet have become manufactured in pediatric sizes, allowing even the longest of residual limbs to be fit with this technology (**Figure 11**). This is especially beneficial to those with unilateral Syme and Boyd amputations, who historically have been limited to low-profile or even custom-made prosthetic feet because of lack of clearance for more advanced componentry.

As children near teenage years, they will transition to adult componentry with more options to match their activity levels and recreational needs.

Regardless of the technology used distally, a comfortable, well-fitting, and supportive socket is of paramount importance in the pediatric patient. As previously stated, sockets should be designed to accommodate growth and last approximately 12 to 18 months before replacement. Often self-suspending sockets can be used for Syme and Boyd amputations, whether through a silicone bladder socket or a pelite segmented socket. By using socks, children can increase or decrease sock ply to accommodate slimming down with longitudinal growth or increased circumference with weight gain. For growing children, suction sockets should be avoided until growth has slowed.

Boyd and Syme amputations for distal congenital deficiencies can provide excellent end-bearing capabilities both with and without a prosthesis. It is important to carefully evaluate the proximal segments for skeletal deficiencies such as a shortened femur or hypoplastic hemipelvis. In these cases, the reference lines for alignment of the prosthesis are not as they would be for an adult-acquired amputation at the same level.

It is important to note that the lateral femoral condyle is often hypoplastic, leading to valgus at the knee, and the knee axis is canted so that it is higher on the lateral side. Careful attention must be paid to alignment to minimize gait deviations and normalize stresses across the knee joint. The foot is often inset in relation to the distal end to ensure even weight bearing through the knee. Proximal design should be patellar tendon bearing so that the inset of the foot does not introduce a varus moment if weight bearing through the distal end. Supracondylar trim lines provide knee stability and rotational control of the prosthesis.

When disarticulation amputation is not an option and a through-bone amputation is done, provisions should be made to accommodate bony overgrowth, because this is a common occurrence. Although this is generally best managed by a surgical revision, overgrowth can often recur in close succession, so being able to delay a revision by socket modifications is often desired. Distal end padding that is removable can extend the life of the socket when using a patellar tendon bearing design. A locking liner can also help elongate the distal soft tissue to reduce pain and skin rupture from bony overgrowth.

Traumatic amputations can often have associated asymmetrical proximal tibial physis trauma due to injury or disease. This can cause angular growth of the tibia. The patient should be monitored closely because this angulation will get progressively worse over time and the socket and alignment will require adjustment to ensure that the forces across the knee are not contributing to the angulation. The alignment may vary greatly from the typical alignment of an adult prosthesis because of these factors.

Children with Syme, Boyd, and transtibial amputations can have excellent functional outcomes, mirroring those of their peers, with appropriately fitting prostheses and regular follow-ups with their healthcare team to accommodate growth and physiologic changes. The activities of daily living for a child will put even the most durable components to the test and the socket design and alignment can have a great effect on the underlying growing skeleton.

SUMMARY

Syme and Boyd ankle disarticulations are commonly used in pediatric patients with both congenital and acquired limb deformities or deficiencies. Each procedure has both short-term and long-term potential complications, which must be taken into consideration at the time of surgery and when counseling patients and families. Transtibial amputations are not typically performed in growing children because of the likelihood of bony overgrowth. However, several surgical options have been described in an attempt to minimize this complication. In contrast with adult patients, pediatric patients generally have similar function, energy expenditure, and patient satisfaction compared with their peers who have not undergone amputation, and regardless of level of transtibial amputation.

References

1. Krajbich JI: Lower-limb deficiencies and amputations in children. *J Am Acad Orthop Surg* 1998;6(6):358-367.
2. Hall M, Cummings D, Welling R, et al: Essentials of pediatric prosthetics. *JPOSNA* 2020;2(3).
3. Sutherland DH, Olshen R, Cooper L, Woo SL: The development of mature gait. *J Bone Joint Surg Am* 1980;62(3):336-353.
4. Ranade A, McCarthy JL, Davidson RS: Angular deformity in pediatric transtibial amputation stumps. *J Pediatr Orthop* 2009;29(7):726-729.
5. Abraham E, Pellicore RJ, Hamilton RC, Hallman BW, Ghosh L: Stump overgrowth in juvenile amputees. *J Pediatr Orthop* 1986;6(1):66-71.
6. Aitken GT: Surgical amputation in children. *J Bone Joint Surg Am* 1963;45:1735-1741.
7. Davids JR, Meyer LC, Blackhurst DW: Operative treatment of bone overgrowth in children who have an acquired or congenital amputation. *J Bone Joint Surg Am* 1995;77(10):1490-1497.
8. O'Neal ML, Bahner R, Ganey TM, Ogden JA: Osseous overgrowth after amputation in adolescents and children. *J Pediatr Orthop* 1996;16(1):78-84.
9. Waters RL, Perry J, Antonelli D, Hislop H: Energy cost of walking of amputees: The influence of level of amputation. *J Bone Joint Surg Am* 1976;58(1):42-46.
10. Jeans KA, Browne RH, Karol LA: Effect of amputation level on energy expenditure during overground walking by children with an amputation. *J Bone Joint Surg Am* 2011;93(1):49-56.
11. MacKenzie EJ, Bosse MJ, Castillo RC, et al: Functional outcomes following trauma-related lower-extremity amputation. *J Bone Joint Surg Am* 2004;86(8):1636-1645.
12. Herbert LM, Engsberg JR, Tedford KG, Grimston SK: A comparison of oxygen consumption during walking between children with and without below-knee amputations. *Phys Ther* 1994;74(10):943-950.
13. Jeans KA, Karol LA, Cummings D, Singhal K: Comparison of gait after Syme and transtibial amputation in children: Factors that may play a role in function. *J Bone Joint Surg Am* 2014;96(19):1641-1647.
14. McQuerry J, Gammon L, Carpiaux A, et al: Effect of amputation level on quality of life and subjective function in children. *J Pediatr Orthop* 2019;39(7):e524-e530.
15. Louer CR, Scott-Wyard P, Hernandez R, Vergun AD: Principles of amputation surgery, prosthetics, and rehabilitation in children. *J Am Acad Orthop Surg* 2021;29(14):e702-e713.
16. Varni JW, Setoguchi Y, Rappaport LR, Talbot D: Effects of stress, social support, and self-esteem on depression in children with limb deficiencies. *Arch Phys Med Rehabil* 1991;72:1053-1058.

17. Harris RI: Syme's amputation. The technical details essential for success. *J Bone Joint Surg* 1956;38-B:614-639.
18. Davidson WH, Bohne WH: The Syme amputation in children. *J Bone Joint Surg Am* 1975;57(7):905-909.
19. Scaduto AA, Bernstein RM: Syme and Boyd amputations for fibular deficiency, in Weisel SW, ed: *Operative Techniques in Orthopaedic Surgery*, ed 2. Lippincott Williams & Wilkins, 2016, pp 1630-1638.
20. Westin GW, Sakai DN, Wood WL: Congenital longitudinal deficiency of the fibula: Follow-up of treatment by Syme amputation. *J Bone Joint Surg Am* 1976;58(4)492-496.
21. Eilert RE, Jayakumar SS: Boyd and Syme ankle amputations in children. *J Bone Joint Surg Am* 1976;58(8):1138-1141.
22. Anderson L, Westin GW, Oppenheim WL: Syme amputation in children: Indications, results, and long-term follow-up. *J Pediatr Orthop* 1984;4(5):550-554.
23. Braaksma R, Dijkstra PU, Geertzen JH: Syme amputation: A systematic review. *Foot Ankle Int* 2018;39(3):284-291.
24. Birch JG, Walsh SJ, Small JM, et al: Syme amputation for the treatment of fibular deficiency. An evaluation of long-term physical and psychological functional status. *J Bone Joint Surg Am* 1999;81(11):1511-1518.
25. Smith NC, Stuck R, Carlson RM, Dux K, Sage R, Pinzur M: Correction of varus heel pad in patients with Syme's amputations. *J Foot Ankle Surg* 2012;51(3):394-397.
26. Bibbo C: Modification of the Syme amputation to prevent postoperative heel pad migration. *J Foot Ankle Surg* 2013;52(6):766-770.
27. Osebold WR, Lester EL, Christenson DM: Problems with excessive residual lower leg length in pediatric amputees. *Iowa Orthop J* 2001;21:58-67.
28. Morrison SG, Thomson P, Lenze U, Donnan LT: Syme amputation: Function, satisfaction, and prostheses. *J Pediatr Orthop* 2020;40(6):e532-e536.
29. Boyd HB: Amputation of the foot with calcaneotibial arthrodesis. *J Bone Joint Surg* 1939;21:997-1000.
30. Blum CE, Kalamchi A: Boyd amputations in children. *Clin Orthop Relat Res* 1982;165:138-143.
31. Westberry DE, Davids JR, Pugh LI: The Boyd amputation in children: Indications and outcomes. *J Pediatr Orthop* 2014;34(1):86-91.
32. Pfeil J, Marquardt E, Holtz T, Niethard FU, Schneider E, Carstens C: The stump capping procedure to prevent or treat terminal osseous overgrowth. *Prosthet Orthot Int* 1991;15(2):96-99.
33. Fedorak GT, Watts HG, Cuomo AV, et al: Osteocartilaginous transfer of the proximal part of the fibula for osseous overgrowth in children with congenital or acquired tibial amputation: Surgical technique and results. *J Bone Joint Surg Am* 2015;97(7):574-581.
34. Benevenia J, Makley JT, Leeson MC, Benevenia K: Primary epiphyseal transplants and bone overgrowth in childhood amputations. *J Pediatr Orthop* 1992;12(6):746-750.
35. Swanson AB: Bone overgrowth in the juvenile amputee and its control by the use of silicone rubber implants. *Interclin Inform Bull* 1969;8:9-18.
36. Tenholder M, Davids JR, Gruber HE, Blackhurst DW: Surgical management of juvenile amputation overgrowth with a synthetic cap. *J Pediatr Orthop* 2004;24(2):218-226.
37. Ertl J: Operationstechnik. Über Amputationsstümpfe. *Chirurgie* 1949;20:218-224.
38. Firth GB, Masquijo JJ, Kontio K: Transtibial Ertl amputation for children and adolescents: A case series and literature review. *J Child Orthop* 2011;5(5):357-362.
39. Drvaric DM, Kruger LM: Modified Ertl osteomyoplasty for terminal overgrowth in childhood limb deficiencies. *J Pediatr Orthop* 2001;21(3):392-394.
40. Taylor BC, Poka A: Osteomyoplastic transtibial amputation: The Ertl technique. *J Am Acad Orthop Surg* 2016;24(4):259-265.
41. Frick SL, Shoemaker S, Mubarak SJ: Altered fibular growth patterns after tibiofibular synostosis in children. *J Bone Joint Surg* 2001;83:247-254.
42. Segal LS, Crandall RC: Tibia vara deformity after below knee amputation and synostosis formation in children. *J Pediatr Orthop* 2009;29(2):120-123.
43. Ng VY, Berlet GC: Evolving techniques in foot and ankle amputation. *J Am Acad Orthop Surg* 2010;18(4):223-235.
44. Pinzur MS, Beck J, Himes R, Callaci J: Distal tibiofibular bone-bridging in transtibial amputation. *J Bone Joint Surg Am* 2008;90(12):2682-2687.
45. Dougherty PJ: Transtibial amputees from the Vietnam War: Twenty-eight-year follow-up. *J Bone Joint Surg Am* 2001;83:383-389.
46. Eldridge JC, Armstrong PF, Krajbich JI: Amputation stump lengthening with the Ilizarov technique. A case report. *Clin Orthop Relat Res* 1990;256:76-79.
47. Bowen RE, Struble SG, Setoguchi Y, Watts HG: Outcomes of lengthening short lower-extremity amputation stumps with planar fixators. *J Pediatr Orthop* 2005;25(4):543-547.

Partial Foot Deficiencies in Children

Robin C. Crandall, MD, FAAOS

ABSTRACT

Childhood partial foot amputations are commonly seen and occur from a variety of etiologies. Treatment plans for congenital as well as acquired partial foot amputations may be both surgical and nonsurgical. To achieve the best possible patient outcomes, it is helpful to be aware of treatment options, possible complications, and prosthetic choices.

Keywords: children; congenital foot loss; partial foot deficiencies; pediatric partial foot amputation

Introduction

There has been a steady increase in the percentage of partial foot amputations (PFAs) seen in pediatric limb deficiency clinics. With improved limb salvage techniques, including wound vacuum-assisted closure, free flap techniques, and improved infection control, a higher percentage of trauma patients have successful PFAs. Similarly, improved foot reconstruction techniques have yielded durable long-term partial foot survival in patients with congenital and neoplastic foot deficiencies.[1-5]

It is important to focus on pediatric patients with congenital or acquired partial foot deficiencies and review etiology, nonsurgical and surgical treatment, and prosthetic management.

Etiology

The etiologies of partial foot deficiencies in children are broad reaching. Based on data gathered at multiple limb deficiency centers, approximately 60% of amputations in children are caused by congenital factors and 40% result from other causes.[6] The exact incidence of childhood partial foot loss in the United States from trauma or congenital causes is unknown.

Acquired Partial Foot Loss

Acquired partial foot loss can result from trauma and amputation related to reconstructive procedures for syndromes associated with limb deficiencies, infection, and congenital or in utero causes. Acquired PFAs can result from vascular and ischemic causes secondary to cardiac or major vessel catheterization in young children or umbilical vessel catheterization in newborns.[7] Iatrogenic injury to blood vessels during foot reconstructive procedures in children can result in PFA. Traumatic foot amputations are usually caused by injuries from powered lawn mowers (PLMs), farm equipment or animals, machinery, motor vehicle crashes, train-related trauma (such as falling from a moving train or injury during boarding), and thermal damage (burn or frostbite). Another class of partial foot deficiency includes loss related to reconstructive procedures for focal gigantism syndromes such as neurofibromatosis, Proteus syndrome, vascular arteriovenous malformation syndrome, Klippel-Trénaunay-Weber syndrome, and macrodystrophia lipomatosa. Infection-related causes of limb loss include purpura fulminans and insensate foot with chronic ulceration or osteomyelitis, which often occur in individuals with diabetes, spinal cord injury, or myelomeningocele. Congenital or in utero causes of partial foot deficiency include transverse deficiencies (mid to proximal tarsal loss), longitudinal (medial or lateral) deficiencies, split-hand/split-foot syndrome, and fetal alcohol syndrome.

General Principles of Treatment

Greene and Cary[8] reported that functional results of PFA are better than amputation at a higher level if a sensate plantigrade foot can be achieved. The authors showed that a Chopart amputation with equinus contracture is functionally inferior to an ankle disarticulation (Syme) procedure. The goal of surgery should be pain-free ambulation and the ability to wear durable, realistic footwear. A composite tissue free flap is an excellent method for covering massive foot wounds, but it is useless if the foot is in a fixed equinus position and the patient is unable to walk. Delicate, nondurable split-thickness skin grafts over weight-bearing areas can allow wound closure, but a lack of durability is an important issue that may require revision to a higher level. Without the expertise of a prosthetist capable of fitting complex partial foot prostheses, amputation at these levels can often result in prosthetic failure.

Neither Dr. Crandall nor any immediate family member has received anything of value from or has stock or stock options held in a commercial company or institution related directly or indirectly to the subject of this chapter.

Traumatic Injuries

PLM Injuries

The perceived benefit of PFA can be lost if the patient requires a prosthesis that rigidly immobilizes the ankle.[9] Careful consideration must be used when planning how the remnant foot can be used functionally to prevent breakdown caused by pressure or shear stresses. Because children are usually very active, reinjury is a possibility. A team approach to care by surgeons and prosthetists is often required.

Many PFAs result from injuries caused by a PLM. PLM injuries, however, have gone down in a 25-year study of US emergency departments.[10] In a multicenter review of 144 children with traumatic injuries caused by a PLM, Loder et al[11] reported that the toes were the most often injured part of the foot (63%), with most of the injured children being bystanders or passengers on riding mowers. The injury resulted in an amputation present on admission in 59 children, with an additional 8 children requiring an amputation before hospital discharge. Of the 67 amputations, 51 were PFAs (40 at the toe level, 5 at the transmetatarsal level, and 6 at the Chopart level). Children injured by riding mowers were generally younger than those injured by push mowers (mean, 5.4 versus 11.0 years, respectively). It has been established that in pediatric patients a bimodal pattern of PLM injury rates exist, with a peak around 2 to 3 years and a second peak around 14 to 15 years. Back-over trauma is characteristic of the first peak, operator trauma the second.[10] Adult operators of riding or push mowers often use hearing and eye protection and are unaware of the presence and impending danger to a nearby child. Loder et al[11] reported that 85% of foot injuries in children could be prevented if children younger than 14 years were not permitted to operate a push or riding PLM or be present in the immediate mowing area. The Amputee Coalition of America has compiled a checklist of precautions to prevent PLM trauma.[12]

Complications and unsatisfactory results are common after a PLM injury. Nearly 10% of the patients in the Loder et al[11] study had residual infection or osteomyelitis, and a 50% complication rate was reported. Infection from PLM trauma commonly involves multiple organisms, including bacteria, fungi, and mycobacteria.[13] Daley and McIntyre[14] reported that infecting organisms such as *Stenotrophomonas maltophilia* are common in PLM injuries, making it difficult to use empiric antibiotic therapies. Repeated surgical débridement is usually needed. Skin breakdown and amputation at a higher level occur at high rates.[15,16]

The surgical team should evaluate the injured foot to determine the options for skin coverage and plan the final shape and functionality of the residual limb. Durable plantar skin should be saved whenever feasible (**Figure 1**). Physeal damage should be objectively assessed. Dormans et al[17] proposed a simple classification system of lower limb PLM injuries. Type I is a shredding-type injury, and type II is a paucilaceration. All of the shredding-type injuries required amputation because of the difficulty of limb salvage. In the group with a paucilaceration injury, excellent results were achieved with more minimalistic procedures. In all groups, 4.9 procedures per patient were required.

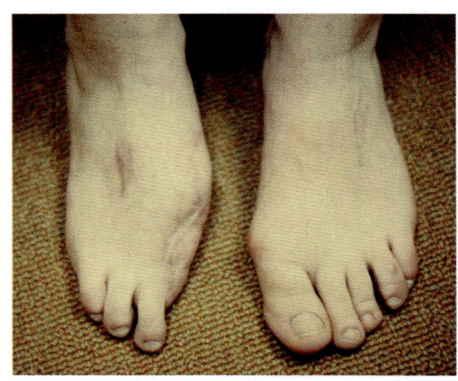

FIGURE 1 Photograph of the feet of a patient treated with a partial right foot amputation. Durable plantar skin is folded dorsally. Ray amputation was necessary in this patient to allow a smooth foot contour and easy fitting of a prosthetic shoe.

Microvascular free flap reconstruction and composite tissue grafting have been successfully used in the distal lower limbs; however, these procedures have a complication rate of at least 62%.[1] Children treated with reconstruction involving free flaps within 2 days of injury had lower complication rates.[1] PFA with free flap reconstruction in pediatric patients is problematic because children have small blood vessels. It is important to recognize that donor-site composite grafts may increase in bulk as the child ages, creating a residual limb that cannot be placed in a shoe (**Figure 2**).

Negative-pressure wound therapy has been shown to be valuable in management of large, soft-tissue injuries to the foot and ankle.[2,3] Shilt et al[3] specifically showed its effectiveness in PLM injuries in children. Incisional negative-pressure wound therapy has also been advocated.[18] However, shredding-type foot and ankle injuries should be managed with a high degree of caution. Families should be advised of the high complication rates and the possibility that revision at a higher amputation level may be needed.

Attempting to salvage a foot that will not allow plantigrade ambulation

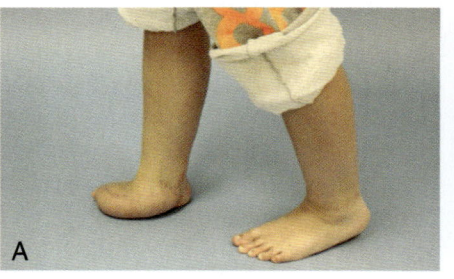 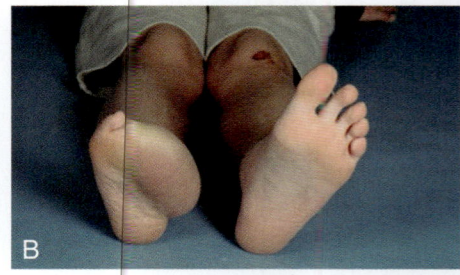

FIGURE 2 **A**, Photograph of the foot of a child with an injury caused by a PLM that necessitated a partial amputation of the right foot, with latissimus dorsi free flap coverage. **B**, Photograph showing the increase in the bulk of the latissimus dorsi free flap, which occurs with the child's growth and weight gain. Further revision surgery was needed.

is a substantial problem in reconstruction of traumatic partial foot injuries. If the foot is in severe equinus, painful, and unusable after a successful composite free flap procedure, amputation at a higher level may be needed. This scenario is particularly common with traumatic PLM injuries. With loss of dorsiflexors, the need to immobilize the residual limb in a weight-bearing position is important. This becomes increasingly difficult in more-proximal foot amputations, such as those at the Lisfranc (tarsometatarsal) or Chopart (midtarsal) levels. If functional ankle dorsiflexion cannot be achieved, a Boyd amputation or Syme ankle disarticulation may be preferable at the initial surgery as opposed to later when additional subjective issues may play a role. A limb that heals in equinus can be one of the most difficult limbs to fit with a prosthesis (**Figures 3** and **4**).

A massive, shredding traumatic injury to the hindfoot can be a particularly difficult injury to manage when caused by a PLM or other machinery (**Figure 5**). Extensive hindfoot and intercalary loss can be managed successfully with a calcanectomy and a subsequent ankle-foot orthosis with a spacer block to substitute for heel loss.[19] High failure rates can be expected with severe hindfoot salvage surgery.[20] Failure of a calcanectomy with an intact forefoot may require a Syme disarticulation with an anterior flap.

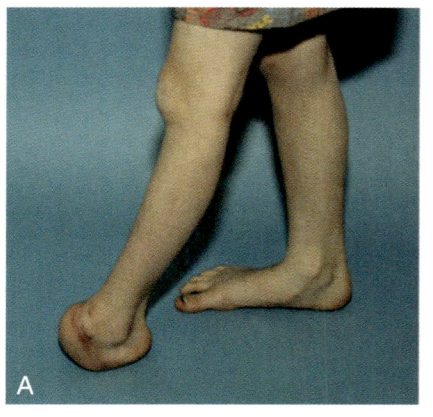
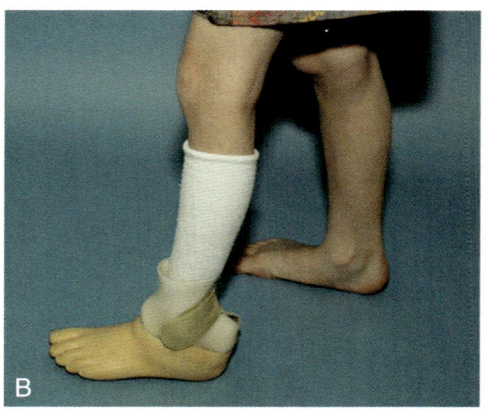
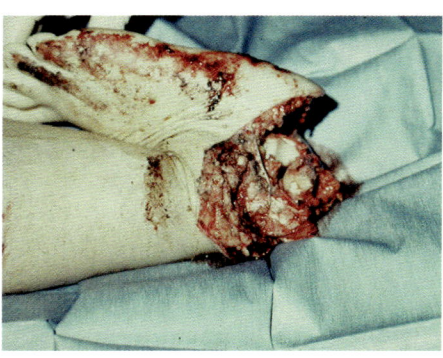

FIGURE 3 Photographs of the foot of a child who has undergone a PFA at the Chopart level. **A**, Equinus contracture developed in the postoperative interval. **B**, Because equinus contracture makes it difficult to obtain a good prosthetic fit, the perceived benefit of a Chopart-level PFA may be inferior to the functionality that could be obtained with amputation at a higher level.

FIGURE 5 Photograph of the lower limb of an adolescent with massive shredding hindfoot trauma. This type of injury can occasionally be managed with calcanectomy and intercalary bone excision, but multiple débridements and a high complication rate should be expected.

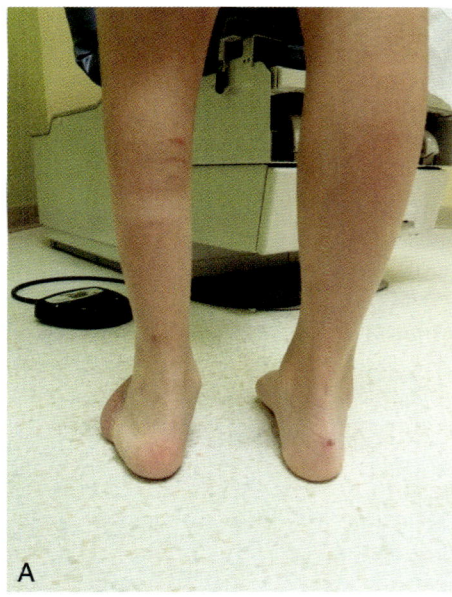
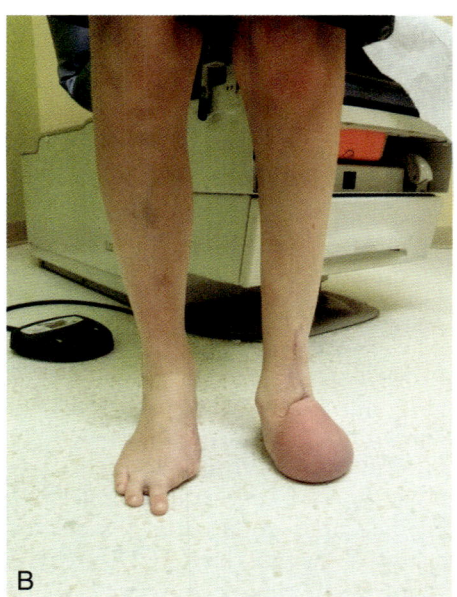
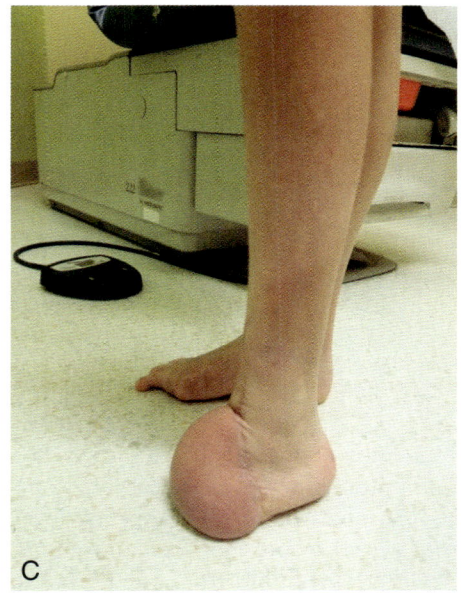

FIGURE 4 Photographs from an 11-year-old patient 5 years after bilateral PLM trauma treated with primary distal PFA on right and two separate free flap procedures on left for PFA Chopart salvage (**A** through **C**). Final latissimus free flap side has required several debulking procedures and Achilles tendon release and is insensate. In addition, significant postinjury calf atrophy brings into question long-term risk and benefits of this level selection versus primary Syme or Boyd level.

Farm-Related Injuries

PFA in children frequently results from injuries sustained on a farm. In a series of farm-related injuries analyzed by Cogbill et al,[21] 46% of the injuries were related to machinery and tractors, with the remaining injuries caused by animals or falls. In the Borne et al[22] review of all pediatric amputations over a 5-year period, machinery was listed as the second most common mechanism with 18% being toe injuries. In a study by McClure and Shaughnessy[23] of farm injuries in children requiring amputation, all the injuries were open type IIIC Gustilo fractures and had polymicrobial contamination. In a 3-year study of farm injuries in 292 children, Lubicky and Feinberg[24] noted that most of the injuries occurred in the lower limbs and that the average age of the injured children was 11.9 years. Although the authors did not specify how many of the children required a PFA, they noted that 41 of 127 open fractures (32%) occurred in the tarsal or metatarsal toe areas.

The general principles of managing foot injury from farm-related causes are similar to those used in managing PLM trauma. The wounds are often infected with multiple contaminants, and multiple procedures are needed to achieve a successful residual limb. It is important to achieve durable skin coverage. Polfer et al[25] noted that split-thickness skin grafts may be successful in salvaging limb length but should be regarded as staging procedures. For farming families with limited financial resources, those who live in certain ethnic communities, and those with limited access to tertiary care centers, the ability to wear normal footwear is of utmost importance.[26]

Motor Vehicle and Train-Related Injuries

In a study by Loder[27] of 256 traumatic amputations in children, the third and fourth most common injuries involved motor vehicle and train-related trauma. Train-related injuries often occur in the process of boarding or jumping from a moving train. Although Loder[27] did not specify the incidence of PFAs from train-related trauma, 10 of 24 train-related injuries in his study occurred in the lower limbs. Because wounds from train-related injuries tend to be sharper and cleaner than injuries from PLM and farm-related trauma, fewer débridements may be needed and wound closure may be easier.

Jawadi[28] recently reported on 21 cases of PFA in young children related to all-terrain vehicle injuries. These children often had bare or sandaled feet, which offered little protection from injury. Loder[27] reported substantial seasonal variation in pediatric amputations caused by motor vehicle injuries, with more amputations occurring in June and July and many involving young drivers. Specific data and follow-up regarding PFAs from motor vehicle trauma in children are unknown, but skin breakdown and traumatic PFA have been reported in the adult population after motor vehicle injuries.[15,16]

Thermal Injuries

Frostbite injuries can result in PFA in children because they are particularly vulnerable to these injuries, along with elderly people, individuals with alcoholism, and drug users. Very young children often cannot or do not communicate that they are very cold, do not recognize the symptoms of impending frostbite, and may stay outside for long periods with improper footwear for protection from the cold. Boles et al[29] noted that in older children, lack of supervision and intoxication played major roles.

In a review by Miller and Chasmar[30] of 101 patients admitted to hospitals with frostbite injuries in Canada, it was found that rapid rewarming and adequate delay before conservative débridement or surgical amputation were important treatment principles. The authors reported on the need to allow demarcation to occur to clearly show the location of the full-thickness injury. Other studies have indicated that after 5 days, scintigraphy and MRI may be useful in determining viable tissue.[31,32] Golant et al[33] recommended rewarming of the affected limb at 104° to 107.6° for 15 to 30 minutes and avoidance of rewarming until definitive medical care is involved. In a study of young adults, frostbite that occurred at high altitude was the best predictor of amputation outcome.[34]

Sharp demarcation between viable and nonviable tissue may indicate that a PFA is necessary. Imray et al[35] thought that the unwillingness to delay surgery was a major cause of avoidable morbidity. The authors suggested that no surgical intervention should occur without a waiting period of 6 to 12 weeks after injury.

It is important to carefully follow the pediatric patient for possible evidence of physeal damage that can occur with thermal injury. Frostbite injuries in the foot can look similar to injuries from purpura fulminans. The physician should wait at least several weeks before débridement and amputation. The management of acute frostbite injury to prevent possible amputation includes thrombolytic agents, hyperbaric oxygen, and prostacyclin.[36-39] Databases are needed to extract the exact incidence of PFAs caused by frostbite injuries in children.[40]

Burns from either electrical or thermal sources also can result in severe tissue damage necessitating PFA. A PFA was reported in a patient with neurologic loss caused by a third-degree burn from a laptop computer.[41]

Nontraumatic Partial Foot Amputation

Focal Gigantism Syndromes

Focal gigantism syndromes involving portions of the foot and the toes can necessitate PFA. In children, these syndromes include vascular arteriovenous malformation syndrome, neurofibromatosis, Proteus syndrome, Klippel-Trénaunay-Weber syndrome, and macrodystrophia lipomatosa. It is important that all abnormal tissue be removed in a soft-tissue or bony reduction to prevent the growth of residual abnormal tissue as the child grows. Central ray PFA is often needed in patients with these syndromes (**Figure 6**). Khan et al[42] reported on four cases of macrodystrophia lipomatosa, which is characterized by enlargement of the second or third digits of the hands or

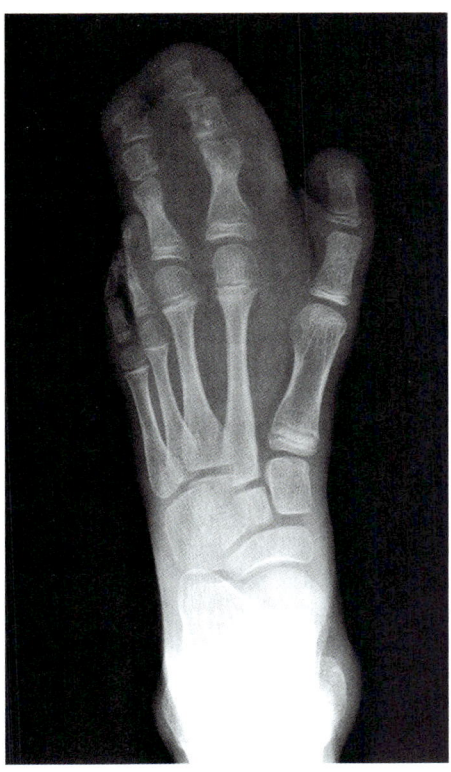

FIGURE 6 Standing radiograph of the foot of a patient with classic macrodystrophia lipomatosa. The second and third toes are enlarged and the remainder of foot is normal. A distal toe amputation with physeal ablation of metatarsal heads two and three can allow successful shoe wear. Central ray PFA may become necessary.

feet. MRI is useful in the diagnosis of this syndrome because it shows adipose tissue in subcutaneous areas without encapsulation. A diagnosis of macrodystrophia lipomatosa can be difficult to make because the symptoms are similar to those of Proteus syndrome.[43-45] The visual manifestations of any of the focal gigantism syndromes can be nearly identical.

Treatments of focal gigantism syndromes involving the foot are similar to each other. Often, inequalities occur that require physeal manipulation at a later time as the child ages. Physeal growth arrest of metatarsals and even phalanges are sometimes used together with distal phalangeal amputation to maintain a reasonable foot size. The child will need a shoe similar in size to the contralateral unaffected side. Tissue debulking with segmental ray resection or PFA is frequently required.

In children with Proteus syndrome, tissues that initially appear relatively normal may enlarge, and amputation at a higher level may be required. In focal gigantism syndromes, it is important to carefully evaluate the child's limb length to allow planning for physeal manipulation as needed.

Infection

Purpura fulminans represents an important cause of PFA in children. Many children with this infection have quadrimembral involvement. Purpura fulminans generally occurs in children younger than 5 years after an acute bacterial or a viral infection; the rate of amputation is 60%.[46] Neonatal purpura fulminans is rare and is associated with congenital protein C deficiency.[47] Risk factors for purpura fulminans include age younger than 5 years and the presence of factor V *G1691A* mutation. Gürgey et al[46] suggest that all patients with purpura fulminans be screened for this mutation and receive anticoagulation therapy to prevent further necrosis. Purpura fulminans has been associated with *Meningococcus*, *Streptococcus*, *Pneumococcus*, *Staphylococcus aureus*, and varicella and rubella viral diseases. The thrombosis that occurs in purpura fulminans is widespread and microvascular. Large amounts of tissue necrosis and loss are common.

The orthopaedic surgeon is often consulted when the child has severely swollen limbs. This clinical appearance can suggest that a transtibial amputation may be needed; however, at this stage of the disease the problem is not the infection but the associated underlying tissue necrosis and substantial swelling. Viable tissue is often present despite the swelling and edema. Waiting for demarcation to occur is critically important. A child who appears to need a transtibial amputation may eventually require only a PFA (**Figure 7**). Amputation at a higher level may be needed, but it should be performed only after a minimum of 4 to 6 weeks of observation. The skin and subcutaneous tissues of residual limbs after purpura fulminans are generally thin, somewhat dystrophic, and often have multiple split-thickness skin grafts. Consultation with an experienced prosthetist is important for achieving the best functional outcome for the child.

PFA in a child can occur because of infections involving failed foot reconstruction; insensate feet, as seen in spinal cord injury; and myelomeningocele. Deep heel ulcers in patients with spinal cord injury and myelomeningocele may require hindfoot amputation and calcanectomy.[2] In a study of 36 ambulatory patients with sacral-level myelomeningocele, 11 of the patients required a total of 14 amputation procedures.[48] Nine of these procedures were PFAs. In this particular population, ambulation on insensate feet can be a significant problem. Although this study involved adult patients, the treatment principles also apply to pediatric patients who are active community ambulators.

Neoplasms

Neoplasms involving the soft tissue or bone of the foot are rare. The most common neoplasm is rhabdomyosarcoma, which occurs more often in boys than girls. In younger children, rhabdomyosarcoma more commonly occurs in the head, the neck, and the pelvis. In adolescents, tumors are most commonly seen in the limbs. Synovial sarcoma can occur in teenagers, with lower-grade lesions generally found around the hands and feet. Chou et al[49] reported that in 2,660 surgically treated musculoskeletal tumors in children and adults, only 5.7% involved the foot or ankle.

Local radiation therapy with surgical resection of the lesion to retain function of the foot has been recommended rather than primary amputation at a higher level.[4] Local radiation, however, is controversial because of complications and adverse side effects seen at long-term follow-ups. Its use in children's feet largely has been abandoned in favor of wider surgical excision. It is important to note that surgical resection with adequate margins in the foot can be difficult to obtain without underlying ray or combined ray amputation.

Children with a neoplastic foot lesion should have a thorough evaluation at a tertiary oncology care center

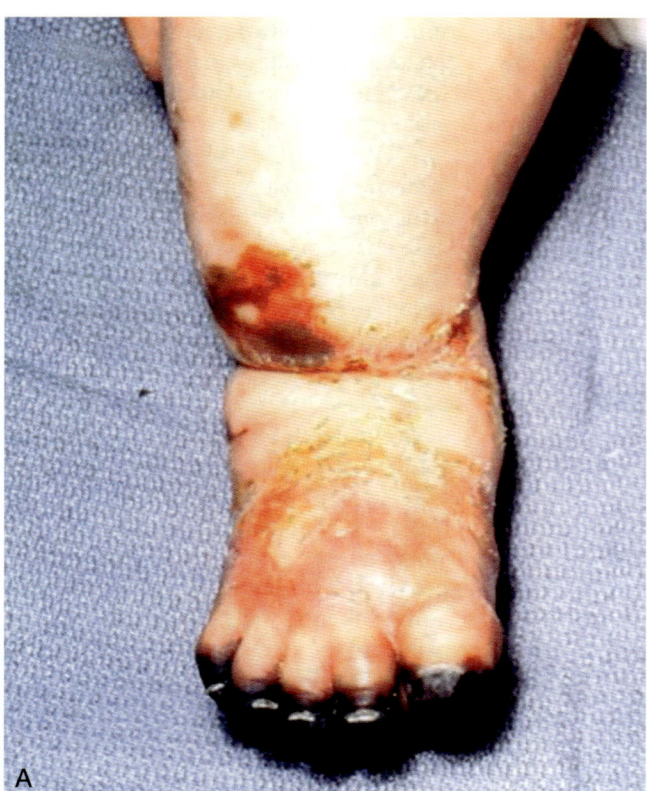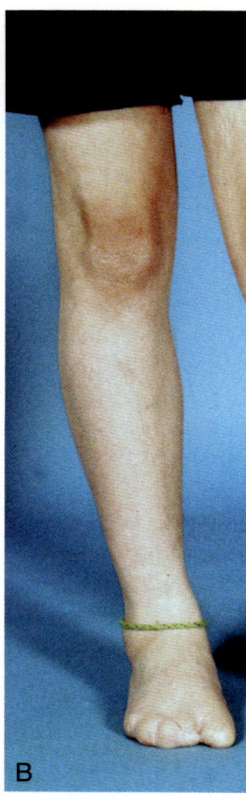

FIGURE 7 **A**, Photograph of the distal lower limb of a child with purpura fulminans. In the early stages of the disease, it may appear that a transtibial amputation is necessary. **B**, Photograph of the limb at a later age. By waiting for full demarcation before choosing the definitive amputation level, the child was treated with a PFA and had only minimal functional loss.

and should be referred to an oncology center for treatment. A diagnosis of rhabdomyosarcoma is made in approximately 250 pediatric patients each year, with 65% of the tumors occurring in children younger than 6 years.[50]

Many types of malignant osseous tumors have been reported in the foot. The most common osseous tumor in children involving the foot may be Ewing sarcoma.[51] Management of pediatric and adolescent bone tumors in the foot has greatly evolved. Long-term survivability has increased, with amputation and limb salvage having similar long-term outcomes.[5] Partial foot salvage in these individuals may fail, however, if a plantigrade, sensate residual foot cannot be achieved.

Congenital Causes of Partial Foot Deficiencies

Transverse Deficiencies of the Foot

Transverse deficiencies of the foot not associated with constriction band syndrome are decidedly more rare than transverse defects in the upper limb. The most common transverse deficiency occurs in the forearm. The International Organization for Standardization describes limb deficiencies by stating the missing elements. For example, a transverse deficiency of the foot is described as phalanges all, metatarsals 1 through 5 incomplete. Because this method is somewhat cumbersome, this deficiency also may be described as a transverse partial foot deficiency. Deficiency can occur at the phalangeal, tarsal, or metatarsal level.

The skin covering the partial foot in children tends to be robust, and prosthetic intervention often is not needed. Limb length inequality should be evaluated. Children with transverse deficiencies may have dysplasia of the entire lower limb; failure to address the difference in limb length can result in an awkward and cosmetically displeasing partial foot prosthesis (**Figure 8**).

In a small study, Jain and Lakhtakia[52] found that hindfoot transverse defects were less common than forefoot transverse defects. Transverse deficiencies are sporadic in nature and not generally associated with other visceral defects. Transverse deficiencies of the foot can occur if the apical ectodermal ridge is removed during embryogenesis.[53] This ridge is one of the three signaling centers that affect limb development. These limb defects are thought to be caused by mechanical and vascular factors, with no specific heritability patterning. Partial foot deficiency can be seen with coagulation deficiency and sometimes after prenatal sampling of chorionic villi.[54,55] As with many congenital limb defects, these deficiencies can often be detected prenatally with fetal ultrasonography.[56]

The exact incidence of transverse foot defects not associated with constriction band or chorionic villi sampling is unknown. Drugs that may create vascular-related partial foot defects include ergotamine and misoprostol. In a study by McGuirk et al[57] of 161,252 births in the Boston area, the prevalence rate of limb reduction defects as a result of presumed vascular disruption was 0.22 per 1,000 births. In this large series, eight children had partial foot deficiencies, three of these children had constriction band syndromes, and one had split-hand/split-foot syndrome.

Longitudinal Deficiencies of the Foot

Longitudinal deficiencies of the foot are generally associated with longitudinal long bone deficiency. This is particularly true with all types of fibular deficiencies with associated lateral ray loss. Some of these patients are considered to have partial foot deficiencies because of minimal limb-length discrepancy and the use of leg lengthening procedures; however, most of these patients are treated with foot ablation if leg length is projected to be short. An exception is a child with bilateral plantigrade feet and similar leg lengths (**Figure 9**). Medial longitudinal deficiencies of the foot that are not associated with long bone deficiency are extremely rare and may be associated with constriction band syndromes. It is important to carefully examine hindfoot function in any longitudinal foot deficiency to evaluate for limb-length discrepancies and tarsal coalitions. Some isolated longitudinal medial foot deficiencies can be seen with Goltz syndrome and fetal alcohol syndrome.[57-59]

Bilateral longitudinal fibular deficiency often is associated with lateral PFA. Because the feet are plantigrade, no higher amputation level is needed, and the patient is fitted with a partial foot prosthesis.

Amniotic Band Syndrome

Amniotic band syndrome is a relatively common cause of PFA. This syndrome occurs in 1 in 10,000 births.[60] These patients may have numerous other organ system involvements, and all four limbs often are affected. Although each manifestation of the syndrome is essentially different, involvement of the lower limbs is common. Digital ring constrictions, distal atrophy, intrauterine transverse or longitudinal deficiencies, syndactyly, and clubfoot can occur in the lower limbs.[61] Digital amputation is frequently necessary in these patients. Constriction band release, however, may salvage a foot or a partial foot.[62] Although not generally considered an inherited condition, many predisposing factors, including maternal smoking, drug use, hyperglycemia, hypertension, amniocentesis, and first-degree relatives with the syndrome, have been identified in patients with constriction band syndrome.[63] Some theories suggest that amniotic band syndrome is the result of a vascular insult early in embryogenesis.[54]

Split-Hand/Split-Foot Syndrome

Split-hand/split-foot syndrome, also known as ectrodactyly-ectodermal dysplasia, is thought to be an autosomal dominant condition in which a variety of systems can be involved.[64] Recently, using chromosomal mapping, 12 different types of split-hand/split-foot syndrome have been identified.[65] If the degree of foot involvement allows the use of normal footwear, surgical intervention may be unnecessary. Often, however, one limb may be more involved than the other, creating the need for reconstruction and possible PFA. The goal is to allow the patient to use normal footwear (**Figure 10**).

Prosthetic Choices

Prosthetic choices for children with a PFA or deficiency have evolved considerably over the past 2 decades. Custom-made leather, lacing-type prostheses

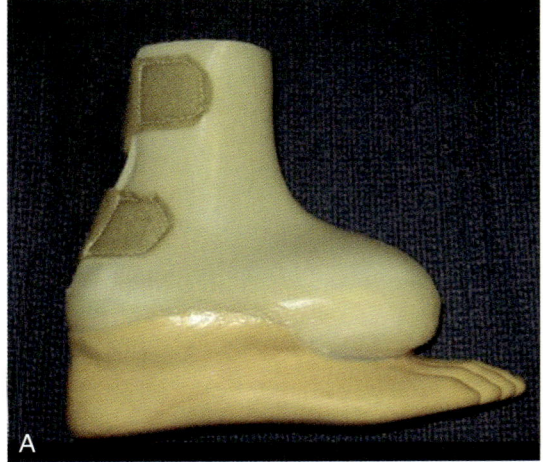
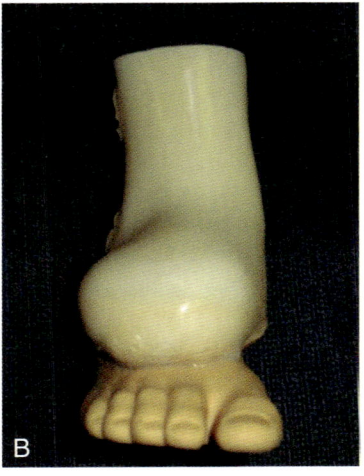

FIGURE 8 Careful observation of limb-length discrepancy is important in children to prevent the necessity for a cosmetically displeasing prosthesis. Lateral (**A**) and AP (**B**) views of a foot prosthesis for a patient with a limb-length discrepancy.

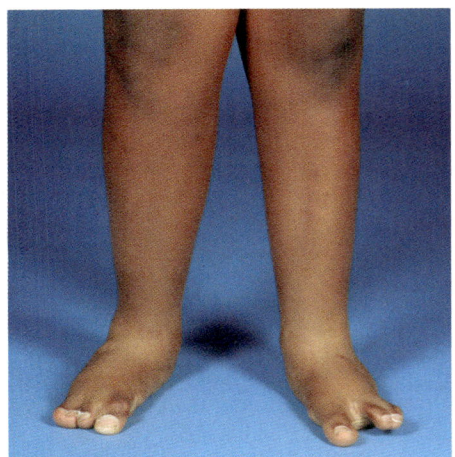

FIGURE 9 Clinical photograph of the lower limbs of a child with a bilateral longitudinal fibular deficiency and lateral ray loss. Because the child has plantigrade feet, amputation at a higher level is not necessary.

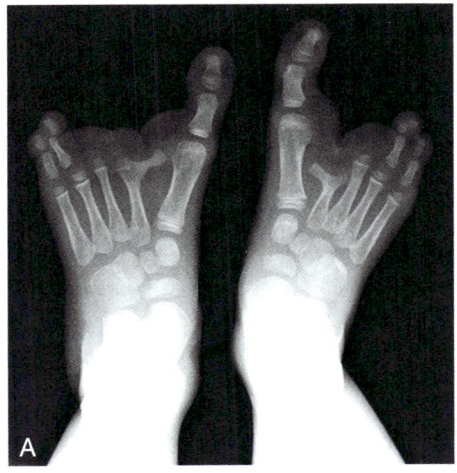
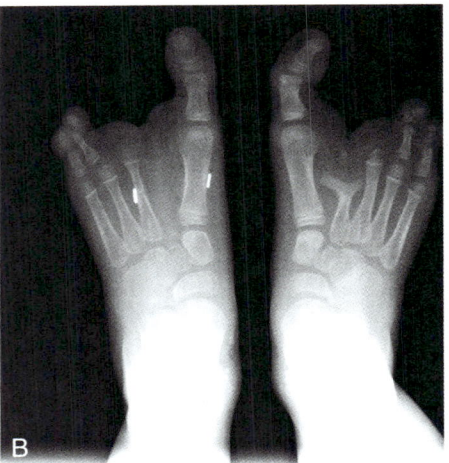

FIGURE 10 A, Standing preoperative radiograph of the feet of a patient with split-hand/split-foot syndrome. The left foot is wider than the right foot. **B,** Postoperative radiograph taken after intercalary resection of the second metatarsal of the foot, with use of a cross metatarsal suture anchor. The procedure narrowed the left foot, allowing easier shoe wear.

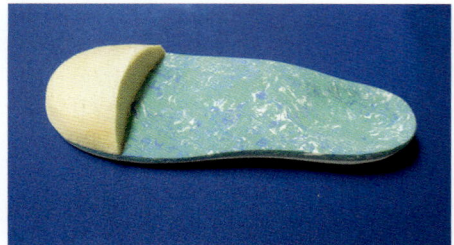

FIGURE 11 Photograph of a simple foam filler, which can be attached to an orthotic device in a patient with partial foot loss.

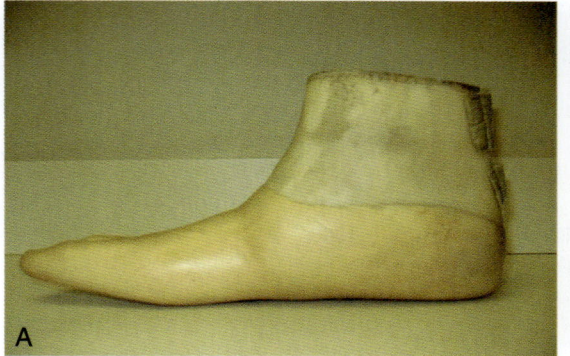

FIGURE 12 Lateral (**A**) and AP (**B**) views of a prosthetic foamer foot, which is used in midlevel to proximal level PFAs.

have been replaced with sophisticated, lifelike molded synthetic constructs. In children with simple metatarsophalangeal loss, toe spacers and foam shoe fillers may suffice (**Figure 11**). Most children with simple toe loss or even multiple toe loss can ambulate with no observable gait abnormalities.[9] Dillon and Fatone[66] reported that after metatarsal heads are compromised, foot length becomes an issue, and the center of pressure remains behind the residual limb until after contralateral heel contact. Patients with very short PFA levels may benefit from ankle immobilization with a relatively stiff forefoot prosthesis.

At the institution of this chapter's author (Twin Cities Shriners Hospital, Minneapolis, MN), success has been reported with a "foamer foot" construct, using a prosthetic foot shell alone without rigid ankle immobilization (unpublished data) (**Figure 12**). Impregnation of fabric within the plastic foot shell has markedly increased its durability. In this construct, the residual limb is placed in an alginate mold in a semi–weight-bearing seated position with the knee in 90° of flexion. The plaster impression is then modified by building up plaster over bony prominences and removing plaster around the ankle circumference. This results in more space over bony prominences, with less space around the ankle to accommodate stretching of the prosthesis. The final prosthesis has proven extremely durable in 12 pediatric patients fitted with a foamer foot construct after PFA (unpublished data). This prosthesis is less expensive than typical prostheses used for ankle disarticulation or Chopart-level amputations and offers excellent cosmesis and function. In an analysis of 141 clinical visits, only two patients required a visit more than once per year (unpublished data). During molding and construction, Zarezadeh et al[67] have incorporated force-pressure sensors facilitating the use of different silicone densities to improve function of the PFA prosthesis. Additional objective data are needed for prosthetic models for PFA. More objective data are needed regarding different prosthetic models for PFA.

SUMMARY

Various etiologies, such as traumatic, syndrome-related, congenital, infectious, and vascular, are often the reason for PFA in children. Durable skin coverage and obtaining a plantigrade foot are essential for a successful PFA. In patients with congenital deficiency or gigantism syndrome, leg-length inequality must be assessed. An experienced prosthetist is needed to fabricate pediatric prosthetic devices for amputations and deficiencies at more proximal levels of the lower limb. An experienced prosthetist is needed to fabricate PFA prosthetic devices that are comfortable and durable in highly active pediatric patients.

References

1. Rinker B, Valerio IL, Stewart DH, Pu LL, Vasconez HC: Microvascular free flap reconstruction in pediatric lower extremity trauma: A 10-year review. *Plast Reconstr Surg* 2005;115(6):1618-1624.
2. Lee HJ, Kim JW, Oh CW, et al: Negative pressure wound therapy for soft tissue injuries around the foot and ankle. *J Orthop Surg Res* 2009;4:14.
3. Shilt JS, Yoder JS, Manuck TA, Jacks L, Rushing C, Smith BP: Role of vacuum-assisted closure in the treatment of pediatric lawnmower injuries. *J Pediatr Orthop* 2004;24(5):482-487.
4. La TH, Wolden SL, Su Z, et al: Local therapy for rhabdomyosarcoma of the hands and feet: Is amputation necessary? A report from the Children's Oncology Group. *Int J Radiat Oncol Biol Phys* 2011;80(1):206-212.
5. Nagarajan R, Neglia JP, Clohisy DR, Robison LL: Limb salvage and amputation in survivors of pediatric lower-extremity bone tumors: What are the long-term implications? *J Clin Oncol* 2002;20(22):4493-4501.
6. Tooms RE: Acquired amputations in children, in Bowker JH, Michael JW, eds: *Atlas of Limb Prosthetics: Surgical, Prosthetic, and Rehabilitation Principles*, ed 2. Mosby-Year Book, 1992, pp 735-742.
7. Alpert J, O'Donnell JA, Parsonnet V, Brief DK, Brener BJ, Goldenkranz RJ: Clinically recognized limb ischemia in the neonate after umbilical artery catheterization. *Am J Surg* 1980;140(3):413-418.
8. Greene WB, Cary JM: PFAs in children: A comparison of the several types with the Syme amputation. *J Bone Joint Surg Am* 1982;64(3):438-443.
9. Dillon MP, Barker TM: Comparison of gait of persons with PFA wearing prosthesis to matched control group: Observational study. *J Rehabil Res Dev* 2008;45(9):1317-1334.
10. Ren KS, Chounthirath T, Yang J, Friedenberg L, Smith GA: Children treated for lawn mower-related injuries in US emergency departments, 1990-2014. *Am J Emerg Med* 2017;35(6):893-898.

11. Loder RT, Brown KL, Zaleske DJ, Jones ET: Extremity lawn-mower injuries in children: Report by the Research Committee of the Pediatric Orthopaedic Society of North America. *J Pediatr Orthop* 1997;17(3):360-369.
12. PLM accidents are the leading cause of major amputations for children under 10. Available at: http://www.cirsop.com/news/lawn-mower-accidents-are-leading-cause-major-amputations-children-under-10. Accessed April 7, 2015.
13. Harkness B, Andresen D, Kesson A, Isaacs D: Infections following lawn-mower and farm machinery-related injuries in children. *J Paediatr Child Health* 2009;45(9):525-528.
14. Daley AJ, McIntyre PB: Stenotrophomonas maltophilia and PLM injuries in children. *J Trauma* 2000;48(3):536-537.
15. Lange TA, Nasca RJ: Traumatic PFA. *Clin Orthop Relat Res* 1984;185:137-141.
16. Mueller MJ, Allen BT, Sinacore DR: Incidence of skin breakdown and higher amputation after transmetatarsal amputation: Implications for rehabilitation. *Arch Phys Med Rehabil* 1995;76(1):50-54.
17. Dormans JP, Azzoni M, Davidson RS, Drummond DS: Major lower extremity PLM injuries in children. *J Pediatr Orthop* 1995;15(1):78-82.
18. Zayan NE, West JM, Schulz SA, Jordan SW, Valerio IL: Incisional negative pressure wound therapy: An effective tool for major limb amputation and amputation revision site closure. *Adv Wound Care* 2019;8(8):368-373.
19. Crandall RC, Wagner FW Jr: Partial and total calcanectomy: A review of thirty-one consecutive cases over a ten-year period. *J Bone Joint Surg Am* 1981;63(1):152-155.
20. Penn-Barwell JG, Bennett PM, Gray AC: The 'could' and the 'should' of reconstructing severe hind-foot injuries. *Injury* 2018;49(2):147-148.
21. Cogbill TH, Busch HM Jr, Stiers GR: Farm accidents in children. *Pediatrics* 1985;76(4):562-566.
22. Borne A, Porter A, Recicar J, Maxson T, Montgomery C: Pediatric traumatic amputations in the United States: A 5-Year Review. *J Pediatr Orthop* 2017;37(2):e104-e107.
23. McClure SK, Shaughnessy WJ: Farm-related limb amputations in children. *J Pediatr Orthop* 2005;25(2):133-137.
24. Lubicky JP, Feinberg JR: Fractures and amputations in children and adolescents requiring hospitalization after farm equipment injuries. *J Pediatr Orthop* 2009;29(5):435-438.
25. Polfer EM, Tintle SM, Forsberg JA, Potter BK: Skin grafts for residual limb coverage and preservation of amputation length. *Plast Reconstr Surg* 2015;136(3):603-609.
26. Land M: Ethical dilemmas in the health care of the pediatric amish population. Available at: https://med.uth.edu/mcgovern/files/2014/10/land.pdf. Accessed April 7, 2015.
27. Loder RT: Demographics of traumatic amputations in children: Implications for prevention strategies. *J Bone Joint Surg Am* 2004;86(5):923-928.
28. Jawadi AH: Traumatic foot amputation in young children secondary to all-terrain vehicles: A case series. *Injury* 2011;42(11):1380-1383.
29. Boles R, Gawaziuk JP, Cristall N, Logsetty S: Pediatric frostbite: A 10-year single-center retrospective study. *Burns* 2018;44(7):1844-1850.
30. Miller BJ, Chasmar LR: Frostbite in Saskatoon: A review of 10 winters. *Can J Surg* 1980;23(5):423-426.
31. Bhatnagar A, Sarker BB, Sawroop K, Chopra MK, Sinha N, Kashyap R: Diagnosis, characterisation and evaluation of treatment response of frostbite using pertechnetate scintigraphy: A prospective study. *Eur J Nucl Med Mol Imaging* 2002;29(2):170-175.
32. Barker JR, Haws MJ, Brown RE, Kucan JO, Moore WD: Magnetic resonance imaging of severe frostbite injuries. *Ann Plast Surg* 1997;38(3):275-279.
33. Golant A, Nord RM, Paksima N, Posner MA: Cold exposure injuries to the extremities. *J Am Acad Orthop Surg* 2008;16(12):704-715.
34. Carceller A, Javierre C, Ríos M, Viscor G: Amputation risk factors in severely frostbitten patients. *Int J Environ Res Public Health* 2019;16(8):1351.
35. Imray C, Grieve A, Dhillon S, Caudwell Xtreme Everest Research Group: Cold damage to the extremities: Frostbite and non-freezing cold injuries. *Postgrad Med J* 2009;85(1007):481-488.
36. Cauchy E, Cheguillaume B, Chetaille E: A controlled trial of a prostacyclin and rt-PA in the treatment of severe frostbite. *N Engl J Med* 2011;364(2):189-190.
37. Bruen KJ, Ballard JR, Morris SE, Cochran A, Edelman LS, Saffle JR: Reduction of the incidence of amputation in frostbite injury with thrombolytic therapy. *Arch Surg* 2007;142(6):546-551.
38. Twomey JA, Peltier GL, Zera RT: An open-label study to evaluate the safety and efficacy of tissue plasminogen activator in treatment of severe frostbite. *J Trauma* 2005;59(6):1350-1354.
39. Cauchy E, Chetaille E, Marchand V, Marsigny B: Retrospective study of 70 cases of severe frostbite lesions: A proposed new classification scheme. *Wilderness Environ Med* 2001;12(4):248-255.
40. Cochran A: *Coming in From the Cold: Management of Frostbite*. University of Utah Grand Rounds, 2011. Available at: http://www.slideshare.net/amaliacochran/frostbite-grand-rounds-2011. Accessed March 4, 2015.
41. Paprottka FJ, Machens HG, Lohmeyer JA: Third-degree burn leading to PFA: Why a notebook is no laptop. *J Plast Reconstr Aesthet Surg* 2012;65(8):1119-1122.
42. Khan RA, Wahab S, Ahmad I, Chana RS: Macrodystrophia lipomatosa: Four case reports. *Ital J Pediatr* 2010;36:69.
43. Kwon JH, Lim SY, Lim HS: Macrodystrophia lipomatosa. *Arch Plast Surg* 2013;40(3):270-272.
44. Blacksin M, Barnes FJ, Lyons MM: MR diagnosis of macrodystrophia lipomatosa. *AJR Am J Roentgenol* 1992;158(6):1295-1297.
45. Biesecker L: The challenges of Proteus syndrome: Diagnosis and management. *Eur J Hum Genet* 2006;14(11):1151-1157.
46. Gürgey A, Aytac S, Kanra G, Secmeer G, Ceyhan M, Altay C: Outcome in children with purpura fulminans: Report on 16 patients. *Am J Hematol* 2005;80(1):20-25.
47. Jafarri SA, AlAttas KM, Bajawi SM, et al: Neonatal purpura fulminans in newborn with severe congenital protein C deficiency: Case report. *J Dermatol Dermatol Surg* 2017;21(2):104-106.
48. Brinker MR, Rosenfeld SR, Feiwell E, Granger SP, Mitchell DC, Rice JC: Myelomeningocele at the sacral level: Long-term outcomes in adults. *J Bone Joint Surg Am* 1994;76(9):1293-1300.
49. Chou LB, Ho YY, Malawer MM: Tumors of the foot and ankle: Experience with 153 cases. *Foot Ankle Int* 2009;30(9):836-841.
50. Dagher R, Helman L: Rhabdomyosarcoma: An overview. *Oncologist* 1999;4(1):34-44.
51. Ruggieri P, Angelini A, Jorge FD, Maraldi M, Giannini S: Review of foot tumors seen in a university tumor institute. *J Foot Ankle Surg* 2014;53(3):282-285.

52. Jain S, Lakhtakia PK: Profile of congenital transverse deficiencies among cases of congenital orthopaedic anomalies. *J Orthop Surg* 2002;10(1):45-52.
53. Kozin SH: Upper-extremity congenital anomalies. *J Bone Joint Surg Am* 2003;85(8):1564-1576.
54. Hunter AG: A pilot study of the possible role of familial defects in anticoagulation as a cause for terminal limb reduction malformations. *Clin Genet* 2000;57(3):197-204.
55. Chitayat D, Silver MM, O'Brien K, et al: Limb defects in homozygous alpha-thalassemia: Report of three cases. *Am J Med Genet* 1997;68(2):162-167.
56. Ermito S, Dinatale A, Carrara S, Cavaliere A, Imbruglia L, Recupero S: Prenatal diagnosis of limb abnormalities: Role of fetal ultrasonography. *J Prenat Med* 2009;3(2):18-22.
57. McGuirk CK, Westgate M-N, Holmes LB: Limb deficiencies in newborn infants. *Pediatrics* 2001;108(4):E64.
58. Pauli RM, Feldman PF: Major limb malformations following intrauterine exposure to ethanol: Two additional cases and literature review. *Teratology* 1986;33(3):273-280.
59. van Rensburg LJ: Major skeletal defects in the fetal alcohol syndrome: A case report. *S Afr Med J* 1981;59(19):687-688.
60. Orioli IM, Ribeiro MG, Castilla EE: Clinical and epidemiological studies of amniotic deformity, adhesion, and mutilation (ADAM) sequence in a South American (ECLAMC) population. *Am J Med Genet* 2003;118A(2):135-145.
61. Walter JH Jr, Goss LR, Lazzara AT: Amniotic band syndrome. *J Foot Ankle Surg* 1998;37(4):325-333.
62. Gabos PG: Modified technique for the surgical treatment of congenital constriction bands of the arms and legs of infants and children. *Orthopedics* 2006;29(5):401-404.
63. Cignini P, Giorlandino C, Padula F, Dugo N, Cafà EV, Spata A: Epidemiology and risk factors of amniotic band syndrome, or ADAM sequence. *J Prenat Med* 2012;6(4):59-63.
64. Buss PW, Hughes HE, Clarke A: Twenty-four cases of the EEC syndrome: Clinical presentation and management. *J Med Genet* 1995;32(9):716-723.
65. Umair M, Hayat A: Nonsyndromic split-hand/foot malformation: Recent classification. *Mol Syndromol* 2020;10(5):243-254.
66. Dillon ME, Fatone S: Deliberations about the functional benefits and complications of PFA: Do we pay heed to the purported benefits at the expense of minimizing complications? *Arch Phys Med Rehabil* 2013;94(8):1429-1435.
67. Zarezadeh F, Arazpour M, Bahramizadeh M, Mardani MA, Head J: Design and construction of a new partial foot prosthesis based on high-pressure points in a patient with diabetes with transmetatarsal amputation: A technical note. *J Prosthet Orthot* 2018;30(2):108-113.

The Child With Multiple Limb Deficiencies

Chinmay S. Paranjape, MD, MHSc • Anna D. Vergun, MD, FAAOS

CHAPTER 82

ABSTRACT

A child with multiple limb deficiencies requires special consideration. A complete physical examination with careful attention to other organ systems is warranted. Most children are extremely adaptive and can be psychologically well adjusted when they are provided with a supportive environment. Treatment should be pursued at centers dedicated to the challenges of integrating occupational therapy, physical therapy, and individualized prosthetic components throughout the child's intellectual and physical development. Because of the increased size and weight of multiple prostheses and associated issues of heat retention and difficulty with donning and doffing equipment, the child with multiple limb deficiencies may achieve optimal functioning using assistive devices, such as a wheelchair with a lift and adaptive computers. Technologic advances such as computerized devices with voice recognition systems hold great promise for improving functional independence.

Keywords: acquired limb amputation; congenital limb amputation; multimembral limb deficiency; multiple limb deficiency; pediatric; prosthesis

Introduction

Children with limb deficiencies have problems distinct from those of adult amputees. Difficulties increase exponentially for children with multiple limb involvement (**Figure 1**). These children should be cared for in special treatment facilities.

The term multiple limb deficiencies covers many possibilities, ranging from a child missing two minor toes and a single finger on the nondominant hand to a child born with no arms or legs. Children may have multiple limb deficiencies, either because they were born with the deficiencies or as a result of an accident or illness. Common sense and a creative team approach are needed to recognize and appropriately treat the varied needs of these children.

Congenital Multiple Limb Deficiencies

The incidence of congenital limb deficiencies is approximately 1 in 2,000 births. In the United States, approximately 1,500 infants annually are born with upper limb reductions and approximately 750 have lower limb reductions.[1] Reports in the literature from British Columbia range from 0.31% per 1,000% to 0.79% per 1,000 births. The variability in incidence likely results from differences in gene pools and reporting methods in different locations.[2-4] Approximately 30% of these infants have deficits in more than one limb (15% with two limbs, 5% with three limbs, and 10% with all four limbs).[5-7] The most common deficit for all congenital deficiencies is digital reductions, which account for approximately 50% of all reported cases. In approximately one-third to one-half of patients, other organs systems also are involved.

Etiology and Presentation

The etiology of congenital limb deficiency is briefly reviewed here in the

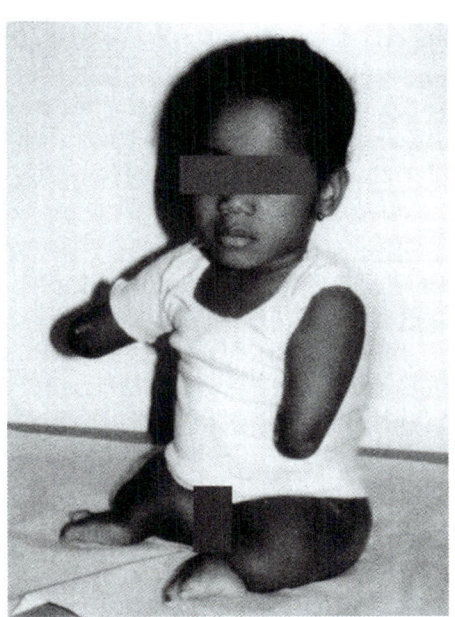

FIGURE 1 Photograph of a child with multiple limb deficiencies.

Dr. Paranjape or an immediate family member has stock or stock options held in Alphatec Spine, OrthoPediatrics, and Stryker. Dr. Vergun or an immediate family member serves as a board member, owner, officer, or committee member of Association of Children's Prosthetic and Orthotic Clinics.

This chapter is adapted from Cuomo A, Watts HG: The child with multiple limb deficiencies, in Krajbich JI, Pinzur MS, Potter BK, Stevens PM, eds: *Atlas of Amputations and Limb Deficiencies: Surgical, Prosthetic, and Rehabilitation Principles*, ed 4. American Academy of Orthopaedic Surgeons, 2016, pp 953-960.

context of multiple limb deficiencies. Vascular disruptions remain the most common etiology and include disorders such as amniotic band syndrome, which accounts for approximately 35% of cases. Other congenital causes include gene mutation, familial occurrence, and known syndromes (24%); chromosomal abnormalities (6%); teratogenic causes (4%); and unknown causes (32%).[8] In general, digits are more often affected than long bones, longitudinal defects are more common than transverse defects, intercalary deficits are rare, and upper limb deficits are either reported slightly more frequently or occur at an equal frequency as lower limb deficit. Both the upper and lower limbs are affected in approximately 8% of infants.[8,9] Amelia (complete absence of limb) is reported to be 1.41 in 100,000, and phocomelia (malformation of limb) is 0.62 per 100,000 births.[10,11]

Limb deficiency can refer to the absence of a limb as well as to limb anomalies that might require a prosthesis or modified prosthesis for one or more of the involved limbs. For example, a child with the most severe form of thrombocytopenia-absent radius syndrome may have phocomelic upper limbs and fusion of both knees caused by congenital synchondroses. These children cannot effectively use their feet to replace limited hand function because their knees do not bend sufficiently to allow the foot to reach the mouth. If bilateral knee disarticulations are performed, the child would be able to sit in a chair more easily but would be unable to rise from the floor after a fall because their short arms could not provide adequate assistance.

Approximately 60% of children treated in amputee clinics have congenital conditions.[5,12] In addition, 10% of children with acquired amputations have a loss of more than one limb, although underreporting may occur because these children are generally treated in the community and not in pediatric amputee centers. This is particularly true of children with lower limb amputations, which are easier to manage in a less-specialized facility than are upper limb amputations.[13] Among children who have acquired amputations, 40% involve the upper limb; however, in children treated at amputee clinics, congenital upper limb involvement is twice as likely as lower limb involvement.[5]

Associated Anomalies

The reader is encouraged to review the embryology of limb bud formation. Limbs form concurrently with other organs such as the heart and kidneys between gestational weeks 4 to 7. Therefore, a thorough examination for associated anomalies is mandatory in a child with one congenital anomaly. The clinician should begin the examination at the head and work downward, checking the cranial nerves (especially cranial nerve VII) to test for associated Möbius syndrome, the palates (soft and hard), and the eyes and ears for placement and formation. The chest should be checked for the proper number and location of nipples, and the pectoral muscles should be examined. The heart should be examined for heart murmur, the anus for normal formation, and the spine for curvature and sacral dimples. The other limbs should be carefully evaluated for the presence of even minor abnormalities that could change the diagnostic (and possibly prognostic) category from single-limb to multiple-limb involvement. The presence of petechiae or bruises can suggest thrombocytopenia-absent radius syndrome because of low platelet counts. The infant's mother and their nurses should be questioned regarding the infant's sucking and swallowing to assess for tracheoesophageal abnormalities.

Additional studies may be indicated. Renal ultrasonography and radiography should be used to evaluate the spine and heart for all infants with a limb deficiency. A complete blood count and differential, including a platelet count, should be obtained for a child with a radial deficiency. Because upper limb deficiency syndromes, such as Holt-Oram syndrome, can have a particularly high association with cardiac defects, echocardiography should be strongly considered. Currently, there are no recommendations for a screening echocardiogram, specifically for a child with multiple limb reductions or anomalies; however, the most recent appropriate use criteria from multiple societies list clinically suspected syndrome or extracardiac congenital anomaly known to be associated with congenital heart disease as an appropriate indication for a newborn screening echocardiogram.[14]

Anomalies in the central nervous system or one of the receptive senses (vision or hearing) are of particular importance. Children are generally extremely adaptable, but if the central nervous system is involved, the child's adaptive capacity may be compromised.[15]

Acquired Multiple Limb Deficiencies

Not all multiple limb loss results from congenital causes. Purpura fulminans, commonly caused by meningococcal disease, results in disseminated intravascular clotting. In the case of neonatal meningococcemia, children can end up with quadrimembral deficiency. Although the incidence of *Meningococcus* is declining secondary to vaccination efforts,[16] other bacterial strains such as *Pneumococcus* and *Streptococcus* may also result in limb gangrene and subsequent loss. Furthermore, purpura fulminans can have long-term sequelae causing cognitive impairments. These include cerebral lesions, hearing loss, and learning difficulties in 10% to 20%, deafness in 3% to 15%, and severe cognitive deficits, cerebral palsy, or epilepsy in 3% to 5%.[17,18] Viremia (eg, chickenpox) can also necessitate the amputation of multiple limbs.[19] Incidents involving trains are another cause of multiple limb loss. A common scenario is that of a child trying to hop a train at the after-end ladder, losing their grip, and being spun around the back end of the railway car and thrown on the tracks in front of the following car. This commonly results in the loss of two or more limbs. Lawnmower injuries,[20] automobile collisions, electrical burns, and injuries caused by explosive devices[21] are other traumatic causes of multiple limb loss.

Special Needs

Children with multiple limb loss present special challenges to the professionals who work with them, and each patient has unique needs and abilities. The knowledge gained by treating one child may not be applicable to another child with limb loss.

Role of Surgery

Multiple limb deficiency is best managed by a multidisciplinary team in a center or group experienced with such children. Children with multiple limb deficiencies substitute other body parts to compensate for missing function of the residuum and affected limbs. Surgery requires very careful consideration because it can create secondary loss of function that is vital for the child. As an example, amputation or surgical correction of remnants of feet should not be done if they substitute for hands. This trade-off must be considered even if surgery could improve gait mechanics or lower limb prosthesis use.

Clearly, care must be individualized for each patient and their family. A few general principles do guide care. The first is to preserve length with split-thickness skin grafts and ideally prevent adherence to the bone to minimize hindrance in any prosthesis. The second is to preserve upper extremity sensation wherever possible. Experience demonstrates that many of these patients will forego even well-fitting prostheses if the residuum is long enough and sensate to allow them compensatory motion and function. For transverse deficiencies of the forearm, the Krukenberg procedure involves separation of the radius and ulna to create a pincer, and can be performed as early as age 2 years.[22] The procedure is capable of restoring up to 4 mm of two-point discrimination and 10 kg of pincer carrying ability, but is less used in the modern setting because of cosmesis concerns.[23] The third is to offer only surgery, which maximizes function—this often implies waiting for the extent of full extremity function to be determined. In children with bilateral upper extremity deficiency, this then necessitates waiting to perform any lower extremity surgery until it is clear how children are using their lower extremities to accomplish their activities of daily living. Finally, consideration of how spinal mechanics may assist the child in accomplishing activities of daily living is paramount. Children often use spinal motion to compensate for deficient extremities. As such, management of scoliosis should use minimal fusion when absolutely necessary.

Prosthetic Components

Children with multiple limb deficiencies have a greater need for specialized prosthetic components than do those with single limb deficiencies. Several characteristics of prosthetic components should be considered in relation to the special needs of the child with multiple deficiencies.

Size and Weight

Prosthetic components for adults are usually available in large, medium, and small sizes, with perhaps an extra small size that is appropriate for smaller women. Children, however, need an array of sizes, ranging from those that can fit a tiny 1-year-old toddler up to devices for a teenager of nearly adult proportions. Although competition has encouraged many manufacturers to address this niche market, it is not economically feasible for manufacturers of prosthetic components to fabricate and store large stocks of multiple-sized items because of the relatively low demand. Therefore, some components may need to be individually crafted. The weight of prosthetic components is an issue not only because of the smaller muscle mass available to move the prostheses but also because children with multiple limb deficiencies find that minor difficulties with one prosthesis can adversely affect the functioning of another.[24]

Heat Retention

Wearing a prosthesis can be hot, especially in warm climates. The limbs provide an increase in total surface area of the skin, which is the primary source of cooling the core body temperature.[25] Children who wear two, three, or even four prostheses may not have enough bare skin to disperse heat adequately. In addition, prostheses for higher levels of limb deficiency demand greater energy expenditure by the child, compounding the heat problem. This is a particular problem if the child has a hip or shoulder disarticulation requiring a prosthesis that covers a considerable area of the trunk. Body temperature may become substantially elevated. Reasonable, normal activities may be prohibitive in any season but especially in the summer, and the child may understandably refuse to wear the prostheses as a result.

Integration of Prosthetic Components

Children with multiple limb deficiencies frequently require custom-designed components, which often require custom fabrication. For example, an 8-year-old boy who was born with bilateral hip disarticulations and an absent left hand was able to walk on bilateral lower limb prostheses by using a regular forearm crutch with his normal right arm and using a custom-made crutch as the terminal device of the left upper limb prosthesis. When the boy was not walking, the left arm prosthesis included a quick-disconnect wrist that allowed him to easily exchange the crutch for a hook. Fabrication of such special items is labor intensive and expensive; however, the challenge of helping these complex patients stimulates creative solutions and provides satisfaction to both the patient and the treatment team.

Donning and Doffing

Independent donning and doffing are paramount to prosthesis design. The child with multiple limb deficiencies may wear such an array of devices that it can be difficult for a parent, let alone the child, to apply them. If the child is to become an independent adult, this aspect must be considered. The need to achieve independence depends on the child's age and psychosocial development, and the relationships within the family. Many parents are reluctant to relinquish their own need to assist the child and must be encouraged by the clinical staff to allow the child to gain independence. Prostheses appropriately designed for easy donning and doffing may be helpful. For example, pull tabs with a fabric hook-and-loop fastener system can be used on belts and harnesses to allow easy grasping with a prosthetic hook for donning a suction socket or a total elastic suspension belt.

Wheelchair Use

Various factors need to be considered if wheelchair use is required. If a powered wheelchair is not necessary, a standard chair is preferable because the exercise it requires can help with the common problem of obesity.[26] If a powered chair is necessary, its size and weight must be considered. It will usually be necessary for the parents to have a van modified with a lift or ramp to accept the chair because power chairs are heavy. For adolescents of driving age, a van will need to be modified to allow the wheelchair user to operate the vehicle.

For children with severe deformity, such as those missing both arms and both legs, the wheelchair may need to be adjustable to almost floor level. This allows the child to crawl or roll onto the seat, and then raise the seat to a level more functional for table activities. Such wheelchairs are individually fabricated and often are expensive.

Gadget Tolerance

Members of the rehabilitation team or the family may devise a complicated mix of equipment, especially electronics, to allow the child to perform an array of activities. Often, these devices outstrip the child's needs and desires. Despite their adaptability, children often will not tolerate having a large number of highly technical mechanical devices applied to them. This is commonly called poor gadget tolerance (**Figure 2**). Children often function much better without highly sophisticated equipment. An electronic replacement for an upper limb often does not have long-term acceptance by a child with multiple limb deficiencies. Many reasons have been given for this lack of acceptance, but factual information is lacking. Many children find it difficult to articulate why they prefer not to wear upper limb prostheses. It has been speculated that the excessive heat buildup, high energy consumption, discomfort,

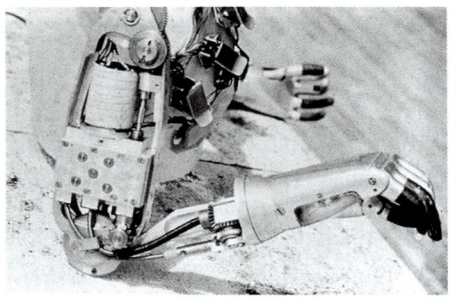

FIGURE 2 Photograph of a prosthesis developed for a bilateral high-level upper limb amputee. This type of prosthesis is unlikely to be worn by a child born with the absence of both upper limbs because it will be hot, heavy, and provide little sensory feedback. It also exceeds a child's gadget tolerance.

and, most importantly, the lack of sensory feedback are important factors in prosthesis rejection. Other clinicians have speculated that children born with a limb deficiency may lack an appropriate representation in the brain for the absent limb. This theory has been supported in recent brain mapping studies comparing individuals with congenital and traumatic upper limb loss.[27] The lack of willingness among children to wear upper limb prostheses provides a difficult challenge for those working to develop and improve upper limb prosthetic components for this population.

Economic Implications

Given the need for multiple prostheses, a special wheelchair, and a customized van for the child's transportation, the major limitation experienced by the family of a child with multiple limb deficiencies is likely to be the ability to pay for the ancillary equipment. Some financial help may be available from government agencies and charitable organizations. Accessibility to the classroom and assistants to help these children (especially with toileting while they are at school) are more commonly available since the passage of legislation ensuring educational opportunities for all children in many countries.

Developmental Capabilities

As is true of able-bodied children, the developmental capabilities of children with limb deficiencies are constantly changing. Unlike able-bodied children, however, those with multiple limb deficiencies face greater challenges, and the adaptation required may be overwhelming. Although there have been reports of successful fittings of toddlers with a unilateral prosthesis incorporating an articulated knee, the child with multiple limb loss faces a greater challenge. Mastering two articulated lower limb prostheses is very difficult, and, if upper limb deficiency is present, the child's ability to avoid injury in a fall is compromised. It is much simpler for these children to learn to use nonarticulated limbs. The child's intellectual development and physical coordination and strength are important in planning the prosthetic program. Prosthetic components for children should be appropriate for the developmental age of the child and for the degree of multiple challenges faced by a particular child. Typically, children function best with simple and durable prosthetic devices. However, as electronic devices become more intuitive with pattern recognition technology and material science affords decreasing weight with increasing durability, the appropriate upper age limit for myoelectric prostheses will change.

Age of First Fitting

The child with multiple limb deficiencies may be limited in their ability to fulfil experiences important for normal intellectual and motor development, such as mobility to explore surroundings, the ability to manipulate objects, and obtaining tactile and proprioceptive feedback. However, most children will naturally seek to substitute other methods for gaining these experiences, and this should be encouraged. It has been proposed that directional sense, such as up and down, left and right, and rotation, is impaired in children with limb deficiencies because they cannot easily explore their surroundings. However, a study by French and Clarke[15] found no difference in directionality test scores between patients with congenital or traumatic amputation, who presumably had the opportunity and ability for normal development before limb loss. There was a trend, however, toward poorer scores with increased severity of the pattern of deficiency. Every effort should be made to help children with multiple limb deficiencies reach appropriate milestones to aid their intellectual and motor development.

Some care clinicians have advocated fitting children younger than 6 months with upper limb prostheses so the children can be trained to develop bimanual eye-hand coordination. A recent study by Toda et al found the rate of rejection for powered upper extremity prosthesis in children fitted after 2 years of age was 21.6%, with rejection occurring between 5 and 19 years of age. They found that children fitted before 2 years of age tended to have higher acceptance than those fitted after 2 years of age.[28] Current practice is to wait until a child is beginning to develop sitting balance, usually at approximately 5 to 6 months of age. The first fitting may occur later in a child with multiple limb loss; however, developmental delay or other health needs may intervene.

Age of Activation of Terminal Devices

A terminal device refers to the component of a prosthesis that replaces the person's hand. Devices can be active where they dynamically open and close or be passive where they assist with cosmesis and statically holding items. The age at which the terminal devices in a child's prostheses should be activated will depend on the child's psychomotor development. Ordinarily, the terminal device is mounted at the time the prosthesis is first applied. At first, the therapists and parents open the device and place objects in it so that the child can understand the principle of the device. If a myoelectric prosthesis is to be used, some clinics will fit the child very early (at age 12 to 24 months) with a simpler single-electrode system, which alternately controls opening and closing. If a body-powered prosthesis is to be used, the activating cable is usually connected at approximately 18 to 24 months of age, when the child is more developmentally ready. The major factor in the timing of these decisions is the child's developmental readiness. In children with multiple limb deficiencies, the timetable may need to be extended.

Sports and Recreational Activities

As is the case with able-bodied children, those with multiple limb deficiencies learn by playing. These children may have an even greater psychological and physical need for active play than able-bodied children because they have few activities to help them burn calories and because food is often offered to these children in sympathy by parents and siblings. This is especially true for children with multiple high-level deficiencies, in whom the propensity for obesity should be counteracted with exercise and caloric limitation. Children with distal deficiencies who wear prostheses and are very active may burn calories at a high rate and need additional calories to maintain a normal weight.

Although parents may worry that swimming is not safe for children with multiple limb deficiencies, swimming is a good sport for amputees, and it can be readily done by those with no legs. Even children with missing arms and legs can perform a porpoise-like trunk motion that will propel them through the water. Although supervision is imperative, many groups welcome the challenge of helping these children learn to swim.

Skiing is also a favorite sport among many amputees because it gives them an opportunity to experience the exhilaration of speed. The child will need help, and prostheses may need to be modified. An extra socket may be needed to protect the residual limb and keep it warm when no prosthesis is worn. For ski poles, modified forearm crutches are fitted with small ski tips (outriggers). Instruction is important to teach the child how to use new equipment. If tritrack or three-track skiing is unrealistic, a child with multiple limb deficiencies can learn to ski seated in a special frame mounted over a single ski.

Special centers are available at which amputees can learn to participate in a variety of sports. Parents should be encouraged to allow their children to participate because it is natural for them to be overprotective. This may require an active effort on the part of the clinical team to reassure parents. A referral to a recreational therapist may be beneficial.

Sexuality

Children with multiple limb deficiencies will undergo normal sexual maturation and have normal concerns about sex. These children face many of the same issues as their able-bodied peers, but their sexual development is often complicated by added concerns about their altered body image and how they will be accepted by a potential partner. Adult amputees discuss issues of sexuality among themselves. Clinic team members are often reluctant to discuss sexuality, but they must provide the developing child with appropriate information and/or counseling. Adult men without arms or legs have fathered children, limbless women have given birth to children, and parents with limb deficiency have successfully raised children. Studies examining sexual dysfunction in amputees tend to focus on adult populations who underwent amputation in adulthood. In these studies, sexual dysfunction is highly prevalent and more common in males who had recently undergone amputation.[29,30] However, similar studies in children who have undergone an amputation as they mature into adulthood are lacking. It is likely that such individuals have a different emotional and physical constitution.

Adolescents with congenital deficiencies commonly worry about passing their condition on to potential offspring. Such worries are generally unfounded, but a referral to a genetic counselor may provide valuable insight and, in most cases, will relieve anxiety.

Psychological Needs of the Child and Family

It might be expected that multiple limb deficiency would exact a heavy toll on a child's psyche, but studies have shown that these children do well psychologically.[31-35] These studies have found that the effect of perceived physical appearance on psychological distress is mediated by general self-esteem, not by the severity of the physical involvement. There is also empiric evidence that coping mechanisms are tied to perceived social support from parents, teacher, and classmates and to the level of family/marital conflict and organization. In essence, the child's self-perception reflects the attitudes of those with whom they interact. This is an important point for parents and caregivers to learn early in the process of caring for their child, because they will have a great influence on the child's self-esteem.

A long-term prosthetic treatment plan may be easier to accomplish in a child than in an adult who is employed and cannot miss work. However, intervening during childhood means that more people (the patient, the parents, and sometimes grandparents) are involved with prosthetic management decisions. To ensure the best care for the child, all concerned parties should be informed of their rights, and treatment options should be explained and discussed. If a conversion amputation is being considered, there is usually no need to rush into an elective conversion amputation until everyone is comfortable with the need to proceed.

The need for cultural sensitivity has assumed more importance in recent decades. Some cultures are much more resistant to conversion amputation, although the clinical team may see the need as obvious. These cultural differences can be compounded because of misunderstandings caused by language translation. Putting the child's family in contact with other families who share the same cultural traditions can often be very beneficial.

Special Aspects of Upper Limb Absence

Scoliosis

Children with upper limb deficiencies have an increased chance for the development of scoliosis, either congenital or idiopathic.[36-40] If the scoliosis becomes progressive, the curves are very resistant to bracing, if for no other reason than braces are difficult to wear for a child with upper limb absence. If spinal fusion is being considered, the possible effects on the child's ability to reach the mouth with the feet should be carefully considered, because most of these children choose to use their feet rather than prostheses. Decisions should be made based on advantages and disadvantages to the child's lifetime functioning rather than on the basis of radiographic findings alone.

Use of Upper Limb Prostheses

Children born without one or both upper limbs can have extraordinary functional capability. James et al[41] concluded children with unilateral transradial transverse deficiencies have nearly normal function and quality of life regardless of whether they wear a prosthesis. The effect of an upper limb prosthesis on quality of life and function in children with multiple limb deficiencies is not well studied; however, it is acknowledged that they can readily be taught to feed themselves and perform many tasks using their feet and toes (**Figure 3**). Objects can be grasped between the chin and shoulder or between a very short residual humerus and the chest wall.[42] The sensory feedback provided by using feet or residual limbs is advantageous over prostheses use. The increased energy consumption required to manipulate a prosthesis can be problematic for a child with a multiple limb deficiency. The recent focus on

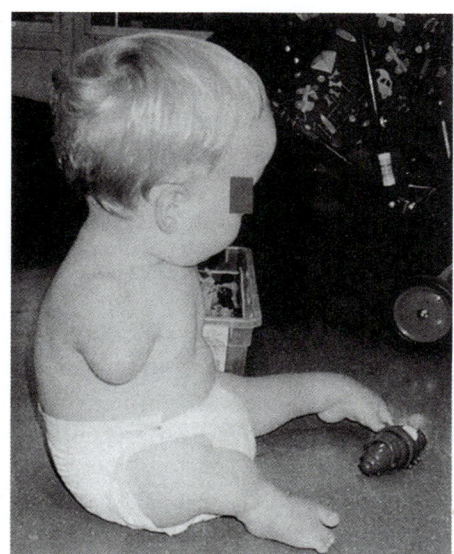

FIGURE 3 Photograph of a child with bilateral upper limb loss using his feet to replace hand function.

highly technical components for adults has not had a substantial effect in the field of prosthetic devices for children because of the high costs. These factors can lead to difficulty when trying to convince a child to wear an upper limb prosthesis because the child may be more facile, especially initially, without the prosthesis. Most children who are born without arms will not wear prostheses throughout their lifetime.[43-45] The percentage of such children who use prostheses may depend on the enthusiasm of the clinic team for fitting such children and the age at which such children are first fitted.[46]

Although there are notable exceptions, many children born with upper limb deficiency function better without prosthetic help. By the time they reach adulthood, they are able to do almost everything for themselves, including driving an automobile with their feet. In contrast, children who lose their arms because of trauma are much more likely to struggle with the limb loss.

There are other factors that may influence intermittent use of prostheses. For example, at some point in the patient's life, especially during adolescence, an individual born without arms may request simple cosmetic arms to be used for special occasions.

Initially, most parents want their child to be fitted with prosthetic arms. As a consequence, a trial of prosthetic fitting may be a necessary stage that a family must go through so that they can personally experience the rejection of the prostheses by the child. Consequently, the prescription of a set of arm prostheses with expensive myoelectric components may not be a practical decision. There may be a temporary need, however, to provide lifelike passive hands for an infant so that a parent will not reject the child.

Because these children will probably not use prosthetic arms and will function by using the feet in place of the hands, it is important to know the status of the motion and muscle control of the hips, knees, ankles, and toes. Careful examination is essential, because congenital anomalies are frequently associated with other anomalies.

The skill of the occupational therapist in upper limb prosthetic training may play only a limited role in the child's care if the child rejects long-term prosthesis use. The therapist's most important role may be to teach the child how best to substitute the feet for the missing arms and how to use adaptive equipment creatively. The ability to shrug the shoulders can be useful for grasping objects between the side of the neck and the upper scapula. The use of assistive devices (eg, a mouth stick for typing or touch screen control) can help the older child interact with the world. Toileting is a major problem for the child without arms, especially if the child wants to use public restrooms.

Computers may change the lives of children with upper limb absence. Computers can be used as controllers to activate remote switches (eg, turning lights on and off or answering a telephone), although control of a computer keyboard is still a problem. There are mouth-controlled stick devices available for keyboards as well as touch-screen devices.

Voice-controlled technology holds great future promise for children with limb deficiency because it is an intuitive means of interacting with devices, does not require prior training with the device or additional technical effort to extract a control signal (eg, from a muscle), and may be cheaper than custom systems that integrate with the peripheral nervous system.[47] Voice recognition systems for adults have improved dramatically over the past decade because of larger databases of training data, which result in more accurate models of human speech. National Institutes of Health-funded trials are currently ongoing for adult upper extremity voice-controlled prostheses.[48] Faster computers and improved algorithms have resulted in better accuracy of speech-to-text systems and have improved overall accuracy for all users. A few issues contribute to the lag for children: (1) voice properties change as children age, (2) children speak with a higher pitch (fundamental frequency), (3) with more irregular prosody (the "tune" of how someone talks), (4) uneven loudness (including shouting-type speech that itself has different characteristics), (5) uneven or unusual durations of words and syllables (both too long or too short), and (6) with unusual word choice (covering both mispronunciations such as "aminal" and ungrammatical utterances such as "I goed there") (Brian Langer, PhD, Senior Speech Scientist, Toy Talk, San Francisco, CA, personal communication, 2015). Recent work has demonstrated that noncommercially developed algorithms perform comparably with adult voice recognition software.[49] However, these algorithms may be costly and are not currently incorporated into any commercially available prostheses for children.

In the future, children are likely to embrace more technology as computer interfaces become more playful and devices become more like toys. Recently, there has even been concern over how intuitively interactive these devices can be and how they may affect marketing to children when used in toys.[50] However, the devices must not detract from the child's own agility or sensation and must provide immediate positive feedback to maintain the child's interest. Small devices that are playful, durable, and have responsive voice recognition software will likely revolutionize the world for a child with multiple limb deficiencies.

SUMMARY

Multiple limb deficiency is rare in children, but those affected often require care at a specialized center that is equipped with a creative team to assist the child in gaining independent function. The needs of children change over the course of their intellectual and physical development. Because congenital limb reductions are often associated with other organ system anomalies, a thorough physical examination and strong consideration of other specialized tests are required. Care clinicians must resist the temptation to simply replace the multiple limb deficits with multiple prostheses, which may result in problems with decreased agility, heat retention, and difficulty with component integration. Instead, there should be a focus on optimizing function and independence. For children with profound deficits, this is often achieved with assistive devices, such as wheelchairs with an elevator platform and computers with a mouth-controlled stick for typing. Voice recognition systems may play an important role in the future. As technology improves, there may be an increasing role for assistive devices at earlier ages if the interfaces are playful and provide immediate positive feedback.

References

1. Canfield MA, Honein MA, Yuskiv N, et al: National estimates and race/ethnic-specific variation of selected birth defects in the United States, 1999-2001. *Birth Defects Res Part A Clin Mol Teratol* 2006;76:747-756.

2. Froster UG, Baird PA: Congenital defects of lower limbs and associated malformations: A population based study. *Am J Med Genet* 1993;45:60-64.

3. Froster UG, Baird PA: Upper limb deficiencies and associated malformations: A population-based study. *Am J Med Genet* 1992;44:767-781.

4. Froster-Iskenius UG, Baird PA: Limb reduction defects in over one million consecutive livebirths. *Teratology* 1989;39:127.

5. Krebs D, Fishman S: Characteristics of the child amputee population. *J Pediatr Orthop* 1984;4:89-95.

6. Wilson JG, Brent RL: Are female sex hormones teratogenic? *Am J Obstet Gynecol* 1981;141:567.

7. Bowen RE, Otsuka NY, Doty SA: The child with a limb deficiency, in Flynn J, Weinstein S, Crawford H, eds: *Lovell and Winter's Pediatric Orthopaedics*. Wolters Kluwer Health, 2020, pp 1465-1536.

8. Gold NB, Westgate MN, Holmes LB: Anatomic and etiological classification of congenital limb deficiencies. *Am J Med Genet* 2011;155:1225-1235.

9. Makhoul IR, Goldstein I, Smolkin T, Avrahami R, Sujov P: Congenital limb deficiencies in newborn infants: Prevalence, characteristics and prenatal diagnosis. *Prenat Diagn* 2003;23:198-200.

10. Bermejo-Sánchez E, Cuevas L, Amar E, et al: Amelia: A multi-center descriptive epidemiologic study in a large dataset from the International Clearinghouse for Birth Defects Surveillance and Research, and overview of the literature. *Am J Med Genet Part C Semin Med Genet* 2011;157:288-304.

11. Bermejo-Sánchez E, Cuevas L, Amar E, et al: Phocomelia: A worldwide

descriptive epidemiologic study in a large series of cases from the International Clearinghouse for Birth Defects Surveillance and Research, and overview of the literature. *Am J Med Genet Part C Semin Med Genet* 2011;157:305-320.

12. Kay HW, Fishman S: *1018 Children With Skeletal Limb Deficiencies.* Prosthetics and Orthotics, New York University Post-Graduate Medical School, 1967.

13. Davies E, Clippinger F: Children with amputations. *Inter Clin Info Bull* 1969;9:6-19.

14. Campbell RM, Douglas PS, Eidem BW, et al: ACC/AAP/AHA/ASE/HRS/SCAI/SCCT/SCMR/SOPE 2014 appropriate Use criteria for initial transthoracic echocardiography in outpatient pediatric cardiology. *J Am Coll Cardiol* 2014;64:2039-2060.

15. French R, Clarke S: The directional senses of the child amputee. *Inter-Clinic Information Bulletin* 1975;14:9-13.

16. Borrow R, Alarcón P, Carlos J, et al: The Global Meningococcal Initiative: Global epidemiology, the impact of vaccines on meningococcal disease and the importance of herd protection. *Expert Rev Vaccines* 2017;16:313-328.

17. Viner RM, Booy R, Johnson H, et al: Outcomes of invasive meningococcal serogroup B disease in children and adolescents (MOSAIC): A case-control study. *Lancet Neurol* 2012;11:774-783.

18. des Portes V: Quel suivi à long terme pour quels patients? Séquelles des méningites bactériennes chez l'enfant et chez l'adulte: Incidence, types, modes d'évaluation. *Med Mal Infect* 2009;39:572-580.

19. Canavese F, Krajbich JI, LaFleur BJ: Orthopaedic sequelae of childhood meningococcemia: Management considerations and outcome. *J Bone Joint Surg Am* 2010;92:2196-2203.

20. Garay M, Hennrikus WL, Hess J, Lehman EB, Armstrong DG: Lawnmowers versus children: The devastation continues. *Clin Orthop Relat Res* 2017;475:950-956.

21. Villamaria CY, Morrison JJ, Fitzpatrick CM, Cannon JW, Rasmussen TE: Wartime vascular injuries in the pediatric population of Iraq and Afghanistan: 2002-2011. *J Pediatr Surg* 2014;49:428-432.

22. Swanson AB: The Krukenberg procedure in the juvenile amputee. *J Bone Joint Surg Am* 1964;46:1540-1548.

23. Kleeman LT, Shafritz AB: The Krukenberg procedure. *J Hand Surg Am* 2013;38:173-175.

24. Nichols PJ, Rogers EE, Clark MS, Stamp WG: The acceptance and rejection of prostheses by children with multiple congenital limb deformities. *Artif Limbs* 1968;12:1-13.

25. González-Alonso J: Human thermoregulation and the cardiovascular system. *Exp Physiol* 2012;97:340-346.

26. Brzeziński M, Czubek Z, Niedzielska A, Jankowski M, Kobus T, Ossowski Z: Relationship between lower-extremity defects and body mass among polish children: A cross-sectional study. *BMC Musculoskelet Disord* 2019;20(1):84.

27. Reilly KT, Sirigu A: Motor cortex representation of the upper-limb in individuals born without a hand. *PLoS One* 2011;6(4):e18100.

28. Toda M, Chin T, Shibata Y, Mizobe F: Use of powered prosthesis for children with upper limb deficiency at Hyogo Rehabilitation Center. *PLoS One* 2015;10(6):e0131746.

29. Verschuren JEA, Geertzen JH, Enzlin P, Dijkstra PU, Dekker R: Sexual functioning and sexual well-being in people with a limb amputation: A cross-sectional study in the Netherlands. *Disabil Rehabil* 2016;38:368-373.

30. Woods L, Hevey D, Ryall N, O'Keeffe F: Sex after amputation: The relationships between sexual functioning, body image, mood and anxiety in persons with a lower limb amputation. *Disabil Rehabil* 2018;40:1663-1670.

31. Pruitt SD, Varni JW, Seid M, Setoguchi Y: Prosthesis satisfaction outcome measurement in pediatric limb deficiency. *Arch Phys Med Rehabil* 1997;78:750-754.

32. Varni JW, Setoguchi Y: Perceived physical appearance and adjustment of adolescents with congenital/acquired limb deficiencies: A path-analytic model. *J Clin Child Psychol* 1996;25:201-208.

33. Tyc VL: Psychosocial adaptation of children and adolescents with limb deficiencies: A review. *Clin Psychol Rev* 1992;12:275-291.

34. Bryant PR, Pandian G: Acquired limb deficiencies. 1. Acquired limb deficiencies in children and young adults. *Arch Phys Med Rehabil* 2001;82:S3-S8.

35. Varni JW, Rubenfeld LA, Talbot D, Setoguchi Y: Determinants of self-esteem in children with congenital/acquired limb deficiencies. *J Dev Behav Pediatr* 1989;10:13-16.

36. Makley JT, Heiple KG: Scoliosis associated with congenital deficiencies of the upper extremity. *J Bone Joint Surg Am* 1970;52:279.

37. Heyman HJ, Ivankovich AD, Shulman M, Millar E, Choudhry YA: Intraoperative monitoring and anesthetic management for spinal fusion in an amelic patient. *J Pediatr Orthop* 1982;2(3):299-301.

38. Herring J, Goldberg M: Instructional case: Amelia and Scoliosis. *J Pediatr Orthop* 1985;5:605-609.

39. Lester DK, Painter GL, Berman AT, Skinner SR: 'Idiopathic' scoliosis associated with congenital upper-limb deficiency. *Clin Orthop Relat Res* 1986;202:205-210.

40. Samuelsson L, Hermansson LL, Norén L: Scoliosis and trunk asymmetry in upper limb transverse dysmelia. *J Pediatr Orthop* 1997;17:769-772.

41. James MA, Bagley AM, Brasington K, Lutz C, McConnell S, Molitor F: Impact of prostheses on function and quality of life for children with unilateral congenital below-the-elbow deficiency. *J Bone Joint Surg Am* 2006;88:2356-2365.

42. Herring JA: Functional assessment and management of multilimb deficiency, in Herring JA, Birch JG, eds: *The Child With a Limb Deficiency*. American Academy of Orthopaedic Surgeons, 1998, pp 437-445.

43. Crandall RC, Tomhave W: Pediatric unilateral below-elbow amputees: Retrospective analysis of 34 patients given multiple prosthetic options. *J Pediatr Orthop* 2002;22:380-383.

44. Davidson J: A survey of the satisfaction of upper limb amputees with their prostheses, their lifestyles, and their abilities. *J Hand Ther* 2002;15:62-70.

45. Kruger LM, Fishman S: Myoelectric and body-powered prostheses. *J Pediatr Orthop* 1993;13:68-75.

46. Scotland TR, Galway HR: A long-term review of children with congenital and acquired upper limb deficiency. *J Bone Joint Surg Br* 1983;65:346.

47. Alkhafaf OS, Wali MK, Al-Timemy AH: Improved hand prostheses control for transradial amputees based on hybrid of voice recognition and electromyography. *Int J Artif Organs* 2021;44:509-517.

48. Mcdonald B, Johansson J, Lambrecht S, Latour D, Rozell B, Farrell T: Voice recognition control of a multi-articulating hand for improved grasp selection, in *Myoelectric Controls and Upper Limb Prosthetics Symposium*. University of New Brunswick, 2020.

49. Purnapatra S, Das P, Holsopple L, Schuckers S: Longitudinal study of voice recognition in children, in *Proceedings of the 15th International Conference of the Biometrics Special Interest Group*, 2020, pp 1-10.

50. Steeves V: A dialogic analysis of Hello Barbie's conversations with children. *Big Data Soc* 2020;7(1):1-12.

Lumbosacral Agenesis

Charles d'Amato, MD, FRCSC • Todd DeWees, MHA, CPO • Joseph Ivan Krajbich, MD, FRCS(C)

ABSTRACT

Lumbosacral agenesis is a rare congenital disorder resulting in the failure of formation of one or more vertebral segments and part or all of the sacrum. There is a wide spectrum of severity ranging from partial absence of the sacrum, with otherwise normal function, to absence of the lumbar and lower thoracic vertebrae and sacrum resulting in severe motor impairment and orthopaedic deformity. There are also frequent visceral abnormalities (such as imperforate anus, upper and lower urinary tract anomalies, and incontinence) and neural anomalies (such as tethered spinal cord, lipomeningocele, and diastematomyelia). When treating a patient with this condition, it is helpful to be familiar with the literature on the prevalence, etiology, and orthopaedic management of lumbosacral agenesis. An illustrative case is presented that describes the surgical and prosthetic management of a child with severe knee flexion contractures, absence of the lumbar vertebrae, and spinopelvic instability.

Keywords: lumbrosacral agenesis; severe knee flexion contracture; spinopelvic instability

Introduction

Lumbosacral deficiency is a disorder consisting of absence of one or more vertebral segments and partial or complete absence of the sacrum. Sacral agenesis and lumbosacral agenesis have been variably called vertebral agenesis, sacral-coccygeal agenesis, caudal regression syndrome, caudal dysplasia, caudal dysplasia sequence, and sacral regression.[1,2] The conditions described by these terms represent a rare, complex disorder with partial or complete absence of the sacrum and partial or complete absence of the lumbar spine. At one end of the spectrum, the condition may be mild and discovered as an incidental radiographic finding (**Figure 1**). At the extreme end of the severity spectrum, the sacrum and lumbar spine are completely absent, and the corresponding neural elements are also absent, causing weakness or complete paralysis of motor function, usually at the level of the last radiographically visible pedicles. In some instances, several more distal segments will be preserved or there will be asymmetric motor function. There is usually comparative sparing of sensation, which is preserved more distally or may even be normal.[3] Visceral deficiencies include renal anomalies, such as absent kidney, horseshoe kidney, and ectopic kidney, and anal-rectal abnormalities such as imperforate anus. Neurogenic bladder, urinary incontinence, and bowel incontinence are common and almost universally present in more severely affected patients. A substantial number of children have associated neurologic abnormalities such as myelodysplasia, tethered spinal cord, lipomeningocele, or diastematomyelia. Any of these abnormalities may affect neurologic function.[4] Fortunately, upper limb function and intelligence are usually normal.[5,6]

The management of more severely affected children presents substantial challenges to the treating orthopaedic surgeon, prosthetist, and rehabilitation team. The orthopaedic management of spinopelvic instability, hip dysplasia, hip dislocation, knee contractures, and foot deformities in more severely affected children has been controversial.

Children with partial sacral agenesis may have a normal appearance and motor function, although urinary incontinence or dribbling may occur. With total absence of the sacrum, dimpling of the buttocks may be present, and there is often substantial disproportion between the trunk and the lower limbs. When multiple lumbar spinal segments are absent, the trunk frequently has a funnel shape (**Figure 2**). Orthopaedic abnormalities include spinosacral instability, upper cervical instability, scoliosis, external rotation and flexion contractures of the hip, hip dislocation, and knee contractures.

Dr. Krajbich or an immediate family member serves as a board member, owner, officer, or committee member of the Scoliosis Research Society. Neither of the following authors nor any immediate family member has received anything of value from or has stock or stock options held in a commercial company or institution related directly or indirectly to the subject of this chapter: Dr. d'Amato and Todd DeWees.

Section 5: Pediatrics

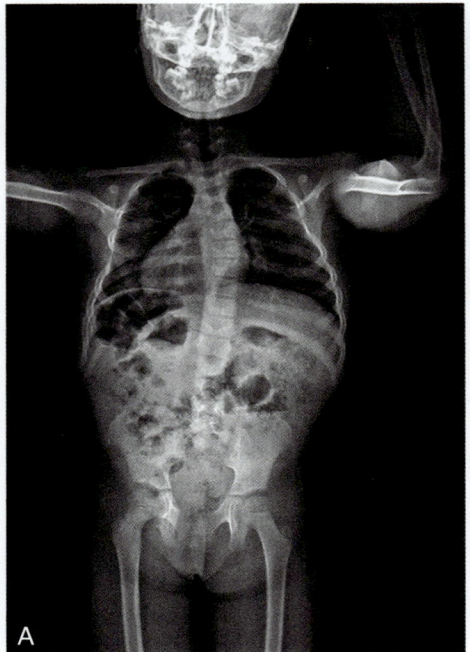
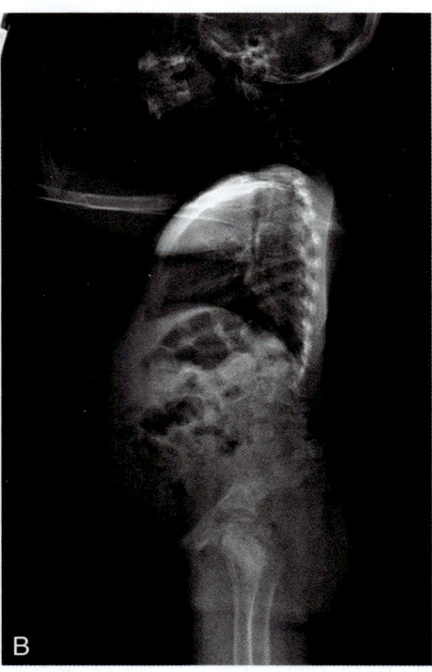

FIGURE 1 AP (**A**) and lateral (**B**) radiographs from a 10-year-old girl with partial sacral agenesis and normal motor, sensory, bladder, and bowel function.

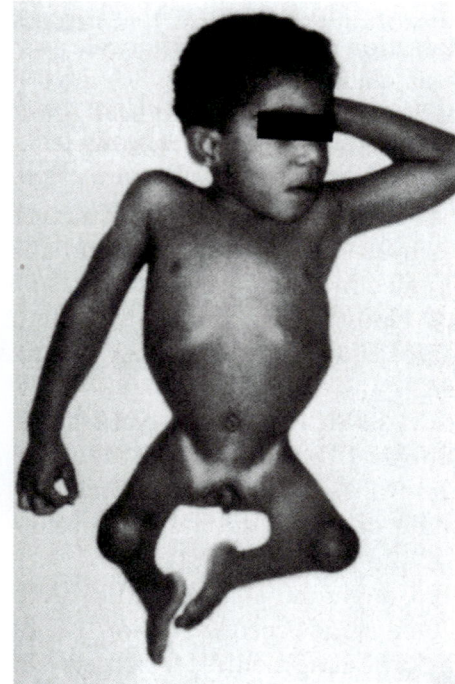

FIGURE 2 Photograph of a child with lumbar sacral deficiency shows the typical funnel-shaped trunk, knee flexion contractures, and popliteus webbing. (Reproduced with permission from Herring JA: Lower extremity injuries, in Herring JA, ed: *Tachdijian's Pediatric Orthopaedics*, ed 5. Elsevier Saunders, 2013, vol 2, pp 1467-1472.)

Severe popliteus webbing may occur in more severely affected patients with a higher-level neurologic abnormality. With weak or absent quadriceps power, the management of knee flexion contractures is difficult, and contracture recurrence is quite common. Foot deformities, such as clubfoot and congenital vertical talus, are frequently present.[3,6-8]

Prevalence and Etiology

Sacral agenesis was first reported by Hohl in 1850.[9] In 1961, Duhamel[10] coined the term caudal regression to describe a spectrum of lumbosacral deficiencies. The incidence of caudal regression has been reported as 0.1 to 0.25 live births.[1] The etiology of this deficiency is likely multifactorial, but its association with diabetes has been recognized by many authors.[3,6,7,11] In a study of 22 patients with lumbosacral agenesis, Phillips et al[6] reported that mothers of 11 of the patients had diabetes. Banta and Nichols[3] reported insulin-dependent maternal diabetes in five of seven patients with sacral agenesis, Guille et al[7] found a maternal history of diabetes in 6 of 18 patients, and Andrish et al[11] in 2 of 17 patients. Women with insulin-dependent diabetes have a 200 to 400 times greater risk of giving birth to an infant with caudal regression syndrome than mothers without diabetes.[1] Although much work needs to be done to establish a causative effect, insulin injections are known to cause embryonic malformations in developing chickens.[12] Nonetheless, the large number of affected patients without a history of maternal diabetes makes the exact role of diabetes unclear.

A genetic cause of lumbosacral agenesis has been postulated. The autosomal dominant *HLXB9* homeobox gene located on chromosome 7q36 has been identified in Currarino triad syndrome. This condition involves sacral agenesis, imperforate anus, perianal fistulas, and a presacral mass.[13] Postma et al[14] recently discovered a mutation in the *T* (brachyury) gene, a member of the T-box family of transcription factors, that causes a syndrome of sacral agenesis, abnormal ossification of vertebral bodies, and a persistent notochordal canal. In four patients from three consanguineous families, homozygosity mapping was used to find a common 4.1-Mb homozygous region on chromosome 6q27 containing the *T* (brachyury) homolog. Sequencing of the *T* gene in affected individuals led to the discovery of a missense mutation, pH171R. The mutation results in diminished DNA binding and increased cell growth, and it interferes with the expression of genes involved in ossification and notochord and axial mesodermal development.

More recent studies involving whole exome sequencing and copy number studies have led to the discovery of multiple genetic features common among patients with sporadic caudal regression patients.[15]

The complex deformities affecting patients with lumbosacral agenesis or caudal regression are understood to be because of the interaction of multiple genetic and environmental factors such as metabolic regulation of retinoic acid metabolism affecting embryonic cell migration, differentiation, and organ development in both animal models and patients. The overlap of syndromes with similar embryologic defects, for example, VACTERL (vertebral defects, anal atresia, cardiac defects, tracheaesophageal fistula, renal anomalies, and limb abnormalities), is recognized.[16]

Classification

In 1978, Renshaw[8] recognized four consistent morphologic patterns of sacral deformity. Type I is partial or total unilateral sacral agenesis. Type II is partial sacral agenesis with a partial but bilaterally symmetrical defect and a stable articulation between the ilia. In type III, there is variable lumbar and total sacral agenesis. The ilia articulate with the sides of the lowest vertebra present. In type IV, there is variable lumbar and total sacral agenesis. The caudal end plate of the most distal vertebra rests above either fused ilia or an iliac amphiarthrosis.

More recently, Guille et al[7] proposed a classification that attempts to predict the potential for ambulation and identifies individuals who might benefit from treatment of their lower limb deformities. Guille et al[7] reviewed 18 patients, 13 with lumbosacral agenesis only (group I) and 5 who also had myelomeningocele (group II). The authors identified three types of spinal deformity (**Figure 3**). In the patients with a type A deformity, the ilia were fused in the midline or there was a slight gap between the ilia. The caudal spine articulated with the pelvis in the midline, and vertical alignment with the pelvis was maintained. One or more lumbar vertebrae were absent. Seven of eight patients in group I with a type A deformity were capable of community ambulation and, with one exception, had motor function below L3 or L4. In patients with a type B deformity, the pelvis was fused in the midline but the spinal articulation was not centered in the midline with respect to the pelvis and articulated with one of the ilia. One patient in group I with a type B deformity was a household ambulator. In patients with a type C deformity, there was agenesis of the lumbar spine and a gap was radiographically visible between the thoracic spine and the pelvis, suggesting spinopelvic instability. All of the ambulatory patients had normal or near-normal sensation. No patient with a type B or C deformity was a community ambulator. No group II patients with myelomeningocele were ambulatory.

Guille et al[7] recommended surgery for patients with type B and C deformities only if the lower extremity deformities interfered with sitting, footwear use, or brace treatment. None of the patients in that study had been treated with spinal stabilization.

Orthopaedic Management

Most patients with an intact lumbar spine and complete or partial deficiency of the sacrum will be able to achieve independent community ambulation with minimal orthopaedic interventions because motor and sensory impairments are not severe.[3,6-8] However, in a patient with myelomeningocele or other untreated intraspinal anomalies, community ambulation may not be possible.[4,6,7]

Deformity in the lower extremity is related to the neurologic level, which often does not correspond to the anatomic level. Phillips et al[6] reviewed 22 patients with lumbosacral agenesis, but with no myelomeningocele or congenital amputations, and focused on the level of neurologic impairment in those with more severe involvement. The patient's anatomic level of lumbosacral agenesis was classified based on the lowest radiographically visible lumbar pedicles. Detailed physical examinations were performed to record motor and sensory levels. Orthopaedic problems related to the level of spinal agenesis and neural levels included hip

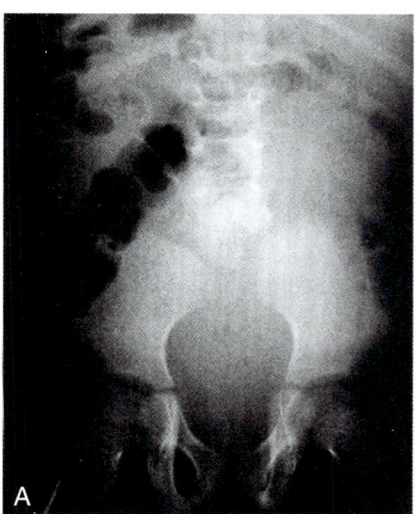
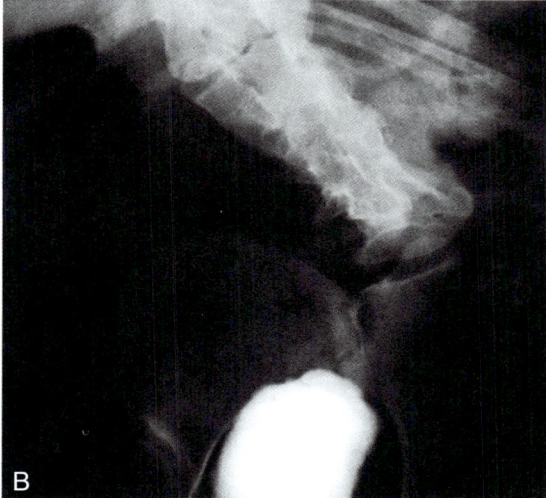
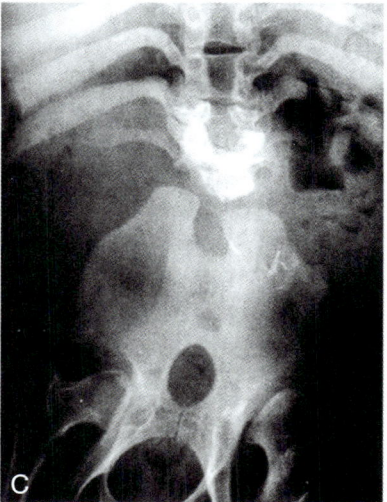

FIGURE 3 Radiographs demonstrating the Guille et al[7] classification of lumbosacral agenesis. This system correlates spinal deformity with ambulatory function. **A**, The vertebral column articulates with the pelvis in the midline in a patient with a type A deformity. These patients have the best potential for ambulation. **B**, In type B deformity, the vertebral column articulates with one of the ilia shifted away from the midline. **C**, In type C deformity, the vertebral column does not articulate with the pelvis. (Reproduced with permission from Guille JT, Benevides R, DeAlba CC, Siriram V, Kumar SJ: Lumbosacral agenesis: A new classification correlating spinal deformity and ambulatory potential. *J Bone Joint Surg Am* 2002;84[1]:32-38. Copyright © The Journal of Bone and Joint Surgery, Incorporated.)

dislocation, hip flexion contractures, knee flexion contractures, and spinopelvic instability. However, foot abnormalities and scoliosis were not related to the functional neurologic level. The 12 patients with spinal agenesis at the T11, T12, or L1 levels (called the first-lumbar group) all had similar findings. This group exhibited the frequently described Buddha-like sitting posture, with abducted flexed hips and flexed knees. For patients in the first-lumbar group, treatment of substantial foot deformity was not needed. Ten of these 12 patients had such severe contractures and popliteus webbing that bilateral lower limb knee disarticulation was performed in nine of the patients and subtrochanteric amputation in one patient. None of the patients with these neurologic levels had hip dislocations, although severe hip flexion contractures were often present.

In patients with lumbar agenesis at the second and third lumbar neurologic levels, hip dislocation occurs in most patients. In the foot, equinus, varus, equinovarus, and calcaneovarus deformities are seen. These patients may require manipulation, casting, or surgery to treat their foot deformities; however, these deformities seldom interfere with ambulation. Knee flexion deformities can be managed with simple bracing treatment or surgery, and these patients do not require limb ablation.

In the study by Phillips et al,[6] scoliosis was identified in 11 of 21 patients for whom there were adequate spinal radiographs. Two of these patients had deformity associated with hemivertebrae. One patient had a 72° curve and back pain, and one had a gibbus deformity; these patients were surgically treated. The other patients with scoliosis had mild curvatures of less than 25°. In their study, Guille et al[7] reported atlantoaxial instability from odontoid hypoplasia and congenital fusions of the upper cervical spine.

The major orthopaedic controversies in the management of patients with lumbosacral agenesis are knee flexion contracture, spinopelvic instability, and, to a lesser extent, hip dislocation. The severity of knee flexion contracture is related to weakness of the quadriceps. In patients with neurologic involvement at the T11, T12, or L1 levels, attempts at reconstruction because of severe contractures associated with popliteus webbing are likely to fail and often result in multiple futile correction attempts and repeated surgeries and hospitalizations. For these patients, bilateral knee disarticulation facilitates sitting. Because the distal femoral epiphyseal plate remains intact, normal femoral length occurs. This greatly facilitates prosthetic fitting. If spinopelvic stabilization is being considered, the tibiae can be used as a structural bone graft.[17,18] Subtrochanteric amputation, which in the past was done to address this problem, is now of historical interest only.[8,19] This procedure sacrifices the distal femoral growth physis in the child, which leads to an extremely short femur, a disfigured body habitus, and requires a more complex and less efficient hip disarticulation prosthesis. It is worthwhile to preserve the lower limbs in patients with intact quadriceps function. When sensation and proprioception are preserved, successful ambulation is more likely.[3,11]

Surgery to treat bilateral hip dislocation may be worthwhile, but it can result in stiff, painful hips if complications such as osteonecrosis occur. In the past, aggressive management of hip dislocations had been recommended in the literature, with the aim of avoiding skin breakdown, pain, gait deterioration, and increased pelvic obliquity.[8] However, in the study by Phillips et al,[6] six patients with bilateral hip dislocation who were not treated were capable of community ambulation.

There are differing opinions on the need to surgically stabilize spinopelvic instability. Patients with complete absence of the sacrum sit on the posterior ilia, which are typically joined at the midline. The associated absence of several lumbar segments results in severe trunk flexion, with unphysiologic compression of the abdominal viscera and crowding of the diaphragm. This can potentially impair respiratory function. Spinopelvic instability also can lead to seating discomfort and positioning difficulties. However, some patients depend on the mobility between the spine and the pelvis to facilitate sitting and movement. This is particularly true when the hips are stiff and contracted. Thus, spinopelvic stabilization should be recommended only after careful functional assessment of the adaptive needs of the individual patient.[20]

Perry et al[21] reported on four patients treated with Harrington rod fixation and grafting to fuse the vertebrae to the pelvis. Success was reported in enabling sitting without dependency on upper extremity support, along with relief of unphysiologic compression of the abdominal viscera. Winter[17] published a case report of spinopelvic stabilization in a girl age 5 years and 11 months with absent vertebrae below T10 and complete absence of the sacrum. The child's lower limbs were drawn up and fixed under her buttocks, with severe flexion contractures of the hip and knees. There was no motor function in the lower limbs, but protective sensation was present. At the time of the spinopelvic stabilization surgery, bilateral knee disarticulation was performed. The patient was placed into halo femoral traction on the operating table to achieve trunk lengthening, and both tibiae were used as structural bone grafts along with Harrington compression instrumentation. Postsurgically, the patient was placed in a halo pantaloon spica cast for 5 months and then into a plastic orthosis for an additional 16 months to achieve solid fusion. To maintain spine and trunk lengthening during growth, lengthening was performed again twice, at age 10 years, 6 months and at age 12 years, 6 months. The lengthening and reinstrumentation was done because of crowding of the internal organs. After osteotomy and distraction through the fusion mass, a more robust modern segment fixation was used; this eliminated the need for a brace or cast immobilization.

Dynamic compression plates, polysegmental fixation with Cotrel-Dubousset instrumentation, and modern transpedicular fixation are currently used for spinal fusion.[22] However, in patients without a sacrum, fixation with sacral screws, Dunn-McCarthy hooks, and Fackler transforaminal or Jackson intrasacral rods is not possible. In those patients, the ilia can be instrumented with Galveston or iliac screw fixation. Yazici et al[18] recently described their technique of using screws and rods anchored in the ilia, along with anterior tibial autograft and bone morphogenetic protein to achieve a solid connection between the trunk and the pelvis, with preservation of the limbs.

Orthotic and Prosthetic Management

Patient Evaluation

The orthotic and prosthetic management of sacral agenesis presents unique challenges and requires a comprehensive patient evaluation. Knowledge of the lowest intact vertebra alone is insufficient to fully understand a patient's motor, sensory, and proprioceptive limitations. This point is well illustrated by an example from a 2002 study by Guille et al.[7] In one of the patients in this study, the lowest vertebra was at the T12 level, and motor and sensory function was at the L5 level. This patient achieved community ambulation with the use of orthotic devices. In contrast, in another patient, the lowest vertebra was at the L1 level; however, this patient had no neurologic function in the lower limbs. Neither of these presentations would be expected based solely on knowledge of the lowest complete vertebral level. It is imperative to perform a thorough physical evaluation to assess range of motion, muscle strength, proprioception, and protective sensation before a treatment plan can be formulated. The stability of the spine in the region of the defect as well as the status of hip contractures also should be determined because these factors have a substantial effect on mobility potential.

Orthotic Management

Generally, the orthotic management of patients with sacral agenesis is similar to the orthotic management of any patient with loss of nervous innervation in the lower extremity, such as those with myelomeningocele or spinal cord injury; however, a patient with sacral agenesis is likely to retain greater protective sensation and proprioception. The retention of protective sensation reduces the risk of unnoticed skin breakdown from an improperly fitting brace.

Orthotic intervention for patients with sacral agenesis can be broadly classified as functional or positional. Functional orthoses are used to aid in mobility and can include ankle-foot orthoses, ground-reaction ankle-foot orthoses, and knee-ankle-foot orthoses (**Figure 4**). Some patients can ambulate over short distances using an orthosis but will choose a wheelchair for longer distances to conserve energy. Positional orthoses, which are typically knee-ankle-foot or ankle-foot orthoses, are used at night and are important for maintaining range of motion to allow continued ambulation or for comfort in sitting. The loss of range of motion leads to the loss of functional ambulation, decreases the ability to sit comfortably, and causes difficulty with hygiene. The orthotic device is used to maximize the functional independence of an individual, whether this means independent ambulation or wheelchair mobility. With proper orthopaedic and orthotic management, most patients can achieve a satisfactory functional status.[11] This highlights the need for an integrated team approach in the treatment of these highly complex patients.

Prosthetic Management

Nearly all patients with lumbosacral agenesis who undergo amputation have neurologic levels at T11, T12, or L1. Hip flexion contractures and severe knee flexion contractures associated with popliteus webbing can interfere with sitting and accomplishing the activities of daily living and should be treated with knee disarticulation and prosthetic fitting. In the past, amputation at the subtrochanteric level was primarily done to facilitate sitting balance. Although these patients technically had transfemoral amputations, the prosthetic fitting was performed as if they had a bilateral hip disarticulation because of the short femoral segments resulting from sacrifice of the distal femoral physis. Prosthetic management of patients with sacral agenesis who are treated with knee disarticulation is far more successful than subtrochanteric or transfemoral amputation because the longer resulting residual limb segment is easier to fit into a prosthesis and much more energy efficient. It

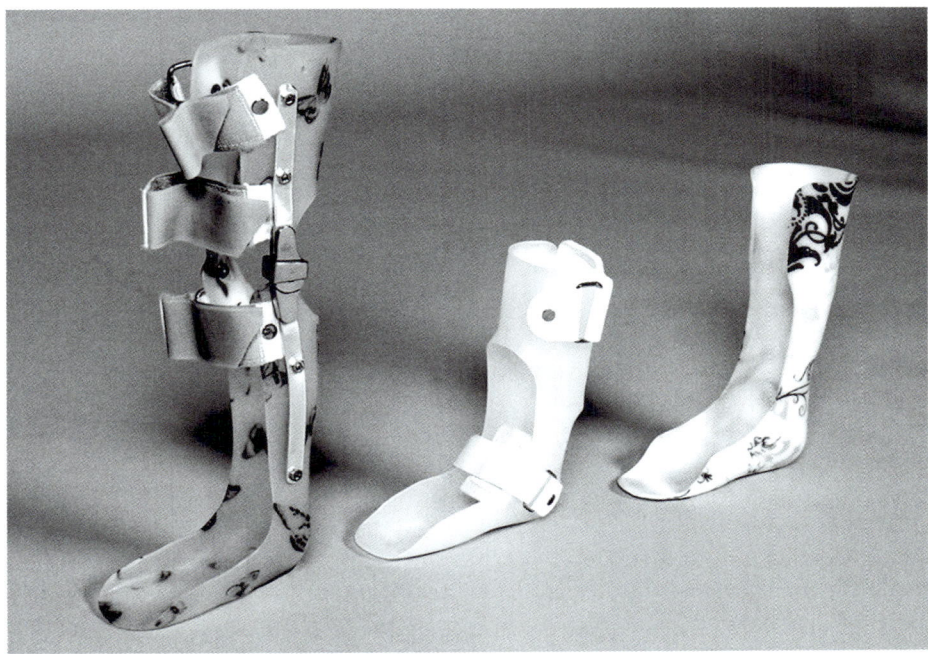

FIGURE 4 Photograph showing (left to right) a knee-ankle-foot orthosis, a ground-reaction ankle-foot orthosis, and an articulated ankle-foot orthosis.

should be noted that the prosthetic fitting can be complicated by limitations in hip range of motion.

Treatment Example

Although the treatment of patients with lumbosacral agenesis varies depending on the status of the individual patient, the following case example illustrates some of the problems, challenges, and potential treatments involved in caring for a patient with lumbosacral agenesis, spinal instability, and severe contractures of the knees and hips.

A male infant with myelomeningocele and Renshaw type IV sacral agenesis was first seen for orthopaedic treatment at the age of 9 months. Over the next 6 years, he was treated with serial casting, orthotic management, and physical therapy in an attempt to manage severe knee contractures. During this time, he also was treated with multiple medical and surgical procedures, including cephalad and peritoneal shunt revisions, bowel resection, cecostomy, bilateral hernia repair, and treatment for pathologic fractures of the femurs and tibiae. His mother reported that the contractures of the child's knees and feet prevented him from being placed in a car seat or in a sitting position on the school bus.

On physical examination, the child was able to ambulate on his hands while sliding his lower body along the floor. Substantial hyperextension of the elbows was present, and he had large callouses on the palmar aspects of both hands. He could ambulate with a walker, bearing all of his weight on his hands and using a swing-through gait. His trunk was short, and there was marked spinopelvic instability. The right hip had no voluntary motion, and the left hip had a range of motion between 35° and 75° of flexion. Both hips were abducted 20° and externally rotated to 90°. Fixed knee flexion contractures, severe popliteus webbing, and fixed cavovarus deformities of both feet were present. Light touch sensation was preserved to the level of the knee. The child's spine collapsed when sitting because of the unstable connection of the spine and pelvis (**Figures 5** through **7**).

At the age of 7 years, after extensive discussion of the proposed treatment with the patient's family, the child underwent bilateral knee disarticulation with fusion of the spine from T12 to the ilium; the harvested tibia was used as a structural bone graft (**Figure 8**). A knee disarticulation prosthesis with a reciprocating gait system was fitted. The primary goal of the device was to provide standing stability, with the possibility of reciprocating gait. A substantial challenge with this approach was the limited range of motion of the hips as well as the fact that this patient had never taken steps and had previously only stood in a standing frame for limited periods of time. The device was fabricated with two-part sockets to allow the patient independent donning in the seated position (**Figure 9**). Manual locking knees were used for stability during stance. A posterior thoracic shell for trunk support incorporated a hooped-style cable reciprocating gait system. After the device was fabricated, the patient was allowed to stand and take his first steps with the use of a walker.

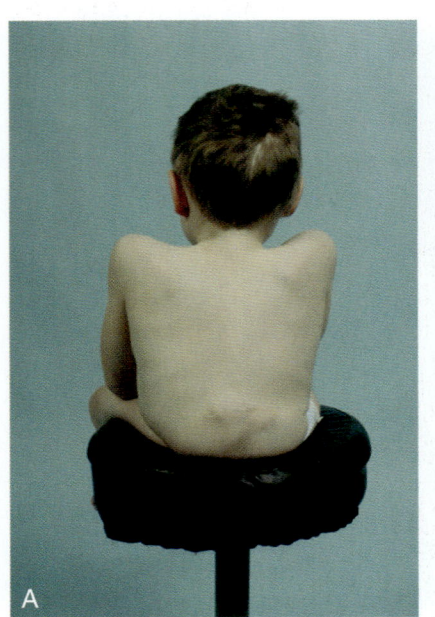 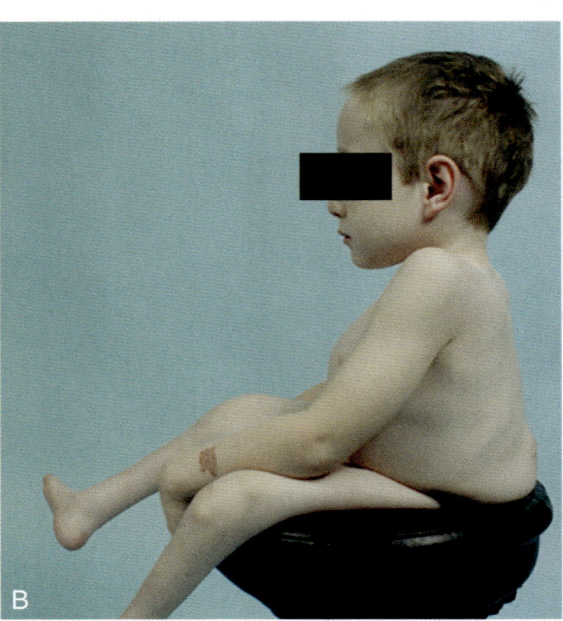 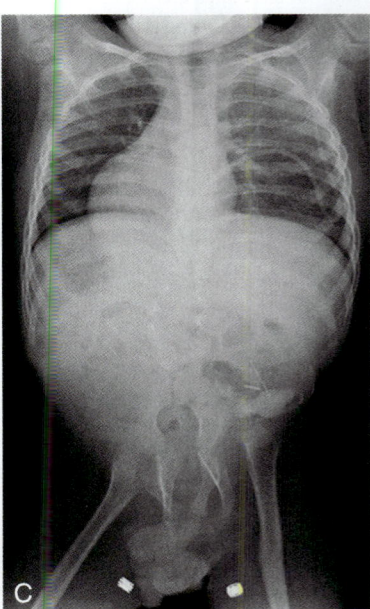

FIGURE 5 Clinical and radiographic images of a child with lumbosacral agenesis. Posterior (**A**) and lateral (**B**) photographs show collapse of the trunk onto the pelvis and thighs when sitting. **C**, Radiograph shows the L2 vertebra perched above the pelvis, with complete absence of the sacrum.

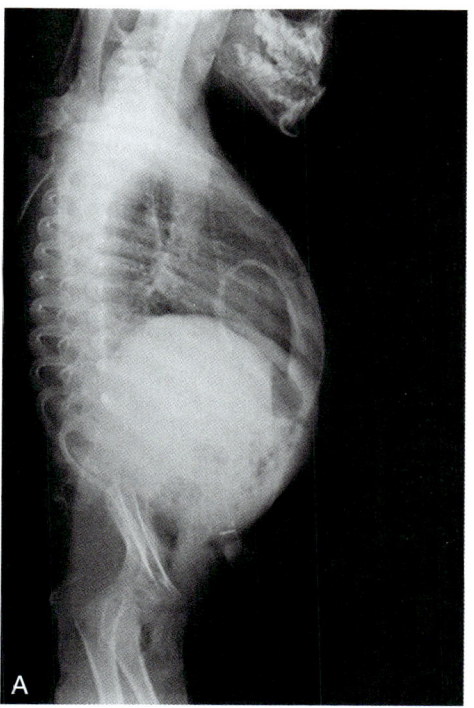 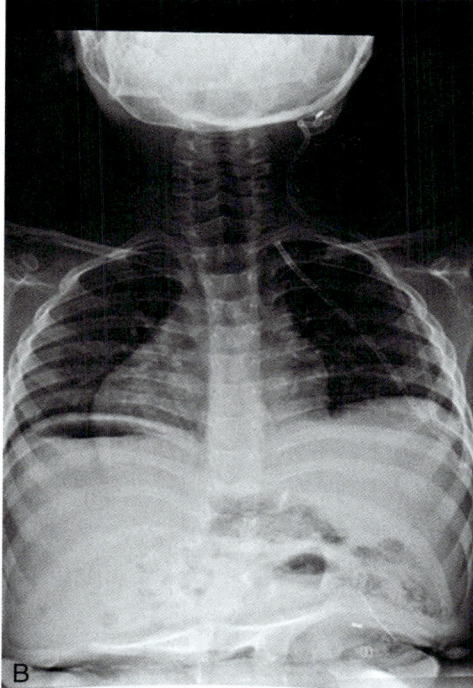 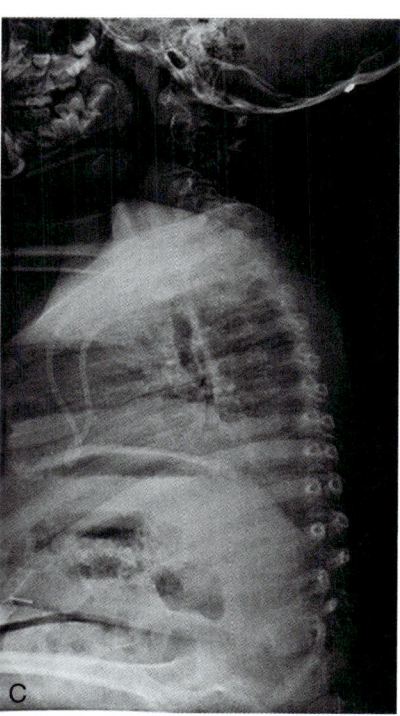

FIGURE 6 Additional radiographic images from the child described in Figure 5. **A**, Lateral radiograph shows the second lumbar vertebra posterior to the pelvis with an unstable articulation. AP (**B**) and lateral (**C**) radiographs show collapse of the trunk onto the pelvis. The patient is sitting on the posterior aspect of the pelvis.

The walker proved to be an impediment to the patient, who preferred to use forearm crutches (**Figure 10**). The attempts at ambulation were performed in a motion analysis laboratory so that a video of the patient's gait could be used to assist in optimizing balance and function. Within 30 minutes of transitioning to crutches as an assistive device, the patient was able to ambulate safely without the need for close supervision. The patient preferred a reciprocating gait.

One obstacle to the patient's functional independence was getting in and out of his wheelchair while wearing the device. His excellent upper body strength allowed him to achieve this goal with relative ease, but his limited hip flexion tended to push him out of the wheelchair. This problem was resolved by tilting the seat and back of the wheelchair into

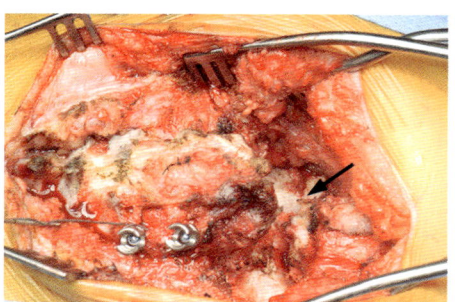

FIGURE 7 Intraoperative photograph of the patient described in Figure 5 showing the unstable spinopelvic articulation (arrow).

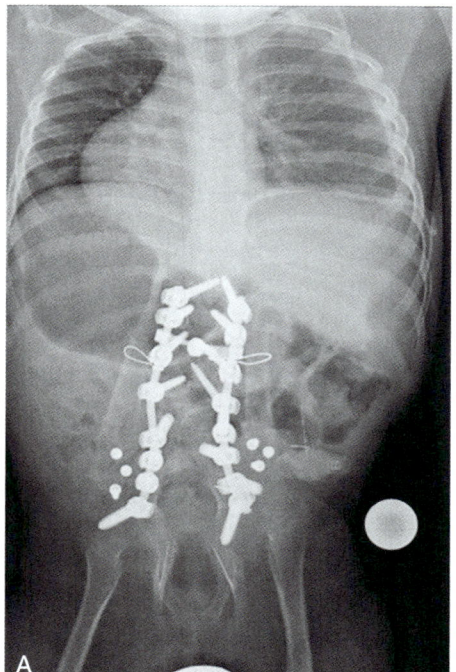 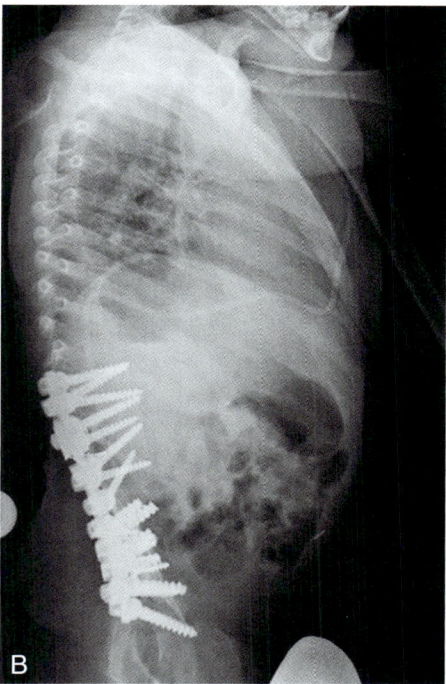

FIGURE 8 PA (**A**) and lateral (**B**) radiographs of the patient in Figure 5 after spinopelvic reconstruction using the patient's tibiae for structural bone graft.

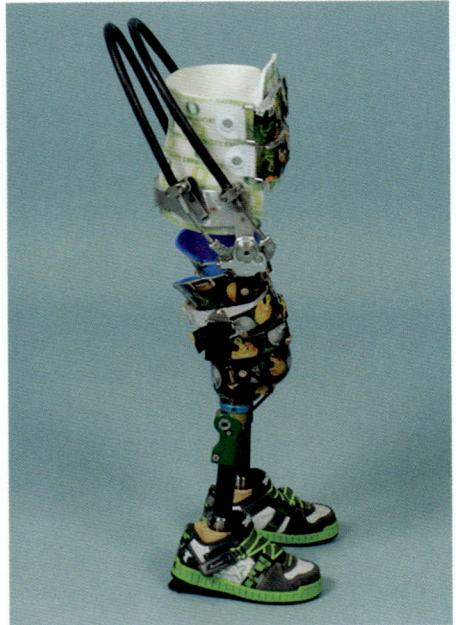

FIGURE 9 Photograph of a knee disarticulation prosthesis with an incorporate reciprocating gait orthosis.

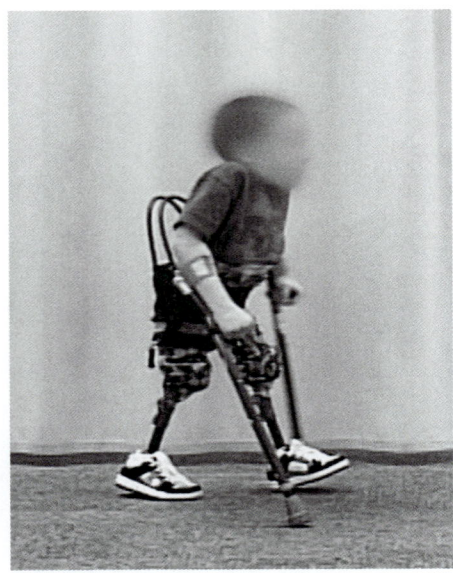

FIGURE 10 Photograph of the patient in Figures 5 and 6 using a knee disarticulation prosthesis and forearm crutches for ambulation.

a slightly more recumbent position. Within weeks of obtaining the device, he was using it as his primary means of mobility within his home and classroom environments, although he continued to use his wheelchair for traveling greater distances.

SUMMARY

Independent function after skeletal maturity is the overarching treatment goal for patients with lumbosacral agenesis. Certain clinical features have an influence on patient outcomes. When motor function is preserved, especially with good quadriceps function, the management of knee flexion contractures is likely to be successful, and independent ambulation can often be achieved. With compromised quadriceps power, the management of contractures is more difficult. Without useful quadriceps function, the ability to achieve community ambulation is very unlikely. When knee contractures cannot be managed, knee disarticulation and prosthetic fitting are the best options, even if community ambulation is improbable after skeletal maturity. This treatment greatly facilitates sitting and accomplishing the activities of daily living. When knee contractures are not present or can be successfully treated, foot deformities can be managed with casting and surgery. Hip dislocation, especially bilateral hip dislocation, can remain untreated if contractures can be accommodated with prosthetic fitting. Spinopelvic stabilization with spinal instrumentation and structural grafts can be performed in selected patients.

References

1. Boulas MM: Recognition of caudal regression syndrome. *Adv Neonatal Care* 2009;9(2):61-69.
2. Chervenak F: Caudal regression syndrome. Available at: https://www.rarediseases.org/rare-disease-information/rare-diseases/byID/898/viewFullReport. Accessed June 10, 2015.
3. Banta JV, Nichols O: Sacral agenesis. *J Bone Joint Surg Am* 1969;51(4):693-703.
4. Emami-Naeini P, Rahbar Z, Nejat F, Kajbafzadeh A, El Khashab M: Neurological presentations, imaging, and associated anomalies in 50 patients with sacral agenesis. *Neurosurgery* 2010;67(4):894-900.
5. Caird MS, Hall JM, Bloom DA, Park JM, Farley FA: Outcome study of children, adolescents, and adults with sacral agenesis. *J Pediatr Orthop* 2007;27(6):682-685.
6. Phillips WA, Cooperman DR, Lindquist TC, Sullivan RC, Millar EA: Orthopaedic management of lumbosacral agenesis: Long-term follow-up. *J Bone Joint Surg Am* 1982;64(9):1282-1294.
7. Guille JT, Benevides R, DeAlba CC, Siriram V, Kumar SJ: Lumbosacral agenesis: A new classification correlating spinal deformity and ambulatory potential. *J Bone Joint Surg Am* 2002;84(1):32-38.
8. Renshaw TS: Sacral agenesis. *J Bone Joint Surg Am* 1978;60(3):373-383.
9. Blumel J, Evans EB, Eggers GW: Partial and complete agenesis or malformation of the sacrum with associated anomalies; etiologic and clinical study with special reference to heredity: A preliminary report. *J Bone Joint Surg Am* 1959;41(3):497-518.
10. Duhamel B: From the mermaid to anal imperforation: The syndrome of caudal regression. *Arch Dis Child* 1961;36(186):152-155.
11. Andrish J, Kalamchi A, MacEwen GD: Sacral agenesis: A clinical evaluation of its management, heredity, and associated anomalies. *Clin Orthop Relat Res* 1979;139:52-57.
12. Duraiswami PK: Insulin-induced skeletal abnormalities in developing chickens. *Br Med J* 1950;2(4675):384-390.
13. Horton WB, Steiner MA, Khan MA: Complete Currarino triad presenting with diarrhea in a 7-month-old girl. *South Med J* 2010;103(8):815-818.
14. Postma AV, Alders M, Sylva M, et al: Mutations in the T (brachyury) gene cause a novel syndrome consisting of sacral agenesis, abnormal ossification of the vertebral bodies and a persistent notochordal canal. *J Med Genet* 2014;51(2):90-97.
15. Porsch RM, Merello E, DeMarco P, et al: Sacral agenesis: A pilot whole exon sequencing and copy number study. *BMC Med Genet* 2016;17(1):98.
16. Warner T, Scullen TA, Iwanaga J, et al: Caudal regression syndrome – A review focusing on genetic associations. *World Neurosurg* 2020;138:461-467.
17. Winter RB: Congenital absence of the lumbar spine and sacrum: One-stage reconstruction with subsequent two-stage spine lengthening. *J Pediatr Orthop* 1991;11(5):666-670.
18. Yazici M, Akel I, Demirkiran HG: Lumbopelvic fusion with a new fixation technique in lumbosacral agenesis: Three cases. *J Child Orthop* 2011;5(1):55-61.

19. Russell HE, Aitken GT: Congenital absence of the sacrum and lumbar vertebrae with prosthetic management. *J Bone Joint Surg Am* 1963;45(3):501-508.
20. Lubicky JP: Congenital absence of the lumbar spine and sacrum: One-stage reconstruction with subsequent two-stage spine lengthening. *J Pediatr Orthop* 1992;12(5):675.
21. Perry J, Bonnett CA, Hoffer MH: Vetebral pelvic fusions in the rehabilitation of patients with sacral agenesis. *J Bone Joint Surg Am* 1970;52(2):287-294.
22. Rieger MA, Hall JE, Dalury DF: Spinal fusion in a patient with lumbosacral agenesis. *Spine* 1990;15(12):1382-1384.

Terminal Bone Overgrowth

Joseph Ivan Krajbich, MD, FRCS(C)

CHAPTER 84

ABSTRACT

Terminal bone overgrowth occurs in transosseous amputations in skeletally immature individuals. It is an appositional growth at the end of the transected bone. It causes trauma to the overlying soft tissues, leading to pain and inability to use a prosthesis. The treatment focuses on prevention whenever possible. Once the condition is established, treatment options include excision of the overgrowth spike with soft-tissue reconstruction and capping of the distal part of the transected bone or osteoplasty.

Keywords: amputation revision; capping; Earth procedure; prevention; terminal bone overgrowth

Introduction

Terminal bone overgrowth is a phenomenon affecting amputated limbs of juvenile amputees. It is an appositional bony growth on the terminal end of transosseous amputation. The overgrowth has a tendency to taper into a pointy end, which can cause significant injury to the overlying soft tissues. Any practitioner, whether an orthopaedic surgeon, prosthetist, or physical therapist, treating young children with limb deficiencies will encounter this phenomenon. It occurs both in acquired and congenital amputations (**Figure 1**). It only occurs in skeletally immature young children. The incidence diminishes with age and as a rule does not occur in adult, skeletally mature individuals. The treatment likely represents a significant portion of surgical procedures in pediatric orthopaedic surgical practice, which specializes in limb deficiencies.

Dr. Krajbich or an immediate family member serves as a board member, owner, officer, or committee member of Scoliosis Research Society.

Etiology

A number of theories have been advanced as to the etiology of the condition. Some theories, such as unchecked proximal epiphyseal growth, have been discarded as wrong. More recently, the idea of bone healing disorder on the molecular level had gained some interest. However, it is not known whether a definitive explanation, which would explain the clinical experience encountered, has been advanced. Until such time, treatment of these patients needs to reflect the current clinical knowledge of the phenomenon. Possible prevention and, in the case of established condition, treatment options are described.

Clinical Presentation

By far the most common presentation is pain at the terminal aspect of the residual limb. Both acquired and congenital deficiencies are affected. The pain can be felt with or without prosthesis use. Sometimes, the pain initially can be

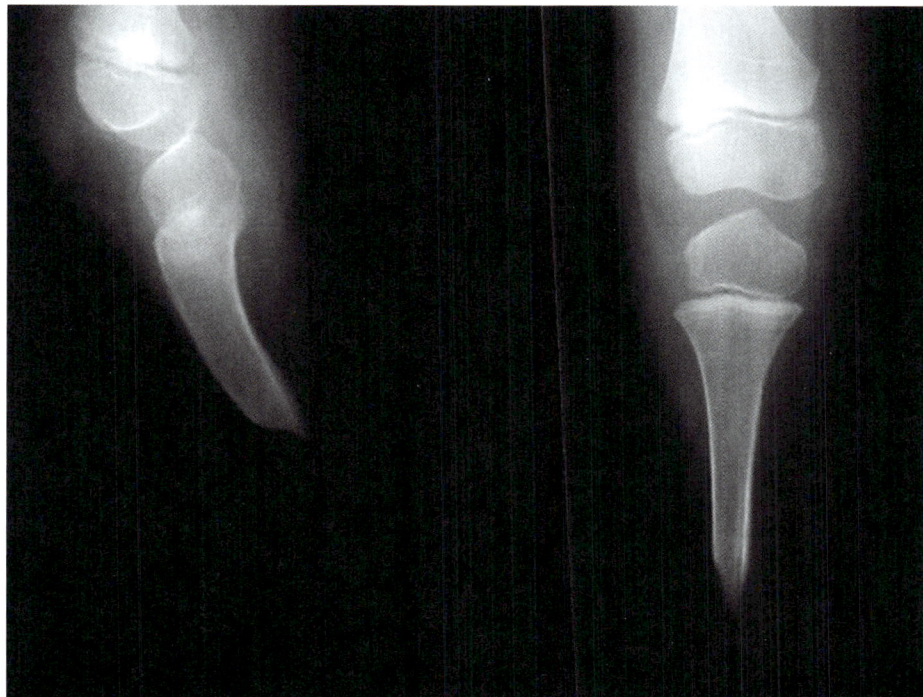

FIGURE 1 Radiographs show a terminal overgrowth of the tibia in a child incorrectly treated by transtibial amputation for underlying fibular hemimelia.

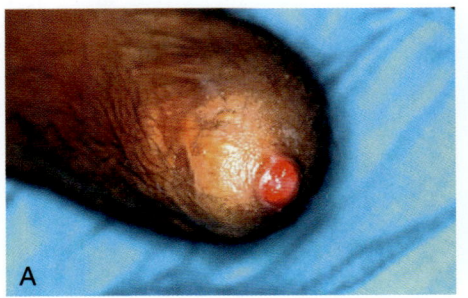 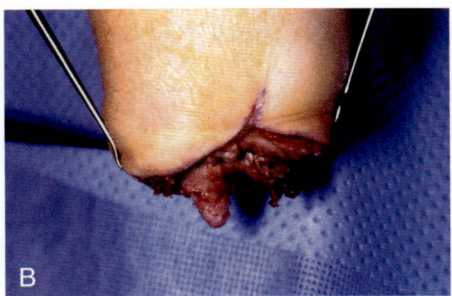 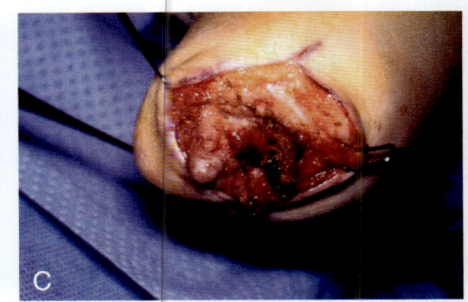

FIGURE 2 **A,** Photograph showing spike produced by terminal overgrowth protruding through the skin. **B** and **C,** Photographs showing surgical exposure of the terminal overgrowth during surgical correction.

temporarily addressed by prosthetic modification to relieve pressure on the end of the limb in children who use a prosthesis. It is likely that this will only be a temporary stopgap measure. More likely the pain will continue/recur with progressive swelling of the affected area. This usually represents a bursa formation around the offending spike. If left untreated, prosthetic use becomes impossible and in severe cases the bone spike will protrude through the soft tissues and skin, causing drainage and possible infection[1,2] (**Figure 2**).

Any long bone can be affected, yet not with the same frequency. Fibula, humerus, tibia, and femur, in this order, are the most frequently involved. The fibula is particularly prone for overgrowth and should be carefully examined when symptoms of terminal overgrowth in a transtibial transosseous amputation are present. It is not rare that the overgrowth spike on the fibula is missed when the surgeon only concentrates on the tibia.

The phenomenon is less likely encountered in the bones of the forearm despite congenital transtibial amputations being the most frequently encountered congenital amputation in a specialty pediatric limb deficiency clinic. Symptomatic distal radius or ulna overgrowth occurs only in the situation of acquired amputation—either postnatally (trauma, neoplasm) or prenatally (amniotic band syndrome).

Prevention

Because terminal bone overgrowth occurs only in transosseous amputations, this type of amputation should be avoided whenever possible. Not surprisingly it is one of the principles of amputation surgery in children. Joint disarticulation is much more preferable to a transosseous amputation. The most obvious example is preference for Boyd or Syme amputation (true ankle disarticulation) over transtibial amputation whenever possible. This is so even in situations where there is an abnormality in the tibia and the temptation on the part of an inexperienced surgeon for a transtibial amputation is high. An example is congenital fibula deficiency (fibular hemimelia) where the tibia can be significantly bowed and misshapen. Another example is a persistent nonunion in the congenital tibial pseudarthrosis where attempts to obtain union have failed and amputation is contemplated. Generally in a skeletally immature individual, amputation should not be performed through the pseudarthrosis or proximal to it. The Syme amputation (ankle disarticulation) is the much

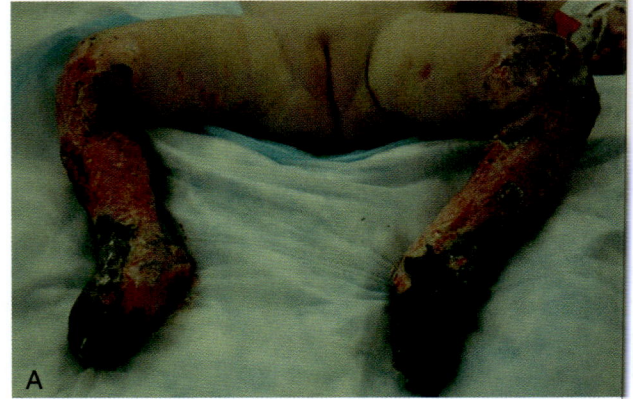 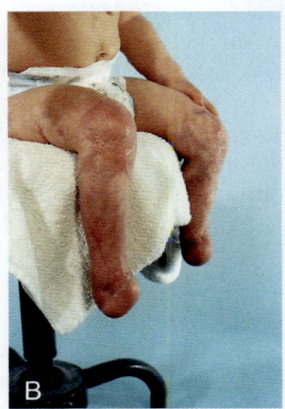

FIGURE 3 **A,** Photograph showing gangrenous extremities treated by Syme amputation, débridement, vacuum dressing application, and skin grafts. **B,** Photograph showing the final appearance of the extremities.

preferred procedure. In this situation, the persistent pseudarthrosis can be stabilized with a well-fitting prosthesis and it is not uncommon for union to eventually occur without any further intervention. Similarly, an ischemic insult such as purpura fulminans gangrenous foot can be removed by ankle disarticulation and soft-tissue débridement as needed, then allowing new granulation tissue to proliferate over the extremity and eventually covering it with a skin graft (**Figure 3**).

In situations when transosseous amputation is inevitable, several strategies can be used to prevent future overgrowth or at least make its treatment less complicated. The two most common reasons for transosseous amputations in children are trauma and malignant tumors. Neither is particularly common in first-world countries. Improved safety features of various machinery, in particular motor vehicles, have decreased the incidence of severe extremity trauma, and modern limb-sparing tumor surgery likewise has decreased the need for routine extremity ablation in the case of sarcoma of the extremity. The situation is clearly different in developing countries, war-torn areas, and earthquake zones. These conditions can present very different scenarios to the treating surgical team. In the case of trauma, the emergency surgical team may or may not be versed in principles of amputation surgery in children, and the child may have other organ injuries for which treatment can be critical to the child's survival and by necessity take precedence over an orthopaedic extremity procedure. Dealing with a severe, complex extremity trauma in the middle of the night with less-than-optimal support staff introduces yet another confounding factor. Simple transosseous amputations can be the simplest and fastest procedure to move the child and also the surgical team out of the operating room. However, there can be alternatives. The level of amputation is frequently determined not by osseous injury but by the injury to the soft tissues. In such a situation early débridement of all clearly necrotic tissue, thorough cleansing of any contamination, and planning to have a second look at a 24- to 48-hour interval may allow for a more sophisticated procedure with functional benefit down the road. At the second look, intercalary shortening saving the distal epiphysis and joint surface to optimize soft-tissue coverage or using some parts of the otherwise-to-be-discarded distal part of the extremity to cap the transosseous amputation with a cartilage-covered epiphyseal/metaphyseal transplant or some other length-sparing or joint-saving procedure can be used. In the lower extremity, parts of the tarsal or metatarsal bones or even proximal phalanges can be used. A similar strategy can be used in the case of infection and/or malignancy (**Figure 4**).

In the case where the transosseous amputation is inevitable and the previously described strategy cannot be used, it is important to preserve as much length of the extremity as possible rather than perform standard adult-level amputations. This is to allow for easier management of the terminal overgrowth without worrying about leaving the extremity too short for effective prosthetic fitting and use.

Management of Established Conditions

The simplest and likely one of the most commonly used treatment options is simple residual limb revision. The end of the bone or bones in the case of transtibial amputations is exposed, bursa if present is excised, and bone is foreshortened approximately 1 cm proximal to the spike. An attempt should be made to close the soft tissues over the distal end in several layers—periosteum, muscle, and fascia if available before skin closure. Some advocate plugging the medullary cavity with muscle, fat, or other available soft tissue to prevent future overgrowth. The exception is a fibula overgrowth, where the bone can be shortened by several centimeters

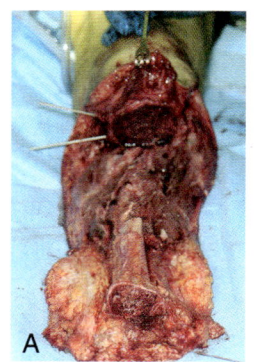
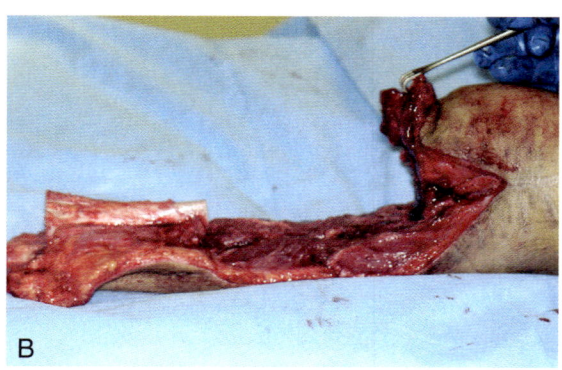
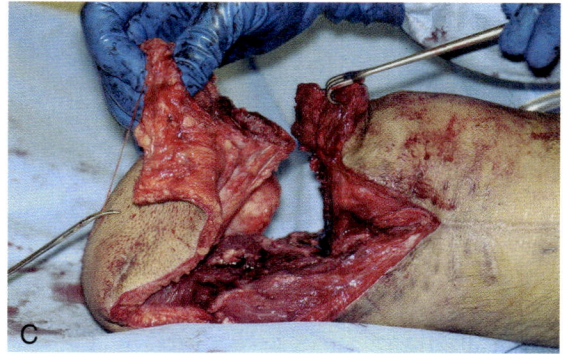
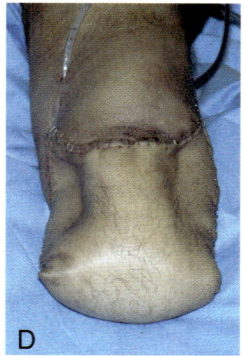
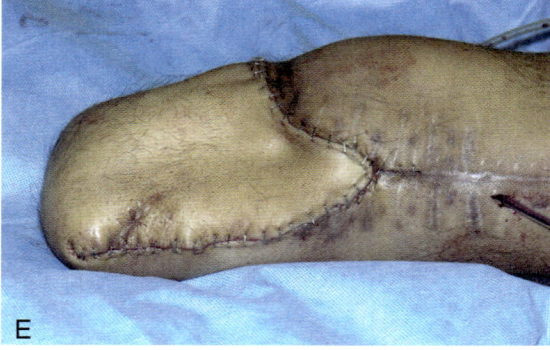

FIGURE 4 **A** and **B**, Intraoperative photographs showing a large defect in the proximal tibia due to infected allograft used in a limb salvage procedure to manage osteosarcoma. **C**, Intraoperative photograph showing upside-down distal tibia being used to reconstruct the defect in the proximal tibia. **D** and **E**, Photographs showing resultant functional transtibial-like amputation.

without compromising the length of the residual extremity.

The procedure is quite effective in the short term; however, recurrence of the overgrowth is quite common and the patient's family needs to be made aware that additional intervention will likely be required in the future. The younger the age of the child, the higher the chance of recurrence and likely the shorter the interval between recurrences. The issue is usually resolved when the child reaches skeletal maturity. Although the advantages of this procedure are its simplicity and low complication rates, its disadvantages are also significant. Shortening of the residual limb and need for likely revision surgeries in the future have led many surgeons to seek alternative solutions.[2,3] These can roughly be divided into capping procedures and osteotomy/osteoplasty procedures. The capping can be by a biologic implant or artificial cap. A variety of metal and synthetic materials were used for caps.[4,5] Unfortunately, relatively high complication rates, particularly infection and loosening, led to procedure abandonment. These implants are no longer used; however, with development of new biologically friendly materials, the procedure may yet be resurrected.

The capping procedure most commonly used is a biologic capping using ipsilateral proximal fibula head with adjacent metaphysis in the situations where the fibula is present or a bicortical graft with cartilaginous apophysis harvested from iliac crest in the case of absent fibula (associated longitudinal fibular deficiency or transfemoral amputation). Iliac crest graft has mixed reviews in the literature but can be successful if adequate cartilage cap and overlying perichondrium is part of the graft.[6] The biologic capping procedure was first popularized in Heidelberg.[5] It was based on the observation that terminal growth does not occur in bones in which the end is covered by cartilage, as is the case of joint disarticulation. Biologic capping and its various modifications have been described by several authors.[3,5,7-11]

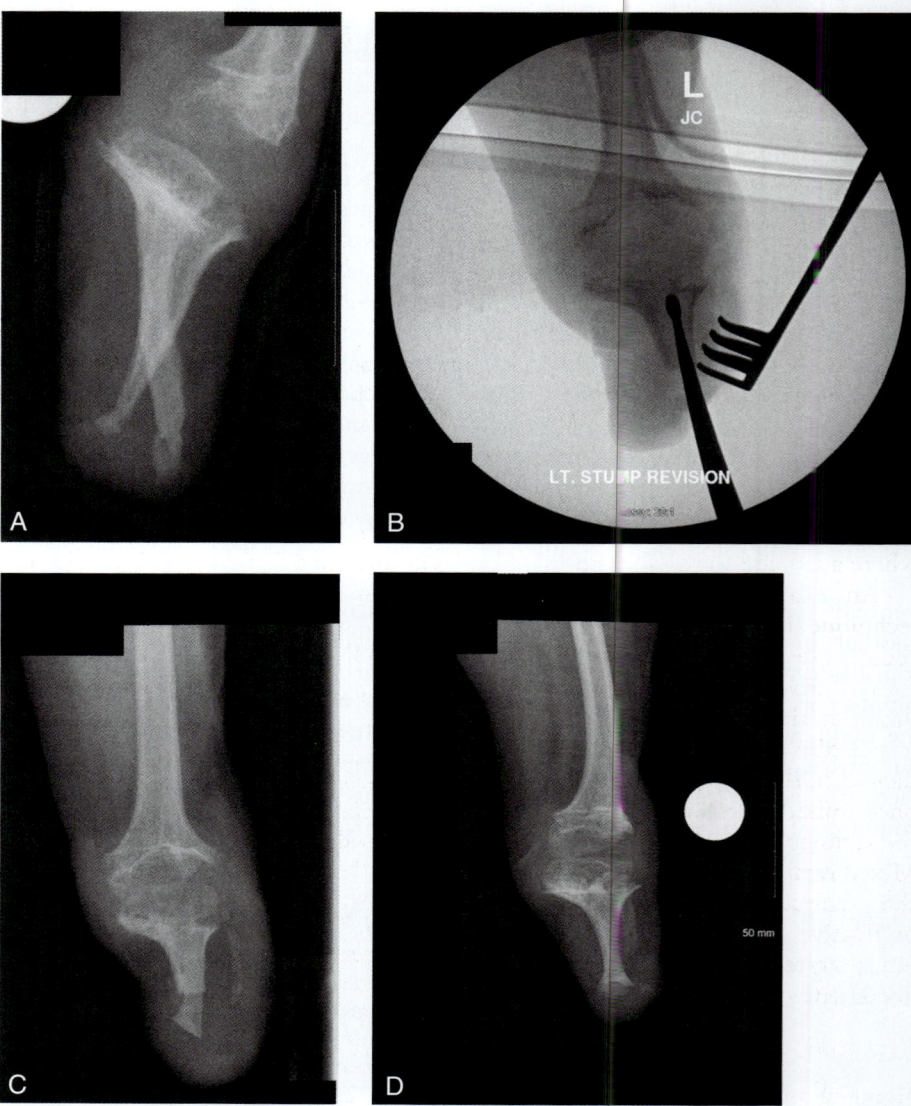

FIGURE 5 Radiographs show transfer of the proximal fibula into the terminal end of the tibia. **A**, Preoperative radiograph shows both tibia and fibula overgrowth. Radiographs show preparation of the recipient site (**B**) and transfer of the proximal fibula into the recipient site in the distal tibia (**C**). **D**, Radiograph 2.5 years after the index procedure shows preservation of epiphysis.

In most instances, the transplanted graft can be fashioned to fit into the medullary cavity of the recipient bone with no minimal need of additional internal fixation (**Figure 5**). Fully vascularized graft is also an option, particularly if used as a composite graft, not only to address the overgrowth but also to reconstruct deficient soft tissues and perhaps even provide some additional length to the residual limb (**Figure 6**).

The use of the proximal fibula from the contralateral otherwise healthy extremity is not recommended because of potential complications, such as risk of peroneal nerve injury or alignment disturbance at the ankle of an otherwise healthy extremity. Similarly, it is best avoided in the case of transhumeral amputation.

Vascularized proximal fibula graft may also be an option. If based on the anterior tibial artery pedicle with blood supply to the proximal fibula epiphysis preserved, it may allow for additional epiphyseal longitudinal growth at the distal end of tibia. It may be of potential use in a case of a very short

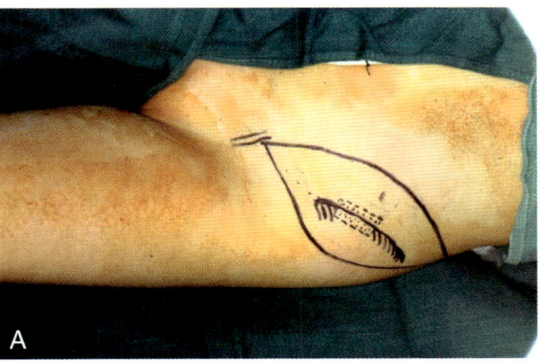 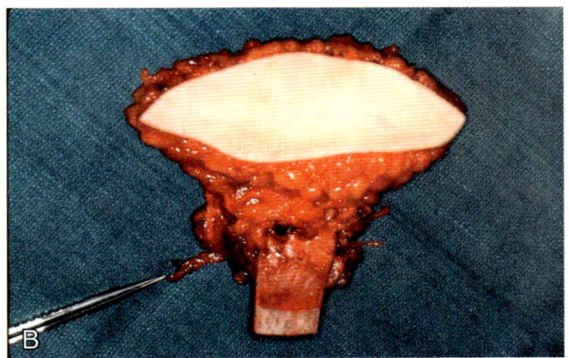 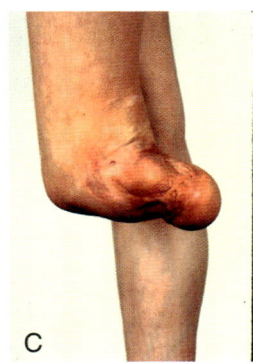

FIGURE 6 Photographs showing the use of composite vascularized free graft. **A**, Harvest site of composite vascularized graft from an iliac crest. **B**, Harvested composite graft with vessel pedicle. **C**, Resolution of overgrowth issue and acquiring additional length in a very short tibial residual limb.

proximal tibial segment in a situation where adequate soft tissue is present.[12]

An example of osteoplasty is a technique described by Ertl.[13] The procedure uses a portion of the fibula to form a cross union between tibia and fibula at the distal end. The osteotomized fibula is oriented near perpendicular to the long axis of the tibia and once united, the fibular cortex forms the terminal element of the extremity. Mixed reviews of the Ertl procedure in the literature can be partially explain by relatively limited numbers reported, but long-term good results are well documented.[14]

SUMMARY

Terminal bone overgrowth is a well-recognized, common phenomenon associated with transosseous amputations in young children. It occurs in both congenital and acquired deficiencies. Prevention in acquired deficiencies is the best treatment. Using distal joint disarticulation, preserving cartilage-covered epiphysis, is the best way of preventing the occurrence of terminal bone overgrowth. Once established, amputation revision, capping the transected bone with cartilage-covered graft, and osteoplasty (Ertl procedure) are the treatment options. The recurrences diminish with age and the condition does not, as a rule, occur in skeletally mature individuals.

References

1. Aitken GT: Overgrowth of the amputation stump. *Inter Clinic Bull* 1962;1:1-8.
2. Marquardt E, Correll J: Amputations and prosthesis for the lower limb. *Int Orthop* 1984;8(2):139-146.
3. Davids JR: Terminal bony overgrowth of the residual limb: Current management strategies, in Herring JA, Birch JG, eds: *The Child with a Limb Deficiency.* American Academy of Orthopaedic Surgeons, 1998, pp 269-280.
4. Swanson A: Silicone-rubber implants to control the overgrowth phenomenon in juvenile amputee. *Interclinic Info Ball* 1972;11:58.
5. Marquardt E: The multiple limb deficiency child, in Bowker JH, Michael JW, eds: *Atlas of Limb Prosthetics: Surgical, Prosthetic and Rehabilitation Principles,* ed 2. Mosby-Year Book, 1992, pp 839-884.
6. Fedorac GT, Cuomo AV, Watts HG, Scaduto AA: Management of terminal osseous overgrowth of the humerus with simple resection and osteocartilagenous graft. *J Pediatr Orthop* 2017;37(3):e216-e221.
7. Bernstein R, Watts H: Modified Marquardt procedure for terminal overgrowth in children, in *69th Annual Meetings Proceedings.* American Academy of Orthopaedic Surgeons, 2002.
8. Davids JR, Meyer LC, Blackhurst DW: Operative management of bone overgrowth in children who have an acquired or congenital amputation. *J Bone Joint Surg Am* 1995;77:1490-1497.
9. Benevenia J, Makley JT, Leeson MC, Benevenia K: Primary epiphyseal transplants and bone overgrowth in childhood amputation. *J Pediatr Orthop* 1992;12:74.
10. Ertl J: About amputation stumps. *Chirurg* 1949;20:218-224.
11. Fedorak GT, Watts HG, Cuomo AV, et al: Osteocartilagenous transfer of the proximal part of the fibula for osseous overgrowth in children with congenital or acquired tibial amputation: Surgical technique and results. *J Bone Joint Surg Am* 2015;97(7):574-581.
12. Taylor GI, Wilson KR, Rees MD, Corlett RJ, Cole WG: The anterior tibial vessels and their role in epiphyseal and diaphyseal transfer of fibula: Experimental study and clinical applications. *Br J Plast Surg* 1988;41:451-469.
13. Drvaric DM, Kruger LM: Modified ertl osteotomy for terminal overgrowth in childhood limb deficiencies. *J Pediatr Orthop* 2001;21:392-394.
14. Firth GB, Masquijo JJ, Kontio K: Transtibial Ertl amputation for children and adolescents: Case series and literature review. *J Child Ortho* 2011;5(5):357-362.

Athletics and Sports Programs for the Child With Limb Difference

CHAPTER 85

Kevin Quinn, MSPO, CPO • Zach Harvey, CPO

ABSTRACT

Positive introduction to athletics and sports programs is important for a child with limb difference. However, there can be physical and social challenges the child or parent encounters along the way. Through awareness of what is possible and in knowing what resources are available, these challenges can become easier to work through. The right adaptations to technique or adaptive equipment are often all that is needed for a successful outcome.

Keywords: adaptive; amputation; prosthesis; sports

Introduction

When it comes to sports, the playing field is not always equal for a child with a limb difference, and participation might feel intimidating. That is why parents, coaches, and health care workers need to pay special attention to the child's potential limitations and help to figure out ways of making participation more inclusive. Participation in sports has shown to have a positive influence on the individuals with disabilities in quality of life as well as physical and psychosocial realms.[1] This applies to team sports as well as to individual sports. Challenges might come up during different developmental stages in a child's life or as interests change, so it is good to be ready to assist when needed.

A caretaker should inspire confidence in a child's introduction to a new sport. The question should not be if it is possible, but how. It is also important to be cognizant of any difficulty that a child might have, so that helpful intervention can be achieved. Intervention can come in the form of adapting technique, adapting the piece of equipment, or provision of an activity-specific prosthesis. A child with limb difference often figures out ways of adapting technique on their own but may also benefit from some instruction. Adaptive equipment can involve simply modifying existing equipment to fit or function better or it might involve different or specialized equipment altogether. An activity-specific prosthesis may be ideal for performance for an avid athlete, but may be unnecessary, especially for someone just starting out.[2]

Adapting equipment should be made with safety and performance in mind. It is important to prevent entrapment, the connection of the child to the piece of equipment if something such as a fall were to occur. For certain sports in which the prosthesis is being used, an auxiliary form of suspension, such as a sleeve or belt, is advised to prevent the prosthesis from falling off, which could cause injury to the child or others. Following these considerations, the child may often participate in sports not specifically organized for individuals with disabilities.[3]

Team Sports

For a child with limb difference, team sports are commonly integrated with nondisabled peers. Padding over the prosthesis is sometimes mandatory for sports with potential contact with other players. If the prosthesis is just getting in the way or is painful to wear, adapting technique is sometimes necessary. Examples include competing on the swim team without a prosthetic leg, or throwing the ball from the sidelines using one hand instead of two. When a prosthesis is not being worn, a residual limb protector may be devised to protect against impact or joint injuries.

For larger groups of children with disabilities, team sports could be played in a seated position. Such examples of events that may be modified in this way and are often included in the Paralympic games include seated volleyball, sled hockey, wheelchair basketball, and wheelchair rugby. Team sports could also be played standing, but with modified rules and equipment. One such example is amputee football or soccer. This is a sport played using Lofstrand crutches for lower extremity amputees and upper extremity amputees playing goalkeeper positions.

Strength and conditioning are part of many team sports. Adaptive needs can be unique to the level of amputation as well as the specific exercise. For those with upper limb differences,

---

Kevin Quinn or an immediate family member serves as a paid consultant to or is an employee of Össur. Zach Harvey or an immediate family member serves as a paid consultant to or is an employee of Hanger Clinic.

strengthening the affected side can be particularly challenging, and alternative tools should be considered, including resistive bands, cables, and cuffs. Exercises can be performed with or without the use of a prosthesis. For lower limb differences, a common problem is that the heel of the prosthetic foot comes off the ground when squatting during certain leg exercises. A good solution is to position a weight underneath the heel to bring it into a more natural athletic stance position.

Running and Jumping Sports

Innovations in prosthetic design have opened up possibilities in performance that were previously limited. One such example is running blades. When Van Phillips first invented and personally used the Flex-Foot in 1984, it opened up doors for many amputees to run more efficiently and with less impact to the residual limb.[4-7] Since then, various manufacturers have created increasingly improved designs.

The biomechanical requirements for running differ compared with walking for lower extremity amputees.[8] The primary difference between walking-specific and running-specific feet is the presence of a heel.[7] Although running on a foot prosthesis designed for walking is possible, and some newer foot designs intend to satisfy both requirements, a foot prosthesis that includes a heel is not optimal for running.[8] Some prosthetic feet such as the Össur Cheetah Xplore JR and Fillauer Pediatric formula (Figure 1) offer a good transitional prosthetic foot that can walk well for day-to-day use and provide adequate energy storage for running in short bursts for field sports. Running prosthetic feet designs incorporate C-shaped (distal mount) or J-shaped (posterior mount) carbon blades with excellent spring-like properties.[5] Although distally mounted prosthetic feet have more adjustability for height and alignment, they do require a larger amount of space available between the ground and socket. Height of the running prosthesis should be slightly higher than the sound side to factor in compression of the carbon fiber spring.[5] Alignment of the toe of the blade should fall in line with the bisection of the socket in the sagittal plane (Figure 2).

For transfemoral designs, the inclusion of a knee is optional. Without a knee joint, circumduction is required to clear the foot during swing phase. For a transfemoral running prosthesis, which includes a prosthetic knee, the prosthetist must ensure stable knee alignment and optimal swing-resistant settings for safety and efficiency. Also, with a prosthetic knee, more learning is required on behalf of the patient, and training with a skilled physical therapist is advised.

Access to prosthetic running legs is a challenge with the expense and lack of coverage by most insurance providers. Fortunately, some nonprofit organizations exist in the United States, such as the Challenged Athletes Foundation, Amputee Blade Runners, Never Say Never Foundation, and High Fives Foundation.[2] These organizations award grants for prosthetic running feet and sometimes other adaptive equipment. Those children fortunate enough to have a dedicated prosthetic running leg may find it useful for team sports, gymnastics, dance, or simply keeping up with peers on the playground.

Snow Sports

Skiing and snowboarding include a wide array of options for a child with limb difference, and many ski resorts offer adaptive lessons with access to various adaptive equipment. Adaptive instructors teach proper technique, match equipment needs, assist the skier, and help with getting on and off the lift. Skiing can be done standing with the

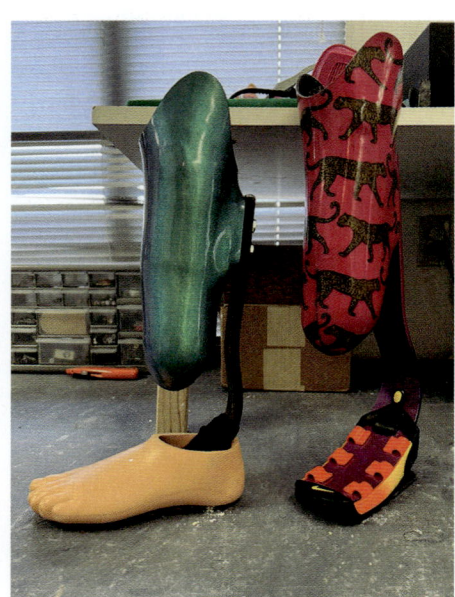

FIGURE 1 Photograph shows posterior-mounted prosthetic feet designed for walking and short-distance running.

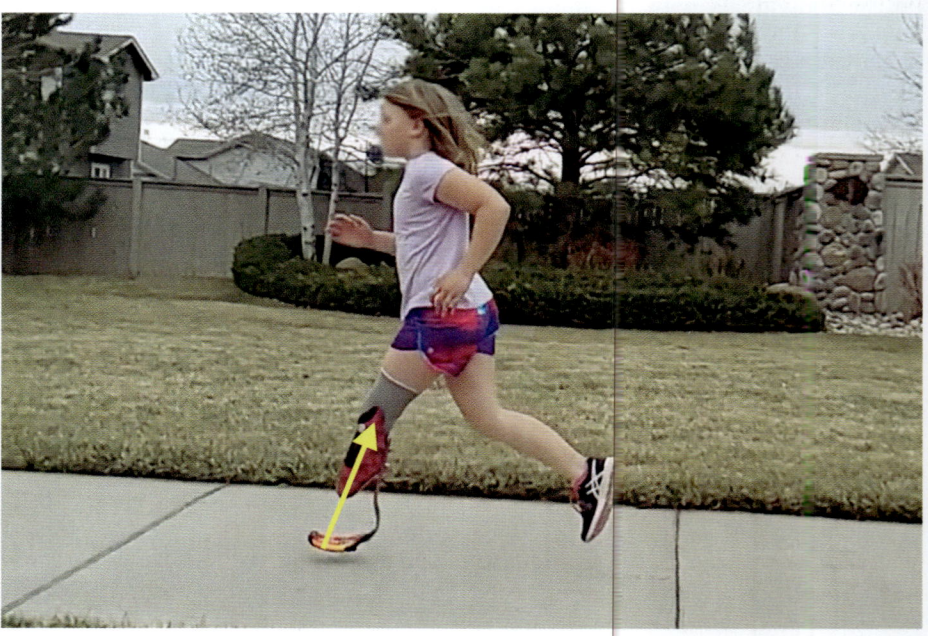

FIGURE 2 Photograph shows running blade designed and aligned specifically for running.

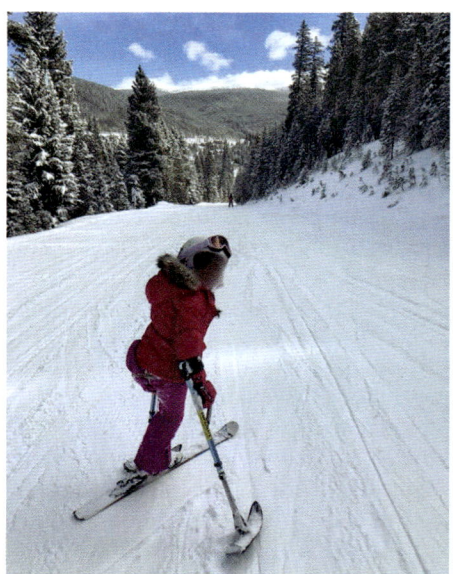

FIGURE 3 Photograph of a three-tracking skier using outriggers. Outriggers are a type of adaptive ski equipment that can benefit standing and seated skiers with balance.

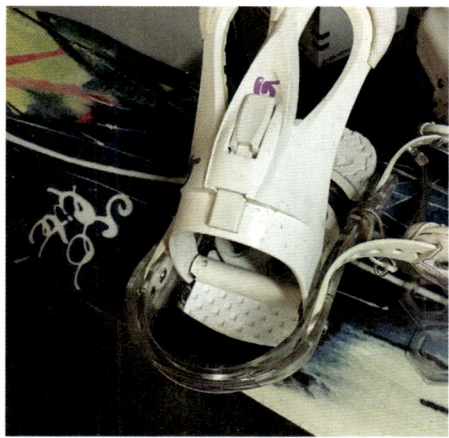

FIGURE 4 Photograph shows wedges are a useful tool for sports such as snowboarding. Wedging can be used inside or outside of a shoe or boot to better improve athletic stance and alignment. Here, a polyvinyl chloride pipe was used as a heel wedge on a snowboard binding.

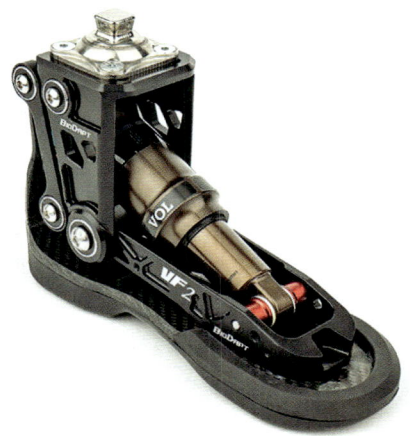

FIGURE 5 Photograph shows the Biodapt Moto knee and Versa foot that incorporate gas shocks and help with various sport performance for avid athletes. (Reproduced with permission from Biodapt. All rights reserved.)

use of a prosthesis, standing without a prosthesis (three tracking), or sitting down. Special poles with small skis, called outriggers, can help skiers of all types with balance (**Figure 3**).

Ski or snowboard boots can be difficult to put on a prosthetic foot, but the use of a plastic grocery bag can help to break the friction. A heel wedge and foam pieces inside the boot can be used to prevent movement inside the boot and to optimize athletic stance and alignment.[9] In order to improve athletic stance and increase comfort while snowboarding, a heel wedge and a lateral cant improve prosthetic alignment. This tilts the prosthesis forward and medially to accommodate a flexed and wide stance (**Figure 4**). Foam pieces inside the boot can reduce movement and can be strategically positioned inside the boot to tilt a ski to one side or the other if needed. With these changes in prosthetic alignment to a more athletic stance, it should be noted that walking can be difficult.

Specialized prosthetic feet and knees, which use mountain bike shocks, can benefit an avid standing skier or snowboarder (in addition to other sports), but are not entirely necessary when learning.[10] Mike Schulz is a decorated snowboarding Paralympic athlete who invented such examples of these components (**Figure 5**).

Sit skiing can use a biski or monoski. These buckets are connected to the ski with a shock absorber and can be positioned in a high position for the lift and then lowered when skiing. The outriggers have small skis that can be flipped up to reveal spikes, which can help the skier navigate lift lines and push themselves on flat surfaces. Two adaptive instructors are needed to assist with lift transfers until the child gains independence. Custom ski buckets can be made for avid sit skiers when required.

Water Sports

Whether to swim with a prosthesis on or off is a matter of preference. If the child chooses to use a prosthesis, it is important to understand if the components are waterproof.[9] The use of auxiliary suspension is recommended so that an expensive prosthesis does not end up at the bottom of a lake.[9] For competitive swimming or triathlon, rules often state that a prosthesis may not be used to be award-eligible.[11] For triathlon, the athlete is allowed a handler, someone to help them out of the water to a place nearby to dry off and put their prosthesis back on so that they can transition to the next event.

Certain water-related sports, such as water skiing, wakeboarding, and surfing, can be easier while wearing the prosthesis for some levels of amputation. Paddle sports, such as kayaking or canoeing, could require some adaptation to equipment or a specialized terminal device for an individual wearing an upper limb prosthesis.[9] Adaptations to technique could also be considered. For example, the prosthesis could be taken off and waterskiing performed on one leg. Knee boarding without the prosthesis could be another alternative to wakeboarding with a prosthesis on (**Figure 6**). Surfing can be done in several different ways with or without a prosthesis. The nonprofit organization, AmpSurf, hosts the International Surfing Organization's World Para Surfing Championship annually with six different divisions of athletes. These divisions include standing, kneeling, visually impaired, upright, prone, and assisted.

Cycling and Riding Sports

Learning to ride a Big Wheel or bicycle may introduce some challenges to children with limb differences. Adaptations to technique may be required for a child with an upper extremity limb absence who may be learning to ride with only one hand. Adaptations to equipment could also be solutions for this child, such as using a prosthesis or adapting a handlebar, as long as it allows for easy detachment from the bike in case of a fall. Something as simple as a cup attached to polyvinyl chloride fittings can suffice to extend the residual limb out to the bike handle (**Figure 7**). For children using leg prostheses, there may be some difficulty keeping the prosthetic foot on the pedal or the heel from hitting the crank arm. Toe clips or straps may be helpful, but only if the child's prosthetic foot can easily come off the pedal if falling to that side.[9] Research has shown that at a recreational level, no significant difference was found between a sports-specific prosthetic foot and an everyday walking prosthetic foot, making cycling an excellent option for the child amputee.[12]

Other difficulties may include socket impingement in the back of the knee (for transtibial amputations) or socket impingement in the groin (for transfemoral amputations).[12] If there is an anatomic knee center difference, as commonly occurs with longitudinal deficiency, there may be some asymmetry expected in pedaling on the left and right sides. Use of a crank arm shortener (**Figure 8**) on the prosthetic side only (or both for bilateral) can be a solution to address socket impingement issues or biomechanical asymmetry because less range of motion is required to generate power through the pedal stroke.[3,12]

For sports such as horseback riding or riding motorcycles and all-terrain vehicles, it is important for the prosthetist to position the lock and valve release buttons on the outside of the socket so that inadvertent release of suspension does not occur, causing loss of suspension. If special boots are required for a riding activity, special considerations to alignment may be necessary. A heel height adjustable foot is ideal when switching between a flatter shoe and a boot with a higher heel.[8,10] Also, boots may be adapted with a zipper in the back or outside to facilitate donning (**Figure 9**).

Peer Support and Adaptive Sports Programs

Amputee support groups have long been a means to offer peer and sometimes professional support to those adjusting to limb loss. Youth camps such as Camp No Limits (Wales, ME), NubAbility camp (Du Quoin, IL), the Paddy Rossbach youth camp (Knoxville, TN), and Living in Motion (LIM) 359 youth camp (Denver, CO) (**Figure 10**) provide similar peer support for children with limb differences. LIM359 has devised a unique model of an activities-based support group for adults and children. Each month, participants of all ages dine out or participate in a new adaptive sport. For some members, this might be the first time since amputation or first time ever doing a sport. Some of the past sport events include archery, indoor skydiving, fencing, snow sports, adaptive cycling, bowling, rock climbing, miniature golf, kayaking, stand up paddle boarding, and hiking. Often, events are coordinated with adaptive sports programs such as the National Sports Center for the Disabled (Winter Park, CO) or Adaptive Adventures (Denver, CO). These partnerships have proven to benefit the programs

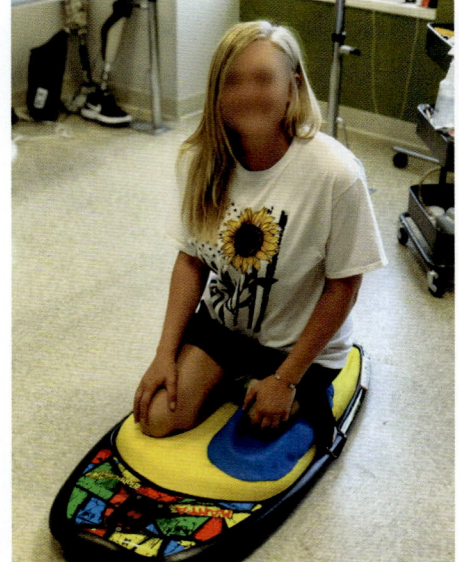

FIGURE 6 Clinical photograph shows creative adaptation to equipment is sometimes an option to still make a sport fun. This kneeboard was adapted by gluing a yoga block and foam for this young woman for water skiing.

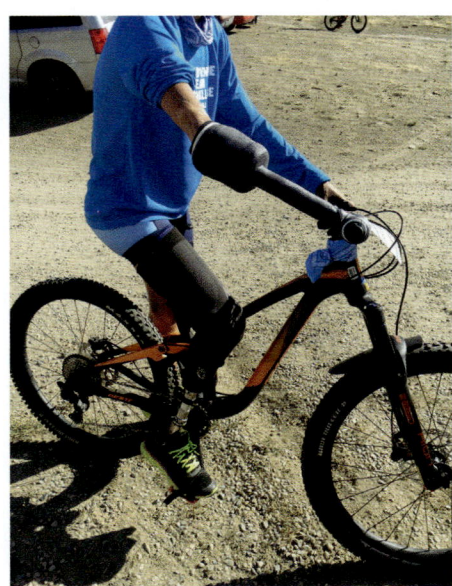

FIGURE 7 Photograph shows how polyvinyl chloride pipe fittings were used to allow this woman to ride a mountain bike. Because her arm is not attached to the pipe, it allows her to release from the bike in case of a fall.

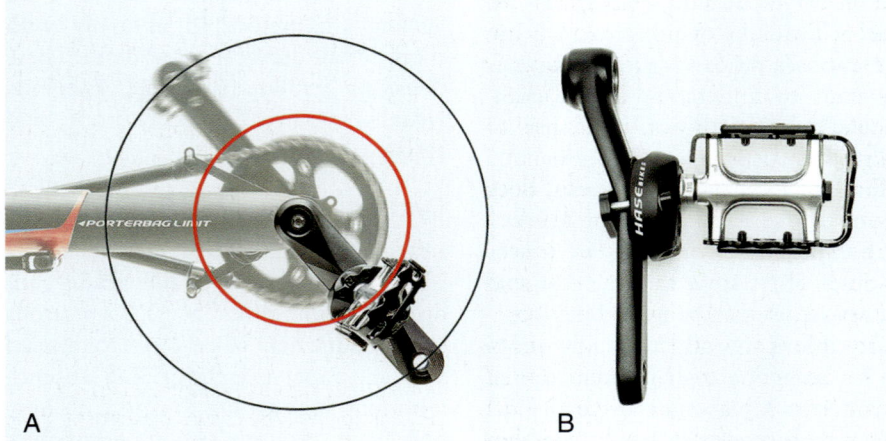

FIGURE 8 Photograph (**A**) and illustration (**B**) show by shortening the crank arm, a more comfortable pedal stroke is possible when cycling. This Ride2 crank arm shortener allows for various pedal positions. (Reproduced with permission from RAD-Innovations LLC.)

Chapter 85: Athletics and Sports Programs for the Child With Limb Difference

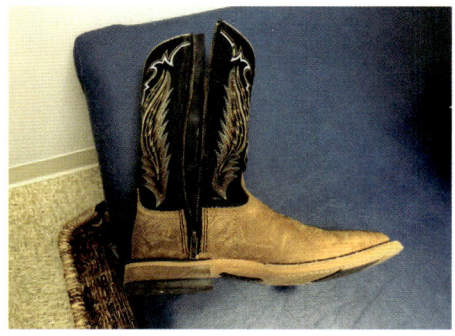

FIGURE 9 Photograph shows boots for various sports can be modified to facilitate donning and doffing of the prosthesis.

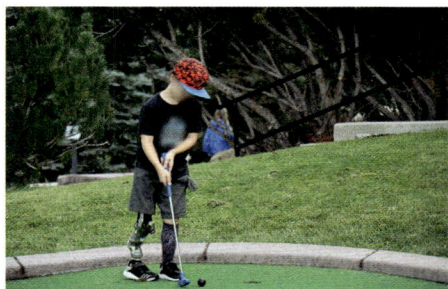

FIGURE 10 Photograph shows the Living in Motion (LIM) 359 youth camp in Colorado as an example of an organization that uses peer support and activity as a method to help children with limb differences normalize their experiences.

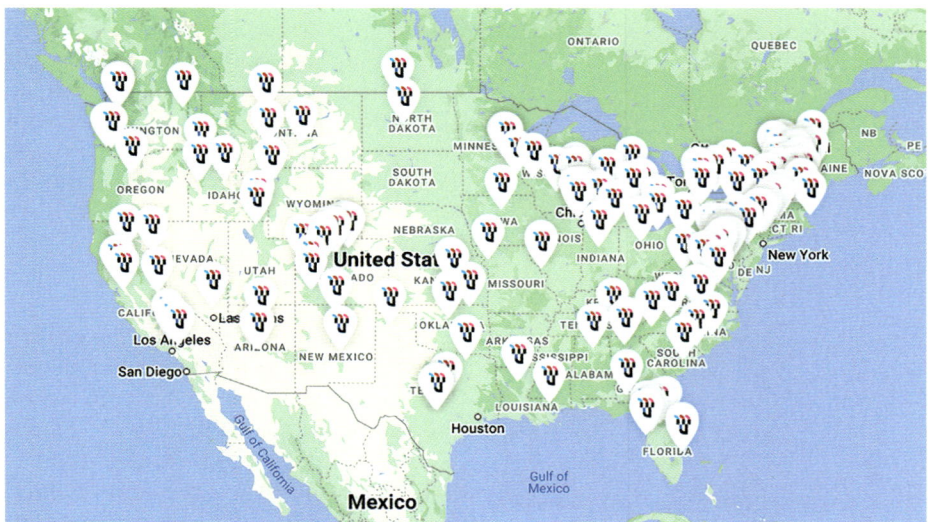

FIGURE 11 Map of Move United Active chapters for Adaptive Sports Programs.

that want more participants and also ensure that the LIM359 group receives proper professional instruction in a safe environment.

Some cities have unique adaptive programs for boxing, skateboarding, climbing, and yoga. B-Bold (Ft. Collins, CO) teaches group classes in boxing and mixed martial arts specifically for persons with disabilities. These classes often include individuals with a wide array of mobility levels including those in wheelchairs. Adaptive Action Sports (Copper Mountain, CO) and Adaptive Skate Kollective (Kansas City, MO) are two resources for adaptive skateboarding. Paradox Sports (Eldorado Springs, CO) offers opportunities for guided adaptive climbing trips including children. These trips include rock climbing, ice climbing, and mountaineering. Adaptive yoga classes are starting to become more prevalent. A good instructor recognizes the needs of the individuals and can adapt the classroom with chairs and possibly assistants. If standing or seating is not possible, the motions can be adapted to a lying-down position.

Finding the right resources both nationwide and locally can be key to involvement in adaptive sports. Although it starts with the child and goal setting with the prosthetist, community plays a large role in adoption of adaptive sports. Move United (Rockville, MD) and Team USA (Colorado Springs, CO) have wonderful website directories of more than 600 clubs (**Figure 11**) and organizations involved with adaptive sports.

SUMMARY

A child with limb difference should not be left on the sidelines when it comes to athletics and sports programs. In fact, the challenges that may be encountered are best approached as opportunities for creative innovation and resourcefulness. There are plenty of inspiring role models who have paved the way and shown what is possible through hard work, determination, and having the right equipment. For a caretaker of a child with limb difference, it is beneficial to be aware of the various forms of adaptive equipment, adaptive sports programs, and peer support. Understanding how to adapt the sport and the equipment and potentially access specialized prostheses, prosthetists should be able to help all children find a way to participate in the sport or sports of their choice regardless of any challenges presented by limb difference. This effort has the potential to bring joy to children who will experience joy through involvement in athletics and sport.

References

1. Yazicioglu K, Yavuz F, Goktepe AS, Tan AK: Influence of adapted sports on quality of life and life satisfaction in sport participants and non-sport participants with physical disabilities. *Disabil Health J* 2012;5(4):249-253.
2. Sayed Ahmed B, Lamy M, Cameron D, et al: Factors impacting participation in sports for children with limb absence: A qualitative study. *Disabil Rehabil* 2017;40(12):1393-1400.
3. Bragaru M, Dekker R, Geertzen JHB, Dijkstra PU: Amputees and sports. *Sports Med* 2011;41(9):721-740.
4. Boonstra AM, Rijnders LJ, Groothoff JW, Eisma WH: Children with congenital deficiencies or acquired amputations of the lower limbs. *Prosthet Orthot Int* 2000;24(1):19-27.
5. Groothuis A, Houdijk H: The effect of prosthetic alignment on prosthetic and total leg stiffness while running with simulated running-specific prostheses. *Front Sports Act Living* 2019;1:16.
6. Phillips V: The Brian Blatchford Prize acceptance speech. *Prosthet Orthot Int* 1998;22(2):90-91.
7. Hobara H: Running-specific prostheses: The history, mechanics, and

controversy. *J Soc Biomechanisms* 2014;38(2):105-110.

8. Hadj-Moussa F, Ngan CC, Andrysek J: Biomechanical factors affecting individuals with lower limb amputations running using running-specific prostheses: A systematic review. *Gait Posture* 2022;92:83-95.

9. Bragaru M, Dekker R, Geertzen JHB: Sport prostheses and prosthetic adaptations for the upper and lower limb amputees. *Prosthet Orthot Int* 2012;36(3):290-296.

10. Curran SA, Lyle DK: Adaptive sports ankle prosthetics. *Prosthet Orthot Int* 2012;36(3):370-375.

11. L: International Paralympic Committee. Swimming Rules and Regulations 2011-2014. Available at: www.ipc-swimming.org/export/sites/ipc_sports_swimming/Rules_Regulations/IPC_Swimming_Rules_and_Regulations_2011_-_2014_FINAL.pdf. Accessed December 3, 2022.

12. Poonsiri J, Dekker R, Dijkstra PU, Hijmans JM, Geertzen JH: Bicycling participation in people with a lower limb amputation: A scoping review. *BMC Muscoskelet Disord* 2018;19(1):398.

Index

Note: Page numbers followed by '*f*' indicate figures and '*t*' indicate tables.

A

Acetabular dysplasia, 932
Acquired multiple limb deficiencies, 990
Acquired partial foot loss, 979
Acute postoperative evaluation, adult lower limb
   assistive devices, potential ambulation with, 607
   bed mobility, 607
   cardiopulmonary status, 606
   sensation, 606–607
Adaptive sport, 726
   adaptive cycling, 727–728, 727*f*–728*f*
   adaptive skiing and snowboarding, 728–729, 729*f*
   functional fitness, 727
AFO. *See* Ankle-foot orthosis (AFO)
Amniotic band syndrome, 985
AMP. *See* Amputee Mobility Predictor (AMP)
Amputation. *See also* individual amputation types
   adaptive sport, 726
      adaptive cycling, 727–728, 727*f*–728*f*
      adaptive skiing and snowboarding, 728–729, 729*f*
      functional fitness, 727
   in children, 10–11
      congenital tibial pseudarthrosis, 784
      disarticulation *vs.* cartilage capping, 781–782
      growth, 780
      ipsilateral proximal limb abnormalities, 782–783
      joint function, 782
      limb length, 780
      multiple limb deficiencies, 784
      perisurgical pain control, 783
      psychologic considerations, 783
      soft-tissue grafting, 780–781
      surgical timing, 783
      Syme *vs.* Boyd amputation, 783–784
      upper limb deficiencies, 783
      Van Nes procedure, 784, 785*f*
   elbow disarticulation, 240, 241*f*
      prosthesis, 248, 248*f*
      rehabilitation, 244
      socket designs, 257–258, 258*f*
      surgical technique, 241, 242*f*–243*f*
   health-related quality of life and, 3
   level selection for, 5
   vs. limb salvage, 4, 21–39
   lower limb amputation, 721–722
      activities and participation, 722
      body functions and structure, 722
      health services, systems, and policies, 723
      legal and social security services, 723
      personal factors, 723
      prosthesis, 722
      skin, 722
      transportation services, 723
   metabolic cost, walking after, 4
   partial hand, 191–200, 193*f*–199*f*
      prosthetic management, 201–208, 202*f*–208*f*
   postoperative prosthetic management, 249–250, 250*f*
   recreation, 729
   resources, 729–730
   shoulder, 261–263, 261*f*–262*f*, 264*f*–273*f*, 265–273
   socket interface, 7, 8*f*
   soft-tissue considerations, 250, 250*f*
   transhumeral amputation, 239, 242–244, 243*f*–244*f*
      control strategies, 258–259, 258*f*–259*f*
      distal humeral shaft, 248–249, 249*f*
      endoskeletal transhumeral prosthesis, 253, 253*f*
      interface construction, 256–257
      interface modification and evaluation, 256, 256*f*
      interfaces, 250, 251*f*
      limb length, 251
      limb shape, 252–253
      limb volume, 251–252, 251*f*–252*f*
      liner suspension, 257, 257*f*
      load-bearing tolerance, 253–254, 253*f*
      osseointegration, 249
      prosthesis acceptance rates, 247
      rehabilitation, 244
      rotational stability, 248, 248*f*
      shoulder mobility, 254
      substructure, 253
   transhumeral casting impression
      limb lengths, 255–256
      mediolateral compression, 255
      proximal contours, 254–255, 255*f*
      volume management, 254, 254*f*
   transradial amputation, 213–215, 215*f*–216*f*
   upper limb
      body functions and structure, 724
      body-powered control activation, 247
      clinical outcomes, 211, 217–219
      complications, 217, 218*f*, 244
      concomitant fractures, 212
      elastomer liners, 233, 233*f*
      environmental factors, 724
      health services, systems, and policies, 725
      humeral amputation levels, 239, 240*f*
      incidence of, 211, 223
      injury, 239, 240*f*
      interface evaluation, 232–233, 232*f*–233*f*
      legal and social security services, 725
      neuroma control, 215–217
      Northwestern design, 230, 230*f*–231*f*
      Otto Bock Muenster interface, 230, 231*f*–232*f*, 232
      postoperative prosthetic management, 224–225, 225*f*
      regenerative peripheral nerve interfaces, 217
      targeted muscle reinnervation, 217
   wartime
      clinical problem for, 75
      definitive care, 81
      evacuation care, 81, 82*f*
      in-theater care, 81
      Iraqi freedom operations, 80–81
      rehabilitation, 81
      revision surgery, 82
      US military care, 76–77
      Vietnam experience, 77–80
   war veterans, 725–726
   wrist disarticulation, 212–213, 214*f*
Amputee Mobility Predictor (AMP), 626, 643
Amputee rehabilitation
   full-length prosthesis, 597, 597*f*–598*f*
   OPRA Axor II device, 597, 597*f*–598*f*
   outcomes, 597–598
   short training prosthesis, 596–597, 596*f*
   stage 1 surgery, 595
   stage 2 surgery, 596, 596*f*
   weight bearing, 596, 596*f*
Angular deformities, 898, 898*f*
Ankle disarticulation
   anticipated outcomes, 469–470
   clinical considerations, 470–471, 471*f*
   clinical outcomes, 464–466, 467*f*
   component and alignment considerations, 473–475, 474*f*–475*f*
   distal heel tissue, 469, 470*f*
   gait, 475
   hindfoot amputations, 466
   indications, 464, 464*f*–465*f*
   primary socket-suspension, 471–473, 471*f*–474*f*
   surgical technique, 464, 465*f*–466*f*
   Syme amputation, 463
   transtibial amputations, 463

Index

Ankle-foot orthosis (AFO), 456–457, 456f–457f
Arthritis, 688–689
Assistive devices
    ambulation with, 608–609
    potential ambulation with, 607
Athletic assessment and training, 637–638

B

Bacterial infections, in adults, 27
Benign growths
    cyst, 665
    neuromas, 664–665
    seborrheic keratoses, 664
Bilateral lower limb amputation
    causes of, 568, 569f
    clinical consideration, 568
        wheelchair selection, 570
        wound care and early function, 568–570, 569f
    component consideration
        definitive feet and shoes, selecting and fitting, 575–576
        definitive knees, selecting and fitting, 574–575
        prosthetic knee joints, 575
        socket design, 576
        suspension options, 576–577
    donning bilateral prostheses
        direct suction systems, 577, 578f
        gel suspension systems, 577
        osseointegrated prostheses, 577
    prosthetic care
        balancing support and independence, 571–572
        gender-based issues, 571
        graduated length prosthetic protocol, 572–574, 572f–574f
        mixed and full-time users, 571–572
        motivation, 571
        partial prosthesis users, 571
        prostheses, candidates for, 570
        prosthesis nonusers, 570–571
        psychological considerations, 572
        slipper prostheses, 574
        transtibial amputation, 574
Bilateral lower limb deficiencies, 898–899, 899f
Bilateral transfemoral amputation, 80
Bilateral upper limb amputation
    control systems, 293, 293t
        body-powered control, 294–295
        hybrid control, 295
        multifunctional prosthesis, 293, 294f
        myoelectric control, 295
    elbows, 292, 292f
    harnessing, 289, 289f–290f
    humeral rotation, 292, 293f
    partial hand, 295–296, 296f–297f
    patient care, 287, 287f
    patient evaluation, 285–286, 286f
    prosthetic rehabilitation, 285
    prototype prostheses, 295, 296f
    shoulder disarticulation, 298–299
    shoulder joints, 293, 293f
    socket design, 287–288, 287f
        shoulder disarticulation sockets, 288–289
        transhumeral sockets, 288, 288f
        transradial sockets, 288
    terminal devices, 289–291, 290f
    transhumeral level, 297–298, 298f
    transradial level, 296–297, 297f
    wrists, 291–292, 291f–292f
Body-powered prostheses, 129
    active prehensor devices, 130–131, 131f
        voluntary-closing hooks, 134, 134f
        voluntary-opening hooks, 131–133, 131f–134f
    elbow disarticulation and transhumeral prostheses
        elbow flexion assists and counterbalances, 144–145, 145f
        elbow units, 143
        friction elbows, 143–144, 144f
        inside-locking elbows, 144, 144f–145f
        outside-locking hinges, 143, 144f
    endoskeletal systems, 147, 148f
    finger prostheses
        Metacarpal Phalangeal Driver, 149–150
        Partial M-Fingers, 150, 151f
        PIP Driver, 149
        Thumb Driver, 150
        X-Finger, 150
    hands, 134–135, 135f
        cosmetic gloves, 136–137, 137f
        voluntary-closing hands, 135–136, 136f
        voluntary-opening hands, 135, 136f
    partial hand prostheses
        figure-of-8 harness, 150, 152f
        M-Fingers, 150, 151f
        Minnesota split-hand prosthesis, 150, 151f
    passive prostheses, 129–130, 130f–131f
    shoulders, 145–146, 145f–147f
        disarticulation applications, 162–164, 162f–164f
    socket components, 146–147, 147f–148f
    transhumeral applications
        anterior suspensor strap, 159, 160f
        bilateral transhumeral applications, 161–162, 162f
        Biomechanically Aligned Harness Anchor, 159, 160f
        double harness ring, 160, 160f
        mechanism of control, 157
        sequence of actions, 157–158, 158f–159f
        shoulder saddle, 161, 161f
        transhumeral amputation, 160, 160f
        Triple Control Harness, 161
        Y split, 161, 162f
    transradial applications
        activation of, 154, 155f–156f
        American Civil War era, 151, 152f
        cable-controlled prosthesis, 151, 153f
        chest strap, 155–156, 156f–157f
        figure-of-9 harness, 156, 157f
        figure-of-8 harness system, 152–153, 155f
        force transmission, 151–152
        glenohumeral flexion, 153
        Götz artificial arm, 151, 152f
        power generation, 153, 155f
        shoulder saddle harness, 154–155, 156f
    transradial prostheses
        flexible hinges, 141–142, 141f
        polycentric hinges, 142, 142f
        residual limb-activated locking hinges, 143, 143f
        rigid hinges, 142
        single-axis hinges, 142, 142f
        step-up hinges, 142–143, 143f
    wrists, 137, 137f
        constant-friction wrists, 138, 139f
        flexion units, 139–141, 140f–141f
        friction wrists, 137–138, 138f
        multifunction wrists, 141, 141f
        quick-disconnect wrists, 138–139, 139f–140f
        rotational wrists, 139, 140f
Bony overgrowth, 898, 898f
Boyd amputation, 971–973, 972f
Brachial plexus injury (BPI)
    amputation
        glenohumeral arthrodesis, 386, 387f
        isolated transhumeral amputation, 386
        isolated transradial amputation, 386
    computed tomography, 378, 380f
    electromyography, 378, 380, 380t
    epidemiology, 375, 376f
    pathoanatomy, 375–378, 376f–377f
    physical examination, 378, 379f–380f, 380t
    primary brachial plexus reconstruction
        direct nerve repair, 381
        free-functioning muscle transfer, 382, 385f
        nerve grafting, 381
        nerve transfers, 381–382, 382f–384f
        neurolysis, 381
    secondary brachial plexus reconstruction
        derotational humeral osteotomy, 384–385
        glenohumeral motor function, 382
        hand, 385–386
        shoulder arthrodesis, 385
        shoulder soft-tissue release, 382–383
        shoulder tendon transfers, 383–384, 386f
        wrist, 385–386
    surgical management, 380–381
Bursitis, 699–700, 700f

C

Cancer, limb salvage and, 32–33
Charcot neuroarthropathy, 31–32, 35f
Children
    acquired upper limb deficiency, 882
    activity-specific prostheses, 882–883, 883f
    amputation in, 10–11
    bilateral transhumeral body-powered prostheses, 881
    bilateral transradial body-powered prostheses, 881, 881f
    bilateral upper limb deficiency, 879–880, 880f
    functional activity training, 875–876, 876f
    passive prosthetic fitting, 880–881
    prosthesis, 883–884, 883f
    shoulder level, 881–882
    subsequent prostheses and changing control strategies, 874–875
    transcarpal and partial hand deficiencies, 878–879
    unilateral transhumeral and shoulder disarticulation-level deficiencies
        body-powered prostheses, 876–878, 878f
        externally powered prostheses, 877–878, 878, 878f
        first active prosthesis, 876
        first passive prosthesis, 876
        fitting, 876

Index

shoulder disarticulation level, 878
training, 876
unilateral transradial deficiency
  first active prosthesis, 870
  first passive prosthesis, 869–870, 869f
  prosthetic considerations, 868–869
  young children
    body-powered prostheses for, 870–871, 871f
    control training, 872–874, 873f–874f
    externally powered prostheses for, 871
    myoelectrode site selection, 871–872, 872f
Chronic pain, after amputation
  assessment, 675–676, 676f
  complementary and integrative medicine therapies, 679, 679f
  epidemiology, 674
  mechanism of pain, 674, 675f
  neuromodulation, 680–681
  peripheral interventional techniques, 679–670
  pharmacologic therapies, 677–678
  surgical treatments, 680
  treatment, 676–677, 677f
Compression dressings, 15–16, 16f–17f
Congenital limb deficiencies
  genetics and associated syndromes, 742
  limb development control, 742
  lower extremity, longitudinal deficiencies of
    femur and fibula, 743–744
      postaxial, 743–744
      preaxial, 744
      tibia, 744
    transverse terminal deficiencies, 744–746, 745f–746f
  upper limb, longitudinal deficiencies of
    Fanconi anemia, 743
    Holt-Oram syndrome, 743
    thrombocytopenia-absent radius syndrome, 743
    VACTERL and VACTERL-H association, 743
Congenital multiple limb deficiencies, 989
Congenital tibial pseudarthrosis, 784
Contact dermatitis, 655–656, 656f–657f
Coxa vara correction, 932
Cycling, 635, 635f
  riding sports, 1015–1016, 1016f

D

Diabetes mellitus
  Charcot neuroarthropathy with, 31–32, 35f
  foot infection with, 30–31, 34f–35f
Diabetic ulcers, 30
Direct suction systems, 577, 578f
Distal femoral focal deficiency, 936
Distance running, 633–634, 633f–634f
Distraction osteogenesis, 790, 790f
Double ray amputation
  complications, 194
  malignant neoplasm, 194, 197f
  preoperative physical examination, 194
  radiosensitive lesions, 192
  rehabilitation, 194
  soft-tissue tumor, 194, 198f
Dressings
  compressive, 15–16, 16f–17f
  hydrofiber, 15, 16f
  negative-pressure wound, 14–15, 14f–15f
  protective, 16
  rigid, 16–17, 17f
    removable, 18, 18f
  soft, 13–14

E

Elbow
  bilateral upper limb amputation, 292, 292f
  disarticulation and transhumeral prostheses
    elbow flexion assists and counterbalances, 144–145, 145f
    elbow units, 143
    friction elbows, 143–144, 144f
    inside-locking elbows, 144, 144f–145f
    outside-locking hinges, 143, 144f
  kinesiology of, 68–69
  upper limb externally powered prostheses, 176–177, 176f
Elbow disarticulation, 240, 241f
  prosthesis, 248, 248f
  rehabilitation, 244
  socket designs, 257–258, 258f
  surgical technique, 241, 242f–243f
Embryologic limb development, 749–750
Endo-exo-femur-prosthesis, 598
Endoskeletal systems, 147, 148f
Energy expenditure, 530
Evidence-based amputee rehabilitation, 625–626
  amputee mobility predictor, 626
  single-limb standing balance, 627
  stairs, 627–628
  turning, 627

F

Fanconi anemia, 743
Farm-related injuries, 982
Femoral lengthening, 933–935
Femur, 743–744, 793, 794f
  congenital deficiencies of
    acetabular dysplasia, 932
    classification systems, 924–926, 925f–927f, 927t
    clinical examination, 927, 928f
    coxa vara correction, 932
    delayed presentation, 924
    distal femoral focal deficiency, 936
    etiology, 923
    femoral lengthening, 933–935
    foot ablation, 931, 931f
    hip reconstruction, 932–933, 933f
    knee fusion, 933, 934f
    knee valgus, 931–932
    postnatal presentation, 924, 924f
    prenatal presentation, 924, 924f
    radiographic features, 927–928, 930f
    rotationplasty, 935–936
    tibial lengthening, 933
    treatment planning, 928–931, 930f–931f
Fibula, 743–744
  congenital longitudinal deficiencies of
    associated abnormalities, 949–950
    classification, 950–951
    clinical findings, 951
    decision-making factors, 951–954, 953f–954f
    etiology, 949
    incidence, 949
    orthotic considerations, 954, 954f
    prosthetic considerations, 954–956, 955f–956f
    treatment, 951
Figure-of-9 harness, 156, 157f
Figure-of-8 harness system, 152–153, 152f, 155f
Finger prostheses
  Metacarpal Phalangeal Driver, 149–150
  Partial M-Fingers, 150, 151f
  PIP Driver, 149
  Thumb Driver, 150
  X-Finger, 150
Focal gigantism syndromes, 982–983
Folliculitis, 659–660, 660f
Foot prosthesis
  ablation, 931, 931f
  abnormalities, 961, 963f
  articulated dynamic response, 421–422, 422f
  diabetes mellitus, 30–31, 34f–35f
  dynamic pylons, 422
  hydraulic ankle feet, 422–423, 422f
  less-resourced setting in, 89–90, 90f
  longitudinal deficiencies of, 984–985, 985f
  mechanical characterization and taxonomy, 424–426, 425f–426f
  microprocessor feet, 422–423, 423f
  nonarticulated dynamic response, 418–421, 419f–420f
  passive-elastic, 417–418, 418f
  propulsive microprocessor feet, 423–424, 424f
  transverse deficiencies of, 984, 985f
Forearm, 792–793, 793f
  kinesiology of, 69, 69f
Forequarter/interscapulothoracic amputation
  adjuncts for, 267
  anterior cervical triangle, 266
  deep dissection, 263
  disarticulation, 263, 263f–264f
  en bloc chest wall excision, 266–267
  incision, 263
  indications, 261–262
  posterior vascular isolation, 263, 265–266
Friction, 661–662, 662f
Fungal infections, in adult, 27, 27f–28f
Furuncle, 660

G

Gait analysis, limb deficiency, 760
  adult *vs.* pediatric populations, 764
  ankle rockers, 763–764, 764f
  clinical assessment, 760
  clinical practice, 766–767
  clinical study, 766
  evaluation, 760
  impact, 764
  kinematics, 760–762, 760f–761f
  kinetics, 762–763, 762f
  transfemoral amputation, 765–766
  transtibial amputation, 765
Gait training skills
  disarticulation and bilaterally affected patients, 619–620
  intact and prosthetic limb training, 615–616
  pelvic motion, 616

Index

Gait training skills *(Continued)*
  prosthetic training program, 616–619, 617f–618f
  stairs, 620
  transtibial amputee step-over-step technique, 621
Gel suspension systems, 577

H
Hand
  body-powered prostheses, 134–135, 135f
    cosmetic gloves, 136–137, 137f
    voluntary-closing hands, 135–136, 136f
    voluntary-opening hands, 135, 136f
  kinesiology of, 70
    pathologic hand deformity, 73–74
    as sensory probe, 71–72
  partial hand prostheses
    figure-of-8 harness, 150, 152f
    M-Fingers, 150, 151f
    Minnesota split-hand prosthesis, 150, 151f
  prehension with, 3–4
  sensation with, 3–4
  transplantation
    clinical outcomes, 396–397
    complications, 396
    distal forearm level, 394, 394f
    donor procurement, 393, 393f
    immunotherapy, 396
    indications, 392
    midforearm level, 395, 395f
    postoperative care, 396
    premedication, 394
    proximal forearm level, 395
    solid organ transplantation, 392
    transhumeral level, 395–396
    vascularized composite allotransplantation, 391–393, 392f, 397
Heat rash, 658–659, 659f
Hemipelvectomy, 903f
  biomechanics, 905–906
  casting and modification, 907–908
  complications, 553
  pediatric considerations, 906–908
  postoperative care, 552–553
  prosthetic alignment, 905–906
  prosthetic design, 908–910
  prosthetic management, 905
  rehabilitation, 553
  surgical technique, 549–552, 550f–552f
  terminology and classification, 902, 902f
  transpelvic amputation, 907–908
  young children, 904, 905f
Heterotopic ossification and bone spurs, 702
Hindfoot-level amputations
  transcalcaneal (Boyd) amputation, 449–450
  transtarsal (Chopart) disarticulation, 448–449
Hip disarticulation
  biomechanics, 905–906
  casting and modification, 907–908
  complications, 549
  etiology, 902
    congenital defects, 904
    neoplasms, 903–904
    phocomelia, 904
    separated conjoined twins, 904
    sepsis, 904
    trauma, 902–903
    whole limb, unilateral congenital absence of, 904
  indications, 547–548
  pediatric considerations, 906–908
  preoperative planning, 548
  prosthetic alignment, 905–906
  prosthetic management, 557–565, 905
  surgical management, 901–902, 902f
  surgical technique, 548, 548f
  terminology and classification, 902, 902f
  transpelvic amputation, 906, 908
Hip flexion contractures, 48
Hip reconstruction, 932–933, 933f
Holt-Oram syndrome, 743
Hybrid recreational prostheses, 637, 638f
Hydraulic ankle, 422–423, 422f
Hydrofiber dressings, 15, 16f
Hyperhidrosis, 668–669
Hypermobile myoplasty, 700–701, 700f

I
Immediate postoperative prosthesis (IPOP), 18–19, 18f
Infection, limb salvage for, 26–28, 27f–29f, 28t
  Charcot neuroarthropathy, 31–32, 35f
  with diabetes, 30–31, 34f–35f
  physiologic reserve and comorbidities, 32
  in upper limb, 28, 30, 30f–33f
Instrumented gait analysis (IGA), 43
Intact and prosthetic limb training, 610–611, 615–616
Interphalangeal thumb disarticulation, 196, 198, 199f
Intertrigo, 658, 658f
Ipsilateral proximal limb abnormalities, 782–783

J
Joint contractures, 697–698
Jones system, 960
  type 1a deficiency, 964
  type 3 deficiency, 965
  type 4 deficiency, 965–966
  types 1b and 2 deficiencies, 965, 965f

K
Kalamchi and Dawe system, 960–961
Knee disarticulation, 964
  active child, 917, 917f
  adult components, transitioning to, 917–918, 918f
  alignment considerations, 513–514, 514f
  anticipated outcomes, 507
  clinical considerations, 507–508, 508f
  complications, 504–505, 914
  component considerations, 511–513, 514f
  congenital anomalies, 918–919, 919f–920f
  distal residual limb, 499
  growing child, 916–917, 917f
  outcome considerations, 499–501, 500f–502f
  primary socket and suspension approaches, 509–511, 510f–511f
  prosthetic management
    begin prosthetic care, 915, 915f
    early suspension, 915–916, 915f–916f
  rehabilitation, 504
  socket considerations, 509, 509f
  suction suspension options, 511, 511f–513f
  surgical technique, 501–504, 502f–504f, 914–915
Knee fusion, 933, 934f
Knee prosthesis
  hybrid mechanical knees, 437
  less-resourced setting in, 90
  manual lock feature, 436–437, 436f
  mechanical stance stability, 431
  microprocessor knees, 437–438, 437f
    ankle-foot mechanisms, 438, 438f
    myoelectric control, 439–440
    positional rotators, 440, 440f
    propulsive microprocessor knee-ankle-feet, 439, 439f
    propulsive microprocessor knees, 439, 439f
  polycentric knees, 434–435, 434f–435f
  polycentric stance flexion features, 435, 435f–436f
  resistance mechanisms, 432–433, 433f
  single-axis constant-friction knee, 433, 433f
  weight-activated stance control, 433–434, 434f
Knee valgus, 931–932

L
Less-resourced setting (LRS)
  in foot, 89–90, 90f
  human resources, 87–88, 87t
  in knees, 90
  policy and funding, 86–87
  prosthetic services, 85–86
  prosthetic systems, 90, 91f
    International Committee of the Red Cross, 90–92, 91f–93f
    Jaipur foot, 92–94, 94f
  prosthetic technologies in, 88–89, 88f–89f
Limb amputation, psychological adaptation to
  amputation, 707–708
  anxiety, 708–709
  depression, 708, 710–711
  pain, 711
  peer support, 715
    self-management, 714
  posttraumatic stress disorder, 709–710
  psychological considerations, in osseointegration, 714
  psychosocial consequences, 713
  self-management, 714–715
  social stigma, 711
Limb deficiencies, 749–750
  body image and self-perception, 771–772
  health-related quality of life, 770–771
  prosthesis use, 771
  psychological functioning, 769–770
  psychosocial adjustment, health care clinicians in, 776
  romantic relationships, 772
  social dynamics, 772
  socioeconomic status, 772–773
  youth and families
    academics and activities, 774
    developmental considerations, 774–776, 775t
    parental/caregiver support, 773–774
Limb mobility, kinesiology of, 67
Limb salvage

amputations, 4, 892, 892t
  in adults, 21–39
  burn injuries, 889, 891–892
    chemical burns, 889
    electric injuries, 889
    frostbite, 889
    nonfreezing cold injuries, 889
    thermal burns, 889
  contraindications, 890
  etiology, 888, 888t
  indications, 890
  infections, 26–28, 27f–29f, 28t, 890
    Charcot neuroarthropathy, 31–32, 35f
    with diabetes patients, 30–31, 34f–35f
    physiologic reserve and comorbidities, 32
    in upper limb, 28, 30, 30f–33f
  malignant tumors, 889, 890–891
  multidisciplinary resources for, 26
  musculoskeletal tumors, 32–34
  nerve injury and, 24–26, 24f–27f
  peripheral vascular arterial disease and, 22, 23t, 24, 24f, 888
  physiologic reserve and medical comorbidities for, 22, 22t
  psychological and psychiatric conditions, 24–26, 24f–27f
  purpura fulminans, 891
  quality of life and, 26
  rehabilitation, 944–945
  trauma amputations, 34–38, 36f–39f, 888–890
  vascular status for, 22, 23f
Locomotor systems
  childhood development
    early development, 750–751
    middle childhood and adolescence, 751
  embryologic limb development, 749–750
  limb deficiency, 749–750
  psychosocial development, 751–752
Lower extremity
  children
    adolescents, medical-legal issues with, 813
    psychological issues in, 812–813
  decision making, 800–802, 801f–802f
  etiology and incidence, 799–800
  pediatric patient with, 812
  through-knee amputation level, 808–809, 810f–811f
  transfemoral amputation levels, 809–812, 810f–811f
  transtibial amputation levels, 805–808, 806f–808f
  traumatic ankle-level amputations, 802–805, 802f–804f
  weight bearing, 4
Lower limb amputation, 721–722
  acute postoperative evaluation
    assistive devices, potential ambulation with, 607
    balance/coordination, 607
    bed mobility, 607
    sensation, 606–607
    setting goals, 607
  advanced gait-training activities
    stairs, 620
    step-by-step method, 620–621, 621f
    transtibial amputee step-over-step technique, 621
  body functions and structure, 722
  evidence-based amputee rehabilitation, 625–626
    amputee mobility predictor, 626
    single-limb standing balance, 627
    stairs, 627–628
  gait training skills
    disarticulation and bilaterally affected patients, 619–620
    intact and prosthetic limb training, 615–616
    pelvic motions, 616
    prosthetic training program, 616–619, 617f–618f
  immediate postoperative treatment, 607
    assistive devices, ambulation with, 608–609
    positioning, 608
    postoperative dressing, 607–608
    transfers, 608
    wheelchair propulsion, 608
  legal and social security services, 723
  patient education
    desensitization, 609–610
    intact limb, issues pertaining to, 610–611
    prosthesis, care of, 610
    prosthesis, donning and doffing of, 610
    residual limb compression dressing, 610
    skin care, 609
    sock regulation, 610
    strategies to, 611
  pregait training
    balance and coordination, 614
    orientation, 614, 614f–615f
    single limb, standing on, 614–615, 615f
  preoperative care, 605–606
  preprosthetic exercises
    cardiopulmonary endurance, 611
    functional activities, 614
    strengthening, 611–613, 612f–613f
  prosthetic ankle and foot performance
    agility drills, 625
    lateral speed weave, 625
    toe-box jumps, 625
  socket, maximizing stability within, 623–625, 624f
  transfemoral amputees
    curbs, 621
    falling, 622–623
    ramps and hills, 621–622
Lower limb amputation (LLA), 118f
  body structure/residual limb
    body functions, 119, 119f
    participation, 120–122
    physical activity, 119–120, 120t
    preoperative and postoperative pain, 118
    risk factors, 118–119
  health-related targets, 117, 118t
  human health parameters, 117, 118t
  incidence of, 117
  minor amputations, 123
  rehabilitation methods
    service dogs, 122–123, 123f
    virtual reality, 122, 123f
Lower limb fitting strategies, 895–897, 896f, 897t
Lower limb prosthetics
  HRQOL and multidomain measures
    EuroQol 5 Dimension 5 Level, 646
    Orthotics Prosthetics User Survey, 646
    PROMIS-29, 646
    prosthesis evaluation questionnaire, 646
  measurement properties, 642–643
  mobility/physical function
    Amputee Mobility Predictor, 643
    prosthetic limb user survey of mobility, 644
    six-minute walk test, 644
    ten-meter walk test, 644
    Timed Up and Go test, 644–645
    timed walk tests, 643–644, 643f
    two-minute walk test, 644
  pain and comfort measures
    Comprehensive Lower-Limb Amputee Socket Survey, 646
    Numerical Pain Rating Scale, 645
    socket comfort score, 645
LRS. *See* Less-resourced setting (LRS)
Lumbosacral agenesis
  classification, 999, 999f
  orthopaedic management, 999–1001
  orthotic management, 1001, 1001f
  patient evaluation, 1001
  prevalence and etiology, 998–999
  prosthetic management, 1001–1002
  treatment, 1002–1004, 1003f–1004f

M
Malignant tumors, 665
  scar formation, 666
  squamous cell carcinoma, 665
  Steward–Treves syndrome, 666
Marginal necrosis, 695–696
Metacarpophalangeal disarticulation, 198–199
M-Fingers, 150, 151f
Microprocessor feet, 422–423, 423f
Microprocessor knees, 437–438, 437f
  ankle-foot mechanisms, 438, 438f
  myoelectric control, 439–440
  positional rotators, 440, 440f
  propulsive microprocessor knee-ankle-feet, 439, 439f
  propulsive microprocessor knees, 439, 439f
Minnesota split-hand prosthesis, 150, 151f
Multiple limb deficiencies, 784
  acquired multiple limb deficiencies, 990
  child and family, psychological needs of, 993–994
  clinical presentation, 989–990
  congenital multiple limb deficiencies, 989
  developmental capabilities, 992
  donning and doffing, 991–992
  economic implications, 992
  etiology, 989–990
  gadget tolerance, 992, 992f
  heat retention, 991
  prosthetic components, 991
  scoliosis, 994
  sexuality, 993
  size and weight, 991
  sports and recreational activities, 993
  terminal devices, activation age of, 993
  upper limb prostheses, 994–995, 994f
  wheelchair use, 992
Muscle strength, kinesiology of, 73

Index

N

Negative-pressure hyperemia, 661, 662f
Negative-pressure wound dressings, 15
Neoplasms, 983–984
Neuromata and neurogenic pain, 698–699, 699f
Neuromodulation, 680–681
Nontraumatic partial foot amputation
    amniotic band syndrome, 985
    focal gigantism syndromes, 982–983
    infection, 983, 984f
    longitudinal deficiencies of, 984–985, 985f
    neoplasms, 983–984
    split-hand/split-foot syndrome, 985, 985f
    transverse deficiencies of, 984, 985f
Numerical Pain Rating Scale (NPRS-11), 645

O

Orthotics Prosthetics User Survey (OPUS), 646
Osseointegration
    amputee rehabilitation
        full-length prosthesis, 597, 597f–598f
        OPRA Axor II device, 597, 597f–598f
        outcomes, 597–598
        short training prosthesis, 596–597, 596f
        stage 1 surgery, 595
        stage 2 surgery, 596, 596f
        weight bearing, 596, 596f
    OPL system, 588–589, 588f–589f
        clinical management, 589
        postoperative management, 591–592, 593t
        preoperative preparation, 589–590, 590f
        surgical procedure, 590–591, 590f, 592f
    OPRA system, 583–584, 584f
        clinical management, 584–585
        postoperative management, 587–588
        preoperative preparation, 585
        surgical procedure, 585–587, 586f–587f
    outcomes, 581–583, 582f, 583t–584t
    press-fit implants
        BADAL X, 599
        compress, 601–602
        endo-exo-femur-prosthesis, 598
        osseointegrated prosthetic limb, 598–599
        percutaneous osseointegrated prosthesis, 600, 600f
        prosthetic attachment, 599–600, 599f–600f
    press-fit intramedullary stem, 588–589
    prosthetic alignment considerations, 602
    prosthetic limb, 577, 598–599
    prosthetic management, 595–603
    spring-loaded constant compression implant, 592
    threaded screw implant, 583–584, 584f
Osteomyelitis, 21
Osteopenia, 689
Osteoporosis, 689

P

Partial foot amputation (PFA)
    complications, 450–451
    hindfoot-level amputations
        transcalcaneal (Boyd) amputation, 449–450
        transtarsal (Chopart) disarticulation, 448–449
    incidence, 453
    interventions, 454–455
        above-ankle prostheses, 457
        ankle-foot orthoses, 456–457, 456f–457f
        effectiveness, 457–459
        silicone cosmetic prostheses, 456, 456f
        toe fillers and insoles, 455–456, 455f
    partial amputation level, 444, 444f, 454
    preoperative evaluation, 444–445
    ray resection, 445–446, 446f
    rehabilitation, 450
    surgical considerations, 445
    tarsometatarsal (Lisfranc) disarticulation, 448
    transmetatarsal amputation, 443–444, 446–447, 447f
Partial foot deficiencies
    acquired partial foot loss, 979
    etiology, 979
    nontraumatic partial foot amputation
        amniotic band syndrome, 985
        focal gigantism syndromes, 982–983
        infection, 983, 984f
        longitudinal deficiencies of, 984–985, 985f
        neoplasms, 983–984
        split-hand/split-foot syndrome, 985, 985f
        transverse deficiencies of, 984, 985f
    prosthetic choices, 985–986, 986f
    traumatic injuries, 980–981, 980f–981f
        farm-related injuries, 982
        motor vehicle and train-related injuries, 982
        thermal injuries, 982
    treatment, 979–980
Partial hand amputations
    clinical outcomes of, 200
    double ray
        complications, 194
        malignant neoplasm, 194, 197f
        preoperative physical examination, 194
        radiosensitive lesions, 192
        rehabilitation, 194
        soft-tissue tumor, 194, 198f
    neuroma management, 199–200
    prosthetic management
        activity-specific prostheses, 202–203, 204f
        aesthetic restoration, 202, 203f
        body-powered prostheses, 203, 204f–205f
        clinical considerations, 201–202, 202f
        externally powered prostheses, 203–205, 205f–206f
        force-sensitive resistors, 205–206, 206f
        incidence of, 201, 202f
        limb loss, 206
        myoelectrodes, 205–206, 206f
        opposition prostheses, 202, 203f
        prosthesis design, 206, 206f
        three-dimensional printing technology, 206–208, 207f–208f
    prosthetic usage, 200
    single ray
        complications, 192
        index ray, 191–192, 193f
        middle finger ray, 192, 194f
        rehabilitation, 192
        ring finger ray, 191–192, 195f
        small finger ray, 191–192, 196f
    thumb amputation
        interphalangeal thumb disarticulation, 196, 198, 199f
        metacarpophalangeal disarticulation, 198–199
        thumb-sparing procedures, 196
    transmetacarpal amputation, 194, 195
Pediatric hand deficiencies
    classification, 830–831, 831t–832t, 832f–833f
    clinical presentation, 830
    early amniotic rupture sequence
        clinical presentation, 837
        complications, 837
        surgical treatment, 837
    polydactyly
        classification, 837–838, 837f
        clinical presentation, 838
        surgical treatment, 838–839
    prostheses, 830
    short transradial amputation, 839
    symbrachydactyly, 831–833, 833f, 834t
        associated findings, 834
        classification, 833
        differential diagnosis, 834
        functional deficits, 834
        imaging studies, 833
        surgical treatment, 834–835, 835f
    syndactyly
        classification, 835–836
        clinical presentation, 835–836
        surgical treatment, 836–837, 836f
    timing of management, 839
    upper limb kinesiology, 829–830
    wrist disarticulation, 839
Pediatric limb deficiencies
    classification, 736–739, 737f–739f, 737t
    embryology, 735–736
    etiology
        acquired, 736
        congenital, 736
    prosthetic advances, 755–757, 756f
    scientific advances, 753–755, 754f
    surgical advances, 753–755, 754f
    technologic advances, 753–755, 754f
Pediatric lower limb amputee
    bilateral lower limb deficiencies, 898–899, 899f
    bony overgrowth and angular deformities, 898, 898f
    growth management, children, 897–898, 897f
    lower limb fitting strategies, 895–897, 896f, 897t
Pediatric physical therapy
    neurologic impairments, multiple limb loss with and without, 864
    physical therapy treatments, 857, 858t
        adolescence, 862–864
        elementary years, 861
        infants, 857–859, 859f
        limb lengthening, 862
        preschool and young childhood years, 860–861
        rotationplasty, 861–862
        sports and recreation, 864
        toddlers, 859–860, 861f
    postoperative considerations, 856–857, 856f–857f
Peer Support and Adaptive Sports Programs, 1016–1017, 1017f
Pelvic motions, 616
Percutaneous osseointegrated prosthesis, 600, 600f
Peripheral vascular disease (PVD), 22
Perisurgical pain control, 783

Index

PFA. *See* Partial foot amputation (PFA)
Phantom limb pain, 312
Phantom limb syndrome (PLS), 100
Physiologic stress, limb salvage and, 25–26
Polycentric knees, 434–435, 434*f*–435*f*
Polydactyly
    classification, 837–838, 837*f*
    clinical presentation, 838
    surgical treatment, 838–839
Postamputation pain, 100
    allograft reconstruction, 313
    central sensitization, 312
    management and prevention, 312–313
    phantom limb pain, 312
    prevalence of, 311
    regenerative peripheral nerve interface, 315–316, 315*f*–316*f*
    targeted muscle reinnervation
        hyperreinnervation process, 313
        neuroma management, 314, 314*f*
        neuroma prevention, 314
        unrepaired nerve transection, 312
Postaxial longitudinal deficiency, 743–744
Power grip, kinesiology of, 72–73
Pneumatic postamputation mobility (PPAM), 16
Postoperative residual limb management
    dressings for, 13–18
    immediate postoperative prosthetic limb fitting, 18–19
    postoperative pneumatic systems, 19
Postoperative pneumatic systems, 19
Preaxial longitudinal deficiency, 744
Pregait training
    balance and coordination, 614
    orientation, 614, 614*f*–615*f*
    single limb, standing on, 614–615, 615*f*
Preprosthetic exercises
    cardiopulmonary endurance, 611
    functional activities, 614
    strengthening, 611–613, 612*f*–613*f*
Press-fit implants
    BADAL X, 599
    compress, 601–602
    endo-exo-femur-prosthesis, 598
    osseointegrated prosthetic limb, 598–599
    percutaneous osseointegrated prosthesis, 600, 600*f*
    prosthetic attachment, 599–600, 599*f*–600*f*
Press-fit intramedullary stem, 588–589
Propulsive microprocessor feet, 423–424, 424*f*
Prosthetic gait
    alignment adjustments, toe and heel levers, 57, 57*t*–63*t*
    analysis tools, 56
    dynamic alignment, 56
    dynamic walking model, 45–46, 46*f*
    gait cycle, phases of, 44–45, 45*f*
    gait deviations, 43
    human locomotion
        efficiency, 44
        kinematic chain, 43
        progression, 44
        stability, 44
    instrumented gait analysis, 43
        electromyography, 47
        temporal and spatial characteristics, 47, 47*f*
    kinetic and kinematic asymmetries, 43
    during loading phase, 49, 50*f*, 51*t*
    aberrant stance flexion, 49, 51
    prosthetic foot rotation, 49
    patient factors, 56
    propulsion phase, 53–54
    step length asymmetries, 48–49, 50*f*
    support phase, 51–52, 52*t*
        coronal plane knee instability, 53
        knee instability, 52–53
        lateral trunk bending, 53
    swing phase, 52*t*, 54
        excessive heel rise, 55
        excessive pistoning, 54–55
        excessive terminal impact, 55
        toe clearance strategies, 55
        whips, 55–56
    vertical ground reaction force, 46, 46*f*
Prosthetic limb user survey of mobility (PLUS-M), 644
Prosthetic management, 595–603, 974–976, 975*f*
Prosthetic socket, 530
Prosthetic training program, 616–619, 617*f*–618*f*
Protective dressings, 16
Pruritus, 666
Psoriasis, 657–658, 657*f*–658*f*
PVD. *See* Peripheral vascular disease (PVD)

Q

Quality of life
    amputation effect on, 3
    limb salvage and, 22

R

Radial longitudinal deficiency
    classification, 820, 820*t*–821*t*
    clinical features, 819
    diagnostic studies, 820
    etiology, 819–820, 820*t*
    treatment, 820–823
Regenerative peripheral nerve interface, 327
    postamputation pain, 315–316, 315*f*–316*f*
Rehabilitation
    less-resourced settings, 85–94, 89*f*–94*f*
    lower limb amputation
        service dogs, 122–123, 123*f*
        virtual reality, 122, 123*f*
    upper limb amputee, 97, 103, 104*f*–105*f*
        healing, 104–105
Removable rigid dressings, 18, 18*f*
Repetitive stress disorder (RSD), 98–99
Residual limb complications, surgical management of
    early complications
        delayed wound healing, 695–696
        infection, 696–697
        joint contractures, 697–698
        marginal necrosis, 695–696
        myodesis failure, 698, 698*f*
        wound dehiscence, 695–696
    late complications and residual limb pain
        bursitis, 699–700, 700*f*
        evaluation, 698
        fractures, 702–703, 703*f*
        heterotopic ossification and bone spurs, 702
        hypermobile myoplasty and redundant soft tissues, 700–701, 700*f*
        inadequate soft-tissue coverage and skin problems, 701–702
        neuromata and neurogenic pain, 698–699, 699*f*
        tibiofibular instability and radioulnar convergence, 703
Residual limb compression dressing, 610
Residual limb length (RLL)
    arm, 792
    complications
        contractures, 795, 797*f*
        fixation, 795, 795*f*
        soft-tissue strategies, 796
    distraction osteogenesis, 790, 790*f*
    femur, 793, 794*f*
    forearm, 792–793, 793*f*
    lengthening, 791
        external fixation technical considerations, 791, 791*f*
        motorized nail technical considerations, 791–792
    tibia, 793–795
Rigid dressings, 16–17, 17*f*
    removable, 18, 18*f*
RLL. *See* Residual limb length (RLL)
Rotationplasty, 935
    components, 947
    diagnostic socket, 946
    dynamic alignment, 946–947
    finished prosthesis, 947
    limb salvage procedure rehabilitation, 944–945
    model modification, 946
    prosthesis, 935–936
    prosthesis molding, 945–946
    surgical considerations
        absolute contraindications, 938
        indications, 937–938
        prerequisites, 938
        relative contraindications, 938–939
RSD. *See* Repetitive stress disorder (RSD)
Running/jumping sports, 1014, 1014*f*

S

Scoliosis, 994
Secondary health effects, amputation
    arthritis, 688–689
    cardiovascular complications, 685–686
    diabetes, 686–687
    economic effects, 689–690
    low back pain, 687–688
    musculoskeletal complications, 687
    obesity, 687
    osteopenia and osteoporosis, 689
    skin problems, 687
Shoulder
    bilateral upper limb amputation, 293, 293*f*
    body-powered prostheses, 145–146, 145*f*–147*f*
    claviculectomy, 273
    complications, 269–270, 269*f*
    disarticulation applications, 162–164, 162*f*–164*f*
    forequarter/interscapulothoracic amputation
        adjuncts for, 267
        anterior cervical triangle, 266
        deep dissection, 263
        disarticulation, 263, 263*f*–264*f*

Index

Shoulder *(Continued)*
    en bloc chest wall excision, 266–267
    incision, 263
    indications, 261–262
    posterior vascular isolation, 263, 265–266
  intercalary shoulder resections, 270, 271f
  kinesiology of, 67–68, 68f
  limb salvage indications, 270, 270f
  magnetic resonance imaging, 261, 261f
  modified shoulder disarticulation, 267–268, 268f
  postoperative management, 269
  prosthetic management
    adaptive prostheses, 279, 279f
    amputation levels, 275, 276f
    bilateral shoulder, 281, 282f
    body-powered prostheses, 279–280, 280f
    elbow alignment, 278
    externally powered prostheses, 280–281
    hybrid prostheses, 280, 280f–281f
    incidence of, 275
    passive oppositional restoration prostheses, 278–279, 279f
    patient evaluation, 275–276
    protective shoulder caps, 278, 278f
    rehabilitation, 281–282
    socket design, 276–277, 276f–277f
    socket material selection, 277, 277f
  saddle harness, 154–155, 156f
  scapulectomy, 272–273, 273f
  surgical neuromodulation, 261
  Tikhoff-Linberg resection, 262, 262f, 270–271, 272f, 281, 281f–282f
  upper limb externally powered prostheses, 177–178
Shoulder disarticulation
  bilateral upper limb amputation, 298–299
  socket design, 288–289
  targeted muscle reinnervation, 306–308, 306f–308f, 324–326, 325f–326f
Single ray amputation
  complications, 192
  index ray, 191–192, 193f
  middle finger ray, 192, 194f
  rehabilitation, 192
  ring finger ray, 191–192, 195f
  small finger ray, 191–192, 196f
Skin pathologies, amputation
  clinical presentations, 666
    classification systems, 669, 669t
    dry skin, 666–667
    hyperhidrosis, 668–669
    odor, 669
    pruritus, 666
    scar, 667–668, 667f
    sweating, 668
  dermatitis
    contact dermatitis, 655–656, 656f–657f
    heat rash, 658–659, 659f
    intertrigo, 658, 658f
    nonspecific eczematization, 656–657
    psoriasis, 657–658, 657f–658f
    urticaria, 659, 659f
  epidemiology, 654, 654t
  hygiene, 654–655
  infection, 659
    folliculitis, 659–660, 660f
    furuncle, 660
    infection treatment and prevention, 660
    superficial fungal infections, 660, 661f
  tumor, 664
    benign growths, 664–665
    malignant tumors, 665
  volume change, 660–661
    friction, 661–662, 662f
    negative-pressure hyperemia, 661, 662f
    verrucous hyperplasia, 663, 664f
    volume-related ulceration, 662–663, 663f
Socket construction, 533, 533t
  flexible inner sockets, 534
  hard sockets, 533–534
Socket designs, 534, 535t
  ischial containment designs, 534–536
  subischial designs, 536
Sock regulation, 610
Soft dressings, 13–14
Soft-tissue envelope, 5–7, 7f
Soft-tissue grafting, 780–781
Spinal cord injuries, 26
Split-hand/split-foot syndrome, 985, 985f
Sports and recreation, adaptive lower limb prostheses for
  athletic assessment and training, 637–638
  hybrid recreational prostheses, 637, 638f
  physical health, 631–632
  psychological determinants, 632
  sport-specific prostheses
    cycling, 635, 635f
    distance running, 633–634, 633f–634f
    sprinting, 634, 634f
    swimming, 635–636, 635f–636f
    water sports, 636, 636f
    winter sports, 636–637, 637f
  technical aids and prostheses, 632
    prosthetic component choice and alignment, 632–633
    prosthetic sockets, 632, 632f
    suspension system, 632
Sport-specific prostheses
  cycling, 635, 635f
  distance running, 633–634, 633f–634f
  sprinting, 634, 634f
  swimming, 635–636, 635f–636f
  water sports, 636, 636f
  winter sports, 636–637, 637f
Spring-loaded constant compression implant, 592
Superficial fungal infections, 660, 661f
Suspension systems, 536, 537t–538t
  belt-type/auxiliary suspension, 540
  hypobaric and vacuum-assisted suspension, 539–540, 540t
  locking mechanisms, 539
  roll-on gel liners, 539–540
  skin-fit, 538–539
  subatmospheric suspension, 536–538
  suction suspension, 538–539
Symbrachydactyly, 831–833, 833, 833f, 834t
  classification, 833
  differential diagnosis, 834
  functional deficits, 834
  surgical treatment, 834–835, 835f
Syme amputation, 970–971, 970f–972f
Syndactyly
  classification, 835–836
  clinical presentation, 835–836
  surgical treatment, 836–837, 836f

T

Targeted muscle reinnervation (TMR), 8–9
  clinical characteristics, 301
  electrode placement and socket designs, 321–322, 322f
  muscle recovery period, 320
  myoelectric control, 302
    osseointegration, 302, 302f
    sensory feedback, 303
    surgical planning, 303–304, 303f
  myotesting, 320, 321f
  pattern recognition control, 320, 322–323, 322f
  postamputation pain
    hyperreinnervation process, 313
    neuroma management, 314, 314f
    neuroma prevention, 314
  prosthetic fittings, 323
  prosthetic rehabilitation, 301
  residual limb musculature, 302
  sensory feedback, 326, 327f
  shoulder disarticulation, 306–308, 306f–308f, 324–326, 325f–326f
  transhumeral, 304–306, 305f, 319, 324, 324f–325f
  transradial fittings, 323–324, 324f
Tarsometatarsal (Lisfranc) disarticulation, 448
Ten-meter walk test, 644
Terminal bone overgrowth
  clinical presentation, 1007–1008, 1008f
  etiology, 1007
  prevention, 1008–1009, 1008f–1009f
Terminal devices, activation age of, 993
Terminal organ, weight bearing, 5, 6f
Thermal injuries, 982
Threaded screw implant, 583–584, 584f
Through-knee amputation level, 808–809, 810f–811f
Thumb amputation
  interphalangeal thumb disarticulation, 196, 198, 199f
  kinesiology of, 70–71, 70f–71f
  metacarpophalangeal disarticulation, 198–199
  thumb-sparing procedures, 196
Tibia, 744, 794–795
  classification
    Jones system, 960
    Kalamchi and Dawe system, 960–961
    Paley classification, 961
    Weber system, 961
  clinical presentation, 959, 960f
  etiology, 962–963
  foot abnormalities, 961, 963f
  history, 959–960
  surgical planning, 963–964
  treatment options
    Brown procedure, 964–965
    Jones type 1a deficiency, 964
    Jones type 3 deficiency, 965
    Jones type 4 deficiency, 965–966
    Jones types 1b and 2 deficiencies, 965, 965f
    knee disarticulation, 964
Tibial lengthening, 933
Tibiofibular instability and radioulnar convergence, 703
TMR. *See* Targeted muscle reinnervation (TMR)
Train-related injuries, 982
Transcalcaneal (Boyd) amputation, 449–450

Index

Transfemoral amputation, 79–80, 809–812, 810f–811f
    adult components, transitioning to, 917–918, 918f
    anticipated outcomes, 529–530
    biomechanics, 518–520, 518f–519f
    body image, 530
    complications, 525, 914
    congenital anomalies, 918–919, 919f–920f
    with distal soft-tissue loss, 517, 518f
    energy expenditure, 530
    Gritti-Stokes amputation, 523–524, 525f
    incidence of, 517
    indications, 520–521, 520f
    modified adductor myodesis, 523, 524f
    postoperative care, 524–525
    prosthetic foot considerations, 541
    prosthetic knee considerations, 540–541
    prosthetic management, 529
        begin prosthetic care, 915, 915f
        early suspension, 915–916, 915f–916f
    prosthetic socket, 530
    socket construction, 533, 533t
        flexible inner sockets, 534
        hard sockets, 533–534
    socket designs, 534, 535t
        ischial containment designs, 534–536
        subischial designs, 536
    surgical technique, 521–522, 521f–524f, 913–914
    suspension systems, 536, 537t–538t
        belt-type/auxiliary suspension, 540
        hypobaric and vacuum-assisted suspension, 539–540, 540t
        locking mechanisms, 539
        roll-on gel liners, 539–540
        skin-fit, 538–539
        subatmospheric suspension, 536–538
        suction suspension, 538–539
    transfemoral socket, 530
        coronal plane, 531–532, 532f
        orientation, importance of, 531
        sagittal plane, 531
        socket stability, 531
        total contact socket fit, 531
        transverse plane, 532–533, 532f
    voluntary control, 530
Transfemoral amputees, 621–622
Transfemoral socket, 530
    coronal plane, 531–532, 532f
    orientation, importance of, 531
    sagittal plane, 531
    socket stability, 531
    total contact socket fit, 531
    transverse plane, 532–533, 532f
Transhumeral amputation, 239, 242–244, 243f–244f, 319
    control strategies, 258–259, 258f–259f
    distal humeral shaft, 248–249, 249f
    endoskeletal transhumeral prosthesis, 253, 253f
    interface construction, 256–257
    interface modification and evaluation, 256, 256f
    interfaces, 250, 251f
    limb length, 251
    limb shape, 252–253
    limb volume, 251–252, 251f–252f
    liner suspension, 257, 257f
    load-bearing tolerance, 253–254, 253f
    osseointegration, 249
    prosthesis acceptance rates, 247
    rehabilitation, 244
    rotational stability, 248, 248f
    shoulder mobility, 254
    substructure, 253
Transhumeral prostheses
    anterior suspensor strap, 159, 160f
    bilateral transhumeral applications, 161–162, 162f
    Biomechanically Aligned Harness Anchor, 159, 160f
    double harness ring, 160, 160f
    mechanism of control, 157
    sequence of actions, 157–158, 158f–159f
    shoulder saddle, 161, 161f
    transhumeral amputation, 160, 160f
    Triple Control Harness, 161
    Y split, 161, 162f
Transmetacarpal amputation, 194, 196
Transpelvic amputation, hip disarticulation, 906
    complications, 549
    indications, 547–548
    preoperative planning, 548
    surgical technique, 548, 548f
Transradial amputation, 213–215, 215f–216f
    additive manufacturing, 234–235, 235f
    amputation level, 224, 224f
    harness suspension, 227–228, 227f–228f
    Muenster design, 229–230, 229f
    prosthetic interface, 225–227, 226f–227f
    self-suspended interface designs, 228–229, 229f
    socket designs, 233–234, 234f–235f
Transradial prostheses
    activation of, 154, 155f–156f
    American Civil War era, 151, 152f
    cable-controlled prosthesis, 151, 153f
    chest strap, 155–156, 156f–157f
    figure-of-9 harness, 156, 157f
    figure-of-8 harness system, 152–153, 155f
    flexible hinges, 141–142, 141f
    force transmission, 151–152
    glenohumeral flexion, 153
    Götz artificial arm, 151, 152f
    polycentric hinges, 142, 142f
    power generation, 153, 155f
    residual limb-activated locking hinges, 143, 143f
    rigid hinges, 142
    shoulder saddle harness, 154–155, 156f
    single-axis hinges, 142, 142f
    step-up hinges, 142–143, 143f
Transtarsal (Chopart) disarticulation, 448–449
Transtibial amputation, 805–808, 806f–808f, 973–974, 973f–974f
    alignment, 493–494, 494f–495f
    anatomic suspension systems, 488–490, 489f
    atmospheric pressure suspension systems, 491, 491f
    clinical outcomes, 477
    complications, 481
    contraindications, 478
    enhanced socket fit, 494, 494f
    Ertl technique, 479–480, 480f
    fibulectomy, 479, 480f
    hybrid designs, 493
    indications, 477–478
    mechanical suspension systems, 490–491, 490f
    moisture management, 496
    patellar tendon–bearing socket, 492, 492f
    patient-reported outcome measures, 485
    prosthetic gel liners, 487–488, 487f
    prosthetic socket, 485, 486f
    prosthetic socks, 486–487
    rehabilitation, 480–482
    socket design, 492, 495–496, 496f
    socket insert design, 486, 486f–487f
    surgical technique, 478–479, 478f–479f
    suspension design, 488
    suspension system performance, 491–492
    total surface-bearing socket, 492–493, 493f
Transtibial amputations, 79
Traumatic ankle-level amputations, 802–805, 802f–804f
Traumatic injuries, 980–981, 980f–981f
    farm-related injuries, 982
    motor vehicle and train-related injuries, 982
    thermal injuries, 982
Trunk stability, kinesiology of, 67, 68f

U

Ulnar longitudinal deficiency
    classification, 824
    clinical features, 823–824
    diagnostic studies, 824
    incidence and etiology, 824
    transverse deficiencies, 825
    treatment, 824–825, 825f
Upper extremity
    amputation, socket interface in, 7, 8f
    prehension, 3–4
    sensation, 3–4
Upper limb, 994–995, 994f
    adaptive prostheses, 341–343, 343t
    activity-specific (avocational) technology, 346–347
    activity-specific (vocational-domestic) technology, 345–346, 346f
    archery and bowhunting, 352–353, 353f
    ball sports, 347–348, 348f
    canoeing, kayaking, paddling, crew, 354–355, 355f
    equestrian sports, 359
    firearms and shooting, 357–358, 357f–358f
    fishing, 353–354, 354f–355f
    golf, baseball, and lacrosse, 348–349, 349f–350f
    hockey, 355–356, 356f
    motorcycling, 359
    mountaineering and technical rock climbing, 356–357, 357f
    musical instrument adapters, 360, 360f
    partial hand, 360, 360f–361f
    preprosthetic exercise, 347, 347f
    prosthetic interfaces and limb design, 343–345, 344f–345f
    road and mountain bicycling, 358–359, 358f–359f
    snow skiing, water skiing, and trekking, 356, 356f–357f
    swimming and swimming pool-based therapeutic exercise, 350–351, 351f

Index

Upper limb *(Continued)*
- tumbling, gymnastics, floor exercise, and yoga, 349–350, 350f
- weight training and conditioning, 351–352, 351f–352f
- wrestling and martial arts, 359, 359f

amputation, 724–725
- abnormal positioning, 101, 102f
- activity analysis, 108
- clinical assessment, 111
- exercise and desensitization, 106
- independent training, 110–111
- integration phase, 111
- limb-loss patient evaluation, 103, 103f
- musculoskeletal conditions, 98–99
- pain assessment, 101–103
- patient education, 104, 105t
- phantom limb syndrome, 100
- physical examination, 103, 104t
- postamputation pain, 100
- prosthesis acceptance, 99–100
- prosthesis preferences, 99
- prosthesis preparation, 106–107
- prosthesis training, 107–108
- prosthesis usage, 99
- prosthesis wear adaptations, 111, 112t–113t
- prosthetic devices, linear approach, 111, 113f
- prosthetic limbs, 98
- prosthetic options, 111, 114f
- prosthetic RX evaluation, 103, 104f
- rehabilitation, 97, 103–105, 104f–105f
- repetitive stress disorders, 98–99
- residual limb, 100–101, 101f, 105–106, 105f–106f
- self-healing, 110
- surgical innovations, 114, 114f
- therapeutic relationship, 108
- timeline for, 111, 114t
- unilateral upper extremity amputation, rating guide, 108, 109f

bilateral involvement, 368
bilateral shoulder disarticulation, 853
body-powered components, 129–148, 130f–148f
- harnessing and controls, 149–164, 150f–164f

Community Reintegration of Injured Services Members, 410
congenital deficiencies, 368, 369f
deficiencies, 783
digital absence, 844
digits remaining, 844–845, 845f
externally powered prostheses
- ancillary equipment, 168, 168f
- anthropomorphic prehensors, 171–173, 172f–173f
- component selection, 166–168
- control strategies for, 186–187, 187f
- direct control strategies, 184–185
- elbow components, 176–177, 176f
- force-sensing resistors, 186, 186f
- hybrid configurations, 168
- joint impedance, 168–169
- joint types, 168, 169f
- linear potentiometer, 185–186, 185f
- movement quality, 169
- multiarticulating hands, 187–188
- myoelectric control, 183–184, 184f, 187
- nonanthropomorphic prehensors, 172
- orthoses, 178–179, 178f
- power sources, 169–170, 170f
- prehensors, 170–171, 170f–171f
- preparatory fitting, 168
- 3D-printed prosthetic hands, 173–174, 174f
- prosthetic components, 165
- shoulder components, 177–178
- wrist components, 174–176, 174f–175f

finger amputation, 365–366, 365f
full hand prostheses, 367, 368f
hair, 369, 369f
implications for, prosthetic prescription, 74
infants, 845–846
infection in, 26
internal armatures, 366
kinesiology of, 67–74, 829–830
- elbow, 68–69
- forearm, 69, 69f
- hand, 70–72
- limb mobility, 67
- muscle strength, 73
- nonprehensile activity, 72
- pathologic hand deformity, 73–74
- power grip, 72–73
- prehensile activity, 72
- pulmonary dysfunction, 71
- shoulder, 67–68, 68f
- thumb, 70–71, 70f–71f
- trunk stability, 67, 68f
- wrist, 69–70, 70f

life-care planning, 339
nails, 368–369
oppositional prostheses, 364, 364f
outcome measures, 406t–408t
- clinical evaluation, 402–403, 404t
- in prosthetics, 402
- psychometric attributes, 401, 402t
partial hand prostheses, 366–367, 366f–367f
patient-reported measures, 405, 408
Patient-Reported Outcomes Measurement Information System, 410
pediatric performance measures, 408
pediatric self-report, 408–409
performance measures, 403, 405, 409f
postoperative considerations
- edema reduction, 330
- pain reduction, 330–331, 331f
- residual limb shaping, 330, 331f
- wound care, 329–330
preprosthetic program
- hand dominance, 332
- home assessment, 332
- limb and core assessment and treatment, 331–332, 331f–332f
- perceptual motor skills, 332
- preprosthetic self-care training, 332, 333f
- sleep patterns, 332
- support system, 332
preprosthetic therapy, 329
prostheses and prosthetic control
- body-powered prosthesis, 333
- hybrid prosthesis, 333
- myoelectric prosthesis, 333
- targeted muscle reinnervation, 333–334
- terminal devices, 334, 334f
prosthetic compliance, 365
prosthetic training, 334–338, 335f–339f
- outcomes, 338–339
proxy-reported measures, 408–409
psychological considerations, 364
radial longitudinal deficiency
- classification, 820, 820t–821t
- clinical features, 819
- diagnostic studies, 820
- etiology, 819–820, 820t
- treatment, 820–823
rehabilitation therapy, 364–365, 365f
restoration options, 370, 370f–372f, 372
school-age children, adolescents, and young adults, 847–848
shoulder disarticulation level, 852
- adolescents, 853
- infants, 852
- school-age children, 853
- toddlers and preschoolers, 852–853
- young adults, 853
skin color, 369–370, 370f
Socket Comfort Score, 410
Southampton Hand Assessment Procedure, 410
thumb prostheses, 366, 366f
toddlers, 846–847, 846f–847f
transhumeral level, 850–851
- adolescents, 852
- infants, 851
- preschoolers, 851–852
- school-age children, 852
- toddlers, 851–852
- young adults, 852
transhumeral prostheses, 367–368
transradial level
- adolescents and young adults, 850, 851f
- infants, 848, 849f
- preschoolers, 849–850, 849f–850f
- school-age children, 850
- toddlers, 849–850, 849f–850f
transradial prostheses, 367, 368f
ulnar longitudinal deficiency
- classification, 824
- clinical features, 823–824
- diagnostic studies, 824
- incidence and etiology, 824
- transverse deficiencies, 825
- treatment, 824–825, 825f
wrist disarticulation, 844–845, 845f

V
Verrucous hyperplasia, 663, 664f
Volume-related ulceration, 662–663, 663f

W
Wartime amputations
- clinical problem for, 75
- definitive care, 81
- evacuation care, 81, 82f
- in-theater care, 81
- Iraqi freedom operations, 80–81
- rehabilitation, 81
- revision surgery, 82
- US military care
  - mechanisms of injury, 76
  - prosthetic devices, 77
  - surgical indications, 76

surgical techniques, 76–77
Vietnam experience
 bilateral transfemoral amputations, 80
 incidence of, 77–78
 transfemoral amputations, 79–80
 transtibial amputations, 79
 Valley Forge Army General Hospital, 78–79
War veterans, 725–726
Water sports, 636, 636f, 1015, 1016f
Wheelchair propulsion, 608
Winter sports, 636–637, 637f
Wound care, dressings for, 13–18
Wound dehiscence, 695–696
Wrist disarticulation (WD), 212–213, 214f, 839
 harness suspension, 227–228, 227f–228f
 prosthetic interface, 226, 226f
 residual limb lengths, 223, 224f
 self-suspended interface designs, 228–229, 229f
Wrists, 137, 137f
 bilateral upper limb amputation, 291–292, 291f–292f
 constant-friction wrists, 138, 139f
 flexion units, 139–141, 140f–141f
 friction wrists, 137–138, 138f
 kinesiology of, 69–70, 70f
 multifunction wrists, 141, 141f
 quick-disconnect wrists, 138–139, 139f–140f
 rotational wrists, 139, 140f
 upper limb externally powered prostheses, 174–176, 174f–175f

X

X-Finger, 150